Contents

ALEXANDER'S
CARE
of the PATIENT
in SURGERY

ALEXANDER'S
CARE
of the PATIENT
in SURGERY

16th Edition

JANE C. ROTHROCK
PhD, RN, CNOR, FAAN
Adjunct Professor, Perioperative Programs
Delaware County Community College
Media, Pennsylvania

Associate Editor
Donna R. McEwen, RN, BSN, CNOR(E)
Instructional Designer Consultant
Optum Operations Training
Optum/UnitedHealthCare
San Antonio, Texas

ELSEVIER

ELSEVIER

3251 Riverport Lane
St. Louis, Missouri 63043

Notices

Knowledge and best practice in this field are constantly changing. As new research and experience broaden our understanding, changes in research methods, professional practices, or medical treatment may become necessary.

Practitioners and researchers must always rely on their own experience and knowledge in evaluating and using any information, methods, compounds, or experiments described herein. In using such information or methods they should be mindful of their own safety and the safety of others, including parties for whom they have a professional responsibility.

With respect to any drug or pharmaceutical products identified, readers are advised to check the most current information provided (i) on procedures featured or (ii) by the manufacturer of each product to be administered, to verify the recommended dose or formula, the method and duration of administration, and contraindications. It is the responsibility of practitioners, relying on their own experience and knowledge of their patients, to make diagnoses, to determine dosages and the best treatment for each individual patient, and to take all appropriate safety precautions.

To the fullest extent of the law, neither the Publisher nor the authors, contributors, or editors, assume any liability for any injury and/or damage to persons or property as a matter of products liability, negligence or otherwise, or from any use or operation of any methods, products, instructions, or ideas contained in the material herein.

Previous editions copyrighted 2015, 2011, 2007, 2003, 1999, 1995, 1991, 1987, 1983, 1978, and 1972.

Library of Congress Cataloging-in-Publication Data

Names: Rothrock, Jane C., 1948- editor. | McEwen, Donna R., editor.
Title: Alexander's care of the patient in surgery / [edited by] Jane Rothrock; associate editor, Donna McEwen.
Other titles: Care of the patient in surgery
Description: 16th edition. | St. Louis, Missouri : Elsevier, [2019] | Includes bibliographical references and index.
Identifiers: LCCN 2017051710 | ISBN 9780323479141 (pbk. : alk. paper)
Subjects: | MESH: Perioperative Nursing–methods | Nursing Care–methods | Surgical Procedures, Operative–nursing
Classification: LCC RD99.24 | NLM WY 161 | DDC 617/.0231–dc23 LC record available at
  https://lccn.loc.gov/2017051710

Executive Content Strategist: Kellie White
Content Development Manager: Lisa Newton
Senior Content Development Specialist: Laura Selkirk
Publishing Services Manager: Catherine Jackson
Book Production Specialist: Kristine Feeherty
Design Direction: Amy Buxton

Printed in Canada

Last digit is the print number: 9 8 7 6 5 4 3 2 1

Working together
to grow libraries in
developing countries

www.elsevier.com • www.bookaid.org

Contributors

Sheila L. Allen, BSN, RN, CNOR, CRNFA(E)
Clinical Educator
Self-employed
Baton Rouge, Louisiana
Chapter 27: Geriatric Surgery

Jacqueline R. Bak, MSN, RN, CNOR, RNFA
Allied Health and Nursing
Delaware County Community College
Media, Pennsylvania;
Nursing, Paoli SurgiCenter
Paoli, Pennsylvania
Chapter 9: Wound Healing, Dressings, and Drains

Kay A. Ball, PhD, RN, CNOR, CMLSO, FAAN
Professor, Nursing Department
Otterbein University
Perioperative Consultant
Lewis Center
Westerville, Ohio
Chapter 8: Surgical Modalities

Barbara A. Bowen, BSN, MSN, CRNP, CRNFA
President
Perioperative Consulting and Surgical Services, LLC
Collegeville, Pennsylvania;
Consultant
Stryker Performance Solutions
Chicago, Illinois
Chapter 20: Orthopedic Surgery

Brian D. Campbell, BS, BSN, CRNA, COL (USA Ret.)
Chief Nurse Anesthetist, Anesthesiology
Winchester Hospital
Winchester, Massachusetts;
Colonel, retired
USAR, 804th Med BDE
Devens, Massachusetts
Chapter 5: Anesthesia

Susan A. Carzo, BSN, RN, CNOR, RNFA
Staff Nurse/RFNA, Operating Room
Winchester Hospital
Winchester, Massachusetts
Chapter 14: Gynecologic and Obstetric Surgery

Mary Michaela Cromb, BSN
Retired
Optum Operations Training
Optum/UnitedHealthCare
San Antonio, Texas
Chapter 7: Sutures, Sharps, and Instruments

Richard G. Cuming, EdD, MSN, RN, NEA-BC, FAAN
Senior Vice President, Patient Care Services and Chief Nurse
 Executive
Administration
Christiana Care Health System
Wilmington, Delaware
Chapter 1: Concepts Basic to Perioperative Nursing

Cateria Davis-Bruno, MSN, CNOR
OR/CVOR Manager, Perioperative Services
Lakeland Regional Health Systems
Adjunct Clinical Instructor, Nursing
Polk State College
Lakeland, Florida
Chapter 25: Cardiac Surgery

Britta E. DeVolder, BSN, MBA, RN, CNOR
Executive Director, Perioperative Services
University Health System
San Antonio, Texas
Chapter 11: Gastrointestinal Surgery

Carmencita Duffy, BSN, RN, CNOR
Surgery
Highland Park Hospital
Northshore University Health System
Highland Park, Illinois
Chapter 16: Thyroid and Parathyroid Surgery

Debra L. Fawcett, MS, PhD
Director of Infection Prevention
Infection Prevention and Control
Eskenazi Health
Indianapolis, Indiana
Chapter 6: Positioning the Patient for Surgery

Beth Fitzgerald, MSN, RN, CNOR
Infection Preventionist
Christiana Care Health System
Newark, Delaware
Chapter 29: Interventional and Image-Guided Procedures

Allison L. Flanagan, MSN, RN, CNOR, RNFA
Specialty Team Coordinator, Operating Room
Paoli Hospital
Paoli, Pennsylvania
Chapter 19: Otorhinolaryngologic Surgery

David P. Gawronski, MSN, RN, CNOR, CST
Nurse Manager, Operating Room, Sterile Processing
Sisters of Charity Hospital, St. Joseph Campus
Cheektowaga, New York
Chapter 28: Trauma Surgery

Cecil A. King, MS, RN
RN Medical Case Manager
Infectious Disease Clinical Services
Cape Cod Healthcare
Hyannis, Massachusetts
Chapter 4: Infection Prevention and Control

Rachael Larner, BSN, MSN, RN
Wexford, Pennsylvania
Chapter 30: Integrative Health Practices: Complementary and Alternative Therapies

Helene P. Korey Marley, BSN, RN, CNOR, CRNFA
Clinical Service Coordinator, Operating Room
Pennsylvania Hospital
Philadelphia, Pennsylvania
Chapter 15: Genitourinary Surgery

Donna R. McEwen, RN, BSN, CNOR(E)
Instructional Designer Consultant
Optum Operations Training
Optum/UnitedHealthCare
San Antonio, Texas
Chapter 22: Reconstructive and Aesthetic Plastic Surgery
Chapter 23: Thoracic Surgery

Eileen Dickson Mielcarek, BSN, RNFA, COE
Practice Administrator, Owner
RNFA, Perioperative, Operating Room
Mielcarek Eye Center
Owner
Premier Medical Facial Aesthetics
Facial Rejuvenation at Mielcarek
Media, Pennsylvania
Chapter 18: Ophthalmic Surgery

Ellen Murphy, BS, MS, JD
Professor Emerita, College of Nursing
University of Wisconsin-Milwaukee
Milwaukee, Wisconsin
Chapter 2: Patient Safety and Risk Management

Maureen P. Murphy, MSN
Certified Registered Nurse Practitioner, Otolaryngology
Registered Nurse, Perioperative
Thomas Jefferson University Hospital
Philadelphia, Pennsylvania
Chapter 21: Neurosurgery

Janice A. Neil, PhD, RN, CNE
Associate Professor, College of Nursing
Department of Baccalaureate Education
East Carolina University
Greenville, North Carolina
Chapter 12: Surgery of the Biliary Tract, Pancreas, Liver, and Spleen
Chapter 17: Breast Surgery

Jan Odom-Forren, PhD, RN, CPAN, FAAN
Associate Professor, College of Nursing
University of Kentucky
Lexington, Kentucky
Chapter 10: Postoperative Patient Care and Pain Management

Susan M. Scully, MSN, RN, CNOR
Clinical Expert, Perioperative Complex
Children's Hospital of Philadelphia
Philadelphia, Pennsylvania
Chapter 26: Pediatric Surgery

Patricia C. Seifert, MSN, RN, CNOR, CRNF(E), FAAN
Independent Cardiac Consultant, Formerly Educator, Cardiovascular Operating Room
Inova Heart and Vascular Institute
Former Editor-in-Chief, AORN Journal
Association of Perioperative Registered Nurses (AORN)
Denver, Colorado;
Cardiac Surgery
Seifert Consulting
Falls Church, Virginia
Chapter 25: Cardiac Surgery

Christine E. Smith, MSN, RN, CNS, CNOR
Semi-retired, Perioperative CNS/Educator
Home Office/Perioperative Educator
Guerneville, California
Chapter 3: Workplace Issues and Staff Safety

James D. Smith, Jr., BSN
RN First Assistant, Surgery
Missouri Baptist Medical Center
St. Louis, Missouri
Chapter 13: Hernia Repair

Michele Clemens Smith, BSN
Clinical Nurse, Operating Room
Children's Hospital of Philadelphia
Philadelphia, Pennsylvania
Chapter 26: Pediatric Surgery

Lisa Spruce, DNP, RN, CNS-CP, CNOR, ACNS, ACNP, FAAN
Director, Evidence-Based Perioperative Practice
Nurse Practice
Association of Perioperative Registered Nurses (AORN)
Denver, Colorado
Patient Engagement Exemplar boxes

Cynthia Spry, BS, BSN, MS, MA
Independent Consultant
New York, New York
Chapter 4: Infection Prevention and Control

Kathryn J. Trotter, DNP
Associate Professor, School of Nursing
Duke University
Nurse Practitioner, Duke Breast Program
Duke Health
Durham, North Carolina
Chapter 17: Breast Surgery

Dana M. Whitmore, BSN, RN, CNOR
Staff Development Nurse, Operating Room
Thomas Jefferson University Hospital
Philadelphia, Pennsylvania
Chapter 21: Neurosurgery

Patricia Wieczorek, MSN, RN, CNOR
Coordinator of Perioperative Nursing Programs
Perioperative Services
The Johns Hopkins Hospital
Baltimore, Maryland
Chapter 24: Vascular Surgery

Clinical Consultants

Chyna Davison, BSN, RN
Staff Nurse, Operating Room
Pennsylvania Hospital
Philadelphia, Pennsylvania

Glen Dixon, Jr., MD
Chairman of Obstetrics and Gynecology
Winchester Hospital
Winchester, Massachusetts

Lorraine J. Foley, MD, MBA
Clinical Assistant Professor
Tufts School of Medicine
Anesthesiologist, Winchester Anesthesia Associates
Winchester Hospital
President of the Society for Airway Management
Boston, Massachusetts

Arlan F. Fuller, Jr., MD
Clinical Vice President for Oncology Services
Winchester Hospital
Winchester, Massachusetts

Charles L. Getz, MD
Associate Professor
Thomas Jefferson University Hospitals
Rothman Institute
Philadelphia, Pennsylvania

Sean P. Larner, DO
Neurotology Fellow
Pittsburgh Ear Associates
Pittsburgh, Pennsylvania

Maureen Lewis, MSN, CRNP, CNOR, CRNFA
RN First Assistant
Riddle Hospital
Media, Pennsylvania

Jess H. Lonner, MD
Associate Professor of Orthopaedics
Thomas Jefferson University Hospitals
Rothman Institute
Philadelphia, Pennsylvania

Elizabeth B. Pearsall, BSN, RN, CNOR
Adjunct Faculty, Perioperative Programs
Delaware County Community College
Media, Pennsylvania

Kim Russo
Riddle Memorial Hospital
Media, Pennsylvania

Inga Sinyangwe, MSN, RN
Staff Development Specialist
Institute for Leadership, Education and Development
Christiana Hospital
Newark, Delaware

Ariana L. Smith, MD
Assistant Professor of Urology
Director of Pelvic Medicine and Reconstructive Surgery
Pennsylvania Hospital
Philadelphia, Pennsylvania

Joseph H. Viveiros, RN, CNOR, RNFA
RN/RNFA Staff Nurse
Winchester Hospital
Winchester, Massachusetts

David L. Yarbrough, RN, BS, MS, JD
COO, Senior Health Planner
Aspen Street Architects, Inc.
Murphys, California

Kathryn Yarbrough, RN
Retired Healthcare Executive
Murphys, California

Reviewers

Sheila L. Allen, BSN, RN, CNOR, CRNFA(E)
Clinical Educator
Self-employed
Baton Rouge, Louisiana

Andrea Bills, BSN, RN, CNOR, RNFA
Dumont, New Jersey

Dee Anne Boner, BSN, MSN, RN, CNOR
Clinical Staff Leader
Vanderbilt University Medical Center
Nashville, Tennessee

James Bowers, BSN, RN, CNOR, TNCC
Clinical Educator
WVU Healthcare
Morgantown, West Virginia

Amy J. Broadhurst, RN, BS, BSN, CNOR
Staff RN Operating Room
Christiana Care Health System
Newark, Delaware

Susan A. Carzo, BSN, RN, CNOR, RNFA
Staff Nurse/RNFA, Operating Room
Winchester Hospital
Winchester, Massachusetts

Monica Y. Cisneros, BSN, MSN, RN, ANP-BC, CRNFA
Advanced Practice Nurse, Registered Nurse First Assistant
Hackensack University Medical Center
Hackensack, New Jersey;
NYP Lawrence Hospital
Bronxville, New York

Marlene Craden, BSN, RN, CNOR, CRNFA
Registered Nurse First Assistant
Kaleida Health
Millard Fillmore Suburban Hospital
Williamsville, New York

Theresa M. Criscitelli, EdD, RN, CNOR
Assistant Vice President Administration
Perioperative/Procedural Services
Winthrop University Hospital
Mineola, New York

Helen M. Dickson, MSN, RN, CNOR, RNFA
Registered Nurse First Assistant
Delaware County Community College
Media, Pennsylvania

Joanne M. Epstein, BSN, RN, CNOR
Educator, Surgical Services
St. Francis Hospital
Wilmington, Delaware

Debra Eustace, BSN, RN, CNOR, CRNFA
President
Surgifirst LLC
Annandale, New Jersey

Teresa M. Galanaugh-Scarpato, BS
Coordinator, Perioperative Services
Main Line Health
Radnor, Pennsylvania

David P. Gawronski, MSN, RN, CNOR, CST
Nurse Manager—Operating Room, Sterile Processing
Sisters of Charity Hospital, St. Joseph Campus
Cheektowaga, New York

Donna Ginsberg, BSN, RN, CNOR, CRNFA
Owner, Surgical First Assistant Services LLC
Meridian and St. Barnabas Health
Asbury Park, New Jersey

Carol Hager, BSN, RN, CRNFA, MSN, CRNP
Nurse Practitioner
UPMC Hamot—Bayview Breast Care at Hamot
Great Lakes Surgery Specialists
Erie, Pennsylvania

Mark Karasin, BSN, BA, RN
Registered Nurse
New Jersey Spine Specialists LLC
Overlook Medical Center
Summit, New Jersey

Cynthia L. Kildgore, RN, MSHA
Director of Perioperative Services
Vanderbilt University Medical Center
Nashville, Tennessee

Andrew Kiskadden, MSN, CRNA
Nurse Anesthetist, Anesthesia Consultants of Erie
Saint Vincent Health Center
Erie, Pennsylvania

Candice Kiskadden, MSN, RN, CNOR
Instructor of Nursing
Mercyhurst University
Erie, Pennsylvania

Susan Lynch, MSN, CSSM, CNOR, RNFA
Clinical Educator
Main Line Health
Media, Pennsylvania

M. Carolyn Malecka, RN, CNOR, RNFA
Medford, New Jersey

Tanya Marandola, MSN, RN, CNOR
Staff Nurse, Ophthalmology Coordinator
Roxana Cannon Arsht Surgicenter
Christiana Care Health Systems
Wilmington, Delaware

Angela Mercer, BSN, RN, CNOR
Perioperative Staff Nurse
Christiana Care Health Systems
Wilmington, Delaware

Joseph K. Mollohan, MSN, RN, CNOR, CSSM, RNFA
President
Perioperative Management Consultants
Springfield, Tennessee

Claudia Orsburn, BSN, MSN, MS
Director of Surgical Services
Vanderbilt University Medical Center
Nashville, Tennessee

Karen S. Pettit, BSN, CRNFA
Phoenix, Arizona

Sharon S. Pomeroy, BSN, MHA, BS, RN
Manager, Perioperative Services
Vanderbilt University Medical Center
Nashville, Tennessee

Carol R. Ritchie, MSN, RN, CNOR
Supervisor, Perioperative Services
Mayo Clinic
Phoenix, Arizona

Judy Roche, RN, CNOR, CRNFA
Owner, CEO
Freelance Assistants, Inc.
Denver, Colorado

Billie Thomas, BSN, RN, CNOR
Operating Room Staff Nurse
Christian Care Health Services
Wilmington, Delaware

Cynthia Townsend, MTHS, BSN, RN, CNOR
Manager, Perioperative Education and Research
Vanderbilt University Medical Center
Nashville, Tennessee

Susanna S. Walsh, RNFA, BSN, CNOR
Peri-Operative Manager
Nashville, Tennessee

Marion Knapp Wardle, MSM, BSN, RN, CNOR
Director of Nursing Programs/Perioperative Education
Quality and Patient Safety
Ann Bates Leach Eye Hospital/Bascom Palmer Eye Institute
University of Miami Health
Miami, Florida

About the Author

JANE C. ROTHROCK, PhD, RN, CNOR, FAAN

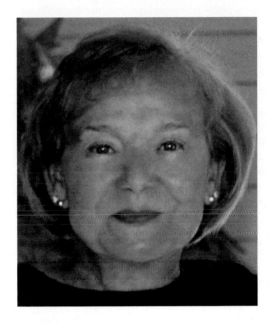

To Brittany Anne Hutt—
an incredible, loving niece
who has energy, motivation, sincere values,
and a passion for creating
a sustainable planet we call home.
You represent who we all
should strive to be.
I love you and everything about you.

Dr. Jane Rothrock has practiced and taught perioperative nursing since 1969. In 1979 she joined the faculty of Delaware County Community College, where she is now an Adjunct Professor in the college's Perioperative Programs. Her current responsibilities include entry-level, postbasic RN education for perioperative nursing. During her 40-year tenure at the college, Jane has helped to educate more than 4500 registered nurses in the professional practice of perioperative patient care.

Jane's decades of experience include not only being a faculty member but also an author, editor, and speaker. She has taught at the University of Pennsylvania, served as an OR director, and acted as preceptor for many graduate students. She has authored five perioperative nursing textbooks, published more than 50 articles, and presented a host of topics to nursing audiences across the United States and internationally. Jane is an AORN past president and chaired AORN's Project Team on Professional Practice Issues, its Project Team on a Professional Practice Model for Perioperative Nursing, and its Perioperative Academic Curriculum Task Force. She also served as an evidence reviewer for AORN's Evidence-based Recommended Practices for Perioperative Patient Care and is currently a research reviewer for the AORN Journal.

Jane has received numerous professional awards and remains very active in both nursing and community organizations. Jane is a past vice chair of NOLF, a past member of the ANCC Magnet Commission, a past president of the ASPAN Foundation, and a past president of the AORN Foundation Board of Trustees. She served on ASPAN's first National Clinical Guideline Panel to develop a Guideline on Prevention of Unplanned Hypothermia in Adult Surgical Patients. In 2000 Jane became a Fellow of the American Academy of Nursing (FAAN). In 2016 she was elected Professor Emerita at Delaware County Community College.

Jane began her nursing education with a diploma from Bryn Mawr School of Nursing. She went on to earn her BSN and MSN from the University of Pennsylvania and became the first recipient of a doctoral degree from Widener University in suburban Philadelphia, earning her PhD in nursing in 1987.

Preface

This updated sixteenth edition of *Alexander's Care of the Patient in Surgery* reflects new and essential key concepts in perioperative nursing practice and an increased sophistication and complexity in surgical procedures. Its multimedia resource, first introduced in the thirteenth edition, strongly enhances the elemental goal of this textbook: to provide a comprehensive foundational reference that will assist perioperative practitioners to meet the needs of patients they care for safely, cost-effectively, and efficiently during surgical interventions.

As the standard in perioperative nursing for more than 50 years, *Alexander's Care of the Patient in Surgery* is written primarily for professional perioperative nurses, but it is also useful for surgical technologists, nursing students, healthcare industry representatives, medical students, interns, residents, and government officials concerned with healthcare issues. Perioperative nurses, RN first assistants, clinical nurse specialists, nurse practitioners, surgeons, and educators from many geographic areas of the United States have served as contributors and reviewers for this text. In doing so, they provide a vast range of perioperative patient care knowledge, procedural information, and wisdom.

This thoroughly revised edition highlights current surgical techniques and innovations. More than 1000 illustrations, including many new photographs and drawings, help familiarize the reader with contemporary procedures, methods, and equipment. Classic illustrations, particularly of surgical anatomy, remain to enhance the text. New to this edition are features highlighting patient engagement and patient-centered communication, the addition of Enhanced Recovery After Surgery protocols, and an expanded emphasis on robotic-assisted surgery. Each chapter contains a summary of Key Points and a Critical Thinking Question. There is a thorough laboratory values appendix in which readers can review normal lab values and ranges. Readers will again find Ambulatory Surgery Considerations; Evidence for Practice; Patient, Family, and Caregiver Education; Patient Safety; Research Highlights; Sample Plan of Care; and Surgical Pharmacology features, updated to reflect changes.

Enhanced in the sixteenth edition is the Evolve website. With its learner resources, readers are able to access animations, The Agency for Healthcare Research and Quality (AHRQ) case studies, answers to the critical thinking questions, interactive study questions, OR Live links, and scenario packets.

Also enhanced in the sixteenth edition are resources for instructors and clinical educators. In addition to the learner resources listed previously, instructor resources contain a lesson plan for each chapter with the following elements: case studies, answers to critical thinking questions, learning objectives, suggested content for lectures and class activities, clinical learning scenarios for each covered surgical procedure, PowerPoint lecture slides with speaker notes, and an image collection of more than 1000 images to use in teaching. Instructors and clinical educators will also find a test bank with more than 750 questions as well as more than 50 customizable

competency assessments for use in clinical settings or simulation laboratories as learners practice new perioperative nursing skills and techniques. Overall, this textbook imparts state-of-the-art information and resources to reflect contemporary practice and to promote delivery of comprehensive perioperative patient care.

Unit I, Foundations for Practice, provides information on basic principles and patient care requisites essential for all recipients of perioperative patient care. The nursing process, a model for developing therapeutic nursing interventional knowledge, reflects a six-step method that includes the identification of desired patient outcomes. Interest in patient outcomes and their improvement continues to be an essential element of nursing. The collection of health data requires clear identification of contributions to patient outcomes and quantification of these contributions. Perioperative nurses must continue to link their interventions to outcomes. This relationship is presented in Chapter 1 and explicated in each Sample Plan of Care throughout the text.

Research Highlights continue to be included in every chapter and reflect the steady increase in the amount and quality of research relevant to perioperative patient care. As current findings of new research are important to use in clinical practice, the editors and authors of *Alexander's Care of the Patient in Surgery* are committed to supporting this research-practice relationship. The Research Highlights will help perioperative nurses implement research findings in their practice and patient care activities.

Chapter 1 also sets the stage for an emphasis on patient, family, and caregiver education and discharge planning throughout the text. Chapters in Units II and III address specific patient, family, and caregiver education and discharge planning relevant for patients undergoing one or more of the respective specialty surgical procedures. As the responsibilities of perioperative nurses become greater with regard to those important care components, it is imperative that we effectively educate patients, their families, and their caregivers. As length of stay in healthcare facilities continues to decrease, patients, families, and caregivers need more and better information to deal appropriately with postoperative needs after discharge. Pain management, addressed in Chapter 10, also appears in many of the chapters on surgical specialties because all perioperative nurses recognize its importance in patient discharge planning.

Chapter 2 focuses on patient safety and risk management, including a review of the use of social media and patient privacy issues. As members of the perioperative team face increasing workloads and workplace stress, this sixteenth edition emphasizes the need for workplace safety in Chapter 3. When pressure in the surgical suite mounts, perioperative staff may feel the need to work faster, even if it means taking shortcuts. The chapter on workplace safety stresses the need for personal safety at work and explores such issues as noise in the OR, active shooter situations, workplace violence, and bullying. The remaining chapters in Unit I focus on perioperative precepts guiding infection prevention; anesthesia; patient positioning;

sutures, sharps, and instruments; surgical modalities; wound healing; and caring for the postoperative patient in the PACU and on the transfer unit.

The chapters in *Unit II, Surgical Interventions,* include more than 400 contemporary and traditional specialty surgical interventions, with descriptions of open approaches, minimally invasive surgical procedures, and robotic-assisted surgery. Each chapter provides a helpful review of pertinent anatomy and details the steps of surgical procedures. Perioperative nursing considerations are again presented within the nursing process framework. Current NANDA International–approved nursing diagnoses and Sample Plans of Care for each surgical specialty aim to help perioperative nurses plan, implement, and evaluate individualized perioperative patient care. Each of these chapters also provides an example of Evidence for Practice related to the surgical specialty. In 2018 and beyond, perioperative nurses can expect to find a continuing emphasis on evidence-based nursing as a means to provide care that is effective and yields improved outcomes. The integration of evidence-based practice with the perioperative nurse's individual clinical expertise leads to optimal care provision, the foundation of perioperative patient care. Improving the quality of patient care and effecting safe outcomes are at the heart of all our efforts to achieve excellence in whatever setting we encounter the patient who is undergoing an operative or other invasive procedure.

Incorporation of Surgical Pharmacology in the sixteenth edition reflects the ongoing emphasis on medication safety in the United States. Medication errors can occur anywhere in the medication use system, from prescribing to administering a drug. *Alexander's Care of the Patient in Surgery* joins the nationwide health professional education campaign that aims to reduce the number of common but preventable sources of medication errors. Providing information about select medications and dosages used in surgical specialties, the Surgical Pharmacology feature is intended to promote safe medication practices and to avoid serious, even potentially fatal, consequences of medication errors by perioperative practitioners.

To further facilitate the perioperative nurse's focus on safe patient care, Patient Safety features in each chapter succinctly review a practice to assist perioperative practitioners in developing a core body of knowledge about safe patient care. We intend for this feature to raise awareness about patient safety applications. We also intend simultaneously to foster communication and ongoing dialogue in perioperative practice settings regarding application of recommended patient safety strategies and use of robust process improvement initiatives. In so doing, we hope to improve quality and safety overall in perioperative patient care.

New to the sixteenth edition is information on Enhanced Recovery After Surgery protocols. These protocols aim to increase efficiency during all phases of perioperative patient care and decrease length of stay for surgery patients and costs of care, while improving outcomes. As applicable to the chapter content, Enhanced Recovery After Surgery features address the evidence-based strategies and merits of such protocols.

The unique needs of pediatric, geriatric, and trauma surgery patients are presented in *Unit III, Special Considerations.* The "Interventional and Image-Guided Procedures" chapter reflects processes of care in sophisticated hybrid OR suites, where enhanced capabilities merge open and interventional surgery in a multidisciplinary environment. The "Integrative Health Practices: Complementary and Alternative Therapies" chapter was introduced in the twelfth edition. Perioperative nurses frequently encounter patients who use such therapies, some of which are nonpharmacologic and some of which involve medications. This chapter explores alternative medical systems, mind-body interventions, biologically based therapies, manipulative and body-based methods, and energy therapies. Treatments and systems within each category are discussed.

Many expert perioperative practitioners, RN first assistants, clinical nurse specialists, and educators have contributed to this sixteenth edition, and I owe a debt of gratitude to all of them for sharing their expertise in the development of this text. I give ongoing thanks to my partner, Alan Zulick, Esquire, for his help during copyediting and page proofs. I also acknowledge the valuable assistance of editors, reviewers, photographers, and illustrators who have contributed their time and expertise to the revision of this text. The team I had the privilege of working with at Elsevier is talented and eager to support perioperative practitioners in their commitment to excellence in patient care. Laura Selkirk, I would clone you and give you as a gift to all of my nurse editor colleagues if I could you walk the entire journey with each edition of this book with supreme aplomb! Donna McEwen, my Associate Editor, is not only a masterful editor but also an instructional design expert. The Evolve website is the elegant and robust feature that it is due to her acumen and talent. Christine Smith is a clinical nurse specialist who developed the competencies. Mickey Cromb is a registered nurse and instructional designer who developed the test bank. Clearly, I work with a team to be admired and esteemed for their contributions to this edition.

Alexander's Care of the Patient in Surgery is written by and for perioperative nurses. Its premise is underscored by the clear understanding that perioperative nursing is a caring and intellectual endeavor, requiring critical thinking, technical acumen, and clinical reasoning and decision-making to improving patient outcomes. With the multimedia package accompanying this sixteenth edition, *Alexander's Care of the Patient in Surgery* invites you to journey with us as we meet the challenges and opportunities of perioperative nursing in the twenty-first century.

Jane C. Rothrock

Contents

UNIT II   Surgical Interventions

UNIT III   Special Considerations

CHAPTER **1**

Concepts Basic to Perioperative Nursing

RICHARD G. CUMING

Overview of Perioperative Nursing Practice

Perioperative nursing is the nursing care provided to patients before, during, and after surgical and invasive procedures. Nurses practice this specialty in surgical suites, ambulatory surgery centers, endoscopy suites, laser centers, interventional radiology departments, mobile surgical units, and physicians' offices across the United States and the world. Perioperative nursing includes a broad array of cutting-edge innovations, such as remote surgery, virtual endoscopy, robotics, computerized navigation systems, transplanted tissue and organs, biologic materials that are absorbed to replace worn-out body parts, radiofrequency identification (RFID), transoral approaches (natural orifice surgery), and electronic health records (EHRs). In this high-tech era, perioperative patient care is very different from the way it was in the past.

In the past, the term *operating room (OR)* nursing was used to describe the care of patients in the immediate preoperative, intra-operative, and postoperative phases of the surgical experience (Fig. 1.1). This term implied that nursing care activities were limited to the physical confines of the OR. The term may have contributed to stereotypic images of the OR nurse who took care of the OR

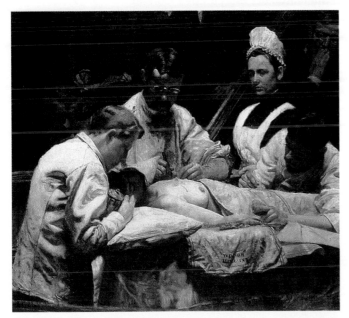

FIG. 1.1 *The Agnew Clinic,* by Thomas Eakins, 1889. In this painting, reforms and advancements in surgical techniques and procedures are apparent. Surgeons wear gowns, instruments are sterilized, ether is used, and the patient is covered. An operating room nurse is a prominent member of the team.

and its equipment but had little, if any, interaction or nursing responsibility for medicated and anesthetized patients in the surgical suite. With such an image, nurses practicing outside the OR had difficulty crediting important elements of the nursing process and patient care accountability to the nurse who practiced "behind the double doors" of the surgical suite.

Today, *perioperative nursing* implies the delivery of comprehensive patient care within the preoperative, intraoperative, and postoperative periods of the patient's experience during operative and other invasive procedures by using the framework of the nursing process. In doing so, the perioperative nurse assesses the patient by collecting, organizing, and prioritizing patient data; establishes nursing diagnoses; identifies desired patient outcomes; develops and implements a plan of nursing care; and evaluates that care in terms of outcomes achieved by and for the patient. Throughout the process, the perioperative nurse functions both independently and interdependently. As with nurses in other specialties, the perioperative nurse collaborates with other healthcare professionals, makes appropriate nursing referrals, and delegates and supervises other personnel in providing safe and efficient patient care.

When nurses practice perioperative nursing in its broadest sense, care may begin in the patient's home, a clinic, a physician's office, the patient care unit, the presurgical care unit, or the holding area. After the surgical or invasive procedure, care may continue in the postanesthesia care unit (PACU), and evaluation of patient outcomes may extend onto the patient care unit, in the physician's office, in the patient's home, in a clinic, or through written or telephone patient surveys.

When nurses practice perioperative nursing in its more limited sense, patient care activities may be confined to the common areas of the surgical suite. Assessment and data collection may take place in the holding area, whereas evaluation may take place on discharge from the OR. Regardless of the way nurses practice perioperative nursing in a healthcare setting, it is based on the nursing process and professional nursing practice.

The perioperative nurse functions as a patient advocate during times of vulnerability. This specialty requires a broad knowledge base, instant recall of nursing science, an intuitive ability to be guided by nursing experience, diversity of thought and action, and great stamina and flexibility. Whether a generalist or a specialist, the perioperative nurse depends on knowledge of surgical anatomy, physiologic alterations and their consequences for the patient, intraoperative risk factors, potentials for and prevention of patient injury, and psychosocial implications of surgery for the patient, family, and caregiver. This knowledge enables the perioperative nurse to anticipate needs of the patient and surgical team and to rapidly initiate safe and appropriate nursing interventions. This too is part of patient advocacy, that is, doing for the patient what needs to be done to provide a safe and caring environment. The Association of periOperative Registered Nurses (AORN) has asserted the significance of such safety by reaffirming that staffing of healthcare personnel must ensure that patients undergoing surgical and invasive procedures have a perioperative nurse as circulator in the OR, and that the core activities of perioperative nursing care (assessment, diagnosis, outcome identification, planning, and evaluation) be completed by a perioperative nurse (AORN, 2014a).

A significant part of perioperative nursing is the delivery of scientifically based care. Such care implies understanding the rationale for certain activities and interventions; knowledge of how and when to implement them; and the skills to evaluate safety, cost-effectiveness, and outcomes of the care delivered. This knowledge empowers the perioperative nurse to anticipate and prepare for steps of the surgical procedure and understand their concomitant implications for the patient and for the surgical team. Scientific nursing interventions; critical thinking and clinical reasoning; and caring, comforting behaviors are at the heart of perioperative nursing. Unit II of this book focuses on surgical procedures common to inpatient and ambulatory settings. Each chapter in Unit II contains a Sample Plan of Care with suggested nursing interventions. A fundamental assumption throughout this textbook is that perioperative nursing is a blend of technical and behavioral care and that critical thinking underpins caring for patients professionally. Quality nursing care is dependent on nurses' ability to think critically (Helzer Doroh and Monahan, 2016). Critical thinking requires purposeful, outcome-directed thought and is driven by patient need. It is based on the nursing process and nursing science. Further, critical thinking requires knowledge, skills, and experience guided by professional standards and ethics and grounded in constant reevaluation, self-correction, and continual striving to improve.

Perioperative Patient Focused Model

AORN has developed a model to describe the important relationship between the patient and the perioperative nursing care provided. The Perioperative Patient Focused Model (AORN, 2015) consists of domains or areas of nursing concern including nursing diagnoses, nursing interventions, and patient outcomes. These domains are in continuous interaction with the health system that encircles the focus of perioperative nursing practice—the patient (AORN, 2015).

Three of these domains (behavioral responses, patient safety, and physiologic responses) reflect phenomena of concern to perioperative nurses and comprise the nursing diagnoses, interventions, and outcomes that surgical patients or their families experience. The fourth domain, the health system, comprises structural data elements and focuses on clinical processes and outcomes.

The model illustrates the dynamic nature of the perioperative patient experience and the nursing presence throughout that process. Working in a collaborative relationship with other members of the healthcare team and the patient, the nurse establishes outcomes, identifies nursing diagnoses, and provides nursing care. The nurse intervenes within the context of the healthcare system to help the patient achieve the highest attainable health outcomes (physiologic, behavioral, and safety) throughout the perioperative experience.

The model emphasizes the outcome-driven nature of perioperative patient care. Perioperative nurses possess a unique understanding of desired outcomes that apply to all surgical patients. In contrast to some nursing specialties in which nursing diagnoses are derived from signs and symptoms of a condition, much of perioperative nursing care is preventive in nature and based on knowledge of risks inherent to patients undergoing surgical and invasive procedures. Perioperative nurses identify these risks and potential problems in advance and direct nursing interventions toward prevention of undesirable outcomes, such as injury and infection. Based on an individual patient assessment, the perioperative nurse identifies risks and relevant nursing diagnoses. This information guides nursing interventions for each patient. From admission through discharge and home follow-up, the perioperative nurse plays a major role in managing the patient's care. Research based on AORN's Perioperative Patient Focused Model continues to test and validate the contributions of perioperative nurses to patient outcomes in the variety of settings in which this nursing specialty is practiced.

Standards of Perioperative Nursing Practice

Perioperative nursing is a systematic, planned process in a series of integrated steps. For professional nursing, national standards establish the full expectations of the professional role within which the nurse practices. In the 1960s, the American Nurses Association (ANA) engaged in standards development. First published in 1973, these standards helped to shape nursing practice. Specialty nursing organizations, including AORN, have worked with the ANA to develop their own standards and guidelines using the ANA framework. This collaboration has resulted in the use of common language and a consistent format for the profession.

Perioperative Nursing Practice Standards

AORN (2015) has developed a set of standards for perioperative nursing (Box 1.1). These standards are authoritative statements that define and enumerate the responsibilities for which perioperative nurses are accountable. The standards represent a comprehensive approach to meeting the healthcare needs of surgical patients and relate to nursing activities, interventions, and interactions. They are

---

BOX 1.1

Standards of Perioperative Nursing

- *Focus:* providing perioperative patient care and performing professional role responsibilities
- *Responsibility:* each perioperative nurse, with appropriate working conditions and resource support
- *Underlying themes:*
  - Perioperative nursing care is individualized to unique patient needs and situations.
  - Care is provided in the broad context of injury prevention.
  - Cultural, racial, and ethnic diversity, along with the patient's preferences and goals, is always taken into account when planning and providing perioperative nursing care.
- *Conceptual framework for practice:* The Perioperative Patient Focused Model
- *Nursing process underpinning:* assessment, diagnosis, planning, implementing the plan of care, and evaluating the patient's progress toward outcomes
- *Quality and appropriateness of practice emphasis:* systematically evaluated
- *Evaluation of own practice:* in the context of current professional standards, rules, and regulations
- *Collegiality:* demonstrated when interacting with peers, colleagues, and others
- *Collaboration:* takes place with the patient and other designated personnel when practicing professional nursing

Modified from the Association of periOperative Registered Nurses: *Guidelines for perioperative practice,* Denver, 2015, The Association.

used to explicate clinical, professional, and quality objectives in perioperative nursing. The *Guidelines for Perioperative Practice* contain recommendations for implementing perioperative patient care based on a comprehensive appraisal of both research and nonresearch evidence (AORN, 2016). They complement the *Standards of Perioperative Nursing*, which are based on and describe the application of the nursing process in perioperative nursing. The guidelines include the collection and analysis of health data, identification of expected outcomes, planning and implementation of patient care, and evaluation of the effects of this care on patient outcomes.

AORN (2015) *Standards of Perioperative Nursing* require, in part, that the perioperative nurse evaluates the effectiveness of nursing practice and the quality of that practice. These standards also require perioperative nurses to evaluate their own practice. Achieving certification (certified nurse, operating room [CNOR]), pursuing lifelong learning, and maintaining competency and current knowledge in perioperative nursing are hallmarks of the professional. The guidelines focus on the importance of evidence-based practice (EBP) and participation in the generation of new knowledge through research. The pace and complexity of advances in surgical procedures, minimally invasive surgery, robotics, new technologies, professional nursing issues, ongoing healthcare reform measures, continuing changes in evidence-based recommendations for practice, and the burgeoning body of nursing research demand constant professional education and development. Perioperative professionals must continue to research patient outcomes, to link nursing interventions to outcomes, and to develop methods that conserve resources when implementing interventions.

Nursing Process

Looking at nursing as a process brings it into perspective as a system of critical thinking that provides the foundation for nursing actions (Fig. 1.2). The focus of the nursing process is the patient, and prescribed nursing interventions are those that meet patient needs. Using the nursing process directs the perioperative nurse's focus on the patient by using clinical skills and knowledge to care for patients and to make independent judgments and clinical decisions. Use of the nursing process, nursing plans of care, clinical pathways, and best practices (discussed later in this chapter) is an integral part of patient care.

In its simplest form, the nursing process consists of the following six steps: assessment, nursing diagnosis, outcome identification, planning, implementation, and evaluation. The process is dynamic and continual. Certain responsibilities are inherent in the nursing process: (1) providing culturally and ethnically sensitive, age-appropriate care; (2) maintaining a safe environment; (3) educating patients and their families; (4) ensuring continuity and coordination of care through discharge planning and referrals; and (5) communicating information.

Assessment

Assessment is the collection and analysis of relevant health data about the patient. Sources of data may be a preoperative interview with the patient and the patient's family; review of the planned surgical or invasive procedure; review of the patient's medical record; examination of the results of diagnostic tests; and consultation with the surgeon and anesthesia provider, unit nurses, or other personnel. Data collection focuses on these major elements: (1) the patient's current diagnosis, physical status, and psychosocial status (including literacy, language skills, and spiritual, ethnic, cultural, and lifestyle information relevant to the delivery of patient-specific care); (2) previous hospitalizations

Assessment...	Review medical record, validate important findings, corroborate with patient. Analyze, interpret, and prioritize information.
Nursing Diagnosis...	Synthesize data collected; then label clinical judgment about the patient as a nursing diagnosis. Can be actual or risk for. Based on patient assessment and perioperative nurse's clinical reasoning and critical thinking.
Outcome Identification...	Because perioperative nursing is largely preventive, generic outcomes have been identified that apply to all patients undergoing an operative or other invasive procedure. Additional outcomes are identified based on individual patient assessment and nursing diagnosis. Some outcomes are mutually formulated by the nurse and patient. Guide implementation of nursing interventions. Should be specific, realistic, and measurable.
Planning...	Incorporate information into a plan for the patient's care. Identify nursing interventions to achieve identified outcomes.
Implementation...	Carry out nursing plan of care. Gather equipment and supplies; participate in/guide/supervise patient preparation, transfer to OR bed, anesthesia induction, antimicrobial skin preparation, draping, patient positioning, time-out, monitoring of physiologic alterations during surgery, and patient discharge (transfer from OR bed, hand off to PACU or other postoperative unit).
Evaluation...	Determine whether outcomes were met; use outcome statements. Incorporate outcomes that have been met and those that are pending in hand-off report to nurse in PACU discharge area.

FIG. 1.2 The steps of the nursing process are interrelated, forming a continuous cycle of thought and action. *OR,* Operating room; *PACU,* postanesthesia care unit.

or surgical interventions and serious illnesses; and (3) the planned surgical or invasive procedure and the patient's understanding of this plan. Implementing patient-centered care requires the perioperative nurse to encourage the patient's active involvement in his or her care as part of patient safety. Of primary importance are the understanding of the scheduled procedure by the patient and patient's family and the patient's participation in activities such as marking the surgical site (Patient Safety) (the Universal Protocol for correct site surgery, along with other National Patient Safety Goals, is discussed in Chapter

Involving Patients in Marking the Surgical Site

Perioperative nurses value the goal of patient safety. One way to facilitate this goal is to improve involvement of patients in their care through information and education. TJC NPSGs and its Speak Up campaigns are safety initiatives that encourage patients to take an active role in their health care. *Help Avoid Mistakes in Your Surgery* offers a patient the following information about marking the surgical site and the time-out:

- A healthcare professional will mark the spot on your body on which the surgeon will operate. Make sure that only the correct part and nowhere else is marked. This helps avoid mistakes.
- Marking usually happens when you are awake. Sometimes you cannot be awake for the marking. If this happens, a family member or friend or another healthcare worker can watch the marking. They can make sure that your correct body part is marked.
- Your neck, upper back, or lower back will be marked if you are having spine surgery. The surgeon will check the exact place on your spine in the OR after you are asleep.
- Ask your surgeon if he or she will take a "time-out" just before your surgery. This is done to make sure the surgeon does the right surgery on the right body part on the right person.

NPSG, National Patient Safety Goals; *OR,* operating room; *TJC,* The Joint Commission.
Modified from The Joint Commission: *2017 hospital national patient safety goals* (website), 2016. https://www.jointcommission.org/hap_2017_npsgs/. (Accessed 26 December 2016).

2) (TJC, 2016a). The perioperative nurse also assesses risk factors that may contribute to negative outcomes.

The perioperative nurse proactively reports any concerns (e.g., abnormal laboratory values, or issues related to the patient's lack of understanding of the planned procedure) to the surgeon, documents all data collected, and notes any referrals that he or she makes.

Assessment formats vary from institution to institution but always include the physiologic and psychosocial aspects of the patient. In some settings the assessment is done in stages by one or more perioperative nurses. A perioperative nurse may perform an assessment in the presurgical care unit or by telephone before the day of surgical admission. In such cases the nurse in the OR verifies parts of the assessment previously done and completes the remainder. For a perioperative nurse caring for a healthy patient, assessment may mean only a thoughtful, brief review of the assessments previously done; a short patient interview; review of the medical record and surgical procedure; and a mental rehearsal of the resources and knowledge necessary to support the patient successfully through an operative procedure or any other invasive procedure. At other times, the perioperative nurse assesses all aspects of the patient and the patient's condition thoroughly.

When developing guidelines for preoperative assessment; patient, family, and caregiver education; and discharge planning, the perioperative nurse considers the following:
- What is the best EBP?
- Is relevant, concise patient information already available to the perioperative nursing staff?
- Is enough information available for perioperative nurses to consider patient care needs when preparing the OR room (e.g., special equipment, accessory items, instruments, sutures)?

- Is sufficient time available to initiate a meaningful perioperative nurse–patient interaction?
- Are surgical patients satisfied with their perioperative nursing care (do they express feelings of comfort and satisfaction regarding their care in the surgical setting)? Do they have knowledge of the perioperative nurse's role?
- Is there continuity of care between the perioperative unit and other nursing care units?

Being able to exchange information about patients in face-to-face meetings, by telephone, or by written messages is helpful for unit and perioperative nurses. A thorough assessment made and recorded by the preoperative nurse can accompany patients to the OR and serve as a guide for the perioperative nurse, who then completes a more focused preoperative patient assessment. With the burgeoning number of ambulatory surgery procedures, preoperative assessment is often integrated with preadmission testing. Some institutions hold group preoperative sessions. These not only help nurses get to know the patients, but also permit nurses to impart information on common routines, reactions, sensations, and nursing procedures that will take place preoperatively, intraoperatively, and postoperatively. The perioperative setting determines the type of interaction that occurs. The use of preoperative phone calls and online questionnaires has gained wide acceptance. The important point is that some form of assessment; patient, family, and caregiver education; and discharge planning is done. The particular facility and nursing staff determine how to accomplish it.

Assessment requires that the nurse know and understand the patient as a feeling, thinking, and responsible individual who is a candidate for a surgical or invasive procedure. Data identified through assessment help the perioperative nurse meet unique patient needs throughout the surgical intervention. Based on data collected, recorded, and interpreted during patient assessment, the perioperative nurse then formulates a nursing diagnosis.

Nursing Diagnosis

Nursing diagnosis is the process of identifying and classifying data collected in the assessment in a way that provides a focus for planning nursing care. Nursing diagnoses have evolved since they were first introduced in the 1950s. Today they are identified, named, and classified according to human response patterns and functional health patterns. The authoritative organization responsible for delineating the accepted list of nursing diagnoses is the North American Nursing Diagnosis Association International (NANDA-I) (Box 1.2). Each NANDA-I–approved nursing diagnosis has a set of components including a definition of the diagnostic term, its defining characteristics (i.e., the pattern of signs and symptoms or cues that make the meaning of the diagnosis clear), and its related or risk factors (i.e., causative or contributing factors that are useful in determining whether the diagnosis applies to a particular patient). For perioperative patients, many nursing diagnoses are "risk" diagnoses, which means they are not evidenced by signs or symptoms because the problem has yet to occur. Nursing interventions are directed at preventing the problem, vulnerability, or risk.

Not all patient problems encountered in the perioperative setting can be described by the list of accepted NANDA-I nursing diagnoses. Perioperative nurses can participate in describing and naming new nursing diagnoses that characterize unique perioperative patient problems. NANDA-I has established a "to be developed" category to designate nursing diagnoses that are partially developed and deemed useful to the nursing profession. Perioperative nurses may develop unique diagnostic labels and definitions

---

BOX 1.2

Selected Perioperative Nursing Diagnoses

- Ineffective airway clearance
- Anxiety
- Risk for allergy reaction
- Risk for aspiration
- Readiness for enhanced comfort
- Ineffective coping
- Risk for electrolyte imbalance
- Impaired urinary elimination
- Risk for imbalanced fluid volume
- Impaired gas exchange
- Hyperthermia
- Risk for hypothermia
- Risk for infection
- Risk for injury
- Risk for perioperative positioning injury
- Deficient knowledge
- Acute pain
- Risk for impaired skin integrity
- Risk for delayed surgical recovery
- Ineffective peripheral tissue perfusion

From NANDA International, Inc: *Nursing Diagnoses: Definitions and Classification 2018-2020,* © 2017 NANDA International. Used by arrangement with the Thieme Group, Stuttgart/ New York.

BOX 1.3

Selected Perioperative Nursing Data Set Desired Patient Outcomes

- O.10 Patient is free from signs and symptoms of injury related to thermal sources.
- O.20 Patient is free from signs and symptoms of unintended retained objects.
- O.30 Patient's procedure is performed on the correct site, side, and level.
- O.40 Patient's specimen(s) is managed in the appropriate manner.
- O.50 Patient's current status is communicated throughout the continuum of care.
- O.60 Patient is free from signs and symptoms of injury caused by extraneous objects.
- O.80 Patient is free from signs and symptoms of injury related to positioning.
- O.130 Patient receives appropriately administered medication(s).
- O.280 Patient is free from signs and symptoms of infection.
- O.290 Patient is at or returning to normothermia at the conclusion of the immediate postoperative period.
- O.300 Patient's fluids, electrolyte, and acid-base balances are maintained at or improved from baseline levels.
- O.310 Patient's respiratory status is consistent with or improved from baseline levels established preoperatively.
- O.320 Patient's cardiovascular status is maintained at or improved from baseline levels.
- O.500 Patient or designated support person demonstrates knowledge of the expected psychosocial responses to the procedure.
- O.550 Patient or designated support person demonstrates knowledge of the expected responses to the operative or invasive procedure.
- O.700 Patient or designated support person participates in decisions affecting his or her perioperative plan of care.
- O.720 Patient's value system, lifestyle, ethnicity, and culture are considered, respected, and incorporated in the perioperative plan of care.
- O.740 Patient's right to privacy is maintained.

Modified from Association of periOperative Registered Nurses (AORN): *PNDS—perioperative nursing data set,* ed 3, Denver, 2011, The Association.

---

and work to develop and validate them further through this process.

Outcome Identification

Outcome identification describes the desired or favorable patient condition that can be achieved through nursing interventions (Box 1.3). To be useful for assessing the effectiveness of nursing care, patient outcomes should be "nursing-sensitive"; they should be influenced by nursing and describe a patient state that can be measured and quantified. Nursing-sensitive patient outcomes derive from nursing diagnoses and direct the interventions that resolve the nursing diagnoses. They are the standards or criteria by which the effectiveness of interventions is measured. Outcomes are stated in terms of expected or desired patient behavior and must be specific and measurable. The appropriate time to measure perioperative nursing sensitive outcomes varies.

Some outcomes from intraoperative nursing interventions can be measured or evaluated immediately. Others occur over a longer period. In this textbook, the use of the phrase "the patient will" indicates an outcome that is expected to occur over time. Identification of expected and desired outcomes unique to the surgical patient provides the opportunity to prioritize care, becomes a basis for continuity of care, and directs evaluation (outcomes research). In this type of research, the relationship between patient characteristics, the processes of care (i.e., what the perioperative nurse does, which is described later in the Implementation section), and the outcomes of that care are studied, enhancing the perioperative nurse's ability to improve care. By using EBP, patient care can be standardized and perioperative nurses can support their choice of interventions that result in improved patient outcomes (Spruce, 2015).

Planning

After collecting and interpreting patient data, identifying appropriate nursing diagnoses, and establishing desired outcomes, the perioperative nurse begins *planning* the nursing care for the patient. Planning requires use of nursing knowledge and information about the patient and the intended surgical or invasive procedure to prepare the surgical environment and to plan patient care. Perioperative nurses check equipment for proper functioning; ensure that requisite supplies and positioning devices are available; and use their knowledge of anatomy to have proper instruments, sutures, accessory items, and surgical supplies on hand for the procedure to be performed. They also modify routines based on unique patient information such as allergies, transmissible infections, risk for perioperative hypothermia, deep vein thrombosis (DVT), infection, or pressure injury. They know the sequence of steps in the operative or other invasive procedure and use surgeons' preference cards, nursing care guides, and other resources, such as computerized data sheets, to prepare the room and equipment for the patient and surgical team.

Planning is preparing in advance for what will or may happen and determining the priorities for care. Planning based on patient assessment results in knowing the patient and the patient's unique needs so that alterations in events, such as positioning requirements

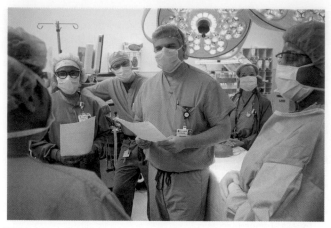

FIG. 1.3 A surgical team at Christiana Care Health System's Christiana Hospital (Newark, Delaware) conducts a briefing before surgery. This briefing allows team members to finalize the plan for the patient's care, anticipate potential changes in the patient's needs, and discuss potential safety concerns effectively.

or the surgical process, are anticipated and readily accommodated. Planning also requires knowledge of the patient's psychosocial state and feelings about the proposed operation so that the perioperative nurse can provide explanation, comfort, and emotional support.

Effective communication with other members of the healthcare team is essential, and improving communication among team members improves patient safety (Cabral et al., 2016). Briefings before the procedure allow for opportunities to improve safety and efficiency of care by ensuring that team members understand the plan of care, are prepared for potential changes, and discuss any safety concerns (Fig. 1.3). Debriefings at the end of the procedure provide an opportunity to discuss changes that should be made based on lessons learned. Coaching the surgical team has been shown to improve the quality of briefings and debriefings (Research Highlight).

Implementation

Implementation is performing nursing care activities and interventions that were planned as well as responding with critical thinking and orderly action to changes in the surgical procedure, patient's condition, or emergencies (Box 1.4). Implementation uses established standards of nursing care, recommendations for practice, clinical practice guidelines, and best practices. During this phase of the nursing process the perioperative nurse continues to assess the patient to determine the appropriateness of selected interventions and to alter interventions as necessary to achieve desired outcomes of care. Interventions are the "work of nursing." Many interventions used in perioperative nursing address patient safety issues (Patient Safety). The study of nursing interventions links nursing diagnoses with interventions and outcomes, and leads to validation of selected interventions or the development of new ones. Likewise, clinical practice, decision-making, and EBP are enhanced by their study. The study of nursing interventions also helps deliver cost-effective care by quantifying resource allocation.

Finally, implementation also means being the patient's advocate by recognition of patient concerns and unmet needs. Advocacy, a part of nurse caring, encompasses caring behaviors that promote

---

RESEARCH HIGHLIGHT

Coaching to Improve Quality of Surgery Briefings and Debriefings

Communication failures are identified as a root cause of many sentinel events occurring during surgery, including such failures as wrong-patient, wrong-site, and wrong-procedure events. To reduce communication failures and make the surgical environment safer for patients, many teams have adopted CRM training. CRM has been shown to improve communication and teamwork in the aviation industry and has been successfully applied to healthcare in many settings. The OR is thought to be an ideal setting for CRM training because effective communication of each team member is essential to improve safety and teamwork.

The purpose of this research was to determine whether or not communication in the OR was improved through coaching. Specifically, the researchers sought to leverage a coaching intervention to improve the quality and quantity of OR briefings and debriefings.

Using a preintervention/postintervention evaluation design, researchers in a large Midwestern hospital used trained observers to evaluate the frequency and quality of communication before and after surgical procedures. On completion of preintervention observations, a retired orthopedic surgeon, highly skilled in the use of CRM techniques, conducted coaching over a 4-week period. This particular surgeon was well known to the OR team, having developed strong relationships with them during the previous 5 years when he participated in their initial CRM training. Postintervention observations were then conducted using the same trained observers and tools with documented reliability and validity.

The frequency of briefings and debriefings was 100% both preintervention and postintervention. The authors, although pleased with these results, suspect that the finding may be attributable to the Hawthorne effect (i.e., staff knew that briefings and debriefings were being observed). When examining the quality of the communication that occurred during briefings and debriefings, there was a significant difference in briefing preintervention scores (mean [M] = 3.478, standard deviation [SD] = 0.70) and postintervention scores (M = 3.644; SD = 0.76; $t = -2.01$; $p = .044$). Likewise, there was a significant difference in the scores for debriefings preintervention (M = 2.377, SD = 1.10) and postintervention (M = 2.991, SD = 1.18; $t = -4.608$; $p < .0001$).

Although there was no difference in the frequency of briefings and debriefings observed in this study, there were significant differences in the quality of the communication observed. Coaching appeared to be an effective intervention, improving the quality of communication among team members.

CRM, Crew resource management; *OR,* operating room.
Modified from Kleiner C et al: Coaching to improve the quality of communication during briefings and debriefings, *AORN J* 100(4):358–368, 2014.

emotional and physical comfort. Caring behaviors include establishing a "connection" with the patient, responding to each patient's individuality, and meeting patient, family, and caregiver expectations (Patient Engagement Exemplar). The role of patient advocate is especially important in surgical settings when patients are sedated or unconscious and unable to speak for themselves. As caring patient advocates, perioperative nurses advance the best interests of their patients.

BOX 1.4

Selected Perioperative Nursing Data Set Perioperative Nursing Interventions

- A.10 Confirms patient identity.
- A.20 Verifies operative procedure, surgical site, and laterality.
- Im.60 Uses supplies and equipment within safe parameters.
- E.10 Evaluates for signs and symptoms of physical injury to skin and tissue.
- Im.20 Performs required counts.
- E.50 Evaluates results of the surgical count.
- Im.330 Manages specimen handling and disposition.
- E.40 Evaluates correct processes have been performed for specimen handling and disposition.
- Im.500 Provides status reports to designated support person.
- E.800 Ensures continuity of care.
- Im.10 Implements protective measures prior to operative or invasive procedure.
- Im.80 Applies safety devices.
- Im.160 Maintains continuous surveillance.
- A.280.1 Identifies physical alterations that require additional precautions for procedure-specific positioning.
- Im.120 Implements protective measures to prevent skin/tissue injury due to mechanical sources.
- Im.210 Administers prescribed solutions.
- Im.220 Administers prescribed medications.
- Im.300 Implements aseptic technique.
- Im.300.1 Protects from cross-contamination.
- Im.270 Performs skin preparations.
- Im.280 Implements thermoregulation measures.
- Im.370 Monitors physiologic parameters.
- E.260 Evaluates response to thermoregulation measures.
- A.520.1 Preserves and protects the patient's autonomy, dignity, and human rights.

Modified from Association of periOperative Registered Nurses (AORN): *PNDS—perioperative nursing data set*, ed 3, Denver, 2011, The Association.

Delegation. A team delivers perioperative patient care, and different categories of team members assist in a host of direct and indirect patient care activities. The surgical team usually consists of a surgeon and assistants at surgery (e.g., residents, interns, physician assistants [PAs], registered nurse first assistants [RNFAs], certified nurse practitioners [NP-Cs], or certified first assistants [CFAs]); an anesthesia provider; a circulating nurse; and a scrub person, who may be either a surgical technologist (ST) or an RN. Other members of the healthcare team, such as nursing assistants, orderlies, environmental services personnel, and patient care technicians, support the surgical team. During implementation of patient care the perioperative nurse may delegate certain nursing activities to these personnel, which are often called *unlicensed assistive personnel (UAP)*. As the use of UAP grows, questions and concerns arise about the proper scope of delegated activities. Each state's board of nursing defines the scope of practice for registered nurses, based on the nursing process. Further, each state's nurse practice act (a state law that protects the health and safety of the public) establishes legal qualifications for who can practice nursing. Implementation of the plan of care and the interventions to accomplish it are part of the nursing process. Therefore guidelines for proper delegation of some of these interventions are necessary. Delegation transfers to a competent person the authority to perform a selected nursing task in a selected situation according to the "five rights" of delegation

PATIENT SAFETY

Perioperative Patient Safety Issues

Much of the work of perioperative nursing involves patient safety including protecting patients from risks and vulnerabilities related to the procedure, positioning, equipment, and the environment. It is essential that perioperative nurses proactively assess risks to their patients and implement interventions to minimize those risks. Steelman and colleagues (2013) surveyed perioperative nurses to identify what safety issues they considered their highest priority. They obtained 3137 usable responses. The majority of nurses considered preventing wrong site, procedure, or patient surgery (69%) and preventing retained surgical items (61%) to be high-priority safety issues in need of heightened attention. More than one-third of respondents identified preventing medication errors, failures in instrument reprocessing, pressure injuries, and surgical fires to be high-priority issues as well.

The top rated issues include the following:

1. Preventing wrong site/procedure/patient surgery
2. Preventing retained surgical items
3. Preventing medication errors
4. Preventing failures in instrument reprocessing
5. Preventing pressure injuries
6. Preventing specimen management errors
7. Preventing surgical fires
8. Preventing perioperative hypothermia
9. Preventing burns from energy devices
10. Responding to difficult intubation/airway emergencies

From Steelman VM et al: Priority patient safety issues identified by perioperative nurses, *AORN J* 97(4):402–418, 2013.

PATIENT ENGAGEMENT EXEMPLAR

Basic Concepts for Engaging Patients

An important aspect of perioperative nursing is actively engaging patients and families in their own care. Patient-centered care and patient engagement is a key strategy for improving safety and efficacy in health care systems.

The NAQC defines patient engagement as "the involvement in their own care by individuals (and others they designate to engage on their behalf) with the goal that they make competent, well-informed decisions about their health and health care and take action to support those decisions" (Sofaer and Schumann, 2013). NAQC has highlighted major assumptions about patient engagement that every nurse should know and practice. First and foremost of these is that nurses establish a relationship with patients and families to form a partnership with them so they are able to participate in decisions about their care. Perioperative nurses form this relationship at the first meeting of the patient; it is based on ethical behavior and respecting patient's privacy. Partnerships with surgical patients should begin at the time a patient decides on surgery, and at that time they should be informed of the risks, benefits, and alternatives to having surgery. Education is offered regarding strategies to optimize surgical outcomes such as smoking cessation, nutrition, preoperative bathing, and exercise. NAQC guiding principles are used throughout this book as important patient-centered care concepts and exemplars are highlighted.

NAQC, Nursing Alliance for Quality Care.
Modified from Sofaer S, Schumann MJ: *NAQC guiding principles. Nursing Alliance for Quality Care. Fostering successful patient and family engagement: nursing's critical role* (website), 2013. http://www.naqc.org/WhitePaper-PatientEngagement. (Accessed 26 December 2016).

(Box 1.5). The perioperative nurse who delegates a task retains accountability for that delegation. Nursing functions of performing assessments, determining nursing diagnoses, establishing patient outcomes, developing the plan of care, and evaluating patient outcomes, as well as nursing interventions that require independent nursing knowledge, skills, or judgment, cannot be delegated (ANA/NCSBN, 2016). Perioperative nurses need to understand that institutional policy cannot contradict the nurse practice act of their state. Although tasks and procedures may be delegated to UAP members of the surgical team, the perioperative nurse remains responsible for supervising care because supervision cannot be delegated. Accordingly, the perioperative nurse assesses the patient and the competency level of personnel to determine which team member has the skill to provide the necessary care. Using UAP appropriately assists the profession of perioperative nursing to maintain high-quality patient care services.

Documenting Interventions. Accurate documentation of nursing care is integral to all phases of the nursing process, especially implementation of the plan of care. A description of the patient, nursing diagnoses and desired patient outcomes, nursing care given, and the patient's response to care (outcomes) should be included in the patient record. Documentation of the nursing care given should include more than technical aspects of care, such as counts or application of the electrosurgical unit (ESU) dispersive pad. Nursing care documentation should be associated with assessment and nursing diagnoses, with preestablished outcomes against which appropriateness and effectiveness of care may be judged. The form for this documentation may include standardized protocols and interventions; space should be provided to add interventions that are unique to individual patients or to describe variances in care. Documentation should require little time to complete, be specific to the perioperative setting, and provide continuity across the various areas in surgery, from presurgical holding areas to the PACU. Most facilities incorporate computerized documentation systems to enhance retrievability of data for evaluation of care and patient outcomes.

Syntegrity. In 1993 AORN recognized the need to describe and define the unique contributions of perioperative nurses to patient outcomes. After 6 years of research and validation, the Perioperative Nursing Data Set (PNDS) was recognized as a specialty nursing language, which provided a uniform and systematic method to document the basic elements of perioperative nursing care (AORN, 2011). The third edition of the PNDS has since been incorporated into an electronic framework called Syntegrity. Similar to the Perioperative Patient Focused Model, the PNDS begins with desired patient outcomes. Each outcome is defined and interpreted and presents criteria by which to measure outcome achievement. Subsequently, nursing interventions to achieve the desired patient outcomes are noted, along with suggested nursing activities to support the interventions. Of special import is the opportunity for perioperative nurses to use Syntegrity to document assessments, interventions, and outcomes electronically, enabling Syntegrity to compare clinical outcomes from large patient populations within an institution and even across institutions. Syntegrity can be used to guide research, develop best practices, and support EBP.

Evaluation

Evaluation is checking, observing, and appraising the results of what was done. Although evaluation is traditionally listed as the last phase of the nursing process, it is an integral, systematic, and ongoing component of providing safe, effective, and good perioperative patient care. Evaluation focuses on the patient's progress in attaining identified

---

BOX 1.5

The Five Rights of Delegation

- **The Right task.** The perioperative nurse determines that this task is delegable for a specific patient, taking into consideration such factors as potential for harm, complexity of the task, necessary problem-solving, and predictability of the outcome. Routine tasks performed according to a standardized procedure and which have predictable outcomes are safest to delegate.
- **The Right circumstances.** The perioperative nurse considers the patient care setting, resources available, and other relevant factors. Tasks delegated must not require independent nursing judgment.
- **The Right person.** The perioperative nurse is the right person to delegate the right task to the right person to be performed on the right patient. The perioperative nurse must be familiar with institutional and state board policies on delegation, along with the job description of the UAP; the person's capabilities, knowledge, and skill level; and learning needs to ensure that safe, quality patient care is provided. In this way the nurse matches tasks to the UAP's skills, qualifications, and competence.
- **The Right communication and direction.** The perioperative nurse provides a clear, specific, and concise description of the task, with key information relating to its objectives, rationale, limits, and expectations. There should be an opportunity for questions and clarifying instructions. Information that the perioperative nurse needs to know from the person performing the task must be identified. Communication should be direct and not provided through others.
- **The Right supervision and evaluation.** The perioperative nurse appropriately monitors the task or person performing it, evaluates results or patient outcomes or both, intervenes if necessary, and provides feedback. Providing immediate feedback or identifying a problem with performance as it occurs is essential to upholding standards of care and performance expectations.

Perioperative nurses must be involved actively in providing the assessment, evaluation, and judgment needed to coordinate and supervise perioperative patient care. When delegating care activities, perioperative nurses retain accountability for analyzing and evaluating the outcomes of delegated tasks. Activities that rely on the nursing process, such as performing assessments; making nursing diagnoses; establishing plans of care; providing extensive patient, family, and caregiver education; and planning for patient discharge, cannot be delegated.

UAP, Unlicensed assistive personnel.
Modified from the *National Council of State Boards of Nursing response to the PEW taskforce principles and vision for health care workforce regulation,* Chicago, 1996, The Council; Cherry B, Jacob SR: *Contemporary nursing: issues, trends and management,* ed 7, St Louis, 2016, Elsevier; Taylor C et al: *Fundamentals of nursing: the art and science of person-centered nursing care,* ed 8, Philadelphia, 2015, Wolters Kluwer.

---

outcomes. When feasible and appropriate, the patient, family, and caregiver should participate in the evaluation process. The attainment of outcomes, any revisions to nursing diagnoses or desired outcomes, and the plan of care are documented. Because perioperative patient care processes and interventions often are interdisciplinary, healthcare facilities may need to use additional evaluation methods.

Evaluation of the patient's progress toward desired outcomes extends throughout the postoperative period and beyond. It is essential

RESEARCH HIGHLIGHT

Transitions in Care

Transitions in care (patient handoffs) should be considered high-risk activities. During a single surgical intervention there are numerous transitions in care, with the first occurring in the preoperative area. Using a qualitative descriptive design, this study aimed to identify the role of the preoperative assessment in the patient's transition and to identify the contributions nursing made in the surgical patient's first transition of care.

Researchers in a large medical center in the northeastern United States used a semistructured interview guide to conduct focus groups with a total of 24 nurses. Four themes emerged:

1. Understanding vulnerabilities
2. Multidimensional communication
3. Managing expectations
4. Connecting the disconnected

The authors conclude that the role of the nurse in the preoperative assessment and transition of care is one of advocate. As an advocate, nurses identify risk factors, vulnerabilities, and patient needs that may be significant during the surgical experience. Additionally, results from this study suggest that the nursing preoperative assessment may be a valid tool to help define and identify risk factors potentially affecting the patient during the entire perioperative experience.

Modified from Malley A et al: The role of the nurse and the preoperative assessment in patient transitions, *AORN J* 102(2):181.e1–181.e9, 2015.

that critical information be shared with nurses responsible for care postoperatively. Communication during this transition of care, referred to as a handoff or handover, is critical to patient safety and continuity of care (Research Highlight).

Performance improvement (PI) activities, notably by monitoring important aspects of care, problem identification, problem-solving, and peer review, may be part of the overall system evaluation. Often referred to as *quality improvement (QI) programs,* overall system evaluations by interdisciplinary teams address areas for improvement in patient care, identify problems, propose solutions, and monitor and evaluate the effectiveness of improvements. This topic is discussed in more detail later in the chapter.

Institutional Standards of Care

Healthcare facilities have developed additional standards to communicate expectations of performance. Perioperative departments have the responsibility, delegated through administrative governance of the institution, to develop policies and procedures, which is often called the *surgical services standards of care.* Policies are written statements that outline responsibilities and appropriate actions in specific circumstances. To be effective, a policy should be consistent with national and state practice standards, be realistic and achievable, be consistently followed except where prior approval of deviation has been obtained, and be based on evidence and reasoned and rational thinking.

Procedures are written guides to implementing policies. They describe detailed chronologic sequences of activities as they relate to particular policies. Policies and procedures are usually combined in the department's *Standards of Care Manual,* which is kept readily available as a perioperative care resource. Many facilities have moved to an online manual as well to provide easy access in multiple patient care locations. Participation of staff members in policy and procedure

development increases their knowledge of the subject matter and generates a sense of ownership. This results in meaningful and authoritative interpretation of approved policy and procedure to peers and furthers successful implementation.

Evidence-Based Practice

Perioperative nursing relies on a strong foundation of traditions designed to provide excellent patient care. These traditions include many aspects of direct patient care as well as control of the environment in which care is provided. Perioperative nurses have an ethical responsibility to review practices and to modify them, based on the best available scientific evidence (Evidence for Practice). This process can be used proactively to evaluate alternative ways of providing care, such as using different patient positioning surfaces or developing patient education materials. EBP can also be used to problem-solve, such as when investigating a serious adverse event or other clinical problems including perioperative hypothermia, a pressure injury, or a retained surgical item. EBP allows the perioperative nurse to base care decisions on the best available research rather than tradition (Spruce, 2015).

EBP, a systematic process, identifies clinical issues and collects and then evaluates the best evidence. It is frequently used to design and implement clinical practice changes after thoroughly evaluating the practice of interest. Early and important changes that were implemented through the EBP process and the work of nurses are double-gloving to reduce sharps injuries (Stebral and Steelman, 2006), asking patients to shower preoperatively twice with chlorhexidine gluconate (Pottinger et al., 2006), administering antibiotics within 60 minutes before the surgical incision (Spalter and Wyatt, 2006), and administering a combination of blood products (massive transfusion protocol) for control of hemorrhage (Enticott et al., 2012).

When there is not enough evidence to guide practice, perioperative nurses can collaborate with a nurse researcher in a research study to address the practice issue or to identify, review, and evaluate evidence about it. One model used in many healthcare facilities is the Iowa Model of Evidence-Based Practice to Promote Quality Patient Care (Fig. 1.4).

EBP has become an integral part of many national quality initiatives. The Surgical Care Improvement Project (SCIP) began as a national quality partnership endorsed by many organizations and focused on improving care of surgical patients by using EBP to significantly reduce surgical complications. SCIP measures address, among other important care aspects, timely administration of preoperative prophylactic antibiotics and the expeditious removal of urinary catheters postoperatively (TJC, 2016b).

Performance Improvement

Continuing trends in health care have seen increased control of costs, more efficient use of resources and supplies, decreased length of stay for surgical patients, and a shift of many surgical procedures from inpatient to ambulatory surgery settings (Ambulatory Surgery Considerations). Concomitantly, there is a keener awareness of the need for continued improvement in delivery of perioperative patient care. TJC has taken a strong position on the need to monitor and evaluate the quality and appropriateness of care delivery continually to resolve any identified problems while striving constantly to improve delivery systems and processes. In 1994 TJC instituted performance assessment, measurement, and improvement as the core of its standards. This represented an evolution from quality assurance to continuous QI, and finally to PI. Such a transition underscored the belief that measuring outcomes and improving care are essential

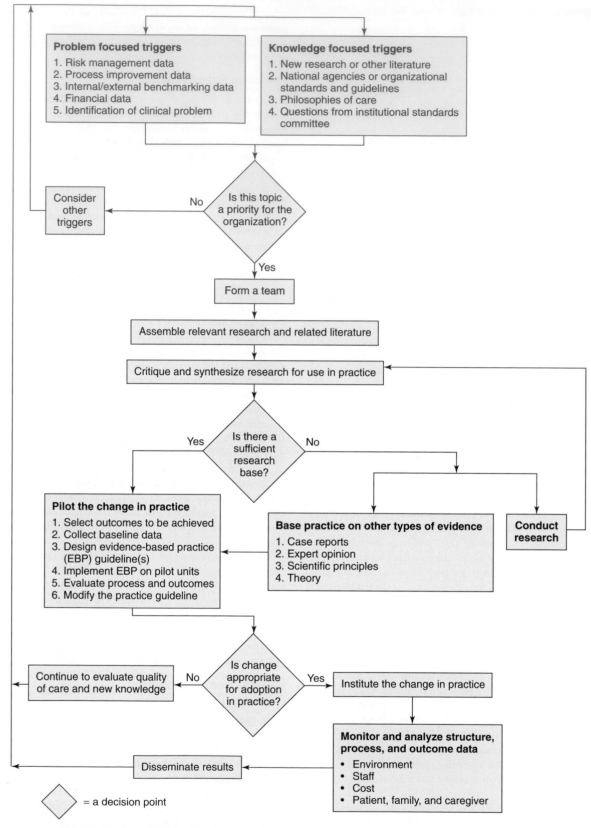

FIG. 1.4 The Iowa Model of Evidence-Based Practice to Promote Quality Patient Care is used in many healthcare settings to identify opportunities to improve care; evaluate evidence; and design, implement, and evaluate evidence-based practice changes.

EVIDENCE FOR PRACTICE

Evidence-Based Practice and Association of periOperative Registered Nurse's Guidelines for Perioperative Practice

Patient care decisions based on scientifically sound evidence rather than the opinion of healthcare providers are known as evidence-based practice (EBP). At times, staff nurses base practice decisions on what they were taught in nursing school or from other nurses rather than on what has been scientifically validated. AORN's *Guidelines for Perioperative Practice* are a collection of evidence-based recommendations to promote patient safety during operative and invasive procedures. These guidelines represent one way that AORN supports perioperative RNs, advances the nursing profession, and promotes excellence in perioperative nursing practice. The guidelines illustrate how the perioperative RN ensures a safe work environment, provides safe perioperative patient care, and reflects the RN's scope of practice. Illustrating optimal levels of workplace safety and patient care, the guidelines are achievable, evidence-based statements of professional practice, which are meant to serve as foundational documents in the development of policies, procedures, and competency validation tools.

Representing AORN's official position on perioperative practice, the guidelines are created by AORN's perioperative nursing specialists in collaboration with the AORN Guidelines Advisory Board and liaisons from a number of related professional organizations such as the American College of Surgeons and the Association for Professionals in Infection Control and Epidemiology. The guidelines help perioperative nurse leaders synthesize and translate a large amount of literature into manageable recommendations. AORN's guidelines meet the National Academy of Medicine's (formerly the Institute of Medicine [IOM]) definition of clinical practice guidelines and are based on a thorough review of both research and nonresearch evidence. Each recommendation is rated based on the quality and strength of the evidence supporting it. Through the application of EBP, the guidelines support cost-effective, scientifically sound, and safe approaches to patient care.

For perioperative nurses to implement an evidence-based approach to problem-solving, it is most useful to adopt a model that helps focus clinical decision-making and solution implementation. Evidence-based models generally include step-by-step direction for addressing clinical problems and pairing them with research-based interventions so that practice changes, supported by the best evidence, occur. There are a number of widely used models, such as the Johns Hopkins Nurse Evidence-Based Practice Model, the Stetler Model of Research Utilization, the ACE Star Model of Knowledge Transformation, and the Iowa Model of Evidence-Based Practice to Improve Quality of Care (see Fig. 1.4). Regardless of the model selected and implemented, communication is essential to ensure that practice changes are understood and adopted.

Providing care that is patient centered, evidence based, and data driven is the responsibility of all nurses. Evidence-based perioperative nursing care results in improved patient outcomes and increases the patient's satisfaction with care delivered. Through the adoption and implementation of an evidence-based model, practice changes are grounded in science.

AORN, Association of periOperative Registered Nurses; *RN*, registered nurse.
Modified from the Association of periOperative Registered Nurses (AORN): *Guidelines for perioperative practice*, Denver, 2016, The Association; White S, Spruce L: Perioperative nursing leaders implement clinical practice guidelines using the Iowa Model of Evidence-Based Practice, *AORN J* 102(1):51–56, 2015.

AMBULATORY SURGERY CONSIDERATIONS

Timely Patient Discharge

Approximately 70% of all surgeries are now performed as ambulatory procedures. This shift from inpatient to outpatient has been facilitated by the development of minimally invasive surgical techniques and the improvement of anesthesia techniques and medications. Performing procedures on an ambulatory basis provides cost efficiencies to the facility and improves patients' experiences, allowing them to recover in their own home. Ambulatory surgery also places additional pressures on the perioperative team, which must ensure that quality care and patient safety are maintained while preparing the patient for a timely discharge.

To ensure that patients are best prepared for a timely discharge after their procedure, a number of strategies are required, and coordinated perioperative team efforts are essential. Preparing for a safe, efficient discharge begins at the time the surgery is planned. Enhanced recovery after surgery (ERAS) protocols are often implemented. Preoperative patient preparation includes nutritional assessment and optimization, smoking cessation, and improved physical fitness. Patient education related to the postoperative course and expected recovery take into account the patient's health literacy level. Because low levels of health literacy are increasingly common, patient education is important. In addition to appropriate thromboprophylaxis and antibiotic prophylaxis, ERAS protocols minimize prolonged fasting and often eliminate routine bowel preparation.

During the intraoperative phase, ambulatory surgical procedures require close attention to a number of surgical and anesthetic issues. The use of minimally invasive techniques is preferable, and close attention to ensuring hemostasis is important. Early ambulation is facilitated if drains and nasogastric tubes are not used. Opiates are avoided for pain management, perioperative hypothermia is prevented, and any intraoperative vascular volume loss is replaced.

Postoperatively early mobilization, early oral intake, and avoidance of opiate analgesics all contribute to a safe and efficient recovery period. The overall aim of performing procedures on an ambulatory surgery basis is to return patients to their optimal state of health, in their natural environment, as quickly as possible. This can be accomplished by a coordinated interprofessional team effort when careful planning and attention are focused around a shared goal.

Modified from Clifford T: Enhanced recovery after surgery, *J Perianesth Nurs* 31(2):182–183, 2016; Ead HM: Ensuring a smooth discharge home after ambulatory surgery, *J Perianesth Nurs* 31(3):254–256, 2016; Liebner LT: I can't read that! Improving perioperative literacy for ambulatory surgical patients, *AORN J* 101(4):416–427, 2015; Maurice E: Timely patient discharge from the ambulatory surgical setting, *AORN J* 102(2):185–191, 2015; Slim K et al: How to implement an enhanced recovery program? Proposals from the Francophone Group for enhanced recovery after surgery (GRACE), *J. Visc Surg* 153(6S):S45–S49, 2016.

elements of effective healthcare delivery. PI efforts encompass improvements in quality and effectiveness based on ethical and economic perspectives.

A surgical services PI program is based on established standards of care, and the intent of each standard is reflected in realistic and measurable outcomes. A plan to measure and improve care, including the scope of care and important aspects of that care, should be in place. Specific quality indicators are identified that reflect important aspects of care. Thresholds that identify the level of acceptable variance for each indicator are then established. Measurement methods include retrospective or concurrent review of medical records, review of adverse event reports, utilization review, patient surveys and interviews, and peer review. Emphasis is on structure, process, and outcome indicators. Some facilities have implemented multiple programs used in industry, such as Six Sigma and Lean process improvement methodologies, to assess and refine processes to improve efficiency and improve processes and outcomes of care.

PI approaches facilitate the delivery of safe, high-quality perioperative patient care. When processes are understood, they can be improved through a systematic plan of action. Involvement of teams that perform the surgical services performance assessments and create improvement plans strengthens the staff's commitment to meet standards and enhance program effectiveness. TJC supports the evolution to an information technology infrastructure (i.e., EHRs) in which performance measurement becomes an integral part of the care delivery process. As current uses of data expand and improve, objectives will still include the use of data for research activities directed at improving quality of care and identifying and disseminating EBPs. Perioperative nurses can anticipate that measurement requirements and performance expectations will change over time with new technologies and care practices as they affect the quality and safety of care. TJC also expects healthcare organizations to evaluate patients' perceptions of care and to use this information to improve the system of care delivery. The objectives of future TJC activities are likely to focus on the following:

- Continued expansion and coordination of nationally standardized core measurement capabilities
- Increased use of measurement data for QI, benchmarking, accountability, decision-making, accreditation, and research.

Perioperative Nursing Roles

The nursing profession and the healthcare culture in the United States continue to change rapidly in response to many elements. An aging population continues to create significant increases in demands for health services (see Chapter 27 for a discussion of the aging perioperative patient). New ambulatory settings for the delivery of health services, including operative and other invasive procedures, continue to develop, as well as community-based clinics, school-linked clinics, mobile clinics, and drive-in health centers. Healthcare organizations that are able to respond quickly to change will have an edge in the healthcare industry of the future. Likewise, perioperative nurses who understand the need for clinical and service quality, cost-effectiveness, information management, coordinated patient-centered care, efficiency, the special needs of an aging surgical population, and the importance of patient satisfaction will be able to anticipate and position themselves for this future. Roles in case management, care coordination, informatics, the healthcare industry, consulting, management, advanced practice nursing, and research are all very real possibilities for future-oriented perioperative nurses.

Traditional Perioperative Roles

There are two traditional perioperative nursing roles: the circulating nurse and the scrub person. *The circulating nurse* remains "non-scrubbed" and uses the nursing process to assess the patient, identify desired outcomes, formulate nursing diagnoses, choose a plan of care, implement or delegate interventions, and evaluate outcomes of the care provided. Among many other responsibilities, the circulating nurse manages patient positioning, antimicrobial skin preparation, medications, implants, specimens, warming devices, and surgical counts. AORN (2014a) reaffirmed its position advocating the

requirement that there be an RN circulator for every patient undergoing surgery or other invasive procedure and that this nurse manage the care of only one patient at a time.

The *scrub person*, working at a sterile field, assembles needed instruments and supplies in a manner to maximize safety and efficiency. This role requires an in-depth knowledge of each step of the surgical procedure and the certain ability to anticipate each instrument and supply that will be needed. Many instruments are complex and require assembly. Instruments are positioned on the sterile table so that the scrub person can prepare each instrument as it will be used and quickly transfer it to the surgeon, often without being asked. This role is highly technical and either an RN or an ST may assume it. The ST who functions as the scrub person may be certified (CST). The certifying agency for STs is the National Board of Surgical Technology and Surgical Assisting (NBSTSA). Surgical technology students who graduate from an accredited surgical technology program are eligible for and must sit for the certification exam. Many of these programs result in an associate degree.

The scrub person and circulating nurse form an important partnership in ensuring patient safety. They work closely and effectively together throughout the procedure. Close teamwork keeps communication open, minimizes the risk of errors, and promotes the cost-effective use of supplies. Based on mutual respect, teamwork enhances quality and safety in the workplace.

The CNOR credential is available to perioperative nurses who function in traditional or nontraditional roles. This credential represents demonstrated knowledge of clinical practices and standards as well as a marked level of professional achievement. It also demonstrates proficiency in support of quality patient care and sets a standard of commitment to the profession of perioperative nursing (CCI, 2015a).

Registered Nurse First Assistant

The role of the perioperative RNFA in surgery is an expanded perioperative nursing role that requires formal academic education (AORN, 2013). The RNFA works collaboratively with the surgeon (and the patient and surgical team) by handling and cutting tissue, using instruments and medical devices, providing surgical site exposure and hemostasis, suturing, and assisting with wound management—all as components of assisting-at-surgery behaviors. AORN has developed standards for RNFA educational programs (AORN, 2014b), and certification is available for this role (CRNFA) (CCI, 2015b). Many experienced perioperative nurses have obtained this education. Effective January 1, 2020, the education level for entry into an RNFA program and subsequent RNFA practice will be the baccalaureate degree. AORN recommends RNs who were practicing as RNFAs before 2020 and do not have a baccalaureate degree be permitted to continue to practice as RNFAs. Performing as an RNFA allows an experienced perioperative nurse to expand clinical knowledge and skills and to assume additional responsibility for preoperative and postoperative patient management while still remaining directly involved with intraoperative patient care. The RNFA has gained wide professional acceptance as a highly skilled member of the surgical team. Functioning in this role is another way perioperative nurses can develop professionally to meet the changing needs of healthcare delivery.

Advanced Practice Registered Nurse

Advanced practice registered nurses (APRNs) include NP-Cs, certified registered nurse anesthetists (CRNAs), certified nurse-midwives (CNMs), and clinical nurse specialists (CNSs). Acute-care NP-Cs fill gaps in providing care for patients who are more acutely ill and whose medical-surgical problems are more complex. In an era of rapid healthcare change, opportunities for APRNs are continually evolving. NP-Cs are employed in acute care hospitals and ambulatory surgery centers across the country. Some NP-Cs focus primarily on the preoperative phase of patient care and use their advanced knowledge to assess patients and order preoperative medications and treatment. Other NP-Cs combine this role with that of the first assistant, allowing them to use their advanced practice skills throughout the perioperative care continuum. Some CNSs also provide licensed independent care to individual patients. However, the traditional role of the CNS involves primarily indirect care within the perioperative leadership team. As part of the management team, the CNS provides support for the care of groups of patients through leadership, education, consultation, management, and research. CNSs have assumed a significant leadership role in adopting and demonstrating the implementation of AORN's "standards of perioperative nursing practice" (AORN, 2014c).

APRNs must have a graduate nursing education (at least a master's degree). In 2004 the American Association of Colleges of Nursing (AACN) advocated for the doctor of nursing practice (DNP) degree as the minimum educational preparation for APRNs. These educational programs are available across the country (AACN, 2015).

Emerging Roles

As patient needs change and technology advances, new perioperative nursing roles develop. Some of these roles include care coordinator, family liaison, robotics coordinator, and informatics specialist. Some healthcare organizations have established the role of care coordinator in specific programs such as trauma, bariatrics, cardiac care, and organ transplant to meet the unique challenges and complexities of these specific patient populations, allowing the perioperative nurse to develop more in-depth skills to meet the needs of a specific population of surgical patients.

As early as the late 1990s the perioperative nursing role of family or surgical liaison evolved to serve as a communication link between the OR and the family during surgery. The liaison translates information from the surgical team to the family, often serving to clarify and answer questions that require an understanding of events in the OR. Hospitals and ambulatory surgery centers have implemented this perioperative nursing role to enhance the patient, family, and caregiver experience of care.

Another emerging role in perioperative nursing is that of robotics coordinator. Both the number and the types of procedures performed with surgical robots have increased dramatically. Robots are now commonly used for general, cardiovascular, pediatric, gynecologic, and urologic surgery. The complexity of the equipment and requisite troubleshooting demand additional specialized skills, create many challenges for the perioperative team, and often lead to the need for a robotics coordinator to oversee this technology, provide complex troubleshooting, and train personnel (Neel, 2014). The robotics coordinator may also serve as a public liaison by providing marketing and public educational opportunities about the robotics surgery program.

Informatics is another specialty in which some perioperative nurses are focusing. Nursing informatics systems have applications for practice, administration, education, and research (McGonigle et al., 2014). More efficient management of fiscal, material, and human resources has stimulated the development of electronic information systems for diverse functions in perioperative patient care settings. A well-designed information system can synthesize large volumes of data efficiently into meaningful reports to support decision-making. Nursing applications include point-of-care clinical systems, EHRs, web-based patient education, research, and telemedicine and telenursing. "Nursing informatics provides the tools and capabilities necessary to enrich the data, information, knowledge, and wisdom pathway and, therefore, literally puts the information and knowledge nurses need at their fingertips" (McGonigle et al., 2014, p. 325). Perioperative nurse informatics specialists have the opportunity to develop clinical nursing systems that incorporate nursing care protocols, critical paths, EBP, the PNDS, and patient education materials. Such systems allow sharing information across wide networks as patients access healthcare at different points and times. Technology systems are developing that include interactive computer/television by which perioperative nurses can remotely communicate with their patients over phone or cable lines, allowing the perioperative nurse to view the patient's wound or discuss recovery and rehabilitation from surgery.

Perioperative nursing is an exciting, ever-changing specialty. The opportunities for continual learning and challenges are endless. As the field of perioperative nursing moves into the future, these opportunities will continue to grow and evolve. Perioperative nurses need to identify their professional goals and develop strategic plans to accomplish those goals, including enhancing their skill sets and education. This strategy will position the perioperative nurse well for exciting roles in the future.

Key Points

- Perioperative nursing is a complex specialty that uses the nursing process to provide high-quality patient care.
- The Perioperative Patient Focused Model provides a framework for perioperative nursing care.
- PNDS is a standardized language used to document patient care to enhance retrievability of data for evaluation of patient care.
- EBP is a systematic process by which to identify an issue, collect and evaluate the best evidence, and make the best clinical decisions.
- Perioperative nurses work with a team to provide patient care; effective, extensive, and ongoing communication within the team is essential to accomplish safe patient care.
- There are a variety of perioperative nursing roles, including circulating nurse, scrub nurse, RNFA, APRN, and emerging roles such as robotics coordinator and informatics specialist.

Critical Thinking Question

When reviewing your assignment for the day, you note that you are caring for a 45-year-old male patient undergoing a left nephrectomy. When you interview him in the preoperative area, you note that he is otherwise healthy. He is approachable, pleasant, and cooperative. As you begin to develop your plan of care, you identify interventions that are delegable to other members of the nursing team. What questions will you ask yourself as you consider the "rights" of delegation? What questions will you ask nursing team members when determining if you can safely delegate an intervention in your plan of care to them?

⊖volve *The answer to the Critical Thinking Question can be found at http://evolve.elsevier.com/Rothrock/Alexander.*

References

American Association of Colleges of Nursing (AACN): *The doctor of nursing practice: current issues and clarifying recommendations*, Washington, DC, 2015,

The Association. http://www.aacn.nche.edu/aacn-publications/white-papers/DNP-Implementation-TF-Report-8-15.pdf. (Accessed 29 October 2016).

American Nurses Association, National Council of State Boards of Nursing (ANA/NCSBN): *Joint statement on delegation* (website), 2016. https://www.ncsbn.org/Delegation_joint_statement_NCSBN-ANA.pdf. (Accessed 26 December 2016).

Association of periOperative Registered Nurses (AORN): *PNDS—perioperative nursing data set*, ed 3, Denver, 2011, The Association.

Association of periOperative Registered Nurses (AORN): *Position statement: registered nurse first assistants*, Denver, 2013, The Association.

Association of periOperative Registered Nurses (AORN): *Position statement: one perioperative registered nurse circulator dedicated to every patient undergoing a surgical or other invasive procedure*, Denver, 2014a, The Association. http://www.aorn.org/aorn-org/guidelines/clinical-resources/position-statements. (Accessed 21 August 2016).

Association of periOperative Registered Nurses (AORN): *AORN: RN first assistant resources*, Denver, 2014b, The Association. http://www.aorn.org/aorn-org/guidelines/clinical-resources/rn-first-assistant-resources. (Accessed 26 December 2016).

Association of periOperative Registered Nurses (AORN): *Position statement: APRNs in the perioperative environment*, Denver, 2014c, The Association. http://www.aorn.org/aorn-org/guidelines/clinical-resources/position-statements. (Accessed 21 August 2016).

Association of periOperative Registered Nurses (AORN): *AORN standards: standards of perioperative nursing* (website), 2015. www.aorn.org/guidelines/clinical-resources/aorn-standards. (Accessed 26 December 2016).

Association of periOperative Registered Nurses (AORN): Quality and performance improvement standards for perioperative nursing. In: *Guidelines for perioperative practice*, Denver, 2016, The Association.

Cabral RA et al: Use of a surgical safety checklist to improve team communication, *AORN J* 104(3):206–216, 2016.

Competency and Credentialing Institute (CCI): *CNOR certification and recertification candidate handbook* (website), 2015a. http://info.cc-institute.org/cnor-certification-handbook-download. (Accessed 7 June 2017).

Competency and Credentialing Institute (CCI): *CRNFA certification and recertification candidate handbook* (website), 2015b. http://www.cc-institute.org/docs/default-source/handbooks/crnfa-candidate-handbook-2017.pdf?sfvrsn=2. (Accessed 7 June 2017).

Enticott JC et al: A review on decision support for massive transfusion: understanding human factors to support the implementation of complex interventions in trauma, *Transfusion* 15(12):2692–2705, 2012.

Helzer Doroh HM, Monahan JC: Student nurses in the OR: improving recruitment and retention, *AORN J* 103(1):89–94, 2016.

McGonigle D et al: Why nurses need to understand nursing informatics, *AORN J* 100(3):324–327, 2014.

Neel D: *Robotic surgery trends create new career options for nurses* (website), 2014. http://www.oncologynurseadvisor.com/oncology-nursing/robotic-surgery-trends-create-new-career-options-for-nurses/article/341748/. (Accessed 29 October 2016).

Pottinger J et al: Skin preparation, *Periop Nurs Clin* 1:203–210, 2006.

Sofaer S, Schumann MJ: *NAQC guiding principles. Nursing Alliance for Quality Care. Fostering successful patient and family engagement: nursing's critical role* (website), 2013. http://www.naqc.org/WhitePaper-PatientEngagement. (Accessed 26 December 2016).

Spalter AW, Wyatt DA: Antibiotic prophylaxis and surgical site infection: are we doing enough to ensure quality? *Periop Nurs Clin* 1:211–222, 2006.

Spruce L: Back to basics: implementing evidence-based practice, *AORN J* 101(1):107–112, 2015.

Stebral LL, Steelman VM: Double gloving for surgical procedures: an evidence-based practice project, *Periop Nurs Clin* 1:251–260, 2006.

Steelman VM et al: Priority patient safety issues identified by perioperative nurses, *AORN J* 97(4):402–418, 2013.

The Joint Commission (TJC): *2017 national patient safety goals* (website), 2016a. https://www.jointcommission.org/hap_2017_npsgs/. (Accessed 26 December 2016).

The Joint Commission (TJC): *Surgical care improvement project* (website), 2016b. http://www.jointcommission.org/assets/1/6/Surgical%20Care%20Improvement%20Project.pdf. (Accessed 7 June 2017).

CHAPTER 2

Patient Safety and Risk Management

ELLEN MURPHY

Think about what happens in the perioperative setting. Patients' natural pain, communication, reflex, and infection defenses are purposefully diminished or obliterated. Their bodies are positioned on firm flat surfaces and frequently in unnatural positions. Then their bodies are further traumatized with instruments, fibers, drugs, and other foreign materials. It is no wonder that nearly one-half of the sentinel events reported to The Joint Commission (TJC) through the second quarter of 2016 could have occurred in the perioperative setting (TJC, 2016). Retained surgical items (RSIs) and wrong-site–patient-procedure events alone comprise about one-quarter of the total reported events. Patient safety, a paramount concern to nurses in all settings, is a critical consideration in perioperative patient care settings.

This chapter briefly describes the evolution of perioperative patient safety, then focuses on management of injury risks as a collective responsibility of the entire surgical team, the concept of "value" as a quality and cost concern, and the emergence of patient safety as a financial risk management and quality compliance consideration. Risk management directors are safety partners with the surgical team for patient safety promotion. The chapter ends with various ethical principles that underlie perioperative patient safety.

Evolution of Perioperative Patient Safety

Patient safety is a primary concern for surgical team members. *Primum non nocere* or "First, do no harm," is a long-standing imperative. Early operating room (OR) nursing textbooks written by OR nurses included counting sponges among nursing duties (e.g., Smith, 1924). Perioperative nursing textbooks and curricula continued to include substantial content on infection control, positioning, safe medication practices, and counts through World War II. The first edition of this very textbook by Edythe Alexander included content on asepsis, the importance of correct side surgery, proper blood handling, and proper tourniquet application. Alexander did not use the word "safety"; rather, she described the purpose of "perfecting every detail…to insure that patients…have every chance to overcome the disease or injury with which they are afflicted" (Alexander, 1943, p. 7).

After World War II, safety activities increased and became more formalized. The Joint Commission for the Accreditation of Hospitals, now The Joint Commission (TJC), emerged. Nursing groups and publications increasingly emphasized patient safety features. The American Nurses Association (ANA) published its *Code for Nurses,* which included provisions on patient safety and privacy, and the Association of Operating Room Nurses (now, the Association of periOperative Registered Nurses [AORN]) organized in the early 1950s. From the beginning, AORN's conferences and publications were replete with patient safety information. Its first conference in 1954 included programs on methods improvement, explosion prevention, bacteria destruction, the surgeon–nurse relationship, and positioning (Glass and Murphy, 2002). AORN annually publishes *Guidelines for Perioperative Practice,* which is evidence-based, using research, evidence-based, and nonresearch studies as a fundamental authority and resource for perioperative safety practices.

Safety as an Individual Responsibility

Throughout the 1980s, healthcare authorities viewed professionals' errors and their effects on patient safety primarily as the individual practitioner's responsibility. Legal cases, statutes and administrative rules, and professional licensure systems tended to reinforce this approach. Any finding of negligence required that at least one individual had failed to do what a similarly situated, reasonable, and prudent professional would have done under similar circumstances and that failure caused the patient's injury. Likewise, professional licensure discipline was related to the abilities and behavior of the individual licensee.

In 1991 Brennan and colleagues proposed that despite individual best efforts by professionals, mistakes continued and were, in fact, more common than previously thought. Their findings, combined with James Reason's influential book *Human Error* (1990), spawned a plethora of new safety-related groups (Box 2.1), as well as fresh research and literature based on the role of systems, human factors, and their relationship to human error in healthcare. Researchers and authorities began to recognize that human errors leading to patient injuries are not so much as a result of an individual's shortcoming, deserving of blame or punishment, but more as a result of *system failures* in patient care areas such as the perioperative setting. Leape (1994) urged that continued focus on individual error was misplaced if adverse patient events were to be effectively prevented. Prominent researchers began urging an emphasis on transparent systems that require open reporting, investigation, innovation, and dissemination. The aviation and nuclear systems' parallel examination of human factors served as models for ideas (e.g., surgical checklists) that led to relative success in preventing healthcare-related injury attributable to human error. Communication and teamwork were identified as key factors to promote patient safety.

Concentrated Emphasis on Systems

This work took on urgency in 1999. The Institute of Medicine (IOM) landmark work, *To Err Is Human,* spurred major additional safety initiatives when it reported that at least 44,000, and perhaps as many as 98,000, patients had died in US hospitals every year as a result of preventable adverse events (IOM, 1999). The IOM report did not focus solely on perioperative errors. However, it did refer to Reason's (1990) theory that complex, tightly coupled systems are most prone to accidents, and specified the surgical suite, along with emergency departments and intensive care units, as examples of complex, tightly coupled systems. Moreover, when one considers

---

BOX 2.1

Safety-Related Entities

CAPS (Consumers Advancing Patient Safety) is a consumer-led nonprofit organized as a voice for individuals, families, and healthcare professionals (www.patientsafety.org).

CPS (Citizens for Patient Safety) is another patient advocacy group (www.citizensforpatientsafety.org).

ECRI Institute is a nonprofit organization dedicated to using applied scientific research to discover which medical procedures, devices, drugs, and processes best improve patient care (www.ecri.org).

HIMSS (Healthcare Information and Management Systems Society) is a global, cause-based, not-for-profit organization focused on better health through information technology (www.himss.org).

IHI (Institute for Healthcare Improvement) works with healthcare providers and leaders throughout the world to enhance delivery of safe and effective healthcare (www.ihi.org).

IOM (Institute of Medicine) has the mission to serve as adviser to the nation to improve health by providing unbiased, evidence-based, and authoritative information and advice on health and science policy (http://www.nationalacademies.org/hmd/).

ISMP (Institute for Safe Medication Practices) is the nation's only nonprofit organization devoted entirely to medication error prevention and safe medication use (www.ismp.org).

Leapfrog Group is a voluntary program aimed at mobilizing employer purchasing power by noting "big leaps" in healthcare safety, quality, and customer value (www.leapfroggroup.org).

NoThing Left Behind is a voluntary surgical patient safety initiative started in 2004 to understand why RSIs are such a persistent problem and to develop practices to ensure RSIs become a never happen event (www.nothingleftbehind.org).

NPSF (National Patient Safety Foundation) partners with patients and families, the healthcare community, and key stakeholders to advance patient safety and healthcare workforce safety and disseminate strategies to prevent harm (www.npsf.org).

NQF (National Quality Forum) is a public-private partnership created to develop and implement a national strategy for healthcare quality measurement and reporting. This group's 27 Safe Practices are widely accepted (www.qualityforum.org).

Office of the National Coordinator for Health Information Technology provides information on mobile devices and health information privacy and security and managing mobile devices in healthcare.

SCIP (Surgical Care Improvement Project) is a national quality partnership interested in improving surgical care by significantly reducing surgical complications (www.cms.gov).

In addition, many states have state-based coalitions that encourage cost-effective, safe, quality healthcare.

RSI, Retained surgical item.

---

the incredibly complex highly invasive surgical procedures and number of team members and disciplines involved, juxtaposed with anesthetized patients who are unable to detect pain or otherwise defend themselves, patient vulnerability and the consequent need for protection by all team members are strikingly apparent.

Brennan and colleagues (1991) found adverse events occurred in 3.7% of hospitalizations. They concluded that substandard care had caused a substantial number of patient injuries. In part 2 of that study, Leape and colleagues (1991) found that nearly half (48%) of adverse events were associated with surgery. Their results were consistent with those of earlier investigators, who had found half of all hospital-based, potentially compensable events (i.e., injuries from substandard care) arose from treatment in the OR. More than 4000 surgical "never events" occurred each year between 1990 and 2010 in the United States, according to the findings of a retrospective study of national malpractice data (Johns Hopkins Medicine, 2012). TJC findings are consistent with those findings. Individual efforts of the best nurses, surgeons, and anesthesia providers, combined with a recognized need for teamwork communication and checklists, remain insufficient to prevent injury, and are especially not sufficient in the perioperative setting.

The shift away from emphasis on individual responsibility to a broader systems approach continues to accelerate. Advances in surgical instrumentation, robotics, and electronic health information systems have combined to change the locus and delivery of perioperative care dramatically. Social media and an acute rise in consumerism have made patient safety a popular issue. Federal statutes and Centers for Medicare and Medicaid Services (CMS) regulations have added financial incentives to safe care and placed indirect financial disincentives to unsafe care. Continued federal and state governments' involvement in healthcare can be anticipated. Current and future

changes in the context of healthcare require a new and more inclusive, comprehensive, and expansive approach to safety.

Checklists and tools for measuring safety practices have multiplied. Safety scholars have published influential treatises for the professions and the public that have raised everyone's awareness of checklist initiatives (Makary and Daniel, 2016) and their effectiveness (Salzwedel et al., 2015).

Despite the impressive initial effectiveness of checklists, barriers and variations in their adoption (Russ et al., 2016; Mayer et al., 2016) are emerging along with a parallel need for flexibility, leadership, and teamwork different from current practice. Makary and Daniel (2016) analyzed the scientific literature on medical errors to identify their contribution to US deaths. They concluded that if medical error was a disease, it would rank as the third leading cause of death. Kachelia and colleagues (2016) noted that the heterogeneity and complexity of errors in healthcare are reflected in multifaceted and wide-ranging initiatives to improve safety. They grouped legal and policy interventions promulgated by professional groups and government regulations into four approaches: greater transparency, financial incentives, forms of professional and legal regulation, and reforms in the liability systems (Austin and Pronovost, 2015; Kachelia et al., 2016; Nguyen and Moffat-Bruce, 2016).

Major Professional Association and Government Regulatory Safety Activities

TJC and TJC International, especially their 2017 National Patient Safety Goals (NPSGs), are excellent sources for safety information applicable to systems and facilities wherever invasive procedures take place. TJC modifies some goals depending on procedure location (i.e., hospitals, ambulatory clinics, acute access hospitals, physician offices). The AORN *Guidelines for Perioperative Practice* (2017) are

PATIENT SAFETY

Root Cause Analysis

The Joint Commission (TJC) Root Cause Analysis and Action Plan tool has 24 analysis questions. TJC framework is intended to provide a template for organizing and answering analysis questions. Not all questions are listed here:

1. What happened?
2. Why did that happen?
   - What was the intended process flow? List pertinent steps in the process; use those identified in policy, procedure, protocols, or guidelines in effect at time of event. In the OR these might be, for example, the site verification protocol, procedures for soft goods, sharps counts, patient identification protocols, or fall risk/fall prevention guidelines for perioperative patient positioning.
   - Were there steps in the policy, procedure, protocol, or guideline that did not occur as intended?
   - What human factors are relevant? Consider staff-related factors such as fatigue, inattention, lack of clinical reasoning/critical thinking skills, and rushing to complete a task. Disruptions in the flow of a surgical procedure, such as teamwork and communication failures, may contribute significantly to the event.
   - Were there problems with equipment that affected the outcome?
   - What factors in the environment were controllable? These factors should be specific to the event.
   - What external factors in the environment were uncontrollable (these are factors that cannot be changed)?
3. What other factors are involved?
   - Was the staff properly qualified and competent for their responsibilities at the time of the event? Address staffing levels and staff performance in this part of the analysis.
   - To what degree was all necessary information available when needed?
   - Was communication among participants adequate for this situation?
   - How does the organization's culture support risk reduction? Are there barriers to communicating potential risk factors?
   - How is the prevention of adverse outcomes communicated as a high priority?

Root cause analysis involves an action plan addressing "what can be done to prevent this?" Root cause analysis concentrates on systems and processes, not individuals. It is characterized by a structured "sense-making conversation."

Modified from Cassin BR, Barach PE: Making sense of root cause analysis investigations of surgery-related adverse events. *Surg Clin North Am* 92(1):101–115, 2012; The Joint Commission (TJC): *Framework for conducting a root cause analysis and action plan* (website), 2013. www.jointcommission.org/Framework_for_Conducting_a_Root_Cause_Analysis_and_Action_Plan. (Accessed 15 June 2017).

the best source for information specific to perioperative nursing practices. Major government agencies that provide financial and research resources for patient safety are also useful sources for safety information for facilities and individual professionals. Federal and state regulations have proliferated to promote safety, including through financial incentives.

The Joint Commission

TJC has long been involved with quality and safety. It sharpened its systems-based safety focus in the mid-1990s when it established its Sentinel Event Policy. That policy first encouraged and then required self-reporting of medical errors and root cause analyses of them. TJC published its first NPSGs in 2003. These goals are revised annually. TJC also recognized the need for standardized methods of patient identification and established the Universal Protocol for preventing wrong-site, wrong-procedure, and wrong-person surgery (TJC, 2017) (discussed later in this chapter). By 2005, the World Health Organization (WHO) formed the Collaborative Centre for Patient Safety Solutions, comprised of TJC and TJC International. TJC also is a founding member of the National Patient Safety Foundation (NPSF), collaborates with the National Quality Forum (NQF), and is an affiliate of Consumers Advancing Patient Safety (CAPS).

Sentinel Events

TJC designated unexpected occurrences involving death or risk of serious physical or psychologic injuries as "sentinel events." It chose the word *sentinel* to indicate that these events signal the need for immediate investigation and response. Investigation includes root cause analysis, which is a systematized process to identify variations in performance that cause or could cause a sentinel event. Suggested steps in such an analysis are briefly summarized in the Patient Safety box. While TJC data collection focuses on sentinel events, it also recognizes the value of analyzing "close calls" and "near misses" to improve patient safety.

TJC categorizes sentinel event errors reported to it and publishes their frequencies. Examples of perioperative care errors are those that (1) are related to anesthesia; (2) are caused by medical equipment; (3) are caused by medication error; (4) result in infection, fires, and transfusion reactions; (5) are operative or postoperative complications; or (6) give rise to unintended RSIs or (7) wrong site/patient/procedure surgery. The summary of sentinel events published in 2016 reveals that of total incidents reviewed from 2005 through the second quarter of 2016, nearly 25% of all incidents reviewed most likely occurred in an operative setting (RSI, referred to by TJC as retained foreign body or object [RFO], and wrong-site procedures). Add in the number of events that could have occurred in the perioperative setting (e.g., falls, fires, medical equipment-related problems, transfusion and medication errors) and the percentage might reach the 50% figure that Leape and Brennan found in the early 1990s.

National Patient Safety Goals

Another TJC initiative relates to NPSGs for hospitals, critical access hospitals, and ambulatory and office-based surgery derived from reported sentinel events. NPSGs are reviewed, updated, or retired each year. Perioperative-related goals for patients in each setting are almost the same. Although initially surprising, this similarity is understandable. Even though patients in office-based surgery settings tend to be of healthier physical status classifications as set out by the American Society of Anesthesiologists (ASA) (see Chapter 5), one could argue that error prevention procedures in office-based surgery facilities, nevertheless, must be rigorous because these

AMBULATORY SURGERY CONSIDERATIONS

Telephone Follow-up Calls

The combination of regional anesthesia and minimally invasive surgery is moving more patients from inpatient to outpatient surgical treatment. Patient/family education is critical for a safe preoperative experience. Postoperative follow-up after discharge is receiving more attention as a critical component of perioperative patient care.

Postoperative telephone follow-up (TFU) has joined the cadre of healthcare interventions that not only provide safer patient care, but also save financial resources of patients and provider systems. Nurses and physicians at a large academic facility recognized that day surgery required a comprehensive postdischarge plan. Even with complete preoperative teaching about this plan, they wondered if working memory recovery resulted in poorly remembered or forgotten discharge teaching instruction which, in turn, could compromise the recovery experience. Although their facility had already instituted TFU for day surgery patients, they determined that a more structured study was in order to ascertain whether there was a significant difference with a standardized questionnaire that included questions about common postoperative complaints such as nausea, vomiting, postoperative pain, and concerns about the surgical site. The investigators aimed to achieve a reduction in postoperative concerns and identify whether patients perceived the call as helpful and left them more satisfied with their discharge care.

Of the 856 participants who consented to participate in the study, 313 received the TFU call and 541 missed it despite three failed call attempts. Investigators decided a control group would be formed by day surgery patients who did not experience a TFU. All participants were asked whether they experienced any pain or nausea and vomiting, had problems with mobility or wound care, or had other issues postoperatively and about their satisfaction with discharge care. The investigators used both Chi squared and independent t-tests to determine if differences existed between the two groups.

Most of the full sample had no postoperative concerns and were fully satisfied with their care. Among participants who did report concerns, the TFU group reported significantly fewer postoperative concerns (19% versus 28%) and higher patient satisfaction. The authors noted that this is consistent with several other published studies. However, they did not find a significant difference in returns to the emergency room between the two groups due to the small number of patients who did so (about 2%). Postoperative pain was the most frequently reported postoperative concern; it was reported less in the TFU group than the control group. After speculating on several limitations (e.g., this was patient-derived feedback on perceptions of care following same-day surgery for their healthcare team), they concluded their project reinforces the need for more patient-experience studies and TFU initiation.

Modified from Daniels SA et al: Call to care: the impact of 24-hour post discharge telephone follow-up in the treatment of surgical day care patients. *Am J Surg* 211(5):963–967, 2016.

smaller facilities are less likely to have available the hospitals' wider array of emergency and corrective equipment and personnel. In addition, office-based and ambulatory perioperative staff provides most patient, family, and caregiver discharge education and preparation, unlike inpatient care settings (Ambulatory Surgery Considerations). Finally, causes of infection and patient defenses against infection do not differ based on the venue of the surgical procedure.

Universal Protocol

TJC has a required safety practice, referred to as the Universal Protocol, as part of the 2017 NPSGs. Key features of the Universal Protocol are performing a preoperative verification process, such as marking the operative site and conducting a time-out immediately before starting the procedure. A properly performed time-out includes information about the patient and procedure, as discussed in more detail later in this chapter.

The Association of periOperative Registered Nurses

For over 60 years AORN has addressed perioperative patient safety issues. AORN provides an array of standards, guidelines, publications, videos, and tool kits that specifically address patient safety from the perioperative team's point of view. Tool kits include subjects such as fire safety, correct site surgery, sharps safety, hand-off communications, safe patient handling, and cultural and human factors. Guidelines include those addressing aseptic practice, equipment and product safety, patient and worker safety, patient care, and sterilization and disinfection. Guidelines and tool kits are as evidence-based as possible. These AORN undertakings aim to develop real-world strategies to implement perioperative patient care practices. Along

with TJC and WHO recommendations, AORN guidelines should be reflected and adopted within institutional policies and procedures, and educational curricula.

Federal Agencies

The federal agencies most relevant to patient safety are found within the Department of Health and Human Services (DHHS). Some of the 12 agencies within the DHHS include the following: Agency for Health Resources and Quality (AHRQ), The Centers for Disease Control and Prevention (CDC), CMS, the Food and Drug Administration (FDA), Health Resources and Services Administration (HRSA), and the National Institutes of Health (NIH). The most relevant are discussed in the following sections.

Centers for Medicare and Medicaid Services

CMS is the federal agency charged with the administration (including regulations for payment) of Medicare, multiple state Children's Health Insurance Programs (CHIP), and part of Medicaid. It also administers the Health Insurance Portability and Accountability Act (HIPAA) and several other health-related federal programs. Significant to patient safety is the decision by CMS to impose financial *disincentives* for selected unsafe patient care outcomes by refusing to pay for the extra cost of treatment to correct those outcomes. Conversely stated, the agency responsible for paying Medicare claims now provides a financial *incentive* for safe patient care. The Deficit Reduction Act of 2005 mandated a quality adjustment to payments for certain healthcare-acquired conditions (HACs) when the condition was not present on admission (POA) to the hospital. Box 2.2 contains a list of nonreimbursable claims that are most relevant to perioperative

BOX 2.2

Nonreimbursable Claims Most Relevant to Perioperative Patient Care

- Foreign object retained after surgery
- Air embolism
- Blood incompatibility
- Stage 3 and 4 pressure injuries
- Falls and trauma
  - Fractures
  - Dislocations
  - Intracranial injuries
  - Crushing injuries
  - Burn
  - Other injuries
- Catheter-associated urinary tract infection
- Central line-associated bloodstream infection
- Surgical site infection, mediastinitis, following coronary artery bypass graft
- Surgical site infection following bariatric surgery for obesity
  - Laparoscopic gastric bypass
  - Gastroenterostomy
  - Laparoscopic gastric restrictive surgery
- Surgical site infection
- Following certain orthopedic procedures
  - Spine
  - Neck
  - Shoulder
  - Elbow
- Surgical site infection following cardiac implantable electronic device
- Deep vein thrombosis/pulmonary embolism following certain orthopedic procedures:
  - Total knee replacement
  - Hip replacement
- Iatrogenic pneumothorax with venous catheterization

Modified from Centers for Medicare and Medicaid Services (CMS): *Hospital-acquired conditions* (website), 2015. www.cms.gov/medicare/medicare-fee-for-service-payment/hospitalacqcond/hospital-acquired_conditions.html. (Accessed 9 January 2017).

patient care, CMS regularly reviews and adds conditions pursuant to its federal rule-making process; the 2017 program includes *Clostridium difficile* infection (CDI) and methicillin-resistant *Staphylococcus aureus* (MRSA) healthcare-acquired infections (ACEP, 2016).

CMS notes that it does not consider listed patient safety concerns more important than others. Rather, it has chosen the selected concerns to emphasize that the facilities deemed responsible must now bear directly otherwise avoidable financial costs of insufficient patient safety controls. Furthermore, CMS regulations prohibit passing these costs on to patients. Most private insurance companies have adopted similar provisions. Thus from a purely risk management standpoint, in addition to potential indirect costs arising from negligence awards and settlements (which can be insured against), facilities now bear the risk of direct, uninsurable, and potentially severe cost disincentives if they fail to avoid the listed conditions through the initiation of facility-based safe practices.

Agency for Healthcare Research and Quality

AHRQ's mission is to improve the quality, safety, efficiency, and effectiveness of healthcare for all Americans. This agency is committed to improve healthcare safety and quality by developing successful partnerships and generating the knowledge and tools required for long-term improvement. The central goal of its research is measurable improvements in healthcare in the United States, including improved quality of life and patient outcomes, lives saved, and value gained.

AHRQ provides substantial clinical support and offers nurses and other providers extensive evidence-based resources related to patient safety on its website (see Box 2.1). For example, an estimated 17% reduction in HACs from 2010 to 2014 indicates that hospitals have made substantial progress in improving safety. An estimated 2.1 million fewer harms were experienced by patients from 2010 to 2014 than would have occurred if the rate of harm had remained at the 2010 level. The reasons for this progress are not fully understood. Likely contributing causes are financial incentives created by CMS and other payers' payment policies, public reporting of hospital-level results, assistance offered by the Quality Improvement Organization (QIO) program to hospitals, and technical assistance and catalytic efforts of the Partnership for Patients (PfP) initiative led by CMS. Numerous other public and private initiatives to improve healthcare quality and patient safety were implemented during these years (e.g., the widespread implementation and improved use of electronic health records [EHRs] under meaningful use programs).

Centers for Disease Control and Prevention

The CDC is no longer limited to disease prevention. It also publishes widely on patient safety topics such as infection prevention, medication safety, consumer education regarding how patients can protect themselves, and patient safety cultures.

The World Health Organization

The United Nations (UN) created WHO to function as its health oversight and coordination authority for all UN member nations who in turn have joined WHO. In 2004 WHO launched the World Alliance on Patient Safety, by which it began to examine patient safety in acute as well as in primary care settings relevant to all WHO member nations. Over 140 countries have worked to address the challenges of unsafe care. WHO estimates that 1 in 10 patients are harmed while in the hospital in developed countries. The World Alliance on Patient Safety's action initiatives include Clean Care is Safer Care and Safe Surgery Saves Lives. The focus of the Clean Care campaign is hand hygiene (also referenced in TJC's NPSGs), which resulted in the release of a 2009 WHO guideline for surgical hand preparation (WHO, 2009) (Evidence for Practice: World Health Organization Hand Hygiene).

WHO estimates 234 million surgical operations are performed globally every year and that 50% of surgical care complications are avoidable. WHO's Safe Surgery Saves Lives initiative led to the publication of its Surgical Safety Checklist (SSC). Similar in content to TJC's Universal Protocol, the WHO checklist adds a third phase, the Sign Out. The Sign Out phase includes team reviews of outcomes and concerns to be included in the handover (the international term for "hand-off") to postanesthesia recovery caregivers (Evidence for Practice: Surgical Safety Checklist). A cluster randomized control trial from Norway compared 2212 control procedures with 2263 procedures using the SSC. The complication rates decreased from 19.9% to 11.5%. Mean length of stay decreased by 0.8 days with SSC. In-hospital mortality decreased from 1.6% to 1.0%. This study is further described in the Research Highlight box.

Despite these substantial health improvements from hand hygiene and use of the WHO SSC, perhaps the most notable fact about WHO's entry into surgical patient safety is the recognition that perioperative adverse events causing complications before, during, and after surgery are a *public health* problem worldwide.

EVIDENCE FOR PRACTICE

World Health Organization Hand Hygiene

Steps before starting surgical hand antisepsis (scrub).

Key Steps

- Keep nails short and pay attention to them when washing your hands; most microbes on hands come from beneath the fingernails.
- Do not wear artificial nails or nail polish.
- Remove all jewelry (rings, watches, and bracelets) before entering the OR.
- Wash hands and arms with a nonmedicated soap before entering the OR and/or if hands are visibly soiled.
- Clean under the nails with a nail file. Nail brushes should not be used because they may damage the skin and encourage shedding of cells. If used, nail brushes must be sterile and used once only (single use). Reusable nail brushes may be resterilized for each use.

Procedural Steps

- Start timing. Scrub each side of each finger, between the fingers, and the back and front of the hand for 2 minutes.

- Proceed to scrub the arms, keeping the hand higher than the arm at all times. This helps avoid recontamination of the hands by water from the elbows and prevents bacteria-laden soap and water from contaminating the hands.
- Wash each side of the arm from wrist to elbow for 1 minute.
- Repeat the process on the other hand and arm, keeping hands above the elbows at all times. If the hand touches anything at any time, the scrub must be lengthened by 1 minute for the area that has been contaminated.
- Rinse hands and arms by passing them through the water in one direction only, from fingertips to elbow. Do not move the arm back and forth through the water.
- Proceed to the OR holding hands above the elbows.
- At all times during the scrub procedure, care should be taken not to splash water onto surgical attire.
- Once in the OR, hands and arms should be dried using a sterile towel and aseptic technique before donning gown and gloves.

Modified from the World Health Organization (WHO): *WHO guidelines on hand hygiene in healthcare* (website), 2009. http://whqlibdoc.who.int/publications/2009/9789241597906_eng .pdf. (Accessed 10 January 2017).

EVIDENCE FOR PRACTICE

World Health Organization — SURGICAL SAFETY CHECKLIST (FIRST EDITION)

Before induction of anaesthesia ▶▶▶▶▶▶▶▶   Before skin incision ▶▶▶▶▶▶▶▶▶▶▶▶   Before patient leaves operating room

SIGN IN

- ☐ PATIENT HAS CONFIRMED
  - IDENTITY
  - SITE
  - PROCEDURE
  - CONSENT

- ☐ SITE MARKED/NOT APPLICABLE

- ☐ ANAESTHESIA SAFETY CHECK COMPLETED

- ☐ PULSE OXIMETER ON PATIENT AND FUNCTIONING

DOES PATIENT HAVE A:

KNOWN ALLERGY?
- ☐ NO
- ☐ YES

DIFFICULT AIRWAY/ASPIRATION RISK?
- ☐ NO
- ☐ YES, AND EQUIPMENT/ASSISTANCE AVAILABLE

RISK OF >500ML BLOOD LOSS (7ML/KG IN CHILDREN)?
- ☐ NO
- ☐ YES, AND ADEQUATE INTRAVENOUS ACCESS AND FLUIDS PLANNED

TIME OUT

- ☐ CONFIRM ALL TEAM MEMBERS HAVE INTRODUCED THEMSELVES BY NAME AND ROLE

- ☐ SURGEON, ANAESTHESIA PROFESSIONAL AND NURSE VERBALLY CONFIRM
  - PATIENT
  - SITE
  - PROCEDURE

ANTICIPATED CRITICAL EVENTS

- ☐ SURGEON REVIEWS: WHAT ARE THE CRITICAL OR UNEXPECTED STEPS, OPERATIVE DURATION, ANTICIPATED BLOOD LOSS?

- ☐ ANAESTHESIA TEAM REVIEWS: ARE THERE ANY PATIENT-SPECIFIC CONCERNS?

- ☐ NURSING TEAM REVIEWS: HAS STERILITY (INCLUDING INDICATOR RESULTS) BEEN CONFIRMED? ARE THERE EQUIPMENT ISSUES OR ANY CONCERNS?

HAS ANTIBIOTIC PROPHYLAXIS BEEN GIVEN WITHIN THE LAST 60 MINUTES?
- ☐ YES
- ☐ NOT APPLICABLE

IS ESSENTIAL IMAGING DISPLAYED?
- ☐ YES
- ☐ NOT APPLICABLE

SIGN OUT

NURSE VERBALLY CONFIRMS WITH THE TEAM:

- ☐ THE NAME OF THE PROCEDURE RECORDED

- ☐ THAT INSTRUMENT, SPONGE AND NEEDLE COUNTS ARE CORRECT (OR NOT APPLICABLE)

- ☐ HOW THE SPECIMEN IS LABELLED (INCLUDING PATIENT NAME)

- ☐ WHETHER THERE ARE ANY EQUIPMENT PROBLEMS TO BE ADDRESSED

- ☐ SURGEON, ANAESTHESIA PROFESSIONAL AND NURSE REVIEW THE KEY CONCERNS FOR RECOVERY AND MANAGEMENT OF THIS PATIENT

THIS CHECKLIST IS NOT INTENDED TO BE COMPREHENSIVE. ADDITIONS AND MODIFICATIONS TO FIT LOCAL PRACTICE ARE ENCOURAGED.

From the World Health Organization (WHO): *WHO surgical safety checklist* (website), 2009. www.who.int/patientsafety/safesurgery/checklist/en. (Accessed 10 January 2017).

RESEARCH HIGHLIGHT ||

Outcomes of World Health Organization Surgical Safety Checklist Implementation

A research team from Norway hypothesized that reduction of 30 days' in-hospital morbidity, mortality, and LOS would result after implementation of the WHO SSC. They noted that other researchers had reported reductions in morbidity and mortality after SSC implementation in prestudies/poststudies but without the usually accepted research controls. Thus they conducted a stepped wedge cluster randomized controlled trial in two hospitals. They chose Norwegian hospitals because the SSC had not yet been mandated there. Their dependent variables were effects on in-hospital complications, using ICD-10 codes, LOS, and mortality. The SSC intervention was randomly introduced to five clusters: cardiothoracic, neurosurgery, orthopedic, general, and urologic surgery. Data were prospectively recorded in control and intervention stages over 10 months.

They compared a total of 2212 control procedures with 2263 SCC procedures. Among their findings was that complication rates decreased from 19.9% to 11.5% ($p < .001$). Adjusted for possible confounding factors, the SSC effect on complications remained significant. The mean LOS decreased by 0.8 days with SCC utilization (95% confidence interval, 0.11–1.43).

In-hospital mortality decreased significantly from 1.9% to 0.2% in one of the two hospitals post-SSC implementation, but the overall reduction (1.6%–1.0%) across hospitals was not significant.

They concluded that the WHO SSC implementation was associated with reduction in morbidity and length of in-hospital stay and some reduction in mortality.

LOS, Length of stay; *SSC,* surgical safety checklist *WHO,* World Health Organization. Modified from Haugen AS et al: Effect of the World Health Organization checklist on patient outcomes: a Stepped Wedge Cluster Randomized Controlled Trial. *Ann Surg* 261(5):821–828, 2015.

Other Patient Safety Groups/Coalitions/Companies

Major professional associations representing other perioperative team members (e.g., American College of Surgeons [ACS], ASA, American Association of Nurse Anesthetists [AANA], American Society of PeriAnesthesia Nurses [ASPAN], and the Association of Surgical Technologists [AST]) have also issued multiple position statements and clinical recommendations related to patient safety. Many of these are coissued or mutually endorsed with AORN. This reflects the increasing systems approach to perioperative safety.

Nonprovider Members of the Perioperative Patient Safety Team

Promoting perioperative patient safety is within the expertise of the perioperative care provider team. Coping with the deluge of state and federal statutes, regulations and other legal and professional initiatives are beyond direct care providers' time and expertise. As more and more healthcare records are electronic, so too is the Information Technology (IT) director needed on the safety team. Risk managers, compliance officers, and IT directors are three nonprovider professionals who can serve as indispensable resources to the provider members within a safety team in a facility culture of safety.

Healthcare risk management is a broad and diverse field within a rapidly evolving and changing healthcare landscape. The American Association for Healthcare Risk Management (ASHRM) has described risk management as a broad-based discipline that works to contribute to the delivery of safe and trusted healthcare. Risk manager duties generally include risk financing and event and incident management. Their expertise and varying job descriptions include psychology and human factors, statistical analysis, and insurance and claims management (ASHRM, 2016).

Compliance officers implement programs to prevent knowing or unknowing illegal, unethical, or otherwise improper individual or group conduct. Doing so necessarily requires awareness of laws, regulations, and other professional mandates related to the facility's patient care providers, human resources, security, and IT as well as all privacy, ethical practice issues, and services. Compliance officers serve as staff to the chief executive officer (CEO) and the Board of Directors' Compliance Committee. This means the compliance officer interacts directly with the CEO and these Board Committees (American College of Healthcare Executives, 2016).

Health IT is a broad concept that encompasses an array of technologies to store, share, and analyze health information. In today's EHR imperative environment, nearly every perioperative facility has IT professional(s) on staff.

Perioperative Nursing Safety Issues

Communication and Teamwork

Communication underpins many patient safety issues. Implementation of both the Universal Protocol and the WHO SSC requires enhanced communication within a culture of teamwork. Hand-off/handover protocols have joined traditional clinical written documentation records to improve communication further in perioperative settings. Research continues in the use of perioperative patient care checklists in a variety of settings and situations. Most articles show that checklists alone cannot improve outcomes, but checklists do enhance meaningful communication and teamwork. With equal commitment to teamwork, trust, and respect, outcomes improve. Improved communication is imbedded in human factors, culture, and social systems. Researchers have demonstrated that the use of a preinduction checklist significantly improves information exchange, knowledge of critical information, and perception of safety in anesthesia teams, all of which are parameters contributing to patient safety. Clearly, there is a trend indicating improved perception of teamwork (Tscholl et al., 2015; Singer et al., 2016). With improved communication, Lau and Chamberlain (2016) found that the use of the WHO SSC is associated with a significant reduction in postoperative complication rates and mortality. They concluded that the WHO SSC is a valuable tool that should be universally implemented in all surgical settings and used with all surgical patients.

Clinical Documentation

The written or digital clinical record communicates perioperative patient information. Evidence suggests, however, that a digital or written clinical record is inadequate as the sole perioperative communication tool. Enhanced communication initiatives such as safer surgery briefings, thorough time-outs, and handoffs augment the digital or written record. Whether documented on paper or digitally, the clinical record is foundational in ensuring a safer patient experience and providing information to other care areas.

Facilities in which operative and other invasive procedures occur maintain records of each operation. Each record must comply with state and federal regulations as well as with accreditation requirements. Operative records include preoperative diagnosis, surgery performed, a description of findings, specimens removed, postoperative diagnosis, and names of all individuals participating in intraoperative care. Additional key components include positioning and stabilizing devices, electrosurgical unit (ESU) number and settings, medications, and evidence of ongoing assessment and additional actions taken. The operative record is a permanent part of the patient's medical record. Note that nearly all components of perioperative clinical documentation relate directly or indirectly to patient safety and injury prevention.

Proper perioperative nursing documentation describes assessment, planning, and implementation of perioperative patient care reflecting individualization of care and evaluation of patient outcomes. It also includes any intraoperative patient care orders. Any and every unusual or significant incident pertinent to patient outcomes must be documented as well as all remediation efforts related to the patient's care. The facility's risk manager may require additional documentation. Only objective information directly related to the specific patient is included in the patient's record. It is inappropriate to record personal opinions or to describe circumstances surrounding an event except as they appear to affect the patient directly.

Thoughtfully designed perioperative nursing documentation tools include defined elements in a format that minimizes time needed for documentation (e.g., checklists). Ideally, collaboration with the preoperative, postanesthesia care unit (PACU), and postoperative nursing units will produce one documentation tool used across all areas, which avoids duplication of patient data by different nursing staff. Increasingly, settings in which operative and other invasive procedures are performed use EHRs to enter and track patient care information. Coordination of the content included in the intraoperative record with that in the surgeon's and anesthesia provider's intraoperative records reduces documentation time and provides a more integrated record that streamlines workflow and reduces documentation errors.

Documentation of perioperative patient care in the clinical record simultaneously serves risk management functions. Documentation templates serve as reminders of actions needed to provide safe care, thus prompting risk reduction strategies and preventing injury. Information in the clinical record also enhances continuity of care, reducing future injury. If a patient injury does occur, documentation that preventive measures or other actions to mitigate risks were taken may lessen the likelihood of a successful lawsuit. Conversely, confusion and contradiction in the patient care record enhances the likelihood of a successful lawsuit by demonstrating that team members involved were not acting as reasonable and prudent caregivers.

Handoffs/Handovers

As noted, digital or written documentation alone, however crucial, is insufficient to ensure patient safety when care responsibility passes from one team or individual caregiver to another. Standardized approaches to hand-off communication further reduce risk for error.

TJC, AORN, and WHO uniformly recommend that time-outs (or "safer surgery briefings"), as well as preoperative and postoperative handoffs, be formalized. In perioperative settings, occasions for transfer-of-care processes, such as handoffs, include nursing shift changes, temporary relief or coverage, nursing and physician handoffs from one department to another, and various other transfers of information in inpatient settings and interhospital transfers. The purpose of hand-off communication and reports is to provide essential, up-to-date, and specific information about the patient. Standardized hand-off communication must include an opportunity to ask and respond to questions.

There is no one prescribed hand-off script. Situation, Background, Assessment, and Recommendation (known as SBAR) remains popular. Other authors have suggested the I-PASS methodology (illness severity, patient summary, action list, situational awareness and contingency planning, and synthesis), a TeamSTEPPS (AHRQ, 2016b), or a perioperative PEARLS format (Fig. 2.1) (Garrett, 2016; Robinson, 2016).

More recently, electronic tools with direct communication have been described (Clarke et al., 2016). Although the implementation of SSCs has facilitated hand-off communication and improved the reliability of OR and postanesthesia handoffs (Boat and Spaeth, 2013), checklists are not sufficient for hand-off communication per se (Caruso et al., 2015). Although data indicate that multimedia time-outs result in improved participation by and satisfaction of all surgical team members (Dixon et al., 2016), the search for better hand-off tools continues (Schoenfeld and Wachter, 2016).

For identification of critical elements for handoffs from preoperative to intraoperative, see Box 2.3; for handoffs intraoperatively

---

BOX 2.3

Elements of the Preoperative to Intraoperative Hand-off Communication Using Situation, Background, Assessment, and Recommendations, or SBAR

Situation
- Name of patient and date of birth
- Name of operative or invasive procedure to be performed, including modifiers and site
- Pertinent documents present and consistent

Background
- Elements of patient history pertinent to surgery
- Medical clearance
- Patient allergies and nothing per mouth status
- Patient's vital signs and pain level
- Medication profile and medications taken today
- Specific laboratory results
- Code status of patient

Assessment
- Patient's current level of understanding of the surgery
- Special patient needs or precautions
- Pertinent aspects of the patient's emotional and spiritual status
- Pertinent cultural implications
- Anesthesia requests

Recommendations
- State whether the patient has been seen preoperatively by the surgeon and anesthesia care provider.
- Determine whether the patient is ready for surgery.
- Allow an opportunity for preoperative and intraoperative staff members to ask questions or voice concerns.

From Amato-Vealey EJ et al: Hand-off communication: a requisite for patient safety, *AORN J* 88(5):766–770, 2008.

P	**Patient name:** _____ **Age:** _____**Allergies:**_____ **Procedure performed**_____ **Primary language spoken:** □ English □ other: _____ **Past medical history:** □ Diabetes □ HTN □ COPD □ Asthma □ OSA □ Renal Disease □ Seizures □ Cardiac □ CAD □ PVD □ CVA □ Liver Disease □ETOH □ Smoking (ppd____) □ Arthritis □ MRSA □ VRE □ TB □ C Diff □ Deaf □ HOH □ Blind **Position during surgery:** □ supine □ prone □ lithotomy (type of stirrups: □ candy cane □ Allen) □ jack knife □ Other _____ **Precautions:** □ Falls □ Seizure □ Aspiration □ Decubitus □ Isolation: □ Contact □ Droplet **Personal Items:** □ Dentures □ Glasses □ Hearing Aids □ Prosthesis :(_____) **Pain management:** □ PCA pump □ Epidural □ On-Q pump □ Other:_____
E	**Extremities:** □ Ted hose □ SCDs □ Pulses **Adverse events intraoperative:** _____ **Equipment needs:** □ CPM □ Ventilator □ Wound Vac □ NGT □ Cell saver **Elimination:** □ Foley □ Suprapubic tube □ I&O □ Straight cath
A	**Assessment:** □ Skin □ Incision □ Packing □ Musculoskeletal □ Neuro **Drains:** □ JP □ Hemovac: location_____ □ Penrose □ Blake tube □ Chest tubes: □ Rt □ Lt □ Urology stents: □ Rt □ Lt □ G tube **Dressings:** Location _____ Number____ Drainage: □ Yes: Type _____ □ No **Antibiotic:** □ Yes: Time last dose_____ □ No
R	**Relationships:** Family location: _____ Contact phone #:_____ **Radiology:** □ CXR □ Other
L	**Labs due:** □ H&H □ BMP □ CBC □ PT/PTT □ T&C □ Accuchek □ Blood sugar □ ABG □ Critical values: _____ **Lines:** □ Central □ Arterial □ Peripheral: location:_____ □ Swan-Ganz □ CVP □ PICC line □ Port: location:_____ **Blood products:** _____
S	**Special devices:** □ Pacemaker □ AICD □ Insulin pump □ Other _____ **Special needs:** □ DVT protocol □ Specialty bed:_____ **Spiritual needs:** _____ **Special communication needs:** □ Sign language interpreter □ Interpreter **Surgical Unit:** □ SCU □ OSU □ CVICU □ PCU □ IMCU □ MSU □ TMU

FIG. 2.1 PEARLS format to guide perioperative handovers.

between scrub persons, see Box 2.4; and for handoffs from intraoperative to PACU or another postanesthesia recovery area, see Box 2.5.

Wrong Site, Person, or Procedure Surgery

Surgery that is the wrong procedure or surgery performed on the wrong site or person includes any operative or other invasive procedure performed on the wrong patient, wrong body part, wrong side of the body, or at the wrong level of the otherwise correctly identified anatomic structure, such as in spinal surgery. Wrong-site surgery not only devastates the patient, family, and caregiver but also negatively affects the entire perioperative team (Makar et al., 2015).

All institutions accredited by TJC must comply with the Universal Protocol (TJC, 2017) including these activities: conduct a preprocedure verification process, mark the procedure site, and perform a time-out before the procedure begins.

- *Preprocedure verification process* ensures that all relevant documents (e.g., the history and physical examination, surgical consent, required laboratory studies) and imaging studies (properly labeled and displayed) are available before the start of the procedure. Preprocedure verification is best conducted when the patient and/or guardian can be involved and should be complete before the patient leaves the preprocedure area. The surgical team must agree that this is the correct patient and the planned procedure

---

BOX 2.4

Elements of the Intraoperative Hand-off Communication Between Scrub Persons Using Situation, Background, Assessment, and Recommendations, or SBAR

Situation
- Name of patient
- Name of procedure being performed
- Pertinent information about the procedure (What is the progress of the surgery, have any additional/different surgical procedures been discussed?)

Background
- Elements of patient history pertinent to surgery (e.g., allergies)
- Who are the members of the surgical team (names, roles)?
- Special instruments, suture, other items being used
- What is the blood loss and will hemostatic adjuncts be needed?
- What medications and fluids are on the sterile field? (Quietly but audibly review each label together.)
- Specifics about any equipment issues/special needs/back table and Mayo setup

Assessment
- What is the status of specimens?
- Have any counts been done? Which ones? Do a transfer of care count together quietly.
- What is the anticipated amount of time remaining in the procedure?
- Have any complications been discussed/anticipated?
- Have there been any problems with anesthesia?

Recommendations
- Note any special requests for closure/dressings/drains noted by the surgical team or special requests noted by the anesthesia provider.
- Prepare to introduce the relief scrub person.
- Allow an opportunity for relief scrub person to ask questions or voice concerns before "breaking scrub" by person being relieved.

Modified from Amato-Vealey EJ et al: Hand-off communication: a requisite for patient safety, *AORN J* 88(5):763–770, 2008.

BOX 2.5

Elements of the Intraoperative to Postanesthesia Care Unit Hand-off Communication Using Situation, Background, Assessment, and Recommendations, or SBAR

Situation
- Name of patient and date of birth
- Full name of operative or invasive procedure performed, including modifiers and site

Background
- Type of anesthesia administered and name of anesthesia care provider
- Intraoperative medications administered, including dose and time
- Intravenous fluids administered
- Estimated blood and urine loss
- Pertinent information related to the surgical site such as dressings, tubes, drains, or packing
- Any significant perioperative operating room events

Assessment
- Hemodynamic stability
- Airway and oxygenation status

- Thermal status (e.g., presence of hypothermia or hyperthermia)
- Urine output
- Presence or absence of surgical complications
- Level of pain
- Method of pain management

Recommendations
- Assist with transfer of lines and equipment.
- Ensure that immediate postoperative orders have been completed.
- Discharge from the PACU when stable.
- Allow opportunity for intraoperative and PACU staff members to ask questions or voice concerns, especially when equipment and information handoff occur simultaneously.

PACU, Perianesthesia care unit.
From Amato-Vealey EJ et al: Hand-off communication: a requisite for patient safety, *AORN J* 88(5):766–770, 2008; van Rensen et al: Multitasking during patient handover in the recovery room, *Anesth Analg* 15(6):1183–1187, 2012; Robinson N: Promoting patient safety with perioperative hand-off communication, *J Perianesth Nurs* 31(3):245–253, 2016.

---

on the specified side and site. The preprocedure verification process also includes confirming availability of necessary equipment, implants, and prostheses, which is reconfirmed during the time-out.

- *Marking the surgical site* must occur so that the intended site of incision or insertion is clear and unambiguous. Procedures that involve left/right distinction, multiple structures, or multiple levels (spinal surgery) require specific marking. The marking also must be unambiguous; initials, a "yes," or a line at or near the incision site are all acceptable. The marking methodology should be consistently used throughout the facility. The person performing the procedure, who is accountable for it, and who will be present

when the procedure is performed, must personally mark the site; the patient should be involved in the marking if possible (Patient Engagement Exemplar). The marking must remain visible after the patient has been prepped and draped. Facilities should have a provision in place for patients who refuse site marking.

- *Taking the time-out.* Facilities must have a procedure to implement the time-out before starting the procedure or making the surgical incision. The surgeon or other physician who is conducting the procedure must be present for the time-out. If separate teams are performing distinct segments of a multiple procedure surgery, there must be a time-out *before each procedure.* This does not apply to patients in whom the same surgical team is performing multiple aspects of a single procedure. Specific situations requiring two time-outs are those in which hospital policy or law/regulation requires two separate consents (e.g., for a cesarean birth followed by tubal ligation). During the time-out, active involvement and communication among all surgical team members is expected. All participants confirm and agree that they have the correct patient, correct side and site, and the correct procedure to be performed. Many facility procedures include verification that the patient is in the correct position and that any needed equipment, supplies, or implants are correct and available and sterile, if indicated; of the presence and review of relevant imaging studies; that all prep solutions have dried; and that all electrical equipment is properly calibrated to minimize surgical fire and burn risks.

Since establishment of the Universal Protocol and WHO's Safe Surgery Saves Lives Checklist, the professional literature has asserted wide acceptance and general success in reducing errors (Treadwell et al., 2014). Literature has also identified barriers to implementation acceptance and a need for a broader systems approach if the checklist is to achieve its desired potential (Berry et al., 2016; Mayer et al., 2016).

Electronic SSCs have impressive results. Gitelis and colleagues (2017) found that an SSC increased compliance and reduced the number of adverse events. Furthermore, 76% of surgeons, 86% of anesthesia providers, and 88% of the perioperative nurses believed the electronic SSC would have a positive effect on patient safety. Comprehensive safety systems depend on compliance for effectiveness. Despite the attributes of checklists, wrong surgeries can and do still happen; randomized controlled clinical trials are not possible to confirm this (Algie et al., 2015).

Retained Surgical Items

RSIs are a concern of AORN, TJC, WHO, and all facilities in which surgery is performed. The physiologic, financial, and public relations consequences from RSIs are potentially severe. In ORs, conducting count processes according to evidence-based policies (audible, visual, and concurrent) are considered a key risk reduction and patient safety strategy (AORN, 2017). The Patient Safety box reviews key components to prevent RSIs. Although a standardized safe surgery program that addresses both wrong-site surgery and RSIs can reduce serious reportable events (SREs) by 52% (Loftus et al., 2015), RSIs remain a problem yet to be solved.

PATIENT ENGAGEMENT EXEMPLAR

Marking the Surgical Site

An active partnership with patients and families before surgery fosters an environment of safety. When patients and families are involved in the surgical site marking process they are taking an active role in prevention of wrong site, person, or procedure surgery. Involve patients and families during all steps of the patient identification and verification process, giving them time to state their understanding of the procedure and surgical site. Most patients and/or families know where and what type of surgery they are having and are a good resource to confirm correct site/procedure. If patients and families are unclear about the scheduled procedure, give them an opportunity to voice concerns and answer their questions, consulting the surgeon if necessary. The perioperative nurse should establish what the patient's main concern is preoperatively and pass on this concern to the next care provider at each phase of care. Having discussions with patients during this process allows them to gather the information needed to make informed decisions about their care and prepares them for what is to come. Patients and families should be involved in the site marking process, indicating the correct side and site of their surgery while it is marked by the provider.

PATIENT SAFETY

Key Components of Counts to Prevent Retained Surgical Items

Research indicates that a discrepancy of a count at any time during a surgical procedure is a safety variance associated with elevated RSI risk. Counts of soft goods such as radiopaque sponges, sharps, and instruments should be performed, reported to the surgical team at each count in Step 4, and recorded:

1. Before the procedure to establish the baseline number of soft goods, sharps, and instruments (record soft goods, sharps, and miscellaneous items in a visible location, such as the count board and use preprinted count sheets for instruments)
2. When new items are added to the field
3. At time of permanent relief of either the scrub person or the circulator (although items within the body cavity may not be directly visible)
4. When cavity (e.g., heart, uterus, peritoneum) closure begins; when wound closure begins; and at the end of procedure when counted items are no longer used; as the first layer of wound closure begins, the scrub person and circulating nurse count all items consecutively in a standardized routine such as proceeding from sterile field to Mayo stand to back table and then off the field, or vice versa; the count is done audibly, visibly, and concurrently; this is referred to as the "second" count; any time a discrepancy is suspected, recount
5. At time of instrument assembly for sterilization

Methods
- Items should be counted audibly and viewed concurrently by two people, one of whom is the circulating nurse for each count.
- The circulating nurse informs the surgeon of the results of the closing counts.
- Individual pieces of assembled units should be accounted for separately; account for all pieces of a broken item.
- Team members should be aware of risk factors associated with retained surgical items (RSIs).
- Preprinted sheets/preformatted screens should be used to record the counts.
- To the extent possible, procedure setup should be standardized with the minimum number of counted items needed.

Modified from Association of periOperative Registered Nurses (AORN): Guidelines for prevention of retained surgical items. In: *AORN guidelines for perioperative practice*, Denver, 2017, The Association; Spruce L: Back to basics: counting surgical soft goods, *AORN J* 103(3):298–301, 2016; Wood A: Use of count boards, *AORN J* 103(1):118–119, 2016.

Soft goods, such as surgical sponges, are one of the most frequent inadvertently retained items (AORN, 2017). In many retained sponge cases, counts are reported as "correct" at the conclusion of the procedure. Physiologic consequences of an RSI include possible infection, obstruction, fistula formation, perforation or consequent pain, suffering, and possible death, along with the likely need for additional surgery.

Increased RSI risk by patient or by procedure can be caused by obesity, complexity of procedure, increased number of personnel, and emergency procedures, but these only partially explain incorrect surgical counts. The OR culture and environment in which the patient has the procedure is also a major risk determinant. Thus prevention of RSIs, once thought of as a straightforward matter of counting to 5 or 10, has joined the human factors/systems analysis research cadre that focuses on perioperative patient safety issues.

As noted, CMS and many private insurers now refuse payment for remedial treatment such as otherwise unnecessary surgery to remove an RSI or to treat the physiologic consequences of its inadvertent retention. The healthcare facility must absorb the costs of extended hospitalization and required corrective treatment; it also may be deemed responsible for the entire cost of care for patients whose condition requires readmission within 30 days of discharge. As with wrong-site surgery, additional financial losses may arise from defending any resultant malpractice litigation, impaired public reputation, and the need to respond to licensing and regulatory body inquiries.

Prevention of Retained Surgical Items

Facilities should have an established system to prevent RSIs that reflects AORN's Guideline. Note that the guideline recommends that facility policy should also incorporate human factors and keep interruptions, distractions, and repetition-induced attention deficits to their minimum (Fencl, 2016).

Two persons counting aloud, combined with the surgeon's visual and manual exploration of the wound and the scrub person's mental tracking of sponges and other counted objects in the wound (situational awareness), have long been mainstay approaches to prevent RSIs. Situational awareness requires that both the perioperative nurse and scrub person perceive relevant clinical cues in the count environment, comprehend the importance of those cues, and identify required interventions based on those cues. New sponge-tracking technologies have emerged to enhance risk reduction strategies to prevent inadvertent retention of RSIs. These include sequentially numbered sponges, bar coding, and radiofrequency identification (RFID) products. Typically, sequentially numbered sponge products are prepackaged, presterilized sponges in groups of 5 or 10 in sequentially numbered packages. When using such numbered systems, surgical teams are more likely to detect a missing/retained sponge because they must account for each individual numbered sponge rather than account for an aggregate number. The usual tenets of counting remain: counts are performed *audibly, concurrently, and visibly.* Count policies and practices in the institution should be standardized with little variability among staff members (AORN, 2017). Distractions are minimized; some institutions take a "pause for the cause," aka "pause for the gauze" and other rubrics while counts are in progress.

An "incorrect" or unreconciled count occurs when the number of items on the count record or worksheet fails to match the number of items recovered during a closing count. All incorrect closure counts must be reported immediately and attempts made to resolve every discrepancy. If a count remains unresolved, the circulating nurse must again notify the surgeon of the unresolved count, and a search must be made for the missing item, including the surgical wound, field, floor, linen, and trash (this is the rationale that linen and trash must not leave the OR until the end of the procedure). All personnel must direct their immediate attention to locating the missing item. If it is not found, an x-ray film may be taken and read by the radiologist or surgeon as specified in institutional policy. If the x-ray is negative, the count is recorded as incorrect or unreconciled and the x-ray results noted on the patient's intraoperative record. An incident/occurrence/event report should be initiated according to institution policy. Accurate counting and recording of soft goods, sharps, and instruments are essential for the protection of the patient, personnel, and the institution, and they are integral to effective risk management.

RFID and bar-code technologies are also incorporated into equipment to prevent RSIs. RFID systems tag instruments, soft goods such as sponges, and other items likely to enter the body during a procedure and use a scanning wand through tissues to ascertain the location of these items before the procedure ends. Bar-code scanning systems require the scanning of items as a procedure begins and/or as they are put into the body and again as they are removed from the body and/or as a procedure ends.

Other technologic approaches continue to emerge. No matter which RSI prevention system a facility adopts, none is a cure-all or infallible. All technologies require precise use, as designed, and in accordance with the manufacturer's instructions. Failure to invest in RSI prevention devices is not without its own costs (Steelman et al., 2015). As with any new technology or approach, all team members must be alert to possible unintended consequences of its use (e.g., electrical interference with other equipment or overreliance on the additional margin of safety provided by an approach, which may lead to less vigilance).

Care and Handling of Specimens

During the many years perioperative patient care has included safe handling of surgical specimens, laboratory medicine's safety practices focused on the analysis of the surgical specimen. The WHO World Alliance on Patient Safety now recognizes that to improve patient safety further in laboratory medicine, the preanalytic and postanalytic stages are equally important. Care of specimens is a multidisciplinary, multistage, and multisystem strategy. Like other areas of patient safety, laboratory errors occur more frequently than commonly believed. Bixenstine and colleagues (2013) found specimen errors in 2.9% of cases they reviewed. The errors included problems with specimen containers (1.2% of containers with errors) and specimen requisitions (2.3% of requisitions with errors). Their analysis of errors only included specimens before they reached the pathology laboratory (from the OR to pathology). There is a wide potential for errors in surgical specimens, including unlabeled and mislabeled specimens (Brent, 2015), empty containers, incorrect side designation (called wrong "laterality"), incorrect or no identified tissue site, or incorrect or no patient names or numbers. As with preventing RSIs, technologies (e.g., bar coding and RFID chips) may reduce the frequency of specimen labeling errors.

TJC (2014) addresses specimen handling, which requires use of at least two patient identifiers when collecting specimens for clinical testing. It also requires action to improve timeliness of reporting critical laboratory results. Accurate and timely communication and delivery of specimens are presumptively necessary for timely reporting of results. The care and handling of specimens raise considerations unique to perioperative settings, and AORN's (2017) guidelines

RESEARCH HIGHLIGHT ||

Key Points in Handling Specimens in the Perioperative Environment

Current research finds that the most common events are reported during the prelaboratory phase, specifically, with specimen labeling, transport and/or storage, and collection/preservation. The most common contributing factors in this study were failures in hand-off communication, staff inattention, knowledge deficit, and environmental issues. The researchers conclude that extra attention must be paid to perioperative specimen handling. The top three activities leading to adverse events and near misses in their study were the following:

1. *Specimen labeling* procedures for correct patient and specimen identification should include consistent and accurate information on labels and forms. Specimen labels should include at least two identifiers and include the correct indicating information (site or side, diagnosis, etc.).
2. *Specimen transporting and/or storing* is best accomplished by hand rather than vacuum tube. Admittedly, hand delivery adds to the opportunity for delay, but hand delivery eliminates electronic tube system issues; makes spillage, leakage, or breakage less likely; and should facilitate delivery to the correct place, thus avoiding specimen loss.
3. *Assessment of specimen collecting and handling needs* begins when the procedure is scheduled. The perioperative nurse and surgeon should discuss specimen information such as anticipated specimens, particular needs, specific information that needs to be communicated to pathology, and specimen identifiers. This should reduce the specimen being placed in the wrong container or solution, or absence of solution when indicated.

Other concerns when handling specimens include:

4. Instituting methods to prevent transmissible infection/contamination of personnel and specimens including the use of tight, appropriate-sized lids for specimen containers.
5. Forensic specimens that may require unique handling to preserve the chain of evidence.

As with most safety issues, communication remains key. Communication begins with the surgeon and follows this pathway:

- The surgeon hands a specimen to the scrub person and tells him or her what the specimen is, what process is needed in the lab, and whether there are any special labeling needs or information to include on the requisition slip for the pathology laboratory.
- The scrub person hands off the specimen to the circulating nurse, repeating what the surgeon said.
- The circulating nurse receives the specimen, places it in the container, and labels the specimen container according to information provided by the surgeon and scrub person, repeating back the label information.
- The circulating nurse completes the necessary laboratory requisition and follows institution-prescribed steps for sending the specimen to the laboratory.
- During the debriefing at the procedure's end, the circulating nurse announces all specimens obtained; if no specimens were obtained, that is also announced.

Data from Steelman VM et al: Surgical specimen management: a descriptive study of 648 adverse events and near misses. *Arch Pathol Lab Med* (129):1390–1396, 2016.

---

provide the best recommendations. The Research Highlight box explores key points in safe specimen care and handling.

Proper management of specimens is critical to the outcome of a patient's surgery. It is the responsibility of the entire surgical team to identify, document, and care properly for specimens. Common specimens include blood, soft tissue, bone, body fluids, and removed foreign bodies. Complete and accurate identification and labeling of specimens and timely delivery to the proper laboratory for analysis are imperative. A mislabeled specimen may result in misdiagnosis and consequent inappropriate treatment of the patient. At a minimum, each specimen must bear a label with the correct patient name and identification number, specific origin of the specimen, and laterality (e.g., Jane Doe, 100001, right breast biopsy). The surgeon provides descriptive information about the specimen (e.g., "suture tag at 6 o'clock"). The nurse "repeats back" to the surgeon information being sent to the laboratory (e.g., patient name, type of specimen, source/location, required tests, special handling needs). All specimens and their disposition are documented in the patient's intraoperative record. Hey and Turner (2016) suggest that any team member can request an intraoperative pause; the perioperative nurse can do so, requesting clarification of any questions or concerns about surgical specimens.

Handling of each specimen occurs according to specific protocols established by the receiving laboratory. Generally the surgical team handles all tissue to preserve its integrity, keeping specimens moist and transporting them to the laboratory as soon as possible. Standard transmission-based precautions govern specimen transport to protect individuals who must handle the specimen (see Chapter 4). Labels

should identify the need for precautions and the presence of biohazardous material.

Formalin is frequently used to preserve specimens if they are not taken to the laboratory immediately. Formalin fumes are a hazardous substance that can cause watery eyes and respiratory irritation. Direct contact will injure human tissue. Gloves are worn and adequate ventilation provided in areas in which formalin is handled. Institutional policy should describe procedures to follow in case of spills. Safer, alternative fixatives have been sought for decades and only recently have complements been identified (Stefanitis et al., 2016).

Specimens for Frozen Section

When immediate tissue identification or identification of malignancy is needed, specimens are quick-frozen, sliced, stained, and examined in the laboratory under a microscope. This method of tissue examination is called *frozen section*. Specimens for frozen section usually are placed on moistened Telfa or into a clean, covered specimen container to prevent drying. They are *never* placed in saline solution or formalin *nor are they ever* transported on a counted sponge. The results of frozen-section analysis are communicated to the surgeon intraoperatively. If the hospital has no system for direct pathologist–surgeon communication, the perioperative nurse receives the telephone report of a frozen section. Because this is considered an especially critical test result, the nurse "reads back" the test result to the pathologist and surgeon and receives a repeat-back from the pathologist and surgeon to verify accurate communication of the results (Smith and Raab, 2016).

Risks for Burns: Electrical Hazards

Electrical hazards in the OR include electric shock, fire, burns, and explosions. Electrical burns result from current flowing through the body and emerging in a concentrated area. They can occur from touching an uninsulated wire, a damaged plug, or an ungrounded piece of metal equipment. ESUs (sometimes called the "Bovie") send a specified current from the ESU through the active electrode (often referred to as a "pencil") to create sufficient heat to cut or coagulate the vessel touched by the pencil or other instrument. The current then exits the body through a dispersive electrode (sometimes called the "ground pad") and returns to the ESU. Chapter 8 contains a thorough discussion of the ESU and electrical safety.

Fires and Explosions

The incidence of OR fires has decreased as less flammable anesthetic agents are being used (Akhtar et al., 2016). Nonetheless, surgical fires are a technology hazard identified by the ECRI Institute (2016). Fires and explosions in all settings require three components: (1) an ignition source/heat, (2) fuel, and (3) an oxidizer (oxygen or another source of oxygenation [e.g., H_2O_2]). Perioperative nurses can decrease risks of burns from fires by considering these "fire triangle" requirements during procedures and working with the surgical team to reduce each to no more than necessary. Elimination of any single component of the triangle prevents fire. The Patient Safety: Surgical Fire Prevention box discusses surgical fire prevention.

Ignition/heat sources serve to provide the energy to initiate the oxidation chemical reaction, that is, ignition. In the OR, concentrated sources of energy such as sparks from static electricity, ESUs, and lasers are key sources of heat and ignition. Oxygen or an oxygen-nitrogen composition, such as nitrous oxide (N_2O), administered via prong or mask, is the usual oxygen source. Room air (21% O_2) can serve as the oxygenation source but only if there is a sufficiently fine fuel (e.g., powders) (Joint Commission Perspectives, 2016). Surgical drapes are a common fuel source (which can also trap oxygen in folds); fuels can literally be anything that burns.

Fire and explosion prevention strategies involve separation of ignition/heat sources, fuel, and oxygen in time and/or space. Speed of ignition depends on temperature, particle size, and the concentration of the reactant fuel. Space separation strategies involve keeping (or eliminating) possible sources of igniting sparks (e.g., static electricity, ESUs, and lasers) as far from anesthesia and the patient's head and throat as possible. The anesthesia provider should use room air rather than more concentrated oxygen or N_2O as much as possible; supplemental oxygen is used cautiously. Nitrous oxide, like free oxygen, is an oxidizing agent but only in the presence of a fire or explosion, which then breaks down its chemical bonds. An explosion, however, can be even more violent when N_2O is present than with

---

PATIENT SAFETY

Surgical Fire Prevention

At the Start of Each Surgery:
- Enriched O_2 and N_2O atmospheres can vastly increase flammability of drapes, plastics, and hair. Be aware of possible O_2 enrichment under drapes.
- Do not apply drapes until all flammable preps have fully dried; remove spilled or pooled prep agent.
- Fiberoptic light sources can start fires; complete all cable connections before activating the source, and place the source in standby mode when disconnecting cables.
- Moisten sponges to make them ignition resistant in oropharyngeal and pulmonary surgery.
- Include fire assessment risk and prevention status in briefing/time-out.

During Head, Face, Neck, and Upper Chest Surgery:
- Use medical-grade air for open delivery to the face if the patient can maintain a safe blood O_2 saturation without supplemental O_2.
- If the patient cannot maintain a safe blood O_2 saturation without extra O_2, secure the airway with a laryngeal mask airway or tracheal tube. *Exceptions:* When patient verbal responses may be required during surgery (e.g., carotid artery surgery, neurosurgery, pacemaker insertion) and when open O_2 delivery is required to keep the patient safe.
- At all times, deliver the minimum O_2 concentration necessary (titrate O_2 to patient's needs) for adequate oxygenation and increase only as necessary.
- Stop supplemental O_2 at least 1 minute before and during use of electrosurgery and other energy-generating devices such as

a laser (if possible). Surgical team communication is essential for this recommendation.
- Keep fenestration towel edges as far from the incision as possible.
- Arrange drapes to minimize O_2 buildup underneath.
- Coat head hair and facial hair (e.g., eyebrows, beard, mustache) within the fenestration with water-soluble surgical lubricating jelly to make them nonflammable.
- For coagulation, use bipolar electrosurgery, not monopolar electrosurgery.

During Oropharyngeal Surgery (e.g., Tonsillectomy):
- Scavenge deep within the oropharynx with a metal suction cannula to catch leaking O_2 and N_2O.
- Moisten gauze or sponges and keep them moist, including those used with uncuffed tracheal tubes.

When Using Electrosurgery Units, Electrocautery, or Laser:
- The surgeon should be made aware of open O_2 use.
- Activate the unit only when the active tip is in view (especially if looking through a microscope or endoscope).
- Deactivate the unit before the tip leaves the surgical site.
- Place electrosurgical electrodes in a holster or another location off the patient.
- Place lasers in standby mode when not in active use.
- Do not place rubber catheter sleeves over electrosurgical electrodes.

Modified from Bruley ME: *New recommendations for surgical fire prevention and management.* In: *AORN Congress,* San Diego, CA, 2013; Association of periOperative Registered Nurses (AORN): Guidelines on safe use of energy generating devices and safe environment of care, part 1. In: *Guidelines for perioperative practice,* Denver, 2017, The Association; Spruce L: Back to basics: preventing surgical fires, *AORN J* 104(3):217–224.e2, 2016.

O_2 alone because when a fuel burns in N_2O, it produces more heat than burning in O_2 alone.

Not surprisingly, procedures using ESUs and lasers around the face and neck (i.e., near O_2 or O_2/N_2O) provide the greatest risk. Thus a fire risk assessment conducted before the start of the procedure and reiterated during the time-out (Spruce, 2016) is part of many facility protocols. As with all surgeries, ESU active electrodes should be kept in holsters and not allowed to rest on drapes; lasers and ESU active electrodes should not be allowed to touch fine gauze or sponges, especially alcohol-soaked sponges. All OR team members should know their role in the event of a fire crisis (Fig. 2.2). (See Chapter 8 for additional safe practice specifics with the laser, ESU, and other energy-generating devices.)

Risk for Chemical Burns

Chemical burns most commonly occur during or after surgical site skin preparation (prep). Skin prep solutions should be applied with care to prevent pooling, which can lead to chemical burns to the skin. Towels should be tucked under the patient along the area to be prepped to catch any dripping solution and removed on completion of skin prep (these towels are sometimes called "drip" towels). In addition to being a chemical irritant, prep solution can serve as the fuel component of the fire triangle that may be ignited by a spark from an active electrode of the ESU or even from a discharge of static electricity. Thus inappropriate use of prep solution can also cause thermal burns. Ignition of prep vapors can also occur as solution evaporates. Solutions used for skin prep must dry before application of surgical drapes.

Pressure Injuries

Pressure injuries (PIs) include nerve compression (peroneal and ulnar nerves are particularly susceptible), nerve stretching (e.g., brachial plexus extension); and PIs (especially on the coccyx, heels, or back of head in supine position). Pressure or the lack thereof also may cause venous stasis and deep vein thrombosis (DVT). Each surgical position has its own predictable pressure risks and methods of prevention (see Chapter 6). As a rule, however, the surgical team should remember that increasing the area of contact or reducing the force pushing on that area will decrease pressure. An easy to remember formula is pressure equals force divided by area ($P = F/A$). Thus both increasing area and decreasing force lessen pressure. This formula explains why both thin and obese patients are at risk for PIs during surgery. Thin patients tend to have a smaller area directly in contact with the OR bed or a positioning device. Obese patients, on the other hand, have more force from their increased weight and body mass. Padding typically reduces pressure by increasing the area over which a force is applied. Dynamic support surfaces, patient risk assessment for PI, and length of surgery (and its type) are all considered when initiating additional protective measures (Spruce, 2017). Reminding scrubbed personnel not to lean on the patient reduces force applied to an area, thus also avoiding PIs.

Medication Administration

Like all perioperative safety concerns, medication administration safety must be examined within the context of its multidisciplinary system (Cochran et al., 2016). That system includes medication prescribing, transcribing, procurement, and dispensing, as well as administering (AORN, 2017). Medication administration in the OR/invasive procedure room is complicated, compared with that found in other nursing care areas. The OR often requires that the circulating nurse and scrub person jointly prepare a medication that will be administered by a third person, usually the surgeon. Moreover, two potentially lethal medications are frequently used on the field, for example, epinephrine and heparin, and both are clear and come in widely disparate dosages. Checking for allergies, which is important in all areas, takes on new dimensions as well because anesthetics may disguise allergic reactions.

Vigilance in following established safe medication practices is crucial. Consider turning down music to avoid distractions, making sure all needed supplies have been dispensed to avoid interruptions, and requesting a "No interruption zone" or "Do not disturb" time during important activities in medication preparation. Pay particular attention to acknowledging medication name, concentrations, and labeling solutions in syringes and containers on and off the sterile field, and performing read-backs/repeat-backs. Tedious as it may seem, the complete name and concentration of the drug should appear on the administration device; thus "lidocaine 2% with epinephrine 1 : 100,000" and not "epi."

Team members follow policies and procedures strictly to double-check a medication or solution before it is dispensed to the sterile field. Medications and medication containers (e.g., syringes, cups, basins), both on and off the sterile field, are labeled fully and accurately with medication names and concentrations; processes must be established and used to verify labels. Scrub persons should identify medications by announcing the name of the medication being passed to the surgeon, along with its concentration. A repeat-back confirmation from the surgeon ensures the correct dose of medication or solution.

The institution's "Do not use" list of abbreviations must be observed and applied to all medication orders and medication-related documentation that are handwritten or on preprinted forms. TJC no longer maintains a look-alike/sound-alike drug list. Instead it recommends that each facility develop a list of drugs stocked, dispensed, and/or administered in the facility based on findings from the Institute for Safe Medication Practices (ISMP, 2012). A facility-specific list should be readily available to all perioperative personnel.

Federal agencies, TJC, and individual institutions increasingly look to bar-code medication administration (BCMA) systems to reduce medication errors. Adoption of BCMA systems has accelerated because BCMA has become a criterion of the "meaningful use" of health IT (CMS, 2012). Empiric studies have found a reduction in errors after BCMA implementation (Truitt et al., 2016) and concluded that the implementation of electronic medication administration record and BCMA technology improved patient safety and reduced the harmful impact to patients caused by administration errors. Bar-code implementation is associated with fewer medication errors; however, medication errors are not eliminated (Cochran et al., 2016; Truitt et al., 2016). Bar-code implementation may also be more difficult intraoperatively (Redman, 2017).

Robotic-Assisted Surgery

Despite, or perhaps because of robotic surgery's rapid and ongoing evolution, data are not conclusive relating to its safety issues. Robotic-assisted surgery safety concerns are usually imbedded in specialty, subspecialty, and individual procedure books and articles. Only very recently have researchers begun a more comprehensive look at safety concerns.

Loftus and colleagues (2015) found that implementation of a standardized safe surgery program led to a significant reduction in SREs, but robotic procedures in their study were seven times more likely to incur an SRE event than were more traditional approaches.

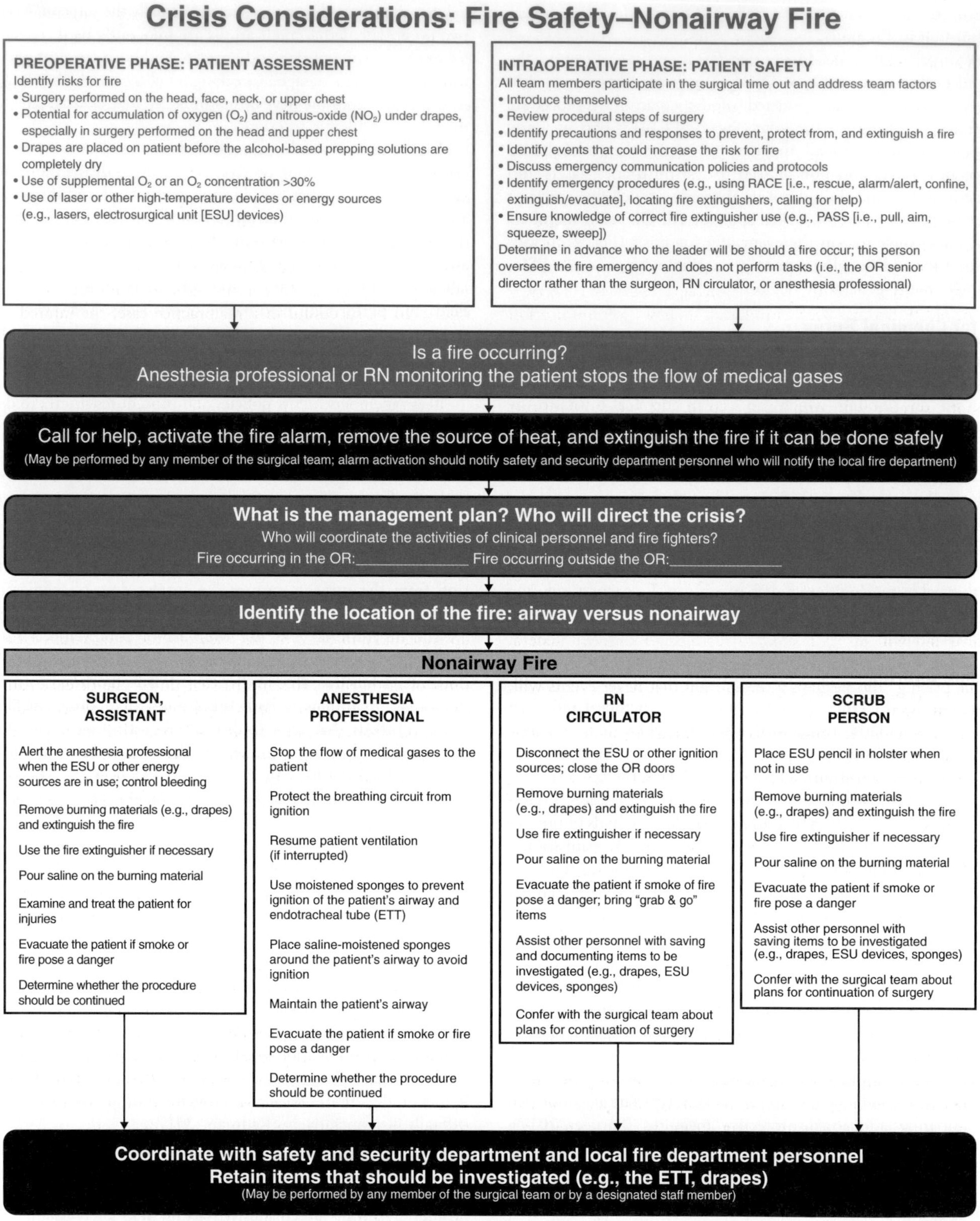

Crisis Considerations: Fire Safety–Nonairway Fire

PREOPERATIVE PHASE: PATIENT ASSESSMENT

Identify risks for fire

- Surgery performed on the head, face, neck, or upper chest
- Potential for accumulation of oxygen (O_2) and nitrous-oxide (NO_2) under drapes, especially in surgery performed on the head and upper chest
- Drapes are placed on patient before the alcohol-based prepping solutions are completely dry
- Use of supplemental O_2 or an O_2 concentration >30%
- Use of laser or other high-temperature devices or energy sources (e.g., lasers, electrosurgical unit [ESU] devices)

INTRAOPERATIVE PHASE: PATIENT SAFETY

All team members participate in the surgical time out and address team factors

- Introduce themselves
- Review procedural steps of surgery
- Identify precautions and responses to prevent, protect from, and extinguish a fire
- Identify events that could increase the risk for fire
- Discuss emergency communication policies and protocols
- Identify emergency procedures (e.g., using RACE [i.e., rescue, alarm/alert, confine, extinguish/evacuate], locating fire extinguishers, calling for help)
- Ensure knowledge of correct fire extinguisher use (e.g., PASS [i.e., pull, aim, squeeze, sweep])

Determine in advance who the leader will be should a fire occur; this person oversees the fire emergency and does not perform tasks (i.e., the OR senior director rather than the surgeon, RN circulator, or anesthesia professional)

Is a fire occurring?
Anesthesia professional or RN monitoring the patient stops the flow of medical gases

↓

Call for help, activate the fire alarm, remove the source of heat, and extinguish the fire if it can be done safely
(May be performed by any member of the surgical team; alarm activation should notify safety and security department personnel who will notify the local fire department)

↓

What is the management plan? Who will direct the crisis?
Who will coordinate the activities of clinical personnel and fire fighters?
Fire occurring in the OR:_____ Fire occurring outside the OR:_____

↓

Identify the location of the fire: airway versus nonairway

↓

Nonairway Fire

SURGEON, ASSISTANT	ANESTHESIA PROFESSIONAL	RN CIRCULATOR	SCRUB PERSON
Alert the anesthesia professional when the ESU or other energy sources are in use; control bleeding	Stop the flow of medical gases to the patient	Disconnect the ESU or other ignition sources; close the OR doors	Place ESU pencil in holster when not in use
Remove burning materials (e.g., drapes) and extinguish the fire	Protect the breathing circuit from ignition	Remove burning materials (e.g., drapes) and extinguish the fire	Remove burning materials (e.g., drapes) and extinguish the fire
Use the fire extinguisher if necessary	Resume patient ventilation (if interrupted)	Use fire extinguisher if necessary	Use fire extinguisher if necessary
Pour saline on the burning material	Use moistened sponges to prevent ignition of the patient's airway and endotracheal tube (ETT)	Pour saline on the burning material	Pour saline on the burning material
Examine and treat the patient for injuries	Place saline-moistened sponges around the patient's airway to avoid ignition	Evacuate the patient if smoke of fire pose a danger; bring "grab & go" items	Evacuate the patient if smoke or fire pose a danger
Evacuate the patient if smoke or fire pose a danger	Maintain the patient's airway	Assist other personnel with saving and documenting items to be investigated (e.g., drapes, ESU devices, sponges)	Assist other personnel with saving items to be investigated (e.g., drapes, ESU devices, sponges)
Determine whether the procedure should be continued	Evacuate the patient if smoke or fire pose a danger	Confer with the surgical team about plans for continuation of surgery	Confer with the surgical team about plans for continuation of surgery
	Determine whether the procedure should be continued		

↓

Coordinate with safety and security department and local fire department personnel
Retain items that should be investigated (e.g., the ETT, drapes)
(May be performed by any member of the surgical team or by a designated staff member)

Adapted from the Fire Crisis Checklist [2013] with permission from Ariadne Labs, Brigham and Women's Hospital and Harvard School of Public Health, Boston, MA. Copyright © 2014, AORN, Inc, All reasonable precautions have been taken to verify the information contained in this publication. The responsibility for the interpretation and use of the materials lies with the reader.

FIG. 2.2 Flowchart use for educating operating room team in managing nonairway fire crisis.

However, Park and colleagues (2017) conducted a meta-analysis and concluded that robotic hysterectomy "appears" to reduce overall complications compared with an open hysterectomy. Both studies concluded with the need for more rigorous prospective studies.

Alemzadeh and colleagues (2016) retrospectively studied 14 years of FDA data related to adverse events in robotic surgery. They extracted data related to injuries (e.g., burns, cuts, organ damage, deaths), surgical specialty, and major types of device or instrument malfunction (e.g., electrical arcing, burned or broken instruments falling into patient bodies). They concluded that despite widespread use of robotics, difficulties and complications still exist. To overcome one difficulty, that of the need to extract the robotic arms from the patient for repositioning the patient during a complex surgery, a new type of OR bed has been introduced. It allows communication between the robot and OR bed so that, as the bed (and patient) moves, the robotic arms automatically reposition while remaining in the patient's body (ECRI Institute, 2017a).

Robotic surgery will continue to evolve. The future of robotic surgery involves cost reduction, development of new platforms and technologies, creation and validation of curricula and virtual simulators, and the conduct of randomized controlled trials to determine its best applications (Ghezzi and Corleta, 2016). Many chapters in Unit II of this textbook discuss robotic applications in the surgical specialty being addressed.

Risk Management In the "Near" Future

Like robotic surgery, perioperative risk management will continue to evolve and will do so related to repealed or different federal statutes and administrative rules; changes in state law; cost reduction via value pricing; and perhaps a recognition that never events will, nevertheless, occur.

Even though much progress has been made in patient safety, there is still more work to be done.

"Let's recognize the progress that we've made…but there's absolutely no room for complacency," said Derek Feeley, CEO of IHI during a December 2016 keynote speech at the IHI National Forum on Quality Improvement in Healthcare in Orlando, Florida (Punke, 2016). Mr. Feeley urged the adoption of a new paradigm for patient safety thinking and described ways to do so, such as positively; proactively; and as systems, not projects. Feeley noted that learning from mistakes is important, but it is not sufficient to rely on hindsight alone. He encouraged provider organizations to learn from and build on successes instead of solely focusing on correcting failures. The ECRI Institute (2017b) does this by emphasizing potential hazards in its top ten hazard alert, rather than reposting what errors have happened.

Feeley also recommended changing from a reactive position to a proactive one. The question should be "Is care safe today and will it be tomorrow?" in addition to asking if care was safe yesterday.

As has been noted previously, and emphasized by Feeley, many safety issues cannot be solved by singular projects. Instead, healthcare organizations need to focus on systems, creating feedback loops so every improvement project builds on the other, until safety is viewed through a system lens. Such systems thinking promotes an environment of transparency and trust and establishes a culture that encourages reporting adverse events and near misses and protects those who report them.

Patient Rights

Protection of patients' personal, ethical, and legal rights underlies patient safety and risk management. Many nurses and other healthcare providers equate patients' legal rights with negligence, malpractice, and informed consent, and equate patient safety with safety from physical injury. These are only some of the many legal and ethical concerns in a myriad of perioperative settings, although legal and ethical issues interrelate as well as all components in healthcare.

Freedom From Negligent Treatment

Malpractice is negligence by a professional in the performance of a professional act that causes patient injury. Provision of safe care to the patient is the best protection for the nurse and facility from malpractice claims. This is because it is rarely possible to sue healthcare providers for malpractice without an injury. Despite emergence of other types of harm, there almost always must still be a physical injury. To be successful in a malpractice case, the injured patient must prove that the member(s) of the surgical team departed from the standard(s) of care applicable to their profession and that this breach of applicable standard(s) caused the injury.

If an injury occurs, both the professional licensure and civil legal systems require the team to act to prevent it from worsening. Risk management should be notified and become involved immediately after injury occurs to minimize the likelihood of the patient or his or her representative bringing suit and, if that fails, to prepare a defense.

Many injuries that do occur in the immediate perioperative period are extremely difficult to defend successfully. Injuries resulting from RSIs, wrong-site surgery, wrong-patient surgery, wrong-side surgery, fires and other burns, and intraoperative PIs are all subject to a legal doctrine, in Latin called *res ipsa loquitur* ("the thing speaks for itself"), because these injuries ordinarily do not occur in the absence of some form of negligence. This means that unless the defense can prove there was no negligence (proving a negative is always difficult, if not impossible), the injured party will prevail. Even in potential *res ipsa loquitur* cases, patients who feel they have been treated with respect and dignity may be likely to accept less than perfect results, may be less inclined to litigate, and may be more likely to cooperate with postinjury treatment, regardless of fault.

Privacy

A patchwork of state statutes attempts to protect confidentiality, to ensure patients' access to their healthcare records, and to preserve healthcare data privacy. Simultaneously, federal law provides that patients must consent for their health information to be used for other than treatment, payment, or business purposes. HIPAA imposes privacy and security rules that limit use or disclosure of protected health information. Legal action for privacy infringement can be brought against the individual producing the infringement all the way up through corporate dissemination (Rosin, 2016). Healthcare facilities accordingly must have administrative procedures to protect the privacy and confidentiality of all patient information. Facility policies should include protocols specific to perioperative settings, such as those governing or limiting the presence of healthcare industry representatives or other visitors in the OR. These policies must include provisions requiring patient consent.

Another federal statute, the Patient Safety and Quality Improvement Act (PSQIA), established a voluntary medical error reporting system to enhance the data available to assess and resolve patient safety and quality issues. To encourage reporting and analysis of medical errors, PSQIA created federal confidentiality protections for patient safety information. That law also sets forth an exception to HIPAA rules requiring patients' consent to disclose information about an error that occurred in the course of their treatment. Many states also have mandatory medical error reporting systems that likewise make exceptions to their confidentiality rules.

Perioperative nurses ethically must protect patient privacy even if HIPAA, state laws, or facility protocols do not specifically address a privacy issue. Team members exercise care to protect patients' bodies from more exposure than is required by a procedure. Likewise, comments made in or out of patient care areas about patient appearance, lifestyle, or social status, for example, are never appropriate unless required for safe care of that patient.

Privacy and Social Media

Widespread use of social media has raised a new challenge for patient privacy protection. Use of social media provides many benefits, including patient access to their records and facilitating patient partnerships in their care and shared decision making. However, confidentiality pitfalls are rife. Inappropriate discussions of patient information in elevators, in cafeterias, or in social settings after work can now wind up being "overheard" worldwide. In that light, all healthcare professionals, employees, and facilities themselves must recognize that they have a heightened obligation to protect patient privacy by avoiding such inappropriate discussions entirely and absolutely. A general rule for all staff who work in healthcare settings is to not use any of their private devices for anything related to work or patient relationship postings. If use of private devices is absolutely necessary, the facility should install encryption and the strongest possible antivirus protection on each. Box 2.6 presents some social media myths and recommendations for safe use.

Nurses must precisely follow the facility policy and procedures related to electronic communication. Care providers cannot be expected to know everything the IT director, compliance officer, security officers, risk managers, attorneys, and so forth, know about

---

BOX 2.6

Social Media Myths and Recommendations for Use

Common myths about social media:
- A post or communication is accessible only by the intended recipient.
- Once a post is deleted it is no longer accessible.
- Posting private information is okay as long as the patient is otherwise unidentified.
- Setting privacy settings is sufficient to ensure privacy.

How to avoid problems:
- Remember that legal and ethical obligations to protect privacy and confidentiality apply at all times and places, not just to care settings and care hours.
- Do not post any patient image or any other information that might degrade or embarrass a patient, even if otherwise unidentified.
- Do not disclose any information gained within the nurse–patient relationship unless there is a patient-related need to disclose.
- Do not take photos or videos of patients on personal devices. Follow facility policy for taking same on facility-provided devices.
- Follow facility policies precisely for work-related postings and use of personal and facility computers, cameras, and other electronic devices in the workplace.

Modified from National Council of State Boards of Nursing (NCSBN): *White paper: a nurse's guide to the use of social media* (website), 2011. www.ncsbn.org/Social_Media.pdf. (Accessed 10 January 2017).

---

patient privacy requirements in this electronic age, but nurses and all staff can and must know and follow the policies and procedures promulgated by safety committees that include these team members. A refinement of HIPAA was passed in 2009 called the Health Information Technology for Economic and Clinical Health Act (HITECH). Later, HIPAA was given stronger enforcement power with the passage of the Omnibus Act of 2013. This act required that facilities proactively conduct risk assessments and develop policies and procedures to train all staff about privacy challenges. Students, unlicensed and licensed healthcare workers, and retired healthcare workers uniformly have a continuing duty to observe and protect patient privacy rights under HIPAA and HITECH. The consequences of violating patient privacy rights via inappropriate use of social media may result in both employer and employee licensure disciplinary actions, possibly including termination of employment, suspension and revocation of license, fines, and other serious penalties.

Photography of even unidentified patients poses a special case. The finite issue regarding the need for patient consent to use a photograph revolves around recognition of the patient's identity (Harting et al., 2015). Identity may be established by the patient's face, obviously, but also other features such as jewelry, tattoos, scars, or venue. Identity can also be established by type of injury and facility location.

In addition to violating federal and state patient privacy laws, posting anonymous patient photographs on social media can also violate another federal statute, the Video Voyeurism Prevention Act of 2004. This Act provides criminal penalties: whoever photographs, films, or records (by any means), and disseminates an image of a private area of an individual who has a reasonable expectation of privacy without the individual's consent shall be fined or imprisoned up to 1 year or both.

As noted previously, every healthcare facility must have a social media use policy, and those policies must include photography. Several professional associations also have developed or are developing such a policy. In addition to legal and ethical considerations, inappropriate postings can harm the reputation of the facility and the student/professional posting them as well as jeopardize future graduate program admission and employment prospects.

Despite such caveats, nurses can use social media when done knowledgeably. Steele and colleagues (2015) urged surgeons to embrace the use of social media to stay in meaningful and timely contact with their patients and other healthcare providers.

Patient Autonomy

Courts in the United States have long recognized that every adult has the right to determine what happens to his or her body (*Schloendorff v. Society of New York Hospitals*, 105 N.E.92 [N.Y., 1914]). This legal right is also an ethical right recognized under the principle of respect for persons as autonomous beings. In perioperative settings, these rights enjoy protections via the informed consent process for the procedure itself and/or for any research interventions along with patient wishes expressed in advance directives for healthcare.

Informed Consent

Courts continue to affirm the patient's right to informed consent in cases involving physical injury. Usually, the informed consent case involves a physical injury caused by other lapses in the safety system, but both aspects of such cases are equally important in the respectful treatment of patients. Except in emergencies, surgical procedures should not be performed without documentation of the patient's consent in the medical record. How to document this informed consent should be described in facility policy. Documentation is typically accomplished by means of a signed consent form and/or the primary surgeon's entry into the progress notes, which may or may not also be signed by the patient. The surgeon or provider performing the procedure is legally responsible to inform the patient about the proposed operation or other invasive procedure and its inherent risks, benefits, alternatives, and complications before obtaining the patient's oral and documented consent. Although this seems straightforward, whether the patient should be told what a reasonable surgeon would tell the patient, or what a reasonable patient should know, or what this patient should know remains unclear.

Increasingly, states are adopting a "reasonable patient" standard as a better reflection of involvement in decision making. The patient must receive this information in terms that he or she can understand. To meet health literacy needs, consent materials should be written at a fifth-grade or lower reading level, subjected to readability tests, designed with bullet points to divide complex material, and translated into the patient's preferred language whenever possible.

The patient also must be informed about who will perform the procedure and when practitioners other than the primary surgeon will perform important parts of the procedure, even when under the primary surgeon's supervision. Nurses with concerns about the adequacy of the patient's understanding should report their concerns to the operating surgeon, or to the anesthesia provider if the concerns involve the anesthesia consent.

Combine these uncertainties about informed consent generally and how it applies to surgical procedures specifically and the need for a facility-wide policy generated by a committee of all relevant disciplines, and the challenge, if not the details, is clear. The good news for most nurses is that the person who performs the procedure, the surgeon, is responsible for informing the patient and obtaining the consent, and not the perioperative nurse. Nurses ensure that consent has been obtained via documentation in the patient's record.

Consent documentation must be complete before administration of preoperative medications. On the patient's arrival in the OR, the circulating nurse and anesthesia provider are responsible to verify that consent documentation is in the chart and is correct, properly signed and dated, and witnessed before administration of anesthesia. Traditionally, consent documentation encompasses at least the following:

- The patient's name (and legal guardian, if applicable)
- Name of the facility in which the procedure is being performed
- Specific name of the surgical procedure (or when multiple procedures are being done, the names of those procedures) in terms the patient understands
- Site/side of the planned procedure
- Name of the practitioner(s) performing the procedure or important aspects of it
- Risks of the procedure
- Alternative procedures, treatments, or therapies
- Signature of the patient (or legal guardian, if applicable)
- Date and time consent is obtained
- Statement that the procedure was explained to the patient (or legal guardian or both if applicable)
- Name and signature of the person who explained the procedure, usually the primary surgeon or physician performing the procedure
- Signature of person witnessing the consent

Nurses who are involved as witnesses to the signing of the consent form attest only to the validity of the patient signature, time, and date, and not to the adequacy of the patient's understanding because that assurance remains the duty of the surgeon or other credentialed professional performing the procedure.

Advance Directives and Do Not Resuscitate Orders

Many of the 50 states have statutes to allow patients to make their wishes regarding their future known in a legally recognized fashion if they were unable to do so when a life-threatening situation arose. Then, in the wake of the first US Supreme Court case to deal with the issue (*Cruzan v. Director, Missouri Department of Health,* 497 U.S. 261 [1990]) Congress passed the Patient Self-Determination Act (PSDA) in 1991. The PSDA extended self-determination protection to all US citizens and residents. Patients have the legal right to accept or refuse medical treatment, including resuscitation, even if refusal will likely result in death. This law also provides that all patients admitted to Medicare and Medicaid recipient providers must be asked whether they have executed, or wish to be given information about, such an advance healthcare directive, and that information must be included in the patient's healthcare record. If a patient arrives in a preoperative area with such a directive, the perioperative nurse should immediately clarify with the surgeon and/or anesthesia provider if there has been a discussion with the patient as to the effect the directive should have in the OR. The law does not address this issue, but an automatic suspension or continuation of advance directives or do not resuscitate (DNR) orders is not justified under either legal or ethical analysis. Facility policy should describe a perioperative protocol that preserves the patient's right to legal and ethical self-determination.

Veracity and Fidelity

These are ethical principles that underlie the respect for persons and autonomy. Veracity includes providing accurate information. Fidelity (or loyalty) carries with it an implicit promise of truth-telling and promise keeping. Both principles relate to the respect for patients and their autonomy (that patients are entitled to full and accurate information and disclosure); both principles are likewise inherent in trust, which also is foundational for patient safety. Within the patient safety and risk management context, veracity and fidelity demand transparency in disclosure of adverse events to the patient/family.

Transparency and disclosure after an error has occurred can minimize the consequences of litigation. Articles encouraging full disclosure often do so more as a risk management issue than as an issue concerning patient rights. One consequence of the renewed emphasis on patient safety and patient rights has been to merge the heretofore separate systems of perioperative care provision, risk management, and quality improvement under a patient safety rubric that enhances the effectiveness of each. Despite these findings, the implementation of transparency regarding medical errors has proven elusive.

In 2016 Elway and colleagues surveyed and completed an observational study of surgeons (Elway et al., 2016). Those who were less likely to follow nationally recommended elements of disclosure noted they were more likely to report being negatively affected by the adverse event. They found that while open disclosure programs are being implemented nationwide, without training on disclosing adverse events using specific communication elements, surgeons may experience negative effects when disclosing such information.

The AHRQ (2016a, 2016b) released a process and tool kit called the Communication and Optimal Resolution (CANDOR) process. It claims that CANDOR is a process that healthcare institutions and practitioners can use to respond in a timely, thorough, and just way when unexpected events cause patient harm. Key learning points for hospitals implementing the CANDOR process in their institutions include how to engage patients and families in disclosure communication following adverse events and a program for providers involved in adverse events. Boothman (2016) editorialized that unintended adverse outcomes can happen even with the best of care; treating patients only as a financial threat leaves them feeling abandoned. He supported the AHRQ CANDOR program's tool kit. He explained that CANDOR is a "deliberate strategy intent on normalizing honesty, transparency, and accountability" (p. 2488) and asserted that healthcare organization leaders insist that clinicians, not lawyers and risk managers, provide honest and transparent responses to patients harmed in their organization. He said this was important not just because it is a moral and ethical imperative, but because honesty serves a true culture of safety that is indispensable to the organization's core mission. Boothman did not use the words "honesty" or "fidelity" but they underlie the more operationally explained need for these principles in patient care.

Key Points

- Management of patient safety and prevention of injury risks is a collective responsibility of the entire perioperative care team.
- Major government, regulatory, and accrediting agencies, and associations address key elements of patient safety. Compliance officers can serve as an excellent resource in patient safety endeavors.
- AORN guidelines are the best source for evidence-based information specific to safe perioperative nursing practices.
- Meaningful communication and a commitment to teamwork, trust, and respect are characteristic in workplace cultures that emphasize patient safety.
- Enhanced communication initiatives such as safer surgery briefings, clinical perioperative records (written or digital), and handoffs are foundational to ensure a safer patient experience and care transitions between providers and units responsible for perioperative patient care.
- Communication for safety in perioperative settings includes a wide array of protocols, checklists, and topics (such as the time-out, counts, surgical specimens, electrical and chemical safety, and proper positioning) to prevent patient harm.
- Protection of a patient's personal, ethical, and legal rights underlie patient safety, compliance, and risk management in perioperative care settings.

Critical Thinking Questions

At 1600, Nurse Steve tweeted: awful day. fat guy fell off table. busted shoulder. MD blames me! Strap on!!!! pooled prep. 2d degree burns! allergic to I !!!!!! Camouflaged d/t drape fire.

Earlier that day:

Mike Jones, a 56-year-old construction worker enters the OR for removal of a suspicious mass of his left upper scapular area under monitored anesthesia care. His history and physical examination review reveals a 40-year history for smoking, chronic obstructive pulmonary disease (COPD), and hypertension. His height is 70 inches and his weight 120 kg.

Mr. Jones was not yet sedated and able to move himself onto the OR bed and lay supine. He is attended by Carole, the anesthesia provider. When the surgeon came in, Carole says, "I note you suggested prone; I'd rather do this right lateral—OK with you?" The surgeon responded, "Sure, whatever," and left to scrub.

Steve, the circulating nurse, gathers the pillows and axillary roll, then stands by Jones's side and loosens the safety strap. Carole, the anesthesia provider, tells Mr. Jones to lie on his right side and bend his knees up until comfortable. She positions his right arm extended on an armboard. Steve places the axillary roll, a pillow between Jones's legs and under left elbow, and reattaches the safety strap across Jones's upper thighs. He looks at Carole to say, "OK?" "Yup, thanks" was the response. Steve then proceeds with the prep; there was a little pooling of the iodine-based solution, but because the procedure was so short and the surgeon was already gowning and gloving and ready to drape, Steve just left it. After draping finished, Steve helped the scrub move the Mayo stand and back table to the left of the surgeon and the incision site as Carole adjusted the oxygen mask on the patient's face and announced she was now injecting the fentanyl and midazolam (Versed). Steve rolled the ESU unit next to the back table and reminded everyone to avoid ESU use when the patient was receiving enriched oxygen. He then called the time-out and read the checklist. All checked out, except Steve's heart sank when Carole answered "Iodine" to the allergies question. But everything was ready for the local injection and it was a short case.

Steve returned to his computer, facing the wall, to document. He glanced over to check for incision time and as he did so he heard a thump. He immediately checked the field and saw Mr. Jones's legs sliding down the other side of the table. He said, "What?" and ran to the patient's side. Carole had been turned away from the patient documenting her sedatives and drawing up a sustaining dose. The surgeon and scrub tech were looking at each other at the Mayo stand, discussing whether the deeper incision required a 10 or 15 blade. Everyone's attention immediately turned to Jones. First they assessed breathing, then alignment, and an orthopedic surgeon came from the next room to assess Jones's shoulder. Then the incision site and a second-degree skin burn was noted. A team was called to safely get the patient back on the OR bed. His shoulder was x-rayed; he was repositioned, reprepped, and the surgery proceeded.

Mr. Jones required extra sedative but was still hyperventilating. Carole began bagging with enriched O_2 under the drape so as not to interfere with the sterile field. The mass involved more bleeding than anticipated. The surgeon requested the ESU. In the confusion of the fall everyone forgot the time-out warning to avoid ESU use when the patient was receiving enriched oxygen. The surgeon activated the ESU tip and ignited a flame flashback from under the drape.

1. Could this fall have been prevented?
   - If not, why not?
   - If yes, by whom?
   - If yes, by doing what?
2. Could these burns have been prevented?
   - By whom?
   - Doing what?
3. What did the team do correctly immediately after the fall?
4. Was lateral really the indicated position for this patient?
5. What should Steve have done differently throughout Mr. Jones's perioperative care and why? Are there ethical and privacy issues that should be addressed with Steve?

evolve *The answers to the Critical Thinking Questions can be found at http://evolve.elsevier.com/Rothrock/Alexander.*

References

Agency for Healthcare Research and Quality (AHRQ): *Communication and optimal resolution (CANDOR) toolkit: patient safety tools and training materials* (website), 2016a. www.ahrq.gov/professionals/quality-patient-safety/patient-safety-resources/resources/candor/introduction.html. (Accessed 8 January 2017).

Agency for Healthcare Research and Quality (AHRQ): *TeamSTEPPS® 2.0* (website), 2016b. www.ahrq.gov/teamstepps/instructor/index.html. (Accessed 8 January 2017).

Akhtar N et al: Airway fires during surgery: management and prevention, *J Anaesthesiol Clin Pharmacol* 32(1):109–111, 2016.

Alemzadeh H et al: Adverse events in robotic surgery: a retrospective study of 14 years of FDA data, *PLoS ONE* 11(4):e0151470, 2016.

Alexander EL: *Operating room technique*, St Louis, 1943, CV Mosby.

Algie CM et al: Interventions for reducing wrong-site surgery and invasive clinical procedures, *Cochrane Database Syst Rev* (3):CD009404, 2015.

American College of Emergency Physicians (ACEP): *Health care-acquired & provider preventable conditions FAQ* (website), 2016. www.acep.org/Clinical---Practice-Management/Health-Care-Acquired---Provider-Preventable-Conditions-FAQ/. (Accessed 8 January 2017).

American College of Healthcare Executives: *Position description: chief compliance officer* (website), 2016. www.ache.org/newclub/career/comploff.cfm. (Accessed 9 January 2017).

American Society for Healthcare Risk Management (ASHRM): *Overview of the healthcare risk management profession* (website), 2016. www.ashrm.org/resources/hrm-week/pdfs/HRM-Week-Overview.pdf. (Accessed 9 January 2017).

Association of periOperative Registered Nurses (AORN): *Guidelines for perioperative practice*, Denver, 2017, The Association.

Austin JM, Pronovost PJ: Never events and the quest to reduce preventable harm, *Jt Comm J Qual Patient Saf* 41(6):279–288, 2015.

Berry W et al: The surgical checklist: it cannot work if you do not use it, *JAMA Surg* 151(7):647, 2016.

Bixenstine PJ et al: Developing and pilot testing practical measures of preanalytic surgical specimen identification defects, *Am J Med Qual* 28(4):308–314, 2013.

Boat AC, Spaeth JP: Handoff checklists improve the reliability of patient handoffs in the operating room and postanesthesia care unit, *Pediatric Anesthesia* 23(7):647–654, 2013.

Boothman RC: CANDOR: the antidote to deny and defend?" (Editorial) *Health Serv Manage* 51(S3):2487–2490, 2016.

Brennan T et al: Incidence of adverse events and negligence in hospitalized patients: results of the Harvard Medical Practice Study I, *N Engl J Med* 324(6):370–376, 1991.

Brent MAZ: OR specimen labeling, *AORN J* 103(2):164–176, 2015.

Caruso TJ et al: Implementation of a standardized post anesthesia care handoff increases information transfer without increasing handoff duration, *Jt Comm Qual Patient Saf* 41(1):35–42, 2015.

Centers for Medicare and Medicaid Services (CMS): *Stage 2 overview tipsheet* (website), 2012. www.cms.gov/Regulations-and-Guidance/Legislation/EHRIncentivePrograms/Downloads/Stage2Overview_Tipsheet.pdf. (Accessed 11 January 2017).

Clarke CN et al: *Implementation of a standardized electronic tool improves compliance, accuracy, and efficiency of trainee-to-trainee patient care handoffs after complex general surgical oncology procedures.* Presented at the 11th Annual Academic Surgical Congress in Jacksonville, FL, February 2–4, 2016. www.sciencedirect.com/science/article/pii/S0039606016304925. (Accessed 9 January 2017).

Cochran GL et al: Comparison of medication safety systems in critical access hospitals: combined analysis of two studies, *Am J Health Syst Pharm* 73(15):1167–1173, 2016.

Cruzan v. Director, *Missouri Department of Health*, 497 U.S. 261 (1990).

Dixon JL et al: Enhancing surgical safety using digital multimedia technology, *Am J Surg* 211(6):1095–1098, 2016.

ECRI Institute: *2017 top 10 hospital C-suite watch list* (website), 2017a. www.ecri.org/Resources/Whitepapers_and_reports/2017_Top_10_Hospital_C-Suite_Watch_List.pdf. (Accessed 9 January 2017).

ECRI Institute: *Executive brief: top 10 health technology hazards for 2017* (website), 2016. www.ecri.org/Resources/Whitepapers_and_reports/Haz17.pdf. (Accessed 9 January 2017).

ECRI Institute: *ECRI Institute preps hospital leaders on top 10 technology issues to watch in 2017* (website), 2017b. https://www.ecri.org/press/Pages/ECRI-Institute-2017-Top-10-Hospital-C-suite-Watch-List.aspx. (Accessed 9 January 2017).

Elway A et al: Surgeons' disclosures of clinical adverse events, *JAMA Surg* 151(11):1015–1021, 2016.

Fencl JL: Guideline implementation: prevention of retained surgical items, *AORN J* 104(1):37–45, 2016.

Garrett JH: Effective perioperative communication to enhance patient care, *AORN J* 104(2):112–117, 2016.

Ghezzi TL, Corleta OC: 30 years of robotic surgery, *World J Surg* 40(10):2550–2557, 2016.

Gitelis M et al: Increasing compliance with the World Health Organization surgical safety checklist—a regional health system's experience, *Am J Surg* 214(1):7–13, 2017.

Glass LK, Murphy EK: *AORN emergence and growth*, Denver, 2002, The Association.

Harting MT et al: Medical photography: current technology, evolving issues and legal perspectives, *Int J Clin Pract* 69(40):401–409, 2015.

Hey LA, Turner TC: Using standardized OR checklists and creating extended time-out checklists, *AORN J* 104(3):248–252, 2016.

Institute for Safe Medication Practices (ISMP): *Side tracks on the safety express. Interruptions lead to errors and unfinished… wait, what was I doing?* (website), 2012. www.ismp.org/newsletters/acutecare/showarticle.aspx?id=37. (Accessed 9 January 2017).

Institute of Medicine (IOM): *To err is human: building a safer health system*, Washington, DC, 1999, National Academy Press.

Johns Hopkins Medicine: *Johns Hopkins Malpractice Study: Surgical 'never events' occur at least 4,000 times per year* (website), 2012. www.hopkinsmedicine.org/news/media/releases/johns_hopkins_malpractice_study_surgical_never_events_occur_at_least_4000_times_per_year. (Accessed 9 January 2017).

Joint Commission Perspectives: Testing and maintaining hoses, dampers, doors, and other fire safety equipment, *Jt Comm Perspect* 36(6):13–15, 2016.

Kachelia A et al: Legal and policy interventions to improve patient safety, *Circulation* 133:661–671, 2016.

Lau CSM, Chamberlain RS: The World Health Organization surgical safety checklist improves post-operative outcomes: a meta-analysis and systematic review, *Surgi Sci* 7:206–217, 2016.

Leape L: Error in medicine, *JAMA* 272(23):1951–1957, 1994.

Leape LL et al: The nature of adverse events in hospitalized patients: results of the Harvard Medical Practice Study II, *N Engl J Med* 324(6):377–384, 1991.

Loftus T et al: Implementing a standardized safe surgery program reduces serious reportable events, *J Am Coll Surg* 220(1):12–17, e3, 2015.

Makar A et al: Never events in surgery, *Eur Urol* 68(6):919–920, 2015.

Makary MA, Daniel M: Medical error: the third leading cause of death in the U.S., *BMJ* 353:i21369, 2016.

Mayer EK et al: Surgical checklist implementation project: the impact of variable WHO checklist compliance on risk-adjusted clinical outcomes after national implementation: a longitudinal study, *Ann Surg* 263(1):58–63, 2016.

Nguyen NC, Moffat-Bruce SD: What's new in academic medicine? Retained surgical items: is 'zero incidence' achievable?, *Int J Acad Med* 2(1):1–4, 2016.

Park DA et al: Surgical and clinical safety and effectiveness of robot-assisted laparoscopic hysterectomy compared to conventional laparoscopy and laparotomy for cervical cancer: a systematic review and meta-analysis, *Eur J Surg Oncol* 43(6):994–1002, 2017.

Punke H: *Redefining patient safety in 2017—6 thoughts from IHI CEO Derek Feeley* (website), 2016. www.beckershospitalreview.com/quality/redefining-patient-safety-in-2017-6-thoughts-from-ihi-ceo-derek-feeley.html. (Accessed 9 January 2017).

Reason J: *Human error*, Cambridge, United Kingdom, 1990, Cambridge Press.

Redman DD: Reducing medication errors in the OR, *AORN J* 105(6):106–109, 2017.

Robinson NL: Promoting patient safety with perioperative hand-off communication, *J Perianesth Nurs* 31(3):245–253, 2016.

Rosin T: *Man sues CNN for airing images of him in hospital: 6 things to know* (website), 2016. www.beckershospitalreview.com/legal-regulatory-issues/man-sues-cnn-for-airing-images-of-him-in-hospital-6-things-to-know.html. (Accessed 9 January 2017).

Russ S et al: Measuring variation in use of the WHO surgical safety checklist in the operating room: a multi-center, prospective cross-sectional study, *J Am Coll Surg* 220(1):1–11, 2016.

Salzwedel C et al: The effect of a checklist on the quality of patient handover from the operating room to the intensive care unit: a randomized controlled trial, *J Crit Care* 32:170–174, 2015.

Schoenfeld AJ, Wachter RM: The search for better patient handoff tools, *JAMA Intern Med* 176(9):1402–1403, 2016.

Singer S et al: Relationship between operating room teamwork, contextual factors, and safety checklist performance, *J Am Coll Surg* 223(4):568–580, 2016.

Smith AA: *The operating room: a primer for pupil nurses*, ed 2, Philadelphia, 1924, Saunders.

Smith ML, Raab S: Quality assurance and regulations for anatomic pathology. In Cheng L, Bostwick D, editors: *Essentials of anatomic pathology*, ed 3, New York, 2016, Springer.

Spruce L: Back to basics: preventing perioperative pressure injuries, *AORN J* 105(1):92–99, 2017.

Spruce L: Back to basics: preventing surgical fires, *AORN J* 104(3):218–221, 2016.

Steele SR et al: Social media is a necessary component of surgery practice, *Surgery* 158(3):857–862, 2015.

Steelman VM et al: The hidden costs of reconciling surgical sponge counts, *AORN J* 102(5):98–506, 2015.

Stefanitis H et al: KINFix—a formalin-free non-commercial fixative optimized for histological, immunohistochemical and molecular analyses of neurosurgical tissue specimens, *Clin Neuropathol* 35(1):3–12, 2016.

The Joint Commission (TJC): *Advancing effective communication, cultural competence, and patient-and family-centered care: a roadmap for hospitals* (website), 2014. www.jointcommission.org/roadmap_for_hospitals/. (Accessed 9 January 2017).

The Joint Commission (TJC): *Summary data of sentinel events reviewed by The Joint Commission* (website), 2016. www.jointcommission.org/assets/1/18/Summary_2Q_2016.pdf. (Accessed 11 January 2017).

The Joint Commission (TJC): *2017 hospital national patient safety goals* (website), 2017. www.jointcommission.org/assets/1/6/2016_NPSG_HAP.pdf. (Accessed 9 January 2017).

Treadwell J et al: Surgical checklists: a systematic review of impacts and implementation, *BMJ Qual Saf* 23(4):299–318, 2014.

Truitt E et al: Effect of the implementation of barcode technology and an electronic medication administration record on adverse drug events, *Hosp Pharm* 51(6):474–483, 2016.

Tscholl DW et al: An anesthesia preinduction checklist to improve information exchange, knowledge of critical information, perception of safety, and possibly perception of teamwork in anesthesia teams, *Anesth Analg* 121(4):948–956, 2015.

World Health Organization (WHO): *WHO guidelines on hand hygiene in healthcare* (website), 2009. http://whqlibdoc.who.int/publications/2009/9789241597906_eng.pdf. (Accessed 10 January 2017).

CHAPTER 3

Workplace Issues and Staff Safety

CHRISTINE E. SMITH

The perioperative care environment is designed to save lives, cure disease, reconstruct deformity, and manage pain, while supporting safe patient care, workplace safety, and security. Advances in surgical science and technology bring high complexity to once basic procedures. Financial pressures drive challenging measures and reductions to save time and money and comply with increasing requirements in regulatory standards. Work hazards challenge the safety of the nursing workforce (Phillips and Miltner, 2015). Hospitals are facing an increasing number of patients of size (AORN, 2014a) and are installing bariatric and architectural retrofittings and renovations for those patients with high body mass indexes (Kumpar, 2014). The more mobility-dependent the patient is, the greater the risk is for injury for those providing care. Although bariatric patients account for less than 10% of the patient census in acute care facilities, they accounted for 29.8% of staff-reported injuries (Kumpar, 2014). Staff safety is a concern as musculoskeletal disorders (MSDs), slips, trips, and falls (STFs) are a major source of workplace injuries (Fitzpatrick, 2014; Rice, 2014). Evidence exists to guide best practices to design a safer work environment and develop better patterns for nursing work (Phillips and Miltner, 2015). Many organizations, including the National Patient Safety Foundation, believe worker safety should be included as a component of patient safety (Simon and Canacari, 2017).

Factors that affect a worker's safety climate include leadership and management commitment to safety, healthcare worker involvement in safety decisions, implementation of measures to reduce safety hazards in the work environment (Press Ganey, 2016), opportunity for feedback on safety improvements, and individual accountability (Research Highlight).

Operating room (OR) staff regularly face low-level but repeated exposure to numerous hazardous materials, including residues from medications, anesthetic gases, sterilization chemicals, radiation, latex, cleaning chemicals, and disinfecting agents. They also risk injuries from sharps and exposure to bloodborne pathogens (BBPs), surgical smoke, fatigue, noise, incivility, bullying, and workplace violence. Risks specific to the perioperative environment are biologic, ergonomic, chemical, physical, psychosocial, and cultural.

If the goals of healthcare are to reduce the burden of illness, injury, and disability and to improve the health and functioning of patients, then unsafe working environments must be corrected to achieve these goals. Perioperative nurses play a critical role in making the workplace environment safer. Many elements of perioperative

RESEARCH HIGHLIGHT ▮▮

The Role of Workplace Safety and Surveillance Capacity in Driving Nurse and Patient Outcomes

The nurse work environment is complex and multidimensional with various processes, traits, and cultures that influence performance outcomes. Key insights of strategic significance from this 2016 Nursing Special Report highlight the importance of creating a work environment in which nurses believe their physical and emotional safety is an organizational priority. Researchers collected data from Press Ganey's NDNQI and data on the patient experience from the CMS (released July 2016). They examined associations between patient, nurse, patient experience, and payment outcomes plus predictors of RN perception of workplace safety and RN surveillance capacity composite. The concept of nurse safety covers factors and practices designed to minimize the risk of physical or psychologic injury in the workplace. *The RN safety composite* is a measure of specific practices such as safe patient handling, RN-to-RN interaction, appropriate patient care assignments, shift duration, and meal-break practices. *Nurse surveillance capacity* is a measure of multiple variables in the practice environment that reflect nurses' autonomy to observe, monitor, collect, interpret,

and formulate patient data to make relevant patient care decisions. Surveillance composite may also include specific RN characteristics such as clinical competence, years of experience, education, and certification.

Analysis of the data, when compared with hospitals in the lower quartile of perceived workplace safety, showed that hospitals in the higher quartile had a

- 52% lower rate of RN-perceived missed care (patient falls, pressure injuries)
- 27% higher RN job enjoyment, intent-to-stay, and nurse-perceived quality of care scores
- 22% higher CMS Overall Hospital Quality Star Rating
- 3% higher average "likelihood to recommend" scores

The safety of the work environment plays a key role in how nurses perceive their jobs, their ability to care for their patients, and their intent to stay. Improving environmental factors that drive and enable nurse safety and surveillance can sustain and support nursing practice excellence.

CMS, Centers for Medicare and Medicaid Services; *NDNQI,* National Database of Nursing Quality Indicators; *RN,* registered nurse.
Modified from Press Ganey: *2016 nursing special report the role of the workplace safety and surveillance capacity in driving nurse and patient outcomes* (website). www.pressganey.com/about/news/2016-nursing-special-report. (Accessed 24 February 2017).

patient safety are parallel with those of workplace safety. A healthy and positive perioperative work environment promotes safe patient care and optimal patient outcomes while creating a desirable workplace (AORN, 2015). This chapter addresses potential risks and challenges of the perioperative workplace and reviews practice guidelines aimed at workplace safety.

Ergonomics

Perioperative staff routinely face a wide array of occupational hazards that place them at risk for work-related MSDs (also called "ergonomic" or "overexertion" injuries), which is a frequent and costly occupational issue in nursing (Stokowski, 2014). More than any other work-related injury or illness, MSDs, repetitive motion injuries, STFs, and fatigue are responsible for the most lost time from work, the need for protracted medical care, and permanent disability among healthcare workers (Phillips and Miltner, 2015). Nurses are known to be at risk for work-related injuries, and many nurses accept musculoskeletal pain as part of their job. The extent of MSDs among nurses should be no surprise, given that nurses lift and turn patients and move heavy equipment every day, often relying on time-honored, but outmoded, body mechanics practices.

The high incidence of MSDs among nurses is the cumulative effect of repeated patient handling events, often involving unsafe loads. OR staff often lift, transfer, or reposition patients on OR beds and transport vehicles, and assist with prepping with arms outstretched or bodies bent forward in awkward postures and positions. Several factors influence the level of ergonomic risk, including patient weight, transfer distance, extent of the workspace, instrument temperature, unpredictable patient behavior, and awkward positions such as stooping, bending, and reaching.

Attention to proper ergonomics when using computers or workstations is important to ensure correct posture to avoid repetitive motion and straining injuries (Box 3.1). Working in the same posture or sitting still for prolonged periods is unhealthy. Working positions should change periodically by making small readjustments to your chair or backrest, stretch fingers, hands, arms, torso, and periodically walk around for a few minutes (OSHA, 2017).

Work activities in perioperative settings present an unavoidable constant—moving; sliding; pushing; and carrying and lifting patients, patient care equipment, and instrumentation. Staff risks injury from sustained standing on hard floors, step stools, and platforms while holding instruments and equipment. An ergonomically healthier

workplace can decrease or prevent injury and support a culture of safety.

Safe Patient Handling and Movement

Collaborative efforts to address workplace safety for perioperative staff have been under way for years. As early as 2005, the American Nurses Association (ANA) partnered with the Association of peri-Operative Registered Nurses (AORN), the National Institute for Occupational Safety and Health (NIOSH), and the James A. Haley Veterans Administration Medical Center (VAMC) in Tampa, Florida, to form the Workplace Safety Task Force. Its aim was to prepare a safe patient handling "algorithm" guidance document to support ergonomically healthy workplaces (ANA, 2013; VAMC, 2016). The task force began by identifying high-risk tasks specific to perioperative nurses that specific ergonomic tools could address. These tasks included transferring patients on and off OR beds, repositioning patients on the OR bed, lifting and holding patients' extremities, standing for long periods, holding retractors for long periods, lifting and moving equipment, and sustaining awkward positions. Using current ergonomic safety concepts, scientific evidence, and technology, such as safe patient handling equipment, the task force developed seven ergonomic tools, or *algorithms,* to guide workplace safety and movement in the perioperative setting. These clinical tools are incorporated in AORN's Safe Patient Handling Tool Kit (AORN, 2012).

The Nurse and Health Care Worker Protection Act of 2015 was a bill before Congress to require the Department of Labor to establish a standard on safe patient handling, mobility, and injury prevention to prevent MSDs for healthcare staff. This standard would require the use of engineering and safety controls to handle patients. The standard would also require healthcare employers to (1) develop and implement a safe patient handling, mobility, and injury prevention program; (2) train workers on safe patient handling, mobility, and injury prevention; and (3) post a notice that explains the standard, procedures to report patient handling-related injuries, and workers' rights under this Act. Labor would have to conduct unscheduled inspections to ensure compliance with the standard (the bill remains in Congress awaiting passing approval) (US Congress, 2015).

An algorithm is a set of rules for solving a problem in a finite number of discrete steps. In this case the algorithm is an ergonomic tool designed to guide decision-making in performing various healthcare tasks (AORN, 2012). The tool directs the worker through a series of questions (diamond boxes in Fig. 3.1) and provides optimal responses for action—specifically, whether assistive equipment should be used, what type of equipment would best support the task, and how many caregivers are needed to perform the task safely. Algorithms are designed to standardize practice based on research and task analysis, rather than allowing each caregiver to rely solely on his or her own training and experience to make decisions.

The ergonomic tools discussed in the following section are designed in the context of an assessment and plan of care for each patient to communicate decisions about safe patient handling practices among all staff likely to participate in these tasks.

Seven Ergonomic Tools for Safe Patient Handling and Movement

Ergonomic Tool #1: Lateral transfer from stretcher to and from the OR bed is shown in Fig. 3.1. Lifting and moving patients occur frequently in perioperative settings, with patients transferring to and from a transport vehicle and the OR bed. Many patients completely or partially depend on help with moving because of

---

BOX 3.1

Principles of the Ergonomic Workstation

- Top of monitor at or just below eye level
- Head and neck balanced and in line with torso
- Shoulders relaxed
- Elbows close to body and supported
- Lower back supported
- Wrists and hands in line with forearms
- Adequate room for keyboard and mouse
- Feet flat on floor or footrest

Modified from Occupational Safety and Health Administration (OSHA): *Computer workstations eTool: checklist* (website). www.osha.gov/SLTC/etools/computerworkstations/checklist.html. (Accessed 26 February 2017).

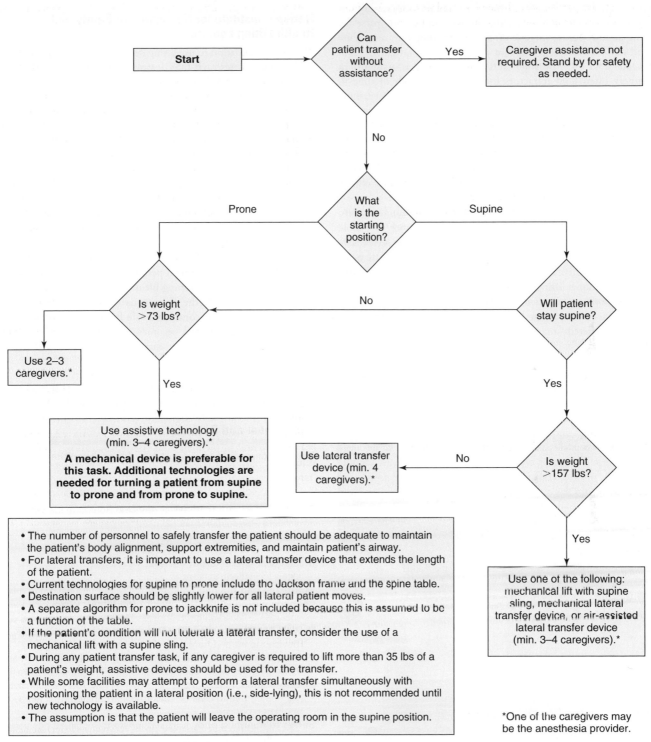

FIG. 3.1 Lateral transfer from stretcher to and from the OR bed.

sedation and/or anesthesia. Lifting and moving patients is a hazardous patient care activity (see Figs. 6.20 and 6.21 for examples of lateral transfer devices).

Ergonomic Tool #2: Positioning and repositioning the patient on the OR bed into and from the supine position. The surgical team often repositions patients once they are on the OR bed to provide appropriate exposure of the surgical site. They frequently lift and maneuver the patient while simultaneously placing a positioning

device. Ergonomic Tool #2 provides guidelines for repositioning the patient in a safe manner.

Ergonomic Tool #3: Lifting and holding legs, arms, and head for prepping in a perioperative setting. OR nurses often lift or hold patients' limbs during skin prep. Ergonomic Tool #3 is a table that provides calculations to determine whether it is safe for only one caregiver to lift the weight of various limbs and the safe length of time the limbs can be lifted.

Ergonomic Tool #4: Prolonged standing. This tool provides suggestions for relief for OR staff when they must stand in one place for long periods during surgery. Prolonged standing can cause acute and chronic back, leg, and foot pain, as well as fatigue.

Ergonomic Tool #5: Retraction. OR staff who act as assistants in surgery often hold retractors for sustained periods of time to expose the surgical site. This tool considers whether a self-retaining retractor can be used safely and, if not, how to determine an optimal working height and posture for the retracting staff member.

Ergonomic Tool #6: Lifting and carrying supplies and equipment. OR staff lift and carry many types of supplies, instrument trays, and equipment. This tool uses the NIOSH lifting index (LI: described later) to predict the risk for back pain from lifting specific objects in the OR.

Ergonomic Tool #7: Pushing, pulling, and moving equipment on wheels. This tool makes recommendations on the number of people required to safely push or pull equipment on wheels; it is especially useful for prescribing safe movement of facility and OR beds. The use of assistive devices is highly recommended for situations in which manual lifting puts the staff at substantial risk of injury.

The development of patient care ergonomics programs that include the use of assistive patient handling equipment and devices has essentially rendered "manual body mechanics" patient handling unnecessary and dangerous to both patient and staff (Stokowski, 2014). A growing selection of equipment and assistive devices have been designed for the variety of patient handling tasks performed by nurses. Box 3.2 lists patient handling devices. Fig. 3.2 illustrates a ceiling lift device in use in the OR.

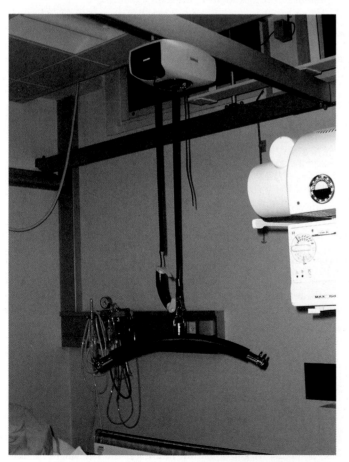

FIG. 3.2 Ceiling lift.

National Institute for Occupational Safety and Health Lifting Equation

The recommendation to use lifting devices for moving patients arises from a body of research that demonstrates that mechanical lifting equipment, as part of a program to promote safe patient handling, can significantly reduce MSDs among healthcare staff. By 1994, NIOSH had revised their 1981 lifting equation to calculate recommended weight limits (RWLs) for specified two-handed, manual lifting tasks (Waters et al., 1994). Although NIOSH did not originally recommend the equation for the lifting of humans, it has revised the equation and now recommends it for many patient lifting activities under certain conditions (e.g., when the patient can follow directions or when an estimate of the weight the staff must handle is possible). The revised NIOSH lifting equation (RNLE) provides a mathematical equation to determine the RWL and LI for selected two-handed manual lifting tasks. RWL is defined for a specific set of task conditions and represents the weight of the load that nearly all healthy staff can perform over a substantial period (e.g., up to 8 hours) without an increased risk of developing lifting-related low back pain.

The concept behind the lifting equation is to start with a recommended weight that is considered safe for an ideal lift and then to reduce the weight as the task becomes more stressful (e.g., the distance of the load from the worker increases, the duration of the task

---

BOX 3.2

Categories and Descriptions of Safe Patient Handling Equipment and Devices

Bed improvements to support transfer or repositioning: Beds that convert directly into chairs or are equipped with a shearless pivot that minimizes slipping toward the foot of the bed when the head is raised

Friction-reducing lateral-assist devices: Boards made with smooth, low-friction material used for patient transfer

Inflatable lateral-assist transfer devices: Flexible mattress inflated with air to create a cushioned layer for patient transfer

Mechanical lateral-assist devices: Height-adjustable stretchers used for patient transfer

Motorized bed moving equipment: Transferring patient in a bed

OR beds with documented weight load limit: Weight load also includes articulation limit

Powered full-body sling lifts: Portable or ceiling-mounted lift devices to lift and transfer highly dependent patients

Powered stand-assist and repositioning lifts: Lift with arm and/or back slings to assist patients with some weight-bearing ability

Sliding boards: Boards made of smooth, rigid, low-friction material for seated bed-to-chair or chair-to-toilet transfers that act as a supporting bridge

Slings to maintain body part suspension: Sustained position for prepping and procedural positioning

Stand-assist and repositioning aids: Secure devices, either free-standing or attached to beds, to help support patients to lift themselves

Transfer chairs: Chairs that convert into a stretcher, eliminating the transfer from a horizontal plane (bed or stretcher) to a seated position

Modified from Bliss M, Gruden M: *Beyond getting started: a resource guide for implementing a safe patient handling program in the acute care setting*, ed 3, 2014 (website). https://aohp.org/aohp/Portals/0/Documents/ToolsForYourWork/free_publications/Beyond%20Getting%20Started%20Safe%20Patient%20Handling%20-%20May%202014.pdf.pdf. (Accessed 23 February 2017).

increases, the type of handhold varies). Generally, the revised equation yields a recommended 35-pound maximum weight limit for use in patient handling tasks. When the weight to be lifted exceeds this limit, assistive devices should be used.

The formula produces an RWL that can be used to determine the LI. This LI may then be used to identify potentially hazardous lifting jobs or to compare the relative severity of two jobs to select the better and safer option. The equation has also been used to provide recommendations for lifting objects such as lead aprons, sterile packs, body positioning devices, and instrument pans or trays. Reliance on body mechanics is not a safe practice and cannot be relied on to prevent MSDs. Safe patient handling programs are more effective.

Slips, Trips, and Falls

Although STFs may occur in many places throughout a hospital or ambulatory surgery center, the OR is of special focus because it is an environment in which critical patient care occurs. An STF that disables a worker is expensive in terms of direct and indirect costs, but a disabling fall of an OR staff member may adversely affect a patient as well. A fall in the OR can cause direct patient injury, disrupt the surgical procedure, contribute to surgical errors, impair equipment, and delay the current surgery as well as other scheduled surgeries while other staff attend to or replace the injured staff member. STFs remain a leading cause of serious injury among healthcare workers and lost time from work.

Slips, Trips, and Falls: Causes and Prevention

STFs have the potential to be a major cause of injury. There is a common misconception that these injuries "just happen" and there is little that can be done to prevent them. STFs arise from many factors, including wet floors, uneven floor surfaces, low-profile equipment and cords, cluttered or poorly lit walkways, dimly lit ORs, and improper footwear. A comprehensive STF-prevention program can significantly reduce workers' compensation claims. To a large degree, STFs are preventable.

Wet Floors

STFs resulting from liquids (e.g., water; fluid; slippery, greasy, and slick spots) are a common cause of staff injury and compensation claims. Providing lids for all cups or other open containers being transported, for example, helps avoid spills. Using high absorptive mats and fluid-reclaiming suction devices for arthroscopy and other wet procedures reduces the potential hazard. Installing paper towel dispensers in high-spill areas, such as near scrub sinks, nursing stations, specimen preparation areas, and elevators promotes opportunities for staff to clean up spills easily and promptly.

Wet floors should be signaled by placing highly visible "Caution: Wet Floor" signs, preferably 4 feet tall and with flashing lights, in areas that have been recently mopped. Housekeeping staff should be equipped with technology to receive alerts to quickly respond to spill areas.

Liquids on an OR floor can make an otherwise slip-resistant surface hazardous. Using a dripless, brush-free gel solution for surgical hand scrubs minimizes water splashes. When used at the surgical site, gel-based skin preps are less likely to drip and run than liquid prep solutions. They are also less likely to pool under patients or to drip and pool on the floor or OR bed. High-absorbent mats can be used to temporarily cover a spill that occurs in an OR. Fluid solidifiers are composed of a granulated substance that can be sprinkled onto a spill or poured into a container with fluid. Fluid solidifiers absorb liquid and solidify the fluid into gel. Adding a fluid solidifier in a liquid medical-waste container or on a fluid spill on the floor serves to control fluid and to reduce the risk of STFs. Care must be taken to avoid spilling dry fluid solidifier powder on a dry floor surface because it is extremely slippery in its dry state. Effective containment also includes adequate waste containers for the planned procedure and readily available waste-control supplies, including absorptive products.

Uneven Floor Surfaces

Falls on the same level also occur at transition areas, such as from dry to wet, on uneven surfaces, or from one type of floor surface to another. Healthcare facilities must ensure that there are no uneven surfaces, including thresholds, on floors. In stairwells with potentially low visibility, the nosing on the top and bottom steps can be painted to provide visual cues.

Obstructed Pathways

Pathways must be kept clear, particularly of low-profile equipment and cords that can be overlooked easily in patients' rooms, hallways, ORs, or other care areas. Keeping pathways clear is difficult in the OR, where multiple cables and cords are used in surgical procedures. Newer ORs are equipped with articulated ceiling-mounted booms that help keep cords off the floor and systems that integrate cables into the OR bed. Cords and cables in older ORs should be routed so that they do not stretch across walking paths, and they should be secured by bundling, taping, or braiding. Routing and securing cords makes it easier to check that all necessary cords are properly connected and less likely that a patient will be injured or the procedure prolonged because someone trips on a cord.

Low-standing equipment and supplies are potential trip hazards. These include buckets, rolling stools or stepstools, support structures for equipment, and supply containers. OR staff often must navigate around intravenous (IV) tubing and poles. Consider marking mobile equipment such as stools with a bright color or a taped X to make them more visible and distinguishable from the floor. Even though protective and absorptive mats play a safety role, they too can pose a trip hazard. Slip-resistant absorptive mats should be used, and soiled absorptive mats should be removed because a mat that is oversaturated can swell and become a STF hazard.

Inadequate Lighting

Lighting throughout a healthcare facility must be adequate to visualize pathways, particularly stairways, when supplies or other items are being carried. Adequate lighting is of specific and critical importance in the OR. Advances in surgical technology, including minimally invasive surgery (MIS), have increased the use of light-emitting diode (LED) monitors in the OR. This requires dimming general room lighting while leaving the surgical site highly illuminated. Not only does this leave the rest of the OR dimly lit, but the high illumination on the surgical site makes adapting one's vision to the dimmer room lighting more difficult. Dimmer lighting tends to heighten the risks of not noticing STF hazards or fluids on the floor. High-quality monitors used during MIS have surface material that minimizes reflected light. Green filters on ambient lighting during MIS procedures minimize reflection of light off the monitors, provide some illumination for other perioperative team members, and reduce ocular fatigue.

Improper Footwear

Improper footwear increases the risk of STFs. Lessons can be learned from industries, such as food service and commercial fishing, where antislip footwear is standard. AORN suggests that shoes worn in the OR have closed toes and backs, low heels, nonskid soles, and meet Occupational Safety and Health Administration (OSHA) standards as well as the healthcare facility's safety requirements (AORN, 2017).

Programmatic Slips, Trips, and Falls Prevention and Reduction

Given the diverse age, job duties, and experience of perioperative staff, an STF program is critical to create a safe work environment. During program development, each healthcare facility should conduct a hazard vulnerability analysis to study its unique hazards so they can be appropriately addressed in a workplace safety program that includes targeted STFs.

A comprehensive prevention program can significantly reduce injuries. One key component of a successful STF prevention program is to educate staff about the importance of STF prevention and to encourage every employee to take personal responsibility for eliminating STF hazards. Whether this involves personally cleaning spills or cordoning off an area to alert fellow employees while waiting for housekeeping staff to arrive, a successful STF program requires that all staff share responsibility for prevention. Regularly scheduled environmental rounds that include a representative of each healthcare worker category is a valuable opportunity to inspect the unit for unsafe conditions, evaluate recent improvements, elicit recommendations from staff, and demonstrate that workplace safety is a critical component of the safety culture.

Sharps Safety and Bloodborne Pathogens

Scope and Significance of Problem

In the high-risk perioperative environment, staff routinely face exposure to BBPs and percutaneous injuries (PIs). Decades ago, a needlestick or sharps injury was the most feared workplace hazard in nursing. Over the past few decades, legislative and regulatory measures have been enacted (Daley, 2017). The Needlestick Safety and Prevention Act (NSPA) of 2000 increased protection to healthcare workers from human immunodeficiency virus (HIV), hepatitis B virus (HBV), hepatitis C virus (HCV), and other BBPs (Stokowski, 2014). This law mandated employers to introduce work practice controls and safe needle and sharps technologies to protect healthcare workers from BBP injuries.

Although HBV, HCV, and HIV are the BBPs most commonly transmitted during patient care, injuries from needles and other sharp devices used in healthcare and laboratory settings are associated with the transmission of many different pathogens. Exposure to BBPs occurs during all phases of perioperative care, although cuts or needlestick injuries are more likely during the intraoperative phase of patient care. Risk of a sharps injury increases during more invasive, longer procedures that result in higher blood loss. Fatigue resulting from working extended hours coupled with the fast pace of the perioperative environment may also contribute to increased risk of PIs (AORN, 2017). Other factors that may contribute to surgical PIs include frequent handling of sharp instruments and items, prolonged contact with open surgical sites, the presence of relatively large quantities of blood, unsafe needle handling techniques (e.g., using sharp rather than blunt needles), and failure to use a neutral zone for passing sharps between perioperative team members.

Although injuries from hollow-bore needles constitute the most common PIs in the healthcare field overall, the pattern of injuries inside the OR is somewhat different. Suture needle injuries (SNIs) are considered the predominant cause of PIs in the surgical setting. They account for as many as 77% of PIs (AORN, 2017) and are a primary cause of occupational exposure to BBPs among OR professionals.

Sharps safety is a priority in the perioperative environment and includes considerations for standard precautions, healthcare worker vaccination, postexposure protocols and follow-up treatment, and treatment for healthcare workers infected with a BBP pathogen. Staff should receive initial and ongoing education and competency verification on their understanding of the principles and performance of processes for sharps safety. Refer to Chapter 7 for more information on sharps safety.

Personal Protective Equipment

Personal protective equipment (PPE) refers to protective clothing, gloves, face shields, goggles, facemasks, and/or respirators or other equipment designed to protect the wearer from injury or the exposure to infection or illness. When used properly, PPE acts as a barrier between infectious materials such as viral and bacterial contaminants and skin, mouth, nose, or eyes (mucous membranes). When used properly and with other infection control practices such as handwashing, using alcohol-based hand sanitizers, and covering coughs and sneezes, spread of infection from one person to another is minimized. Effective use of PPE includes properly removing and disposing of contaminated PPE to prevent exposing both the wearer and other staff to infection. All PPE that is intended for use as a medical device must follow Food and Drug Administration (FDA) regulations and meet specific performance standards for protection. This includes surgical masks, N95 respirators, medical gloves, and gowns (FDA, 2016b). PPE must be selected based on the potential for exposure during the intended procedure or activity (SGNA, 2016). The N95 respirator mask is measurably superior in protection to high-filtration and surgical masks when perioperative staff are exposed to surgical smoke. N95 respirator masks certified by NIOSH provide secondary protection from residual surgical smoke that evades smoke evacuation (Stanton, 2016).

The conjunctivae can serve as a transmission route for bacteria and viruses. Eye protection devices include goggles, glasses with solid side shields, and chin-length face shields and must be worn to protect staff from injury or exposure to blood, tissue, body fluids, and aerosols (AORN, 2017). All OR staff, regardless of proximity to the surgical site or the patient's upper body, should wear eye protection as routinely as a surgical mask.

Double-Gloving

Glove barrier failure commonly occurs in the perioperative setting. Glove failures can be caused by punctures, tears by sharp devices, or spontaneous failures exposing the wearer to BBPs.

Strong evidence supports that scrubbed staff should wear two pairs of gloves, one over the other, during surgical and other invasive procedures with the potential for exposure to blood, body fluids, or other potentially infectious substances (AORN, 2017). The addition of the second pair of surgical gloves can significantly reduce perforations to the inner glove.

Perforation indicator systems should be used where a colored glove is worn beneath the regular surgical gloves. When a glove perforation occurs, moisture seeping into the defect between the glove layers permits easy visualization of the puncture. Strong evidence supports changing gloves after each patient procedure; immediately after direct contact with methyl methacrylate (MMA); when a visible defect or perforation is noticed; or when a suspected, or actual perforation occurs from a suture, needle, bone, or any other sharp object. Gloves should be changed every 90 to 150 minutes (AORN, 2017).

Responding to Exposure

As early as 2012, OSHA mandated a requirement for healthcare organizations to protect their workers and have a sharps injury and BBP exposure control plan (ECP). The plan must be written, communicated to all workers in the perioperative setting, regularly updated, and uniformly supported and enforced by perioperative leadership. At a minimum, the ECP must include the following:

- Determination of employee exposure
- Implementation of exposure control methods, including:
  - Standard precautions
  - Engineering and work-practice controls
  - PPE, using a biohazard risk assessment to determine type of PPE for at-risk employees
  - Written protocols for cleaning and decontamination
  - HBV vaccination
  - Postexposure evaluation and follow-up
  - Communication of hazards to employees and training
  - Recordkeeping
  - Procedures to evaluate exposure incidents

If You Sustain an Injury

If a needlestick, sharps injury, or other occupational contact (e.g., splashing or spraying) that could result in a BBP exposure occurs, the injured person must begin these following procedures *immediately*.

Immediate Response

- Wash all wounds and skin sites that have been contacted by blood or body fluids with soap and water. Flush mucous membranes with water (ANA, 2010).
- Irrigate eyes with clean water, saline, or sterile irrigants.
- Report the incident to your supervisor.
- Immediately seek medical treatment; initiate the injury reporting system used in your workplace.
- Identify the source patient; this patient should be tested for HIV, HBV, and HCV infections. Your workplace will begin the testing process by seeking patient consent.
- Immediately report to employee health, the emergency department, or the designated facility site.
- Get tested immediately and confidentially for HIV, HBV, and HCV infections.
- Get postexposure prophylaxis (PEP) using the Centers for Disease Control and Prevention (CDC) guidelines when the source patient is unknown or tests positive for HIV or HBV (there is no PEP for HCV). PEP medications for HIV should be started within 2 hours of exposure. PEP can be started after 2 hours from exposure; however, you should be evaluated as soon as possible after injury (CDC/NIOSH, 2016).
- Document the exposure in detail, for your own records as well as for the employer and for workers' compensation purpose.
- Obtain an immediate evaluation and risk assessment.
- Initiate a postexposure treatment plan to include counseling, education, and follow-up testing.

Follow-Up

- Obtain confidential postexposure testing at 6 weeks, 3 months, 6 months, and (depending on the risk), 1 year.
- Undergo monitoring of PEP toxicity.
- Prevent exposing others until follow-up testing is complete.

Exposure Prevention Information Network and Stop Sticks Campaign

The Exposure Prevention Information Network (EPINet) is a voluntary surveillance system used to record and track PIs and blood and body fluid contacts. Since its introduction, many hospitals throughout the United States and overseas have acquired EPINet. The federal NSPA 2000 and the 2001 revised BBP Standards require healthcare facilities to maintain a sharps injury log. The log must include, at a minimum, the type and brand of device involved in the exposure incident, the department in which the exposure occurred, and an explanation of how it occurred. EPINet data can be used to help facilities target high-risk devices and products, identify injuries that may be prevented with safer medical devices, and evaluate new technology designed to prevent needlesticks. Data can also be used by institutions to share and compare information and successful prevention measures (UVA, 2017).

The Stop Sticks campaign is a community-based information and education program used in many hospitals. Its goal is to raise awareness about the risk of exposure to BBPs from needlesticks and other sharps-related injuries. Campaign target audiences include clinical and nonclinical healthcare staff and healthcare administrators in multiple settings. Campaign resources are based on CDC and NIOSH standards. In this sharps injury campaign, the key message is "STOP STICKS" (CDC/NIOSH, 2013).

A Culture of Safety

A culture of safety is one in which core values and behaviors stem from a collective and sustained commitment by the organization's leadership, managers, and staff to promote safety over competing challenges and goals. The attributes of a positive safety culture include the following:

- Openness and mutual trust when discussing safety issues and solutions without placing individual blame
- Assembling appropriate resources, such as safe staffing and skill-mix levels
- Creating and sustaining a collaborative learning environment in which staff members learn from errors and proactively identify weaknesses
- Promoting and demonstrating transparency, accountability, and teamwork (ANA, 2016)

These powerful elements are part of the foundation of a high-reliability organization and a center for excellence, which is also a place where nurses want to work; they perceive they are respected; they plan to stay and have the autonomy to assess, formulate, and make decisions about their patient care and feel safe (Research Highlight). Perioperative nurses can and should individually and collectively work toward creating a culture of safety in their workplaces, which means ensuring not only the safety of their patients, but also their own safety. They can contribute to a culture of safety in their practice environments, including summoning the courage to give feedback on workplace issues that could negatively impact their patients or themselves.

Protecting Yourself

You have the responsibility to use habits and measures that can significantly protect you from exposure to hazards and prevent of injury by doing the following:

- Adopt and incorporate safe practices into daily work activities when preparing and using sharp devices.

RESEARCH HIGHLIGHT

Differences in Hospital Managers', Unit Managers', and Healthcare Workers' Perceptions of the Safety Climate for Respiratory Protection

Respiratory ailments are a prominent cause of work-related illness among HCWs. In 2014 OSHA identified respiratory protection standards as the fourth most frequently cited violation during worksite inspections. Safety culture is an aspect of an organization that demonstrates its commitment to staff well-being and influences safety behavior and compliance with standards. The safety climate is the collective perception of how the staff feels about the work environment. When workers perceive a strong safety climate, they are more likely to practice safe workplace behaviors, using PPE such as gloves, gowns, eye protection, and high-filtration and N95 respiratory masks when dealing with potentially infectious body fluids. Management commitment to staff safety is a significant predictor of a strong safety climate. Five key dimensions of a safety climate include managerial commitment to safety, management feedback on safety procedures, coworkers' safety norms, staff involvement, and staff safety.

This study explored differences in safety climate perceptions of HCWs in 98 acute care hospitals in six states in the United States based on nurses' hospital roles. The research question was Do perceptions of safety climate vary by type of healthcare provider? The researchers examined differences among three categories of healthcare providers: HCWs, HMs, and UMs in their responses to 10 agree/disagree questions, using data from a REACH II study. The core purpose was to understand how well the organizations were implementing the OSHA respiratory protection program requirements and the CDC guidelines for infection control.

In-person interviews were conducted with the HMs, UMs, and HCWs. Of the 98 participating hospitals, 33% were small, 26.5% were medium, and 39.8% were large. The researchers compared the HM, UM, and HCW perceptions for the dimensions of safety climate. Two questions assessed management commitment, two questions assessed the perception of managers' feedback on safety, two questions assessed coworkers' safety norms, two questions assessed staff involvement in health and safety issues, and two questions assessed staff training.

Significant differences were revealed among perceptions of safety climate. HCWs' perceptions differed greatly from the perceptions of the UMs and the HMs for 7 of the 10 safety climate items. The HCWs had a less positive opinion of management's commitment to safety, staff involvement in health and safety, staff safety training, the safety climate, and their involvement in respiratory protection policy decisions. HCWs perceived that their input was not formally requested on policy decisions. HCWs had the least positive perceptions, whereas HMs had the most positive, and UMs were somewhere in between. One exception to the pattern was management feedback on safety procedures because UM perceptions were markedly more positive than HMs and HCWs. This may be because UMs are more likely to be responsible for employee feedback. HCWs had the least positive opinions of coworker norms than all three groups. Hospital size was a significant predictor for management commitment to the safety model, leading the authors to suspect that manager communication and feedback are greater in larger hospitals. Education and tenure were predictive of management feedback and worker training questions. The data suggest that, although HCWs rarely question management commitment to safety, they did not feel that they received sufficient feedback on the use of respirators from their managers. The authors recommended that UMs should focus communication on how and when to use respirators. Hospitals can develop formal educational opportunities to teach, reinforce, and provide feedback. There were several primary limitations noted in this study. Survey samples were convenience samples, the study was considered exploratory in nature, all 10 questions were framed in positive terms, and the final study did not include the HCWs' work shift.

Findings from this study recommend that hospitals put in place control strategies to minimize risk of hazards that HCWs encounter in their workplace. Policies and procedures must support a safety climate that engages all staff through training, feedback, monitoring, collaboration, and practicing a culture of safety.

Implications for perioperative practice call attention to the hazards of surgical smoke and the need for collaborative measures among and between all perioperative staff to create and maintain a safety culture and climate as well as awareness of risk and the need for appropriate respiratory protection.

CDC, Centers for Disease Control and Prevention; *HCW,* healthcare workers; *HM,* hospital manager; *OSHA,* Occupational Safety and Health Administration; *PPE,* personal protective equipment; *REACH II,* Respirator Use Evaluation in Acute Care Hospitals; *UM,* unit manager.
Modified from Peterson K et al: Differences in hospital managers', unit managers', and health care workers' perceptions of the safety climate for respiratory protection, *Workplace Health Saf* 64(7):326–336, 2016; Occupational Safety and Health Administration: *Ten most frequently cited standards for Fiscal 2015* (website). www.osha.gov/Top_Ten_Standards.html. (Accessed 24 February 2017).

- Be constantly observant and clearly aware of your environment. Work smart and refrain from multitasking activities. Pay attention and be poised to respond to changes in the environment.
- Observe local, state, and federal (e.g., CDC, FDA, NIOSH, OSHA) regulations.
- Comply with methods to protect yourself from disease transmission (e.g., maintain HBV and influenza prophylaxis).
- Disinfect personal phones with hospital disinfectant wipe after each use.
- Participate in education about BBPs, and comply with recommended infection control and prevention practices.
- Know the location in your department of the exposure control plan.

- Follow the exposure control policy if injured, including *immediately* reporting the incident and commencing exposure response procedures.
- Engage in annual appropriate disaster education and simulations if your workplace is in an area prone to wildfires, floods, hurricanes, tornados, earthquakes, or other natural or human-made events.

Waste Anesthetic Gases

Scope and Significance of Problem

Waste anesthetic gases (WAGs) are small amounts of gases that may leak either from the patient's anesthetic breathing circuit into the OR air while anesthesia is being administered or from exhalation of the patient during emergence and recovery. Both mechanisms of exposure create risks for OR staff. Early research on the effects of WAG exposure appeared in the literature in 1967. Short-term exposure can cause headaches, irritability, nausea, drowsiness, lethargy, impaired judgment and coordination, and fatigue. Long-term exposure may be linked to spontaneous abortion, congenital abnormalities, infertility, premature births, cancer, and renal and hepatic disease. Today, perioperative staff members are exposed to trace amounts of WAG, and although this exposure cannot be eliminated, it can be controlled.

OR staff are more prone to be exposed to WAGs in facilities with no automatic scavenging systems or automated ventilation, in facilities with anesthesia systems in poor working order, or in recovery areas such as the postanesthesia care unit (PACU) with inadequate systems. Where scavenging and ventilation systems are in place, OR staff, nevertheless, can be exposed when leaks occur in anesthesia breathing circuits because of poor maintenance of tubing, connectors, or valves, or because of circuits with loose connections. Gases can also escape during connection and disconnection of the system. Poor-fitting patient masks or endotracheal tube connections can cause gases to escape into the air, making induction of anesthesia another occasion when gas leakage places OR staff at risk. Other mechanisms of potential exposure include defects in tubing and hoses; certain anesthesia techniques; improper practices such as gas flow control valves being left open after use; liquid anesthetic spills; and improperly inflated tracheal tubes, which can allow WAGs to escape into the ambient OR air.

PACU staff are exposed to WAGs from patients who have received anesthetics and then are admitted to the PACU or another postanesthesia recovery area. Postoperative patients eliminate anesthetics through their respiratory tracts by simply exhaling. The nurse's close proximity to the patient on admission to the PACU puts them at risk for exposure of varying concentrations of anesthetic agents. In contrast to the OR, ambient air in the PACU may contain multiple WAGs. Detection of the levels of WAGs without monitoring air samples in the breathing zone is deceiving because PACU nurses may be unable to detect the presence of agents until concentrations are greater than the NIOSH-recommended exposure limit.

Healthcare facilities are required to develop, implement, and measure control practices to reduce WAG exposure to the lowest practical level. Exposure levels must be measured every 6 months and maintained at less than 25 parts per million (ppm) for nitrous oxide and 2 ppm for halogenated agents to be compliant with NIOSH and OSHA standards.

As early as 2011, the NIOSH Health and Safety Practices Survey of Healthcare Workers was conducted among anesthesia providers, examining self-reported use of controls to minimize exposure to WAGs. The use of scavenging systems was universal; however, adherence to other recommended controls was lacking to varied degrees and differed between providers giving anesthesia to pediatric or adult patients. Examples of measures that increase WAG exposure risk include high, fresh gas flows; not routinely checking anesthesia equipment for gas leaks; starting gas flow before placing mask on the patient; using a funnel-fill system to fill vaporizers; lack of prompt attention to spills; and lack of safe handling procedures and awareness training. Interestingly, adherence to safety practices was highest among nurse anesthetists compared with other anesthesia providers (Boiano and Steege, 2016).

Chemicals and Drugs

Chemicals are used in OR settings for many purposes, including sterilization and disinfection of equipment, cleaning, specimen preservation, and anesthesia. Some commonly used chemicals include disinfectants and sterilants (e.g., glutaraldehyde, ortho-phthalaldehyde [OPA], ethylene oxide [ETO], hydrogen peroxide, peracetic acid), tissue preservatives (e.g., formalin, formaldehyde), antiseptic agents (e.g., hand hygiene products, surgical prep solutions), and MMA. The FDA has also raised a concern about the long-term effects of antiseptics and hand sanitizers. Research suggests that as many as 30 different ingredients used in antiseptics have higher levels of absorption and systemic exposure, particularly triclosan and triclocarban. In the absence of soap and water, hand sanitizers are a valuable tool in preventing hospital-associated infections (HAIs) and protecting healthcare workers; however, alcohol-based hand rubs are not as effective as soap and water on visibly soiled skin (Nania, 2016). (For detailed information on hand hygiene, refer to Chapter 4.)

Exposure to chemicals occurs through several routes. Toxic exposure effects can be limited to the site of exposure or result in a systemic effect. The following are three main routes of exposure to toxic chemicals:

1. *Inhalation* is the introduction of toxic chemicals, radioisotopes, or pathogens via the respiratory tract. Gases or vapors of volatile liquids are the most commonly inhaled chemicals, although it is possible to inhale chemicals as aerosols or dusts. Inhaled chemical agents are generally quickly absorbed because of lung vascularity and large surface area, with exposure symptoms manifesting within 1 to 3 days after exposure.

2. *Skin contact or absorption through mucous membranes* is slower than inhalation. Mucous membranes include the mouth, eyes, and nose. Nonintact skin (exposed skin that is chapped, abraded, or afflicted with dermatitis) can also lead to exposure.

3. *Ingestion* is the least common route of exposure. Ingestion may be the result of unintentional exposures from the hand (including cuticle tears and nail biting) or mouth, such as swallowing saliva containing trapped airborne particles.

The amount of chemical absorbed by the body varies, depending on duration of exposure, concentration of the chemical, and various environmental factors. Toxicity can be acute or chronic. Acute toxicity usually results from an accidental spill of a chemical. Exposure is sudden and results in an emergency. Chronic toxicity can result from repeated exposure to low levels of a chemical over a prolonged period (CDC/NIOSH, 2016).

Exposure limits for many chemicals used in healthcare help to provide a safer environment. Exposure limits published by OSHA are the only legally recognized regulatory limits. OSHA defines a permissible exposure limit (PEL) as the amount of exposure to a chemical permitted as a time-weighted average (TWA). Recommended exposure limits (RELs) are occupational exposure limits developed and recommended by NIOSH, providing protection over a working lifetime. NIOSH uses a TWA for up to a 10-hour workday during a 40-hour workweek. A short-term exposure limit (STEL) is a designated value that should not be exceeded anytime during the workday, based on a 15-minute TWA. For example, for glutaraldehyde, the NIOSH REL is 0.2 ppm, with an OSHA PEL of zero (NIOSH, 2016).

The responsibility to inform staff about chemical hazards and to use control measures, including providing PPE, rests with the employer. The OSHA Hazard Communication Standard requires all manufacturers and importers of hazardous chemicals to develop safety data sheets (SDSs) for all chemicals and mixtures of chemicals. Employers must make these data sheets readily available to all staff who could be exposed to hazardous products.

The purpose of the OSHA standards is to ensure evaluation of all hazardous chemicals produced or imported and dissemination of information concerning such hazardous chemicals to employers and staff. Dissemination occurs by comprehensive hazard communication programs that must include container labeling and other forms of warning, SDSs, and employee training. SDSs initially arose as tools for workers with health and safety roles in the chemical industry. With the expansion of federal and state right-to-know laws and regulations, however, the need for information on SDSs expanded to the healthcare industry.

A typical SDS includes the following sections:

- Material identity, including chemical and common names
- Hazardous ingredients
- Cancer-causing ingredients
- List of physical and chemical hazards and characteristics
- List of health hazards, including acute and chronic effects
- Whether OSHA, the International Agency for Research on Cancer, or the National Toxicology Program lists the material as a carcinogen
- Limits to which a worker can be exposed
- Routes of entry
- Specific target organs likely to be damaged with exposure, and medical problems exacerbated by exposure
- Precautions and safety equipment
- Emergency and first aid procedures
- Firefighting information
- Procedures for cleanup of leaks and spills
- Safe handling precautions
- Identity of the organization responsible for the SDS, date of issue, and emergency phone number

The *NIOSH Pocket Guide to Chemical Hazards* offers useful information about several hundred chemicals (NIOSH, 2016). It is important that healthcare staff are aware of chemicals they are exposed to in their work settings and take necessary precautions to use PPE and other means to eliminate or reduce their occupational risks. Measures may include attending training provided by the employer and being familiar with information about occupational exposures, such as the chemicals inventoried on their work unit. These inventories should be located on each unit and be easily accessible.

Another form of chemical exposure in perioperative settings is exposure to hazardous drugs. Exposure can result from handling hazardous drugs as well as working near sites in which they are used. The drugs can be in the air, on surfaces in the work area, on medical equipment, or in the urine or feces of patients. NIOSH defines a hazardous drug as having one or more of the following characteristics: carcinogenicity, teratogenicity or other developmental toxicity, reproductive toxicity, organ toxicity at low doses, genotoxicity or structure, and toxicity profile in a new drug that mimics an existing drug considered hazardous by the same criteria. Examples of drugs considered hazardous include chemotherapy, some anticonvulsants, antivirals, some estrogens, progestins, some contraceptives, cell stimulants, and bone resorption inhibitors (Stokowski, 2014). Nursing units should maintain a current list of hazardous drugs that are used; staff should know how to protect themselves with specific practices and PPE. Work practices and training are critical to minimize occupational risks of hazardous drug exposure.

Surgical procedures that generate surgical smoke and aerosols, also known as plume, from the thermal destruction of tissue place perioperative staff at risk of inhaled toxic gases, along with viable cellular, bacterial, and viral material and chemicals in the plume

---

BOX 3.3

Surgical Smoke Safety Advocacy

Research findings to raise awareness and protect OR staff from the dangers of surgical smoke include the following:

- Inhaling smoke produced when using an ESU device to vaporize 1 g of tissue is like smoking six unfiltered cigarettes in 15 minutes.
- Being passively exposed to 1 day of surgical smoke in the OR exposes nurses to an equivalent mutagenicity of smoking 27 to 30 unfiltered cigarettes a day.
- Long-term exposure to PAHs such as benzene, along with particles and volatile organic compounds found in surgical smoke, may have synergistic and additive effects.
- Even when researchers found levels of benzene, xylene, ozone, and other toxins in surgical smoke measured within permissible exposure limits, they cautioned that repeated exposure to a combination of these substances increases the possibility of developing adverse effects. Adverse health effects of benzene exposure include respiratory irritation, dizziness, headache, nausea, and fatigue.
- Infective and malignant cells found in the plume of surgical smoke are sufficiently small enough to inhale.

ESU, Electrosurgery unit; *PAH,* polycyclic aromatic hydrocarbons.
Modified from Association of periOperative Registered Nurses (AORN): *Go Clear Award™, surgical smoke free-recognition program* (website), December 1, 2016. www.aorn.org/education/facility-solutions/aorn-awards/aorn-go-clear-award. (Accessed 24 February 2017); Trosman S: Inside surgical smoke, *Am Nurse Today* 12(2):26–27, 2017.

(Evidence for Practice). These substances, when inhaled, are associated with upper respiratory irritation and mutagenic effects (Stokowski, 2014). Any procedure that generates plume should use a smoke evacuation device with the suction wand placed as close as possible to the area of activation. All perioperative staff present in the procedure must wear respiratory protection that is as effective as a fit-tested N95 filtering respirator facemask. High-filtration facemasks must not be used as the first line of protection from the airborne contaminant (AORN, 2017). If you smell it, you are inhaling it (Box 3.3).

Standard Precautions

The CDC's Standard Precautions aim to reduce transmission of microorganisms from both recognized and unrecognized sources of infection. Standard Precautions apply to all patients receiving care, regardless of diagnosis or presumed infection status. They are considered the first and most important tier of precautions; as such, they are the primary strategy for successful infection prevention and control. Standard precautions apply to (1) blood; (2) all body fluids, secretions, and excretions (except sweat), regardless of whether they contain visible blood; (3) mucous membranes; and (4) nonintact skin. Consistent application of these precautions and frequent handwashing by all members of the perioperative team serve to protect the healthcare provider and to minimize cross-infection of pathogens among patients (refer to Chapter 4 for further discussion of standard- and transmission-based precautions).

Cell Phone Hygiene

Cell phones and portable devices that are frequently handled must be disinfected after each use. Strategies for protecting patients and

EVIDENCE FOR PRACTICE

Promoting Guidelines and Workplace Practices for Surgical Smoke Safety

Unpleasant odors, gases, vapors, aerosols, and particulates are generated and emitted as by-products of surgical smoke (also known as plume) during surgical procedures that require the use of energy-generating devices, such as the electrosurgery unit (ESU), tissue-ablating lasers, ultrasonic scalpels and high-speed drills, burrs, and saws. Surgical smoke puts the OR staff at risk for potentially hazardous inhalation of chemical, bacterial, viral, carcinogenic, mutagenic, malodorous, and cytotoxic agents. Efforts have been launched to improve surgical smoke safety awareness and provide education and competency verification, guidance, and evidence-based practices. New guidelines for electrosurgery, lasers, and MIS techniques include the following:

- Promote buy-in among leadership
- Assemble a multidisciplinary team to evaluate and purchase systems based on unit needs
- Conduct education and competency verification
- Perform gap analysis on smoke reduction processes to identify areas for improvement
- Wear N95 respirator surgical masks rather than high-filtration surgical masks
- Use a smoke evacuator; one smoke evacuator should be available for each OR; ensure the evacuator capture device is positioned at the sight of tissue activation
- Use a smoke filter during MIS procedures
- Evacuate and filter smoke during the procedure and at pneumoperitoneum release
- Use in-line filters for wall suction
- Change and dispose of filters per manufacturer recommendations
- Handle filters during removal using Standards Precautions and PPE

Modified from Association of periOperative Registered Nurses (AORN): *Go Clear Award™: surgical smoke free-recognition program* (website). December 1, 2016. www.aorn.org/education/facility-solutions/aorn-awards/aorn-go-clear-award. (Accessed 24 February 2017); Okoshi K et al: Health risks associated with exposure to surgical smoke for surgeons and operation room personnel, *Surg Today* 45(8):957–965, 2015; Ogg MJ: Implementing surgical smoke evacuation practices, *AORN J* 105(2):233–235, 2017; Stanton C: Guideline first look: guideline for surgical smoke safety, *AORN J* 104(4)10–12, 2016.

healthcare staff from contamination from cell phones include the following:

- Wash your hands, and keep your hands away from your eyes, nose, and mouth.
- Do not take your phone into the bathroom.
- Wipe your phone with an alcohol-based wipe periodically.
- Cover your mouth when you cough or sneeze.
- Do not place your phone on germy surfaces (APIC, 2017).

Immunizations and Infectious Disease Exposure

Contact with infected patients or infectious material puts healthcare staff at risk for occupational-acquired infection. Many diseases and infections are preventable through immunizations and vaccines. It is therefore essential for nurses and other healthcare staff to establish and maintain their immunity in cooperation with their employers. Healthcare organizations providing direct patient care should develop a comprehensive immunization program for staff.

HBV is a major infectious risk for healthcare staff from percutaneous and permucosal exposure to blood or other potentially infectious material. Through a joint advisory notice in 1987, the Departments of Labor and Health and Human Services initiated standards to regulate exposure to HBV. The federal standard, issued in December 1991, mandated that HBV vaccine be made available at the employer's expense to all healthcare staff occupationally exposed to blood or other potentially infectious materials. It is important for healthcare staff to have an HBV antibody titer to evaluate their immune response to a vaccine series. Once immunity is documented, there is no need for booster doses even if titer levels drop.

Seasonal influenza and its complications are responsible for many deaths and hospitalizations each year. Despite the well-documented seriousness of seasonal influenza cases, too many healthcare staff fail to receive vaccination annually. Patients transmit influenza to healthcare staff and, in turn, healthcare staff who are clinically or subclinically infected with influenza can transmit seasonal influenza to patients or others. By receiving the seasonal influenza vaccination, healthcare staff protect themselves, their patients, and their families.

HAIs with measles, mumps, and rubella are well documented. Previously, birth before 1957 was considered acceptable evidence of measles immunity. Serologic studies of healthcare staff, however, conclude that many of those born before 1957 are not immune to measles.

HAIs from varicella zoster virus (VZV) are also well documented. Patients who are at increased risk for varicella infection are pregnant women; premature infants born to susceptible mothers; infants born at less than 28 weeks' gestation or who weigh less than 1000 g, regardless of maternal immune status; and immunocompromised people of all ages (including individuals undergoing immunosuppressive therapy, that have malignant disease, or are immunodeficient). Sources of healthcare-associated varicella infection include patients, facility staff, and visitors who are infected with either varicella or zoster. Generally, a reliable history of chickenpox is a valid measure of VZV immunity.

Recent increases in rates of pertussis (an acute, infectious cough illness) among healthcare staff have led to a recommendation that they receive one dose of tetanus toxoid, reduced diphtheria toxoid, and acellular pertussis vaccine (Tdap). Should an exposure to an infectious or communicable disease occur in the clinical area, chemoprophylaxis may be available. Healthcare staff should report an exposure to their occupational health department or other provider in compliance with the facility's procedures and receive proper follow-up. Infectious exposures outside the workplace should also be reported for the protection of patients and coworkers. Postexposure work restrictions may range from restricting contact with high-risk patients to furlough for healthcare staff without immunity.

Exposure of healthcare staff to diphtheria, pneumococcal disease, or tetanus is not significantly more than that of the general population; staff therefore should elect to receive these immunizations from their primary care providers. In addition to immunization records maintained by their employers, healthcare staff should also maintain accurate *personal* records of all their immunizations and exposures, including any prophylaxis or laboratory studies.

Immunizations are part of a comprehensive workplace infection control program. Guidance for development of a program is available from OSHA, the CDC, and the Department of Health in the state in which the facility is located. Recommended and required vaccinations vary by state and depend on legislation at either the state or the federal level. To further evaluate compliance with recommended or required vaccinations, healthcare staff should consult with the occupational or employee health department at their workplace.

Radiation Safety

Radiologic imaging studies are invaluable diagnostic and treatment tools. However, radiation presents environmental safety concerns for patients and staff. Many surgical procedures use radiologic studies performed immediately before, during, or after surgery, increasing the potential for radiation exposure. X-rays of all frequencies can damage tissues and may produce long-term effects. The effects of radiation are dose dependent and cumulative: the larger the dose or the more frequent the exposure, the greater the risk of toxic effects of radiation.

Sources of radiation exposure in the OR include (1) ionizing sources, such as portable x-ray machines and portable fluoroscopy units (C-arm), and (2) nonionizing sources, such as lasers (laser safety discussion appears more extensively in Chapter 8). Ionizing radiation is used in diagnostic, interventional, and therapeutic procedures, but can damage living tissues and may produce long-term effects (AORN, 2017). Expanding use of x-ray imaging during interventional surgery has dramatically increased exposure of many OR personnel to ionizing radiation in recent years. Acute exposure to ionizing radiation can result in dermatitis and reddening of the skin (erythema) at the point of exposure, and large, full-body exposures can lead to radiation poisoning, the symptoms of which may include nausea, vomiting, diarrhea, weakness, and death.

The guiding philosophy of radiation safety and protection is represented by the idea of As Low as Reasonably Achievable (ALARA). Typically, reducing the patient dose also reduces the dose to healthcare staff. Therefore performing optimized procedures is an important aspect of radiation protection. Optimization includes performing only necessary studies and performing them sufficiently well that they do not need to be repeated.

In OR settings, the main source of occupational doses is radiation that scatters as the x-ray beam passes through the patient, particularly from fluoroscopically guided procedures. Healthcare staff who do not protect themselves from scatter radiation are especially at risk when performing interventional procedures, given significantly increased exposure time and proximity during the procedure (AORN, 2017). Personnel may stand near patients for sustained amounts of time, and angulated geometries with C-arm equipment may result in high staff doses from backscatter.

Guidelines for radiation safety are based on the principles of time, distance, and shielding effect from dose levels sustained. When exposed to radiation at a constant rate, the total dose equivalent received depends on the length of time exposed. If the distance from the point source of radiation doubles, then exposure quarters. Passage through shielding materials also reduces the amount of radiation.

Surgical staff should avoid unnecessary exposure to radiation sources and comply with practices that reduce potential exposure. Maintain the greatest practical distance (at least 6 feet) from the radiation source or remain behind leaded shielding when ionizing radiation use occurs during surgery. Personnel assisting with radiologic procedures should not hold the patient manually during a study because of the risk of exposure by the direct beam (AORN, 2017). Members of the sterile scrub team should wear protective devices and move as far from the radiation source as possible while still adhering to aseptic technique. Nonessential personnel should leave the room.

Protective equipment reduces the intensity of radiation exposure. Radiation safety devices include mobile rigid shields on wheels; ceiling-suspended transparent barriers; flexible leaded aprons (e.g., wraparound), vests, skirts, thyroid shields, and gloves; and leaded safety eyeglasses with side shields (AORN, 2017). AORN recommends that personnel who may have to stand with their back to the radiation beams wear wraparound aprons to decrease their risk of exposure, and that personnel nearest to the radiation beam shield their upper chest, neck, and upper legs.

OSHA has established mandatory, health-based limits on occupational exposure to ionizing radiation and provides a series of guidelines that healthcare facilities can use to protect staff from excess radiation exposure. OSHA requires that staff working with radiation sources be monitored for exposures and be informed of their levels of exposure at least once a year (Stokowski, 2014).

OSHA also recommends that film badges, or an equivalent, be used for long-term monitoring. A film badge is a passive dosimeter for personal exposure monitoring that should be worn whenever an employee works with x-ray equipment, radioactive patients, or radioactive materials. During the preprocedure or radiation time-out, it should be confirmed that every team member is wearing their dosimeter. Dosimeters should be worn in a consistent location for each procedure. Staff who work in high-dose fluoroscopy settings wear two badges for additional monitoring. For staff members who know or suspect they are pregnant, it may be required by their facility, or may be prudent, to submit an official voluntary declaration of pregnancy, which includes an estimated date of conception, to establish safety protocols monitoring monthly radiation exposure. Radiation exposure should not exceed 0.5 rem during the entire gestational time frame. An additional dosimeter should be worn under the apron at the waist and read monthly. A maternity or double-thickness apron or wraparound apron should be worn that provides coverage for the entire abdomen (AORN, 2017).

Leaded garments should be handled carefully and examined regularly to ensure the integrity of shielding. They should not be folded during storage, they should be wiped down after every procedure with a recommended antiseptic solution or wipe, and they should undergo regular radiologic testing to ensure effective shielding. Staff-development programs on radiation safety should occur periodically to reinforce radiation safety practices and to correct misconceptions or unrealistic practices relating to radiation exposure and monitoring.

The American College of Radiology (ACR, 2017) recommends that facilities adopt the following safety measures to protect personnel:

- Implement a radiation-exposure monitoring program, as required by the Nuclear Regulatory Commission or appropriate state agencies.
- Perform systematic inspection of interlock systems.
- Provide appropriate room shielding.
- Perform routine leak testing of all sealed sources, as required by regulatory agencies.
- Furnish appropriate safety equipment for use of sealed sources. For further information on radiation safety, see Chapter 29.

Latex Allergy

Natural rubber latex allergy is a serious medical problem for a growing number of patients and a disabling occupational disease among healthcare workers. Latex allergy develops from exposure to natural rubber latex and plant cytosol, which is used extensively to manufacture medical gloves and other devices, as well as numerous consumer products. Allergic reactions to latex range from skin disease to asthma and anaphylaxis, which can result in chronic illness, disability, career loss, and death.

Latex has been the material of choice for surgical gloves because it is flexible and maintains tactile sensitivity for the wearer. Although natural rubber latex has been a common component in thousands of medical and consumer products for many years, latex sensitivity is a relatively new problem for patients and healthcare staff. Clinicians were aware of contact dermatitis from chemicals in rubber as early as the 1930s; they did not recognize, however, systemic allergic reactions to latex proteins until the 1970s. Latex allergy erupted in the United States shortly after the CDC introduced Universal Precautions in 1985. Researchers hypothesize that the latex allergy outbreak is the result of multiple factors, including increased latex exposure and deficiencies in manufacturing, among others. Latex allergy affects a larger number of staff in all health disciplines than in the general population.

Certain foods are potential problems for people with latex allergy and can provide significant assessment trigger questions during the preoperative patient assessment. Foods of concerns are apples, avocadoes, bananas, carrots, celery, chestnuts, kiwi, melons, papaya, raw potato, and tomato (American College of Allergy, Asthma and Immunology, 2014).

Individuals can experience three reactions to latex. *Irritant contact dermatitis* is the most common reaction, characterized by dry, reddened, itchy, or cracked hands. Irritant contact dermatitis is not a true allergic reaction. *Allergic contact dermatitis* (also called *chemical contact dermatitis*) is a delayed cell-mediated, type IV localized allergy caused by chemicals used to manufacture rubber products. The most common contact sensitizers are the accelerators thiurams, mercaptobenzothiazoles (MBTs), and carbamates. Allergic contact dermatitis is a delayed reaction, usually appearing 6 to 48 hours after exposure. Symptoms are similar to those from irritant contact dermatitis (i.e., pruritus, edema, erythema, vesicles, drying papules, crusting and thickening of the skin), except that the reaction may extend beyond the actual point of contact.

The most serious is a true latex allergy, a type I, immunoglobulin E (IgE)–mediated hypersensitivity reaction that involves systemic antibody formation in reaction to proteins in products made from natural rubber latex. Natural rubber latex contains up to 240 potentially allergenic protein fragments, and different people may be sensitized to different combinations of latex allergens. Synthetic latexes are not involved in latex allergy. A true latex allergic response is immediate, IgE mediated, and anaphylactic. The onset of anaphylaxis may occur within minutes of contact with the proteins, with symptoms that may include generalized urticaria, wheezing, dyspnea, laryngeal edema, bronchospasm, tachycardia, angioedema, hypotension, and cardiac arrest. Many serious anaphylactic reactions have occurred when a latex product (e.g., surgical gloves) directly contacts mucous membranes during surgical procedures. This situation permits a rapid introduction of latex antigen directly into the vascular circulation.

Traditionally it was assumed that sensitization to latex resulted only from cutaneous absorption in healthcare staff or from direct mucosal contact during clinical treatment. Studies have confirmed that latex protein allergens, when airborne, can remain suspended for prolonged periods. Inhalant exposure is an additional risk factor for sensitization to latex allergens.

Healthcare professionals should use the following strategies to reduce their risk of allergic reaction to latex:
- Use powder-free gloves (FDA, 2016a).
- Use nonlatex gloves for activities that are not likely to involve contact with infectious materials.
- Be aware that hypoallergenic gloves do not reduce the risk of latex allergy, although they may reduce reactions to chemical additives in the latex.
- When wearing latex gloves, do not use oil-based hand creams or lotions because they can cause glove deterioration.

- After removing latex gloves, wash hands with a mild soap and dry thoroughly.
- Learn to recognize the symptoms of latex allergy, which may include skin rashes; urticaria; flushing; pruritus; nasal, eye, or sinus symptoms; asthma; and shock.

Institutions need to develop strategies to limit the occupational exposure of healthcare staff to latex. If a latex-free environment cannot be created, the goal is to create a latex-safe environment, one in which the facility makes all reasonable efforts to remove high-allergen and airborne latex. This includes switching to powder-free gloves to reduce airborne latex allergen sources. In addition, appropriate latex-free gloves should be provided for healthcare staff with known latex sensitivity or for procedures in which patients have known sensitivity or allergy. See Box 3.4 for valuable information on latex allergy.

Fatigue and Burnout

Prolonged work hours can negatively impact patient outcomes and pose dangers to nurses' personal health (Ambulatory Surgery Considerations). Shift work and long working hours have been linked with sleep disturbances, injury, obesity, and many other serious occupational based disorders (Brown, 2014, 2015). Sleep deprivation has long been associated with impairment of various cognitive functions including mood, motivation, response time, initiative, and cognitive function. Acute and chronic sleep deprivation may cause cumulative deficits in executive function and irritability and impaired communication and coordination. Fatigue and sleep deprivation are prime risks for occupational injuries that can affect healthcare staff at work, at home, and while driving. This condition

---

AMBULATORY SURGERY CONSIDERATIONS

Compassion Fatigue in Ambulatory Surgery Settings

Compassion is an emotion of empathy or kind concern for others who may be suffering or experiencing distress. Nursing is a profession that typically attracts individuals for whom compassion and consideration for others comes easily. Perioperative settings can present stressful experiences at many levels for patients and their families. The ambulatory surgical setting is a fast-paced and busy environment of care focused on efficiency, minimizing waste, and saving time. Ambulatory surgery nurses care for many patients and may perform multiple roles during the course of their day. The fast-paced, efficiency-focused care delivery model can put nurses at risk for feeling disconnected from their patients' needs, ability to deliver quality care, and avoid errors (Garton, 2016).

Compassion fatigue (CF) may develop when a nurse feels overwhelmed with emotional challenges or a sense of chronic distress. Signs and symptoms of CF may present as a loss of ability to nurture, lack of feeling of fulfillment in a job well done, sleep deprivation, anxiety, moodiness, feelings of burnout, headaches, impaired immune system, and other stress-response–mediated conditions. CF may come from long hours, unreasonable workload or time restraints, other work-related stressors, and pressures and challenges outside of the workplace. Prevention and treatment of CF include using healthy and effective coping strategies that involve physical, emotional, and spiritual healing in a supportive environment.

Modified from Garton D: Compassion fatigue in ambulatory surgery settings, *AORN J* 104(3):244–247, 2016.

BOX 3.4

Latex Allergy

Latex allergy is an IgE-mediated reaction to proteins retained in finished natural rubber latex products.

Etiology and Incidence

Latex is the milky sap of the rubber tree *Hevea brasiliensis*. This natural rubber product contains proteins. Latex allergy is the reaction to certain proteins in the latex rubber. It remains a serious problem, and healthcare staff are at increased risk to acquire latex allergies. Children with spina bifida and individuals with chronic illnesses who require frequent operations are especially susceptible to latex allergy.

Pathophysiology

The amount of latex exposure necessary to produce sensitization or an allergic reaction is unknown. Increased exposure to latex proteins increases the risk of developing allergic symptoms. The precise protein responsible for causing allergic contact dermatitis latex type I hypersensitivity remains unknown and may differ among individuals.

Risk Factors by Occupational Status

- Healthcare professionals such as surgery personnel, emergency care workers, dentists, and obstetrics staff are at highest risk
- Children with spina bifida or others with conditions requiring frequent operations
- People with congenital urogenital abnormalities requiring indwelling catheters
- Employees in the rubber industry
- Individuals with history of other IgE-dependent allergies (e.g., rhinitis, asthma, food allergies, hyperpnea) with a positive skin test

Clinical Manifestations: Immediate Type I Hypersensitivity

Clinical signs include local skin redness, dryness, and itching after contact with latex. Inhalation of particles results in respiratory symptoms, such as rhinitis, sneezing, itchy eyes, scratchy throat, or asthma. More severe systemic manifestations include anaphylaxis with bronchospasm, laryngeal edema, respiratory distress, or respiratory failure. Consider using an anaphylactic crisis response checklist in perioperative settings.

Complications

Complications may include anaphylactic shock and respiratory and cardiac arrest, leading to death.

Diagnostic Tests

History

Diagnostic significance in an individual's history includes atopic history, hives under latex gloves, hand dermatitis related to gloves, allergic conjunctivitis after rubbing eyes after hand contact with latex, swelling around mouth after dental procedures or inflation of a balloon, and vaginal burning after pelvic examination or contact with latex condoms.

Immunologic Evaluation

Immunologic evaluation comprises skin prick, intradermal, and patch contact skin tests and serologic testing (e.g., RAST or ELISA). The FDA has approved a standardized latex reagent for skin testing for research only; it is not for public use.

Therapeutic Management

Medications

Medications include epinephrine for reaction (may be autoinjector carried by allergic individual), β-agonist inhaler, prednisone, and other anaphylactic life-supporting medications.

General

Immediate assessment and interventions for acute reaction include cardiac monitoring and, if needed, respiratory support.

Prevention and Education

Latex-sensitive individuals should do the following:

- Avoid all items containing latex.
- Avoid environments with high levels of circulating aeroallergens (e.g., ORs, emergency departments, blood banks).
- Wear a medical alert bracelet or tag.
- Carry epinephrine autoinjector for use at first signs of anaphylaxis.
- Communicate latex allergy to all healthcare staff, especially when having surgery.

ELISA, Enzyme-linked immunosorbent assay; *FDA*, US Food and Drug Administration; *IgE*, immunoglobulin E; *RAST*, radioallergosorbent test.
Modified from American College of Allergy Asthma and Immunology: *Latex allergy* (website). http://acaai.org/allergies/types/skin-allergies/latex-allergy. (Accessed 27 February 2017); Seifert PC: Crisis management of anaphylaxis in the OR, *AORN J* 105(2):219–227, 2017.

has serious implications for patient safety as well. Fatigue is also often associated with burnout.

The term *burnout* has been used to describe the chronic work stress symptoms of people who work in complex and stressful environments. The concept of burnout is described as a syndrome characterized by emotional exhaustion and a sense of depersonalization (Ross, 2016). Burnout is frequently seen in the nursing profession because of the emotional demands and the high-stress workplace. Burnout can develop into depression, excessive fatigue, cardiac disease, anxiety, and substance abuse (Ross, 2016). Individuals may not recognize that they are experiencing burnout and need help. Ross (2016) suggests that therapeutic tips for dealing with burnout may include the following:

- Talk to someone about how you are feeling.
- Get adequate sleep, at least 7 to 9 hours per night/day.
- Tune out the rat race and take a break from electronics.
- Immerse yourself in self-care, yoga, exercise, art, and/or walking.

The ANA Position Statement on Nursing Fatigue recommends evidence-based steps for enhancing performance and safety and patient outcomes. The statement emphasizes that employers and registered nurses (RNs) should work together to reduce the risks related to nurse fatigue (ANA, 2014) by doing the following:

- Employers should include nurse input when designing work schedules and implement a "predictable schedule" that allows nurses to plan for work and personal obligations.
- Nurses should work no more than 40 hours in a 7-day period and limit work shifts to 12 hours in a 24-hour period, including on-call hours worked.
- Employers should not use mandatory overtime as a staffing solution.
- Employers should encourage frequent, uninterrupted rest breaks during work shifts.
- Employers should adopt an official policy that gives the RN the right to accept or reject a work assignment to prevent risks from

fatigue. The policy should be clear that rejecting an assignment under these conditions is not patient abandonment and that RNs will not be retaliated against or face negative consequences for rejecting such an assignment.

- Employers should encourage nurses to be proactive about managing their health and rest, including getting 7 to 9 hours of sleep per day; managing stress effectively; developing healthy nutrition and exercise habits: and using naps in compliance with employer policy.

Noise

Excessive noise in the workplace environment may negatively affect patient and staff safety. Communication is difficult during periods of high noise levels, which can potentially lead to clinical errors, distraction, poor concentration, and impaired problem-solving. Distraction and noise can divert the team's attention from the current task, causing errors in patient care and leading to mental lapses and care omissions (AORN, 2014b). Staff can become desensitized, or immune, to the continuous barrage of clinical noise (e.g., alarm fatigue) (Appold, 2015). AORN supports and advocates for a multidisciplinary team approach to reduce noise and distractions, particularly those that do not serve a clinical purpose, to promote a safer environment of care for patients and perioperative staff (Wright, 2016). Examples of nonclinical noise may be music, phones, conversation, laughter, unnecessary overly loud instruments, alarms, and machinery sounds. The creation of a no interruption zone (NIZ) is a care environment in which there is minimal or no nonessential conversation and activities during critical phases including surgical time-outs and briefings, anesthesia induction and emergence, surgical counts, surgical specimen management, medication preparation and administration, critical phases of the procedure, and hand-off reports.

Education for all staff should focus on keeping noise to a minimum through acknowledging the critical phases of surgery and promoting concentration on the task at hand for delivery of high-quality care. Education should include the following ways to reduce noise (Wright, 2016):

- Discuss the appropriate use of NIZ in the preprocedure time-out.
- Eliminate nonessential conversation.
- Reduce or turn off noise volume on electronic devices.
- Silence mobile devices.
- Avoid use of instruments or devices that increase noise levels if unnecessary at the time.
- Monitor compliance with noise reduction practices.

Distractions and noise must be managed to maintain the primary focus on both patient and workplace safety (AORN, 2014b).

Workplace Violence

Disrespectful behavior and hesitation to, or lack of, speaking up are hallmarks of a dysfunctional safety culture, which can be resistant to change. Discord in the workplace affects patient care and healthcare staff and undermines a culture of safety. The OSHA Act of 1970 ensures every working person a safe and healthy workplace, free from recognized hazards that may cause death or serious physical harm. Workplace violence may be any physical assault, threatening behavior, or verbal abuse occurring in the workplace.

Workplace violence can occur in various forms, from bullying and verbal abuse to physical abuse, assault, and even homicide.

As early as 2008, The Joint Commission (TJC) noted that medical errors can arise from intimidating and disruptive behaviors. Such behaviors can also decrease patient satisfaction, foster preventable adverse outcomes, increase cost of care, and lead staff to seek new positions in more professional environments. Despite such an early warning, various disruptive behaviors are still evident in many healthcare settings. Key disruptive behaviors and their descriptive definitions include incivility, bullying, and horizontal/lateral violence. Incivility is disrespectful, rude, or inconsiderate conduct with an intent to be hurtful. Such an individual may demonstrate eye-rolling, screaming, name-calling, rude comments, and public shaming. Bullying is a repetitive and long-term targeted and abusive behavior that is demonstrated by persistent taunting in front of others, verbal attacks, physical threats, and acts of being reported to management (TJC, 2016). Horizontal/lateral violence is characterized by unkind and discourteous divisive backbiting and infighting. This individual may complain to others without directing his or her insults and condescending comments to the intended target. This disruptive behavior may also manifest itself with sarcastic or patronizing comments, withholding support, or ignoring one's input or worth (Clark, 2017; Lachman, 2015). The 2001 *ANA Code of Ethics for Nurses* considers disruptive behaviors a violation of the code of ethics (Lachman, 2015).

Uncivil and bullying nurses will often report they are unaware that they are responsible for this disruptive behavior; however, studies support that they essentially know exactly what they are doing and probably engage in this behavior to meet a neurotic need (Quinlan, 2016).

Harmful effects of bullying include a decline in the quality of patient care delivery; poor staff relations; low morale; increases in stress and stress-related illness; feelings of shock, disbelief, shame, guilt, anger, fear, and powerlessness; depression; self-blame with decreased self-confidence that can endanger patients; sleeplessness and loss of appetite; increased cost to employers and the healthcare system; increased absenteeism and use of sick time; poor performance; reduced productivity; loss of creative problem-solving capacity; and attrition. Bullying risk factors in the workplace include stress, tension, and frustration; poor management skills; inadequate or nonexistent prevention policies; lack of training to recognize or cope with bullying; shift work and demanding workloads; working alone; and lack of reporting systems or punishment of perpetrators. Most healthcare facilities have a code of conduct defining acceptable and disruptive or inappropriate behaviors that undermine a culture of safety. Leaders are expected to create and implement a process to manage behaviors that undermine this culture of safety. Perioperative nurses should be able to practice in an environment in which they communicate, collaborate, and respect each other's role and skill set.

Workplace violence in any form negatively affects healthcare staff and patients. It harms staff professionally and personally, and it alters the quality of care provided to patients. The perioperative area is not excluded from the effect or incidence of workplace violence. Nurses and other healthcare staff in this setting need education and training to recognize workplace violence in all forms, including lateral violence, to create, support, and sustain a safe working environment that promotes teamwork and collaboration in the perioperative setting. Unit-level leadership and structural empowerment play key roles in creating healthy work environments and supporting a culture of safety.

Practical intervention strategies, along with terminating the offender, may provide opportunities for improvement in counseling and changing the disruptive behaviors of an employee. Such strategies may involve the organization's Employee Assistance Program (EAP) and focus on the following:

- Standards and code of conduct
- Skill development
- Empowerment
- Addressing practitioner/employee impairment (Lachman, 2015).

Perioperative staff and leadership share the responsibility to create and maintain a culture of safety and respect by implementing these evidence-based strategies:

- Promote healthy interpersonal relationships and be aware of their own interactions.
- Participate in training on effective communication, diversity, and conflict negotiation.
- Establish an agreed on code signal to alert others when/if harmful actions are taking place.
- Practice cognitive rehearsal techniques for deflecting incivility, learn and rehearse phrases to use in uncivil encounters, and reinforce instructions (Clark, 2017).
- Promptly report incidents through appropriate channels.
- Keep detailed records of incivility or bullying incidents with names, dates, and witnesses.
- Support coworkers (Brown, 2015).
  Employers/leadership should:
- Develop a comprehensive violence prevention program from federal guidelines.
- Educate staff on incivility/bullying prevention guidelines.
- Encourage staff to participate in policy/procedure programs.
- Provide direction for those who need support.
- Encourage staff to report incidents.
- Establish a "zero tolerance" policy that treats all cases in the same manner.
- Inform staff about available conflict resolution strategies and respectful communication (Brown, 2015).

Active Shooter

It is an unfortunate fact that terroristic violence can occur in healthcare facilities. TJC has received reports from its accredited organizations of violent criminal events including assault, rape, homicide, and suicide (TJC, 2014). Victims of an active shooter can be randomly selected, and they often are facility staff. These situations are unpredictable and evolve quickly. Since active shooter situations may be over within 15 minutes, before law enforcement arrives, healthcare organizations must prepare their staff for an active shooter situation (TJC, 2014).

Preventative environmental solutions include controlled access doors, metal detectors, alarm systems, panic buttons, handheld noise devices and cell phones; lockable staff areas, such as lounges and bathrooms; curved mirrors and adequate lighting; and well-lit parking areas. Work practices that help prevent workplace violence include identification of high-risk patients, including flagging charts, both hard copy and electronic; proper training of staff; avoidance of employees working alone, particularly in secluded areas; easy and effective processes to report suspicious behavior, harassment, threats, or violent assaults; careful supervision of the movement of psychiatric and prisoner patients within the facility; and use of a team approach to prevent workplace violence. Team training should include review of prevention policies, reporting procedures, support systems, and action plans; identification of risk factors that cause or contribute to violence; early identification of warning signs of escalating behavior; tools to diffuse violent situations; and review of system and policy failures. Organizations should be prepared to respond as safely as possible to the potential active shooter event. Good practices for coping with an active shooter situation include, in this order: escape, hide, and fight (US State Department of Homeland Security [USDHS], 2017; TJC, 2014). Response measures include the following:

- Be aware of your environment and any possible dangers.
- Take note of the two nearest exits in any facility you visit.
  - If the shooter is in your vicinity, evacuate and help others.
  - If you cannot escape, find a place to hide out of the shooter's view and help others.
- If you are in an office, stay there and secure the door, silence your cell phone.
- If you are in a hallway, get into a room and secure the door, turn off all noise sources, block the door with furniture, hide behind large objects, and remain silent.
- As a last resort, attempt to take the active shooter down. When the shooter is at close range and you cannot flee, your chance of survival is much greater if you try to incapacitate the shooter.
- When evacuation and hiding are not possible, remain calm. Dial 911 when it is safe to do so to alert police to the location. If you cannot speak, leave the line open and allow the dispatcher to listen (US State Department of Homeland Security, 2017; TJC, 2014).

Key Points

- Collaborative patient safety and workplace safety programs share a common goal and are the foundation of a culture of safety and a strong perioperative safety climate.
- Perioperative staff routinely face a wide array of occupational hazards that place them at risk for work-related musculoskeletal injuries.
- Ergonomic tools for safe patient movement and handling help the nurse determine whether assistive equipment should be used, what type of equipment would best support the task, and how many caregivers are needed to perform the task safely.
- STFs are caused by many factors, including wet floors, uneven floor surfaces, low-profile equipment and cords, cluttered or poorly lit walkways and ORs, and improper footwear.
- Surgical smoke is a serious and harmful by-product of various energy-generating devices.
- During perioperative patient care, healthcare workers routinely face exposure to BBPs and PIs.
- Observing safety precautions during all phases of surgery, from setup to cleanup, reduces the number of injuries and exposures for all OR staff.
- OSHA regulations require healthcare organizations to protect their workers and to have a sharps injury and BBP exposure control plan.
- Smoke evacuation devices and N95 filtration respirator masks must be used when surgical smoke is generated in a surgical procedure.
- Incivility, bullying, and horizontal/lateral violence are not tolerated in the perioperative workplace.
- In the event of an active shooter situation in your vicinity, escape, hide, and/or fight.
- A nurturing work environment in which nurses believe their physical and emotional safety is a high priority leads to higher job satisfaction, the ability to make meaningful contributions to patient care, and a demonstrated intent to stay.

Critical Thinking Question

David and Kathy, the orthopedic surgery team leaders, will devote the day to updating and revising the procedural pick lists. They will be sitting at a computer workstation most of the day. What ergonomic principles must they use to demonstrate healthy sitting and workstation positioning practices?

⊖volve *The answer to the Critical Thinking Question can be found at http://evolve.elsevier.com/Rothrock/Alexander.*

References

American College of Allergy, Asthma and Immunology: *Latex allergy* (website), 2014. http://acaai.org/allergies/types/skin-allergies/latex-allergy. (Accessed 27 February 2017).

American College of Radiology (ACR): *Radiology safety* (website), 2017. www.acr.org/Quality-Safety/Radiology-Safety. (Accessed 27 February 2017).

American Nurses Association (ANA): *Seven things to do in response to needlestick injury* (website), 2010. www.nursingworld.org/DocumentVault/Occupational Environment/Needles/7-Responses.pdf. (Accessed 23 February 2017).

American Nurses Association (ANA): *Safe patient handling and mobility*, Silver Spring, MD, 2013, ANA.

American Nurses Association (ANA): *Addressing nurse fatigue to promote safety and health: joint responsibilities of registered nurses and employers to reduce risks* (website), 2014. www.nursingworld.org/MainMenuCategories/Policy-Advocacy/Positions-and-Resolutions/ANAPositionStatements/Position-Statements-Alphabetically/Addressing-Nurse-Fatigue-to-Promote-Safety-and-Health.html. (Accessed 23 February 2017).

American Nurses Association (ANA): *Creating a culture of safety* (website), 2016. www.nursingworld.org/CreatingSafetyofCulture. (Accessed 23 February 2017).

Appold K: Noise complaint, *Hospitalist* 19(6):1, 20–22, 2015.

Association of periOperative Registered Nurses (AORN): *AORN bariatric tool kit*, Denver, 2014a, The Association.

Association of periOperative Registered Nurses (AORN): *AORN position statement on managing distractions and noise during perioperative patient care*, Denver, 2014b, The Association.

Association of periOperative Registered Nurses (AORN): *AORN position statement on a healthy perioperative practice environment*, Denver, 2015, The Association.

Association of periOperative Registered Nurses (AORN): *AORN safe patient handling and movement tool kit*, Denver, 2012, The Association.

Association of periOperative Registered Nurses (AORN): *Guidelines for perioperative practice*, Denver, 2017, The Association.

Association of Practitioners in Infection Control and Epidemiology (APIC): *Cell phones and germs* (website), 2017. http://consumers.site.apic.org/infection-prevention-in/everywhere-else/cell-phones-and-germs/. (Accessed 23 February 2017).

Boiano JM, Steege AL: Precautionary practices for administering anesthetic gases: a survey of physician anesthesiologists, nurse anesthetists and anesthesiologist assistants, *J Occup Environ Hyg* 13(10):782–793, 2016.

Brown T: *ANA releases new position statement on nurse fatigue, medscape medical news* (website), 2014. www.medscape.com/viewarticle/835281. (Accessed 23 February 2017).

Brown T: *ANA: 'zero tolerance' for workplace violence, bullying* (website), 2015. www.medscape.com/viewarticle/850383. (Accessed 18 June 2017).

Centers for Disease Control and Prevention (CDC)/NIOSH: *Stop sticks: campaign user's guide and resources* (website), 2013. www.cdc.gov/niosh/stopsticks. (Accessed 23 February 2017).

Centers for Disease Control and Prevention (CDC)/NIOSH: *Bloodborne infectious diseases: HIV/AIDS, hepatitis B, hepatitis C* (website), 2016. www.cdc.gov/niosh/topics/bbp/emergnedl.html. (Accessed 23 February 2017).

Clark CM: Promoting civility in the OR: an ethical imperative, *AORN J* 105(1):60–66, 2017.

Daley KA: Sharps injuries: where we stand today, *Am Nurse Today* 12(2):23–24, 2017.

Fitzpatrick MA: *Safe patient handling and mobility: a call to action. Current Topics in Safe Patient Handling and Mobility, September 2014. Supplement to Am Nurse Today* 1-3, 2014.

Food and Drug Administration (FDA): *Banned devices; powdered surgeon's gloves, powdered patient examination gloves, and absorbable powder for lubricating a surgeon's glove* (website), 2016a. www.federalregister.gov/documents/2016/12/19/2016-30382/banned-devices-powdered-surgeons-gloves-powdered-patient-examination-gloves-and-absorbable-powder. (Accessed 25 February 2017).

Food and Drug Administration (FDA): *Personal protective equipment for infection control* (website), 2016b. www.fda.gov/medicaldevices/productsandmedicalprocedures/generalhospitaldevicesandsupplies/personalprotectiveequipment/default.htm. (Accessed 24 February 2017).

Garton D: Compassion fatigue in ambulatory surgery settings, *AORN J* 104(3):244–247, 2016.

Kumpar D: *Prepare to care for patients of size. Current topics in mobility. Supplement to Am Nurse Today*, September, 20–22, 2014.

Lachman VD: Ethical issues in the disruptive behaviors of incivility, bullying and horizontal/lateral violence, *Urol Nurs* 35(1):39–42, 2015.

Nania P: Concerns regarding long-term effects of antiseptics and hand sanitizers, *AORN J* 104(3):4, 2016.

National Institute of Occupational Safety and Health (NIOSH): *NIOSH pocket guide to chemical hazards* (website), 2016. www.cdc.gov/niosh/npg/default.html. (Accessed 24 February 2017).

Occupational Safety and Health Administration (OSHA): *Computer workstation eTool* (website), 2017. www.osha.gov/SLTC/etools/computerworkstations/. (Accessed 24 February 2017).

Phillips JA, Miltner R: Work hazards for an aging nursing workforce, *J Nurs Manag* 23(6):803–812, 2015.

Press Ganey: *2016 nursing special report: the role of workplace safety and surveillance capacity in driving nurse and patient outcomes* (website), 2016. www.pressganey.com/about/news/2016-nursing-special-report. (Accessed 24 February 2017).

Quinlan P: *Incivility vs. bullying: know the difference* (website), 2016. www.aorn.org/about-aorn/aorn-newsroom/periop-insider-newsletter/2016/2016-articles/incivility-versus-bullying. (Accessed 24 February 2017).

Rice S: *Retrofitting hospitals for obese patients* (website), 2014. www.modernhealthcare.com/article/20140208/MAGAZINE/302089980. (Accessed 24 February 2017).

Ross J: The connection between burnout and patient safety, *J Perianesth Nurs* 31(6):539–541, 2016.

Simon RW, Canacari EG: *Workplace safety in healthcare* (website), 2017. https://psnet.ahrq.gov/perspectives/perspective/214. (Accessed 24 February 2017).

Society of Gastroenterology Nurses and Associates (SGNA): SGNA standards of practice: standards of infection prevention in the gastroenterology setting, *Gastroenterol Nurs* 39(6):487–496, 2016.

Stanton C: Guideline first look: guideline for surgical smoke safety, *AORN J* 104(4):10–12, 2016.

Stokowski LA: *The risky business of nursing* (website), 2014. www.medscape.com/viewarticle/818437. 850437. (Accessed 18 June 2017).

The Joint Commission (TJC): *Quick safety: preparing for active shooter situations* (website), Issue 4, 2014. www.jointcommission.org/assets/1/23/Quick_Safety_Issue_Four_July_2014_Final.pdf. (Accessed 18 June 2017).

The Joint Commission (TJC): *Workplace violence prevention—Joint Commission Newsletters: bullying has no place in healthcare* (website), Issue 24, 2016. www.jointcommission.org/wpv_healthcare_joint_commission_newsletters/. (Accessed 24 February 2017).

University of Virginia (UVA): *Exposure prevention information network (EPINet)* (website), 2017. www.medicalcenter.virginia.edu/epinet/about_epinet.html. (Accessed 24 February 2017).

US Congress: *United States Congress: H.R.4266—Nurse and Health Care Worker Protection Act of 2015* (website), 2015. www.congress.gov/bill/114th-congress/house-bill/4266/all-actions. (Accessed 3 February 2017).

US Department for Homeland Security: *Active shooter preparedness* (website), 2017. www.dhs.gov/active-shooter-preparedness. (Accessed 24 February 2017).

Veterans Administration Medical Center (VAMC): *Safe patient handling toolkit* (website), 2016. www.tampavaref.org/safe-patient-handling.htm. (Accessed 24 February 2017).

Waters TR et al: *Application Manual for the Revised NIOSH Lifting Equation* (website), 1994. www.cdc.gov/niosh/docs/94-110/pdfs/94-110.pdf. (Accessed 24 February 2017).

Wright MI: Implementing no interruption zone in the perioperative environment, *AORN J* 104(6):536–540, 2016.

CHAPTER 4
Infection Prevention and Control

CECIL A. KING AND CYNTHIA SPRY

Advancements in surgical interventions and the science of infection prevention and control continue to evolve and have become increasingly complex. The complexity is derived from the changes in the healthcare environment; the advancements in minimally invasive and advanced surgical procedures; and the development of new, highly technical instrumentation and equipment. This chapter provides an overview of the etiology of surgical site infection (SSI), including emerging multidrug-resistant organisms (MDROs), and identifies various methods to control infection in the perioperative environment. Use of Standard Precautions along with engineering and work-practice controls assist perioperative practitioners in reducing the transmission of pathogenic organisms. Perioperative patient care is based on surgical aseptic principles. Careful adherence to these principles supports infection prevention and control, ultimately improving surgical patient safety and outcomes. Each member of the surgical team must demonstrate the highest integrity in the application of this knowledge. Finally, the potential for bioterrorism and infectious disease threats posed by recent endemics has forced the United States along with the rest of the world to strengthen security and emergency readiness. Threats of a bioterrorist attack and endemic infectious disease outbreaks have resulted in massive exposure and illness. Perioperative personnel need to be prepared to mobilize to serve in a variety of locations and need to be familiar with the most likely biologic threats and the levels of precautions required for patient and personnel safety.

Causes of Infection

Before the mid-nineteenth century it was commonplace for surgical patients to develop what was then referred to as postoperative "irritative fever" with subsequent purulent wound drainage, sepsis, and most often death. It was Louis Pasteur's experiments in 1862 with putrefaction that established the fundamental principle of germ theory and the concepts of sepsis (i.e., the presence of harmful bacteria, toxins) and asepsis (i.e., the absence of infectious organisms). In 1865 Joseph Lister, after learning of Pasteur's theory that germs cause infection, introduced the use of phenol as an antiseptic. His introduction of the antiseptic process decreased surgery-related deaths by 15% and paved the way for the common practice of asepsis. Yet despite the fundamental benefits of antisepsis it became apparent that antisepsis alone did not eliminate SSI. The 1940s provided for a highly successful era of modern surgery with the introduction of antibiotics. However, the use of antibiotic prophylaxis was not consensually accepted until the discovery that *Staphylococcus aureus* could be isolated from the surgical field under "sterile" conditions. However, a consensus on the use of perioperative antibiotics was not established until 1963. The importance of timing in the administration of the antibiotic was noted as early as 1946 when Howe noted a correlation between the development of infection, the interval between wound contamination, and the administration of the

antibiotics. In 1963 Burke demonstrated that antibiotics given shortly before or at the time of incision resulted in notably less wound induration (Burke, 1963).

Despite the tremendous advancements in infection prevention and control, aseptic practices, and antibiotics, SSIs continue to present substantial burden to patients and the healthcare system with associated increased length of stay and a 2- to 11-fold increase in associated mortality. Although the estimated annual incidence of SSI in the United States varies, the rate of SSI reported among patients undergoing inpatient surgery is 2% to 5% or 160,000 to 300,000 annually. The financial burden of SSI has been estimated between $3.5 and $10 billion per year. Because 60% of SSIs are preventable with the use of evidence-based practices, SSIs have become a major pay-for-performance and a quality of improvement metric (Ban et al., 2016) (Evidence for Practice).

Additional challenges in the prevention and treatment of SSIs have been complicated by minimally invasive procedures with highly technologic instrumentation and equipment, adding an additional challenge to cleaning, disinfecting, and sterilization in an environment with emerging MDROs (e.g., methicillin-resistant *S. aureus* [MRSA], vancomycin-resistant enterococci [VRE]). Following the published "Guideline for Prevention of Surgical Site Infection, 1999" (Mangram et al., 1999) and the inconsistent implementation of these guidelines, the Centers for Medicare and Medicaid Services (CMS) collaborated with the US Centers for Disease Control and Prevention (CDC) on the Surgical Care Improvement Project (SCIP) with the goal of standardizing quality improvement measures that would be implemented nationally. These guidelines have become part of The Joint Commission's (TJC) National Patient Safety Goals (NPSGs). NPSG.07.05.01, "Implement Evidence-Based Practices for Preventing Surgical Site Infections," specifically provides elements of performance for standard operating room (OR) suites, ambulatory care, and office-based surgery centers as it relates to the prevention of SSIs. These elements of performance outline education, policy, and procedural practices aimed at reducing the risk of SSI. Given the seriousness of this problem and to increase the incentive for compliance, CMS has required reporting by hospitals if they are to receive full Medicare payment (mandatory reporting went into effect in 2012). Over 150 years after the discovery of the role microorganisms play in sepsis and the knowledge of asepsis, SSIs remain a common healthcare-associated infection (HAI) justifying the need for a vigilent sterile conscience and implementation of evidence-based perioperative guidelines (TJC, 2013).

Pathogenesis of Surgical Site Infection

The development of an SSI is dependent on a complex interaction between patient-related factors that are modifiable or nonmodifiable, and extrinsic factors (e.g., procedure, facility, preoperative preparations)

▐ EVIDENCE FOR PRACTICE

Prevention of Surgical Site Infections: 2016 Update

Many studies suggest that SSIs are among the most common complications of surgical patient care. SSIs increase morbidity and consume additional resources. The CMS considers SSIs to be largely preventable and therefore do not reimburse healthcare facilities when SSIs occur after coronary artery bypass; bariatric surgery; and orthopedic surgery involving the spine, neck, shoulder, or elbow.

SSIs include superficial incisions, deep incisions, and organ/space infections. These have been defined in the CDC NNIS system and are recognized worldwide. Surgical patients often receive some form of antibiotic prophylaxis. SCIP is a national partnership of organizations committed to improving the safety of surgical care through the reduction of postoperative complications. In 2005 the SCIP launched a multiyear campaign to reduce surgical complications. It is somewhat controversial if SCIP measures have reduced the national rate of SSI. A systematic review of outcomes associated with SCIP measures reported a 4% decrease in SSIs after introduction of SCIP interventions; however, this 4% decrease in SSIs did not correlate with increased compliance with SCIP measures. It is of interest that the list of chart-based SCIP measures (SCIP-INF-4) was retired by TJC as of December 31, 2015. The American College of Surgeons and Surgical Infection Society released new guidelines for the prevention and treatment of surgical site infections on December 1, 2016.

Evidence for Practice Identified by This Consensus to Reduce Surgical Site Infections

Although some surgical complications are unavoidable, surgical care can be improved through decisions and subsequent care focusing on evidence-based practice recommendations. Research shows that delivering antibiotics to a patient within 1 hour before incision can dramatically decrease SSI rates, yet this practice is not followed in all situations.

Postoperative complications impose a substantial mortality to morbidity ratio on patients. The cost to the healthcare community is overwhelming. One approach to improving outcomes from surgery is to promote adherence to process of care measures such as administering prophylactic antibiotics specific to the common pathogens as well as the patterns of resistance within different organizations. This methodology supports the practice of using hospital-specific antibiograms and diverse antibiotics to decrease resistant organisms. For example, in elective colorectal procedures a combination of oral antibiotics, bowel preparation, and intravenous antibiotics are recommended.

Key measures identified to reduce SSIs and affect outcomes are the following:

- A prophylactic antibiotic should be administered 1 hour before surgical incision, or within 2 hours for vancomycin or fluoroquinolones. Vancomycin should not be routinely used in MRSA-negative patients.
- Antibiotics should be discontinued at the time of incision closure, except in procedures involving breast reconstruction with implants, joint arthroplasty, and cardiac surgery during which the optimal duration of antibiotic prophylaxis is unknown at this time.
- Perioperative antibiotics should be weight based and a subsequent dose administered based on the antibiotics half-life or for every 1500 mL of blood loss.
- Target blood glucose should be between 110 and 150 mg/dL, regardless of the patient's diabetic status.
- Preoperative warming is recommended, and intraoperative normothermia is recommended for all surgical procedures.
- Hair removal should be avoided. If removal is necessary hair clippers should be used.
- An alcohol-containing skin prep should be used unless contraindicated.
- A waterless chlorhexidine surgical hand scrub is as effective as the traditional soap and water scrub.
- There is limited evidence to support recommendations regarding surgical attire. However, TJC and AORN guidelines recommend facility-laundered scrub attire and the use of a disposable bouffant hat. The ACS guidelines support the use of a skull cap when there is minimal hair that could be exposed. All jewelry should be moved or contained with the scrub attire.
- The use of an impervious plastic wound protector may prevent SSIs during open abdominal surgery. The strongest evidence supporting this practice is during elective colorectal and biliary tract procedures.
- Triclosan antibacterial suture is recommended for wound closure during clean and clean-contaminated abdominal procedures.
- Double-gloving is recommended.
- For colorectal procedures: gloves should be changed before beginning surgical closure, and new or clean instruments should be used for closure.

ACS, American College of Surgeons; AORN, Association of periOperative Registered Nurses; CDC, Centers for Disease Control and Prevention; CMS, Centers for Medicare and Medicaid Services; MRSA, methicillin-resistant Staphylococcus aureus; NNIS, National Nosocomial Infections Surveillance; SCIP, Surgical Care Improvement Project; SSI, surgical site infections; TJC, The Joint Commission.

Modified from Ban KA et al: American College of Surgeons and Surgical Infection Society: Surgical site infection guidelines, 2016 update, J Am Coll Surg 224(1):59–74, 2016; The Joint Commission (TJC): Surgical Care Improvement Project (SCIP) Measure Information Form (Version 2.1c) (website), 2006 www.jointcommission.org/surgical_care_improvement_project_scip_measure _information_form_version_21c. (Accessed 4 February 2017).

---

that may or may not be modifiable. Nonmodifiable patient-related factors include increased age, prior surgical site radiation, and a history of skin or soft tissue infection. Some modifiable patient-related factors are glycemic control, obesity, alcoholism, tobacco smoking, preoperative albumin <3.5 mg/dL, total bilirubin >1.0 mg/dL, and immunosuppression. Extrinsic related factors include emergent procedures; inadequate OR ventilation, cleaning, disinfecting, and sterilization processes; increased OR traffic; hair removal method; inadequate skin preparation; inappropriate antibiotic choice; timing; or dosing, preexisting infection, wound classification II or greater,

perioperative hypothermia, perioperative hypoxia, surgical technique (e.g., poor hemostasis, tissue trauma), lapses in sterile technique, longer and more complex procedures, and blood transfusion. SSIs are influenced by the interaction of these numerous risk factors, only some of which are under the perioperative nurse's control. Strategies to decrease SSIs involve numerous practices occurring across the perioperative continuum under the supervision of numerous providers (Ban et al., 2016).

The human body has three lines of defense to combat infection. The first line of defense consists of *external barriers*, such as the skin and mucous membranes, which are usually impervious to most pathogenic organisms. The second line of defense is the *inflammatory response*, which prevents an invading pathogen from reproducing and possibly involving other tissue. The third line of defense, the *immune response*, is triggered after the inflammatory response. When a break in this defense mechanism occurs, the possibility for infection increases (Box 4.1 lists term definitions).

Surgery by its inherent nature violates the first, if not all, lines of the body's natural defense mechanisms with inevitable bacterial contamination of the surgical wound. Major advances in aseptic technique have been associated with a dramatic decrease in bacteria, yet even under the strictest conditions (e.g., laminar flow) bacteria have been isolated from the wound. Historically surgical wounds have been classified based on the expectation that there are typical

---

BOX 4.1

Definition of Terms

Aeration: Method by which absorbed ethylene oxide (EO) is removed from EO-sterilized items.

Aerobes: Microorganisms unable to live and reproduce without access to free atmospheric oxygen, such as *Mycobacterium tuberculosis*.

Anaerobes: Bacteria able to survive only in the absence of molecular oxygen, such as *Clostridium perfringens*.

Bioburden: Amount of microbial load and organic debris on an item before sterilization.

Biofilm: A thin coating containing biologically active organisms that have the ability to grow in water, solutions, or in vivo and coat the surface of structures or devices. Biofilms may contain viable and nonviable microorganisms that may adhere to a surface and are trapped within organic matter.

Biologic indicator: A sterilization process–monitoring device commercially prepared with a known population of highly resistant spores to test the effectiveness of the sterilization process being used.

Cohorting: Practice of grouping patients who are colonized or infected with the same pathogen.

Colony-forming unit (CFU): Term used in microbiology to estimate the number of viable bacteria or fungal cells in a sample.

Contamination: Presence of pathogenic microorganisms on or in animate or inanimate objects. This term generally is used in reference to a specific object, substance, or tissue that contains microorganisms, especially disease-producing microorganisms.

Deep incisional surgical site infection (SSI): Infection involving deep soft tissue, fascia, and muscle.

Dynamic air removal: Mechanically assisted air removal from a sterilizer's chamber. This includes prevacuum and steam flush, pressure pulsed steam sterilizers.

Flash sterilization: See Immediate-use steam sterilization (IUSS).

Gram stain: A procedure for staining bacteria that is the first step in classifying and differentiating them into two large groups (gram-positive and gram-negative) based on the chemical and physical properties of their cell walls.

Healthcare-associated infections (HAIs): Infections acquired by patients during hospitalization, with confirmation of diagnosis by clinical or laboratory evidence. The infective agents may originate from endogenous sources, as from one tissue to another within the patient (self-infection), or from exogenous sources, as acquired from objects or other patients within the hospital (cross-infection). HAIs, which are often referred to as hospital-acquired or nosocomial infections, may not become apparent until after the patient has left the hospital.

Immediate-use steam sterilization (IUSS): Steam sterilization process of instruments intended to be used immediately. Items subject to IUSS may not be stored for use at a later time.

Immediate use is the shortest time possible between the time the item(s) is removed from the sterilizer and aseptically transferred to the sterile field.

Immunity: Resistance to infection.

Infection: Invasion and multiplication of microorganisms in body tissues, causing cellular injury attributable to competitive metabolism, toxins, intracellular replication, or antigen-antibody response.

Infectious agent: Parasite (bacterium, spirochete, fungus, virus, or any other type of organism) that is capable of producing infection.

Microorganisms: Microscopic, living, single-celled organisms such as bacteria and viruses.

Opportunists: Microorganisms of low virulence and requiring large numbers to produce infection.

Organ or space SSI: Infection involving any part of the anatomy other than the incision.

Pathogen: Any disease-producing agent or microorganism.

Primary pathogens: Highly virulent organisms that are capable of producing disease in low numbers.

Resident microorganisms (flora): Organisms that habitually live in the epidermis, deep in the crevices and folds of the skin.

Reuse: Repeated or multiple uses of any medical device whether marketed as a reusable or single-use device. Repeated/multiple uses may be on the same patient or on a different patient with applicable reprocessing of the device between each use.

Source: Object, substance, or individual from which an infectious agent passes to a host. In some cases transfer is direct from the reservoir, or source, to the host.

Spore: Dormant stage of some bacteria that is reversible under favorable conditions. Common spore-forming bacteria include *Clostridium perfringens, C. botulinum, C. tetani,* and *Bacillus anthracis*.

Sterilization process–monitoring device: Device used to monitor specific sterilization processes. These devices can be biologic, physical, or chemical.

Superficial SSI: Infection involving skin and subcutaneous tissue as opposed to deep tissue.

Surgical site (incisional) infection: Infection involving body-wall layers that have been incised.

Toxins: Protein molecules released by bacteria to affect host cells at a distant site.

Transient microorganisms: Organisms with a very short life span, such as the normal flora present on the skin surface of humans. Gram-negative bacteria are transient on the hands of hospital personnel and account for 60% of infections.

Virulence: Potency of a pathogen measured in the numbers required to kill the host.

Virus: Ultramicroscopic infectious agent that replicates itself only within cells of living organisms.

organisms within the patient's bodily structures (e.g., skin, mucous membranes, bowel) that pose an inherent risk to developing an SSI. Although wound classification has some predictive value, patient- and procedure-related determinants contribute a great deal to determining if an infection will develop.

Microorganisms That Cause Infection

The pathogen(s) most commonly associated with SSIs are the patient's endogenous skin flora. Various organisms have been described as typical surgical wound pathogens, whereas the source of infection for most SSIs may not be established with a great deal of certainty. The patient's endogenous skin organisms, gram-positive organisms in general (e.g., staphylococcal species), are a principal cause of infection of clean surgical procedures. Over the last decade, the microbiology of SSIs reflects the current evolution of various MDROs. Although the CDC reported a decline in SSIs caused by MRSA, there is a concerning increase in SSIs from multidrug-resistant (MDR) gram-negative organisms. A major risk factor for developing a *S. aureus* infection exists in those patients whose nares are colonized with *S. aureus,* especially those patients with patient-related risk factors, such as diabetes and hemodialysis, who have *S. aureus* colonization rates of 50% or more. Just as a patient's colonization poses an increased risk for SSI, so does staff in which wound infections have been reported in clusters of infection related to a nurse or surgeon colonized with *S. aureus* or *S. epidermidis* (Talbot, 2015).

Modern methods of disinfection and sterilization reduce but do not eliminate the skin-related organisms endogenous to the surgical patient. This is because up to 20% of patient's skin resident microorganisms reside in the hair follicles and sebaceous glands. Because these organisms are below the skin's surface, topical antiseptic skin preparations have no bactericidal effect. The surgical incision transects these structures and may carry the resident microorganism into the surgical wound, setting the stage for infection. The microbes most frequently associated with SSIs are those species considered normal flora of the body's structures entered during the surgical procedure. For example, enteric gram-negative organisms and anaerobic bacteria (e.g., *Escherichia coli*) are common causes of infection after procedures of the gastrointestinal (GI) tract. However, infection by an organism does not correlate directly with the resident microorganisms, but by the virulence of a bacteria and its potential to manifest as a wound pathogen. The Surgical Pharmacology box lists typical microorganisms associated with commonly performed surgical procedures in adults (Talbot, 2015).

Virulence Factors

Although various sources and risk factors related to bacterial contamination of surgical wounds have been identified, it is extremely difficult to identify with any degree of certainty the source and route of contamination. It is the direct inoculation by the patient's normal (i.e., endogenous) flora that is believed to be the most common source of contamination. Whereas transmission from contaminated surgical instruments is an obvious concern, contamination by seeding from a preexisting infection from another area of the patient's body is more of a concern in procedures involving prosthetic implants. Another long-held belief is that the shedding from the skin, mucous membranes, or clothing of perioperative personnel is a potential source of surgical wound contamination. Streptococcal wound infections have been traced to the carriage of organisms by perioperative personnel. Infections with *Candida albicans* osteomyelitis and diskitis have been traced to the wearing of artificial fingernails by staff, leading organizations to prohibit the wearing of artificial nails

by those involved in direct patient care. Studies using *S. aureus* have demonstrated that an inocula as low as 1 colony-forming unit can produce a wound infection, provided the organism is inoculated into a suitable microenvironment. This dismissed previously held theories that a large inocula was required to cause an infection. Staphylococcal species possess enzymes and toxins with the ability to adhere to the cellular matrix of blood clots and subendothelium, damaging the patient's tissues and reducing antibody-mediated phagocytosis. The virulence of other species is similar in that given a suitable microenvironment coliform gram-negative rods may cause abdominal sepsis by producing a variety of tissue-damaging enzymes. Studies suggesting that the efficacy of preoperative antibiotics is limited to only a few hours after the moment of bacterial contamination suggest that the microenvironment of the surgical wound is not static, but wound-related changes occur, diminishing tissue perfusion and antibiotic delivery brought about by the effect of the inflammatory response. The introduction of foreign material (e.g., suture, drains, implants) has been shown to potentiate wound infection. Operative tissue trauma from mechanical injury (e.g., pressure from tissue retractors), electric cautery, and devitalized tissue distal to ligated vessels may allow for a small inocula of bacteria to develop into an infection during clean and clean-contaminated procedures. Anesthesia alters the body's ability to regulate normothermia, resulting in hypothermia that diminishes the body cell-mediated chemotaxis. Hypothermia also causes vasoconstriction, which results in tissue hypoxia, and both are risk factors for SSIs. Perioperative blood transfusion is associated with decreased cell-mediated immunity and an increased risk of infection. These virulence factors contribute to potentiating an SSI (Talbot, 2015).

Bloodborne Pathogens

Bloodborne pathogens are infectious microorganisms found in blood that can cause disease in humans. The bloodborne pathogens of perioperative significance include hepatitis B virus (HBV), hepatitis C virus (HCV), and human immunodeficiency virus (HIV). These diseases are caused by a virus and most often transmitted by blood or other potentially infectious body fluids such as semen, vaginal secretions, cerebrospinal fluid, synovial fluid, pleural fluid, peritoneal fluid, amniotic fluid, saliva (in dental procedures), and any body fluid that is visibly contaminated with blood. Within the perioperative setting these pathogens are more commonly transmitted parenterally, such as by a needlestick and other sharps-related injury, or by a splash exposure to a mucous membrane (e.g., eyes or mouth). As the understanding of the transmission of HIV grew in the late 1980s so did the development of methods for preventing the transmission of bloodborne disease in healthcare settings. To reduce or eliminate the hazards of occupational exposure to bloodborne pathogens, an employer must implement an exposure control plan that details employee protective measures. The plan must also describe how an employer implements engineering and work-practice controls, personal protective equipment (PPE), employee training, medical surveillance, hepatitis B vaccination, and other provisions as required by the Occupational Safety and Health Administration (OSHA) Bloodborne Pathogens Standard (OSHA, 2012a). HBV vaccine is strongly recommended for healthcare workers who may be exposed to blood and body fluids. OSHA mandates that all healthcare workers report blood and body fluid exposures, and perioperative personnel should follow their employer's protocol for exposure reporting. It is important to remember that although these viruses, especially HIV and HCV, are commonly associated with sexual transmission and injection drug use, they are bloodborne and therefore pose

SURGICAL PHARMACOLOGY

Typical Microbiologic Flora and Recommended Antimicrobial Drugs for Surgical Prophylaxis for Commonly Performed Surgical Procedures in Adults

Procedure	Typical Microorganism[a]	Recommended Antimicrobials
Cardiac	Staphylococcus aureus, CoNS, (GNR less common)	
Coronary artery bypass		Cefazolin, cefuroxime
Cardiac device insertion (e.g., pacemaker)		Cefazolin, cefuroxime
Ventricular assist device placement		Cefazolin, cefuroxime
Thoracic	S. aureus, CoNS	Cefazolin, ampicillin-sulbactam
Gastroduodenal (involving entry into the lumen of the gastrointestinal tract or without entry into lumen in high-risk patients)	Coliform GNR, streptococci, staphylococci	Cefazolin
Biliary	GNR (less commonly, anaerobes and enterococci)	
Open		Cefazolin, cefoxitin, cefotetan, ceftriaxone, ampicillin-sulbactam
Laparoscopic, high risk		Cefazolin, cefoxitin, cefotetan, ceftriaxone, ampicillin-sulbactam
Appendectomy	GNR, anaerobes	Cefoxitin, cefotetan, cefazolin + metronidazole
Colorectal	GNR, anaerobes (especially Bacteroides fragilis and Escherichia coli)	Cefazolin + metronidazole, cefoxitin, cefotetan, ampicillin-sulbactam, ceftriaxone + metronidazole, ertapenem; IV agent used along with mechanical bowel preparation and oral antimicrobial (neomycin sulfate + erythromycin base or neomycin sulfate + metronidazole)
Neurosurgery (craniotomy, CSF shunting, intrathecal pump implantation)	S. aureus, CoNS	Cefazolin
Cesarean section	S. aureus, streptococci, enterococci, vaginal anaerobes	Cefazolin
Hysterectomy (vaginal or abdominal)	S. aureus, streptococci, enterococci, vaginal anaerobes	Cefazolin, cefoxitin, cefotetan, ampicillin-sulbactam
Orthopedic	S. aureus, CoNS, streptococci, GNR (Propionibacterium spp. in shoulder procedures)	
Clean procedure of hand, knee, and foot without implantation of foreign materials		None
Spinal procedures, hip fracture repair, internal fixation procedure, total joint arthroplasty		Cefazolin
Urologic	GNR (E. coli), rarely enterococci	
Lower tract instrumentation (includes transrectal prostate biopsy)		Fluoroquinolone, trimethoprim-sulfamethoxazole, cefazolin
Clean procedure (with or without entry into urinary tract		Cefazolin (single-dose aminoglycoside may be added for placement of prosthetic material)
Clean contaminated		Cefazolin + metronidazole, cefoxitin
Vascular	S. aureus, CoNS	Cefazolin

[a]Staphylococci will be associated with SSIs after all types of operations.

CoNS, Coagulase-negative staphylococci; *CSF,* cerebrospinal fluid; *GNR,* gram-negative rods/bacilli; *IV,* intravenous.

From Talbot TR: Surgical site infections and antimicrobial prophylaxis. In Bennett JE et al, editor: *Mandell, Douglas, and Bennett's principles and practice of infectious diseases,* ed 8, Philadelphia, 2015, Elsevier.

appreciative risk to perioperative personnel. There is no risk of hepatitis B infection in persons who have been vaccinated and developed immunity. For an unvaccinated person, the risk from a single needlestick or cut is 6% to 30%, depending on the hepatitis B e antigen (HBeAg) status of the source patient. Persons who are both hepatitis B surface antigen (HBsAg) and HBeAg positive have more circulating virus in the blood and carry a greater chance of transmitting HBV. Although there is limited research concerning the transmission risk of HCV, it is estimated at 1.8% after a needlestick or cut. The projected risk of HIV transmission is 0.3% (1 in 300) or more simply, 99.7% of needlesticks or cut exposures do *not* result in HIV infection. If exposure occurs, appropriate postexposure management should take place as a part of the workplace safety program. The source patient should be informed of the incident. Serology testing should be done per institutional policy and governmental requirements. Policies should be established for instances in which source patient consent cannot be obtained. The healthcare worker should be counseled about the risk of infection, and he or she should be evaluated clinically using serology testing for evidence of HIV infection and baseline hepatitis B and C serology as soon as possible after exposure. Postexposure prophylaxis (PEP) regimens should be supervised by an expert in the management of exposures (e.g., infectious disease provider); follow-up should be provided for adherence to PEP and adverse events, including serological testing for seroconversion. Postexposure management should be treated as an urgent medical condition given the window of opportunity for PEP medication to be effective in preventing the transmission of HIV (CDC, 2017).

The US Public Health Service has made the following recommendations for the management of healthcare workers who have had occupational exposure to blood and/or other potentially infectious body fluids that may contain HIV. Summary of recommendations: PEP is recommended when occupational exposure occurs and should be started as soon as possible after the exposure (i.e., within 72 hours) and continued for 4 weeks postexposure. The newer antiretroviral raltegravir (Isentress), 400 mg, orally, twice daily and tenofovir DF/emtricitabine, 300 mg/200 mg (Truvada) once daily by mouth is the preferred HIV PEP regimen, in addition to updating tetanus vaccine as indicated. An expert consultation should be arranged within 72 hours (e.g., with an infectious disease specialist) and with postexposure follow-up testing for HIV and HCV at baseline, 6 weeks, 12 weeks, and 6 months postexposure (Kuhar et al., 2013).

Multidrug-Resistant Organisms

Over the last decade, the microbiology of SSIs changed because of the emergence of MDROs. MDROs are defined as bacteria that are resistant to one specific antibiotic (e.g., MRSA or VRE). Although the names are specific to a single antibiotic, MDROs, as the name implies, are usually MDR, and it is not uncommon for these microorganisms to be resistant to most available antibiotics. Although the percentage of SSIs caused by MRSA declined from 48% in 2007 to 43.7% in 2010 (the latest date for which data are available), a concerning proportion of SSIs were caused by MDR gram-negative organisms (Table 4.1) (CDC, 2006).

Perioperative Considerations

About 7% of patients screen positive for MRSA, and although the incidence of MRSA-SSI is 1%, MRSA colonization is associated with worse outcomes and a higher risk of both MRSA-SSI and SSI overall. Patients colonized with MRSA pose a greater risk of MRSA-SSI; therefore both the use of a MRSA preoperative decolonization protocol and the use of vancomycin intraoperatively have been explored. The most recent guidelines from the American College of Surgeons and the Surgical Infection Society recommend the use of MRSA bundles, including MRSA screening, decolonization, contact precautions, and vancomycin antibiotic prophylaxis. Decolonization protocols must take place close to the time of surgery to be effective. Usual decolonization protocols include the application of 2% nasal mupirocin twice daily for 5 days and bathing with chlorhexidine gluconate (CHG) on days 1, 2, and 3 preoperatively. It is important to note that the use of vancomycin in a patient who is MRSA negative places him or her at higher risk for a methicillin-sensitive *S. aureus* SSI. Conversion of a MRSA-negative status to positive and the development of an SSI have been reported among patients of advanced age from the use of vancomycin antibiotic prophylaxis (Ban et al., 2016).

A primary reason for concern about MDROs is that options for treating patients with these infections are often extremely limited, and MDRO infections are associated with increased lengths of stay, increased costs, and increased mortality. Many of these traits associated with MDROs have also been observed for *Clostridium difficile* infection *(C. diff.)*. In most cases, MDRO infections present the same as infections by susceptible pathogens; however, although antibiotics are now available for the treatment of MRSA and VRE, resistance to each new generation of antibiotics has already emerged. Higher case fatalities have been associated with MRSA infections such as bacteremia, poststernotomy mediastinitis, and SSIs. In the past patient acquisition of MRSA, VRE, or *C. diff.* was more prevalent among intensive care patients, patients in tertiary care facilities, and patients in long-term care facilities. However, because of the selective pressure

TABLE 4.1

Percentage of Surgical Site Infection Pathogen Isolates Resistant to Selected Antimicrobial Agents, National Healthcare Safety Network, 2009–2010

Pathogen	No. of Isolates Tested	Percentage of Isolates Resistant (%)
Staphylococcus aureus		
Resistant to oxacillin/methicillin (MRSA)	6304	43.7
Enterococcus faecium		
Resistant to vancomycin (VRE)	509	62.3
Escherichia coli		
Extended-spectrum cephalosporin resistant	1627	10.9
Carbapenem resistant	1330	2.0
Multidrug resistant	1390	1.6
Pseudomonas aeruginosa		
Extended-spectrum cephalosporin resistant	1097	10.2
Fluoroquinolone resistant	1111	16.9
Carbapenem resistant	872	11.0
Multidrug resistant	1053	5.3
***Enterobacter* spp.**		
Extended-spectrum cephalosporin resistant	816	27.7
Carbapenem resistant	594	2.4
Multidrug resistant	648	1.7
***Klebsiella* spp.**		
Extended-spectrum cephalosporin resistant	710	13.2
Carbapenem resistant	582	7.9
Multidrug resistant	621	6.8
***Acinetobacter* spp.**		
Carbapenem resistant	102	37.3
Multidrug resistant	114	43.9

MRSA, Methicillin-resistant *Staphylococcus aureus; VRE,* vancomycin-resistant enterococci. From Talbot TR: Surgical site infections and antimicrobial prophylaxis. In Bennett JE et al, editors: *Mandell, Douglas and Bennett's principles and practice of infectious diseases,* ed 8, Philadelphia, 2015, Elsevier.

by exposure to antibiotics, particularly fluoroquinolones outside of the intensive care unit (ICU) and in the community, there are increasing community-acquired MRSA colonization and infections. The primary mode of transmission for MDROs is most likely direct contact transmission from the hands of healthcare personnel. The organism has been recovered from the hands of personnel after they touched contaminated material and before they washed their hands. It also has been shown that MRSA can be carried in the nares of personnel and transferred to patients by hand contact. The importance of hand hygiene cannot be overemphasized (AORN, 2016i; CDC, 2006). Because MDROs and *C. diff.* are transmitted by contact, perioperative protocols should be used when caring for these patients. They should include the following:

• Segregate the patient, using Contact Precaution guidelines.
• Wear a gown and gloves whenever there is potential for contact with contaminated fluids or materials.

- Implement strict hand hygiene practices.
- Limit patient transportation to essential movement only.
- Clean and disinfect patient care equipment as close as possible to the time of use (AORN, 2016i).

The threat of emerging MDROs continues to grow with the emergence of a truly pan-drug–resistant strain of *E. coli*. In August 2016 a strain of *E. coli* was identified to be resistant to polymyxin E (colistin). Colistin is one of the last resort antibiotics for the treatment of highly resistant bacteria (McGann et al., 2016). *E. coli* is frequently a cause of bacteremia and urinary tract infections. Most of the MDR strains are community acquired from food and water. There seems to be a direct link between the misuse of antibiotics in food animals and the emergence of this resistant strain of *E. coli* (Johnson et al., 2009). Regulatory and accrediting agencies have taken steps to force healthcare organizations to take responsibility for antibiotic stewardship.

Antibiotic Stewardship

Although antibiotics have transformed the practice of medicine, there is no mistake that the misuse and overuse of antibiotics has created an international problem of MDR bacteria. All antibiotic use carries a risk of contributing to the development of antibiotic resistance. It is well known that the use of antibiotics increases the potential risk for a patient to develop *C. diff.*, which may result in life-threatening diarrhea. In 2009 the CDC launched a campaign to promote improved use of antibiotics in acute care hospitals. In the United States alone about 2 million people will acquire serious antibiotic-resistant infection each year. In 2014 the CDC recommended that all acute care hospitals implement an antibiotic stewardship program. This is a multidisciplinary approach in establishing strategies to improve antibiotic use, while decreasing the potential for further antibiotic resistance. Of specific concern to the perioperative registered nurse (RN) is the use of antibiotics in irrigation solutions. Three major concerns have been raised as it relates to antibiotic irrigation (AORN, 2016a).

1. The mixing of antibiotics with prosthetic cement may slowly leach out depositing subtherapeutic levels of the medication in the surrounding tissue, as a precursor to antimicrobial resistance.
2. Antibiotics used in irrigation and/or prosthetic cement may be absorbed in the patient's surrounding tissue or into the bloodstream with the potential to result in acute renal failure.
3. The mixing of irrigation solutions with a medication should not be performed in the OR but compounded by a pharmacist under a pharmacy compounding hood under strict sterile conditions. Solutions for irrigation mixed in the OR could more easily become contaminated with an infectious pathogen.

The CDC has outlined the following core elements of an antibiotic stewardship program.

- *Leadership Commitment:* Dedicating necessary human, financial, and information technology resources.
- *Accountability:* Appointing a single leader responsible for program outcomes. Experience with successful programs shows that a physician leader is effective.
- *Drug Expertise:* Appointing a single pharmacist leader responsible for working to improve antibiotic use.
- *Action:* Implementing at least one recommended action, such as systemic evaluation of ongoing treatment need after a set period of initial treatment (i.e., antibiotic stop time after 48 hours).
- *Tracking:* Monitoring antibiotic prescribing and resistance patterns.

- *Reporting:* Regular reporting information on antibiotic use and resistance to doctors, nurses, and relevant staff.
- *Education:* Educating clinicians about resistance and optimal prescribing (CDC, 2014).

Multidrug-Resistant Mycobacterium Tuberculosis (MDR-TB). Outbreaks of tuberculosis (TB) have heightened concern about healthcare-associated transmission of this disease. Transmission is most likely to occur from patients with unrecognized pulmonary or laryngeal TB and those who do not take their TB medication regularly. Populations at greatest risk of developing TB or MDR-TB are the elderly, indigent, minorities, immigrants from countries in which TB and MDR-TB are prevalent, and HIV-infected individuals (CDC, 2016c). Transmission also occurs because of procedures such as bronchoscopy, endotracheal intubation, endotracheal suctioning, and open abscess irrigation, inclusive of inadequate equipment disinfection. Extensively drug-resistant (XDR) TB (XDR-TB) is now a threat in many Asian countries and the former Soviet Union. This strain of TB is very difficult to treat because of its resistance to the primary medications used to treat TB (e.g., isoniazid and rifampin) as well as many of the secondary medications used (e.g., fluoroquinolone, amikacin, kanamycin, and capreomycin) (Mase et al., 2013).

The CDC's *Guidelines for Preventing the Transmission of Mycobacterium Tuberculosis in Health-Care Settings* (last published in 2005) emphasized the following:

- Importance of control measures, including engineering controls and personal respiratory protection, including fit-tested, personal respirators when indicated
- Use of risk assessment to develop a TB-control plan
- Early detection and treatment of patients with TB
- Screening programs for healthcare workers
- Training and education for healthcare workers
- Evaluation of the TB-control program (CDC, 2005)

Management of New and Emerging Microorganism of Perioperative Significance

Prions: Creutzfeldt-Jakob Disease. Creutzfeldt-Jakob disease (CJD) is an infectious, human prion disease that is a fatal neurodegenerative disease of the central nervous system. CJD is one of a group of encephalopathies known as *transmissible spongiform encephalopathies (TSEs)*. Other human forms of TSE are Gerstmann-Sträussler-Scheinker syndrome and *new variant CJD (nvCJD)* or *variant CJD (vCJD)* (CDC, 2015a).

CJD is caused by a self-replicating prion. Prions are a unique class of organisms that have no detectable DNA or RNA. These small proteinaceous agents are abnormal isoforms of normal cellular proteins. The incubation period for CJD varies from months to years to decades. Symptoms include rapidly progressing dementia, memory loss, rapid physical and mental deterioration, and a distinctive electroencephalogram reading. Positive diagnosis can be made only by direct examination of affected brain tissue. Most cases occur randomly and for unknown reasons when the patient is between 50 and 75 years old. Death typically occurs within 1 year of symptom onset. In contrast, vCJD has an earlier onset (between 18 and 41 years of age). Patients exhibit initial psychiatric symptoms and then neurologic symptoms differing from those of CJD, and the course of illness averages 14 months. The disease is always fatal. According to the CDC, there is strong epidemiologic and laboratory evidence to support a causal association between vCJD and bovine spongiform encephalopathy (also known as *mad cow disease*).

CJD can be familial (i.e., inherited in the form of a mutant gene) or sporadic (no family history and no known source of transmission).

Approximately 90% of cases are sporadic. Only about 1% of cases result from person-to-person transmission, and those are primarily the result of iatrogenic (medically related) exposure. Exposures have occurred via transplantation of contaminated central nervous system tissue, such as dura mater or corneas, from injections of pituitary hormone extracts, and by use of contaminated surgical instruments or stereotactic depth electrodes (CDC, 2015a).

CJD and other TSEs are unusually resistant to conventional chemical and physical decontamination methods. The causative prions are resistant to steam autoclaving, dry heat, ethylene oxide (EO) gas, and chemical disinfection with formaldehyde or glutaraldehyde as normally used in the healthcare environment (AORN, 2016d). Glutaraldehyde and formaldehyde act as fixatives, causing the prions to become more stable and less susceptible to normal sterilization/disinfection protocols. Special protocols for instrument care after exposure to prions should be followed (AAMI, 2013a). Some institutions use disposable instrument sets for diagnostic brain biopsies to rule out CJD or TSE. Processes being investigated for cleaning and sterilizing devices contaminated with prions include the use of an alkaline cleaning agent and vaporized hydrogen peroxide (VHP) sterilization. Protocols for handling CJD are evolving as researchers learn more about prions and their destruction. Table 4.2 lists options from which an acceptable protocol for care of instruments and equipment exposed to the CJD prion can be developed (Rutala and Weber, 2010).

Carbapenem-Resistant Enterobacteriaceae. The OR is a unique practice setting demanding that perioperative nurses also function as infection preventionists. This requires meticulous care when it

TABLE 4.2

Care of Items Exposed to the Creutzfeldt-Jakob Disease Prion

Tissue Infectivity	Item/Device (Using Spaulding Classification System)	Cleanable	Heat/Moisture Stable	Disposition
High infectivity	Critical/semicritical instruments/devices	If easily cleaned	If yes	1. Thoroughly clean with detergent germicide 2. Autoclave at 272°F (134°C) prevacuum sterilizer for 18 min (extended cycle) *or* 3. Autoclave instruments at 121°C (250°F) in gravity sterilizer for 1 h *or* 4. Immerse in 1N NaOH (1 normal sodium hydroxide) for 60 min at room temperature After 60 min, remove items from 1N NaOH, rinse, and steam sterilize at 250°F (121°C) in gravity sterilizer or 273°F (134°C) for 1 h 5. After processing, according to one of previous options, prepare instruments in usual fashion and sterilize for future use
			If no	Discard
	Critical/semicritical instruments/devices	If impossible to clean	NA	Discard
	Noncritical instruments/devices	If cleanable	NA	1. Clean according to routine procedures 2. Disinfect with a 1:5–1:10 dilution of sodium hypochlorite (bleach) or 1N NaOH, choosing solution that would be least damaging to items 3. Continue processing according to routine procedures
		Noncleanable	NA	Discard
	Environmental surfaces	NA	NA	1. Cover surface with plastic-backed sheet 2. Incinerate material after use 3. Clean with detergent then spot decontaminate with a surface with 1:5–1:10 dilution of sodium hypochlorite (bleach), preferable 15-min contact time 4. Wipe entire surface using routine facility decontamination procedures for surface decontamination
Medium/low/no infectivity	Critical/semicritical/noncritical instruments/devices	Cleanable	NA	Clean, disinfect, or sterilize according to routine procedures
		Noncleanable	NA	Discard
	Environmental surfaces	NA	NA	1. Cover surface with disposable, impermeable material 2. Dispose of material according to facility policy 3. Disinfect surface with OSHA-recommended agent for decontamination of blood-contaminated surfaces (e.g., 1:10 or 1:100 dilution of sodium hypochlorite [bleach])

Note: Research into processing of medical devices contaminated with prions is ongoing, and institutional policies relating to processing of prion-contaminated devices should periodically consult the World Health Organization and the Centers for Disease Control and Prevention to determine whether recommendations have changed.

NA, Not applicable; *OSHA*, Occupational Safety and Health Administration.

Modified from Rutala W, Weber D: Guideline for disinfection and sterilization of prion-contaminated medical instruments, *Infect Control Hosp Epidemiol* 31(2):107–117, 2010.

comes to environmental cleaning; disinfection and sterilization; use of antiseptics and antibiotics; equipment reprocessing; adherence to the principles of sterile technique; surgical attire; and competent performance in the application of perioperative guidelines, principles, and policy. There has been an increased focus on the reprocessing of endoscopes and equipment with reports linking failed disinfection and sterilization processes to clustered outbreaks of carbapenem-resistant Enterobacteriaceae (CRE) in patients undergoing endoscopic retrograde cholangiopancreatography (ERCP). This and similar outbreaks linked to transmission of hepatitis C have resulted a collaboration between infection control practitioners, perioperative personnel, endoscopists, and sterile processing personnel working with the industry to improve reprocessing and explore the development of disposable endoscopes (O'Horo et al., 2016).

Mycobacterium chimaera. A more recent emerging infectious agent of concern has been the transmission of a nontuberculous *Mycobacterium* (NTM) associated with the Stöckert heater-cooler units used during open-heart surgery. The CDC issued an alert October 13, 2016, warning healthcare providers and patients about the risk of infection with *Mycobacterium chimaera* from this specific device. The heater-cooler units are thought to have been contaminated with *M. chimaera* during the manufacturing process. *M. chimaera* is commonly found in the environment (e.g., soil, water) and rarely is a cause of infection. It is believed that the device aerosolized the bacteria into the OR during surgery with subsequent contamination of the surgical wound. The CDC issued a Health Alert Notice that patients who have had open-heart surgery using the Stöckert heater-cooler device and are having symptoms (e.g., night sweats, muscle aches, weight loss, fatigue, unexplained fever) should seek further medical evaluation. The risk of contracting an infection from *M. chimaera* is between 1 in 100 and 1 in 1000. Both the CDC and equipment manufacturers recommend performing routine bacterial cultures as a means of monitoring the cleaning and disinfection of this equipment. Further information to help organizations and healthcare providers identify and inform patients who might be at risk is available online at the CDC's website (CDC, 2016b).

Ebola. In this era of global transportation it is most likely that an infectious pathogen can be spread across the globe in a matter of hours or within a day by an infected traveler. Such was the scenario in 2003 with severe acute respiratory syndrome (SARS) and more recently with the threat posed by Ebola. Although the natural reservoir of Ebola is not clearly understood, scientists believe a human becomes infected through contact with an infected animal such as a fruit bat or primate. This mode of transmission is called a "spillover event." Once an infection occurs in humans it can be spread from one human to another through direct contact with blood or body fluids. Ebola is not airborne or spread by water or by food. However, in Africa, Ebola may be spread by the ingestion of wild animals, or bushmeat, whose meat is partially cooked, which allows the live virus to be ingested. Healthcare providers caring for Ebola patients are at risk if they come in close contact with infected patients' blood or body fluids. The CDC recommends focusing on PPE and environmental infection control measures that include a single patient room, dedicated, preferably disposable medical equipment, limited use of needles and sharps with heightened awareness to sharp safety, avoiding aerosol-generating procedures, and vigilant hand hygiene. Meticulous application and removal of PPE has been the cornerstone of preventing the transmission of Ebola within the healthcare setting (CDC, 2015b).

Zika. Zika is a mosquito-borne disease that gained international attention in 2015 when it was linked to severe birth defects (e.g.,

microcephaly). Again, because of the ease of international travel, what was once confined to South America was soon reported in the southern United States. Although Zika is primarily spread though the bite of an infected *Aedes* mosquito, it can be transmitted sexually or from a pregnant woman to her fetus. Healthcare workers exposed to the blood or body fluids of an infected person may be at risk. Many people who have Zika may be asymptomatic or present with mild symptoms of fever, rash, joint pain, red eyes, muscle pain, and headache. Both the symptoms and the infection are self-limiting. The best treatment is prevention and mosquito control. Zika is not a surgical disease, and typically patients with Zika will not require any surgical intervention. Perioperative personnel caring for patients with Zika should follow standard blood and body fluid precautions. There have been no confirmed cases of Zika virus transmission in healthcare settings in the United States (CDC, 2016a).

Preventing Infection

Asepsis

The term *asepsis* means the absence of infectious organisms. Asepsis is directed at cleanliness and the elimination of all infectious agents. Surgical asepsis is designed to exclude all microbes, whereas medical asepsis is designed to exclude microbes associated with communicable diseases. Practices that restrict microorganisms in the environment and on equipment and supplies and that prevent normal body flora from contaminating the surgical wound are termed *aseptic techniques.* The goal of each aseptic practice is to optimize primary wound healing, prevent surgical infection, and minimize the length of recovery from surgery. For perioperative practitioners, surgical aseptic principles and practices are the foundation for infection control efforts in the perioperative arena.

Infection control practices should primarily focus on prevention. Transmission of infection involves a chain of events, including the presence of a pathogenic agent, reservoir, portal of exit, transmission, portal of entry, and host susceptibility. Prevention occurs when there is a break in the chain of transmission. Infection control practices involve personal and administrative measures. Personal measures should include fitness for work and application of aseptic principles. Administrative measures should include provision of adequate physical facilities, appropriate surgical supplies, and operational controls in the perioperative area. Standards for inpatient and outpatient settings should be established and followed (Ambulatory Surgery Considerations).

As new organisms emerge, and known organisms become more resistant, the importance of patient education as a risk-reduction strategy cannot be minimized. In addition to practicing sound infection control practices, nurses partner with the patient through effective education about infection control measures to maximize the potential for perioperative safe care (Patient, Family, and Caregiver Education).

Universal, Standard, and Transmission-Based Precautions
Universal Precautions

In 1987, in response to the growing concern over the occupational risk posed by HIV, and a better understanding of the occupational risk posed by other bloodborne pathogens (e.g., HBV, HCV) the CDC published recommendations for the use of Universal Precautions (CDC, 1987, 1988).

With knowledge that many patients with bloodborne infections are undiagnosed, Universal Precautions, for the first time, placed emphasis on applying Blood and Body Fluid Precautions universally

AMBULATORY SURGERY CONSIDERATIONS

Infection Prevention in Ambulatory Settings

The CDC notes that more than three-quarters of all operations in the United States are performed on an outpatient basis. Care provided in outpatient settings must minimize or eliminate the risks of HAIs. In response to outbreaks of the transmission of gram-negative and gram-positive bacteria, mycobacteria, viruses, and parasites in ambulatory settings, the CDC published the *Guide to Infection Prevention for Outpatient Settings: Minimum Expectations for Safe Care*. The document represents the absolute minimum for safe care in ambulatory care settings. The fundamental elements needed to prevent the transmission of infectious agents in ambulatory care settings include the following:

- Implement administrative measures.
  - Develop and maintain infection prevention and occupational health programs.
  - Ensure sufficient and appropriate supplies necessary for adherence to Standard Precautions (e.g., hand hygiene products, PPE, use safe injection practices).
  - Ensure at least one individual with training in infection prevention is employed by or regularly available to the facility.
  - Develop written infection prevention policies and procedures appropriate for the services provided by the facility and based on evidence-based guidelines, regulations, or standards.
- Educate and train healthcare personnel.
  - Provide job- or task-specific infection prevention education and training to all HCP.

- Ensure training focuses on principles of both HCP safety and patient safety and they are presented at employee orientation and repeated regularly (e.g., annually).
  - Complete initial and repeated documented competencies as appropriate for the specific HCP positions.
- Monitor and report HAIs.
  - Adhere to local, state, and federal requirements regarding HAI surveillance, reportable diseases, and outbreak reporting.
  - Perform regular audits and competency evaluations of HCP adherence to infection prevention practices:
    - Adherence to Standard Precautions.
    - Observation of sound practices for hand hygiene.
    - Utilization of PPE.
    - Observation of safe injection practices.
    - Observation of respiratory hygiene/cough etiquette.
- Provide for cleaning and disinfection of environmental surfaces.
- Provide for cleaning, disinfecting, and/or sterilizing medical equipment.

A wealth of information regarding infection prevention in ambulatory settings is available from a variety of sources, including a checklist published by the CMS. The checklist captures all the elements of a sound infection prevention program and is a valuable resource for establishing and maintaining a program.

CDC, Centers for Disease Control and Prevention; *CMS,* Centers for Medicare and Medicaid Services. *HAI,* healthcare-associated infection; *HCP,* healthcare personnel; *PPE,* personnel protective equipment.
Modified from Centers for Disease Control and Prevention (CDC): *Guide to infection prevention in outpatient settings: minimum expectations for safe care* (website), 2016. www.cdc.gov/hai/settings/outpatient/outpatient-care-guidelines.html. (Accessed 4 February 2017). Centers for Medicare and Medicaid Services (CMS): *Ambulatory surgical center infection control surveyor worksheet* (website), 2015. www.cms.gov/Regulations-and-Guidance/Guidance/Manuals/downloads/som107_exhibit_351.pdf. (Accessed 4 February 2017). Oregon Patient Safety Commission: *Oregon Ambulatory Surgery Center Infection prevention and control toolkit* (website), 2016. http://oregonpatientsafety.org/healthcare-professionals/infection-prevention-toolkit/. (Accessed 4 February 2017).

to all individuals regardless of their presumed transmissible status. Universal Precautions expanded the Blood and Body Fluid Precautions by recommending masks and eye protection to prevent mucous membrane exposures in addition to the routine use of barrier protection, such as gowns and gloves. Universal Precautions also emphasized the prevention of needlestick injuries and the use of ventilation devices when resuscitation was performed. The CDC continued to recommend the use of Universal Precautions until 1988, when a new system of isolation precautions called *Body Substance Isolation* (BSI) was proposed. BSI directed isolation of *all* moist and potentially infectious body substances (e.g., blood, feces, urine, sputum, saliva, wound drainage, other body fluids) for all individuals regardless of their infectious status. This was accomplished primarily with the use of gowns and gloves. Because of the similarities yet differences between Universal Precautions and BSI, confusion reigned. In 2007 the CDC further expanded the "Guidelines for Isolation Precautions" (CDC, 1988).

The OSHA Bloodborne Pathogens Standard 29 CFR 1910.1030(d)(1) is intended to reduce or eliminate the probability of an occupational exposure to a bloodborne pathogen. Employers are required to implement an exposure control plan that details policies and procedures for employee safety. This plan must explain how the employer will use engineering and work-practice controls, provide

PPE, training and education, surveillance, hepatitis B vaccine, and postexposure follow-up. These standards are based on the concept of Universal Precautions. OSHA's Bloodborne Pathogens Standard requires employees to practice Universal Precautions to prevent direct contact with blood or other potentially infectious materials (OPIM), to consider *all* body fluids as potentially infectious with the use of gloves, masks, and gowns, if blood or OPIM exposure is indicated, and by using engineering and work-practice controls (OSHA, 2012a). The following is a summary of the requirements of the OSHA's Bloodborne Pathogens Standard:

1. Each facility must develop and implement an exposure control plan that defines exposure and implements the requirements of the final rule. This plan is to be reviewed and revised annually with information provided to all employees. The plan must reflect changes in available technology to reduce exposure to bloodborne pathogens and implementation of appropriate technology to that end. Nonmanagerial employee input must be solicited in selecting technology to be implemented in the practice setting.
2. Engineering and work-practice controls must be used to eliminate or minimize employee exposure. The following are examples:
   a. The employer must provide necessary equipment, soaps, and antiseptics for proper hand hygiene.

PATIENT, FAMILY, AND CAREGIVER EDUCATION

Patient Education for Surgical Site Infection Prevention

TJC has established several NPSGs to provide organizational guidance for key patient safety issues. One of these goals, NPSG 7, focuses on how organizations reduce the patient's risk for developing an HAI. In addition to implementing hand hygiene measures and other evidence-based practices to prevent HAIs and SSIs, organizations are also required to provide adequate education about SSI prevention to patients having surgical procedures as well as their families. Education can be provided by any means the organization chooses (e.g., printed materials, verbal teaching, classes), but there must be some documentation within the patient's record that the education occurred. Items that might be included in a patient handout are included below.

Millions of people have surgery each year. Every surgery has risks, but some can be prevented. One way for patients to help lower their risk for problems from surgery is to learn about some of the things that can cause infection and talk with a member of their surgical care team before surgery about the type of care they should receive. The following are some questions that patients often ask about SSIs.

What Is a Surgical Site Infection?

An SSI is an infection that occurs after surgery in the part of the body where the surgery took place. Most patients who have surgery do not develop an infection. However, infections develop in about 1 to 3 out of every 100 patients who have surgery.

The following are some of the common symptoms of an SSI:
- Redness and pain around the area where you had surgery
- Drainage of cloudy foul-smelling fluid or pus from your surgical wound
- Fever

Can Surgical Site Infections Be Treated?

Yes. Most SSIs can be treated with antibiotics. The antibiotic given to you depends on the bacteria (germs) causing the infection. Sometimes patients with SSIs also need another surgery to treat the infection.

What Are Some of the Practices Performed in Healthcare Facilities to Prevent Surgical Site Infections?

To prevent SSIs, physicians, nurses, and other healthcare providers do the following:
- Clean their hands and arms up to their elbows with an antiseptic agent just before the surgery.
- Clean their hands with soap and water or an alcohol-based hand rub before and after caring for each patient.
- May remove some of your hair immediately before surgery (if necessary) using electric clippers if the hair is in the same area where the procedure will occur. Personnel should not shave you with a razor. Using a razor to remove hair before surgery can lead to an infection because of the risk of leaving small cuts on the skin in which bacteria can grow and possibly gain access to the surgical wound.

- Wear special hair covers, masks, gowns, and gloves during surgery to keep the surgery area clean.
- Administer antibiotics before your surgery starts. In most cases, antibiotics are given within 60 minutes before the surgery starts and should be stopped within 24 hours after surgery. Given properly, antibiotics can greatly lower your chances of getting an infection after surgery.
- Clean the skin at the site of your surgery with a special soap that kills germs.

What Can I Do to Help Prevent Surgical Site Infections?

Before your surgery:
- Tell your physician about other medical problems you may have. Health problems such as allergies, diabetes, and obesity could affect your surgery and your treatment.
- Quit smoking. Patients who smoke get more infections. Talk to your doctor about how you can quit before your surgery.
- Do not shave near where you will have surgery. Shaving with a razor can irritate your skin and make it easier for bacteria to proliferate and to develop an infection.

At the time of your surgery:
- Speak up if someone tries to shave you with a razor before surgery. Ask why you need to be shaved and talk with your surgeon if you have any concerns.
- Ask if you will get antibiotics before surgery.

After your surgery:
- Make sure that your healthcare providers clean their hands before examining you; either with soap and water or with an alcohol-based hand rub. *If you do not see your providers clean their hands, please ask them to do so.*
- Do not let family and friends who visit you touch the surgical wound or dressings.
- Ask family and friends to wash their hands with soap and water or an alcohol-based hand rub before and after visiting you. If you do not see them clean their hands, ask them to do so.

What Do I Need to Do When I Go Home From the Healthcare Facility?

- Make sure you understand how to care for your wound before you leave the hospital. Your physician or nurse should explain everything you need to know about taking care of your wound.
- Always clean your hands before and after caring for your wound.
- Make sure you know who to contact if you have questions or problems after you get home.
- Call your physician immediately if you have any symptoms of an infection, such as redness and pain at the surgery site, drainage, or fever.

If you have additional questions, please ask your physician or nurse.

HAI, Healthcare-associated infection; *NPSGs,* National Safety Patient Goals; *SSI,* surgical site infection; *TJC,* The Joint Commission.
Modified from Centers for Disease Control and Prevention (CDC): *Frequently asked questions about surgical site infections* (website), 2016. www.cdc.gov/hai/ssi/faq_ssi.html. (Accessed 14 January 2017). Centers for Disease Control and Prevention (CDC): *What you should know before your surgery* (website), 2016. www.cdc.gov/features/safesurgery/index.html. (Accessed 14 January 2017).

b. Contaminated needles must not be recapped or removed unless such action is required by a specific medical procedure. Such recapping or removal must be accomplished using a mechanical device or one-handed technique.

c. A clamp or other mechanical device should be used to disassemble a knife blade and handle.

d. Sharps are to be placed in labeled or color-coded, puncture-resistant, leakproof containers for disposal.

e. Specimens of blood or body fluids must be placed in containers that prevent leakage and are labeled or color coded. Warning labels must be affixed to containers of regulated waste, refrigerators and freezers containing blood or potentially infectious materials, and other containers used to transport blood or potentially infectious materials (Fig. 4.1). The labels must be fluorescent orange or orange-red.

f. Food and drink are not to be kept in the same storage area where blood or OPIM is present.

g. PPE must be provided by the employer at no cost to the employee. Appropriate PPE shall include but is not limited to gloves, gowns, face shields or masks, and eye protection. Protective eyewear must have solid side shields. Gloves are to be worn when contact with blood or body fluids is anticipated. Disposable gloves are to be replaced as soon as possible after contamination occurs. Disposable gloves are not to be washed or decontaminated for reuse. Some facilities may have educational signs posted to assist employees in recognition of appropriate PPE (Fig. 4.2).

h. Signs must be posted at the entrance to work areas of potential contamination. These signs are to bear the biohazard legend with the following information: name of infectious agent, special requirements for entering the area, and name and telephone number of the responsible individual.

i. Housekeeping provisions are to ensure that the workplace is clean and sanitary. A written schedule for cleaning and a method of decontamination must be established. All equipment and working surfaces must be cleaned and decontaminated after contact with blood or OPIM.

j. Contaminated laundry must be placed in a labeled or color-coded container that is recognized by all employees.

k. All employees are to receive education and training about safe handling of hazardous substances and materials. Information must be provided to all occupationally exposed employees at no cost to them. Individuals must receive training at the time of employment and annually thereafter. Individual employee training records are to be maintained by the employer for the duration of employment plus 30 years. The healthcare worker is highly encouraged to receive the HBV vaccine after obtaining the required information about the risk of exposure and about the vaccine. If the employee chooses not to accept the vaccination, the employer must have the employee sign a letter of declination.

l. Employees should report all exposures to blood and body fluids for postexposure evaluation.

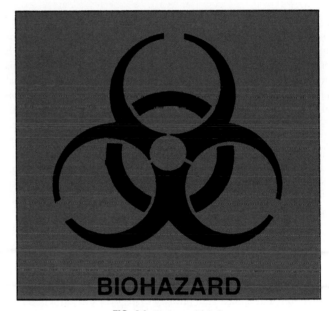

FIG. 4.1 Biohazard label.

BODY SUBSTANCE ISOLATION IS FOR ALL PATIENT CARE | BODY SUBSTANCES INCLUDE ORAL SECRETIONS, BLOOD, URINE AND FECES, WOUND OR OTHER DRAINAGE.

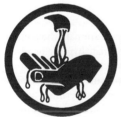
Wash hands.

Wear gloves when likely to touch body substances, mucous membranes or nonintact skin.

Wear plastic apron when clothing is likely to be soiled.

Wear mask/eye protection when likely to be splashed.

DO NOT RECAP
Place intact needle/syringe units and sharps in designated disposal container. **Do not** break or bend needles.

© 1987 San Diego Forms

FIG. 4.2 Example of universal symbols for blood and body fluid protection.

m. Employers who are required to maintain a log of occupational injuries and illnesses must maintain a sharps injury log that acts as a tool for identifying high-risk practice areas and for evaluating various devices in use. This log must protect the confidentiality of the injured employee. Log information should include the type and brand of the device, the practice area in which the injury occurred, and an explanation of how the incident occurred.

The Bloodborne Pathogen Standard is enforceable by OSHA at the federal and state levels. This regulation is based on the concept of Universal Precautions to serve and protect healthcare providers and to minimize the transfer of pathogens from one patient to another. Surveyors for OSHA may engage in onsite visits to healthcare facilities. Unannounced visits may occur at any site in which an employee exposure occurs. The visit may be a result of a verbal or written employee concern, referral from another regulatory agency, or random inspection (OSHA, 2012a).

Standard Precautions

By the early 1990s the controversy regarding Universal Precautions and BSI had escalated. There was considerable confusion about which body fluids required special care under either Universal Precautions or BSI. There were also concerns about the need for additional precautions to prevent airborne, droplet, and contact transmission of other infectious agents. The CDC developed a single set of precautions incorporating the major features of Universal Precautions and BSI. These precautions are called *Standard Precautions,* and they are designed to reduce the transmission risk of bloodborne and other pathogens. Additional precautions based on routes of transmission for patients known or suspected to be infected or colonized with highly transmissible or epidemiologically significant pathogens are included in the document.

Standard Precautions are intended to reduce the transmission of microorganisms from recognized and unrecognized sources of infection. Standard Precautions should be applied to all patients receiving care regardless of their diagnosis or presumed infection status. They are considered the first, and most important, tier of precautions and as such are a primary strategy for successful infection prevention and control. Standard Precautions apply to (1) blood, (2) all body fluids and secretions and excretions (except sweat) regardless of whether they contain visible blood, (3) mucous membranes, and (4) nonintact skin. Standard Precautions include the following:

1. *Hand hygiene.* Hand hygiene is the most important factor in preventing the spread of infection. Hands are to be washed whenever they are in contact with blood, body fluids, secretions, excretions, and contaminated items, whether or not gloves are worn. Hands are washed immediately after gloves are removed, between patient contacts, and when otherwise indicated to avoid transfer of microorganisms to other patients or environments. Sometimes it is necessary to wash hands between tasks and procedures on the same patient to prevent cross-contamination of different body sites. A plain (nonantimicrobial) soap should be used for routine handwashing. When special circumstances such as hyperendemic conditions occur, an antimicrobial soap or an antiseptic hand rub (waterless antiseptic agent) should be used. The hand rub antiseptic agent is most effective if the hands are clean before the antimicrobial agent is applied. For effectiveness, a sufficient amount of the agent must be used for the hand rub. Manufacturers' written instructions should be followed. An additional amount of hand rub agent may be necessary.

2. *Gloves.* Clean, nonsterile gloves should be worn when touching blood, body fluids, secretions, excretions, and contaminated items. Freshly donned gloves should be worn when touching mucous membranes and nonintact skin. Gloves should be changed between tasks and patient procedures and after contact with material that may contain high concentrations of organisms. Gloves should be removed immediately after use and hands washed before engaging in another task or giving care to another patient.

3. *Masks, eye protection, face shields.* A mask and eye protection or a face shield is to be worn at any time patient care activities are likely to generate sprays or splashes of blood or body fluids, secretions, and excretions. These protective devices help protect the mucous membranes of the nose, mouth, and eyes.

4. *Gowns.* Clean, nonsterile gowns are to be worn at any time patient care activities are likely to generate sprays or splashes of blood or body fluids, secretions, and excretions. Gowns help protect the skin and prevent soiling of clothing. The activity to be performed and the amount and type of fluid likely to be encountered dictate the degree of protective barrier necessary in the gown. Gowns should be removed immediately after use and hands washed before engaging in other activities or giving care to another patient.

5. *Sharps.* Needles, scalpels, and other sharps should be handled in a manner to avoid injury. Needles should never be recapped using any technique that directs the point of the needle toward any body part. If recapping is necessary, it should be done using a mechanical device or a one-handed scoop technique. Used needles should not be removed from disposable syringes, and they should not be bent, broken, or otherwise manipulated by hand. Used disposable sharps should be placed in puncture-resistant containers located as close as possible to the point-of-sharps use. Reusable sharps should be contained in a puncture-resistant container for transport to the point of decontamination.

6. *Patient care equipment.* Single-use items should be discarded after use. Reusable equipment must be cleaned and reprocessed to ensure safe use for another patient. Equipment soiled with blood, body fluids, secretions, and excretions should be handled carefully to prevent exposure of skin and mucous membranes, contamination of clothing, and transfer of organisms to patients, personnel, and the environment.

7. *Linens.* Linens soiled with blood, body fluids, secretions, or excretions should be handled in a manner to avoid skin and mucous membrane exposure; clothing contamination; and transfer of microorganisms to other patients, personnel, and the environment.

8. *Environmental control.* Adequate procedures for routine care and cleaning of environmental surfaces, beds, and associated equipment are to be developed, and the use of these procedures is monitored on a regular basis.

9. *Patient placement.* Patients who contaminate the environment or who are unable to maintain appropriate hygiene or environmental control are to be housed in a private room with appropriate air handling and ventilation. If a private room is unavailable, the infection control professional may determine a method for cohorting patients with similar infectious organisms (Siegel et al., 2007).

Transmission-Based Precautions

Transmission-Based Precautions are the second tier of infection prevention, designed for patients known or suspected to be infected by epidemiologically important pathogens spread by airborne or droplet transmission or by direct contact or indirectly by contaminated surfaces. They may be used singly or in combination with one another if the patient has a disease that has multiple routes of transmission and are to be used in addition to Standard Precautions.

Airborne Precautions. Airborne transmission occurs when disseminated small particles that contain pathogens that remain infectious over a prolonged time are inhaled (e.g., *M. tuberculous*). These particles can remain suspended in the air for long periods or by dissemination of dust particles that contain the infectious agent. This is specific to infectious particles 5 μm or smaller in size. Airborne microorganisms can be dispersed widely depending on air currents and can be inhaled by or deposited on a susceptible host. In addition to Standard Precautions, Airborne Precautions include the following:

1. Patients are to be placed in private, negative-pressure rooms. The air exchange should be at a rate of 6 to 12 exchanges per hour with air discharged to the outdoors or circulated through high-efficiency particulate-arresting (HEPA) filters before being circulated to other areas of the facility.
2. Caregivers must wear OSHA-specified respiratory protection when caring for patients with known or suspected TB. If susceptible personnel care for patients with rubeola (measles) or varicella (chickenpox), respiratory protection should be worn. If the caregiver is immune to rubeola and varicella, respiratory protection is unnecessary.
3. All precautions for preventing transmission of TB should be implemented if the patient is known or suspected to have TB.
4. A surgical mask should be placed over the patient's nose and mouth for Airborne Infection Isolation Precautions when the patient must be transported from one location to another. Patient transport should be limited to essential purposes only.

Droplet Precautions. Droplet Precautions are used for patients known or suspected to be infected with microorganisms that are transmitted by large droplets (>5 μm). These droplets can be generated when the patient sneezes, coughs, or talks. Droplet Precautions are used in addition to Standard Precautions. Droplet Precautions include the following:

1. Patients are to be placed in private rooms when available. If this is not possible, the patient should be placed in a room with another patient who is infected with the same organism and with no other infection. If this is not possible, a 3-foot spatial separation should be maintained between the infected patient and other patients in the same room. For Droplet Precautions no special air handling is required.
2. Caregivers should wear a mask when working within 3 feet of the patient.
3. Patients should be transported only for essential purposes. When transport is necessary, a mask should be placed over the patient's nose and mouth to minimize dispersal of droplets (Siegel et al., 2007).

Contact Precautions. In addition to Standard Precautions, Contact Precautions should be used for patients known or suspected to be infected or colonized with epidemiologically important organisms that can be transmitted by (1) direct contact, as occurs when the caregiver touches the patient's skin, or (2) indirect contact, as occurs when the caregiver touches patient care equipment or environmental surfaces in the patient's room. Contact Precautions include the following:

1. Patients should be placed in private rooms. If this is not possible, the patient should be placed in a room with another patient who is infected with the same organism and with no other infection.

If this is not possible, patient placement must be determined on an individual basis, depending on the organism involved.

2. Gloves should be worn on entering the patient's room. Gloves should be changed after handling infective material that might contain a high concentration of microorganisms. When patient care activities have been completed, gloves should be removed before leaving the patient's room. Hands should be washed after glove removal. To avoid transferring microorganisms to others, no environmental surfaces in the patient's environment should be touched after the hands have been washed.
3. Gowns should be worn on entering the patient's room if there is a probability that the caregiver's clothing will be in contact with the patient or the environmental surfaces or if the patient is incontinent, has diarrhea, or has an ileostomy or colostomy. The gown should be removed before leaving the patient's room, and care should be exercised to avoid contact with environmental surfaces.
4. Patient transportation should be limited to essential transport only and Contact Precautions maintained to avoid contamination of personnel, visitors, or the environment.
5. Patient care equipment should be dedicated to a single patient and not be shared between patients. If this is impossible, equipment must be cleaned and disinfected thoroughly before being used for another patient (Siegel et al., 2007).

Perioperative staff members traditionally have relied on numerous types of precautions to protect themselves and others from bloodborne pathogens and other infectious diseases. Implementing these precautions within the surgical environment requires critical thinking skills and sound nursing judgment. Consistent application of these precautions by all members of the perioperative team serves to protect the healthcare provider and to minimize cross-infection of pathogens among patients (AORN, 2016i).

Infection Control and Bioterrorism

The potential for bioterrorism is a reality. The CDC has identified agents that may pose a risk to the national security because of their (1) easy dissemination or transmission from person to person, (2) potential to cause high mortality and have a major public health impact, (3) potential to cause public panic and social disruption, and (4) necessity for special action for public health preparedness (Table 4.3) (CDC, 2016d). Perioperative personnel should have a basic knowledge and understanding of the agents most likely to be encountered and the levels of precautions required for patient and personnel safety. Communication, collaboration, and coordination are required in the face of any bioterrorist event or natural disaster. Communities need emergency plans for such matters, such as guarding patient data and protecting information systems, linking quickly and easily with state and federal resources, ensuring culturally competent communication and care, accessing mental health resources, and identifying agencies that can partner with one another to provide services. Each institution must be compliant with TJC's requirements for periodic testing of emergency management systems and their associated plans.

Engineering Practices to Prevent Infection

Environment of Care

The surgical suite should be designed in such a way as to minimize and control the spread of infectious organisms. Either a central-core, race track, or a single-corridor design may be used. With the central-core design, sterile equipment and supplies should be contained within the central-core area, which is surrounded by ORs and a peripheral corridor. The single-corridor design places the ORs on either side of a single corridor, with separate storage rooms, usually

TABLE 4.3

Bioterrorism Agents[a]

Agent	Transmission	Incubation	Symptoms	Management
Anthrax (Bacillus anthracis)	Cutaneous: Direct contact Inhalation: Droplet, aerosolization	Cutaneous: 1–7 days Inhalation: 1–6 days on average, may be as late as 2 months	Cutaneous: Itching, progressing to papular and vesicular lesions, eschar, edema, ulceration, and sloughing If untreated may spread to lymph nodes and bloodstream Fatality: 5%–20% Inhalation: Influenza-like with progression to high fever dyspnea, stridor, cyanosis, and shock Chest-wall edema and hemorrhagic meningitis may be present Death is universal in untreated cases and may occur in 95% of cases not treated within 24–36 h	Standard Precautions Special attention should be given to protection and containment of any draining wounds, inclusive of cutaneous lesions
Smallpox (variola major/ variola minor viruses)	Usually prolonged face-to-face contact is required Also spread through direct contact with infected body fluids or contaminated objects Rarely spread by virus carried in the air	Typically 12–14 days	High fever, malaise, head and body aches, and sometimes vomiting Rash develops over face and spreads to extremities Rash soon becomes vesicular and then pustular All lesions progress at same rate Fever continues throughout course of disease, and growing and expanding pustules are very painful Historical, variola major fatality rate is at 30%	Standard, Droplet, Airborne, and Contact Precautions for patients with vesicular rash pending diagnosis Avoid contact with organism while handling contaminated bedding Wear protective attire to include gloves, gown, and N95 respirator Vaccine does not give reliable lifelong immunity Previously vaccinated persons are considered susceptible After exposure, initiate Airborne Precautions and observe for unprotected contact (from days 10–17) Vaccinate within 2–3 days of exposure One case is a public health emergency because of highly communicable nature of this disease Consult CDC and local health agencies at earliest opportunity
Plague (Yersinia pestis)	Pneumonic plague: Aerosolized bacteria carried on respiratory droplets from infected person Bubonic plague: Bites from fleas or infected rodent Does not spread from person to person	Pneumonic plague: 1–3 days Bubonic plague: 2–8 days	Pneumonic: Fever, headache, and weakness, with rapid progression to pneumonia with dyspnea, chest pain, cough, and bloody or watery sputum Respiratory failure and shock may follow within 2–4 days Bubonic: Symptoms include swollen, tender lymph nodes (buboes), fever, headache, chills, and weakness	Standard and Droplet Precautions Patients should be placed in private rooms or cohorted with "like" patients Transport should be limited to essential movement only, and patient should wear mask during transport Contact Precautions until decontamination is complete

TABLE 4.3

Bioterrorism Agents[a]—cont'd

Agent	Transmission	Incubation	Symptoms	Management
Tularemia (*Francisella tularensis*)	Bites of ticks, deerflies, and other arthropods that have eaten infected animal tissue; by handling infected animal carcasses; by eating or drinking contaminated food or water; or by inhaling infected aerosols	1–14 days (average 3–5 days)	Depending on route of exposure, skin ulcers, inflamed eyes, sore throat, oral ulcers, swollen and painful lymph nodes, and pneumonia. When bacteria are inhaled, symptoms include sudden fever, chills, headache, muscle aches, joint pain, cough, and progressive weakness. Symptoms may progress to chest pain, dyspnea, bloody sputum, and respiratory failure	Standard Precautions
Botulism (*Clostridium botulinum*)	Foodborne: Ingestion of preformed toxin. Wound: When wounds are infected with *C. botulinum* that secretes toxin; injection drug users are at risk for wound botulism	Foodborne: Within hours of ingesting food, but can occur up to 8 days later	Early symptoms of botulism include gastrointestinal distress, nausea, and vomiting. Symptoms progress to diplopia, blurred vision, drooping eyelids, slurred speech, difficulty swallowing, dry mouth, and muscle weakness. If not treated, the disease progresses to respiratory paralysis and paralysis of arms and legs. Botulinum toxin is the most poisonous substance known	Standard Precautions

[a]The information about bioterrorism and the identified biologic weapons presented in this table represents current knowledge at the time of publication. The CDC updates its website with the most current information from throughout the world. Practitioners are encouraged to update their knowledge continually by consulting the CDC website (www.cdc.gov) and other experts in the field. The Health Alert Network (HAN) is the CDC's surveillance system. It connects local, state, and national public agencies with high-speed and satellite Internet access. The extent of precautions necessary can be quickly determined by using this system.

Modified from Centers for Disease Control and Prevention (CDC): *General fact sheets on specific bioterrorism agents* (website), 2016. https://emergency.cdc.gov/bioterrorism/factsheets.asp. (Accessed 15 January 2017).

---

along the corridor, to house sterile equipment and supplies. If a single-corridor design is used, sterile and contaminated items must be separated by either space or time. That is, sterile, wrapped, or containerized items can pass contaminated items in the corridor when the contaminated items are covered or otherwise contained.

Floors in the ORs should be hard, seamless, easily cleaned, and contiguous with the walls. This design eliminates the sharp angle where the floor and walls meet, in which bacteria can become lodged and proliferate. Floors should be monolithic and joint free. Walls may be constructed of any hard surface that is easily cleaned and hard enough to withstand the impact of surgical equipment that may accidentally be pushed into the wall during transport. If ceramic tile is used, smooth-surface grouting mortar should be used. This grout provides a surface nearly as smooth as the tile itself, eliminating concerns that surface roughness may attract and retain bacteria. Painted walls are less desirable because the paint flakes and peels, particularly in areas of higher humidity. If a hard-finish epoxy paint is used, it is only as good as the surface beneath it. Equipment banged into a wall may cause damage and expose construction material to the environment. A soft-colored, matte-finished wall may be preferred to reduce reflectance and glare (AIA, 2010).

Doors in the ORs may swing or slide. If sliding doors are used, they should not recess into the wall but should slide over the adjoining wall to facilitate housekeeping. Cabinets should be recessed into the wall if possible. This configuration allows for maximum use of open floor space in ORs. Size and configuration of ORs are discussed in detail by the American Institute of Architects (AIA)/Academy of Architecture for Health. Stainless steel cabinets are preferred because the surfaces remain smooth and are easily cleaned. Wooden cabinets quickly become damaged with cracks and crevices in which bacteria can collect and proliferate. Wooden cabinets are difficult to clean and disinfect and should be avoided in ORs. Cabinet doors may be of either the swinging or the sliding type. A cleaning protocol should be established for the tracks if sliding doors are used. For noncabinet shelving, open wire shelves are preferred because dust and bacteria do not accumulate, and air can circulate freely around shelf contents (AIA, 2010).

Scrub sinks should be located adjacent to each OR, with a single area serving two ORs if possible. Ideally, scrub sinks are located in a room or alcove adjacent to the peripheral or single corridor of the OR. Scrub sinks should not be within the central-core area because aerosolization and splashing may occur where sterile items are stored, contaminating the environment.

Each surgical suite must contain an enclosed soiled workroom exclusive for its own use. The workroom should contain a flushing hopper, receptacles for waste and soiled linen, a handwashing sink, and a work counter. If the area is used as a holding area as part of a larger system for collection and disposal of soiled materials, the flushing hopper is not required (AIA, 2010).

Heating, Ventilation, Air Conditioning

To control bioparticulate matter in the OR environment, ventilating air should be delivered to the room at the ceiling and exhausted near the floor and on walls opposite to those containing inlet vents. Airflow should be in a downward directional flow, moving down and through the location with a minimum of draft, to the floor and exhaust portals (AIA, 2010).

Air pressure in the OR should be greater than that in the surrounding corridor; this is called "positive pressure" in relation to corridors and adjacent areas. This positive pressure helps maintain the unidirectional airflow in the room and minimizes the amount of corridor air (less clean area) entering the OR (more clean area). Each OR should have a minimum of 15 total air exchanges per hour, with the equivalent of at least three replacements being of outside air to satisfy exhaust needs of the system. No recirculating devices, such as cooling fans or room humidifiers or dehumidifiers, are to be used. These units create a turbulent airflow and may recirculate settled bacteria. Doors to ORs should be kept closed to maintain correct ventilation, airflow, and air pressure. To minimize static electricity and to reduce the potential for bacterial growth, relative humidity in the OR should be maintained between 30% and 60%. A lower relative humidity may support accumulation of static electricity, whereas the presence of a higher humidity may cause condensation of ambient moisture, which may result in damp materials and supplies. This dampness supports bacterial growth. Temperatures in ORs should be maintained at 68°F to 73°F (20°C to 23°C) (AIA, 2010). Specific policies and procedures related to temperature and humidity should be developed in collaboration with the organization's infection preventionist and made in accordance with Association for the Advancement of Medical Instrumentation guidelines.

Practices to Prevent Infection

Preparing items for use in surgery and other invasive procedures requires thorough cleaning and drying of the items followed by either sterilization or high-level disinfection process. The efficacy of the sterilization or high-level disinfection process depends in part on cleaning to lower or limit the amount of bioburden present on the item to the lowest level possible.

Preparation of Items/Instruments for Sterilization and High-Level Disinfection

Cleaning. To prevent infection, all items that come into contact with the patient or sterile field, whether or not they were used, should be considered contaminated and should be systematically decontaminated after a surgical procedure. Decontamination consists of cleaning and disinfection. Handling, transport, and decontamination methods must be selected to prevent cross-contamination to other patients, exposure of personnel to bloodborne and other pathogens, and damage to instruments. The cleaning and disinfection methods chosen should be economical and of demonstrated effectiveness (Research Highlight). Cleaning is the first step in the decontamination process. Items may be cleaned manually, by mechanical means, or by a combination of the two (AAMI, 2013a). Increased productivity, consistency in the cleaning process, greater cleaning effectiveness, and increased employee safety may result from use of mechanical cleaning methods. Although some mechanical cleaning

RESEARCH HIGHLIGHT

Medical Device Cleaning

Cleaning is critical to subsequent successful disinfection and sterilization. There is a growing appreciation, not only for the importance of cleaning, but also because as lumens have become increasing narrow and devices more complex, cleaning has become significantly challenging. The tenet that items that are not clean cannot be sterilized and debris that remains inside or outside of a surgical instrument poses a threat to patient safety is basic to the core of infection control in the perioperative environment. In light of a number of patient infections and deaths resulting from inadequately cleaned duodenoscopes, the FDA issued the following statement: "Inadequate cleaning between patient uses can result in the retention of blood, tissue and other biologic debris (soil) in certain types of reusable medical devices. This debris can allow microbes to survive the subsequent disinfection or sterilization process, which could then lead to Healthcare-Associated Infections" (FDA, 2015b). There is a growing appreciation for the importance of cleaning and the associated difficulties. In a study to determine whether despite strict adherence to cleaning guidelines endoscopes may be contaminated after cleaning, testing was performed after cleaning from 60 encounters with 15 colonoscopes and gastroscopes used for GI procedures. Surface swabs were used to sample distal ends, control heads, ports, caps, and buttons. Water samples were obtained from suction-biopsy and water auxiliary channels. Postcleaning samples were tested for blood, protein, and ATP. Results were that after cleaning 46% of the samples exceeded ATP benchmarks. Residue was seen on swabs of effluent for 31%. Cleaning is critical to subsequent successful disinfection and sterilization. The researchers concluded that this study demonstrates the need for improved processing guidelines.

ATP, Adenosine triphosphate; *FDA,* Food and Drug Administration; *GI,* gastrointestinal. From Ofstead C: Persistent contamination on colonoscopes and gastroscopes detected by biologic cultures and rapid indicators despite reprocessing performance in accordance with guidelines, *Am J Infect Control* 43(8):794–801, 2015; Maisel W: *Bacterial infections associated with duodenoscopes: FDA's actions to better understand the problem and what can be done to mitigate it* (website), 2015. http://blogs.fda.gov/fdavoice/index.php/2015/02/bacterial-infections-associated-with-duodenoscopes-fdas-actions-to-better-understand-the-problem-and-what-can-be-done-to-mitigate-it/. (Accessed 4 February 2017); US Food and Drug Administration (FDA): *FDA-cleared sterilants and high level disinfectants with general claims for reprocessing reusable medical and dental devices* (website), 2015. www.fda.gov/MedicalDevices/DeviceRegulationandGuidance/ReprocessingofReusableMedicalDevices/ucm437347.htm. (Accessed 4 February 2017).

equipment does not include a disinfection phase, most mechanical cleaning equipment includes a cleaning and rinsing phase followed by either a thermal or a chemical disinfection phase. The most commonly used mechanical cleaners are ultrasonic cleaners, washer disinfectors/decontaminators, and cart washers.

All workers handling soiled surgical instruments, whether in the OR, a substerile room, or a decontamination area, must wear PPE sufficient to prevent contact with any blood or other body fluid. This generally means scrub attire covered with a liquid-resistant gown, coverall, or sleeved apron; hair covering; surgical facemask; eye protection; and gloves suitable to the task. In the event that fluids may pool on the floor, liquid-proof boots or shoe covers are recommended.

Instruments should be kept as free as possible from gross soil and other debris during the surgical procedure. Throughout the surgical procedure, the scrub person, who may be a surgical technologist or RN, should wipe used instruments with sponges moistened with sterile water. When blood is allowed to dry on an instrument, it may cause pitting, rusting, or corrosion. Sterile water should be used rather than saline, which can cause pitting and damage to instrument surfaces. Initial decontamination should begin immediately on completion of the surgical procedure (AAMI, 2013a; AORN, 2016d). All instruments that can be immersed are disassembled, and box locks are opened to allow solution to contact all soiled surfaces. These instruments should be placed in a basin, solid-bottom container system, or bin with a lid. Scissors and lightweight instruments should be placed on top. Heavy retractors should be placed in a separate tray.

Some instruments have sharp or pointed edges, such as scissors, forceps with teeth, perforating towel clamps, curettes, and rongeurs. These items can penetrate gloves and skin, creating a portal of entry for infectious organisms. Sharp instruments must not be placed in a basin or tray in such a way that a worker would have to reach into the container to retrieve the instrument, risking injury. To prevent debris from drying on instruments until they are cleaned an enzyme solution, foam, or spray, or a towel moistened with water can be added to the instruments. An enzyme spray or foam intended for surgical instruments may be used to begin the process of breaking down any proteinaceous materials that may remain on the instruments and is useful in preventing debris from drying and preventing the formation of biofilms. Biofilms are densely packed communities of microbial cells that attach themselves to a surface and surround themselves with slimy self-secreting polymers that make removal difficult. Biofilms are thought to be responsible for up to 80% of device and tissue infections (Edmiston et al., 2015). Instrument sprays or foam should be used strictly according to the product's instructions for use (IFU). Soiled instruments should be contained within leakproof containers, or trays inside plastic bags, when they are transported from the OR for cleaning and decontamination. Soiled instruments should never be cleaned in a sink used for handwashing or a surgical scrub. Contaminated instruments should be transported to and cleaned only in a dedicated decontamination area. If sharps are being transported, the container should be puncture resistant. Means of containing instruments include plastic, rubber, or metal bins with lids; solid-bottom sterilization container systems with the lids and filters in place; or simply placement of the instrument tray in a plastic bag. All soiled containment packages should be labeled with the biohazard symbol to warn handlers as to the nature of the contents. Liquids used to soak instruments at point of use should be discarded before transport. Transporting instruments while they are soaking is discouraged because of the possibility of a liquid spill and its associated cleanup problems as well as the difficulty of safely disposing the contaminated liquid (AAMI, 2013a; AORN, 2016l).

In the decontamination area, an initial cold water rinse with tap water or a soak in cool water with a protein-dissolving and blood-dissolving enzyme helps remove blood, tissue, and gross debris from device lumens, joints, and serrations. After completion of this pretreatment, the instruments should be processed in a mechanical washer or manually washed if a mechanical system is not available (AAMI, 2013a) or if the device cannot tolerate mechanical washing. It is critical to successful cleaning to follow the detergent manufacturer's IFU including temperature, concentration, and contact time. The final rinse should be with sterile or treated water (AAMI 2013a; AORN 2016d).

Mechanical processing is usually accomplished with an ultrasonic cleaner and a washer disinfector/decontaminator. Washer disinfector/decontaminator cycles vary to some degree and may include an initial cool water rinse to remove protein debris, an enzymatic-solution soak, a detergent wash, ultrasonic cleaning, a hot water rinse, a liquid chemical germicide rinse, a lubrication cycle, and drying phase. Soiled utensils such as basins, rigid sterilization containers, and trays should also pass through a mechanical washer. Some washers provide cycles specific to delicate or specialty instruments. When endoscopic devices or other items with a lumen are cleaned, a cleaning apparatus for these items can be attached. Many ultrasonic cleaners and washer disinfectors/decontaminators provide such attachments (AAMI, 2013a; CDC, 2016e).

The ultrasonic cleaning process is designed to remove fine soil from crevices and lumens of complex devices and from box lock areas and serrations of instrumentation. It should be used only after gross debris has been removed. Ultrasonic energy occurs in waveforms and is generated by transducers on the sides or bottom of a specially constructed chamber that is filled with water or a water and detergent solution. The ultrasonic waves pass through the water, creating tiny bubbles that collapse or implode. This creates a negative pressure, which pulls debris away from surfaces. This process is known as *cavitation.* Some ultrasonic cleaning equipment includes a disinfection process. Instruments should be rinsed to remove the loose debris.

Not all items tolerate the energy waves of the ultrasonic process. For example, lensed instruments should not be subject to ultrasonic cleaning because the energy can compromise the integrity of the lens seal. Dissimilar metals, such as stainless steel, titanium, copper, and lead, should not be ultrasonically processed at the same time. The energy waves, combined with the heat and detergent solution, can cause electrolysis to occur, plating one metal onto others, potentially ruining the instruments. Some manufacturers recommend that microsurgery instruments should not be subjected to ultrasonic cleaning because of their delicate design and because they may contain several types of metal. The detergent or enzyme cleaner used in the ultrasonic machine should be selected in accordance with the device and ultrasonic manufacturer's written IFU. The instructions should be consulted to determine compatibility with the ultrasonic cleaner machine and with the device. The corrosiveness and overall effectiveness of some solutions can be dramatically affected by the combination of heat and ultrasonic energy in such a machine. The water in the ultrasonic cleaner should be replaced when it is visibly soiled or at regularly scheduled intervals. Ultrasonic cleaners should be cleaned according to the manufacturer's written IFU.

Some instruments, such as air-powered and some microsurgical instruments, do not tolerate immersion in water or cannot tolerate the heat or pressures involved in mechanical processes. These items must be manually cleaned using an appropriate detergent for the type of material and the type of soil on the item. A neutral pH detergent is often recommended. A detergent that is highly alkaline or acidic can be damaging to instruments. Written instructions from the instrument manufacturer should be consulted to determine appropriate cleaning products and procedures (AAMI, 2013a). If instruments are manually cleaned, they should be submerged in warm water with an appropriate detergent and then cleaned and rinsed while submerged. Cleaning in this fashion helps protect personnel from aerosolization or splashing of infectious material. Unless indicated in the device manufacturer's written IFU, abrasive cleaners should not be used because these can damage the surface of instruments and potentially create imperfections that can trap debris. Brushes used to clean lumens should be long enough to exit the distal end of the lumen. Brush diameter should be appropriate to lumen diameter. Brushing should be done under the surface of the water to prevent aerosolization and splashing of contaminants. Bristle diameter should be large enough to allow consistent contact with the inner walls of the lumen but small enough to not collapse when inserted. Brushes should be either single-use disposable or should be decontaminated at least daily.

Items that were soiled with blood or body fluids and that have been cleaned only may not have been sufficiently decontaminated to allow safe handling by workers not wearing protective attire and may require a microbicidal process, such as soaking in a liquid chemical germicide or liquid chemical sterilant. The device manufacturer's written IFU should be consulted to determine whether decontamination using a microbicidal process is required after cleaning and before packaging and sterilization. If there is no method suitable to further decontamination of the item, because of damage to the item, cost, or unavailability, workers in the preparation area should wear protective gloves when handling, inspecting, assembling, and packaging these items for sterilization.

The final steps before sterilization for reuse include instrument inspection, function testing, and packaging. These activities should occur in a clean area, separate from the area in which decontamination occurs. Instruments should be inspected under lighted magnification for cleanliness and tested for functionality. Soiled instruments should be returned to the decontamination area for further cleaning. Instruments with movable parts may be treated with a water-soluble lubricant solution if indicated in the device manufacturer's written IFU. Broken or worn instruments should be set aside for repair. Instruments are then assembled into sets according to set content lists prepared by perioperative nursing staff.

Packaging and Sterilizer Loading. Packaging of surgical supplies and their arrangement in loads in the sterilizer are factors that govern the effectiveness of sterilization. The prime function of a package containing a surgical item is to permit sterilization of the contents and to ensure the sterility of the contents up to the time the package is opened. Provision must be made for the contents to be removed without contamination. All packaging systems should have FDA clearance for its intended use. To be effective, packaging material should have the following characteristics:

- Is suitable to the items being packaged and sterilized
- Allows for adequate air removal and sterilant penetration and contact
- Maintains sterility of contents until opened
- Resists tearing or punctures
- Protects contents from damage
- Allows for aseptic delivery of package contents
- Is free of toxic ingredients
- Is low-linting
- Has a favorable cost-benefit ratio (AORN, 2016l)

Rigid sterilization container systems are one method of packaging instrumentation. Rigid containers can be sterilized, stacked, and stored. Because of the rigid material of the container, they cannot be punctured, abraded, or easily contaminated by environmental microbes. Rigid sterilization containers are subject to wear and tear through repeated use. Containers should be cleaned and inspected after each use in accordance with the container manufacturer's written IFU. Preventive maintenance and strict adherence to the container manufacturer's written IFU is critical to the ability of the container to maintain sterility of the contents until opened (Research Highlight).

Written instructions for sterilizing should be obtained from the container manufacturer. Before purchase, performance testing should be performed in the sterile processing department of the healthcare

RESEARCH HIGHLIGHT

Evaluation of Rigid Sterilization Containers

Rigid sterilization containers are commonly used packaging systems. They are durable, protect instruments from damage, may contain templates to identify and secure instruments, and facilitate neat storage. Like all terminal packaging systems their intent is to provide a sterile barrier indefinitely. Rigid sterilization containers, however, must be maintained to function as intended. In this study to evaluate the ability of rigid sterilization containers and wrapped instrument trays to prevent bacterial ingress the researchers challenged containers with aerosolized bacteria under dynamic environmental conditions. One hundred eleven containers of varying duration of use and 161 polypropylene wrapped trays were challenged with 10^2 colony-forming units per liter of air containing *Micrococcus luteus*. Eighty-seven percent of the containers demonstrated ingress into the containers. Contamination rates increased with duration of container usage. None of the wrapped trays demonstrated ingress of bacteria. More research is needed to determine barrier effectiveness of packaging systems including rigid sterilization containers. The fact, however, that older containers experienced greater bacterial ingress than packaging highlights the need for robust inspection and maintenance of containers.

From Shaffer HL et al: Sterility maintenance study: dynamic evaluation of sterilized rigid containers and wrapped instrument trays to prevent bacterial ingress, *Am J Infect Control* 43(12):1336–1341, 2015.

facility to ensure that all conditions essential for sterilization and drying can be achieved. See AAMI ST79 (AAMI 2013b) for information on prepurchase performance testing. The container manufacturer should be consulted for information regarding set preparation and the most challenging areas within the container for placement of chemical indicators. Chemical indicators serve to verify that the sterilant has reached the interior of the container and is evidence that one or more of the parameters of the sterilization process were sufficient to cause a color change (see Quality Monitoring Practices, p. 76). Many in-hospital packaging materials (woven and nonwoven, reusable and disposable) are marketed and should be evaluated carefully before a product is chosen.

If textile wrappers are used, they must be laundered between sterilization exposures to ensure sufficient moisture content of the fibers. This prevents superheating, which can result in a process failure during steam sterilization. Rehydrated materials also deteriorate at a slower rate. All wrappers must be checked for holes or tears before use for packaging. The manufacturer's IFU should be consulted to determine acceptable size, weight, and density of textile packs. Wrappers should be held at room temperature (68°F–73°F [20°C–23°C]) at least 2 hours before sterilization. Temperature and humidity equilibration of packaging materials are needed to prevent superheating and possible sterilization failure. When textiles are used for wrapping, the items should be wrapped sequentially in two barrier-type wrappers, which may be disposable or reusable. A single-textile reusable wrapper is defined as one layer of 270- to 280-thread count woven fabric. Sequential double-wrapping creates a package within a package, providing for ease in presenting the wrapped item to the sterile field. A commonly used envelope wrap is made by placing the article diagonally in the center of the wrapper. The near corner, which should point toward the worker, is brought over the item, and the triangular tip is folded back to form a cuff.

The two side flaps are folded to the center in like manner. The far corner of the wrapper is then folded on top of the other three. Careful wrapping to prevent tenting and gapping of the package is essential (Fig. 4.3). The process is repeated with the second wrapper, and the package is secured with autoclave indicator tape.

When the pack is opened for use, the flaps at the corners are used to form a protective cuff over the person's hands during dispensing of the sterile contents.

Single-use disposable nonwoven wrappers made of synthetic materials have largely replaced textiles for wrap. These wrappers are available in a variety of sizes and may be supplied as a single sheet or a double wrap that is bonded together. Double-wrap sheets provide a bacterial barrier at least equivalent to the sequential double wrap and allow for safe and easy presentation of the package contents to the sterile field, providing an alternative to the sequential double-wrapping procedure. Wrapping technique is the same as when using a textile wrapper. Nonwoven, single-use wrappers should not be reused (AAMI, 2013a). Instrument sets, including the packaging, should not exceed 25 pounds (AAMI 2013a, 2013b).

Sterilization process (chemical) indicator tape should be used to hold wrappers in place on packages and to indicate that the packages have been exposed to the physical conditions of a sterilization cycle. When packages are opened, these tapes should be first torn so that the package cannot be retaped and then removed from reusable wrappers because they create laundry problems, such as occluding screens and filters. Tapes also may leave an adhesive residue that can interfere with future sterilization of the fabric.

Sterilization pouches, commonly manufactured from a combination of paper or Tyvek and plastic films, provide an option for the packaging of single (or small groups) or lightweight instruments or other objects (e.g., medicine cups). Pouches are selected based on material compatibility with the intended sterilization technology.

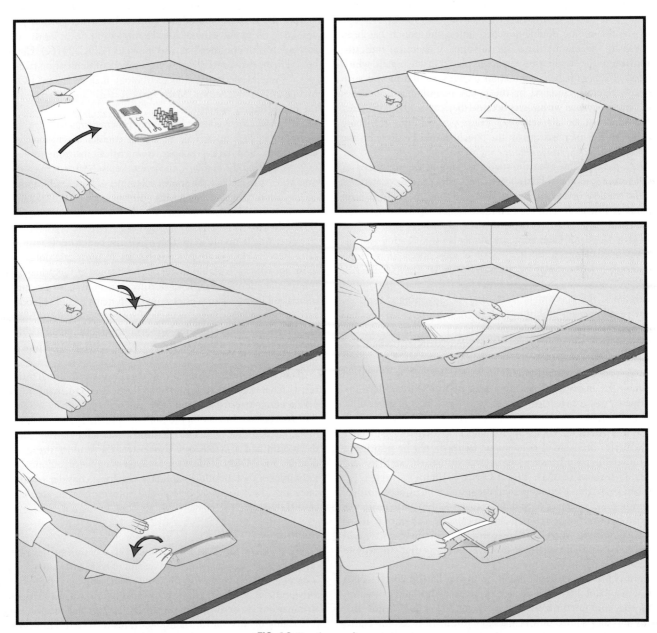

FIG. 4.3 Envelope-style wrapping.

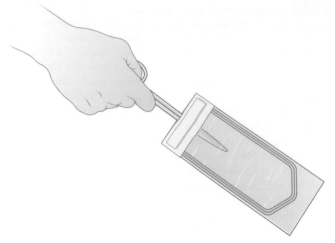

FIG. 4.4 Sterilization pouch.

Items should not be double-pouched unless the pouch has been validated by the manufacturer for this use. A chemical indicator appropriate to the sterilization method is placed in the pouch, which is sealed either with heat lamination or with a self-adhesive strip (Fig. 4.4). Unless validated by the pouch manufacturer, pouches should not be placed within sets because they cannot be positioned to ensure adequate air removal, steam penetration, or drying (AAMI, 2013a). Any writing on the pouch should be done on the plastic side.

Every package intended for sterile use should be imprinted or labeled with a load-control number that identifies the date of sterilization, the sterilizer used, and the cycle or load number. Load-control numbers facilitate identification and retrieval of supplies, inventory control, and appropriate rotation to ensure that dated packages are used first (AAMI, 2013a). Some instruments or packaging systems may present challenges to the sterilization process. Special preparation or loading procedures may be necessary to meet these challenges. Hinged instruments must be arranged so that the sterilant can contact all surfaces of the instrument, including the tips, hinged surfaces, and ratchets. To accomplish this, these instruments must be sterilized in the open position. If the instruments have ringed handles for the fingers, the instruments may be placed on a "stringer," which is a U-shaped metal rod made especially for this purpose. When using container systems for sterilization, basket attachments may be used to immobilize instruments in the proper position for sterilization. Instruments with concave or other surfaces that can hold water must be carefully placed on edge to facilitate removal of air, which may become trapped in the concave surface. Placing the package on edge also facilitates drainage of condensate. Items should be positioned with sufficient space between all surfaces so that the sterilant can contact all surfaces (AAMI, 2013a; CDC, 2016e).

When packaging is complete and the sterilizer chamber is loaded, the bundles and packages should be arranged to minimize resistance to sterilant contact or penetration and to enhance air removal. Items capable of holding water, such as basins or medicine cups, should be positioned, usually arranged on their sides, so that condensate can drain.

Rigid container systems should be placed flat on the sterilizer shelf. These containers should not be stacked during sterilization unless the container manufacturer specifically recommends this practice and then should only be stacked in the manner recommended by the manufacturer's written instructions. Stacking may interfere with air removal and sterilant penetration. Rigid sterilization containers should not be placed above absorbent packed items as condensate, which can occur when the sterilizer door is opened and cooler air contacts the container, may cause wetting of packages below (AAMI, 2013a; CDC, 2016e).

Pouches should be positioned on edge in a rack. They should be placed paper to plastic, all facing in the same direction.

The Spaulding Classification System. Items to be sterilized or high-level disinfected are classified as critical, semicritical, and noncritical, based on the risk of infection for the patient. This classification system, known as the *Spaulding classification system* (CDC, 2016e) and named for its developer, Earle Spaulding, has withstood the passage of time and continues to be used today to determine the correct processing method for preparing instruments and other items for patient use. According to the Spaulding system, the level of disinfection required is based on the nature of the item and the manner in which it is to be used.

Critical items are those that enter sterile tissue or the vascular system. These items should be subjected to a sterilization process and be sterile at the time of use. Examples of critical items include surgical instruments, needles, and implants (CDC, 2016e). Unsterile critical items may be sterilized using a variety of sterilization technologies. Examples of sterilization technology include steam, EO, and hydrogen peroxide vapor. Many critical items are purchased from the manufacturer as sterile.

Semicritical items contact but do not penetrate mucous membranes. Examples include anesthesia breathing circuits, thermometers, GI endoscopes, and laryngoscopes. Semicritical instruments require high-level disinfection; that is, these items must be free of microorganisms other than all bacterial spores. Examples of high-level disinfecting agents include glutaraldehyde, ortho-phthalaldehyde (OPA), stabilized hydrogen peroxide, peracetic acid, and chlorine or chlorine compounds (FDA, 2015b).

Noncritical items are items that come into contact only with intact skin. Because skin is an effective barrier to most microorganisms, most noncritical, reusable items can be cleaned at the point of use. Intermediate-level or low-level disinfectants may be used to process noncritical items. Examples of noncritical items include blood pressure cuffs, bedpans, linens, utensils, furniture, and floors. Examples of low-level disinfectants include alcohols, sodium hypochlorite, phenolic solutions, iodophor solutions, and quaternary ammonium solutions.

Since development of the Spaulding classification in 1939 instruments have become increasingly sophisticated and many modern devices currently classified as semicritical enter sterile tissue secondarily (i.e., through a mucous membrane). Examples of such items are a bronchoscope that enters sterile lung tissue after passing through the mouth and a cystoscope that enters the bladder through the urethra. The AORN "Guideline for Processing Flexible Endoscopes" recommends that a multidisciplinary task force consider whether to categorize these items as critical and subject them to sterilization (AORN 2016j).

Sterilization

Sterilization is defined as the complete elimination or destruction of all forms of microbial life. The concept of what constitutes "sterile" is measured as the *probability* of sterility for each item to be sterilized. This probability is known as the *sterility assurance level* (SAL). For terminal steam sterilization processes, 10^{-6} is the recommended probability of survival for microorganisms on a sterilized device. A probability of microorganism survival of 10^{-6} means that there is less than or equal to a 1 in 1 million chance that any viable micro-organisms remain after sterilization. The SAL of 10^{-6} is considered appropriate for items to be used on compromised body tissue (AAMI, 2013a; CDC, 2016e).

Steam Sterilization. Steam sterilization is the oldest, safest, most economical, and most commonly used method of sterilization available in healthcare. It is the preferred method of sterilization for items that are heat and moisture tolerant (AORN, 2016n). The efficacy of steam sterilization depends on lowering and limiting bioburden on the item to be sterilized, using effective sterilization cycles, and preventing recontamination of sterile items before delivery to the point of use.

Theory of Microbial Destruction. Microorganisms are believed to be destroyed by moist heat through a process of denaturation and coagulation of the enzyme-protein system within the bacterial cell. Microorganisms are killed at a lower temperature when moist heat is used as opposed to when dry heat is used. This fact is based on the theory that all chemical reactions, including coagulation of proteins, are catalyzed by the presence of water.

Principles and Mechanisms. A steam sterilizer is referred to as an autoclave. Sterilization is achieved in an autoclave in which items are exposed to direct steam contact. There are four parameters of steam sterilization described in Perkin's classic work that are still relevant to modern practice: water quality, steam pressure, temperature, and time. Steam quality describes the amount of steam vapor or liquid water in the steam. Steam quality should be 97% or greater, which means there should be no more than 3% of liquid water in the steam. A common cause of sterilization failure is poor steam quality often caused by improper boiler function and/or poorly maintained steam distribution lines to the sterilizer. At atmospheric pressure steam is 100°C (212°F). Minimum temperature necessary to kill microorganisms is 121°C (250°F) (Perkins, 1969). Pressure greater than atmospheric pressure is necessary to raise the temperature of steam to a temperature sufficient to kill microorganisms. An autoclave is a vessel in which higher than atmospheric pressure can be achieved. Standard required temperatures to achieve sterilization are 121°C (250°F) and 132°C (270°F). To achieve kill of all micro-organisms temperatures must be maintained for a specified time, typically 30 minutes at 121°C (250°F) and 4 minutes at 132°C (270°F). The higher the temperature the shorter the required exposure time. Actual exposure time does not begin until the required preset temperature is reached (AAMI, 2015).

Sterilizing. When steam enters the autoclave, it is at the same pressure as the atmosphere. As the valves and doors to the outside close, steam pressure rises inside the chamber, increasing the temperature of the steam. As pressure rises air is evacuated from the sterilizer and steam penetrates packaging and contacts the items to be sterilized. Evacuation of air from the sterilizer is necessary to permit proper permeation of steam. If a sterilizer is improperly loaded, mixing of air with steam acts as a barrier to steam penetration and prevents attainment of the sterilization temperature.

The microbial destruction period is based on the known time and temperature necessary to accomplish sterilization in saturated steam. If the temperature is increased the time may be decreased.

The length of exposure varies with the type of sterilizer; cycle design; altitude; bioburden; packaging; and size, design, and composition of items to be sterilized. Written instructions for sterilization parameters should be obtained from the device and the sterilizer manufacturer. If a closed-container system is used as packaging for items to be sterilized, the container manufacturer's written instructions for exposure times should be consulted and reconciled with those of the sterilizer and the device manufacturer (AAMI, 2013a). When the IFU for a device specifies a time or temperature not identified in the sterilizer IFU, the device and the sterilizer manufacturer should be consulted to attempt reconciliation. If reconciliation cannot be achieved, the IFU for the device should be followed. The device manufacturer has validated the cycle that must be used to achieve sterilization.

The configuration of some instruments or medical devices may hinder air removal and steam penetration, making sterilization more difficult. In such circumstances the device manufacturer must be able to specify the necessary parameters to achieve sterility. Typical minimum cycle times for gravity-displacement steam sterilization and typical minimum cycle times for dynamic air-removal steam sterilization are provided in Table 4.4. Certain instruments, instrument sets, and implants require extended time cycles, however. The manufacturer's written instructions for extended cycle times must be followed.

The recording mechanism on the sterilizer gives information about the run of the load and to what temperature the goods were exposed and the exposure time. To achieve sterilization the temperature inside the chamber must be maintained throughout the determined time of exposure. The sterilizer recording device (e.g., printout) documents the come-up time (time to reach required temperature), temperature, exposure time, and exhaust time (AAMI, 2013a).

Drying, Cooling, and Storing. On completion of the sterilization exposure time, the steam inside the chamber is exhausted immediately so that it does not condense and produce wet packs. When the chamber has been exhausted and the pressure reduced, the door may be opened slightly to permit vapor to escape. Drying time can vary according to load contents.

After removal from the sterilizer, freshly sterilized packs should be left untouched on the loading carriage until they have cooled to room temperature. This is usually accomplished in 30 to 60 minutes but may take up to 2 hours, depending on the load contents (AAMI,

---

TABLE 4.4

Common Time-Temperature Parameters for Steam Sterilization

Type of Sterilization Cycle	Load Configuration	Temperature [°F (°C)]	Time (Minutes)
Gravity displacement	Porous or nonporous	250–254 (121–123)	15–30
		270–275 (132–135)	10–25
Prevacuum	Porous or nonporous	270–275 (132–135)	3–4 or manufacturer's instructions
Steam flush/pressure pulse	Porous or nonporous	250–254 (121–123)	20
		270–275 (132–135)	3–4

2013a). If freshly sterilized packages are placed on cool surfaces such as metal tabletops, vapor still inside the essentially dry package may condense to water. This water may dampen the package from the inside to the outside. When the outside is wet, bacteria may follow the moist tract into the contents of the package. Because bacteria are capable of passing through layers of wet material, any packages that are wet must be considered unsterile. Touching a hot pack may result in strikethrough in which any condensate that has not evaporated and is touched may cause microorganisms to be wicked into the package and cause contamination.

A record of existing conditions during each sterilization cycle should be maintained. It should include the sterilizer number, the cycle or load number, the time and temperature of the cycle, the date of sterilization, the contents of the load, and the initials of the operator. These records should be retained for the length of time designated by the statute of limitations in each state. Records may be provided in the form of a paper printout or a digital recording.

Sterile packages must be handled carefully and only as necessary. They should be stored in clean, dry, limited-access areas that are well ventilated and have controlled temperature and humidity. Closed cabinets are preferred to open shelves for sterile storage. If open shelves must be used, the lowest shelf should be a solid bottom and 8 to 10 inches from the floor to avoid floor contamination. The highest shelf should be at least 18 inches from the ceiling or the sprinkler head to allow for circulation around the stored items. All shelves should be at least 2 inches from outside walls to facilitate air circulation and avoid any condensation that might accumulate on the walls during periods of severe temperature change (AAMI, 2013a). Shelving should be smooth, with no projections or sharp corners that might damage the wrappers. Their arrangement on the shelves should provide for air circulation on all sides of each package. Excessive handling, crowding, and dropping of sterile packs may cause loss of package integrity and possible subsequent contamination of package contents. Sterile items should not be stored in any area in which they can become wet.

Shelf life refers to the length of time a pack may be considered sterile. Loss of package sterility is event related as opposed to time related; that is, what happens to the package after sterilization determines its continued sterility, not the length of time the package remains on the shelf ready for use. Variables that must be considered in determining shelf life are the type and number of layers of packaging material used, the presence or absence of impervious protective covers, the number of times a package is handled before use, and the conditions of storage. Impervious protective covers known as *dust covers* may extend shelf life by protecting the sterile package from a contaminating event. When used to protect sterilized items, impervious covers should be designated as such to prevent their being mistaken for a sterile wrap. They should be applied only to thoroughly cooled, dry packs at the time of removal from the sterilizer cart, after the required cooling period (AORN, 2016l).

A large number of commercially sterilized packages carry an expiration date after which the product should not be used. Expiration dating in these instances is usually related to product degradation not sterility.

Supply standards should be planned to maintain adequate stock with prompt turnover. Appropriate volume and proper rotation of supplies reduce the need for concern about shelf life. The longer an item is stored, the greater the chances of contamination. For proper rotation, the most recently dated sterile packages should be placed behind those already on the shelves.

Quality Monitoring Practices. Physical, chemical, and biologic monitors are used for quality monitoring of the sterilization process. These monitors assist in identifying process failures that may be a result of equipment malfunction or operator errors. Physical monitoring is accomplished with temperature and pressure recorders, digital printouts, electronic recordings, and gauges. Types; classification; and application of physical, chemical, and biologic monitors are described in Table 4.5.

Most sterilizers provide a digital readout or printout. Older and tabletop sterilizers that do not supply a recording of the sterilization cycle should be replaced or retrofitted to include recording or print out capability. The readout records the time the sterilizer reaches the desired temperature and the duration of each exposure. It can be determined whether a decrease in temperature occurred, warning of sterilizer failure. These recordings verify that the exposure time of loads has been correct and proper temperature limits have been maintained. The daily record should identify the sterilizer, the number of cycles run, the time, and the date. Physical monitoring devices provide real-time assessment of sterilizer-cycle conditions and permanent records. This evidence can be used for detection of malfunctions as soon as possible so that alternative procedures can be implemented while the cause of the malfunction is identified and corrective action is taken. Chemical controls, also known as *chemical indicators,* integrators, or emulators, include devices such as pellet-containing, sealed glass tubes; sterilizer indicator tapes; and color-change cards or strips. Common chemical indicators used in healthcare facilities are indicator tape and color-change cards or strips. Chemical indicators are used to detect exposure to the sterilant and failures in packaging, loading, or sterilizer function, such as presence of cool air pockets inside the sterilizing chamber. Chemical indicators, such as tape or labels that are impregnated with a material that changes color when steam initiates a chemical reaction, are placed on the outside of instrument trays or other packages and indicate contact with the sterilant. Chemical integrators are so named for their ability to integrate time, temperature, and the presence of steam. Chemical emulators are cycle specific. They are designed to react to all the critical variables of a specified sterilization cycle (AAMI, 2013a). Chemical integrators or emulators are placed inside every package. They indicate that one or more of the parameters necessary for sterilization have been achieved. Chemical indicator color changes and wording vary for each type of sterilization modality to denote that an instrument set or other item is acceptable for use. As a result, perioperative nurses and scrub persons should always refer to the manufacturer's written IFU for proper use and interpretation of results (AORN, 2016n).

An external chemical indicator should be used on all packages to be sterilized except those that allow direct visualization into the package, where an internal indicator is used (e.g., paper/plastic pouches). The primary purpose of the external indicator is to differentiate between processed and nonprocessed packages. It indicates whether exposure to the sterilant has occurred; it does not indicate the items are sterile. This indicator should be checked after the sterilization process and before a package is distributed or opened to determine that the package has been exposed to a sterilization process.

Each package requiring sterilization should have one or more chemical integrators or emulators placed within the area most challenging or least accessible to the sterilization process. The chemical indicator should be located and interpreted by the user at the time the package is opened and before use of the contents (AORN, 2016n).

TABLE 4.5

Physical, Chemical, and Biologic Sterilization Monitors

Type	Classification	Application
Temperature and pressure recording devices Time recording devices Digital recording devices	Physical monitors	Steam EO Low temperature: • Low-temperature H_2O_2 • Ozone • Peracetic acid
External strips/tape Bowie-Dick type indicators Internal CI strips	Chemical monitors	Used on outside of packages Used for dynamic air removal in steam sterilizers Used for: • Steam • EO • Low-temperature H_2O_2 • Ozone
Geobacillus stearothermophilus	Biologic monitors (indicator)	Used for routine load release, efficacy monitoring, qualification testing, product quality assurance, etc. Used for: • Steam • Low-temperature H_2O_2 • Ozone sterilizers • Liquid peracetic acid sterilant systems (spore strip only) Should be done weekly, preferably daily, and according to sterilizer manufacturer's written instructions Each load that contains implantable devices should be monitored with a BI; load should be quarantined until BI test results are obtained
Bacillus atrophaeus (formerly *Bacillus subtilis*)	Biologic monitor	EO monitoring Should be performed on every load to be sterilized

BI, Biologic indicator; *CI*, chemical indicator; *EO*, ethylene oxide.

Modified from Association for the Advancement of Medical Instrumentation (AAMI): *AAMI comprehensive guide to steam sterilization and sterility assurance in health care facilities*, Arlington, VA, 2013, The Association; Association of periOperative Registered Nurses (AORN): Guideline for sterilization. In: *Guidelines for perioperative practice*, ed 16, Denver, 2016, The Association.

A biologic indicator (BI) is the most accurate method of checking lethality of the sterilization process. Commercially prepared BIs should be stored and used according to the manufacturer's written IFU. BIs used for monitoring steam sterilization contain a known population of *Geobacillus stearothermophilus* spores. *G. stearothermophilus* is a spore-forming microorganism that does not produce toxins, is nonpathogenic, and is resistant to moist heat sterilization. Some BIs contain spores with an enzyme-based early readout capability. These indicators provide an enzymatic reaction that is highly correlated to biologic kill. Reaction times range from 30 minutes to 3 hours. The length of time necessary for an initial reading depends on the type of sterilization cycle and the type of BI used. Because early readout biologic indicators do contain spores, it is possible, if desired, to incubate them for a longer time to demonstrate actual spore growth and to verify the enzyme-based result.

Biologic testing should be done after initial installation of steam sterilizers, after any major repair of the sterilizer, and with all loads containing an implant. Except in defined emergencies, implantable devices should be quarantined until the results of the biologic testing are available (AORN, 2016n).

Sterilizer efficacy testing using a BI should be conducted weekly and preferably daily. The BI should be placed in a process challenge device (PCD), sometimes referred to as a test pack, that is positioned in the most challenging location within the sterilizer. The most challenging location is usually the front bottom over the drain. Except with immediate-use steam sterilization, the BI test should be run with a full load. Although users may make the PCD using towels according to AAMI instructions (AAMI, 2013a), commercially prepared test packs are more commonly used. For immediate-use steam sterilization, the PCD is the "flash" container itself, and testing is done in an empty chamber.

After the sterilization cycle, the BI is removed from the PCD and incubated according to the manufacturer's written IFU. Negative reports (failure to recover any spores from the indicators in the test pack) indicate that the sterilizer is functioning properly. Results of these tests should be available as a permanent record. A positive report does not indicate sterilizer failure because false-positive results sometimes occur. If the cause for the failure is immediately identified or confined to an item in the load, the cause should be corrected and the load reprocessed. If a sterilizer malfunction is found, all items prepared in the suspect load should be considered unsterile. They should be retrieved if possible and cleaned, repackaged, and resterilized in another sterilizer. All items in any load processed since the last negative result also should be considered suspect and should similarly be retrieved if possible (AAMI, 2013a). A malfunctioning sterilizer should be repaired and the sterilizer retested. AAMI ST79 Comprehensive Guide to Steam Sterilization and Sterility Assurance in Health Care Facilities should be consulted to determine appropriate testing protocol.

When a dynamic air removal sterilizer (see Types of Steam Sterilizers) is used, a test designed to detect residual air in the chamber should be run daily before the first load of the day. The test, generally known as a *Bowie-Dick* test, is run with an otherwise empty chamber. The Bowie-Dick test determines the efficacy of the air removal system of the sterilizer. Air that is not removed can prevent contact of the sterilant with an item.

Types of Steam Sterilizers. For sterilization to occur, steam must contact all surfaces of the item to be sterilized. To accomplish this, the air in the sterilizer chamber must be evacuated. The terms *gravity displacement* and *dynamic air removal* describe the methods by which air leaves the sterilizer chamber. Dynamic air removal sterilizers use preconditioning techniques to remove air from the sterilizing chamber. This may be through a vacuum pump (prevacuum) or by an above atmospheric pressure process, such as the steam-flush pressure-pulse process. In a gravity displacement cycle the air is removed by the force of gravity.

At the beginning of the cycle in a gravity displacement sterilizer, steam enters the chamber after the door is closed and locked (Figs. 4.5 and 4.6). An initial burst of steam enters the chamber and forces out much of the free air in the chamber. Air is heavier than steam, and the two do not mix well. As more steam enters the chamber, the air that is held by gravity at the bottom of the chamber exits through the drain, which is at the bottom of the sterilizer, hence the name *gravity displacement sterilizer*.

In a dynamic air removal (e.g., prevacuum) cycle, rather than passive air removal as is the case with the gravity sterilizer, air is removed through a vacuum pump mechanism that evacuates the air from the chamber (Fig. 4.7). This is referred to as the preconditioning phase. When steam enters the sterilizer the force of the vacuum causes the steam to make instant contact with the items. In a steam-flush-pressure-pulse sterilizer air is removed from the chamber through a series of repeated steam, flush, and pressure pulses above atmospheric pressure. A vacuum is not drawn and therefore an air-removal test (Bowie-Dick) is not used in this type of sterilizer.

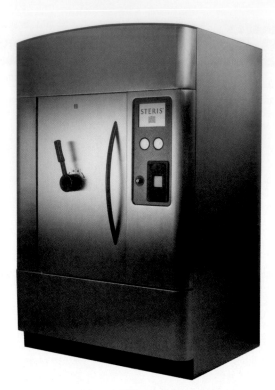

FIG. 4.5 Large unit general-purpose steam sterilizer. This type of sterilizer has gravity or dynamic air removal cycles and can be used for terminal or immediate-use steam sterilization of instruments and utensils, linen packs, and solutions in specially designed vented flasks. These units are available in several sizes, from small less than 2 cubic feet or tabletop sterilizers, to large floor-loading units. Some units have sophisticated microprocessor controls that allow maximum flexibility in selecting sterilization and drying times and help in troubleshooting if a problem occurs during a cycle.

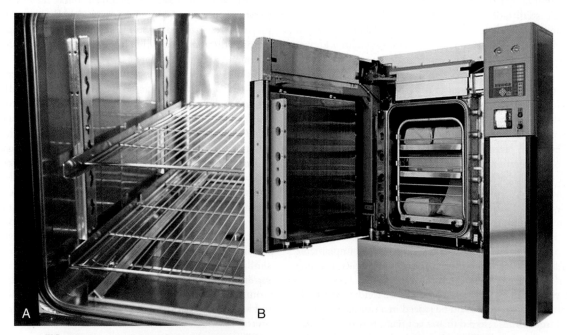

FIG. 4.6 (A) Adjustable racks used within sterilizers are designed to permit maximum loading efficiency. (B) Instrument baskets or trays should have either wire-meshed bottoms or a sufficient number of perforations in the sheet metal to allow for air removal and drainage of condensate during the sterilization cycle.

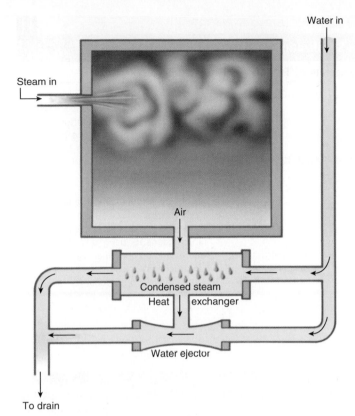

Steam in

Water in

Air

Condensed steam

Heat | exchanger

Water ejector

To drain

FIG. 4.7 Dynamic air removal/prevacuum steam sterilizer. This type of sterilizer features active, aggressive removal of air rather than relying on the passive action of gravity. When the cycle is initiated, steam is injected with force into the chamber. At the same time, the drain at the bottom of the chamber is automatically closed. As more steam enters the chamber, pressure increases and the steam and air form a turbulent mixture. When a specific pressure is reached, the drain opens, and the pressurized steam and air rush from the chamber, aided by a water ejector or a vacuum pump. This sudden rush of gas from the chamber creates a vacuum within the chamber. This process is repeated several times and deepens the level of vacuum drawn with each pulse. The effect of this pulsing cycle is to displace any air in the load and rapidly increase the chamber and load temperatures. At the conclusion of this conditioning phase, steam flows into the chamber and raises the temperature to sterilization levels, usually 270°F to 275°F (132°C to 145°C). Steam is removed from the chamber to draw a partial vacuum again. Heated, filtered air is introduced into the chamber to dry the load. Drying times are selected and set by the user, depending on the nature of the load. Some units have a special cycle designed for rapid sterilization of an instrument tray in a single wrapper. This express cycle has fewer conditioning pulses, a 4-minute exposure time, and 1 or 2 minutes of dry time, for a total cycle time of approximately 12 minutes. Although the wrapper feels warm and dry to the touch, the contents may not be totally dry. This package should be handled by individuals wearing sterile gloves and using sterile towels for protection from burns. The instruments sterilized in this express cycle must be used immediately. Because the contents are not dry, the package is not suitable for storage.

Some sterilizers can run only gravity displacement cycles. These sterilizers are referred to as gravity displacement sterilizers. Historically gravity displacement sterilizers were the only type of sterilizer available and were located in the OR suite where they were used to "flash" instruments. Hence, they became known as "flash sterilizers." With the exception of tabletop sterilizers, most sterilizers today can run either a dynamic air removal cycle or a gravity displacement cycle. To ensure selection of the cycle indicated in a device IFU the person operating the sterilizer needs to know whether the sterilizer cycle is set for gravity or for dynamic air removal. The device manufacturer's IFU should be consulted to determine the preferred or required cycle type, time, and temperature parameters.

All sterilizers should be serviced and maintained according to the sterilizer manufacturer's written IFU. This may include daily or other periodic inspection of components and cleaning and periodic preventive maintenance. Preventive maintenance should be performed by a qualified individual such as a biomedical engineer or a sterilizer service employee. Records of maintenance and repair should be maintained and readily retrievable.

Immediate-Use Steam Sterilization. Immediate-use steam sterilization (IUSS) (formerly known as flash sterilization) is a process used to sterilize items that are not intended to be stored for use at a later time. The cycle used for IUSS has a very minimal or no dry time, which decreases the total time for processing. Items processed using IUSS should be used as soon as possible after they are removed from the sterilizer. They should not be stored for later use or held for a later procedure (AAMI et al., 2011). IUSS sterilization can be accomplished using either a gravity displacement or a dynamic air removal cycle. IUSS is most frequently used in the OR for sterilizing urgently needed instruments for which there is no terminally sterilized replacement. Terminal sterilization is the process by which items are packaged and sterilized using a cycle that includes dry time and after which the packages can be stored in a sterile state until needed. Items subject to IUSS are not packaged but should not be sterilized in an open pan or tray. Containers validated for IUSS should be used for this process. The IUSS container IFU should be consulted to determine required cycle type and time and temperature parameters. IUSS should not be used for implantable devices except in cases of emergency when no other option is available. In an emergency, when IUSS of an implant is unavoidable, a BI and a chemical integrating indicator should run with the load (AORN, 2016n). Results of the BI may not be known until after completion of the surgery. Documentation should reflect patient follow-up if the BI result indicates a failure. If available, an early readout BI should be used because results may be known before the implant must be used in surgery. Appropriate perioperative planning along with communicating and working with implant manufacturers may help decrease unplanned IUSS. Devices subject to IUSS should be meticulously cleaned in a dedicated decontamination area. IUSS containers should be used, cleaned between each use, and maintained according to the manufacturer's written IFU. Containers intended only for IUSS should be differentiated from other types of containers (AORN, 2016n). Routine cycle parameters for IUSS sterilization are shown in Table 4.6. Meticulous recordkeeping must be implemented for IUSS. At a minimum, facilities should document the date and time, patient's name, surgery or procedure performed, item(s), cycle parameters (the printout), and the name of the sterilizer operator. Additional information to document includes the reason IUSS was necessary. Analysis of the frequency of and the reasons for IUSS can be used as an impetus for process improvements (i.e., reducing the incidence of IUSS).

Chemical Sterilization. There are many critical devices that require sterilization but cannot tolerate the heat and/or moisture of steam sterilization. Sterilization for heat- and moisture-intolerant devices is accomplished using chemical sterilization, which is most often referred to as *low-temperature sterilization.*

Ethylene Oxide. *EO* is an alkylating agent that results in microbial death under controlled parameters. EO has had application for heat-labile and moisture-sensitive items, such as flexible GI endoscopes,

TABLE 4.6

Time-Temperature Parameters for Immediate-Use Steam Sterilization

Type of Sterilizer/Cycle	Load Configuration	Temperature [°F (°C)]	Time (Minutes)
High-speed gravity displacement	Metal or nonporous items only (no lumens)	270–272 (132–135)	See device, container, and sterilizer manufacturer's instructions for use (follow manufacturer's instructions for express cycle to determine number of items permitted and cycle time)
	Metal items with lumens and porous items (e.g., rubber, plastic), which are sterilized together	270–272 (132–135)	See device and container manufacturer's instructions for use
Prevacuum (dynamic air removal)	Metal or nonporous items only (no lumens)	270–272 (132–135)	See device and container manufacturer's instructions for use
	Metal items with lumens and porous items, which are sterilized together	270–272 (132–135)	See device and container manufacturer's instructions for use
Pulsing gravity	All loads	Manufacturer's instructions	See device and container manufacturer's instructions for use; also see sterilizer manufacturer's instructions

some lensed instruments, delicate surgical instruments, and electrical devices. EO is colorless at ordinary temperatures, has an odor similar to that of ether, and has inhalation toxicity similar to that of ammonia gas. EO is a known carcinogen and must be used carefully because of its toxicity. It is highly explosive and very flammable in the presence of air.

Destruction of microorganisms takes place by alkylation by which the DNA of the microorganism is destroyed, inactivating the reproductive process of the cell. As with all sterilization and disinfection processes, items to be sterilized with EO must be thoroughly cleaned and dried. Ethylene oxide in combination with water forms ethylene glycol (antifreeze). Drying inhibits the formation of ethylene glycol (antifreeze) during the sterilization cycle. Items should be disassembled before placement within sets or trays and should be configured to permit the gas to circulate throughout the items. The packaging material used should possess the characteristics described previously in this chapter and should be compatible with EO.

Proper loading of the sterilizer is essential to ensure adequate gas circulation and penetration. Distribution and arrangement of items should be in accordance with the sterilizer manufacturer's instructions. An excessively large load or a load that is tightly packed interferes with proper air removal, load humidification, sterilant penetration, and sterilant evacuation at the conclusion of the cycle. An EO-sensitive chemical indicator should be used on the outside of every package as a means to indicate that the package was exposed to the gas. As with all external indicators this only indicates that exposure has occurred. It does not confirm sterility. Factors affecting sterilization with EO are time of exposure, gas concentration, temperature, humidity, and penetration. The exposure time required depends on temperature, humidity, gas concentration, the ease of penetrating articles to be sterilized, and the type of microorganisms to be destroyed. Gas concentration is affected by the temperature and humidity inside the sterilizing chamber. Temperature and humidity are important in gaseous sterilization with EO because they affect penetration of the gas through bacterial cell walls and through wrapping and packaging material (Table 4.7). The adequacy of every EO cycle should be verified using a PCD containing a BI consisting of a known population of *Bacillus atrophaeus* spores.

TABLE 4.7

Common Parameters for Ethylene Oxide Sterilization

Time (Minutes)	Temperature [°F (°C)]	Humidity (%)	Gas Concentration (mg/L)
105–300	99–145 (37–63)	45–75	450–1200

EO has been identified by OSHA as a human carcinogen (OSHA, 2012b). EO-sterilized items must be aerated to make them safe for personnel handling and patient use. The length of aeration for each item should be based on the device and the sterilizer manufacturer's written IFU. Aeration is a lengthy process and may take up to 8 hours or more.

Because of the highly explosive and flammable nature of EO, it is commonly available in small cartridges that contain enough gas to sterilize a single load. The sterilizer should be installed in a well-ventilated room and be vented to the outside atmosphere as recommended by the manufacturer and by the requirements of the National Institute for Occupational Safety and Health (NIOSH). Only authorized personnel are allowed access, and hazard signs should be posted. Compliance with other administrative controls to ensure safety is essential.

Excessive exposure to EO represents a health hazard to personnel. It is a known carcinogen and has been linked to reproductive problems. Exposure to EO should be avoided. OSHA has issued standards regulating personnel exposure to EO (OSHA, 2012b). These standards set the permissible exposure level (PEL) (the amount of EO in the air) at 1 part per million (ppm) and the action level (AL) (monitored value at which corrective action should occur) at 0.5 ppm. These are calculated as time-weighted averages (TWAs) over an 8-hour period. OSHA requires that monitoring and surveillance be performed to ensure that exposure levels do not exceed 1 ppm over an 8-hour period (OSHA, 1984). In addition, occupational exposure level to EO may not exceed 15 ppm in any 15-minute period. This is known as the *excursion level* (EL). Beginning June 1,

2016, a sign must be posted demarcating regulated areas and entrances or accesses to the regulated area (Fig. 4.8).

Personnel with the potential for EO exposure should wear an EO-monitoring badge that meets the NIOSH accuracy standards. Butyl rubber, nitrile, or neoprene gloves should be worn if it becomes necessary to handle items that have not been fully aerated (AORN, 2016n).

Because of the long cycle and aeration time and the many safety requirements EO sterilizers are not located in the OR. In addition, many facilities have replaced EO sterilizers with other low-temperature sterilization technologies with short cycles and few safety concerns.

Low-Temperature Hydrogen Peroxide Gas Plasma Sterilization. Low-temperature hydrogen peroxide gas plasma sterilization may be used for moisture- and heat-sensitive items and when indicated by the device manufacturer. Plasma is the fourth state of matter, with the sequence being solid, liquid, gas, and plasma. During the process a vacuum is created in the sterilization chamber, liquid hydrogen peroxide is injected into a cap and enters the chamber as a vapor or gas, which is effective at killing pathogenic microorganisms.

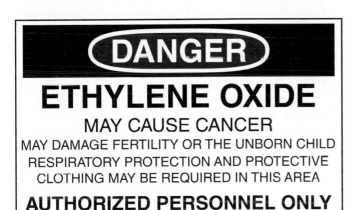

FIG. 4.8 Ethylene oxide warning sign.

To create a plasma hydrogen peroxide is charged with radiofrequency energy. The plasma breaks down the hydrogen peroxide into a cloud of free radicals that recombine into oxygen and water in the form of humidity. There are no toxic residuals, and packages are dry at the end of the cycle.

Cycle times for hydrogen peroxide gas plasma sterilization vary depending on the model of sterilizer. The cycle time can be as short as just less than 30 minutes. At the completion of the sterilization process, no toxic residues remain on the sterilized items and no aeration is necessary. Device manufacturer's IFU should be consulted to determine compatibility of devices with sterilization in hydrogen peroxide gas plasma. Instrumentation preparation for sterilization includes cleaning and decontaminating procedures, drying, packaging, and wrapping with nonwoven polypropylene wraps, Tyvek/Mylar pouches, or containers validated for use with hydrogen peroxide gas plasma (Fig. 4.9). Cellulosic-based products, such as paper and linen, are not recommended for use with plasma systems because they tend to absorb the vapor and cause the sterilization cycle to abort. Lumen restrictions prevent use for sterilization of long-channeled devices. Manufacturer's written IFU should always be followed (AORN, 2016n).

Biologic and chemical indicators for process verification are used in the same manner as indicators for steam and EO sterilization procedures. Plasma sterilization processes should be tested with BIs containing *G. stearothermophilus* spores. These spores show the greatest resistance to kill in hydrogen peroxide gas plasma. Efficacy testing of the sterilization cycle should be performed daily, preferably with every load (AORN, 2016n).

Hydrogen Peroxide Vapor. Low-temperature hydrogen peroxide vapor is suitable for devices that cannot tolerate high temperature or moisture and that are indicated as compatible by the device manufacturer. In this process hydrogen peroxide vapor is the sterilant. This is an oxidative process that inactivates microorganisms. The byproducts at the end of the cycle are oxygen and water vapor. Packages are dry at the end of the cycle. The process is nontoxic and no aeration is required.

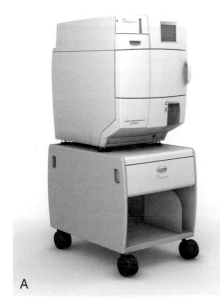
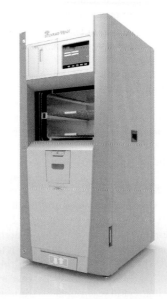
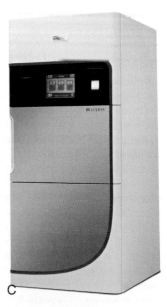

FIG. 4.9 Low-temperature gas plasma sterilizers. (A) Tabletop model. (B) Floor standing model. (C) V-PRO Max sterilizer.

Items must be cleaned, dried, and packaged as with other sterilization processes. Compatible packaging includes nonwoven polypropylene wraps, Tyvek/Mylar pouches, trays, and containers validated for use with hydrogen peroxide sterilization; cellulose-based products are not recommended. One or more chemical indicators should be placed within each package to be sterilized. Sterilizer efficacy monitoring with a BI containing *G. stearothermophilus* spores should be performed with every load.

Liquid Peracetic Acid Sterilant Systems. Many facilities use a liquid peracetic acid sterilant processing system. Liquid peracetic acid systems are used for devices that are heat sensitive, can be immersed, and have been validated by the device manufacturer for use in these systems. Items with lumens are connected to irrigation adaptors that permit contact within the lumens with the peracetic acid. Liquid peracetic acid is suitable for devices that cannot be sterilized with terminal sterilization methods. Terminal sterilization includes packaging and a sterilization process that permits storage of the package for an indefinite period. A liquid peracetic acid processing system is a just-in-time process. At the end of the process items are wet, are not wrapped or containerized, and cannot be stored for use at a later time. Cycle time is approximately 30 minutes. Peracetic acid is an oxidizing agent. Parameters are measured with microprocessors and a printout is provided. A chemical indicator is available and should be used with each cycle. A spore strip containing *G. stearothermophilus* spores is used to test the sporicidal activity of the sterilant dilution. Items processed in these systems should be taken to the point of use and used immediately. The circulating nurse will open the lid of the tray in which the items were processed and the scrub person will remove the items and place them on the sterile field.

Managing Loaned Instruments. Loaned instruments are instruments that are loaned to a facility by a vendor. Depending on the specific agreement between the healthcare facility and the vendor there may be a fee for this service. Loaned instruments and equipment are commonly referred to as "loaners." Use of loaned instruments and equipment is common practice in spine and orthopedic specialties where the facility purchases the implant but not the instrumentation. Problems associated with loaned instruments have included lack of inventory control, delivery to the facility with insufficient lead time to process using a terminal sterilization process, and pressure to use an IUSS process to prevent delay of the surgery schedule. In recent years facilities have taken steps to better manage loaners to prevent these problems; however, the process is not always problem free. A policy for loaners should cover the entire process from the time the decision is made to use the instruments or equipment through the time the instruments and equipment leave the facility. Policies and procedures should include defining the person responsible for each step in the process (Burlingame, 2015). Management of loaners should include the following:

- Responsibilities of the facility and the vendor
- Identification of delivery location
- Delivery with enough lead time to be able to decontaminate and process using terminal sterilization (this is typically a minimum of 24 hours)
- Delivery of IFU and inventory list to the responsible person
- Procedure for inventory of set contents, equipment, and documentation of same
- Inspection of instruments
- Decontamination, inspection, packaging, and terminal sterilization
- Decontamination of instruments before return to the vendor

Disinfection

Disinfection is a process that destroys microorganisms either through a liquid chemical or a thermal process. Liquid chemical germicides are used to destroy microorganisms on environmental surfaces and on medical devices. The term *disinfection* also may refer to treatment of body surfaces that have been contaminated with infectious material. Chemicals used to disinfect inanimate objects are referred to as *disinfectants*. Chemicals used for body surfaces are known as *antiseptics*. The term *germicide* refers to any solution that destroys microorganisms. Some germicides are disinfectants and antiseptics.

Disinfectants vary in their ability to kill microorganisms. A variety of liquid chemical germicide disinfectants are used in healthcare settings. Disinfectants are categorized as high level, intermediate level, or low level, depending on their disinfecting capability.

- High-level disinfectants kill all microorganisms except high numbers of bacterial spores.
- Intermediate-level disinfectants may kill tubercle bacilli, vegetative bacteria, and most viruses and fungi but not bacterial spores.
- Low-level disinfectants kill most vegetative bacteria and some viruses and fungi.

Low-level and intermediate-level disinfectants are generally used on environmental surfaces such as floors and counter tops. High-level disinfectants are used to disinfect medical devices to render them safe for handling and for use on a patient. High-level disinfectants play a key role in the processing of semicritical medical devices.

In healthcare facilities, a semicritical item intended to be disinfected with a high-level disinfectant is usually either soaked in a liquid chemical for a specified period or processed in an automated disinfecting system, such as an automated endoscope processor, to achieve disinfection of the item. The disinfection process may destroy tubercle bacilli and inactivate hepatitis viruses and enteroviruses but usually does not kill resistant bacterial spores. As with sterilization, an item must be cleaned before it is disinfected.

Types of Disinfectants. Many disinfectants are used alone or in combination, such as hydrogen peroxide and peracetic acid, in healthcare settings. These include alcohols, chlorine and chlorine compounds, glutaraldehyde, OPA, hydrogen peroxide, iodophors, peracetic acid, phenolics, and quaternary ammonium compounds. In healthcare the commercial products are considered unique and must be registered with the Environmental Protection Agency (EPA) or in the case of high-level disinfectants, cleared by the FDA. FDA-cleared high-level disinfectants include glutaraldehyde solutions, OPA, hydrogen peroxide, peracetic acid, and hydrogen peroxide solutions. A complete listing may be found on the FDA website (FDA, 2015b). In most cases a given product is designed for a specific purpose and should be used accordingly. Disinfectants are not interchangeable, and incorrect use can compromise effectiveness of the disinfection process. The disinfectant manufacturer's written IFU should be followed and precautions should be taken to minimize exposure to these products. Instructions include concentration, temperate and contact time requirements, product shelf life, use life, activation instructions if activation is needed, the disposal process, spill cleanup instructions, and quality control processes.

High-level disinfectants should be tested for minimum effective concentration (MEC) before each use. A chemical indicator designed for testing the MEC and specific to the disinfectant product is used for this purpose. The indicator is supplied as a paper or plastic strip that must be dipped into the solution for a specified amount of time and checked for the appropriate color change. MEC chemical indicator strips are not interchangeable. High-level disinfectants state an expiration date on their label. This is usually 2 to 4 weeks;

however, the MEC could fail before the stated expiration date. Factors that impact the MEC include amount of time the solution is used and dilution that can occur when items are immersed before they are dried. Results of the MEC test should be documented. In addition, the date the solution is first opened and the expiration date should be documented. The expiration date should also be visible on the solution container. Other documentation includes the name of the person performing the disinfection, the date and time, the item(s) being disinfected, and the patient on whom the item(s) will be used. Some high-level disinfectant solution instructions include a quality control requirement before the first use of the solution. Results of this testing should be documented.

Chemical disinfectants can irritate skin and mucous membranes and precautions should be taken to minimize personnel exposure to these chemicals. High-level disinfection should be performed in a well-ventilated area. A vapor control system can help to protect personnel from irritation. The following are various types of disinfectants used in healthcare facilities (CDC, 2016e).

High-Level Disinfectants Commonly Used for Instrument Processing

Glutaraldehyde Solutions. Glutaraldehyde is a saturated dialdehyde that has gained wide acceptance as an overall effective high-level disinfecting agent and chemical sterilant. Aqueous solutions of glutaraldehyde are acidic and in this state not sporicidal. The solution is said to be "activated" when alkalizing agents are added to make the solution alkaline. Glutaraldehyde is widely used for high-level disinfection of semicritical items. Glutaraldehyde is actually a chemical sterilant because it is capable of sterilization at extended contact times of up to 10 hours' immersion. Because of the lengthy time required to achieve sterilization, and because the device is wet at the end of the process, is unpackaged, and cannot be stored in a sterile state, it is rarely, if ever, used for sterilization. However, depending on the formulation and temperature, high-level disinfection with glutaraldehyde can be achieved in many cases in 10 minutes or less. Immersion times of 20 to 45 minutes may be found on some glutaraldehyde instructions. Glutaraldehyde products are more commonly used in the GI lab for processing GI endoscopes than in the OR or sterile processing department. Glutaraldehyde is not corrosive to endoscopes and has a wide range of materials compatibility. Glutaraldehyde can irritate skin and mucous membranes and has been associated with asthma symptoms. It should be used in a well-ventilated area or under a fume hood. NIOSH has established a recommended exposure limit of 0.2 ppm (CDC, 2016f). Personnel working with glutaraldehyde should wear PPE, which may include nitrile gloves, eye protection, masks, and moisture-repellent gowns. To achieve high-level disinfection, instruments must be free from bioburden, dried, and completely immersed in activated aqueous glutaraldehyde solution. During immersion all surfaces of the instrument must be in contact with the liquid chemical. After immersion, instruments must be rinsed thoroughly with sterile water before being used.

Ortho-Phthalaldehyde. Ortho-phthalaldehyde is a 0.55% solution in an aqueous buffer with a pH of 7.5 and is considered a high-level disinfectant. It is a nonglutaraldehyde disinfectant. It is tuberculocidal at a minimum exposure time of 12 minutes at room temperature. It has excellent stability over a wide pH range and is odorless. Because OPA has a very low vapor pressure it is less irritating than glutaraldehyde. As a result, many facilities no longer use glutaraldehyde and have switched to OPA.

As with any high-level disinfectant, PPE should be used with OPA. It should be used in a well-ventilated area and start-of-use date and expiration date should be documented. The expiration date of the solution remaining in the bottle differs from the expiration date once it is put into use. Both expiration dates should be noted and documented. OPA can be used for most applications for which glutaraldehyde is used and has broad materials compatibility. It is commonly used in automated endoscope processing systems. Several manufacturers produce OPA and their IFUs may vary. As with all chemical disinfectants the manufacturer's written IFU should always be followed.

Peracetic Acid Solutions. Peracetic acid is rapid acting and has excellent antimicrobial activity. Automated systems using peracetic acid are commonly used in the GI lab for processing flexible endoscopes. Users should check the endoscope manufacturer's written IFU to determine compatibility with peracetic acid. Peracetic acid in combination with hydrogen peroxide is commonly used to disinfect hemodialyzers.

Other Disinfectants

Alcohols. For disinfection in healthcare, the term *alcohol* refers to either 70% or 90% isopropyl alcohol. Both of these compounds are water soluble and have a high degree of germicidal activity. They are bactericidal as opposed to bacteriostatic against vegetative forms of bacteria. They also are tuberculocidal, fungicidal, and virucidal. Isopropyl alcohol (*n*-propanol) and ethyl alcohol (*n*-ethanol) at concentrations of 60% to 80% are potent virucidal agents that can inactivate lipophilic viruses such as herpes and the influenza virus along with many hydrophilic viruses such as rhinovirus and rotaviruses. Studies have demonstrated the ability of ethyl and isopropyl alcohol to inactivate HBV and to inactivate HIV (CDC, 2016e). The alcohols do not destroy spores or kill certain hydrophilic viruses. Alcohols are flammable and must be stored in a well-ventilated area. Because they evaporate rapidly, extended contact time is difficult to achieve unless items are immersed. Alcohols lack residual effect and are easily inactivated by protein material. Alcohols tend to damage the coating on lensed instruments and may cause hardening of certain rubber and plastic tubing after repeated exposure to the compound. Alcohols are considered intermediate-level disinfectants. They are often used to disinfect thermometers and rubber stoppers on medication vials. Alcohol also is used in processing flexible endoscopes. After high-level disinfection and a tap water rinse, alcohol is effective in inactivating water contaminants. Its speed of evaporation also assists in rapid drying of the endoscope channels.

Chlorine Compounds. In healthcare facilities, hypochlorites are the most widely used of the chlorine compounds. Hypochlorites are available in a liquid form (sodium hypochlorite [liquid household bleach]) and in a solid form (calcium hypochlorite). Hypochlorites have a broad spectrum of antimicrobial activity. They are inexpensive and fast acting. Low concentrations of free chlorine (50 ppm) are effective against vegetative bacteria and *Mycoplasma*. Free chlorine at 50 ppm inactivates HIV, whereas a 500-ppm concentration is needed to inactivate HBV. Concentrations of 1000 ppm are recommended for inactivation of bacterial spores. Household bleach contains 5.25% sodium hypochlorite. A dilution of 1:1000 provides 50 ppm of available chlorine. A dilution of 1:50 provides 1000 ppm of available chlorine, which is considered adequate to achieve high-level disinfection. The CDC recommends a 1:10 solution, which provides 5000 ppm of available chlorine. Hypochlorite solutions are stable for 30 days in opaque containers. Beyond that time a new solution should be prepared. Hypochlorites are inactivated in the presence of organic matter. All organic material should be removed before application of the disinfecting solution. Hypochlorites are not routinely used for disinfection of surgical instruments because of the corrosive action of the compound. Hypochlorites are most often used for countertops, floors, and other surfaces to be disinfected. Hypochlorites are recommended for environmental disinfection of surfaces suspected of being contaminated with *C. diff.*

Hydrogen Peroxide. Hydrogen peroxide is active against a wide range of microorganisms, including bacteria, yeasts, fungi, viruses, and spores (CDC, 2016e). Unstable and low concentrations of hydrogen peroxide (<3% solution) may be used as a low-level disinfectant for work-surface cleaning and disinfection. Stabilized 6% hydrogen peroxide is sporicidal and can be used as a liquid sterilant with sufficient exposure time. The solution is corrosive, however, to copper, zinc, and brass. It also can damage rubber and plastic.

Iodine and Iodophors. Iodine solutions have been used widely by health professionals, primarily as antiseptics on skin or tissue. An iodophor is a water-soluble combination of iodine and a solubilizing agent or carrier that allows for a slow but continuous release of free iodine over time. Iodophors may be used as disinfectants or antiseptics, depending on the concentration of free iodine. The most widely used iodophor is povidone-iodine, although its use as a skin cleanser or surgical scrub agent has largely been replaced with CHG, an antibacterial agent with efficacy against a wide range of pathogenic microorganisms. As disinfectants, iodophors have the advantage of having the germicidal efficacy of iodine without the disadvantages of toxicity and surface irritation. Iodophors are usually nonstaining and effective against vegetative bacteria, *M. tuberculosis,* and most viruses and fungi. Iodophors are not considered suitable for high-level disinfection or for use as hard-surface disinfectants because they have no sporicidal capability (CDC, 2016e).

Phenolics. Phenol (carbolic acid) was first used by Lister in the mid-1800s. Since then, many phenol derivatives (phenolics) have been developed. Phenolics are not sporicidal, and they are not considered effective as high-level disinfectants. They are used primarily as intermediate-level and low-level disinfectants for environmental cleaning. They are known to have toxic effects, however, and their use has been associated with depigmentation and hyperbilirubinemia in newborns. Because of this, phenolics are not recommended for cleaning incubators or infant bassinets (CDC, 2016e).

Quaternary Ammonium Compounds. Quaternary ammonium compounds ("quats") have been used for many years as a result of their reputation for microbicidal activity, good detergent action, and low-level toxicity. In more recent times, it has been noted that environmental factors, such as hard water, soap residues, and protein soils, reduce or nullify the efficacy of these compounds. Quaternary compounds kill a wide range of microorganisms with the exception of spores. They are used most often for noncritical surfaces such as floors, walls, and furniture.

Pasteurization

Pasteurization is a process that uses hot water at a temperature generally at 158°F (70°C) for 30 minutes to achieve high-level disinfection. Pasteurization can be accomplished using a commercial washer or pasteurizer. The actual time/temperature relationship depends on the items to be disinfected. Contact time is inversely related to temperature. For equivalent microbial destruction, longer exposure times are required when the temperature is decreased. Pasteurization is intended to kill all pathogenic vegetative microorganisms. Pasteurization does not kill spores. Pasteurization of respiratory and anesthesia equipment is recognized as an alternative to chemical disinfection. Semicritical items, such as respiratory therapy and anesthesia devices, are ready for patient use after cleaning and pasteurization (CDC,

2016e). Advantages of pasteurization include absence of toxic residues and the associated need for postprocess rinsing. After pasteurization, and before storage, items are typically dried in a hot-air drying cabinet.

Reprocessing/Reuse of Items Labeled for Single Use Only

Devices that are labeled as single use should not be reprocessed unless the FDA guidelines for reprocessing can be met. The guidelines are the same as those for the original device manufacturer, and most healthcare facilities cannot meet them (FDA, 2015c). Reprocessing can, however, offer an opportunity for reduced costs. Facilities considering reprocessing of single-use devices should investigate the feasibility of contracting with a commercial reprocessing company that can meet these requirements. Requirements include registration as a reprocessing firm, listing all devices reprocessed, submitting reports of device adverse events, tracking devices, correcting or removing unsafe devices from the market, and compliance with all manufacturing and labeling FDA requirement (FDA, 2015c) (Patient Safety).

Aseptic Practices to Prevent Infection

Surgical Aseptic Principles

Asepsis has been defined as the absence of infectious organisms. Surgical aseptic practices are based on the premise that most infections are caused by organisms exogenous to the surgical patient's body. To avoid infection, surgical procedures must be performed in a manner that minimizes or eliminates the patient's exposure to exogenous pathogenic organisms. Opening sterile supplies as close to the time of their use as possible, using sterile drapes to create a sterile field around the incision site, using sterile instruments for the surgical procedure, and placing the operative team in sterile attire after their hands and arms have been cleansed of surface bacteria are examples of helping to avoid infection.

Aseptic technique stems from the principles of asepsis derived over time from microbiologic and epidemiologic concepts. Although some investigators may believe that current aseptic practices and techniques have become too ritualistic or lack scientific research to support their use, present-day infection-control statistics support the application of aseptic principles for safe perioperative nursing practice. Until empiric research shows that a technique is unnecessary or ineffective, the basic aseptic principles should be followed. These principles are as follows:

1. Only sterile items are used within the sterile field. Individuals dispensing sterile items to the sterile field must look at the sterilization indicator on or visible in the package, check for package integrity, and check for the package expiration date (or appropriate marking for event-related shelf life) before dispensing the item to the field.

2. Items of doubtful sterility must be considered unsterile. Examples include sterile items found in unsterile work areas, sterilized packages wrapped in pervious materials that have become wet, sterilized items without an integrator or other internal chemical indicator, or packages in which integrity has been compromised.

3. Whenever a sterile barrier is permeated, it must be considered contaminated. This principle applies to packaging materials and to draping and gowning materials. Obvious contamination occurs from direct contact between sterile and unsterile objects. Other less apparent modes of contamination are the filtration of airborne microorganisms through materials, passage of liquids through materials, and undetected perforations in materials. Moisture

PATIENT SAFETY

Considerations for Reprocessing of Single-Use Devices

Three ways to handle used single-use medical and surgical devices are identified in the following manner:

- Dispose of them after use.
- Reprocess the device according to the stringent FDA guidelines.
- Contract with a reprocessing specialty company to collect, reprocess, and reship the product to the healthcare facility.

The FDA became involved in the issue of reprocessing products labeled as single use when they were alerted by the original manufacturers of devices that facilities were reprocessing without ensuring the efficacy, effectiveness, and sterility of the original product. In 2000 the FDA published a guidance document, which is still in use, called *Enforcement Priorities for Single-Use Devices Reprocessed by Third Parties and Hospitals*. It concerned the reprocessing of single-use devices. A facility that chooses to reprocess single-use devices must meet the same requirements as the original device manufacturer. Because these requirements are almost impossible to meet within healthcare facilities, the practice of reprocessing single-use devices within healthcare facilities has essentially stopped.

The FDA publishes an extensive listing of single-use devices that have been identified for reprocessing. The FDA has been monitoring this situation since 2001, with vigorous oversight as well as the development of stringent guidelines and their subsequent enforcement. They have clearly identified those devices that penetrate the mucosa as high risk and do not endorse reprocessing these devices. These guidelines for reprocessing single-use devices include processes that almost no healthcare facility is able to comply with. For example, required validation studies necessitate the use of equipment not found in healthcare facilities. This does not mean that certain single-use devices cannot be effectively and safely reprocessed by commercial enterprises engaged in this activity or more commonly referred to as third-party reprocessors. FDA requirements include the following:

- Submitting documents for premarket notification of approval
- Registering reprocessing firms and listing all products
- Submitting adverse event reports
- Tracking devices whose failure could have serious outcomes
- Correcting or removing from the market unsafe devices
- Meeting manufacturing and labeling requirements (FDA, 2015c)

Each requirement has associated resource needs. An in-depth discussion of these requirements is beyond the scope of this textbook. Details of the FDA requirements for reprocessors can be found in the *Code of Federal Regulations* (FDA, 2015a).

If a user facility chooses to engage a third-party reprocessor it is the facility's responsibility to assess the quality of the services provided under the contractual arrangement with the third-party reprocessor. The user facility must review the processes used by the contracted agency and determine whether correct procedures are being followed (AORN, 2016n; CDC, 2016e).

FDA, Food and Drug Administration.
Modified from Association of periOperative Registered Nurses (AORN): Guideline for sterilization. In: *Guidelines for perioperative practice*, ed 16, Denver, 2016, The Association; Centers for Disease Control and Prevention (CDC): *Infection control: disinfection and sterilization* (website), 2016. www.cdc.gov/infectioncontrol/guidelines/disinfection/index.html. (Accessed 9 August 2017); US Food and Drug Administration (FDA): *Reprocessing of reusable medical devices* (website), 2015. www.fda.gov/MedicalDevices/ProductsandMedicalProcedures/ReprocessingofReusableMedicalDevices/ucm20081513.htm. (Assessed 4 February 2017).

soaking through a drape, gown, or package is considered a strikethrough, and the item must be considered contaminated.

4. Sterile gowns are considered sterile in front from the chest to the level of the sterile field and at the sleeves from 2 inches above the elbow to the cuff. The cuff should be considered unsterile because it tends to collect moisture and is not an effective bacterial barrier. The sleeve cuffs should always be covered by sterile gloves. Other areas of the gown that must be considered unsterile are the neckline, shoulders, axillary area, and back (AORN, 2016m). These areas may become contaminated by perspiration or by collar and shoulder surfaces rubbing together during head and neck movements. Wraparound gowns that completely cover the back may be sterile when first put on. The back of the gown must not be considered sterile, however, because it cannot be observed and protected from contamination. The sterile area of the front of the gown extends to the level of the sterile field because most scrub personnel work adjacent to a sterile table. For this reason the scrub person should avoid changing levels, as would occur while moving from footstool to floor. To maintain sterility, scrub persons should not allow their hands or any sterile item to fall below the level of the sterile field. Scrub persons should neither sit nor lean against unsterile surfaces because the threat of contamination is great. The only time scrub persons may be seated is when the entire surgical procedure is performed at that level. Self-gowning and gloving should be done from a sterile surface separate from the sterile field. This method eliminates reaching over the sterile field to retrieve the sterile towel and then the sterile gown. It also eliminates the potential for water to be dripped on sterile items or on any part of the sterile field, preventing inadvertent contamination. When prepared, the scrub person's hands should be kept in sight at or above waist level. Elbows should be kept close to the body, and the hands should be kept away from the face. Hands should not be folded under the arms because axillary perspiration may permeate the bacterial barrier of the gown.

5. Sterile drapes are used to create a sterile field. When placed, a drape should not be shifted or moved. Items should be dispensed to a sterile field by methods that preserve the sterility of the items and the integrity of the sterile field. Good judgment must be used when dispensing items by presenting them to the scrub person or by placing them securely on the sterile field. A sterile field should be created as close as possible to the time of use. Sterile drapes also are used to create a sterile field when placed over the patient and operative bed. Any item that extends beyond the sterile boundary is considered contaminated and cannot be returned to the sterile field. Interpretation of sterile areas versus unsterile areas on a draped patient requires astute observation and use of good judgment. When contamination of the sterile field occurs, corrective action should immediately be taken unless this will put the patient at risk (AORN, 2016m). A contaminated

item must be lifted clear of the operative field without contacting the sterile surface and must be dropped with minimal handling to a nonscrubbed surgical team member, an unsterile area, or a designated receptacle.

6. Items should be dispensed to the field in a manner that preserves the sterility of the item and the integrity of the sterile field. When opening a sterile wrapper, the top flap is first opened away from the operator; the side flaps then follow. The inside or proximal flap is opened last. All flaps are secured in the hand by the operator so they do not dangle and contaminate other items. When removing an item from a sterile package, the scrub person should lift it straight up from the package. Peel pouches should be presented to the scrub person to maintain sterility. The edges of peel pouches have a tendency to curl so that care must be taken to prevent the contents from sliding across an unsterile edge. Interpreting sterile boundaries requires good judgment based on an understanding of aseptic principles.

7. Sterile individuals touch only sterile items or areas; unsterile individuals touch only unsterile items or areas. All members of the surgical team must understand which areas are considered sterile and which are considered unsterile. Everyone must maintain a continual awareness of these areas. Scrubbed individuals must guard the sterile field to prevent any unsterile item from contaminating the field or the individuals themselves. Unsterile individuals must not touch or reach over a sterile field or allow any unsterile item to contaminate the field. When a perioperative nurse opens a package, hand and arm motions are always from unsterile to sterile objects. The nurse avoids contact with the sterile area by placing the hands under the cuff to provide a protected wide margin of safety between the inside of the pack (sterile) and the hands (unsterile) (Fig. 4.10). As the unsterile

nurse opens a sterile article that is wrapped sequentially in two wrappers with the corners folded toward the center of the article, the corner farthest from the body is opened first and the corner nearest the body opened last. When a scrub person opens a sterile wrapper, the side nearest the body is opened first. This portion of the wrapper then protects the gown and enables the individual to move closer to the table to complete opening of the wrapper (Fig. 4.11). If a solution must be poured into a sterile receptacle on a sterile table, the scrub person holds the receptacle away from the table or sets it near the edge of a waterproof-draped table (Fig. 4.12). This procedure eliminates the need for the unsterile nurse to reach over the sterile field. Maintaining a safe margin of space can reduce accidental contamination when items are passed between sterile and unsterile fields.

8. Movement within or around a sterile field must not contaminate the field. The patient is the center of the sterile field during an operative procedure; additional sterile areas are grouped around the patient. If contamination is to be prevented, patterns of movement within or around this sterile grouping must be established and rigidly practiced. Scrub persons stay close to the sterile field. If they change positions, they turn face to face or back to back with another individual while maintaining a safe distance between themselves and other objects. Accidental contamination is a threat to any scrub person who wanders into a traffic pathway or out of the clean area of the OR. Perioperative nurses approach sterile areas facing them and do not walk between two sterile fields. Keeping sterile areas in view during movement around the area and maintaining a safe distance from the sterile field assist in preventing accidental contamination. Bacterial fallout from the body or clothing is a source of potential contamination when an unsterile individual leans over a sterile field. All perioperative personnel must maintain vigilance over sterile areas and identify contamination immediately. All personnel moving within or around the sterile field should do so in a manner that prevents contamination of the sterile field (AORN, 2016m).

Close adherence to principles of asepsis and consistent observance of the boundaries established in the principles provide protection against infection. Application of the basic principles of aseptic technique depends primarily on the individual's understanding and conscience. Every person on the surgical team must share the responsibility for monitoring aseptic practice and initiating corrective action when a sterile field is compromised.

Traffic Control

The surgical suite should be designed to minimize the spread of infectious organisms and to facilitate movement of patients and personnel within that framework (AORN, 2016c). Ideally, the suite is divided into three areas, each defined by the activities occurring within the area. The *unrestricted* area includes areas outside of the surgical suite and a control point to monitor the entrance of patients, personnel, and materials. Street clothes are appropriate attire in this area, and traffic is not limited, but provisions must be made for isolation of patients with communicable conditions. The *semirestricted* area comprises the peripheral support areas within the surgical suite. These may include storage areas, work areas, and corridors leading to restricted areas of the surgical suite. Traffic in the semirestricted area is limited to appropriately attired personnel and patients. Personnel must wear surgical attire and cover all head and facial hair when in this area. Patients should have their hair covered, wear clean hospital attire, and be covered with clean hospital linens. The *restricted* area includes the OR, procedure rooms (if any), the central core,

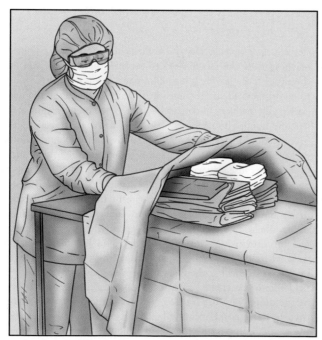

FIG. 4.10 The perioperative nurse is shown opening the cover of a pack containing sterile drapes for surgery. The cover is cuffed to provide protection for the sterile contents. The nurse avoids contact with the sterile area by keeping all fingers under the cuff as the cover is drawn back over the table to expose the pack contents.

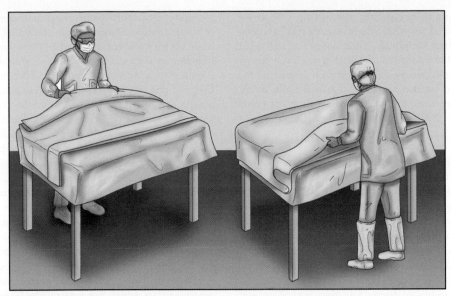

FIG. 4.11 The circulator creates a sterile field opening on one side of the drape. Then the nurse walks around the table to open the opposite side while taking care not to contaminate the drapes.

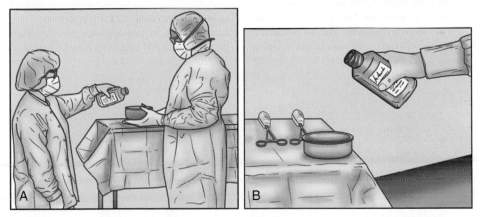

FIG. 4.12 (A) When pouring solution into the receptacle held by the scrub person, the perioperative nurse maintains a safe margin of space to avoid contamination of sterile surfaces. (B) Care must be used when pouring solution into a receptacle on a sterile field to avoid splashing fluids onto the sterile field. Placement of the receptacle near the edge of the table permits the nurse to pour solution without reaching over any portion of the sterile field.

and the scrub sink area. Personnel must wear surgical attire including hair coverings when in the restricted area. Masks are worn where open sterile supplies or scrub persons may be present. Except for patients on droplet precautions masks are not required for patients entering this area because a mask could hinder access to the patient's face and airway and cause additional patient anxiety (AORN, 2016c).

Personnel entering semirestricted or restricted areas of the surgical suite should do so through prescribed routes. These routes contain vestibular areas, which serve as transition zones between the outside and inside of the suite. Offices, holding rooms, and locker rooms act as transition zones. Personnel entering the OR should access the locker room via the unrestricted area. After donning clean, hospital-laundered surgical attire, personnel should exit directly into the OR suite without retracing steps through the unrestricted area.

Air is a potential source of pathogenic microorganisms. Airborne contamination increases with movement of the surgical team. This movement should be kept to a minimum during operative procedures. Each OR door should remain closed except during movement of patients, personnel, supplies, and equipment. The positive-pressure gradient of air in the OR is disrupted if the door remains open. The turbulent flow occurring as the pressure equalizes can increase airborne contamination (AORN, 2016m).

Surgical equipment and supplies also are potential sources of contamination. Clean and sterile supplies should be separated from contaminated items by space, time, or traffic patterns. Clean and sterile items delivered to the surgical suite should be transported in a manner that preserves package integrity and protects the packaged items from contamination along the travel route. Because external shipping containers may collect dust, debris, and insects during shipment, contents should be removed in the unrestricted area before delivery to the surgical suite. External shipping containers should be removed in the unrestricted area. Within the suite, supplies should move from the clean core or storage area through the OR to the peripheral or semirestricted corridor. Soiled instruments, supplies, and equipment should not reenter the clean core. Instead, soiled items should be covered or contained in closed carts or containers, labeled as biohazard, and transported to an area designated for decontamination. This decontamination area, as well as the soiled linen and trash collection areas, should be separate from personnel and patient traffic areas (AORN, 2016d, 2016l).

Surgical Attire

Every surgical department should have a written policy and procedure regarding proper attire in the surgical suite. According to OSHA regulations and institutional policy and to prevent transmission of organisms from the patient to personnel, personnel are required to wear PPE when it can be reasonably anticipated that the individual may come into contact with blood or OPIM. PPE, which includes protective eyewear; gloves; and fluid-resistant gowns, aprons, and shoe covers, must be included as part of the surgical attire policy as determined by OSHA regulations (OSHA, 2012a).

People are a major source of bacteria in the surgical setting. To reduce bacterial and skin shedding (scurf) and promote environmental control and cleanliness, all persons entering the semirestricted and restricted areas of the surgical suite should wear clean, facility-laundered, not previously worn, surgical attire (Fig. 4.13). Attire should be made of multiuse fabric or limited-use nonwoven material. Multiuse surgical attire should be laundered in a healthcare-accredited laundry facility. Controlled laundering of surgical attire, also known as scrub attire, can reduce the risk of spreading contamination to the home environment if laundered at home. Multiuse surgical attire should be made of tightly woven fabric (AORN, 2016o). A variety of fabric combinations are available including antibacterial fabric. Surgical attire should be constructed of a low-linting material that minimizes bacterial shedding, is comfortable, and provides a professional appearance. If a two-piece pantsuit is worn, the top of the pantsuit should be tucked into the trousers or fit close to the body. Care should be taken when donning scrub pants to avoid dragging the pant legs on the floor. A head cover, facial hair covering, mask, and, if required, shoe covers complete the surgical attire ensemble. Shoe covers are required if there is a risk of blood or body fluid contamination, as described in OSHA regulations (OSHA, 2012a). To protect the patient and the healthcare worker, surgical attire must be changed whenever it becomes soiled or wet with blood; any body fluid, including perspiration; or food. Nonscrubbed personnel should wear long-sleeved freshly laundered or disposable warm-up jackets that are buttoned or snapped closed during wear. These jackets help decrease bacterial and skin shedding from bare arms. Closing the jackets helps prevent inadvertent contamination, which can occur if the loose fabric brushes against a sterile area. All jewelry should be confined within scrub attire or removed when personnel enter the semirestricted or restricted areas of the surgical suite. This includes any visible jewelry associated with body piercing. Confinement reduces the possibility of jewelry falling or shedding bacteria into a sterile field or wound. Before handwashing, rings, watches, and bracelets should be removed because organisms can be harbored beneath these pieces of jewelry (AORN, 2016o).

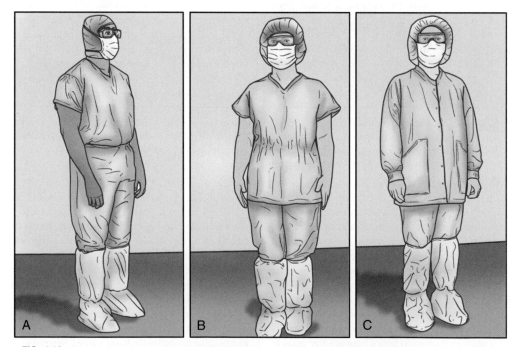

FIG. 4.13 Proper surgical attire consists of a two-piece pantsuit, a scrub dress, or a one-piece coverall suit. Shoe covers should be worn when it is reasonably anticipated that spills or splashes will occur. If worn, they should be changed whenever they become wet, torn, or soiled. In semirestricted and restricted areas, all head and facial hair should be covered. In restricted areas, all personnel should wear masks. Jewelry should be removed or totally confined. Artificial nails should not be worn. (A) When a two-piece scrub suit is worn, loose-fitting scrub tops should be tucked into pants. (B) Tunic tops that fit close to the body may be worn outside of pants. (C) Nonscrubbed personnel should wear long-sleeved jackets that are buttoned or snapped closed.

Individuals entering the restricted or semirestricted area of the surgical suite should wear a clean, lint-free surgical hat or hood that completely covers all head and facial hair. The head cover should confine all hair, the ears, sideburns, and the nape of the neck (AORN, 2016o). Head covers should always be worn in areas in which equipment and supplies are processed and stored. Disposable bouffant and hood types of head covers are preferred. Disposable head covers are discarded in a designated receptacle immediately after use. Skullcaps that fail to cover the side hair above the ears and hair at the nape of the neck should not be worn in the OR. If reusable hats or hoods are worn, they should be laundered daily. If they become contaminated with blood or body fluids, they must be laundered according to OSHA (2012a) regulations.

Ideally perioperative personnel should wear shoes that are dedicated to use within the perioperative area. Shoes worn outdoors have been shown to be significantly more contaminated than dedicated shoes (AORN, 2016o). Dedicated shoes can decrease the amount of bacteria brought into the OR. It is possible that bacteria on the floor may be dispersed into the air by walking, by wheelchair, or by stretcher wheels (Koganti et al., 2016). For personnel safety, shoes that provide protection should be worn. Shoes should have closed toes and backs and should be low heeled and nonskid. Cloth shoes and open-toe shoes provide little protection against spilled liquids or sharp items that may be accidentally dropped to the floor. Shoe covers may be worn to help keep shoes clean and may decrease the amount of soil and bacteria tracking throughout the suite. It is easier to change a shoe cover than to stop to clean or change a shoe that has become soiled. If it is reasonably expected that the feet may become contaminated with blood or body fluids, shoe covers are required as part of personal protective attire. Shoe covers should be kept in an area adjacent to the semirestricted area entrance. They should be removed and discarded in the appropriate receptacle when leaving the restricted area (AORN, 2016o). Removing shoe covers can cause transfer of microorganisms from the shoe cover to one's hands. Hand hygiene should follow removal of shoe covers. Shoe covers are required as part of PPE and must be worn where gross contamination is expected (OSHA, 2012a) (such as in vascular or orthopedic surgery).

A single surgical mask is worn to reduce the dispersal of microbial droplets expelled from the mouth and nasopharynx of personnel and to protect healthcare workers from aerosolized pathogenic organisms and particles from the surgical environment. Surgical masks in combination with eye protection devices, such as glasses with solid sides, or a chin length face shield, must be worn whenever splash, spray, or splatter or droplets of blood can be anticipated. OSHA regulations mandate the use of surgical masks as part of personal protection (OSHA, 2012a).

Single, high-filtration surgical masks are worn in ORs and other designated areas in which open sterile supplies or scrub persons may be located. Masks should cover the nose and mouth and should be secured to prevent venting at the sides (AORN, 2016o). Individual practice settings need to develop polices based on OSHA (2012a) and state-mandated recommendations on mask use. Masks with a microbial filtration efficiency of 95% or greater should be selected. The filtration efficiency of masks should ensure protection against aerosol particles that are 0.1 μm or larger. These masks, however, should not be used as protection against surgical smoke or as protection from chemical or particulate contaminants smaller than 0.1 μm as may be found in surgical smoke plume, such as during a laser procedure (AORN, 2016g). Mask selection should be based on the anticipated contaminants (AORN, 2016o).

The most effective filter mask is relatively useless if worn incorrectly. Fig. 4.14 illustrates the proper application and removal of a surgical mask.

The mask must cover the mouth and nose entirely and have facial compliance, fitting comfortably around the contours of the nose and cheeks. The mask is tied securely without crossing the strings. Crossing strings allows the sides of the mask to gap (tenting) and consequently permits nonfiltered air to escape through venting. Air should pass only through the mask's filtering system (the faceplate). A pliable metal or adhesive strip in the top hem of some masks provides a firm, contoured fit over the bridge of the nose. This strip may help prevent fogging of protective eyewear. Masks should be either on (properly) or off. They should not be reused for different procedures (e.g., by allowing the mask to hang from the neck or by tucking it into a pocket). Bacteria that have been filtered by the mask become dry and airborne if the mask is worn in a necklace fashion. Only the string should be touched when removing the mask. Touching only the strings during removal of the mask reduces contamination of the hands. Masks should be changed between procedures and sometimes during a procedure if they become wet or soiled. The faceplate, which is contaminated with droplet nuclei, should not come into contact with the hands of personnel. Immediately after removal, masks should be discarded directly into a designated covered waste receptacle. After discarding the mask, the wearer should perform hand hygiene (AORN, 2016o).

Gloves should be selected according to the task to be completed: sterile gloves for sterile procedures, and medical, unsterile gloves for nonsterile activities. Gloves should be changed between patient and patient surroundings contacts and after contact with any infectious material. Hand hygiene should be performed after gloves are removed. To reduce the risk of mouth, nose, and eye mucous membrane exposure, protective eyewear, masks, or face shields are worn whenever there is an opportunity for contamination by splash or aerosols. When the protective devices become contaminated, they should be discarded or decontaminated as soon as possible to prevent contamination to the wearer. Other protective equipment such as liquid-resistant attire, including gowns and shoe covers, should be worn whenever there is a reasonable expectation of exposure to infectious materials (AORN, 2016o).

Identification badges should be securely fastened to the scrub top of jacket and should not be worn attached to a lanyard. Lanyards can harbor bacteria and can be difficult to clean.

Institutional policy should govern the use of cover gowns. Reusable cover gowns should be laundered in a healthcare accredited laundry after each daily use. AORN guidelines state that healthcare personnel should change into street clothing when exiting the building (AORN, 2016o).

Surgical Hand Antisepsis

The normal skin flora on hands includes bacteria and other microorganisms that can be a source of infection if transmitted to a patient. It is well known that hand hygiene is a critical factor in preventing transmission of pathogenic microorganisms and decreasing potential for healthcare associated infections. The term *hand hygiene* is used to describe measures related to the physical hand condition and decontamination. Routine hand hygiene, other than in preparation for participation in surgery, is performed with either soap and water or use of an alcohol-based hand rub. Hand hygiene in preparation for participation in surgery is referred to as *surgical hand antisepsis*. Surgical hand antisepsis is performed before gowning and gloving. Skin harbors both transient and resident microorganisms. Transient

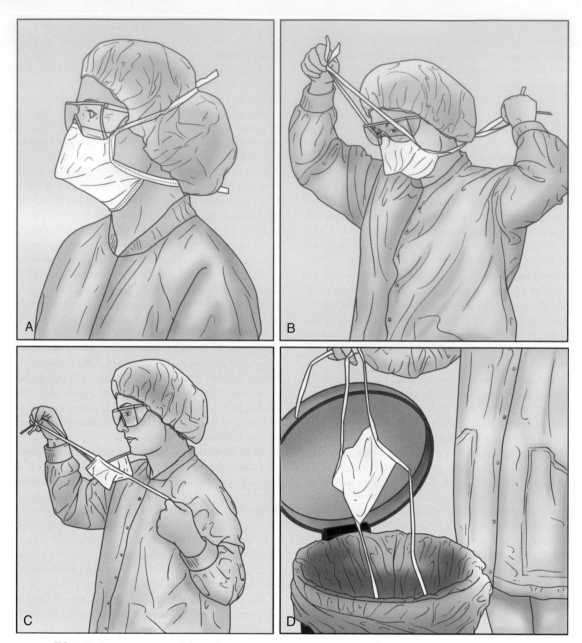

FIG. 4.14 Proper handling of a mask. (A) Edges of a properly worn mask conform to facial contours when the mask is applied and tied correctly. (B and C) Personnel should avoid touching the filter portion of the mask when removing it. (D) Masks should be discarded on removal.

microorganisms are microorganisms that colonize the superficial layers of the skin and can be removed with hand hygiene. Resident microorganisms are found under the superficial layers of the skin and are harder to remove. The purpose of surgical hand hygiene is to reduce the risk of SSIs by removing transient microorganisms and suppressing growth of resident microorganisms. Although members of the surgical team at the sterile field wear sterile gowns and gloves the skin of their hands and forearms should be cleaned preoperatively to reduce the number of microorganisms in the event of glove failure. The skin can never be rendered sterile, but it can be made surgically clean by reducing the number of microorganisms present.

Personnel with breaks in hand skin integrity, infection of the nails, exudative lesions, and nonintact skin on hands and arms may be at risk of transmitting infection and their work activities, such as scrubbing, should be restricted to activities that do not put patients at risk for infection. Because microorganisms may be harbored by jewelry (e.g., rings, watches, and bracelets), these items should be removed before scrubbing (AORN, 2016f). Fingernails of scrub persons should be short, clean, and healthy. The subungual region of the nails harbors most microorganisms on the hands. Soap, running water, and a nail-cleaning device are necessary to clean under the fingernails. Nails that extend beyond the tips of the fingers may harbor higher numbers of microorganisms than shorter nails, be more difficult to clean, and can increase the risk of glove tears. Longer nails also may scratch patients during the positioning or transfer process. Artificial nails or nail extenders should not be worn by personnel in the perioperative environment. Gram-negative organisms have been cultured from the nails of individuals wearing artificial nails or nail polish (World Health Organization, 2009). Old (more than 4 days) and chipped nail polish has been associated with higher numbers of microorganisms than freshly applied nail polish. Further research on the quality of nail polish and correlation with SSI is lacking. A multidisciplinary committee should review the available research and perform a risk analysis to determine related policies and procedures. Facility infection control procedures govern the selection of materials and the methods used for surgical hand hygiene. This may be accomplished by a surgical scrub or with the use of an approved hand rub agent (AORN, 2016f).

Surgical Hand Rubs

Alcohol-based hand rubs are easy to use and fast acting, and they provide activity against most bacteria, viruses, and fungi. Not all hand rub products that are alcohol based are indicated for use in place of the traditional surgical hand scrub. Rubs come in many forms, combinations, and concentrations of alcohols, which may influence the antimicrobial strength and kill factor. Surgical hand hygiene products should be selected after a thorough analysis of each product's efficacy, effectiveness, application processes, cost-to-benefit ratio analysis, and acceptance by its users. When hand rubs are used for surgical hand antisepsis, the only acceptable products are alcohol-based antiseptic surgical hand rubs with documented persistent and cumulative activity that have met FDA regulatory requirements for surgical hand antisepsis. The manufacturer's written instructions for product use, including time and amount, should be followed. The basic steps of a surgical rub are as follows:

1. Remove jewelry from hands and wrists
2. Apply the amount of alcohol-based hand rub recommended by the manufacturer to cover all surfaces of the hand
3. Rub hands together covering all surfaces of the hands and fingers until dry.

If hands are visibly soiled they should be washed with soap and water before performing a surgical hand rub (AORN, 2016f).

Surgical Hand Scrub

A surgical hand scrub should be performed by healthcare personnel before donning sterile gloves for surgical or other invasive procedures. Use of a sponge is recommended for performing a surgical hand scrub. A brush should not be used as it may cause skin damage, increase bacterial shedding from hands, and is not less effective than a sponge. Sponges are available with a variety of antimicrobial soap or antiseptic solutions impregnated into the sponge (AORN, 2016f).

A multidisciplinary team should evaluate and select surgical scrub hand agents that meet FDA requirements. Products should be evaluated for safety and efficacy (FDA, 2015c).

Surgical hand scrub agent selection should be based on the efficacy and effectiveness of the product, application requirements, contact time, and user friendliness. Surgical hand scrub products should have the following attributes:

- Reduce microorganisms on the skin
- Be fast acting
- Have a broad range of activity
- Not depend on cumulative action
- Have a minimally harsh effect on skin
- Inhibit regrowth of microorganisms

CHG is commonly used for surgical hand scrubs, although some facilities may prefer povidone-iodine complex. These agents are broad-spectrum, rapid-acting antimicrobials that are effective against many gram-positive and gram-negative microorganisms. Moisturizing agents are often incorporated into various surgical scrub agents to reduce the potential of skin irritation resulting from multiple scrubs.

An anatomic scrub, using a prescribed amount of time or number of strokes plus friction, is used to effectively cleanse the skin. The fingers, hands, and arms should be visualized as having four sides; each side must be scrubbed effectively. Individual attention to detail is essential. When using the timed approach, the product IFU and the institution's policies and procedures should be followed. Surgical hand scrub procedures should be documented and available within the perioperative practice setting.

Scrub Procedure. Before beginning the surgical hand scrub, members of the surgical team should inspect their hands to ensure that their nails are short, their cuticles are in good condition, and no cuts or skin problems exist. The procedure may include but not be limited to the following steps:

- Remove all jewelry, including rings, watches, and bracelets, from the hands and forearms.
- Cover all head and facial hair. Don a surgical mask. If other personnel are at the scrub sink, a surgical mask should be worn in the presence of hand scrub activity. Protective eyewear, such as goggles with side shields or a full-face shield, should be adjusted to ensure clear vision and to avoid lens fogging. Scrub shirts are tucked into the trousers to prevent potential contamination of the scrubbed hands and arms from brushing against loose garments. The basic steps of the scrub procedure follow:

1. Wash hands and forearms with soap and running water immediately before beginning the scrub procedure, if visibly soiled. Bring water to a comfortable temperature. Most scrub sinks have automatic or knee controls for the faucets.
2. Moisten hands and forearms with water. Using a foot control, dispense the manufacturer's recommended amount of the antimicrobial agent into the palms, adding small amounts of water to create lather if necessary.
3. Wash hands and forearms using the antimicrobial soap or detergent. Rinse before beginning the surgical hand scrub. The amount of time needed varies with the amount of soil and the effectiveness of the cleansing agent.

This may be followed with a surgical hand scrub using either an antimicrobial surgical scrub agent or an alcohol-based antiseptic surgical hand rub.

For a surgical hand scrub:

1. Open the sponge package, remove the sponge and nail cleaner, and discard the package. Hold the sponge in one hand; clean the subungual areas of both hands under running water, and then complete the nails on the other hand (Fig. 4.15).
2. Rinse the hands and arms thoroughly, exercising care to hold the hands higher than the elbows. Avoid splashing water onto the surgical attire because this moisture may cause subsequent contamination of the sterile gown.
3. Moisten the sponge (if the sponge is impregnated with antimicrobial soap) and begin scrubbing. If the sponge is not impregnated with soap, apply antimicrobial soap or detergent solution to hands according to the manufacturer's written IFU. Starting at the fingertips, scrub the nails vigorously, holding the sponge perpendicular to the nails. Visualize each finger, hand, and arm as having four sides all of which must be scrubbed. Scrub all sides of each digit, including the connecting webbed

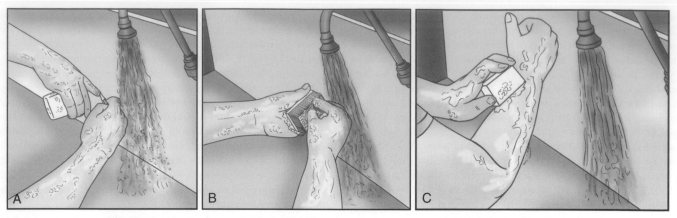

FIG. 4.15 Traditional surgical scrub technique. (A) Cleaning nails with plastic nail cleaner. (B) Holding sponge perpendicular to nails facilitates thorough scrubbing of underside of nails. (C) Holding sponge lengthwise along arm covers maximum area with each stroke.

spaces. Next scrub the palm and back of the hand. Repeat on the other hand and arm.

4. Scrub each side of the forearm with a circular motion (see Fig. 4.15) up to the elbows. Scrub for the length of time indicated in the manufacturer's IFU.
5. Conserve water by turning off water when not in use.
6. Discard sponges.
7. Rinse hands and arms under running water in one direction from fingertips to elbows.
8. Hold hands higher than elbows and away from scrub attire allowing the water and detritus to flow away from the first-scrubbed and cleanest area.
9. Rinse the hands and arms thoroughly.
10. Turn off the faucet by using the knee control or by using the edge of the sponge on a hand control.
11. Discard the sponge.
12. Hold the hands and arms up in front of the body with elbows slightly flexed, and enter the OR.

If the timed method is used, the policies and procedures of the facility should be followed.

If using an alcohol-based surgical hand rub after handwashing, apply the product to hands and forearms according to the manufacturer's IFU.

Drying the Scrubbed Area. Moisture remaining on the cleansed skin after the scrub procedure should be dried with a sterile towel before donning a sterile gown and gloves. The gown and gloves should be opened on a flat surface before the surgical scrub is completed. A small sterile field is created by the gown wrapper, which is opened over the flat surface. The gown and gloves should not be opened on the sterile back table because of the increased chance of contamination to the field. The towel must be used with care to avoid contaminating the clean skin. The folded towel is grasped firmly near the open corner and lifted straight up and away from the sterile field without dripping contaminated water from the skin onto the sterile field. The person steps away from the sterile field and bends forward slightly from the waist, holding the hands and elbows above the waist and away from the body. The towel is allowed to unfold downward to its full length and width (Fig. 4.16). If the towel contacts an unsterile surface the towel is considered contaminated.

The top half of the towel is held securely with one hand, and the opposite fingers and hand are blotted dry ensuring that they are

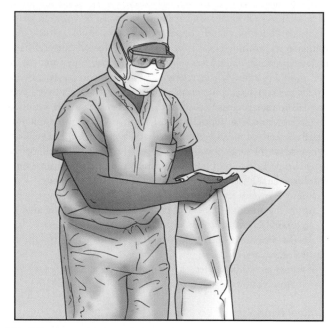

FIG. 4.16 Drying hands and forearms. Fingers and hand are dried thoroughly before forearm is dried. Extending arms reduces the possibility of contaminating towel or hands.

thoroughly dry before moving to the forearm. A rotating motion is used while moving up and down the arm to avoid contamination; areas are not retraced. The lower end of the towel is grasped with the dried hand, and the same procedure is used for drying the second hand and forearm. Care must be taken to prevent contamination of the towel and hands. On completion, the towel is discarded without dropping the hands below waist level. The hands of scrubbed sterile team members should be completely dry before gowning or gloving.

Gowning

Before scrub personnel touch sterile equipment or the sterile field, they must put on sterile gowns and surgical gloves to prevent microorganisms on their hands and clothing from being transferred to the patient's wound during surgery. The sterile gowns and gloves also protect the hands and clothing of personnel from microorganisms present in the patient or in the atmosphere. The surgical gown should be made of a combustion-resistant material that establishes an effective barrier to minimize the passage of microorganisms, particulate matter, and fluids between unsterile and sterile areas. Reusable fabrics must allow complete penetration of steam during the sterilization process and should withstand multiple launderings and other processing. Tightly woven textiles eventually lose their barrier quality when subjected to multiple laundering and sterilizations. Users should follow the manufacturer's written IFU to determine the useful life of the barrier material. The manufacturer must provide the facility with instructions for testing the material at periodic intervals during the life cycle of the product to ensure continued barrier quality. The particular item should be removed from circulation when the maximum number of processing cycles has been reached. Before each use reusable materials must be examined to determine their integrity. Gowns should be evaluated for efficacy and cost (AORN, 2016m). Regardless of the gown material, the shape and size should fit personnel and allow freedom of movement. To provide extra protection, the gown's front from the waist upward and the forearms of the sleeves can be reinforced with additional or different water-repellent material. Each sleeve should be finished with a tight-fitting cuff that prevents the inner side of the sleeve from slipping down onto the outer side of the sterile glove. Cotton tapes, snaps, or Velcro fasteners are attached to the back of the gown to hold it closed. A wraparound gown may be used to achieve better coverage of the back. Once donned, however, the back of the gown is not considered sterile.

Because the outer side of the front and sleeves of the gown come into contact with the sterile field during surgery, the gown must be folded so that the scrub person can put it on without touching the outer side with bare hands. For in-house wrapping and sterilization, the gown is folded with the inner side out and the back edges together. The sleeves are not turned inside out; consequently, they remain within the folded gown. The side folds of the gown are folded lengthwise toward the center back opening, overlapping slightly at the center. With the open edges of the gown remaining on the inside, the bottom third of the gown is folded upward and the top third of the gown is folded over the bottom portion. The gown is then folded in half widthwise so that the inside front neckline of

the gown is visible on top. Gowns with wraparound backs are prepared in the same manner, with care taken to tie the tape securely on the wraparound back flap to the external side tie of the gown before initial folding. A folded hand towel with its free corners facing up is usually placed on top of the folded gown before the gown is wrapped and sterilized. Surgical gowns should be selected for use according to the barrier quality of the item and the wearers' anticipated exposure to blood and body fluids in accordance with OSHA's guidelines for the use of PPE, as found in the OSHA Bloodborne Pathogens Standard (OSHA, 2012a).

Self-Gowning Procedure

The procedure for donning a wraparound sterile surgical gown is as follows (Figs. 4.17 and 4.18). The scrub person should do the following:

1. Grasp the sterile gown at the neckline with both hands and lift from the wrapper. Step into an area where the gown may be opened without risk of contamination.
2. Hold the gown away from the body, and allow it to unfold with the inside toward the wearer.
3. Keep hands on the inside of the gown while it completely unfolds.
4. Slip both hands into the open armholes, keeping the hands at shoulder level and away from the body.
5. Push the hands and forearms into the sleeves of the gown, advancing the hands only to the proximal edge of the cuff.

The perioperative nurse in the circulating role should then do the following:

1. Pull the gown over the scrub person's shoulders, touching only the inner shoulder and side seams.
2. Tie or clasp the neckline and tie the inner waist ties of the gown, touching only the inner aspect of the gown. The neck and back of the gown should be completely fastened by the perioperative nurse before the scrub person dons gloves to prevent contamination from flapping of the gown.
3. Secure the gown around the body and prepare to tie the belt. After gloving the scrub person hands the cardboard tab that is attached to one of the gown ties to the circulating nurse. The circulating nurses takes hold of the tab without contaminating

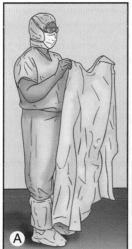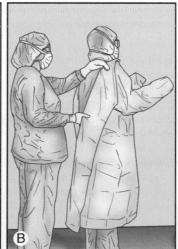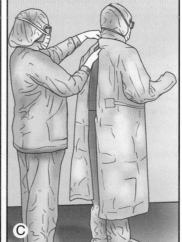

FIG. 4.17 Gowning procedure. (A) Scrub person keeps hands on inside of gown while unfolding it at arm's length. (B) Circulating nurse reaches under flap of gown to pull sleeves on scrub person. (C) Circulating nurse snaps neckline of gown, touching only snap section of neckline.

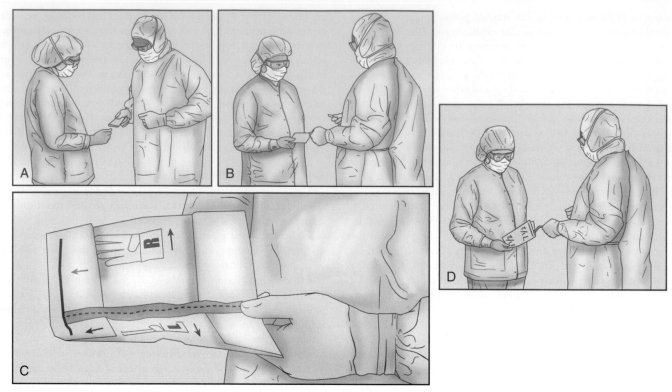

FIG. 4.18 Methods of tying a wraparound gown. (A) After handing tab on back tie of gown to perioperative nurse, scrub person makes a three-quarters turn toward the left. (B) Sterile back panel now covers previously tied unsterile ties; scrub person retrieves back tie by carefully pulling it out of the tab held by the nurse and ties it securely with other tie. (C) For gowns having no tab on back tie: using sterile inner glove wrapper, scrub person places the end of the back tie in the crease of the wrapper. (D) After closing the wrapper, scrub person hands tie to the nurse, who grasps it carefully, touching neither the tie nor the gloved hand of the scrub person. The scrub person makes a three-quarters turn to the left, carefully pulls back tie from wrapper, and ties it to other tie.

the glove of the scrubbed person and holds it while the scrubbed person makes a three-quarter turn in a manner that causes the gown to wrap around the body and cover the inner waist ties that the circulating nurse used to secure the gown on the scrub person. The scrubbed person then pulls the belt so that the tab is freed and remains in the hand of the circulating nurse. The scrub person then ties the two ends of the belt.

When a reusable gown is used, the absence of a tab on the back tie necessitates use of an alternate procedure for securing the gown (see Fig. 4.18C–D). If the closed-gloving technique and commercially prepared, double-wrap gloves are used, the inner wrap can be used as a protective extension for the gown tie when the perioperative nurse assists with tying a wraparound gown. After gloving, the scrub person unties the exterior gown ties (which were tied at the front of the gown before it was folded, wrapped, and sterilized) and holds both ties. The end of the back tie is placed in the center crease of the empty glove wrapper, approximately two-thirds of the way up to the edge of the opened wrapper. The glove wrapper is then closed so that the tie is concealed. The closed wrapper is handed to the perioperative nurse, who firmly grasps the folded edge of the wrapper without touching the tie or the scrubbed person's hand. The scrub person pivots in the opposite direction from the nurse, who extends the back tie to its full length. The scrub person grasps the exposed portion of the back tie, pulls it out of the glove wrapper while taking care to avoid touching the glove wrapper or the perioperative nurse,

and ties both ties. If a sterile glove wrapper is unavailable, a sterile hemostat or ringed forceps may be clamped to the back tie and used in the same manner as a glove wrapper. After the gowning procedure has been completed, the perioperative nurse retains the instrument in the room to avoid problems with the subsequent instrument count.

If another scrub person is gowned and gloved, that individual, instead of the circulating nurse, may assist with the wraparound procedure. The assisting individual must extend the back tie to its fullest length before the scrub person turns, to avoid any potential contamination.

Assisted-Gowning Procedure

A gowned and gloved individual may assist another individual in donning a sterile gown (Fig. 4.19). The scrub person, who is already gowned and gloved, hands the newly scrubbed person a towel to dry his or her hands and forearms unless an alcohol-based surgical hand rub was used in which case a towel is not necessary. The scrubbed person picks up the sterile gown. The gown is opened in the manner previously described. The inner side with the open armholes is turned toward the individual who is to be gowned. A cuff is made of the neck and shoulder area of the gown to protect the gloved hands. The gown is held until the person's hands and forearms are in the sleeves of the gown. The circulating nurse assists in pulling the gown onto the shoulders, adjusting the back, and

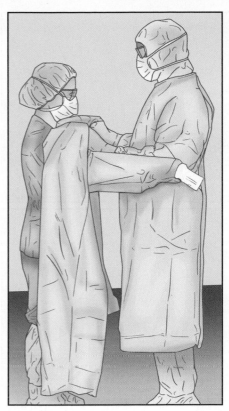

FIG. 4.19 Gowning another person. Gowned and gloved scrub person cuffs neck and shoulder area of gown over gloved hands to prevent contamination as scrub person puts hands and forearms into sleeves.

tying the tapes. The wraparound back of the gown is fixed into position by the scrub person after gloving is completed by using the same procedure for final closure of the gown as used when self-gowning.

Gloving

Scrubbed personnel wear sterile surgical gloves to provide a protective barrier between the patient and healthcare personnel to decrease the probability of exposing the patient to exogenous organisms with a resulting SSI. Gloves also decrease the chance of the healthcare provider being exposed to blood or OPIM. Nonetheless, many surgeons, first assistants, and perioperative scrub personnel have encountered blood on their hands at the conclusion of a surgical procedure without being aware of any breech in the glove barrier (glove puncture, tear, or rip). Increasing evidence supports and recommends the practice of double-gloving to offer a degree of protection from this and other common events. The evidence for wearing two pairs of gloves during surgical procedures is compelling. According to Copeland (2009, p. 325), "Two layers of surgical gloves can reduce the number of breaks to the innermost glove that might allow cross-infection between the surgical team and patient.... A second pair of gloves does protect the first set, without apparently lessening surgical skill." Two gloves are better than one, and although this may be considered optional, all evidence points to double-gloving as being the best practice that can protect both the healthcare provider and the patient (Copeland, 2009). Although a breech may occur in the outer glove, the inner glove remains intact and continues to serve as a barrier. These conclusions are supported in a recent study in

which 141 of 512 double-glove sets used in surgery were perforated but only six double-glove sets were perforated through both layers. The researchers concluded that double-gloves offered 90% protection from perforation through both layers and that double-gloving should be encouraged (Makama et al., 2016). Some surgeons who work in areas in which perforation risk is high, such as orthopedics or thoracic surgery, opt to wear double-layer gloves, with the inside glove being a colored glove, which allows the wearer to recognize perforations to the outer glove. In orthopedic surgery, surgeons may wear a glove liner between two layers of gloves to reduce perforations to the inner glove. On completion of the procedure both pairs of gloves should be removed and discarded and hand hygiene should be performed.

Powdered gloves should not be used. Aerosolized powder from natural latex gloves can disperse and carry latex proteins, and individuals sensitive to latex may experience an allergic reaction. Latex gloves have been associated with adverse events including airway inflammation, wound inflammation, and postsurgical adhesions. Because of the safety risks the FDA published a final rule banning powdered gloves as of January 17, 2017, stating they pose an unreasonable and substantial risk of injury, illness, or injury to individuals exposed to powered gloves (National Archives and Records Administration, 2016).

Latex Allergies and Sensitivities

The increased reporting of latex sensitivity continues to be a concern among perioperative personnel. Individuals can experience three types of reactions to latex. *Irritant contact dermatitis* is the most common type of reaction and is characterized by dry, reddened, itchy, or cracked hands. Irritant contact dermatitis is not a true allergic reaction. *Allergic contact dermatitis* is considered a type IV allergic reaction and is an allergic response caused by chemicals used in the manufacture of gloves. Allergic contact dermatitis is a delayed reaction, usually appearing 6 to 48 hours after exposure. Symptoms are similar to those of irritant contact dermatitis except that the reaction may extend beyond the actual point of contact. *True latex allergies* are classified as type I allergic responses. This is an allergy to water-soluble natural rubber latex (NRL) proteins. True latex allergies are usually seen within minutes of contact with the proteins. Symptoms range from skin redness and itching to hives, dyspnea, GI upset, hypotension, tachycardia, and anaphylaxis. Reactions to latex rarely progress to anaphylaxis because the wearer is treated with appropriate drugs to interrupt the allergic response. Appropriate latex-free gloves should be provided for healthcare workers with known latex sensitivity or for procedures in which patients have known sensitivity or allergy. Some personnel claim allergy to the starch powder in latex gloves. Although this is possible, it is more likely that individuals are allergic to the latex proteins that bind with the starch powder and become aerosolized (AORN, 2016b; FDA, 2016).

Closed-Gloving Technique

The closed method of gloving (Fig. 4.20) is the technique of choice when initially donning a sterile gown and gloves. When using this technique, the gloves are handled through the fabric of the gown sleeves. The hands are not extended from the sleeves and cuffs when the gown is put on. Instead, the hands are pushed through the cuff openings as the gloves are pulled into place. The woven cuff should remain in the natural wrist area. Because the cuffs of a sterile gown collect moisture, become damp during wearing, and are considered unsterile, the closed-gloving technique is used only for initial gloving. Cuffs may not be pulled down over the wearer's hand for subsequent

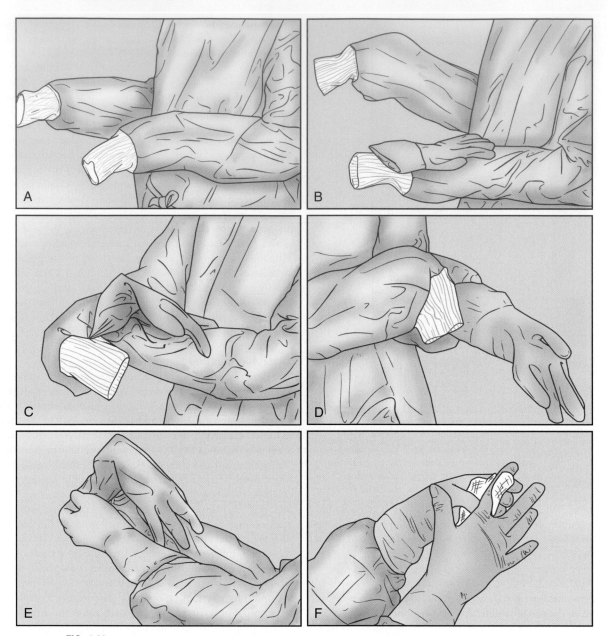

FIG. 4.20 Closed-gloving procedure. (A) When donning gown, scrub person does not slip hands through gown cuffs. Hands are not extended from sleeves. (B) First the glove is lifted by grasping it through the fabric of the sleeve. The glove's cuff facilitates easier handling of the glove. The glove is placed palm down along the forearm of the matching hand, with thumb and fingers pointing toward elbow. Glove cuff lies over gown cuff. If the scrub person is double-gloving, the larger size gloves are donned first. (C) The glove cuff is held securely by the hand on which it was placed, and with the other hand the cuff is stretched over the opening of the sleeve to cover the gown cuff entirely. (D) As the cuff is drawn back onto the wrist, fingers are directed into their cots in the glove, and the glove is adjusted to the hand. (E) Gloved hand is used to position remaining glove on opposite sleeve in the same fashion. Glove cuff is placed around gown cuff. The second glove is drawn onto the hand, and the cuff is pulled into place. (F) Fingers of gloves are adjusted, and gloves are wiped with wet gauze sponge or commercially prepared sterile, disposable glove wipe to remove any powder that may be on them.

gloving. For subsequent gloving, an alternative technique must be used, such as assisted gloving or open gloving.

Open-Gloving Technique

With the open-gloving technique, the everted cuff of each glove permits a gowned individual to touch the glove's inner side with ungloved fingers and to touch the glove's outer side with gloved fingers (Fig. 4.21). Keeping the hands in direct view, no lower than waist level, the gowned individual flexes the elbows. Exerting a light, even pull on the glove brings it over the hand, and using a rotating movement brings the cuff over the wristlet. Extreme caution is necessary when using the open method to prevent contamination

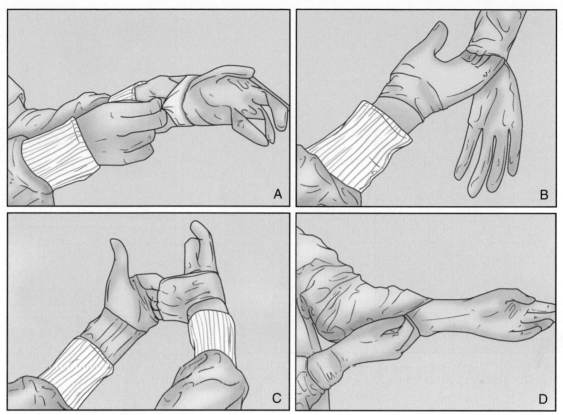

FIG. 4.21 Open-gloving procedure. (A) Scrub person takes one glove from the inner glove wrapper by placing the thumb and index finger of the opposite hand on the fold of the everted cuff at a point in line with the glove's palm and then pulls the glove over the hand, leaving the cuff turned back. If the scrub person is double-gloving, the larger size gloves are donned first. (B) Scrub person takes the second glove from the inner glove wrapper by placing gloved fingers under the everted cuff. (C) Scrub person, with arms extended and elbows slightly flexed, introduces free hand into glove and draws it over gown cuff by slightly rotating arm externally and internally. (D) To bring turned-back cuff on other hand over cuff of gown, scrub person repeats step C.

by the exposed hands. The open-gloving technique is useful for gloving in instances in which it is not necessary to don a gown in preparation for participation in surgery.

Assisted-Gloving Technique

A gowned and gloved individual may assist another gowned individual with gloving. To assist another individual, grasp the glove under the everted cuff. Ensure the palm of the glove is turned toward the ungloved individual's hand with the thumb of the glove directly opposed to the thumb of the individual's hand. Using fingers, stretch the cuff to open the glove. The ungloved individual can insert his or her hand into the glove. Repeat the procedure for the other hand (Fig. 4.22).

Process When a Team Member's Gown and/or Glove Becomes Contaminated

In the event that a sterile team member's glove becomes contaminated the team member should step away from the sterile field and extend his or her hand to the circulating nurse who will remove the contaminated glove. Using a gloved hand the circulating nurse will grasp the glove and remove it without allowing the stockinette cuff of the scrubbed person's gown, which is not considered sterile, to slip over the hand. Another scrubbed team member may then facilitate regloving using the assisted-gloving technique. Closed gloving is not

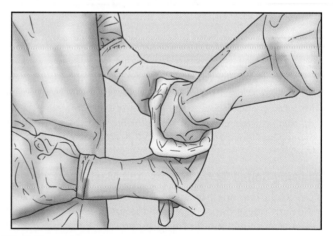

FIG. 4.22 Gloving another person. Gowned and gloved scrub person places fingers of each hand beneath everted cuff, keeping thumbs turned outward and stretching cuff as gowned person slips hand into sterile glove, using firm downward thrust. If other person is double-gloving, the larger size gloves are donned first.

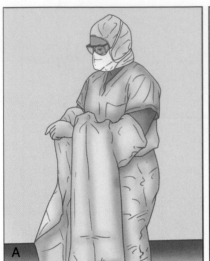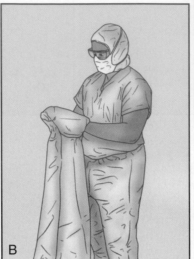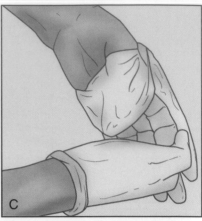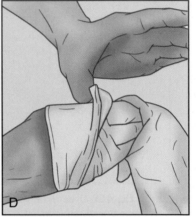

FIG. 4.23 Removing soiled gown and gloves. (A) To protect scrub suit and arms from bacteria that are present on outer side of soiled gown, the gown is grasped without touching the scrub clothes. (B) Scrub person turns outer side of soiled gown away from body, keeping elbows flexed and arms away from body so that soiled gown will not touch arms or scrub suit. (C) To prevent outer side of soiled gloves from touching skin surfaces of hands, the scrub person places gloved fingers of one hand under everted cuff of other glove and pulls glove off hand and fingers. (D) To prevent ungloved hand from touching outer side of soiled glove, the scrub person hooks bare thumb on inner side of glove and pulls glove off.

acceptable for regloving because the stockinette cuff is considered contaminated and the closed-gloving technique would cause the sterile glove to contact the unsterile stockinette cuff. Open gloving is not recommended because of the risk of contamination. In the event that assisted gloving is not possible AORN recommends regowning and gloving using the closed-gloving technique (AORN, 2016m).

Removing Soiled Gown, Gloves, and Mask

To protect the forearms, hands, and clothing from contacting bacteria on the outer side of the used gown and gloves, members of the scrub surgical team should use the following procedure to remove soiled gowns, gloves, and masks (Fig. 4.23):
- Wipe gloves clean with a wet, sterile towel.
- Untie surgical gown; the circulating nurse must unfasten back closures.
- Grasp gown at one shoulder seam without touching scrub clothing.
- Bring the neck and sleeve of the gown forward, over, and off the gloved hand, turning the gown inside out and everting the cuff of the glove.

- Repeat the previous two steps for the other side.
- Keep arms and gown away from body while turning the gown inside out and discarding carefully in the designated receptacle.
- Using the gloved fingers of one hand to secure the everted cuff, remove the glove, turning it inside out. Discard appropriately.
- Using the ungloved hand, grasp the fold of the everted cuff of the other glove and remove the glove, inverting the glove as it is removed. Discard appropriately.
- After leaving the restricted area, remove the mask by touching the ties or elastic only.
- Discard in the designated receptacle.
- Perform hand hygiene and include the forearm

Patient Skin Antisepsis

To prevent bacteria on the skin surfaces from entering the surgical wound, the skin area at and around the proposed incision site must be cleaned and disinfected. Skin preparation methods vary, but all are based on the same principles and share the same objectives: to remove dirt and transient microbes from the skin, to reduce the resident microbial count as much as possible in the shortest time and with the least amount of tissue irritation, and to prevent rapid rebound growth of microbes. Factors to be considered in skin disinfection are as follows:

1. Condition of the involved area
2. Number and kinds of contaminants
3. Characteristics of the skin to be disinfected
4. General physical condition of the patient

There is conflicting evidence as to which antiseptic is most effective in preventing SSIs. AORN recommends that a multidisciplinary team (e.g., RNs, physicians, and infection preventionists) make decisions about product selection based on a review of the current evidence and professional guidelines. Equally important, an effective antimicrobial agent should be used to achieve skin antisepsis; it should be selected according to its ability to decrease the microbial count of the skin rapidly, be applied quickly, and remain effective throughout the operation. The agent should not cause irritation or sensitization or be incompatible with or inactivated by alcohol, organic matter, soap, or detergent (AORN, 2016h). While which active ingredient in the prep solution is debated, there is evidence that alcohol-based solutions are more effective than aqueous solutions and should be used unless specific patient contradictions exist (Ban et al., 2016).

Preoperative bathing removes organic and inorganic debris and reduces the bacterial count on the patient's skin. Although current evidence fails to support a direct correlation between preoperative bathing and SSI, the benefits of preoperative bathing outweighs the harm. The most recent guidelines for the prevention of SSI from the American College of Surgeons recommends preoperative bathing with chlorhexidine reduces transient and resident skin flora and may lower the patient's risk of developing an SSI (Patient Engagement Exemplar). The use of preoperative bathing as part of a formal decolonization protocol for MRSA differs from using preoperative bathing to lower transient normal flora from the patient skin preoperatively. Research is being conducted using chlorhexidine-impregnated cloths to determine whether they produce a more sustainable bacterial reduction when used in conjunction with chlorhexidine bathing (Ban et al., 2016) (Research Highlight).

Hair should not be removed from the surgical site unless it is required. The necessity for hair removal depends on the amount of hair, the location of the incision, and the type of surgical procedure to be performed. Preoperative shaving of the surgical site increases the risk of SSI (Ban et al., 2016). If hair is to be removed, clipping with an electric or battery-operated clipper, or using a depilatory, is recommended. Shaving is not recommended. Clipping immediately before surgery is the simplest and least irritating method of hair removal. Use of a depilatory requires a pretest to ascertain that the patient is not sensitive to the depilatory product. The specific manufacturer's written instructions should be carefully followed. If a shave is desired by the surgeon, some institutions require a written order. The patient should be shaved as close to the time of surgery as is possible. The shave should be performed in an area within the surgical suite that affords privacy and is equipped with good lighting. Clipping the morning of surgery as opposed to the day before may reduce the incidence of SSI. Hair removal should be performed by skilled personnel, with great care taken to avoid scratching, nicking, or cutting the skin because cutaneous bacteria proliferate in these areas and increase the chances of infection. The method of hair removal and the condition of the skin before and after removal should be documented (AORN, 2016h).

The surgical principle followed when preparing the patient's skin for surgery ("prepping") is to prepare ("prep") the cleanest area first

---

PATIENT ENGAGEMENT EXEMPLAR

Preventing Surgical Site Infections

Educating patients about SSI prevention is just one step in the prevention process. Patients have to comply with the instructions given. SSI prevention strategies are a bundled approach with interventions that include actions by surgeons, anesthesia care providers, perioperative nurses, and patients. Part of an SSI bundle can include preoperative bathing or showering, but many times patients fail to complete the showering or bathing process, putting themselves at risk for an SSI. A study done by Edmiston and colleagues (2014) tested an electronic notification process to remind patients to complete their preoperative shower or bathing. Notifications were sent by either voice mail, email, or a text message, Eighty percent of the patients in the study group received a text message and were compared with a group that did not receive a reminder. The study found that the patients who did not receive an electronic reminder were significantly less compliant with preoperative showering or bathing compared with those who received the electronic reminders. Engaging patients in this manner empowers them to become involved in their own care and helps them to understand that they are helping to prevent their risk of SSI.

SSI, Surgical site infection.
From Edmiston CE et al. Empowering the surgical patient: randomized, prospective analysis of an innovative strategy for improving patient compliance to the preadmission showering protocol, *Am J Infect Control* 219(2):256–264, 2014.

---

and then move to the less clean areas (clean to dirty). The skin at the surgical site should be exposed and inspected before beginning the skin prep. Patients should have been instructed to remove any body jewelry before cleansing the site. Jewelry harbors microorganisms and traps them in adjacent skin. Jewelry should also be removed to reduce the risk of injury when positioning the patient or from using electrical devices. Surgical departments often stock snap-ring pliers to remove jewelry from piercings for emergency situations or when a patient has neglected to remove body jewelry. A variety of skin prepping products are available. A two-step product will include a scrub (clean) and paint and others are one step only. The skin prep usually begins at the point of the incision and continues to the periphery of the area (Fig. 4.24). When prepping the surgical site, the nurse dons sterile gloves and applies the antimicrobial agent using commercially prepared devices or applicators that have handles to provide distance between the nurse's hand and the area being prepared. A soiled applicator is never brought back over a previously prepped surface. On completion of the skin prep, the nurse may or may not, depending on manufacturer's instructions, blot the area with dry, sterile sponges or a sterile towel. Depending on the surgeon's preference, a topical antimicrobial solution or "paint" may be carefully applied to the prepped area, using care to avoid any solution pooling beneath the patient. All wet drapes should be removed from the patient area after the skin preparation is complete (AORN, 2016h).

When an intestinal or urinary stoma or other contaminated area is involved within the surgical field and during the prep procedure, a sponge soaked in the antimicrobial agent of choice is placed over the stoma when the prep is initiated. The area should be cleansed separately from the rest of the prepped area. At the completion of

RESEARCH HIGHLIGHT

Evidence for a Standardized Chlorhexidine Shower

The recommendation to have patients shower or bathe with chlorhexidine preoperatively to reduce skin microbial counts is included as a risk prevention measure in the CDC guidelines for prevention of SSIs (Anderson et al., 2014); however, meta-analysis failed to establish a corresponding decrease in SSI with the use of chlorhexidine (Webster et al., 2015). In a recent study by Edmiston and colleagues (2015), a randomized prospective study was undertaken to evaluate the efficacy of skin surface concentrations of 4% CHG, using a protocol of two to three sequential showers with a 1-minute pause before rinsing. It was determined that a shower with 118 mL of aqueous CHG 4% per shower, at a minimum of two sequential showers and a 1-minute pause before rinsing resulted in a skin-surface concentration of 16.5 µg/cm CHG, which is considered adequate to inhibit or kill gram-positive and gram-negative organisms. In spite of providing patients with instructions and a bottle of CHG for showering, the practice of preoperative bathing by the patient at home comes with inherit variability as to the patient's understanding, ability, and compliance with any preoperative bathing regimen. Although this study supports the current approach to skin antisepsis of reducing the microbial burden at the incision site, these findings do not directly correlate the use of 4% CHG preoperative showers with a reduction in SSIs.

CDC, Centers for Disease Control and Prevention; *CHG,* chlorhexidine gluconate; *SSI,* surgical site infection.

From Anderson DJ et al: Strategies to prevent surgical site infection in acute care hospitals: 2014 update, *Infect Control Hosp Epidemiol* 35(6):605–627, 2014; Webster J, Osborne S; The Cochrane Collaborative. Perioperative bathing or showering with skin antiseptics to prevent surgical site infection (website), 2015. www.cochrane.org/CD004985/WOUNDS_preoperative-bathing-or-showering-with-skin-antiseptics-to-prevent-surgical-site-infection. (Accessed 26 January 2017). Edmiston CE Jr, Lee CJ, et al: Evidence for a standardized preadmission showering regimen to achieve maximal antiseptic skin surface concentrations of chlorhexidine gluconate, 4%, in surgical patients, *JAMA Surg* 150(11):1027–1033, 2015.

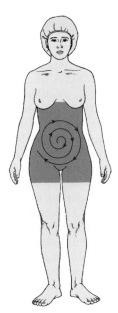

FIG. 4.24 Principles of starting at the intended incision site and working toward the periphery are illustrated on this example of an abdominal prep. *Shaded areas* indicate the area to be cleaned with antiseptic; *arrows* show direction of motion for the prep. (Always refer to manufacturer's instruction for prep application. Some instructions may indicate a different pattern to follow.)

the prep, the sponge is discarded. Sponges used to cleanse or disinfect an open wound, sinus, ulcer, intestinal stoma, the vagina, or the anus are applied once to that area and discarded. In contrast to the principle of working from the proposed incision to the periphery, open wounds and body orifices are potentially contaminated areas and as such are prepared after the peripheral intact skin is cleansed. The surgical principle is to work from the cleanest to the least clean area (AORN, 2016h).

The nurse should document the area prepped and the antiseptic solution used in the perioperative record. Documentation is an effective way to promote safe, continuous patient care. Although at times it may seem time consuming, periodic audits of the documentation of skin preparation help the perioperative nurse assess the effectiveness of the process, while protecting patients from possible SSIs (AORN, 2016h).

Creating the Sterile Field With Surgical Drapes

To create a sterile field, sterile sheets and towels, known as surgical drapes, are strategically placed to provide a sterile surface on which sterile instruments, supplies, equipment, and gloved hands may rest. The patient and OR bed is covered with sterile drapes in a manner that exposes the prepared incision site and isolates it from surrounding areas. Objects normally draped and composing the sterile field include instrument tables, trays, basins, the Mayo stand, some surgical equipment, and the patient. Within this defined sterile area, the actual operative procedure takes place.

Today, reusable and single-use (disposable) drapes are widely used. There are advantages and disadvantages for reusable (fabric) and single-use (disposable, nonwoven) drapes. Regardless of the type of material used, surgical drapes should have the following characteristics (AORN, 2016m):

- Create an appropriate barrier to microorganisms, particulate matter, and fluids
- Withstand methods of sterilization
- Maintain integrity
- Sustain durability
- Withstand physical conditions
- Resist tears, punctures, fiber strains, and abrasions
- Be free of toxic ingredients
- Be low-linting
- Be free of holes or other defects
- Achieve positive cost-to-benefit ratio

In addition, draping materials should meet or exceed the current requirements of the National Fire Protection Association.

Reusable Drapes

Chemically treated cotton or cotton-polyester fabrics provide a barrier to liquids and are abrasion resistant. Quantitative data verifying the barrier quality of any textile drape must be provided by the manufacturer. Care should be taken with reusable drapes to eliminate pinholes caused by towel clamps, needles, or other sharp objects. Only nonpenetrating towel clamps should be used. Should breaks in the fabric occur, a heat-sealed patch may be used for repair after laundering. An abundance of heat-sealed patches on any surgical drape may interfere with the sterilization process and render the barrier ineffective. Manufacturer's written instructions on the use of patching should be followed. The exact percentage of any item that may be successfully patched is unknown. As with reusable gowns, laundering eventually impairs the barrier quality of the drape. Most manufacturers report a loss of barrier quality after 75 to 100 laundry or sterilization cycles. The process of laundering and steam sterilization swells the fabric fibers, whereas drying and ironing shrink the fibers. Over time these processes loosen fabric fibers, altering the fabric structure and decreasing the barrier properties and fluid impermeability of the fabric. As with surgical gowns, a system to monitor the number of times an item has been processed is essential for quality control of the barrier and fluid impermeability.

Single-Use (Disposable) Drapes

Commercially packaged and sterilized synthetic single-use disposable drapes are widely used. They reduce the hazards of contamination in the presence of known infectious microorganisms from body fluids and excretions and in situations in which laundering of grossly contaminated textiles may be problematic. They prevent bacterial penetration and fluid breakthrough, also known as *strikethrough*. When considering the purchase of single-use drapes, the perioperative team must determine whether the drapes will meet the needs of the surgical procedure, be acceptable to the perioperative team, and be cost-effective (versus laundering and processing of reusable drapes). A cost-to-benefit ratio analysis may warrant their use in the healthcare facility. Availability of items, storage facilities, and disposal methods must be analyzed (AORN, 2016k).

The environmental effect of disposable items can be only roughly estimated. Each facility must carefully evaluate its capabilities and restrictions for handling single-use and reusable supplies and equipment to make an informed decision about the products it will use in the practice setting.

Compactors provide a relatively inexpensive method of discarding disposable drapes. They accept any material and reduce its volume substantially. Storage, collection, and transportation of compacted waste materials can be a problem. Hospital engineers must establish methods of controlling odor and maintaining sanitation in the compactor area. Because a portion of the compacted material may be grossly contaminated, city or county codes may prohibit transporting this potentially infectious material through city streets or dumping it at landfills. Incineration is an alternative method for destroying waste disposables. If hospital incinerators are used, they must be managed properly to prevent environmental contamination. Facilities choosing to incinerate must follow specific state and local guidelines established for medical waste incinerators and must meet federal standards (EPA, 2016).

In addition to commercially prepared drapes, commercially prepared preassembled sterile, disposable custom packs are used in many healthcare facilities. These packs are specific to a surgical procedure and contain the items needed for a particular procedure. The contents of the pack are determined by the surgeon/facility. Advantages of these packs include reduced setup and room-turnover times resulting from fewer individually wrapped items that must be opened. Other advantages include less waste resulting from fewer individually wrapped items, improved inventory control, and fewer lost charges. Although custom packs may be more expensive than multiple separate items, indirect savings related to increased efficiency can offset those costs.

Drape Configurations

Careful planning by perioperative personnel helps determine the desired types and sizes of surgical drapes required for groups or individual surgical procedures. Standardized draping methods provide management control that ensures patient safety, simplifies staff education, and conserves human and material resources.

A whole, or plain, sheet is used to cover instrument tables, operating tables, and body regions. The sheet should be large enough

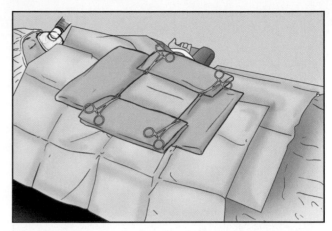

FIG. 4.25 Abdomen may be draped with four sterile towels, which are secured with nonperforating towel clamps. Standard method of placement of disposable towels is used.

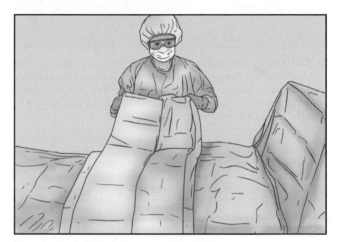

FIG. 4.26 Placement of laparotomy sheet. Identification of top portion of the laparotomy sheet helps the scrub person readily determine correct placement of the drape. After placing the folded laparotomy sheet on the patient, with fenestration of sheet directly over site of incision outlined by sterile towels, the scrub person unfolds drape over sides of patient and bed.

to provide an adequate margin of safety between the surrounding physical environment and the prepared operative field. Surgical towels should be available in several sizes to drape the operative site. Four surgical towels of woven or nonwoven material are usually sufficient (Fig. 4.25).

Fenestrated, or slit, sheets are used for draping patients. They leave the operative site exposed. A typical fenestrated (laparotomy) sheet is large enough to cover the patient and operating bed in any position, extend over the anesthesia screen at the head of the bed, and extend over the foot of the bed (Figs. 4.26–4.28). The typical fenestrated laparotomy sheet can be used for most procedures on the abdomen, chest, flank, and back. Other types of fenestrated sheets with small or split fenestrations may be used for the limbs, head, and neck when the patient is in the supine or prone position. The size of the fenestration is determined by the use for which the sheet is intended. The fenestrated sheet is fan-folded and handled as a typical laparotomy sheet. A perineal drape is needed for procedures on the perineum and genitalia when the patient is in the lithotomy

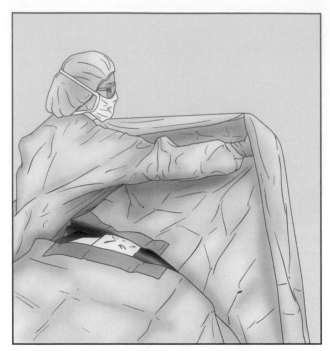

FIG. 4.27 Laparotomy draping continued. Scrub person protects gloved hands under cuff of fan-folded laparotomy sheet and draws the upper section above fenestration toward the head of the bed, draping it over the anesthesia screen. The bottom portion of the fan-folded sheet is extended over the foot of the bed in a similar manner.

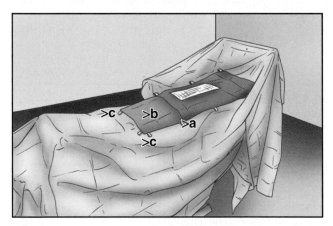

FIG. 4.28 Laparotomy draping completed. Fenestration provides exposure of prepared operative site: >*a*, Reinforced area around drape fenestration provides greater protection and fluid control; >*b*, built-in instrument pad prevents instrument slippage, and >*c*, perforated tabs provide means of controlling position of cords and suction tubes.

position. A lithotomy drape consists of a fenestrated sheet and two triangular leggings.

Several types of impermeable polyvinyl chloride (PVC) sheeting are available in the form of sterile, prepackaged surgical drapes. Plastic, adherent incisional drapes are available as a plain impermeable drape or impregnated with an antimicrobial. These plastic drapes are useful adjuncts to the conventional draping procedure. They can be applied after the fabric drape, alleviating the need for towel clamps. They obviate the need for skin towels and sponges to separate

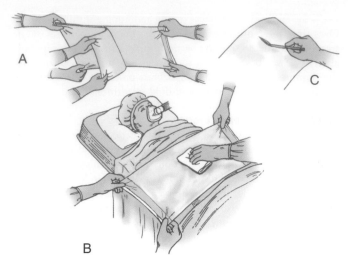

FIG. 4.29 Sterile, impermeable adhesive drape. For maximum sealing to prevent wound contamination, prepared skin must be dry, and the drape must be applied carefully, preventing wrinkles and air bubbles. (A) Surgeon and assistant hold plastic drape taut while another assistant peels off back paper. (B) Surgeon and assistant may apply plastic drape to operative site and, using folded towel, apply slight pressure to eliminate air bubbles and wrinkles. (C) Surgeon would then make incision through plastic drape.

the surgeon's gloves from contact with the patient's skin. Skin color and anatomic landmarks are readily visible, and the incision is made directly through the adherent plastic drape. These materials facilitate draping of irregular body surfaces, such as neck and ear regions, extremities, and joints (Fig. 4.29).

Draping Procedure
Drapes should be folded so that the gowned and gloved members of the team can handle them with ease and safety. The larger, regular sheet is usually fan-folded from bottom to top. The bottom folds may be wider than the upper ones. The small sheet is folded in half and quartered, with the top corners of the sheet turned back or marked for easy identification and handling. To provide for safe, easy handling and a wide margin of safety between the unsterile item and the scrub person's gloved hands, the open end of the Mayo stand cover should be cuffed or folded back on itself (Fig. 4.30). Most fenestrated sheets are fan-folded to the opening from the top and the bottom, and the folds are rolled or fanned toward the center of the opening. The drape fenestration is place over the incision site and the fan folds are drawn away from the incision site. The edges of the top and bottom folds of the sheet are fanned to provide a cuff under which the perioperative scrub person may place his or her gloved hands. The top and lower sections should be identified by markings to facilitate easy handling.

When applying drapes to create the sterile field, these principles should be followed:
- Allow sufficient time and space to permit careful draping and proper aseptic technique.
- Handle sterile drapes as little as possible. Rapid movement of draping materials creates air currents on which dust, lint, and other particles can migrate (AORN, 2016m).
- Carry the folded drape to the operative site. Carefully unfold the drape, and place it in the proper position. Do not move the drape after it has been placed. Shifting or moving the drape may

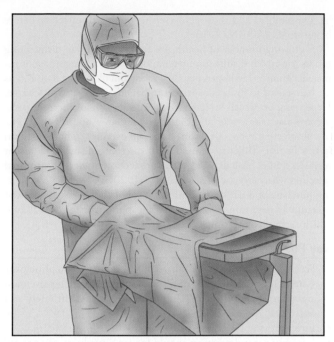

FIG. 4.30 Draping Mayo stand. Folded cover is slipped over the frame. Scrub person's gloved hands are protected by the cuff of drape. Cover is unfolded to extend over upright support of stand.

transport bacteria from an unprepared area of the patient's skin into the surgical field.

- Hold the sterile drape above the level of the OR bed and place it moving from the surgical site to the periphery. Do not allow the drape to fall below the level of the waist because this may increase the risk of contamination. A drape should be carefully unfolded and allowed to fall gently into position by gravity.
- Consider the drape contaminated any time the sterility is questionable and immediately discard a drape that becomes contaminated during the draping procedure.
- Protect the gown by distance. During draping, gloved hands should be protected by cuffing the draping material over the gloved hands to reduce potential contamination. Control all parts of the drape at all times during placement, using precise and direct motions.
- Drape the incisional area first and then the periphery. Always drape from a sterile area to an unsterile area by draping the near side first. Never reach across an unsterile area to drape. When draping the opposite side of the OR bed, go around the bed to drape. The low portion of a sheet that falls below the safe working level should never be raised or lifted back into the sterile area.
- Use nonperforating towel clamps or devices to secure tubing and other items on the sterile field.

After the patient is positioned, prepared, and draped, a time-out is conducted to verify patient identification, correct position, and correct surgical site (and side if applicable) and that required equipment is available.

Environmental Cleaning

Contamination in the OR can occur from various sources. The patient, healthcare workers, and inanimate objects are all capable of introducing potentially infectious material onto the surgical field. The patient should be provided a clean, safe environment. Techniques

have been established to prevent the transmission of microorganisms into the surgical area, such as wearing proper surgical attire and establishing controlled traffic patterns in the surgical suite. During the surgical procedure, traffic within and through the room should be kept to a minimum to reduce air turbulence and to minimize human shedding. All doors in and out of the OR should be kept closed to decrease air agitation and the potential for contamination. HEPA filters placed between outside air processing and the OR vents are used in many facilities and are recommended for newly constructed systems/facilities. HEPA filters are capable of screening out particles larger than 0.3 μm (AORN, 2016e; CDC, 2016e). The perioperative RN should assess the perioperative environment frequently for cleanliness and take action to implement cleaning and disinfection procedures if needed (AORN, 2016e).

All surgical patients should be considered to be potentially infected with bloodborne or other infectious material. For patient and personnel safety, cleaning procedures should be uniform throughout the OR and for all patients. Policies and procedures should be in place that clearly identify what needs cleaning, how it should be cleaned, what it should be cleaned with, how often it should be cleaned, and who is responsible for cleaning it. In addition, there should be a procedure for ongoing monitoring and evaluation of cleaning processes.

Using a uniform procedure designed to protect persons from visible or invisible contamination eliminates the need for special cleaning procedures for so-called dirty cases. Cleaning procedures should be performed in a manner that protects patients and personnel from exposure to potentially infectious microorganisms. Cleaning measures are needed before, during, and after surgical procedures and at the end of each day. A safe, clean environment should be reestablished after each surgical or invasive procedure. Overall housekeeping procedures, such as wall and ceiling washing, should be completed on a defined, regular basis, and terminal cleaning and disinfection of operating and invasive procedure rooms should be performed when scheduled procedures are completed for the day or each regular 24-hour period (AORN, 2016e).

Transmission-Based Precautions, as described earlier, are designed for patients who have a documented infection or who are suspected to be infected with a highly transmissible pathogen for which additional precautions are necessary. The CDC (2016e) guidelines should be followed when all facility policies and guidelines for cleaning are developed.

Before beginning the first procedure of the day, horizontal surfaces in the ORs should be dusted with a cloth dampened with a facility-approved disinfecting agent. Dust and lint deposited on horizontal surfaces during the night can become airborne vectors for organisms if not removed. During surgery, efforts should be made to confine contamination to as small an area as possible around the patient. Sponges should be discarded in plastic-lined containers. As they are counted, they should be contained in an impervious receptacle. The perioperative nurse must use protective eyewear and gloves, instruments, or both when collecting and counting sponges or handling contaminated items. Spills should be cleaned immediately, and the cleaned area should be disinfected with a broad-spectrum disinfectant or germicide. Specimens of blood or other potentially infectious tissues or materials should be placed in a container that prevents leakage. The container must be color coded or labeled using the biohazard symbol (see Fig. 4.1). If the outside of the container becomes contaminated, the primary container must be placed within a second container that prevents leakage and is labeled or color coded. Some facilities use biohazard-labeled impervious bags to transport blood or OPIM (AORN, 2016e; CDC, 2016e).

Environmental cleaning including removal of trash and laundry should not begin until the patient has left the room (AORN, 2016e). Soiled linens should be discarded in fluid-impervious bags to eliminate potential contamination from wet linen soaking through to the outside of the bag. Contaminated items should be placed in leakproof, color-coded, or labeled containers. Sharps (e.g., needles, scalpels, electrosurgical tips) are considered infectious and should be placed in special puncture-resistant containers (OSHA, 2012a). Bulk blood or suctioned fluid may be poured carefully down a drain connected to a sanitary sewer unless prohibited by environmental regulations. Local and state environmental regulations may exist and should be consulted before establishing guidelines for waste disposal. Wall suction units should be disconnected to eliminate contamination of the wall outlet. Suction contents should be disposed as soon as possible on completion of the procedure. Depending on local and state regulations, powder treatments of a chlorine compound are available to solidify liquid material before transport. This chemical also may be tuberculocidal, virucidal, and bactericidal. Suction tubing should be discarded. Personnel should remove their gowns and gloves and place them in the proper receptacles before leaving the OR, and then perform hand hygiene. Instruments and supplies should be contained, labeled with a biohazard label, and taken to the decontamination area, where personnel wearing personal protective attire begin the instrument decontamination process. Care should be taken to arrange sharp instruments in such a manner that personnel need not reach into basins where sharp instruments are unexposed and could cause injury. Equipment and furniture in the OR should be cleaned with an EPA-approved hospital disinfectant. It is important to follow manufacturers' instructions. Some disinfectants may require an extended contact time. If the disinfectant dries quickly, meeting the contact requirements may require several applications. Between-case cleaning should include cleaning of the anesthesia cart and equipment, such as IV poles, anesthesia machine, patient monitors, OR bed, attachments and positioning equipment, transfer device, table strap, overhead lights, and mobile and fixed equipment (AORN, 2016e).

The floor should be cleaned as necessary and should be wet-vacuumed with an EPA-registered disinfectant after scheduled cases are completed (AORN, 2016e). A standard practice of cleaning helps prevent SSI and maintains a clean and safe environment (AORN, 2016e; CDC, 2016e).

At the end of each day's operative schedule, all rooms in which procedures may be performed should be cleaned by qualified, trained, supervised personnel. Areas to be cleaned include the following:

- Surgical lights and external tracks
- Fixed and ceiling-mounted equipment
- All furniture and equipment including wheels and casters
- Equipment
- Handles of cabinets and push plates
- Ventilation faceplates
- Horizontal surfaces (e.g., countertops, fixed shelving, autoclaves)
- Floor
- Kick buckets
- Scrub sinks

If refillable liquid soap dispensers are used, they should be disassembled and cleaned before being refilled because they can serve as reservoirs for microorganisms. At the conclusion of the housekeeping protocol, cleaning equipment and supplies should be properly cleaned, disinfected, and stored. If a wet vacuum has been used, it should

be disassembled and thoroughly washed with a disinfectant before being stored (AORN, 2016e).

A growing number of healthcare facilities are using disinfecting robots (no-touch disinfection technology) as an adjunct to environmental cleaning. Hydrogen peroxide vapor and ultraviolet light robots are being used to disinfect surfaces in patient rooms after discharge. Depending on which system is used and the size of the room, the process may take under an hour or more than 3 hours. Some ORs use disinfecting robots to disinfect a room overnight when the room is not in use. These systems do kill microorganisms, and recent research studies have demonstrated a reduction of hospital-acquired infection when they are used (Weber et al., 2016). Facilities considering purchase and use of a disinfecting robot should review current literature to determine whether they are appropriate for the OR and which technology to purchase.

Key Points

- Perioperative patient care is based on surgical aseptic principles. Careful adherence to these principles supports infection prevention and control and ultimately improves surgical patient safety and outcomes.
- Infection may be caused by bacteria, viruses, or prions.
- Infection control practices should focus primarily on prevention. Transmission of infection involves a chain of events, including the presence of a pathogenic agent, reservoir, portal of exit, transmission, and portal of entry, and host susceptibility. Prevention occurs when there is a break in the chain of transmission.
- Standard Precautions are intended to reduce the transmission of microorganisms from recognized and unrecognized sources of infection. Standard Precautions should be applied to all patients receiving care regardless of their diagnosis or presumed infection status.
- Cleaning is a critical precursor to successful sterilization. Instruments should be decontaminated as soon as possible after surgery.
- Preparing items for use in surgery and other invasive procedures requires thorough cleaning and drying of the items followed by either sterilization or high-level disinfection process.
- Sterilization is defined as the complete elimination or destruction of all forms of microbial life.
- Disinfection is defined as the process that kills all microorganisms with the exception of high numbers of bacterial spores.
- A variety of methods are available for sterilization. Perioperative personnel choose the appropriate method based on the item to be sterilized and manufacturer's recommendations.
- Aseptic technique stems from the principles of asepsis derived over time from microbiologic and epidemiologic concepts.

Critical Thinking Questions

A 42-year-old female is scheduled for an outpatient wound debridement to her right ankle. The perioperative nurse phones the patient the day before her procedure to begin the preoperative assessment. During the course of the assessment, the patient tells the nurse that her surgeon called and told her that her recent wound culture was positive for MRSA.

1. Why is this information important for the perioperative nurse to consider in planning care?
2. What nursing interventions should the nurse plan for after the patient arrives?

ℰvolve *The answers to the Critical Thinking Questions can be found at http://evolve.elsevier.com/Rothrock/Alexander.*

References

American Institute of Architects Academy of Architecture for Health (AIA): *FGI guidelines for design and construction of hospital and outpatient facilities,* Washington, DC, 2010, AIA.

Anderson DJ et al: Strategies to prevent surgical site infection in acute care hospitals: 2014 update, *Infect Control Hosp Epidemiol* 35(6):605–627, 2014.

Association for the Advancement of Medical Instrumentation (AAMI): *AAMI comprehensive guide to steam sterilization and sterility assurance in health care facilities,* Arlington, VA, 2013a, The Association.

Association for the Advancement of Medical Instrumentation (AAMI): *Containment devices for reusable medical device sterilization,* Arlington, VA, 2013b, The Association.

Association for the Advancement of Medical Instrumentation (AAMI): *Sterilization equipment design and use,* Arlington, VA, 2015, The Association.

Association for the Advancement of Medical Instrumentation (AAMI) et al: *Multi-disciplinary position paper on immediate use steam sterilization,* Arlington, VA, 2011, The Association.

Association of periOperative Registered Nurses (AORN): *Antibiotic resistance: are these OR risks on your radar? Periop Insider Newsletter* (website), 2016a. www.aorn.org/about-aorn/aorn-newsroom/periop-insider-newsletter/2016/2016-articles/antibiotic-resistance-are-these-or-risks-on-your-radar?utm_source=Informz&utm_medium=Email&utm_campaign=AORN+Informz+Emails&utm_term=Periop+Insider+%2D+October+12%2C+2016&utm_content=Antibiotic+Resistance%3A+Are+These+OR+Risks+on+Your+Radar%3F. (Accessed 4 February 2017).

Association of periOperative Registered Nurses (AORN): Guideline for a safe environment of care, part 1. In *Guidelines for perioperative practice,* ed 16, Denver, 2016b, The Association.

Association of periOperative Registered Nurses (AORN): Guideline for a safe environment of care, part 2. In *Guidelines for perioperative practice,* ed 16, Denver, 2016c, The Association.

Association of periOperative Registered Nurses (AORN): Guideline for cleaning and care of surgical instruments. In *Guidelines for perioperative practice,* ed 16, Denver, 2016d, The Association.

Association of periOperative Registered Nurses (AORN): Guideline for environmental cleaning. In *Guidelines for perioperative practice,* ed 16, Denver, 2016e, The Association.

Association of periOperative Registered Nurses (AORN): Guideline for hand hygiene. In *Guidelines for perioperative practice,* ed 16, Denver, 2016f, The Association.

Association of periOperative Registered Nurses (AORN): Guideline for laser safety. In *Guidelines for perioperative practice,* ed 16, Denver, 2016g, The Association.

Association of periOperative Registered Nurses (AORN): Guideline for preoperative patient skin antisepsis. In *Guidelines for perioperative practice,* ed 16, Denver, 2016h, The Association.

Association of periOperative Registered Nurses (AORN): Guideline for prevention of transmissible infections in the perioperative practice setting. In *Guidelines for perioperative practice,* ed 16, Denver, 2016i, The Association.

Association of periOperative Registered Nurses (AORN): Guideline for processing flexible endoscopes. In *Guidelines for perioperative practice,* ed 16, Denver, 2016j, The Association.

Association of periOperative Registered Nurses (AORN): Guideline for product selection. In *Guidelines for perioperative practice,* ed 16, Denver, 2016k, The Association.

Association of periOperative Registered Nurses (AORN): Guideline for selection and use of packaging systems for sterilization. In *Guidelines for perioperative practice,* ed 16, Denver, 2016l, The Association.

Association of periOperative Registered Nurses (AORN): Guideline for sterile technique. In *Guidelines for perioperative practice,* ed 16, Denver, 2016m, The Association.

Association of periOperative Registered Nurses (AORN): Guideline for sterilization. In *Guidelines for perioperative practice,* ed 16, Denver, 2016n, The Association.

Association of periOperative Registered Nurses (AORN): Guideline for surgical attire. In *Guidelines for perioperative practice,* ed 16, Denver, 2016o, The Association.

Ban KA et al; American College of Surgeons and Surgical Infection Society: Surgical Site Infection Guidelines, 2016 update, *J Am Coll Surg* 224(1):59–74, 2016.

Burke JF: Identification of the sources of staphylococci contaminating the surgical wound during operation, *Ann Surg* 158(5):898–904, 1963.

Burlingame B: Clinical issues: loaned instruments, *AORN J* 102(1):90–97, 2015.

Centers for Disease Control and Prevention (CDC): Recommendations for prevention of HIV transmission in health-care settings, *MMWR Recomm Rep* 36(SU02):001, 1987. www.cdc.gov/mmwr/preview/mmwrhtml/00023587.htm. (Accessed 4 February 2017).

Centers for Disease Control and Prevention (CDC): Perspectives in disease prevention and health promotion update: universal precautions for prevention of transmission of human immunodeficiency virus, hepatitis B virus, and other bloodborne pathogens in health-care settings, *MMWR Recomm Rep* 37(24):377–388, 1988. https://wonder.cdc.gov/wonder/prevguid/p0000255/p0000255.asp. (Accessed 4 February 2017).

Centers for Disease Control and Prevention (CDC): Guidelines for preventing the transmission of *Mycobacterium tuberculosis* in the healthcare settings, 2005, *MMWR Recomm Rep* 54(RR17):1–141, 2005. www.cdc.gov/mmwr/preview/mmwrhtml/rr5417a1.htm. (Accessed 4 February 2017).

Centers for Disease Control and Prevention (CDC): *Management of multidrug-resistant organisms in healthcare settings* (website), 2006. www.cdc.gov/hicpac/pdf/MDRO/MDROGuideline2006.pdf. (Accessed 2 January 2017).

Centers for Disease Control and Prevention (CDC): *Core elements of hospital antibiotic stewardship programs* (website), 2014. www.cdc.gov/getsmart/healthcare/implementation/core-elements.html. (Accessed 4 February 2017).

Centers for Disease Control and Prevention (CDC): *About CJD* (website), 2015a. www.cdc.gov/prions/cjd/about.html. (Accessed 4 February 2017).

Centers for Disease Control and Prevention (CDC): *Ebola (Ebola virus disease): U.S. healthcare workers and settings* (website), 2015b. www.cdc.gov/vhf/ebola/healthcare-us/index.html. (Accessed 4 February 2017).

Centers for Disease Control and Prevention (CDC): *About Zika, what we know* (website), 2016a. www.cdc.gov/zika/about/index.html. (Accessed 4 February 2017).

Centers for Disease Control and Prevention (CDC): *Contaminated heater-cooler devices* (website), 2016b. www.cdc.gov/hai/outbreaks/heater-cooler.html. (Accessed 7 January 2017).

Centers for Disease Control and Prevention (CDC): *Drug-resistant TB* (website), 2016c. www.cdc.gov/tb/topic/drtb/default.htm. (Accessed 4 February 2017).

Centers for Disease Control and Prevention (CDC): *Emergency preparedness and response: bioterrorism* (website), 2016d. https://emergency.cdc.gov/bioterrorism/index.asp. (Accessed 15 January 2017).

Centers for Disease Control and Prevention (CDC): *Infection control: disinfection and sterilization* (website), 2016e. https://www.cdc.gov/infectioncontrol/guidelines/disinfection. (Accessed 9 August 2017).

Centers for Disease Control and Prevention (CDC): *NIOSH pocket guide to chemical hazards* (website), 2016f. www.cdc.gov/niosh/npg/. (Accessed 4 February 2017).

Centers for Disease Control and Prevention (CDC): *Get smart for healthcare in hospitals and long-term care: core elements of hospital antibiotic stewardship programs* (website), 2017. https://www.cdc.gov/getsmart/healthcare/implementation/core-elements.html. (Accessed 23 August 2017).

Copeland JT: Do surgical personnel really need to double-glove?, *AORN J* 89(2):322–330, 2009.

Edmiston CE et al: Clinical and microbiological aspects of biofilm-associated surgical site infections, *Adv Exp Med Biol* 830:47–67, 2015.

Johnson JR et al: Molecular analysis of *Escherichia coli* from retail meats (2002-2004) from the United States National Antimicrobial Resistance Monitoring System, *Clin Infect Dis* 49(2):195–201, 2009.

Koganti S et al: Evaluation of hospital floors as a potential source of pathogen dissemination using a nonpathogenic virus as a surrogate marker, *Infect Control Hosp Epidemiol* 37(11):1374–1377, 2016.

Kuhar DT et al: *Updated U.S. Public Health Service guidelines for the management of occupational exposures to HIV and recommendations for postexposure prophylaxis* (website), 2013. https://stacks.cdc.gov/view/cdc/20711. (Accessed 4 February 2017).

Makama JG et al: Glove perforation rate in surgery: a randomized, controlled study to evaluate the efficacy of double gloving, *Surg Infect (Larchmt)* 17(4):436–442, 2016.

Mangram AJ et al: Guideline for prevention of surgical site infection 1999. Hospital Infection Control Practices Advisory Committee, *Infect Control Hosp Epidemiol* 20(4):250–278, 1999.

Mase S et al: Provisional CDC guidelines for the use and safety monitoring of bedaquiline fumarate (Sirturo) for the treatment of multidrug-resistant tuberculosis, *MMWR Recomm Rep* 62(RR09):1–12, 2013. www.cdc.gov/mmwr/preview/mmwrhtml/rr6209a1.htm. (Accessed 12 January 2017).

McGann P et al: Erratum for McGann et al, *Escherichia coli* harboring *mcr*-1 and ^bla^CTX-M on a novel IncF plasmid: first report of *mcr*-1 in the United States, *Antimicrob Agents Chemother* 60(8):5107, 2016.

National Archives and Records Administration: *Department of Health and Human Services, Food and Drug Administration, 21 CFR Parts 878, 880, and 895 [Docket No. FDA-2015-N-5017] RIN 0910-AH02* (website), 2016. https://s3.amazonaws.com/public-inspection.federalregister.gov/2016-30382.pdf. (Accessed 4 February 2017).

Occupational Safety and Health Administration (OSHA): Occupational exposure to ethylene oxide, final standard, *Fed Regist* 49(122):25737–25768, 1984. www.osha.gov/pls/oshaweb/owadisp.show_document?p_table=FEDERAL_REGISTER&p_id=12438. (Accessed 4 February 2017).

Occupational Safety and Health Administration (OSHA): *Bloodborne pathogens standard (29 CFR 1910.1030)* (website), 2012a. www.osha.gov/pls/oshaweb/owadisp.show_document?p_table=STANDARDS&p_id=10051. (Accessed 4 February 2017).

Occupational Safety and Health Administration (OSHA): *Ethylene oxide, 29 CFR 1910.1047* (website), 2012b. www.osha.gov/pls/oshaweb/owadisp.show_document?p_table=STANDARDS&p_id=10070. (Accessed 4 February 2017).

O'Horo JC et al: Carbapenem-resistant Enterobacteriaceae and endoscopy: an evolving threat, *Am J Infect Control* 44(9):1032–1036, 2016.

Perkins JJ: *Principles and methods of sterilization*, Springfield, IL, 1969, Charles C Thomas.

Rutala WA, Weber DJ: Guideline for disinfection and sterilization of prion-contaminated medical instruments, *Infect Control Hosp Epidemiol* 31(2):107–117, 2010.

Siegel JD et al: Guideline for isolation precautions: preventing transmission of infectious agents in healthcare settings (2007), *Am J Infect Control* 35:S65–S164, 2007. www.cdc.gov/hicpac/2007IP/2007isolationPrecautions.html. (Accessed 4 February 2017).

Talbot TR: Surgical site infections and antimicrobial prophylaxis. In Bennett JE et al, editors: *Mandell, Douglas, and Bennett's principles and practice of infectious diseases*, ed 8, Philadelphia, 2015, Elsevier.

The Joint Commission (TJC): *The Joint Commission's implementation guide for NPSG.07.05.01 on surgical site infections* (website), December 3, 2013. www.jointcommission.org/implementation_guide_for_npsg070501_ssi_change_project/. (Accessed 4 February 2017).

US Environmental Protection Agency (EPA): *Hospital, Medical, and Infectious Waste Incinerators (HMIWI): New Source Performance Standards (NSPS), emission guidelines, and federal plan requirements regulations* (website), 2016. www.epa.gov/stationary-sources-air-pollution/hospital-medical-and-infectious-waste-incinerators-hmiwi-new-source. (Accessed 4 February 2017).

US Food and Drug Administration (FDA): *FDA cleared sterilants and high level disinfectants with general claims for reprocessing reusable medical and dental devices* (website), March 2015a. www.fda.gov/MedicalDevices/DeviceRegulationandGuidance/ReprocessingofReusableMedicalDevices/ucm437347.htm. (Accessed 4 February 2017).

US Food and Drug Administration (FDA): *Reprocessing of reusable medical devices* (website), August 2015b. www.fda.gov/MedicalDevices/ProductsandMedicalProcedures/ReprocessingofReusableMedicalDevices/ucm20081513.htm. (Accessed 4 February 2017).

US Food and Drug Administration (FDA): Safety and effectiveness of health care antiseptics; topical antimicrobial drug products for over-the-counter human use; proposed amendment of the tentative final monograph: reopening of administrative record, 21 CFR, Part 310, *Fed Regist* 81(126):2015c. www.federalregister.gov/documents/2015/05/01/2015-10174/safety-and-effectiveness-of-health-care-antiseptics-topical-antimicrobial-drug-products-for. (Accessed 25 January 2017).

US Food and Drug Administration (FDA): *Safety and effectiveness for health care antiseptics; topical antimicrobial drug products for over-the-counter human use; proposed amendment of the tentative final monograph; reopening of administrative record* (website), 2016. https://www.fda.gov/downloads/AboutFDA/ReportsManualsForms/Reports/EconomicAnalyses/UCM447035.pdf. (Accessed 4 February 2017).

Weber DJ et al: "No touch" technologies for environmental decontamination: focus on hydrogen peroxide devices and ultraviolent systems, *Curr Opin Infect Dis* 29(4):424–431, 2016.

Webster J et al. *Perioperative bathing or showering with skin antiseptics to prevent surgical site infection* (website), 2015. www.cochrane.org/CD004985/WOUNDS_preoperative-bathing-or-showering-with-skin-antiseptics-to-prevent-surgical-site-infection. (Accessed 26 January 2017).

World Health Organization: *WHO guidelines on hand hygiene in health care* (website), 2009. http://www.who.int/gpsc/5may/tools/9789241597906/en/. (Accessed 23 August 2017).

CHAPTER 5
Anesthesia

BRIAN D. CAMPBELL

The first medical report of anesthesia was announced to the world on November 18, 1846, by Henry J. Bigelow in the *Boston Medical and Surgical Journal*. An era had ended during which successful surgery depended largely on the surgeon's speed while working on a struggling, distressed patient. Anesthetic techniques gave the surgeon more time to operate and permitted new procedures to be undertaken that would have been impossible before. Many modern surgical techniques are now feasible because of advances in the art and science of anesthesia.

As integral members of the patient care team in operative and other invasive procedure settings, perioperative nurses need to be familiar with the principles and practices of anesthesia and the perioperative functions of the anesthesia provider. This chapter presents an overview of the practice of anesthesia, factors involved, and interrelationships with the perioperative nurse. It discusses major types of anesthesia, introduces commonly used medications, reviews standards of anesthesia care, and summarizes problems that can occur during the perioperative period. The anesthesia machine and monitoring equipment are described so that perioperative nurses can become familiar with their basic functions because the nurse may use them during local anesthesia or conscious sedation/analgesia procedures. To provide a single reference source for the student or novice perioperative nurse, most abbreviations are defined in Box 5.1.

BOX 5.1

Abbreviations Used in This Chapter

AA: Anesthesiologist's assistant

AANA: American Association of Nurse Anesthetists

ACLS: Advanced cardiac life support, a protocol for resuscitation from the American Heart Association

APL: Adjustable pressure-limiting valve; a valve on anesthesia machines that limits the maximum pressure in the patient breathing circuit; frequently referred to as the "pop-off valve"

ASA: American Society of Anesthesiologists

ASA PS: ASA physical status classification system

cm: Centimeter; 1×10^{-3} m; 2.54 cm = 1 inch

CRNA: Certified registered nurse anesthetist

CSF: Cerebrospinal fluid; the fluid surrounding the brain and spinal cord; for spinal anesthesia, local anesthetics are injected into the CSF

EGTA: Esophageal (gastric tube) airway; a cuffed tube that is inserted blindly into the esophagus and connected to a mask; this permits ventilation through the mask and gastric suctioning through the cuffed tube

ERAS: Enhanced recovery after surgery

ETco₂: End-tidal carbon dioxide reported as a partial pressure; see Capnography section

ETT: Endotracheal tube

FIo₂: Fraction of inspired oxygen; this is a fraction (0.00 to 1.00) that corresponds to the percent (0% to 100%) of inspired oxygen

FO: Fiberoptic

kg: Kilogram; 1 kg = 2.2 lb

LMA: Laryngeal mask airway or laryngeal airway

MAC: Monitored anesthesia care; see Monitored Anesthesia Care section, also the *minimum alveolar concentration* (MAC) as the inhaled anesthetic atmospheric pressure required to prevent movement in response to a defined noxious stimulus in 50% of subjects

mcg: Microgram

mg: Milligram; 1×10^{-3} g

MH: Malignant hyperthermia; see Malignant Hyperthermia section

MHAUS: Malignant Hyperthermia Association of the United States

MMS: Master of medical science degree

MRI: Magnetic resonance imaging

nm: Nanometer; 1×10^{-9} m

NMS: Neuroleptic malignant syndrome; see Malignant Hyperthermia section

N₂O: Nitrous oxide

NSAID: Nonsteroidal antiinflammatory drug

Paco₂: Partial pressure of arterial carbon dioxide; lowercase "a" denotes "arterial"; an uppercase "A" denotes "alveolar"

Pao₂: Partial pressure of arterial oxygen, lowercase "a" denotes "arterial"; an uppercase "A" denotes "alveolar"

PCA: Patient-controlled analgesia; see Pain Management section

PNB: Peripheral nerve block

POCD: Postoperative cognitive dysfunction

ppm: Parts per million; 1 ppm = 1×10^{-6}

psi: Pounds per square inch; a measurement of pressure

QA: Quality assurance; this function also may be identified as quality improvement (QI), continuous quality improvement (CQI), or similar names

RSI: Rapid-sequence induction

SGA: Supraglottic airway device

Spo₂: Saturation (pulse) of oxygen or in a pulsating vessel, expressed as a percentage; see Pulse Oximetry section

Svo₂: Saturation of mixed venous oxygen in percentage; this measurement is made from a special pulmonary artery catheter

torr: A unit of pressure, which is necessary to support a column of mercury 1 mm high at 0°C and standard gravity

---

Anesthesia Providers

In the United States anesthesia care usually is provided in one of three ways: (1) by an anesthesiologist; (2) by a certified registered nurse anesthetist (CRNA) working alone, in collaboration with, or under the direction of an anesthesiologist or a physician; or (3) by an anesthesiologist's assistant (AA) working under direct supervision of an anesthesiologist.

An anesthesiologist is a licensed physician with 4 or more years of specialty training in anesthesiology. Nurse anesthesia programs last a minimum of 2 years and require a bachelor of science (BS) degree in nursing or other appropriate field and a minimum of 1 year of critical care experience before acceptance. Nurse anesthesia programs range from 24 to 36 months, depending on university requirements. All nurse anesthesia programs are at the master's degree level at a minimum. On completion, graduates must successfully complete a national certification examination. By 2025, it is projected that all CRNAs will graduate with a doctor of nursing practice (DNP) degree (AANA, 2016).

Since 1969 AAs have been used as assistants to anesthesiologists. Acceptance into an AA program requires a BS degree that includes college-level "premed" education. AAs are graduate students within a medical school and typically receive a master of medical science (MMS) degree from the medical school. They also take a national certification examination administered by the National Commission on Certification of Anesthesia Providers' Assistants under the supervision of the National Board of Medical Examiners.

In this chapter the term *anesthesia provider* denotes the individual *providing* the continuous anesthesia care for the patient. Depending on practice in a given hospital or surgical setting, this may be an anesthesiologist, a CRNA, or an AA. In many settings an *anesthesia care team* includes CRNAs, with or without AAs supervised by anesthesiologists. In small rural hospitals, an anesthesiologist may not be present, and a CRNA may be the sole anesthesia provider.

The anesthesia provider is the patient's advocate in the perioperative period; as such, he or she must be concerned with many divergent factors when the patient's own sensory and cerebral functions are obtunded by anesthesia. The field of anesthesia has become so complex that in many large hospitals an anesthesia provider may specialize further in obstetric, neurosurgical, pediatric, cardiovascular, regional, or ambulatory anesthesia. The anesthesia provider also may subspecialize in acute and chronic pain management or in critical care medicine.

Patient Safety

Patient safety is a primary concern during surgery and anesthesia. Over 40 million anesthetics are administered each year in the United States. With advances in medications, monitoring technology, and safety systems, as well as highly educated anesthesia providers, the risk caused by anesthesia to a patient undergoing routine surgery is very small. Mortality attributable to general anesthesia is said to occur at rates of less than 1:100,000.

The most common minor complication is postoperative nausea and vomiting (PONV) (35.53%), and the most common major complication is medication error (11.71%). Patient age, sex, ASA PS (see Box 5.1), facility type, type of anesthesia, time the surgery occurs, and duration of surgery are associated with higher complication rates. Procedures that occur during evening hours and the holidays are not associated with increases in adverse event rates. Patients age 50 and over or classified as ASA PS 4 exhibit the highest major

adverse event rates, whereas minor complications are more common in healthier patients (ASA PS 1–2) undergoing elective daytime procedures (Liau and Havidich, 2014).

The public still considers anesthesia a major risk of surgery. This may be attributable to sensationalized reports in the media, magazine articles, and in movies. In addition, people may have a heightened awareness of anesthesia-related deaths because these often occur in the perioperative period; problems unrelated to anesthesia may not result in death until days after the procedure.

Environmental Noise

Many studies demonstrate the effects that noise has on humans. Multiple conversations, loud music, and other noises can create or worsen patient anxiety, as well as make communication difficult among team members and between the patient and team members. Noise can also cause distraction, increasing the potential for miscommunication and errors (AORN, 2017). One study of patients recovering during the immediate postoperative period showed that 10% of the patients perceived noise levels in the operating room (OR) as very high and experienced the noise as annoying, disruptive, and stressful (Hasfeldt et al., 2014). Although the patient is in the OR, *especially* during induction and emergence, every effort is made to maintain a calm, quiet environment. This is especially true when caring for pediatric patients.

Awareness During Anesthesia

Remaining conscious during anesthesia is a concern of both patients and anesthesia providers. Some patients are so anxious about being aware of anything during surgery that it may affect their reasoning when discussing options for anesthesia. Many procedures, such as biopsies, inguinal hernias, or procedures on the lower extremities, can be done under regional anesthesia or monitored anesthesia care (MAC). Some patients may want general anesthesia, however, because they do not want to be aware of anything during the procedure.

In rare cases, during general anesthesia for emergent procedures or trauma, the patient may be paralyzed, aware of what is occurring, but unable to tell anyone. Intraoperative awareness (IOA) is reported with multiple and differing anesthetic techniques. Several factors may contribute to its occurrence. An incidence of 1 to 2 cases per 1000 is a reproducible finding and should be used both to inform patients and guide future studies (Avidan and Mashour, 2013). Incidence of IOA may increase to 1% to 1.5% in higher risk patient populations, such as patients requiring anesthesia for obstetrics, major trauma, and cardiac surgery (Duke, 2016).

The bispectral index system (BIS) analyzes the relationship and frequency of brain signals using an algorithm to generate a composite, numeric value that seems to correlate with the cerebral state. Four electrodes, positioned across the forehead, connect to a monitor that gives an index (0–100) of the patient's hypnotic state or sedation level; an index of 40 to 60 is considered optimal anesthesia. The system monitors the effects of anesthetics and sedatives on the hypnotic status of the brain, but is less informative about the level of analgesia. Motion artifacts and mental changes cause erratic changes under lighter levels of sedation commonly used with MAC. The BIS monitor is not a predictor of motor depression; it also lags by 3 to 5 seconds, leading to a potential for the anesthesia provider to not anticipate a sudden rise in the depth of anesthesia. Nonetheless, use of the BIS monitor to alert the anesthesia provider to IOA with recall (AWR [awareness with recall]) using a BIS-based protocol can be effective.

Preoperative Preparation

Patient Evaluation

Preoperative evaluation is often done one or more days before the scheduled surgical procedure in a preadmission clinic (sometimes called *preadmission testing [PAT], preanesthesia clinic,* or *anesthesia-assessment unit*). Preadmission staff secures admission data, appropriate consent forms, and a preoperative history; they also perform a physical examination, complete a preanesthesia evaluation and examination, obtain an airway history and patient's weight, and process appropriate diagnostic or laboratory tests. Selective testing is recommended when test results may change perioperative management (Breyer and Gropper, 2014). Patients with higher than average risk based on history are those who usually require more extensive testing. An anesthetic preoperative evaluation clinic (PEC) enhances OR efficiency, decreases day-of-surgery cancellations or delays, reduces hospital costs, and enhances quality of patient care (Miller, 2015). After assessing the patient's physical status (PS), the anesthesia provider in the preadmission setting selects the most appropriate anesthetic technique. Resolving the patient's questions and concerns follows, as well as instructions aimed to expedite admission on the day of surgery. Before elective surgery, the patient should be in optimal medical condition. Preoperative testing aims to identify patients at risk for perioperative complications so that appropriate perioperative therapy can foster a return to functional status. The morbidly obese patient is at greater risk for cardiopulmonary aberrations, sleep-disordered breathing, and abnormal airway issues (Marley and Calabrese, 2014).

Anesthesia, even in healthy patients, presents particular risks. A goal in risk assessment is to inform patients so that they can weigh options and identify opportunities to alter that risk. In a recent study of PECs, the authors found a reduction in mortality for patients seen in a PEC versus patients not seen. However, there was little difference between the groups in failure to rescue (FTR) cases of unanticipated surgical complications (Blitz, 2016). If it is determined that the patient's PS should improve to reduce the risks involved, the patient's primary physician or surgeon discusses this with the patient, and, if necessary, elective surgery is deferred until the patient's condition optimizes. In emergent surgery, however, any benefits gained from a delay must be weighed carefully against the hazards of deferral.

The assignment of a PS classification depends on the patient's physiologic condition independent of the proposed surgical procedure. The PS classification was developed by the American Society of Anesthesiologists (ASA) to provide uniform guidelines. It is an evaluation of the severity of systemic diseases, physiologic dysfunction, and anatomic abnormalities. The ASA classification system is widely used to estimate perioperative risk (Table 5.1).

Although many hospitals and ambulatory surgery centers (ASCs) use PECs, nurses may conduct preoperative telephone interviews with patients in reasonably good health, posing questions relating to pulmonary and cardiac disease; medication (prescription, over the counter, herbal, and homeopathic remedies) and alcohol use; medication, latex, or anesthetic allergies; personal or family history of anesthetic reactions; and pregnancy. Use of anesthetic agents and sedative medications, especially for procedures lasting more than 3 hours, should be balanced against potential risks in women in their third trimester of pregnancy (FDA, 2016).

The preadmission interview, whether by phone or in person, provides an opportunity for patient education as it relates to the proposed procedure (Patient, Family, and Caregiver Education).

On the day of surgery, patients arrive 1 to 2 hours before the scheduled surgery to complete other preoperative processes. In some facilities certain ambulatory patients are evaluated further just before surgery. These are usually healthy patients having minor procedures or patients with stable, chronic conditions about to undergo a procedure

---

TABLE 5.1

American Society of Anesthesiologists Physical (P) Status Classification

Status[a,b]	Definition	Description and Examples
P1	Normal healthy patient	No physiologic, psychologic, biochemical, or organic disturbance
P2	Patient with mild systemic disease	Cardiovascular disease with minimal restriction of activity; hypertension, asthma, chronic bronchitis, obesity, diabetes mellitus, or tobacco abuse; mild asthma or well-controlled hypertension; no significant impact on daily activity; unlikely impact on anesthesia and surgery
P3	Patient with a severe systemic disease that limits activity, but is not incapacitating	Cardiovascular or pulmonary disease that limits activity; severe diabetes with systemic complications; history of myocardial infarction, angina pectoris, poorly controlled hypertension, or morbid obesity; renal failure on dialysis or class 2 congestive heart failure; significant impact on daily activity; likely impact on anesthesia and surgery
P4	Patient with a severe systemic disease that is a constant threat to life or requires intensive therapy	Severe cardiac, pulmonary, renal, hepatic, or endocrine dysfunction, acute myocardial infarction, respiratory failure requiring mechanical ventilation; serious limitation of daily activity; major impact on anesthesia and surgery
P5	Moribund patient who is not expected to survive 24 h with or without operation	Surgery is done as last recourse or resuscitative effort; major multisystem or cerebral trauma, ruptured aneurysm, or large pulmonary embolus
P6	Patient declared brain dead whose organs are being removed for donor purposes	—

[a]In statuses P2–P4, the systemic disease may or may not be related to the reason for surgery.
[b]For any patient (P1–P5) requiring emergency surgery, an E is added to the physical status, such as P1E, P2E. ASA1–6 or I to VI is often used for physical status.

Modified from American Society of Anesthesiologists (ASA): *Physical status classification system* (website). www.asahq.org/resources/clinical-information/asa-physical-status-classification-system. (Accessed 5 January 2017).

PATIENT, FAMILY, AND CAREGIVER EDUCATION

Preanesthesia Preparation

During preoperative assessment the patient is interviewed, and it is important to discuss the following topics:

Preoperative fasting: Explain why it is important. Review differences in materials consumed (clear versus solid), and when they may or may not be consumed to prevent possible vomiting and gastric aspiration.

Medications: Patients take necessary medications (such as antihypertensive, cardiac, seizure, and asthma medications) with sips of water, preferably before they leave their homes to come to the facility. Patients with diabetes continue taking oral hypoglycemic agents until the evening before surgery. If the patient takes insulin, it is common to administer a fraction (one-fourth to one-half) of the usual morning dose. Aspirin and aspirin-containing products are discontinued 1 week before surgery. Nonsteroidal antiinflammatory drugs are discontinued 4 days before surgery. If the patient is taking warfarin, it is usually discontinued 3 days before major surgery, but continued for minor surgery. The prescribing clinician may need to be consulted to ensure it is safe to discontinue these medications or switch to alternative medications, especially if the patient has recently undergone heart valve replacement surgery or has other serious conditions.

Herbal supplements: Many herbal supplements can interact with anesthetics. It is important to ask about any supplements the patient is taking; some authors recommend discontinuation of all supplements (see Chapter 30).

Recent upper respiratory tract infections: A patient with a reactive airway has an increased risk of respiratory complications (e.g., bronchospasm, laryngospasm).

Family-centered preanesthesia preparation for children and their families: Such preparation aims to reduce anxiety and improve cooperation without the adverse effects of pharmacologic intervention. A Cochrane review of nonpharmacologic interventions for children found that the presence of either one or both parents did not diminish the child's anxiety. Potentially promising nonpharmacologic interventions are parental auricular acupuncture, clowns/clown doctors, playing of videos, cartoons of the child's choice, and handheld video games. There is insufficient evidence to determine comparative effectiveness of different educational interventions or to recommend specific ones, but the diversity of patient needs and patient preferences supports the need for individualized approaches. When the elements of modeling, parental involvement, and child life preparation are provided in the context of supportive healthcare relationships, even though fear and anxiety may not disappear completely, the child and family may feel more empowered to manage the demands of upcoming surgery.

Anesthesia options: Anesthesia providers also discuss the anesthesia options appropriate for that patient/procedure after reviewing pertinent history and physical information and pertinent diagnostic studies and consultations. The American Association of Nurse Anesthetists (AANA) has a number of patient education brochures available on its website. These brochures can be printed and offered to patients and their families, or the perioperative nurse can simply direct the patient, family, and caregiver to the AANA website (www. aana.com/forpatients/pages/Brochures-and-Resources.aspx).

Modified from Cohn S: Preoperative evaluation. In Goldman L, Schafer A, editors: *Goldman–Cecil medicine*, ed 25, Philadelphia, 2016, Saunders; Manyande A: Non-pharmacological interventions for assisting the induction of anesthesia in children, *Cochrane Database Syst Rev* 7, CD006447, 2015; Chou R: Practice Guideline From the American Pain Society, the American Society of Regional Anesthesia and Pain Medicine, and the American Society of Anesthesiologists' Committee on Regional Anesthesia, Executive Committee, and Administrative Council, *J Pain* 17(2):131–157, 2016; Boles J: Preparing children and families for procedures or surgery, *Pediatr Nurs* 42(3):147–149, 2016.

(e.g., cataract removal, skin lesion excision) under MAC. These preadmission processes reduce healthcare costs, decrease risk of healthcare-associated infections (HAIs), increase use and efficiency of healthcare resources, improve patient relations, and enhance the chances of having a well-informed patient in optimal health status both before and after the procedure. In larger hospitals and ASCs, the patient evaluator in the preanesthesia clinic is often not the anesthesia provider for the patient's surgical procedure. Preoperative histories, physical examinations, and assessments performed by medical specialists often fail to address specific anesthesia-related concerns, such as risk for postoperative cognitive dysfunction (POCD) in older patients (Wijeysundera and Sweitzer, 2015) (Research Highlight). Immediately before surgery, therefore, the anesthesia provider (1) reviews the patient's chart, laboratory data, and diagnostic studies, such as electrocardiogram (ECG) and chest x-ray if ordered and necessary; (2) confirms that the appropriate consent forms (surgery, anesthesia, use of blood products) have been signed and dated; (3) identifies the patient; (4) verifies the surgical procedure; (5) reviews the choice of anesthesia; (6) examines the patient; and (7) administers preoperative medications as indicated (Miller, 2015). As ambulatory surgery becomes increasingly common, other factors are taken into consideration (Ambulatory Surgery Considerations).

Choice of Anesthesia

The patient, anesthesia provider, and surgeon make the choice of anesthesia for a given surgical procedure. Many factors influence this choice, including the following:

1. Patient's wishes and understanding of the types of anesthesia that could be used (Patient Engagement Exemplar)
2. Patient's physiologic status
3. Presence and severity of coexisting conditions
4. Patient's mental and psychologic status
5. Postoperative recovery from various kinds of anesthesia
6. Options for management of postoperative pain
7. Type and duration of surgical procedure
8. Patient's position during surgery
9. Surgeon's particular requirements

Premedication

The primary purpose of premedication before anesthesia is to sedate the patient and reduce anxiety. Medications that may be given preoperatively include sedatives and hypnotics, anxiolytics, amnestics, tranquilizers, narcotics or other analgesics, antiemetics, and anticholinergics. A single medication may possess the properties of several medication classes. Midazolam (Versed) is administered frequently

RESEARCH HIGHLIGHT ||

Postoperative Cognitive Dysfunction

Postoperative cognitive dysfunction (POCD) is defined as a decline in cognitive function that occurs after surgery. The function of the brain is altered after anesthesia and surgery as evidenced by depressed consciousness, attention, memory, and reaction time; some patients have complete amnesia for several hours after emergence from anesthesia despite the appearance of being completely awake. The time to return of normal brain function after anesthesia is not clear, and it is reasonable to assume that if the anesthetic agents were responsible, full function should return soon after discontinuation of the agents involved. It has also been shown that the type of anesthetic technique, whether general or regional anesthesia, does not demonstrate a significant advantage beyond the first week after surgery. The one recurring factor noted in several studies identifying POCD risk was increasing age, with seven studies noting this risk factor especially in patients over the age of 60 years of age. One case of POCD in a 65-year-old male after total knee arthroplasty lasting 19 days has been reported. In their investigation of this case, the researchers noted that the patient had underlying predisposing factors such as depression, mild memory deficit, and generalized brain volume loss, leading them to recommend a preoperative evaluation of cognitive function, and other risk factors when dealing with the geriatric patient population undergoing elective surgery. Another study found a reduced incidence of POCD in aged patients when dexmedetomidine was used, suggesting inflammation suppression may be the underlying mechanism of action.

The incidence of POCD after cardiac surgery (coronary artery bypass, valve replacement or repair, or both) has been reported at 50% to 70% in the first postoperative week, 30% to 50% after 6 weeks, and 20% to 40% at 6 months and 1 year. There were multiple factors examined to understand POCD in this patient population including use of arterial filters, temperature management, types of oxygenators, and whether the surgery was performed on or off pump (see Chapter 25).

A significant issue is how POCD affects patient's lives. Several studies show that patients over the age of 60 with POCD also have a significant effect on their activities of daily living. As a result, many patients sought early retirement, social security type financial support, and in long-term follow-up had significantly higher mortality rates regardless of type of surgery.

Modified from Chen W et al: The effects of dexmedetomidine on post-operative cognitive dysfunction and inflammatory factors in senile patients, *Int J Clin Exp Med* 8(3):4601–4605, 2015; Paredes S et al: Post-operative cognitive dysfunction at 3 months in adults after non-cardiac surgery: a qualitative systematic review, *Acta Anaesthesiol Scand* 60(8):1043–1058, 2016; Rasmussen LS et al: Cognitive dysfunction and other long-term complications of surgery and anesthesia. In Miller RD, editor: *Miller's anesthesia*, ed 8, Philadelphia, 2015, Elsevier; Yap KK, Joyner P: Post-operative cognitive dysfunction after knee arthroplasty: a diagnostic dilemma, *Oxf Med Case Reports* (3):60–62, 2014.

AMBULATORY SURGERY CONSIDERATIONS

Patient Selection

Ambulatory surgery is increasingly common, accounting for nearly two-thirds of all surgery visits. Ambulatory surgery may be a "same-day" procedure in the hospital, in an office, or in an ASC. Patients usually enjoy an earlier return to their preoperative physiologic state and fewer complications with ambulatory surgery compared with inpatient surgery. Ambulatory procedures also offer a reduced chance of HAIs. Advances in medical technology and pain control are allowing increasingly complex procedures, such as total joint replacements, to be performed in ambulatory settings. Advances in medical devices and pharmaceuticals have also contributed to reduced recovery times, furthering the preference for ambulatory surgery. Although a small percentage of patients have health conditions that require ambulatory surgery to be performed in proximity to a full-service hospital should complications arise, most patients receive the same level of care at lower cost by seeking treatment in an ASC.

Patient selection for ambulatory procedures is extremely important. The procedure should have neither a significant incidence of perioperative or postoperative problems, nor require intensive postoperative management. The patient should be in general good health or have well-managed existing conditions. Patients with a significant history are interviewed before the day of surgery to determine how well coexisting conditions are controlled and what tests or consultations may be needed before the day of surgery.

The following are some patient conditions for which ambulatory surgery is unacceptable:

- Ex-premature infants younger than 60 weeks post conceptual age requiring general anesthesia with endotracheal intubation
- Full-term infants with a history of respiratory difficulties, apneic episodes, or feeding difficulties
- Unstable physical status (ASA PS 3 or 4) (see Table 5.1)
- Active substance or alcohol abuse
- Poorly controlled seizures
- Previously unevaluated and unmanaged moderate to severe obstructive sleep apnea
- Uncontrolled diabetes
- Infectious process requiring isolation
- Anticipation of postoperative pain not controllable with oral analgesics or regional anesthesia blocks
- Inability to care for self and without access to assistance
- Noncompliance

Anesthetic technique is based on the surgical procedure, surgeon and patient preference, and skill of the practitioner. Goals for anesthesia in an ambulatory setting include minimal physiologic changes secondary to the anesthetic, fast induction, rapid emergence while maintaining patient comfort, intraoperative amnesia and analgesia, suitable operating conditions, minimal perioperative side effects, and minimized postoperative side effects, such as PONV. Use of an LMA, BIS awareness monitoring, and certain anesthetics (such as propofol, sevoflurane, and desflurane) contribute to attaining these goals.

ASA, American Society of Anesthesiologists; *ASC*, ambulatory surgery center; *BIS*, bispectral index system; *HAI*, hospital-associated infection; *LMA*, laryngeal mask airway; *PONV*, postoperative nausea and vomiting.
Modified from Marley RA, Calabrese T: Outpatient anesthesia. In Nagelhout JJ, Plaus KL, editors: *Nurse anesthesia*, ed 5, St Louis, 2014, Saunders; Healthcare Bluebook: *Commercial insurance cost savings in ambulatory surgery centers* (website). https://healthcarebluebook.com/files/ascsavings.pdf. (Accessed 5 January 2017).

PATIENT ENGAGEMENT EXEMPLAR

Decision Making and Anesthesia

NAQC guiding principal number 2 states "Patients are the best and ultimate source of information about their health status and retain the right to make their own decisions about care" (Sofaer and Schumann, 2013). The anesthesia provider, as a partner with the patient, reviews pertinent health history to ensure that anesthesia risks are identified. If there is a choice of sedation or type of anesthesia, present those options with benefit and risks and allow the patient to make the decision. Anesthesia providers and perioperative nurses interview the patient and identify allergies, malignant hyperthermia risk, and if there is a living will or power of attorney present. If there is a possibility of blood product use make sure the patient's wishes are known and documented. With children, the elderly, or patients who need an interpreter, the perioperative team considers allowing parents or family members to accompany patients to the OR or procedure room and being present during the induction of anesthesia. This engagement strategy helps alleviate patient anxiety and fear and has not proven to be a detriment to care (Perel et al., 2007).

NAQC, Nursing Alliance for Quality Care.
Modified from Sofaer S, Schumann MJ: *Fostering successful patient and family engagement: nursing's critical role* (website), 2013. www.naqc.org/WhitePaper-PatientEngagement. (Accessed 17 June 2016); Perel A, Mishuk Y, Matot I: Family member presence during induction of anesthesia in elderly patients–a feasibility study, *Eur J Anaesthesiol* 24(Supplement 39):190, 2007.

TABLE 5.2

Nothing by Mouth Fasting Guidelines[a]

Ingested Material Allowed	Minimal Fasting Period Recommended
Food and fluids as desired	Up to 8 hours
Light meal (e.g., toast and clear liquids, infant formula, and nonhuman milk)	Up to 6 hours
Breast milk	Up to 4 hours
Clear liquids only, NO solid food or foods with fat content[b]	Up to 2 hours
No solids or liquids	During the 2 hours until surgical time

[a]These guidelines are recommended for healthy patients undergoing elective procedures. They are not intended for women in labor. They do not guarantee complete gastric emptying. The fasting periods noted above apply to patients of all ages.
[b]Clear liquids include water, fruit juices without pulp, black coffee, clear tea, and carbonated beverages. Patients should also be instructed not to chew gum or eat any candies or mints. The type of fluid is more important than the amount and should never include alcohol.
Modified from The American Society of Anesthesiologists (ASA): Practice guidelines for preoperative fasting and the use of pharmacologic agents to reduce the risk of pulmonary aspiration: application to healthy patients undergoing elective procedures, an updated report by the American Association of Anesthesiologists Task Force on Preoperative Fasting and the Use of Pharmacologic Agents to Reduce the Risk of Pulmonary Aspiration, *Anesthesiology* 126(3):376-393, 2017.

to relieve apprehension and provide amnesia. An analgesic or narcotic may be ordered if preoperative discomfort is anticipated during invasive procedures or during the administration of a regional anesthetic. An anticholinergic, such as atropine or glycopyrrolate, may be used to prevent bradycardia in pediatric patients, to control secretions in patients undergoing oropharyngeal procedures, or to control cardiac reflex that may cause bradycardia (e.g., during ophthalmic procedures) (Miller, 2015).

To decrease the incidence of aspiration for at-risk patients, metoclopramide (Reglan) may be given to empty the stomach and to reduce PONV. In addition, an antacid or an H_2-receptor–blocking medication, such as cimetidine (Tagamet), ranitidine (Zantac), or famotidine (Pepcid), may be given to decrease gastric acid production or the acidity of the gastric contents, or both. Using medications such as these is part of safe airway management.

Before administering premedication, the anesthesia provider answers any last-minute questions from the patient concerning surgery and anesthesia, and completes the preoperative verification process, or "anesthesia time-out," to ensure that all relevant documents (e.g., history and physical examination, consents) and imaging studies (properly labeled and displayed) are available before the start of the procedure. The anesthesia provider reviews these documents, which must be consistent with the patient's stated expectations (when the patient is awake and aware, the patient should actively participate in the verification process). During the surgical time-out, the entire surgical team must agree that this is the correct patient and the correct procedure on the correct side and site. Any additional special equipment, supplies, or implants also are confirmed as correct and available. The surgical site must be marked before administering premedication.

Administration of premedication(s) may be intramuscular (IM), intravenous (IV), intranasal, or oral (PO) with 15 to 30 mL of water.

Patients usually prefer oral premedication, and the small amount of water is readily absorbed directly across the gastric mucosa. Except for the small amount of water needed to swallow any medications, adult patients traditionally must maintain a nothing-by-mouth (NPO) status for a minimum of 4 to 6 hours before elective surgery. More recent data suggest, however, that clear liquids are acceptable up to 2 hours before surgery (ASA, 2017) (Table 5.2). Alternatively, IV premedication is administered 30 to 90 minutes before surgery in preoperative holding or after the patient arrives in the surgical suite.

Although premedication use is common, studies have shown that visits before surgery by the anesthesia provider and the perioperative nurse are similarly important to relieve patient anxiety and concern. Major patient concerns include fear of the unknown, relinquishing control of one's life to someone else, being awake during surgery, not awakening from anesthesia, and concerns related to the surgery itself (e.g., diagnosis, prognosis). Premedication may be unnecessary for older patients because their anxiety levels are lower, their responses to medications are unpredictable, and IV sedation can be given in the OR if required.

Types of Anesthesia Care

Anesthesia care standards apply when patients receive, in any setting, moderate or deep sedation or general, spinal, or other major regional anesthesia. Descriptions of frequently used classifications of anesthesia care are detailed in the following sections.

General Anesthesia

General anesthesia is a reversible, unconscious state characterized by amnesia (sleep, hypnosis, or basal narcosis), analgesia (freedom from pain), depression of reflexes, muscle relaxation, and homeostasis or specific manipulation of physiologic systems and functions. Most patients think of general anesthesia when they are scheduled to have a surgical procedure; that is, they expect to be "put to sleep." As such, they experience a medication-induced loss of consciousness during which they are not arousable. Their ability to maintain ventilatory function is often impaired, requiring assistance maintaining a patent airway. Positive-pressure ventilation may be required, given the possibility of decreased spontaneous ventilation or medication-induced depression of neuromuscular function.

Regional Anesthesia

Regional anesthesia is defined broadly as a reversible loss of sensation in a specific area or region of the body when a local anesthetic is injected to block or anesthetize nerve fibers in and around the operative site. Common regional anesthesia includes spinal (also called "subarachnoid block" or SAB), epidural, caudal, and major peripheral nerve blocks (PNBs). The use of ultrasound guidance significantly reduces the risk of local anesthetic systemic toxicity (LAST) as well as the incidence and intensity of hemidiaphragmatic paresis, but has no significant effect on the incidence of postoperative neurologic symptoms (Neal et al., 2016).

Monitored Anesthesia Care

MAC is infiltration of the surgical site with a local anesthetic and is performed by the surgeon (*local standby* and *anesthesia standby* are older, less accurate terms used interchangeably with MAC) wherein the anesthesia provider supplements the local anesthesia with IV medications that provide sedation and systemic analgesia, monitors the patient's vital functions, and may use additional medication to optimize the patient's physiologic status. MAC is often used for healthy patients undergoing relatively minor surgical procedures. It also may be used for some procedures for critically ill patients who will tolerate a general anesthetic poorly.

Moderate Sedation/Analgesia

Moderate sedation/analgesia (conscious sedation) is administered for specific short-term surgical, diagnostic, and therapeutic procedures performed within a hospital or ambulatory center. The Association of periOperative Registered Nurses (AORN) defines moderate sedation/analgesia as "a level of sedation in which the patient maintains adequate spontaneous ventilation, protective reflexes, and the ability to communicate verbally but experiences a mitigated perception of pain" (Putnam, 2015). Patients maintain a patent airway and require no airway interventions; spontaneous ventilation remains adequate. Cardiovascular function is usually maintained.

The demand for appropriate providers to administer and monitor the patient receiving conscious sedation/analgesia has grown and now exceeds the supply of anesthesia providers. This demand has resulted in increased use of registered nurses with additional training in administering moderate sedation/analgesia medications and monitoring these patients. Various medications and techniques are used to achieve conscious sedation/analgesia, each with advantages and disadvantages. Competency-based education programs and assessment should be established for nurse-monitored sedation. AORN publishes recommendations for managing patients undergoing moderate sedation/analgesia that should be used by healthcare facilities to develop such programs (Fencl, 2016).

Local Anesthesia

Local anesthesia refers to the administration of an anesthetic agent to one part of the body by local infiltration or topical application, usually administered by the surgeon. Local anesthesia is used (1) for minor procedures, (2) if the patient's cooperation is necessary for the procedure, or (3) if the patient's physical condition warrants its use. An anesthesia provider is not involved in the patient's care. During the procedure, a perioperative nurse monitors the patient's vital signs and evaluates for symptoms of a LAST reaction (Fencl, 2015). Monitoring is done according to institution policy and at a minimum should include pain level, anxiety level, and level of consciousness, as well as assessment of the patient's pulse, blood pressure, heart and respiratory rates, and pulse oximetry level. AORN (2017) recommendations for managing patients undergoing local anesthesia and documenting patient care should be used to establish policies and procedures in operative and other procedure settings.

Perioperative Monitoring

Significant advances continue in perioperative monitoring. Anesthesiology has been a pioneer in review and analysis of perioperative mishaps and implementation of improved monitoring techniques and guidelines. These monitors include pulse oximetry, which measures oxygen saturation in a pulsating vessel (SpO_2), and capnography, which measures end-tidal carbon dioxide ($ETCO_2$) level (Kossick, 2014). These monitors markedly increase the probability of a successful anesthesia outcome (Hernandez and Sherwood, 2017).

The ASA amended its Standards for Basic Anesthetic Monitoring (Patient Safety) as guidelines for patient care. Perioperative nurses should be familiar with these standards and understand their significance in patient safety. If routine or frequent deviations from such standards occur, a quality assurance and performance improvement (also known as *quality assurance* [QA]) review along with a risk management analysis sets the goals and processes for measuring, improving, and ensuring safety in patient care (Fenner, 2016).

PATIENT SAFETY

Standards for Basic Anesthetic Monitoring

These standards apply to all anesthesia care, although in emergency circumstances appropriate life support measures take precedence. The standards may be exceeded at any time based on the judgment of the responsible anesthesiologist. They are intended to encourage quality patient care, but observing them cannot guarantee any specific patient outcome. They are subject to revision from time to time, as warranted by the evolution of technology and practice. They apply to all general anesthetics, regional anesthetics, and MAC. This set of standards addresses only the issue of basic anesthetic monitoring, which is one component of anesthesia care. In certain rare or unusual circumstances, some of these monitoring methods may be clinically impractical, and their appropriate use may fail to detect untoward clinical developments. Brief interruptions of continual monitoring may be unavoidable. These standards are not intended to apply to the care of the obstetric patient in labor or in the practice of pain management.

Standard I
Qualified anesthesia personnel shall be present in the room throughout administration of all general anesthetics, regional anesthetics, and MAC.

Continued

PATIENT SAFETY

Standards for Basic Anesthetic Monitoring—cont'd

Objective

Given the rapidity of possible changes in patient status during anesthesia, qualified anesthesia personnel shall be continuously present to monitor the patient and to provide anesthesia care. In the event there is a direct known hazard (e.g., radiation to anesthesia personnel that might require intermittent remote observation of the patient), some provision for patient monitoring is made. In the event that an emergency requires the temporary absence of the person primarily responsible for the anesthetic, the best judgment of the anesthesiologist is exercised in comparing the emergency with the anesthetized patient's condition and in the selection of the person left responsible for the anesthetic during a temporary absence.

Standard II

During administration of all anesthetics, patient oxygenation, ventilation, circulation, and temperature shall be evaluated continually.

Oxygenation

Objective

To ensure adequate oxygen concentration in the inspired gas and the blood during all anesthetics.

Methods

1. *Inspired gas:* During every administration of general anesthesia using an anesthesia machine, the concentration of oxygen in the patient breathing system shall be measured by an oxygen analyzer with a low-oxygen concentration limit alarm in use.*[a]
2. *Blood oxygenation:* During all anesthetics, a quantitative method of assessing oxygenation such as pulse oximetry shall be used.* When the pulse oximeter is used, the variable pitch pulse tone and the low-threshold alarm shall be audible to the anesthesiologist or anesthesia care team personnel.* Adequate illumination and exposure of the patient are necessary to assess color.*

Ventilation

Objective

To ensure adequate ventilation of the patient during all anesthetics.

Methods

1. Every patient receiving general anesthesia shall have adequacy of ventilation continually evaluated. Qualitative clinical signs such as chest excursion, observation of the reservoir breathing bag, and auscultation of breath sounds are useful. Continual monitoring for the presence of expired carbon dioxide shall occur unless invalidated by the nature of the patient, procedure, or equipment. Quantitative monitoring of the volume of expired gas is strongly encouraged.*
2. When an ETT or LMA is inserted, its correct positioning must be verified by clinical assessment and by identification of carbon dioxide in the expired gas. Continual end-tidal carbon dioxide analysis ($ETCO_2$), in use from the time of ETT/LMA placement, until extubation/removal or initiating transfer to a postoperative care location, shall be performed using a quantitative method such as capnography, capnometry, or mass spectroscopy.* When capnography or capnometry is used, the $ETCO_2$ alarm shall be audible to the anesthesiologist or anesthesia provider.*

3. When a mechanical ventilator controls ventilation, there shall be in continuous use a device capable of detecting disconnection of components of the breathing system. The device must sound an audible signal when it exceeds the alarm threshold.
4. During regional anesthesia (with no sedation) or local anesthesia (with no sedation), the adequacy of ventilation shall be evaluated by continual observation of qualitative clinical signs. During moderate or deep sedation, the adequacy of ventilation shall be evaluated by continual observation of qualitative clinical signs and monitoring for the presence of exhaled carbon dioxide unless precluded or invalidated by the nature of the patient, procedure, or equipment.

Circulation

Objective

To ensure the adequacy of the patient's circulatory function during all anesthetics.

Methods

1. Every patient receiving anesthesia shall have an ECG continuously displayed from beginning of anesthesia to preparing to leave the anesthetizing location.*
2. Every patient receiving anesthesia shall have arterial blood pressure and heart rate determined and evaluated at least every 5 minutes.*
3. Every patient receiving general anesthesia shall have, in addition to that previously mentioned, circulatory function continually evaluated by at least one of the following: palpation of a pulse, auscultation of heart sounds, monitoring of a tracing of intraarterial pressure, ultrasound peripheral pulse monitoring, or pulse plethysmography or oximetry.

Body Temperature

Objective

To aid in the maintenance of appropriate body temperature during all anesthetics.

Methods

Every patient receiving anesthesia shall have temperature monitored when clinically significant changes in body temperature are intended, anticipated, or suspected.

Note that "continual" is defined as "repeated regularly and frequently in steady rapid succession," whereas "continuous" means "prolonged without any interruption at any time."

---

[a]Under extenuating circumstances, the responsible anesthesiologist may waive requirements marked with an asterisk (*); it is recommended that when this is done, it should be so stated (including the reasons) in a note in the patient's medical record.

ECG, Electrocardiogram; *ETCO2,* end-tidal carbon dioxide analysis, *ETT,* endotracheal tube; *LMA,* laryngeal mask airway; *MAC,* monitored anesthesia care.

Modified from The American Society of Anesthesiologists (ASA), Park Ridge, IL: Approved by the ASA House of Delegates on October 21, 1986, last amended on October 20, 2010, and last affirmed on October 28, 2015.

Monitors and basic anesthetic monitoring include the following:

- Inspired oxygen analyzer (FIO_2), which is calibrated to room air on a daily basis
- Low-pressure disconnect alarm, which senses pressure in the expiratory limb of the patient circuit
- Inspiratory airway pressure
- Respirometer (these first four devices are an integral part of most anesthesia machines)
- Electrocardioscope
- Blood pressure (usually measured with a noninvasive automated unit)
- Heart rate
- Precordial or esophageal stethoscope
- Temperature
- Peripheral nerve stimulator if muscle relaxants are used
- SpO_2
- $ETCO_2$

Newer models of anesthesia machines have basic monitors integrated into a computerized system. These generally include FIO_2; inspired and expired CO_2; inspired and expired volatile agents; airway pressure and disconnect alarms; tidal volume, respiratory rate, and minute ventilation; noninvasive blood pressure (systolic, diastolic, and mean); SpO_2 and pulse rate; temperature; and an event marker. A sophisticated, prioritized system displays caution or alarm conditions in one location, making it unnecessary to scan numerous individual monitors with a variety of displays when an alarm sounds. Perioperative nurses ensure that all appropriate monitor alarm systems are on and active, and that issues of "alarm fatigue" have not induced the anesthesia provider to shut off these alarms (Ruskin and Hueske-Kraus, 2015).

Based on the cardiovascular and pulmonary status of the patient, scheduled surgical procedure, and chance of significant physiologic changes, additional invasive monitors may prove necessary. These include direct arterial and venous pressure measurements, a pulmonary arterial catheter (PAC), and continuous mixed venous O_2 saturation (SvO_2) measured with a special PAC. One type of PAC provides a continuous measurement of cardiac output, using pulsed thermodilution to provide intermittent heat along a distal segment of the catheter. Small changes in the temperature of the blood are proportional to blood flow (cardiac output). These changes are sensed by a thermistor on the tip of the catheter (Contrera et al., 2014).

For certain conditions, equipment such as transcutaneous O_2 and CO_2 monitors, evoked potentials, electroencephalography (EEG), cerebral or neurologic function monitors, and transesophageal echocardiography (TEE), may be required. TEE is the most sensitive method of detection, but may also be the most expensive (Ranalli and Taylor, 2014). An indwelling urinary catheter is frequently inserted to provide a useful indication of renal function and hemodynamic status.

For procedures posing a risk of venous air embolism, a Doppler probe may be used. A central venous catheter is inserted, and the probe is placed over the right side of the heart, along the right sternal border between the third and sixth intercostal spaces. Positioning is confirmed if there is a change in Doppler signal after a 10-mL bolus of saline is rapidly injected through the catheter. The signal is monitored for the sound of a "mill-wheel" murmur.

Somatosensory evoked potential (SEP) monitoring is widely used during neurosurgery procedures (Fan et al., 2016) to assess the integrity of the spinal cord during surgery in which the spinal cord is manipulated. Upper and lower extremities may be monitored. Electrodes are usually placed preoperatively, but occasionally may be placed in the OR, before administration of anesthesia. Ischemia of ascending somatosensory pathways produces a drop in amplitude or loss of waveforms, thus warning the surgeon to take corrective action. Ischemic changes are usually widespread. Rarely, however, is motor function lost when somatosensory pathways have not been affected.

Despite some controversy, most anesthesia providers believe that the monitoring used depends on the physiologic status and stability of the patient, the surgical procedure planned and its potential for sudden changes in cardiopulmonary functions, the anticipated blood loss and major fluid shifts, and the anticipated monitoring needs for postoperative management. Although not yet a standard of care, many facilities use the BIS monitor to provide a measure of the sedative and hypnotic effects of anesthetic medications on the central nervous system (CNS). Monitoring of some parameters may be negated by the anesthetic technique selected (Clark and Curdt, 2014).

Pulse Oximetry

Pulse oximetry works by analyzing the pulsatile arterial component (AC) of blood flow, ensuring that arterial saturation (SpO_2) rather than venous saturation is being measured. Two wavelengths of light are used, usually 660 nm (red) and 940 nm (infrared), because oxygenated and deoxygenated blood absorbs light quite differently at these wavelengths. At 660 nm, HbO_2 (oxygenated hemoglobin) absorbs less light than HbR (reduced hemoglobin, or deoxyhemoglobin) does, whereas the opposite is observed with infrared light. Two diodes emitting light of each wavelength are placed on one side of the probe, and a photo diode that senses the transmitted light is placed on the opposite side. The amount of light absorbed at each wavelength by the pulsatile AC of blood flow differentiates itself from baseline absorbance of the nonpulsatile component and surrounding tissue (Miller, 2015). Given that absorption by other tissue components is essentially constant, the major variable is saturation of hemoglobin with O_2. An internal microprocessor analyzes variations in absorption of light emitted from both diodes and provides a readout of the percent saturation of hemoglobin with O_2. Pulse rate also is given. The pulse oximeter converts the detected light to a plethysmographic signal that measures the drop in light intensity with each beat (Bozimowski, 2014).

The O_2 dissociation curve indicates the percentage of totally saturated hemoglobin with O_2. The following values are approximations (the O_2 saturation [SpO_2] values are percentages and the PaO_2 levels are in torr): 98% to 100% ($\geq$95 torr), 90% (60 torr), 75% (39 torr), 50% (26 torr), and 25% (16 torr). Most pulse oximeters are accurate to within $\pm$2% greater than 70% and $\pm$3% from 50% to 70% but correlate poorly at less than 50%. When breathing room air, the SpO_2 for a young, healthy individual should be 98% to 100%; the SpO_2 percentage for an elderly patient may be in the low 90s, whereas the percentage for a heavy smoker or a patient with severe lung disease may be in the 80s. It is wise to establish a baseline SpO_2 value of a patient before any O_2, medications, or stimulation is introduced. Maintenance of SpO_2 levels greater than 90% corresponds to a PaO_2 value of 60 torr or greater (Miller, 2015).

Pulse oximeter readings (often referred to as "pulse ox") can be adversely affected by any event that significantly reduces vascular pulsations, such as hypoperfusion, hypotension, hypovolemia, vasoconstriction, or hypothermia. Electrosurgery, motion, or ambient light may also cause artifacts that falsely decrease the readout. Carboxyhemoglobin (carbon monoxide bound to hemoglobin) falsely elevates indicated SpO_2 saturation, whereas methemoglobin (hemoglobin that has an oxidized iron molecule and cannot reversibly combine with O_2) falsely lowers SpO_2 measurements. IV dyes may affect pulse oximetry. Methylene blue may cause a drop to 65% for 1 to 2 minutes; indigo carmine, a very slight decrease; and indocyanine green, a slightly greater decrease. Nail polish also can decrease SpO_2 values. Blue, black, or green polish significantly decreases the SpO_2 value, whereas red polish has only a slight effect. Opaque, acrylic nail coverings may block the light beam. Studies suggest the more advanced monitors have eliminated these effects (Bozimowski, 2014). If nail polish or coverings seem to cause problems, turn the sensor sideways so that the fingernail is parallel to the light path.

The sensor usually is placed on a finger or a toe. Some manufacturers have sensors for the earlobe and the bridge of the nose, as well as smaller ones for soles and palms of infants and children. Care must be taken to prevent localized neurovascular or ischemic damage. For example, a hard-cased sensor placed on a finger may cause ischemia when the arms are tightly secured at the patient's side during a long procedure.

If trouble with the pulse oximeter arises with use of a local anesthetic, the perioperative nurse should evaluate the patient's ventilatory status, verify proper placement of the sensor, and rule out the factors just listed that may adversely affect unit operation. Pulsatile blood flow in the extremity may be inadequate because of hypovolemia, decreased cardiac output, malpositioning, constriction by the blood pressure cuff, or hypothermia. As a final step the nurse can place the sensor on his or her own finger to verify satisfactory function of the pulse oximetry unit, cable, and sensor.

Capnography

A capnometer measures CO_2 concentration; it produces a capnograph that displays the CO_2 waveform. The capnograph provides a continuous display of the CO_2 concentration of gases from the airway. CO_2 concentration at the end of normal exhalation ($ETCO_2$, $P_{ET}CO_2$) is a reflection of gas from the distal alveoli; therefore it represents an estimate of alveolar concentration (P_ACO_2). When ventilation and perfusion are well matched, the P_ACO_2 closely approximates the $PaCO_2$, and $P_ACO_2 \cong PaCO_2 \cong P_{ET}CO_2$ (where $PaCO_2$ is partial pressure arterial, P_ACO_2 is alveolar partial pressure, and $P_{ET}CO_2$ is end-tidal partial pressure). The normal gradient between $PaCO_2$ and $P_{ET}CO_2$ is more than 6 mm Hg. The gradient between $PaCO_2$ and $P_{ET}CO_2$ increases when pulmonary perfusion is reduced or ventilation is maldistributed (Hagberg, 2013). Under general anesthesia the gas is sampled at the point where the ETT connects to the patient breathing circuit. During other types of anesthesia, in which oxygen is administered via a nasal cannula, a small-bore tube is connected to the cannula, which is then attached to the anesthesia machine so that $ETCO_2$ levels can be measured. CO_2 analyzers use various principles to measure CO_2 in the inspired and exhaled gases on a breath-to-breath basis and display the CO_2 waveform by mass spectrometry, infrared absorption spectrometry, or Raman scattering. Although capnography typically distinguishes tracheal from esophageal intubation, false-negative results (i.e., ETT in trachea, absent waveform) and false-positive results (i.e., ETT in esophagus or pharynx, present waveform) have been reported (Hagberg, 2013).

Compact units that provide a continuous indication of the $ETCO_2$ level are the most widely used. These units measure the amount of infrared light absorbed by CO_2 in the sample of gas. Two types of monitors are in use. In the *mainstream* unit all respired gas passes through the detector, whereas in the *sidestream* unit a portion of the gas is aspirated at a constant rate (50–250 mL/min) through small-bore tubing into the unit. Each design has advantages. Most units display a waveform of expiratory CO_2 partial pressure relative to

time after a short sampling and processing delay. The waveform is important to interpret output data correctly. Digital readouts usually give $ETCO_2$ and respiratory rate. Daily user calibration is rarely required with newer units. The units confirm proper endotracheal intubation and are useful to detect anesthesia circuit disconnection, alveolar ventilation, early return of respiratory function after muscle relaxants are used, and acute alterations in metabolic functions, such as malignant hyperthermia (MH) or thyrotoxicosis (see Chapter 16) (Bozimowski, 2014).

Anesthesia Machines and Anesthetic Gases

Anesthesia machines look complicated, but the basic functions are similar and simple to understand. Perioperative nurses should be familiar with the basic function of anesthesia machines (Fig. 5.1) because they may need to administer O_2 during procedures with local anesthesia or conscious sedation/analgesia.

Facility pipelines usually supply oxygen, nitrous oxide (N_2O), and air to the anesthesia machine at pressures of 50 to 55 pounds per square inch (psi). Gas hoses connected to the machine are color coded as green (O_2), blue (N_2O), and yellow (medical air). Connectors are specific for each gas so that they cannot be inadvertently cross-connected. If a central gas supply is not available or the hospital piping system fails, machines are equipped with E-size cylinders of O_2 and N_2O. One or two cylinders of each gas are connected to yokes on the machine. These yokes are pin-indexed so that only the correct gas can be connected in that position. In the pin-indexing safety system, two steel pins are in a unique location on the yoke assembly. The mating gas cylinder (e.g., the O_2 tank) has two matching holes in the same locations so that cylinders must be mounted correctly and cannot be mounted in the wrong place (Dosch, 2014).

O_2 stores as a compressed gas in cylinders. A full E-size cylinder contains about 660 L of O_2 at approximately 2000 psi. As the O_2 is used, the pressure decreases in direct proportion to the remaining volume. Because the E-size cylinder is used to provide O_2 while patients are being transported, one must know how much O_2 remains in a partially used tank; 1000 psi indicates 330 L remaining, and 500 psi indicates 165 L remaining or sufficient O_2 at 5 L/min flow for about 30 minutes. When pressure decreases to about 250 psi, the cylinder should not be used because it no longer has an adequate reserve (Dosch, 2014).

N_2O stores as a liquid in cylinders, and pressure above the liquid is 745 psi. A full E-size cylinder contains about 1600 L of N_2O. As the N_2O is used, the pressure above the liquid remains constant. Only when the liquid has been completely vaporized does pressure begin to decrease. The N_2O cylinder can be nearly empty but still show the same pressure. In contrast to O_2, the amount remaining in the N_2O tank cannot be readily determined (Dosch, 2014).

Gases in the cylinders flow through regulators that reduce pressure to about 45 psi as gas enters the machine. Hoses from hospital gas sources are connected to the machine at the outlet of these regulators. A safety interlock device either shuts off the N_2O flow if O_2 pressure is not present or proportionally lowers the O_2 and N_2O flow rates to maintain 30% O_2. The gases flow through individual flowmeters (or rotameters) on the front of the machine so that the anesthesia provider can select gas flows and the ratio of O_2 to N_2O or air. From the top of the flowmeters, the gases are mixed and then flow through a vaporizer in which the inhalational anesthetic of choice is vaporized and added to the gas mixture. The total gas flow is delivered from the machine to the patient. With a flow-through vaporizer, all the fresh gas moving from the anesthesia machine to the patient flows through the vaporizer. The control dials usually are located on top

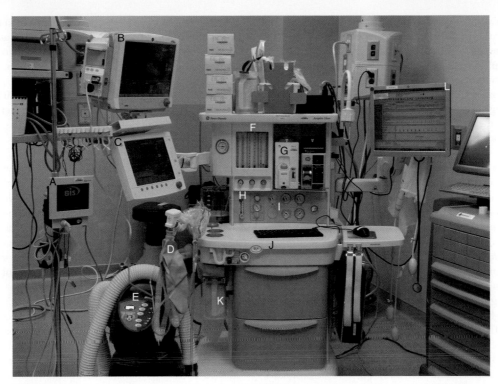

FIG. 5.1 Modern anesthesia machine. *(A)* Bispectral index system monitor. *(B)* Patient vital signs display monitor. *(C)* Ventilator display monitor. *(D)* Patient breathing circuit. *(E)* Bair Hugger patient warmer. *(F)* Gas flowmeters. *(G)* Anesthetic vaporizers. *(H)* Supplemental oxygen supply. *(I)* Oxygen, air, and nitrous oxide gauges. *(J)* Oxygen flush valve. *(K)* Carbon dioxide absorber. *(L)* Electronic recordkeeping screen.

of these vaporizers and are calibrated in percentages. The filling ports on the vaporizers are usually key-indexed so that personnel can use only the appropriate volatile agent. Newer vaporizers are reasonably accurate at all flow rates and temperatures (Dosch, 2014).

Desflurane (Suprane) is a unique inhalational anesthetic because it boils at 22.8°C, near room temperature, and its vapor pressure (669 mm Hg) approximates atmospheric pressure (760 mm Hg). The vaporizer for desflurane is pressurized and contains an electric heater. Desflurane also has several other unique characteristics: (1) its solubility in blood (blood-gas partition coefficient) is lower (0.42) than those of N_2O (0.47), sevoflurane (0.63–0.69), isoflurane (1.41), and halothane (2.30), which means that it has a faster "wash-in" (induction) and "wash-out" (emergence) than the other agents; (2) metabolism is far less (0.02%) than that of isoflurane (0.2%), sevoflurane (5%), and halothane (15%–20%); (3) emergence and recovery from general anesthesia and discharge from the postanesthesia care unit (PACU) are significantly faster than when other agents are used; (4) the cardiovascular effects are similar to those of isoflurane; and (5) muscle relaxation is similar to that which occurs with other inhalational agents. Because desflurane is pungent, it is not used as an induction agent.

Sevoflurane (Ultane) is the most recent volatile agent available in the United States. Its pleasant odor and low solubility in blood make it a popular volatile agent for rapid and pleasant inhalational induction in both adult and pediatric patients.

Another important feature of the anesthesia machine is the O_2 flush valve. Pushing the O_2 flush valve allows 100% O_2 from the 50 psi line to flow directly to the *fresh gas outlet* on the machine and to the patient. This O_2 flow completely bypasses flowmeters and vaporizers. *Caution must be exercised, however, when using the O_2 flush valve because the pressure is 35 to 50 psi, and the flow rate is 35 to 75 L/min.*

In most hospitals and ASCs in the United States, a *semiclosed-circle system* is used to deliver fresh gas flow (including anesthetic gases) to patients. The circle system is composed of a container filled with a CO_2-absorbing material (e.g., soda lime or calcium hydroxide lime), two one-way (unidirectional) valves, an adjustable pressure-limiting (APL) valve, a reservoir bag, an inlet connection for fresh gas flow, and two connections to the patient through corrugated breathing (or anesthesia circuit) tubing. As the patient inhales, gases are drawn through the CO_2 absorber and from the fresh gas supply through the inspiratory limb of the corrugated tubing. As the patient exhales, the one-way valve on the inspiratory limb prevents backflow, and the exhaled gases flow into the expiratory limb and through the expiratory one-way valve. The expiratory limb and valve are easily identified by the condensation of water vapor along this portion of the circuit. The reservoir bag absorbs the peak flow of expired gases and allows the anesthesia provider to force gas through the CO_2 absorber, along the inspiratory limb of the circuit, and to ventilate the patient. The expired gases flow through the CO_2 absorber, in which CO_2 is removed. Substances used in the CO_2 absorbent include an indicator that changes color as exhaustion of the soda lime or calcium hydroxide lime occurs. The soda lime may turn from white to blue, indicating a required change of the absorbent material to prevent a buildup of CO_2 in the patient. Any excess gas vents through the APL valve into the gas-scavenging system. The APL valve usually mounts just ahead of the CO_2 absorber (Dosch, 2014).

The FIO_2 sensor usually is mounted in the inspiratory limb just after the one-way valve. It measures the FIO_2 and can be set to alarm if a low concentration is detected. A low-pressure sensor usually is mounted in the expiratory limb near the one-way valve to detect a ventilator malfunction or a circuit disconnection.

Volumeters are mounted in the inspired and expired limbs where the patient breathing circuit is connected. When using the ventilator, electronic circuitry measures inspiratory and expiratory volumes to ensure that they correspond with the tidal volume and respiratory rate selected. With a cuffed ETT, the ventilator compensates for changes in fresh gas flow or small leaks in the breathing circuit and alarms if a disconnection or inadequate flow occurs (Dosch, 2014).

The advantage of the circle system is that it enables the use of much lower flows of O_2, N_2O, and anesthetic gases; this conserves the patient's body heat and respiratory moisture, and reduces the cost of expensive, volatile agents.

With a *closed-circle system,* all CO_2 is absorbed. No gas vents from the system, and only enough O_2 is added to meet the basal requirements of the patient (approximately 3.5 mL/kg/min). A *semiopen circuit* (e.g., Ayres T-piece, Magill, Bain T-piece circuits) uses a relatively high flow of fresh gas, and most exhaled gas vents from the circuit. The fresh gas flow rate per minute varies from about two-thirds of the patient's minute volume with the Magill circuit to at least 100 mL/kg with the Bain T-piece circuit. The semiopen circuit system is commonly used for newborns, infants, and small children (Dosch, 2014). With all these circuits, the final connection to the patient is by mask, ETT, or LMA.

General Anesthesia

Mechanism of Action

Our understanding of the nature of the anesthetic state continues to evolve. Whereas the anesthesia provider can induce a coma-like state of general anesthesia by inhaled anesthetics administered at appropriate concentrations, use of high concentrations is fraught with short-term and possibly long-term side effects. It is now clear that anesthesia consists of separable and at least partially independent components or substrates, each of which involves distinct, but possibly overlapping, mechanisms at different sites in the CNS and with variations in relative potencies between specific agents. Immobilization, the core measure of the anesthetic state, is mediated largely at the level of the spinal cord by inhaled anesthetics but not by barbiturates. The spinal cord, however, is unlikely to be the major site of other anesthetic actions, which produce phenomena such as amnesia, sedation, and unconsciousness; these are associated with cerebral cortical function. A functional separation between amnesia and sedation has been demonstrated for IV anesthetics and is likely for inhaled anesthetics as well. These and similar findings have led to the concept that general anesthesia consists of multiple independent components that are experimentally and clinically identifiable. Theoretically, each component can be preferentially induced in a concentration and agent-specific manner using individual cellular/molecular pathways in various regions of the CNS. Thus general anesthetics produce separate identifiable anesthetic substrates via agent-specific actions at discrete anatomic sites in the CNS by different molecular targets. An important consequence of this complexity is that the anesthetic state, based exclusively on the motor response, might not proportionately reflect other components of anesthesia. Although this heterogeneity of anesthetic action complicates a mechanistic understanding, it does open the possibility of developing substrate-specific medications.

Numerous proposed theories explain the action of general anesthetics. Investigations have involved inhalation anesthetics (*volatile anesthetic, potent agent,* and *inhaled* or *inhalational anesthetic* are virtually synonymous with *inhalation anesthetic* and used interchangeably). Although no single theory explains all phenomena, a few theories explain many of the actions (Miller, 2015). The following two theories are some of those more widely suggested.

Protein Receptor Theory

This theory proposes that hydrophobic areas of specific proteins in the CNS act as receptor sites. Today, there is widespread (but not universal) acceptance of the notion that critical signaling proteins (e.g., ion channels or ligand-gated receptors) are the relevant molecular targets of anesthetic action, even though the submolecular mechanisms of their modulation by anesthetics are debated. The exact identity of proteins contributing to specific anesthetic endpoints continues to be sought, with research addressing not only the "where" (target) but also the "how" (process) of anesthetic mechanisms (Miller, 2015).

Endogenous Endorphins

Endogenous endorphins, or opiate-like substances, suppress various pain pathways. Several classes of endorphins have been identified. The action of β-endorphins is antagonized by naloxone or nalmefene, which are specific narcotic antagonists, but the relative potency of inhaled anesthetics remains unaltered. Although this mechanism explains some degree of analgesia, it does not correlate well with the level of anesthesia achieved by inhaled anesthetics.

IV anesthetics also may function using some of the same mechanisms proposed for inhaled anesthetics. Factors involved in the pharmacokinetics of IV anesthetics include the volume of distribution, biotransformation, and clearance of the medication by metabolism, excretion, or elimination of the medication and its metabolites (Miller, 2015).

No single theory posited to explain the mechanism of anesthetic action explains all effects observed with anesthetic agents. The range of anesthetic activity varies with different anesthetics; the effects on the CNS and skeletal muscles are similar but not identical, structural and spatial differences exist among agents, changes at the membrane and cellular levels occur, and optical isomers produce different responses. Although similar in many respects, anesthetic agents are individually unique and probably work through numerous mechanisms and at multiple sites to produce their multiple effects.

Levels of General Anesthesia

Arthur Ernest Guedel was an American anesthesiologist noted for his work on the uptake and distribution of inhaled anesthetics, and various stages of anesthesia. Although Guedel's system (Stages 1–4) gave us an appreciation for the interrelationships of numerous signs during anesthesia, the variety of medications and anesthetic techniques used today do not provide uniform responses suitable to estimate the exact depth of anesthesia. Premedication such as narcotics and anticholinergic medications alter pupillary responses. Evaluation of respiratory responses and muscle tone is not valid when controlled ventilation and muscle relaxants are used. General anesthesia usually is induced with IV injection of a rapid-acting medication, such as propofol (Diprivan), which takes the patient rapidly to stage 3 and eliminates the untoward responses often seen during stage 2.

For optimal anesthesia and good surgical conditions, several different but interrelated factors occur. These include hypnosis (sleep); analgesia (freedom from pain); amnesia (lack of recall or awareness); appropriate surgical conditions, including muscle relaxation and positioning of the patient; and continued homeostasis of the patient's vital functions. Different medications and anesthetic agents possess various properties that facilitate these factors. Combinations of medications are used to obtain the desired effects. Hypotensive or hypertensive medications and cardioactive agents also may be used to achieve optimal depth of anesthesia while affecting physiologic homeostasis as little as possible. The Surgical Pharmacology box briefly describes medications commonly used in anesthesia.

Phases of General Anesthesia

General anesthesia consists of three phases: *induction, maintenance,* and *emergence. Induction* begins with administration of anesthetic agents and continues until the patient is ready for positioning or surgical prepping (surgical prep), surgical manipulation, or incision. Surgical prep often starts after administration of induction medications. The endpoint of induction varies with the surgical procedure.

SURGICAL PHARMACOLOGY

Commonly Used Anesthetic Gases and Drugs

	Common Usage	Advantages	Disadvantages	Comments
Inhalation Gases				
Air	Maintenance with O_2; laser surgery near airway	Less support of combustion than N_2O	No anesthetic qualities	Can use as supplemental assist for FIO_2 control for fire prevention (Miller, 2015)
Oxygen (O_2)	Essential for life	Can slightly ↑ O_2 available to tissues in low cardiac output states	Can cause retinopathy in premature infants	Concentrations should be at minimum to avoid hypoxia with lasers in surgery of head, neck, and pulmonary areas (Apfelbaum et al., 2013)
Nitrous oxide (N_2O)	Maintenance; frequently for induction	Rapid induction and recovery; additive effects to other anesthetics, more analgesia than other inhalation agents	No relaxation; can depress myocardium; expands within closed spaces	Hypoxia if overdose given; ↑ uptake of other volatile agents, only nonhalogenated agent used today (Brenner, 2013)
Desflurane (Suprane)	Maintenance in surgical procedures	Rapid emergence; good relaxation; lowest 0.02% biotransformation to metabolites	May cause transient ↑ HR and ↓ BP, airway irritation; requires heated vaporizer	Rapid recovery phase; no need for high gas flows (Miller, 2015)
Isoflurane (Forane)	Maintenance	Good relaxation; maintains cardiac output; 0.2% metabolized; inexpensive	Reduced SVR, ↑ respiratory depression; slightly irritating odor	Pungent order; airway irritant; trigger for malignant hyperthermia (Kossick, 2014)
Sevoflurane (Ultane)	Induction and maintenance	Rapid induction and emergence; good relaxation; ~5% metabolized	Caution using sevoflurane with fresh gas flows below 1 L/min for procedures lasting longer that 1 h; is nephrotoxic in rats; effect in humans unknown (Sevoflurane, 2016)	Rapid uptake and elimination; nonpungent; excellent for inhalation induction (Kossick, 2014)
Opioid Analgesics				
Morphine sulfate	Perioperative pain; premedication	Inexpensive; duration of action 4–5 h; euphoria; good cardiovascular stability	Nausea and vomiting; histamine release; postural ↓ BP (↓ SVR); caution with renal failure patients	Used intrathecally and epidurally for postoperative pain; elimination half-life 3 h (Nagelhout, 2014)
Alfentanil (Alfenta)	Surgical analgesia in ambulatory patients	Duration of action 0.5 h; used as bolus or infusion	Possible truncal rigidity (Brenner, 2013)	Potency: 750 mcg = 10 mg morphine sulfate; elimination half-life 1.6 h (Nagelhout, 2014)
Fentanyl (Sublimaze)	Surgical analgesia; epidural infusion for postoperative analgesia; add to SAB	Good cardiovascular stability; duration of action 0.5 h	Possible truncal rigidity (Brenner, 2013)	Most commonly used opioid; potency: 100 mcg = 10 mg morphine sulfate; elimination half-life 3.6 h (Nagelhout, 2014)
Remifentanil (Ultiva)	0.25–1 mcg/kg/min infusion for surgical analgesia; small boluses for brief, intense pain	Easily titratable; metabolized by blood and tissue esterases; short duration; good cardiovascular stability	Requires mixing; increased cost	Potency: 25 mcg = 10 mg morphine sulfate; 20–30× potency of alfentanil; elimination half-life 3–10 min (Nagelhout, 2014)

Continued

SURGICAL PHARMACOLOGY

Commonly Used Anesthetic Gases and Drugs—cont'd

	Common Usage	Advantages	Disadvantages	Comments
Sufentanil (Sufenta)	Surgical analgesia	Good cardiovascular stability; duration of action 0.5 h; prolonged analgesia	Prolonged respiratory depression	Potency: 15 mcg = 10 mg morphine sulfate; elimination half-life 2.7 h (Nagelhout, 2014)
Hydromorphone (Dilaudid)	Surgical and postoperative pain relief	Long duration of action 3–5 h; can switch to PO form for postoperative pain management; high ceiling effect limited only by increased adverse side effects	Caution with seizure history and biliary tract surgery; addiction potential, not approved for epidural or intrathecal use in United States	Not metabolized by cytochrome P-450 enzyme pathway, which reduces its drug–drug interaction (Gregory, 2013)
Morphine liposomal (DepoDur)	For epidural use only	Single dose provides analgesia for up to 48 h; decreased requirements for supplemental opioids	Potential for respiratory depression; avoid other epidural medications ≈ 48 h	10–15 mg epidural, one dose for lower abdominal or major lower limb surgery (Miller, 2015); 6–10 mg post C-section delivery (Carvalho and Butwick, 2014)

Depolarizing Muscle Relaxants

	Common Usage	Advantages	Disadvantages	Comments
Succinylcholine (Anectine, Quelicin)	Intubation; short procedures	Rapid onset; short duration	Requires refrigeration; may cause fasciculations, postoperative myalgias, and dysrhythmias; ↑ serum K^+ with burns, tissue trauma, paralysis, and muscle diseases; slight histamine release	Prolonged muscle relaxation with serum cholinesterase deficiency and certain antibiotics; trigger agent for MH (Nagelhout, 2014)

Nondepolarizing Muscle Relaxants: Intermediate Onset and Duration

	Common Usage	Advantages	Disadvantages	Comments
Atracurium (Tracrium)	Intubation; maintenance of relaxation	No significant cardiovascular or cumulative effects; good with renal failure	Requires refrigeration; slight histamine release	Breakdown by Hofmann elimination and ester hydrolysis (Nagelhout, 2014)
Cisatracurium (Nimbex)	Intubation; maintenance of relaxation	Similar to atracurium	No histamine release	Similar to atracurium (Nagelhout, 2014)
Rocuronium (Zemuron)	Intubation; maintenance of relaxation	Rapid onset, dose dependent; elimination via kidney and liver	Vagolytic; may increase HR	Duration similar to atracurium and vecuronium (Nagelhout, 2014)
Vecuronium (Norcuron)	Intubation; maintenance of relaxation	No significant cardiovascular or cumulative effects; no histamine release	Requires mixing	Mostly eliminated in bile, some in urine (Nagelhout, 2014)

Nondepolarizing Muscle Relaxants: Longer Onset and Duration

	Common Usage	Advantages	Disadvantages	Comments
Pancuronium (Pavulon)	Maintenance of relaxation	Increased duration	May cause ↑ HR and ↑ BP	Mostly renal elimination (Nagelhout, 2014)

Intravenous Anesthetics

	Common Usage	Advantages	Disadvantages	Comments
Etomidate (Amidate)	Induction	Minimal effects on cardiovascular system; rapid acting, smooth induction and recovery	May cause pain with injection and myoclonus with induction dose	Administer through large vein to decrease pain and thrombophlebitis on injection (Brenner, 2013)
Diazepam (Valium, Dizac)	Amnesia; hypnotic; preoperative medication	Good sedation	Prolonged duration	Residual effects for 20–90 h; alcohol, and other CNS depressants potentiate effects (Brenner, 2013)
Ketamine (Ketalar)	Induction, occasional maintenance (IV or IM)	Short acting; fast onset IV; patient maintains airway; good in small children and burn patients, hypovolemic shock; bronchospastic disease	Large doses may cause hallucinations and respiratory depression; not indicated in patients with increased ICP	Increased use with subanesthetic doses; often used in trauma procedures (Garcia et al., 2013)

SURGICAL PHARMACOLOGY

Commonly Used Anesthetic Gases and Drugs—cont'd

	Common Usage	Advantages	Disadvantages	Comments
Midazolam (Versed)	Hypnotic; anxiolytic; sedation; often used as adjunct to induction	Excellent amnestic; water soluble (no pain with IV injection); short acting	CNS depression along with respiratory depression	Often used for anterograde amnesia for stressful procedures; insertion of invasive monitors or regional anesthesia (Brenner, 2013)
Propofol (Diprivan)	Induction and maintenance; sedation with regional anesthesia or MAC	Rapid onset; awakening in 5–10 min, even after prolonged infusion	May cause pain when injected; lipid based: can support bacterial growth if aseptic technique is compromised	Short elimination half-life (34–64 min); patients >80 years of age can require only 50% of dose for equal level of sedation (Miller, 2015)
Sodium methohexital (Brevital sodium) Oxybarbiturate	Induction	Ultrashort-acting barbiturate; low cardiac toxicity; minimal anticonvulsant properties	May cause hiccups; less amnestic effects than benzodiazepines; central respiratory system depressant	Can be given rectally (Miller, 2015)

Local Anesthetics

	Common Usage	Advantages	Disadvantages	Comments
Bupivacaine (Marcaine, Sensorcaine)	Epidural, spinal, or local infiltration; good wound infiltration	Good relaxation; long acting; can constrict blood vessels to reduce bleeding at site	Overdose can cause cardiac collapse	Epidural or caudal: 2.5 mg/kg; duration: 120–240 min (Nagelhout, 2014)
Chloroprocaine (Nesacaine)	Epidural anesthesia	Ultrashort acting; good relaxation	May cause neurotoxicity if injected into CSF unless preservative free	Maximum dose 11 mg/kg not to exceed 800 mg; with epinephrine 14 mg/kg, maximum dose 1000 mg (Nagelhout, 2014)
Lidocaine (Xylocaine)	Epidural, spinal, peripheral IV anesthesia, and local infiltration anesthesia	Short acting; good relaxation; low toxicity	Overdose can cause convulsions; possible transient neurologic changes with spinal anesthesia	Also used for ventricular dysrhythmias; maximum dose 7 mg/kg and 5 mg/kg with and without epinephrine; duration 60–120 min (Nagelhout, 2014)
Ropivacaine (Naropin)	Local infiltration anesthesia, peripheral nerve block, epidural	Long duration; less cardiotoxic than bupivacaine	Hypotension and bradycardia are prominent adverse effects when ropivacaine is used epidurally, particularly with concentrations of ropivacaine over 0.5% (Aronson, 2016)	200–300 mg single doses for duration up to 5 h achieved by various regional techniques, both minor and major nerve blocks (Miller, 2015)
Tetracaine (Pontocaine)	Spinal anesthesia	Long acting; good relaxation	Not appropriate for short procedures because of the long duration of action	Dose 5–20 mg (epinephrine rarely used); duration 60–180 min for SAB (Miller, 2015)

Anticholinergics

	Common Usage	Advantages	Disadvantages	Comments
Atropine	Blocks effects of acetylcholine; ↓ vagal tone; reverse muscle relaxants; treat sinus bradycardia	↑ HR; suppresses salivation, bronchial and gastric secretions	Depresses sweating; may cause dry mouth, flushing, dizziness, CNS symptoms	Quite selective at muscarinic receptors in smooth and cardiac muscle and exocrine glands (Nagelhout, 2014)
Glycopyrrolate (Robinul)	Similar to atropine	Slightly ↑ HR; does not cross blood-brain barrier; can increase gastric pH more than atropine	Prolonged duration of effects	Lower incidence of dysrhythmias than atropine (Nagelhout, 2014)

Cholinergic Agent

	Common Usage	Advantages	Disadvantages	Comments
Neostigmine (Prostigmine)	Reverses effects of nondepolarizing neuromuscular blocking agents	Prevents breakdown of acetylcholine by inhibiting acetylcholinesterase	The need to wait until evidence of spontaneous recovery (TOF ratio of >0.9) before administering. (Miller, 2015)	Given with either atropine or glycopyrrolate (Nagelhout, 2014)

Continued

SURGICAL PHARMACOLOGY

Commonly Used Anesthetic Gases and Drugs—cont'd

	Common Usage	Advantages	Disadvantages	Comments
Other				
Sugammadex (Bridion)	First SRBA to antagonize a muscle relaxant's effects	Rapidly terminates the neuromuscular block of rocuronium, vecuronium, and pancuronium by diffusion of medication away from neuromuscular junction; choice of anesthetic does not affect efficacy of sugammadex	No effect on succinylcholine or benzylisoquinolinium relaxants, can affect hormone-based oral contraceptives; recommend alternative method if used on female patients of child-bearing age for 7 days; not recommended for severe renal impaired patients on dialysis (Miller, 2015)	If need to reestablish muscle relaxation arises after administration of sugammadex, then using a benzylisoquinolinium or succinylcholine is recommended; cases of marked bradycardia have been observed, some resulting in cardiac arrest, monitor hemodynamic changes (Merck & Co, 2015)
Dexmedetomidine (Precedex)	Selective α_2-agonist; sedation in the ICU	Produces centrally mediated sympatholytic, sedative, and analgesic effects; hemodynamic stability, potentiates anesthetics, reduces anesthetic requirements, preserved drive (Garcia et al., 2013)	Limited amnestic effect; avoid as sole anesthetic agent with patients in which neuromuscular blockade is used; risk of bradycardia; use with caution in patients with heart block (Garcia et al., 2013)	Even at high doses does not produce general anesthesia, but is a valuable sedative in a number of settings (Garcia et al., 2013)

BP, Blood pressure; *CNS*, central nervous system; *CSF*, cerebrospinal fluid; *HR*, heart rate; *ICP*, intracranial pressure; *ICU*, intensive care unit; *IM*, intramuscular; *IV*, intravenous; *MAC*, monitored anesthesia care; *MH*, malignant hyperthermia; *PO*, oral; *SAB*, subarachnoid block; *SRBA*, selective relaxant binding agent; *SVR*, systemic vascular resistance, *TOF*, train-of-four.

Maintenance continues from this point until near completion of the procedure; the anesthesia provider achieves this phase either with inhalation agents, with IV medications given in titrated doses, or by continuous infusion. *Emergence* varies in length and depends on the patient's state and the depth and duration of anesthesia. Emergence starts as the patient begins to "emerge" from anesthesia and usually ends when the patient is ready to leave the OR; however, recent court cases have determined that this phase is fluid, and can continue until discharge from PACU (*US ex rel Donegan v. Anesthesia Associates of Kansas City*, 2015 WL 3616640 [W.D. Mo., June 9, 2015]). Intubation occurs during the induction phase, and extubation usually is performed during emergence. Recovery from anesthesia amounts to a fourth phase of general anesthesia.

Types of General Anesthesia

The types of general anesthesia used often are described as IV technique, inhalation technique (with a volatile anesthetic agent), or a combination of IV and inhalation techniques. *IV technique* traditionally includes (1) an induction agent such as propofol, combined with 30% to 40% O_2 and N_2O; (2) an amnestic/anxiolytic, such as midazolam or diazepam; (3) an analgesic such as fentanyl or hydromorphone; and (4) a muscle relaxant, if required for airway management or surgical necessity.

In contrast, an *inhalation technique* may use propofol to facilitate rapid induction or patients may "breathe themselves down" with a potent agent, such as sevoflurane, plus N_2O and O_2. Inhalation induction is often used with children to avoid inserting an IV catheter while they are awake. Depending on the surgical procedure, maintenance of anesthesia may be accomplished with only inhalation agents and spontaneous, assisted, or controlled ventilation. Effects of volatile agents are dose related and provide differing levels of

anesthesia, amnesia, analgesia, muscle relaxation, and hemodynamic responses. If supplemental muscle relaxation is needed, the relaxant dose required is significantly less than the dose necessary during IV anesthesia. Use of anesthetic agents and sedative medications, especially for procedures lasting more than 3 hours or if multiple procedures are necessary, is balanced against potential risks in children under 3 years; single, short exposure is unlikely to have negative effects (FDA, 2016).

Balanced anesthesia is often used to describe a combination of IV medications and inhalation agents used to obtain specific effects tailored to each patient and procedure.

Anesthesia providers also may use *total IV anesthesia* (TIVA). TIVA may be used in the OR but more commonly is used for pediatric, uncooperative, or trauma patients in locations outside of the OR, such as in magnetic resonance imaging (MRI), radiology, or surgical laser suites, in which waste-gas evacuation systems are not available. TIVA use also occurs with enhanced recovery after surgery (ERAS) (Evidence for Practice), in the expanding area of office-based surgery, and with robotic-assisted surgery (Robotic-Assisted Surgery). With TIVA, providers use short-acting medications such as propofol with remifentanil or alfentanil for induction and maintain anesthesia by infusion plus O_2 alone or with either air or N_2O. They may also give an intermediate-acting muscle relaxant (cisatracurium, atracurium, rocuronium, or vecuronium). As surgery nears completion, the anesthesia provider titrates off the maintenance medications, and emergence from anesthesia follows.

Muscle Relaxants

Muscle relaxants (also referred to as neuromuscular blocking drugs [NMBDs]) are used to facilitate intubation and provide good operating conditions at lighter planes of general anesthesia. Muscle relaxants

EVIDENCE FOR PRACTICE

Enhanced Recovery After Surgery for Major Surgery

Enhanced recovery after surgery (ERAS) is a multimodal, evidence-based approach to perioperative care that combines a range of interventions to enable early mobilization and feeding after surgery. Its widespread implementation challenges anesthesia providers, and others, to implement changes in a timely fashion. The anesthesia provider has a role in five main areas of ERAS: (1) preoperative assessment and optimization; (2) conducting anesthesia with minimal residual effects and ensuring intraoperative compliance with all ERAS elements; (3) optimizing intravascular blood volume, cardiac output, oxygen delivery, and tissue perfusion using a combination of fluids and vasopressors; (4) using, where appropriate, central neuraxial blockade, regional/truncal blocks, or local anesthetic techniques in combination with multimodal analgesia to control postoperative pain; and (5) immediate postoperative optimization of fluids and analgesia to restore homeostasis and function at a time when there are significant physiologic changes for the patient.

Perioperative nurses have a role in implementing these five areas. They are the agents who bring evidenced-based practice to the patient level of care and need the rationale of why the program does what it does. For example, understanding the issue of a multimodal approach to pain management versus the old ways of using opioids and their increased risk of side effects, makes it more understandable for nurses when nurses implement the change. Nurses educate patients in understanding the requirements of enhanced recovery protocols and provide hands-on support as patients mobilize early and begin their nutritional course to restore bowel function postsurgery. All patient care providers need education about ERAS protocols to see the complete vision of initiating evidence-based change that benefits their patients.

Modified from Bloomstone, JA: Overcoming challenges—anesthesiologists. In Tong JT et al, editors: *Enhanced recovery for major abdominopelvic surgery*, ed 1, New York, 2016, Professional Communications, Inc.; Scott MJ: Overview for anesthesiologist and CRNA. In Tong JT et al, editors: *Enhanced recovery for major abdominopelvic surgery*, ed 1, New York, 2016, Professional Communications, Inc.; Gan TJ et al: *Enhanced recovery after major abdominal surgery*, West Islip, 2016, Professional Communications, Inc.

ROBOTIC-ASSISTED SURGERY

Anesthetic Concerns

RAS arose from the evolution of minimally invasive surgery, and the historical need for remotely controlled surgical interventions on the battlefield. Because the patient benefits from less surgical trauma, less pain, and shorter overall length of stay, RAS expanded to multiple surgical specialties. Positioning (see Chapter 6) is a major concern for anesthesia providers during robotic procedures with steep Trendelenburg position, such as for radical prostatectomy and hysterectomy. In thoracoscopic surgery, prolonged one-lung anesthesia can be a risk factor.

In RAS, the anesthesia provider starts the anesthetic in the supine position. All appropriate monitors are placed, including invasive monitoring (if needed). After induction, the eyes are protected, an orogastric tube and urinary catheter are placed, and convective-air body warmers are used, when possible (Goswami et al., 2015). In many surgical procedures, arms are tucked at the patient's side. Once the robot "docks" beside the patient, the body position cannot be changed unless it is an emergency.

Therefore it is often necessary to place a second IV line, as a backup in the event a primary IV line fails. The OR team is trained to quickly disengage the robot to assist in any airway, or other emergency, situation. The patient can be maintained with a volatile anesthetic, or TIVA with awareness monitoring. Neuromuscular blockade is essential to prevent patient movement while the robotic instruments are in the surgical site. During otorhinolaryngeal surgery, the anesthesia provider is near the foot of the bed to monitor and care for the patient. Fluid management may need to be restricted, especially in longer procedures with steep Trendelenburg in which edema can accumulate in the face and eyes; resulting swollen sclera can cause patients to scratch their eyes on awakening. When the surgery is finished, the surgeon or assistant sutures the multiple small incisions. The anesthesia provider removes the orogastric tube, antagonizes the muscle relaxant, and readies the patient for transfer to the PACU.

IV, Intravenous; *PACU*, postanesthesia care unit; *RAS*, robotic-assisted surgery; *TIVA*, total IV anesthesia.

affect skeletal muscle and have little effect on cardiac or smooth muscle. Although not always dose dependent, many of these medications have adverse side effects. The route of metabolism and elimination varies, and this may be important for patients with hepatic or renal disease. Muscle relaxants are classified as *depolarizing* or *nondepolarizing*.

The standard *depolarizing* agent is succinylcholine (Anectine). It has a chemical structure similar to that of acetylcholine (ACh) and depolarizes the postjunctional neuromuscular membrane. Administration is followed by a brief period of muscle fasciculations (random generalized muscle contractions that may be associated with painful myalgias [Duke, 2016]) that corresponds to initial membrane depolarization and muscle fiber activation. Unlike ACh, which is released in minute amounts and hydrolyzed in milliseconds, succinylcholine requires several minutes for breakdown. During this time the neuromuscular junction remains depolarized, but the muscles relax and will not contract again until the neuromuscular endplate and adjacent sarcoplasmic reticulum return to the resting state and are again depolarized. Relaxation proceeds from small, distal, rapidly moving muscles to proximal, slowly moving muscles. The diaphragm is one of the last muscles to relax. To prevent fasciculations and associated postoperative myalgia, a small dose of nearly any nondepolarizing relaxant is given 2 minutes before administering the intubating dose of succinylcholine. Onset of paralysis (30–90 seconds) is faster, and duration of action (5–10 minutes) is shorter than with other relaxants. The speed of onset makes it a preferred medication for rapid-sequence induction (RSI). Adverse side effects associated with use of succinylcholine include cardiac dysrhythmias, hyperkalemia, myalgia (particularly in young and muscular patients), and increases in intraocular, intracranial, and intragastric pressures. It also can trigger MH in susceptible patients. It can be infused for longer procedures, but an excessive dose may cause prolonged relaxation (known as *phase II blockade*). Succinylcholine is hydrolyzed by plasma cholinesterase, and the rare patient with an abnormal or absent enzyme (plasma cholinesterase) has prolonged muscle paralysis (Nagelhout, 2014).

Nondepolarizing muscle relaxants competitively block the depolarizing action of ACh at the neuromuscular junction, which results in skeletal muscle paralysis. Fasciculations do not occur. Nondepolarizing agents can be subdivided by duration of action into intermediate-acting (atracurium, cisatracurium, rocuronium, and vecuronium) and long-acting (pancuronium, pipecuronium, and doxacurium) (Duke, 2016; Nagelhout, 2014). Potency, duration, and side effects of these medications vary and may be individually altered in patients with hepatic or renal dysfunction, electrolyte imbalance, or hypothermia or when used in combination with other perioperative medications (inhalation and local anesthetics, aminoglycoside antibiotics, calcium-entry blockers, magnesium, and cardiac antidysrhythmics). Generally, nondepolarizing relaxants can be used for patients with MH or plasma cholinesterase deficiencies. Side effects vary with individual medications, are dose dependent, and include alterations in blood pressure and heart rate. The neuromuscular blockade of muscle relaxants can be monitored with a peripheral nerve stimulator. Paralysis caused by nondepolarizing relaxants may be antagonized (reversed) by IV anticholinesterases, such as edrophonium, neostigmine, or rarely pyridostigmine. Sugammadex (Merck & Co, 2015) is a selective relaxant binding agent (SRBA) that encapsulates the steroidal neuromuscular agents rendering them inert, and is excreted in the urine. Antagonism with sugammadex occurs even with deep block because of the rapid fall of muscle relaxant concentration, and appropriate doses can antagonize within 3 minutes. Other antagonists allow ACh to accumulate and compete for receptor sites at the neuromuscular junction and may be associated with bradycardia, arrhythmias, hypotension, bronchoconstriction, and hypersalivation, for which atropine or glycopyrrolate is routinely given (Nagelhout, 2014). Because sugammadex does not affect acetylcholinesterase or stimulate cholinergic receptors, the administration of an anticholinergic is not necessary (Duke, 2016). Sugammadex does have the potential for bradycardia.

Typical Sequence of General Anesthesia

After arriving in the preoperative area or OR, the anesthesia provider again identifies the patient; verifies consents; reviews current laboratory tests, diagnostic studies, and pertinent medical history; and confirms there have been no interval changes in the patient's status. An IV infusion may be started in the preoperative area or after the patient is transferred to the OR. After the patient arrives in the OR and is transferred to the OR bed, monitors are connected.

Before induction the anesthesia provider usually preoxygenates the patient using a mask with 100% O_2 for 3 to 5 minutes. This practice permits wash-out of most gaseous nitrogen from the body and provides a large reserve supply of O_2 in the lungs. Next, administration of opioids and benzodiazepines are given. If succinylcholine is to be used for intubation, a small pretreatment dose of a nondepolarizing muscle relaxant (e.g., 0.04 mg/kg of rocuronium [Kim et al., 2014], or 7.5 mcg/kg of pancuronium [Motamed and Duvaldestin, 2014]) usually occurs next. If the patient can be safely ventilated with a mask, the anesthesia provider may opt to avoid the adverse effects of succinylcholine and use a nondepolarizing muscle relaxant to intubate the patient.

To induce anesthesia, a short-acting barbiturate, such as propofol (1.5–2.5 mg/kg), is given. When the patient becomes apneic and the eyelash reflex is absent, the anesthesia provider checks the airway

for patency by ventilating the patient with a mask. At this time eye protection is applied, and depending on several factors, O_2 and anesthetic gases may be delivered to a spontaneously breathing patient through a mask held in place with a head strap. Repositioning of the head or insertion of an oral or nasal airway may help to maintain a patent airway. If spontaneous or assisted ventilation is planned, an LMA may be inserted without a muscle relaxant. The anesthesia provider may use a mask or LMA for a patient with a good airway, at minimal risk of aspiration, and undergoing a relatively short procedure as long as the surgical site is not compromised in the head or neck area.

If mask anesthesia or an LMA is inappropriate, an ETT is used to facilitate ventilation and to prevent aspiration. Typical equipment for intubation, and airway control and monitoring, appear in Fig. 5.2. An "intubating dose" of a muscle relaxant is administered, resulting in temporary paralysis. When the patient is paralyzed, ventilation is controlled during the procedure.

To facilitate intubation, the patient's head is placed in a "sniffing" position. The laryngoscope is held in the left hand. The clean laryngoscope blade is inserted into the right side of the mouth and moved to the midline, "sweeping" the tongue to the left. The ETT is introduced on the right side of the mouth and gently inserted into the trachea so that the cuff is approximately 1 cm below the vocal cords. The cuff is inflated just enough to occlude any air passage with the peak pressures used for ventilation. Location of the ETT in the trachea is verified by an appropriate level and waveform of $ETCO_2$, bilaterally equal breath sounds and absence of sounds over the stomach (determined using a stethoscope), symmetric movement of the thorax with positive-pressure ventilation, and condensation of moisture from expired air in the ETT and breathing circuit. Proper placement of the ETT appears in Fig. 5.3. The vocal cords are the narrowest portion of an adult trachea; however, the smallest portion of a child's airway is below the vocal cords at the cricoid cartilage. Uncuffed ETTs have been traditionally selected for children up to age 8; newer designs for ETTs with microcuffs, however, allow use of cuffed tubes down to age 1 (Armendi et al., 2015; Miller, 2015). After initial paralysis from the muscle relaxant has worn off, the patient may be allowed to breathe spontaneously with intermittent assistance, or additional muscle relaxant is given and ventilation controlled mechanically.

If the procedure is emergent or the patient is at risk for aspiration (as in cases of a full stomach, intestinal obstruction, hiatal hernia, or significant esophageal reflux), an RSI or an "awake" fiberoptic intubation may be planned. In these instances, the perioperative nurse may be asked to assist by applying cricoid pressure (Fig. 5.4). The nurse exerts downward pressure on the cricoid cartilage, the only complete ring in the trachea, with the thumb and index finger of one hand (Sellick maneuver). Correctly applied downward pressure occludes the esophagus, which lies immediately posterior (or dorsal) to the trachea. Such downward pressure can enhance the view required for intubation. The pressure is not released until proper placement of the ETT has been confirmed and the cuff inflated. Although this procedure previously had wide acceptance among anesthesia providers, research suggests that the maneuver is difficult to do correctly and effectively (Barak et al., 2015; Miller, 2015; Heiner and Gabot, 2014). Thus use of cricoid pressure is controversial and is no longer a class I recommendation (Miller, 2015).

The perioperative nurse provides additional assistance if an unexpected difficult intubation occurs or the patient cannot be ventilated adequately via mask (Research Highlight). The difficult-airway cart should be brought into the room immediately. The

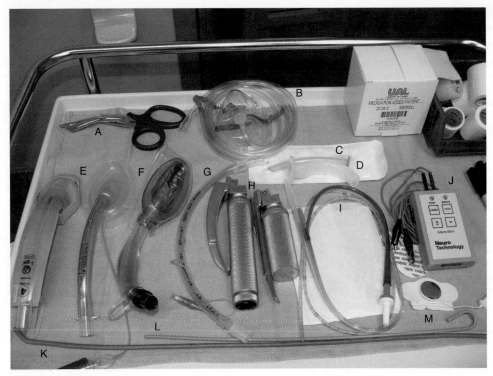

FIG. 5.2 Commonly used anesthesia equipment. *(A)* Scissors. *(B)* Supplemental oxygen mask. *(C)* Nasal trumpet airway. *(D)* Guedel oral airway. *(E)*, Supraglottic airway I-gel laryngeal mask airway "Unique." *(F)* Cook intubating LMA. *(G)* Endotracheal tube. *(H)* Long- and short-handled laryngoscopes with curved Macintosh and straight Miller blades. *(I)* Nasogastric/orogastric tube. *(J)* Peripheral nerve stimulator. *(K)* Elastic bougie endotracheal tube (ETT) introducer. *(L)* ETT malleable stylet. *(M)* Skin temperature probe.

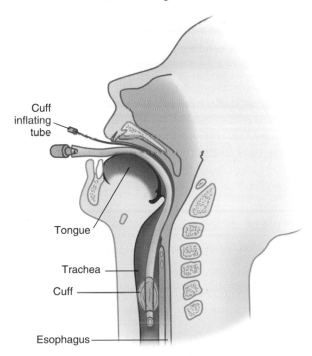

FIG. 5.3 Endotracheal tube in position.

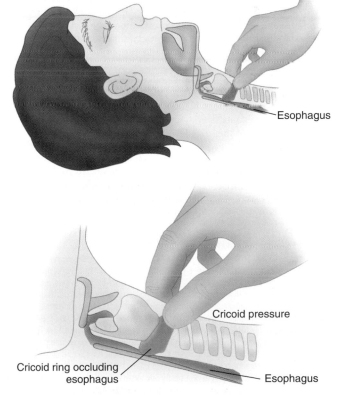

FIG. 5.4 Applying cricoid pressure.

RESEARCH HIGHLIGHT

Obstructive Sleep Apnea: Perioperative Risks, Complications, and Risk for Difficult Intubation

OSA is a sleep breathing disorder characterized by periodic, partial, or complete obstruction of the upper airway. OSA is associated with many comorbidities, especially hypertension, cardiovascular disease, cerebral vascular disease, and metabolic syndrome. In OSA, upper airway function of both anatomical and neuromuscular control is imbalanced. Anatomical imbalance occurs between upper airway soft tissue volume and bony enclosure size, resulting in pharyngeal airway obstruction during sleep and anesthesia. The incidence of moderate to severe OSA is 23.4% in women and 49.7% in men; this may be the result of central fat deposition pattern around the neck, trunk, and abdominal viscera of men. In bariatric surgical patients, incidence of OSA has been reported to be greater than 70%. Age is another OSA risk factor; risk increases until age 65 and then plateaus off. OSA may be on the rise as members of our society live longer and as obesity continues to occur at high rates.

The gold standard for diagnosis of OSA is a PSG sleep study, measuring the number of episodes of apnea and hypopnea per hour of sleep (the AHI). The American Academy of Sleep Medicine (AASM) measures severity of OSA by the AHI. Mild AHI range is >5, moderate is >15, and severe >30. As the PSG is expensive, time consuming and not readily available, a simple and rapid clinical questionnaire is often used to assess and identify patients with OSA before or at the time of surgery. There are multiple clinical screening tools. Pataka's retrospective study of five different questionnaires found that the STOP BANG questionnaire had high sensitivity and low specificity. The STOP BANG questionnaire is an easy and rapid tool to help identify patients with OSA. With each positive answer, the likelihood of moderate to severe OSA increases.

Research shows that OSA patients have increased risk for postoperative complications. The incidence of adverse respiratory events in OSA patients is greater than in non-OSA patients; hypoxemia is also significantly higher. In addition, cardiac complications including dysrhythmias, abnormal heart rate, myocardial infarction and ischemia, hypotension, and congestive heart failure are prevalent risks in OSA patients. Neurologic complications such as delirium, agitation, confusion, and excessive drowsiness are also significantly increased, as are the number of unplanned ICU transfers in patients with OSA.

The ASA has developed practice guidelines for perioperative management of patients with OSA. It is important to advise surgical patients of their risk for OSA. There are three types of OSA patients: those diagnosed with OSA and treated with CPAP, those diagnosed and not using CPAP, and those undiagnosed. The latter two patient groups are at a higher risk of postoperative complications.

Once a patient is identified with OSA, intraoperative measures are taken. The anesthesia provider prepares for difficult airway management. Because of the high closing pressure of the pharyngeal airway, there is an increase in difficult mask ventilation. Difficult intubation is more prevalent in severe OSA than mild to moderate OSA. Obese patients with OSA are more likely to have a decreased FRC. Therefore, during induction, the use of apneic oxygenation to prolong or prevent desaturation is considered.

Anesthesia and surgical pain exacerbates upper airway collapse in OSA patients. ASA guidelines recommend considering benefits of alternative anesthesia techniques and postoperative pain management. OSA patients may be more susceptible to opioid respiratory depression via obstructive and central apnea. The use of opioids is avoided whenever possible. In one study, the severity of preoperative sleep disorder breathing, aging, and postoperative opioid dose were associated with postoperative AHI and central apnea.

CPAP is the gold standard for treatment of OSA. Postoperative CPAP for OSA patients has been shown to decrease cardiovascular complications. Chung's review examined the use of CPAP in the preoperative and postoperative period for surgical patients with diagnosed OSA and undiagnosed OSA. He concluded that use of CPAP may be an effective intervention to reduce the incidence of postoperative adverse events. The ASA Guidelines for OSA also recommend (if possible) perioperative use of CPAP with OSA patients. Positioning patients postoperatively is important, as well; Semi-Fowler's position is recommended.

The ASA guidelines recommend discharging OSA patients to an unmonitored bed, or home, *only when* they are no longer at risk for postoperative respiratory depression. If admitted, a patient is placed in a monitored bed with continuous pulse oximetry and an alarm system. A Dartmouth study reported that OSA patients who were on continuous pulse oximeter monitoring showed a decrease in rescue events and ICU transfers because of early recognition of deterioration.

As OSA rises to epidemic proportions, anesthesia providers will encounter an increase in diagnosed and undiagnosed OSA patients with perioperative risks of morbidity and mortality. To decrease such events, hospital protocols and policies for OSA patients are now standard.

AHI, Apnea-hypopnea index; *ASA,* American Society of Anesthesiologists; *ASSM,* American Academy of Sleep Medicine; *CPAP,* continuous positive airway pressure; *FRC,* functional residual capacity; *ICU,* intensive care unit; *OSA,* obstructive sleep apnea; *PSG,* polysomnography.

Modified from: Abrishami A et al: A systematic review of screening questionnaires for obstructive sleep apnea, *Can J Anaesth* 57(5):423–438, 2010; AASM: *Clinical practice guidelines for diagnostic testing for adult obstructive sleep apnea: an update for 2016* (website). www.aasmnet.org/resources/pdf/DTOGuideline.pdf. (Accessed 19 December 2016); Brousseau C et al: A retrospective analysis of airway management in patients with obstructive sleep apnea and its effects on postanesthesia care unit length of stay, *Can J Respir Ther* 50(1):23–25, 2014; Chung F et al: Factors associated with postoperative exacerbation of sleep disorder breathing, *Anesthesiology* 120(2):299–311, 2014; Chung F et al: CPAP in the perioperative setting: evidence of support, *Chest* 149(2):586–597, 2016; Doyle A et al: Preoxygenation and apneic oxygenation using trans nasal humidified rapid insufflation ventilation exchange for emergency intubation, *J Crit Care* 36:8–12, 2016; Gaddam S et al: Postoperative outcomes in adult obstructive sleep apnea patients undergoing non-upper airway surgery: a systematic review and meta-analysis, *Sleep Breath* 18(3):615–633, 2014; Lam K et al: Obstructive sleep apnea, pain and opioids: is the riddle solved? *Curr Opin Anaesthesiol* 29(1):134–140, 2016; Loke Y et al: Association of obstructive sleep apnea with risk of serious cardiovascular events; a systemic review and meta-analysis, *Circ Cardiovasc Qual Outcomes* 5(5):720–728, 2012; Muller J: Perioperative opioids aggravate obstructive breathing in sleep apnea syndrome: mechanisms and alternative strategies, *Curr Opin Anaesthesiol* 29(1):129–133, 2016; Mutter TC et al: A matched cohort study of postoperative outcomes in obstructive sleep apnea: could preoperative diagnosis and treatment prevent complications? *Anesthesiology* 121(4):707–718, 2014; Pataka A et al: Evaluation of five different questionnaires for assessing sleep apnea, *Sleep Med* 15(7):776–781, 2014; Peppard P et al: Increased prevalence of sleep disordered breathing in adults, *Am J Epidemiol* 177(9):1006–1014, 2013; American Society of Anesthesiologists Task Force on Perioperative Management of Patients with Obstructive Sleep Apnea: Practice Guidelines for the Perioperative Management of Patients with Obstructive Sleep Apnea: an updated report by the ASA Task Force on perioperative management of patients with obstructive sleep apnea, *Anesthesiology* 120(2):268–286, 2014; Reed K et al: Screening for sleep disordered breathing in a bariatric population, *J Thorac Dis* 8(2):268–275, 2016; Sato S et al: Mask ventilation during induction of general anesthesia, *Anesthesiology* 126(1):28–38, 2017; Singh M et al: Proportion of surgical patients with undiagnosed obstructive sleep apnea, *Br J. Anaesth* 110(4):629–636, 2013; Schwartz A et al: Obesity and obstructive sleep apnea: pathogenic mechanism and therapeutic approaches, *Proc Am Thoracic Soc* 5(2):185–192, 2008; Tsuiki A et al: Anatomical balance of upper airway and OSA, *Anesthesiology* 108(6):1009–1015, 2008.

perioperative nurse should be familiar with the location of the various pieces of equipment on the cart, know how to assemble the equipment for use, and assist the anesthesia provider in securing the airway. Securing the airway in an emergency situation requires a concerted team effort. The contents of a typical difficult-airway cart are listed in Box 5.2. If invasive monitors (e.g., an arterial line) are to be placed after induction, the perioperative nurse may assist by properly

---

Fiberoptic Equipment
Flexible FO bronchoscopes (adult and pediatric); FO light source (newer models have their own battery-powered source); Bullard scope (FO); and siliconized spray

Laryngoscope Equipment
Assorted pediatric and adult laryngoscope handles and blades; extra alkaline batteries, or chargers for FO handles; and video laryngoscope (GlideScope, etc.)

Endotracheal Tubes
Regular ETT: uncuffed, 2.5–6 mm; regular ETT: cuffed, 5–9 mm; oral RAE ETT: uncuffed, 3–7 mm; oral RAE ETT: cuffed, 6–8 mm; nasal RAE ETT: uncuffed, 3–7 mm; nasal RAE ETT: cuffed, 6–8 mm; reinforced ETT: cuffed, 7–8 mm; controllable-tip ETT (Endotrol); Combitube

Airways
Regular oral: assorted pediatric and adult; regular nasal: assorted adult; intubating airways: assorted (e.g., Ovassapian, Williams); nasopharyngeal airway with inflatable introducer; assorted sizes of supraglottic airways (e.g., LMAs, ILMA; tongue blades; and water-soluble lubricant (K-Y)

Intubating Equipment
Intubating stylets; McGill forceps: pediatric and adult; EGTA; hollow ETT changers with removable Luer-Lok connectors for O_2 insufflation

Suction Equipment
Assorted flexible suction catheters to fit ETT and LMA as well as stiff suction catheters (Yankauer suction catheters)

Topical Anesthesia Equipment
Atomizers and pressurized topical anesthetic spray; long cotton-tipped swabs; lidocaine 4%; lidocaine 4% with phenylephrine; lidocaine 2%, viscous; lidocaine 5%, ointment; lidocaine 10%; tetracaine 1%

Transtracheal Airway Equipment
Transtracheal O_2 jet ventilator with pressure regulator, manual control valve, and Luer-Lok male connector; assorted large IV catheters; and assorted long guidewires, epidural needles, and epidural catheters (for retrograde intubation)

Miscellaneous
Safety glasses; heat-moisture exchanger (Humidivent); assorted facemasks with port for FO scope; right-angled connector (for facemasks) with port for FO scope; exhaled carbon dioxide detector; $ETCO_2$ chemical indicators (Easy Cap); twill tape (to secure ETT); skin adhesive (Mastisol)

EGTA, Esophageal (gastric tube) airway; *ETT,* endotracheal tube; *FO,* fiberoptic; *ILMA,* intubating laryngeal mask airway; *IV,* intravenous; *LMA,* laryngeal mask airway; *RAE,* Ring-Adair-Elwyn.

---

positioning the patient or extremity; prepping the area or areas with antimicrobial solution; and assisting with placement, connection, and calibration of the monitors. If the procedure is emergent, the perioperative nurse also may assist by obtaining additional IV access, connecting fluid-warming or patient-warming units, double-checking blood products, and "pumping" IV fluids as needed. If the anesthesia provider faces a critical procedure, such as a difficult airway/airway emergency, the perioperative nurse can perform a valuable service by ensuring provision of 100% O_2, having suction available, observing monitors, recording data (SpO_2 and $ETCO_2$ values), and communicating significant changes to the anesthesia provider.

The LMA (also called "supraglottic airway," or SGA) is a good airway device in many settings (Bosson, 2016). Placement is relatively simple and does not require laryngoscopy or muscle relaxation. When comparing ease of use, invasiveness, and airway protection, the LMA ranks between the facemask and an ETT. It is ideal for a supine patient under general anesthesia with spontaneous ventilation. The LMA also may be useful in a difficult-airway situation in which tracheal intubation cannot be achieved.

The recommended technique for insertion of the LMA appears in Fig. 5.5, and correct placement is seen in Fig. 5.6. Placement of devices follow the manufacturer's instructions and recommendations. For adults, it is recommended that a 2.5- to 3-cm diameter roll of gauze sponges be used as a "bite-block" and inserted beside the LMA tube. The LMA and gauze roll can be secured with tape. Some, like the LMA Supreme, have a bite-block integrated within the device (Teleflex Medical, 2015).

The anesthesia provider achieves anesthesia maintenance with IV or inhalational anesthetic techniques, or a combination of both, with or without additional muscle relaxation, and considers a variety of factors when selecting the anesthesia technique for each patient.

Whichever technique is selected for general anesthesia (or for any other anesthesia types discussed subsequently), the entire surgical team participates in a time-out just after the patient is anesthetized, positioned, prepped, and draped, and before starting the surgical procedure. The entire surgical team ceases other activity and verifies the patient's identity, the procedure to be done, operative side and site, and correct surgical position. The patient must be positioned such that the marking of the operative site is visible on the patient's skin. The mark is unambiguous and is used consistently throughout the organization. The mark is made at or near the procedure site. It is sufficiently permanent to be visible after skin prep and draping. Implants, special equipment, and any other requirements (e.g., blood or blood products, if ordered) are verified. Any special concerns about the patient or procedure are shared by team members. When complete, the procedure can begin. The time-out is documented according to institutional protocol.

Many factors influence emergence. The objective is to move the patient from the OR bed to the PACU bed as soon as the dressing is applied. During emergence, the anesthesia provider suctions the oropharynx before extubation to decrease the risk of aspiration and laryngospasm after extubation, reverses any residual neuromuscular blockade, and allows the wash-out of N_2O and volatile agents by giving 100% O_2 for several minutes before extubation. After extubation the patient is transported to PACU to awaken. In some situations the patient may be transferred to PACU before extubation and the ETT removed when the patient is fully awake.

Untoward events that can occur with general anesthesia include hypoxia; respiratory, cardiovascular, or renal dysfunction; hypotension; hypertension; fluid or electrolyte imbalance; residual muscle paralysis; dental damage; neurologic problems; hypothermia; and MH. The

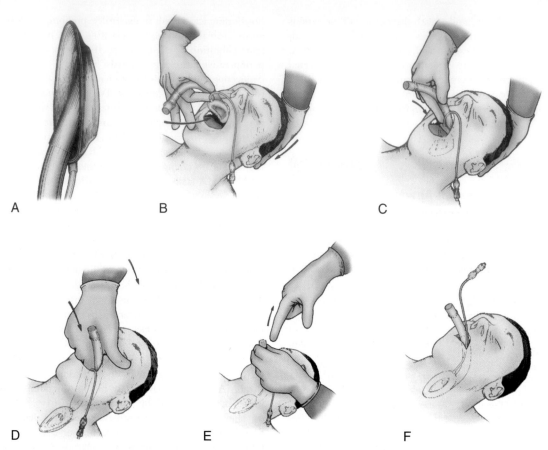

FIG. 5.5 Insertion of the laryngeal mask airway (LMA). Select the appropriate-size LMA (1, neonates ≤5 kg; 1.5, infants 5–10 kg; 2, infants and children 10–20 kg; 2½, children 20–30 kg; 3, children and small adults >30 kg; 4, normal size to large adults; 5, large adults). (A) Carefully deflate the LMA as flat as possible so that the rim faces away from the mask aperture as shown. There should be no folds near the tip. (B) Under direct vision, press the tip of the LMA cephalad against the hard palate to flatten it out. Using the index finger, continue pressing the LMA against the palate as the LMA is advanced into the pharynx to ensure that the tip remains flattened and avoids the tongue. (C) Keeping the neck flexed and the head extended, use the index finger to press the LMA into the posterior wall. (D) Continue pushing with the ball of the index finger, guiding the LMA posteriorly into position. By withdrawing the other fingers and slightly pronating the forearm, it is usually possible to push the LMA fully into position in one fluid movement. (E) Firmly grasp the tube with the other hand; then withdraw the index finger from the pharynx. Gently press the LMA posteriorly to ensure that it is fully inserted. (F) Carefully inflate the LMA with the recommended volume of air for size (1, 2–4 mL; 2, ≤10 mL; 2½, ≤14 mL; 3, ≤20 mL; 4, ≤30 mL; 5, ≤40 mL). Do not overinflate. Do not touch the LMA tube while inflating, unless it is obviously unstable (as with elderly edentulous patients with loose oropharyngeal tissues). Usually the LMA moves slightly forward out of the hypopharynx as it is inflated. Insert a bite-block (roll of gauze) alongside the LMA tube to minimize occlusion of the tube as the patient is awakening.

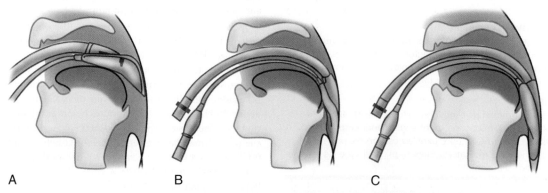

FIG. 5.6 Sagittal views of insertion and proper placement of the laryngeal mask airway (LMA). (A) Insertion of LMA. (B) Proper location of LMA (deflated). (C) Properly placed and inflated LMA.

anesthesia provider usually directs the treatment and management of such events.

Regional Anesthesia

Regional anesthesia (also called *conduction anesthesia*) is accomplished by injecting a local anesthetic along the pathway of a nerve from the spinal cord, providing anesthesia to a region of the body (referred to as a "block"). Preoperative preparation for regional anesthesia is essentially the same as that for general anesthesia. Preoperative medication frequently is used to ease any discomfort that may be experienced during placement of the block. The criteria for monitoring during regional anesthesia are similar to those during general anesthesia. Whenever regional anesthesia is performed, resuscitative equipment and medications are immediately available. During preparation and placement of the regional anesthetic, the perioperative nurse can provide valuable assistance. This assistance may include placing appropriate monitors, such as pulse oximetry, ECG, and blood pressure; providing supplemental O_2 if indicated; reassuring the patient; administering sedation, such as midazolam, as directed; and properly positioning the patient, which is crucial for a successful block.

Peripheral blocks on lower or upper extremities or on the head frequently occur in a preoperative holding area to allow adequate time for the local anesthetic to penetrate the peripheral nerve before transfer to the OR. For peripheral blocks the perioperative nurse may need to perform aspiration during needle placement (to detect vascular puncture) and inject the local anesthetic while the anesthesia provider stabilizes the needle in the precise location. After an initial period of evaluation by the anesthesia provider, the nurse monitors the patient for any substantial change in vital signs or untoward reactions until transfer of the patient to the OR.

Spinal Anesthesia

A local anesthetic (usually lidocaine, tetracaine, or bupivacaine) injected into the cerebrospinal fluid (CSF) in the subarachnoid space is termed a *spinal anesthetic* or an *SAB*. To provide additional analgesia, fentanyl or preservative-free morphine often is added to the local anesthetic. The anesthesia provider inserts a spinal needle into a lower lumbar interspace with the patient either lying on one side or in a sitting position. The local anesthetic, generally mixed with a dextrose solution for a total of 1 to 4 mL, results in a *hyperbaric* (heavier than the CSF) solution. These hyperbaric mixtures settle in a gravity-dependent manner after injection into the CSF. By changing the patient's position, the block can be directed up, down, or to one side of the spinal cord. With prostate surgery, the patient may remain in the sitting position for about 1 minute after injection of the local anesthetic to achieve a bilateral block of the S1–S5 dermatomes.

For surgery in the upper abdomen, the patient may be placed in a slight 5- to 10-degree head-down position to allow the anesthetic to move cephalad while the anesthesia provider carefully checks the level of sensory block. After reaching an adequate level, the bed is leveled to minimize further extension of the sensory block. After 10 to 15 minutes, the block usually "sets" or stabilizes, and does not extend farther. The sympathetic nervous system usually is blocked two dermatomes higher and the neuromuscular system two dermatomes lower than the sensory block. The patient is then positioned for surgery.

If the local anesthetic is mixed with a larger volume of sterile water, the solution is *hypobaric,* and the medication moves to the nondependent area. Hypobaric spinal anesthesia usually is done after the patient is positioned and the surgical site exposed (with the site of injection above the surgical site, as in perianal surgery in the prone position).

By mixing the local anesthetic with some CSF withdrawn from the subarachnoid space, the solution becomes *isobaric.* Distribution of this solution is minimally affected by gravity.

Spinal anesthesia may cause several physiologic responses, which are outlined in the following sections, which can result in major problems if not properly managed.

Hypotension

Hypotension may occur rapidly after an SAB. It results from vasodilation because the sympathetic nerves that control vasomotor tone are blocked. Peripheral pooling of blood occurs, resulting in reduced venous return to the heart and decreased cardiac output. A hypotensive response usually can be avoided by infusing 750 to 1500 mL of balanced salt solution immediately before the block and placing the patient in a 5-degree head-down position to improve venous return to the heart. A vasopressor, such as ephedrine, also may be appropriate.

Total Spinal Anesthesia

Total spinal anesthesia (or inadvertent high spinal block) may cause paralysis of the respiratory muscles and necessitate immediate intubation and ventilation. Any sign or symptom of respiratory distress occurring shortly after instituting spinal anesthesia should alert the anesthesia provider to the possibility of a high spinal block.

Positioning Problems

Positioning problems can occur because pain and sensory inputs to a portion of the patient's body are blocked. Care is taken to position the surgical patient to avoid neurologic damage, pressure injury, loss of skin integrity, or respiratory compromise. Positioning is a collaborative effort among the anesthesia provider, surgeon, assistant, and perioperative nurse.

Postdural Puncture Headache

Postdural puncture headache (PDPH) (also called *postspinal cephalgia* or *spinal headache*) is a frequent postoperative complaint after spinal anesthesia. It occurs more commonly in young parturients (new mothers) or other patients younger than 40 years. With use of a 25- or 27-gauge blunt-bevel needle, incidence is about 1% (Olson et al., 2014). PDPH is unrelated to how soon the patient ambulates postoperatively. Current belief suggests the headache results from leakage of CSF through the hole in the dura and typically occurs when the patient assumes an upright position. Incidence, severity, and duration of the headache appear to correlate with the size of the hole left in the dura. The headache usually occurs in the occipital area and generally resolves over 1 to 3 days but may last 2 weeks. Several treatments have been used to relieve the headache: strict bed rest for 24 to 48 hours, vigorous hydration, abdominal binders, PO or IV caffeine, and injection of 5 to 20 mL of autologous blood into the epidural space at the puncture site ("blood patch"). Although rare, a repeat dose can be given within 24 hours (Olson et al., 2014).

Many anesthesia providers use different spinal needles that have a tip shaped like a sharpened wood pencil with holes on the side of the needle. These 24- to 26-gauge spinal needles presumably separate or go between the dural fibers as opposed to cutting the fibers, which may occur when a blunt-bevel spinal needle is used. With these "pencil-point" needles, the incidence and severity of PDPH lower substantially (Olson et al., 2014).

Epidural and Caudal Anesthesia

The epidural space is between the ligamentum flavum and the dura, and extends from the foramen magnum to the sacrococcygeal membrane. In it are epidural veins, fat, and loose areolar tissue. For *epidural* anesthesia, the anesthesia provider usually injects local anesthetic through the intervertebral spaces in the lumbar region (lumbar epidural), although injection also can be into the cervical or thoracic regions. The anesthetic spreads cephalad and caudad from the site of injection. A comparative location of the needle points and injected anesthetic appears in Fig. 5.7.

For *caudal* anesthesia, local anesthetic also is injected into the epidural space, but the approach is through the caudal canal in the sacrum. Compared with a lumbar epidural, this approach requires a greater volume of anesthetic to fill the epidural space. Caudal anesthesia has a 5% to 10% technical failure rate. Given its ease of administration, however, it is often used for perineal procedures or pediatric surgery on the lower extremities along with a light general anesthetic (Olson et al., 2014).

Several techniques may be used for epidural or caudal anesthesia. A "single-shot epidural" involves administration of a local anesthetic through the needle before its removal. For intermittent injections or continuous infusions, a small catheter is inserted into the epidural space for administration of local anesthetic.

For combined spinal and epidural anesthesia, the anesthesia provider first inserts the epidural needle (dual-conduit needles are available to reduce possible complications from a one-channel Tuohy needle) into the epidural space, and then inserts a special, long 25-, 27-, or 29-gauge spinal needle through the epidural needle into the CSF. A small amount of fentanyl or preservative-free morphine may be injected, which provides good analgesia for several hours. Removal of the spinal needle follows, and an epidural catheter inserted. Using a dual-channel needle, the epidural catheter is inserted first, and then the spinal needle is placed. This technique is especially useful for obstetric anesthesia (Olson et al., 2014).

Techniques to identify the epidural space include the "hanging drop" and the "loss of resistance" to injection of either air or liquid (saline or local anesthetic) as the needle is advanced slowly through the ligamentum flavum. With the hanging-drop technique, the needle is filled with liquid to form a meniscus at the needle hub. As the needle is slowly advanced into the epidural space, negative (less than atmospheric) pressure draws the liquid inward toward the epidural space. Location of the needle tip within the epidural space is verified by injection of an additional 1 to 2 mL of air or saline.

When local anesthetics are injected into the epidural space, the major sites of action are the nerve roots as they leave the spinal cord and proceed out the intervertebral foramina beyond the meningeal sheath. Some anesthetic diffuses into the subarachnoid space to the spinal cord. As local anesthetics diffuse away from the site of injection, segmental anesthesia is possible in specific areas. In contrast to spinal anesthesia, much larger volumes of local anesthetic are needed with epidural anesthesia; the head-up, head-down, or lateral position of the patient does not affect the level of the epidural anesthetic as much, and onset of anesthesia is much slower. Hypotension can occur with epidural anesthesia, but a previously taught technique of using a preload regime of 250 to 2000 mL of hydration has not been shown to prevent the hypotension; therefore using ephedrine, a mixed adrenergic agonist, is appropriate (Miller, 2015).

Local anesthetics most frequently used for epidural anesthesia are lidocaine, bupivacaine, and chloroprocaine. Ropivacaine and levobupivacaine may prove to be less cardiotoxic than bupivacaine and possess a larger therapeutic ratio. Although much of their pharmacologic profile is similar to that of bupivacaine, levobupivacaine and ropivacaine seem to possess more selective action for neural blockade (Olson et al., 2014). Depending on the concentration of the anesthetic agent, effects can range from loss of sensory input to complete motor blockade. To verify that the anesthetic is not being injected into the subarachnoid space or into an epidural vein, a test dose of 3 to 5 mL of 1.5% lidocaine with a 1:200,000 concentration of epinephrine is frequently used. Injected intravascularly, this test dose causes a transient tachycardia. If injected into the subarachnoid space, it produces a low level of spinal anesthesia.

Complications associated with the use of local anesthetics in the epidural and subarachnoid spaces are unique to the agent used. Permanent neurologic sequelae have been reported when chloroprocaine with a preservative was injected into the subarachnoid space. Bupivacaine is associated with pronounced cardiac toxicity if injected intravascularly (Olson et al., 2014). With epidural anesthesia several complications can occur, including inadvertent dural puncture, subarachnoid injection, and vascular injection.

Inadvertent Dural Puncture

Inadvertent dural puncture with the epidural needle (a wet tap) can cause a PDPH. This headache is significant in about 50% of patients, and its intensity can incapacitate. Treatment is essentially the same as that discussed under the section Spinal Anesthesia earlier in this chapter.

Subarachnoid Injection

Subarachnoid injection occurs if the needle or catheter is unintentionally inserted into the subarachnoid space. If a large volume of local anesthetic is injected as a bolus, it causes "total spinal" anesthesia. This condition is associated with a rapid onset of hypotension caused by vasodilation and profound bradycardia as the sympathetic nerves

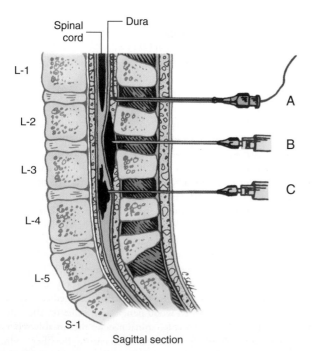

FIG. 5.7 Location of needle point and injected anesthetic relative to dura. (A) Epidural catheter. (B) Single injection epidural. (C) Spinal anesthesia. (Interspaces most commonly used are L4–L5, L3–L4, and L2–L3.)

to the heart are blocked, causing a totally paralyzed patient. Treatment includes intubation, control of ventilation, support of blood pressure and the cardiovascular system, and administration of amnestic medications until the block resolves. If properly managed this problem is not life-threatening.

Vascular Injection

Injection of local anesthetic into an epidural vein may occur inadvertently with the initial dose or with subsequent injections. IV-injected bupivacaine is associated with cardiac arrest (Research Highlight). Toxicity from other local anesthetics can cause sudden and profound hypotension, convulsions from effects on the CNS, and tachycardia if the solution contains epinephrine. The airway is supported/managed for oxygenation and ventilation, seizures are treated, then lipid emulsion infusion is begun to reverse signs and symptoms of toxicity. Basic life support measures are used when indicated to ensure tissue perfusion and circulation of resuscitation medications, including lipid emulsion.

Convulsions usually dissipate rapidly as local anesthetic redistributes throughout the body. An IV benzodiazepine may be given to reduce these effects. A vasopressor (e.g., ephedrine or phenylephrine) can be used to restore blood pressure. If the patient becomes paralyzed, intubation and ventilation are required until the toxic effects are gone. Use of a test dose with each injection usually prevents these problems.

Peripheral Nerve Blocks

Peripheral nerves can be blocked effectively by injecting local anesthetic around them to provide adequate surgical anesthesia. Onset and duration of the block depend on the medication used and its concentration and volume, addition of epinephrine, and site of injection. Complications usually arise from an inadvertent intravascular injection or an overdose of the local anesthetic. Rarely, trauma caused by the needle or compression from the volume of local anesthetic injected may cause nerve damage.

PNBs are an effective method to deliver analgesia and anesthesia. With the exponential growth of ambulatory surgery, there are many benefits of PNBs. Local anesthetics have quick onset of action, provide prolonged analgesia, and often do not require administration of powerful anesthetics that have undesired side effects. Patients often leave with less pain, and less PONV, report greater satisfaction with the quality of care received, and avoid the undesirable side effects of excess opioids. PNBs are an essential part of contemporary multimodal anesthesia.

Peripheral Nerve Anatomy and Physiology

The peripheral nervous system consists of 31 pairs of spinal nerves that exit between the vertebrae on each side of the body. These spinal nerves traverse the torso and innervate specific regions to coordinate CNS ability to perceive cutaneous sensation and respond

---

RESEARCH HIGHLIGHT

Lipid Infusion for Local Anesthetic Systemic Toxicity and Cardiac Resuscitation

IV local anesthetics work by blocking voltage-gated sodium ion channels that are essential for normal nerve impulse conduction. This impedes transmission of pain stimuli. However, voltage-gated sodium ion channels are found in cardiac nerve cells. Bupivacaine, a commonly used local anesthetic agent, has been implicated as a causative agent for patients experiencing cardiac arrest after accidental intravascular injection during a PNB. Research findings and case reports suggest that lipid infusion is an effective adjunct to standard cardiac resuscitation procedures for bupivacaine toxicity. Additionally, a 20% lipid emulsion (Baxter Pharmaceuticals, Deerfield, IL) should be administered (1.5 mL/kg bolus followed by a continuous infusion at 0.25 mL/kg/min for 10–60 min). Although propofol is formulated in a lipid emulsion, the formulation is only 10% lipid; therefore it is not used as a substitute for lipid emulsion. Cardiovascular suppression associated with use of propofol may worsen the ability to resuscitate the patient. In some cases, patients have been placed on cardiopulmonary bypass until cardiac toxicity resolves.

The use of lipid emulsion early in the sequence of rapidly worsening toxicity appears to attenuate or prevent progression of cardiac toxicity. This suggests that early lipid infusion might prove an advantage, presumably by interrupting the vicious cycle of low-output, tissue acidosis, and worsening toxicity, preventing progression to cardiac arrest. The infused intravascular lipid mass binds the offending toxin in sufficient quantity to pull drug from the target tissue, reversing the toxicity.

There is a generally accepted approach: establish an airway as the first priority to ensure optimal oxygenation and ventilation; then seizure suppression, preferably with a benzodiazepine; and then lipid emulsion infusion to reverse signs and symptoms of toxicity. A single bolus has been used in most case reports; however, this should be repeated or the infusion increased for failure of return of spontaneous circulation or declining blood pressure (respectively). Given that the lipid infusion must circulate to the coronary vascular bed, *high-quality basic life support* is a necessary element of lipid resuscitation in the setting of a low output state.

Monitor the patient during and after completing injection because clinical toxicity can be delayed up to 30 minutes. Weinberg (2012) suggests making a lipid rescue kit for every area in a facility in which regional anesthesia blocks are administered. He suggested a box or bag containing a 500-mL bag of 20% lipid solution, IV tubing, 60-mL syringes (2), and needles. A treatment protocol and LAST checklist should be included in the kit. Weinberg (2012) also recommends ready availability of 20% lipid emulsion in any site in which local anesthetics are administered.

IV, Intravenous; *LAST,* local anesthetic systemic toxicity; *PNB,* peripheral nerve block.
Modified from American Society of Regional Anesthesia and Pain Medicine: *Checklist for treatment of local anesthetic systemic toxicity* (website). www.asra.com/advisory-guidelines/article/3/checklist-for-treatment-of-local-anesthetic-systemic-toxicity. (Accessed 5 January 2017); McGee DL: Local and topical anesthesia. In Roberts JR, editor: *Roberts and Hedge's clinical procedures in emergency medicine,* ed 6, Philadelphia, 2014, Elsevier Saunders; pp 519–540.e2; Neal JM et al: ASA practice advisory on local anesthetic systemic toxicity, *Reg Anesth Pain Med* 35(2):152–161, 2010; Sirianni AJ et al: Use of lipid emulsion in the resuscitation of a patient with prolonged cardiovascular collapse after overdose of bupropion and lamotrigine, *Ann Emerg Med* 51(4):412–415, 2008; Turabi, AA: Toxicity of local anesthetic agents. In Murray MJ et al, editors: *Faust's anesthesiology review,* Philadelphia, 2015, Elsevier Saunders, pp 272–273; Weinberg G: Lipid emulsion infusion: resuscitation for local anesthetic and other drug overdose, *Anesthesiology* 117(1):180–187, 2012.

with synchronized motor reflexes. Peripheral sensory nerve impulses initiate by noxious stimuli, such as surgical incision. This stimulus creates an "action potential" that changes the electrical voltage traveling across the axonal membrane of the nerve by allowing an influx of sodium ions (referred to as cellular depolarization). This creates a propagating electrical wave that conducts a sensory nerve impulse to the brain, which interprets it as pain. Local anesthetics block sodium channels, by physically plugging the transmembrane pore, interacting with various amino acid residues, and preventing the nerve impulse to allow pain perception (Rang et al., 2016).

Common Peripheral Nerve Blocks

Upper Extremity: The Brachial Plexus. Spinal nerves leaving the cervical vertebrae, C5–T1, converge to form a bundle of nerves known as the brachial plexus. Each bundle of nerves innervates the right and left side of the neck and axilla. The brachial plexus divides further into branches that eventually terminate in the radial, ulnar, and median nerves.

PNBs of the brachial plexus are performed for surgery of the shoulder, forearm, or hand. The different anatomic sites that anesthesia providers use to perform a brachial plexus nerve block are the interscalene, supraclavicular, infraclavicular, or axillary sites. The choice of anatomic site for a PNB depends on (1) the area of the arm undergoing surgery and (2) the specific surgical procedure. As an example, a shoulder arthroscopy dictates an interscalene brachial plexus block as appropriate, whereas for carpal tunnel surgery, an infraclavicular or axillary block is proper.

Lower Extremity. Lumbar and sacral spinal nerves, also exiting through each side of the vertebrae, eventually separate into the sciatic, femoral, popliteal, and tibial nerve roots that innervate the lower extremities. PNBs for the lower extremities are often performed for knee and foot procedures. For example, a femoral nerve block is effective for a knee arthroscopy or for pain management after total knee arthroplasty, whereas an ankle block (essentially a block of the deep and superficial peroneal, tibial, and sural nerve branches of the sciatic nerve) is useful for a wide variety of procedures on the feet and toes (Shastri et al., 2014).

Peripheral Nerve Block Equipment

To identify the correct injection site for the PNB, the anesthesia provider typically uses a nerve stimulator, often with ultrasound guidance (Vacchiano and Biegner, 2014). The nerve stimulator creates an electrical current. The goal is to elicit a motor response from the nerve while applying the correct amount of voltage. Once the anesthesia provider isolates the desired nerves to be "blocked," the appropriate local anesthetic is carefully injected into tissue close to the nerve. The local anesthetic then inhibits the propagation of nerve impulses to the CNS. Depending on the desired site of action, PNBs can take from a few minutes to as long as an hour to achieve complete effect. The duration of the nerve block depends on the local anesthetic used.

Important Perioperative Nursing Considerations

Expected Side Effects and Special Care Concerns. PNBs often have side effects. For example, with an interscalene block, patients may experience Horner syndrome (miosis, ptosis, and increased salivation) and may also have a unilateral phrenic nerve paralysis that causes breathing difficulty. These side effects may need special anesthesia attention. All perioperative staff must remember that the patient with a PNB has lost the protective reflex of pain sensation. Therefore special care is required for proper patient positioning as

well as for postoperative patient education regarding the risk of burns or falls.

Preparation for Adverse Events. PNB is a safe method of anesthesia and analgesia delivery. It does, however, pose serious potential complications that all perioperative staff must anticipate in advance of emergencies.

LAST results when a patient absorbs an unsafe amount of a local anesthetic into the bloodstream (see Research Highlight: Lipid Infusion for Local Anesthetic System Toxicity and Cardiac Resuscitation). This can occur either slowly from systemic absorption of a local anesthetic correctly injected into tissue, or immediately and catastrophically if injected accidentally directly into a blood vessel. Signs of systemic local anesthetic toxicity often progress in a stepwise manner. Patients may initially report perioral numbness, a metallic taste in the mouth, ringing in the ears, visual disturbances, and/or dizziness. If toxicity progresses, or is immediate, the patient will likely have seizures, respiratory arrest, and/or cardiac arrest.

Performance of PNB is appropriate only in areas well equipped to handle emergencies, that is, areas having access to an external oxygen source; vacuum suction; ventilation bag and mask; laryngoscope; ETT tubes; monitoring equipment; and resuscitation medications to treat hypotension, bradycardia, and seizures. The increased use of PNBs has occasioned increased reports of cardiac arrest from accidental intravascular injection; however, actual incidence has dropped to 4 per 10,000 epidurals (Nagelhout, 2014).

Intravenous Regional Anesthesia

IV regional anesthesia was first described by Bier in 1908 and is frequently called a *Bier block*. IV injection of a local anesthetic using a tourniquet creates a high venous pressure gradient that encourages the flow of the anesthetic to the smaller nerve endings of the extremity (Shilling et al., 2015). Although it can be used on a lower extremity, it is used more often on the upper extremities. A larger volume of medication is necessary for a lower limb block, which increases the risk for the most common complication of this block—local anesthetic toxicity. The block is highly reliable and straightforward to accomplish.

A small IV catheter is inserted as distal to the surgical site as feasible, and a single-cuffed or double-cuffed pneumatic tourniquet placed around the limb proximal to the surgical site. The limb is raised and exsanguinated by wrapping it with an Esmarch bandage. The tourniquet is inflated to approximately 100 mm Hg above the patient's systolic blood pressure, and the Esmarch bandage removed. About 50 mL of 0.5% lidocaine is injected through the catheter. Anesthesia onset is rapid, lasting until the tourniquet is deflated (Vacchiano and Biegner, 2014).

When a double-cuffed pneumatic tourniquet is used, the proximal cuff is initially inflated. When the patient experiences discomfort from the cuff pressure (usually about 35–40 minutes after cuff inflation), the distal cuff, which is located over an anesthetized area, is inflated and the proximal cuff deflated. The proximal cuff remains inflated until the distal cuff has been inflated to prevent loss of the IV anesthetic from the limb. Two single-cuffed tourniquets can substitute for a double-cuffed tourniquet. If the patient experiences pain from the tourniquet, an IV analgesic or sedative can supplement the block; ketorolac (15–30 mg in the local anesthetic) has been found to provide postoperative analgesia without increased risk of bleeding (Vacchiano and Biegner, 2014).

Ensuring excellent tourniquet occlusion for a minimal time interval can minimize the risk of toxicity. With a lidocaine Bier block, 45 minutes is recommended for a sufficient amount of the drug to bind to tissues, which ensures safe serum levels before cuff release (Shilling et al., 2015).

Monitored Anesthesia Care

For sicker, unstable patients, surgeons and anesthesia providers weigh the relative risks and benefits of MAC versus general anesthesia. During MAC, the anesthesia provider usually supplements a local anesthetic with an IV analgesic (e.g., fentanyl) and with sedative and amnestic medications (e.g., midazolam or propofol). Vital signs, respiratory and cardiovascular status, and positioning are carefully monitored, and supplemental low-flow O_2 often administered. Depending on the clinical situation, the anesthesia provider may have to induce general anesthesia or use one of the regional techniques described previously if a greater degree of anesthesia becomes necessary.

Moderate Sedation/Analgesia

Moderate sedation/analgesia refers to IV administration of certain sedatives and analgesics that produce a condition in which the patient exhibits a depressed level of consciousness but retains the ability to maintain a patent airway independently and respond appropriately to verbal commands or physical stimulation. It is also referred to as "conscious sedation." An anesthesia provider may not be involved in the patient's care. Perioperative nurses who have additional training and demonstrated competencies in (1) administering medications to achieve moderate sedation/analgesia and (2) patient monitoring perform these functions (AORN, 2017). Objectives for a patient receiving moderate sedation/analgesia include mood alteration, continued consciousness, enhanced cooperation, elevated pain threshold, minimal variation of vital signs, some degree of amnesia, and rapid and safe return to activities of daily living.

Selection of patients for moderate sedation/analgesia depends on established criteria developed by an interdisciplinary team. Patients undergo thorough assessment before the procedure. Assessment includes a review of physical examination findings: age; height; weight; body mass index (BMI); medication use; allergies; test results; vital signs, and NPO status (Fencl, 2016). Assessment also includes specific elements regarding the administration, and patient perceptions of, moderate sedation/analgesia. Monitoring methods for patients receiving moderate sedation, medications administered, and interventions initiated must be within the scope of nursing practice as defined by the respective state board of nursing. If the nurse does not feel comfortable managing the care and monitoring a particular patient, the attending physician and an anesthesia provider should be consulted. During the past few years, advocates have supported propofol administration by nurses. The US Food and Drug Administration (FDA) continues, however, to include a "black box" warning that only trained anesthesia providers should administer propofol. The American Association of Nurse Anesthetists (AANA) and the ASA continue to support the FDA view for patient safety reasons (FDA, 2016). Even in the hands of an anesthesia provider, propofol can affect respirations, possibly requiring advanced airway management.

When monitoring a patient receiving moderate sedation/analgesia, the nurse should have no other responsibilities that would leave the patient unattended or compromise continuous patient monitoring. The nurse must be clinically competent in the use of monitoring equipment and oxygen-delivery devices, medications used for moderate sedation/analgesia and resuscitation, and airway management. Advanced cardiac life support (ACLS) certification of nurses responsible for monitoring patients receiving moderate sedation/analgesia

is usually required. If not, healthcare professionals with ACLS skills should be readily available to render support if needed in an emergency (AORN, 2017).

The nurse who administers moderate sedation/analgesia medications should know usual dosages, contraindications, interactions with other medications, onset and duration of action and desired effects, adverse reactions, and emergency management techniques. Benzodiazepines (e.g., diazepam, midazolam) and opioids (e.g., fentanyl, meperidine hydrochloride) are used for moderate sedation/analgesia (AAMSN, 2016). Equipment in the room in which moderate sedation/analgesia is administered includes a noninvasive blood pressure device, an ECG, a pulse oximeter, oxygen-delivery devices, and suction. An emergency cart with appropriate resuscitative medications and equipment (e.g., a defibrillator) is kept immediately available.

Establish an IV access line to administer medications, along with any emergency medications and fluids. Monitor respiratory rate, cardiac rate and rhythm, blood pressure, oxygen saturation, level of consciousness, and skin color/condition. Document preprocedure assessment; dosage, route, time, and effects of all medications administered; type and amount of fluids administered; physiologic data from continuous monitoring at 5- to 15-minute intervals and on significant events; level of consciousness; nursing interventions initiated and patient responses; and any significant patient reactions and their resolution (Fencl, 2016).

Postprocedure monitoring is provided until the patient returns to baseline parameters. Patients and family members or significant others receive appropriate, health-literate oral and written discharge instructions; have them verbalize understanding (i.e., teach-back in their own words).

Discharge criteria should be established by an interdisciplinary team and include adequate respiratory function, stable vital signs, return to preprocedure level of consciousness, intact motor reflexes, return of motor and sensory control, absence of protracted nausea, acceptable skin color and condition, absence of significant pain, and satisfactory surgical site and dressing condition (when present). A responsible adult must accompany and drive the patient home.

Local Anesthesia

The terms *local anesthesia, local,* and *straight local* are used interchangeably to describe the administration of an anesthetic agent to a specific area of the body by topical application, local infiltration, regional nerve block, or "field" block. The surgeon administers local anesthetics. Other physicians, such as cardiologists, pulmonologists, proctologists, and gastroenterologists, may perform local procedures in the OR suite. No anesthesia provider is involved.

Hospitals and ASCs establish interdisciplinary guidelines for selecting patients who are appropriate for local anesthesia procedures and for patient monitoring criteria. Decisions to monitor the patient receiving local anesthesia, parameters that need to be monitored, and frequency of observation and monitoring are tailored to the patient, the surgical procedure, and medications used. Patients receiving local anesthetics require preoperative assessment and monitoring by the perioperative nurse during the procedure.

Local anesthesia usually is used for minor, short-term surgical, diagnostic, or therapeutic procedures. Because the patient does not lose consciousness, local anesthesia is frequently preferred when the patient's cooperation is necessary for the procedure. Local anesthesia is economical and eliminates the undesirable effects of general anesthesia. Adverse reactions, however, may occur from large doses of local agents. If the agent enters the bloodstream directly, convulsions, circulatory and respiratory distress, cardiovascular collapse, or even death can result.

The surgeon chooses local anesthetics based on desired duration of action, surgery site, potency potential, and the patient's PS. Topical agents, such as cocaine hydrochloride, tetracaine, or lidocaine, may be applied to mucous membranes of the nose, throat, trachea, and urethra. Lidocaine 0.5% to 2%, with or without epinephrine, is the medication most commonly used for local anesthesia, although bupivacaine (Marcaine) may also be selected. Epinephrine may be added to the local anesthetic agent for its vasoconstricting properties in the area injected, slower rate of absorption and longer duration of the local anesthetic agent (by reducing blood flow to the area injected), and lower incidence of toxicity. Epinephrine is used with caution in patients with hypertension, diabetes, or heart disease. A general recommendation for a local anesthetic such as lidocaine is that no more than 50 mL of a 1% solution, or 100 mL of a 0.5% solution, should be injected per hour (for maximum adult dosages, see the earlier Surgical Pharmacology box). All local anesthetic containers or syringes should be clearly labeled, both on and off the sterile field. Medication safety practices are initiated.

Preoperatively, the perioperative nurse reviews the patient's history, physical examination findings, and results of any ordered laboratory or other diagnostic tests. Patients undergo careful assessment to determine physiologic baselines, allergies (to medications, latex, adhesive tape, or other substances), and emotional status. IV infusion begins before the procedure because adequate venous access is crucial in life-threatening emergent situations, when resuscitative medications must be given immediately (see Research Highlight: Lipid Infusion for Local Anesthetic System Toxicity and Cardiac Resuscitation).

The perioperative nurse must be clinically competent to use monitoring equipment, to make equipment connections, and to interpret data. Monitoring includes heart rate and regularity, respiratory rate, and mental status. Additional monitoring parameters depend on the patient's condition and include blood pressure, skin condition, and oxygen saturation status (AORN, 2017). Any change in the patient's condition is communicated immediately to the surgeon.

The perioperative nurse also must be familiar with medications administered during the procedure, usual dosages, limits on rate of injection and maximum dosage (usually stated on a per-kilogram basis), duration of action, physiologic and psychologic changes expected, normal and abnormal reactions, and appropriate action to take if untoward reactions occur. The nurse observes the patient for side effects such as CNS disturbances, cardiovascular problems, hypersensitivity to medication, and toxic reaction resulting from high levels of local anesthetic. Emergency medications, suction apparatus, and resuscitation equipment are kept readily available. Symptoms of adverse medication reactions include restlessness, unexplained anxiety or fearfulness, diaphoresis, nausea, palpitations, disturbed respiration, pallor or flushing, syncope, and convulsive movements. Signs and symptoms of allergic reaction include urticaria, tachycardia, laryngeal edema resulting in breathing difficulties, nausea, vomiting, and elevated temperature. In some instances, anaphylactic symptoms, including severe hypotension, can occur. If a significant change occurs in the patient's status, the nurse notifies the surgeon immediately. As the patient is awake during the procedure, conversation and noise are minimized.

Documentation of care provided to a patient receiving a local anesthetic should be consistent with the AORN's evidence-based guidelines and recommendations (AORN, 2017). This includes medications administered, including dosage, route, and time of administration; patient monitoring; and any untoward reactions.

After the procedure the patient's postoperative status undergoes careful assessment. This evaluation and any special patient needs are documented, and the receiving unit receives a report before the patient's transfer (if the patient is going to a recovery area). The hand-off report includes types and amount of medications given and any adverse reaction noted, site and condition of the IV (if applicable), type and amount of solution infused in the OR, intraoperative vital signs, procedure performed, and condition of any dressing. Included are any special postoperative orders, allergies, and a general statement of the patient's tolerance of the procedure. The patient may transfer to the ambulatory surgery discharge area or return directly to a hospital room. Transfers of local anesthesia patients to PACU for recovery or observation are rare.

Pain Management

Many anesthesia providers have applied their expertise in analgesia and regional anesthesia to acute and chronic pain management. Chronic pain is often multifactorial and may occur after a discrete injury, trauma, or surgical procedure. It also may result from prolonged repetitive stress, such as "low back pain." Chronic pain frequently has complex psychologic components unrecognized by patients or by individuals closely associated with them. Diagnosis and treatment of such chronic pain usually involve multiple medical disciplines and prolonged management.

Acute perioperative pain is a different problem. Traditionally, postoperative pain has been treated with IM narcotics every 3 to 6 hours as needed. This treatment is often associated with undesirable side effects, including oversedation, respiratory depression, deep vein thrombosis (DVT) secondary to decreased mobility, and variable degrees of pain relief. Use of pain management modalities are now multimodal. Patient-controlled analgesia (PCA) uses a programmable electronic pump that can continuously infuse a small amount of IV narcotic (at a basal rate); in addition, the patient can administer a predetermined bolus "on demand." Safety interlocks limit the frequency of boluses and total dose per hour (Bordi, 2014).

With spinal or epidural anesthesia, a small amount of preservative-free narcotic, such as fentanyl, sufentanil, or morphine, may be added to the local anesthetic mixture. The narcotic acts via central opiate receptors and provides analgesia for 24 to 36 hours.

Continuous epidural analgesia may be appropriate for managing prolonged postoperative pain. Physicians may use this technique for extensive procedures, including total hip or knee replacements; knee reconstruction; and major abdominal, thoracic, or gynecologic operations. In addition, it can be useful for acute trauma, such as multiple rib fractures. Typically a lumbar or thoracic epidural catheter is inserted before surgery, covered with a transparent occlusive dressing, and injected with local anesthetic. Given the duration, manipulation, or positioning required for the operative procedure, general anesthesia is often used for patient comfort. The epidural greatly reduces analgesic requirements of general anesthesia. This allows for the avoidance of systemic opioids, making regional anesthesia a superb method of pain control (Rieker, 2014). After surgery the infusion rate is adjusted to provide analgesia during early recovery. As the level of pain decreases over time, reduction of the infusion rate follows. Catheter removal occurs after 2 to 5 days to minimize infection risk. Benefits of epidural analgesia for acute postoperative pain include good analgesia with minimal sedation, early ambulation and physical therapy, and excellent patient satisfaction. Possible side effects include nausea, pruritus, and areas of slight numbness. These are controlled by using medications such as diphenhydramine (Benadryl) or naloxone

(Narcan) and by adjusting the infusion rate. A nonsteroidal antiinflammatory drug (NSAID), such as ketorolac (Toradol), is given for any "breakthrough pain" instead of increasing the epidural infusion (Rieker, 2014).

A single caudal injection is often used in pediatric patients who have surgery of the lower abdomen, pelvis, or lower extremities. It usually follows induction of general anesthesia, with selection typically of a long-acting local anesthetic such as bupivacaine with epinephrine. This injection provides good analgesia for 8 to 24 hours postoperatively and greatly decreases intraoperative requirements for general anesthesia. If the procedure requires prolonged recovery, a lumbar epidural catheter can be placed intraoperatively. Postoperatively, management is similar to that with an epidural catheter (Olson et al., 2014).

Fluid Management

Blood Loss

Measuring blood loss is a vital procedure in the surgical management of critically ill or elderly patients, patients undergoing complex procedures, trauma and organ transplant patients, patients with abnormal bleeding or clotting time or with extensive renal/liver disease, and infants. Some anesthesia providers prefer to estimate blood loss via visual inspection of drapes, suction canisters, and used soft goods such as sponges. When blood loss estimates must be more accurate, weighing sponges provides a reliable means of judging the amount of blood lost and of gauging the need for transfusion. The weight of dry, unused sponges and the weight of the plastic bag for soiled sponges must first be determined and then excluded from the weight tally. Grams (g) measured are converted to milliliters (mL) on a 1:1 basis, and blood loss estimates are reported to the anesthesia provider. The setup to weigh sponges requires a gram scale and plastic bags to hold soiled sponges. The estimated blood loss (EBL) may be part of the hand-off report in ORs that use a surgical Apgar score.

Blood and Blood Products

Maintaining circulating blood volume is crucial during surgical procedures; this is accomplished with administration of whole blood or blood components. Blood products are literally lifesavers but can be fatal if improperly stored or administered. AABB (formerly known as the American Association of Blood Banks) standards and technical manuals should be incorporated into facility policy and must be followed exactly (Carson et al., 2016). Whole blood is rarely administered unless the patient has an acute, massive loss (often empirically determined as a loss greater than 15% of estimated blood volume, or approximately 1000 mL for an adult [Elkins et al., 2017]). Instead, packed red blood cells (PRBCs) that improve oxygen-carrying capacity and oxygen transport to tissues, with or without crystalloid or colloid solutions, are administered to maintain intravascular blood volume. Crystalloid solutions include normal saline and lactated Ringer's solution; colloid solutions include albumin, purified protein factors, dextran, and hydroxyethyl starch (hetastarch). If coagulopathy is an issue, as in the case of massive transfusion protocols, fresh frozen plasma (FFP), platelets, and cryoprecipitate are considered. When blood or any blood product is given, appropriate precautions are taken to reduce administration hazards.

Methods to decrease the need for blood transfusions include preoperative autologous donation, intraoperative blood retrieval and reinfusion, and isovolemic hemodilutions. Such methods allow withdrawing a patient's blood at the start of surgery, replacing it with volume expanders, and then, at the end of surgery, retransfusing the patient with his or her donated blood (Rhee and Bellal, 2017).

Elective surgery patients who may need blood products during surgery have a pretransfusion sample taken 1 to 7 days (facility policy and patient history dependent) before surgery to ensure compatibility and to avoid antibodies that may emerge in response to exposure through blood transfusions, pregnancy, or environmental factors, or as a consequence of the patient's disease process. *Type* refers to the test to determine the ABO and Rh blood type. *Screen* refers to the test for unexpected antibodies. *Crossmatching* refers to the test for the compatibility of the recipient's serum and the donor's red blood cells (RBCs). It is crucial to correctly identify the patient before the pretransfusion blood sample is drawn and then to ensure that the sample is properly labeled. Improperly identified pretransfusion blood samples can result in acute hemolytic transfusion reactions at the time of transfusion, and death.

Patients having elective surgical procedures for which blood has been requested should not be anesthetized without verification that the requested blood products are typed, crossmatched, and available, and that informed consent to receive blood products has been documented. This is part of the preoperative verification process; it is reverified during the time-out. A blood requisition form, with complete and accurate patient identification information, is sent to the blood bank when blood or blood products are requested. Included on or with this requisition is the number of units desired. Computerized ordering requires the same information.

If the patient is sent to the OR directly from the emergency department or trauma admitting area without a chart, all patient identification information must be printed plainly on a piece of paper. The perioperative nurse should contact the blood bank to explain the emergency situation and facilitate release of the needed blood products. RBC transfusions should be fully crossmatched if possible; however, the patient should not suffer adversely for want of serologically compatible RBCs. Transfusion can be started with group O uncrossmatched RBCs. If the patient's Rh type is unknown, Rh(D)-negative RBCs are preferable, especially for females with childbearing potential (Elkins et al., 2017).

Precise and accurate blood product storage conditions are important to ensure patient safety and to avoid wasting improperly stored products. Whole blood and blood products are stored under continuously monitored conditions in accordance with AABB rules and FDA regulations. Storage temperatures are documented, and all storage equipment for blood products properly maintained and tested, including function checks on alarms. The return of unused blood products complies with facility policy; further, each component presents specific requirements for proper maintenance and return (e.g., thawed cryoprecipitate and platelets must be maintained at room temperature [22°C]; red cells and thawed plasma must be kept refrigerated at 4°C).

Before administration of any blood product, the perioperative nurse and anesthesia provider (or a second licensed individual) confirm that a signed consent is in the medical record, and then proceed to confirm the following:

- The unit number on the blood product corresponds with the unit number on the blood requisition. Facilities using electronic records will return a "transfusion card" or "crossmatch card" as verification that this unit can be given to this patient in lieu of the requisition.
- The name, birth date, and number on the patient's identification band agree with the name, birth date, and number on the slip with the blood product.
- The patient's name on the slip with the blood product corresponds with the name on the requisition.

- The blood group indicated on the blood product corresponds with that of the patient.
- The date and time of expiration have not been reached.
- The blood product bag is free of leaks, damage, or signs of possible bacterial contamination (e.g., presence of fine gas bubbles, discoloration, clots, or excessive air in the bag).

Both individuals who verify this information must sign the slip that comes with the blood product. If a discrepancy arises with any of these checks, the blood product is not infused until and unless resolution of the discrepancy occurs.

When it becomes apparent that more blood products will be needed than originally anticipated, the perioperative nurse should request the blood bank prepare a specified number of units in advance of the actual need to transfuse. This procedure allows the blood bank time to crossmatch the units carefully, without rushing and jeopardizing patient safety. Crossmatch requisitions should be sent for any additional units requested. If a significant amount of blood product has been required, a new, properly labeled sample with a blood grouping requisition may be needed to have an adequate sample for crossmatching.

Rapid blood transfusion requires warming of blood products to prevent hypothermia, which may induce cardiac arrest. Blood products should be warmed during passage through the transfusion set. The warming device must incorporate a temperature sensing device and a warning system to detect malfunction to prevent hemolysis or other damage to blood components (Carson et al., 2016). Blood must *never* be warmed in a microwave because its uneven, rapid heating can cause hemolysis. The probability of a transfusion reaction increases in direct proportion to the number of units transfused. The perioperative nurse should remain alert for any signs of reaction, including the following:

- Hyperthermia
- Increased intraoperative bleeding
- Weak pulse
- Hypotension
- Visible hemoglobinuria
- Vasomotor instability
- Greatly decreased or no urinary output

If any such suspicious signs of reaction occur, the perioperative nurse should assist the anesthesia provider to do the following:

- Stop the transfusion. The tubing is disconnected and a new infusion of fluid such as 0.9% sodium chloride is begun to maintain venous access.
- Report the reaction to the surgeon and blood bank immediately.
- Anticipate possible order for stat antihistamines.
- Return the unused portion of the blood product, the IV tubing used during the transfusion, and a properly labeled sample of the patient's blood to the blood bank.
- Send a urine sample to the laboratory if requested.
- Monitor the patient's reaction carefully.
- Complete an incident/occurrence/event report covering the suspected reaction. The report might include time and date of reaction, type and amount of blood/blood product infused, and time the transfusion started and stopped. Signs and symptoms, in the order of occurrence, along with the patient's vital signs, any urine or blood samples sent to the laboratory for analysis, any treatment given, and the patient's response should all be noted. A suspected transfusion reaction report must be sent to the blood bank.

Any unused blood product is returned to the blood bank as soon as the patient leaves the OR. Returned blood can be reissued if it has not been allowed to warm to a temperature greater than 10°C. External blood bag thermometers (e.g., HemoTemp II; Biosynergy, Inc., Elk Grove Village, IL), similar to a skin contact tape thermometer, are used on blood product bags by many blood banks to quickly identify blood that has exceeded safe storage temperatures.

Autotransfusion, the reinfusion of a patient's own blood intraoperatively, once comprised as many as 6% of blood units transfused, but this practice has largely fallen out of favor. Reasons include the difficulties associated with storage and the need to ultimately discard many units (O'Keefe and Rhee, 2014). During intraoperative autotransfusion (cell salvage), blood is collected as it is lost during the surgical procedure and reinfused to the patient after it is filtered or washed. This technique can be lifesaving in emergency situations, as with major trauma, or in procedures with major blood loss, as in liver transplantation. It may also be used for patients who refuse blood based on religious beliefs.

Maintaining Fluid and Electrolyte Balance

The body's fluids and electrolytes play a key role in maintaining homeostasis, transporting necessary oxygen and nourishment to cells, removing waste products of cellular metabolism, and helping to maintain body temperature. Electrolytes are also essential to transmission of nerve impulses, regulation of water distribution, contraction of muscles, generation of adenosine triphosphate (ATP; needed for cellular energy), regulation of acid-base balance, and hemostasis. The intake, distribution, and output of water and electrolytes, regulated by the renal and pulmonary systems, normally maintain fluid and electrolyte balance.

Fluid and electrolyte imbalances may occur rapidly in the surgical patient, and can be caused by numerous factors, including preoperative fluid and food restrictions, intraoperative fluid loss, or the stress of surgery. The surgical patient is unable to regulate body fluid and electrolyte requirements by normal activities of drinking, eating, excreting, and breathing unaided. The perioperative nurse collaborates in monitoring intraoperative fluid and electrolyte status.

Body Fluids

The adult human body is approximately 60% water, although water content varies by age, gender, and body mass. In the elderly, body water content averages 45% to 55% of body weight, whereas it ranges from 70% to 80% in infants. Older adults are at higher risk for fluid imbalance because they have less fluid reserve, whereas the very young are at risk for fluid problems because a greater percentage of their body weight is water. Both age groups have a decreased ability to compensate for fluid loss. Muscular tissue contains more water than the same amount of adipose tissue; men generally have higher water content because they usually have more lean muscle mass than women.

Body fluids are distributed in two main functional compartments, intracellular and extracellular. *Intracellular fluids (ICFs)* are within cell membranes that contain dissolved substances essential to fluid and electrolyte balance and metabolism. ICFs constitute approximately 70% of the body's fluid. Consequently, anything that affects water loss at the intracellular level has significant implications for the entire body. *Extracellular fluids (ECFs)* (30% of the body's fluid) are in compartments outside the cells, including plasma, intravascular fluids, fluids in the gastrointestinal (GI) tract, and CSF.

It has been argued that surgical trauma leads to a shift of fluid volume between the fluid compartments, creating a loss of ECF to a nonanatomical compartment named "the third space." This previously led to recommendations to give up to 15 mL/kg/h the first hour of surgery and thereafter declining amounts of fluid in accordance with algorithms. However, this hypothesis is based on few studies using a specific but flawed method of measurement of the extracellular volume. More recent studies using sounder methods cannot demonstrate any such fluid loss. The concept of a loss to the third space may be abandoned (Voldby and Brandstrup, 2016).

Electrolytes

Electrolytes are found in both ICFs and ECFs. When dissolved in water, electrolytes dissociate into ions and are able to carry an electric charge. Positively charged ions are called cations, and negatively charged ions are called anions.

The electrolytes found in ICFs and ECFs are essentially the same, but concentrations in each compartment differ. The primary ICF cation is potassium, and the primary ECF cation is sodium. The primary ICF anion is phosphate, and the primary ECF anion is chloride. Fluids and electrolytes move between the ICF and ECF spaces to facilitate body processes, such as acid-base balance, tissue oxygenation, response to drug therapies, and response to illness. Diffusion, active transport, and osmosis control these movements.

Diffusion, Active Transport, and Osmosis

Diffusion is movement of molecules from an area of high concentration to one of low concentration. It takes place with or without a membrane separating the concentration gradient. Movement continues until there is an equal concentration of molecules. Diffusion across membranes is particularly important in regulating fluid transport and balance in the body.

Active transport is a process by which molecules move across a cell membrane against a concentration gradient (i.e., from an area of low concentration to an area of high concentration) with the impetus of external energy. A "sodium-potassium pump" moves sodium out of the cell and potassium into the cell to maintain the intracellular and extracellular concentration differences of sodium and potassium. ATP is the energy source for this sodium-potassium pump.

Osmosis is movement of a fluid through a semipermeable membrane from a solution that has a lower solute concentration to one that has a higher solute concentration. The semipermeable membrane prevents movement of solute particles. The concentration of these particles is measured in a unit called the osmole (osm). *Osmolality* is the term used to express the concentration of a solution in milliosmoles per kilogram (mOsm/kg) of water. A solution with the same osmolality as blood plasma is called *isotonic*. Isotonic solutions, such as 0.9% normal saline or lactated Ringer's solution administered IV, prevent the shift of fluid and electrolytes from intracellular compartments. A *hypotonic* IV solution (0.45% saline or 2.5% dextrose) has a lower concentration of solutes than that found in plasma; it moves water into the cells. Administration of a *hypertonic* IV solution (5% dextrose in normal saline or 5% dextrose in lactated Ringer's solution) with a greater concentration of solutes than that of plasma moves water out of the cells.

Preoperative Considerations

Preoperative laboratory analysis of electrolyte levels are checked and abnormalities corrected to within normal limits before surgical procedures, unless the surgery is needed to correct a life-threatening problem. Preexisting conditions, such as diabetes mellitus, liver disease, or renal insufficiency, may worsen with surgical stress, increasing a patient's risk of fluid and electrolyte imbalances. Diagnostic procedures that require the administration of IV dyes may produce osmotic diuresis, with resulting urinary excretion of water and electrolytes. Preoperative steroids or diuretics affect the excretion of water and electrolytes; diuretics, used in the management of hypertension, may cause loss of potassium. Preoperative surgical regimens, such as bowel-cleansing routines, when indicated, may increase fluid loss from the GI tract. Medical management, such as nasogastric (NG) suction, can also affect fluid and electrolyte balance in the surgical patient, as can preoperative fluid restriction (nil per os [NPO]).

Preoperative fluid restrictions are used to reduce nausea, vomiting, and aspiration risks. Many providers are changing this practice as newer anesthetic agents tend to cause less PONV than in the past. Prolonged fluid restrictions may not be necessary in healthy patients before surgery; black coffee or pulp-free juice may be ingested safely 2 to 3 hours before surgery, without an increase in gastric volume. Preoperative carbohydrate drinks are now part of ERAS protocols.

Deficient Fluid Volume

The most common patient problems associated with fluid and electrolyte imbalances during surgery include deficient fluid volume (DFV), water imbalance, and potassium imbalance. DFV is an imbalance in isotonic body fluids related to decreased intravascular, interstitial, or intracellular fluid. Very young and very old surgical patients are affected most rapidly by fluid losses from bleeding; inadequate intake because of NPO status; inadequate IV fluid replacement; excessive cutaneous losses from fever and sweating; fluid losses attributable to bowel obstructions, ascites, or peritonitis; excessive GI losses resulting from diarrhea, vomiting, GI suctioning, or fistulas; evaporation of fluid from the exposed peritoneum during open abdominal surgery; shifting of intravascular fluid into the surgical site; and inhalation of dry gases. Insensible fluid losses cannot be measured directly, and have been overestimated even after extensive dissection of tissue. Intraoperative use of an electrolyte solution, such as lactated Ringer's solution, for fluid replacement can help to correct intraoperative fluid losses when used with a tightly managed protocol. Colloid therapy is the preferred fluid replacement therapy when acute blood loss is below transfusion threshold levels. As much as possible both hypovolemia, and hypervolemia, are avoided to the maximum extent.

The effect of fluid loss on a surgical patient depends on the amount of fluid lost and the speed at which the fluid is lost. A patient who loses a large amount of fluid (>500 mL) or loses fluid rapidly exhibits symptoms of shock; immediate fluid replacement therapy is required. A slow loss of fluid may be compensated through albumin synthesis and erythropoiesis.

Sodium and Water Imbalances

Sodium is a cation in ECF; it plays a major role in maintaining the osmolality and water balance of ECF. Because cell membranes are permeable to water, sodium also affects ICF volume and helps maintain acid-base balance in the body. The sodium-potassium pump plays a vital role in neuromuscular activity.

Hyponatremia (serum sodium level <135 mEq/L) can be caused by increased excretion of sodium with diuretic therapy and the abnormal loss of sodium through NG suctioning. Patients undergoing procedures such as transurethral resection of the prostate (TURP) or similar procedures are at risk for dilutional hyponatremia and volume overload caused by absorption of the irrigation solution used. Given that saline is a good conductor of electrical current, fluids that contain no electrolytes (e.g., glycine, sorbitol, and mannitol) are used to irrigate when using electrical current in tissue dissection during these procedures.

Potassium Imbalances

Potassium is the major ICF cation; it is necessary for contraction of skeletal, smooth, and cardiac muscle. It is also necessary for cardiac contractions and for peristaltic movements of the GI tract. Potassium plays a major role in the transmission of nerve impulses by regulating neuromuscular excitability and in the formation of muscle protein by transporting glucose into the cells with insulin. It is also elemental in maintaining acid-base balance and ICF osmotic pressures.

Hypokalemia (serum potassium concentration <3.5 mEq/L) can occur intraoperatively as a result of suctioning of large amounts of body fluids or using diuretic therapy and other drugs (e.g., mannitol) that increase renal flow. Signs and symptoms of hypokalemia include cardiac effects, such as ectopy, dysrhythmias, conduction abnormalities, and altered sensitivity to digitalis. The neuromuscular effects of hypokalemia include muscle weakness; its smooth muscle effects include gastric distention, paralytic ileus, and urinary retention.

Treatment of hypokalemia includes IV replacement when the deficit is severe, as in the development of cardiovascular or other serious symptoms. Potassium irritates veins on infusion; the infusion site therefore requires monitoring for redness, heat, swelling, and site pain, which are all signs of chemical phlebitis. Overcorrection and subsequent hyperkalemia are avoided by monitoring serum potassium levels at frequent intervals (often every 2–4 hours).

Hyperkalemia (serum potassium level of more than 5 mEq/L) can arise during surgery via massive transfusions of stored blood; decreased excretion of potassium caused by hypovolemia or renal failure; and shifting of potassium from the cells into the ECF caused by acidosis, tissue breakdown from surgery, crush injuries, or burns. Drugs infused during surgery can also induce hyperkalemia; such drugs include antiinflammatory agents, β-adrenergic receptor blockers, digitalis, succinylcholine, heparin, and the penicillins.

Signs and symptoms of hyperkalemia include neuromuscular symptoms such as weakness and paresthesias in the arms and legs. Smooth muscle symptoms include diarrhea and abdominal distention. Excess potassium can cause serious cardiac symptoms such as ventricular dysrhythmias, heart block, and asystole. Cardiac side effects of hyperkalemia are treated by calcium gluconate infusion. Sodium bicarbonate or insulin-glucose infusions can shift ECF potassium into the cells, reducing the plasma's potassium level.

Temperature Control

Monitoring body temperature is an important part of anesthesia monitoring. Standards of care of both the AANA and ASA support monitoring a patient's temperature as essential (Bozimowski, 2014) in maintaining normal ranges (normothermia) for pediatric and adult patients. Hypothermia is the most common disorder of temperature homeostasis and may be intentional or unintentional. Unintentional hypothermia can cause patient discomfort, untoward cardiac events, adrenergic stimulation, impaired platelet function, altered medication metabolism, delayed emergence from anesthesia, and impaired wound healing (Odom-Forren, 2014).

Risk factors for developing unintentional hypothermia include age extremes (elderly and pediatric patients), comorbidity, surgical duration, cachexia, fluid shifts, cold irrigating fluids, and general and regional anesthesia. Agents such as skeletal muscle relaxants interfere with shivering mechanisms. Agents that depress the CNS decrease autonomic reflexes that ordinarily autoregulate body temperature. Vasodilation, which accompanies use of various anesthetic agents, including inhalation agents, enhances heat transfer from the core to the periphery, where it is lost to the atmosphere. Cold,

unhumidified inhalation gases further promote hypothermia through convection and evaporation.

Room temperature can be increased and infrared warming lamps used for pediatric patients. Fresh-gas flow rates of cool, dry anesthetic gases can be lowered. A heat and moisture exchanger (e.g., Humidivent, Hudson-Teleflex Medical, Morrisville, NC) helps maintain the heat and moisture of inspired gases. A variety of IV fluid warmers are available to warm crystalloid solutions or refrigerated blood products. Some warmer units heat fluids at flow rates of 500 mL/min. Forced-air warming devices applied to the upper or lower body are commonly used to keep patients warm and maintain normothermia. Forced-air warming devices must be used according to manufacturers' instructions. They must be used with an appropriate disposable blanket and should *not* have the hose inserted under surgical drapes to warm the patient (this directs the heat on the patient, with the risk of a burn, rather than filtering it through the blanket). The blanket air temperature is typically a few degrees lower than that coming from the hose because heat dissipates as it moves through the blanket.

Malignant Hyperthermia

MH is a rare, life-threatening complication that may arise from medications commonly used in anesthesia. Inhalational anesthetics and succinylcholine are the most frequently implicated triggering agents. Trauma, strenuous exercise, or emotional stress also may induce MH. MH has an autosomal dominant pattern of inheritance, with clinical heterogeneity and variable expression in affected individuals (Wedel, 2015). The incidence of MH increases in patients with central core disease (a congenital myopathy) and some muscular dystrophies; it complicates 1:100,000 adult cases, and 1:30,000 pediatric cases (Karlet and Cahoon, 2014; MHAUS, 2017).

The MH syndrome begins with a hypermetabolic condition in skeletal muscle cells that involves altered mechanisms of calcium function at the cellular level. Characteristics include cellular hypermetabolism resulting in hypercarbia, tachypnea, tachycardia, hypoxia, metabolic and respiratory acidosis, cardiac dysrhythmias, and elevation of body temperature at a rate of 1° to 2°C every 5 minutes. Increase in body temperature is a late manifestation of MH. These signs may occur during induction or maintenance of anesthesia, although MH can occur postoperatively or even after repeated exposures to anesthesia. The signs and symptoms associated with MH appear in Box 5.3.

BOX 5.3

Signs and Symptoms Often Seen With Malignant Hyperthermia

- Hypercarbia
- Tachycardia
- Tachypnea (may not be seen in a paralyzed patient)
- Muscle stiffness or rigidity
- Hypoxia and dark (desaturated) blood in operative field
- Unstable or elevated blood pressure
- Cardiac dysrhythmias
- Changes in CO_2 absorbent (temperature, color)
- Metabolic and respiratory acidosis
- Peripheral mottling, cyanosis, or sweating
- Rising body temperature (1°C–2°C every 5 minutes)
- Myoglobinuria
- Hyperkalemia, hypercalcemia, lactic acidemia
- Pronounced elevation in creatine kinase level

It is important to remember that MH is a rare, multifaceted syndrome and can have variable clinical presentations. Many of the signs and symptoms associated with MH can have other causes. Other disorders, such as neuroleptic malignant syndrome (NMS), may have similar presentations. NMS occurs after use of neuroleptic medications, such as haloperidol, and is characterized by muscular rigidity, akinesia, hyperthermia, and autonomic dysfunction. Because MH is such a life-threatening disorder, many anesthesia providers initiate a treatment protocol when some of these early signs and symptoms occur that cannot otherwise be readily explained.

Time is crucial when MH is diagnosed. All OR and anesthesia personnel should be familiar with the protocol for its management. Immediate infusion of dantrolene (Dantrium, Ryanodex) and proper treatment reduce mortality to about 5%. Dantrolene is a hydantoin skeletal muscle relaxant that also has effects on vascular and heart muscle. In addition to dantrolene, the major modalities of treatment include cooling the patient with ice packs and cold IV solutions, administering diuretics, treating cardiac dysrhythmias, correcting acid-base and electrolyte imbalances, and monitoring fluid intake and output and body temperature.

Many hospitals maintain an emergency MH kit or cart that contains medications, laboratory tubes, other supplies, and instructions to treat MH in the OR area. The location of the iced or cold saline and other equipment also should be listed in the emergency kit. Chilled saline is often kept in the refrigeration unit for blood products (Karlet and Cahoon, 2014; MHAUS, 2017). MHAUS has names of on-call physicians available for consultation in MH emergencies at 1-800-MH-HYPER (1-800-644-9737). For patient-referral or nonemergency calls, 1-607-674-7901 is used.

Patients known or suspected to have MH can be anesthetized with minimal risk if appropriate precautions are taken. If the syndrome is suspected, a muscle biopsy specimen is obtained to make a diagnosis before elective surgery. For their own safety, relatives of persons with MH should be evaluated for the presence of the syndrome (MHAUS, 2017).

Perioperative Nursing Considerations

Care of surgical patients is a cooperative effort, and perioperative personnel function as a smooth, well-coordinated team. As part of conducting the preoperative patient assessment and developing the plan of care, the perioperative nurse participates with the anesthesia provider in the preoperative verification process. As part of this process, the nurse verifies the patient, the surgeon, and the scheduled procedure; confirms that the operative and anesthesia consents are properly signed and dated; identifies and communicates patient allergies; ensures that the surgical site is marked; and ensures that current reports of laboratory tests and diagnostic studies are complete and in the medical record.

In many ORs a preoperative preparation or *holding area* is used for insertion of arterial, central venous, or PACs and placement of epidural catheters or PNBs. Nursing personnel from the OR, PACU, or anesthesia department may staff this area. Its purpose is to improve patient care delivery, optimize flow of patients, and provide supportive patient care.

A patient is never to be left alone in the OR. When an anesthetized patient is in the OR, a perioperative nurse is always immediately available to provide assistance if needed. During insertion of IV, arterial, central venous, or PACs, the nurse assists as required.

During induction of anesthesia, particularly with urgent and emergency surgical procedures, the patient presumptively has a "full stomach." The perioperative nurse should be ready to apply cricoid pressure to prevent regurgitation of stomach contents and to assist the anesthesia provider in visualizing the vocal cords. When cricoid pressure is used to prevent aspiration, it should not be released until completion of intubation, inflation of the cuff on the ETT, and proper placement of the ETT. When two anesthesia providers are present, one usually provides this support.

The OR team never moves an unconscious patient without first coordinating the positioning or move with the anesthesia provider. When the patient is positioned for surgery, the perioperative nurse collaborates with the anesthesia provider to check the arms and legs to ensure that no pressure points exist and that the extremities are appropriately positioned and padded (see Chapter 6). After positioning, prepping, and draping, the time-out is conducted and documented.

Before transporting the patient from the OR to the PACU, the circulating nurse often calls the PACU to give a preliminary status report. This report, like the anesthesia provider's hand-off report, includes the surgical procedure performed, type of anesthesia provided, information specific to the patient's preoperative diagnosis and subsequent outcome(s) related to intraoperative interventions, and any special equipment required (e.g., ventilator, T-piece, arterial pressure monitor). PACU care and functions are described in Chapter 10.

Key Points

- Without anesthesia, most modern surgical procedures would not be feasible.
- In the United States, anesthesia care may be provided by (1) an anesthesiologist; (2) a CRNA working alone, in collaboration with, or under the direction of an anesthesiologist or a physician; or (3) an AA working under direct supervision of an anesthesiologist.
- Patient safety is always a primary concern during anesthesia.
- IOA has been reported with multiple and differing anesthetic techniques.
- POCD is an emerging issue for mature patients.
- Preoperative evaluation for anesthesia is done in advance of the scheduled procedure.
- The patient, anesthesia provider, and surgeon make the choice of anesthesia for a given surgical procedure. Many factors influence this choice.
- Premedication is given before anesthesia to lightly sedate the patient and reduce anxiety.
- Patients may receive, in any setting, moderate sedation/analgesia, general, spinal, major regional anesthesia, or local anesthesia.
- There are many theories as to how general anesthesia works.
- Patients are monitored with various devices during anesthesia.
- Muscle relaxants (also referred to as NMBDs) are used to facilitate intubation and provide good operating conditions at lighter levels of general anesthesia.
- Patients with OSA who are undergoing procedures that require sedation, anesthesia, and/or analgesia are at higher risk for complications than patients who do not have OSA.
- Perioperative nurses have many important responsibilities when assessing and monitoring patients undergoing any type of anesthesia.

Critical Thinking Questions

Your next patient for surgery is listed as a 67-year-old male for laparoscopic-assisted sigmoid resection for diverticulitis. He has a history of OSA and prior difficult intubation noted in his medical record. Your preoperative interview reveals that he has not been compliant with his CPAP therapy. You also elicit information that he finds himself sleeping a lot during the day, has trouble focusing on his work, and is more forgetful than before. He is 5'9" and weighs 265 lb for a BMI of 39. What factors would you consider in your plan of care that is influenced by this history? How will your plan address potential issues that the anesthesia provider will face when inducing this patient before attempting an intubation? What equipment and supplies will be needed in the OR and on an "kept ready" basis to prepare for this procedure? What other nursing interventions will you consider and how will the actual surgical procedure affect your patient's care?

℮volve *The answers to the Critical Thinking Questions can be found at http://evolve.elsevier.com/Rothrock/Alexander.*

References

American Association of Moderate Sedation Nurses (AAMSN) *Registered nurse (CSRN) scope of practice* (website), 2016. http://aamsn.org/resources/pdfs/sedation-related-pdfs/registered-nurse-csrn-scope-of-practice. (Accessed 5 January 2017).

American Association of Nurse Anesthetists: *AANA announces support of doctorate for entry into nurse anesthesia practice by 2025* (website), 2016. www.aana.com/newsandjournal/News/Pages/092007-AANA-Announces-Support-of-Doctorate-for-Entry-into-Nurse-Anesthesia-Practice-by-2025.aspx. (Accessed 5 January 2017).

American Society of Anesthesiologists (ASA): Practice guidelines for preoperative fasting and the use of pharmacologic agents to reduce the risk of pulmonary aspiration: application to healthy patients undergoing elective procedures: an updated report by the American Society of Anesthesiologists Task Force on Preoperative Fasting and the Use of Pharmacologic Agents to Reduce the Risk of Pulmonary Aspiration, *Anesthesiology* 126(3):376–393, 2017.

Apfelbaum JL et al: Practice advisory for the prevention and management of operating room fires: an updated report by the American Society of Anesthesiologists Task Force on Operating Room Fires, *Anesthesiology* 118(2):271–290, 2013.

Armendi A et al: A randomized, single-blinded, prospective study that compares complications between cuffed and uncuffed nasal endotracheal tubes of different sizes and brands in pediatric patients, *J Clin Anesth* 27(3):221–225, 2015.

Aronson JK: *Meyler's side effects of drugs*, ed 16, Waltham, MA, 2016, Elsevier.

Association of periOperative Registered Nurses (AORN): *Guidelines for perioperative practice*, Denver, 2017, The Association.

Avidan MS, Mashour GA: Prevention of intraoperative awareness with explicit recall: making sense of the evidence, *Anesthesiology* 118(2):449–456, 2013.

Barak M et al: Airway management of the patient with maxillofacial trauma: review of the literature and suggested clinical approach, *Biomed Res Int* 724032:2015, 2015.

Blitz JD: Preoperative evaluation clinic visit is associated with decreased risk of in-hospital postoperative mortality, *Anesthesiology* 125(2):280–294, 2016.

Bordi SK: Pain management. In Nagelhout JJ, Plaus KL, editors: *Nurse anesthesia*, ed 5, St Louis, 2014, Saunders.

Bosson N: *Laryngeal mask airway* (website), 2016. www.emedicine.medscape.com/article/82527-overview. (Accessed 5 January 2017).

Bozimowski G: Clinical monitoring II: respiratory and metabolic systems. In Nagelhout JJ, Plaus KL, editors: *Nurse anesthesia*, ed 5, St Louis, 2014, Saunders.

Brenner G: *Pharmacology*, ed 4, Philadelphia, 2013, Saunders Elsevier.

Breyer K, Gropper M: Preparation of the surgical patient. In Cameron J, editor: *Current surgical therapy*, ed 11, Philadelphia, 2014, Saunders.

Carson JL et al: Clinical practice guidelines from the AABB: red blood cell transfusion thresholds and storage, *JAMA* 316(19):2025–2035, 2016.

Carvalho B, Butwick A: Postoperative analgesia. In Chestnut D et al, editors: *Chestnut's obstetric anesthesia: principles and practice*, ed 5, Philadelphia, 2014, Saunders.

Clark GD, Curdt NC: Clinical monitoring III: neurologic system. In Nagelhout JJ, Plaus KL, editors: *Nurse anesthesia*, ed 5, St Louis, 2014, Saunders.

Contrera MA et al: Anesthesia for cardiac surgery. In Nagelhout JJ, Plaus KL, editors: *Nurse anesthesia*, ed 5, St Louis, 2014, Saunders.

Dosch M: Anesthesia equipment. In Nagelhout JJ, Plaus KL, editors: *Nurse anesthesia*, ed 5, St Louis, 2014, Saunders.

Duke J: *Anesthesia secrets*, ed 5, St Louis, 2016, Mosby.

Elkins M et al: Transfusion medicine. In McPherson R, Pincus M, editors: *Henry's clinical diagnosis management by laboratory methods*, ed 23, St Louis, 2017, Elsevier.

Fan B et al: An intelligent decision system for intraoperative somatosensory evoked potential monitoring, *IEEE Trans Neural Syst Rehabil Eng* 24(2):300–307, 2016.

Fencl JL: Guideline implementation: moderate sedation/analgesia, *AORN J* 103(5):500–511, 2016.

Fencl JL: Local anesthetic systemic toxicity, *AORN J* 101(6):111–116, 2015.

Fenner K: *Nine common traits of organizations experiencing CMS scrutiny* (website), 2016. www.beckershospitalreview.com/quality/nine-common-traits-of-organizations-experiencing-cms-scrutiny.html. (Accessed 5 January 2017).

Food and Drug Administration (FDA): *FDA Drug Safety Communication: FDA review results in new warning about using general anesthetics and sedation drugs in young children and pregnant women* (website), 2016. www.fda.gov/Drugs/DrugSafety/ucm532356.htm. (Accessed 5 January 2017).

Garcia P et al: Intravenous anesthetics. In Hemmings H, Talmage D, editors: *Pharmacology and physiology for anesthesia*, Philadelphia, 2013, Saunders.

Goswami S et al: Anesthesia for robotically conducted surgery. In Miller RD, editor: *Miller's anesthesia*, ed 8, Philadelphia, 2015, Saunders.

Gregory TB: Hydromorphone: evolving to meet the challenges of today's health care environment, *Clin Ther* 35:2007–2027, 2013.

Hagberg CA: *Benumof and Hagberg's airway management*, ed 3, Philadelphia, 2013, Elsevier Saunders.

Hasfeldt D et al: Patients' perception of noise in the operating room—a descriptive and analytic cross-sectional study, *J Perianesth Nurs* 29(5):410–4177, 2014.

Heiner JS, Gabot MH: Airway management. In Nagelhout JJ, Plaus KL, editors: *Nurse anesthesia*, ed 5, St Louis, 2014, Saunders.

Hernandez A, Sherwood E: Anesthesiology principles, pain management, and conscious sedation. In Townsend CM et al, editors: *Sabiston textbook of surgery*, ed 20, Philadelphia, 2017, Elsevier.

Karlet MC, Cahoon TM: Musculoskeletal system anatomy, physiology, pathophysiology, and anesthesia management. In Nagelhout JJ, Plaus KL, editors: *Nurse anesthesia*, ed 5, St Louis, 2014, Saunders.

Kim KN et al: Optimal precurarizing dose of rocuronium to decrease fasciculation and myalgia following succinylcholine administration, *Korean J Anesthesiology* 66(6):451–456, 2014.

Kossick MA: Clinical monitoring: cardiovascular system. In Nagelhout JJ, Plaus KL, editors: *Nurse anesthesia*, ed 5, St Louis, 2014, Mosby.

Liau A, Havidich J: *An overview of adverse events in the National Anesthesia Clinical Outcomes Registry (NACOR)* (website), 2014. www.asaabstracts.com/strands/asaabstracts/searchresults.htm?base=1&index=1&display=10&highlight=true&highlightcolor=0&bold=true&italic=false. (Accessed 5 January 2017).

Malignant Hyperthermia Association of the United States (MHAUS): *Homepage* (website), 2017. www.mhaus.org. (Accessed 5 January 2017).

Marley RA, Calabrese T: Outpatient anesthesia. In Nagelhout JJ, Plaus KL, editors: *Nurse anesthesia*, ed 5, St Louis, 2014, Saunders.

Merck & Co: *Sugammadex (Bridion) injection package insert* (website), 2015. www.merck.com/product/usa/pi_circulars/b/bridion/bridion_pi.pdf. (Accessed 5 January 2017).

Miller RD: *Miller's anesthesia*, ed 8, Philadelphia, 2015, Saunders.

Motamed C, Duvaldestin P: The effect of defasciculating doses of pancuronium and atracurium on succcinylcholine neuromuscular blockade, *Anesth Pain Med* 4(4):e18488, 2014.

Nagelhout JJ: Neuromuscular blocking agents, reversal agents and their monitoring. In Nagelhout JJ, Plaus KL, editors: *Nurse anesthesia*, ed 5, St Louis, 2014, Saunders.

Neal JM et al: The Second American Society of Regional Anesthesia and Pain Medicine Evidence-Based Medicine Assessment of Ultrasound-Guided

Regional Anesthesia: executive summary, *Reg Anesth Pain Med* 41(2):181–194, 2016.

Odom-Forren J: Postanesthesia recovery. In Nagelhout JJ, Plaus KL, editors: *Nurse anesthesia*, ed 5, St Louis, 2014, Saunders.

O'Keefe T, Rhee P: Blood transfusion therapy in trauma. In Cameron J, editor: *Current surgical therapy*, ed 11, Philadelphia, 2014, Saunders.

Olson RL et al: Regional anesthesia: spinal and epidural anesthesia. In Nagelhout JJ, Plaus KL, editors: *Nurse anesthesia*, ed 5, St Louis, 2014, Elsevier Saunders.

Perel A, et al: Family member presence during induction of anesthesia in elderly patients—a feasibility study, *Eur J Anaesthesiol* 24(Suppl 39):190, 2007.

Putnam K: Guideline for care of the patient receiving moderate sedation, *AORN J* 102(5):P10–P12, 2015.

Ranalli LJ, Taylor GA: Neuroanatomy, neurophysiology and neuroanesthesia. In Nagelhout JJ, Plaus KL, editors: *Nurse anesthesia*, ed 5, St Louis, 2014, Saunders.

Rang HP et al: Local anaesthetics and other drugs affecting sodium channels. In Rang HP et al, editors: *Rang & Dale's pharmacology*, ed 8, Philadelphia, 2016, Elsevier.

Rhee P, Bellal J: Shock, electrolytes, and fluid. In Townsend CM et al, editors: *Sabiston textbook of surgery*, ed 20, Philadelphia, 2017, Elsevier.

Rieker M: Anesthesia for thoracic surgery. In Nagelhout JJ, Plaus KL, editors: *Nurse anesthesia*, ed 5, St Louis, 2014, Saunders.

Ruskin KJ, Hueske-Kraus D: Alarm fatigue: impacts on patient safety, *Curr Opin Anaesthesiol* 28(6):685–690, 2015.

Sevoflurane (website), 2016. www.drugs.com/pro/sevoflurane.html. (Accessed 5 January 2017).

Shastri U et al: Lower extremity nerve blocks. In Benzon HT et al, editors: *Practical management of pain*, ed 5, Philadelphia, 2014, Mosby.

Shilling AM et al: Anesthesia and perioperative medicine. In Miller MD, Thompson SR, editors: *DeLee & Drez's orthopaedic sports medicine*, ed 4, Philadelphia, 2015, Saunders.

Sofaer S, Schumann MJ: *Fostering successful patient and family engagement: nursing's critical role* (website), 2013. www.naqc.org/WhitePaper-PatientEngagement. (Accessed 17 June 2016).

Teleflex Medical. *Instructions for use—LMA Supreme* (website), 2015. www.lmaco-ifu.com/sites/default/files/node/440/ifu/revision/3596/ifu-lma-supreme-paj2100002buk.pdf. (Accessed 5 January 2017).

Vacchiano A, Biegner A: Regional anesthesia: upper and lower extremity blocks. In Nagelhout JJ, Plaus KL, editors: *Nurse anesthesia*, ed 5, St Louis, 2014, Saunders.

Voldby AW, Brandstrup B: Fluid therapy in the perioperative setting—a clinical review, *J Intensive Care* 4:27, 2016.

Wedel DJ: Malignant hyperthermia. In Murray MJ et al, editors: *Faust's anesthesiology review*, ed 4, Philadelphia, 2015, Elsevier.

Weinberg G: Lipid emulsion infusion: resuscitation for local anesthetic and other drug overdose, *Anesthesiology* 117(1):180–187, 2012.

Wijeysundera DN, Sweitzer BJ: Preoperative evaluation. In Miller RD, editor: *Miller's anesthesia*, ed 8, Philadelphia, 2015, Elsevier Saunders.

CHAPTER 6

Positioning the Patient for Surgery

DEBRA L. FAWCETT

Proper patient positioning is imperative for safe, successful surgery. The surgical team pays close attention to the physiologic and physical consequences of the position the patient is placed in for the procedure. Given that surgery may be performed on all anatomic areas, patient positioning may result in multiple and sometimes unnatural body positions to provide optimal exposure to a surgical site. Positioning, combined with anesthesia and its physiologic effects, can yield undesirable changes if safety factors are not considered a paramount patient safety outcome. This chapter discusses major risks and preventive strategies associated with standard surgical positions.

The goals of surgical positioning include providing optimal exposure and access to the surgical site, maintaining body alignment, supporting circulatory and respiratory function, protecting neuromuscular and skin integrity, and allowing access to intravenous (IV) sites and anesthesia monitoring devices. Meeting these goals while ensuring patient comfort and safety is the responsibility of every member of the surgical team.

Anatomic and Physiologic Considerations

The perioperative nurse must understand the anatomic and physiologic changes associated with positioning the patient. These changes are affected by numerous factors, including the type of surgical position; the length of time the patient is in that position; the operating room (OR) bed, padding, and positioning devices used; the type of anesthesia given; and the operative procedure. These changes most frequently affect (1) the skin and underlying tissue; (2) the musculoskeletal system; (3) the nervous system; (4) the cardiovascular system; (5) the respiratory system; and (6) other vulnerable areas, such as the eyes, breasts, perineum, and fingers.

Skin and Underlying Tissue

Physical forces used to establish and maintain a surgical position can injure the skin and underlying tissue. These forces include *pressure, shear, microclimate,* and *friction.* Additionally, OR conditions such as *moisture, heat, cold,* and *negativity* further increase the vulnerability of the skin and underlying tissues to injury.

Pressure is the force placed on underlying tissue. Pressure comes from the weight of the body as gravity presses it downward toward the surface of the OR bed. Pressure can also come from the weight of equipment resting on or against the patient, such as drills, Mayo stands, surgical instruments, rigid edges of the OR bed or its attachments, or vertical posts for self-retaining retractors. Positioning devices, such as stirrup bars, leg or arm holders, and edges of laminectomy frames, can rest or press against the patient. Team members can also put pressure on the patient by leaning or pressing down during the procedure.

Shear is the folding of underlying tissue when the skeletal structure moves while the skin remains stationary. A parallel force creates

shear while a perpendicular force creates pressure (Fig. 6.1). This can happen when the head of the bed is raised or lowered and when the patient is placed in Trendelenburg (head down, supine) or reverse Trendelenburg (head up, supine) position. As gravity pulls the skeleton, the stretching, folding, and tearing of the underlying tissues as they slide with the skeleton occlude vascular perfusion, which can lead to tissue ischemia.

Microclimate is defined as the external climate between the patient and support surface. It includes the amount of moisture and temperature between the skin/body and the surface it is on (NPUAP, 2014).

Friction is the force of two surfaces rubbing against one another. Friction on the patient's skin occurs when the body is dragged across the OR bed linen instead of being lifted. Friction can denude the epidermis and make the skin more susceptible to higher stages of pressure injury (PI), pain, and infection.

Moisture weakens the cell wall of individual skin cells and begins to change the pH of the skin, leading to potential weakness of the skin and underlying tissues. Maceration can occur when prolonged moisture on the skin saturates the epidermis to the point that the connective tissue fibers dissolve and can be torn apart easily. As the epidermis erodes, it leaves the dermis at risk and more likely to incur PI. In surgery, skin maceration occurs if the patient perspires or is allowed to lie in a pool of prep solution, blood, irrigation solution, urine, or feces. If friction occurs on macerated skin, it becomes more vulnerable to denuding into the dermal layer. Every effort should be made to avoid pooling of fluids under the patient. Prolonged

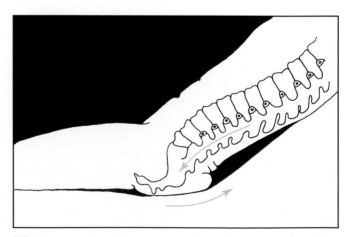

FIG. 6.1 Shearing force. As gravity forces the vertebral column downward, skin adhering to the surface counters and resists that force. The result is folding and compression of tissue in between.

exposure to chemicals in the skin prep solution under the pressure area also can increase the likelihood of chemically induced contact dermatitis.

Heat on the body surface increases tissue metabolism and increases oxygen and nutritional demands. If tissue is also under pressure, constriction of vessels tends to impede blood flow enough so that those demands are not met. Preexisting vascular impairment and the hypotensive effects of anesthesia may harm tissue further and lead to cellular tissue damage. Excessive heat can cause thermal damage as well, resulting in burns.

Cold environmental conditions, such as those found in the OR, can lead to perioperative hypothermia. Major surgery can cool the patient further by exposing the core of the body to cold air. A cold core temperature can reduce peripheral circulation, reducing oxygen delivery to the skin and underlying tissue.

Negativity occurs when layers of materials, such as extra sheets or blankets, are placed over the OR mattress or padding. Extra linen can add rigidity and diminish the pressure-reducing properties of the mattress or padding. Such linen is absorbent and abrasive and can produce high and inconsistent pressure. Eliminating extra layers of material between the patient and the OR bed can reduce sacral pressure readings.

Interface pressure refers to the force per unit area that acts perpendicularly between the body and a support surface (NPUAP, 2014).

Pressure Injury

In 2016 the National Pressure Ulcer Advisory Panel (NPUAP) revised the definition and stages of a PI (Edsberg et al., 2016) (Table 6.1). The term *pressure ulcer* was replaced with the term *pressure injury*. This revision was undertaken to incorporate current understanding of the etiology of pressure injuries as well as to clarify the anatomical features present or absent in each stage of the injury (Edsberg et al., 2016). The change more accurately reflects injuries to both intact and ulcerated skin from undue pressure. In the OR a PI may occur but not be visible for several days after the surgical procedure.

NPUAP defines a PI as localized damage to the skin and/or underlying soft tissues, usually over a bony prominence or related to a medical or other device (NPUAP, 2016). The injury can present as intact skin or as an open ulcer, and it may be painful. The injury occurs as a result of intense and/or prolonged pressure or pressure in combination with shear. The tolerance of soft tissue for pressure and shear may also be affected by microclimate, nutrition, perfusion, comorbidities, and the condition of the soft tissues before the procedure (Edsberg et al., 2016).

The incidence of PI in the OR is difficult to measure with certainty in both inpatient and ambulatory surgery settings (Ambulatory Surgery Considerations). Reported ranges vary from under 1% up to 57%. The reason for the large span in ranges of PI incidence is that the actual rates are unknown. Many facilities do not yet track

---

TABLE 6.1

National Pressure Ulcer Advisory Panel Guidelines for Staging Pressure Injuries

Stage/Category	Definition
DTPI	Purple or maroon localized area of discolored intact skin or blood-filled blister caused by damage of underlying soft tissue from pressure and/or shear; the area may be preceded by tissue that is painful, firm, mushy, boggy, warmer, or cooler compared with adjacent tissue; DTPI may be difficult to detect in individuals with dark skin tones; evolution may include a thin blister over a dark wound bed; the wound may further evolve and become covered by thin eschar; evolution may be rapid, exposing additional layers of tissue even with optimal treatment
Stage 1	Intact skin with nonblanchable redness of a localized area usually over a bony prominence; darkly pigmented skin may not have visible blanching; its color may differ from the surrounding area; the area may be painful, firm, soft, warmer, or cooler compared with adjacent tissue; stage I may be difficult to detect in individuals with dark skin tones; may indicate "at-risk" persons
Stage 2	Partial-thickness loss of dermis presenting as a shallow open ulcer with a red-pink wound bed, without slough; may also present as an intact or open/ruptured serum-filled or serosanguineous-filled blister; presents as a shiny or dry shallow ulcer without slough or bruising[a]; this category should not be used to describe skin tears, tape burns, incontinence-associated dermatitis, maceration, or excoriation
Stage 3	Full-thickness tissue loss; subcutaneous fat may be visible, but bone, tendon, or muscle is *not* exposed; slough may be present but does not obscure the depth of tissue loss; *may* include undermining and tunneling; the depth of a stage 3 PI varies by anatomic location; the bridge of the nose, ear, occiput, and malleolus do not have (adipose) subcutaneous tissue, and stage 3 PIs can be shallow; in contrast, areas of significant adiposity can develop in extremely deep category/stage 3 PIs; bone/tendon is not visible or directly palpable
Stage 4	Full-thickness tissue loss with exposed bone, tendon, or muscle; slough or eschar may be present; often includes undermining and tunneling; the depth of a category/stage 4 PI varies by anatomic location; the bridge of the nose, ear, occiput, and malleolus do not have (adipose) subcutaneous tissue, and these PIs can be shallow; stage 4 PIs can extend into muscle and/or supporting structures (e.g., fascia, tendon, joint capsule) making osteomyelitis or osteitis likely to occur; exposed bone/muscle is visible or directly palpable
Unstageable pressure injury	Full-thickness tissue loss in which actual depth of the PI is completely obscured by slough (yellow, tan, gray, green, or brown) and/or eschar (tan, brown, or black) in the wound bed; until enough slough and/or eschar is removed to expose the base of the wound, the true depth cannot be determined, but it will be either a stage 3 or 4; stable (dry, adherent, intact without erythema or fluctuance) eschar on the heels serves as the body's natural (biologic) "cover" and should not be removed

[a]Bruising indicates deep tissue pressure injury.
DTPI, Deep tissue pressure injury; *PI*, pressure injury.
Modified from National Pressure Ulcer Advisory Panel (NPUAP): *NPUAP pressure injury stages* (website), 2016. www.npuap.org/resources/educational-and-clinical-resources/npuap-pressure-injury-stages/. (Accessed 30 December 2016). Used with permission of the National Pressure Ulcer Advisory Panel.

Hospital-Acquired Pressure Injuries in Ambulatory Surgery Settings

There is an increasing number of traditionally complex surgical procedures previously performed in inpatient settings that have moved to ambulatory surgery settings. Because of this increase, patients may present with more comorbidities, higher ASA physical status scores, and surgery may last longer. Data on the development of HAPIs note that they may not manifest until days after surgical procedures. Ambulatory surgery patients are most often discharged on the day of surgery, making collection of data on HAPI rates difficult.

In this quality improvement strategy, the authors proposed a three-prong approach to identifying ambulatory surgery patients at risk for PI and following up with them regarding HAPI. The preoperative risk factor score, using the Munro Pressure Ulcer Risk Assessment Scale for Adult Perioperative patients, is determined (see Table 6.2) as the first component. The second is provision of patient, family, and caregiver discharge instructions that delineate how to identify PIs and what information should be reported to a healthcare provider. Third, patients previously identified as high risk for PI are queried about their skin condition at areas subject to pressure during intraoperative and postoperative positioning during postoperative telephone calls. This allows an additional opportunity to identify early problems and make appropriate referrals.

ASA, American Society of Anesthesiologists; *HAPI,* hospital-acquired pressure injury.
Modified from Fuzy KM, Vega RA: Hospital-acquired pressure ulcers in the ambulatory surgical setting, *AORN J* 103(2):224–228, 2016.

incidence of PIs originating in the OR. As early as 2008, the Centers for Medicare and Medicaid Services (CMS, 2008) decided to end reimbursement to hospitals for many preventable hospital-acquired conditions broadly described as "never events." These never events are classified as adverse events that are clearly identifiable and measurable, serious, and usually preventable. Among these conditions are stage 3 or 4 PIs that develop after admission (AHRQ, 2016). It has been estimated the cost of PIs to the US healthcare system is about $11 billion per year (Lupe et al., 2013). That cost does not include the cost of the pain and suffering that the patient undergoes after developing a PI.

Risk Factors for Pressure Injury. During surgical procedures, the patient is immobile, unable to reposition for comfort or complain of discomfort. Further, the surgical team positions the patient and preps and drapes the patient so that areas of pressure are not visible. There are both extrinsic and intrinsic risk factors associated with the development of PIs in the OR.

Extrinsic Factors. PI in the OR usually results from undesirable, but usually necessary, body positioning, extended length of time on the OR bed, inadequate padding/protection, and possibly from use of positioning devices (Black et al., 2014). Other factors that may increase the risk of PI include heat, shear, microclimate, friction, and mechanical pressure (Black et al., 2014). As duration of pressure increases, the likelihood of PI also increases.

One source of mechanical pressure includes the OR bed because it is made for utility and not for comfort. The perioperative nurse, therefore, must have an understanding of the OR mattress/surface on which a patient is lying and its abilities to redistribute and reduce pressure. OR mattresses/surfaces should allow some concavity of

the patient into the surface. In other words, the perioperative nurse needs to confirm that a patient lying on the mattress surface does or does not sink into the surface so that more body is touching the surface, therefore, increasing the ability to reduce/redistribute pressure. In years past, the OR mattress/surface for the most part was made of 2-inch thick material covered with a black elastic covering that could withstand multiple cleanings and uses. Newer surfaces are often made of a combination of materials that have a greater ability to reduce and redistribute pressure. Another factor when looking at mattresses/surfaces in the OR is the age of the surface. The older the surface being used, the more likely that pressure redistribution/reduction will be less than optimal. Installing new OR mattresses/surfaces in the OR is an added expense, but the cost of treatment of an OR-acquired PI can be even more expensive (Scott, 2016).

Many positioning devices have not been tested for pressure redistribution or the ability to sustain pressure for extended periods of time. Devices such as the Bookwalter retractor can cause deep tissue pressure injury (DTPI) because it is pressed into the side of the patient by the support bars. Mayo stands can cause pressure to the legs, knees, and feet if they rest on them for long periods of time. The surgical position can lead to increased risk of a PI and indeed surgical team members can contribute to a PI if they lean on the patient during a procedure.

Microclimate is the temperature of the body and the amount of moisture between the skin/body and the mattress/support surface it is on. Moisture develops both from perspiration of the patient and from the use of fluids. Temperature and moisture changes in the OR occur through radiation, conduction, convection, and evaporation. It is important to remember this because in the OR, anesthesia providers partly maintain thermoregulation of the patient. Body temperature can be influenced through artificial means such as forced-air warming devices, cooled/warmed IV fluids, mechanical ventilation, and temperature of the room, and possibly by impermeable surgical drapes on the patient. There are also sources of moisture to consider such as irrigation fluids, wound drainage, and blood loss. Moisture, such as from prep solutions, weakens the cell wall of the skin and changes the pH of the skin (Giachetta-Ryan, 2015). Shear and friction forces may increase when the skin is overhydrated. Exposure to one or a combination of these factors can cause skin injury (Campbell et al., 2016).

Intrinsic Factors. Intrinsic factors can lower a patient's tissue tolerance to pressure and decrease the time and pressure required for tissue breakdown. Certain preexisting conditions are regarded as intrinsic risk factors for OR-induced PI development. These conditions include diabetes mellitus, age, peripheral vascular disease, cerebrovascular disease, malignancy, sepsis, hypotension, malnutrition (serum albumin levels <3.5 g/dL), body size (obesity as well as thin, frail build; body mass index [BMI] <19 or >40), weight loss in the 2 weeks before surgery, impaired mobility, certain medications (such as vasopressors and corticosteroids), smoking, fractures, and low hemoglobin or hematocrit levels (Black et al., 2014; Giachetta-Ryan, 2015; Minnich et al., 2014; Scott, 2016).

The first step in preventing a PI in a surgical patient is to assess risk. When patients are identified as "at risk" for a PI, additional interventions may reduce the risk (Black et al., 2014) (Research Highlight).

Two tools developed for the perioperative setting are the Munro Scale and the Scott Triggers tool. The Munro Scale can be used to identify patients at risk for PI and is geared toward the adult population. The Munro Scale is a standardized risk assessment tool. It

RESEARCH HIGHLIGHT ▎▎

Predisposing Factors for Intraoperative Pressure Injuries

In this study, researchers reported on their retrospective review of the charts of 222 surgical patients who underwent surgery of at least 2 hours' duration. The authors isolated the following factors: (1) length of procedure, (2) comorbidities, (3) intraoperative position, (4) surgery type, and (5) pressure ulcer (hereinafter called "pressure injury" or "PI" to conform to current, accepted terminology) location. Their overall conclusions were that PIs are overly costly, debilitating, and potentially avoidable surgical complications.

First discussing "materials and methods," the authors noted that they isolated and analyzed 812 unique patients, of whom they deemed 222 to meet the inclusion criteria. Those criteria were (a) PI appraised as related to the intraoperative period, (b) age less than 80 years (to avoid "general frailty" as the main cause of PI development as opposed to surgical environment), and (c) procedure length longer than 2 hours. The procedure length chosen avoided those thought to be too brief to form a PI.

Next, the authors outlined their results and discussed each. Their study cohort of 222 surgical patients included 68% men and 32% women; mean age was 57.5 years; age range was 18 to 80 years; and the racial composition was 68.5% white, 6.8% African American, and 20.3% unknown.

The *length of procedure* was the first factor addressed. As time increases, there is a greater impact on PI development because there is a greater potential for pressure on vulnerable bony prominences. PIs can develop in as little as $2\frac{1}{2}$ hours of surgery as reported in the literature. In the data of these 222 patients, PIs developed in a mean surgical time of just short of 4 hours, with a range of 2 to 15 hours (2 hours' surgery duration was the minimum time for the inclusion criteria). The highest number of procedures saw development of PIs between 2 and 4 hours (42.3%). Both the literature and the study recommend repositioning every 2 to 3 hours when possible.

Second, the effect of *patient comorbidities* on PI development remained unclear. Some literature reviewed suggested that there was no meaningful correlation between comorbidities and PI development. Other studies hypothesized that diabetes, hypertension, respiratory disease, and vascular disease predispose patients to PI development caused by tissue hypoperfusion. The authors noted their own review results for the four highest incidences of comorbidities as hypertension (67 or 30%), cardiac disease (62 or 28%), diabetes (55 or 25%), and respiratory disease (49 or 22%). Cancer, malnutrition, and paraplegia/

quadriplegia made up the remainder of comorbidities (64 or 29%). The numbers and percentages of comorbidities total more than 222 patients and 100% because many patients presented with more than one comorbidity, each of which counted as a comorbidity.

Third, the *intraoperative positions* of the patients were supine, prone, lateral, lithotomy, and sitting. In the literature, the supine position was most implicated in PI development, mainly in the occiput (back of head), hips, sacrum/coccyx, and heels. For the authors, supine position was consistent with this view: 189 of 222 patients (85%) developed PIs intraoperatively after supine-positioned surgery; most patients were supine positioned in surgery in their sample.

Fourth, the *types of surgery* most implicated in the literature for the development of PIs were cardiac, thoracic, orthopedic, and general vascular procedures. The most prevalent as reported by the researchers was abdominal surgery (98 or 44%), followed by much smaller numbers for noncardiac thoracic, orthopedic, trauma/burn, neurologic, and cardiac surgeries. The authors linked the high prevalence of abdominal surgeries to tissue hypoperfusion at the bony prominences of the occiput, hips, sacrum/coccyx, and heels over extended time while in supine position.

Last, the *location of PIs* depends on type of surgery, length of surgery, and surgical position, per the authors. Areas of vulnerability are tissues over bony prominences directly exposed to pressure over long periods. Most often found in this study were PIs at the sacrum/coccyx (86 of 222 or 39%). Other PIs in descending order of frequency included buttocks, penile, heels, scrotal area, head, lower extremity, and other areas. It correlated well with other studies that highly implicated the sacrum/coccyx and buttocks regions as PI locales.

The authors concluded with the following recommendations. The OR team should develop a scoring algorithm to identify major PI risks. This would be based on age (>50), length of surgery (>4 hours), relevant comorbidities (diabetes, hypertension, nonspecific cardiac disease, and respiratory disease), and type of surgery (abdominal, cardiac, and orthopedic). The OR team should identify at-risk patients during the time-out and all handoffs. There should be improved follow-up of PIs because lesions can develop up to 48 hours postoperatively. When possible, the OR team should implement physical interventions to alleviate continuous pressure during surgery.

Modified from Lumbley JL et al: Retrospective review of predisposing factors for intraoperative pressure ulcer development, *J Clin Anesth* 26(5):368–374, 2014.

scores patient risk during each phase of the surgical procedure and aims to enhance communication at each level of care through a cumulative score for each phase. The risk factors are noted in Table 6.2. General intraoperative factors include type of anesthesia, hypotension, length of surgical procedure, and blood loss. Specific intraoperative risk factors include use of positioning accessories, moisture under or on the patient, and friction and sheer during transfers (Mathias, 2015). The Munro Scale has undergone several rounds of Delphi study to reach consensus on its content. It has completed an implementation study and is undergoing validity studies.

The Scott Triggers tool identifies high-risk patients by evaluating four nurse-designed, evidenced-based predictors of perioperative PI:

(1) age ≥62, (2) serum albumin level <3.5 g/dL, (3) ASA physical status score ≥3 (see Chapter 5), and (4) a surgical procedure lasting longer than 3 hours (Meehan et al., 2016; Scott, 2016).

Although not specifically developed for the perioperative setting, the Braden Scale may also be used as a preoperative baseline for predicting at-risk perioperative patients (Research Highlight).

Assessment for PI risk factors and development should be done consistently and be aimed at three periods: *preoperative, intraoperative,* and *postoperative.* Assessments should accompany the hand-off report to the nurse in the postanesthesia care unit (PACU) (see Chapter 10) or the nurse on the receiving patient care unit. Postoperative assessment includes inspection for changes in skin temperature, color, moisture level, turgor, and integrity. This inspections starts in the

RESEARCH HIGHLIGHT

Nurse-Initiated Perioperative Pressure Injury Risk Assessment and Prevention Protocol Using Braden Scale Scores

HAPIs are problematic for many reasons, but two major reasons stand out. First, they afflict hospital patients who enter the hospital to become healthy, but instead wind up with new injuries. Second, since 2008, the CMS have refused to reimburse acute care facilities for stage 3 or 4 HAPIs. The result is that while still exceedingly costly, HAPIs today are increasingly the focus of health researchers to help patients avoid these injuries.

Three such nurse-researchers, aware that surgical patients undergoing general anesthesia were at heightened risk to develop HAPIs, began studies of selected surgical patient groups at Cleveland Clinic Akron General in Akron, Ohio. The researchers reported in December 2016 that they had completed retrospective and prospective statistical studies aimed at development and validation of a perioperative risk assessment metric. They also wanted to apply their validated risk assessment metric and evidence-based preventive interventions prospectively to lessen the number of HAPIs in surgical patients, and they succeeded.

They began their research by creating a perioperative PI risk assessment measure and applying it retrospectively to a sample of 350 past surgical patients, and validated their measure. They then applied the risk assessment and intervention measures

prospectively to 350 incoming surgical patients who would be in supine or lateral positions, with a resulting 60% reduction in PIs.

The essential elements of the risk assessment measure as validated and applied were (1) previous surgery during the same admission, (2) diabetes, (3) a Braden score ≤16, (4) preexisting PI, and (5) surgical time ≥5 hours. If a patient met a single element, five specific interventions were to be implemented. If a patient had a Braden score of ≤16, or surgery was expected to last 5 hours or more, then a second, more extensive set of interventions was applied. Suggested interventions included a range of options including counseling the patient, repositioning, confirmation of pressure-relieving OR bed surfaces, heel relief options, foam border dressings to the sacrum or nonoperative greater trochanter, and use of a head donut to relieve occipital pressure, as well as others.

These nurse-researchers concluded that their findings supported a multipronged approach for prevention of HAPIs in surgical patients, including risk assessment, use of evidence-based interventions for at-risk patients, and continuation of prevention measures beyond surgery and into the nursing care unit. Additional research continues.

CMS, Centers for Medicare and Medicaid Services; *HAPI,* hospital-acquired pressure injuries; *PI,* pressure injury.
Modified from Meehan A et al: A nurse-initiated perioperative pressure injury risk assessment and prevention protocol, *AORN J* 104(6):554–565, 2016.

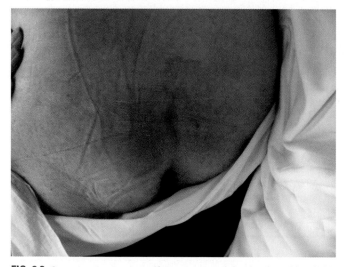

FIG. 6.2 Stage 1 pressure injury. Skin is intact with localized nonblanchable redness over the bony prominence (sacrum).

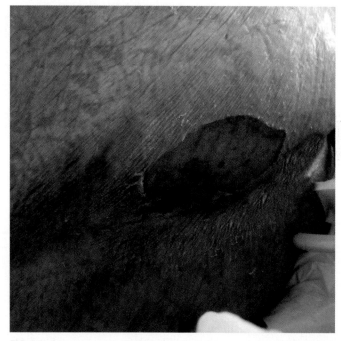

FIG. 6.3 Stage 2 pressure injury. Note the shallow open ulcer with red-pink wound bed showing partial thickness loss of dermis.

preoperative area and OR, continues in the PACU, and goes beyond, to discharge. It is in the early postoperative phase that many small problems picked up by astute assessments can be treated to avert bigger problems later.

Stage 1 or stage 2 PIs (Figs. 6.2 and 6.3) may appear immediately after surgery. These areas must be kept free from additional pressure for healing to occur and to stop them from worsening. Such PIs are sometimes misidentified and treated inappropriately. Stage 1 PIs can look like normal erythema, which is a reaction to pressure in which the healthy tissue blanches when compressed. The erythema generally fades on its own in one-half to three-quarters of the time that the area was under pressure, with little or no permanent tissue damage.

Stage 1 PIs do not blanch when compressed. Failure to blanch is a serious sign, indicating that the compromised tissue is not receiving adequate oxygen and nutrients. The blistering or partial dermal loss seen in stage 2 PIs is often misidentified as a chemical or thermal burn. The lack of contact with a chemical or thermal agent in that area and its location under a bony prominence or near where a hard surface had been during surgery can help identify the PI as a stage 2 PI.

Full manifestation of PIs may not occur for hours to days after the triggering injury. Given such delayed manifestation, the connection to the triggering event (the surgical experience) may be overlooked. Lack of awareness of an early PI can lead to a delay of pressure relief and treatment.

DTPI (Fig. 6.4) must also be differentiated from a stage 1 or 2 PI. Stage 1 injuries present with discolored, nonblanchable, but intact skin, which is also true of a DTPI. Instead of pink or red, however, the DTPI is deep red, maroon, or purple, or evidences as an epidermal separation revealing a dark wound bed or blood-filled blister (NPUAP, 2016). Stage 2 PIs present a partial-thickness loss of skin with exposed dermis. The wound bed is viable, pink or red,

---

TABLE 6.2

Munro Pressure Ulcer Risk Assessment Scale for Perioperative Patients: Adult

The Munro Pressure Risk Assessment Scale evaluates the patient's risk factors, for pressure ulcer development. The risk assessment and score is cumulative and evaluates three phases of care: **Preoperative, Intraoperative** and **Postoperative**. Each assessment phase will result in a risk score of low, medium or high. The level of risk may change throughout the perioperative period based on accumulation of risk factors. As part of the patient's health record, the risk score is communicated to each perioperative phase of care continuing to the inpatient unit as part of care coordination.

Preoperative Risk Assessment evaluates six risk factor categories to determine a score of 1, 2 or 3. The sum of the risk factors results in the Preoperative Munro Score Total to determine the Level of Risk.

		Preoperative Risk Factor Score			Total
Mobility		**1**	**2**	**3**	**1**
		Not limited, or slightly limited, moves independently	Very limited, requires transfer assistance	Completely immobile, requires full assistance	
Nutritional State		**1**	**2**	**3**	**1**
Length of NPO status		12° or <	> 12° but < 24°	> 24°	
BMI		**1**	**2**	**3**	**1**
		< 30kg/m^2	30kg/m^2–35kg/m^2	> 35kg/m^2	
Weight Loss		**1**	**2**	**3**	**1**
Weight loss in 30–180 days		Up to 7.4% weight loss, no change or unknown	Between 7.5% to 9.9% weight loss	≥ 10% weight loss	
Age		**1**	**2**	**3**	**1**
Years		39 or less	40-59	60 or greater	
Co-morbidity		Each co-morbidity/grouping equals a score of 1. A minimum score of 0 and a maximum score of 6 is possible.			
	Smoking (current)				**1**
	Prehypertension or high BP levels (BP > 120/80)				
	Vascular/Renal/Cardio-vascular/Peripheral-vascular Disease				
	Asthma/Pulmonary/Respiratory Disease				
	Prior History of Pressure Ulcer/Existing Pressure Ulcer				
	Diabetes/IDDM				
				Preoperative Munro Score Total:	**6**
5–6 = Low Risk	7–14 = Moderate Risk	15 or greater = High Risk		**Level of Risk:**	Low Risk

(Left vertical label: Preoperative Assessment)

Risk assessment performed by:

RN Signature:		Date:	Time:

Munro Score level of risk communicated to: _____

by:

RN Signature:		Date:	Time:

Continued

TABLE 6.2

Munro Pressure Ulcer Risk Assessment Scale for Perioperative Patients: Adult—cont'd

Intraoperative Risk Assessment evaluates seven risk factor categories to determine a score of 1, 2 or 3. The sum of the risk factors plus the Preoperative Munro Score Total results in the Intraoperative Munro Score Total to determine the Level of Risk.

		Intraoperative Risk Factor Score			Total
Intraoperative Assessment	**Physical Status / ASA Score**	1	2	3	3
	As per anesthesia provider	Healthy & mild systemic disease, no functional limitations	Moderate to severe systemic disease, some function limitation	Moderate to severe systemic disease, constant threat to life and functionally incapacitating or ASA >3	
	Anesthesia	1	2	3	3
		MAC, Local	Regional	General	
	Body Temperature	1	2	3	3
	Calculate high/low change as per anesthesia provider	36.1°–37.8° C Body T° maintained	<36.1° or >37.8° (+ or - 2°) T° fluctuated + or - 2°	<36.1° or >37.8° (+ or - >**2**°) T° fluctuated + or - >**2**°	
	Hypotension	1	2	3	2
	Calculate SBP high/low percentage change as per anesthesia provider	Absent or ≤10% change in BP	Fluctuating or 11% to 20% change in BP	Persistent or 21% to 50% change in BP	
	Moisture	1	2	3	3
	Skin under patient	Remains dry	Some moisture	Pooled or heavy fluid	
	Surface/Motion	1	2	3	3
	Positioning aids, warming blanket, position change	None/use of blanket over/stationary	Use of aids/blanket under/stationary	Shearing force/added pressure/variable position	
	Position	1	2	3	1
	For procedure	Lithotomy	Lateral	Supine/Prone	
				Intraoperative Score Subtotal:	18
				Add **Preoperative** Munro Score Total for a cumulative total:	6
				Intraoperative Munro Score Total:	24
	13 = Low Risk	14–24 = Moderate Risk	25 or greater = High Risk	Level of Risk:	Moderate Risk

Cumulative risk assessment performed by:

RN Signature:	**Date:**	**Time:**

Munro Score level of risk communicated to: _____

by:

RN Signature:	**Date:**	**Time:**

TABLE 6.2

Munro Pressure Ulcer Risk Assessment Scale for Perioperative Patients: Adult—cont'd

Postoperative Risk Assessment evaluates two risk factor categories to determine the score of 1, 2 or 3. The sum of the risk factors plus the Intraoperative Munro Score Total results in the Postoperative Munro Score Total to determine the Level of Risk.

		Postoperative Risk Factor Score			Total
Postoperative Assessment	**Length of Perioperative Duration**	1	2	3	**3**
	Total time from arrival to preoperative and departure from postoperative units	Up to 2°	>2° but <4°	>4°	
	Blood loss	1	2	3	**3**
	Intraop plus PACU sanguinous fluid via wound, orifice &/or drain as per LIP	Up to 200cc	201–400cc	>400cc	
				Postoperative Score Subtotal:	**6**
				Add **Intraoperative** Munro Score Total for a cumulative total:	**24**
				Postoperative Munro Score Total:	**30**
	15 = Low Risk	16–28 = Moderate Risk	29 or greater = High Risk	**Level of Risk:**	**High Risk**
	Final cumulative risk assessment performed by:				
	RN Signature:			Date:	Time:
	Final cumulative Munro Score level of risk communicated to: _____				
	by:				
	RN Signature:			Date:	Time:

©The Munro Scale.

moist. and may also present as an intact or ruptured fluid-filled blister. Adipose and deeper tissues are not visible. Granulation tissue, slough, and eschar are not present. Stage 2 injuries commonly result from adverse microclimate and shear in the skin over the pelvis and sheer in the heel (Edsberg et al., 2016).

Pressure alopecia (pressure-induced hair loss on the scalp) is a complication not typically classified as a PI, but can result from prolonged local pressure to the scalp during and after surgery. Symptoms can occur between postoperative days 3 and 28. Occipital scalp pain, swelling, exudate, crusting, or focal ulceration may precede the actual loss of hair. Pressure alopecia most commonly occurs in procedures that require prolonged intubation and head immobilization. The longer the time, the greater the risk is that alopecia may be permanent. Periodically repositioning the patient's head during prolonged procedures (if possible) and using ample cushioning (Cassorla and Lee, 2015) such as soft, contoured head padding, can reduce the potential for pressure alopecia.

Musculoskeletal System

The musculoskeletal system may be subjected to unusual stress during surgical positioning. Ordinarily the alert patient maintains normal range of motion by pain and pressure receptors that warn against overstretching and twisting of ligaments, tendons, and muscles. The tone of opposing muscle groups also acts to prevent strain and stretch to muscle fibers. In surgery, however, when pharmacologic agents,

such as anesthetics and muscle relaxants, depress pain and pressure receptors and muscle tone, a patient's normal defense mechanisms cannot guard against joint and nerve damage and muscle stretch and strain (Chard, 2016). The perioperative team aims to maintain the body's natural alignment as much as possible, while still providing adequate access to the surgical site. The team needs to be aware of the limits to range of motion and refrain from joint extension beyond what is necessary.

On each transfer to or from the OR bed, alignment of the patient's body needs to be maintained. This is especially true when transfer involves moving the patient from a supine position to lateral or prone. During positional changes, extremities are gently supported; quick, jerky movement of unsupported limbs can cause strain to the muscles and ligaments.

Nervous System

Nervous system depression accompanies the administration of anesthetic agents and other drugs (see Chapter 5). The degree of depression depends on the type of regional anesthesia or the level of general anesthesia. Pain and pressure receptors may be affected regionally or systemically. The most important factor for perioperative nurses to remember is that when nervous system depression occurs, the body's communication and command system becomes totally or partially ineffective. Compensatory reactions to changes in physical status no longer occur normally.

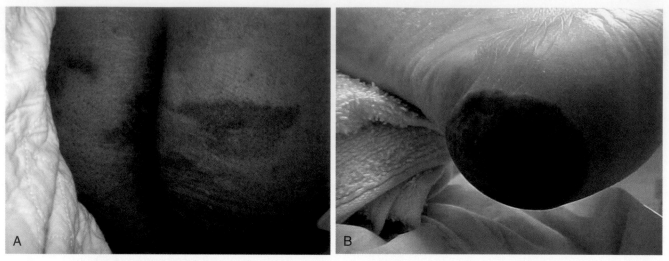

FIG. 6.4 Deep tissue pressure injury (DTPI). (A) Note intact discolored skin localized over bony prominence (sacrum); skin color, however, is deep purple or maroon compared with nonblanchable erythema stage 1 PI. (B) DTPI over bony prominence (heel) presenting as a blood-filled blister.

Peripheral Neuropathies

Peripheral nerves can suffer injury during positioning, resulting in impaired sensory function or motor function, or both. Although precise mechanisms of injury often cannot be determined, principle mechanisms for nerve injuries include compression (mechanical pressure), ischemia, and stretch (Cassorla and Lee, 2015). Prolonged stretching from hyperabduction of an extremity or compression from pressure in areas known to carry nerves prone to injury can result in ischemia. In addition, collateral damage to the surrounding tissue and capillaries can affect circulation and nourishment to nerves. These pathologic forces can combine to result in structural or functional damage to the nerves.

Using the Seddon classification, there are three degrees of nerve injury (Chhabra et al., 2014). Depending on the degree, subsequent injuries may be temporary or permanent. The first degree of injury, neurapraxia, is a response to compression and has the best prognosis. There is only slight demyelination and no axonal degeneration. Full recovery can be expected within 6 weeks without residual loss of function. The second degree of injury, axonotmesis, manifests as the destruction of the axons within a nerve sheath that remains intact. The distal axons degenerate, but proximal axons are able to use the intact sheath to guide regeneration at a rate of 1 mm per day. The third and most severe degree of nerve injury is neurotmesis in which the axon, sheath, and connective tissue covering are disrupted. Again, the distal axon degenerates. Without an intact sheath to guide regeneration, regrowth is disorganized, sometimes forming painful neuromas. Surgical intervention is required for repair of this nerve injury (Chhabra et al., 2014).

During surgery all patients are at risk for nerve injury if sustained compression is placed on nerves. Numerous patient characteristics have been identified, however, which potentially increase the risk for intraoperatively acquired neuropathies. These include diabetes mellitus, peripheral vascular disease, electrolyte imbalances, vitamin B_{12} deficiency, alcoholism, smoking, malnutrition, advanced age, previous nerve injuries or neuropathies (e.g., carpal tunnel syndrome, thoracic outlet syndrome), arthritis, obesity, thin body habitus, and male gender (for ulnar nerve injuries [Goodman and Spry, 2017]). Possible risk factors associated with the patient's surgical experience

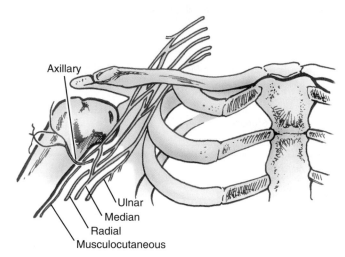

FIG. 6.5 Brachial plexus on the right with associated bone structures and nerve branches that extend down the right arm.

include lengthy surgical procedures, the use of abdominal pelvic self-retaining retractors, long duration in the lithotomy position, sternal retraction from a median sternotomy, surgical procedures in which shoulder braces are used for support while the patient is in steep Trendelenburg, improper arm placement, tight arm restraints, improperly placed blood pressure cuff, prolonged hospitalization, hypotension, hypothermia, and prolonged bed rest postoperatively (ASA, 2011). Damage usually remains undiscovered until the patient reaches the PACU or even days or weeks after the suspected insult. This delay can lead to some confusion as to whether the injury occurred during surgery or convalescence. Although the incidence is relatively low, allegations of peripheral nerve injuries are a significant source of professional liability claims (Cassorla and Lee, 2015).

Upper Extremity Neuropathies. Upper extremity neuropathies generate from lesions to the brachial plexus and the nerves that emerge from it. The brachial plexus consists of a bundle of nerve cords that run through the shoulder and innervate the lower shoulder, arm, and hand (Fig. 6.5). This bundle originates from cervical spinal

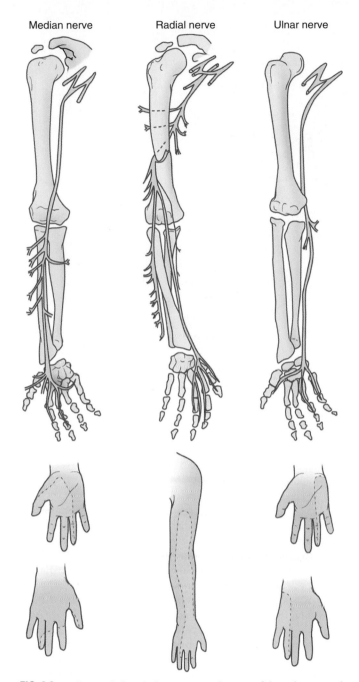

FIG. 6.6 Median, radial, and ulnar nerves and nerves of the right arm with areas of sensory distribution shaded.

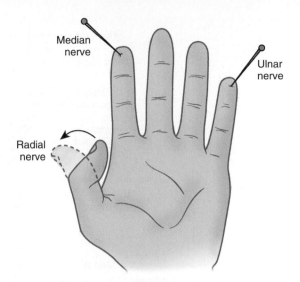

FIG. 6.7 A quick way to check for injuries to major peripheral nerves of the upper extremity. Ability to actively extend the thumb indicates an intact radial nerve. A normally perceived pinprick to the distal palmar surface of the index finger indicates an intact median nerve. A normally perceived pinprick to the distal palmar surface of the fifth finger indicates an intact ulnar nerve.

nerves C5–C8. The nerve cords emerge to form peripheral nerves. The axillary nerve innervates the deltoid muscle, and the musculoskeletal nerve innervates the biceps muscle. Three main peripheral nerves run down the arm to the fingers: median, radial, and ulnar (Fig. 6.6).

The *median nerve* runs through the antecubital space to the fingers and provides sensory and motor ability to the distal and palmar surfaces of the thumb and adjacent two fingers. A normally perceived pinprick to the palmar surface of the distal index finger generally shows that the median nerve is intact (Fig. 6.7).

The *radial nerve* loops around the posterior humerus before it runs through the antecubital space to the fingers. It provides motor and sensory function to the triceps and the muscles of the posterior forearm and hand. Injury to this area can cause difficulty extending the wrist and thumb. If the distal thumb can be actively extended, this generally indicates an intact radial nerve (see Fig. 6.7).

The *ulnar nerve* runs behind the elbow and innervates the third, fourth, and fifth fingers and the muscles of the medial forearm. It is responsible for wrist flexion and, along with the radial nerve, enables the thumb to oppose the other four fingers. A normally perceived pinprick over the plantar surface of the distal fifth finger generally indicates an intact ulnar nerve (see Fig. 6.7).

The most common OR-related nerve injuries are to the ulnar nerve and brachial plexus (Cassorla and Lee, 2015), and there is a good reason for this. As the ulnar nerve circles behind the elbow, it lies superficially in the shallow cubital tunnel of the humerus, where it is subject to pressure and to stretching from flexion of the elbow (Fig. 6.8). The brachial plexus resides in the shoulder, which is subject to abduction, manipulation, and sometimes pressure, depending on position. The use of shoulder braces to reduce sliding while in the Trendelenburg position should be avoided; braces can compress proximal nerve roots and stretch the brachial plexus. Arm abduction on armboards should be limited to 90 degrees or less. Avoid excessive head rotation, especially away from the abducted arm (Cassorla and Lee, 2015) because doing so can stretch and compress the nerves between the clavicle and the first rib (Fig. 6.9).

The brachial plexus can also suffer injury by the separation of the sternum during open cardiac procedures that require a median sternotomy. When splitting the sternum, a retractor is used to separate it, allowing access to the heart. This separation forces the ribs to move laterally. If internal mammary artery dissection occurs as part of the procedure, there is additional asymmetric retraction of the rib cage. The first rib compresses the brachial plexus nerve bundles and, in particular, the nerve cord that emerges into the ulnar nerve. If neuropathies develop as a result, they generally are not preventable by proper positioning of the patient's arm.

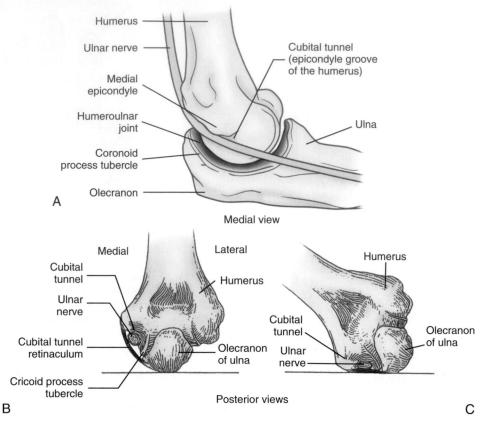

FIG. 6.8 Ulnar nerve at cubital tunnel. (A) Medial view. (B) Posterior view. Note cubital tunnel retinaculum over ulnar nerve in the cubital tunnel. (C) Posterior view with elbow tilted on the medial side. Note compressed ulnar nerve.

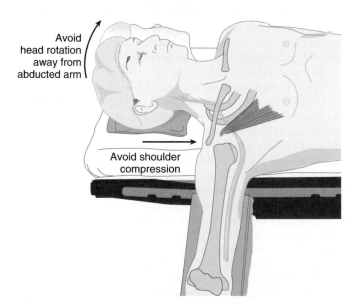

FIG. 6.9 Vertical compression on the shoulder can injure the brachial plexus. Rotating the head away from an abducted arm can stretch the brachial plexus between the clavicle and first rib.

Isolated ulnar nerve injuries arise primarily from pressure on the vulnerable location of that nerve. The ulnar nerve becomes superficial as it runs behind the elbow, nesting in the epicondyle groove of the humerus, which makes up the cubital tunnel. Ulnar nerve injuries occur primarily in male patients, most likely because of the following:

1. The tubercle of the coronoid process is larger in men than in women, creating a smaller cubital tunnel around the ulnar nerve.
2. Men generally have less adipose tissue over the medial aspect of the elbow compared with women with similar body fat composition; this results in less natural padding.
3. Men likewise have a thicker, more developed cubital tunnel reticulum, which can reduce further the space for the ulnar nerve in the cubital tunnel; this increases the risk of injury when the elbow is flexed.

The main goal in protecting the ulnar nerve is to eliminate pressure on it. Pressure on the medial aspect of the elbow may compress the ulnar nerve (see Fig. 6.8C). Fig. 6.10 illustrates ways to prevent this pressure. Supination (palms up) of the forearms on an armboard (see Fig. 6.10A) places the olecranon of the elbow on the flat surface instead of the cubital tunnel, which contains the ulnar nerve. When the arm of a supine patient rests on the trunk, direct trauma can occur to the ulnar nerve as the weight of the arm presses the flexed elbow against the surface of the bed. Padding placed under the upper arm, proximal to the elbow, leaves a free space under the elbow, eliminating pressure on the nerve (see Fig. 6.10B). When a patient is prone (abdomen facing down) with arms pronated on armboards, the ulnar nerve is vulnerable to pressure from the elbow. Padding

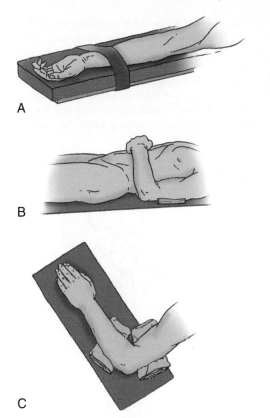

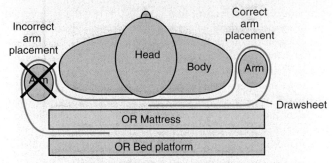

FIG. 6.11 Correct method for tucking arms in at patient's side.

FIG. 6.10 Three ways to protect ulnar nerve. (A) Arm of supine patient on armboard with palms up. (B) Elbow lifted free from bed surface by padding the upper arm when the arm is resting on the trunk. (C) Arm of prone patient pronated on armboard. Padding above and below elbow frees the ulnar nerve from the pressure of armboard surface.

placed proximal and distal to the elbow frees the nerve from pressure (see Fig. 6.10C).

Ulnar neuropathy symptoms may appear in the immediate postoperative period. Sometimes, however, symptoms are delayed until 2 to 7 days after surgery, making it difficult to isolate the exact event that triggered the complication. The postoperative course cannot be completely ruled out as a possible cause or contributing factor. Some patients are forced to lie on their backs for prolonged periods postoperatively because of devices such as endotracheal tubes (ETTs) and abdominal drains. Often they rest with elbows flexed and hands on their chest. This may place pressure on that superficial section of the ulnar nerve under the elbow, which may in turn cause or contribute to injury to the nerve during the postoperative period.

Many OR-induced peripheral upper extremity nerve injuries can be avoided by properly securing the arms when they are tucked at the patient's side. The arms should be tucked in a way that prevents them from sliding down the side of the OR bed and contacting the bed edge or rigid bed attachments. An effective technique to prevent arm slippage during surgery is to wrap the drawsheet smoothly around the arm and then tuck the drawsheet under the patient's body instead of under the mattress (Fig. 6.11). This technique is useful in the supine and prone positions. It is best accomplished when an assistant on the other side of the OR bed moves the patient's body over enough to tuck the drawsheet underneath it. Care should be taken to ensure that the drawsheet is not tucked so tightly it causes pressure to the arms. A tight fold pressing on the elbow could cause an isolated ulnar nerve injury.

Complete and thorough documentation of intraoperative measures taken to protect vulnerable nerves should include the following:

- How the arms were secured and by whom (name and role of person [AORN, 2017])
- Location of padding
- Angle of armboards (approximate degree of extension from body), the position of the palms, and the location of arm straps
- Times and type of repositioning or passive range of motion (PROM) performed
- Presence of distal pulses, color, and temperature of arms and hands when the procedure is long

The upper extremities should also be evaluated postoperatively. Any changes from the preoperative condition should be verbally reported and documented.

Lower Extremity Neuropathies. Lower extremity neuropathies result most frequently from prolonged lithotomy positioning and tend to manifest symptoms within hours after surgery. The common peroneal, sciatic, and femoral nerves are most frequently implicated.

Intraoperative risk factors include the length of time in lithotomy, high or exaggerated lithotomy, and positioning the extremities beyond their comfortable range of motion when awake. Different types of stirrups vary in the degree to which they control hip flexion. Hip extension should be limited to the minimum amount required for adequate access to the surgical site.

The *common peroneal nerve* branches from the sciatic nerve behind the knee and becomes superficial as it wraps around the lateral head of the fibula (Figs. 6.12–6.14). At this level, it is vulnerable to direct compression by stirrup bars. This risk may be increased in extremely thin patients who have minimal overlying tissue in this area. It is important to ensure that the lateral head of the fibula does not rest against stirrup bars or any other rigid surface. Compressive leg wraps (i.e., intermittent pneumatic compression devices [IPCDs], graduated compression stockings) also can put pressure on this nerve if the wrapping is too tight in this area. In addition, pressure behind the knee can compress the common peroneal and tibial nerves where they run through the popliteal fossa, so only *soft* padding or pillows should be used for knee support. The patient's ability to dorsiflex the great toe (point it upward) indicates that the common peroneal nerve is intact.

The *sciatic nerve* originates from the L4–S3 spinal nerve roots and travels down the buttock and posterior thigh before it divides into the common peroneal and tibial nerves (see Fig. 6.12). The stretching that occurs during hyperflexion of the hip may injure it. A patient who has had a total hip replacement may have some preexisting sciatic nerve damage as a result of the excessive rotation of the femur that is part of that operative procedure. Additionally, patients with a history of hip trauma who have required surgery, such as open reduction and internal fixation (ORIF), may be at increased risk for sciatic neuropathy because of the potential presence of scar tissue around the nerve area. As the branches of the sciatic nerve run from the thigh to the hamstring, the patient's ability to flex the thigh generally indicates an intact sciatic nerve.

The *femoral nerve* arises from the L2–L4 spinal nerve roots and runs through the medial thigh. Injury to the deep femoral nerve may occur more as a result of inappropriate placement of abdominal pelvic retractors and vaginal retractors in the pelvic cavity rather than inappropriate positioning. The femoral nerve and obturator

nerve can be subjected to excessive stretching and injury, however, as a result of inappropriate lithotomy positioning (see Fig. 6.14). The patient's ability to flex the thigh to the trunk generally indicates an intact femoral nerve.

The *obturator nerve* originates from the L2–L4 nerve roots. It runs through the obturator foramen of the ischium to innervate the adductor group of muscles in the inner thigh (see Fig. 6.14). It can be subjected to excessive stretching when the patient is in the

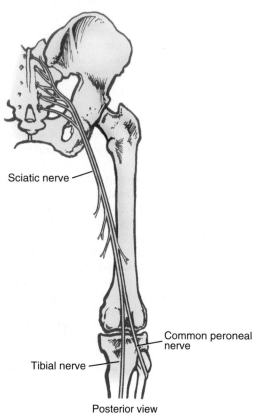

FIG. 6.12 Right sciatic nerve and right thigh and upper leg, posterior view. Note division of sciatic nerve into the tibial and common peroneal nerves.

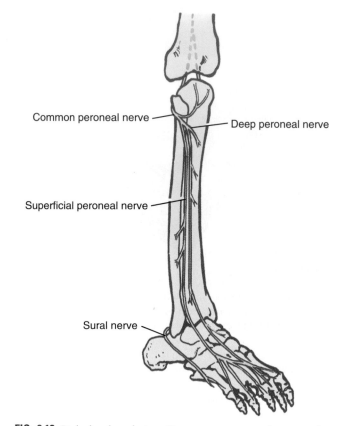

FIG. 6.13 Right leg, lateral view. Note common peroneal nerve pathway around the lateral fibular head. The nerve is very susceptible to injury when patient is in the lateral position. Also, note sural nerve in the heel area. This nerve is susceptible to injury from stirrup straps.

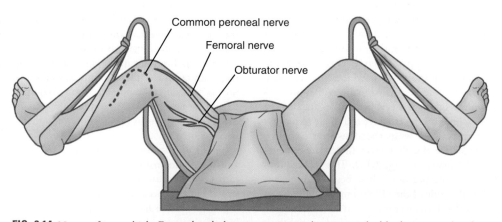

FIG. 6.14 Nerves of inner thigh. Femoral and obturator nerves can be overstretched by hyperextending hips or by team members leaning against thighs. If the lateral knee rests against a stirrup bar, the common peroneal nerve can be compressed.

lithotomy position. Scrubbed personnel may lean against the inner thigh while holding vaginal or anal retractors, causing additional stretching and compression of the nerve. The patient's ability to adduct the leg generally means the obturator nerve is intact.

The *tibial nerve* branches from the sciatic nerve behind the knee and runs along the posterior tibia to the foot (see Fig. 6.12), and from there it branches into the medial and lateral plantar nerves. The patient's normal sensation at the plantar surface of the foot and ability to curl the toes downward generally indicate an intact tibial nerve.

The perioperative nurse should document measures taken to protect the lower extremities from injury, including the following:

- Location and type of padding used (i.e., pillow to support knees or calves, padding under heels)
- Type of stirrups used; names and roles of persons placing legs in stirrups (AORN, 2017)
- Type of lithotomy position (low, standard, high, or exaggerated)
- Presence of distal pulses, color, and temperature of legs and feet
- Use of IPCDs or graduated compression stockings

The lower extremities should be evaluated postoperatively. Any changes from the preoperative condition should be verbally reported and documented.

The use of intraoperative neurophysiologic monitoring is an effective method to prevent peripheral nerve injuries in the upper and lower extremities during procedures in which there is otherwise a high risk of such injuries. A common method of this type of monitoring in the OR is somatosensory-evoked potential (SSEP). Its goal is to establish a baseline of the patient's normal nerve function along selected pathways and then to monitor those pathways at continual intervals during the procedure. The median nerve (at the wrist) is most commonly used as the stimulation site for upper extremity monitoring. For the lower extremity, most commonly the posterior tibial nerve just posterior to the medial malleolus is used. The ulnar and peroneal nerves can also be used (Liem, 2016).

The Association of periOperative Registered Nurses (AORN, 2017) offers specific recommendations to prevent nerve injuries during surgery. They are listed in the Evidence for Practice box.

▌ EVIDENCE FOR PRACTICE

Prevention of Perioperative Peripheral Neuropathies

- When arms are tucked at the side of body, the palms and wrists should be in neutral position (facing inward).
- Armboards for a supine patient should be at less than a 90-degree angle on the OR bed with palms facing up or in neutral position.
- Unless contraindicated by the surgical procedure, the patient's head should be placed in a neutral position.
- Avoid positioning arms above the patient's head.
- Prevent the lateral aspect of the knee from resting on the vertical post of a candy cane stirrup when patient is in lithotomy position.
- Avoid using shoulder braces to prevent patient from sliding in Trendelenburg position.

Modified from Bouyer-Ferullo S: Preventing perioperative peripheral nerve injuries, *AORN J* 97(1):111–121, 2013; AORN: *Guidelines for perioperative practice*, Denver, 2017, The Association.

Vascular System

General anesthesia causes peripheral vessels to dilate by depressing the sympathetic nervous system. This dilation decreases overall blood pressure because blood pools in dependent areas of the body. In general anesthesia, these effects are systemic; in regional anesthesia, such as spinal and epidural, these effects are more limited to the areas anesthetized.

Position changes affect where blood pooling occurs. Muscle tone and peripheral vascular resistance are no longer as effective in counteracting the forces of gravity on blood pooling. Blood pools to whatever part of the body is lowest. For example, if the head of the OR bed is raised, the lower torso has increased blood volume. Conditions such as hypovolemia and cardiovascular disease may compromise the patient's status further.

The anesthesia provider can treat some of the hypotensive effects of positioning through pharmacologic agents and increased IV infusion. Vital signs, IV intake, and urinary output need to be monitored closely. Position changes may need to be delayed until blood pressure stabilizes.

Deep vein thrombosis (DVT) is a serious complication of surgical positioning. Compression to deep and peripheral vessels (e.g., resulting from tight safety strap or wrist restraints) may predispose the patient to venous thrombosis. When the legs are in a dependent position (i.e., legs lowered during knee arthroscopy, sitting position, reverse Trendelenburg), venous return slows and venous stasis can occur (AORN, 2017). Graduated compression stockings or IPCDs can reduce this risk (Goodman and Spry, 2017); interventions such as these are collectively referred to as "mechanical prophylaxis" (AORN, 2017), and they are used according to the manufacturer's written instructions. Thrombosis also can occur as a result of hyperabduction of the arms beyond 90 degrees. Subclavian and axillary vessels pass through the brachial plexus, and vessel constriction can occur by compression between the clavicle and the first rib. Radial pulses require monitoring when arms are extended to ensure that the radial pulse is not obliterated.

Vascular assessment of upper and lower extremities should occur preoperatively. Document measures taken to reduce assessed risks and evaluate vascular status intraoperatively and postoperatively. Any changes from the preoperative condition require verbal reports and documentation.

Acute compartment syndrome is a serious complication that may arise from excessive constriction to, or improper positioning of, extremities. It is characterized by ischemia, hypoxic edema, and elevated tissue pressure within the fascial components of the extremity, leading to further damage to the muscles and nerves. This process occurs at a cellular level, and distal pulses and capillary refill may initially appear normal; then, however, the process may rapidly escalate to a dangerous condition. The syndrome may progress to rhabdomyolysis with resulting renal damage, permanent nerve damage, or loss of limb. The most effective means to end this syndrome is a decompressive fasciotomy.

Respiratory System

Positioning can compromise the respiratory system. In almost all positions, except semi-Fowler, sitting, and reverse Trendelenburg, the abdominal viscera shift upward toward the diaphragm. Subsequently, the diaphragm shifts upward and outward such that it contributes only about two-thirds of the ventilatory force and significantly reduces tidal volume. Obese or pregnant patients or those who have pulmonary disease have additional respiratory compromise in these positions. Patients who experience dyspnea should have the head of the bed elevated during transport and during local, regional, or spinal anesthesia if this does not interfere with surgical access. During general anesthesia, the anesthesia provider normally ventilates these patients mechanically.

External chest movement during surgery needs to be as unrestricted as possible to avoid further reduction in tidal volume. Avoid placement of arms across the chest because arms resting on the chest restrict chest expansion and add pressure on the ulnar nerve at the elbow area. Some positions (e.g., lateral, fracture bed) require the placement of straps around the chest area to secure the patient to the OR bed without obstructing the surgical site. Such strapping requires efforts to ensure against excessive tightness. These positions are not maintained any longer than necessary. Anesthesia personnel closely monitor the respiratory status of these patients.

Positioning also affects the portions of the lungs perfused with blood. As blood pumps into the lungs, the areas of the lung that are most dependent have a greater pulmonary arterial pressure as the blood pools. The greater the pressure, the greater is the perfusion. Perfusion is slightly higher and ventilation is generally highest in the alveoli in the bases of the lungs. An even distribution of ventilation and perfusion (ventilation-perfusion ratio) is needed for efficient gas exchange. If the position causes a pathologically compromised area of the lung to be dominant and more perfused, the balance between perfusion and ventilation may be disrupted and respiratory status may diminish. The rest of the lung fields may or may not have the capacity to compensate. Positive-pressure ventilation along with the use of muscle relaxants may ameliorate ventilation-perfusion mismatches during general anesthesia. Adequate minute ventilation can be maintained and atelectasis limited (Cassorla and Lee, 2015).

Monitoring of respiratory status includes pulse oximetry. In some cases, intraoperative arterial blood gas monitoring is also necessary.

Obesity

Obesity is an important consideration in the perioperative environment because its incidence has risen steadily. The upward trend exists among children, teens, and adults. The degree of obesity is based on BMI. Obesity and morbid obesity are considered to be BMI of ≥ 30 kg/m^2 or ≥ 40 kg/m^2 (weight)/m^2(height), respectively (see Chapter 11 for a discussion of obesity and bariatric surgery). Morbid obesity is a complex medical disorder that frequently coexists with numerous other medical problems. These include arthritis and degenerative joint disease, sleep apnea, hypertension, type 2 diabetes, and esophageal reflux. The incidence of these conditions increases with the age of the patient and the duration of severe obesity. Morbid obesity is associated with some considerable perioperative risks (Patient Safety). Obese patients (referred to as "persons of size") have a diminished respiratory reserve and become distressed quickly and easily when lying flat in supine. Trendelenburg is even more poorly tolerated and should be avoided until the patient is intubated and mechanical ventilation can assist with breathing. With excess fat distribution around the patient's back, neck, and shoulders, positioning interventions are necessary to gain control of the patient's airway in the supine position. This is done by what has been called "ramping," that is, building a ramp of cushioning materials (e.g., pillows, linens, foam wedges) to elevate the head, neck, and shoulders above the chest into alignment with the airway. To create the correct plane, an imaginary horizontal line can be drawn between the earlobe and the sternum, as noted in Fig. 6.15. This ramped position enables the anesthesia provider to gain control of the patient's airway by

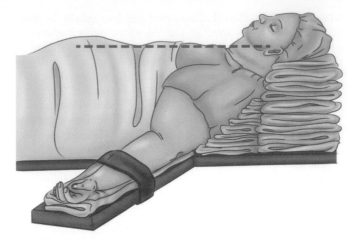

FIG. 6.15 This figure illustrates "ramping" an obese patient's torso to facilitate optimal airway alignment. Imaginary horizontal line between earlobe and sternum *(dashed line)* references proper position.

aligning the oral, laryngeal, and pharyngeal axes. It has also been called the head-elevated laryngoscopy position (HELP) because it facilitates laryngoscopy and intubation (Brodsky, 2013).

Obese patients are at a high risk for DVTs. Thromboembolism prophylaxis is used in these patients, especially if their lower extremities will be bent or in a dependent position. When applying graduated compression stockings or IPCDs, they must be large enough not to restrict circulation, which might otherwise risk compartment syndrome development.

In addition to being at higher risk for PIs from long periods of immobility during surgery, obese patients are also at risk for rhabdomyolysis. Pressure from their large body mass can crush dependent tissue causing muscle fiber breakdown, releasing myoglobin into the bloodstream.

Beds and accessories must accommodate the width and weight of morbidly obese patients. Available products specifically enhance the safety of the obese patient in surgery. They are discussed in the Operating Room Beds and Accessories section of this chapter.

Eye Injuries and Perioperative Vision Loss

Perioperative vision loss (PVL, also referred to as "postoperative visual loss" [POVL]), although rare, has become the subject of a substantial number of medical publications because it is so devastating to the patient and is now an important medicolegal issue. Direct pressure on the eye, especially coupled with systemic hypotension, may cause central retinal artery occlusion, which in turn may result in temporary or permanent blindness. Direct pressure can also displace the implanted intraocular lens in a patient who has had cataract surgery. Care needs to be taken to constantly monitor the eyes when using any prone head positioner, especially the horseshoe type (Fig. 6.16), because poor placement can put direct pressure on the globe of the eye (American Society of Anesthesiologists Task Force on Perioperative Visual Loss, 2012). The prone position itself, even without pressure on the eyes, may increase intraocular pressure, which may then lead to ischemic optic neuropathy (Hartley, 2015), particularly with prolonged prone Trendelenburg position, any position that brings the head lower than the heart (e.g., prone on a Wilson frame), and steep Trendelenburg, such as that used in certain robotic-assisted procedures (Freshcoln and Diehl, 2014).

Key Considerations in Positioning Morbidly Obese Patients

The following complications may occur more frequently in surgery patients who are morbidly obese:

- DVT and PE
- Pressure injuries and rhabdomyolysis
- Ventilation impairment with diminished pulmonary functional residual capacity in all surgical positions except sitting
- Higher rates of perioperative ulnar nerve palsies and brachial plexus neuropathies
- Lower limbs falling off OR bed causing lateral femoral cutaneous nerve injuries
- Sciatic nerve palsies from tilting the bed sideways
- Postoperative back pain from buttocks acting as a fulcrum for legs, extending the lumbar spine
- Skin breakdown from moisture and prep solutions trapped in tissue folds

  The following interventions may enhance the morbidly obese patient's safety:

- Provide an OR bed made to accommodate patient's size and weight; know the weight limit of each OR bed.
- Use mattress padding (identify the mattress padding rating) and positioning accessories (bariatric stirrups, longer and wider safety straps [two straps may be necessary: one for the upper legs and one for the lower legs], side bed attachments, foam and gel supports, etc.) specifically designed and sized for bariatric patients.
- Elevate the head, upper body, and shoulders to facilitate the airway when supine. A wedge, placed under the right flank, can alleviate pressure on the vena cava.
- Have difficult-airway cart immediately available.
- Pad armboards to match the higher elevation of the shoulders to avoid stretching of the brachial plexus.
- As directed by the anesthesia provider, apply cricoid pressure to facilitate intubation and prevent aspiration from esophageal reflux. Be prepared to assist with inability to establish an airway.
- Support the knees with pillows to reduce strain on back.
- Use graduated compression stockings or IPCDs on lower extremities.
- Use appropriate transfer devices (air-cushioned transfer pads, pneumatic lifts, etc.) to reduce friction and shear in patients and protect team members from injury.

DVT, Deep vein thrombosis; *IPCDs*, intermittent pneumatic compression devices; *PE*, pulmonary embolism.
Modified from Goodman T, Spry, C: *Essentials of perioperative nursing*, ed 6, Burlington, MA, Jones & Bartlett Learning, 2017; Hortman C, Chung S: Positioning considerations in robotic surgery, *AORN J* 102(4):435–439, 2015.

Additional risk factors identified include male gender, obesity, long anesthetic duration, high blood loss, low percentage of colloid fluid replacement, decreased systemic blood pressure, anemia, diabetes, chronic hypertension, and use of vasopressors (Postoperative Visual Loss Study Group, 2012).

PVL may be complete or partial and unilateral or bilateral. It is typically painless and noticed by the patient on awakening from general anesthesia or soon afterward. Sometimes, however, it can take a day or more for the patient to notice vision changes, and the optic nerve can slowly atrophy over a period of several weeks.

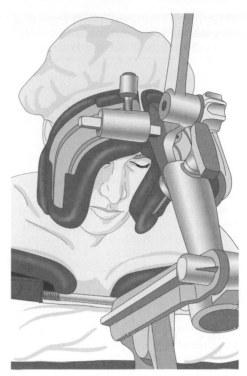

FIG. 6.16 Horseshoe head positioner must be carefully adjusted to avoid putting pressure on eyes.

Regardless of onset of symptoms, presently there is no cure and no effective treatment. The emphasis, therefore, is on prevention.

Perioperative Nursing Considerations

Assessment

Assessment for positioning needs should be made before the patient transfers to the OR bed. The perioperative nursing assessment includes a patient interview, and review of the physical examination and pertinent medical records. Key assessment points related to surgical positioning include age, height, and weight; risk assessment for PI; nutritional status; comorbid conditions (e.g., conditions of the vascular, respiratory, circulatory, neurologic, or immune system); and physical/mobility limits (e.g., prostheses, implants, range of motion) (Goodman and Spry, 2017). It also should be determined if there are any particular areas of discomfort that a particular position may cause and what interventions might alleviate or reduce that discomfort (AORN, 2017) (Patient Engagement Exemplar).

The assessment should alert the perioperative nurse to patient circumstances and problems that could be worsened during surgical positioning. The assessment should be reported to all team members that will continue the care of the patient during the surgical experience. Vulnerable patients include the following:

- Geriatric patients, whose thinner skin layer makes them more prone to skin breakdown from pressure
- Pediatric patients, whose size and weight must be considered when selecting positioning aids
- Patients who have respiratory and circulatory disorders, diabetes mellitus, malnutrition, advanced age, and anemia because they are more prone to skin breakdown caused by pressure

Shared Responsibility in the Positioning Process

NAQC guiding principle number 3 states "In this relationship, there are shared responsibilities and accountabilities among the patient, the family, and clinicians that make it effective."

Both patient and nurse are accountable in the positioning process. Nurses assess the patient's limitations and skin before positioning, and patients must share information about skin or musculoskeletal issues that patient positioning could affect. Consider the following scenario:

You are doing your preoperative interview with a 72-year-old woman who will be undergoing a uterine D&C for postmenopausal bleeding. As part of your interview, you assess her mobility and flexibility for lithotomy positioning and she shares her limitations with you.

Nurse: "Mrs. Chen, we plan to place your legs into stirrups after you get medicine that makes you sleepy so that you will be in a similar position as you were during your gynecology exam in your doctor's office. Did that position cause you any discomfort?"

Mrs. Chen: "Well, like I told my doctor, my legs aren't what they used to be. I'm not doing too well on stairs these days. She helped me get up into those stirrups, but I can't bend my knees very far or it hurts."

Nurse: "Would it be OK with you if we help you get into the stirrups before you get the medicine that makes you sleepy? We will keep your lower body completely covered with a blanket. You can let us know how much we can bend your knees so that you will stay as comfortable as possible."

D&C, Dilation and curettage; *NAQC,* Nursing Alliance for Quality Care.
From Nursing Alliance for Quality Care: *Fostering successful patient and family engagement: nursing's critical role* (website). www.naqc.org/WhitePaper-PatientEngagement. (Accessed 17 June 2016).

- Patients with limited mobility because of congenital anomalies, preexisting injuries, arthritis, or prosthetic implants, who need special considerations during positioning
- Patients with edema, infection, cancer, or conditions of lowered cardiac or respiratory reserves and who have poor general health, making them vulnerable to tissue injury
- Patients with demineralizing bone conditions such as malignant metastasis or osteoporosis, putting them at higher risk for skeletal fractures
- Patients who will be subjected to anticipated high-risk surgical situations, such as
  - Lengthy surgical procedures (≥2 hours) because there is increased risk of pressure-related injuries
  - Lengthy time in the lithotomy position because of increased risk of lower extremity nerve injury
  - Vascular surgery because optimal blood perfusion already may be compromised as a result of the patient's disease process
  - Excessive sustained pressure to certain body areas caused by the surgical procedure or retraction
  - Cool environment or exposure of large body surfaces, or both, because there is risk of perioperative hypothermia and its related complications

Nursing Diagnosis

The encompassing nursing diagnosis related to the care of the patient during surgical positioning is the risk for perioperative positioning injury. Other potentially applicable nursing diagnoses include the following:

- Impaired Comfort
- Impaired Transfer Ability
- Risk for Falls
- Risk for Impaired Skin Integrity
- Risk for Impaired Tissue Integrity
- Risk for Perioperative Hypothermia
- Impaired Physical Mobility
- Risk for Peripheral Neurovascular Dysfunction

Outcome Identification

The outcome identified for safe surgical positioning may be stated as "the patient is free from signs and symptoms of perioperative positioning injury." Primary outcome indicators mandate a review of the skin condition and cardiovascular and neuromuscular status, along with other considerations. The perioperative nurse may define freedom from injury, noting that the patient will do the following:

- Experience a safe transfer to and from the OR bed.
- Be warm and comfortable.
- Experience no tingling, numbness, or pain unrelated to the surgical procedure.
- Maintain skin and tissue integrity consistent with preoperative status.
- Maintain a respiratory status consistent with preoperative status.
- Regain normal baseline physical mobility postoperatively.
- Maintain normal baseline peripheral neurovascular function.

Planning

The perioperative nurse plans activities that will protect the patient from injury and provide physiologic support and comfort, while allowing for optimal exposure and access to the surgical site. Although safe surgical positioning involves all members of the surgical team, the circulating nurse plans and coordinates this teamwork. Knowledge of any preexisting risk factors that may affect positioning strategies (e.g., obesity, diabetes, paralysis, advanced age, preexisting PI) should be considered when planning for additional staff assistance for positioning and support devices or padding needed.

It is imperative that the exact location of the operative site be identified so that access to that site is not obstructed. If a secondary surgical procedure is involved, such as a graft donor site, the area needs to be exposed and accessible as well. On occasion, all anticipated incision sites cannot be exposed during initial positioning. Plans need to be made for repositioning an anesthetized patient (i.e., additional: personnel, padding devices, and sterile drapes) so that repositioning occurs quickly and smoothly without unnecessarily prolonged anesthesia time.

Planning for physiologic support involves collaborating with the anesthesia provider. Sometimes chest rolls are needed for adequate lung expansion while the patient is in the prone position. If the patient is in the prone position and chest rolls are used, make sure breasts are gently placed between the chest rolls and not under pressure. Supports and padding for the head, arms, hands, and axilla should be anticipated and easily accessible.

Planning for the patient's comfort can involve communicating with the patient as to potential areas for discomfort and possible remedies. An awake patient receiving local anesthesia can give feedback on the comfort of the position before, during, and immediately after the procedure. In some cases, all or part of the positioning for a patient who is to undergo general anesthesia can be done before induction if it does not interfere with the anesthesia process. A patient could be placed in the lithotomy position before induction if he or she has a history of discomfort with leg abduction or lower back pain. If this is done, privacy and patient dignity must be ensured by covering the patient with a sheet or blanket and covering or pulling the blinds on room windows. A Sample Plan of Care for the patient undergoing surgical positioning is shown on this page.

Implementation

Perioperative nurses involved in positioning should have an individualized plan of care designed to prevent injury while maintaining optimal surgical access, patient comfort, and physiologic support. Patient comfort measures need to include physical and emotional aspects. Patient safety measures include verifying that the patient has removed all jewelry, including body piercings (Patient, Family, and Caregiver Education). Talking with the patient about any positioning concerns reassures the patient and provides the nurse with insight into possible comfort issues (see Patient Engagement Exemplar). Providing the patient with personal warmth and privacy may help the patient to feel more comfortable and relaxed, and to feel respected and cared for.

Assemble all necessary positioning aids, such as padding, pillows, OR bed accessories, and stirrups, before induction because the patient is generally positioned immediately after anesthesia administration. Ensure that all positioning devices are clean and in proper working order. Ensure that extra staff members are available when needed to lift or turn the patient.

Institutional procedures to prevent wrong-site, wrong-procedure, and wrong-person surgery are followed. When the patient enters the OR suite, the circulating nurse identifies the patient using two identifiers and verifies the correct person, procedure, and operative site. The patient is prepared for transfer onto the OR bed, which should be positioned in the room in such a way that relocation after

SAMPLE PLAN OF CARE

Nursing Diagnosis
Risk for Perioperative Positioning Injury

Outcome
The patient will be free from injury related to perioperative positioning.

Interventions
- Identify surgical site and determine appropriate position.
- Identify and document specific risk factors that may predispose the patient to position-related injuries.
- Identify areas of potential discomfort/limitations in mobility and possible remedies. Note condition of patient's skin and presence of peripheral pulses, as applicable.
- Check OR bed for proper functioning.
- Obtain needed positioning aids, OR bed attachments, and padding materials; verify these are clean and in working order.
- Ensure a safe transfer from the transport vehicle to OR bed and document mode of transfer.
- Safely secure the patient to the OR bed without compromising circulation underneath restraining straps.
- Provide the patient with warmth, privacy, and reassurance.
- Include correct position and any positioning concerns in the time-out.
- If the patient is repositioned after being anesthetized, support all body parts and maintain body alignment throughout the move. Consider a "pause" during the procedure for change in surgical position (Mathias, 2015).
- Use slow, smooth movements in making all position changes, using a team approach.
- Avoid pulling or dragging the patient; use lifting techniques instead.
- Pad or suspend bony prominences and all pressure-prone areas in contact with a solid surface.
- Protect the eyes and anatomic areas containing superficial vessels and nerves.
- Secure the patient to the OR bed to prevent falls or slippage of extremities over the OR bed's edge.
- Collaborate with the anesthesia provider in monitoring physiologic effects of position changes, and be prepared to intervene when necessary.

- Ensure access to airway, IV lines, and monitoring devices.
- Prevent pooling of fluids under dependent areas or any area under pressure by placing towels, impervious pads, or an impervious barrier under or around area to be prepped. Remove the towels, pad, or barrier at the conclusion of prepping and before draping.
- During long procedures, periodically perform passive range of motion (PROM) on accessible extremities when possible; this intervention cannot interfere with the surgical procedure, integrity of the sterile field, or anesthesia administration.
- Use strategies to maintain normothermia.
- Ensure that no equipment or personnel create or impose pressure on the patient throughout the procedure.
- Periodically recheck position, straps, and padding to ensure that nothing has slipped or moved; this intervention cannot interfere with the surgical procedure, integrity of the sterile field, or anesthesia administration.
- At the end of the procedure, reposition slowly to allow for patient's hemodynamic accommodation.
- Secure patient and remain at patient's side during emergence from anesthesia.
- Transfer patient using a team approach with a secured transport vehicle.
- Protect the patient against friction or shear during transfers.
- Reassess tissue integrity; document and verbally communicate any changes during hand-off report.

Document in detail patient position, including the following:
- Names and roles of surgical team members participating in positioning
- Surgical position used
- Position of extremities
- Type and location of restraints, positioning aids, and padding materials
- Frequency of PROM performed (if possible) and other injury prevention interventions
- Use and location of warming or cooling devices
- Positional changes made during procedure (e.g., supine to lithotomy to supine)
- Adverse physiologic responses to positions and interventions taken

Perioperative nurses strive to ensure that patients they care for are free from signs and symptoms of a positioning injury. Assessment, combined with patient, family, and caregiver education, assists in achieving this outcome. During assessment, perioperative nurses routinely ask patients if they have removed all of their jewelry and explain the risk of infection, electrical burns, trauma (e.g., catching a piece of jewelry or body piercing on equipment as the patient is transferred and positioned), or airway obstruction. It is important, in this discussion, to recognize and respect cultural implications of body piercing. Cultures from various geographic locations in the world embrace the piercing of specific body sites.

A more difficult issue is dealing with dermal implants. Transdermal and microdermal implants may have posts on them that protrude from the skin. In addition to getting caught on equipment, these posts create a risk for pressure at the site of the implant from the position or positioning accessories. Educate the patient, family, and caregiver about the reasons you are asking about dermal implants. Invite them to be frank with you about their location. Jewelry like this that cannot be removed should be identified and documented; noting the presence of all dermal implants becomes part of the hand-off report and intraoperative plan of care. Part of that plan ensures that prolonged pressure against the implant is avoided by using supportive foam or other devices and that external transdermal and microdermal implant pins are protected with gauze or tape.

Modified from Delaisse J et al: Peri-operative management of the patient with body piercings. *J Dermatol Clin Res* 2(1):1009–1013, 2014; Smith FD: Caring for surgical patients with piercings, *AORN J* 103(12):584–593, 2016; Wanzer LJ, Hicks RW: Identifying and minimizing risks for surgical patients with dermal implants, *OR Connections* 96(4), C5–C6, 2012.

the patient is anesthetized is kept to a minimum. During transfer the OR bed and transport vehicle should be next to each other and locked. At least one individual should stand on either side to assist the patient in the transfer. If the patient is unable to assist in the transfer, perform a four-person lift using a drawsheet or a transfer device, being sure to support the head and feet.

Falls are an important consideration during all patient transfers and positioning. Falls can occur during transfers if the two beds are not locked. They also can occur while the patient is on the OR bed, whether awake or anesthetized. An awake patient may not fully appreciate the narrowness of the OR bed and can continue to move beyond the bed edges. Someone needs to stand on either side of the patient until a safety strap is applied. Falls also are a risk during induction and emergence from anesthesia. Lighter stages of anesthesia can result in patient movement. Movement may be strong enough that safety straps alone do not offer adequate security. Infants and toddlers are particularly at risk because standard safety straps frequently are not used on them because of their small stature. Other means to secure a pediatric patient may be used, depending on the area needed for surgical access. Constant personnel presence immediately at the patient's side and the use of safety straps or portable cushioned side rails minimize the risk of patient falls during vulnerable times.

When the patient is on the OR bed, the safety strap is placed 2 inches above the knees. The strap should be snug but not so tight that it places pressure on nerves or restricts venous return. To ensure snugness without tightness, two fingers should slide comfortably beneath the strap. The patient's ankles must not be crossed because vessel and nerve constriction and skin pressure may result. The patient should be reminded of this because some patients automatically cross their ankles while lying down.

Movement of the patient should be slow and smooth, ensuring that the entire body is supported during movements. Quick, jerky movements can cause musculoskeletal injury and put the patient at risk for bruises, pinches, abrasions, fractures, or falls. Any lateral, anterior, or posterior movement of the patient on the OR bed should be done by lifting the patient with the drawsheet rather than by pulling or dragging the patient. Make sure all personnel know how to correctly use transfer devices.

When in the desired position, the patient should be secured so that movement off the OR bed cannot occur from any direction. Check safety straps and other support accessories for pressure against the patient, particularly in areas adjacent to bony prominences. Padding or adjustment needs to happen at this point because it is the last opportunity before prepping and draping. In addition, consider how the position may cause certain body parts to sustain more gravitational weight. If a pillow elevates the knees, the heels bear additional weight from the calves; heels should be totally off the surface of the bed. Placing the pillow under the calves elevates the knees and lifts the heels off the surface of the OR bed at the same time.

During the procedure, the circulating nurse monitors and assists with any modification to the position that is required. Periodically, the circulator checks pressure points that are accessible and adjusts the patient or padding as needed. PROM can be done to accessible extremities. This is particularly important during long procedures (≥2 hours). The position, all padding, positioning devices, and methods used to secure the patient to the OR bed are documented. If the patient needs to be repositioned during the procedure, the circulating nurse coordinates the move by calling additional personnel to the OR to assist, ensuring additional positioning devices and padding are available, and protecting the patient from injury as the move commences. Interventions for repositioning are documented.

Evaluation

After the surgical procedure ends, check all pressure sites, especially those under bony prominences, before transfer to the PACU. Remember that the occurrence of a PI during the surgical procedure may not be evident immediately after surgery. Document any changes in skin integrity, mode of transfer, time of discharge, and patient status on discharge as well as actions, observations, and patient responses to treatment. Evaluation of the plan of care concludes with a hand-off report to the PACU nurse. The outcome of successful implementation of the plan of care may be measured by the positive patient outcomes listed in the later section Outcome Identification.

Operating Room Beds and Accessories

Operating Room Beds

As designed, modern OR beds support and accommodate various positions required in surgery. Their height is adjustable, they can tilt laterally, and they adjust to Trendelenburg or reverse Trendelenburg position. Generally, OR beds operate electrically or by battery with manual, mechanical backup. They have roller wheels to allow them to move easily and brakes to lock them in place. They consist of a flat platform divided into three major sections: head, torso, and leg sections. Each section has a corresponding removable mattress pad, which usually attaches to the main platform by Velcro or straps.

The area between each section is called a "break." Raising or lowering sections is called "breaking the bed."

Along the edges are side rails that separate at each break and run horizontally along both sides of the entire OR bed. Armboards lock directly on the side rails at any level of the OR bed. The side rails also accommodate sockets, straps, and clamps that can secure a multitude of attachments, including stirrups, anesthesia screens, armboards, and various retractors. Underneath the OR bed platform is a tunnel that runs under the entire body and leg sections to support x-ray cassettes. In newer models, the entire OR bed platform is radiopaque to accommodate the use of intraoperative fluoroscopy.

The typical OR bed is relatively narrow to allow easy access to the operative site. Wider beds or side extensions that lock into the side rails of the bed are available for obese patients. All OR beds have weight limitations. Many newer OR beds are designed to accommodate more weight than earlier models, given the increase in the bariatric patient population. Some can hold up to 1000 pounds. The weight limitations should be marked on the bed. Make sure that the bed you use accommodates your patient's weight.

The torso section is attached to the base of the OR bed because this section supports the heaviest parts of the body: the chest, abdomen, and pelvis. This section also has a break in the center at the hip level that can be flexed or lowered to allow the head and chest areas to be elevated or lowered. At this central break in the torso section is a crossbar, called a *kidney bridge* (body elevator), which can be raised or lowered for kidney or gallbladder exposure. The kidney bridge is concave and can accommodate lateral braces that slide vertically onto the bridge to maintain the patient in a lateral position. The distal portions of the torso section's platform and mattress have a concave perineal cutout to accommodate access to the perineum when the patient is in the lithotomy position. Drainage trays may be fitted into this section for gynecologic, urologic, and proctologic procedures.

The head section of the OR bed can be flexed, lowered, or removed. It connects to the bed by two horizontal posts that fit into corresponding grooves in the front of the torso section as well as the bottom of the leg section. Special headrests, such as a craniotomy or ophthalmic headrests, substitute for the head section and slide into these grooves for specific procedures.

Switching the head section to the leg section allows for movement of C-arm fluoroscopy around the patient's chest and abdomen because the leg section protrudes farther away from the base than the head section does. This configuration can also provide support for the feet when a patient is positioned low on the bed for lithotomy. Once the patient's legs are placed in stirrups that are connected to the side rails of the torso section, the head section (now supporting the feet) can be removed and the leg section lowered to give the surgeon direct access to the perineal area.

The grooves at the bottom of the leg section can also accommodate a distal platform that can be used as a foot extension for tall patients or folded up at 90 degrees and padded to support the feet and ankles when the patient is in steep reverse Trendelenburg.

Specialty OR beds are available for specific types of procedures. The orthopedic fracture bed (Fig. 6.17) has multiple movable and removable parts and suspended frames. Special orthopedic extensions and accessories that duplicate the functions of the features on traditional orthopedic fracture beds are available for some OR beds. Although urologic procedures can be done on a general OR bed set up in the lithotomy position, specialty urology beds remain useful in the OR because they have built-in drainage trays and radiologic equipment. Special beds are made specifically for spinal procedures (Fig. 6.18). These beds support the prone patient's torso so that the abdomen falls freely. This prevents the abdominal contents from compressing the aorta, inferior vena cava, and diaphragm. This allows for better circulation and ventilation and reduces venous constriction, which in turn reduces bleeding during spinal surgery. The leg supports are open at the knees, thus eliminating knee pressure.

Multiple positioning accessories help to achieve desired positions and cushion pressure points. Examples include various headrests, stirrups, arm supports, hand tables, and footboards. Foam and gel pads and overlays come in various shapes and sizes for specific areas of the body (Fig. 6.19).

Mattress Materials and Their Pressure-Reducing Properties

OR mattresses should meet certain basic requirements. They should be durable; versatile for many uses; nonflammable; resistant to bacterial growth; radiolucent with low x-ray attenuation; compatible with

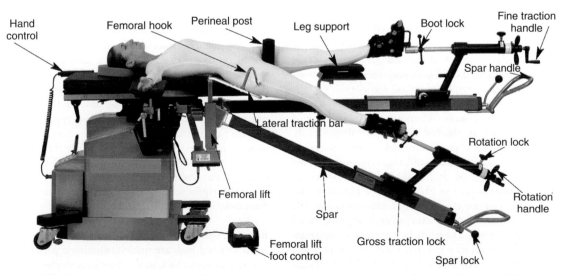

FIG. 6.17 Model on fracture bed. Unaffected leg may be also raised, abducted, and supported in a padded leg rest.

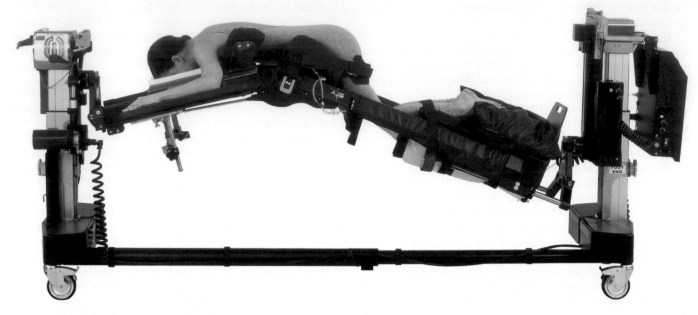

FIG. 6.18 Axis Jackson system uses hinged technology to position patient in various prone and semikneeling positions for spinal surgery.

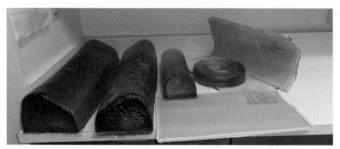

FIG. 6.19 Various positioning pads and supports made with dry viscoelastic gel. *Left to right*, Chest rolls for prone positioning, small flat bottom roll used as a bolster or axillary roll (two could be used as pediatric chest rolls), donut headrest, arm sled/toboggan, small pad *(right front)*.

warming and cooling devices; and covered with flexible, nonallergenic, antistatic fabric. Mattresses also should be able to withstand many cleanings with bactericidal agents. Many mattress pads are now made without latex. OR mattresses should also have pressure-reduction capabilities.

Pressure-reduction and pressure redistribution are primary considerations in OR mattress pads. When neither the position of the patient nor time spent on the OR bed can be altered easily during surgery, using effective pressure-reducing mattresses and positioning devices along with initial and ongoing perioperative assessment of the patient's PI risk and tissue integrity may be the most appropriate methods to prevent PI. With more attention paid to optimal pressure reduction, manufacturers are improving OR mattresses to be more protective of tissue integrity. As mentioned earlier, distributing pressure over a larger surface of the body decreases the force of that pressure. Pressure refers to the distribution of forces on the individual's body surface that is in contact with the device (NPUAP, 2014). As a person sinks or settles into the surface of the mattress pad, the weight of the body is distributed over a larger

surface area, spreading out the pressure. Overall interface pressure can be reduced by providing even pressure distribution without "bottoming out" (i.e., flattening or collapsing such that parts of the body rest on the underlying hard surface, defeating the purpose of the mattress). Mattress pads are generally constructed from a combination of materials, possibly a combination of foam, gel, air, and/or fluid. Mattress pad materials vary in their pressure-reducing characteristics. Ideal characteristics include low average interface pressure, low peak interface pressure, and a high skin contact area (Kirkland-Walsh et al., 2015). Following are some examples of available materials.

Standard Foam Operating Room Mattress Pads

Standard foam OR mattress pads have greatly improved in quality over the years. They are usually purchased with OR beds, and replacement pads can be purchased as needed. Years ago these mattresses were about 2 inches thick; made of standard foam; and covered with a relatively rigid, vinyl covering. Many of today's mattresses are more than 2 inches thick and have greater protection against the effects of pressure, and have a soft, pliable waterproof cover. With more pliable covers, patient benefit increases from the pressure-reducing properties of the mattress. Many pads are now made with advanced foam technology that reduces bottoming out. Higher specification foams should be used whenever possible (NPUAP, 2014); they have contouring properties, which allow the bony prominences to settle into the surface of the foam. As the body weight spreads over the surface, more pressure is redistributed, thus reducing interface pressures and less injury is likely to occur. The many benefits of these newer products have allowed manufacturers to offer them as their new "standard" OR pads.

Bariatric Operating Room Bed Pads

Some OR bed pads are made for bariatric patients. These pads are 4 or more inches thick, and manufacturers claim the foam contours to the patient's body in all areas it contacts to "immerse" the patient in the foam, distributing pressure forces over more of the body surface. Different products accommodate patients of varying weight and offer side attachments that also accommodate varying widths.

Products

Gel products made of viscoelastic polymer are used as overlays to mattress segments and positioning devices. Some OR mattress pads are made with a layer of gel over the foam, under a pliable cover. Gel products seem to reduce the effects of shear forces because they are pliable and similar to body fat. They support weight and prevent shearing and "bottoming out."

Other available products include a static air surface applied to the OR bed when assessment suggests a higher risk. A static air pad may allow offloading pressure points caused by the position of the patient. Also, a static air product on the OR surface may better redistribute the patient's weight, decreasing overall risk for PI.

Positioning Accessories

Many accessories are available to achieve and maintain surgical positions. Some are made of viscoelastic polymer gels (see Fig. 6.19), whereas others have specific uses and can be used in multiple ways. Table 6.3 provides a list of some common positioning devices and their typical uses.

Transfer devices enable lateral transfers ergonomically and protect patients from shear and friction. Slide boards and rollers are the most often used lateral transfer devices (Fig. 6.20). However, bariatric patients present a greater risk of injury to both patient and staff during transfers. Special air-assisted transfer devices (Fig. 6.21) enable the patient to float on a small cushion of forced air. These devices, placed deflated under the patient, can be inflated and used to transfer the patient onto the OR bed; at the conclusion of the procedure, they can be reinflated for transfer to the PACU bed. This prevents friction on the patient's skin as well as injury from a fall or trauma from a rough move. This also protects the healthcare team from back and muscle injuries; lateral moves of even morbidly obese patients are smoother and safer for everyone.

Standard Surgical Positions

This section discusses standard positions and variations for most surgical procedures, unique risks, and nursing interventions that diminish patient risks.

Supine

The supine (dorsal recumbent) position is most common. The patient lies with the back flat on the OR bed. The arms may be tucked at the side (adducted) if surgically necessary or placed on armboards. Supine is the most natural position of the body at rest and is the position in which the patient usually undergoes anesthesia.

The supine position allows access to the major body cavities (peritoneal, thoracic, pericardial). It also allows access to the head, neck, and extremities. Vulnerable pressure areas in the supine position are the occiput, scapulae, olecranon, thoracic vertebrae, sacrum, coccyx, and calcaneus (Fig. 6.22).

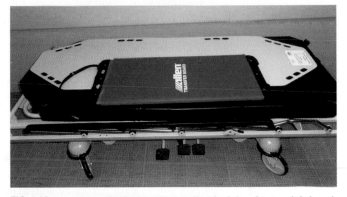

FIG. 6.20 Lateral transfer devices. *Front*, roller; *back*, low friction slide board.

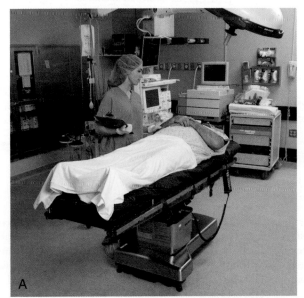

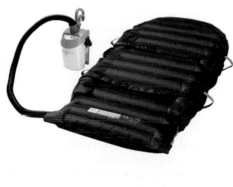

A   B

FIG. 6.21 (A and B) HoverMatt air transfer system allows for easy lateral transfers of bariatric patients because patient floats on a small cushion of air.

TABLE 6.3

Positioning Accessories: Their Purpose and Uses

Accessory Device	Purpose	Types of Procedures	Corresponding Figure
Headrests; donut, contoured	Used to support head in alignment with body	Most general and plastic procedures, ENT, vascular, orthopedic in all positions except prone	Figs. 6.19, 6.22, 6.37
Prone head positioners	Support head in prone, enabling space for and support to endotracheal tube	Spinal, posterior craniotomies, anal/rectal, Achilles tendon surgery	Figs. 6.16, 6.32, 6.35
Mayfield head device	Totally immobilizing head without putting pressure on facial structures	Craniotomies, spinal surgery	Figs. 6.31, 6.36
Pillow	Used for a variety of padding needs, including under knees to reduce back strain in supine; supporting head in supine; between knees, ankles, and arms in lateral positions	Most general and plastic supine procedures Lateral kidney, chest, shoulder, and craniotomies	Figs. 6.31, 6.36
Heel pads	Used to protect heels from pressure in supine and dependent foot in lateral positions	Most lengthy general and plastic supine procedures, especially when pillow is placed under knees Lateral kidney, chest, shoulder, and craniotomies	Fig. 6.25
Wedge	Placed under right flank in supine to shift weight of pregnant uterus or abdominal panniculus off vena cava	C-section, general or plastic surgery done on bariatric patient; for prone and semilateral positions	Not pictured
Chest rolls	Used to provide space for diaphragm and chest expansion and to ↓ compression on abdominal cavity while in prone	Posterior craniotomies, anal/rectal, Achilles tendon, liposuction of flank and hips	Figs. 6.19, 6.33, 6.34
Axillary roll	Placed under dependent lateral ribs to create enough space to prevent compression of vessels and nerves in the brachial plexus	Procedures on kidney, chest, shoulder, and craniotomies in lateral position	Fig. 6.38A–B
Shoulder roll	Placed horizontally under shoulder blades to hyperextend the neck	Tonsillectomy, bronchoscopy, esophagoscopy, thyroid procedures in supine	Fig. 6.25
Wilson frame	To arch back to separate and expose vertebrae during laminectomies and to allow for diaphragm and chest expansion and to ↓ compression on abdominal cavity while in prone	Posterior cervical, thoracic, and lumbar laminectomy procedures in prone	Fig. 6.32
Perineal post	To counteract the tension on tibia, femur, or hip during; also to stabilize patient on fracture bed	ORIF of lower extremity fractures in modified supine on fracture bed	Fig. 6.17
Stirrups	To support legs while providing access to the perineal and rectal area	Gynecologic, obstetric, urologic, and rectal procedures in lithotomy	Figs. 6.14, 6.23, 6.28, 6.29
Beach chair attachment	To provide access to the shoulder and upper chest while in semi-Fowler position	Shoulder, posterior arm, and anterior chest surgery in Fowler or semi-Fowler	Fig. 6.30
Bean bag	Support chest and trunk in lateral position; prevents sliding in steep Trendelenburg	Kidney, lateral chest, hip, elbow, shoulder procedures	Figs. 6.23, 6.36
Lateral braces	Used as support in lateral position; one round pad placed at abdomen, and vertical pads placed at lumbar area and buttocks	Kidney, lateral chest, hip, elbow, shoulder procedures	Fig. 6.37
Foam and/or folded linen	To elevate or pad selected areas of the body to provide support and/or protection from pressure	Any procedure	Figs. 6.10, 6.15, 6.22, 6.24, 6.31, 6.32, 6.34, 6.35, 6.36, 6.38

ENT, Ear, nose, and throat; *ORIF,* open reduction internal fixation.

A safety strap is placed 2 inches above the knees, with a sheet or blanket placed between the safety strap and the patient's skin. Applied with enough tension to secure the patient to the OR bed, the strap must not compromise circulation. The patient's head rests on a small pillow or head cushion to support cervical alignment, reduce occipital pressure, and minimize neck muscle strain.

Tuck arms at the side only when necessary for surgical reasons. Arm tucking subjects the patient to the risk of PI to the tissue and nerves of the arms, hands, and fingers from team members leaning against the arms or from being tucked too tight against the body, further risking compartment syndrome. If the arms must be tucked for procedural reasons, follow the safety steps discussed previously in the Upper Extremity Neuropathies section and illustrated in Fig. 6.11.

Place arms palms up on padded armboards that are at the same level as the OR bed. Abduction should be less than a 90-degree

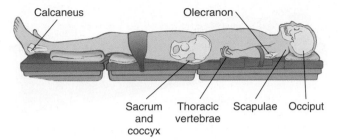

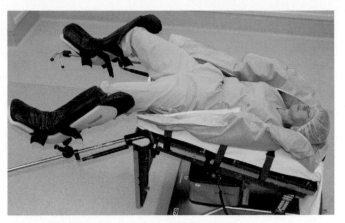

FIG. 6.22 Potential pressure areas: supine position. Pillow under calves frees popliteal areas and heels from pressure.

FIG. 6.23 Model demonstrates proper positioning in a vacuum-packed positioning device (i.e., beanbag) for lithotomy position with steep Trendelenburg.

angle to prevent stretching and compression of the brachial plexus (Cassorla and Lee, 2015). Wrist restraints should be soft and nonocclusive.

Sometimes the patient's legs must be flexed frog-leg fashion to provide access to the groin, perineum, and medial aspects of the lower extremities. To accomplish this, flex the hips and knees, externally rotate the hips, and face the feet together (Cassorla and Lee, 2015). Support the knees with a pillow under each leg or a specially contoured positioning pad. Use of this position occurs when access to the genitals is required for abdominal gynecologic and urologic procedures. During coronary artery bypass graft procedures, this position allows access to harvest the saphenous vein.

In supine position, blood volume to the heart and lungs increases compared with the standing position because venous blood from the lower body flows back to the heart without the counterforce of gravity. This increased blood volume increases cardiac output and workload. The weight of the chest in obese patients can cause increased intrathoracic pressure and increase cardiac workload further. If a patient has cardiovascular deficiencies, supine position can further increase risk for cardiac workload.

Increased pressure on the inferior vena cava from abdominal viscera, abdominal masses, or a fetus in a pregnant woman may decrease blood return to the heart; blood pressure would then lower. The inferior vena cava lies slightly to the right of the vertebral column. Tilting the patient slightly to the left by placing a small roll or wedge under the right flank can divert the weight away from the vena cava. An example is tilting a supine cesarean section patient slightly to the left until the fetus delivers.

The supine position can compromise respiratory function because tidal volume is less than when standing. The position does allow a more even distribution of ventilation from the apex to the base of the lungs. Anterior and upward excursion of the chest during inspiration is not greatly impeded except in an obese patient, whose chest wall weight significantly compresses the rib cage. The abdominal viscera lessen diaphragmatic excursion, particularly when an abdominal retractor is used and packs are placed toward the diaphragm.

Trendelenburg

Trendelenburg position is a variation of supine in which the upper torso is lowered and the feet are raised. This position facilitates pelvic organ visualization during open, laparoscopic, or robotic-assisted surgeries in the lower abdomen or pelvis (Robotic-Assisted Surgery). Trendelenburg can improve circulation to the cerebral cortex and basal ganglia when blood pressure suddenly lowers. In this position, the knees are often bent by flexing the leg section of the bed to keep the patient from sliding. The patient's knees must be over the break in the bed to maintain safe anatomic positioning.

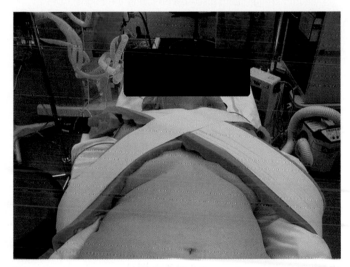

FIG. 6.24 Cross-chest strap stabilization technique for steep Trendelenburg.

Sometimes the legs are placed in stirrups during steep Trendelenburg, which is frequently used during laparoscopic and robotic gynecology or urology procedures (Fig. 6.23). Shearing is a significant risk in this position. The skeletal structure slides upward to the head of the bed. If the patient is draped, lifting the patient to realign the tissue cannot be done. Shoulder braces historically were used to limit upward sliding; however, such braces pose a risk to the brachial plexus (as described in the Upper Extremity Neuropathies section earlier in this chapter) and should not be used. In robotic-assisted laparoscopic procedures, even the slightest movement caused by sliding can negatively affect the delicate steps of such procedures done under high magnification. To prevent sliding while protecting the nerves of the brachial plexus, consider using a vacuum-packed positioning device (i.e., beanbag) that is approved for use in lithotomy position with steep Trendelenburg (see Table 6.3) or placing the patient directly on a gel overlay (without a sheet) to create a high friction coefficient. This may counteract some of the effects of shear and pressure. Additionally, padded cross-chest straps secured to the bed after the arms have been padded and tucked at the sides (Fig. 6.24) can further secure the patient. Some manufacturers offer

ROBOTIC-ASSISTED SURGERY

Positioning Considerations in Trendelenburg

As robotic-assisted procedures encompass nearly all surgical specialties, the surgical team is required to understand the unique challenges in positioning patients for robotic surgery. Basic robotic surgery positioning considerations focus on patient safety and include (1) maintaining circulation; (2) protecting from PI and injury from contact with robotic arms; (3) ensuring adequate exposure; (4) protecting the airway; and (5) affording the anesthesia provider access to monitoring equipment and IV lines. Although basic positioning prevention strategies apply to all robotic-assisted procedures, in steep Trendelenburg with severe head-down position, the following need to be considered:

- Strategies to prevent the patient from slipping toward the head of the OR bed: use accessories such as beanbag positioning systems (avoid abducting the arm), memory-foam positioners designed for steep Trendelenburg, and padded cross-torso straps.
- Methods to protect the ulnar nerve: tuck patients' arms in anatomic alignment; place palms facing the thighs; use protectors on the elbows and under the arms.
- Techniques to protect the brachial plexus: keep head in neutral positon; avoid dorsal extension or lateral flexion.
- Discussions of risk of POVL caused by increased intraocular pressure with the perioperative team. Address any assessment findings predisposing the patient to POVL. The anesthesia provider may consider administration of dorzolamide hydrochloride maleate ophthalmic solution after 2 hours of steep Trendelenburg position. If so, the perioperative nurse should verify this ophthalmic solution is readily available.
- Protocols to limit time spent in position: evaluate the need for repositioning "supine rests" at time-limited intervals.
- Discussions of the supine rest intervention during the preoperative briefing or time-out so all team members are prepared for their respective roles.
- Perform a vision check in the immediate postoperative period

IV, Intravenous; *PI,* pressure injury; *POVL,* postoperative visual loss.
Modified from Freshcoln M, Diehl, MR: Repositioning during robotic procedures to prevent postoperative visual loss, *OR Nurse* 8(4):37–40, 2014; Hortman C, Chung S: Positioning considerations in robotic surgery, *AORN J* 102(4):435–439, 2015.

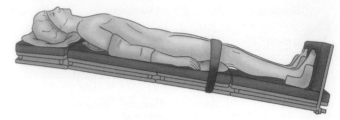

FIG. 6.25 Reverse Trendelenburg position with soft roll under the shoulder for thyroid, neck, and shoulder procedures.

access to the head and neck and to facilitate gravitational pull on the viscera away from the diaphragm and toward the feet during laparoscopic and robotic surgery in the upper abdomen. When the foot of the bed tilts toward the floor, a padded footboard supports the patient's body.

For thyroid, neck, or shoulder surgery, a pillow or soft roll is placed horizontally under the patient's shoulders to hyperextend the neck. Slightly flexed knees counteract sliding forward and minimize shearing. Arms tucked at the side allow for closer access to the surgical site.

In reverse Trendelenburg position, respiratory function is similar to that while standing. Venous circulation may be compromised by extended time in the legs-downward position. When this is anticipated, preoperative application of graduated compression stockings, elastic bandages, or IPCDs can aid superficial venous return. If the legs are wrapped, avoid compression of the common peroneal nerve at the head of the fibula. Return to the supine position from reverse Trendelenburg is slow and smooth to avoid overloading the cardiovascular system.

Fracture Bed Position

The orthopedic fracture bed allows patient positioning for hip fracture surgery or closed femoral nailing (see Fig. 6.17). The patient may be brought into the OR in the hospital bed with traction applied. Before transfer, the patient can be anesthetized. During transfer to the fracture bed, manual traction to the injured leg can be applied. Distal lower extremity pulses should be evaluated before, during, and after fracture bed positioning.

The fracture bed stabilizes the pelvis by use of a vertical post placed close to the perineum. This post should be placed between the genitalia and the uninjured leg so that pressure is not directly on the genitalia. If the post is not well padded, the intense pressure placed on the pelvis during traction of the injured leg can crush and severely injure the genitalia and pudendal nerve. Injury to the perineal and pudendal nerves can cause fecal incontinence and loss of perineal and penile sensation.

Traction occurs by securing the foot of the injured leg in a well-padded bootlike device connected to the traction bar so that the leg may be rotated, pulled into traction, or released, as surgery requires. One method to secure the foot in this device is to use a boot-shaped cuff that wraps around the entire foot and connects to the traction device. It is inflated with air to secure the foot. Another method is to cushion the foot and secure it to the device with restraining straps, elastic bandages, or a self-adhering wrap. Whatever method is used, excessive pressure on the foot and ankle, especially while traction is being applied, must be avoided and adequate padding must be used. If the boot-shaped cuff is used, do not inflate it beyond the manufacturer's recommendations. The unaffected leg rests on a well-padded, elevated leg holder or is secured in a well-padded bootlike device.

Trendelenburg positioning kits with padded cross-chest straps and arm padding.

Any variation of Trendelenburg position should continue only as long as necessary. In this position, blood pools in the upper torso, increasing central venous pressure, intraocular pressure, and intracranial pressure (Cassorla and Lee, 2015). Although the head-down position facilitates drainage of secretions from the bases of the lungs and the oropharyngeal passages, the weight of the abdominal viscera impedes diaphragmatic movement; as abdominal viscera push the diaphragm up and compress the lung bases, pulmonary compliance and tidal volume diminish. Fluid shifts into the alveoli and can cause edema, congestion, and atelectasis. Slow, smooth postural transitions allow sufficient time for the body to adjust to physiologic changes. Hypotension may result if the patient is not returned slowly to the supine position.

Reverse Trendelenburg

Reverse Trendelenburg position is described as the head-up, feet down, supine position (Fig. 6.25). It is frequently used to provide

C-arm fluoroscopy examinations can be done during surgery because the unaffected leg is abducted out of the field of the machine.

The arm on the operative side is generally secured over the patient's body in a padded sling or a postsupported arm holder to reduce obstruction of the operative area. Avoid pressure on the ulnar nerve. The edges of the sling should not be on the bend of the elbow. If a post supports the arm holder, the post and arm holder should be distal to the elbow, freeing the cubital tunnel from pressure.

Lithotomy

The lithotomy position is used for gynecologic, rectal, and urologic procedures. With the patient supine, the legs are raised and abducted to expose the perineal region. The legs are placed in stirrups to maintain this position. There are four levels of lithotomy: low, standard, high, and exaggerated (Fig. 6.26). *Low lithotomy* is used for most urologic procedures and for procedures that require access to the perineum and abdomen simultaneously. The thighs are elevated approximately 30 to 45 degrees. *Standard lithotomy* is most commonly used for gynecologic procedures. The thighs are flexed approximately 90 degrees from the trunk, and the calves remain horizontal. For improved perineal access, some surgeons prefer a *high lithotomy* position. The hips are often flexed beyond 90 degrees, and the legs are suspended high toward the ceiling. The *exaggerated lithotomy* position is sometimes used for transperineal access to the retropubic area. This extreme position moves the legs completely out of the way of the surgical field. The thighs are flexed toward the abdomen; the calves are suspended vertically; and the pelvis is flexed vertically at the spine, propped upward on a pillow or pad. Compartment syndrome is a rare complication of lithotomy position. It is more likely to occur in long procedures (greater than 2–3 hours); in these circumstances, the surgical team may consider periodically lowering the legs to the level of the body. Additional risks factors have been noted to be high BMI, blood loss, peripheral vascular disease, hypotension, and reduced cardiac output (Cassorla and Lee, 2015). Although the hips must be flexed beyond 90 degrees, care should be taken that the knees are not flexed beyond 90 degrees as well. No pressure should be placed on the legs from stirrup edges or leaning surgical staff. The amount of time in these positions should be as limited as possible. If the patient will be in this position for longer than 2 hours, graduated compression stockings/IPCDs are usually applied to the patient's legs.

Stirrups should be checked before use to see that they are securely fastened to the side rails of the OR bed. Slippage of the stirrups or dropping the legs during stirrup adjustments could cause hip dislocation, muscle or nerve injury, or bone fractures. Both stirrups should be at equal height, attached to the OR bed at the same level. The legs should be raised simultaneously to prevent strain on the patient's lower back; this requires two people so that both legs are supported throughout the move. Each person grasps the sole of a foot with one hand and supports the calf near the knee with the other. They then raise the legs simultaneously and flex the knees, all in slow, smooth movements.

When the legs are secured in the stirrups, the mattress of the leg section of the OR bed is removed, and the leg section platform is lowered. The buttocks should be even with the edge of the perineal cutout section of the OR bed, not hanging beyond the edge, to reduce the risk of lumbosacral strain.

Arms rest on armboards, or across the trunk, or tucked at the patient's side. If tucked, caution must be taken when the leg section of the bed is elevated back to a horizontal position at the conclusion of the procedure. Otherwise, the hands and fingers can be caught in the break of the bed and crushed (Fig. 6.27).

Several stirrup types are used for lithotomy positioning (Fig. 6.28). The most common include posts with knee crutches, candy cane–shaped bars with straps that wrap around the ankles and plantar surface of the foot, and boot-type stirrups that cradle the lower foot and heel and extend to the midcalf area. Each type can create unique hazards.

Knee crutch stirrups (see Fig. 6.28B), in which the weight of the leg rests solely on the knee supports, may put pressure on the posterior tibial and common peroneal nerves, and the popliteal artery, in the popliteal fossa. This pressure predisposes the patient to complications, such as neuropathies and compartment syndrome.

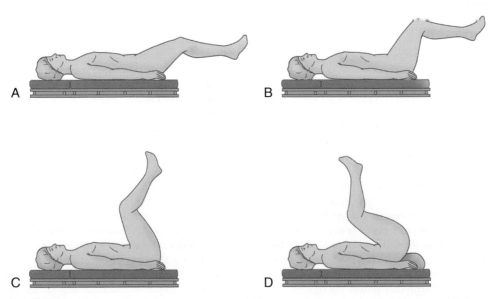

FIG. 6.26 Four basic types of lithotomy position with progressively increasing leg elevation. (A) Low. (B) Standard. (C) High. (D) Exaggerated.

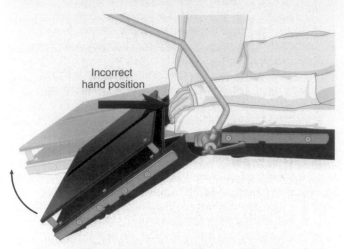

FIG. 6.27 Improper placement of arms puts fingers at risk for crush injuries when the lower section of the bed is raised.

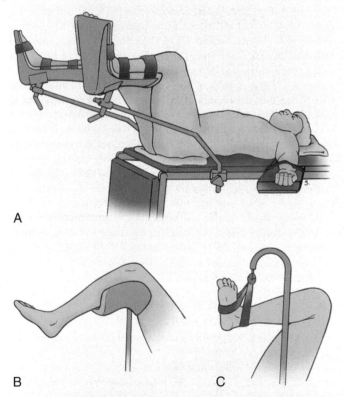

FIG. 6.28 (A) Lithotomy position using boot-type stirrups. (B) Knee crutch stirrup. (C) Candy cane stirrup.

When using candy cane stirrups (see Fig. 6.28C), the knees can drop close enough to the vertical stirrup bars that the lateral or medial side of each knee or calf may rest against the bars. This can put pressure on the common peroneal nerve as it curves laterally over the fibula, which may cause footdrop and a lack of sensation below the knee. If the medial aspect of the knee or calf rests against a stirrup bar, the saphenous branch of the femoral nerve may compress against the tibia. Padding the stirrup bars softens the rigidity of the bars, but will not eliminate pressure totally if the legs rest against the stirrup bars.

Hips should not be flexed more than 90 degrees. When the legs of an anesthetized patient hang freely in candy cane stirrups, the relaxed hips may separate further than they comfortably would if the patient were awake. There is a risk of hyperabduction of the hips, which can stretch the sciatic and obturator nerves as well as strain the hip joint and muscles.

When relatively thin ankle straps support the weight of the entire leg, such straps put pressure on the ankles and distal sural and plantar nerves. Neuropathies of the foot and PIs at the ankle support sites may result. Heavier leg weight in obese patients adds to the pressure on the ankle supports. Using wide straps or cradling the feet with gel or foam padding before placing them in the stirrup straps reduces localized pressure to the nerves in the foot. This is especially important when legs are highly elevated and so maintained for a long time. Compartment syndrome may be an undesired outcome of a patient kept in high or exaggerated lithotomy for many hours.

Boot-type stirrups (see Fig. 6.28A) allow for controlled and limited abduction, support the foot and calf, and distribute pressure more evenly, reducing the risk of extreme localized pressure on any one area of the foot or leg. The foot and calf must be well cradled in the padding of the stirrup. Slightly angle each stirrup outward to align with the shoulder. Ensure that the upper edge of the boot puts no pressure on the lateral and medial aspects of the calf and knee.

Special care is needed for the patient who has a limited range of motion attributable to a hip prosthesis. Avoid severe hip flexion and abduction of the joint. The stirrup should be as low as possible.

Preexisting lumbar backache may worsen in lithotomy position if the buttocks or lower back are not adequately supported. Likewise, elevating the legs may aggravate the pain of a herniated nucleus pulposus. Such a patient may be placed in lithotomy position before anesthesia induction to assess areas of discomfort and to implement therapeutic measures (e.g., additional padding under the lumbar area).

The weight of the legs in the morbidly obese patient may be too great for safe use of any stirrups discussed here. The thighs need to separate enough for surgical access to the perineum while safely supporting the weight of the legs. This may be achieved by using two pneumatic lifts, with pillows placed in the slings to reduce their concave shape and thick gel pads extending beyond the sling edges to cradle the feet, calves, and knees (Fig. 6.29). Egg crate foam further protects any additional pressure areas on the legs.

Lithotomy position poses significant risks for respiratory and circulatory compromise. Risks increase as the position is exaggerated for radical surgery of the groin, vulva, or prostate. Extreme flexion of the thighs impairs respiratory function by increasing intraabdominal pressure against the diaphragm, decreasing tidal volume. Interference with gravity flow of blood from the elevated legs causes pooling in the trunk of the body during the operative procedure. This effect is greater when hip and knee flexion is extreme, as in high or exaggerated lithotomy positions. This increased trunk volume may mask blood loss during surgery. When the legs are lowered, however, trunk volume returns to the general circulation, circulating volume reduces, and blood pressure may decrease. Effects of anesthesia on the nervous system depress normal compensatory mechanisms, and hemodynamic adjustment may not return easily.

Releasing the patient from lithotomy position must be done slowly and with adequate assistance. Both legs are taken out of stirrups and lowered simultaneously, giving support to the joints to prevent strain on the lumbosacral musculature. Lower the legs slowly to allow for gradual hemodynamic adjustment as more blood shifts

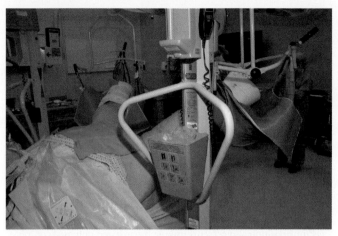

FIG. 6.29 Securing morbidly obese patient's legs in lithotomy using pneumatic lifts.

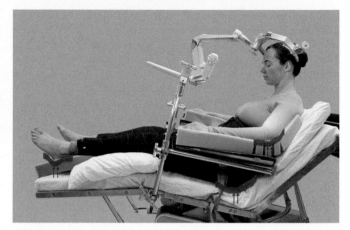

FIG. 6.31 Model demonstrates the sitting position with the head secured with a Mayfield pin device.

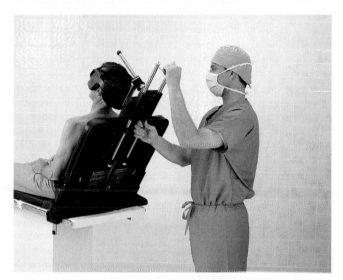

FIG. 6.30 Shoulder chair with drop-away shoulder support panels to allow surgical access to the shoulder while maintaining torso support. Padded U-shaped head restraint with adjustable Velcro straps holds the head secure and reduces undue stress on the neck when the back section is positioned.

into the lower extremities. Distal lower extremity pulses should be evaluated before, during, and after this position.

Semi-Fowler

Semi-Fowler (beach chair) position may be used for some cranial, shoulder, nasal, abdominoplasty, or breast reconstruction procedures. This position begins with the patient supine. The upper body section of the bed is flexed 45 degrees, and the leg section is lowered slightly, flexing the knees. The arms may rest on a pillow in the lap or be secured on armboards parallel to the OR bed. A footboard may be flexed at the bottom of the OR bed to act as a footrest and to prevent footdrop. The entire OR bed tilts back so that the head of the bed is not so erect.

When using semi-Fowler for shoulder surgery, a shoulder chair attachment placed at the patient's torso allows for a segment of the back support to be removed on the affected side to expose the entire shoulder area (Fig. 6.30). A head holder wraps around the head,

supports it in neutral position, and moves vertically as the head of the bed is raised and lowered. The affected arm and shoulder are prepped and draped to allow for intraoperative shoulder manipulation. They can then be placed in a sterile draped pneumatic arm holder that the surgeon repositions as needed throughout the procedure. The opposite arm is bent at about 90 degrees and rests in an arm holder secured to the bed. A large padded bolster placed under the patient's legs allows the knees to bend and secures the patient in position.

Diaphragmatic excursion improves in this position compared with supine. Although pressure points remain similar to those of the supine position, additional pressure occurs on the ischial tuberosities, calcanei, and coccyx. The risk of shear increases as the head of the bed is raised and lowered.

Fowler

Fowler (sitting) position is used for some ear and nose procedures, posterior cervical spine surgery, and craniotomies involving a posterior or occipital approach (Fig. 6.31). This position begins with the patient supine. Slowly, the upper body section of the OR bed is raised 90 degrees, while the knees are slightly flexed and the legs lowered. A padded footrest is used to prevent footdrop. The arms either rest in the lap on a pillow with elbows flexed 90 degrees or less or remain at the sides on padded armboards. Cervical, thoracic, and lumbar sections of the spine should be in alignment. When this position is used for posterior fossa craniotomy or cranial ventricular procedures, a special craniotomy headrest secures and immobilizes the head.

The main pressure points in the Fowler position include the scapulae, ischial tuberosities, calcanei, and coccyx, and pressure increases on the sciatic nerve. Padding should be adequate at the lumbar area and under the elbows, knees, buttocks, and heels. Check the popliteal space to ensure that the edge of the mattress imposes no pressure at the bottom of the torso section.

This position poses circulatory compromises and risks. Blood pooling occurs in the lower torso and legs, which in turn causes significant orthostatic hypotension and diminished perfusion to the brain. Venous return from the lower extremities also lessens, and such hindrance increases the threat of venous thrombosis. Graduated compression stockings or IPCDs assist in supporting venous return.

With the operative site elevated compared with the heart, gravity causes a negative venous gradient between the operative site and the right atrium; this negative gradient creates the potential for an air embolism if a venous sinus is opened. During a craniotomy, this potential increases when the surgeon dissects tissue free from the cranium, removes bone, tacks up the dura, or enters a highly vascular tumor bed. Monitoring for venous air embolism includes central venous catheter insertion into the pulmonary artery or right atrium, and placement of a Doppler probe over the chest wall. If air embolism is diagnosed, the scrub person irrigates the area quickly with normal saline to prevent further aspiration of air into the vein. The exposed area is then packed with saline-soaked sponges or cottonoids. If air embolism occurs during bone entry, then placing bone wax immediately over the exposed bone seals it. The anesthesia provider may aspirate air from the right atrium through the central venous line. The perioperative nurse assists and supports the anesthesia provider and scrub team.

Respiration is probably least impeded in Fowler position compared with other surgical positions. It is important, nevertheless, to ensure that if arms are resting on a pillow in the lap and secured with tape, they do not restrict chest movement. Avoiding head and neck flexion prevents kinking of the ETT and airway obstruction.

When the procedure ends, repositioning the patient back to supine happens slowly so that the patient can make hemodynamic adjustments gradually. Evaluate distal lower extremity pulses before, during, and after Fowler position.

Sometimes the Fowler position is used intermittently in short durations during breast augmentation to check the size and symmetry of the breasts under gravity and in an upright position. Although these short intervals carry none of the risks of longer durations in this position, care is taken to ensure that the arms do not fall off the armboards when raising the head of the bed. Wrapping the arms loosely, but securely, in Webril before draping keeps them in place during position changes.

Prone

In prone position, the patient lies with the abdomen toward the surface of the OR bed (Fig. 6.32). Modifications of the position allow approaches to the posterior cranium, posterior spine, perirectal area, and dorsal areas of the extremities. Pressure points include the cheeks, eyes, ears, female breasts, male genitalia, knees, and toes. Range of arm and cervical motion, as well as positional neck and arm pain, should be assessed before anesthesia induction.

Anesthesia is induced with the patient in supine position, usually on the transport vehicle. Before the patient is turned, the anesthesia provider secures the ETT with tape, applies eye ointment in each eye, and tapes the eyelids closed to prevent corneal abrasions. The

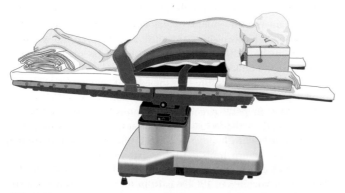

FIG. 6.32 Prone position using Wilson laminectomy frame for spinal procedures and face pillow head support.

transport vehicle is locked adjacent to the locked OR bed. Four people using the log-roll technique turn the supine patient to prone position safely, smoothly, and gently. The anesthesia provider supports the head and neck during the turn. A second person stands at the side of the transport vehicle with hands at the patient's shoulders and buttocks to initiate the roll of the patient. A third person stands at the opposite side of the OR bed, with arms extended to support the chest and lower abdomen, as the patient is rolled laterally onto the abdomen. The fourth person stands at the foot of the transport vehicle to support and turn the legs. At the completion of the turn, the transport vehicle is removed.

The respiratory system is vulnerable in prone position because normal anterior lateral respiratory movement is restricted, and the compressed abdominal wall and rib cage inhibit normal diaphragmatic movement. This position generally requires ventilator assistance.

Prone position also presents unique hazards and potential complications. As the anesthetized patient is turned from supine to prone, ETTs, IV lines, and monitoring devices can dislodge easily. In prone position, normal compensatory mechanisms are depressed, and the patient cannot readily adjust to imposed hemodynamic changes and resulting hypotension. Crush injuries can occur to the extremities during the roll from supine to prone and back. Pressure necrosis can injure the skin, peripheral nerves, and brachial plexus. Pressure on the eyes can cause PVL. Venous air embolism can occur when the surgical site is above the level of the heart. If an airway problem occurs as a result of a kinked, dislodged, or obstructed ETT, reintubation, and emergency airway management are extremely difficult from this position. Also, the position can result in swelling of the tongue, causing macroglossia.

Arm Support

Proper arm placement requires care to avoid injury: the arms may be secured alongside the torso, placed on armboards, or brought alongside the head in a "surrender" pose. If the patient has symptomatic thoracic outlet syndrome, the arms are best placed alongside the torso. Arms need to be secured so that they do not hang over the edge of the OR bed; if allowed to do so, the weight of the humerus against the OR bed side rails can compress the radial nerve quickly. Arms and palms should be neutral, close to the body, and secured with the drawsheet pulled smoothly, but not tightly, around the arms and tucked under the patient's body. The elbows face outward in this position, so there is less risk of pressure on the ulnar nerve from the mattress. Compression still can occur, however, from a too-tight drawsheet or from scrub personnel inadvertently leaning on the elbow. Padding the elbow minimizes this risk. An alternative is to wrap foam padding around the arms and to secure them to the sides of the OR bed with arm sleds.

If the arms are placed on armboards, bring the arms down and forward slowly, with minimal abduction to prevent shoulder dislocation and brachial plexus injury. Armboards should be at the same height as the OR bed or at a lower line parallel to the OR bed, arms resting with elbows flexed 90 degrees or less and hands pronated. Pads are placed distal and proximal to the elbow so that the ulnar nerve cannot make contact with the armboard (see Fig. 6.10C). If using the "surrender" position, abduct the arms less than 90 degrees without tension to the musculature of the shoulders, and pad the elbows. Check wrist pulses; they should be strong and full.

Chest and Trunk Support

If a patient were to lie flat on the OR bed surface in prone position, blood return from the inferior vena cava would be impaired between the compressed abdomen and the weight of the spine and back structures. This could cause decreased cardiac output, venous stasis, and thrombotic complications. Blood return would divert through the epidural plexus, increasing the potential for bleeding during spinal surgery. Allowing the abdomen to hang free by using a ventral support or frame can counteract this. These devices also raise the chest and permit the diaphragm to move more freely and the lungs to expand. The choice of support depends on the requirements of the procedure, the physique of the patient, and the availability of equipment. One type of ventral support consists of two parallel rolls of linen or cylindrical flat-bottomed gel pads (see Fig. 6.19) extending lengthwise from the clavicle to the iliac crest; these are often called "chest rolls." The Wilson laminectomy frame (see Fig. 6.32) also uses two parallel pads, but they are on an arched frame to facilitate spinal access. With both of these supports, female breasts may be compressed between the weight of the body and the ventral chest supports. If the breasts displace laterally, their medial borders can be stretched and injured. If the patient has a mammary prosthesis, direct pressure can rupture the implant. Gently diverting the breasts inward, toward the midline (Fig. 6.33), prevents compression from the frame.

A bolster or pillow under the pelvis can further decrease abdominal pressure on the inferior vena cava, especially in obese patients with large abdominal girths. Care should be taken, however, that a bolster rests at the iliac crest, and not at the lower anterior groin, where it can compress femoral nerves and vessels or crush male genitalia. Female breasts and male genitalia should be checked after final positioning to ensure freedom from pressure. A cushion or pillow is placed under the ankles to prevent pressure on the toes.

Another type of ventral support uses four pillar-type padded frames, two to support the chest and two to support the hips (Relton-Hall frame) or a single horizontal pad on the superior chest at the sternum and two pads supporting each side of the hip (Jackson spinal bed or Axis Jackson system, pictured in Fig. 6.18). The legs are either supported with thigh pads and a padded foot support or are placed in a padded suspension sling.

Head Support

Protection of the head and neck while positioning in prone is critical to prevent serious complications. The head of the anesthetized patient should be kept in a neutral position (Hartley, 2015). Avoid inadvertent rotation of the head and neck, hyperextension, hyperflexion, and lateral flexion or rotation.

Face pillows and facial helmet devices enable positioning with the head facing straight down while in the prone position, establishing natural spinal alignment. Such devices consist of foam or gel contoured to reduce pressure to the eyes, nose, and mouth (see Figs. 6.18 and 6.32). Openings on the side of the devices allow access to the ETT. Some come with mirrors to enable the anesthesia provider to see the facial structures during surgery. The weight of the head is supported by foam or gel at the forehead, cheeks, and chin. These areas require monitoring for signs of undue pressure.

A horseshoe headrest is another device used to stabilize the head in prone position (see Fig. 6.16). It attaches to the OR bed and replaces the removable head section, and stabilizes the head by supporting the cheeks and forehead. Its advantage is that the anesthesia provider can access and observe the entire head, face, and airway without obstruction by the OR bed. Its disadvantage is that the head is not fixed in place, so it can move. The head may become unstable during adjustments to the OR bed, which can make it difficult to keep pressure off the eyes.

Pin fixation of the head (e.g., Mayfield head device for sitting patient, as in Fig. 6.31) is frequently used for craniotomies in the prone position (as well as other positions). Three pins are tightened into the skull to support the head. This has the advantage of providing complete access to the head, face, and airway, yet, unlike the horseshoe headrest, allows for complete stabilization of the head without the risk of pressure to the eyes or other facial structures.

Tightening of the pins on the scalp, however, has a profound stimulating effect and may cause tachycardia and hypertension. Such a hemodynamic effect could be detrimental to the patient with increased intracranial pressure or a cerebral aneurysm. For these patients, a local anesthetic is injected into the skin before pin fixation (regardless of whether the patient is awake or anesthetized). Patients under general anesthesia should have their anesthesia deepened before the application of pins. Additional complications include entering veins within the skull during placement causing an air embolism; therefore the pin sites should be lubricated. Perforation of the skull can occur in patients with thin skulls (especially children) or if overtightening occurs. Special pins are used for children. Perforation of the skull can injure the middle meningeal artery, which can cause an epidural hematoma or a middle meningeal arteriovenous fistula. In patients who have had previous cranial surgery or shunts, care is required to not reenter previous pin or burr hole sites, strike craniotomy plates, or puncture a shunt valve or tubing.

Use of both the horseshoe headrest and pin fixation device risks dropping the head before it is stabilized in these devices. One designated team member holds the head until it is secured into the device. This team member should have no other responsibility than to support the head until it is safely secured in the head-positioning device.

After completion of a procedure done in prone, returning the patient to supine position on the transport vehicle requires a four-person log-roll technique. If a laminectomy frame was used, it can be tilted in the direction of the transport vehicle to initiate the

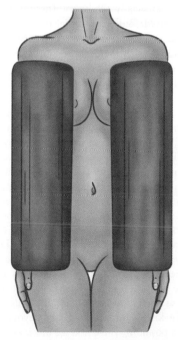

FIG. 6.33 Breasts diverted inward toward midline while using chest rolls in prone position (posterior view).

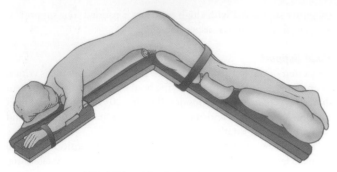

FIG. 6.34 Jackknife (Kraske) position.

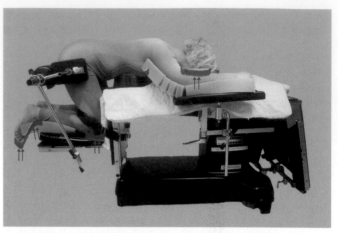

FIG. 6.35 Kneeling position with pressure points highlighted in red.

move. Skin integrity is checked over all pressure-point areas. Distal extremity pulses should be evaluated before, during, and after prone position.

Prone Jackknife

The jackknife (or Kraske) position is a modification of the prone position often used for hemorrhoidectomy or pilonidal sinus procedures (Fig. 6.34). The patient's hips are placed on a bolster or pillow over the break in the lumbar section of the OR bed, and the bed is flexed at a 90-degree angle, raising the hips and lowering the head and trunk. The patient's head, chest, and feet need the usual prone supports in this position. Chest rolls placed from under each shoulder to the iliac crest relieve pressure on the brachial plexus from the clavicle. A pillow is placed under the lower legs to prevent pressure on the toes. The restraint strap is placed across the posterior thighs.

For anal procedures the buttocks may be separated with strips of 3-inch tape secured firmly at the level of the anus a few inches from the midline on either side. These strips are pulled tight simultaneously and are fastened to the underside of the bed surface. The strips are released at the end of the procedure to facilitate approximation of the wound edges.

Jackknife position causes circulatory changes because the head and feet are in dependent positions, causing cephalad and caudad venous pooling. Graduated compression stockings or IPCDs assist in venous return and decrease the risk of venous thrombosis.

This position also severely compromises respirations because it restricts anterior lateral chest movement. In addition, it allows the abdominal viscera to exert pressure on the diaphragm, and that stress exacerbates the pressure from the flexed OR bed. This may pose significant risks to obese patients. Increased intra-abdominal pressure poses increased risk of aspiration; inferior vena cava compression and an increase in cardiac output are also considered risks for obese patients in prone jackknife (Fletcher, 2014).

When the procedure is completed, the patient is placed on the transport vehicle in supine position. The OR bed is first straightened slowly so that the body can adjust hemodynamically. Four people using the log-roll technique turn the patient. Distal lower extremity pulses should be evaluated before, during, and after the prone jackknife position.

Prone Kneeling

Use of the kneeling modification to the prone position occurs primarily for spinal surgeries such as thoracic and lumbar laminectomies and diskectomies, but can also be used for adrenal or rectal surgery (Fig. 6.35). The prone kneeling position requires the hips and knees to be flexed approximately 90 degrees. A padded platform supports the legs, and the feet and toes are supported so they remain free of pressure. Either lateral supports on both sides of the hip or a posterior support at the back of the buttocks stabilize the hips and buttocks. Place a safety strap around the posterior area of the thighs, avoiding compression of the nerves and vessels in the popliteal fossa. If a female patient's breasts are large, a flat-bottomed gel bolster placed above the breasts supports the chest. If the breasts are small, the bolster is placed immediately below the breasts. Male genitalia are checked to ensure that they are not compressed between the pelvis and OR bed. The head is supported in a neutral position with a head positioner. The arms are supported on armboards placed parallel to the OR bed. The prone kneeling position can be achieved on a regular OR bed with the support accessories described here or on a spinal surgery bed (Andrews) designed specifically for this position.

Pressure points are a vital consideration for this position. They include the eyes, ears, chin, anterior rib cage, female breasts, anterior iliac crests, male genitalia, anterior tibial aspects of the calves, dorsal feet, and toes, and, especially, the knees. These areas need to be well padded and supported. Pedal and radial pulses should be assessed before, during, and after prone kneeling positioning to ensure adequate perfusion of all four extremities.

The advantage of this position is that it enables the abdomen to hang free, reducing pressure on the abdomen and the inferior vena cava. This eases ventilation and reduces bleeding by minimizing pressure on the epidural veins. It also provides good exposure and access to the posterior spine. Complications associated with this position are similar to those of prone, but also raise concern for the effects of legs being lower than the body and the weight of the hips and thighs resting on bent knees. The knees sustain significantly more pressure in prone kneeling than in any other position. Injury to the knee joint and necrosis to the skin and muscles around the knee may result. Hypotension is caused by the pooling of blood into the lower extremities. This can be somewhat counteracted by the use of graduated compression stockings or IPCDs placed on the patient before anesthesia induction. The longer this position continues, however, the greater is the risk for thrombosis and pulmonary embolism. There have been reports of compartment syndrome and rhabdomyolysis as complications of prone kneeling position, particularly when the knees and hips are flexed beyond 90 degrees (the tuck or knee-chest position). These risks are increased in obese patients. A 45/45 suspended position (i.e., hips and knees flexed at 45 degrees and legs suspended in a sling) could reduce the risk of compartment

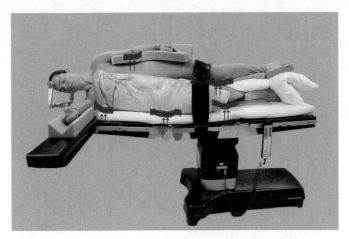

FIG. 6.36 Lateral position with Mayfield pins and beanbag positioner. Pressure points highlighted in red.

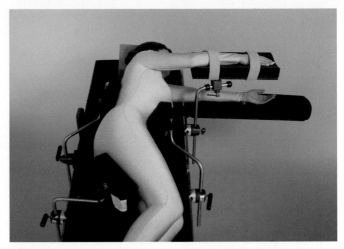

FIG. 6.37 Maintaining lateral position with three lateral braces positioned at the abdomen, lower back, and upper posterior thighs.

syndrome for procedures that require a kneeling or knee-chest position. Some newer specialty spinal bed systems use a hinged frame to place the patient in a 45/45 suspended prone position (see Fig. 6.18), accomplishing the surgical access benefits of the prone kneeling position while limiting some of the associated risks.

Lateral

In the lateral (lateral recumbent, lateral decubitus, or Sims) position, the patient lies on the nonoperative side, providing access to the upper chest, the kidney, or the upper section of the ureter (Fig. 6.36) and the hip. Reference to right or left lateral position depends on the side on which the patient lies: in right lateral position, the patient lies with the right side down; in left lateral, the patient lies with the left side down.

After induction of anesthesia and with the patient in supine position on the OR bed, the patient is turned to the side. A four-person team uses a prepositioned lift-sheet under the patient to facilitate a safe, smooth, gentle turn.

A pillow, cushion, or other head positioner (the Mayfield pin device is pictured in Fig. 6.36), is placed under the patient's head to maintain good alignment with the cervical spine and the thoracic vertebrae; good alignment also helps minimize stretching on the dependent brachial plexus. Bottom leg flexion at the knee and hip stabilizes the patient on the OR bed. The top leg is straight or slightly flexed. A pillow is placed lengthwise between the patient's legs. Padding at the lateral aspect of the bottom knee and ankle prevents pressure on the common peroneal nerve and distal fibula. Designated team members remain at the patient's front and back to steady and support the torso during positioning of the lower extremities.

Pillows, rolled blankets, padded lateral braces (Fig. 6.37), or a surgical positioning system, (sometimes referred to as a "vac-pac," or "beanbag" as shown in Fig. 6.36), support the torso. A beanbag is a soft pad filled with tiny beads. When suction is attached to a port on the pad, it conforms to the shape of whatever it is wrapped around. A valve closes to maintain the vacuum. The beanbag acts as an immobilizer until air is reintroduced and then softens back into its original shape. During the time it is rigid, the beanbag increases the interface pressures on all the tissue it contacts, and risk of PI increases. Some manufacturers offer beanbag positioners with a layer of gel on the surface to reduce interface pressures.

Wide tape fastened to the platform of the OR bed secures the shoulders, hips, and legs. The upper arm is placed on an elevated armboard or rests on a pillow in front of the patient. The lower arm is flexed and rests on an armboard. The lower shoulder is brought slightly forward, and an axillary roll is placed under the rib cage of the down chest, posterior to the axilla (not in the axilla; the axilla is kept clear; Fig. 6.38). This places the weight of the chest on the rib cage instead of compressing the down shoulder and axilla, which could lead to injury to the brachial plexus of the dependent arm. An axillary roll is typically made of rolled linen or a cylindrical gel pad. IV bags should not be used for this purpose because they are not designed to redistribute pressure. They can roll and leak, increasing the risk of tissue trauma, PIs, and electrosurgical burns. After the patient is positioned, radial pulses are checked to confirm adequate circulation in the dependent hand and arm.

Systolic and diastolic pressures decrease in the lateral position because pharmacologic agents and pathophysiologic processes depress normal compensatory mechanisms. The patient may not readily compensate for abrupt postural changes. Respiratory function is compromised by the weight of the body on the lower chest. Chest movements are limited, and the chest size may be decreased. Distal extremity pulses should be evaluated before, during, and after lateral position and all of its modifications.

Lateral Chest

The lateral chest position is a modification that allows operative approach to the uppermost part of the thoracic cavity. A variation in upper arm placement occurs when the arm is flexed slightly at the elbow and raised above the head to elevate the scapula. This provides access to the underlying ribs and widens the intercostal spaces. A raised armboard or pillow supports the uppermost arm. Slanting the upper section of the bed downward places the trachea and mouth at a level lower than the lungs, a position that enables bronchial secretions and fluids from the lung bases to drain into the mouth and not pass into the unaffected side of the chest.

A respiratory effect of lateral chest position is that the dependent lung is more perfused because of gravitational pooling of blood. The nondependent lung is more easily ventilated, however, because it is less compressed. This results in a ventilation-perfusion mismatch. The anesthesia provider applying positive end-expiratory pressure

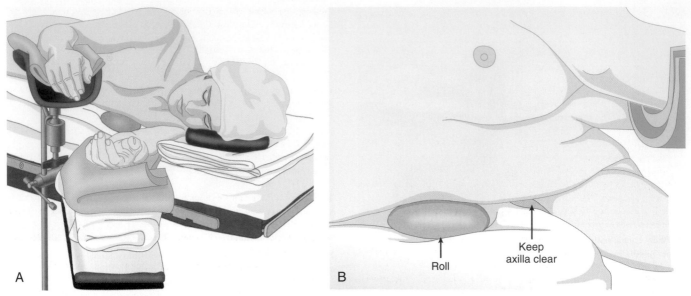

FIG. 6.38 Proper placement of axillary roll in lateral position. (A) Note the placement of arms with additional padding under the head to maintain alignment. Dependent eye is clear of the headrest. (B) The roll is placed under the chest wall, caudal to the axilla, leaving the axilla area free to prevent compression of the brachial plexus.

(PEEP) to both lungs helps compensate for this decrease in functional lung capacity. When the nondependent lung is the site of the operation and decompressed, however, functional lung capacity worsens further.

Lateral Kidney

The lateral kidney position allows the approach to the retroperitoneal area of the flank. While being turned from the supine to lateral kidney position, the anesthetized patient is positioned so that the lower iliac crest is just below the lumbar break on the OR bed where the kidney bridge is. For torso stabilization, well-padded lateral braces can support the abdomen, back, and hips. To render the kidney region readily accessible, the kidney bridge is raised, and the bed flexed so that the area between the 12th rib and the iliac crest elevates. Raising the kidney bridge depends on the cardiovascular response of the body to increased pressure transmitted from this area. It should be raised slowly as the anesthesia provider monitors blood pressure. The OR bed is flexed to lower the patient's head and legs. The patient's affected side thus presents a straight horizontal line from shoulder to hip. In this position the gravitational force on the head and torso opposes that on the extended limb to facilitate operative exposure.

Increased intraabdominal pressure induced by the kidney bridge and by flexion of the lower limbs toward the abdomen limits diaphragmatic movement. The acute angulations of the body in lateral kidney position and the effect of gravity also may decrease blood return to the right side of the heart.

Before wound closure the kidney bridge is lowered and the bed is straightened to facilitate approximation of wound edges.

Key Points

- Positioning is a collaborative effort among the entire surgical team.
- To ensure the safety of patients undergoing surgery, perioperative nurses need to understand the physiologic effects of placing anesthetized patients in their intended surgical positions and assist in taking preventative measures to safeguard them from complications that may arise.
- Physical forces during lengthy surgical procedures predispose patients to skin and tissue injuries related to pressure, shear, friction, moisture, and heat. Perioperative nurses need to identify and protect pressure points, avoid shear and friction producing movements, keep the skin dry, and prevent thermal injuries.
- Nerve injuries can occur in any surgical position. Special care is taken to avoid their occurrence. Perioperative nurses must know the location of commonly injured nerve sites (such as the ulnar nerve and brachial plexus) and use positioning strategies to safeguard nerves in these areas. Not all postoperative neuropathies are explainable or entirely preventable.
- Severely and morbidly obese patients present unique challenges and risks during surgical positioning. Perioperative nurses need to properly prepare for these patients to ensure their safety during transfer and positioning without causing injury to them or to OR personnel.
- The OR bed and accessories need to provide an adequate surface with appropriate padding to protect patient tissue and nerves.
- Perioperative nurses need to understand and accommodate for respiratory and cardiovascular risks in any intended position.

Critical Thinking Questions

A 35-year-old woman is scheduled for an ORIF of a fractured distal fibula. She weighs 305 pounds and is 5′5″ tall. She was recently diagnosed as having type 2 diabetes. You interview her in the preoperative area and note that the head of her bed is elevated about 60 degrees. She is alert and oriented and states she broke her ankle while walking on an uneven sidewalk. What factors would you incorporate in your perioperative plan of care? What critical assessment factors would you include? What perioperative nursing interventions would you use to address them?

ⓔvolve *The answers to the Critical Thinking Questions can be found at http://evolve.elsevier.com/Rothrock/Alexander.*

References

AHRQ Patient Safety Network: *Never events* (website), 2016. https://psnet.ahrq.gov/primers/primer/3/never-events. (Accessed 1 January 2017).

American Society of Anesthesiologists (ASA): Practice advisory for prevention of perioperative peripheral neuropathies, *Anesthesiology* 114(4):741–754, 2011.

American Society of Anesthesiologists Task Force on Perioperative Visual Loss: Practice advisory for perioperative visual loss associated with spine surgery, *Anesthesiology* 116(2):2745–2785, 2012.

Association of periOperative Registered Nurses (AORN): *Guidelines for perioperative practice*, Denver, 2017, The Association.

Black J et al: Ten top tips: preventing pressure ulcers in the surgical patient, *Wounds International* 5(4):14–18, 2014.

Brodsky JB: *Positioning the morbidly obese patient* (website), 2013. www.airwaylearning.com/awel/articles/articles-1.aspx?Action=1&NewsId=1944&PID=71655.(Accessed 2 January 2017).

Campbell JL et al: The skin safety model: reconceptualizing skin vulnerability in older patients, *J Nurs Scholarsh* 48(1):14–22, 2016.

Cassorla L, Lee J-W: Patient positioning and associated risks. In Miller RD, editor: *Miller's anesthesia*, ed 8, Philadelphia, 2015, Saunders.

Centers for Medicare & Medicaid Services: *Hospital-acquired conditions* (website), 2008, www.cms.gov/Medicare/Medicare-Fee-for-Service Payment/HospitalAcqCond/Hospital-Acquired_Conditions.html. (Accessed 1 January 2017).

Chard R: Care of intraoperative patients. In Ignatavicius DD, Workman ML, editors: *Medical-surgical nursing—patient-centered collaborative care*, St Louis, 2016, Elsevier.

Chhabra A et al: Peripheral nerve injury grading simplified on MR neurography: as referenced to Seddon and Sunderland classifications, *Indian J Radiol Imaging* 24(3):217–224, 2014.

Edsberg LE et al: Revised national pressure ulcer advisory panel pressure injury staging system, *J Wound Ostomy Continence Nurs* 43(6):585–597, 2016.

Fletcher HC: Preventing skin injury in the OR, *OR Nurse* 8(2):29–34, 2014.

Freshcoln M, Diehl MR: Repositioning during robotic procedures to prevent postoperative visual loss, *OR Nurse* 8(4):37–40, 2014.

Giachetta-Ryan D: Perioperative pressure ulcers: How can they be prevented?, *OR Nurse* 9(4):22–28, 2015.

Goodman T, Spry C: *Essentials of perioperative nursing*, ed 6, Burlington, MA, 2017, Jones & Bartlett Learning.

Hartley J: *Patient positioning during anaesthesia* (website), 2015. www.aagbi.org/sites/default/files/311%20Patient%20positioning%20during%20anaesthesia[1]_0.pdf. (Accessed 1 January 2017).

Kirkland-Walsh H et al: Pressure mapping comparison of four OR surfaces, *AORN J* 102(1):61, 2015.

Liem LK: *Intraoperative neurophysiological monitoring* (website), 2016. http://emedicine.medscape.com/article/1137763-overview#a4. (Accessed 1 January 2017).

Lupe L et al: Prevention of hospital acquired pressure ulcers in the operating room and beyond: a successful monitoring and intervention strategy program, *Int Anesthesiol Clin* 51(1):128–146, 2013.

Mathias JM: Fine-tuning the Munro Scale for pressure ulcers, *OR Manager* 31(6):4–5, 2015.

Meehan A et al: A nurse-initiated perioperative pressure injury risk assessment and prevention protocol, *AORN J* 104(6):554–565, 2016.

Minnich L et al: partnering for perioperative skin assessment: a time to change a practice culture, *J Perianesth Nurs* 29(5):361–366, 2014.

National Pressure Ulcer Advisory Panel (NPUAP), European Pressure Ulcer Advisory Panel and Pan Pacific Pressure Ulcer Injury Alliance: *Prevention and treatment of pressure ulcers: clinical practice guidelines*, Osborne Park, Western Australia, 2014, Cambridge Media.

National Pressure Ulcer Advisory Panel (NPUAP): *NPUAP announces a change in terminology from pressure ulcer to pressure injury and updates to the stages of pressure injury* (website), 2016. www.npuap.org/national-pressure-ulcer-advisory-panel-npuap-announces-a-change-in-terminology-from-pressure-ulcer-to-pressure-injury-and-updates-the-stages-of-pressure-injury/. (Accessed 1 January 2017).

Postoperative Visual Loss Study Group: Risk associated with ischemic optic neuropathy after spinal fusion surgery, *Anesthesiology* 116(1):15–24, 2012.

Scott S: Perioperative pressure injuries, *Patient Safety and Quality Healthcare* 13(4):21–26, 2016.

CHAPTER 7
Sutures, Sharps, and Instruments

MARY MICHAELA CROMB

Sutures, sharps, and instruments are the tools of the surgical team that are necessary to successfully complete a surgical procedure. It is the responsibility of the perioperative team to understand these tools and be proficient with their preparation for surgery. Although there are many other aspects of the perioperative registered nurse (RN) role that ensure the expected outcome of a surgical intervention, these items are the basis for surgical procedures. This chapter describes and illustrates a basic knowledge for the perioperative RN and scrub person (who may be an RN or a surgical technician), but as the surgical arena continues to evolve, especially technologically, the perioperative team should be receptive to change and develop proficiencies in new surgical devices and techniques.

Suture Materials

Suture is a generic term for all materials used to repair and reapproximate incised or torn tissues. The primary reason to use sutures is to encourage wound healing of the injured tissue to reduce the risk of infection. To *suture* is to stitch together cut or torn edges of tissue. A *ligature* is a strand of suture material used to tie off or occlude blood vessels to prevent bleeding or to isolate a mass of tissue for excision. A variety of suture materials are available for ligating, suturing, and closing the wound. Each type of suture has inherent characteristics, which affect its handling, tying, and stability in tissue. Selection of closure material is determined by lesion location, anticipated wound tension, defect size, type of repair, and patient attributes. An understanding of the characteristics of suture materials, knowledge of the risk factors of wound healing, and awareness of the interactions between tissues and suture materials for proper wound healing is essential for the perioperative nurse, as well as all members of the surgical team.

Characteristics of Suture Material

The naming of suture is guided by diameter and tensile strength. Very large sutures have numbers greater than zero, with the size number of the suture increasing with increased diameter. For sutures below size zero, the nomenclature changes to one of an increasing number of zeros for decreasing size. Thus 00 (2-0) suture has a larger diameter than 000 (3-0) suture (Lear, 2015).

Key features used to evaluate the general properties of suture material are (1) physical characteristics, (2) handling characteristics, and (3) tissue-reaction characteristics (Box 7.1).

The ideal suture material is one that causes minimal inflammation and tissue reaction while providing maximal strength during the inflammatory phase of wound healing (see Chapter 9). There is no ideal suture for every application, and even the best application presents risks of individual suture failure. Perioperative nurses should evaluate the characteristics of sutures to determine the ideal choice for surgical patient care and incorporate research findings into their clinical practice.

Physical Characteristics

The Food and Drug Administration (FDA) uses United States Pharmacopeia (USP) naming, diameter and tensile strength standards in assessing sutures, and sterility and packaging controls to ensure the safety of the public. Physical characteristics of sutures can be measured or visually determined and include the following properties:

- *Physical configuration:* Suture material can be single-strand (monofilament) or multistrand (multifilament), containing numerous fibers rendered into a single thread by twisting or braiding (Fig. 7.1).
- *Coating:* Sutures may be coated with various materials to facilitate passage through tissue. Newer innovations include suture coatings with antibacterial or antitumor qualities (Srivastava et al., 2015).
- *Capillarity:* The ability to transmit fluid along the strand.
- *Diameter (size):* Size is measured in millimeters and expressed in USP sizes with zeros, that is, the smaller the cross-sectional diameter, the more zeros; sizes range from #7, the largest, to 11-0, the smallest. Suture sizes 0 to 4-0 are the most commonly used in general surgery. (The surgeon usually selects the finest suture possible for the tissue being closed. The finer diameter [smaller size] provides better handling qualities and small knots.

BOX 7.1

Characteristics of Suture Material

Physical Characteristics
- Physical configuration
- Coating
- Capillarity
- Diameter (caliber; also referred to as size)
- Tensile strength
- Knot strength
- Elasticity
- Plasticity
- Memory

Handling Characteristics
- Pliability
- Tissue drag (related to the coefficient of friction)
- Knot tying (related to the coefficient of friction)
- Knot slippage (related to the coefficient of friction)

Tissue-Reaction Characteristics
- Inflammatory and fibrous cell reaction
- Absorption
- Potentiation of infection
- Allergic reaction

Modified from Srivastava D et al: Suturing technique and other closure materials. In Robinson JK et al, editors: *Surgery of the skin*, ed 3, Philadelphia, 2015, Elsevier.

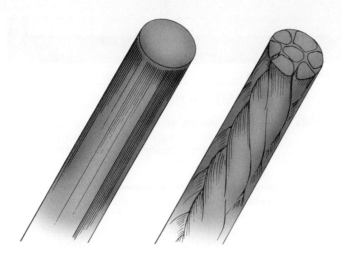

FIG. 7.1 *Left,* Monofilament suture; *right,* multifilament (braided) suture.

Improved suturing techniques are possible with sutures of finer diameter.)
- *Tensile strength:* The amount of weight (breaking load) necessary to break a suture (breaking strength); it varies according to the type of suture material.
- *Knot strength:* The force necessary to cause a given type of knot to slip, either partially or completely.
- *Elasticity:* The suture's inherent ability to regain original form and length after having been stretched.
- *Memory:* The capacity of a suture to return to its former shape after being re-formed, as when tied; high memory yields less knot security.

Handling Characteristics

Handling characteristics of suture material are related to pliability (e.g., how easily the material bends) and the coefficient of friction (e.g., how easily the suture slips through tissue and can be tied). A suture with a high friction coefficient tends to drag through tissue. It is more difficult to tie because its knots do not set easily. Some suture materials are coated to reduce their coefficient of friction. This coating not only improves the way they pull through tissue on insertion but also lessens the force needed to remove the suture after the wound is healed. The coefficient of friction should not be too low, however, because then knots will be loosened too easily.

Tissue-Reaction Characteristics

Because it is a foreign substance, all suture materials cause some tissue reaction. Tissue reaction begins when the suture inflicts injury to the tissue during insertion. In addition, tissue reacts to the suture material itself. This reaction begins with an infiltration of white blood cells into the area; macrophages and fibroblasts then appear; and by about the seventh day, fibrous tissue with chronic inflammation is present. The reaction persists until the suture is encapsulated (nonabsorbable material) or absorbed (absorbable material) by the body.

Types of Suture Material

Suture materials are classified into two main groups: absorbable and nonabsorbable. The suture may then be divided into two subgroups: braided and monofilament. Absorbable sutures have varying lengths of absorption time, which affects healing time and strength of the closure.

Absorbable Sutures

The USP defines an absorbable surgical suture as a "sterile, flexible strand prepared from collagen derived from healthy mammals, or from a synthetic polymer." It is capable of being absorbed by living mammalian tissue but may be treated to modify its resistance to absorption. It also may be modified with respect to body or texture. It may be impregnated with a suitable coating, softening, or antimicrobial agent and/or colored by a color additive approved by the FDA.

Absorbable sutures can be digested (by enzyme activity) or hydrolyzed (broken down by reaction with water in tissue fluids) and assimilated by the tissues during the healing process. Absorbable sutures vary in treatment, color, size, packaging, and resistance to absorption, according to their purpose. Types of absorbable suture include plain or chromic surgical gut and glycolic acid polymers.

Surgical Gut. Surgical gut is obtained from the collagen of the submucosal layer of the small intestine of sheep or the intestinal serosa of cattle or hogs. The processed strands or ribbons of collagen are either plain or treated with chromium salts (chromic, type C).

Plain gut sutures are indicated for use in general soft tissue approximation and/or ligation, including use in ophthalmic surgery, but not in cardiovascular or neurologic surgery.

Chromatization delays absorption of the suture. Proper chromatizing of gut ensures the integrity of the suture and the maintenance of its strength during the early stages of wound healing. It enables a wound with slow healing power to heal sufficiently before the suture is entirely absorbed.

Absorption occurs by digestion of the gut suture by tissue enzymes. The type of body tissue it contacts and, to some extent, the patient's general condition influence the absorption rate of surgical gut. Studies also show that surgical gut is absorbed faster in serous or mucous membranes than in muscular tissues. When fine chromic gut is properly buried in successive layers of the gastrointestinal tract, it retains its strength long enough for primary union to take place.

Surgical gut suture is wet-packaged in an alcohol solution to provide maximal pliability and should be used immediately after removal from the packet. When a gut suture is removed from its packet and is not used at once, the alcohol evaporates, which causes the strand to lose its pliability. If required, the strand's pliability may be restored just before use by immersing it in sterile water or normal saline solution, preferably at body temperature, for only a few seconds. This immersion is recommended only for eye sutures; in other areas, tissue fluids moisten the gut sufficiently as it passes through the tissue when the surgeon sews. Excessive moisture reduces tensile strength.

Synthetic Absorbable Sutures. The only natural absorbable suture available is surgical gut. Synthetic braided materials include polyglycolic acid and polyglactin. Monofilamentous forms include polydioxanone, polytrimethylene carbonate, and poliglecaprone (Table 7.1). The molecular structure of these products has a tensile strength sufficient for approximation of tissues for 2 to 3 weeks, followed by rapid absorption.

Other synthetic polymers provide wound support for longer periods (3 months). They are used when prolonged support for wound healing is desired, as with fascial closure or for elderly or oncology patients. They combine the desirable qualities of extended wound support and eventual absorbability.

Synthetic absorbable sutures are absorbed by slow hydrolysis in the presence of tissue fluids. Hydrolysis is the chemical process in which the polymer reacts with water to cause an alteration of the

TABLE 7.1

Characteristics of Absorbable Suture

	Handling	Knot Security	Tensile Strength	Tissue Reactivity	Uses
Gut	Fair	Poor	Low	High	Mucosal tissues, vessel ligation
Polyglycolic acid	Fair-good	Fair-good	High	High	Buried
Polyglactin	Good	Fair	High	Low-moderate	Buried; in wounds requiring short-term dermal support
Polydioxanone	Poor	Poor	Moderate	Low	Buried; in wounds requiring short-term dermal support
Polytrimethylene carbonate	Good	Good	High	Low	Buried; in wounds requiring short-term dermal support
Poliglecaprone	Excellent	Good	High	Low	Buried

Material sourced with permission from Medscape Drugs & Diseases (http://emedicine.medscape.com/), Materials for Wound Closure, 2017, available at: http://emedicine.medscape.com/article/1127693-overview.

TABLE 7.2

Characteristics of Nonabsorbable Suture

	Handling	Knot Security	Tensile Strength	Uses
Silk	Excellent	Excellent	Low	Mucosal tissues, conjunctiva
Nylon, monofilament	Poor	Poor	High	Percutaneous
Nylon, multifilament	Fair-good	Fair-good	High	Used infrequently in wound closure
Polyester	Good	Good	High	Deep tissue such as tendon or fascia
Polypropylene	Poor	Poor	Moderate	Percutaneous, buried, running subcuticular closures
Polybutester	Good	Fair-good	High	Percutaneous, running subcuticular closures

Material sourced with permission from Medscape Drugs & Diseases (http://emedicine.medscape.com/), Materials for Wound Closure, 2017, available at: http://emedicine.medscape.com/article/1127693-overview.

breakdown of the molecular structure. These sutures are degraded in tissue by this process at a more predictable rate than surgical gut (or collagen) and with less tissue reaction. These sutures are dry-packaged in sizes 10-0 to #3. They should not be dipped in solutions because moisture reduces their tensile strength. Some polymers have additional coatings to reduce drag in tissue.

Nonabsorbable Sutures

Nonabsorbable sutures are strands of material that effectively resist enzymatic digestion in living animal tissue. The USP classifies nonabsorbable surgical suture as follows:

- *Class I* suture is composed of silk or synthetic fibers of monofilament, with a twisted or braided construction.
- *Class II* suture is composed of cotton or linen fibers or coated natural or synthetic fibers, in which the coating significantly affects thickness but does not contribute significantly to strength.
- *Class III* suture is composed of monofilament or multifilament metal wire.

The strand of suture material may be uncoated or coated with a substance to reduce capillarity and friction when passing through the tissue. Several products are used for coating, including silicone, polytef, and various polymers. Fibers may be uncolored, naturally colored, or impregnated with a suitable dye.

Nonabsorbable suture material is encapsulated or walled off by the tissues around it during the process of wound healing. Skin sutures, for which nonabsorbable materials are often the choice, are removed before healing is complete. The most common nonabsorbable suture materials are silk, nylon, polyester fiber, polypropylene (Table 7.2), and stainless steel wire.

Silk. Silk is prepared from thread spun by the silkworm larva while making its cocoon. Top-grade raw silk is (1) processed to remove natural waxes and gum, (2) manufactured into threads, and (3) colored with a vegetable dye. The strands of silk are twisted or braided to form the suture, which gives it high tensile strength and better handling qualities. Silk handles well, is soft, and forms secure knots.

Because of the capillarity of untreated silk, body fluid may transmit infection along the length of the suture strand. For this reason surgical silk is treated to eliminate its capillarity properties (able to resist the absorption of body fluids and moisture). It is available in sizes 9-0 to #5, in sterile packets or precut lengths, and with or without attached needles. Silk should be kept dry. Wet silk loses 20% of its original strength. Silk is not a true nonabsorbable material. When buried in tissue, it loses its tensile strength after about 1 year and may disappear after several years.

Nylon. Surgical nylon is a synthetic polyamide material. It is available in two forms: multifilament (braided) and monofilament strands. Multifilament nylon is relatively inert in tissues and has a high tensile strength. It is used in conditions similar to those in which silk and cotton are used. Monofilament nylon is a smooth material that is particularly well suited for closing skin edges and for tension sutures. Because of its poor knot security, the surgeon usually ties three knots in small sutures and a double square knot in large sutures. It is used frequently in ophthalmology and microsurgery because it can be manufactured in fine sizes. Size 11-0 nylon is one of the smallest suture materials available.

Polyester Fiber. Surgical polyester fiber (polyethylene terephthalate, polyester/Dacron) is available in two forms: an untreated polyester fiber suture and a polyester fiber suture that has been specifically coated or impregnated with a lubricant to allow smooth passage through the tissue. Polyester fiber is available in fine filaments that can be braided into various suture sizes to provide good handling properties.

Polyester material has many advantages over other braided, nonabsorbable sutures. It has greater tensile strength, minimal tissue reaction, and maximal visibility and does not absorb tissue fluids. It is used frequently as a general-closure fascial suture and in cardiovascular surgery for valve replacements, graft-to-tissue anastomoses, and revascularization procedures.

Polypropylene. Polypropylene is a clear or pigmented polymer. This monofilament suture material is used primarily for cardiovascular, general, and plastic surgery. Because polypropylene is a monofilament and is extremely inert in tissue, it may be used in the presence of infection. It has high tensile strength and causes minimal tissue reaction. Sizes range from 10-0 to #2.

Polybutester. The newest monofilament nonabsorbable synthetic suture is polybutester. This suture combines many of the desirable characteristics of polypropylene and polyester. Polybutester has a high tensile strength with good handling qualities. Its memory is lower than that of polypropylene; therefore its knots are more secure. Like polypropylene, polybutester has a low coefficient of friction and is an excellent choice for a running subcuticular closure. Polybutester is available as a clear or blue suture (Stolle Satteson et al., 2015).

Stainless Steel. Surgical stainless steel is formulated to be compatible with stainless steel implants and prostheses. This formula, 316L (L for "low carbon"), ensures absence of toxic elements, optimal strength, flexibility, and uniform size. Monofilament and multifilament surgical stainless steel sutures are known for their strength, inert properties, and low tissue reaction. Stainless steel suturing technique is very exacting, however. Steel can pull or tear out of tissue, and necrosis can result from a suture that is too tight. Barbs on the end of steel can traumatize surrounding tissue or tear gloves. Torn or cut gloves fail to provide an adequate and effective barrier for the patient or the surgeon and assistant and can remain undetected. Kinks in the wire can render it practically useless. For this reason, packaging has played an important part in the development of surgical stainless steel sutures. Surgical stainless steel is available in packets on spools or in packages of straight, precut, sterile lengths, with or without attached needles. This packaging affords protection to the strands and delivery in straight, unkinked lengths.

Before surgical stainless steel was available from suture manufacturers, it was purchased by weight with the Brown and Sharp (B&S) scale for diameter variations. Today the B&S gauge, along with USP size classifications, is used to distinguish diameter ranges.

Suture Packaging and Storage

Types of Packaging

For packaging, the suture material is sealed in a primary inner packet, which may or may not contain fluid; placed inside a dry outer peel-back packet; and sterilized. This method permits easy dispensing onto the sterile field. Various forms of foil, plastic, and special paper are used for the inner and outer packets.

Each primary suture packet is self-contained, and its sterility for each patient is ensured as long as the integrity of the packet is maintained. Some suture packets have expiration dates that relate to stability and sterility. Packages should be stored in moisture-proof and dust-proof containers in units of one size and type.

Suture without needles is packaged as multiple strands and in reels for delivery as free ties. Suture with swaged (e.g., attached) needles can be packaged as single stitches or as multipacks containing several of the same sutures commonly used for the planned procedure. Multipacks may be permanently swaged needles that require being cut for tying or control-release (pop-off) for easy needle detachment. Some sutures may be double-armed, with a needle at each end of the strand. Double-armed sutures are most commonly used for vascular procedures such as anastomoses and vessel repairs.

Color Codes

Most companies use color-coded packaging based on suture fiber to make identification quicker and easier. Each individual packet is color coded, as is the dispenser box.

Trends in Suture Materials

There is a growth in the development of classes of suture materials based on their properties and ability to improve wound closure. Trends include antimicrobial sutures and bioactive sutures, which expand the versatility of sutures from being used just to approximate tissues to a more biologically active component enabling delivery of drugs and cells to the desired site (Dennis et al., 2016).

Barbed suture is another innovative suture type designed to prevent knot-related complications. The suture has many small barbs cut into its monofilament core along its length (Fig. 7.2), and it is

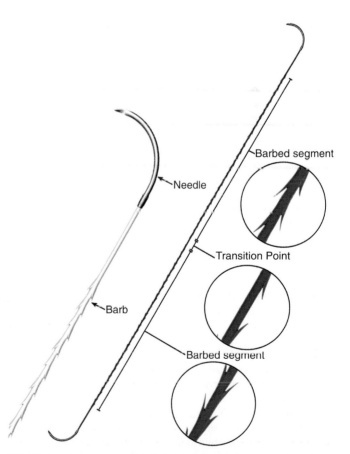

FIG. 7.2 Standard barbed suture is depicted with barbed segments oriented to lock the soft tissues into position and prevent back-tracking or sliding of the suture. The swaged-on needles and transition zone centrally are also shown.

RESEARCH HIGHLIGHT ||

Clinical Applications of Barbed Suture in Aesthetic Breast Surgery

The use of barbed suture applications is growing as surgeons become more familiar with the advantages of this new suture technology. Barbed suture devices were first used by plastic surgeons for use in various minimally invasive techniques but have now surpassed these applications and are much more commonly used in breast and body closures.

This study describes an experience with the use of barbed suture in breast augmentation and other revisional breast surgeries. The authors' longest and most used closure application with barbed suture was the two-layer breast closure in primary augmentation and revisional breast surgery. This specific closure method was used from 2011 to 2016 in more than 1200 breast procedures. The authors have not experienced any wound breakdown, skin dehiscence, or suture track infections since its implementation. The authors also found barbed suture material to be effective in all types of breast reduction patterns, nipple areolar incisions, and pedicle orientations.

Internal cost studies performed by the authors showed that for most breast procedures the net cost of using barbed versus standard sutures is essentially equivalent. For instance, the cost of using one 2-0 polyglactin and two 3-0 Monoderm (i.e., barbed suture) for a bilateral breast augmentation is cost equivalent to using two 3-0 and 4-0 poliglecaprone sutures. Additional advantages, such as time savings and efficiency of closure techniques, are also noted.

The authors noted that although barbed sutures facilitate efficiency and the speed of incision closures and allow for a very well-approximated dermis that is locked together, which may also be done sewing toward the surgeon in two layers (both deeper and more superficial dermis), it is important to use the Monoderm/poliglecaprone type versus the polydioxanone (PDS/PDO) type when superficial in the breast.

In conclusion, there is an emerging new area of surgery that has been termed limited-access surgery. It is in these limited-access applications that barbed technology is extremely useful by facilitating suturing internally in limited spaces without the need for tying knots. This limited-access application and increased speed and efficiency of closures are the main applications and benefits of using these barbed devices.

Modified from Mitchell RT et al: Clinical applications of barbed suture in aesthetic breast surgery, *Clin Plast Surg* 42(4):595–604, 2015.

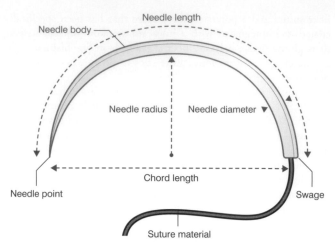

FIG. 7.3 Anatomy of a surgical needle.

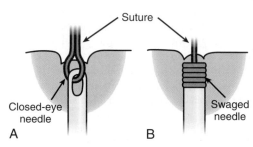

FIG. 7.4 (A) Tissue disruption can be caused by the double-suture strand with a closed-eyed needle. (B) Tissue disruption is minimized by a single-suture strand swaged to needle.

tissue. Stainless steel is the most popular, not only because it provides these physical characteristics, but also because it is noncorrosive.

Surgical needles are composed of three sections: the swage, which permanently connects the suture to the needle, the *body*, and the *point* or *tip* (Fig. 7.3). The use of eyed needles has all but been eliminated in current surgical practice; however, eyed needles may still be seen. Use of the closed eye needle requires the needle to be threaded with the suture strand, resulting in two strands of suture being pulled through the tissue (Fig. 7.4A).

Swage

The swaged suture is a single strand of suture material. When it is drawn through the tissue it is less traumatic to the tissue than an eyed needle and suture (see Fig. 7.4B). The swaged needle may need to be cut off with suture scissors or swaged for controlled release of the suture (semiswaged), which is commonly referred to as a "pop-off." With semiswaged suture, the needle remains attached until the surgeon releases it with a straight tug of the needle holder.

Body

The body, or shaft, of the needle may be round, triangular, or flattened. Surgical needles also may be straight or curved; the curve is described as part of an imaginary circle. As the radius of the imaginary circle increases, the size of the needle also increases. The body of a round needle gradually tapers to a point.

Point

Taper needles, which are round with a point, are the most common needles used and are provided as swaged sutures in many sizes for

available in several absorbable and nonabsorbable polymers. The barbs ensure that the suture stays in place and approximates the tissue without the need to tie knots. If the suture breaks during suturing, the surgeon leaves it in place and begins again rather than removing it to prevent tissue damage. Barbed suture was initially used in plastic surgery and is now used in other specialties such as general and laparoscopic surgery (Research Highlight).

Surgical Needles

Surgical needles vary in shape, size, point design, and wire diameter Needle selection is determined by the type of tissue, suture material, and action to be performed. Surgical needles are made from stainless steel or carbon steel. Various metal alloys used in manufacturing surgical needles determine their basic characteristics. They must be strong, ductile, and able to withstand the stress imposed by tough

TABLE 7.3

Atraumatic Needles

Needle Type	Description of Body	Use
Taper point	Round shaft, straight or curved, taper point, no cutting edge	Soft tissue closure, such as gastrointestinal, fascial, vascular, and most soft tissues below the skin surface
Penetrating point	Taper body with finely sharpened point	Ligaments, tendons, and calcified, fibrous, and cuticular tissue; mostly used for vascular, thoracic, plastic, obstetrics/gynecology, and orthopedic surgery; optimal penetration with less tissue wound Excellent penetration through synthetic grafts and scar tissue during repeat surgeries
Blunt point	Taper body with rounded point, no cutting edge	Friable tissue, fascia, liver, intestine, kidney, muscle, uterine cervix (note recommendations below regarding use of blunt needles)
Protect-point	Taper body with blunted point, no cutting edge	Primarily in fascia and mass closure to minimize potential of needlesticks
Reverse cutting	Triangular point with cutting edge on outer curvature	Skin closure; retention sutures; subcutaneous, ligamentous, or fibrous tissues
Cutting taper	Reverse-cutting tip with taper shaft	In microsurgery for excellent penetration through tough tissue, such as vasovasostomy, tuboplasty
Hand-honed reverse cutting	Same as reverse cutting but hand-honed for added sharpness	Primarily in plastic surgery for delicate work and where good cosmetic result is a priority
Spatula side cutting	Two cutting edges in horizontal plane	Ophthalmic surgery for muscle and retinal repair; also for delicate eyelid or plastic surgery; cutting edges "ride" along scleral layers
Rogular cutting	Triangular point with cutting edge on outer curvature	General skin closure, subcutaneous tissue; sometimes for ophthalmic surgery, plastic, or reconstructive surgery
Lancet, inverted lancet	Spatula needle with cutting edge (lancet) or outer (inverted lancet) curvature	Ophthalmic surgery and microsurgery

Modified from Ethicon: *Wound closure resource center* (website), 2016. http://woundclosure.ethicon.com. (Accessed 6 August 2016).

both absorbable and nonabsorbable materials. The cutting needle, which is round with sharp triangular edges at the objective end of the needle, is most often used for dense or tough tissues such as skin closure, thick scar, or bone (Table 7.3).

Triangular needles have cutting edges along three sides. The cutting action may be conventional or reverse. The cutting edge of the conventional cutting needle is directed along the inner curve of the needle, facing the wound edge when suturing is performed.

The reverse cutting needle is preferred for cutaneous suturing. When it transects the skin lateral to the wound, the outside cutting edge is pointed away from the wound edge, and the inside flat edge is parallel to the edge of the wound. This cutting action reduces the tendency for suture to tear through tissue.

For certain types of delicate surgery, needles with exceptionally sharp points and cutting edges are used. Microsurgery, ophthalmic surgery, and plastic surgery require needles of this type; special honing wheels provide needles of precision-point quality for surgery in these specialties. In some instances the application of a microthin layer of plastic to the needle surface provides for easier penetration and reduces drag of the needle through tissue.

Blunt Suture Needles

Available blunt protect-point needles are recommended as an alternative to taper point needles (Saarto et al., 2011). Interest in blunt needles has evolved because of the risk of bloodborne exposure from percutaneous injuries (PIs). The use of blunt needles represents a key strategy to reduce risk to the surgical team. Blunt needles are associated with a statistically significant reduction in PIs and can be substituted for conventional curved needles in a variety of surgical procedures.

Needlestick injures (NSIs) are the predominant cause of PIs in the surgical setting. Straight suture needles pose the highest risk of injury per needle use, but NSIs occur most often during suturing of fascia or muscles with curved sharp suture needles. According to the American College of Surgeons (ACS), blunt suture needles permit suturing of fascia and other structures with minimal risk of injuring the surgeon, even when the surgeon's glove punctures.

The ACS, the Council on Surgical and Perioperative Safety, National Institute for Occupational Safety and Health (NIOSH), and the FDA have all endorsed the use of blunt suture needles. The Association of periOperative Registered Nurses (AORN) Guideline for Sharps Safety recommends the perioperative team use blunt needles unless clinically contraindicated (Box 7.2).

Suturing Technique and Wound Closure Materials

Suture Selection

The choice of suture material, size, needle, and type depends on the procedure, the tissue being sutured and type of reapproximation required by the general condition of the patient, and the surgeon's preferences. A surgical services committee or project team may be responsible for establishing standard suture uses for various operations. Current guides published by suture manufacturers should be consulted. These guides list the specific suture materials recommended for various wounds and are based on current clinical practice and research. Although the perioperative nurse and scrub person are not responsible for choosing the suture material used, they must be knowledgeable of the suture properties to ensure the best possible outcome for the surgical patient.

The blunt suture needle does not have a sharp point; it dissects tissue as it is used, causing less tissue trauma than a conventional sharp-pointed needle. The risk of needlestick injury significantly lessens. The following organizations support the use of blunt suture needles in surgery:

- The *ACS* issued a statement on blunt suture needles, noting that the ACS supported "the universal adoption of blunt suture needles as the first choice for fascial suturing to minimize or eliminate needlestick injuries from surgical needles" and recommending that "blunt suture needles should be available in various sizes and with a range of suture adequate for different surgical applications."
- The *CSPS* endorses use of blunt suture needles as a recommended sharps safety measure.
- *NIOSH* strongly encourages the use of blunt-tip suture needles to decrease percutaneous injuries to surgical personnel.
- The *FDA* strongly encourages surgeons, OR supervisors, perioperative nurses, infection preventionists and other healthcare professionals to use and promote the use of blunt-tip suture needles instead of standard suture needles to suture fascia and muscle.
- *AORN* in its Guidelines for Perioperative Practice notes that blunt suture needles should be used unless clinically contraindicated.

ACS, American College of Surgeons; *AORN,* Association of periOperative Registered Nurses; *CSPS,* Council on Surgical and Perioperative Safety; *FDA,* US Food and Drug Administration, *NIOSH,* National Institute for Occupational Safety and Health.
Modified from American College of Surgeons (ACS): *Revised statement on sharps safety, Bull Am Coll Surg, October 1, 2016* (website). http://bulletin.facs.org/2016/10/revised-statement-on-sharps-safety/. (Accessed 10 October 2016); Association of periOperative Registered Nurses (AORN): Guideline for sharps safety. In: *Guidelines for perioperative practice,* Denver, 2016, The Association; CSPS: *The CSPS endorses sharps safety measures to prevent injury during perioperative care. Sharps safety measures should include double-gloving, blunt suture needles for fascial closure, and the neutral zone when appropriate to avoid hand to hand passage of sharps* (website), 2009. http://cspsteam.org/sharpssafety/sharpssafety.html. (Accessed 14 July 2016); FDA, NIOSH and OSHA Joint Safety communication: *Blunt-tip surgical suture needles reduce needlestick injuries and the risk of subsequent bloodborne pathogen transmission to surgical personnel* (website), 2012. www.fda.gov/downloads/MedicalDevices/Safety/AlertsandNotices/UCM306035.pdf. (Accessed 14 July 2016). NIOSH: *Use of blunt-tip suture needles to decrease percutaneous injuries to surgical personnel: safety health information bulletin* (website), 2008. www.cdc.gov/niosh/docs/2008-101/default.html. (Accessed 14 July 2016).

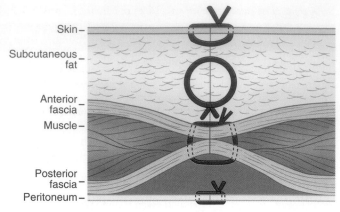

FIG. 7.5 Primary suture line on the abdominal wall, midline incision.

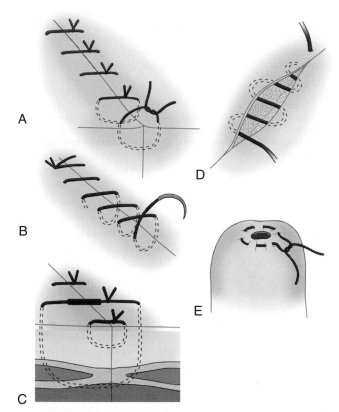

FIG. 7.6 Types of stitches. (A) Interrupted. Each stitch is made with a separate pass or "throw" of suture material, which is tied separately. (B) Continuous or "running." A stitch is made with one uninterrupted length of suture material. (C) Retention. Stitches are used to reinforce the primary suture line; heavy, strong suture material is used. (D) Subcuticular. Stitch is placed completely under the epidermal layer of the skin. (E) Purse-string. A stitch runs parallel to the edge and encircles a circular wound.

Suturing Technique

Surgeons may use suture or other devices to accomplish wound closure. The *primary suture line* refers to sutures that obliterate dead space, prevent serum from accumulating in the wound, and hold the wound edges in approximation until healing takes place (Fig. 7.5).

The *secondary suture line* refers to sutures that supplement the primary suture line. They are placed on each side of the primary suture line, passing through several layers of tissue at once. A secondary suture line helps eliminate tension on the primary sutures and reduces the risk of evisceration or dehiscence. Retention sutures are a type of secondary suture line.

An *interrupted suture* is inserted into tissues or vessels in such a way that each stitch is placed and tied individually. This type of suture is widely used and generally considered the strongest and most secure (Fig. 7.6A). Although wound closure with interrupted

technique is more time consuming, it is intended to distribute stress uniformly along the incision/wound as well as improve strength and encourage better healing. Interrupted closure should be considered when significant preoperative wound healing comorbidities exist, such as chronic obstructive pulmonary disease (COPD), diabetes, infection, and steroid dependence. The interrupted technique is routinely used for bowel and vascular anastomoses and vascular repairs.

A *continuous suture* consists of a series of stitches, of which only the first and last are tied (see Fig. 7.6B). With this type of suture, a break at any point may mean a disruption of the entire suture line. It is used to close tissue layers in which there is little tension but tight closure is required, such as the peritoneum, to prevent the intestinal loops from protruding, or on blood vessels to prevent leakage.

Retention (or *stay*) sutures are placed at a distance from the primary suture line to provide a secondary suture line (see Fig. 7.6C), relieve undue strain, and help obliterate dead space. These sutures are placed in such a way that they include most if not all layers of the wound. A simple interrupted or figure-of-eight stitch is used. Usually heavy, nonabsorbable suture materials, such as silk, nylon, polyester fiber, or wire, are used to close long, vertical abdominal wounds and lacerated or infected wounds. To prevent the suture from cutting into the skin surface, a small piece of rubber tubing (bumper, bolster, or bootie) or other type of device (bridge or button) is passed over or through the exposed portion of the suture. The bridge device allows the surgeon to adjust tension over the wound postoperatively.

Subcuticular sutures, sometimes referred to as *buried,* are sutures placed completely under the epidermal layer of the skin (see Fig. 7.6D). This technique is often used to achieve a cosmetic closure.

A *purse-string suture* is a continuous circular suture placed to surround an opening in a structure and cause it to close (see Fig. 76E). This type of suture may be placed around the appendix before its removal, or it may be used in an organ such as the cecum, gallbladder, or urinary bladder before it is opened so that a drainage tube can be inserted; then the purse-string suture is tightened around the tube. It may also be used in plastic surgery for periareolar reduction.

The Nursing Interventions Classification (NIC) lists suturing as a nursing intervention, defined as "approximating edges of a wound using sterile suture material and a needle" (Bulechek et al., 2013). The NIC was developed to classify nursing interventions so that the work of nursing could be documented and nursing knowledge improved through the evaluation of patient outcomes. In perioperative nursing practice, the act of suturing is considered part of the education and subsequent role of the RN first assistant (AORN, 2013).

General Considerations

In the preparation and use of sutures in surgery, every precaution must be taken to keep the sutures sterile, to prevent prolonged exposure and unnecessary handling, and to avoid waste. Before perioperative personnel prepare any suture materials, they should review the sutures listed on the physician's preference card or in the computerized data/preference sheets. Care should be taken to ensure fiscal responsibility by minimizing the number of sutures on the field when the initial count is performed. The perioperative nurse should have an adequate supply of sutures available for immediate dispensing to the sterile instrument table as needed throughout the procedure.

Customized suture kits that contain a designated number and variety of sutures for particular procedures, surgeons, or both are available for use when suture preferences are consistent. These kits may be more economical than individually packaged sutures because of reduced packaging costs, decreased gathering and dispensing times, and less capital outlay for inventory.

Opening Primary Packets

The scrub person tears the foil packet across the notch near the hermetically sealed edge and removes the suture. Some sutures may be packaged for delivery to the field in their inner folders, ready to load, with no foil wrapper. After opening, all sutures must be examined to ensure that the correct number of sutures is in the packet. The scrub person and perioperative nurse should verify this together.

Handling Suture Materials

To remove suture strands to be used for ties when they are not on a reel or disk, the user pulls the loose end out with one hand while grasping the folder with the other hand. To straighten a long suture, the free end is grasped (using the thumb and forefinger of the free hand) and the kinks, caused by package memory, are removed by gentle pulling with the free ends secured, one in each hand. Then the arms are slowly abducted to straighten the strands.

The scrub person should never remove kinks from suture by running gloved fingers over the strand because this action causes fraying. The tensile strength of a gut suture should not be tested before it is handed to the surgeon. Sudden pulls or jerks may damage the suture so that it will break when in use.

To remove a suture-needle combination from the package, the scrub person grasps the needle with a needle holder and gently pulls (Fig. 7.7). To straighten the suture in a suture-needle combination, the scrub person grasps the suture 1 to 2 inches distal to the needle and pulls gently on the other end of the strand with the other hand to remove kinks. The jaws of the needle holder grasp the flattened surface of the needle to prevent breakage and bending.

To facilitate suturing, the needle is secured about 1/8 inch distal from the tip of the needle holder (Fig. 7.8). The holder is placed

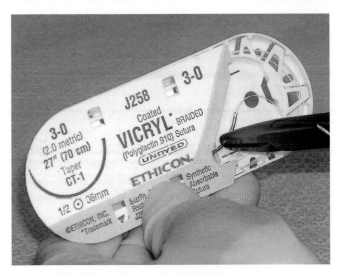

FIG. 7.7 Loading a suture directly from the packet.

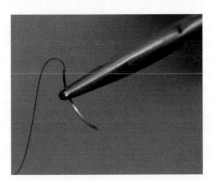

FIG. 7.8 Needle holder with needle in place.

on the needle about one-third of the distance distal from the eye or swaged end.

A suture or free ligature should not be too long or too short. A long suture is difficult to handle and increases the possibility of contamination because it may be dragged across the sterile field or fall below it. A short suture makes tying difficult. The depth and distance to the site of tying or suturing guide the scrub person in preparing ties or sutures of the correct length.

For general surgery, a continuous suture swaged on a needle is usually about 24 inches long, and its short end is 3 to 4 inches long (half lengths). An interrupted suture is 12 to 14 inches long, with 2 or 3 inches threaded through the needle (quarter lengths). To ligate a vessel in the epidermal and subcutaneous layers, the ligature may be quarter lengths. Vessels or structures deep in the wound are ligated with a suture or ligature that is 24 to 30 inches long (third lengths to half lengths). The manufacturer also provides suture in 12- to 60-inch precut lengths along with the more commonly used 54-inch lengths on reels or disks and labyrinth packs, in which precut strands may be removed one at a time from the package rather than all at once.

Knot-Tying Techniques

The successful use of the many varieties of suture materials depends, in final analysis, on the skill with which the surgeon or first assistant ties the knot. The completed knot should be firm to prevent slipping and should be small, with ends cut short, to minimize the bulk of suture material in the wound. Inappropriate handling may weaken the suture. Excessive tension, sawing, friction between the strands, and inadvertent crushing with clamps or hemostats should be avoided.

Endoscopic/Robotic Suturing and Surgical Knot Tying

Suturing endoscopically is a learned skill, not an innate talent. An array of needles and suture materials are available for endoscopic suturing, and research and development of techniques, instruments, needles, and suture materials continue to evolve as the types of procedures done endoscopically and robotically assisted increase and methods are perfected. Knot tying is one of the most challenging aspects of endoscopic surgery. Preformed ligature loops are used in ligating the appendix or blood vessels. Extracorporeal knots are tied outside the abdomen and slid into the abdomen using a knot pusher. They can be tied rapidly and securely; the square knot is commonly tied with braided suture and the slip, or granny knot, is tied when monofilament suture is used. Intracorporeal knotting is done completely within the abdominal cavity whenever fine sutures are being placed in tissues for reconstruction purposes. When the intracorporeal method is required, the suture is generally precut to a significantly shorter length permitting adequate view and easy access of the suture ends for tying. All suturing and knot-tying techniques performed through the endoscope require excellent hand-eye coordination, practice, and the ability to perform these techniques while the operative site is being viewed on a television monitor. Competency in performing surgical tasks that require the surgeon or surgical assistant to perform tasks originating from a three-dimensional (3-D) visual field (extracorporeal) to a two-dimensional (2-D) visual field (intracorporeal via monitor) requires practice, preparation, and focus. Robotic-assisted suturing (Fig. 7.9) is an exceptional example of these skills (Box 7.3).

Skin Staples

Skin staples are one of the most frequently chosen methods of skin closure and can be used on many types of surgical incisions. The

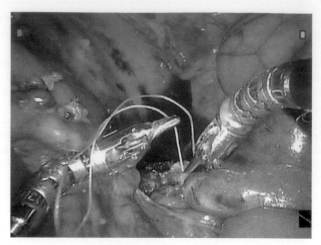

FIG. 7.9 Robotic suturing.

staple appliers are easy to use. They reduce operating time and tissue trauma, allowing uniform tension along the suture line and less distortion from the stress of individual suture points. When properly applied (Fig. 7.10), they provide excellent cosmetic results. Some staplers use bioabsorbable staples that are placed under the skin and absorbed, and the use of this bioabsorbable staple line reinforcement has become more widespread (Frattini et al., 2015). Others use stainless steel staples. With these, the length of time the staples stay in place depends on the part of the body affected; they are usually removed within 5 to 7 days. An extractor is required for their removal.

Most staplers use a similar anvil-type mechanism for forming the staple, but the application device varies from company to company. Device choice usually is determined by the weight, handling characteristics, ease of application, and unobstructed view of the site during application. Staplers are packaged in various assortments of numbers and types of staples, depending on the length of the incision and the type of tissue encountered.

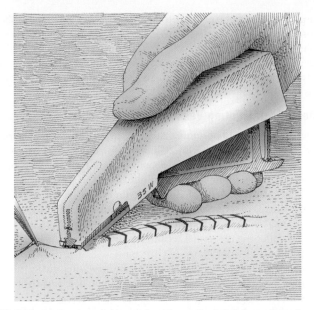

FIG. 7.10 Application of skin staples. The stapler is lightly positioned over everted skin edges. It is not necessary to press the staple, or stapler anvil, into the skin to get a proper "bite" (just "kiss" the skin). Center the staples over the incision line, using the locating arrow or guideline, and place staples approximately ¼ inch apart.

Wound Closure Strips

Wounds that are subjected to minimal static and dynamic tension are easily approximated with sterile wound closure skin tape. The selection of surgical tape for skin closure is based on the tape's adhesive ability, tensile strength, and porosity. The tape must provide a firm tape-to-skin bond to keep the wound edges closely adhered. The tensile strength must be sufficient to maintain wound approximation. A tape that is too occlusive limits moisture or vapor transmission; fluid may accumulate under the tape and lead to maceration and bacterial growth. Microporous tapes prevent this problem. The surgeon must apply the tape to dry skin; an adhesive adjunct (e.g., tincture of benzoin or other skin barrier) may be applied in a thin film to the skin at the wound edges before tape application. If an alcohol-based adhesive adjunct is used, care must be taken to prevent inadvertent surgical fires (e.g., the electrosurgical unit [ESU] must be shut off before the agent is delivered to the field by the perioperative nurse). Edema at the surgical site may cause taped wound edges to invert; supplemental skin sutures may be used to enhance closure. Tapes may be cut to accommodate smaller incisions. Tapes are applied perpendicularly to the wound edge, first on one side and then the other, so that the edges can be pulled together (Fig. 7.11).

Surgical Adhesives

Surgical adhesives may be divided into two categories: cyanoacrylates and fibrin tissue (Toriumi et al., 2016). These adhesives are sometimes

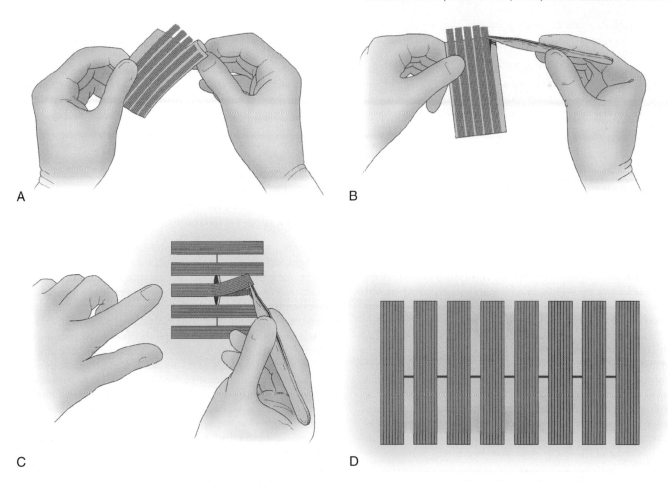

FIG. 7.11 Application of skin tapes. (A) Perforated tab is bent and removed. (B) Tape is peeled from the card. (C) Tape is applied to wound. (D) Completed application.

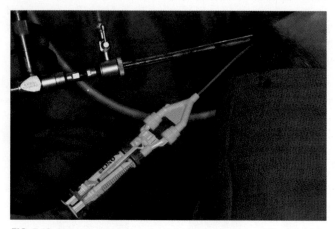

FIG. 7.12 Surgical adhesive application during endoscopic forehead lift.

grouped together and considered the same product, but the inherent properties of each result in separate indications (Box 7.4).

Cyanoacrylates

Cyanoacrylates bond and seal tissue well, but early cyanoacrylates generated a long-lasting inflammatory reaction within the body. By increasing the chain length of the molecule, the tissue reactivity decreased, but foreign body reactions still occur when cyanoacrylates are deposited below the dermis. In addition, this category of surgical adhesive has no hemostatic properties, limiting its application to superficial wound closure.

Fibrin Tissue Adhesives

Fibrin tissue adhesives, however, do have hemostatic properties. Blood clot formation occurs through the coagulation cascade of clotting factors within the blood plasma. The final result of that pathway is the conversion of the inactive fibrinogen to the active fibrin, which is one of the main components of clots. The two components of fibrin tissue adhesives take advantage of this physiology (Fig. 7.12).

Hemostasis

Hemostasis is an ongoing process during surgery. In addition to the damaging physiologic effects of blood loss for the patient, bleeding from cut vessels obscures visualization of the operative site for the surgeon and must be controlled. Hemostasis may be accomplished from direct pressure applied with surgical soft goods (e.g., radiopaque sponges, towels) or by the use of suture materials, electrosurgical devices, lasers, and chemical agents. Before wound closure the surgeon carefully checks the operative site to ensure that all active bleeding has been stopped.

Methods of Ligating Vessels

A ligature is a strand of suture material used to encircle and obstruct the lumen of a vessel to affect hemostasis, block a structure, or prevent leakage of materials. Ties may be on a reel (i.e., a spool or disk containing a long length of suture) that the surgeon may use to ligate several superficial vessels, or they may be free ties (i.e., precut lengths of suture) handed to the surgeon one at a time, usually for bleeders in deeper tissues.

The following are several techniques used to secure a ligature in deep tissues:

- A hemostat is placed on the end of the structure; the ligature is then placed around the vessel. The knot is tied and tightened with the surgeon's fingers or with the aid of forceps.
- A slipknot is made, and its loop is placed over the involved structure by means of a forceps or clamp.
- In deeper cavities, ties are often placed on clamps with the long end extending from the tip. These are sometimes called *ties on a pass* or *bow ties*. The extending long end is held tightly against the rings by the surgeon (creating the bow), who then passes the tip of the clamp under the vessel or duct to be ligated. The first assistant grasps the extending tie with a forceps, the surgeon releases it, and the tie is pulled under and up to the wound surface and tied.
- A forceps or a clamp is applied to the structure, and transfixion sutures are applied and tied. A *suture ligature*, *stick tie*, or *transfixion ligature* is a strand of suture material threaded or swaged on a needle. This is usually placed through the vessel and around it to prevent the ligature from slipping off the end.
- When two ligatures are used to ligate a large vessel, usually a free ligature is placed on the vessel and a suture ligature is placed distal to the first ligature. To ligate a blood vessel situated in deep tissues, the strand must be of sufficient strength and length to allow the surgeon to tighten the first knot.

Ligating Clips

Ligating clips are small V-shaped staple-like devices that are placed around the lumen of a vessel or structure to close it. They may be made of one of several metals, such as stainless steel, tantalum, or titanium. Stainless steel clips are the most economical to use. Although more expensive, titanium clips are used frequently in specific surgical procedures because the starburst reflection on postoperative radiographs is less with titanium than with other metals. Absorbable clips made of synthetic absorbable suture material also are available. Ligating clips are available in several sizes. These clips are available in individual sizes that must be loaded by the scrub person onto the clip applier or as preloaded, disposable, prepackaged units that include the applier. Multiple sizes and lengths of clips can be used in both open and endoscopic procedures. Ligating clips afford a rapid and secure method of achieving hemostasis when arteries, veins, nerves, and other small structures are ligated. Since the introduction of minimally invasive endoscopic surgery, the need for ligating clips that can be applied through a trocar has emerged. These clips are changing frequently, and no one standard has emerged. Regardless of the type of clip, the surgeon applies them similarly.

The surgeon often follows the application of a clip with a request for scissors.

Instruments

Historical Perspective

The history of surgical instruments dates back to 2500 BC. The first instruments were sharpened flints and fine animal teeth. Ancient Greek, Egyptian, and Hindu instruments are amazing in their resemblance to contemporary instruments.

To be equipped for the practice of surgery in the late 1700s, the surgeon had to use various skilled artisans, such as coppersmiths; steelworkers; needle grinders; turners of wood, bone, and ivory; and silk and hemp spinners. The surgeon had to explain the mechanisms of the instruments and supervise their manufacture. The resulting instruments were crude, expensive, and time consuming to make. Each artisan used hand labor exclusively and devoted time to making only one type of instrument, thus, gaining proficiency in the manufacture of a certain kind of instrument. For example, a cutter would keep a small supply of surgical knives. Thus began physicians' supply houses and surgical instrument making.

In the mid-1800s, physicians' principal tools were their eyes and ears. Official records show that amputation, the trademark of the Civil War, was the end result in three of four operations performed. Surgeons were scarce, and medical instruments were almost nonexistent. Kitchen knives and penknives, carpenter saws, and table forks did the job. After the Civil War the advent of the administration of ether and chloroform brought a demand for new ideas and methods in surgery and instruments. The division of general surgery into specialties occurred in the late 1800s and early 1900s. Delicate instruments were seen as more useful than the force of crude and heavy instruments. So that instruments could withstand repeated sterilization, handles of wood, ivory, and rubber were discontinued.

The development of stainless steel in Germany ensured a better material for surgical instruments and other equipment. Today, surgeons and perioperative nurses assist manufacturers in research, design, and development of new and better instrumentation. Most instrument companies design an instrument to a physician's specifications. Advancement in endoscopic surgery continually requires the development of instrumentation specifically designed for this type of surgery.

Throughout the history of surgery, the tools of the surgeon and the manual aspects of the surgical technique have influenced the evolution of practice. Along with innovative wound closure materials and tools in recent decades, there have been unprecedented developments of new and improved instrumentation. The benefits of minimally invasive surgery are well documented, especially in surgical procedures that typically required lengthy hospital stays, required long and sometimes difficult postoperative recovery or rehabilitation, and exposed the patient to increased risk of surgical infection.

Composition of Surgical Instruments

Successful management of instrumentation requires a continual partnership between surgeons, perioperative nurses, surgical technologists, and central processing personnel, each of whom shares responsibility for the use, handling, and care of surgical instruments. A basic knowledge of how these instruments are manufactured can help in their selection and maintenance. Surgical instruments are expensive and represent a major investment for every institution.

The United States does not have an agency that reviews or sets standards for surgical instruments. The individual manufacturer sets the quality. A reputable company endorses its product. An instrument that receives proper care should last 10 years or more.

Most instruments are manufactured from stainless steel. Stainless steel is a compound of iron, carbon, and chromium, which means that stainless steel can have varying qualities. Grading the steel into series by the American Iron and Steel Institute (AISI) designates these qualities. The 400 series stainless steel has some noncorrosive characteristics and good tensile strength. It resists rust, produces a fine point, and retains a keen edge. Handheld ringed instruments, such as scissors and clamps, should be 400 series stainless steel.

For ringed instruments, a machinist making an impression of the piece in a stainless steel blank converts the raw steel into instrument blanks. These blanks are die-forged into specific pieces—male and female halves. The excess metal is trimmed away, and the instrument parts are ready for the final steps.

The two halves are milled to prepare the box lock fittings, jaw serrations, and ratchets, and the jaws and shanks are properly aligned. After this is completed, the halves are assembled by hand. A hole is drilled through the box lock, and a pin or rivet is inserted through the hole. Final grinding and hardening, accomplished by heat-treating, permit the object to attain proper size, weight, spring temper, and balance.

The last part of the process is called *passivation.* The instruments are submerged into nitric acid to remove any residue of carbon steel. The nitric acid also produces a surface coating of chromium oxide. Chromium oxide is important because it produces a resistance to corrosion in the stainless steel instrument. The instrument is then polished.

There are three types of instrument finishes. The first is the bright, highly polished mirror finish, which tends to reflect light and may interfere with the vision of the surgeon. The second is the satin or dull finish, which tends to eliminate glare and lessen eyestrain for the surgeon. The third finish is ebonized, which produces a black finish. Ebonized instruments are used during laser surgery to prevent deflection of the laser beam.

The final inspection and testing are for hardness, proper jaw closure, and smooth lock-and-ratchet action. The instrument is cleaned and ready for sterilization and subsequent use.

Instrument Categories

Although there is no standard nomenclature for specific instruments, there are four main categories: *cutting instruments* (also called *dissectors*), *clamps, retractors,* and *accessory* or *ancillary* instruments.

Cutting Instruments (Dissectors)

Dissectors, which may be sharp or blunt, are instruments used to cut or separate tissue. The largest categories of sharp dissecting instruments are blades and scissors. The combination of blade/knife handle is probably the oldest of all surgical instruments. Most of these instruments are handles (knife handle) with one end suited to the attachment of disposable blades (Fig. 7.13). During an operation, the scrub person may conveniently change the blades as often as necessary. The blades are available prepackaged and sterile and are opened onto the sterile field as needed by the perioperative nurse. Careful handling of blades during the procedure and disposal of blades at the end of a procedure are important in the implementation of Standard Precautions.

Scissors (Fig. 7.14) are designed in various shapes and sizes for different purposes in cutting body tissues and surgical materials. The basic design consists of two blades, each having a chisel-shaped edge with the bevel consistent with the structure or material it has

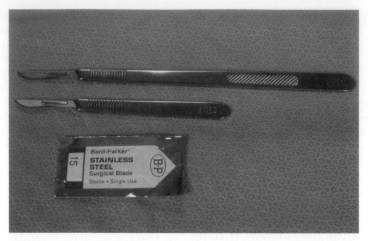

FIG. 7.13 Standard and long blade handles range from 6 to 10 inches in length.

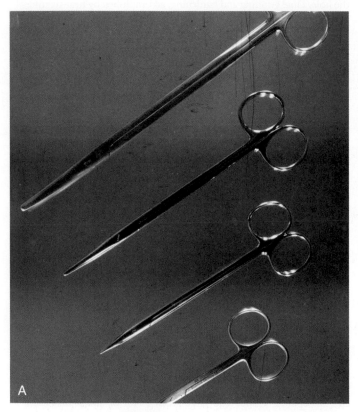

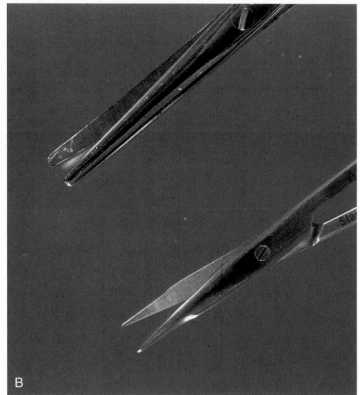

FIG. 7.14 (A) Two general types of dissecting scissors are shown here. The top two are long and standard Metzenbaum scissors. The bottom two are long and short Stevens tenotomy scissors. (B) The differences between Metzenbaum and Stevens scissors are apparent. The latter are finer and are beveled for precision cutting.

to cut. Scissor tips may be blunt or sharp, and the blades may be straight or curved. Conventional scissors require two movements in use: one to open and another to close the jaws. Other scissors may have a spring action in the body design that holds the jaws in an open position. A single movement pressing the spring together closes the jaws to cut. Scissors designed for delicate plastic and eye surgery are often of the latter type. A basic instrument set usually includes a curved Mayo scissors for dissection of heavy tissues, a Metzenbaum

scissors for dissection of delicate tissues, and a straight scissors for cutting suture. For surgery in deep areas of the body, scissors with long handles and short blades are used for better control and easier use.

Other sharp dissectors include drills, saws, osteotomes, rongeurs, and other instruments such as adenotomes and dermatomes. Some instruments in the dissecting category are produced in sharp or blunt form, such as curettes and periosteal elevators. Instruments

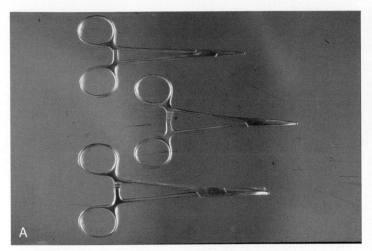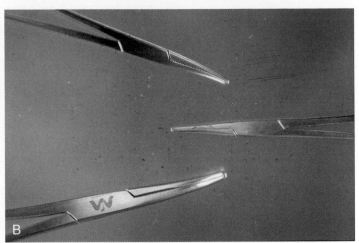

FIG. 7.15 (A) The two upper clamps are Halsted mosquito clamps. A curved Kelly clamp is pictured at the bottom. (B) The detail shows the heavier aspect of the Kelly hemostatic *(bottom)* compared with the finer, tapered Halsted mosquito clamp.

or devices used for blunt dissection include gauze dissectors (e.g., peanuts, pushers, kitners), a sponge on a stick, the back of a knife handle, and the surgeon's finger or hand.

Clamps

Clamps are instruments specifically designed for holding tissue or other materials, and most have an easily recognizable design. They have finger rings, for ease of holding; shanks, whose length is appropriate to the wound depth; ratchets on the shanks near the rings, which allow for the distal tip to be locked on the tissue or object grasped; and a joint, which joins the two halves of the instrument and allows opening and closing of the instrument. Instruments made up of two halves have one of three types of joints.

- The most common joint is the box lock, where one arm has been passed through a slot in the other arm and is riveted or pinned. This joint is needed where accurate approximation of the tips is necessary, and it is basic to most ringed instruments.
- The second type is the screw joint. The two halves are aligned and placed on top of each other, connected only by a screw. The joint must be checked and tightened periodically because the screw may become loose. Screw-joint instruments are easy to make and comparatively inexpensive.
- The final and least common type is the semibox, or aseptic, joint. It has the advantage that the two halves can be separated for easy cleaning.

Clamps also have a jaw, which is the working portion of the instrument and defines its use. Clamps are divided into the following categories.

Hemostats (Fig. 7.15) may be straight or curved and are used to close the severed ends of a vessel with a minimal amount of tissue damage. They prevent the excessive loss of blood in the course of dissection. The jaws have deep transverse cuts so that the bleeding vessels may be compressed with sufficient force to stop bleeding. The serrations must be cleanly cut and perfectly meshed to prevent the tissue from slipping free from the jaws of the clamp.

Occluding clamps usually have vertical serrations or special jaws that have finely meshed, multiple rows of longitudinally arranged teeth to prevent leakage and to minimize trauma when clamping bowel, vessels, or ducts that are to be reanastomosed.

Graspers and *holders* (Fig. 7.16) are used for tissue retraction and generally have jaws of a specific design based on their use. The Kocher (also referred to as an Ochsner) clamp has transverse serrations and large teeth (1 × 2) at its tip to grasp tightly on tough, slippery tissue such as fascia. The Allis clamp has multiple, interdigitating short teeth on the tip, minimizing crushing or damaging tissue. The Babcock clamp has broad, flared ends with smooth tips, and it atraumatically grips or encloses delicate structures, such as bowel, ureters, or fallopian tubes. Other holding forceps have handles like clamps with specialized tips or jaws, which may be triangular, straight, angular, or T-shaped.

Nonclamp graspers and holders are known as *forceps* or *pickups* because they are used to lift and hold tissue (Fig. 7.17). Often, while the surgeon is cutting with scissors or sewing with a needle, forceps are used in the other hand. Forceps are held like a pencil. The most common kinds are the various two-arm spring forceps. Forceps resemble tweezers, vary in length and thickness, and are available with and without teeth. Nontoothed forceps create minimal damage and hold delicate, thin tissues. Toothed forceps hold thick or slippery tissues that need extra grip. Toothed forceps ("rat tooth") have interdigitating teeth that hold tissue without slipping; these are used to hold skin or dense tissue. Adson tissue forceps have small, serrated teeth on the edge of the tips; these are designed for light, careful handling of tissue and are commonly used during skin closure.

Grasper and holder clamps may hold objects as well. Sponge-holding forceps with ring-shaped jaws are available in 7- and 9-inch lengths. They can be used to grasp or handle tissue but are commonly used to hold sponges. The sponge is folded and placed in the jaws and is used to retract tissue, to absorb blood in the field, and occasionally to perform blunt dissection.

Needle holders, because they must grasp metal rather than soft tissues, are subject to greater damage. As a result, needle holders must be repaired and replaced regularly. For maximal usage, needle holders must retain a firm grip on the needle. Many types of jaws have been designed to meet this need. The so-called *diamond jaw* needle holder has a tungsten carbide insert designed to prevent rotation of the needle. In needle holders of standard design, a longitudinal groove or pit in the jaw releases tension, prevents flattening of the needle, and holds the needle firmly. Needle holders

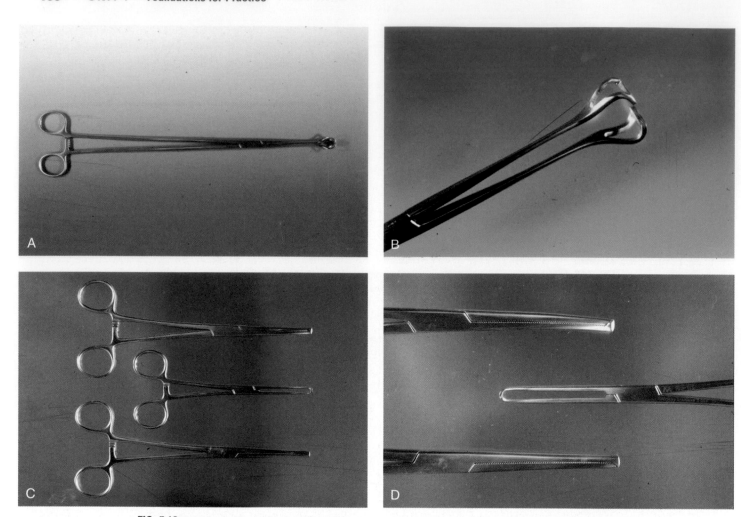

FIG. 7.16 (A) The Babcock clamp, which ranges in length from 8 to 14 inches, is an atraumatic grasping instrument ideal for placing traction on tubular structures while not crushing the tissue. (B) Close-up of the shaft and terminus of the Babcock clamp. (C) The three clamps illustrated here are curved Ochsner *(top)*, Allis *(center)*, and straight Ochsner clamps *(bottom)*. (D) Close-up view of Fig. 7.17C. Note the toothed jaws of the Ochsner clamps *(top)*, which grasp very securely but can be rough on tissue. In contrast, the Allis clamp *(center)* grasps tissue firmly but less aggressively than the Ochsner clamp.

may have a ratchet similar to that of a hemostat, or they may have a spring action that may or may not lock.

Towel clamps also are considered holding instruments. Of the two basic types, one is a nonpenetrating towel clamp used for holding draping materials in place. The other has sharp tips used to penetrate drapes and tissues, and it is damaging to both. The use of sharp towel clamps to secure drapes is highly discouraged because they penetrate the sterile field.

Retractors

Retractors are used to hold back the wound edges, structures, or tissues to provide exposure of the operative site. A surgeon needs the best exposure possible that inflicts a minimal degree of trauma to the surrounding tissue. Retractors are self-retaining or manually held in place by a member of the surgical team (Fig. 7.18). The two types of self-retaining retractors are (1) retractors with frames to which various blades may be attached, and (2) retractors with two blades held apart with a ratchet. Other very large self-retaining retractors are equipped with multiple blades and attachments of varying lengths and sizes. With handheld retractors, the handles

may be notched, hook-shaped, or ring-shaped to give the holder a firm grip without tiring. The blade is usually at a right angle to the shaft and may be a smooth blade, rake, or hook. A malleable (ribbon) retractor is a flat metal ribbon that may be shaped at the field.

Accessory and Ancillary Instruments

Accessory and ancillary instruments are designed to enhance the use of basic instrumentation or to facilitate the procedure. These include suction tips (Fig. 7.19) and tubing; irrigators-aspirators; electrosurgical devices; and special-use devices, such as probes, dilators, mallets, and screwdrivers.

Many miscellaneous instruments or specialty items are particular to a certain specialty but generally fall into one of the categories just mentioned. Microsurgical instruments are delicate and expensive. They are extremely fine and should be handled separately from other instruments. Instruments used in specialty surgery are discussed in each of the chapters under Unit II: Surgical Interventions.

When perioperative team members can analyze the planned surgical procedure and approach and identify each instrument and

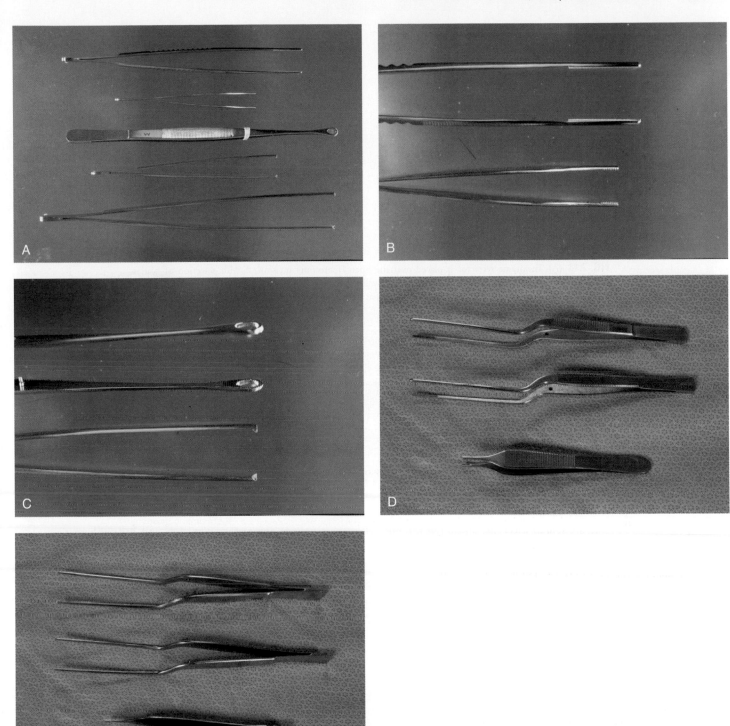

FIG. 7.17 (A) Five surgical forceps are shown. From the top: DeBakey, Adson-Brown, ring, rat-tooth, standard (6-inch), and medium (10-inch) tissue forceps. (B) Close-up view of the atraumatic DeBakey *(top)* and Adson-Brown forceps *(bottom)*. (C) Close-up view of the ring forceps, which are ideal for clearing fatty tissue from the obturator fossa and between large vessels. Below is the grasping end of rat-tooth tissue forceps. (D) Bayonet forceps *(top and center)* and Adson forceps *(bottom)* are ideal for fine tissue handling. (E) Another view of the forceps shown in part D.

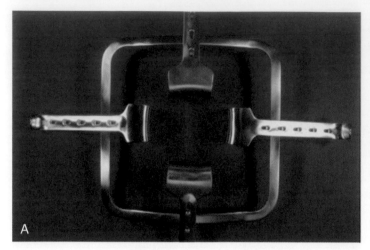
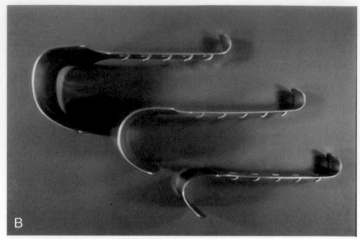

FIG. 7.18 (A) The frame retractor is placed over the open laparotomy incision. A wide selection of blades permits bladder and bowel retraction, as well as sidewall exposure. (B) The ratchets on the undersides of the retractor blades are easily interlocked via a series of spaces located on the underside of the frame retractor.

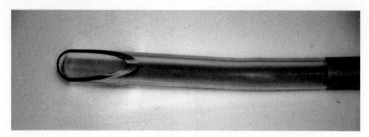

FIG. 7.19 Suction cannulas are available in a variety of diameters, ranging from 6 to 14 mm. The device illustrated here is 12 mm in diameter.

its specific function, they are able to select instrument sets without omitting necessary items and without including items that will not be used. This intelligent, planned approach ensures economy of time and motion, protects instruments from misuse, and prevents unnecessary handling. During the operation the informed scrub person who anticipates instrument needs becomes a more valuable member of the surgical team.

Endoscopic Instrumentation

Laparoscopy has introduced new equipment and instrumentation to the surgical suite. In addition to insufflation equipment, an optical system, and a documentation system, perioperative personnel must be familiar with the instrumentation used by the surgeon when performing a surgical procedure through the endoscope. Basic instrumentation, which may be disposable or reusable, includes trocars, forceps, or graspers; clip appliers; stapling devices; scissors; needle holders; and aspiration-irrigation systems.

Insufflation (Veress) needles and trocars provide access to the peritoneal and thoracic cavities. The Veress needle is a spring-loaded needle developed for gaining intraperitoneal access. After confirming placement, CO_2 gas is attached via tubing for insufflation. After adequate pneumoperitoneum is achieved, the Veress needle is removed and the primary trocar is placed. The primary trocar may also be placed into the abdomen directly, without prior gas insufflation (Soto et al., 2016).

A variety of graspers/forceps (Fig. 7.20) are available, from 2 to 10 mm in diameter, with a variety of functional tips. Atraumatic graspers provide appropriate retraction and little risk to tissues. Bipolar coagulation forceps are used to control bleeding. Biopsy forceps are used for obtaining small superficial samples from the peritoneum or ovary. Scissors may be reusable or disposable. These scissors come with different tips: hook, straight, and microtipped; serrated; and curved. They may also have cautery capability for cutting and coagulation of tissue.

Needle holders come with a variety of handle styles and have a hinged-jaw tip to allow easy positioning of the needle before intracorporeal suturing and using the sliding sheath. The sliding sheath holds the needle in a distal notch and inner spring-loading mechanism. To aid with extracorporeal knot tying, the surgeon may use a knot pusher to deliver tied knots into the abdomen. A slide and cinch pusher also is used to deliver and secure the preformed knot. Intra-abdominal stapling devices have been modified to fit and function through the endoscope. The development and introduction of robotic-assisted surgery has produced a new generation of multiarticulating instruments.

Robotic Instrumentation

Robotic surgery uses a programmable manipulator designed to maneuver specialized instruments to complete a specific task. These are most common in orthopedic and neurosurgery and are used for precise tasks such as drilling and probe insertion. Robotic-assisted surgery involves mechanical devices under partially programmed control that can be controlled or modified by the surgeon. A third type of robot is the telemanipulator. This device mimics the operator's exact or scaled hand motions. A common system is the da Vinci Robotic Surgical System (Fig. 7.21). The FDA has approved this system for use in multiple types of procedures (Goswami et al., 2015).

Robotic surgery instrumentation is similar to laparoscopic instruments; in fact the tips of the instruments are the same as other laparoscopic instrumentation. Near the tip of the instrument is the wrist. The wrist articulates the tip guided by microchips in the instrument base (housing unit). As in other laparoscopic cases, an endoscope is required, but robotic surgery also necessitates a camera that has 3-D capability. A camera adapter connects the scope and camera to each other, with a bifurcated light cord connecting the scope to a high-intensity light source. One can see the similarities to traditional endoscopic cases, but there are key differences with the scope, cameras, and light sources.

As with all surgery, the scrub person should inspect the instrumentation for damage and the perioperative nurse should inspect all connections on the machines. The instruments are maneuvered by a pulley system within the robot's arms, and it is important that the scrub person press the pulleys to confirm they are able to move freely.

Regular instrument sets and a traditional laparoscopy set should be available in the event the surgeon aborts the robotic-assisted procedure. If a robotic-assisted procedure must be quickly converted to an open procedure, the robot's arms are released from the trocars and the robot is undocked or backed out of position.

Stapling Instruments

Surgical staplers are used in gastrointestinal, gynecologic, thoracic, and many other surgeries to remove part of an organ (resection), to cut through tissue (transection), and to create connections between structures (anastomoses). Surgical staplers are examples of devices commonly used during surgery that are in a constant state of developmental evolution (Chekan et al., 2014).

Generally, these instruments may be classified as follows (Medtronic, 2016; Ethicon, 2016):

- Circular staplers
- Curved or radial staplers
- Endo-GIA devices
- End-to-end anastomosis (EEA) staplers
- Laparoscopic staplers
- Linear staplers
- Open staplers

Used in many surgical specialties, the mechanical application of these instruments reduces tissue manipulation and handling. The edema and inflammation that usually accompany anastomoses are minimized because the noncrushing B shape of the staples allows nutrients to pass through the staple line to the cut edge of the tissue.

Mechanical staplers (both nondisposable and disposable) use cartridges of tiny stainless steel staples or absorbable nonmetallic staples that are commercially preloaded, prepackaged, and presterilized. The staples are essentially nonreactive; metal staples remain permanently in the tissue. The staplers may fire individually or lay down multiple rows in a straight or circular pattern. Devices to cut or anastomose bowel and other structures are available for open-wound use or through endoscopic cannulae. The use of staplers significantly decreases operating time and may shorten postoperative stays.

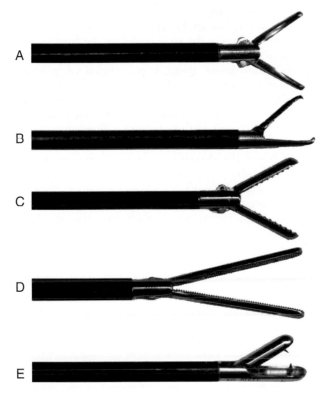

FIG. 7.20 The following graspers are commonly used: (A) Maryland dissector for fine grasping and dissecting tissue planes, (B) Allis graspers for a secure hold during ovarian cystectomy and excision of pelvic sidewall peritoneum endometriosis, (C) general use grasper, (D) bowel grasper for atraumatic manipulation of the bowel, and (E) biopsy forceps for obtaining tissue biopsy specimens.

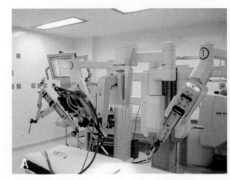
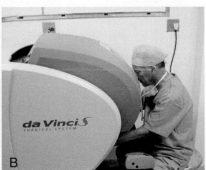

FIG. 7.21 Robotic-assisted endoscopic surgery. (A) Da Vinci surgical system with the ports. (B) Control unit.

Selecting and Preparing Instruments for Patient Use

Designated operating room (OR) or central supply personnel arrange the various instruments into trays or sets. The trays are named according to their functions. Tray/set names and instrument composition vary by institution, but three basic OR instrument sets are the minor/plastic, the basic laparotomy, and the dilation and curettage (D&C). A minor (or plastic surgery) set includes instruments needed for simple superficial incision, excision, and suturing. A basic laparotomy set includes instruments to open and close the abdominal cavity and repair any gross defects in the major body musculature. A D&C set, in addition to its use for D&C, is often used as the basic instrumentation for vaginal surgery.

According to each procedure's needs, more individualized instruments or specialty sets, such as an intestinal set or a vascular set, may be added. In the same way, basic instrument sets may be selected for opening other body cavities, such as the chest and pelvis.

Instruments are selected according to the size of the patient's body structures and the nature of the organs involved. Proper selection requires a general understanding of surgical procedures and approaches and knowledge of anatomy, possible pathologic conditions, and the design and purpose of instruments.

Basic Table Setups

In most ORs the instruments are set up on Mayo stands and back tables in a planned, standardized, organized, functional manner to maintain continuity when the original scrub person is replaced by another. Care is taken on all sterile fields to ensure that all solutions, syringes, and medication cups are clearly labeled to guarantee patient and staff safety. Each facility should create tools as a part of a comprehensive orientation process to ensure standardization of setups.

A proficient scrub person must know the instrument inventory of the department; the instruments routinely needed for each type of operation; the individual surgeon's preferences; and the correct use and handling, method of preparation, and postoperative care of the instruments. Preference cards, the foundation for management of daily OR activities, specify the resources preferred by each surgeon for a specific procedure. Correct preference cards streamline the process of obtaining needed supplies, which allows time to focus on patient care. Electronic management of surgeon preference cards may be used to enhance efficiency, control cost, control inventory, and facilitate charges (Dizon et al., 2016).

Before an operative procedure, the scrub person may assist the perioperative nurse in gathering the needed supplies, equipment, and sutures. The scrub person scrubs; dons gown and gloves; and begins to set up the sterile tables with drapes, instruments, supplies, and sutures. Instruments are arranged with those most frequently used on the Mayo stand.

One or two back tables, according to the number of instruments and supplies, also are set up. The scrub person prepares the sutures and ligatures and places the knife blades on the handles. Other supplies needed are suction tubing and tips, electrosurgical cord and tip, drains, basins, gowns, gloves, drapes, surgical soft goods, and needles, all of which are sterile and set up on the back table according to standardized institutional policy (Fig. 7.22). During the final "time-out" before incision, the scrub person has the responsibility to articulate instrument and equipment readiness to the team to enhance a safe, seamless procedure. When the patient is on the OR bed and is draped, the Mayo stand, set up for instrument use at the immediate operative site, is brought across the lower part of the patient's legs (Fig. 7.23).

The scrub person must be attentive to the sterile field to anticipate the surgeon's needs. Instruments should be passed in a positive and decisive manner. Each instrument is placed or slapped firmly into the surgeon's palm in such a manner that it is ready for immediate use with no wasted motion. When a curved instrument is passed to the surgeon, the curve should be pointing in the direction of intended use, there should be no need for readjustment. It is necessary

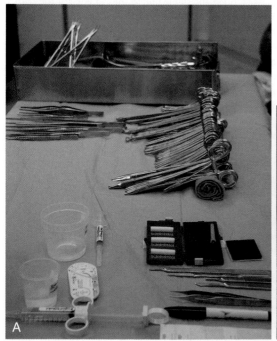
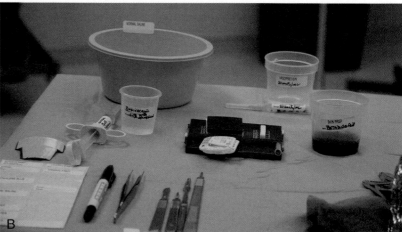

FIG. 7.22 (A) Back table setup. (B) Labeled medications and sharps on table setup.

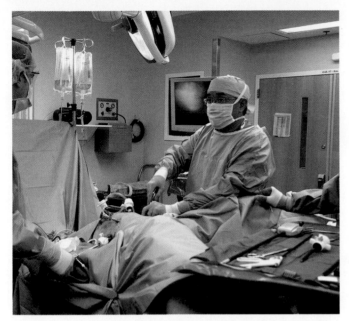

FIG. 7.23 Mayo stand, with instruments required for start of the surgical procedure, is moved into place across the lower part of the draped patient.

to know if a surgeon or assistant is left-handed or right-handed to pass instruments efficiently and in the correct position.

Often the surgeon or assistant uses hand signals for the type of instrument desired, to eliminate unnecessary talking. Scrub persons should become familiar with the basic signals for knife, scissors, suture, forceps, and clamp.

Care and Handling of Instruments

An instrument should be used only for the purpose for which it is designed. Proper use and reasonable care prolong its life and protect its quality. Scissors and clamps, which are most frequently misused, can be forced out of alignment, cracked, or broken when used improperly. Tissue scissors should not be used to cut suture or gauze dressings. Hemostatic clamps should not be used as towel clamps or to clamp suction tubing.

Each instrument should be inspected before and after each use to detect imperfections. An instrument should function perfectly to prevent needlessly endangering a patient's safety and increasing operative time because of instrument failure.

Forceps, clamps, and other hinged instruments must be inspected for jaw and teeth alignment. Instrument jaws and teeth should meet perfectly so that blood flow is occluded without damaging the vein or artery. Ratchets should hold firmly yet release easily. Instrument joints should work smoothly.

All instruments should be checked for worn spots, chips, dents, cracks, or sharp edges. Damaged instruments should be set aside and sent for repair or replacement. An instrument repair service should be selected carefully and used for regular maintenance, such as sharpening and realignment.

Instruments must be handled gently. Bouncing, dropping, and setting heavy equipment on top of them must be avoided. During the procedure the scrub person should wipe the used instruments with a damp sponge or place them in a basin of sterile water to prevent blood from drying on the surfaces and in the box locks. Saline solution should never be used on instruments because the salt is corrosive and accelerates rusting or deterioration of the metal. As time allows during the procedure, the scrub person should rinse and dry the used instruments and replace them on the back table to facilitate closing counts.

At the end of a procedure, during the table breakdown process, the scrub person must handle the instruments in a logical organized fashion, either individually or in small groups. Sharp and delicate instruments should be set aside for individual handling and cleaning to avoid damage and accidental injury. Surgeon-specific instrumentation should be isolated to prevent loss or damage in the cleaning and reassembly process. Standard Precautions should be applied as dictated by institutional policy. All instruments set up for the procedure should be disinfected and terminally sterilized before reassembly. Instruments must be completely clean to ensure effective sterilization. Refer to Chapter 4 for information on instrument decontamination and sterilization.

With today's focus on cost containment, perioperative nurses must assess the care and handling of instrumentation carefully. Instrument sets can be monitored for use, and instruments that are used infrequently can be removed and packaged separately to prevent continued wear from unnecessary resterilization.

Storing Instruments

Instruments should be stored in a manner that keeps them safe and supports the maintenance of the container's integrity (see Chapter 4). Cabinet shelving should be adjustable and properly spaced for storage of various sizes and types of instruments. Most institutions store instruments in presterilized trays or containers. Attached labels and diagrams in cabinets assist personnel. An inventory of all instruments should be taken at periodic intervals.

Perioperative Nursing Considerations

Preventing Sharps Injuries During Surgery

Sharps injuries increase the risk of exposure to bloodborne pathogens in the OR. Eliminating exposure to such hazards is not a "once and done" effort. Often several diverse steps must occur simultaneously. These might be as different as hazard-proofing a room, changing the type of equipment used, and changing staff behavior by asking each team member to wear a particular type of protective garment. Control methods should be based on a hierarchy of impact and include elimination of the risk (removing a sharp device from use), using safety-engineered devices (e.g., safety scalpel), work practice controls (e.g., use of a neutral zone), and proper personal protective equipment (PPE) such as double-gloving (AORN, 2016b).

Surgery involves precise, regimented actions that require planning, communication, and teamwork. Using these same elements can mitigate inherent hazards associated with sharp devices in the perioperative setting. AORN (2016b) has developed a Guideline for Sharps Safety that OR nurses can use to protect themselves and other team members from exposure injuries in surgery. Care in setting up the surgical work area includes placement of sharp items, constant awareness of the location of sharps and other sterile team members during surgery, and careful disposal of sharps after surgery. Such care contributes to ensuring a safe surgical environment for all participants.

Safety-Engineered Devices

AORN's Guideline for Sharps Safety (2016b) states that perioperative personnel must use sharps with safety-engineered devices. These devices include:

- Blunt suture needles
- Safety scalpel devices (Fig. 7.24)
- Alternative wound closure devices such as tissue staplers, tissue adhesives, or adhesive skin closure strips
- Safety-engineered syringes and needles
- Needleless systems for collecting/withdrawing bodily fluids after initial access is established
- Blunt cannulas for withdrawing medication or other fluids from a vial (AORN, 2016b)

Neutral Zone

The neutral zone has been defined as a location on the surgical field on which sharps are placed in a predesignated sterile basin or tray or on a magnetic pad, from which the surgeon or assistant can retrieve them (Fig. 7.25). After use, the items are placed back in the neutral zone, and the scrub person retrieves them. This technique eliminates hand-to-hand passing of sharps between the surgeon and the scrub person, so that no two individuals touch the same sharp at the same time. Because it reduces the chance of accidental needle punctures and cuts, both the ACS and AORN (2016b) recommend

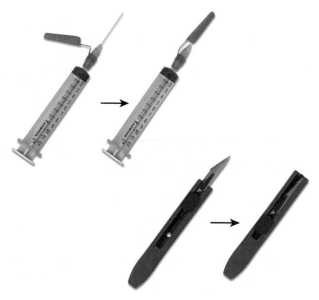

FIG. 7.24 Using safety systems such as retracting scalpels dramatically reduces percutaneous injuries to perioperative team members.

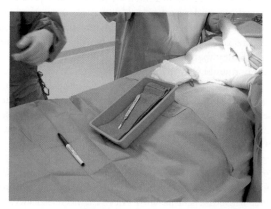

FIG. 7.25 Neutral zone.

use of the neutral zone to transfer sharps as a risk-mitigating strategy. When using the neutral zone:

- Communicate the location of sharps on the sterile field during the procedure and during personnel change
- Use a neutral zone or hands-free technique for passing sharps
- Use a basin, instrument mat, magnetic pad, or designated area on the Mayo stand as the neutral zone
- Place one sharp at a time in the neutral zone
- Place sharp items in the neutral zone after use
- Orient sharps for easy retrieval by the surgeon
- Handle the sharp by one person at a time

No-Touch Technique

AORN's Guideline for Sharps Safety (2016b) recommends a "no-touch technique" to minimize the manual handling of surgical sharps, thus, reducing the risk of injury to the surgical team. In using this technique:

- Do not manipulate suture needles with gloves hands
- Use the suture packet to position the needle holder
- Use a blunt instrument (such as a forceps) to guide the needle through tissue
- Remove suture needle from suture before tying
- Use forceps to turn the suture needle 90 degrees before returning the loaded needle holder to the Mayo stand or neutral zone
- Use an instrument to pick up sharp items that have fallen off the sterile field

Work Practice Controls

Work practice controls change the method of performing a task to minimize the risk of injury (AORN, 2016b). The perioperative team should:

- Use sharp instruments only when clinically necessary
- Use an instrument to load a blade on the knife handle
- Retract tissue with instruments, not hands
- Not recap needles
- Use a one-handed scooping technique when a safe needle device is not available and recapping is necessary
- Use an ampule breaker that covers the neck of the ampule or wrap sterile gauze around the ampule neck before breaking the top

Personal Protective Equipment

Intact surgical gloves provide a barrier that protects both the patient and the wearer. Punctures or tears can cause glove failure. To reduce the risk of glove failure, perioperative staff should:

- Wear two pair of gloves, one over the other (Evidence for Practice)
- Use a perforation indicator system
- Monitor gloves for punctures
- Change gloves when a suspected or actual perforation occurs, or when a visible defect is noted

Preventing Retained Surgical Items

A surgical item unintentionally retained in a patient after surgery or other invasive procedure is a serious, preventable error that can result in patient harm. Perioperative team members have a moral obligation to protect patients by preventing retained surgical items (RSIs) (Patient Engagement Exemplar). The AORN (2016a) Guideline for Prevention of Retained Surgical Items provides guidance for implementing an effective system to prevent RSIs, accounting for surgical items (radiopaque soft goods, sharps, and instruments),

EVIDENCE FOR PRACTICE

Gloves, Extra Gloves, or Special Types of Gloves for Preventing Percutaneous Exposure Injuries in Healthcare Personnel

Healthcare workers are at risk of acquiring diseases such as hepatitis B, hepatitis C, and HIV through exposure to contaminated blood and body fluids at work. Most often infection occurs when a healthcare worker inadvertently punctures the skin of his or her hand with a sharp implement that has been used in the treatment of an infected patient. Such occurrences are commonly known as percutaneous exposure incidents. WHO reports that 2 million healthcare workers across the world experience percutaneous exposure to infectious diseases each year.

There are several strategies available to reduce exposure among healthcare workers and these are widely used. Therefore it is important to know whether these preventive interventions are effective. The authors explored multiple databases to select RCTs with healthcare workers as the participants, extra gloves or special gloves as the intervention, exposure to blood or body fluids as the primary outcome, and dexterity as the secondary outcome. They identified 31 RCTs that included 6890 operations. There were no studies for nonsurgical staff.

The authors found moderate-quality evidence that double gloves reduce the risk of percutaneous exposure incidents compared with single gloves for surgeons and surgical staff. The risk of inner glove perforations was reduced by 71% and the risk

of blood contamination by 65%. Even though loss of dexterity was reported in two studies, based on measurement with visual analogue scales, double gloves were still rated as good in one study and average in another.

Some evidence suggested perioperative team members could achieve a further reduction in the risk of percutaneous exposure by using three pairs of gloves or extra gloves made from a special material. However, the authors rated the evidence for the use of three glove layers or special gloves as low to moderate and pointed out it needs to be balanced against the additional costs and the influence on dexterity, which is unknown. Thicker gloves did not perform better than thinner gloves.

The authors concluded that the prevention of percutaneous exposure incidents could be successfully achieved with an increase in the number of glove layers, rather than by increasing the thickness of gloves. There is low-quality evidence that triple gloving and the use of special gloves can further reduce the risk of glove perforations compared with double gloving with normal material gloves. The preventive effect of double gloves on percutaneous exposure incidents in surgery does not need further research. Further studies are needed to evaluate the effectiveness and cost-effectiveness of special material gloves and triple gloves.

RCT, Randomized controlled trial; *WHO,* World Health Organization.
Modified from Mischke C et al: *Gloves, extra gloves or special types of gloves for preventing percutaneous exposure injuries in healthcare personnel* (website), 2014. http://onlinelibrary.wiley.com/doi/10.1002/14651858.CD009573.pub2/abstract. (Accessed 4 September 2016).

PATIENT ENGAGEMENT EXEMPLAR

Retained Surgical Items

Perioperative team members are accountable for all of the soft goods, instruments, and miscellaneous items used in surgical procedures. All items placed inside the patient for surgery must be removed unless intentionally left in the patient. An retained surgical item (RSI) is a rare but serious patient safety issue, so care must be taken to prevent it from happening. Unfortunately RSIs do occur and can have a profound impact on patients. When an error happens, patients and family members often have these questions:

1. How did this error happen and who was involved?
2. Why did this happen? Can you explain?
3. How will the effects of this error be minimized?
4. What steps will the person or organization take to prevent this from happening again?

Many healthcare providers are fearful of disclosing errors because of the potential for litigation, but there is a growing body of evidence that suggests that being open and honest with patients and family members actually decreases the risk of lawsuits. Patients want to know what happened and they want an apology. Implementing an error disclosure policy will assist facilities with a process to handle error, allow improvement in the quality of healthcare, and allow patients to engage in the improvement process. Giving patients a voice in improving care will help them to feel empowered to help the facility improve processes so errors can be decreased or eliminated.

preventing retention of device fragments, reconciling discrepancies, and using adjunct technologies to augment manual counts (Research Highlight).

Reducing the Risk of Retained Surgical Items

Multidisciplinary Approach

All perioperative team members are responsible for the prevention of RSIs. Improving teamwork and communication is an important aspect to any systems approach to reduce these surgical errors. Distractions, noise, and unnecessary interruptions should be minimized during the count, with the initial count completed before the patient enters the room if possible. Counts, along with events that require counts (such as relief of a team member), should not take place during critical parts of the procedure. Each organization should establish a consistent, logical count sequence (Patient Safety).

Two individuals, one of whom is the RN perioperative nurse, concurrently review items being counted. The counts should be performed audibly and with each sharp, soft good, and instrument visualized by both the scrub person and the perioperative nurse. The number of needles, soft goods, and instruments is recorded. The perioperative nurse records the count immediately after each type of item is counted, on a standardized template that is visible to the surgical team. The documentation of counts should include the items on the instrument table at the beginning of the procedure as well as those added during the procedure. It is possible for packages to contain an incorrect number of items (soft goods, blades, suture, etc.), so it is important to identify any discrepancies immediately.

Anesthesia providers should actively participate in RSI prevention by not using counted items and communicating use (and removal) of throat packs, bite guards, and so forth.

RESEARCH HIGHLIGHT

Risk Factors for Retained Surgical Items: A Meta-Analysis and Proposed Risk Stratification System

Unintentionally RSIs are felt to be completely preventable "never events." Despite numerous case reports and clinical series, many published studies have failed to identify clinically important differences among proposed risk factors for RSIs. In this meta-analysis, the authors examined the best available data for RSI risk factors, seeking to provide a clinically relevant risk stratification system.

The authors performed a search of English language medical literature. Nineteen candidate studies were considered for this meta-analysis. Three retrospective, case-control studies of RSI-related risk were chosen for further analysis. The "common factor" variables compiled from these studies included BMI, emergency procedure, estimated operative blood loss greater than 500 mL, incorrect surgical count, lack of surgical count, more than one subprocedure, more than one surgical team, nursing staff shift change, operation "after hours" (i.e., between 5 p.m. and 7 a.m.), operative time, trainee presence, and unexpected intraoperative factors. Examples of unexpected intraoperative factors included equipment malfunction, unanticipated change in operative course, or other complication not reasonably expected during the course of the surgical case. The authors further stratified resulting RSI risk factors into low, intermediate, and high risk.

Despite the fact that only between three and six risk factors were associated with increased RSI risk across the three studies, the analysis of pooled data demonstrated that seven risk factors are significantly associated with increased RSI risk.

Variables found to elevate the RSI risk were identified as follows:
- Estimated blood loss greater than 500 mL (increased risk)
- An incorrect surgical count (significant risk)
- Lengthy procedures (increased risk)
- Surgical counts not performed (increased risk)
- Unexpected intraoperative factors occurred (high risk)
- More than one operative procedure performed (significant risk)
- Involvement of more than one surgical team (significant risk)

Variables not found to be associated with increased risk were as follows:
- BMI
- Emergency procedures
- Changes of staff or operating afterhours
- Presence of a surgical trainee

Among the "common risk factors" reported by all three case-control studies, seven show elevated RSI risk across the pooled data. Based on these results, the authors proposed a risk stratification scheme and recommended large, prospective, and multicenter studies evaluating effects of specific changes at the institutional level (i.e., universal surgical counts, radiographic verification of the absence of RSI, and radiofrequency labeling of surgical instruments and sponges) on the risk of RSI. Overall, the authors feel the findings provided a meaningful foundation for future patient safety initiatives and clinical studies of RSI occurrence and prevention.

BMI, Body mass index; *RSI*, retained surgical item.
Modified from Moffatt-Bruce SD et al: Risk factors for retained surgical item: a meta-analysis and proposed risk stratification system, *J Surg Res* 190(2):429–436, 2014.

PATIENT SAFETY

Timing of the Surgical Count

Counts Should Be Performed:
- Before the procedure to establish a baseline (initial count)
- When new items are added to the field
- Before closure of a cavity within a cavity
- When incision site closure begins or at the end of the procedure when counted items are no longer in use
- At the time of permanent relief of either the scrub person or perioperative nurse
- For counted items in use when there is relief of the scrub person or perioperative nurse for short durations
- Any time a discrepancy is suspected
- When requested by any perioperative team member

Counts Are Not Performed at Critical Phases of the Procedure, Such as:
- Time-out periods
- Critical dissections
- Confirming and opening of implants

- Anesthesia induction and emergence from anesthesia
- Care and handling of specimens

Subsequent Counts
- Maintain the count running total in one location.
- Immediately record items added to the sterile field.
- Notify the scrub person if an item is passed or dropped from the sterile field. Isolate it from the sterile field and include it in the count.
- Use a pocketed soft goods bag system.
- Do not subtract or remove items from the count.
- Count all items together at the final count for multiple procedures.
- Keep all items that are part of the count within the OR until counts are completed and reconciled.
- Do not remove linen or waste containers until counts are complete and reconciled and the patient has been transferred out of the room.

Modified from Association of periOperative Registered Nurses (AORN): Guideline for prevention of retained surgical items. In: *Guidelines for perioperative practice*, Denver, 2016, The Association.

All counted items should remain in the room until final counts are reconciled. Used or open counted items should be removed only after the patient has left the room.

Surgical Soft Goods

Cotton gauze sponges account for 48% to 69% of RSIs (Williams et al., 2014) and result in more serious tissue reactions than metal items. The abdomen and pelvis are reported to be the most common locations in which RSIs are found. Surgical soft goods can be retained in the smallest of incisions, including in procedures involving natural orifices, such as the vagina or nose, and in minimally invasive surgeries. A variety of surgical radiopaque soft goods are available commercially packed in increments of 5 or 10 (Box 7.5). AORN's (2016a) guideline recommends that all soft goods (including

---

BOX 7.5

Surgical Soft Goods

Surgical soft goods (e.g., radiopaque sponges, towels, other textiles) are used to effect hemostasis via direct pressure, absorb intraoperative blood loss and drainage, act as aids to blunt dissection, pack the viscera from the field, and keep areas of the wound moist. Surgeons may also use soft goods as a filter between a suction tip and delicate tissue. A variety of surgical radiopaque soft goods are available commercially packed in increments of 5 or 10. Any soft goods used during a surgical procedure must contain an x-ray–detectable element to facilitate location of the item if a count discrepancy occurs.

The following is a list of the types of surgical soft goods:

- *Radiopaque 4 × 4s:* This sponge (often referred to as a "raytec" or "radio") is composed of loosely woven gauze folded into a 4-inch square. A radiopaque thread, which may change to a darker color when exposed to fluid, is integrated into the sponge. This type of sponge is useful for superficial small incisions, and may be folded into thirds and mounted onto a sponge stick for use in deeper incisions. Other sizes such as 4 × 8 may also be available.
- *Laparotomy sponges:* Also referred to as "laps," "lap pads," or "tapes," these sponges are either square or oblong and have a loop of colored twill tape with a radiopaque marker sewn to one corner. Used for major surgical procedures with large incisions, laparotomy sponges are presented to the surgeon either moist or dry.
- *Dissectors:* Dissecting sponges have the radiopaque element incorporated into the weave of the material and are generally composed of very tightly rolled cloth tape. They may be referred to as "peanuts," "pushers," or "kitners." Dissecting sponges are *always* presented to the surgeon mounted on a clamp because of their small size.
- *Round sponges:* Often known as "tonsil" or "cherry" sponges, round sponges are gauze-covered cotton balls with strings attached. The radiopaque element is woven into the gauze covering. These sponges are often used in the oropharynx and are presented on the tip of a clamp or sponge stick.
- *Flat neurosurgical patties:* Flat sponges are composed of soft compressed cotton or rayon with an embedded radiopaque element and string attached. Often used in neurosurgical procedures, these sponges are available in a multitude of sizes and widths. They may be used as a filter for a suction tip to prevent damage to the underlying tissue, or as a vehicle for the application of topical anesthetic to the nasal mucosa.

---

towels in the surgical wound) be radiopaque and that team members isolate nonradiopaque sponges (such as those used for skin antisepsis) from counted radiopaque sponges before the beginning of the procedure.

The scrub person places soiled soft goods in a designated container off the sterile field (such as a sponge bucket at the end of the OR bed) for retrieval by the circulating nurse. To facilitate counting, the circulating nurse places the soft goods in visible pocketed bags. The final count should not be considered complete until all surgical soft goods used in closing the wound are removed from the wound by the surgeon and returned to the scrub person.

Sharps and Miscellaneous Items

Sharps and miscellaneous items (such as guidewires) are commonly miscounted and have been retained in patients. Needles are the most likely surgical item to be miscounted (Cole et al., 2013). All suture needles, regardless of size, should be counted in all surgical procedures. Sharps and miscellaneous items used in the surgical incision should be accounted for in their entirety immediately on removal from the surgical site.

The scrub person should account for needles as they are placed in the neutral zone on a one-for-one exchange basis when possible. Needles are retained on the sterile field and counted according to the number indicated on the package; the scrub person verifies this number with the perioperative nurse when the package is opened. Used needles should be kept on a needle pad or counter on the scrub person's table. Broken or missing needles must be reported to the surgeon and accounted for in their entirety.

Instruments

Although individual reports of prevalence vary, evidence indicates (Moffatt-Bruce et al., 2014) that instruments have been retained and are implicated in count discrepancies. Instruments should be counted for all procedures in which a body cavity is entered. The final count should not be considered complete until the instruments used in closing the incision site are removed from the site and returned to the scrub person.

Device Fragments

The useful life of a surgical instrument is not well defined. Instrument failure over time, along with surgical labeling techniques, may increase the risk for RSIs (Ipaktchi et al., 2013). Measures should be taken to prevent instrument breakage to include fragmentation of instrument labels. All instruments (including attached labels), intravascular devices, and hypodermic needles should be used in accordance to manufacturer's instructions and should be inspected before use to identify any defect that may increase the risk of fragmentation. Defective instruments should not be used. Intravascular devices should be accounted for in their entirety by inspection for breakage immediately on removal from the patient.

Count Discrepancies

Each institution should have established policies for dealing with incorrect counts. Unintentional retention of objects during surgery has been identified as a never event; institutions need to adopt a comprehensive strategy to manage the complexity of this issue. The entire perioperative team is responsible for immediately addressing any count discrepancy (AORN, 2016a), and immediate actions must be taken to reconcile the count (Box 7.6). Documentation of these activities should be completed according to institutional policy and procedure. Any unresolved count discrepancies must be documented

BOX 7.6

Management of Surgical Count Discrepancy

Immediate actions to reconcile a count discrepancy include the following:

- Verbally notifying the entire team
- Recounting the item(s) of concern
- Searching the entire room including trash and linen receptacles, kick buckets, the floor, and so forth
- Searching the sterile field including drape folds, back table, and so forth
- Suspending closure of the incision site if clinically feasible
- Exploring the incision site
- Ordering intraoperative imaging to rule out retained surgical items
- Documenting actions and outcomes in the patient record

Modified from Fenci J: Guideline implementation: prevention of retained surgical items, *AORN*, 104(1): 37–48, 2016.

in the patient record including all measures taken to recover the missing item, a description of the item and its location if known, patient notification, and the plan for follow-up care.

Key Points

- Sutures, needles, and instruments are the tools of the surgical team. It is the responsibility of the perioperative nurse to understand these tools and be proficient with their preparation for surgery.
- An understanding of the characteristics of suture materials, knowledge of the risk factors of wound healing, and awareness of the interactions between tissues and suture materials is essential for the perioperative nurse.
- The use of barbed suture applications is growing as surgeons become more familiar with the advantages of this new suture technology.
- Surgical needles vary in shape, size, point design, and wire diameter. Needle selection is determined by the type of tissue, suture material, and action to be performed.
- Available blunt protect-point needles are recommended as an alternative to taper point needles.
- Wound closure materials include suture, skin staples, wound closure strips, and surgical adhesives.
- There are four main instrument categories: cutting instruments (also called dissectors), clamps, retractors, and accessory or ancillary instruments.
- Laparoscopy and robotic-assisted surgery have introduced new equipment and instrumentation to the surgical suite.
- Perioperative team members who handle sharp devices or equipment are at risk for sharps injuries. Because sharps injuries can expose individuals to potentially infectious diseases, safety practices should be followed at all times.
- A surgical item unintentionally retained in a patient after an operative or other invasive procedure is a serious, preventable medical error with the potential to cause the patient great harm. Perioperative RNs play a key role in preventing RSIs.

Critical Thinking Question

You have been assigned to a perioperative team conducting a proactive risk analysis of the management of surgical soft goods, from case preparation through the completion of surgery, with the goal of preventing inadvertent retention of these items. Develop a best practice recommendation for maintaining an accurate count of surgical soft goods.

evolve *The answer to the Critical Thinking Question can be found at http://evolve.elsevier.com/Rothrock/Alexander.*

References

Association of periOperative Registered Nurses (AORN): *AORN position statement on RN first assistants* (website), 2013. www.aorn.org/guidelines/clinical-resources/rn-first-assistant-resources. (Accessed 11 August 2016).

Association of periOperative Registered Nurses (AORN): Guideline for prevention of retained surgical items. In *Guidelines for perioperative practice*, Denver, 2016a, The Association.

Association of periOperative Registered Nurses (AORN): Guideline for sharps safety. In *Guidelines for perioperative practice*, Denver, 2016b, The Association.

Bulechek GM et al: *Nursing interventions classification (NIC)*, ed 6, St Louis, 2013, Mosby.

Chekan E et al: Surgical stapling device-tissue interactions: what surgeons need to know to improve outcomes, *Med Devices (Auckl)* 7:305–318, 2014.

Cole K et al: Finding a needle in the dark, *AORN J* 98(3):532–537, 2013.

Dennis C et al: Suture materials—current and emerging trends, *J Biomed Mater Res A* 104(6):1544–1559, 2016.

Dizon J et al: Factors disrupting the preference card management process: a root cause analysis, *AORN J* 103(1):105e1–105e12, 2016.

Ethicon: *Wound closure resource center* (website), 2016. http://woundclosure.ethicon.com. (Accessed 6 August 2016).

Frattini F et al: Current developments and unusual aspects in gastrointestinal surgical stapling, *Surg Technol Int* 27:99–101, 2015.

Goswami S et al: Anesthesia for robotically conducted surgery. In Miller RD, editor: *Miller's anesthesia*, ed 8, Philadelphia, 2015, Saunders.

Ipaktchi K et al: Current surgical labeling techniques may increase the risk of unintentionally retained foreign objects: a hypothesis, *Patient Saf Surg* 7(1):31, 2013.

Lear W: Instruments and materials. In Robinson JK et al, editors: *Surgery of the skin*, ed 3, Philadelphia, 2015, Elsevier.

Medtronic: *A comprehensive portfolio of wound closure materials and accessories* (website), 2016. www.medtronic.com/covidien/products/wound-closure. (Accessed 6 August 2016).

Moffatt-Bruce SD et al: Risk factors for retained surgical items: a meta-analysis and proposed risk stratification system, *J Surg Res* 190(2):429–436, 2014.

Saarto A et al: *Blunt versus sharp suture needles for preventing percutaneous exposure incidents in surgical staff* (website), 2011. http://onlinelibrary.wiley.com/doi/10.1002/14651858.CD009170.pub2/abstract. (Accessed 15 July 2016).

Soto E et al: Trocar placement. In Baggish M et al, editors: *Atlas of pelvic and gynecologic surgery*, ed 4, Philadelphia, 2016, Elsevier.

Srivastava D et al: Suturing technique and other closure materials. In Robinson JK et al, editors: *Surgery of the skin*, ed 3, Philadelphia, 2015, Elsevier.

Stolle Satteson E et al: *Materials for wound closure* (website), 2015. http://emedicine.medscape.com/article/1127693-overview#a3. (Accessed 6 September 2016).

Toriumi D et al: Surgical adhesives in facial plastic surgery, *Otolaryngol Clin North Am* 49(3):585–599, 2016.

Williams TL et al: Retained surgical sponges: findings from incident reports and a cost-benefit analysis of radiofrequency technology, *J Am Coll Surg* 219(3):354–364, 2014.

CHAPTER 8

Surgical Modalities

KAY A. BALL

Surgery continues to evolve as less invasive procedures and instrumentation are adopted. Modalities have developed to enhance and advance surgical procedures. This chapter examines the evolution of some widely used surgical modalities, including laparoscopy (sometimes referred to as *endoscopy*), other minimally invasive surgery (MIS) technologies, robotic-assisted surgery, video technology, and energies used during surgical interventions.

Minimally Invasive Surgery Overview

In the late 1980s, the "laparoscopy revolution" began in the United States. General surgeons developed techniques to perform procedures using the laparoscope, eliminating the need for a large incision. As surgeons and perioperative nurses kept pace with evolving knowledge and information, the surgical industry worked to accommodate a rapid change from open surgical procedures to the newer techniques of MIS. Perioperative nurses and surgical technologists acquired new competencies. Since the 1990s, equipment, instrumentation, surgical skills, and perioperative nursing knowledge have expanded markedly as MIS has become a safe approach for many surgical interventions. Ongoing changes in surgery that aim to incorporate MIS procedures present complex challenges for the surgical team while offering patients potentially shorter hospital stays, reduced postoperative pain, lower rates of surgical site infections, decreased intraoperative blood loss, and faster recuperation (Arezzo, 2014; Table 8.1). Understanding the goals of endoscopic MIS, clinical competence, and preoperative patient assessment establishes the basis for the perioperative plan of care (Patient Engagement Exemplar).

Endoscopes

An endoscope is a tube inserted into a natural body orifice or through a small incision to access internal organs or structures. Endoscopes are flexible, rigid, or semirigid. Flexible endoscopes include angioscopes, bronchoscopes, choledochoscopes, colonoscopes (Fig. 8.1),

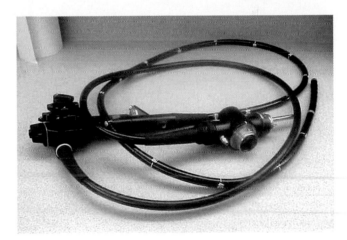

FIG. 8.1 Flexible colonoscope.

cystonephroscopes, hysteroscopes, mediastinoscopes, ureteroscopes, and ureteropyeloscopes. Rigid endoscopes include cystoscopes, laparoscopes, sinuscopes, arthroscopes, bronchoscopes, laryngoscopes, and hysteroscopes (Fig. 8.2). Some endoscopes are manufactured with both flexible and rigid components. A semirigid ureteroscope may appear to be a rigid endoscope but has a deflectable tip to provide a complete field of view from different angles (Fig. 8.3). Hybrid endoscopes have been introduced that are part reusable (eyepiece) and part disposable (shaft and deflection tip). When connecting these two components, take care to ensure proper alignment and proper focusing for image clarity.

Endoscopes (often referred to as "scopes") are diagnostic or operative. *Diagnostic* scopes are for observation only and have no operating channels. The system is sealed at both ends. A diagnostic scope can be used, however, when multiple access sites are planned for the introduction of other instrumentation to perform a surgical procedure. *Operative* scopes are channeled to irrigate, suction, insert, and connect accessory instrumentation (Fig. 8.4). For example, when a potassium titanyl phosphate (KTP) laser is used, the laser fiber is inserted into the operating port of the laparoscope. Advanced laparoscopic techniques may include the use of a flexible endoscope to check for anastomotic leaks, identify bleeding sites, or detect other problems before, during, or immediately after the laparoscopic procedure.

Endoscopes are available in various diameters and lengths, depending on access to the area being visualized and the requirements of the procedure. Optical capability through a rigid scope is controlled by a lens system and can be direct (0-degree angle) or angled (e.g., 30, 70, 120 degrees; Fig. 8.5). Some rigid endoscopes integrate a

TABLE 8.1	
Advantages of Minimally Invasive Surgery Over Open Surgery	
Minimally Invasive	**Open**
Ambulatory or shortened length of stay	Hospital admission
Short postoperative recuperation	4- to 6-week recuperation
Decreased postoperative pain; decreased need for pain medications	Postoperative pain related to surgical site; more analgesics required
Earlier return to normal activities and lifestyle	Return to normal activities and lifestyle varies with recuperation period

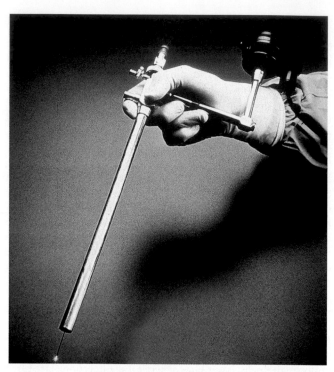

FIG. 8.4 Operative laparoscope.

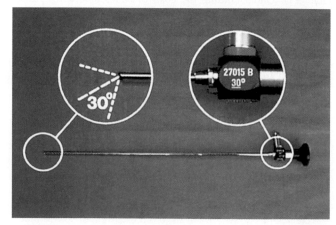

FIG. 8.2 Rigid endoscope.

FIG. 8.5 Lenses inside the endoscope determine the angle of view.

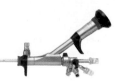

FIG. 8.3 Semirigid ureteroscope.

distally mounted camera chip inside the scope with a rotation dial for proper orientation of the target site. Because flexible scopes are able to be angulated, they allow for a more panoramic view.

There are two types of flexible scopes: fiberoptic endoscopes and videoscopes. Fiberoptic endoscopes have an eyepiece with a lens for visualization; the image is carried through the endoscope via a bundle of tiny glass fibers. Videoscopes have, at their distal end, a video chip that provides an image that is directly viewed on a monitor; a videoscope does not have an eyepiece for direct viewing.

Flexible endoscopes have four distinct components:

1. Control body (e.g., angulation knobs, air-water channels, biopsy port, eyepiece for fiberoptic endoscopes)
2. Insertion tube (e.g., flexible tube containing channels for suction, biopsy, irrigation, air and water, image bundles for the fiberscope, light bundles)
3. Bending section at distal tip (e.g., bending rubber, lenses, air-water nozzle, C-cover, charge-coupled device [CCD] chip for videoscopes)
4. Light-guide connector unit (e.g., suction, air-water channel)

Flexible endoscopes also have three different systems that include some of the various components within the endoscope:

1. Mechanical system (provides ports to introduce accessories to perform treatments and procedures)
2. Angulation system (allows the endoscope's distal tip to be moved in different directions)
3. Illumination system (provides light to view internal structures)

Rigid endoscopes also have four distinct components:

1. Eyepiece (e.g., ocular lenses; rigid videoscopes are also available without an eyepiece)
2. Body (e.g., light-guide connector, valves)
3. Shaft (e.g., rod lenses, spacers)
4. Distal end (e.g., objective lens, negative lens)

Understanding the parts of an endoscope helps assess technical problems that can occur during any endoscopic procedure. Internal components are complex, sophisticated, and sometimes delicate. Scopes must be treated with care.

Light Sources and Fiberoptic Cables

Endoscopic light is often referred to as *cold light,* meaning that the heat from the light source is not transmitted through the length of the scope. Therefore tissue damage from heat at the distal tip of the scope is minimized. When the ends of the fiberoptic cables are disconnected from the scope, however, they may be very hot. The surgical team must use extreme caution to ensure the ends of the cables do not contact the patient's skin or any flammable materials or liquids. If the fiberoptic cable is disconnected from the endoscope during surgery, the scrub person ensures that the cable end is held away from drapes or placed on a moist towel to prevent burns and fires. Ideally the light should be turned off whenever disconnected from the endoscope. The ECRI Institute recommends labeling all fiberoptic light sources with a warning to prevent fires from the hot light source energy (ECRI, 1982). High-intensity fiberoptic light sources and cables can ignite drapes and other materials. To prevent a fire, all cable connections must be completed before activating the light source. The light source must be placed on standby when the cables are disconnected.

Light sources should have adjustable manual and automatic brightness modes. The automatic mode adjusts brightness according to the video image. When the light source is set in this mode, the circulating nurse need not constantly make adjustments.

When selecting a light source, certain options are considered. A light source that can adapt to several rigid endoscopic systems is desirable, such as one with a universal light cable adapter, which enhances flexibility and usage (Fig. 8.6). If a previously purchased unit does not provide this feature, universal light cables with connectors to an interchangeable light source and endoscope adapters are available (Fig. 8.7). A generic cord can be used with most scopes and light sources, but some light cables can only be used with specific sizes of scopes. For example, a 2.5-mm cable is used with a scope less than 4 mm and a 4.5-mm cable is used with a 10-mm scope. Using the incorrect light cable with a scope may overheat or damage the optics. Color coding different cable sizes helps differentiate them. Light sources also must have connection capability with different camera units.

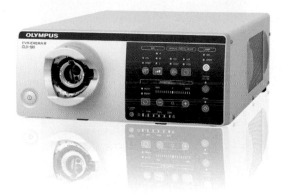

FIG. 8.6 Light source with universal light cable adapter.

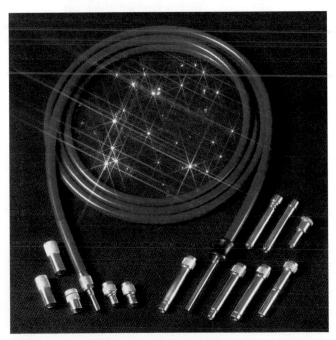

FIG. 8.7 Universal light cable with interchangeable light source connectors and endoscope adapters.

Handle fiberoptic light cables with extreme care. They consist of hundreds of glass fibers that transmit light (Fig. 8.8). These tiny fibers can be broken easily if kinked or dropped. Cables are loosely coiled, never bent, when not in use. After multiple uses, fibers can break. Cables must therefore be checked after each use. To do this, hold one end of the cable pointing toward a bright light while the opposite end is observed for light transmission (Fig. 8.9). Do not test the cable by looking into the end while it is attached to the light source. The visible light and ultraviolet light produced by the light source may harm the eye if directly viewed for extended periods. "Peppering" on the light cable end indicates broken fibers. When

approximately 20% of the fibers are broken, the cable is replaced because adequate light for visualization cannot be transmitted through fractured fibers.

Bulbs within the light source usually are easy to replace. Extra bulbs are stored in lamp-assembly drawers, which are readily accessible. The bulb itself is not touched because (1) it may be very hot and (2) the oils on an individual's hands and fingers can adhere to the bulb, causing the bulb to burn out more quickly. Nonmetal handles usually are built into the light source for bulb removal and replacement.

Three popular types of light sources are available: xenon, metal halide, and halogen. Advantages and disadvantages are associated with each. *Xenon bulbs* are more expensive, but last longer. Xenon light is better for smaller diameter endoscopes (≤2 mm) because the light can be focused to a smaller spot size. Xenon light also is a preferred light for video or picture taking. *Metal halide bulbs* have a shorter life span (about 250 hours) and are less expensive. These bulbs are easier than others to handle and replace, and do not require large fans for cooling. *Halogen light sources* are used for office and some hospital applications. They do not, however, offer the light intensity required for many endoscopic and video applications. Personal preference and conditions for use are two key factors in choosing an appropriate light source for endoscopy. Light sources that incorporate a lamp-life status–testing mode are desirable so bulb replacement can be anticipated.

Given that light sources produce different colors of light whenever a camera is used, *white balancing* must be performed during each procedure. White balancing adjusts the camera to all other optical components (endocoupler, light cable, and laparoscope), enabling the camera to reference white so that it can identify all primary colors properly. White balancing is performed once the scope and light cable are connected, the light source turned on, and the lens held close to a white gauze sponge or white drape (for white color referencing).

Endoscopic Minimally Invasive Surgery Instrumentation

Endoscopic MIS instrumentation is designed to correspond with the surgical site and the technique used while functioning as an ergonomic extension of the surgeon's hand. The length and working end of the instrument must be adequate to perform surgery at the target site.

Because endoscopic MIS and robotic approaches differ from traditional open equivalents, modifications of existing instruments have been made. Some basic patterns have been used for years and continue to be popular, whereas others have been designed to accommodate newer MIS and robotic approaches. This new era in surgery began in the 1990s, and some instrument designs are now in their seventh and eighth generations. As MIS becomes more sophisticated, so do the instruments required for successful, less-invasive techniques. MIS instrumentation is discussed in more detail in the next sections, and insufflation safety and MIS complications and considerations are addressed in the section on Practices and Potential Risks During Minimally Invasive Surgery.

Trocar System

When a natural orifice does not exist for diagnostic or operative procedures, one or several orifices are created. To do so, a trocar system is used, consisting of an obturator and a sleeve (also known as a cannula or sheath). The trocar system provides a mechanism to insert and remove instruments while MIS is performed. The obturator and sleeve are inserted to access the operative site. When the port of entry has been made, the obturator is removed, and the sleeve is

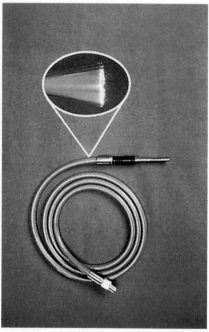

FIG. 8.8 Inside the light cable are hundreds of glass fibers that transmit light.

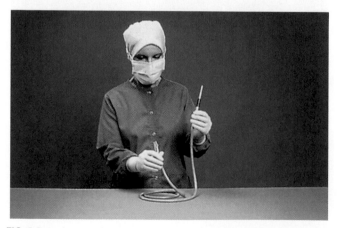

FIG. 8.9 Light cable can be checked for broken fibers by holding one end toward a bright light while looking at the other end.

left in place. More complex procedures may require a greater number of trocar systems and puncture sites.

If a reusable trocar system is used, the obturator tip must be sharpened routinely. The stopcock and trumpet valves are inspected before and after each use to ensure proper functioning. Internal gaskets may need occasional replacement. The obturator and sleeve must fit properly and may not always be interchangeable. Component parts are kept together, but are disassembled completely for cleaning and sterilization.

Disposable trocar systems offer several advantages (Fig. 8.10). One is that the obturator is always sharp. When multiple ports of the same size are used, the same obturator is reused on the same patient. Some manufacturers also package one obturator and two or more sleeves of the same size. The same obturator is used to establish multiple access ports. Disposable units also may provide siliconized obturator tips and safety features when entry has been made. Systems are available that both engage a safety shield to advance automatically over the obturator tip (Fig. 8.11) and provide retraction of the obturator tip when entry is made.

Many disposable sleeves have gripping devices that can reduce the risk of accidental sleeve removal during repeated advancement and withdrawal of instruments. Grippers are incorporated into the

sleeve or as separate entities. Grippers can be used with reusable sleeves as long as the fit is appropriate.

Disposable sleeves have a stopcock assembly for insufflation gas, similar to the reusable system. One-way flapper valves in disposables provide leakproof protection and operate automatically for instrument insertion, specimen removal, or rapid desufflation. Because instrument diameters vary with design and use, different sizes of obturator and sleeve units may be required for one procedure. Reusable and disposable trocar systems are available in a variety of diameters and lengths. To increase flexibility, converters and reducers are used to adapt the size of the instrument. Converters can be separate or built into the sleeve as a diaphragm seal. Both systems are designed to reduce the chance of carbon dioxide (CO_2) leaks so that the pneumoperitoneum can be maintained. Radiolucent disposable sleeves offer the ability to visualize tissue and lesions without obstruction. This feature may be crucial during an endoscopic cholangiogram to avoid obstructing the view during fluoroscopy. During other procedures this design may not be necessary.

Radially expanding dilator systems, consisting of a cannula with blunt obturator and an insufflation/access needle with a radially expandable sleeve, have been shown to cause less traumatic abdominal wall entry and yield smaller fascial defects. Intra-abdominal entry is accomplished using an access needle with a radially expandable sleeve. When insufflation is achieved, the needle is withdrawn, leaving the expandable sleeve in place. While the sleeve and tissue are expanded, a tapered, blunt-tipped dilator is inserted, providing a large working channel for an access port. Because a sharp-tipped obturator is not used, the muscles are spread, not cut, and the risk of abdominal wall or vascular damage is minimized. Bladeless obturators, which separate tissue in a sequential fashion rather than cut or stretch tissue, also are available in an optical version that allows the surgeon to visualize all tissue layers being separated.

Occasionally a procedure is scheduled as an *open laparoscopy*. Patients who have had multiple surgeries or who have developed adhesions, and pediatric patients, can present an added risk and may be candidates for open laparoscopy. A small paraumbilical incision is made and tissues dissected. The peritoneum is opened and a large blunt-tipped obturator-sleeve assembly is inserted (Fig. 8.12). The sleeve is designed to fit snugly against the peritoneum from underneath

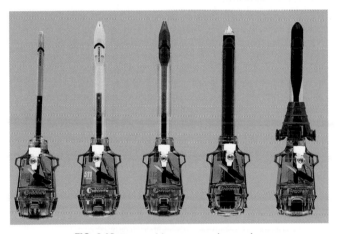

FIG. 8.10 Disposable trocars and cannulae.

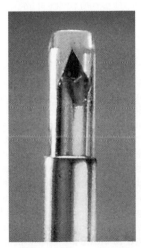

FIG. 8.11 Close-up view of the trocar safety shield in place.

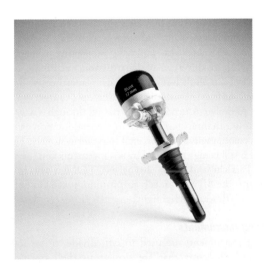

FIG. 8.12 Blunt-tipped trocars can be used to minimize injuries during insertion.

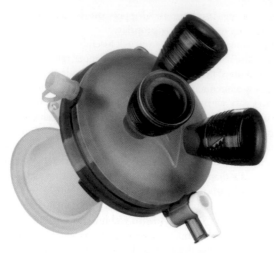

FIG. 8.13 Single-entry access platform that facilitates triangulation of laparoscopy instruments.

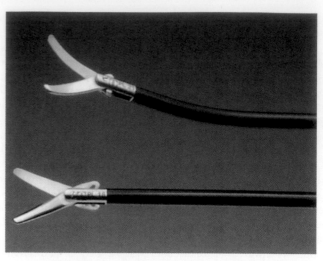

FIG. 8.14 Straight and curved endoscopic scissors.

and against the skin from above. Stay sutures are used to close any excess incision. Wafer seals reduce further loss of CO_2 gas. Pneumoperitoneum is then created and maintained. If a reusable system is used, stay sutures also are used to stabilize the system. Sealed system devices have been developed to introduce not only instrumentation but also the surgeon's hand when direct surgical approaches are necessary during laparoscopy.

When extracorporeal surgery is performed during laparoscopy (i.e., when tissue undergoing surgery is brought outside the body through a small hole), a larger diameter port is used. During certain bowel resections, loops of bowel are brought through a larger port to be resected or sutured.

When the chest is entered, shorter blunt obturators are used with grippers that provide stabilization while in the pleural cavity. This type of obturator does not have insufflation ports. If insufflation is required to assist the anesthesia provider in collapsing the lung, regular obturators with insufflation ports are used.

Single-incision laparoscopic surgery (SILS), in which the surgeon operates through a single-entry port, usually the umbilical area, leaves only a single small scar. There are single-port platforms that provide an airtight fulcrum that assists with access and the triangulation of standard or articulating instrumentation (Fig. 8.13). Single-port laparoscopy is associated with minimal postoperative pain and scarring. Advancements in this type of laparoscopic technique have been made not only in adult but also pediatric laparoscopy.

Natural orifice transluminal endoscopic surgery (NOTES) continues to evolve. An endoscope is passed through a natural orifice (mouth, anus, urethra, etc.) so that an internal incision can be made (stomach, colon, vagina, bladder, etc.) to perform surgery. This scarless procedure is still being challenged by advancements and the resurgence in SILS (Pasriche and Rivas, 2015). NOTES has also been incorporated into the SILS approach to promote precision and surgical effectiveness (Research Highlight).

Dissecting Instruments

Dissecting instruments are used to cut, divide, or separate tissue. Scissors and dissectors that are similar to their open-procedure counterparts (see Chapter 7) have been designed for use in MIS procedures. Scissors are available for blunt or sharp dissection. They

RESEARCH HIGHLIGHT

Hybrid Natural Orifice Transluminal Endoscopic Surgery for Rectal Carcinoma

NOTES has emerged as an innovative surgical approach in treating many types of diseases, including treating rectal cancer. A hybrid approach (hNOTES) that combines the single-incision laparoscopic platform with the transanal endoscopic approach has been used to provide precise dissection of the diseased tissue while requiring fewer staples in the rectal stump. Twenty patients met the criteria for a standardized procedure to excise rectal cancer using both approaches. One case converted to an open procedure because of uncontrolled bleeding, whereas two cases developed abscesses caused by leakage. When compared with conventional surgery, hNOTES has the potential to preserve autonomic nerve function and neurovascular bundles, while promoting less dissection. A simultaneous two-team approach (abdominal and pelvic teams) can significantly shorten the operative time. The hNOTES for rectal cancer was shown to be safe and feasible and may become a viable option for treating rectal cancers.

hNOTES, Hybrid natural orifice transluminal endoscopic surgery; *NOTES,* natural orifice transluminal endoscopic surgery.
Modified from Chen C et al: The evolving practice of hybrid natural orifice transluminal endoscopic surgery (NOTES) for rectal cancer. *Surg Endosc* 29:119–126, 2015.

can be straight or curved (including hook scissors), depending on the location of the target tissue and technique used (Fig. 8.14). Scissors usually have a rounded tip when closed so that they also can be used to manipulate tissue without trauma. When open, both blades of the scissors should be visualized to prevent inadvertent injury. Some scissors are designed to be connected to an electrosurgical energy source so that coagulation can be provided during cutting.

Dissectors are used to separate or divide tissue. Many different tip shapes are available to dissect, spread, divide, grasp, retract, and coagulate structures (Fig. 8.15). Other dissecting instruments, such as balloon dissectors, have been developed for blunt dissection or creation of a space so that surgery can be performed. A balloon dissector may be used to create a preperitoneal space during laparoscopic herniorrhaphy (Fig. 8.16).

Clamping and Grasping Instruments

Clamping instruments are used to grasp and hold tissue or other materials. Ratchets are used in the instrument design to allow the distal tip to be locked onto the tissue being grasped. Graspers, forceps, and biopsy forceps are classified as clamping instruments.

Graspers and forceps can be (1) traumatic, with sharp teeth, or (2) atraumatic, with a smooth, serrated jaw surface (Fig. 8.17). Traumatic graspers and forceps customarily are used to hold tissue that will be excised, whereas the atraumatic versions are used to gently hold structures, such as the bowel or liver. Some clamping instruments are insulated so that electrosurgical energy can be transmitted to provide coagulation.

Suturing and Stapling Instruments

Suturing or stapling instruments deliver sutures, staples, or clips to join, hold, and secure tissue. Needle holders, clip appliers, and staplers are in this category.

Needle holders are designed to deliver and place sutures within body cavities during MIS procedures. Tungsten carbide jaw inserts on needle holders are used to prevent rotation of the suture needle. These inserts can be replaced when they become worn. Some needle holders are designed to transfer the needle from one jaw to the other during suturing (Fig. 8.18). Suture passers and curved needle holders also are available.

A clip applier is used to provide hemostasis and tissue security. Its use represents the safest, easiest, and quickest way to occlude small vessels and structures. Reusable appliers exist, but many must be removed from the cannula each time to be reloaded. This process adds time, contributes to loss of pneumoperitoneum (if used), and causes frustration when the clip is dislodged on reinsertion. For this reason, automatic-feed, reloadable, disposable versions are more desirable (Fig. 8.19).

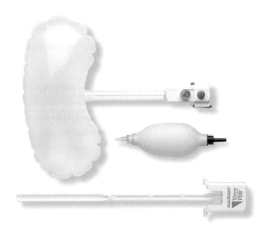

FIG. 8.15 Dissector with jaws open to divide and separate tissue.

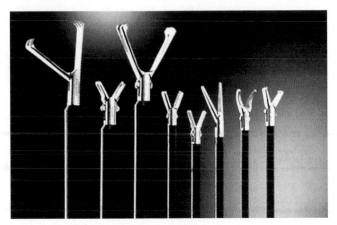

FIG. 8.17 Endoscopic grasping instruments.

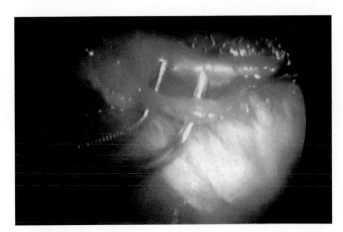

FIG. 8.16 Balloon dissecting instrument.

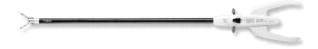

FIG. 8.18 Endoscopic needle holder that transfers the needle from one prong of the jaw to the other.

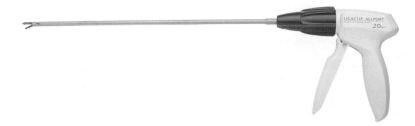

FIG. 8.19 Disposable endoscopic reloading rotating clip applier.

Staplers provide cutting and stapling during MIS resections (Figs. 8.20 and 8.21). Certain structures can be easily resected intracorporeally (within the abdominal cavity), such as the ovary or appendix. Others may necessitate extracorporeal resection (outside the body) or reanastomosis; if this is necessary, traditional stapling devices are used.

The evolution of more complex MIS techniques has challenged traditional suturing and ligation methods. As a result, several devices and techniques have been developed for laparoscopic tissue suturing. When surgical clips and staples cannot be used, a laparoscopic suture may be substituted. Conditions that preclude the use of clips include large arteries and edematous or inflamed ducts. Most general surgeons prefer to use nonabsorbable sutures and ligation materials to prevent rapid absorption. Three basic types of laparoscopic suturing materials are *loop ligatures, extracorporeal sutures,* and *intracorporeal sutures.*

Loop Ligatures. Preknotted suture loops (loop ligatures) are used to ligate pedicle tissues. The suture loop is packaged with an introducer sleeve, which is inserted through one of the obturator sheaths. The loop is passed over the target tissue or pedicle using a grasping forceps to assist. When the loop is in position, the existing suture knot is pushed down the introducer sleeve until it is cinched tightly around the tissue (Fig. 8.22). The suture is then cut with endoscopic scissors.

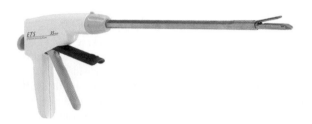

FIG. 8.20 Disposable linear cutter with reloading unit.

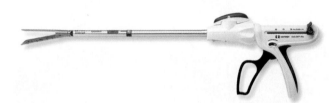

FIG. 8.21 Disposable endoscopic stapling device.

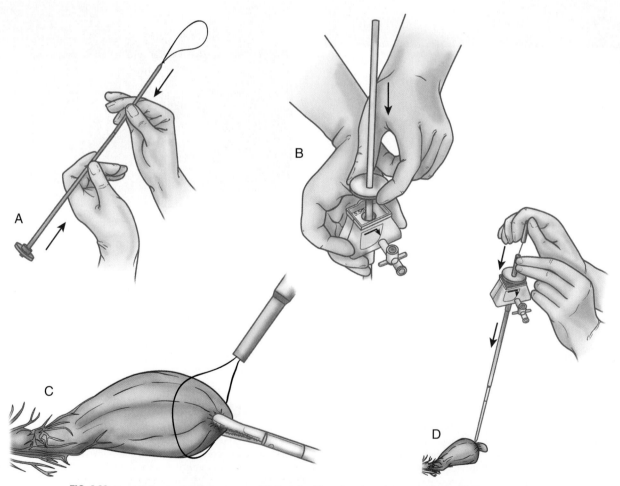

FIG. 8.22 Surgitie ligating loop on an ovary. (A) Back-load loop into introducer completely. (B) Insert introducer into trocar, all the way down. (C) Push suture loop through introducer. Grasp desired tissue with grasping forceps (passed through another trocar) and maneuver loop over tissue. (D) Push down knot by advancing nylon carrier all the way until knot is cinched. Cut suture.

Extracorporeal Sutures. Tissue can be approximated intra-abdominally when the knot is tied extracorporeally. To accomplish this, endoscopic swaged sutures are used. The suture is grasped proximally to the needle, and both are inserted through one of the obturator sleeves into the abdomen. The needle is held with the grasper or laparoscopic needle holder and driven through the desired tissue. A second grasper or needle holder inserted through a second obturator sleeve is used to assist. The needled end of the suture is pulled through the tissue and out through the sleeve. The needle is removed, and a knot is tied extracorporeally. The knot is advanced down the sleeve and onto the tissue (Fig. 8.23). The suture is cut with laparoscopic scissors. The three types of

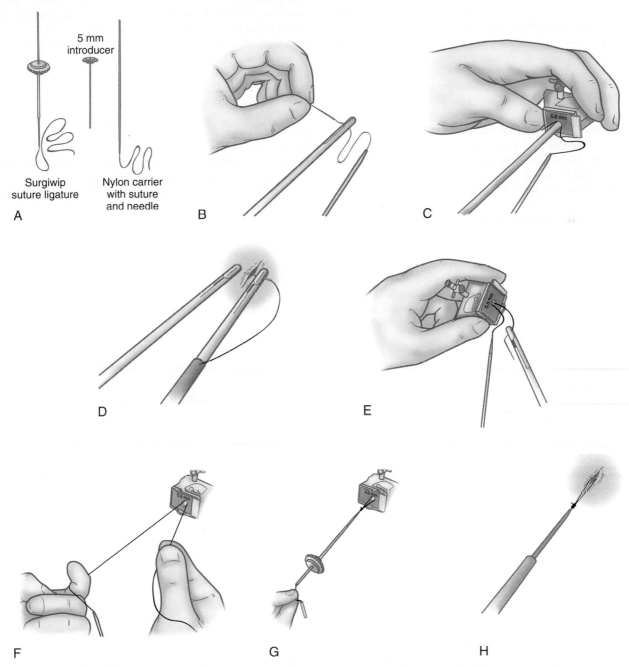

FIG. 8.23 Surgiwip suture ligature application for approximating tissue intra-abdominally by extracorporeal knot tying (outside body). (A) Component pieces. (B) Grasp suture behind swage of needle with tissue grasper or needle holder. (C) Introduce grasper or needle holder and suture through trocar into abdomen. (D) Drive needle through tissue to be approximated. Place instrument close to center of needle for control. Pull needle through tissue using second grasper (introduced through another trocar). (E) Regrasp needle behind swage intracorporeally, and pull it through and out the same trocar. (Allow for slack of suture to avoid tissue tears.) (F) Remove needle. Tie knot. (G) After knot is tied, break end of nylon carrier. (H) Push knot down with nylon carrier and out onto tissue. Cut suture. For additional suturing, repeat steps B through H until tissue is satisfactorily approximated.

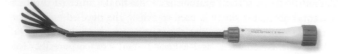

FIG. 8.24 Endoscopic fan retractor with five fingers.

knots tied extracorporeally are the *slip knot, fisherman's knot,* and *surgeon's knot.*

Intracorporeal Sutures. A suture ligature also can be passed through the obturator sleeve to be tied while it is inside the body. The tissue is approximated in the same fashion but tied intracorporeally using grasping forceps or laparoscopic needle holders.

Retractors and Accessory Instruments

Retractors are used to hold tissue and expose the operative target site (Fig. 8.24). Retractors can be traumatic to some structures, such as the bowel and liver, and are used with caution. Mini-retractors and balloon retractors have been designed for use on delicate structures. A miniature version of a surgical clamp with blades that splay the incision open beneath the tissue is available. Other accessory instruments have been designed to enhance the use of basic MIS instruments, provide exposure, and facilitate the procedure. Probes used to manipulate tissue are blunt to minimize tissue trauma. Some probes have centimeter gradations to measure structures within the body. Irrigation-aspirator probes enhance visualization of internal structures, and electrosurgical probes provide hemostasis. Endoscopic specimen bags contain specimens to minimize cross-contamination. Special accessory instruments are continually being designed to enhance MIS procedures.

Care and Handling of Endoscopes and Instrumentation

Endoscopes and instruments must be clean and free from all bioburden (contaminating organisms) before sterilization or high-level disinfection (HLD). The complex design of many endoscopes complicates reprocessing (Brooks, 2015). The ECRI Institute compiles a list of the "Top 10 Patient Safety Concerns for Healthcare Organizations" and for 2016 lists "inadequate cleaning and disinfection of flexible endoscopes" as number four on that list (ECRI, 2016). Patient deaths from carbapenem-resistant Enterobacteriaceae (CRE) gained media attention from inadequate endoscope reprocessing, especially during ECRP procedures using hard-to-clean duodenoscopes (Muscarella, 2014).

During routine use, bioburden accumulates in channels, ports, crevices, and other movable parts of scopes and instruments. Periodically throughout the procedure, gross blood and bioburden must be removed by flushing the channels and wiping the surfaces with sterile water. Saline is never routinely used to remove gross debris during the procedure because this salt solution can leave mineral deposits on or in the device. Keeping instruments and scopes relatively clean during the procedure helps prevent debris from drying, thus facilitating the cleaning process and protecting the instrument.

After each procedure, all instruments and devices are decontaminated thoroughly. Immersible equipment is cleaned or flushed with an enzymatic or other appropriate detergent solution; this loosens organic material and makes it easier to remove. Instruments that can withstand cavitation or ultrasonic cleaning (processes in which high-frequency energy causes microscopic bubbles to assist with debris removal) can be placed in an ultrasonic device. Fiberoptics and endoscopes usually cannot be placed in an ultrasonic machine because the vibratory motion can damage tiny fiberoptic bundles.

Selection of an appropriate cleaning solution or detergent is critical. Detergents consist of various formulations that may include pH builders, buffers, surfactants, and chelants that provide the chemical compositions that clean devices. The amount of cleaning power within a solution is determined by the pH of the formulation. The "potential for hydrogen" is the meaning of pH, which represents the degree of acidity (more hydrogen ions present), neutrality (equal hydrogen and hydroxyl ions), and alkalinity (more hydroxyl ions present). A detergent with a very low pH can cause staining and pitting on the surfaces of stainless steel instruments because they are more susceptible to damage during prolonged exposure of acidic solutions. When detergents are combined with the mechanical or automatic force of a cleaning spray, removal of bioburden is easier.

A low-sudsing detergent is recommended so that the detergent can be completely removed. Cleaning solutions with surfactant are less desirable because they are more difficult to rinse. If surfactant is left on the surface, the device may feel sticky or gummy, which could affect the electrical conductivity of the instrument. Careful attention is paid to the solution used as well as the type of device being cleaned. Certain detergents are not appropriate for cleaning endoscopes or endoscopic instruments.

Careful rinsing and flushing with copious amounts of water follows the cleaning process. Often deionized or demineralized water is recommended for the final rinse to minimize mineral buildup from tap water. The manufacturer's written recommendations for cleaning and processing should always be followed. After the final rinse, instruments are dried before disinfection or sterilization.

Automatic cleaning devices that flush the ports of instruments provide an economic and effective way to clean reusable channeled instruments. Although instruments have flush ports, debris can become lodged distally. Some automatic systems provide a means to flush in a retrograde fashion, forcing debris from the larger proximal port. Sealed instruments also can be tested for seal integrity using this system.

After the device has been thoroughly cleaned, rinsed, and dried, its integrity and functionality are assessed. Personnel involved with reprocessing MIS devices must be aware of instrument composition, design, and use. Any device with electrosurgical capabilities is checked to ensure that the length of the insulation sheath has not been compromised. Equipment is available that scans these instruments for electrical leakage through breaks in insulation.

Often new MIS accessories are purchased and used without educating the staff responsible for their reprocessing. Staff members must be oriented on how instrumentation is assembled, disassembled, and thoroughly cleaned. The perioperative and sterile processing team members, along with the device manufacturer and vendor, should partner to ensure safe reprocessing practices.

The US Food and Drug Administration (FDA) requires that any device purchased as reusable must have written instructions for reprocessing. Staff must understand how the instrument works to ensure that functionality of the device has not changed during reprocessing. Compliance with federal, professional, and regional standards for reprocessing is mandatory.

Instruments and devices that contact sterile tissues and the vascular system must be sterile. Instruments contacting intact mucous membranes can be processed using HLD (Fig. 8.25). This means that sterility is required for all laparoscopy, angioscopy, thoracoscopy, and arthroscopy procedures. HLD (cold soak) may be acceptable for colonoscopy, laryngoscopy, bronchoscopy, cystoscopy, and other

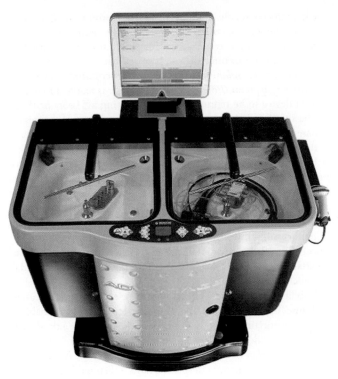

FIG. 8.25 High-level disinfection reprocessor that handles two scopes at one time.

diagnostic procedures in which surgical devices touch intact mucous membranes. Invasive procedures that access the vascular system (biopsies) are performed during many endoscopy procedures. The adequacy of HLD must be evaluated for these procedures. Viruses and microorganisms, such as HIV and hepatitis B and C viruses, *Mycobacterium* (tuberculosis bacteria), and antibiotic-resistant organisms are not easily destroyed during HLD. Even though it has been the accepted primary standard of reprocessing for some endoscopic instrumentation, the concern over viruses and microorganisms has caused debate about the adequacy of using HLD. Therefore sterilization is quickly becoming the standard for reprocessing endoscopes and endoscopic instruments.

Thermal pasteurization, using a heat-automated washer/pasteurizer, may be chosen for thermal HLD for devices that can withstand heat (i.e., 71°C–77°C) for 30 minutes in a water bath (AORN, 2016). This process destroys all microorganisms except bacterial spores (AORN, 2016).

An FDA-approved chemical germicide may be selected for chemical HLD. Glutaraldehyde, used for many years, has hazards for staff that must be considered when this agent is selected for HLD. The maximum recommended exposure level of glutaraldehyde determined by the Occupational Safety and Health Administration (OSHA) is 0.2 parts per million (ppm). When solution is being poured after mixing or when devices are being submerged, the level rises to approximately 0.4 ppm, which is double the recommended maximum exposure level. The odor of glutaraldehyde becomes an irritant at 0.3 ppm, causing tearing, nausea, and other effects. Hooded systems to house glutaraldehyde solutions are designed to remove odor and fumes. When using this or any other chemical germicide, the device must be totally immersed and soaked for the specified contact time, following the manufacturer's recommendations for cleaning protocols, preparing the solution, maintaining contact time, and calculating

expiration dates. Other solutions are available for HLD without the hazards that glutaraldehyde presents. When using a high-level disinfectant, the department's Material Safety Data Sheets (MSDS) Manual must be available for referencing along with the manufacturer's Instructions for Use (IFU) and guidelines. For example, a device may not be fully immersible for HLD.

Institutional policy sets the guidelines from which practitioners work. Insight and coordination are required to provide comparable levels of care when there are too few instruments for the number of scheduled procedures. If sterile instruments are required for a particular procedure, they should be used for all patients undergoing that procedure. Sufficient instruments, accessory items, and equipment must be purchased to accommodate patient volume, and appropriate reprocessing measures must be planned and implemented.

When sterile devices and instruments are needed, multiple options for sterilization include steam, ethylene oxide, gas-plasma, peracetic acid, and ozone sterilization (AORN, 2016). Often steam cannot be used on delicate endoscopes, but accessory instruments may withstand the heat produced during steam sterilization. Some arthroscopes and laparoscopes have been designed to withstand high temperatures of steam sterilization. For items that cannot withstand high temperatures, options include the following (see Chapter 4 for a detailed discussion):

- *Ethylene oxide sterilization:* This process has been used for many years to sterilize endoscopes and instruments. Past decisions to eliminate agents that were combined with ethylene oxide to decrease flammability, such as chlorofluorocarbon (CFC) and halogenated CFC (HCFC), have led to the use of 100% ethylene oxide for safe and effective sterilization. Limitations of ethylene oxide sterilization are the prolonged time needed for aeration of ethylene oxide and the installation and monitoring requirements for this type of sterilizer.
- *Plasma sterilization system:* This system uses hydrogen peroxide gas plasma, which sterilizes within approximately 24 to 75 minutes (depending on the system) and dissociates into nontoxic byproducts. Understanding the advantages and limitations (e.g., lumen restrictions) of this system is important when determining if it meets the needs of endoscope or instrument sterilization.
- *Liquid chemical sterilization:* Powerful chemicals, such as 35% peracetic acid, can provide sterilization for cleaned, immersible, reusable, and heat-sensitive devices. The pH-neutral chemical solution eliminates all microbial life and then can be safely rinsed down the drain. It is gentle on delicate surgical instruments, including flexible endoscopes with multiple channels.
- *Ozone sterilizer:* Oxygen is used in a natural process to produce ozone. When oxygen is exposed to an intense electrical field, the oxygen molecule separates into atomic oxygen (O). Atomic oxygen combines with other oxygen molecules (O_2) to create triatomic oxygen (O_3), which is ozone. Ozone reverts quickly back to its oxygen state while producing no toxic residuals. Ozone is a powerful sterilizing agent because it oxidizes organic matter (fungi, bacterial spores, and viruses). Key features of ozone sterilization include ease of use, low-temperature sterilization, cost effectiveness, and compatibility with anodized aluminum containers. The manufacturer's instructions must be followed regarding operation of the sterilizer, instrument and device preparation, and device limitations.

Single-Use Versus Reusable Instrumentation

Many facilities use a combination of reusable and single-use laparoscopic instruments. Advantages of single-use items include sharpness, reliability related to function, guaranteed sterility, and safety. Indirect advantages include no reprocessing, no repair costs, and comparable levels of patient care. Upgraded designs are more easily brought to market when the device is labeled for single use. Disadvantages include the need for increased storage space, budgetary implications, and environmental concerns related to disposal of biohazardous waste.

Advantages of reusable instruments include less storage space, reduced costs (except for initial purchase and repair), and minimal waste. With reusable instruments, decontamination and reprocessing systems must be reliable, compatible with the devices being processed, and monitored for effectiveness.

Above all, safe and effective patient outcomes should be the major criteria considered when comparing single-use with reusable instrumentation. Advantages and disadvantages of reusable versus single-use devices (SUDs) must be explored by using a risk-to-benefit analysis before purchasing decisions can be made. Institutional policy may dictate whether reusable or single-use items are chosen. The choice between single-use and reusable instrumentation and equipment must be evaluated thoroughly in each individual practice setting and justified accordingly.

Reprocessing Single-Use Devices

Reprocessing SUDs is a practice that has grown in acceptance. In the United States the practice of reprocessing SUDs is highly regulated by the FDA. The first FDA guidance document was published in 2000. The document was updated and published in 2006, titled *Guidance for Industry and FDA Staff: Medical Device User Fee and Modernization Act of 2002, Validation Data in Premarket Notification Submissions (510[k]s) for Reprocessed Single-use Medical Devices* (FDA, 2006). The document outlines regulatory requirements, enforceable by the FDA, for reprocessing previously used SUDs. The FDA continues to provide prescriptive guidelines to control this industry. In 2008 the Government Accounting Office (GAO) published a document stating that there was no elevated risk with reprocessing SUDs (GAO, 2008).

A "reprocessor" is usually a third-party reprocessing company that reprocesses SUDs. Hospitals rarely pursue the challenges of becoming listed as a reprocessor, given the expense involved with this activity. The FDA states that reprocessing SUDs can reduce medical waste and save costs if the reprocessor follows the same requirements as the original manufacturer including (FDA, 2006):

1. *Registration and listing with the FDA:* Any organization reprocessing SUDs must register with the FDA and provide a comprehensive list of all single-use medical devices that it reprocesses.
2. *Medical device reporting (MDR) of adverse events:* Any organization reprocessing SUDs must comply with the FDA's manufacturer reporting requirements and report not only all patient injuries from device malfunctions or failures but also any event that could have led to patient injury or death.
3. *Device tracking whose failure could lead to serious outcomes:* The FDA can issue a tracking order for any specific device, if applicable. These devices are typically high-risk, class III medical devices, such as implants. Reprocessing companies usually refrain from reprocessing class III devices.
4. *Corrections and removals of unsafe devices:* Every reprocessor must have a formal procedure in place to recall or correct affected devices.
5. *Labeling and manufacturing requirements:* Every reprocessor must provide instructions-for-use documents (IFUs) with reprocessed medical devices and must comply with specific requirements for

what appears on the device label. Any reprocessed SUD must be labeled "prominently and conspicuously," with the following statement: "Reprocessed device for single use. Reprocessed by (name of manufacturer that reprocessed the device)."

6. *FDA premarket submission of a premarket notification (510[k]) or premarket approval (PMA):* Every reprocessor is required to register each device to be reprocessed by submitting a 510(k) or PMA. The specific FDA requirements for the regulation of devices are based on the criticality (critical, semicritical, or noncritical) and the risk category/class of the device.

Reprocessors also repackage and resterilize items with an expired shelf life date or when sterility of the outer packaging has been compromised. SUDs that are reprocessed are segregated into two categories for reprocessing: *open/not used* and *open/used*. The devices that have been used are grossly decontaminated before they are sent for reprocessing. If devices are not grossly decontaminated, they are collected in approved containers and transported by a licensed biohazardous material hauler using appropriate packaging materials and labeling.

Liability is an important concern for those engaged in reprocessing single-use items. A hospital or surgery center may be liable if reprocessing occurs within the confines of the facility. If a third-party company provides this service, it may likewise be liable and must document liability insurance coverage for this service. Although the original manufacturer of a device warrants a disposable product for one use, a reprocessing company also warrants the reprocessed device for one additional use.

Questions to ask when determining whether to reprocess SUDs include the following:

- Can the disposable device be adequately cleaned?
- Can the device withstand disinfection or sterilization? Can it be adequately aerated if ethylene oxide sterilization is used?
- Is the device tested and checked for proper form and function after cleaning has been completed?
- Has device integrity been destroyed during reprocessing or is equipment available to test the integrity of the device? How is the integrity of insulation checked on an electrosurgical instrument?
- Can the device be returned to its original intended use?
- Will cost savings be passed on to the patient, if appropriate?
- What is the maximum number of safe reuses, as determined through comprehensive testing? How is the number of reuses indicated on the device?
- Should the patient be informed that a reprocessed device may be used? The FDA does not require informed consent for the use of reprocessed SUDs. Many providers contend that because reprocessing is so highly regulated and the risk of using a reprocessed device is the same as using the device for the first time, there is no need to seek informed consent.

No matter where reprocessing is performed, appropriate equipment must be available to ensure that the form and function of the device have not been compromised. Customers should inquire about reprocessing and quality assurance practices if dealing with a third-party reprocessor. Usually these companies have appropriate equipment to perform comprehensive device and validation testing. They must register with the FDA and comply with the Quality System Regulation (QSR; FDA, 2006). Reprocessors should provide documentation of FDA registration; any reports of FDA inspection, such as an establishment inspection report (EIR); FDA warning letters; all-important 510(k) or PMA documentation; and the limited number of uses for each specific device.

The practice of reprocessing SUDs continues to grow as significant cost savings are realized by all sizes and types of healthcare facilities. Surgical team members must work closely with their purchasing agent, infection control officer, financial administrator, and others to decide if reprocessing SUDs is an appropriate option for their facility.

Video Technology

Evolution of Video Technology

A basic standard medical video system includes the scope, light cable, light source, camera head, camera cord, camera-scope coupler, camera control unit (CCU), video monitor, and recording devices. Additional peripheral equipment is necessary for specific surgical procedures and is discussed later. Given the complexity of video technology, a glossary of terms is provided in Box 8.1.

Setting up a video system in surgery begins with the image source—the camera. A CCU is needed to convert the image signal from the camera into a viewable format. The monitor is then connected as the display device that shows the image signal. Options

can be added to this setup to record the surgical procedure or to take still images. The image recorder and/or printer is positioned before the display device.

Video systems use light energy from a source, convert it into electrical energy, and then convert it back into light energy to provide pictures. The camera head contains a sensor, which is light sensitive. The sensor may be a solid-state unit or chip, called a *charge-coupled device*, which produces the unprocessed video signal. The sensor may be a high-definition (HD) system.

The CCD is composed of small picture elements called *pixels*, which in the presence of light are conductive and in the absence of light remain nonconductive. Each pixel can sense red, blue, or green light. The picture is transformed into a matrix made up of the conductive and nonconductive pixels. This matrix will scan at an extremely rapid rate that generates the signal frequency.

The National Television Standards Committee (NTSC) sets the standard analog video format in the United States, Canada, Japan, and most of South America and Asia. It was established for broadcast purposes. Even though the NTSC format has been used for more than 50 years, most transmissions in the United States were replaced

---

BOX 8.1

Video Glossary

Autoexposure: An electronic circuit built into cameras to eliminate electronically (within the camera) excess light from the picture; sometimes referred to as electronic shutter.

Automatic gain control: Ability to increase or decrease video output levels depending on the average light level of the viewed object.

Blooming: A glaring effect on the monitor caused by excessive light.

Boost: The ability to increase the signal strength of the camera. When used under low light conditions, boost provides increased sensitivity.

CCD: Charge-coupled device.

CCU: Camera control unit.

Chroma: Saturation of a color.

Chrominance: Defines the video camera's ability to handle the color red, which is the most difficult color to reproduce. The more accurate the color reproduction is, the higher the chrominance.

C-mount: Standard thread size and diameter for a standard video camera lens.

Color bars: A test pattern used to adjust controls on the monitor for color, brightness, and contrast.

Color reproduction: Ability of an imaging device to reproduce colors exactly as the human eye perceives them.

Composite video output: Most commonly used video signal; the typical television video signal.

DICOM: Digital Imaging and Communications in Medicine; format for images in healthcare.

DVI: Digital visual interface, a popular system for medical imaging.

Electronic shutter: Ability of a camera to freeze image information within fractions of a second (1/60, 1/125, 1/1000, 1/10,000).

Foot-candle: Standard measure of luminance; the amount of light emitted by a standard candle at a distance of 1 foot from the flame; 10 lux = 1 foot-candle.

HD-SDI: High-definition serial digital interface; a popular medical imaging system.

High-definition television (HDTV): A digital broadcasting system with higher resolution capabilities than traditional television systems, such as standard-definition TV (SDTV). Less bandwidth is needed for transmission because of digital video compression.

Light gain: Another circuit within the camera that amplifies the picture electronically to show a brighter image; sometimes referred to as automatic gain control (AGC), or boost circuit.

Luminance: Intensity or effectiveness of a given light on the eye.

NTSC: National Television Standards Committee; also a designation for a television signal used in the United States.

Orientation: A mark or ridge on the camera head to orient the top portion of the video monitor.

PACS: Picture archiving communication system.

Pixel: A signal sensor element on a solid-state video chip; most solid-state chips used in medical videography have about 400,000 pixels on their surface. Each pixel is light-sensitive and sees its own small part of the total picture.

Resolution: An optical device's ability to separate fine detail; usually expressed in TV lines. Resolution traditionally is measured by aiming the camera at a target chart with squares of fine lines. The maximum resolution of the optical device is determined at the point in which it begins to blur the lines together. If a box showing 400 lines per inch is still clear with spaces between the lines, the optical device has at least 400 lines-per-inch resolution.

Sensitivity: Response to low light levels by a video system.

S-Video: Super Video, used to designate analog video signals.

S-VHS output: Super-Video Home System (Victor Company of Japan, Yokohama, Japan), a signal from the camera that splits the chroma and luminance, allowing for a richer resolution recording.

White balance: Different light sources produce different temperatures of light and different colors of light. White balancing is an adjustment of the camera for various sources of light.

with the Advanced Television Systems Committee (ATSC) format in 2009, and by August 31, 2011, the ATSC format began to be used in Canada.

The three most commonly used video formats are Super-Video (S-Video), HD serial digital interface (HD-SDI), and digital visual interface (DVI). S-Video is a technology used for analog video signals. The information of S-Video is divided into two separate signals, one for color (chroma) and one for luminance (brightness), and carries standard-definition video. Standard-definition displays 720 lines vertically (side to side) and 480 lines horizontally (from top to bottom). This is usually designated as 720×480 resolution, which produces 345,600 pixels. An S-Video cable is needed to support this transmission.

For medical imaging, the two most widely used systems are HD-SDI and DVI. The HD-SDI system was engineered for the highest picture quality (and is most widely used for endoscopic systems), whereas DVI was engineered for copy-protected distribution.

HD systems that produce ultrasharp images with increased levels of contrast have replaced many standard analog video systems. HD systems offer picture quality almost equivalent to what one experiences with the naked eye.

An *HD video system* refers to a system that has higher resolution (greater numbers of lines of resolution) than with the standard-definition analog systems. The HD visual image is much sharper because gaps between the scan lines are either narrower or invisible to the naked eye. This improvement is most evident with larger screens, but on smaller screens there is no noticeable improvement in picture quality. With a higher number of pixels, compared with the old standard analog video signal, HD results in a much clearer picture, with higher quality and greater detail.

Vertical lines are also described with a lowercase "i," meaning interlaced, or lowercase "p," meaning progressive (which also describes the picture refreshment rate). An interlaced scanning format divides the 1080 lines of resolution into pairs, with the first 540 alternate lines on one frame, then another 540 lines on a second frame. The progressive scanning method displays all 1080 lines simultaneously on every frame, which then requires a greater bandwidth. Today's high resolution of $1920 \times 1080p$ is only surpassed by the Ultra HD option of $2160 \times 3840p$ of the 4K systems, which make an image look three-dimensional (3-D) only without the glasses (Rudolph, 2015). HD video systems that use 1080i resolution are appropriate for endoscopy because this procedure targets small areas and uses slow-moving videos.

Advancements in 3-D imaging systems are continuing to be refined. New systems are becoming highly reliable to facilitate intraoperative manipulation and depth perception, especially for complex procedures. New 3-D endoscopes provide 100-degree angulation, which cannot be performed with the rod lens system. Research has shown that when training is done with a simulated 3-D model, the participants can attain proficiency sooner compared with the standard two-dimensional (2-D) model (Ashraf et al., 2015). The 3-D imaging system has also been successfully incorporated into robotic technology for better visualization and articulation (Clements et al., 2014).

Visualization Systems

Endoscopes are used to offer visualization only to the operating physician. The introduction of the teaching arm provided direct visualization not only for the physician but also for the assistant, perioperative nurse, and other surgical team members. Often, however, images seen through the teaching arm were not identical to the images seen through the primary optics. The inability to interact effectively with the physician or to anticipate surgical needs was frustrating and time consuming.

In the late 1960s and early 1970s, medical video and still cameras were continually being introduced to the marketplace, which allowed for still photography and video documentation of select surgical procedures. Tube-style cameras were large, bulky, and heavy, and inadequate for the video needs of surgery. Video technology rapidly changed with the introduction of the chip TV camera. Its lightweight, low-profile design triggered the era of video-guided surgery. Cameras that previously weighed several pounds now weigh only a few ounces.

Rapid developments in video imaging resulted in higher resolution monitors. Today's integrated video systems provide increased visual capabilities. This leads to enhanced participation by assistants and promotes accurate assessment and planning by perioperative staff. Video technology has evolved to the point of being almost mandatory during MIS procedures. All surgical disciplines have been enhanced by the availability and capability of video systems.

Camera, Cable, and Control Unit

The video camera represents the beginning of the optical-electronic chain of the video system. The camera cable transfers the signal frequency from the camera to a CCU (processor), which modifies the signal and then transmits the image to a video monitor, recorder, or hard copy picture, or all three. The camera, being the first in the video chain, is the most important component of the video system. Camera options vary widely according to available technology, specialty, and personal preference.

Cameras have either one or three CCD chips. Three-chip cameras provide enhanced color and image quality, but are larger, can cost three times that of a single-chip camera, and are not as light sensitive. Color and the resulting image are enhanced because each chip is dedicated to one of the primary colors (red, green, or blue). For this reason three-chip cameras are often used with microscopes when higher magnification requires increased resolution.

Newer single-chip cameras are available with digital processing in their control units, which boosts resolution. In essence, this technology incorporates three-chip quality in a single chip. Although signal processing in the control unit may be digital, the video output from most cameras may be an analog signal.

Digital processing refers to the way information is delivered through the various components of the control unit. This processing format allows for image enhancement and manipulation of the video image. It also allows multiple video signals to be shown on one monitor, has electronic zoom capability, and provides the user with freeze-frame capability when using video printers and when using picture-in-picture systems.

Most cameras also feature the ability to adjust to changes in light intensity while in use. This adjustment is done by an automatic shutter (iris), which measures the availability of light and adjusts accordingly. Automatic shutter activation also helps reduce glare from light reflected off instruments and moist viscera. The ability for continuous variable shutter speeds (rather than discrete speeds) allows for instruments to be brought into the field without glare, while still maintaining adequate illumination of background objects. The shutter's response should be rapid, without perceptible stepping of image intensity.

Camera heads have buttons to control certain functions, such as white balancing; light-sensitivity boosting (ability to provide a brighter picture when the image requires more light, especially when a scope less than 3 mm is used during sinusoscopy); starting and stopping the recorder; and taking hard copy prints. The surgeon controls these functions at the camera head instead of requesting the circulating nurse to do so each time at the recording device or with a remote; therefore the surgeon also has the ability to capture events exactly as and when they occur. Zoom and focusing are also available on the camera head for one-hand usage (Fig. 8.26).

White balancing is performed by turning on the light source; holding the camera about 2 inches away from a white surface; and pressing the white balance button, which is usually found on the camera head or CCU. By sensing pure white, the primary colors of red, green, and blue are controlled so that a white image is created without a visible tint or color cast.

All cameras have focusing capability at the camera-coupler interface. Some also have zoom capability, allowing for closer visualization of specific structures or pathologic conditions. A camera cable connects the camera head to the CCU (Fig. 8.27). Most camera malfunctions are cable related, not camera related. For this reason a system that provides field-replaceable cables is optimum (Fig. 8.28). If wires in the cable break, a new cable can be quickly exchanged, reducing downtime from having to ship the camera and cable for repair. Because wires in the flexible cable can break, the cable must be handled with care. Cables should never be twisted, crimped, or kinked. They also must be long enough to allow sufficient space between the sterile field and the visualization system.

Couplers (Adapters)

Endocouplers are optical coupling devices used to connect cameras to various endoscopes. They are usually available in 22- to 35-mm focal lengths, with different optical magnifications.

The specific coupler required depends on the surgery or diagnostic procedure to be performed and endoscope to be used. When the surgeon will view only on a monitor, a direct-link coupler between the telescope and camera head is required or a camera with the appropriate camera attachment can be used (Fig. 8.29). Cameras are also available for the surgeon to look directly through the endoscope, but this technique is quickly losing popularity because of bloodborne pathogen risks. For the surgeon to look directly through the endoscope and also have monitor-viewing capability, a beam-splitter coupler is necessary. Beam splitters often are used with flexible endoscopes. There are rotating beam splitters designed for the surgeon who operates in a sitting position. Zoom couplers provide variable focal lengths, with ranges from approximately 18 to 50 mm.

A videoscope is a camera-to-scope connection designed without using a coupler (Fig. 8.30). As a coupler adds one more link to the chain, coupler connections can cause loss of light and lens fogging. Connecting the camera and scope with a screw-in design instead of a coupler clamp achieves a tighter fit. This design, however, requires that the camera and scope be purchased as a unit; there is

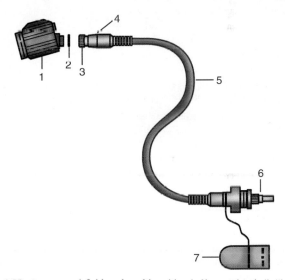

FIG. 8.28 Camera and field-replaceable cable. *1,* Camera head; *2,* O-ring; *3,* knurled ring; *4,* cable connector; *5,* replaceable cable; *6,* camera connector; *7,* soak cap.

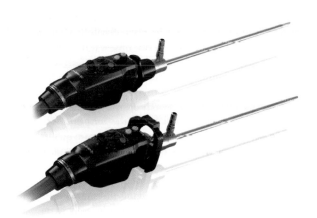

FIG. 8.26 Video zoom and focusing on the camera head for one-hand usage.

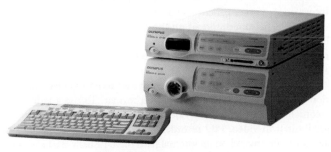

FIG. 8.27 Camera control unit.

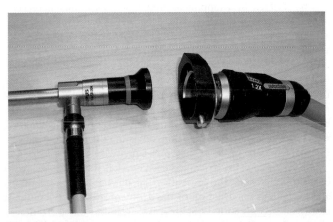

FIG. 8.29 This camera can be directly attached to the endoscope for viewing on the monitor.

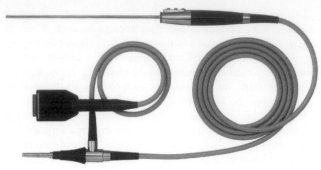

FIG. 8.30 One-piece design with a camera incorporated into the endoscope provides consistent, superior image quality.

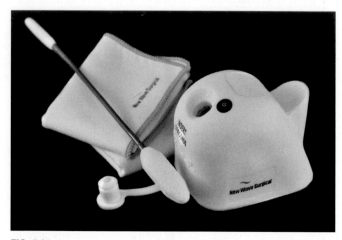

FIG. 8.31 Scope warmer used to decrease lens fogging during laparoscopy.

no interchangeability between systems. It does not allow for sterile bagging of the camera because the camera is part of the endoscope.

Lens fogging can be frustrating. It occurs because a cool metal scope is introduced into a warm body. There are several ways to address this problem. Elimination of a coupler has been discussed. Sterile defogging solutions can be applied to the endoscope and coupler lenses. These provide a coating and reduce the incidence of fogging. Other options on the market include O-ring seals at connections, sapphire lenses, and various water seals. Warming the endoscope before insertion also may reduce fogging. The endoscope can be warmed by wrapping it with lap sponges that have been soaked in warm, sterile water. Also available are scope warmers, such as wraps, sleeves, thermos jugs, and other devices that warm the scope while maintaining sterility (Fig. 8.31).

Another method is to use a CO_2 insufflator that warms the gas (if used) before it enters the body. It may be sufficient to change the insufflation site to a secondary port, after the initial pneumoperitoneum has been achieved. The surgeon also may opt to warm the lens of the endoscope by gently touching an intra-abdominal structure that requires visualization, obviating the need to withdraw the scope to wipe or defog the outer lens.

An advanced video system has been developed that uses the "chip on a tip" technology. This innovative digital imaging system positions a video chip at the distal tip of the endoscope so that the target is clearly and consistently visualized. The seamless one-piece design eliminates couplers that join together the camera head, telescope, and light cable. The distal end can have either a rigid or flexible tip to access hard-to-reach areas. This unique videoscope minimizes problems encountered by other video systems, such as fogging and faulty connections.

Video Monitor

High-resolution video monitors are the end of the chain in video endoscopy. They have become the "windows of observation" during MIS. Monitors should closely match the resolution quality of the camera used. A high-resolution monitor that meets or exceeds the horizontal resolution of the camera is required for optimum visualization. By definition, the camera-monitor system will always have the resolution of the least-detailed element. Determining picture quality of monitors is difficult unless the monitors are side by side. Picture-tube design is the component that alters a monitor's picture quality. Monitors must be able to handle the camera/recorder format (standard analog or HD).

Many operative procedures require two video monitors, one placed on each side of the patient so that the primary surgeon and assistant can view the screen simultaneously. The second monitor is called the *slave monitor.* Abdominal and thoracic procedures are performed in this manner. Certain procedures can be performed with only one monitor. Whenever the monitor can be placed comfortably in a position of visibility to both the surgeon and assistant, only one is necessary. This is usually the method of choice for urologists, endoscopists, gynecologists, and otorhinolaryngologists. Most general surgeons require only one monitor whenever they perform surgery with the endoscope directed toward the patient's feet (as in laparoscopic herniorrhaphy).

Monitors should be at least 19 inches (diagonal measurement of screen) for adequate visualization. When the endoscopic revolution began, most institutions purchased 19- or 20-inch main monitors and 13-inch slave monitors. Today many institutions purchase mainly 24- to 55-inch monitors. This size increases flexibility in usage and provides excellent visibility from most observational angles and distances.

When only one monitor and a composite signal are used, the 75-ohm termination on-off switch must be in the *on* position. When multiple monitors are used, the switch on the last monitor in line to receive the video signal should be in the *on* position, and all others should be in the *off* position to enhance picture quality. Some monitors are self-terminating and do not have termination switches.

Recording Systems

Some recording devices allow for archiving the surgical procedure or selected portions of it. The most commonly used is the video printer, similar to a Polaroid camera in that it takes still pictures instantly. The printer stores the selected image and prints it onto special paper. Many units can be programmed to print 1, 4, 9, or 25 pictures on one piece of $5\frac{1}{2} \times 8$-inch paper in split-screen fashion. Comparisons can then be made as the pathologic condition changes. Information such as patient name, date, time, and operating surgeon usually can be superimposed on top of the print. These prints can be used both for teaching purposes and as part of the permanent record. Some patients are interested in seeing prints of "before and after" images of their condition.

Video disc recorders store and permit easy access to video information and are a popular documentation format. To use a video disc recorder, one also must use a video printer because the images stored are limited to video. HD recorders with touchscreen monitors are available; they record on an internal hard drive (usually 250 gigabytes or more). The images and videos can then be exported via a USB port, burned onto a DVD, or sent to the hospital's server. The optical disc standard, known as Blu-ray, can provide digital storage for up to 10 hours of HD, depending on the encoder settings used.

If a picture or video is sent to the hospital's server, Health Insurance Portability and Accountability Act (HIPAA) regulations must be met. The digital images must be saved in a Digital Imaging and Communications in Medicine (DICOM) format as opposed to JPG or MPG formats used in the consumer market. The digital images are exported from the camera to the hospital's server system, the picture archiving communication system (PACS).

Storage Systems

Space, storage capability, security, and required components determine the type and size of video storage carts needed. Purchasing a cart that can house multiple components of the video system is optimum (Fig. 8.32). Such carts eliminate the clutter of multiple smaller carts and tables. They also eliminate the number of cord connections to wall outlets because most carts have power strips incorporated into their electrical setup. If a cart has a power strip, an on-off main switch usually is located near its base. The power switch must be in the *on* position for the equipment that is plugged into the strip to work. Given the location of the switch, it can be turned off easily during transport and cleaning. Time and embarrassment can be avoided if this switch position is routinely checked before each use.

Articulating arms can be used as monitor mounts. Surgeon preference and room space determine whether this option is necessary or possible. If a surgical or treatment room has been designated for endoscopy, the monitor can be suspended from the ceiling on a swivel mount. The mount should be placed in a location in which the monitor can be easily and comfortably viewed and cleaned. Care

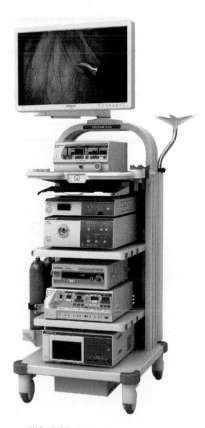

FIG. 8.32 Video laparoscopy cart.

must be taken to ensure the swivel mount can support the weight of the monitor and other equipment.

Carts have either a locked or an open shelf design. Institutional security determines this configuration. Storage, tampering, and key availability are important issues. A locked drawer may be ideal to store HD recording devices, printing paper, and other valuable video supplies. Carts also should be selected for ease of movement, component accessibility, and cleaning. Carts may also include an optional storage bracket for E-cylinders when insufflation is required. Secondary (slave) monitor carts usually do not contain multiple shelving and cabinet components.

Videoconferencing

Videoconferencing is a method to reach distant sites through two-way interactive communications using live audio and video signals. Communications between two or more sites may be live, or one site may play a videotape for the other sites connecting to the videoconference. This technology requires basic videoconferencing equipment and a network mode to transmit the communication signal to multiple sites. The higher the network bandwidth used by the participating sites, the better are audio and video motion-handling capabilities, and the resolution of the video signal that can be transmitted to each. A videoconference can be held between two sites or dozens of sites simultaneously. Videoconferencing applications in healthcare include education, surgical observations, remote assessments and consultation, administrative meetings, and product development.

Some issues remain with videoconferencing. Standardization must be followed so that videoconferencing equipment can communicate and be compatible with each other. Various governmental and professional organization recommendations and mandates guide manufacturers to meet approved criteria so that global interconnectivity occurs more easily. Because patient information, assessment data, and treatment results are being shared among providers by means of videoconferencing, patient confidentiality and privacy must be maintained. HIPAA compliance is vital when transmitting patient records. Private networks, advanced coding systems, and other technology can help address this issue. Practicing across state lines is a concern as videoconferencing in healthcare evolves. A state board of nursing, through the Nurse Licensure Compact (NLC), enables multistate licensure for nurses, providing the ability to practice across state lines physically and electronically. In 2016, there were 25 NLC states (NCSBN, 2015). Reimbursement for remote consultation and assessment is being analyzed by many insurance carriers. Pilot project sites have been established by the Centers for Medicare and Medicaid Services to study reimbursement practices. When reimbursement is consistently provided, more healthcare providers and facilities will embrace videoconferencing.

Robotics

Research and experimentation continue to advance robotic technology to assist with more delicate and precise procedures, such as laparoscopic surgeries. Basic robotic devices were introduced in the late 1990s to assist with holding and maneuvering a laparoscope, freeing team members to perform other roles and attend to other duties. Current surgical robots are computer-based electromechanical devices that are engineered to replicate surgeon movements. Computer-assisted surgery (CAS; also called image-guided surgery, surgical navigation, and 3-D computer surgery) has been integrated into robotic systems. CAS is any computer-based surgery that uses high technology, such as 3-D computer imaging and real-time sensing, to provide ultimate visibility and site targeting in the performance of surgical procedures.

A robotic system consists of a surgeon console, a side-cart with robotic arms that move around fixed pivot points while attached to articulated instrumentation that may have up to 7 degrees of movement, and a vision cart with HD monitoring equipment (Fig. 8.33). The general setup of the robotic system is shown in Fig. 8.34. Patient positioning depends on the surgery being performed while accommodating the robotic system. Docking of the side-cart with the robotic arms at the patient's bedside is facilitated by activating a targeting button and laser beam, which allow the arms to assume the optimal position for the procedure. Newer endoscopes are easier to use with no need for white balancing, calibrating, or draping. The thinner, lightweight robotic arms holding the laparoscope and instrumentation are controlled directly by the surgeon's hand, wrist, and finger movements and are translated into precise and accurate motions of the instruments within the body. Each instrument performs a specific task to coagulate, cut, excise, clamp, manipulate, retract, or suture tissue (Fig. 8.35). These instruments may even have more flexibility and range of motion than that of the human wrist. A quick release connection allows for fast instrument changes during surgery. Safety technology within the robot prevents any inadvertent or independent movement of the instruments or arms that may lead to patient injury.

The 3-D vision allows depth perception of the articulated instrumentation by the surgeon. Computer software is able to filter tremors and motion infarctions through eye-hand alignment that offers intuitive control of the surgical devices (Jung et al., 2015). Such vital advancements have overcome the earlier motion challenges and visual limitations of conventional laparoscopic surgery.

Robotic surgery offers great precision through a "shared-control system" because the procedure is performed by the surgeon through the use of a robot. For example, during a laparoscopic procedure, small incisions are made into the abdomen to insert three to four robotic arms. One arm serves as the camera, two of the arms act as the surgeon's hands, and a fourth may be used to retract structures that are in the way. The surgeon is seated at a nearby console and

through the viewfinder sees a 3-D image of the surgical site. The surgeon manipulates the robotic arms through special devices that direct the instrumentation. Any tremors in the surgeon's hands are filtered out so delicate procedures can be expertly performed.

Single-incision robotic-assisted laparoscopy is gaining popularity as advancements in instrumentation are introduced. A new articulated needle holder for the single-incision approach was developed to facilitate suturing (Jung et al., 2015). Additional laparoscopic platforms have been designed to insert multiple instruments simultaneously through one incision (Fig. 8.36).

Robotic surgery has been accepted in many specialty areas including general, urology, and gynecology (Taylor, 2016). The use of the robot has shown similar results when compared with conventional laparoscopic approaches, even though it is still in its infancy. Robot technology continues to evolve as research demonstrates improved patient outcomes. Some advantages of robotic use for certain procedures include shorter patient length of stay, decreased blood loss intraoperatively, less physical stress and mental strain on the surgeon, and shorter operating room (OR) time (Jung et al., 2015). With robotics, control of the scope is returned to the physician with any quick scope movements being accommodated through a computerized memory, minimizing scope-positioning time and providing a steady image and enhanced video quality. Advances in laparoscope stabilization and movement facilitate the procedure, promote safety, and sometimes minimize the time to perform the procedure. Even though there is limited evidence of its cost-effectiveness, robotic surgery promises to revolutionize surgical techniques and approaches.

With any new technology, negative outcomes and potential risks and complications must be recognized. Although robotic-assisted laparoscopy is recognized as safe and feasible, its risks, complications, and negative outcomes are similar to traditional laparoscopy, thoracoscopy, or transoral endoscopy (Intuitive Surgical, Inc., 2016). The surgeon may have to switch from an endoscopic procedure to an open approach requiring a larger incision. The operating and anesthesia time may be longer. Surgical device injuries to tissue, organs, and nerves may occur. There may be changes in heart rate, blood pressure, or blood values caused by the absorption of the

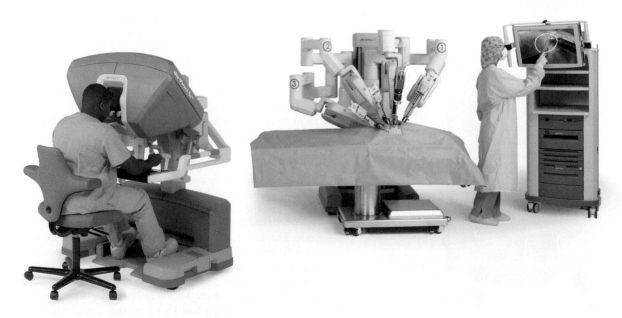

FIG. 8.33 Robotic system with surgeon console, patient side-cart with robotic arms, and vision cart.

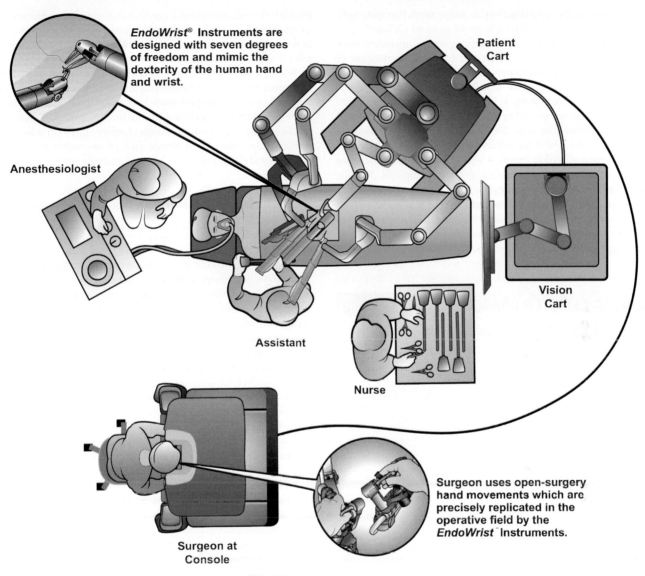

***EndoWrist®* Instruments are designed with seven degrees of freedom and mimic the dexterity of the human hand and wrist.**

Patient Cart

Anesthesiologist

Assistant

Nurse

Vision Cart

Surgeon at Console

Surgeon uses open-surgery hand movements which are precisely replicated in the operative field by the *EndoWrist¨* Instruments.

FIG. 8.34 Setup for robotic system.

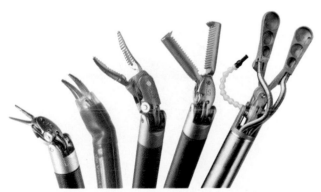

FIG. 8.35 Various robotic instrumentation.

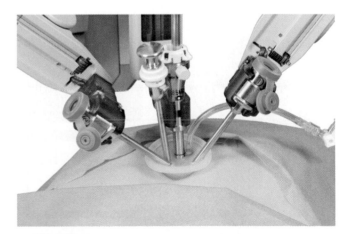

FIG. 8.36 Robotic single-incision port for multiple instruments.

insufflation gas used to create the pneumoperitoneum. Postoperatively, there may be shoulder pain or pain from the gas used for insufflation. The added risks associated with robotic surgery also include robotic system failure or malfunction that could lead to serious injury or the need to convert to another surgical approach. The Robotic-Assisted Surgery box includes initiatives for robotic emergencies.

To develop the mandatory skills needed to become proficient in robotic surgery, the physician ideally participates in a variety of different educational formats. There are product training modules available online along with procedure videos. Surgeons should attend training sessions offered at hospitals or at the robot manufacturing facility where physicians can teach and mentor surgeons. Robotic surgical simulators have been designed to incorporate virtual reality scenarios for physician education and training (Fig. 8.37). The progress and achievement score of the learner is reported and recorded within the simulator. A curriculum to achieve the fundamental skills of robotic surgery is critical to promote learning. In a study conducted to establish the effectiveness of a curriculum focused on achieving basic simulated robotic skills, results confirmed significant improvements in demonstrating basic robotic skills when following the fundamental robotic skills curriculum (Stegemann et al., 2013).

Miniaturized surgical robots are being designed as remotely controlled robots to perform surgery within the patient's body. Currently being developed, these tiny robots may crawl inside of a blood vessel to treat occlusive disease or explore the surface of the epicardia to address malformations (Jung et al., 2015) while being externally controlled. Even though these advancements are just being imagined and developed, unlimited opportunities await within robotic technology.

Practices and Potential Risks During Minimally Invasive Surgery

Insufflation

To help visualize abdominal structures and enhance safety during laparoscopic procedures, a pneumoperitoneum is created. The surgeon makes a paraumbilical incision and inserts an insufflation (Veress) needle into the abdomen (Fig. 8.38). To decrease the risk of bladder perforation when the needle is inserted, the bladder must be empty. Preoperatively the patient is told to empty his or her bladder. A straight catheter is used intraoperatively to ensure the bladder is empty. Trendelenburg position is used to reduce the risk of visceral perforation (see Chapter 6). As the surgeon inserts the needle, he or she lifts up the patient's abdomen by grasping and lifting a fold of tissue on either side of the umbilicus. Preoperative patient education includes the possibility of finger-pinched bruising at the site in which the abdominal tissue is grasped.

The needle safely enters the peritoneum positioned at a 45-degree angle. Placement is confirmed by negative bowel and blood return on aspiration and by saline instillation that meets no resistance. This is a relatively blind procedure because no scope can be introduced until the pneumoperitoneum is established. Newer laparoscopic trocar systems use the obturator tip instead of a needle. When this is inserted, there is less penetration into the peritoneum; then rapid insufflation is provided.

After needle confirmation, insufflation tubing is connected and the process begun. CO_2 gas is used to insufflate because it does not

---

ROBOTIC-ASSISTED SURGERY

Initiatives for Robotic Emergencies

Because of the complexity of robotic technology, proactive plans are developed by a multidisciplinary team of surgeons, nurses, surgical technologists, physician assistants, and anesthesia providers to prevent and manage robotic emergencies. Initiatives include the following:

- A checklist for a quick conversion to an open procedure (defining the tasks to be performed).
- A robotic emergency tray and a service-specific standby cart with instrumentation are readily available for conversion to the open approach.
- A sterile wrench to release robotic instrumentation in an emergency.

Ongoing education and simulation exercises are vital to rehearse robotic emergent conversion by surgical team members to maintain confidence during these critical events.

Modified from Carlos GB: Are you ready for a disaster? Clinical improvement poster, *2016 AORN Surgical Conference & Expo.* Used with permission from Memorial Sloan Kettering Cancer Center.

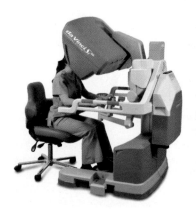
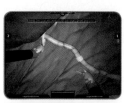
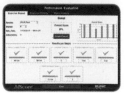

FIG. 8.37 Simulator for education on basic robotic skills.

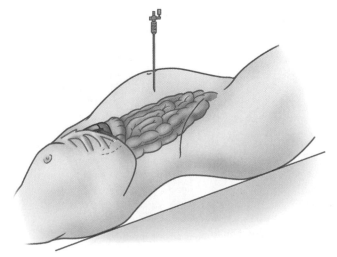

FIG. 8.38 Veress needle insertion into abdomen.

support combustion, can be absorbed at large volumes per minute without serious side effects, and is fairly inexpensive. The peritoneal cavity is filled, first at a low flow rate that is increased to a high flow rate of at least 9 L/min ideally. *Flow rate* refers only to how quickly a predetermined intra-abdominal pressure can be reached. Intra-abdominal pressure is the actual measure that must be closely monitored and should be maintained between 14 and 16 mm Hg. High flow rates are important because during the procedure, the insufflation CO_2 gas can escape through smoke evacuation, instrument changes, and other practices. The quicker the gas can be replaced, the less time is spent waiting for the abdomen to be redistended. Perioperative nurses must demonstrate competence in insufflation and understand how to manage its potential risks.

Insufflator control panels monitor and display flow rate, volume delivered, and intra-abdominal pressure. Selection of an insufflator that accommodates a high flow rate is important. Insufflators delivering 15 to 20 L/min are much more effective than those delivering gas at slower rates. The insufflator must monitor insufflation pressure continuously, stop the insufflation process when the predetermined set pressure has been reached, and release pressure if there is an inadvertent pressure increase (called "taking a breath"). Intra-abdominal pressure can be increased for reasons other than CO_2 insufflation; leaning on the abdomen and additional gas introduction from other sources, such as an argon-beam coagulator or a CO_2 laser with a purge gas system, can inadvertently increase intra-abdominal pressure.

Overpressurization can be extremely hazardous to the patient. Excess pressure can force CO_2 to diffuse into the blood, resulting in hypercarbia. End-tidal CO_2 monitoring is a crucial assessment parameter to detect increased CO_2 absorption. Excess pressure also increases diaphragmatic pressure, which can cause gastric regurgitation and aspiration of stomach contents. It can reduce intrathoracic space, resulting in decreased respiratory effort and cardiac output. The phrenic nerve innervates the diaphragm and is responsible for some motor activity associated with respiration. CO_2 gas can irritate this nerve, causing postoperative pain in the shoulder and neck. Excessive pressure can cause tremendous postoperative discomfort and severe nerve damage. The surgeon or assistant should press on the patient's abdomen to release as much residual CO_2 gas as possible before removal of the last trocar sheath when the procedure is completed. Insufflators that automatically vent excess CO_2 gas into the air ensure that many potential complications can be avoided. Smoke evaluators have been designed to monitor insufflation pressure and also provide a safe and quick method to manually remove the insufflated gas using a closed system so that no gas escapes into the environment when the surgeon is releasing the insufflated gas. This minimizes contaminated air that could be inhaled by the surgical team.

A two-way, single-use disposable filter should be incorporated into the insufflation tubing. This hydrophobic filter provides patient protection from harmful gas-tank contamination, such as chromium particles. It also provides protection from the colonization of organisms in the insufflator itself. Without a filter, when the insufflator is turned on, organisms such as *Klebsiella, Pseudomonas,* and *Staphylococcus aureus* can be blown into the patient. This contamination could be deadly for a very ill, elderly, or immunocompromised patient. The manufacturer's written instructions must be followed when performing CO_2 insufflation. Perioperative nurses should consider the following steps to reduce cross-contamination of the patient and insufflator during CO_2 insufflation:

1. *Before* the procedure, verify that the cylinder is medical-grade CO_2; note the level of gas in the cylinder.

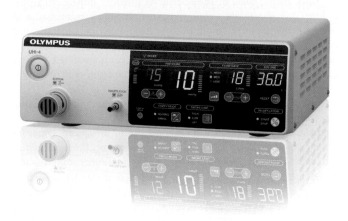

FIG. 8.39 Computerized high-flow insufflator with CO_2 warmer.

2. Flush insufflator and tubing with CO_2 gas before attaching to patient.
3. Use a disposable hydrophobic filter on insufflation tubing. Discard after procedure.
4. *During* the procedure, monitor level of CO_2 remaining in cylinder; have second cylinder readily available.
5. Keep insufflator elevated above the patient to prevent fluid backflow.
6. *At end of the procedure,* disconnect tubing from insufflator before turning off.

An insufflator capable of warning the team of insufflation problems throughout the procedure is vital. Alarms that sound when there is a deviation from predetermined parameters call attention to the need for immediate intervention, such as an alarm ringing and a monitor blinking "Gas supply low." An alarm sounding when overpressurization occurs from a secondary source (e.g., by leaning on the abdomen) also alerts the team to take corrective action.

Insufflators are also available with CO_2 warming devices (Fig. 8.39). Cylinder CO_2 is a liquid, and as it is released, it expands into a gas. During conversion from liquid to gas, energy is lost, and the gas becomes colder. The higher the flow, the colder the gas. Some warming occurs as the gas travels through insufflation tubing. Use of cold CO_2 can cause a decrease in patient temperature, especially with prolonged laparoscopy. Many factors contribute to reduced body temperature during laparoscopic procedures (e.g., cold irrigation, room temperature, surface exposure, length of the procedure, patient's age and medical history, anesthetic choice); cold CO_2 represents an additional one. The best way to reduce patient heat loss and the risk for perioperative hypothermia is to address all variables and intervene wherever possible.

Anesthetic Considerations and Potential Complications During Minimally Invasive Surgery

Although anesthetic technique and delivery are the responsibility of the anesthesia provider, perioperative nurses must anticipate and respond appropriately to associated risks during MIS procedures. Many open surgical procedures are now performed as MIS procedures in ambulatory surgery. With this change, anesthetic technique also has changed. Today emphasis is on minimal anesthesia during surgery. Short-acting drugs are used so that the patient awakens quickly and experiences far fewer side effects (see Chapter 5).

Three major goals of the anesthesia provider during MIS procedures are: *respiratory stability, appropriate muscle relaxation,* and *hemodynamic stability.* In addition, during many laparoscopic and pelviscopic procedures, it is necessary to control diaphragmatic excursion. Patient monitoring includes an electrocardiogram (ECG) and assessment of end-tidal CO_2, blood pressure, oxygen saturation, and temperature.

When Trendelenburg position is used, intra-abdominal pressure increases, and this can cause respiratory complications, including hypoxia. CO_2 absorption from the peritoneal cavity can aggravate this situation. Reverse Trendelenburg position, on the other hand, can cause decreased venous return, reduced cardiac output, and hypotension. CO_2 insufflation in this position can also cause an increase in total peripheral resistance, especially if intra-abdominal pressure is high and the aorta is compressed. The perioperative nurse must be prepared to quickly change the position of the OR bed, decrease the CO_2 flow rate of the insufflator, and assist the anesthesia provider with medications and extra supplies.

CO_2, highly soluble in blood, generally is not hazardous when used during laparoscopic insufflation because it is rapidly absorbed in the splanchnic vascular region. Excessive intra-abdominal pressure or any anesthetic technique that reduces splanchnic blood flow, however, could increase the potential for CO_2 gas emboli. This, in turn, could lead to circulatory collapse. CO_2 also could advance from the heart to pulmonary circulation, causing acute pulmonary hypertension with right-sided heart failure. If these effects are undetected and CO_2 insufflation continues, then cardiac arrest and death may occur. If there are signs of CO_2 embolus, and there is not sufficient assistance, it may be necessary to call a rapid response team.

Intraoperative hypotension can result from excessive bleeding, excessive intra-abdominal pressure, and hypoxia. CO_2 insufflation rates may need to be reduced. Extra intravenous fluids may be needed. Likewise, intraoperative hypertension can result from increased intra-abdominal pressure, and increased CO_2 gas absorption also may be evident. Increased bleeding may result. The perioperative nurse may need to decrease CO_2 insufflation flow rates. Additional hemostatic agents and endoscopic clips may be required.

Gastric reflux may occur if the patient is obese, a hiatal hernia is present, or excessive pneumoperitoneum occurs. A nasogastric or orogastric tube may be inserted after general anesthesia is induced. Postoperative discomfort is less if an orogastric tube is used. During epidural and regional anesthesia, patients are usually awake, and insertion of a gastric tube may be poorly tolerated. For this reason the tube is not inserted unless gastric distention occurs. The perioperative nurse must be quick to respond if assistance is required during gastric tube insertion. Intercostal nerve blocks offer surgical pain relief and abdominal muscle relaxation when the patient is awake during MIS surgery. The perioperative nurse's role during intercostal nerve block induction is to remain at the patient's side and help reduce anxiety. Other risks during MIS procedures include hypercarbia, subcutaneous emphysema, and pneumoscrotum.

The surgical team must always be ready to rapidly convert an endoscopic procedure into an open procedure. Appropriate equipment and instruments must be readily available to provide a seamless transition. Many facilities require nurses to perform counts during the MIS procedure just in case there is a chance the procedure is converted to open. Those policies are followed for counting soft goods, instruments, and sharps to prevent a retained surgical item.

Energies Used During Surgery

Electrosurgery

Electrosurgical units (ESUs) have been used for many years to cut and coagulate tissue, but ESU use also has been associated with numerous patient injuries and accidents. The same laser safety measures used to prevent surgical fires and to evacuate surgical smoke are also used for electrosurgery (see Laser Safety section for detailed information). Education is vital to ensure safe use of electrosurgery by understanding the principles and actions of this surgical energy.

Physics of Electrosurgery

The basic principles of electricity underpin electrosurgery. Electricity involves the motion of subatomic particles that behave in a consistent and predictable manner. Electrons orbit the nucleus of an atom. Once electrons are charged, they jump from one atom to the orbit of another, creating a charged particle or ion, and an electrical current is generated.

Three terms describe the properties of electricity: current, voltage, and impedance. *Current* is the flow of electrons measured in amperes or amps. *Voltage* is the force or push that moves the electrons from one atom to another and is measured in volts. *Impedance* is the opposition to the flow of current and is measured in ohms. As electrons encounter impedance, heat is produced, and a tissue effect results.

Electricity must have a complete circuit or pathway so that electrons can flow. That is, if an electrical current originates from earth, the electricity must be returned to ground to complete the circuit. Two forms of electrical current are used today: direct current (DC) and alternating current (AC). With DC the electrons flow in only one direction, whereas with AC the electrons flow back and forth as polarity changes. During electrosurgery, AC enters the patient's body, causing the patient to become part of the circuit as the energy is returned to the source of the energy.

Frequency is the number of waves passing through a given point over a specified time. This is measured in hertz (Hz) or cycles per second. Electrosurgical systems operate at frequencies greater than 100,000 Hz, which also is the frequency at which nerve and muscle stimulation ceases. In comparison, the electrical current in a normal household wall outlet in the United States alternates at 60 cycles per second, or 60 Hz. An ESU generator takes the 60-cycle current and increases its frequency to greater than 200,000 Hz so that it can pass through the patient's body without muscle or nerve stimulation and with no risk of electrocution (Fig. 8.40).

"Electrocautery" often is misused as a reference for electrosurgery. Electrocautery devices use DC because electrons flow in one direction through a wire. The wire provides resistance and becomes hot. As the hot wire is held in contact with tissue, coagulation results. Electrocautery units are usually battery operated, such as the small disposable units used during ophthalmic procedures to coagulate small blood vessels.

Electrosurgical Modes

The two modes used for electrosurgical cutting or coagulation are *monopolar* or *bipolar.* In a monopolar system, electrical energy flows from the generator through an active electrode to the patient (Fig. 8.41). If energy is concentrated in a small area, and the tissue provides increased impedance, controlled heat is generated and cutting or coagulation is achieved. Electrical energy passes through the patient

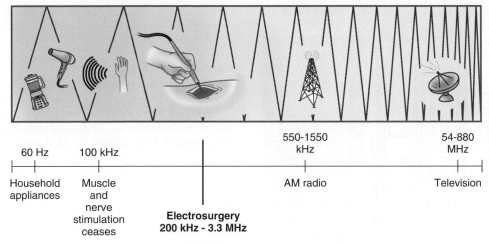

FIG. 8.40 Frequency spectrum.

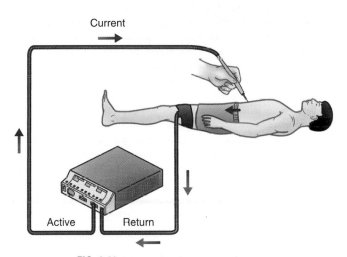

FIG. 8.41 Monopolar electrosurgical circuit.

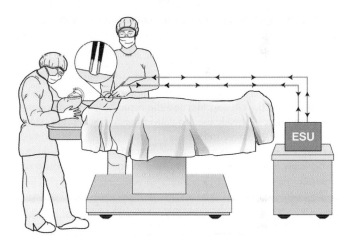

FIG. 8.42 Bipolar electrosurgical circuit. *ESU*, Electrosurgical unit.

to a dispersive electrode (pad) or patient return electrode (PRE) placed on the patient's body. The dispersive electrode surface area is large enough that energy is not concentrated enough to generate significant heat. Energy is then returned to the generator as the circuit is completed. If the dispersive electrode is tented, or only a small part of the pad is in contact with the patient's body, electrical energy becomes concentrated, and a burn can result. With monopolar electrosurgery, the patient completes the electrical circuit; it is the most common mode of electrosurgery used today.

In a bipolar system a dispersive electrode is not needed because electrical energy flows from one tine (or prong or blade) of the bipolar instrument to the other tine as it passes through the tissue located between the tines (Fig. 8.42). Energy returns directly through the instrument to the generator to complete the circuit, eliminating flow of current through the patient. During bipolar electrosurgery, the flow of electricity stops if a certain impedance level is reached. This is frequently 100 ohms but may differ for various bipolar generators available today. Although the ESU seems to be activated because an audible sound is heard while the pedal is depressed, the flow of current significantly decreases when the specified impedance

is met. Impedance meters (or ammeters) are often used to alert the physician when tissue desiccation is occurring or when complete desiccation has occurred.

Tissue Effects
As electrosurgery variables change, different tissue effects can be achieved. Electrosurgery variables, explained next, include the following:
• Waveform
• Power setting
• Length of exposure
• Active electrode size
• Type of tissue
• Eschar presence

As waveform changes, so does the tissue effect. Waveforms range from pure cut to pure coagulation. To produce a pure-cut mode, the generator must be on a 100% duty cycle, meaning that the electrical flow is continually applied, and heat is quickly generated for cutting and tissue vaporization (Fig. 8.43). Current is high, but voltage is low. As less force (voltage) is used to push the current,

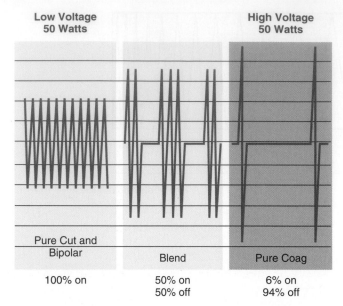

FIG. 8.43 Electrosurgery waveforms: typical examples.

the cut mode may be considered safer than other modes. As the cut mode produces a constant bombardment of electrons on the tissue, heat is produced, cells rupture, and the tissue is cut. For maximum effect the active electrode used to deliver the current should be held slightly above the tissue so that the electrons have to jump through the impedance of the air to reach the target site. This generates even more heat. Most of the heat dissipates as steam when tissue cells vaporize.

In pure coagulation mode, current is decreased but voltage is increased. The duty cycle is on only about 6% of the time, leaving 94% of the time with no flow of electrons to the surgical site (see Fig. 8.43). To compensate for this "off" duty cycle, the voltage, or force of the push, must be increased to produce the desired wattage. During coagulation this intermittent delivery of electrons causes cells to heat and then cool, producing a coagulative effect. Higher voltage allows the active electrode to be held over the area while a fulguration or spraying effect delivers the electrical energy to coagulate a larger area. The tissue effect is superficial, collapsing the cells and producing a coagulum.

Most ESUs have a blend mode that allows the operator to achieve different levels of simultaneous coagulation in the cut mode. Increasing voltage and decreasing the duty cycle provide increased coagulation effects (see Fig. 8.43).

The power setting also influences tissue effect. Higher power settings produce more extensive tissue effects. Long activation of electrical current increases the thermal effects in tissue. Thermal energy can spread from the target site, causing damage to adjacent tissue. Smaller active electrodes concentrate electrical energy and require lower power settings; larger electrodes disperse electrical energy and require higher power settings.

Tissue type also influences tissue effect. Tissue that is not well vascularized, such as adipose tissue, offers more impedance. As a result, electrical energy is not conducted as well, and higher power settings may be required. Muscle tissue is well vascularized and requires less power to achieve a tissue effect. Electrosurgical tips on the active electrode must be kept clean and free from debris (eschar) to function properly. Eschar is less conductive and impedes the flow

of electrons, requiring more power to be used to achieve the desired tissue effect. Electrode tips with nonstick coating make removal of eschar easier.

Electrosurgical Units

Four ESU systems have evolved over the years: grounded, isolated, dispersive electrode monitoring, and tissue response monitoring.

Grounded Electrosurgical Units. The grounded ESU system was the first introduced to the surgical market during the late 1920s. The grounded ESU delivers electrical energy from the generator to the patient and returns energy to ground, which is intended to be the generator. As electricity takes the path of least resistance, current can flow or divide through any grounded alternative path, such as an ECG pad or an intravenous pole that touches the patient, as it returns to a grounded site. Patients have sustained burns at these alternative path sites as the electricity searches for the most conductive object or path to return to ground. When an alternate path is chosen, the current may not be dispersed over a large area, so an alternate site burn may result as current concentrates.

Isolated Electrosurgical Unit. During the late 1960s the isolated ESU was introduced. An isolated ESU has a transformer that causes current to return only to the generator and not use alternate pathways to return to its source. Current flows through the patient's body and must return to the generator to complete the circuit. If this is not possible, the generator shuts down, adding to the safety of this type of unit. An isolated ESU prevents alternative site burns, but not PRE burns. The function of a PRE is to remove electrical current from the patient safely, but this may not always happen. If the PRE is tented, the electrical current arcs from the patient's skin to the pad to complete the circuit. The current concentrates in the reduced PRE-patient interface surface area and may cause a burn at this site. With experience, surgical teams became more focused on proper PRE placement by choosing a well-vascularized site with a secure PRE-patient interface. Monitoring PRE placement with an isolated ESU is a crucial responsibility of the perioperative nurse.

Dispersive Electrode Monitoring. In the 1980s different dispersive electrode monitoring systems were introduced, using a variety of names: dispersive pad monitoring, return electrode monitoring (REM), return electrode contact quality monitoring system (RECQMS), contact quality monitoring system, and patient safety system. Dispersive monitoring protects the patient from dispersive electrode site burns caused by inadequate contact of the dispersive electrode. The system continually monitors impedance under the split pad as it transmits an interrogation circuit to measure impedance levels (Fig. 8.44). The system deactivates current flow when impedance under the pad increases to an unsafe level, thus preventing a burn.

Placement of a dispersive electrode pad is crucial to prevent patient injuries. The pad is placed over an area that is well vascularized, such as a muscle mass. Sites with excessive hair, bony prominences, excessively dry skin, or adipose tissue should be avoided. When a patient is repositioned after the pad has been placed, the pad site is inspected again to ensure proper adherence, whenever possible.

A capacitance pad working on the principle of "bulk resistivity" and "capacitive coupling" is an advanced technology. A capacitor is defined as two conductors separated by an insulator. With an ESU the patient is one conductor (plate), and the conductive mesh (plate) inside the pad is the other conductor. The ability for current flow to be induced from one plate of the capacitor to the other is affected by three primary variables: (1) frequency of current, (2) size of the plates, and (3) distance between the plates. Higher-frequency large

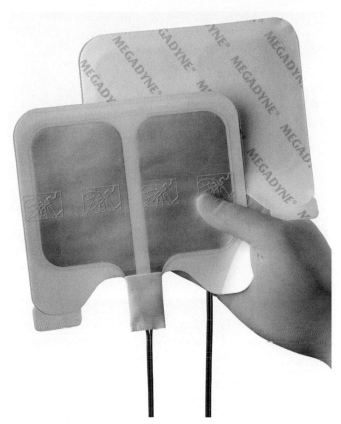

FIG. 8.44 Split pad for dispersive (return) electrode monitoring.

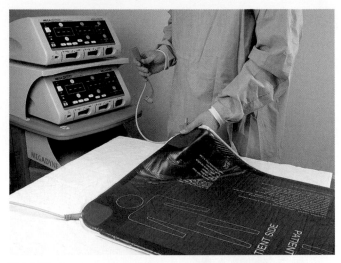

FIG. 8.45 Capacitance pad that provides pressure reduction to prevent skin breakdown.

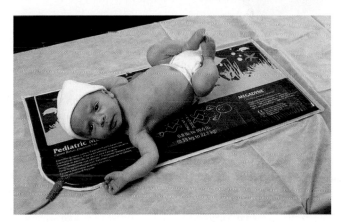

FIG. 8.46 Pediatric capacitive dispersive pad for infants weighing from 0.8 to 50 pounds.

plates and less distance between plates lead to better current flow. One small low-frequency plate or a great distance between the plates yields decreased current flow.

The large capacitive pad, approximately 2 feet by 3 to 4 feet, consists of a flexible conductive fabric surrounded by a nonlatex urethane insulating material. The pressure reduction version of this pad is composed of a dry, viscoelastic polymer.

This large reusable pad is placed on the OR bed (Fig. 8.45) with a linen sheet and drawsheet placed on top of it. When the patient is lying on the OR bed, the electrode pad forms a large capacitor with the patient that capacitively couples or connects the patient into the ESU circuit. When in place, this dispersive electrode completes the circuit by capacitive reactance, allowing the ESU to function. The amount of current transmitted into the pad is directly proportional to the amount of contact with the pad. The pad serves as the gatekeeper for this current. With too little current, there is very little current flow, and it is too low to cause burns.

The capacitive pad can be used for patients in all types of positions. A positioning chart is available from the manufacturer to assist the surgical team with safe and appropriate positioning. This larger pad is inappropriate for patients weighing less than 25 pounds because adequate contact (weight-bearing area) cannot be achieved. Pediatric capacitive pads are available for patients between 0.8 and 50 pounds (Fig. 8.46).

The large capacitive pad eliminates the need for an individual adhesive dispersive electrode pad, which is problematic if an ESU is used without dispersive electrode monitoring capabilities and the pad tents during a procedure. The bulk resistivity of this unique capacitive pad ensures that current densities are kept to a clinically safe level such that pad site burns rarely occur. Adhesive pads can irritate sensitive skin, may require a shaved area for placement, or may become a hazard if not placed on the patient appropriately. As surgical teams learn more about the use and safety features of the capacitance pad, its acceptance continues to grow.

Tissue Response Monitoring. This system represents a substantial advancement in ESU generator technology. It uses a computer-controlled tissue feedback system that senses impedance of the tissue and automatically adjusts current and voltage output to maintain a constant surgical effect. This feedback system eliminates the need to adjust power settings for different tissue types. In addition, improved performance at lower power settings and voltages reduces the risk of patient injury.

Another advanced feedback–controlled generator has been combined with a bipolar instrument to seal vessels and tissue bundles reliably for surgical ligation during open and laparoscopic procedures. The feedback system helps achieve a reliable tissue seal in less time, reducing thermal spread compared with traditional bipolar systems. With a single activation this system combines uniform compression and heat to provide stable seals on tissue bundles or on vessels up to 5 to 7 mm in diameter (Fig. 8.47). The surgeon can assess the

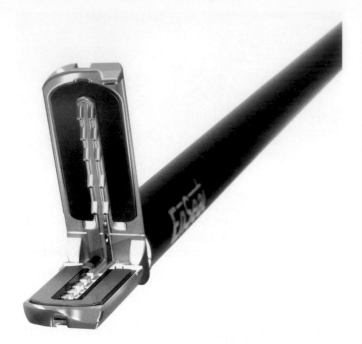

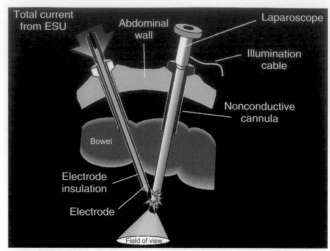

FIG. 8.48 Direct coupling during laparoscopy. *ESU,* Electrosurgical unit.

FIG. 8.47 Advanced bipolar vessel sealing instrument that controls the temperature and provides uniform compression.

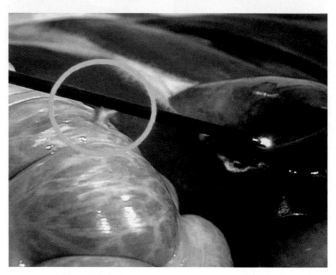

FIG. 8.49 Insulation failure during laparoscopy.

level of hemostasis at the seal site before cutting. The strength of the seal compares favorably with mechanical ligation methods, such as suture or clips, and is significantly stronger than standard bipolar coagulation. It is important to note that tissue response systems use the cut mode, and the new tissue sensing systems give feedback when implementing the coagulation mode of ESU generators.

Special Electrosurgery Considerations During Endoscopic Minimally Invasive Surgery

Three unique problems can occur during MIS procedures involving electrosurgery: direct coupling, insulation failure, and capacitive coupling (Liu and Sun, 2013; AORN, 2016).

Direct Coupling. Direct coupling occurs when the active electrode accidentally touches a noninsulated metal instrument, allowing the electrical energy to flow from one to the other (metal-to-metal sparking; Fig. 8.48). Direct coupling may also occur if an active electrode is activated while in contact with a clip. When the metal instrument or clip receives electrical energy, a burn can easily result. This coupling is often called "pilot error" because it is within the surgeon's control to avoid the burn. The surgeon should not activate the active electrode until the target site is within the field of vision and the active electrode is in proximity or direct contact with target tissue and not a metal object.

Insulation Failure. Insulation failure occurs when the insulation coating of an endoscopic instrument has been compromised. If a crack or break occurs in the insulation along the shaft of the instrument, electrical energy can escape at the point of the defect and burn untargeted tissue (Fig. 8.49). Insulation must be inspected before, during, and after each use of the instrument. A scanning device can be used to ensure that insulation is not compromised during reprocessing. Even an area of insulation that is merely weakened may be penetrated by electrical flow if high voltage, or pure coagulation mode, is being used. Given that the force (or voltage) of electrons is greater in coagulation mode, any weakened area may become an

actual break along the insulation sheath. Insulation failure presents the greatest risk to the patient because the full energy output can be delivered to nontargeted tissue. Insulation failure may result in instantaneous, irreversible death to tissue as a result of the high power density that insulation failure creates on the instrument shaft. The resulting tissue burn may not be observed or realized by the surgeon because it may not be within the field of vision.

Laparoscopic instruments may be purchased with a dual layer of insulation. The outer black insulation layer lies on top of a bright yellow insulation layer. When the top black layer is penetrated, the bright yellow layer can be seen easily and alerts the user that insulation failure may be imminent.

Capacitive Coupling. Capacitive coupling is a natural radiofrequency (RF) electrosurgical energy phenomenon that occurs when energy is transferred through intact insulation on the laparoscopic instrument shaft to nearby conductive materials (Fig. 8.50). A capacitor consists of *two conductors* separated by an *insulator.* The metal active electrode is one conductor, and an adhesion, an adjacent organ, or a conductive trocar/suction irrigation cannula can act as the second conductor. The primary insulation on the instrument represents the insulator. When an electrode is activated within a

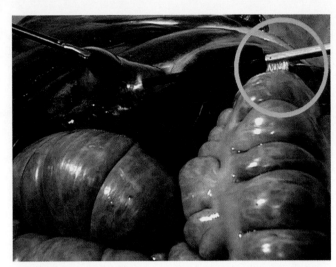

FIG. 8.50 Capacitive coupling occurs when electrical energy flowing from an instrument charges a nearby metal trocar sheath or laparoscope.

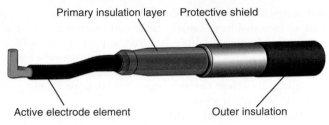

Primary insulation layer   Protective shield

Active electrode element   Outer insulation

FIG. 8.51 Cross section of active electrode monitoring instrument.

narrow suction irrigator, the RF energy can flow from the active electrode through the intact insulation and transfer 20% to 80% of the power displayed on the ESU to the metal suction irrigator. The induced current on the suction irrigator can cause a burn even though the outer insulation on the first instrument has been inspected and determined to be intact.

Monopolar ESUs used in concert with metal suction irrigators or shafts increase the risk of visceral burns through capacitive thermal energy. The laparoscope also can cause alternate-site burns if the ESU electrode is used through a narrow-lumen scope. In addition, long and narrow instruments with thin insulation, combined with high voltage, increase the incidence of capacitive coupling.

An electrical charge remains in the second metal instrument until it finds a path to the dispersive electrode to complete the circuit. Usually this energy disperses safely through the large surface of the abdominal wall from the conductive cannula. However, if a non-conductive device, such as a plastic stability collar, is in this path, energy cannot be safely discharged and will burn any tissue touched by the metal instrument. These burns often are undetected by the surgeon, and the problem is not diagnosed until the patient presents with complications after surgery. Accordingly, surgeons avoid hybrid instruments (combination of plastic and metal) during laparoscopy to minimize capacitive coupling.

To further eliminate the hazard of capacitive coupling and insulation failure, special instruments that provide active electrode monitoring (AEM) and shielding are available to capture stray energy transferred from one conductive device to another (AORN, 2016). AEM laparoscopic instruments are shielded and monitored to detect stray RF current and prevent ESU burns. The protective shield built within an AEM instrument provides the neutral path for capacitive-coupled energy and returns it to the ESU (Fig. 8.51). These safety devices also detect insulation failure and provide a path for stray current back to the generator. AEM is the only fail-safe technology currently designed to address insulation failure and capacitive coupling. AEM ensures that 100% of electrosurgical energy is delivered at the intended site.

Many hospitals that have implemented AEM technology require documentation of its use on the patient's perioperative chart for liability and risk management, much like rationales for documenting needle and soft good counts.

Another phenomenon involving principles of capacitive coupling is known as "antenna coupling." This occurs when high-frequency electric energy, conducted by a monopolar active electrode, is captured by a nonelectrically active device (such as an ECG lead or a nerve electrode), which is in close proximity but not in direct contact with the active electrode (Robinson et al., 2012). AORN's *Guideline for the Safe Use of Energy-Generating Devices* (2017) recommends that precautions, such as these, be taken to prevent antenna coupling to minimize burns in areas not near the surgical site by positioning:

- The monopolar ESU cord as far away as possible or at 90 degrees from other cords (ECG cables, neuromuscular monitoring cords, light cords, etc.) on the sterile field; and
- Patient monitoring electrodes at a distance from the surgical site.

Electrosurgery Safety

AORN's *Guidelines for Perioperative Practice* note that the electrosurgery pencil should be placed in a safety holster when not in use (AORN, 2016). This prevents the device from being inadvertently activated. Longer electrosurgical devices used during laparoscopic procedures require special attention to ensure that they are safely secured on the sterile field when not in use. Electrosurgical devices that are controlled with a foot pedal require the foot pedal to be identified and the handpiece given to the practitioner who will deliver the electrosurgical energy to the tissue during the procedure.

Electrosurgery devices (along with other surgical energy sources) must not be used near flammable liquids (such as alcohol), instruments, and other supplies. The electrosurgery device can serve as an ignition source for a fire if flammables and an oxygen-enriched environment are present. A hot electrosurgery blade after activation can provide the heat source to ignite a flammable material, such as a surgical drape; surgical soft goods, such as sponges; or a plastic instrument.

The size of the electrosurgery blade often determines the amount of energy delivered to the surgical site. The manufacturer often sets cutting and coagulation limits depending on the electrosurgery blade-to-tip size. For example, an insulated needle tip can only conduct limited amounts of energy to tissue. The power settings for cut and coagulation on the ESU are thus adjusted accordingly.

Many physicians have power settings listed on their preference cards depending on the type of procedure to be performed. These power settings must be verbalized to the surgeon at the beginning of each procedure. Before power settings are increased, other factors must be reviewed that could affect these settings (such as the presence of eschar on the blade, the size of the electrosurgery blade, the type of tissue being treated, etc.). The surgical team must always react to an ESU alarm because this indicates that safety parameters are being compromised.

The scrub person removes any charred material from the electrosurgery pencil blade or tip so that the electrical energy can be efficiently delivered to the surgical site. Residual debris on an electrosurgical blade obstructs the delivery of the electrons and can cause an increased heat buildup, causing an unwarranted need to increase the electrosurgical power. Cleaning pads are available to scrape off any charred debris. Some manufacturers provide a coated blade tip for easy cleaning because the coating prevents debris accumulation. To clean nonstick coated ESU tips, use a moistened sponge or instrument wipe.

Patients with piercing jewelry can present a problem when electrosurgery is used. Piercing appliances include earrings, barbells, labrets, captive beads, nose studs or nose screws, or dermal implants and are usually made of metal, which can conduct electricity (Smith, 2016). AORN recommends that body piercing accessories be removed before surgery because they can increase the risk of electrical burns (AORN, 2016). The surgeon should discuss the need to remove piercing appliances before surgery, and the perioperative nurse should remind the patient again during the perioperative phone interview and also document any piercings. During the immediate preoperative assessment, the nurse should inquire about piercings and document the response. If the patient cannot or will not remove the piercing appliance, then an alternate energy-generating device should be used. Preoperative patient education that explains the potential risk for burns may encourage a patient's cooperation in removing piercings.

Argon-Enhanced Electrosurgery

An argon-enhanced ESU device combines argon gas with electrosurgical energy to improve the effectiveness of the electrosurgical current. Because argon gas is heavier than air, inert, and noncombustible, it creates an efficient pathway for electrosurgical energy to travel from an electrode to target tissue. The flow of argon gas also clears the surgical site of blood and fluids, allowing for greater visibility of the bleeding site or target area, and disperses oxygen, decreasing the chance of combustion and formation of surgical smoke.

Benefits of argon-enhanced electrosurgery include the following:
- Rapid coagulation of diffuse bleeding site(s) with reduced blood loss
- Reduced risk of rebleeding
- Noncontact tissue coagulation
- Reduced depth of penetration by electrical energy and less adjacent tissue damage

When an argon-enhanced ESU is used during laparoscopic procedures, care must be taken not to overinsufflate (or overpressurize) the abdomen because the constant flow of argon gas could cause formation of a gas embolism. Often another port is left open during activation of argon-enhanced ESUs to allow excess gas to escape. An insufflator with an audible alarm indicating overpressurization should be used. The patient is monitored closely so that early symptoms of an embolism can be detected and treated.

Laser

A healthcare revolution occurred with the birth and evolution of the laser. Perioperative nurses must be aware of expanded responsibilities associated with laser applications. The laser has significantly affected surgery by making possible less-invasive procedures, decreasing inpatient hospitalization, diminishing postoperative complications, and saving healthcare dollars.

Laser Biophysics

Principles of Light. *LASER* is an acronym that describes a process in which light energy is produced—*l*ight *a*mplification by *s*timulated *e*mission of *r*adiation. The term also refers to the device that generates laser energy.

Light is a form of electromagnetic energy that can be graphically illustrated on a continuum known as the electromagnetic spectrum (Fig. 8.52). The unit of measurement for this continuum is called a wavelength, which is the distance between two successive peaks of a wave. Wavelength determines color and usually is measured in nanometers (10^{-9} m) or micrometers (1000 nm). Various wavelengths of light extend from the shorter waves in the ultraviolet area to the longer waves in the infrared region (Table 8.2). Visible laser wavelengths occupy only a small portion of this continuum. Radiation used in laser technology in healthcare is nonionizing because it does not present the hazard of cellular DNA disruption with continual tissue exposure. Pregnant women, for example, can work with lasers because laser energy produces no harmful ionizing radiation.

Briefly, the laser functions in the following way. A negatively charged electron orbits a positively charged nucleus while the atom is in its ground or resting state, which is its lowest energy level. An outside source of energy (e.g., electricity, flash lamps, other lasers) can excite the atom and cause an electron to jump to a higher, less stable orbit. The electron almost immediately returns to its stable orbit, and the atom resumes its normal resting state. As the unstable electron returns to its ground state, it spontaneously releases a tiny packet of light energy known as a photon, which travels away from the source in the form of waves. If the photon is close to another similar atom while still in the excited state, it interacts with this atom. The photon triggers the excited second atom to return to its resting state, and in this process another photon of laser light is emitted. These two photons of identical energy travel together. The process of stimulated emission has occurred, and laser energy initiated

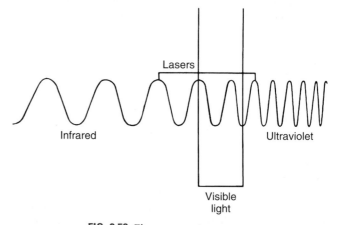

FIG. 8.52 Electromagnetic spectrum.

TABLE 8.2	
Electromagnetic Spectrum Wavelengths	
Type of Light	**Wavelength (nm)**
Ultraviolet (UV)	100–400
Visible	400–750
Near-infrared (NIR)	750–3000
Mid-infrared (MIR)	3000–30,000
Far-infrared (FIR)	30,000 nm–1 mm

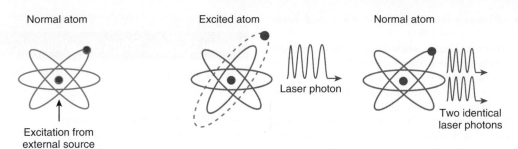

Normal atom   Excited atom   Normal atom

Laser photon

Excitation from external source

Two identical laser photons

FIG. 8.53 Laser energy is produced when an external source excites the atom to emit a photon spontaneously. This photon can "stimulate" the emission of two identical photons.

(Fig. 8.53). This process repeats itself over and over again, creating more photons of laser energy.

This activity occurs in the resonating chamber of the laser, in which the lasing medium is contained. The name of the laser usually is derived from the actual medium that causes the lasing action. The photons generated during the stimulated emission process are reflected back and forth between mirrors at each end of the resonating chamber as the process is amplified, until the number of excited atoms surpasses the number of resting atoms. This is known as population inversion. One of the mirrors in the chamber is partially reflective and, when activated, allows a stream of laser photons to escape the unit. These photons are introduced to the target area by means of a specific delivery system.

Characteristics of Laser Light. Three distinct characteristics distinguish laser light from ordinary light. Laser light is monochromatic, collimated, and coherent.

1. *Monochromatic light* is composed of photons of the same wavelength or color. In contrast, ordinary light consists of many different colors or wavelengths. When white light is passed through a prism, an array of different colors is displayed. White light is the presence of all colors, whereas laser light consists of one color or wavelength.

2. A *collimated* laser beam consists of waves parallel to each other that do not diverge significantly, minimizing any loss of power. When a collimated beam is passed through a lens, the light pattern is changed, allowing the light to be focused into a tiny spot that highly concentrates the energy. In comparison, the light waves from a flashlight are not parallel and lose intensity as they travel away from the source. A lens cannot easily focus these noncollimated waves to concentrate the light into a small area.

3. Laser light is *coherent*—that is, all the waves are orderly and in phase with each other as they travel in the same direction. All peaks and troughs of the waves are opposite each other in time and space. This property provides an additive effect that gives the laser beam power. Ordinary light is incoherent because the waves radiate away from the source without being in phase or in an orderly pattern.

Laser Power. The power, or energy, of a laser beam is measured in watts. An important factor in laser applications is the concept of power density, or irradiance of the beam. *Power density* is the amount of power that is concentrated within an area and is described by the following formula:

$$\text{Power density} = \text{watts/spot size (cm}^2)$$

The spot size of the laser beam can be controlled when the beam is passed through a special lens that causes the beam to converge.

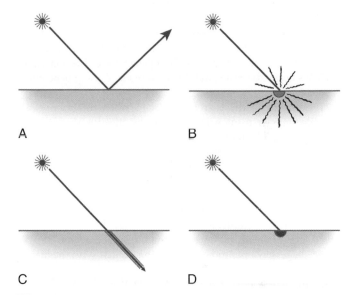

FIG. 8.54 Laser-tissue interaction. (A) Reflection. (B) Scattering. (C) Transmission. (D) Absorption.

The focal configuration of the lens determines at what distance from the lens the beam would be most intense, and this is called the *focal point*. If the beam is defocused into a larger spot size, the laser energy is spread over a greater area, decreasing the intensity or power density of the beam. In contrast, a small spot size of the beam concentrates the laser energy into a smaller area, increasing the intensity or power density of the beam. When power density is increased, the beam has a greater depth of penetration into the tissue.

A *joule* is the unit of measure used to describe total energy used. A joule is expressed by the power multiplied by the time duration of the beam exposure (expressed in the equation joule = watts × time). Often the laser energy used during ophthalmic procedures is expressed in millijoules.

Fluence is a term that expresses the power and duration of exposure of the beam and measures the specific amount of energy delivered to tissue. Fluence is also known as energy density or radiant exposure. The following equation calculates fluence:

$$\text{Fluence} = \text{watts} \times \text{duration time/spot size (cm}^2)$$

Tissue Interaction. When laser energy is delivered to a target site, four different interactions can occur: reflection, scattering, transmission, or absorption (Fig. 8.54). The extent of reaction of the beam on the target depends on laser wavelength, power settings, spot size, length of contact time with target tissue, and tissue characteristics.

Reflection of the laser beam occurs when the direction of the beam is changed after it contacts an area. Specular reflection occurs when the angle of the incoming light is equal to the angle of the reflected light. Laser light can be intentionally reflected in this manner off a reflective mirror to contact hard-to-reach areas. Such reflection also can pose safety problems by inadvertently striking untargeted areas if it is not controlled at all times. The CO_2 laser beam can be reflected off of the surface of a shiny instrument and impact a surgery team member's mask, causing it to ignite. Accordingly, eye and fire safety measures are mandatory when the potential for laser beam reflection is high.

Scattering of laser light occurs when the beam spreads over a large area as tissue causes the beam to disperse. The intensity of the beam decreases as the waves travel in different directions. The Nd:YAG laser beam can backscatter up an endoscope and cause damage to the end of the scope, the optics, or the operator's eye. The noncontact Nd:YAG beam also can scatter through tissue, causing penetration of 3 to 5 mm.

Transmission of the laser beam occurs when the beam passes through fluids or tissue without thermally affecting the area. The argon beam can be transmitted through clear fluids and structures of the front part of the eye and the vitreous to cause thermal photocoagulation on the retina, whereas the cornea, lens, and vitreous are unaffected by transmission of this beam.

Absorption of laser light results when tissue is altered from the absorption of the beam. As the amount of energy delivered to tissue (fluence) increases, different tissue effects can be produced. The lowest level of energy produces a photochemical reaction. Then as fluence increases, a photothermal reaction occurs. With the highest level of fluence, a photoacoustic effect occurs. Reactions from the lowest to highest level of energy occur as follows:

- *Photochemical effect:* Laser energy is selectively absorbed by tissue containing a light-sensitive dye, leading to a chemical change that produces singlet oxygen, which ultimately causes tissue destruction.
- *Photothermal effect:* Laser energy is absorbed by tissue, heating it.
- *Photoacoustic effect:* Laser energy is absorbed, creating kinetic energy that produces a snapping sound, disrupting the tissue without significant thermal effect.

Consistency, color, and water content of the target tissue often determine the rate of absorption of laser energy. Laser wavelength also affects absorption of the beam. Certain laser light, such as that from the argon laser, is highly absorbed by pigmented tissues. The CO_2 laser, however, is independent of color-selective absorption. CO_2 laser light is absorbed superficially by tissue to a shallow depth of approximately 0.1 to 0.2 mm, whereas the holmium laser beam is absorbed to about 0.4 to 0.6 mm. Argon laser light is readily absorbed by pigmented tissue to a depth of approximately 1 to 2 mm, whereas that of the noncontact Nd:YAG laser beam is more readily absorbed by darkened tissue to a depth of 3 to 5 mm.

Photothermal tissue reaction becomes more pronounced as the temperature of the target area increases during absorption of the laser beam (Table 8.3). As laser energy is absorbed, the water within each cell is heated. As temperature increases, intracellular protein is destroyed and water inside the cell turns to steam. Eventually the cellular membrane ruptures from increased pressure, spewing cellular debris and plume (smoke) from the tissue. The surrounding tissue also is heated through conduction because it borders the impingement site. The degree of adjacent tissue damage depends on the duration

TABLE 8.3

Tissue Changes With Temperature Increases

Temperature °F (°C)	Visual Change	Biologic Change
98.6°F–140°F (37°C–60°C)	No visual change	Warming, welding
140°F–149°F (60°C–65°C)	Blanching	Coagulation
149°F–194°F (65°C–90°C)	White/gray	Protein denaturization
194°F–212°F (90°C–100°C)	Puckering	Drying
>212°F (>100°C)	Smoke plume	Vaporization, carbonization

of laser-beam exposure that causes the intended thermal destruction of target tissue.

Laser Systems

New laser systems are introduced into healthcare regularly. Constant efforts by researchers and physicians to explore the use of different wavelengths frequently change surgical approaches in a variety of specialties. Some of the most common lasers are described in Table 8.4, beginning with lasers in the infrared region with long wavelengths, through visible wavelengths, and finally to short ultraviolet wavelengths.

Because lasers are often expensive and technology continues to change, some companies offer laser rentals. Rental contracts need to be created that will quote the agreed charge for use or segment of time. Most rental companies will also provide a laser safety officer (LSO) to operate the laser control panel for the surgeon and oversee laser safety practices during the procedure. Healthcare administrators must request documentation to ensure that training of these laser team members is adequate and that The Joint Commission and other regulations have been met regarding laser rentals. Laser documentation used by rental company members must be approved by the facility if integrated as part of the patient's chart.

Laser System Components. Five major components of a laser system are the laser head, excitation source, ancillary components, control panel, and delivery system. When a laser malfunctions, an organized investigation of each of these parts (Fig. 8.55) usually can determine the source of the problem.

The *laser head,* or resonating chamber, is the component in which laser energy is generated and amplified. The laser head contains the active medium or substance that actually produces the photons that generate laser light. The active medium can be a gas (CO_2 or argon), a solid crystal (Nd:YAG), a liquid (tunable dye), or a semiconductor crystal (diode). As technology continues to advance, laser wavelengths are being combined into a single unit so that a selection of wavelengths, such as the Nd:YAG, erbium:YAG, or holmium:YAG, can be offered easily during a procedure.

The *excitation source* supplies the energy to excite the active medium in the laser head. Different sources include flash lamps, electricity, radio waves, batteries, chemicals, and other laser systems. The CO_2 laser gas mixture is excited by electrical current or radio waves, and the Nd:YAG laser crystal is excited by flash lamps. Diode lasers, such as the gallium arsenide laser, are solid-state lasers that are excited by electrical energy.

Ancillary components are other laser parts needed to help produce laser energy. A cooling system maintains the appropriate temperature of the laser head and keeps the unit from overheating. Usually lasers are air cooled or water cooled. A vacuum pump may be required in a CO_2 free-flowing laser to pull the gas mixture from an external cylinder into the laser head for laser light production. Current

TABLE 8.4

Description of Common Lasers Used

Active Medium	Wavelength	Delivery System	Penetration	Characteristics
CO_2 laser (gas laser)	10,600 nm, infrared	Articulated arm, waveguide, scanner, microscope via microslad	Shallow penetration (0.1–0.2 mm), photothermal effect	Highly absorbed by water; not color selective; helium-neon aiming beam; sometimes the handpiece has a tubing to conduct compressed air to keep plume from coating the lens; CO_2 energy can be delivered in a continuous wave or pulsed mode; when delivery system is attached, the laser must be test fired to ensure the aiming beam is aligned with CO_2 beam; used on soft tissue, ablations, cutting, coagulation, vaporization
Erbium:YAG laser (solid crystal laser)	2940 nm, infrared	Fiber (handpiece, microscope)	Shallow penetration, photothermal effect	Highly absorbed by water; delivered in pulsed mode; helium-neon aiming beam; frequently used in dermatology for skin resurfacing and ablation; also used in dentistry
Holmium:YAG laser (solid crystal laser)	2140 nm, infrared	Fiber (handpiece, microscope)	Shallow penetration (0.4–0.6 mm), photothermal effect	Absorbed by water but can be delivered in a fluid environment within a vapor bubble if fiber is within 55 mm of target site; helium-neon aiming beam; pulse mode; used for sculpting and ablating soft tissue; has also been used on cartilage and to fragment urinary or biliary stones with photoacoustic effect
Neodymium:YAG laser (Nd:YAG) (solid crystal laser)	1064 nm, infrared	Contact and noncontact fibers, contact tips, handpiece for dermatology, slit lamp for ophthalmology, microscope	Scatters in tissue (3–5 mm) with noncontact fiber; shallow penetration (<1 mm) with contact delivery	Transmitted through clear solutions; highly absorbed by pigmented tissue; helium-neon aiming beam usually used; used in continuous or pulsed modes; ophthalmology Nd:YAG lasers (class 3B lasers) use special pulsed mode delivery (Q-switched) to provide photoacoustic effect within the eye to rupture the secondary membrane
KTP (potassium titanyl phosphate) laser (solid crystal laser)	532 nm, visible (frequency doubled YAG)	Fiber (handpiece, microscope)	1–2 mm depth of penetration	An Nd:YAG incident beam (1064 nm) is passed through a KTP crystal, which doubles the frequency and halves the wavelength (532 nm); aiming beam can be a low-power KTP beam or helium-neon beam; highly color selective; transmitted through clear solutions; often used in dermatology, urology, general surgery, and gynecology
Argon laser (gas laser)	Blue-green light of 488 and 514.5 nm (or 457 and 528 nm), visible	Fiber (handpiece, microscope, slit lamp)	1–2 mm depth of penetration	Intense visible blue-green laser light; aiming beam can be a low-power argon beam or a helium-neon beam; highly color selective; transmitted through clear solutions; often used in ophthalmology, dermatology, and soft tissue procedures
Tunable dye laser (liquid laser)	Range of 400–900 nm, visible	Fiber (handpiece, microscope, slit lamp)	Depends on wavelength	Can dial in desired wavelength within limited range of visible light; by changing dyes and other parameters, the wavelength can be altered; laser energy formed by exposing a liquid dye to an intense light source, such as an argon beam; the dye absorbs the laser light and fluoresces over a broad spectrum of colors and with special prisms, diffraction gratings or filters, a specific wavelength is produced; some wavelengths are highly absorbed by pigmented tissues; can be delivered in continuous or pulsed modes; often used in dermatology, ophthalmology, and urology (to fragment stones)
Diode laser (semiconductor crystal laser)	Varies (i.e., 532–910 nm), visible	Fiber (handpiece, microscope, slit lamp)	Depends on wavelength	Compact, reliable laser system; often used for ophthalmology and dermatology
Excimer laser (gas laser)	Ultraviolet (wavelength depends on chemical composition of active medium)	Fiber (handpiece, microscope, slit lamp)	Depends on wavelength (mostly <1 mm); acts by disassociating cellular molecular bonds	"Excited dimer" laser; most popular excimer lasers are argon fluoride (ArF) at 193 nm, krypton fluoride (KrF) at 248 nm, xenon chloride (XeCl) at 308 nm, and xenon fluoride (XeF) at 351 nm; appropriate protective housing needed for laser because gases are extremely toxic; extremely effective ablative capabilities; used for corneal sculpting; also used for other ablative procedures; used experimentally to treat psoriasis and vitiligo

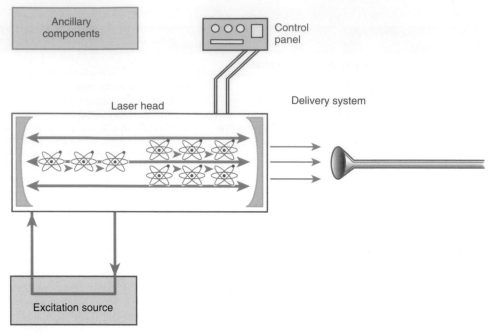

FIG. 8.55 Parts of a laser system.

sealed-tube CO_2 lasers do not require a vacuum pump because the laser gas mixture is catalyzed to regenerate itself for the lasing action to continue, using the same gas mixture over and over again.

The *control panel* consists of a board that regulates delivery of laser energy. Various power settings, modes, durations, and other parameters can be selected. Most laser panels are computerized, allowing the laser to be controlled quickly and accurately.

The *delivery system* is the device or accessory that conducts laser energy from the laser head to the target area. CO_2 laser energy usually is delivered to tissue through an articulated arm (hollow tube) with a series of special mirrors at each joint to reflect the laser energy forward. Care must be taken when moving the laser so that mirrors are not jarred out of alignment. The articulated arm can be attached to a microscope, a special handpiece, or a scanner for the most precise energy delivery. A lens system within these attachments causes the beam to converge at the focal point. A special coating on the lens maintains the beam's integrity and intensity, and must be carefully maintained, following manufacturer's instructions, so that the coating is not disrupted. The focal length of the lens is the distance from the lens to the focal point in which the beam converges and is most concentrated and intense within a small spot. The size of the spot can be changed by focusing or defocusing the lens to allow the spot to become larger or smaller. When the CO_2 handpiece is moved toward and then away from the tissue, the spot size changes.

The articulated arm is connected to a microscope through the use of a microslad (or micromanipulator). Laser energy is conducted through the articulated arm to a mirror within the microslad that directly reflects the beam to tissue. The position of the beam is controlled by moving a joystick. When connected to a scanner, a specific geometric pattern of laser pulses can be delivered to the tissue during ablation (dermatologic) or vaporization (gynecologic) procedures.

The CO_2 laser beam also can be conducted through a narrow wave guide, which consists of a hollow, semiflexible tube that allows energy to "wiggle" down its path by being reflected off the surface of the inner lumen. With this reflection, some beam power is lost

as it exits the delivery device. Flexible fiber waveguides are continually being refined to be more durable, maneuverable, and lighter in weight. These fiber waveguides also provide consistent energy with minimal transmission power loss.

The commonly used argon, KTP, Nd:YAG, and holmium lasers deliver energy through a fiber system. The core fiber, usually made of quartz, is surrounded by a polytetrafluoroethylene (Teflon) silicone coating or cladding that retains the light. This is known as a bare fiber. If the bare fiber is encased by a catheter sheath, a purge gas, air, or fluid can be conducted down the length of the fiber. This purge is used to cool the fiber tip and keep debris from accumulating.

Most laser fibers deliver laser energy to the tissue in a *noncontact mode,* meaning that the fiber does not touch the tissue. If the noncontact fiber contacts the tissue, any debris on the end of the fiber can cause the fiber to heat to the point of destroying the tip. Some fibers can deliver laser energy to the tissue using the *contact method.* For example, a synthetic sapphire contact probe or scalpel that is attached to the end of a fiber with a special connector can deliver Nd:YAG laser energy directly to the tissue in a more concentrated manner. These contact tips are available in a variety of configurations. Depending on the desired tissue effects, the appropriate contact tip is chosen. A scalpel is used to cut; a rounded probe is used to vaporize. A flat probe may be used to coagulate tissue. The end of the quartz fiber also may be sculpted into a configuration that can be used in direct contact with the tissue. Contact technology provides precision because the power output of the beam is confined to a small area and less wattage is needed. It causes less thermal buildup, so adjacent tissue is relatively unaffected.

Benefits of Laser Technology

Laser technology evolves as more surgical applications are explored and introduced. As physicians become more adept in laser applications, use continues to grow. The laser has fostered the development of new minimally invasive procedures and endoscopic techniques along with ophthalmic, dermatologic, and robotic applications. The true potential of the laser has yet to be realized as healthcare practitioners explore different procedures that can benefit from its use. Following are some advantages that have been associated with laser technology, depending on the procedure performed:

- Seals small blood vessels (less intraoperative and postoperative blood loss)
- Seals lymphatics (decreases postoperative edema and potential spread of malignant cells in the lymphatic system)
- Seals nerve endings (on selective procedures, decreases postoperative pain)
- Sterilizes tissue (from the heat generated at the laser-tissue impact site)
- Decreases postoperative stenosis (by decreasing the amount of scarring that could lead to stenosis)
- Produces minimal tissue damage (from precision of the laser beam)
- Reduces operative and anesthesia time
- Allows a shift to more ambulatory surgery procedures
- Allows more use of local anesthetics instead of general anesthetics
- Provides quicker recovery and return to daily activities

Laser Safety

Because laser systems are capable of concentrating high amounts of energy within very small areas, they present hazards. Safe and appropriate use of lasers is the responsibility of the entire healthcare team. Each member must be acutely aware of the many controls needed to prevent accidental injury. The laser team member must be given the responsibility and authority to shut down the laser system if safety policies are not being followed.

The laser is a class III medical device that is subdivided into four subclasses. Lasers designated as subclasses 3 and 4 have the potential to cause injury. Some ophthalmic Nd:YAG lasers that cause a photoacoustic, instead of a photothermal, reaction are classified in the subclass 3B category and can cause injury with sustained interaction. Most of the lasers used in surgical applications are subclass 4 lasers and can cause photothermal reactions that may lead to fire, skin burns, and optical damage by either direct or scattered radiation. Specific safety precautions must be followed to prevent injury from these lasers.

Many agencies address laser safety. Healthcare facilities must develop safety protocols in anticipation of mandates by regulatory agencies as technology advances and grows.

The American National Standards Institute (ANSI), a nongovernmental organization of experts, first published standards (Z136.1: American National Standard for Safe Use of Lasers) in 1973 as safety guidelines for laser use in warfare, industry, and healthcare with the latest revision published in 2014. The standards were expanded and ANSI Z136.3 was published to provide specific recommendations for laser use in healthcare environments (ANSI, 2011). The appendix of ANSI Z136.3 discusses a consensus on laser safety in each of the special areas of medicine and surgery. These standards are reviewed periodically and revised as surgical trends change. The most current versions of both ANSI standards are recommended to be available for referencing because the Z136.3 document often refers to the Z136.1 publication.

Other guidelines have been introduced by the Center for Devices and Radiological Health (CDRH), AORN, American Society for Laser Medicine and Surgery (ASLMS), Laser Institute of America (LIA), FDA, OSHA, and individual state and local regulatory bodies.

Hospitals and other healthcare delivery facilities need to create laser safety policies and procedures using these expert references as

resources. In developing safety guidelines for a facility, protocols should address various situations while being neither too general nor too specific. A policy or procedure must be general enough to address the need, but not so detailed that the surgical team cannot follow it consistently. Staff must realize that they are accountable for following their own safety policies and procedures. Basic education on written laser policies and procedures for all personnel in the surgical environment (including orderlies, aides, and housekeeping personnel) should be mandatory. Topics for policy and procedure development for laser safety should include the following areas, each of which is addressed in more detail below:

- Eye protection
- Controlled access
- Fire safety
- Smoke (plume) evacuation
- Documentation
- Laser team responsibilities
- Skin/tissue protection
- Electrical safety
- Education/training
- Credentialing

Eye Protection. The eye is extremely sensitive to laser radiation and great care must be taken to protect eyes during laser intervention. Even low levels of laser radiation can lead to permanent optical damage. Possible ophthalmologic injuries depend on laser wavelength (Fig. 8.56). The CO_2 laser can damage the cornea because this beam

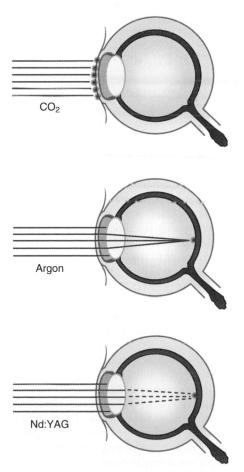

FIG. 8.56 CO_2 laser beam can damage the cornea; the argon and Nd:YAG beams can injure the retina.

PATIENT SAFETY

Eye Safety During Laser Surgery

- Ensure that everyone in the laser room is wearing appropriate eye protection with side shields before activating the laser. Eyewear should have the laser wavelength protection and optical density of the lens material inscribed on it.
- Place a special lens cover over the eyepiece of an endoscope to protect the physician's eye from laser backscatter. Remember that the physician's other eye is unprotected.
- Ensure that everyone in the laser room is wearing eye protection during laser endoscopic procedures.
- Connect an automatic lens shutter to a microscope head, if needed, to provide eye protection for individuals viewing the procedure through the microscope.
- When general anesthesia is used, cover the patient's closed eyes with moistened gauze pads. When the patient is awake, place appropriate glasses or goggles on the patient. Explain the need for eye protection to the patient.
- During laser surgery near the eye, place a special sterile laser eye shield directly on the anesthetized eye surface.
- Ensure that appropriate protective eyewear is available at all entrances to the laser room for anyone entering this area.
- Cover windows in the laser treatment area appropriately, depending on the wavelength of the laser used.
- To prevent reflection of the laser beam, follow special precautions (i.e., using anodized or ebonized instruments near the laser-tissue impact site, covering large reflective retractors with wet towels or sponges).
- When storing protective eyewear, guard against scratches and mishandling. Scratches on the lenses may decrease their effectiveness. Inspect eyewear before use for damage or scratches.

Modified from AORN: *Guidelines for perioperative practice,* Denver, 2016, The Association.

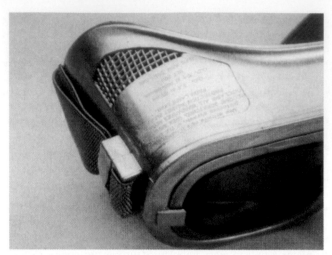

FIG. 8.57 Frame of the protective eyewear displays wavelength and optical density information.

is absorbed readily by water within surface cells, causing a burn. Immediate pain is associated with this corneal injury. Lasers, like the argon and Nd:YAG, in contrast, are transmitted through clear optical structures and fluids and can be refocused by the eye's lens. The beam's intensity after refocusing can permanently damage the retina. No pain may be felt during this injury (Patient Safety).

Adequate eye protection requires understanding the two concepts of maximum permissible exposure (MPE) and nominal hazard zone (NHZ). According to the ANSI Z136.3 standards, the MPE is the level of laser radiation to which a person may be exposed without hazardous effects to the eye or skin. MPE levels are determined through consideration of laser wavelength, power, exposure time, and pulse repetition.

The NHZ is the space in which the level of direct, reflected, or scattered radiation during normal laser operation exceeds MPE; eye, skin, and fire safety precautions must be followed while one is working within this hazard zone. The NHZ can be calculated mathematically to determine the distance from the laser beam emission in which the beam can cause skin and eye damage. With power, operating modes, and other parameters changing frequently during a procedure, this calculation is not always possible. Therefore the area inside the surgical room usually is considered to be within the NHZ so that consistency and simplicity can be maintained when lasers are used.

Protective goggles and glasses must be inscribed with the appropriate filtering capabilities and adequate optical densities for the specific wavelength being used (Fig. 8.57). For example, a pair of Nd:YAG goggles may be inscribed "1064 nm, optical density 5." The optical density of the lens is the capability of the lens material to absorb a specific wavelength. Darker lens shades do not indicate higher optical density, nor do they give more protection than lighter ones. There are lighter lens shades with high optical densities that provide adequate safety. Laser team members must ensure that eyewear is properly labeled, handled, and stored so that hazards are minimized, and scratching and damage of the eyewear avoided.

During surgical procedures using multiple wavelengths, protective eyewear must change as wavelengths change. Some eyewear protects against a limited range of wavelengths. If the range is expanded to block a greater variety of wavelengths, the transparency of the eyewear is reduced.

Controversy exists as to the appropriateness of using personal prescription eyeglasses as CO_2 laser eye protection when the wearer is not in the immediate vicinity of the laser beam emission (e.g., the circulating nurse). Prescription eyeglasses do not have wavelength protection inscribed on them and have not been tested to determine the protective ability of the lens; therefore adequate protection cannot be guaranteed. Proponents state that the NHZ is so limited when the CO_2 beam is passed through the focusing lens that individuals who are not close to the laser emission port are not at high risk for eye damage. Facilities must address this controversy and develop a policy for the surgical team. Contact lenses and half glasses do not offer adequate protection against CO_2 laser energy and should not be used.

During a microscopic procedure, the optics of the microscope provide eye protection against CO_2 laser energy for the operative physician. When other wavelengths are used, such as argon or Nd:YAG, an automatic lens shutter can be connected to the microscope head. During laser activation the shutter allows a lens filter to drop into place to provide a shield from any laser backscatter, protecting the laser operator's eyes. When this device is attached to the microscope head, any observer tube being used must be placed above the filter so that all portal optics offer protection. Others involved with the procedure must wear appropriate eyewear.

A lens filter can be placed over the eyepiece of a rigid or flexible endoscope. The lens must offer appropriate protection for the specific laser being used. Guidelines recommend that other surgical team members also wear eye protection, even though laser energy seems confined within an enclosed cavity. Optical injury is always possible if a fiber or articulated arm separates from the endoscope while the laser is activated, or if a fiber fractures and the beam escapes at the fracture site.

For healthcare professionals who routinely work with laser systems, a baseline eye exam is sometimes recommended, including visual acuity and an assessment of retinal health. Another eye exam can be performed after any ophthalmic accident or on termination of employment. The baseline exam provides a foundation for comparison with abnormal findings from subsequent exams. Performing baseline eye exams merely documents the ocular health of laser team members so that it can be used during a potential workers' compensation claim for retinal damage from accidental beam exposure. Some facilities opt not to follow this expensive and difficult-to-monitor guideline of performing baseline eye exams. Instead they strictly enforce their eye safety policy, minimizing the chance of ophthalmic injury. These facilities state in their eye safety policy that an eye exam will be performed if an ocular accident occurs.

The patient's eyes also must be protected during laser intervention. When general anesthesia is used, patients' eyes are covered with wet eye pads, or a moistened towel; eyelids are taped closed. If awake or under local anesthesia, the patient wears appropriate eye protection. Explanations about this eye protection are provided. If the laser is used in the immediate vicinity of the eye, such as to lighten a port-wine stain on the eyelid, a special laser eye shield can be placed on the eye's surface after instilling a drop of ophthalmic local anesthetic. If the laser eye shields are sterilized with steam, these devices must be cooled completely before being placed on the cornea to prevent burns.

Controlled Access. Inadvertent access to rooms in which laser treatments are being performed should be prevented. Laser warning signs must be placed at all entrances to the treatment area so that access is granted only to individuals who have been appropriately educated in laser safety. The word "Danger" and the universally accepted laser symbol should be present on laser warning signs to indicate the possibility of hazards (Fig. 8.58). Laser signs should be removed when the procedure has been completed.

Windows and ports into rooms in which lasers are used must be covered with appropriate protection for the specific laser being used. The CO_2 laser beam, passed through a lens, and the holmium laser beam, delivered through a fiber, provide a limited NHZ, so window coverage is not required. Argon, Nd:YAG, and certain other laser wavelengths can be transmitted through window glass and have longer NHZs. Windows and ports must be covered with a blocking barrier that stops transmission of specific wavelengths with more extensive NHZs. Many facilities require window coverage for all laser procedures just to provide consistency within the laser program.

The laser key must not be left in the laser during storage. The key should be available only to authorized personnel who have appropriate education and training to operate the laser. Laser keys can be stored in the narcotics cabinet or in a special key lockbox to control access.

Fire Safety. An awareness of laser biophysics and tissue interaction is necessary to understand actions needed to prevent laser fires. A fire can be started by a reflected beam as easily as from direct impact. The laser team responds quickly if a fire occurs. Immediate action is key to minimizing injury to the patient and the surgical team.

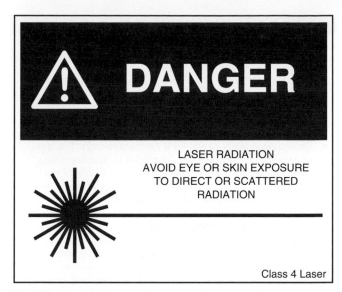

FIG. 8.58 Warning signs should be placed at all entrances to the surgical room to notify personnel that a laser is being used and that appropriate eye protection is needed before entering the room.

The Patient Safety: Fire Safety During Laser Use box provides important detailed measures for fire safety during laser surgery.

Sterile water or saline solution should be readily available to douse a small fire on the patient. A laser-appropriate fire extinguisher should be available to control a fire within the laser system. During surgery, combustibles, such as any soft goods near the laser target site, should be kept wet to prevent ignition. The surgical team should monitor constantly the moisture level of sponges and other materials to prevent drying, which eventually could support a fire.

A laser beam can ignite flammable draping material easily. Some water-repellent drapes and other laser-safe materials are able to withstand laser impact because the flammability of the material is minimal. If the flammability of draping material or any other supplies is questionable (e.g., plastic tooth protectors), the suspect item can be tested in the manufacturer's or researcher's laboratory.

Instruments used in the immediate vicinity of the laser target site should be nonreflective to decrease the chance of the laser beam bouncing off the surface and accidentally impacting another area. The laser beam can easily be reflected off shiny instrument surfaces and can cause skin or eye injury or ignite flammable materials. To decrease reflectivity, an instrument may be ebonized by coating it with a special substance (usually black). The instrument should be inspected regularly to ensure integrity of the coating. Any scratched surface on which ebonization has worn off should be recoated.

Instruments also may be anodized or surfaced with a matte finish to decrease reflectivity. Other coatings and surfaces that cause laser light to scatter and diffuse on impact are being introduced. Large retractors can be covered with wet sponges or towels so that the laser beam cannot accidentally reflect off a shiny surface.

Special instruments have been designed to provide backstops for laser energy to decrease adjacent tissue damage and fire risk. Titanium rods are effective backstops. Quartz rods often are used as backstops for the CO_2 laser beam, but argon and Nd:YAG beams may be transmitted through them. Wet sponges also can be used as backstop material. Glass rods are never to be used with a CO_2 laser because glass material heats and shatters after continuous impact by a laser

PATIENT SAFETY

Fire Safety During Laser Use

- Ensure sterile water or saline is immediately available to douse a small fire near or on the patient.
- Have a laser-appropriate fire extinguisher available in the department in case the laser catches fire. Surgical team members must know how to operate the fire extinguisher.
- Do not place fluids or solutions on the laser unit. The laser system should be protected from spills or splatter, which could cause short-circuiting and fire.
- Do not place dry combustibles in the vicinity of the laser impact site. Use wet towels, nonflammable drapes, or special laser-retardant materials near the laser target area. Moisten dry drapes and soft goods such as radiopaque sponges with sterile saline or water to prevent ignition. Monitor the moisture level constantly throughout the procedure. Remoisten as needed.
- Do not use flammable materials near the laser-tissue impact site.
- Use nonreflective instruments in or near the laser-tissue impact site to decrease accidental reflection of the laser beam. Cover larger instruments, such as retractors, with wet sponges or towels to protect against reflection.
- Do not use flammable skin preparations, such as alcohol, as prepping solutions.
- Insert a wet pack into the rectum as a tampon to prevent methane gas from escaping into the surgical area, according to physician directions. A cleansing bowel prep before surgery also decreases this risk.
- Use appropriate laser-resistant endotracheal tubes during upper airway surgery. Follow directions in product literature and on labels, which typically include information regarding the tube's laser resistance, use of dyes in the cuff to indicate a puncture, use of a saline fill to prevent cuff ignition, and immediate replacement of the tube if the cuff is punctured.
- Protect the endotracheal tube cuff with counted wet gauze sponges.
- Keep oxygen concentrations between 21% and 30% to minimize the possibility of an airway fire during laser procedures of the airway.
- Do not use nitrous oxide, because it supports combustion.
- Place the laser in standby mode when it is not in active use.
- Identify and verify the laser foot pedal with the operating physician to avoid accidental activation. Allow only the individual using the laser to activate it. Only activate the laser when the delivery tip is within the user's direct field of vision.

Modified from AORN: *Guidelines for perioperative practice*, Denver, 2016, The Association.

beam. Teflon backstops are not to be used because they can melt when heated and produce toxic fumes.

Special laser mirrors that directly reflect the beam onto hard-to-reach areas are available. Mirrors may be made of rhodium or stainless steel. Glass-surface mirrors do not withstand laser impact and heat and shatter instead. Using a laser mirror requires skill because the beam must be focused on the target area and not on the mirror to deliver the full impact of laser energy. A laser beam that is misdirected off a mirror can easily cause a fire.

Flammable skin preparations should not be used for laser procedures. During skin cleansing, prep solution can pool underneath

a patient, and ethanol vapors from alcohol-based preparations can be trapped beneath drapes. The volatility of these vapors increases the risk of a surgical drape fire. If flammable skin preps are used, drying must be adequate to allow the flammable vapors to dissipate before drapes are applied. Iodophor or any other tinted prep solution should be wiped before argon or Nd:YAG lasers are used because the tint may increase laser absorption by the skin.

When a laser is used in the rectal area, a wet pack may be used to tamponade the bowel to prevent the escape of methane gas, which could enter the surgical area from the colon and cause an explosion. Wet sponges used for the pack must be counted so that packing is not inadvertently left in place after surgery. Some practitioners disagree with this practice, stating that inserting wet sponges may stretch the colon walls, increasing peristalsis and the movement of methane gas into the surgical area. Whatever method is chosen, a cleansing bowel prep before surgery also helps decrease this potential hazard.

Airway explosion caused by the laser beam igniting the endotracheal tube (ETT) can cause a potentially lethal accident for the patient. A polyvinyl chloride (PVC) ETT is highly flammable, especially when a high concentration of oxygen flows through it during anesthesia administration. Specific laser-retardant ETTs should be used during oral, tracheal, or esophageal laser procedures that require general anesthesia. The laser power limitations of a commercially manufactured ETT must be followed closely to ensure proper protection. The cuff of the ETT should be inflated with sterile saline to provide a heat sink and retard a fire if perforated by the laser beam. Saline may be tinted with methylene blue to note a cuff rupture more quickly as the blue dye escapes. A protocol should be developed to describe the emergency steps needed to control an endotracheal fire. Immediate considerations include the following:

- Remove the ETT, ensuring the entire tube is removed.
- Stop ventilation (disconnect gas flow).
- Extinguish all flames (pour saline or water in the airway).
- Ventilate the patient by mask or reintubate immediately to prevent laryngospasm.
- Examine the airway (mouth, oral cavity, bronchial tree) for burns, foreign bodies, or both.
- Decide on the next course of action (anesthesia provider and surgeon), that is, cancel or continue with procedure.

A nonintubation technique involving jet ventilation also may be used during laser microlaryngoscopy. A jet ventilator is a mechanical ventilation unit that delivers oxygen through a small metal needle used with a rigid laryngoscope. Under pressurization, the jet ventilator is set to deliver a predetermined amount of oxygen with a set rate, pressure (in pounds per square inch [psi]), and percentage of inspiratory time. The needle is positioned between the vocal cords on the side opposite the lesion. The needle extends into the trachea so that the proper amount of oxygen is easily delivered. After surgery the patient may be intubated to maintain an open airway if postoperative edema or tracheal spasm is anticipated.

Other nonintubation techniques, such as apneic methods, can be used to avoid intubation. The patient's oxygen saturation must be monitored closely when these techniques are used.

Endoscope Safety. Special precautions should be followed when using the laser during an endoscopic procedure. When a laser fiber is introduced through the biopsy port of a flexible or rigid endoscope, the operator must view at least 1 cm of the tip of the fiber before activating the laser. If the end of the fiber is still within the sheath of the endoscope and the laser is fired, the heat from the laser energy quickly damages the optics and channel of the endoscope.

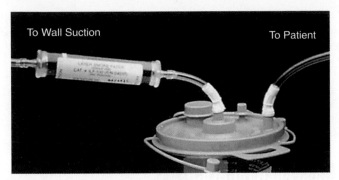

FIG. 8.59 An in-line filter is placed between the suction canister and the wall outlet and is used to evacuate small amounts of surgical smoke.

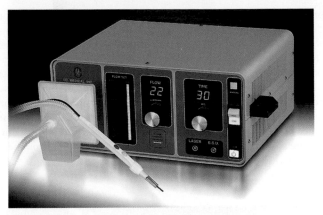

FIG. 8.60 Individual smoke evacuator.

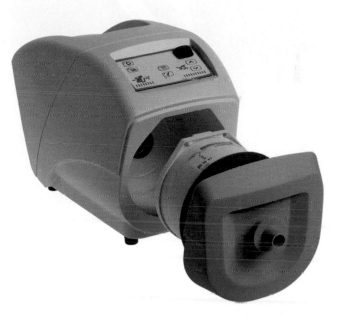

FIG. 8.61 Contaminated filter being removed from smoke evacuator.

When a "bare" fiber is placed down the biopsy channel of a flexible endoscope, the sharp tip can tear the inside lumen of the channel. A length of medical-grade tubing can be placed over the fiber with the tip recessed within the sheath. The entire unit is then passed through the endoscope. When the end of the tubing is observed, the medical-grade tubing is withdrawn sufficiently to expose the end of the fiber. This procedure effectively protects the inside lumen of the endoscope channel during fiber insertion.

Smoke Evacuation. Smoke evacuation and odor control must be adequate whenever a plume is generated, whether it is from the laser, ESU, or other energy devices being used in surgery. When "hot" tools such as these are used to cut, excise, ablate, or coagulate tissue, cells of the target tissue are heated to the point of boiling. This causes cellular membranes to rupture, spewing cell contents into the air and producing surgical smoke.

One of the crucial elements of adequate smoke evacuation is to determine the method of smoke evacuation. The method selected depends on the amount of plume produced.

An *in-line smoke evacuation filter* is appropriate only for small amounts of plume generation, similar to what is produced during microlaryngoscopy vaporization of vocal cord polyps. The in-line filter connects to the existing suction line by positioning it between the wall connection and suction canister (Fig. 8.59). If the filter becomes wet, it loses its effectiveness.

If an in-line filter is not used, particulate matter from surgical smoke can occlude and corrode suction pipes and contaminate the building. Wall suction flow may not be forceful enough to capture the plume adequately. Wall suction usually generates 2 cubic feet per minute (cfm) of air movement, whereas an individual smoke evacuator may move air at 35 to 50 cfm. An in-line filter is changed after each procedure (or according to the manufacturer's instructions).

When greater amounts of surgical smoke are generated, an *individual smoke evacuator* is used. Individual smoke evacuators have filtration systems that include a charcoal filter and an ultra–low-penetration air (ULPA) filter (Fig. 8.60). The charcoal filter removes toxic gases and odor, whereas the ULPA filter removes small particulates with filtration of 0.12 micron size matter at 99.9999% efficiency (Schultz, 2014; Ball, 2016).

Maintenance of a smoke evacuator requires changing the filter per the manufacturer's written instructions (Fig. 8.61). Standard Precautions are used when changing a contaminated filter because of the possibility of bacterial and/or viral contamination (AORN, 2016). Many manufacturers recommend that the contaminated filter be treated as infectious and disposed of as regulated medical waste (biohazardous).

Centralized smoke evacuation systems provide smoke evacuation for several surgical rooms at the same time. The smoke evacuation line needs to be routinely flushed and cleaned to prevent debris buildup and pathogen growth within the system. A central system is convenient because it is always available; however, if it malfunctions, smoke evacuation is not available to multiple surgical areas.

Contamination by surgical plume and tissue splatter is decreased when the surgical team wears gloves, gowns, and masks. The surgical team must ensure that the smoke evacuation wand or suction device is close to the target site so that all plume is evacuated. Devices are available that attach or are built into the ESU or laser delivery system that effectively evacuate surgical smoke as it is generated (Fig. 8.62). Using appropriate smoke evacuation methods (Evidence for Practice) to ensure that all plume is eliminated is the only practice that protects the surgical team from exposure to hazardous surgical smoke. The Research Highlight box describes a study performed to quantitatively measure selected chemical substances found in surgical smoke produced during laparoscopic cholecystectomies and to determine the risk to healthcare personnel.

Compliance studies have been performed to note the acceptance and implementation of smoke evacuation recommendations. Education has clearly been the reason for compliance with using appropriate smoke evacuation practices. The main barriers to compliance have been that the equipment and supplies are not available, the surgeon refuses to allow smoke evacuation to be performed during the procedure, the smoke evacuator is too noisy, and the staff is complacent and just will not use available smoke evacuation equipment and devices (Ball, 2016).

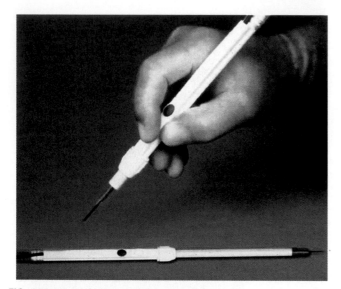

FIG. 8.62 Electrosurgery pencil with the smoke evacuation system built into the device.

Surgical smoke that arises during flexible endoscopic or laparoscopic procedures impairs visibility. Hand control suction devices and valve filters provide gentle movement of plume during laparoscopy without destroying the pneumoperitoneum.

A high-flow insufflator is recommended for continual replacement of CO_2 gas. A special smoke evacuator may be used that automatically provides slow evacuation of plume without destroying the pneumoperitoneum.

RESEARCH HIGHLIGHT

Hazards of Laparoscopic Surgical Smoke to Healthcare Personnel

A study was performed to assess the presence of selected chemical substances released into the surgical suite during laparoscopic cholecystectomies. Air samples were captured from the breathing zones of surgical personnel located near the OR bed. Gas chromatography and mass spectrometry were used to identify the compounds and their concentrations within the air samples. Results showed that the concentrations were lower than the national hygienic standards, but *repeated* exposure to these chemical substances increases the possibility of adverse effects. Most of the compounds in surgical smoke are toxic with over 600 chemical substances being found in surgical smoke, including benzene, dioxins, aldehydes, and other volatile organic substances. Many of these toxins are carcinogenic, mutagenic, or genotoxic. Even at low concentrations, exposure to these compounds can cause a significant risk to healthcare personnel. Therefore adequate smoke evacuation must be used to protect surgical team members even during laparoscopic procedures.

Modified from Dobrogowski M et al: Health risk to medical personnel of surgical smoke produced during laparoscopic surgery, *Int J Occup Med Environ Health* 28(5):831–840, 2015.

EVIDENCE FOR PRACTICE

Smoke Evacuation During Laser Surgery

- Use the appropriate smoke evacuation system, depending on the amount of plume generated. If small amounts of plume are generated and room suction is to be used, an in-line suction filter is positioned between the suction canister and the wall outlet to capture surgical smoke particulate. An individual smoke evacuation system is used if larger amounts of plume are generated.
- Change the smoke evacuation filter(s) according to the manufacturer's written instructions.
- Hold the smoke evacuation suction tube close (<2 inches away) to the tissue interaction site to remove as much plume (odor and particulate matter) as possible.
- Smoke evacuation tubing should have a smooth inner lumen to eliminate any whistling.
- Use a reducer fitting to adapt a large smoke evacuation tube to a smaller suction or evacuation tube.
- The scrub person or first assistant can operate the smoke evacuation foot pedal (if available) to minimize wear and tear on the smoke evacuator motor and to decrease noise. Some smoke evacuators have sensing mechanisms that automatically activate the smoke evacuator when plume is generated.

- Evacuate surgical smoke generated during endoscopic or laparoscopic procedures. Endoscopic smoke evacuation instruments, such as suction tubes, help decrease the presence and retention of plume inside a body cavity or organ. A low-pressure suction valve can be used to remove plume gently during a laparoscopic procedure without destroying the pneumoperitoneum. A high-flow insufflator is recommended to replace any lost insufflation gas quickly. A special smoke evacuator that provides automatic plume removal also can be used to evacuate intra-abdominal smoke without destroying the pneumoperitoneum.
- Wear a surgical mask that provides adequate filtration (0.1-μm filtration) to protect against residual smoke particulate that has not been evacuated. The high-filtration mask must fit snugly around the face. Wearing a high-filtration mask does not replace the use of a smoke evacuation system to remove surgical smoke from the environment.
- Continuing education helps healthcare personnel to understand the hazards of surgical smoke and encourages the use of appropriate methods for evacuation.

Modified from AORN: *Guidelines for perioperative practice*, Denver, 2016, The Association.

```
┌─────────────────────────────────────────────────────┐
│ Date _____ OR Room No. _____ │
│                                                       │
│ PATIENT INFORMATION:                                  │
│ Name _____ Patient ID No. _____  │
│ Zip Code _____ Sex: M F Age _____   │
│ Status: IP OP                                         │
│                                                       │
│ SURGERY INFORMATION:                                  │
│ Physician _____ Anesthesia: General MAC Local    │
│ Procedure _____   │
│                                                       │
│ LASER INFORMATION:                                    │
│ Laser and wavelength_____    │
│ Power _____ Duration _____    │
│ Total spots _____ Total energy _____    │
│ Laser time on _____ Laser time off _____    │
│                                                       │
│ DELIVERY SYSTEM:                                      │
│ Laser fiber _____ _  │
│ Contact tip _____ _  │
│ Microscope handpiece _____    │
│                                                       │
│ LASER SAFETY:                                         │
│ Eye protection_____    │
│ Smoke evacuation _____    │
│ Fire safety_____    │
│ Other safety measures _____    │
│ _____     │
│                                                       │
│ COMMENTS:                                             │
│ _____     │
│ _____     │
│                                                       │
│ Laser team member _____     │
└─────────────────────────────────────────────────────┘
```

FIG. 8.63 Sample laser log.

Other Safety Measures. Foot pedals present safety problems if mistakenly activated. Multiple foot pedals placed on the floor can be confusing and lead to accidents. The laser pedal should be identified clearly and used only by the physician delivering laser energy to the target area.

Laser team members must appreciate potential electrical hazards because the laser, similar to the ESU, is high-voltage equipment. Water and other solutions should not be placed on the laser unit, and the components of the laser should be protected against spills or splatter, which could cause short-circuiting. The outside housing of the laser should never be removed by unauthorized personnel because of the potential for electrical shock or electrocution.

Transportation hazards are always a threat because some laser systems are quite heavy. When these units need to be moved, proper body mechanics must be used to prevent injury to the transporter. The laser unit should be pushed instead of pulled to provide less stress on the transporter's back muscles. The laser should not be bumped against a wall because its internal components can be damaged or become misaligned.

Documentation. Closely following written laser safety procedures is crucial for safety and legal reasons, as with any hazardous equipment. Specific notes about laser safety can be written on a laser log form or as part of the intraoperative nursing note. Either record should be included in the patient's medical record so that safety activities are documented. Safety measures may not be specifically documented if already described and mandated in the facility's policies and procedures. This is referred to as "documentation by exception."

A special laser log can be designed to be a permanent part of the patient's record and might include information such as the laser used, power, pulse duration, and other laser parameters. The use of smoke evacuation, fibers, and contact tips also may be documented, especially if specific charges for these items are made. A sample laser log is shown in Fig. 8.63.

Role of the Laser Team Member. As the use of laser technology grows, the role of the laser team member becomes more important. The backbone of a progressive and successful laser program is the enthusiastic and dedicated laser team. Expanded responsibilities are being assumed by the laser team member to provide consistency and promote a safe environment for the patient and the surgical team. Some roles of the laser team member may include serving as the LSO, serving on the laser/safety committee, becoming actively involved with laser procurement, and promoting the laser program through marketing.

According to ANSI Z136.3 (2011), the definition of the LSO is

the one person in each facility or organization responsible for the laser safety program ... [who] has the training and experience to administer a laser safety program ... is authorized by the health care facility administration and is responsible for monitoring and overseeing the control of laser hazards. (p. 7)

Following are some of the duties of the LSO:
- Ensures all lasers have been labeled by the manufacturer with appropriate hazard classification
- Evaluates potential hazards of the laser
- Serves on the laser committee
- Enforces standard operating procedures (e.g., maintenance, service, perioperative checklists, policies)
- Ensures protective equipment and devices are in good working order (e.g., protective eyewear)

- Ensures laser installation and maintenance are performed by qualified individuals, documented, and performed regularly
- Ensures appropriate training and education on laser safety are conducted and documented
- Documents incidents with lasers that could cause or have caused harm to patients or healthcare providers
- Delegates duties within the laser program as appropriate

Perioperative nurses who are part of the laser team are often involved with patient education. The perioperative nurse reinforces what the physician has described to the patient before a laser procedure. When told that surgery is needed, the patient is often anxious because of the unknown. Anxiety may be compounded because the patient is confronted with two alarming unknowns. Many patients develop uneasiness about laser procedures based on information from science-fiction movies, talk shows, and other such sources. The patient always should have the opportunity to discuss a proposed procedure to allay any worries. The perioperative nurse may provide additional information if the patient has further questions about laser technology. After the physician has explained the procedure, a surgical consent is signed, timed, and dated. Sometimes the consent form reflects that a laser will be used during surgery. Some physicians, however, suggest that a laser is merely a tool used during surgery and do not believe it is necessary to list laser use on the consent form.

Adequate time should be allotted for patient questions before the procedure. If a local anesthetic is used, the patient should understand what to anticipate during surgery, what sounds or odors will arise, why eye protection is needed, and what the patient's role is during the procedure. If the patient understands the application, the role of the laser, and his or her responsibility during and after the procedure, the perioperative nurse can expect better compliance and less anxiety in the patient.

Discharge instructions are required for any ambulatory procedure; laser discharge instructions may be preprinted for each surgical application. These written instructions should be reviewed and given to the patient on discharge. A follow-up phone call helps the perioperative nurse evaluate the care delivered during the laser intervention and the patient's compliance with postoperative instructions.

Sometimes the perioperative nurse is placed in a compromising position by being expected to circulate during the surgical procedure as well as operate the laser. This nurse has the tremendous responsibility of being accountable for two crucial roles in the OR. Because of this the risk of a laser incident may increase. In the traditional setting one nurse circulates while another nurse or a technologist, a member of the laser team, operates the laser. The healthcare facility must determine which procedures require more staffing to deliver safe patient care.

Ultrasonic Device Surgery

Vibrating mechanical energy devices provide a safe option for cutting and coagulation. High-frequency sound waves are propagated to a blade tip to produce ultrasonic energy. These ultrasonic waves have a frequency of greater than 20,000 Hz and cannot be sensed by the human ear.

Production of ultrasonic energy begins with electrical current that generates an electrical signal sent through a coaxial cable to a transducer in a handpiece. The transducer converts electrical energy to mechanical motion through contraction and expansion of piezoelectric ceramic elements. A longitudinal vibratory response that moves the tip at the end of the handpiece from 23,000 Hz to greater than 55,000 Hz is produced. As the power increases, the

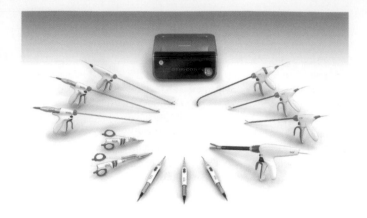

FIG. 8.64 Ultrasonic energy system with different handpieces.

frequency remains the same, but longitudinal excursion of the tip lengthens.

Because the tip is in contact with tissue, mechanical motion causes tissue protein to denature as hydrogen bonds are broken. As protein molecules become disorganized, a sticky coagulum forms that welds and coagulates smaller bleeding vessels. Aerosolization occurs during cellular destruction, consisting of a small amount of water vapor that usually dissipates quickly. Only a small amount of thermal energy is produced and any adjacent tissue damage is minimal.

Different tip configurations include a blade, ball, and hook (Fig. 8.64). To obtain optimal tissue response, countertraction must be applied to the structure being treated. A shear-grasper to hold the tissue between a blade and tissue pad can be used to eliminate the need for countertraction.

The following are advantages of using an ultrasonic device to cut and coagulate:

- No surgical plume or odor is generated; only a small amount of aerosolization is created.
- Less adjacent tissue is damaged compared with laser and ESU devices.
- Tactile feedback is retained.
- No nerve or muscle stimulation occurs because no electrical current is delivered to the target area.
- No stray electrical or laser energy is produced.
- Precise cutting and control are offered.

Neutral Plasma Coagulation

A neutral plasma coagulator is an energy source that produces pure plasma to provide coagulation. Plasma is created when a low flow of argon gas is excited within the handpiece, consisting of an anode (where current enters) and cathode (where current exits). The gas, in the plasma state, emerges from the handpiece tip as an electrically neutral pale blue jet stream that coagulates tissue. When the plasma reaches bleeding tissue, it releases its kinetic energy as heat and causes coagulation of the bleeding surface as well as cutting capabilities. Because the electrodes are contained within the handpiece, no dispersive pad is used. Patient risk is reduced because no electrical current passes through the patient. Thermal conductivity is very limited, so the depth of tissue damage is minimized. This energy can be used near pacemakers, metallic implants, and defibrillators because it is electrically neutral. The plasma flow helps remove liquid from the target site, so the surgeon's visibility is not compromised. The neutral plasma jet can cut all tissues, including bone, while simultaneously providing coagulation. The system consists of a range of disposable handpieces.

Microwave Ablation

Microwave ablation uses frictional heat generated from rotation of water molecules that creates an ablation zone with simultaneous application of one or more antennas. When the antennas are close to each other (i.e., 1.5–2 cm apart), one combined ablation zone is created. No electrical current flows through the patient and no dispersive pad is required. The system automatically shuts off when the set ablation time is achieved. The advantage of microwave ablation is that the desired level of soft tissue coagulation can be reached more quickly compared with other RF ablation devices.

Microwave ablation can be used for treatment during percutaneous, laparoscopic, or open access procedures to treat primary and secondary diseases, such as liver disease, lung malignancies, renal and adrenal tumors, and even bone metastases. Tumor boundaries have been successfully treated using microwave energy. Research in this technology may confirm microwave ablation as a new era in tumor ablation.

Hydrodissection and Irrigation

Hydrodissection and irrigation are essential during most open and endoscopic procedures to provide a clear field of view and even release structures. Hydrodissection is used routinely for cataract extraction through a process called phacoemulsification. Nerve hydrodissection, such as carpal tunnel release, is a relatively new technique performed by using ultrasound guidance to inject a small amount of fluid around the affected nerve. The nerve is then released by using a hydrodissection process, allowing the nerve to glide easier within surrounding structures.

Irrigation is accomplished with irrigation probes for open procedures; via irrigating channels built into endoscopes; or by irrigating systems inserted through an operating port, cannula sheath, or operative endoscope. For endoscopic procedures, irrigating fluid can be introduced manually using a syringe and stopcock attached to irrigation tubing on one end and an irrigation bag and tubing assembly on the other. Fluid flows by gravity and is manually forced through the distal tubing.

A pressure bag can be used to increase flow, if desired. Irrigation through a flexible endoscope also can be delivered directly by a syringe attached to the irrigation port. Fluid travels through a specific channel built into the scope. Rigid scopes, such as ureteroscopes, cystoscopes, and hysteroscopes, also have this capability, as do operative laparoscopes.

Pumps are used for large quantities of fluid and when manual operation is cumbersome and time consuming. Pumps are beneficial when irrigation is used for hydrodissection because more fluid can be introduced to the surgical site under pressurization. More force can be exerted over longer periods, and the pressure is adjustable.

A common pump irrigation system includes the irrigation pump (CO_2 or electric), irrigation bottle caps, irrigation probe with dual trumpet valves, and Y-tubing irrigation set. When a CO_2-controlled system is in use, an E-cylinder of CO_2 gas is attached by means of a tank yoke and input hose. A wrench must be available to turn off the tank when not in use. It is important to check tank pressure before and after each use. The pump usually has an adjustable pressure on-off capability and dual irrigation bottle selection. As one bottle empties, a flip of the switch redirects CO_2 flow to the second bottle. Bottles can be replaced as needed. The system operates by displacement of water or saline with CO_2 gas.

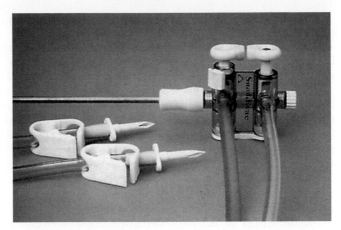

FIG. 8.65 Trumpet valve controls the flow of irrigant and suction.

When an electric setup is used, a carrier bag with an inflatable bladder surrounds the solution bag. When the bladder inflates, adequate pressure can be achieved and controlled to provide irrigation and hydrodissection. Distal tubing attaches directly to an irrigation probe. The length of time and volume of irrigation are controlled by a trumpet valve (Fig. 8.65). Probes are available as reusable, disposable, or a combination of both. All three types incorporate a second trumpet valve for suctioning.

If reusable probes are used, they are completely disassembled for cleaning and sterilization or disinfection. Each trumpet valve has a spring mechanism (similar to that of a ballpoint pen). These springs are under pressure when the trumpet valve is inserted. During disassembly it is important to hold a hand over the valve so that the spring cannot eject, disappear, or cause eye injury. Protective eyewear is worn during disassembly, and extra springs should be available.

Completely disposable units are available; other systems incorporate disposable with reusable components. In the latter, tubing and pistol-grip handles containing the trumpet valves are disposable, but suction and irrigation probes are reusable. The disposable and disposable-reusable units may also incorporate electrosurgical capability, allowing the device to be used for three separate functions.

Choice of irrigation fluid depends on surgeon preference. Traditionally, normal saline has been used. Because saline is a conductive fluid, use of a monopolar ESU presents a safety hazard relating to potential for transfer of heat and current to adjacent tissues. As a result, sterile water or other nonconductive solutions should be considered to prevent ESU energy from transferring to alternative sites when extensive use of a monopolar ESU is anticipated. Sorbitol, also used for irrigation during hysteroscopy, can be absorbed rapidly into the vascular system, especially during excessive venous bleeding. The patient is monitored carefully because of the potential for congestive heart failure from fluid overload.

Cryosurgery

Cryosurgery is used to destroy small quantities of unwanted tissue, such as skin tumors, and to ablate larger tissue targets, such as liver tumors, prostatic cancer, renal tumors, and cervical dysplasia. Cryosurgery causes tumor death by freezing. When internal tumors (e.g., liver cancer) are treated, dead tumor cells eventually are absorbed into surrounding tissue. Cryosurgery often involves cycles or steps during treatment as a tumor is frozen, allowed to thaw, and then refrozen.

To freeze tissue properly a cooling device or cryosurgical probe produces an ice ball capable of destroying tissue at approximately −122°F (−50°C) and colder. Some devices produce temperatures as low as −464°F (−240°C). The cooling source is usually gaseous nitrogen or supercooled liquid nitrogen.

For external tumors, liquid nitrogen is applied directly to the dysplastic tissue either with a cotton swab or with a spraying device. For internal tumors, liquid nitrogen is circulated through the length of a cryoprobe with an insulated shaft to confine freezing to the distal tip. Ultrasound imaging often is used to guide the cryoprobe and monitor tumor freezing. By localizing the freezing effects, nearby healthy tissue is spared. Smaller cryoprobes can be inserted through small trocar sites.

Cryosurgery may be used to treat early-stage skin cancers (basal and squamous cell carcinomas) and retinoblastoma (a childhood cancer that attacks the retina of the eye). Precancerous lesions, such as actinic keratosis and cervical intraepithelial neoplasia, may also be treated with this therapy. Cryosurgery has also been found useful in ophthalmology to reattach detached retinas and to treat other eye problems.

Cryosurgery has been used to treat a variety of cancers, including prostate, liver, breast, bone, brain, spinal, renal, lung, and tracheal. It can be performed using open, laparoscopic, and percutaneous approaches. It may be used in combination with other cancer treatments, such as radiation, hormone therapy, chemotherapy, and surgery. Cryosurgery is used to maximize the effort in nephron-sparing renal tumor surgery by offering another treatment modality, especially in patients who are poor surgical candidates.

The primary advantage of cryosurgery over other therapies for cancer treatment is that it is less invasive. Only a small incision is needed to introduce the cryoprobe through the skin, and less bleeding, pain, and other complications occur. Cryosurgery is also less expensive compared with other treatments and often requires shorter hospital stays and recovery time. The main disadvantage of cryosurgery is the uncertainty of its long-term effectiveness because microscopic cancer cells can spread easily if they are missed during the freezing application. Cryosurgery continues to evolve as new techniques are explored for treatment and palliative therapy.

Like laser technology, there are companies that offer cryosurgical equipment and devices for rent. Facility administrators must ensure that trained personnel are available when rental systems are used in surgery and that all of The Joint Commission and any other regulatory requirements for rentals are met.

Key Points

- The perioperative nurse is responsible and accountable for the safe use of a variety of different devices and pieces of equipment.
- The main components of a flexible endoscope include the control body, insertion tube, bending section with distal tip, and light-guide connector that form the foundation of the mechanical system, angulation system, and illumination system.
- The main components of a rigid endoscope include the eyepiece, body, shaft, and distal end.
- To check the transmission of light within a fiberoptic cable, one end of the cable is held pointing toward a bright light while the other end is checked for any peppering, which indicates broken fibers. When approximately 20% of the fibers are broken, the cable must be replaced.
- White balancing allows the camera to adjust to white light so all primary colors appear properly.

- Instrumentation and port access devices have been introduced to allow single-entry laparoscopic procedures because there is less scarring and increased recovery with this technique.
- Endoscopes and instrumentation must be reprocessed following the manufacturer's written instructions. Devices must be thoroughly cleaned so that sterilization by steam, ethylene oxide, plasma, liquid chemical, or ozone can be accomplished.
- The FDA closely monitors the practice of reprocessing SUDs, enforcing the regulatory guidelines that have been published.
- Nurses must understand the technical components of a video system that include the camera, cable, control unit, couplers (adapters), monitors, recording systems, and storage systems.
- Robotic technology involves computer-based electromechanical devices that are engineered to provide ultimate visibility and precise operative maneuverability (as an extension of the surgeon's hands).
- Nurses must be aware of insufflation hazards and closely monitor the rate of flow and the volume of gas delivered while also monitoring the patient's intra-abdominal pressure.
- Electrosurgery is the most common energy source used in surgery today; therefore nurses must understand the difference between coagulation and cutting settings, monopolar and bipolar systems, and dispersive pad considerations.
- The three hazards associated with electrosurgery used during laparoscopy are direct coupling, insulation failure, and capacitive coupling.
- Laser energy can cause photothermal, photoacoustic, or photochemical reactions.
- When laser energy impacts tissue it can be reflected, scattered, transmitted, or absorbed depending on the laser wavelength.
- Complying with laser safety guidelines is mandatory when laser energy is used during a surgical procedure. Some of these protocols include smoke evacuation, eye safety, fire safety, and controlled access.
- Nurses must be educated on different energies used during surgery to provide a safe environment for both patients and staff.

Critical Thinking Questions

You are the circulating nurse during surgery to excise a patient's vocal cord polyps using a CO_2 laser. You have received specialized laser education required to circulate during laser procedures. You understand the hazards associated with laser technology and when using a laser in the airway. What devices would you gather to provide a safe laser environment for the patient and the surgical team during this procedure? What critical assessment factors would you consider and what would you include as intraoperative nursing interventions as the laser team member?

evolve *The answers to the Critical Thinking Questions can be found at http://evolve.elsevier.com/Rothrock/Alexander.*

References

American National Standards Institute (ANSI): *American national standard for the safe use of lasers in health care facilities*, ANSI Z136.3, New York, 2011, ANSI.

Arezzo A: The past, present, and the future of minimally invasive therapy in laparoscopic surgery: a review and speculative outlook, *Minim Invasive Ther Allied Technol* 23(5):253–260, 2014.

Ashraf A et al: Three-dimensional (3D) simulation versus two-dimensional (2D) enhances surgical skills acquisition in standardized laparoscopic tasks: a before and after study, *Int J Surg* 14:12–16, 2015.

Association of periOperative Registered Nurses (AORN): *Guidelines for perioperative practice*, Denver, 2016, The Association.

Association of periOperative Registered Nurses (AORN): *Guidelines for perioperative practice*, Denver, 2017, The Association.

Ball K: Smoke evacuators, *Outpatient Surgery Magazine* XVII(1):130–131, 2016.

Brooks M: *FDA warns endoscopes may spread drug-resistant bacteria* (website), 2015. www.medscape.com/viewarticle/840057. (Accessed 28 September 2016).

Clements R et al: *Special report: improving precision and accuracy in laparoscopy using the Endoeye Flex 3D articulating videoscope* (website), 2014. www.generalsurgerynews.com/download/SR1316_WM.pdf. (Accessed 24 September 2016).

ECRI Institute: OR fires caused by fiberoptic illumination systems, *Health Devices* 211(7):148–149, 1982. www.mdsr.ecri.org/summary/detail.aspx?doc_id=8182. (Accessed 26 October 2016).

ECRI Institute: *Executive brief: top 10 patient safety concerns for healthcare organizations 2016* (website), 2016. https://www.ecri.org/EmailResources/PSRQ/Top10/2016_Top10_ExecutiveBrief_final.pdf. (Accessed 27 June 2017).

Government Accounting Office (GAO): *Reprocessed single-use medical devices: FDA oversight has increased, and available information does not indicate that use presents an elevated risk* (website), 2008. www.gao.gov/new.items/d08147.pdf. (Accessed 29 September 2016).

Intuitive Surgical, Inc: *Important patient safety information* (website), 2016. www.davincisurgery.com/da-vinci-surgery/safety-information.php. (Accessed 30 September 2016).

Jung M et al: Robotic general surgery: current practice, evidence, and perspective, *Langenbecks Arch Surg* 400(3):283–292, 2015.

Liu Q, Sun XB: Indirect electrosurgical injuries from capacitive coupling: a rarely mentioned electrosurgical complication in monopolar laparoscopy, *Acta Obstet Gynecol Scand* 92(2):238–241, 2013.

Muscarella L: Risk of transmission of carbapenem-resistant *Enterobacteriaceae* and related "superbugs" during gastrointestinal endoscopy, *World J Gastrointest Endosc* 6(10):457–474, 2014.

National Council of State Boards of Nursing (NCSBN): *NCSBN delegate assembly adopts revised nurse licensure compacts* (website), 2015. www.ncsbn.org/7320.htm. (Accessed 29 September 2016).

Pasriche PJ, Rivas H: *Natural orifice transluminal endoscopic surgery (NOTES)* (website), 2015. www.uptodate.com/contents/natural-orifice-transluminal-endoscopic-surgery-notes. (Accessed 30 September 2016).

Robinson TN et al: Antenna coupling—a novel mechanism of radiofrequency electrosurgery complication: practical implications, *Ann Surg* 256(2):213–218, 2012.

Rudolph R: *The highest level of imaging resolution yet* (website), 2015. www.mdtmag.com/article/2015/07/highest-level-imaging-resolution-yet. (Accessed 29 September 2016).

Schultz L: An analysis of surgical smoke plume components, capture, and evacuation, *AORN J* 99(2):289–298, 2014.

Smith FD: Caring for surgical patients with piercings, *AORN J* 103(6):583–593, 2016.

Stegemann AP et al: Laparoscopy and robotics: fundamental skills of robotic surgery: a multi-institutional randomized controlled trial for validation of a simulation-based curriculum, *Urology* 81(4):767–774, 2013.

Taylor D: A reflection on the experiences of implementing gynaecology robotic surgery, *J Perioper Pract* 26(3):36–41, 2016.

US Food and Drug Administration (FDA): *Guidance for industry and FDA staff: medical device user fee and modernization act of 2002, validation data in pre-market notification submissions (510(k)s) for reprocessed single-use medical devices* (website), 2006. www.fda.gov/medicaldevices/deviceregulationandguidance/guidancedocuments/ucm071434.htm. (Accessed 12 October 2016).

CHAPTER 9

Wound Healing, Dressings, and Drains

JACQUELINE R. BAK

The ability to heal wounds is one of the most powerful defensive properties humans possess. Wound healing is a complex, highly organized response by an organism to tissue disruption caused by injury. This process is highly reliable in the absence of endogenous and exogenous infection, mechanical interference, or certain disease processes. Apposition and maintenance of the edges of a cleanly incised wound almost always result in prompt healing. A primary goal of perioperative patient care is the prevention of surgical site (wound) infections. Surgical site infections (SSIs) are a significant cause of illness, death, and excessive healthcare costs. Surgical wounds have the potential for infection from strains of antibiotic-resistant bacteria, such as methicillin-resistant *Staphylococcus aureus* (MRSA), methicillin-sensitive *Staphylococcus aureus* (MSSA), and vancomycin-resistant enterococci (VRE) (Research Highlight).

RESEARCH HIGHLIGHT

Epidemiology of Surgical Site Infections

SSIs have an economic impact and are likely to increase hospital stay, affect admission to the intensive care unit, and impact multiple readmissions. With this in mind it is important to understand and identify the causative pathogens associated with SSIs, the outcomes, and preventative measures. The purpose of this study was to determine whether a preoperative staphylococcus screening and treatment program would decrease the incidence of SSI in elective joint arthroplasty patients. The study was conducted over a 5-year period (2009–2014) and had a total of 9690 patients who met the selection criteria of having an elective joint arthroplasty and were screened before surgery for MRSA and MSSA with nares swabs, with patients from the previous year and 2008 serving as the control. All patients with positive nares colonization for MSSA and MRSA were treated with mupirocin and chlorhexidine gluconate showers for 5 days before surgery. MRSA patients received vancomycin preoperatively and were placed in contact isolation. All elective arthroplasty patients used chlorhexidine gluconate antiseptic cloths the evening prior and the day of surgery.

SSI rates decreased from 1.11% (prescreening) to 0.34% (nasal screening; *p* < .05) after initiation of the process. *Staphylococcus* was identified in 66.7% of the SSI infections before nasal screening and in 33.3% of the SSI patients after routine screening (*p* > .05). The researchers concluded that the addition of the nares screening along with perioperative decolonization protocol resulted in a 69% decrease in SSI rate.

MRSA, Methicillin-resistant *Staphylococcus aureus; MSSA,* methicillin-sensitive *Staphylococcus aureus; SSI,* surgical site infection.
Modified from Sporer SM et al: Methicillin-resistant and methicillin-sensitive staphylococcus aureus screening and decolonization to reduce surgical site infection in elective total joint arthroplasty, *J Arthroplasty* 31(9 Suppl):144–147, 2016.

Postoperative SSIs are a common and serious complication that affects approximately 2% to 5% of the 30 to 40 million individuals undergoing surgery annually in the United States, with SSIs as the second most commonly reported hospital-associated infection (HAI). Patients with SSIs have markedly higher mortality rates, increased lengths of stay, hospital readmission rates, and direct patient costs when compared with patients without an SSI (Rosenberger and Sawyer, 2014).

Although many surgeries are performed on an ambulatory basis and the average number of admissions to hospitals and length of stay have steadily decreased over the last decade, the incidence of HAIs has increased (Ambulatory Surgery Considerations). In response to the Deficit Reduction Act of 2005, the Centers for Medicare and Medicaid Services (CMS) modified payment for selected reasonably preventable complicating conditions known as hospital-acquired conditions (HACs), which have evidence-based prevention guidelines. Examples of these conditions are catheter-related infections and infections associated with coronary artery bypass grafts, certain orthopedic procedures, and certain bariatric surgery procedures. Additions and specifications to surgical procedures noted in 2013 were SSI after cardiac implantable electronic device, foreign object retained after surgery, and deep vein thrombosis/pulmonary embolism after total knee and hip replacement (CMS, 2015). Actions taken by perioperative personnel sometimes can mean the difference between developing an SSI and normal healing. A clear understanding of these actions along with a solid knowledge of wound healing and factors adversely affecting healing are essential to the appropriate management of patients undergoing surgery. It is also imperative in light of the evolving CMS-implemented reduction in payment for an expanding array of avoidable conditions, which include wound-related infections.

Anatomy

The skin is the largest organ of the body and acts as the first line of defense against infection. It provides protection and sensation, regulates fluid balance and temperature, and produces vitamins (e.g., vitamin D) and immune system components. The skin of the average adult covers about 3000 square inches, weighs about 6 pounds, and receives one-third of the body's circulating blood volume. It varies in thickness from 0.5 mm in the tympanic membrane to 6 mm on the soles of the feet and the palms of the hands. Key structures of the skin are the primary layers of the epidermis, the dermis, and the subcutaneous. The *epidermis* is the outermost layer of the skin, lines the ear canals, and is contiguous with the mucous membranes. The epidermis is composed of several layers consisting of keratin and lipids. Keratin is the primary substance that hardens nails and hair and protects the body from fluid loss and invasion by pathogens. The epidermis is supported by the *dermis,* which is thicker than the epidermis and composed of collagen. The dermis is the largest portion

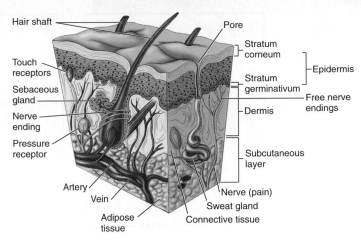

FIG. 9.1 The skin.

of the skin, providing strength and structure. Contained within the dermis are blood vessels, lymph ducts, hair roots, nerves, and sebaceous and sweat glands. The dermis is vascularized and innervated (Fig. 9.1). The innermost *subcutaneous* layer is composed of adipose tissue that merges with the deepest layer of the dermis to provide insulation, shape, and support. Any wound or disruption of the skin can provide a portal for bacteria and possible infection.

Etiology of Wounds

The causes of wounds can be described as follows:
- *Surgical:* caused by an incision or excision
- *Traumatic:* caused by mechanical, thermal, or chemical destruction
- *Chronic:* caused by an underlying pathophysiologic condition (e.g., pressure ulcers or venous stasis ulcers) over time

The amount of tissue loss, the existence of contamination or infection, and the degree of damage to tissue are some factors that determine the type of wound closure selected by the surgeon. The healing process is inherently related to whether the wound is closed or left open. This process occurs in one of three ways: primary intention, second intention (granulation and contraction), and third intention (delayed closure) (Fig. 9.2).

Types of Wound Closure

Primary Intention

Healing through primary intention occurs when wounds are created aseptically, with a minimum of tissue destruction and postoperative tissue reaction. Wounds closed with sutures, staples, tape, or surgical adhesive applied as soon after the time of injury as possible fall into

this category. When wounds are created under sterile conditions, healing is optimized and begins almost immediately. This type of healing is known as primary intention and occurs under the following conditions:
- Edges of an incised wound in a healthy individual are promptly and accurately approximated.
- Contamination is held to a minimum by rigid adherence to aseptic technique.
- Trauma is minimal.
- No tissue loss occurs.
- On completion of closure, no dead space remains to become a potential site of infection.
- Drainage is minimal.

Second Intention (Granulation and Contraction)

When surgical wounds are characterized by tissue loss with an inability to approximate wound edges, healing occurs through second intention (see Fig. 9.2). This type of wound is usually not closed; instead, it is allowed to heal from the inside toward the outer surface. In infected wounds this process allows the proper cleansing and dressing of the wound as healthy collagen tissue expands from the inside. The area of tissue loss gradually fills with granulation tissue, comprising fibroblasts and capillaries. Scar tissue is extensive because of the size of the tissue gap that must be closed. The scar is referred to as a *cicatrix*. Contraction of surrounding tissue also occurs. Consequently this healing process takes longer than primary intention healing. Healing by second intention is often seen in chronic wounds, dirty wounds, and traumatic wounds in which large areas of tissue are lost.

Delayed Primary Closure or Third Intention

As the name *delayed primary closure* implies, this healing process occurs when approximation of wound edges is intentionally delayed by 3 or more days after injury or surgery (see Fig. 9.2). These wounds may require debridement and usually require a primary and secondary suture line, such as when retention sutures are used. The conditions leading to a decision to delay closure are as follows:
- Removal of an inflamed organ
- Heavy contamination of the wound
- The critical nature of the patient's intraoperative condition, such as with hemodynamically unstable trauma patients

▶
Healing
by First
Intention

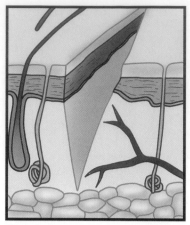
Clean incision

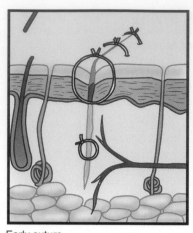
Early suture

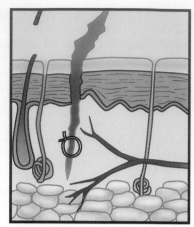
"Hairline" scar

An aseptically made wound with minimal tissue destruction and minimal tissue reaction begins to heal as the edges are approximated by close sutures or staples. No open areas or dead spaces are left to serve as potential sites of infection.

▶
Healing by
Second
Intention
(Granulation)
and
Contraction

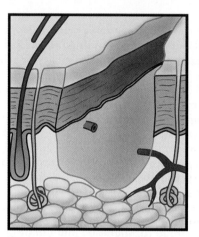
Gaping, irregular wound

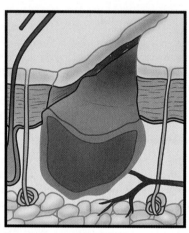
Granulation and contraction

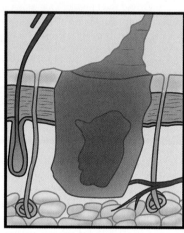
Growth of epithelium over scar

An infected or chronic wound or one with tissue damage so extensive that the edges cannot be smoothly approximated is usually left open and allowed to heal from the inside out. The nurse periodically cleans and assesses the wound for healthy tissue production. Scar tissue is extensive, and healing is prolonged.

▶
Healing by
Third
Intention
(Delayed
Closure)

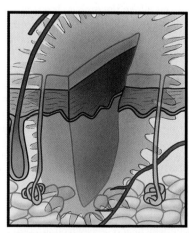
Infected wound

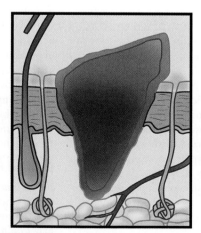
Granulation

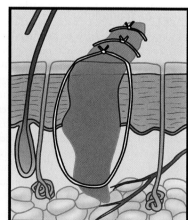
Closure with wide scar

A potentially infected surgical wound may be left open for several days. If no clinical signs of infection occur, the wound is then closed surgically.

FIG. 9.2 Processes of wound healing.

Phases of Wound Healing

Wound healing is the effort of the injured tissue to return to normal integrity after injury. It is an intricate biologic process that occurs in three simultaneous yet overlapping phases: (1) inflammatory (also known as the reactive stage) with increased vascular permeability, (2) proliferative (also known as the regenerative stage) characterized by granulation, and (3) remodeling (also known as the maturational stage) with noted wound contraction (Leong et al., 2017) (Fig. 9.3).

Inflammatory Phase

In the inflammatory phase, an exudate containing blood, lymph, and fibrin begins to clot and loosely binds the cut edges together. Blood supply to the area increases, and the basic process of inflammation begins. Inflammation is a prerequisite to wound healing and is a vascular and cellular response to dispose of bacteria, foreign material, and dead tissue. Leukocytes increase in number to fight bacteria in the wound area and by phagocytosis help to remove damaged tissues. The severed tissue is quickly glued together by strands of fibrin and a thin layer of clotted blood, forming a scab. Plasma seeps to the surface to form a dry, protective crust. This seal helps prevent fluid loss and bacterial invasion. During the first few days of wound healing, however, the seal has little tensile strength. The inflammatory phase normally lasts 1 to 4 days. The skin edges may appear mildly swollen and slightly red in this phase as a result of the inflammatory processes at work. Many chronic wounds "stall" at this phase.

Proliferative Phase

The proliferative phase, beginning within hours of the injury, allows new epithelium to cover the wound. Epithelial cells migrate and proliferate to the wound area, covering the surface of the wound to close the epithelial defect. Epithelialization also provides a protective barrier to prevent fluid and electrolyte loss and to reduce the incidence of infection. While reepithelialization takes place collagen synthesis and wound contraction are occurring. Contraction begins approximately 5 days after the wound onset and peaks at 2 weeks, gradually shrinking the entire wound. Granulation tissue forms under the edges of the incision and can be palpated as a hard ridge, which eventually resolves during the remodeling phase. Epidermal migration is limited to about 3 cm from the point of origin. Larger wounds may require skin grafting because of this limited epidermal migration.

Collagen synthesis produces fiber molecules that crosslink to provide strength to the wound.

Remodeling Phase

Remodeling begins after approximately 2 to 4 weeks, depending on the size and nature of the wound. It may last 1 year or longer. During the remodeling phase, scar tissue formed during fibroplasia changes in bulk, form, and strength. Throughout normal wound healing, new collagen is produced while old collagen breaks down in a balanced fashion. This collagen turnover allows randomly deposited connective tissue to be arranged in linear and lateral orientation. As the scar ages, fibers and fiber bundles become more closely packed and form a crisscross pattern, ultimately creating the final shape of the wound. At best, the tensile strength of scar tissue is never more than about 80% of the tensile strength of nonwounded tissue.

Factors Affecting Wound Healing

Patients should be assessed for factors that may impair wound healing. Important factors in tissue repair and healing to consider are the patient's age, physical status, preexisting conditions, nutritional status, oxygenation level, and overall recuperative power. The inflammatory response and oxygen tension depend on microcirculation to deliver components to the wound. Decreased oxygen tension to the wound area inhibits fibroblast migration and collagen synthesis, resulting in decreased tensile strength of the wound. Nutritional status also has a profound effect on healing because of the need for an adequate supply of protein necessary for the growth of new tissues. Procedural factors that also influence wound healing are very much in the forefront, such as adherence to preoperative infection control measures including skin preparation, surgical scrub, and preoperative hand antisepsis. Other surgical influences include duration of procedure, appropriate antibiotic prophylaxis, operating room (OR) environment, sterilization procedures, sterile technique, and surgical items (Lynden and Dellinger, 2016).

The most common cause of delayed wound healing in a surgical patient is SSI. Box 9.1 lists the types of SSIs and defines criteria for classification. There are many possible causes of SSIs, including patient susceptibility to and severity of illness, microbial contamination by the patient's microflora, and exogenous wound contamination from the OR environment and personnel. Adherence to strict aseptic principles, careful observation of sterile technique, and thorough antimicrobial preparation of the patient and operative site are essential to minimize the risk of postoperative SSIs. Perioperative personnel who are not scrubbed at the sterile field must maintain meticulous hand hygiene during the procedure to decrease the transmission of bacteria to the surgical field or the patient (Patient Safety).

Wound healing also can be impaired by poor surgical technique. Rough handling of tissue may cause trauma that can lead to bleeding and other conditions conducive to infection. Examples of surgical technique promoting wound healing include adequate hemostasis, precise cutting and suturing techniques, efficient use of time to minimize wound exposure to air, elimination of dead spaces, and minimal pressure from retractors and other instruments.

Additional factors affecting wound healing are the patient's age, stress level, immunologic status, and smoking history. Preexisting conditions, such as diabetes, anemia, malnutrition, cancer, obesity, certain drug therapies (e.g., steroid therapy), and cardiovascular or respiratory impairments, also contribute to poor wound healing. Additional terms used in connection with wound healing are shown in Box 9.2.

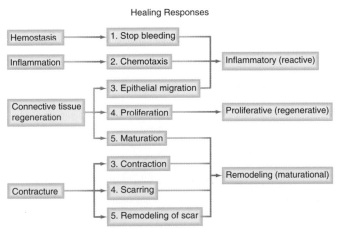

FIG. 9.3 Schematic diagram of the wound-healing continuum.

BOX 9.1

Criteria for Defining a Surgical Site Infection: Reportable Infections

Superficial Incisional Surgical Site Infection
- Infection occurs within 30 days after the procedure.
- Involves only skin or subcutaneous tissue of the incision *and* at least *one* of the following:
  1. Purulent drainage, with or without laboratory confirmation, from the superficial incision.
  2. Organisms isolated from an aseptically obtained culture of fluid or tissue from the superficial incision.
  3. At least one of the following signs or symptoms of infection, such as pain or tenderness, localized swelling, redness, or heat, *and* superficial incision is deliberately opened by surgeon, *unless* incision is culture-negative.
  4. Diagnosis of superficial incisional SSI by the surgeon or attending physician.

Deep Incisional Surgical Site Infection
- Infection occurs within 30 days after the procedure if no implant[a] is left in place or within 1 year if implant is in place and the infection appears to be related to the procedure.
- Infection involves deep soft tissues (e.g., fascial and muscle layers) of the incision *and* at least *one* of the following:
  1. Purulent drainage from the deep incision but not from the organ/space component of the surgical site.
  2. A deep incision spontaneously dehisces or is deliberately opened by a surgeon when the patient has at least one of the following signs or symptoms: fever greater than 100.4°F (>38°C), localized pain, or tenderness, unless site is culture-negative.

3. An abscess or other evidence of infection involving the deep incision is found on direct examination, during reoperation, or by histopathologic or radiologic examination.
4. Diagnosis of a deep incisional SSI by a surgeon or attending physician.

Note:
- Report infection that involves both superficial and deep incision sites as deep incisional SSI.
- Report an organ/space SSI that drains through the incision as a deep incisional SSI.

Organ/Space Surgical Site Infection
- Infection occurs within 30 days after the procedure if no implant[a] is left in place or within 1 year if implant is in place and the infection appears to be related to the procedure.
- Infection involves any part of the anatomy (e.g., organs or spaces), other than the incision, which was opened or manipulated during a procedure *and* at least *one* of the following:
  1. Purulent drainage from a drain that is placed through a stab wound[b] into the organ/space
  2. Organisms isolated from an aseptically obtained culture of fluid or tissue in the organ/space
  3. An abscess or other evidence of infection involving the organ/space that is found on direct examination, during reoperation, or by histopathologic or radiologic examination
  4. Diagnosis of an organ/space SSI by a surgeon or attending physician

[a]National Nosocomial Infection Surveillance definition: a nonhuman-derived implantable foreign body (e.g., prosthetic heart valve, nonhuman vascular graft, mechanical heart, or hip prosthesis) that is permanently placed in a patient during surgery.
[b]If the area around a stab wound becomes infected, it is not an SSI. It is considered a skin or soft tissue infection, depending on its depth.
SSI, Surgical site infection.
Modified from Mangram AJ et al: Guideline for prevention of surgical site infection, 1999, *Am J Infect Control* 27(2):97–132, 1999.

PATIENT SAFETY

Perioperative Handwashing

TJC has made patient safety a priority through annual NPSGs. One NPSG is reducing the risk of HAIs (TJC, 2016). One of the criteria for meeting this goal is for organizations to comply with the current hand hygiene recommendations from the CDC or the WHO. Perioperative nurses are especially vigilant about complying with hand hygiene guidelines. Patients are vulnerable whenever their intact skin barrier is breached. Activities that are not properly conducted in a sterile fashion, such as application of surgical dressings to a fresh incision, provide an opportunity for entry of pathogens. HCWs often have a false sense of security about the protection that gloves offer and may think that frequent hand hygiene is unnecessary. Use of gloves cannot replace routine, faithful adherence to effective hand hygiene. Effective hand hygiene is the easiest, least expensive, and most effective tool that perioperative nurses have when acting as a patient advocate. The goal of hand hygiene is a sufficient reduction of microbial counts on the skin to prevent cross-contamination of pathogens. Good hand hygiene practices also provide safety and protection to the HCW.

After extensive research, the WHO along with the CDC has published guidelines for hand hygiene. The guidelines are ranked by category ratings, which provide direction to facilities for implementation.

Category I rankings (IA and IB) are applicable to all settings and should be adopted; they are listed here.

Rankings
Indications for Hand Hygiene
Category IA
- If hands are not visibly soiled, use an alcohol-based hand rub for routinely decontaminating hands.
- Perform hand hygiene after contact with body fluids or excretions, mucous membranes, nonintact skin, and wound dressings.

Category IB
Perform hand hygiene:
- Before and after having direct contact with patients.
- Before handling an invasive device for patient care; gloved or ungloved.

PATIENT SAFETY

Perioperative Handwashing—cont'd

- When moving from a contaminated body site to another body site during care of the same patient.
- After removing nonsterile gloves.
- After contact with inanimate surfaces, objects, medical equipment in immediate vicinity of patient.
- If alcohol-based hand rub is not obtainable, wash hands with soap and water.
- Wash hands with soap and water when visibly dirty or visibly soiled with blood or other body fluids.
- Handwashing with soap and water is the preferred method if exposure to potential spore-forming pathogens is strongly suggested or proven, including outbreaks of *Clostridium difficile.*
- Use an alcohol-based hand rub or wash hands with plain or antimicrobial soap and water before handling medication or preparing food.

Hand Hygiene Techniques
Category IB
- Apply a palmful of alcohol-based hand rub and cover all surfaces of hands. Rub hands until dry.
- When washing hands with soap and water, wet hands first with water, then apply an amount of product necessary to cover all surfaces. Rinse hands with water and dry thoroughly with a single-use towel. Use clean, running water whenever possible. Avoid using hot water, because repeated exposure to hot water may increase the risk of dermatitis.
- Use a towel to turn off tap/faucet.
- Dry hands thoroughly using a method that does not recontaminate hands. Make sure towels are not used multiple times or by multiple people.

Recommendations for Surgical Hand Preparation
Category IB
- Artificial nails are prohibited.
- Brushes are not recommended for surgical hand preparation.
- Surgical hand antisepsis should be performed using either a suitable antimicrobial soap or suitable alcohol-based hand rub, preferably with a product ensuring sustained activity, before donning sterile gloves.
- When performing surgical hand antisepsis using an antimicrobial soap, scrub hands and forearms for the length of time recommended by the manufacturer, typically 2 to 5 minutes. Long scrub times (e.g., 10 minutes) are not necessary.
- When using an alcohol-based surgical hand rub product with sustained activity, follow the manufacturer's instructions for application times. Apply the product to dry hands only.
- When using an alcohol-based hand rub, use sufficient product to keep hands and forearms wet with the hand rub throughout the surgical hand preparation procedure.
- After application of the alcohol-based hand rub as recommended, allow all hands and forearms to dry thoroughly before donning sterile gloves.

Selection of Hand Hygiene Agents
Category IA
- Do not add soap to a partially empty soap dispenser. If soap dispensers are reused, follow recommended procedures for cleaning.

Category IB
- Provide HCWs with efficacious hand hygiene products that have low irritancy.
- To maximize acceptance of hand hygiene products by HCWs, solicit their input regarding the skin tolerance, feel, and fragrance of any products under consideration. When selecting hand hygiene products:
- Solicit information from manufacturers about the risk of product contamination.
- Ensure that dispensers are accessible at the point of care.
- Elicit and evaluate information from manufacturers regarding any effects that hand lotions, creams, or alcohol-based hand rubs may have on the efficacy of antimicrobial soaps being used in the institution.

Skin Care
Category IA
- Provide HCWs with hand lotions or creams to minimize the occurrence of irritant contact dermatitis associated with hand antisepsis or handwashing.

Category IB
- Include information regarding hand-care practices designed to reduce the risk of irritant contact dermatitis and other skin damage in education programs for HCWs.

Use of Gloves
Category IB
- Using gloves does not replace the need for hand hygiene by either hand rubs or handwashing.
- Remove gloves after caring for a patient. Do not wear the same pair of gloves for the care of more than one patient.
- Reusing gloves is not recommended.

Other Aspects of Hand Hygiene
Category IA
- Do not wear artificial fingernails or extenders when having direct contact with patients.

Category	Ranking System for Evidence
IA	Strongly recommended for implementation and strongly supported by well-designed experimental, clinical, or epidemiologic studies
IB	Strongly recommended for implementation and supported by some experimental, clinical, or epidemiologic studies and a strong theoretic rationale

CDC, Centers for Disease Control and Prevention; *HCW,* healthcare worker; *NPSGs,* National Patient Safety Goals; *TJC,* The Joint Commission; *WHO,* World Health Organization.
Modified from The Joint Commission: *2016 hospital national patient safety goals* (website), 2016. https://www.jointcommission.org/assets/1/6/2016_NPSG_HAP_ER.pdf. (Accessed 26 November 2016); *Hand hygiene in healthcare settings* (website), 2011. www.cdc.gov/Handhygiene. (Accessed 26 November 2016).

Additional Terms Used in Connection With Wound Healing

Adhesions: Adherence of serous membranes to one another, causing fibrous tissue to form; sometimes occur in healing and inflammatory processes; commonly occur in or around gastrointestinal tract, in which adhesions may form bands and cause obstructions and subsequent surgical emergencies.

Chemotaxis: A cellular function, particularly of neutrophils and monocytes, whose phagocytic activity is influenced by chemical factors released by invading microorganisms.

Dead space: Air or empty space between layers of tissue or beneath wound edges that have been approximated.

Dehiscence: Separation of layers of surgical wound (Fig. 9.4).

Evisceration: Extrusion of internal organs or viscera through gaping wound (see Fig. 9.4).

Gangrene: Anaerobic infection process that may occur instead of healing; implies necrosis (death of tissue) and putrefaction (decomposition); usually caused by failure of nutriment or blood to reach a part.

Keloid: Dense, unsightly connective tissue or excessive scar formation that is often removed surgically.

"Proud flesh": A mass of excessive granulation formed when a wound shows no other sign of healing or excessive cicatrization.

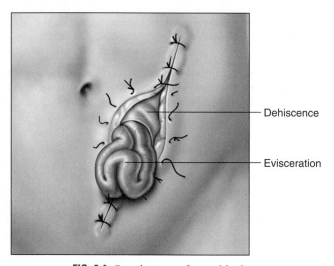

— Dehiscence

— Evisceration

FIG. 9.4 Complications of wound healing.

Wound Classification

The Centers for Disease Control and Prevention (CDC) have long recommended four surgical wound classifications: clean wounds, clean contaminated wounds, contaminated wounds, and dirty or infected wounds. This classification scheme reflects the probability of infection and enables appropriate preventive measures to be taken. The Association of periOperative Registered Nurses (AORN) *Guideline for Prevention of Transmissible Infection* notes the importance of documenting the wound classification in the patient record (AORN, 2017). Following are descriptions of each classification.

Clean Wounds (Class I)

Clean wounds are uninfected wounds in which no inflammation is encountered, and the respiratory, alimentary, and genitourinary tracts are not entered. They are closed with a primary suture line. If required,

they can be drained using a closed wound drainage system. Clean wounds show no sign of infection. Examples are breast biopsy, total hip replacement, and open heart surgery.

Clean Contaminated Wounds (Class II)

Clean contaminated wounds are those in which the respiratory, alimentary, or genitourinary tract is entered under controlled conditions. There is no sign of infection and no break in surgical aseptic technique. Examples of clean contaminated wounds are nonperforated appendectomy, hysterectomy, and thoracotomy.

Contaminated Wounds (Class III)

Contaminated wounds are open, fresh, accidental wounds, such as penetrating trauma, open fractures, or operations with major breaks in aseptic technique, such as the inadvertent intraoperative use of nonsterile instruments or supplies. Incisions with signs of infection or gross spillage from the gastrointestinal tract also are included. Examples are a penetrating abdominal trauma involving bowel and a gunshot wound to the abdomen.

Dirty or Infected Wounds (Class IV)

Infected wounds include old, physically induced (traumatic) wounds with retained devitalized tissue and wounds that involve an existing clinical infection or perforated viscera. Examples are excision and drainage of abscess and delayed primary closure of a wound after appendectomy for ruptured appendix.

Antimicrobial Prophylaxis

The most effective course of action in dealing with SSI is prevention. Appropriate antimicrobial prophylaxis (antibiotic administration) also is an important factor in the prevention of SSI (Evidence for Practice). Major considerations in administering prophylactic antimicrobial therapy include selecting the appropriate agent, properly timing the administration of the agent, and limiting the duration of therapy.

Proper selection of the prophylactic antimicrobial agent is based on clinical efficacy, safety, cost, and whether the agent is broad spectrum. The surgeon commonly considers the nature of the surgical procedure, noting the most common pathogens associated with it (e.g., common pathogens of the small bowel in undertaking a small-bowel resection). Cephalosporins often are used for elective clean or clean contaminated surgical procedures. For these procedures a single dose usually is administered during the immediate preoperative period. It is important to carefully evaluate the need for antibiotics with the emergence of antibiotic-resistant microorganisms.

To enhance the effectiveness of prophylactic antimicrobial therapy, it is necessary for the optimal level of the antibiotic to be present in the tissue at the time of the incision. Equally important is the need to maintain circulating blood levels throughout some procedures. The antibiotic of choice should be administered within 1 hour before the skin incision. The anesthesia provider usually administers the antibiotic intravenously. If the surgical procedure is longer than the half-life of the antibiotic, another dose usually is administered intravenously during the procedure. Antibiotic therapy is usually discontinued within 24 hours; there is little evidence that ongoing administration contributes to decreased SSI rates in clean or clean contaminated procedures.

Nursing Diagnoses

The nursing diagnoses (Risk for Infection, Risk for Impaired Skin Integrity, Imbalanced Nutrition: Less than Body Requirements,

EVIDENCE FOR PRACTICE

Antimicrobial Prophylaxis

According to the Institute for Healthcare Improvement an estimated 40% to 60% of SSIs are preventable with appropriate use of prophylactic antibiotics with an average between 2% and 3% occurring in clean cases (Class I as defined by the CDC). Overuse, underuse, improper timing, or misuse of antibiotics occurs in 25% to 50% of operations. A large number of hospitalized patients develop infections caused by *Clostridium difficile,* and 16% of this type of infection in surgical patients can be attributed to inappropriate prophylaxis use alone. Inappropriate use of broad-spectrum antibiotics or prolonged courses of prophylactic antibiotics puts all patients at even greater health risks because of the development of antibiotic-resistant pathogens. Suggestions for improvements regarding appropriate use of prophylactic antibiotics are described in the following list:

- Use preprinted or computerized standing orders specifying antibiotic, timing, dose, and discontinuation.
- Develop pharmacist-driven and nurse-driven protocols that include preoperative antibiotic selection and dosing based on surgical type and patient-specific criteria (age, weight, allergies, renal clearance, etc.).
- Change operating drug room stocks to include only standard doses and standard drugs, reflecting national guidelines.
- Assign dosing responsibilities to anesthesia or designated nurse (e.g., preop holding or circulator) to improve timeliness.
- Involve pharmacy, infection control, and infectious disease staff to ensure appropriate timing, selection, and duration.
- Verify administration timing duration "time-out" or preprocedural b riefing so action can be taken if not administered.

CDC, Centers for Disease Control and Prevention; *SSI,* surgical site infection.
From Institute for Healthcare Improvement: *How-to guide: prevent surgical site infections.* Cambridge, MA, 2012.

PATIENT ENGAGEMENT EXEMPLAR

Postoperative Wound Care

Wound care requires patient, family, and caregiver knowledge of the process and requires a strategy for successful patient engagement. The teach-back method is a health literacy strategy that serves to improve patient and provider communication and patient understanding. The perioperative nurse instructs the patient on his or her wound care and then asks the patient to recall in his or her own words the information he or she has been given. This permits the patient to process the information in a way that demonstrates understanding and is also meaningful to him or her. Ask Me 3 is often used with the teach-back method and encourages patients to ask three questions of any healthcare provider:

1. What is my main problem?
2. What do I need to do?
3. Why is it important for me to do this?

Allowing patients to ask these three questions engages them in their care and helps them to understand clearly why they need to follow the instructions and what they need to do to care for their own surgical wound.

With these techniques, the perioperative nurse can have a reasonable certainty that the patient, family, and caregiver understand their wound care instructions.

Modified from Teach-Back Toolkit: *Always use teach back! Training toolkit* (website), 2016. www.teachbacktraining.org/. (Accessed 4 December 2016); National Patient Safety Foundation (NPSF): *Ask me 3: good questions for your good health* (website), 2016. www.npsf.org/?page=askme3. (Accessed 4 December 2016).

providers instead of by the hospital nurse. Early planning and teaching about wound care and Standard Precautions are vital in the prevention of SSI and in preparing patients for discharge (Patient Engagement Exemplar). In a convenience sample (Anderson et al., 2013) 50 patients were surveyed to determine awareness and knowledge regarding risks and consequences of prevention of SSI. The researchers found that 26% of respondents thought that education for SSI prevention could be improved and that 16% could not recall discussing SSI risks and prevention with a healthcare worker. Only 60% of patients recalled receiving an informational flyer in the hospital. The results of the study showed that better educational and engagement interventions that incorporated patient preferences were needed to promote awareness and patient engagement regarding the prevention of SSI.

Wound Management

A variety of treatments exist for acute and chronic wound management. Perioperative nurses often care for patients with infected wounds and are familiar with surgical wound debridement and sterile dressing changes performed under anesthesia. Patients also may come to the OR with chronic wounds being managed with a combination of surgical interventions and other treatment modalities. An understanding of adjunct wound therapies is essential to planning perioperative nursing care. These therapies include hyperbaric oxygenation (HBO), negative pressure therapy, hydrotherapy, use of engineered living skin substitutes, and the topical application of growth factors.

Debridement

Debridement is the act of removing dead and devitalized tissue from a wound. It is necessary because dead tissue in the wound provides a nidus for wound infection. Perioperative nurses often care for patients scheduled for surgical wound debridement (i.e., the sharp

Ineffective Peripheral Tissue Perfusion, and Risk for Perioperative Hypothermia) point the perioperative nurse toward strategies that can be used to prevent wound infections and promote healing.

The World Health Organization (WHO) provides SSI prevention guidelines for consideration in planning and implementing nursing interventions to optimize successful patient outcomes (Box 9.3). The nurse assesses the patient's susceptibility for infection; including preexisting conditions, classifies the wound on the intraoperative record, implements and monitors sterile technique, protects the patient from cross-contamination, and collaborates in administration of antibiotic prophylaxis. The perioperative nurse performs other responsibilities to create and control the environment of care such as nursing measures to ensure normothermia and decrease room traffic. Attention is also given to controlling perioperative serum glucose levels in major surgical procedures, to maintaining skin integrity through proper positioning and the use of pressure-reducing mattresses as needed (see Chapter 6), and to using safe practices during electrosurgery (see Chapter 8). The perioperative nurse plays an essential role in preventing adverse events and patient injury by using critical thinking, clinical reasoning, and technical knowledge.

Patient, Family, and Caregiver Education and Discharge Planning

Given that more patients are discharged from the acute care setting to the home care setting much earlier in their recovery, more surgical wound care is delivered by patients, their families, and home care

---

BOX 9.3

Guidelines for Prevention of Surgical Site Infections From the World Health Organization

SSIs account for 14% to 16% of all hospital-acquired infections. An understanding of the guidelines for preventing SSIs enables perioperative nurses to weigh factors that are viewed as effective in preventing SSIs. The following guidelines from WHO are based on a review of evidence and research. They focus on hand hygiene, appropriate and judicious use of antibiotics, antiseptic skin preparation at the surgical site, wound care, and instrument decontamination and sterility. As with many of the recent AORN guidelines, these potentially beneficial practices are classified into categories on the basis of clinical evidence or expert opinion as to their ability to reduce the likelihood of serious, avoidable surgical harm. If adherence was unlikely to introduce injury, was only to "be considered" for surgical procedures, or was of unmanageable cost, it is not included here.

Highly Recommended (Practice That Should Be in Place in Every Procedure)

- Prophylactic antibiotics should be used routinely in all clean contaminated surgical procedures and considered for use in any clean surgical procedure. When antibiotics are given prophylactically to prevent infection, they should be administered within 1 hour of incision (this is also an SCIP infection measure) at a dosage and with an antimicrobial spectrum that is effective against the pathogens likely to contaminate the procedure. During the time-out, and before skin incision, the team should confirm that prophylactic antibiotics were given within the past 60 minutes. (When vancomycin is used, infusion should be completed within 1 hour of skin incision.)
- Every facility should have a routine sterilization process that includes the means for verifying the sterility of all surgical instruments, devices, and materials. Indicators should be used to determine sterility and checked before equipment is introduced onto the sterile field. Before induction of anesthesia, the nurse or other person responsible for preparing the surgical trays should confirm the sterility of the instruments by evaluating the sterility indicators and should communicate any problems to the surgeon and anesthesia provider. (See Chapter 4 for a full discussion of sterilization processes and indicators.)
- Redosing with prophylactic antibiotics should be considered if the surgical procedure lasts more than 4 hours or if there is evidence of excessive intraoperative bleeding. (When vancomycin is used as the prophylactic agent, there is no need for redosing in operations lasting less than 10 hours.)

- Antibiotics used for prophylaxis should be discontinued within 24 hours of the procedure.
- Hair should not be removed unless it will interfere with the procedure. If hair is removed, it should be clipped less than 2 hours before the procedure. Shaving is not recommended because it increases the risk for SSI.
- Surgical patients should receive oxygen throughout the perioperative period according to individual requirements and intraoperative fire safety precautions.
- Measures to maintain core normothermia should be instituted throughout the perioperative period.
- The skin at the surgical site should be prepared with an appropriate antiseptic agent before surgery. The antimicrobial agent should decrease the microbial count of the skin rapidly and have persistent efficacy throughout the procedure.
- Surgical hand antisepsis (rub or scrub) should be performed with an antimicrobial agent approved by the facility. The hands and forearms should be scrubbed for 2 to 5 minutes. If the hands are physically clean, an alcohol-based hand antiseptic agent can be used for antisepsis as long as manufacturer's instructions are followed.
- The OR team should cover all hair and wear sterile gowns and sterile gloves during the procedure.

Recommended (Practice That Is Encouraged for Every Procedure)

- "On call" orders for administration of antibiotic prophylaxis should be discouraged.
- If hair is to be removed, the use of depilatories is discouraged.
- Tobacco use should be stopped at least 30 days before elective surgery if possible.
- Patients should take up to three preoperative showers or baths with antiseptic soap such as CHG.
- Prior infections should be eliminated before a scheduled procedure.
- The operating team should wear masks during the procedure.
- Surgical drapes should be effective barriers to the transmission of microorganisms.
- Sterile dressings should be applied over the surgical wound and maintained for 24 to 48 hours.
- Active surveillance for SSIs should be conducted prospectively by trained infection control practitioners.
- Information on the SSI rate should be provided to surgeons and appropriate administrators.

AORN, Association of periOperative Registered Nurses; *CHG,* chlorhexidine gluconate; *SCIP,* surgical care improvement project; *SSI,* surgical site infection; *WHO,* World Health Organization.
Modified from Allegranzi B et al: New WHO recommendations on preoperative measures for surgical site infection prevention: an evidence-based global perspective, *Lancet Infect Dis* 16(12):e276–287, 2016; Institute for Healthcare Improvement: *How-to guide: prevent surgical site infections* (website), 2012. www.ihi.org/resources/Pages/Tools/HowtoGuidePreventSurgicalSiteInfection .aspx. (Accessed 17 November 2016).

---

excision of dead or devitalized tissue). Debridement also can be accomplished through mechanical means (forceful irrigation), enzymatic action (application of chemical agents), and biologic methods (sterile maggot debridement therapy) (Kwon and Janis, 2013). There are advantages and disadvantages to each method. Surgical debridement may not always be precise and healthy tissue may be sacrificed. Additionally, the act of surgical debridement may shower organisms into the bloodstream, resulting in bacteremia. Mechanical debridement is painful and nonselective in the tissue it removes. Enzymatic debridement may be uncomfortable for the

patient and may macerate surrounding tissue. Biologic debridement, also referred to as biosurgery, may not be accepted by most patients. However, the nonsurgical options may be alternatives for patients who are not candidates for general anesthesia. Patients with chronic, nonhealing wounds may become well known to the perioperative staff as they are scheduled for procedures such as debridement, grafting, flaps, and other wound coverage. Perioperative nurses play a key role in wound care and must be familiar with various wound care treatments to support patients throughout the course of their recovery.

Hyperbaric Oxygenation

Some form of HBO treatment for medical disorders has been used since 1662. HBO increases the capacity of blood to carry oxygen to the tissues. The increased oxygenation assists in cellular restoration, and improves leukocyte migration and phagocytosis fibroblast function. HBO therapy is administered in a pressurized chamber with the patient breathing 100% oxygen at elevated atmospheric pressures. Benefits of HBO therapy to chronic wounds may include reduction in inflammation, edema, and inhibition of infection (Marston, 2014). Chambers may be monoplace to accommodate a single patient or multiplace to allow simultaneous treatment of multiple patients. Patients who undergo HBO therapy may require the insertion of myringotomy tubes to manage pressure changes while in the chamber. Perioperative nurses may be involved in the placement of the tubes and may be involved in wound debridement procedures for these patients.

Negative-Pressure Wound Therapy

Also known as vacuum-assisted closure (VAC), negative-pressure wound therapy (NPWT) is used for difficult to manage wounds that do not respond to traditional wound care methods. NPWT works by using a device to apply constant controlled negative pressure to a wound that is filled with a drainage sponge (polyurethane foam) and sealed with an occlusive dressing. The VAC system has three mechanisms of action that interact to promote wound healing. First, the negative pressure results in mechanical tension on the tissues, causing a reduction in edema and fluid removal, which provides an optimal wound environment. The fluid removal also serves to decrease the bacteria load. The second action is macro-deformation and wound contraction, and the third action is micro-deformation and mechanical stretch perfusion (Huang et al., 2014). VAC therapy may be used for acute and traumatic wounds, subacute wounds, pressure ulcers, chronic open wounds, meshed skin grafts, and skin flaps. NPWT must be used carefully and monitored frequently and evaluated to avoid complications such as bacterial colonization and biofilm generation, which may result in increased wound exudate that is not well managed with the NPWT system. Other potential complications when using NPWT is significant pain, particularly during dressing changes, and problems obtaining an adequate seal in irregularly shaped wounds (Marston, 2014). NPWT may accelerate granulation tissue formation and promote closure in a number of wound types while reducing the number of painful dressing changes (Huang et al., 2014).

According to the Food and Drug Administration (FDA) and manufacturer guidelines, contraindications to NPWT therapy for chronic wounds include, but may not be limited to, exposed vital organs, necrotic tissue with eschar present, untreated osteomyelitis, nonenteric and unexplored fistulas, necrotic tissue with eschar; malignancy in the wound (NPWT may lead to cellular proliferation), exposed nerves, exposed vasculature, exposed anastomotic site, and an allergy to any component required for the procedure (FDA, 2011).

The negative pressure unit may be applied in the OR after wound debridement. All nonviable tissue is first removed to reduce bacterial load in the wound bed. The skin area around the wound is dried and specialized reticulated foam is cut to fit the wound bed, including all tunnels and tracks. The surgeon takes care not to overfill the wound with the sponge because this could cause further mechanical trauma. The sponge is never cut directly over the wound, and all sponge pieces are accounted for and dressing sizes placed in the wound are documented. When the sponge is in place, the surgeon

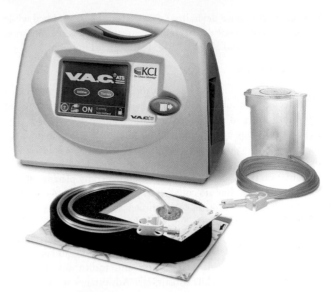

FIG. 9.5 Vacuum-assisted closure pump.

covers the entire sponge, wound bed, and surrounding skin with a transparent occlusive drape, taking care to seal the edges completely. A 2-cm or greater edge of intact periwound skin is left available to ensure an airtight seal of the dressing. A 2-cm cut is made through the occlusive dressing into the sponge for insertion of the drainage tube, which has side and end ports. The tubing is connected to a VAC pump (Fig. 9.5). A portable, battery-operated unit also is available for ambulatory patients. A canister collects the fluid and exudate. The NPWT acts to reduce edema, promote granulation tissue perfusion and formation, and remove exudate and infectious materials. The vacuum pump creates an intermittent or continuous subatmospheric pressure in the range of −80 to −125 mm Hg (Salvo et al., 2016).

When working with an NPWT system, the perioperative nurse assesses the patient and follows all of the manufacturer's instructions on the use of the NPWT system including the prescribed pressure ranges.

Hydrotherapy and Hydrosurgery

Traditionally, hydrotherapy is undertaken via immersion in a whirlpool tank or tub. The mechanism of agitated water and injected air is thought to dilute bacterial loads and remove debris while increasing circulation to the area. Because immersion in a tank is not practical from an intraoperative perspective, the hydrotherapy method most frequently used in the OR is pulsatile lavage. Manufacturers provide a variety of systems to deliver pulsatile lavage. Most systems consist of a motor that creates pressure within tubing set to allow the delivery of fluid at 10 to 15 pounds per square inch (psi) through a handpiece to the wound bed. The handpiece is equipped with a splash shield to help concentrate the spray and minimize droplet aerosolization of the irrigant. While the system is delivering the fluid, it simultaneously suctions it to remove debris and bacteria. Standard Precautions are implemented by all healthcare team members while using pulsatile lavage, and the patient is also protected from aerosolization.

Hydrosurgery is a form of wound debridement and irrigation that uses a powered handpiece system with a narrow nozzle through which pressurized saline (up to 15,000 pounds psi) is used to excise necrotic tissue. The highly pressurized stream creates a vacuum effect that allows the surgeon to remove devitalized tissue from the wound bed while preserving healthy tissue with a confined stream and less aerosolization of bacteria (Levin and Kovach, 2014) (Research Highlight).

Skin Substitutes

An evolving technology for the treatment of wounds is the use of an engineered skin substitute. The skin substitute stimulates wound epithelialization and is capable of producing growth factors. The skin substitute may be used in lieu of a split-thickness skin graft for wound coverage. Skin substitutes are not permanent solutions in most cases, but are a bridge to permanent closure with skin grafts or granulation tissue. Skin substitutes are formed by placing human cells onto matrices that are collagen or synthetic based. As the cells grow and divide, they secrete growth factors and other useful substances to help build a foundation for healing. The substitutes are formed into a variety of shapes and sizes to facilitate wound coverage. They also may be used to cover donor sites from skin graft harvesting. Table 9.1 summarizes the description and indications for some commercially available skin substitutes. Advantages to using skin substitutes are increasing as are the wide variety and availability of these wound treatment products.

Growth Factors

Growth factors are naturally occurring proteins (cytokines and peptides) that are "signaling molecules." They stimulate cycles of mitosis of fibroblasts and epidermal cells, smooth muscle cells, and vascular endothelial cells. Human or recombinant growth factors may be applied to wounds in the OR, but are more typically administered in the clinic setting. Growth factors initiate wound healing by accelerating the formation of granulation tissue and work most effectively in the proliferative phase of wound healing. They improve the cellular or molecular environment of the wound and signal target cells to begin tissue repair. Growth factors generally are

---

RESEARCH HIGHLIGHT

Hydrosurgical Wound Debridement

Surgeons use many techniques to manage wounds and to prepare wound beds for healing or closure, including the use of pressurized fluid delivered via a bulb syringe or pulsed lavage. These hydrosurgery methods have limitations in terms of effectiveness of tissue removal and increased exposure of the patient and surgical team to droplet aerosolization or splashing from irrigant use. Hydrosurgery technology allows surgeons to remove devitalized tissue via the Versajet, a commercially available system that pressurizes an irrigant via a disposable handpiece. As the irrigant is forced through the handpiece, a localized vacuum is created and the dissected tissue is suctioned.

In a retrospective randomized controlled trial, surgeons compared the Versajet hydrosurgery system to conventional debridement in 61 children ≤16 years of age undergoing debridement and skin grafting for partial-thickness burns to prepare the wound beds. Thirty-one children underwent conventional debridement and 30 underwent debridement using Versajet. The researchers noted a significant difference in the amount of viable dermal preservation between the two groups ($p = .02$), with more viable tissue lost in the conventional group versus the Versajet. The researchers concluded that hydrosurgery with the Versajet appears to be a more precise method of burn wound debridement, with no significant differences between scarring at 3 months or 6 months after injury. The researchers noted long-term follow-up of these patients should be considered for further evaluation of these techniques.

Modified from Hyland E et al: Prospective, randomized controlled trial comparing Versajet™ hydrosurgery and conventional debridement of partial thickness paediatric burns, *Burns* 41(4):700–707, 2015.

TABLE 9.1

Permanent and Temporary Skin Substitutes

Category	Trade Name	Description	Indications
Allogeneic dermal	Dermagraft (Advanced Biohealing, Westport, CT)	Fibroblasts seeded and cultured on bioabsorbable mesh, then cryopreserved; delivered on dry ice. 5 × 7.5 cm; applied to either side of wound	Nonhealing full-thickness diabetic foot ulcers >6 weeks' duration, extending through dermis, but without tendon, muscle, joint, or bone exposure
Allogeneic bilayered	Apligraf (Organogenesis, Canton, MA)	Fibroblasts mixed with bovine collagen gel and cultured; keratinocytes seeded and cultured on gel. Delivered fresh; apply to dermal side toward wound	Venous ulcers >1-month duration Full-thickness diabetic neuropathic foot ulcers >3 weeks' duration but without tendon, muscle, capsule, or bone exposure
Cadaver skin	GammaGraft (Promethean LifeSciences, Pittsburgh, PA)	Gamma-irradiated human cadaver skin Stored at room temperature up to 2 years May stay in place until wound heals if it remains adherent to wound bed Left in place while new host skin grows in under dressing Gradually dries out and edges peel away	Chronic wounds and burns
Cadaver skin	TheraSkin (Soluble Systems, Newport News, VA)	Cryopreserved human cadaver skin Delivered on dry ice Available in two sizes and meshed	Chronic wounds and burns

NOTE: The products included in this list are representative of what is available and are not meant to be inclusive.
Modified from Bryant RA, Nix DP, editors: *Acute and chronic wounds: current management concepts*, ed 5, St Louis, 2016, Mosby.

categorized by their source (i.e., if obtained from platelets, they are designated as platelet-derived growth factors [PDGFs]; from the epidermis, epidermal growth factors [EGFs]). To obtain PDGFs, typically 50 to 200 mL of venous blood is withdrawn. The platelets are separated and activated with thrombin to make a gel that is applied to a clean wound bed. The wound is covered with a nonadherent gauze dressing. Debridement may help to speed the wound healing process by exposing viable receptors for proper growth factor–receptor interaction (Robinson et al., 2015).

Wound Scaffolds

Acellular matrix products are used in a wide variety of applications, including burns and reconstructive surgery, soft tissue and abdominal wall repair, and even as internal implants for orthopedic use in joint resurfacing and tendon repair. They are frequently used as scaffolds in hard-to-heal wounds such as diabetic foot ulcers, venous leg ulcers, and pressure ulcers (Table 9.2) (Swanson et al., 2016). Work goes on in research labs to develop extracellular matrix (ECM) from

TABLE 9.2

Acellular Extracellular Matrix Scaffolds

Category	Trade Name	Description	Indications
Allogeneic	AlloDerm (LifeCell, Branchburg, NJ)	Derived from cadaveric human skin from tissue banks. Epidermis and all cellular components removed, leaving dermal matrix; freeze-dried; rehydrate to use. Contains intact collagen fibers to support ingrowth of new tissue, elastin filaments to provide strength, and hyaluronan and proteoglycans for cell attachment and migration	Burns, traumatic or oncologic wounds with deep structure exposure, hernia repair, breast and other tissue reconstruction
Allogeneic	Cymetra (LifeCell)	Injectable micronized particulate form of AlloDerm. Dry form, packaged in syringe, rehydrated before use with either normal saline or lidocaine for injection	Cosmetic soft tissue augmentation and treatment of vocal cord paralysis by injection laryngoplasty
Allogeneic	GraftJacket Regenerative Tissue Matrix (Wright Medical Technology, Arlington, TN)	Same as AlloDerm, but meshed 1:1 to allow wound exudate to pass through; available in two sizes (4 × 4 cm and 4 × 8 cm) and one thickness (0.4–0.8 mm) for chronic wound care. Available nonmeshed and thicker for tendon and ligament repair	Diabetic foot ulcers and other chronic wounds, ligament and tendon repair
Allogeneic	GraftJacket Xpress (Wright Medical Technology)	Same as Cymetra. Available in a prefilled 5-mL syringe. Once rehydrated, is injected to fill the entire dead space of a sinus tract or deep wound	Deep wounds, tunnels or sinus tracts
Allogeneic	DermaMatrix (Synthes CMF, West Chester, PA)	Cadaver human skin from tissue banks. Donor skin is processed to remove all cellular components, including epidermis, and then is freeze-dried. Rehydrate to use	Similar to indications for AlloDerm: soft tissue repair, breast reconstruction, abdominal hernia repair, head and neck reconstruction
Biosynthetic	Biobrane (UDL Laboratories, Sugar Land, TX)	Very thin sheet of semipermeable silicone bonded to a knitted trifilament nylon fabric. Nylon coated with type 1 porcine collagen, which creates hydrophilic coating that facilitates adherence to wound. Silicone membrane has water vapor loss rate similar to that of intact skin; once Biobrane has adhered to a wound, it provides moist, protected environment that minimizes water loss	Partial-thickness burns, skin graft donor sites, superficial wounds after surgery, laser resurfacing, dermabrasion. Lesions secondary to toxic epidermal necrolysis and pemphigus, as coverage for chronic wounds
Biosynthetic	Biobrane-L (UDL Laboratories)	Same as Biobrane, except monofilament nylon is used instead of knitted trifilament nylon, which renders it less adherent to wound bed	Indicated where less adherence is desired (e.g., over meshed autografts)
Biosynthetic	Integra Dermal Regeneration Template (IDRT) (Integra Life Sciences, Plainsboro, NJ)	Bilayered product composed of outer semipermeable silicone sheet (functions as epidermal substitute) and inner ECM scaffold containing bovine crosslinked collagen and chondroitin-6-sulfate. Inner layer facilitates cell migration and tissue ingrowth, which leads to formation of neodermis, usually within 2–3 weeks of application. As neodermis is formed, ECM degrades. Silicone covering is then removed	Deep partial- or full-thickness burns, contracture release procedures, reconstructive surgery of complex wounds and surgical defects

Continued

TABLE 9.2

Acellular Extracellular Matrix Scaffolds—cont'd

Category	Trade Name	Description	Indications
Biosynthetic	Integra Bilayer Matrix Wound Dressing (BMWD) (Integra Life Sciences)	Same product as IDRT but repackaged for chronic wound care Available meshed or unmeshed in multiple sizes	Chronic wounds of various etiologies, surgical wounds, traumatic wound; can be placed over deep structures
Biosynthetic	Integra Matrix Wound Dressing (Integra Life Sciences)	ECM scaffold of the BMWD without silicone membrane Can be used alone or with BMWD for deeper wounds (Matrix Wound Dressing first, then covered with BMWD)	Same indications as BMWD
Biosynthetic	Integra Flowable Wound Matrix (Integra Life Sciences)	Same ingredients (minus silicone layer) as other Integra products ECM is provided in syringe as dry granules that are rehydrated with saline before one-time use Injected directly into wound until filled	Same indications as BMWD but use focuses on application to wounds with deep tunnels or undermining
Synthetic	Suprathel (PolyMedics Innovations, Denkendorf, Germany)	Synthetic epidermal substitute composed of copolymer of polylactide, trimethylene carbonate and ε-caprolactone Completely dissolves within 4 weeks	Used in Germany since 2004 for deep partial-thickness burns, superficial full-thickness burns, skin graft donor sites, abrasions, scar revision
Xenographic porcine	Oasis Wound Matrix (Healthpoint, Fort Worth, TX)	Porcine SIS with complex matrix of collagen, glycosaminoglycans, proteoglycans, cell adhesive glycoproteins, and growth factors Freeze-dried Available multiple sizes, fenestrated, or meshed	Partial- and full-thickness wounds, chronic ulcers, traumatic wounds, superficial and second-degree burns, surgical wounds
Xenographic porcine	MatriStem (Medline Industries, Mundelein, IL)	Derived from porcine UBM with intact basement membrane Composed of collagen matrix, glycosaminoglycans, glycoproteins, and proteoglycans Available as fenestrated sheets of variable sizes or as powder Must be rehydrated before use and cut to size of wound	Partial- and full-thickness wounds, traumatic wounds, surgical wounds, chronic wounds
Xenographic porcine	Mediskin and E-Z Derm (Brennan Medical, St. Paul, MN)	Porcine skin with epidermis and dermis Mediskin is frozen and irradiated, with a shelf life of 24 months; stored in a standard freezer E-Z Derm is chemically crosslinked for durability; stored at room temperature up to 18 months Both are available in multiple sizes, perforated or nonperforated	Temporary coverage of burns, surgical wounds, partial- and full-thickness wounds of variable etiologies
Xenographic equine	Unite Biomatrix (Synovis Orthopedic and Woundcare, Irvine, CA)	Derived from decellularized equine pericardium Available fenestrated, in three sizes Must be rehydrated Apply 2–4 mm larger than wound and staple in place	Partial- and full-thickness wounds, chronic wounds, traumatic wounds, surgical wounds
Xenographic bovine	PriMatrix (TEI Biosciences, Boston, MA)	Derived from fetal bovine dermis, which has been decellularized, freeze-dried, and sterilized Must be rehydrated Available nonfenestrated in various sizes and thicknesses Must fenestrate for high-exudating wounds	Skin ulcers, second-degree burns, surgical wounds

ECM, Extracellular matrix; *SIS,* small intestinal submucosa; *UBM,* urinary bladder matrix.
NOTE: The products included in this list are representative of what is available and are not meant to be inclusive.
Modified from Bryant RA, Nix DP, editors: *Acute and chronic wounds: current management concepts,* ed 5, St Louis, 2016, Mosby.

native cardiac tissue (potential use of acellular cardiac ECM as a biomaterial for heart regeneration) and in tissue engineering of the esophagus.

Dressings

Application of surgical dressings is often the responsibility of the perioperative nurse. The dressing may serve one or more of the following purposes:

- Cushioning and protection of the wound from trauma and gross contamination
- Absorption of drainage
- Debridement of the wound
- Support, splinting, or immobilization of the body part and incisional area
- Assistance in hemostasis and minimization of edema and dead space, as in a pressure dressing

- Promotion of the patient's physical comfort and aesthetic appearance
- Maintenance of a moist environment and prevention of cell dehydration
- Application of medications

Dressings are selected based on the characteristics of the surgical site, depth, and area, and the patient's overall condition (Table 9.3). Questions to ask when choosing a dressing are as follows:

- What does the wound need?
- What is the purpose of the product?

- How well does the product function? Is there evidence to support use of this product?
- What does the patient need?
- What is available?
- What is practical? Is it also cost-effective?

Dressings can be grouped into two main categories: primary and secondary dressings. *Primary* dressings are placed directly over or in the wound. A variety of primary dressing materials are available on the market. Their function is to absorb drainage and then wick it away from the wound edge. Cotton gauze or synthetic dressings

TABLE 9.3

Wound Dressings

Product and Examples	Description	Indications for Use	Instructions for Use
Antimicrobial: Antiseptics, cadexomer iodine, honey, Hydrofera blue, mupirocin ointment, silver cream, silver dressings	Inhibits growth and replication of microorganisms	Partial- or full-thickness wound Critical colonization, infection, or biofilms Odorous wound	Cleanse wound Avoid saline in nanocrystalline silver products Apply to wound Apply appropriate secondary dressing as needed and secure in place
Calcium alginate: Restore CalciCare (Hollister), SeaSorb (Coloplast), Algisite (Smith & Nephew)	Polysaccharide derived from brown seaweed Highly absorbent Converts to viscous, hydrophilic gel Provides moist environment Hemostatic properties	Partial- or full-thickness wound with or without depth Moderate to heavily exudative wound Contraindicated in third-degree burns	Cleanse wound base Place or lightly pack into wound Apply appropriate secondary dressing and secure in place Change as needed, usually every 24–48 h
Charcoal: CarboFlex odor control (ConvaTec), Lyofoam C (Molnlycke, ConvaTec)	Activated carbon (charcoal) Absorbs toxins and wound degradation products Absorbs volatile amines and fatty acids responsible for odor	Malodorous wound (e.g., infected, fungating) Fecal fistula Pressure ulcer	Apply as a "filter" for odor control If absorbing exudate, may need to be changed daily; weekly if no exudate Can be reused if filter only
Collagen: Puracol collagen (Medline), Biostep (Smith & Nephew), Cellerate gel (Hymed Group), CollaSorb (Hartmann)	May enhance deposition of organized collagen fibers Chemoattractant to granulocytes and fibroblasts Bioresorbable Hemostatic properties Most processed from bovine or porcine sources	Full-thickness wound with or without depth Noninfected wound Minimal to moderate drainage Contraindicated in bovine sensitivities and third-degree burns	Packaged as gels, alginates, sheets, powders Cleanse wound as appropriate Apply to wound base Apply appropriate secondary dressing Secure as necessary
Promogran (Systagenix Wound Management)	Some collagens also inactivate matrix metalloproteinases	Chronic wound free of necrotic tissue	Read manufacturer's instructions carefully; some may need to be moistened with saline if wound bed is dry
Composite: Tegaderm absorbent clear acrylic dressing (3M), Alldress (Molnlycke), Covaderm Plus (DeRoyal)	Combine physically distinct components into single dressing Functions as bacterial barrier Absorptive layer distinct from alginate, foam, hydrocolloid, hydrogel Semiadherent or nonadherent	Partial- or full-thickness wound without depth Dry to heavy exudate (depends on dressing components) Product selection varies based on wound characteristics	Cleanse wound as appropriate Dressing application dependent on product selected Can function as either primary or secondary dressing May be used with topical medications
Contact layer: Restore TRIACT technology (Hollister), Mepitel (Molnlycke)	Protects wound bed from direct contact with other agents and dressings Conforms to wound shape Porous to allow exudate to pass or medication to absorb into wound	Partial- or full-thickness wounds with or without depth Infected wounds Donor sites Split-thickness skin grafts	Cleanse wound as appropriate Line wound bed Apply topical agent over contact layer *or* apply secondary dressing for absorption Not intended to be changed with each dressing change

Continued

TABLE 9.3

Wound Dressings—cont'd

Product and Examples	Description	Indications for Use	Instructions for Use
Fiber gelling: Aquacel Hydrofiber (ConvaTec)	Carboxymethylcellulose Absorbs heavy exudate Converts to a gel Keeps wound base moist	Partial- or full-thickness wound with or without depth Moderate to heavily exudative wound	Cleanse wound base Place or lightly pack into wound Apply appropriate secondary dressing and secure in place Change every 24–48 h
Foam: Biatain (Coloplast), Hydrocell (Derma Sciences), PolyMem (Ferris Manufacturing Corp)	Absorptive and nonadherent Consists of hydrophilic polyurethane or film-coated layer	Partial- or full-thickness wound without depth (sheets) or with depth (fillers) Moderate to heavily exudative wound Contraindicated in ischemic wound with dry eschar and third-degree burns Frequently a secondary dressing	Cleanse wound base and dry well Apply topical agent or primary dressing to wound base Place foam dressing in wound Apply appropriate secondary dressing and secure in place Change every 24 h or as needed
Gauze: Hypertonic saline Curasalt (Tyco Healthcare/ Kendall), Mesalt (Molnlycke Health Care)	Gauze impregnated with dry sodium chloride by the manufacturer	Full-thickness, heavily exudating wound and nonviable wound base with or without infection	Cleanse wound, apply to the wound dry, cover with secondary dressing
Hydrocolloid: DuoDERM (ConvaTec), Exuderm (Medline), Replicare (Smith & Nephew)	Contains gel-forming agents (gelatin, pectin, carboxymethylcellulose) Forms gelatinous mass Impermeable to contaminants, reducing risk of infection Promotes autolysis Reduces pain and protects Promotes moist wound Molds to body contours Adhesive	Partial- or full-thickness wound without depth Minimal to moderately exudative wound Avoid acutely infected wound Avoid dry eschar Use with caution in persons with diabetes Contraindicated in third-degree burns	Cleanse wound and dry periwound area well Select dressing 1–2 inches larger than wound Apply light pressure to allow body heat to promote adhesion Change every 3–5 days as needed Use periwound skin preparation product
Hydrogel: Skintegrity (Medline), Elasto-Gel (Southwest Technologies), Vigilon (Bard)	Maintains clean, moist wound Nonadherent Little or no absorption Various formulations: amorphous gel, sheet, impregnated gauze Cool and soothing Decreases pain Aggressive autolytic debridement by autolysis	Partial- or full-thickness wound without depth (sheet or gel) or with depth (impregnated gauze) Dry to minimally exudative wound Sterile gel for every 3-day dressing changes Nonsterile gel can be used for daily dressing changes Contraindicated in third-degree burns	Cleanse wound Apply to cover wound base Do *not* use as wound filler Use appropriate secondary dressing Secure as necessary Change daily
Transparent film: Tegaderm (3M) Suresite (Medline), Opsite (Smith & Nephew)	Permeable to oxygen and water vapor Protects from environmental contaminants—good shield Maintains moist wound Creates "second skin" Reduces friction Nonabsorbent Promotes autolysis	Shallow partial-thickness wound Dry to minimally exudative wound Not recommended for acutely infected wound Contraindicated in third-degree burns	Cleanse wound and dry periwound area Allow for 1- to 2-inch border around wound Apply without stretching or tension Change every 4–7 days *or* as needed Use skin sealant around wound edges
Wound fillers: Flexigel strands (Smith & Nephew), Multidex maltodextrin (DeRoyal)	Pastes, granules, powders, beads, gels	Full-thickness wound with depth Minimal to moderate exudate Infected or noninfected	Cleanse wound as appropriate Apply directly to wound Use appropriate secondary dressing to optimize moist wound environment Change every 1–2 days

NOTE: Examples of product brand names within this formulary are neither inclusive nor intended as a product endorsement.
Modified from Bryant RA, Nix DP, editors: *Acute and chronic wounds: current management concepts*, ed 5, St Louis, 2016, Mosby.

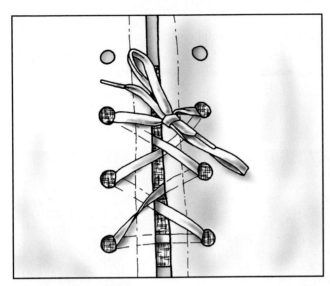

FIG. 9.6 Montgomery straps.

may be used for this purpose. The layer of primary dressing directly contacting the wound should be nonadherent, unless debridement is desired.

Secondary dressings are placed directly over the primary dressing. These function to absorb excessive drainage, provide hemostasis by compression, and protect the wound from further trauma. These functions usually are accomplished with a bulky dressing, such as an abdominal pad. These pads have a cotton filling that provides extra absorbency.

Dressings may be secured with a variety of products, including tape, elastic wrap bandages, or soft roll products. Tape is available with a variety of backing materials (cloth, paper, taffeta, and plastic) and with regular or nonallergenic adhesive. The strength and elasticity required, patient allergies, the condition of the patient's skin, and anticipated frequency of dressing change determine which type is selected. When applying tape to the dressing, the perioperative nurse applies pressure evenly from both sides of the tape and away from the direction of the incision. Applying tape with excessive pressure may result in stretching and trauma to the skin. The tape covers the edges of the dressing and is placed at right angles to the direction of motion when applied over a joint. When frequent dressing changes are anticipated, Montgomery straps can be selected to secure the dressing (Fig. 9.6). When compression of the wound for hemostasis or reduction of edema is desired, a polyurethane dressing, elastic tape, or elastic bandage may be used to secure the secondary dressing. Immobilization is accomplished with the addition of soft padding, elastic bandages, splints, and casting materials (splints and casts are discussed in greater detail in Chapter 20).

In some situations, the wound is not dressed at all. An undressed wound that heals by exposure to air has the following advantages: (1) allows for optimal observation of the incisional area, (2) aids bathing, (3) prevents possible adhesive-tape reactions, (4) increases comfort and maneuverability for many patients, and (5) seems to minimize adverse responses by the patient to the operation.

Drains

Drains control ecchymosis and provide exits through which air and fluids, such as serum, blood, lymph, intestinal secretions, bile, and pus, can be evacuated from the operative site. Drains also may be used to prevent the development of deep wound infections. They usually are inserted at the time of surgery, primarily through a separate small incision known as a *stab wound*, close to the operative site. Drains may or may not be sutured to the skin.

In some instances (e.g., chest, common bile duct, bladder), drainage is directly through the lumen of the tube (as with a Foley retention catheter) or via perforations or fenestrations in the tubing into a closed drainage system. In other instances (e.g., peritoneal cavity or skin wound), drainage of pus or blood is primarily along the outside surface of the drain by capillary action and gravity (as with the simple Penrose drain) into a dressing. The selection of a simple versus a closed drainage system depends on the needs of the site to be drained, patient activity, and overall healing capability. Many types of drains are available. The most common are made of latex, polyvinyl chloride (PVC), silicone, or silver coated (Fig. 9.7). Particular care should be taken to ensure that the patient is not allergic to latex when considering any latex drain. For many wounds, a portable, self-contained closed wound suction unit is selected. These units create a negative pressure in a reservoir attached to the drain. Fluid is gently drawn out of the wound and collected in the reservoir.

The perioperative nurse documents the location and type of drain and ensures the drain is working properly before the patient leaves the OR. This information is important for the hand-off report to nurses caring for the patient in the postanesthesia care unit (PACU) and postoperative nursing units. Some wounds yield significant drainage and must be monitored closely during the postoperative course. A disadvantage of wound drains is that they create a portal for entry and exit of infectious microorganisms. Extreme care must be taken in emptying drain reservoirs to avoid contamination. Closed autologous drains allow for collection of blood from a surgical wound and the return of that blood to the patient; this minimizes the need for transfusion of blood from outside donors, reducing the risk of bloodborne pathogen transmission.

Key Points

- Wound healing and the final surgical result depend on anatomic location, structure of the skin, and functional interaction with underlying elements of the operative region.
- The skin, with its multilayered organization of the epidermis, dermis, and appendages, has unique healing properties.
- In surgical procedures, there are four potential sources of contamination: the surgical team, the surgical environment, the patient, and the instruments/supplies. The patient's normal flora is the most common reservoir of microorganisms.
- Preoperative assessment should include a review of the medical, surgical, and social history; list of current medications; and results of physical examination.
- Wound healing occurs in overlapping phases: the inflammatory, the proliferative, and the remodeling phases.
- Dressings cover the wound, absorb drainage, apply pressure, and provide a moist environment for healing.

Critical Thinking Questions

The perioperative nursing assessment is essential to individualizing your plan of care and communicating information to the surgical team. With surgical infection prevention (SIP) a priority initiative to reduce SSIs, what risk factors would place a patient at an increased risk for an SSI? What nursing interventions would you include in your perioperative plan of care that pertain to antibiotic prophylaxis?

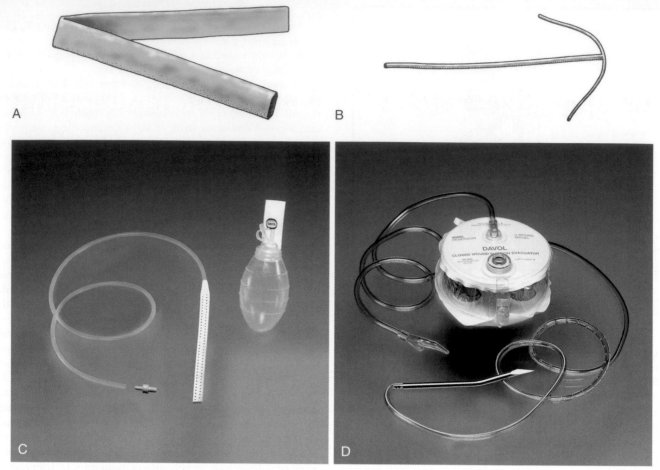

FIG. 9.7 Drains are available in a variety of styles: Penrose (A) and T-tube (B), which drain by gravity, and Jackson-Pratt (C) and Hemovac (D), which represent closed drainage systems.

(e)volve *The answers to the Critical Thinking Questions can be found at http://evolve.elsevier.com/Rothrock/Alexander.*

References

Anderson M et al: A survey to examine patient awareness, knowledge, and perceptions regarding the risks and consequences of surgical site infections, *Am J Infect Control* 41(12):1293–1295, 2013.

Association of periOperative Registered Nurses (AORN): *Guidelines for perioperative practice*, Denver, 2017, The Association.

Centers for Medicare and Medicaid Services (CMS): *Hospital-acquired conditions* (website), 2015. www.cms.gov/medicare/medicare-fee-for-service-payment/hospitalacqcond/hospital-acquired_conditions.html. (Accessed 30 October 2016).

Food and Drug Administration (FDA): *Update on serious complications associated with negative pressure wound therapy systems: FDA safety communication* (website), 2011. www.fda.gov/MedicalDevices/Safety/AlertsandNotices/ucm244211.htm. (Accessed 25 November 2016).

Huang C et al: Effect of negative pressure wound therapy on wound healing, *Curr Probl Surg* 51(7):301–331, 2014.

Kwon R, Janis J: Pressure sores. In Neligan P, editor: *Plastic surgery*, ed 3, New York, 2013, Elsevier.

Leong M et al: Wound healing. In Townsend CM et al, editors: *Sabiston textbook of surgery: the biological basis of modern surgical practice*, ed 20, Philadelphia, 2017, Elsevier.

Levin S, Kovach S: Soft tissue reconstruction for the foot and ankle. In Coughlin M et al, editors: *Mann's surgery of the foot and ankle*, Philadelphia, 2014, Elsevier.

Lynden J, Dellinger E: Surgical site infections, *Hosp Med Clin* 5:319–333, 2016.

Marston WA: Wound care. In Cronenwett JL, Johnston KW, editors: *Rutherford's vascular surgery*, ed 8, Philadelphia, 2014, Saunders.

Robinson JK et al: *Surgery of the skin: procedural dermatology*, ed 3, St Louis, 2015, Elsevier.

Rosenberger LH, Sawyer RG: Surgical site infections. In Cameron JL, editor: *Current surgical therapy*, ed 11, 2014, Saunders Elsevier.

Salvo P et al: A D-optimal design to model the performances of dressing and devices for negative pressure wound therapy, *J Tissue Viability* 25(2):83–90, 2016.

Swanson T et al: *IWII: wound infection in clinical practice* (website), 2016. www.woundsinternational.com/consensus-documents/view/iwii-wound-infection-in-clinical-practice. (Accessed 28 July 2017).

The Joint Commission (TJC): *2016 hospital national patient safety goals* (website), 2016. https://www.jointcommission.org/assets/1/6/2016_NPSG_HAP_ER.pdf. (Accessed 26 November 2016).

CHAPTER 10

Postoperative Patient Care and Pain Management

JAN ODOM-FORREN

The postoperative phase of care begins when the surgical procedure concludes and the patient is transferred to the postanesthesia care unit (PACU). The PACU, in the past, was called the *recovery room* or *postanesthesia room*. Florence Nightingale (1863) first described a postanesthesia area this way:

> *It is not uncommon, in small country hospitals, to have a recess or small room leading from the operating theater in which the patients remain until they have recovered, or at least recovered from the immediate effects of the operation.*

PACUs have flourished since researchers reported that as many as a third of perioperative deaths examined over an 11-year period could have been prevented by improved postoperative nursing care (Odom-Forren and Clifford, 2016).

Technologic innovation has profoundly affected PACU care. The complexity of anesthesia management demands specially trained nurses who have expertise in prompt recognition and management of postoperative complications. Most patients who receive general anesthesia, major regional anesthesia, or monitored anesthesia care are transferred to the PACU. PACU is considered postanesthesia phase I, in which basic life-sustaining needs are of the highest priority. Patients then transition to phase II (preparation for home discharge), an inpatient setting, a critical care unit (CCU), or an intensive care unit (ICU) (ASPAN, 2016). PACU care is the bridge between one-on-one monitoring in surgery to the less acute monitoring on the hospital unit or, in some cases, self-sufficiency of the patient at home (Nicholau, 2015). PACUs are adjacent to the surgical suite with easy access for patient transport. The patient's status is assessed for needs during transfer (e.g., oxygen, manual positive-pressure ventilation device, a patient hospital bed). A perioperative nurse accompanies the patient to the PACU with an anesthesia provider and gives a hand-off report on the status of the patient to a PACU nurse, who assumes care of the patient after an initial assessment report.

Perianesthesia Considerations

Assessment

Admission to the Postanesthesia Care Unit

Initial assessment of the patient begins with an immediate determination of airway and circulatory adequacy. The airway is assessed for patency, humidified oxygen applied, and respirations counted. Pulse oximetry is initiated on all patients, and the quality of breath sounds determined. The PACU nurse connects the patient to the cardiac monitor, and evaluates heart rate and rhythm. Blood pressure (BP) is measured by means of a manual cuff or an automatic cuff. If the patient has an arterial line, the PACU nurse connects it to the

monitor. In some cases, a capnograph to monitor end-tidal CO_2 ($ETCO_2$) is applied.

After the PACU nurse assesses the *ABCs* (*a*irway, *b*reathing, and *c*irculation), the perioperative nurse and anesthesia provider give a comprehensive hand-off report. The hand-off is a real-time process of passing patient-specific information from one caregiver to another or from one team of caregivers to another for the purpose of ensuring continuity and safety. Hand-off communication from the anesthesia provider and perioperative nurse allows the PACU nurse to ask questions, verify any unclear patient information, and anticipate any potential postoperative complications (Garrett, 2016). Standardization of how information is communicated ensures that the information is accurate and complete (Weinger et al., 2015). Box 10.1 includes information on what each surgical team member reports. The patient's American Society of Anesthesiologists (ASA) physical status classification (see Chapter 5) also is provided during the hand-off report. The perioperative nurse provides information about airway status and presence of tubes, drains, catheters, and intravascular lines. Any postoperative orders to be initiated in the PACU are discussed at this time. The anesthesia provider should not leave the patient until the PACU nurse accepts responsibility for the patient's care (AANA, 2013; ASA, 2014).

Initial Assessment

After immediate assessment of the ABCs and completion of the hand-off report, the PACU nurse begins a more thorough assessment. The assessment is performed efficiently and is specific, in part, to the type of operative procedure. Recommended elements of an initial assessment in the PACU are presented in Box 10.2. Some PACUs use a head-to-toe assessment to organize the data obtained (Fig. 10.1). Other PACUs take a major body systems approach (Fig. 10.2). In any case, the PACU nurse assesses admitting vital signs and the ABCs, beginning with the respiratory system. Respiratory assessment comprises rate, rhythm, auscultation of breath sounds for ventilatory adequacy, oxygen saturation level, and capnography level if applicable (Carlisle, 2015). Any artificial airway and type of oxygen delivery system are noted.

The PACU nurse next assesses the cardiovascular system by monitoring heart rate and rhythm. The patient's initial BP is compared with one or more preoperative readings. Body temperature is obtained, skin condition examined, and peripheral pulses checked, if indicated. Next, the PACU nurse assesses neurologic function by asking the following: Has the patient reacted (awakened from anesthesia)? Can the patient follow commands? Is the patient oriented, at least to name and facility? Can the patient move all extremities and lift the head? Are there deviations from preoperative neurologic functioning? Some operative procedures require a more detailed assessment.

BOX 10.1

Suggestions for Hand-Off Report From Anesthesia Provider and Perioperative Nurse to Postanesthesia Care Unit Nurse

Anesthesia Provider May Report:
- Patient name, allergies, surgical procedures performed
- Pertinent medical and/or surgical histories
- Current medications
- Anesthetic delivered
- Medications administered
- Regional anesthetic used
- Intraoperative course (anesthesia-related along with any complications)
- Lines, fluids, losses; the anesthesia provider may include EBL
- Pain and comfort management
- PACU orders
- Questions and answers

Perioperative Nurse May Report:
- Identity of patient
- Preoperative diagnosis

- Procedure performed
- Location of incision(s), dressings, drains, catheters, tubes, packing, stomas
- Surgical complications
- Allergies and reactions
- Medications, fluids, irrigations delivered by surgeon or RN
- Positioning during surgery
- Communication of other pertinent issues:
  - Location/presence of family or significant others
  - Special requests verbalized by the patient preoperatively
  - Special devices
  - Patient deficits
  - Questions and answers

EBL, Estimated blood loss; *PACU,* postanesthesia care unit; *RN,* registered nurse.
Modified from American Society of PeriAnesthesia Nurses: *2017-2018 Perianesthesia nursing standards, practice recommendations and interpretive statements,* Cherry Hill, NJ, 2016, ASPAN; Chard R: Care of postoperative patients. In Ignatavicius DD, Workman ML, editors: *Medical-surgical nursing: patient-centered collaborative care,* ed 87, St Louis, 2016, Saunders; Odom-Forren J: *Drain's perianesthesia nursing: a critical care approach,* ed 7, St Louis, 2017, Elsevier.

BOX 10.2

Initial Assessment in the Postanesthesia Care Unit

Initial assessment in the PACU includes documentation of the following:
1. Integration of data received at hand-off report for transfer of care
2. Vital signs
   a. Respiratory status: airway patent, breath sounds, type of artificial airway, mechanical ventilator settings, oxygen saturation, and $ETCO_2$ if indicated
   b. Blood pressure: cuff or arterial line
   c. Pulse: apical, peripheral
   d. Cardiac monitor, rhythm documented
   e. Temperature/route
   f. Hemodynamic pressure reading if indicated (central venous, arterial blood, pulmonary artery wedge, and intracranial pressure)
3. Pain/sedation/comfort assessment (including emotional comfort)
4. Neurologic function including level of consciousness
5. Position of patient
6. Condition and color of skin
7. Patient safety needs
8. Neurovascular: peripheral pulses and sensation of extremity or extremities as applicable
9. Condition of dressings or suture line, drains, tubes, receptacles
10. Amount and type of drainage
11. Muscular response and strength/mobility status
12. Pupillary response as indicated
13. Fluid therapy: location of lines, condition of IV site, and security and amount of solution given and infusing (including crystalloid, colloid, and blood component therapy)
14. Intake and output
15. Postanesthesia score (if scoring system used)
16. Procedure-specific assessment

IV, Intravenous; *PACU,* postanesthesia care unit.

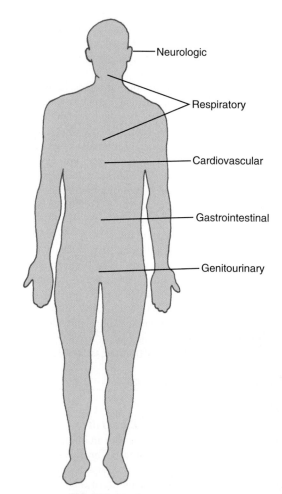

FIG. 10.1 Head-to-toe assessment.

To assess renal function, the PACU nurse measures intake and output (I&O). Total intraoperative fluid intake and estimated blood loss are reviewed. Intravenous (IV) lines, infusions, and irrigation solutions are noted and recorded. Any drains or catheters are listed; their output is noted for color, amount, and consistency.

The surgical site is checked, noting any drainage on the dressing, including amount and color. The area around the incision is inspected so that any future changes may be compared. Patients undergoing

vaginal hysterectomy require that the abdomen is assessed for firmness. A rigid abdomen may indicate hemorrhage. Noting firmness of the abdomen on admission and later findings of a rigid abdomen leads to important comparisons. The patient is also assessed for signs or symptoms of pain, discomfort, or nausea, and medicated appropriately. Information obtained from the admission assessment is documented in the PACU record.

Nursing Diagnosis

Common nursing diagnoses related to the care of postanesthesia patients include the following:
- Ineffective Breathing Pattern
- Risk for Decreased Cardiac Output
- Ineffective Thermoregulation
- Acute Pain

Outcome Identification

Outcomes identified for the selected nursing diagnoses can be stated as follows:
- The patient will demonstrate adequate oxygenation, ventilation, perfusion, and expansion of the lungs on discharge from the PACU.
- The patient will achieve and maintain adequate cardiac output on discharge from the PACU.
- The patient will attain a normal body temperature (96.8°F–100.4°F [36°C–38°C]) on discharge from the PACU.
- Pain will be assessed and, if present, appropriate pharmacologic and nonpharmacologic interventions will be initiated before discharge from the PACU.

Planning

When nursing diagnoses and desired outcomes are identified for the postoperative patient, a plan of care is designed that considers specific patient needs. Some nursing diagnoses are appropriate for all postanesthesia patients. A Sample Plan of Care for a patient in PACU follows.

Implementation

The PACU nurse continually assesses the patient and implements interventions for care. In addition to constant vigilant monitoring discussed under assessment, the nurse often begins a stir-up regimen that helps minimize complications. The stir-up regimen includes deep breathing exercises, coughing, positioning, mobilization, and pain management to facilitate respiratory function (O'Brien, 2017a).

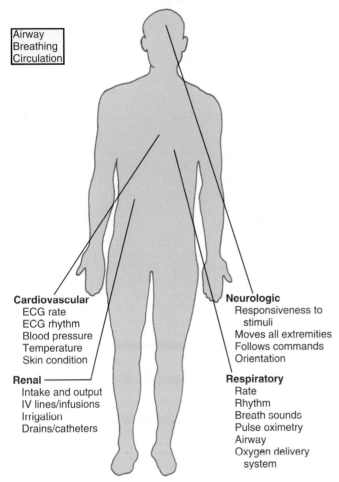

Airway
Breathing
Circulation

Cardiovascular
ECG rate
ECG rhythm
Blood pressure
Temperature
Skin condition

Renal
Intake and output
IV lines/infusions
Irrigation
Drains/catheters

Neurologic
Responsiveness to stimuli
Moves all extremities
Follows commands
Orientation

Respiratory
Rate
Rhythm
Breath sounds
Pulse oximetry
Airway
Oxygen delivery system

FIG. 10.2 Postanesthesia care unit major body systems assessment. *ECG,* Electrocardiogram; *IV,* intravenous.

SAMPLE PLAN OF CARE

Immediate Postoperative Patient Care in the Postanesthesia Care Unit

Nursing Diagnosis
Ineffective Breathing Pattern related to medications associated with anesthesia (e.g., benzodiazepines, opioids), type of surgical procedure, pain, tracheobronchial obstruction

Outcome
The patient will demonstrate adequate oxygenation, ventilation, perfusion, and expansion of lungs on discharge from the PACU as evidenced by regular respiratory rate and pattern, clear and equal bilateral breath sounds, BP and pulse within preoperative range,

oxygen saturation at least 92% or equal to preoperative status, patent airway, and control of pain.

Interventions
- Determine need for chin tilt or jaw thrust if patient is nonreactive without patent airway. Insert artificial airway if needed. Call anesthesia provider for further assistance.
- Assess respiratory status and oxygen saturation level on admission to the PACU and at intervals until discharge.
- Monitor ETCO$_2$ if indicated and ordered.

Continued

SAMPLE PLAN OF CARE

Immediate Postoperative Patient Care in the Postanesthesia Care Unit—cont'd

- Determine level of consciousness (to assess for need to reverse opioid, benzodiazepine, or muscle relaxant).
- Administer humidified oxygen; assess need for continued oxygen after discharge.
- Elevate head of bed (if not contraindicated).
- Encourage patient to take deep breaths or sustained maximal inspiration.
- Note preoperative assessment for sleep apnea. Have patient's own sleep apnea equipment available (if applicable).
- Assess patient for level of comfort. Administer pain medication as needed, per order or protocol.
- Assess patient for opioid-induced ventilatory impairment (OIVI), a depression of the central nervous system associated with opioids.

Nursing Diagnosis

Risk for Decreased Cardiac Output related to anesthetic agents and other medications, fluid or blood loss or replacement, peripheral pooling of blood, alteration in preload or afterload, alterations in rate or rhythm

Outcome

The patient will maintain adequate cardiac output on discharge from the PACU as evidenced by BP within preoperative range, skin warm and dry, oriented to person and place, and pulse strong and regular.

Interventions

- Monitor vital signs, electrocardiogram (ECG), and central venous pressure (CVP), with or without pulmonary artery catheter.
- Assess level of consciousness to determine effect of medication still in circulation.
- Monitor and record any drainage from surgical site.
- Monitor and record I&O.
- Administer fluid or blood replacement therapy if indicated.
- If hypotensive, elevate legs unless contraindicated; increase rate of fluid administration.
- Maintain patency of IV lines.
- Administer medication if needed to improve depressed myocardial contractility, increase cardiac output, and promote diuresis.
- Administer vasodilators, vasoconstrictors, or antidysrhythmics as ordered.
- Warm patient to 96.8°F (36°C).
- Administer humidified oxygen.

Nursing Diagnosis

Ineffective Thermoregulation related to surgical procedure: anesthetic agents, length of surgery, age of patient, OR environment, irrigation, type of surgery, or genetic predisposition to malignant hyperthermia (MH)

Outcome

The patient will attain a normal body temperature (96.8°F–100.4°F [36°C–38°C]) on discharge from the PACU.

Interventions

- Measure body temperature on admission; document temperature and route of measurement.

- Use same route of measurement for each temperature documented.
- Assess peripheral circulation.
- Monitor vital signs and oxygen saturation.
- Observe for shivering.
- Initiate measures to warm patient if hypothermic: place warmed blankets on patient's body and head; use active warming (e.g., forced-air warming device) to rewarm patient.
- Initiate appropriate measures for MH, if indicated (see Chapter 5).
- Maintain ongoing temperature monitoring until discharge.

Nursing Diagnosis

Acute Pain related to operative or other invasive procedures

Outcome

Pain will be assessed and, if present, appropriate pharmacologic and nonpharmacologic interventions will be initiated before discharge from the PACU. The patient will exhibit pain/comfort that is tolerable and be able to meet functional goals (e.g., move, deep breathe).

Interventions

- Assess for subjective signs of pain and comfort: patient reports pain to the PACU nurse; consider a visual analogue or numeric scale to rate pain level.
- Assess for objective signs of pain: protective guarding behavior, moaning, crying, whimpering, restlessness, irritability, diaphoresis, dilated pupils, facial expression of pain, and changes in vital signs (BP, respiratory rate, or pulse).
- Refer to facility protocol for assessing and treating pain based on patient's pain rating.
- Monitor for pain relief and adverse reactions (respiratory depression, oversedation); document significant findings.
- Administer pain medication as prescribed: titrate IV doses; initiate patient-controlled analgesia (PCA) or patient-controlled epidural analgesia (PCEA) as ordered.
- Encourage use of a multimodal approach to pain management (e.g., nonopioid analgesics).
- If epidural analgesia (EA) is used, assess for numbness, leg weakness, pruritus, and respiratory depression. Document findings and notify physician if findings are positive.
- If patient is intubated but conscious, collaborate in pain rating scale by pointing to a number or face and having patient indicate yes or no. If patient is unconscious, be especially attentive to signs such as grimacing.
- Initiate alternate methods of pain relief: transcutaneous electrical nerve stimulation (TENS), music, massage, relaxation, guided imagery.
- Reposition patient for comfort if not contraindicated.
- Assess causes of pain (e.g., surgical site versus chest pain).
- Document medications administered, dose, route, time, and effectiveness of pain relief.
- Assess level of sedation with the use of a sedation scale to detect advancing unwanted sedation during opioid pain management.

Oxygen delivery is monitored and decreased as per patient condition and PACU orders. In some cases, the patient may have entered the PACU with a capnograph in place; if so, the nurse monitors $ETCO_2$ and intervenes when ventilation is inadequate. The PACU nurse monitors BP and heart rate to assess cardiovascular function and cardiac output throughout the patient stay. The nurse also provides interventions to maintain adequate normothermia and manage pain. Throughout PACU care, dangerous and life-threatening changes can occur rapidly (see Perianesthesia Complications, discussed later).

Evaluation

The PACU nurse evaluates the identified patient outcomes before discharge from PACU. For the outcomes presented previously in this chapter, these might be stated as follows:

- The patient demonstrated adequate ventilation, perfusion, and expansion of lungs on discharge from the PACU. Oxygen saturation was adequate while receiving room air.
- The patient maintained adequate cardiac output; BP and heart rate were within normal range.
- The patient was normothermic at discharge from the PACU.
- The patient's pain was assessed at regular intervals and, if present, appropriate pharmacologic and nonpharmacologic interventions were initiated before discharge from the PACU. The patient exhibited pain/comfort that was tolerable; was able to meet functional goals (e.g., moved, took deep breaths) on discharge from the PACU. The patient was relaxed and slept at intervals. The patient verbalized satisfactory pain relief.

Perianesthesia Complications

The following complications are pertinent to the care of all patients during the immediate postoperative period. Three of the most common complications in the PACU are respiratory difficulties, cardiovascular problems, and nausea and vomiting (Nicholau, 2015). Prompt recognition and immediate intervention are imperative for the well-being of PACU patients.

Respiratory

Airway Obstruction

The first priority in the care of the PACU patient is to establish a patent airway. A common cause of airway obstruction is the tongue, which is relaxed because of anesthetic agents, muscle relaxants, and opioids used during surgery (Nicholau, 2015) (Fig. 10.3). The patient may present with snoring, little or no air movement on lung auscultation, retraction of intercostal muscles, asynchronous movements of the chest and abdomen, and a decreased oxygen saturation level. Nursing actions may be simple, such as stimulating the patient to take deep breaths, positioning the patient on the side, or providing supplemental oxygen. If the patient is still unresponsive, the nurse may need to open the airway with a chin tilt or jaw thrust. A chin tilt is accomplished by lifting the chin with one hand while tilting the forehead back with the other. A jaw thrust is accomplished by displacing the temporomandibular joint forward bilaterally. The patient also can be repositioned on the right side. This position is called the recovery position; it allows the tongue to move forward and the airway to remain open.

If these actions do not open the airway, an artificial airway may need to be inserted. An oral or nasal airway may be used. An oral airway is used with an unresponsive patient (Fig. 10.4). A nasal airway is better tolerated by an arousable or awake patient.

Hemorrhage after neck surgery or carotid endarterectomy also can cause acute airway obstruction. The PACU nurse assesses such patients carefully for bleeding. In situations such as apnea, intubation

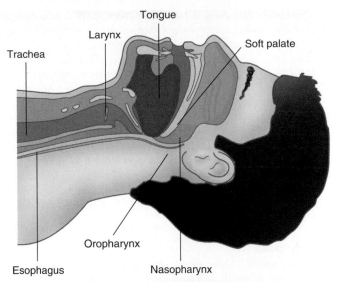

FIG. 10.3 Obstruction of airway by tongue.

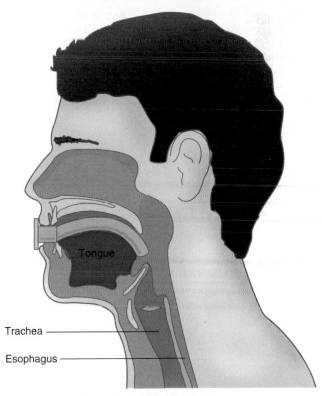

FIG. 10.4 Oropharyngeal airway in place.

with ventilation may be required. If intubation is impossible, the patient may require a tracheostomy, although this rarely is needed.

Laryngospasm

A serious PACU complication is laryngospasm, which is usually the result of an irritable airway. Laryngeal obstruction may occlude the airway as a result of partial or complete spasm of the intrinsic or extrinsic muscles of the larynx. The muscles of the larynx contract and the vocal chords either partially or completely obstruct the airway; the patient can become hypoxemic quickly (Drain, 2017). Symptoms of a laryngospasm include agitation, decreased oxygen saturation/hypoxemia, no breath sounds, and a rocking motion of the chest when attempting to breathe (O'Brien, 2017b). Incomplete obstruction results in a crowing sound or stridor (Odom-Forren, 2014). With laryngospasm, remove the irritating stimulus, suction secretions that may be triggering a glottic response, hyperextend the patient's neck, oxygenate the patient, and prepare to administer an aerosol with racemic (optically inactive) epinephrine. An awake patient experiencing a laryngospasm is terrified and needs reassurance and a calm demeanor from nurses and physicians. During the crisis, an awake patient benefits from a medication for sedation such as midazolam. In many cases, positive-pressure ventilation is delivered by mask and bag. If symptoms last longer than 1 minute and are unrelieved by positive pressure, administration of a muscle relaxant, such as succinylcholine, by the anesthesia provider is required to relax the muscles of the larynx (Drain, 2017). Reintubation is used only as a last resort.

Bronchospasm

Bronchospasm is a lower airway obstruction caused by spasms of the bronchial tubes. These spasms can cause complete airway closure because of lack of cartilaginous support in the bronchioles. The patient presents with wheezing, dyspnea, use of accessory muscles, and tachypnea (Odom-Forren, 2014). Bronchospasm can result from aspiration, pharyngeal suctioning, or histamine release secondary to allergic response or related to medication use. Inhaled bronchodilators are the first choice of therapy for these patients, followed by IV aminophylline. Both IV and inhaled lidocaine can ease bronchospasm induced by histamine. If bronchospasm becomes life-threatening, epinephrine may be administered. Steroids, such as methylprednisolone, also may be administered if the underlying cause is inflammatory disease (e.g., asthma) (O'Brien, 2017b; Schick, 2016).

When obstruction occurs, partial pressure of arterial carbon dioxide ($PaCO_2$) increases significantly and quickly. The PACU nurse makes a quick assessment, rapidly intervenes with airway assistance, and calls for help from the anesthesia provider.

Obstructive Sleep Apnea

Patients in the PACU sometimes present with obstructive sleep apnea (OSA), exhibiting a period of partial or complete obstruction of the upper airway. OSA is related to diminished muscle tone in the airway, which results in obstruction during sleep (ASPAN, 2016). OSA is exacerbated by use of anesthetic agents and opioids. The patient may have a history of OSA or be previously undiagnosed. OSA is often overlooked in the PACU as the cause of airway obstruction because many patients are undiagnosed (Nicholau, 2015). As many as 12 to 18 million adults are estimated as undiagnosed OSA sufferers (Spence et al., 2015). Airway obstruction may cause episodic oxygen desaturation and hypercarbia, and may lead to cardiac dysfunction. It is estimated that 9% of women and 24% of men in the United States show disordered breathing while asleep, and 2% of women and 4% of men show overt symptoms of OSA (Fowler and Spiess, 2013). Perioperative patients with undiagnosed OSA have an increased incidence of morbidity, complications, longer length of stay in the hospital, and a higher rate of admission to the ICU (ASPAN, 2016).

ASA and ASPAN have practice recommendations for postoperative care of the OSA patient (ASA, 2014; ASPAN, 2016). Patient assessment and screening for risk factors should occur preoperatively using standardized screening tools (ASPAN, 2016). The screening instrument with the highest validity and ease of use is the STOP-Bang clinical scale (ASPAN, 2016; Odom-Forren, 2014). Concerns with OSA in the PACU patient include use of analgesia, appropriate oxygenation,

---

▌EVIDENCE FOR PRACTICE

Obstructive Sleep Apnea in the Adult Patient: Recommended Practice

The purpose of this practice recommendation is to promote perianesthesia patient safety in the care of adult patients with known or suspected OSA who have received opioids, procedural sedation, or general or regional anesthesia. The following safety recommendations are not meant to be all-inclusive. Institutions should develop a multidisciplinary guideline or algorithm to meet the needs of their patient population and with consideration of organizational resources.

1. Assess and screen patients for risk factors associated with OSA. Examples in the guideline include, but are not limited to, obesity, cardiovascular disease, and age.
2. Assess and screen undiagnosed patients for signs of OSA such as daytime sleepiness, fatigue, observed snoring, and witnessed apnea.
3. Incorporate the use of a standardized screening tool to identify patients at risk for OSA.
4. Consider preoperative interventions, including preoperative application of the CPAP.
5. Manage patients in PACU with monitoring, positioning, individualized pain management plans, and possible extended monitoring needs.
6. Develop a plan for discharge from PACU.
7. Develop a plan for discharge from Phase II PACU to include the patient having no evidence of hypoxia or obstruction when left undisturbed for 30 minutes.
8. Provide discharge education emphasizing the importance of a reliable individual who is able to report clinical complications. Encourage the patient to sleep on his or her side or in the upright position in a recliner using his or her CPAP therapy (if available).

OSA, Obstructive sleep apnea; *PACU,* postanesthesia care unit.
Modified from American Society of PeriAnesthesia Nurses (ASPAN): Practice recommendation 10: obstructive sleep apnea in the adult patient. In *2017–2018 Perianesthesia nursing standards, practice recommendations and interpretive statements,* Cherry Hill, NJ, 2016, ASPAN.

---

patient positioning, and monitoring. Supplemental oxygen should be used immediately postoperatively. Patients who use continuous positive airway pressure (CPAP) or noninvasive positive-pressure ventilation at home should continue to use these therapies during the postsurgery stay. The patient's position can be changed based on the type of surgery to decrease the chance of airway obstruction. Lateral, prone, and sitting positions result in better airway management for the OSA patient compared with supine. Use of telemetry for monitoring pulse oximetry, ECG, or ventilation can be beneficial in reducing adverse postoperative events and should be used on a patient-need basis (Fowler and Spiess, 2013). Patients with OSA may require extended monitoring in the postoperative period (ASPAN, 2016) (Evidence for Practice).

Cardiovascular

Cardiovascular system instability is a frequent finding after surgery because many anesthetic agents exert a depressive effect on the heart and vascular system. Common problems include hypotension, hypertension, and dysrhythmias. A rare complication in the PACU is cardiopulmonary arrest, which requires early clinical response to signs and symptoms and maintenance of resuscitation skills by PACU nurses.

Hypotension

Hypotension has been defined as a BP that is 20% less than baseline or preoperative BP measurement; it often indicates either relative or absolute hypovolemia (O'Brien, 2017b). Clinical signs of hypotension include a rapid, thready pulse; disorientation; restlessness; oliguria; and cold, pale skin. Because hypovolemia is the most common cause of postoperative hypotension, the initial intervention is to administer IV fluids (physiologic saline or lactated Ringer's solution) at a maximum rate while making a specific diagnosis. Hypovolemia may be caused by inadequate fluid replacement, blood loss during surgery, or continued postoperative blood loss (Seifert and Wadlund, 2015). If no response is observed to administration of fluid, myocardial dysfunction should be ruled out.

Cardiac output and vascular resistance determine BP. Hypotension may be caused by cardiac dysfunction (such as myocardial infarction [MI], tamponade, embolism, ischemia, dysrhythmias, congestive heart failure, valvular dysfunction) or by medications (including anesthetic agents). In such cases, the heart no longer pumps effectively. Hemodynamic monitoring, supplemental oxygen, and cardiac stimulants are used as needed.

Hypovolemia

Hypovolemia reduces cardiac output and may be caused by hemorrhage, dehydration (inadequate fluid replacement), or increased positive end-expiratory pressure (PEEP). Fluid or blood replacement is used to treat hypovolemia. If the patient is hemorrhaging at the surgical site, a return to the operating room (OR) is indicated.

Decreased vascular resistance, which causes relative hypovolemia (interference with venous return to the heart), can be related to medications, general and regional anesthesia, or anaphylaxis (Odom-Forren, 2014). Vasodilation can be treated with fluids, vasopressors, or by elevating the patient's legs. Causative medications should be discontinued. Anaphylactic reactions are treated with epinephrine, antihistamines, and additional fluids.

Hypertension

The normal range for systolic and diastolic BP is generally accepted as <120–<80 mm Hg. Hypertension has been defined as a 20% to 30% increase above baseline BP (O'Brien, 2017b). Hypertension is among the most common postoperative complications and often occurs early in the recovery phase. BP must be verified and rapidity of its change noted. Clinical signs and symptoms are the most important indicators of the severity of the hypertension. Headache, mental status changes, and substernal pain are all indicators of end-organ damage. Hypertension may be caused by volume overload or pulmonary edema, which causes an increase in the cardiac output. In this case the patient is given diuretics, placed on fluid restriction, and hemodynamically monitored. The patient with a history of cardiac disease is more at risk for adverse results.

Asymptomatic hypertension commonly occurs in the PACU and is usually considered harmless. The solution usually is determined by the cause. Patients with a history of essential hypertension are more likely to experience systemic hypertension in the PACU (Nicholau, 2015). Pain is one of the most common causes of hypertension and results in a somatosympathetic reflex when somatic afferent nerves are stimulated (Hall et al., 2016). Analgesics reduce the sympathetic response with a resulting decrease in BP. Other causes of hypertension are anxiety, reflex vasoconstriction from hypothermia, hypoxemia, hypercapnia, and viscous distention, all of which cause increased vascular resistance. Patients in pain are

medicated, and patients with hypothermia are warmed. Patients are oxygenated and ventilated if necessary to improve hypoxemia or hypercapnia. Patients are encouraged to void or are catheterized to empty a full bladder.

Antihypertensive drugs are used as necessary to control BP. A significant number of patients, especially those with a history of essential hypertension, will require pharmacologic BP control in the PACU (Nicholau, 2015). Beta-blockers and α_2-agonists may be used postoperatively when needed. Other agents are available and may include the patient's usual prescription for hypertension (Odom-Forren, 2014). Patients who were on beta-blockers before surgery should be given a beta-blocker on the day of surgery. Giving surgery patients who are on a beta-blocker before surgery a beta-blocker during the perioperative period is a Surgical Care Improvement Project (SCIP) measure (SCIP, 2016). Patients usually are directed to take their prescribed antihypertensives on the day of surgery; they should resume taking prescribed preoperative antihypertensives as soon as possible after surgery.

Dysrhythmias

Most dysrhythmias seen in PACU have an underlying cause that is unrelated to myocardial injury (Odom-Forren, 2014). Hypokalemia, excess fluid administration, anemia, hypoventilation resulting in hypercarbia, altered acid-base status, substance withdrawal, and circulatory instability are postanesthetic and surgical factors that can lead to perioperative dysrhythmias (Nicholau, 2015). A common dysrhythmia after surgery is sinus tachycardia (rate >100 beats/min in an adult). Frequent causes include pain, hypoxemia, hypovolemia, increased temperature, and anxiety. The underlying cause of the dysrhythmia is treated. Propranolol, metoprolol, or esmolol may be given. Sinus bradycardia (heart rate <60 beats/min in an adult) also is a common dysrhythmia in the PACU. Causes include hypoxemia, hypothermia, high spinal anesthesia, vagal stimulation, and some medications commonly given during or after surgery. The underlying cause of the bradycardia is treated. Atropine is the drug of choice to increase heart rate, and usually no other treatment is required, although temporary or permanent pacemakers sometimes are required.

Premature ventricular contractions (PVCs) are represented by wide, bizarre-looking QRS complexes. The most common causes in PACU are hypoxemia and hypokalemia, which are treated. Often, if cardiac disease or hypotension is not present, PVCs do not require medication.

Treatment of dysrhythmias begins with determining and removing the source of the problem. The urgency of treating cardiac dysrhythmias depends on the patient's underlying condition; dysrhythmias are most harmful in patients who have a history of coronary heart disease (Nicholau, 2015). Antidysrhythmic drugs, resuscitation equipment, and monitoring equipment should be immediately available.

Thermoregulation and Temperature Abnormalities

Hypothermia

Postoperative hypothermia, defined as a temperature less than 96.8°F (36°C) (Hooper, 2017), continues to be a widespread PACU problem. While hypothermia may not be life-threatening, it does cause physiologic stress. Hypothermia can prolong recovery time and contribute to postoperative morbidity. Especially vulnerable to the effects of hypothermia are the elderly and children 2 years old or younger. Other risk factors include female gender, burn patients, patients who received general anesthesia with neuraxial anesthesia, low ambient

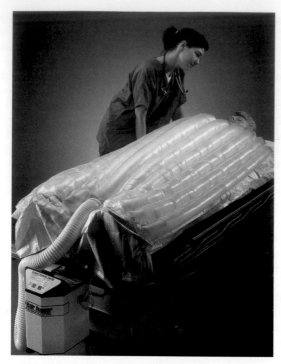

FIG. 10.5 Bair Hugger: focused thermal environment.

temperature of the OR, length and type of surgical procedure, cachexia, significant fluid shift, and use of cold irrigants (Hooper et al., 2016). Patients taking vasodilators, nonsteroidal antiinflammatory agents (NSAIDS), and phenothiazines have changes in thermoregulation that are caused by either vasodilation or inhibition of the thermoregulatory center (Sessler, 2016).

Assessing the need for prewarming begins preoperatively. Preventive warming measures are begun for normothermic patients and active warming measures instituted for hypothermic patients (Hooper, 2017). Prevention of heat loss continues in the OR. A common device to prevent hypothermia in the OR is a forced-air warming device (Fig. 10.5).

In the PACU tremendous demands are made on the body when the patient shivers. Shivering can increase the need for oxygen by 300% to 400%. Shivering affects patient comfort in the PACU and can sometimes lead to more severe complications (Sessler, 2016). As the patient rewarms, small doses of some medications may be indicated in the treatment of shivering during emergence and delivery including meperidine, tramadol, ketamine, dexmedetomidine, granisetron, magnesium sulfate, and clonidine (Golembiewski, 2015). Hypothermic patients should have oxygen therapy initiated immediately on admission. For a patient with a healthy heart, there may be no harmful effects. For a patient with coronary artery disease or cardiomyopathy, however, decompensation can occur. Perioperative hypothermia has been associated with increased incidence of cardiac incidents including myocardial ischemia and MI (Nicholau, 2015).

Other problems associated with hypothermia include intravascular volume loss; the patient can require large amounts of IV fluids to avoid hypovolemia. The central nervous system (CNS) is depressed by hypothermia. A cold postanesthesia patient remains more anesthetized than a warm patient while recovering. Patient discomfort, increased adrenergic stimulation, coagulopathy, impaired wound healing, surgical site infection, and increased hospital costs are other

adverse effects of hypothermia (Sessler, 2016). Hypothermia slows the metabolism and alters the effects of some anesthetic drugs. Of special interest is the prolonged elimination of muscle relaxants in hypothermic patients. Clotting abnormalities can occur. Platelet activity declines, and fibrinolysis increases; both conditions enhance the tendency to bleed (Hooper, 2017).

Rewarming is a postoperative priority. Wet and cold gowns and blankets are removed, and warm, dry gowns and blankets are applied to the head and body. Several external rewarming techniques are available. Application of warm cotton blankets has been a PACU tradition. Warm blankets are applied every 5 to 10 minutes until the patient is normothermic. Cotton blankets gradually increase the patient's temperature. They do not actively heat patients, however, and warming can be a slow process. Forced-air warming devices are effective in rewarming patients. They produce a thermal-focused environment that transfers heat by blowing warm air through a plastic and tissue paper blanket that covers the patient. Forced-air warming devices are standard hypothermia treatment in PACU settings. There is some evidence that continuous fluid-circulating blankets or warm-water mattresses, radiant heat lamps, gel pads, and resistive heating also work (Hooper, 2017). Fluid and blood warmers are useful for large volumes of cool fluids, but not to reverse hypothermia. Single strategies such as forced-air warming were more effective at increasing temperature than passive warming as determined by one systematic review; however, combined strategies, including use of preoperative prewarming, use of warmed fluids, forced-air warming, and other active warming strategies, were more effective in vulnerable groups (Moola and Lockwood, 2011).

Studies have explored the best method to obtain accurate temperatures in the PACU when invasive core temperature measures (e.g., pulmonary artery, distal esophagus, nasopharynx, and tympanic membrane) are unavailable. A study comparing eight noninvasive techniques with bladder temperature (Langham et al., 2009) concluded that the most accurate method for routine postoperative temperature monitoring was via electronic oral temperature devices.

Hyperthermia

Hyperthermia may indicate an infectious process; sepsis; or MH, which is a serious hypermetabolic process. MH is a life-threatening emergency that is genetic in origin (Fiszer et al., 2015). It is triggered by volatile anesthetic agents and the depolarizing muscle relaxant *succinylcholine*. Death may ensue unless MH is immediately recognized and treated (see Chapter 5 for a discussion of MH). Team training and rehearsing appropriate actions are essential to responding quickly and effectively when MH occurs (Seifert et al., 2014).

Disturbances in Cognitive Function

PACU patients may be disoriented, drowsy, confused, or delirious. Delirium is described as an extreme disturbance of arousal, attention, orientation, perception, affect, and intellectual function accompanied by fear and agitation (Viswanath et al., 2015). Attempts have been made to differentiate emergence delirium from agitation, with agitation defined as mild restlessness and mental distress. Delirium is easily confused with agitation, but may actually be the source of agitation (Guenther et al., 2016). Causes of agitation range from residual effects of anesthetics to pain and anxiety. Hypoxemia is ruled out first; it remains the most common cause of postoperative agitation. Chemically dependent patients often awaken in an agitated state. Viscous distention also can contribute to agitation in a drowsy, confused patient. The PACU nurse should identify and eliminate the cause of the agitation or confusion, if possible.

The patient can be engaged in short conversations and reoriented to place and person. Baseline preoperative data are important to determine the cause of agitation. Persistent changes from preoperative status require thorough assessment and possible intervention by the physician.

Aggressive pain management may be the key in facilitating early recovery from delirium. Once hypoxemia is ruled out as the underlying cause of delirium or agitation, sedation may prove useful. Fig. 10.6 provides a summary of factors contributing to emergence delirium and treatment options.

Postoperative Nausea and Vomiting

Postoperative nausea and vomiting (PONV) affects approximately 30% of PACU patients (Apfel, 2015). Primary risk factors associated with PONV are female gender, nonsmoker, history of PONV or motion sickness, use of volatile anesthetics, use of nitrous oxide, postoperative use of opioids, duration of surgery, and type of surgery (Gan et al., 2014). Patients with four or more risk factors have a higher incidence of PONV. Management of nausea and vomiting begins preoperatively and continues into the intraoperative period. Preventive therapy for patients at high risk of PONV is effective in reducing its incidence. There is no single method to prevent or treat PONV. Many causative factors relate to anesthesia and surgery. Pharmacologic prophylaxis improves patient comfort, readiness for discharge, and satisfaction with care (Gan et al., 2014). Apfel (2015) suggested a rule of three for the prevention and management of PONV: (1) assess the need for prevention, (2) titrate preventive measures based on patient need, and (3) use rescue treatment immediately and target mechanisms not tried previously including nonpharmacologic methods.

Two risk assessment tools for PONV commonly are used. Apfel and colleagues (1999) developed their risk assessment tool based on four risk factors: female gender, smoking status, history of PONV or motion sickness, and postoperative use of opioids. Koivuranta and colleagues (1997) identified five risk factors: surgery lasting more than 60 minutes, female gender, history of motion sickness, history of PONV, and nonsmoking status. Table 10.1 presents a simplified algorithm to manage PONV. The Society for Ambulatory Anesthesia (SAMBA) also offers clinical practice guidelines and recommendations for antiemetic prophylaxis and treatment of PONV and postdischarge nausea and vomiting (PDNV) (Gan et al., 2014) (Fig. 10.7).

Receptors that can cause nausea and vomiting when triggered are dopamine type-2, serotonin type-3, histamine type-1, muscarinic cholinergic type-1, and neurokinin type-1. Nausea and vomiting may be induced by various pathways (Fig. 10.8). Patients at risk for PONV receive either one or a combination of agents that block one or more of these receptor sites (Surgical Pharmacology: Antiemetic Pharmacology). Effective medications are aprepitant (Emend), ondansetron (Zofran), dolasetron (Anzemet), granisetron (Kytril), promethazine (Phenergan), prochlorperazine (Compazine), dexamethasone, palonosetron (Aloxi), and transdermal scopolamine. Other medications that can be considered are metoclopramide (Reglan) at a dosage of at least 25 to 50 mg IV, dimenhydrinate

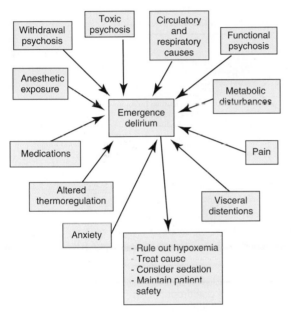

FIG. 10.6 Emergence delirium in the postanesthesia care unit: contributing factors and treatment.

TABLE 10.1						

Algorithm for the Management of Postoperative Nausea and Vomiting[a]

		TIVA Preferred	**Anticipated Rescue**	**1 Risk Factor**	**2 Risk Factors**	**3 Risk Factors**	**4 Risk Factors**
Inpatients		Yes	Ondansetron	Dex	+TIVA	+D₂-RA	+Aprep
			Non-5-HT₃	Dex	+TIVA	+Ond	+Aprep
		No	Ondansetron	Dex	+D₂-RA	+Aprep	+TIVA
			Non-5-HT₃	Dex	+Ond	+Aprep	+TIVA
		TIVA Preferred	**Anticipated Rescue**	**1 Risk Factor**	**2 Risk Factors**	**3 Risk Factors**	**4–5 Risk Factors**
Outpatients		Yes	Palo	Dex	+TIVA+TDS	+D₂-RA	+Aprep
			Non-5-HT₃	Dex	+TIVA+TDS	+Palo	+Aprep
		No	Palo	Dex	+TDS	+Aprep	+TIVA
			Non-5-HT₃	Dex	+TDS	+Palo	+Aprep

[a]Recommended prophylactic strategy based on patient's risk, inpatient or outpatient status, anticipated rescue treatment, and the preference of the anesthesia provider regarding total intravenous anesthesia.

Aprep, Aprepitant; *D2,* dopamine-2; *dex,* dexamethasone; *5-HT,* 5-hydroxytryptamine 3 (serotonin); *Ond,* ondansetron; *Palo,* palonosetron; *RA,* receptor antagonist; *TDS,* transdermal scopolamine; *TIVA,* total intravenous anesthesia.

From Apfel CC: Postoperative nausea and vomiting. In Miller RD et al, editors: *Miller's anesthesia,* ed 8, Philadelphia, 2015, Elsevier.

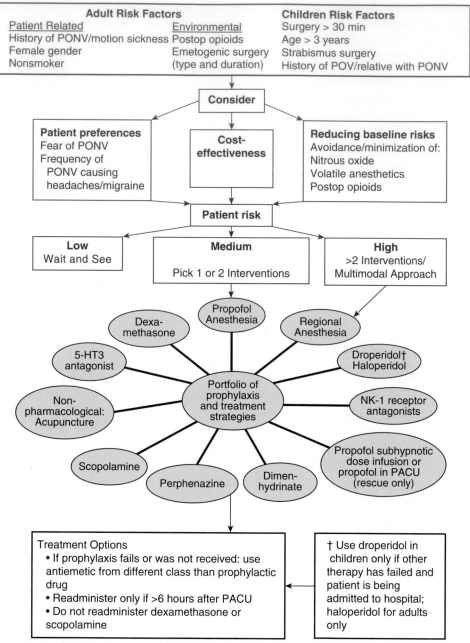

FIG. 10.7 Algorithm for management of postoperative nausea and vomiting *(PONV)*. *POV,* Postoperative vomiting.

(Dramamine), diphenhydramine (Benadryl), or droperidol (Inapsine). Droperidol has a black box warning; the patient must be monitored for QT prolongation/torsades de pointes after administration; however, the droperidol doses used for the management of PONV are low and are unlikely to be associated with significant cardiovascular events (Gan et al., 2014). If the patient is hypotensive with PONV, ephedrine and additional fluids may be administered. PONV rescue medication administered in the PACU should be an antiemetic from a different pharmacologic class than medication given for prophylaxis (Apfel, 2015).

Nonpharmacologic interventions also may be helpful to mitigate symptoms of PONV. Acupuncture, TENS, acupoint stimulation, and acupressure are all effective in reducing the incidence of PONV and need for rescue medication. Aromatherapy (e.g., isopropyl alcohol, peppermint oil) has been used to treat PONV. Controlled breathing

has been found to be as effective alone as in combination with isopropyl alcohol in the treatment of PONV.

Patients may also experience PDNV after ambulatory surgery. Apfel and colleagues (2012) determined that predictors for PDNV were female gender, age less than 50 years, a history of nausea or vomiting, opioid administration, or nausea in the PACU. Depending on the number of factors present, the patient's risk for PDNV can be predicted as 10%, 20%, 30%, 50%, 60%, or 80%. Although postoperative use of opioids is strongly correlated with PDNV, Odom-Forren and colleagues (2015) found significantly more PDNV patients with a higher level of pain than those with lower levels of pain, even when controlling for opioid use in 248 ambulatory surgery patients over 5 days postoperatively; higher levels of pain seemed to exacerbate nausea and vomiting after 48 hours (Research Highlight).

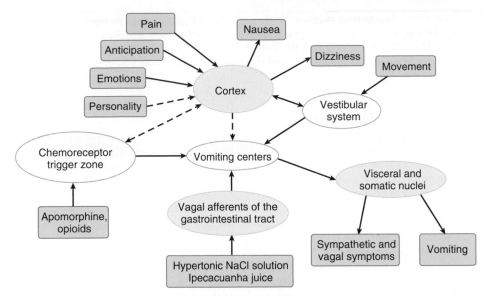

FIG. 10.8 Pathways for nausea and vomiting. Dotted lines are hypothetic pathways with only indirect evidence. *NaCl*, Sodium chloride.

SURGICAL PHARMACOLOGY

Antiemetic Pharmacology

Agent	Receptors Affected	Route and Dosage	Comments
Aprepitant (Emend)	NK$_1$	40 mg PO	Patient should receive 1–3 h before surgery.
Dexamethasone (Decadron)	unknown	4 mg IV	Administer before induction.
Dimenhydrinate (Dramamine)	H$_1$, M$_1$	50–100 mg IV, IM	Side effects include dry mouth, urinary retention.
Diphenhydramine (Benadryl)	H$_1$, M$_1$	12.5–25 mg IM, IV	Side effects include dry mouth, urinary retention.
Dolasteron (Anzemet)	5-HT$_3$	12.5 mg IV	—
Droperidol (Inapsine)	D$_2$	0.625–1.25 mg IV	Use requires ECG monitoring for 3 h after dose.
Granisetron (Kytril)	5-HT$_3$	5 mcg/kg–1 mg IV	—
Metoclopramide (Reglan)	D$_2$	10 mg IV	Increases GI motility; no effective prophylaxis.
Ondansetron (Zofran)	5-HT$_3$	4 mg IV or ODT	Give 15–30 min before end of surgery.
Palonosetron (Aloxi)	5-HT$_3$	0.075 mg IV	Typically given at the start of surgery.
Prochlorperazine (Compazine)	D$_2$	5–10 mg IV, IM	Side effects include dry mouth, urinary retention.
Promethazine (Phenergan)	D$_2$, H$_1$, M$_1$	6.25–12.5 mg IV; 12.5–25 mg IM; PR	Extrapyramidal symptoms possible.
Scopolamine (Transderm Scop)	H$_1$M$_1$	1.5-mg transdermal patch	Apply 4 h before end of surgery; anticholinergic effects.

D$_2$, Dopamine receptor blocker; *ECG*, electrocardiogram; *GI*, gastrointestinal; *H*, histamine blocker; *5-HT$_3$*, serotonin receptor blocker; *IM*, intramuscular; *IV*, intravenous; *M$_1$*, muscarinic receptor blocker; *NK$_1$*, NK receptor blocker; *ODT*, ondansetron dissolving tablet; *PO*, per os, orally; *PR*, per rectum.
Modified from Fetzer SJ: Postoperative nausea and vomiting. In Schick L, Windle P, editors: *Perianesthesia nursing core curriculum: perioperative, phase I and phase II PACU nursing*, ed 2, St Louis, 2016, Saunders; Odom-Forren J: *Drain's perianesthesia nursing: a critical care approach*, ed 7, St Louis, 2017, Elsevier; Odom-Forren J: Postoperative and postdischarge nausea and vomiting. In Stannard D, Krenzischek DA, editors: *PeriAnesthesia nursing care: a bedside guide for safe recovery*, ed 2, Sudbury, CT, 2017, Jones & Bartlett; Gan TJ et al: Consensus guidelines for the management of postoperative nausea and vomiting, *Anesth Analg* 118(1):85–113, 2014.

RESEARCH HIGHLIGHT

The Relationship of Pain and Nausea in Postoperative Patients During the First Week After Ambulatory Surgery

Odom-Forren and colleagues conducted a study to determine whether pain level was associated with demographic or surgery-specific characteristics among patients recovering from ambulatory surgery, and to assess the relationship between pain and nausea over the 7-day postoperative period, controlling for demographic and surgery-related covariates. Participants who had a cumulative pain score of >24 (rated 0–10 each day) over the 7-day period were categorized as having a high pain level. There were significant differences between the two pain groups in age, surgical procedure, cumulative morphine equivalent dose, and use of antiemetics postdischarge. Patients in the high-pain group reported a higher intensity of nausea on the day of surgery and on each of the first 5 postoperative days, controlling for differences in age, sex, education, use of antiemetics presurgery and postsurgery, use of acetaminophen postsurgery, daily morphine equivalent dose, and surgical procedure. Younger patients and those who undergo orthopedic procedures were at a higher risk for postoperative pain. As a majority of surgeries are now conducted in ambulatory surgery settings, it is important to determine pain management regimens and patient education practices that allow for a more comfortable recovery for patients.

From Odom-Forren J et al: The relationship of pain and nausea in postoperative patients for 1 week after ambulatory surgery, *Clin J Pain* 31(10):845–851, 2015.

Less research is available to direct the care of patients after discharge, but use of transdermal scopolamine, promethazine (suppositories or oral), or ondansetron dissolving tablets (ODTs) is supported by small studies. Longer acting antiemetics may be needed (DeJohn, 2013).

Aspiration

Aspiration, the passage of regurgitated material into the lungs, occurs most often during tracheal intubation or extubation. Prevention of aspiration postoperatively includes responding quickly to reports of nausea and vomiting, avoiding conversations that could elicit nausea and vomiting, and preventing rapid movement and head elevation of the patient. Nonreactive patients can be placed on their sides in the recovery position (ASA, 2017).

Volume and acidity of the aspirate determine the extent of damage to the lungs. The most severe damage seems to be in cases in which the pH is less than 2.5 or the volume is greater than 25 mL. Preoperatively, patients may receive clear, nonparticulate antacids, such as sodium citrate (Bicitra), to raise the gastric fluid pH (Fowler and Spiess, 2013). Histamine H_2-receptor antagonists, such as cimetidine, ranitidine, or famotidine, decrease gastric acid production. Metoclopramide speeds gastric-emptying time. Aspiration does not occur in patients with normal protective reflexes. Risk factors can be divided into general and specific (Table 10.2).

Signs and symptoms of aspiration include tachypnea and hypoxemia attributable to a decrease in lung compliance. Wheezing, coughing, dyspnea, hypotension, apnea, and bradycardia may occur. Treatment focuses on promoting tissue oxygenation. Supplemental

TABLE 10.2

Risk Factors for Pulmonary Aspiration

General Risk Factors	Specific Risk Factors
Age (older > younger)	Emergency
Gender (female > male)	Pregnancy
Comorbid diseases	Recent oral intake
Type 1 diabetes	Opioid administration
CNS deficits	Increased gastric residual volume, as with GI obstruction or delayed gastric emptying
Peripheral vascular disease	Obesity
Hepatobiliary or GI diseases	Difficulty in protecting airway, as with depressed level of consciousness
Renal dysfunction	Previous esophageal dysfunction, esophageal cancer, hiatal hernia, gastroesophageal reflux
	Head injury or neurologic dysfunction
	Lack of coordination of swallowing and respiration
	Procedures that increase intra-abdominal pressure (e.g., upper abdominal surgery, straining with ETT)
	Difficult intubation/airway

CNS, Central nervous system; ETT, endotracheal tube, GI, gastrointestinal.
Modified from King W: Pulmonary aspiration of gastric contents (website), 2010. www.frca.co.uk/Documents/192%20Pulmonary%20aspiration%20of%20gastric%20contents.pdf. (Accessed 14 January 2017); Schick L: Perianesthesia complications. In Schick L, Windle P, editors: Perianesthesia nursing core curriculum: perioperative, phase I and phase II PACU nursing, ed 3, St Louis, 2016, Elsevier; Nason KS: Acute intraoperative pulmonary aspiration, Thorac Surg Clin 25(3):301–307, 2015.

oxygen is given. Positive pressure applied by use of a mask or an endotracheal tube may be needed to maintain arterial oxygenation, and a chest x-ray may be performed. If intubated, the trachea can be suctioned. Bronchoscopy is performed if aspirated particles are large and cause airway obstruction. Tracheal secretions can be cultured, and if the results are positive, appropriate antibiotic therapy started (Fowler and Spiess, 2013). Bronchodilators are used as required. Patient recovery depends on recognition of the problem, quantity and pH of aspirate, physical condition before the event, and speed with which interventions begin.

Acute Pain

Pain is a subjective experience and may or may not be verbalized. Often healthcare providers require objective signs of discomfort in addition to subjective reports of pain from the patient, which can lead to undertreatment of pain. The guiding principle in pain care is that pain is whatever the patient says it is via a self-report. All patients may be assessed for pain severity using a verbal descriptor rating scale, numeric rating scale, or a visual analogue scale (Figs. 10.9 and 10.10). A multidisciplinary guideline panel recently recommended that clinicians use a validated pain assessment tool to track responses to postoperative pain treatments and adjust treatment plans accordingly (Chou et al., 2016). However, dosing based on specific pain intensity is dangerous and discouraged (Quinlan-Cowell, 2017). The Joint Commission (TJC) has broader requirements for what should be addressed in organizations' policies including (1) a comprehensive pain assessment that is consistent with scope of care, treatment, and services and the patient's condition; (2) methods to assess pain that are consistent with the patient's age, condition, and ability to understand; (3) the patient's pain is reassessed with an appropriate response; and (4) pain is treated or the patient is referred for treatment (Baker, 2016).

Pain management is one of the highest priorities of PACU. Patients should be assessed for pain on admission to the PACU and at frequent intervals (Box 10.3). It is important to remember that not all patients respond to pain in the same manner, despite comparable surgical procedures. Measures of pain assessment should be correlated with the patient's self-report of pain intensity. Measures to determine pain intensity in a patient who cannot self-report include exposure to a painful procedure or underlying painful conditions; behavioral signs, such as crying or restlessness; using valid and reliable behavioral pain assessment tools; a proxy pain rating by someone who knows the patient well; and physiologic indicators, such as elevated vital signs (Makic, 2013; Pasero and McCaffery, 2011). An analgesic trial can be attempted as a final measure in the hierarchy of importance in assessing the nonverbal patient (Booker and Haedtke, 2016).

Treatment strategies for pain include pharmacologic and non-pharmacologic approaches. A patient-centered approach and consideration of the patient's current condition; the health care providers' clinical judgment; and the risks and benefits associated with the strategies, including potential risk of dependency, addiction, and abuse are the focus of treatment strategies (Baker, 2016). Evidence indicates that early analgesia reduces postoperative problems. Nonopioids, such as acetaminophen, NSAIDs, or cyclooxygenase type 2 (COX-2) inhibitors for patients who have experienced adverse effects from conventional NSAID use, and opiates are the analgesics of choice. Newer nonopioids available in IV format are acetaminophen (paracetamol) and ibuprofen (Chou et al., 2016; Pasero and Stannard, 2012). Onset of analgesia occurs within 5 to 10 minutes of IV administration, with peak analgesic effect occurring within 1 hour and duration of 4 to 6 hours. Availability of these IV nonopioids

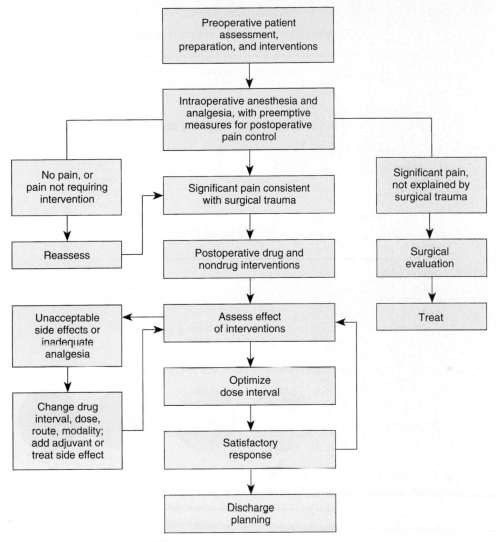

FIG. 10.9 Acute pain management in adults.

for postoperative patients adds an option when developing a multimodal pain management plan in the PACU (Surgical Pharmacology: Dosing Data for Nonopioid Analgesics and Surgical Pharmacology: Dosing Data for Opioid Analgesics). Multimodal pain techniques that use nonopioids as well as opiates can reduce opioid requirements significantly (Chou et al., 2016). The ASA recommends the use of multimodal pain management therapy including central regional blockade with local anesthetics, and unless contraindicated, patients should receive an around-the-clock regimen of COX-2 inhibitors, NSAIDs, or acetaminophen with treatment individualized to each patient. It also suggests that gabapentin and pregabalin can be beneficial in some patients as part of a multimodal therapy (ASA, 2012). Other medications have been suggested as effective in pain medication (Research Highlight)

Inadequate pain relief experienced by postoperative patients using intramuscular (IM) injections is attributable to varying blood levels and is no longer a supported method of analgesic delivery. A common opioid-delivery system is PCA, which allows patients to control their analgesic administration. Dosage, time between doses, and the maximum allowable dosage are programmed into the PCA pump. This form of analgesia also allows for a basal rate of opioids to infuse continuously, if ordered. The PCA pump also can be set to deliver

continuous infusion and patient boluses. The bolus function allows the patient to premedicate before an activity or for breakthrough pain. When PCA devices are started in the PACU, delays in preventing pain are avoided, effectiveness of the PCA in managing pain can be evaluated, and the patient's understanding and ability to use PCA can be monitored.

Other forms of postoperative pain relief may involve use of spinal analgesia, usually in the form of epidural opioid or local anesthetic administration. Patients who have had extensive procedures, including total hip or knee replacements, knee reconstruction, and major abdominal or thoracic operations, have been shown to profit from this method of pain control. Benefits of EA for acute postoperative pain include good analgesia with minimal sedation, early ambulation and physical therapy, and excellent patient satisfaction. An extended-release epidural morphine (DepoDur) that provides pain relief for 48 hours after a single bolus injection is available. Side effects of intrathecal administration of opioids include nausea, pruritus, urinary retention, areas of slight numbness, and respiratory depression. These side effects can be controlled by adjusting the infusion rate or by adding drugs such as diphenhydramine, ondansetron, or naloxone.

Naloxone is the opioid antagonist used most frequently to reduce opioid-induced respiratory depression. It is administered slowly, never

Pain Intensity Scales

Simple descriptive pain intensity scale*

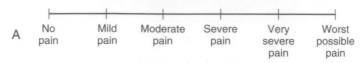

A
No pain | Mild pain | Moderate pain | Severe pain | Very severe pain | Worst possible pain

0–10 Numeric pain intensity scale*

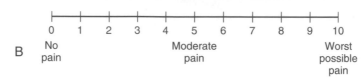

B
0 1 2 3 4 5 6 7 8 9 10
No pain | Moderate pain | Worst possible pain

Visual analogue scale (VAS)†

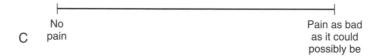

C
No pain | Pain as bad as it could possibly be

* If used as a graphic rating scale, a 10-cm baseline is recommended.
† A 10-cm baseline is recommended for VAS scales.

Which face shows how much hurt you have now?

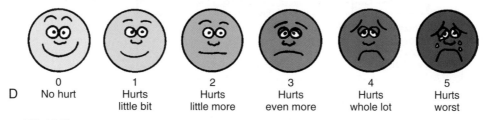

D
0 No hurt | 1 Hurts little bit | 2 Hurts little more | 3 Hurts even more | 4 Hurts whole lot | 5 Hurts worst

FIG. 10.10 (A–C) Examples of pain intensity and pain distress scales. (D) FACES pain rating scale.

RESEARCH HIGHLIGHT

Perioperative Dextromethorphan as an Adjunct for Postoperative Pain

N-methyl-D-aspartate (NMDA) receptor antagonists have been shown to reduce perioperative pain and opioid use. The most commonly used NMDA in the perioperative setting is ketamine, which has been shown to decrease pain when given preemptively, intraoperatively, or postoperatively. Ketamine has possible side effects including hallucinations and nightmares. Dextromethorphan is an NMDA receptor antagonist that is most routinely used as an oral antitussive and has known perioperative analgesic effects. Researchers conducted a meta-analysis of randomized controlled studies to determine whether the use of perioperative dextromethorphan decreases use of opioids or pain scores. The meta-analysis identified 21 studies that were randomized, double-blinded, placebo-controlled trials written in English with patients 12 years of age or older describing effects of dextromethorphan on postoperative pain and opioid consumption. Dextromethorphan was found to reduce pain from 1 to 24 hours postoperatively and was found to reduce morphine requirements 24 to 48 hours after surgery. Side effects for both opioids and dextromethorphan typically consist of nausea, vomiting, dizziness, and lightheadedness. Ten studies reported either no side effects or a nonsignificant difference between groups; however, five studies reported a decrease in side effects in groups receiving dextromethorphan. Only one study found a higher incidence of mild to moderate nausea in the dextromethorphan group. The authors note that larger studies are needed to clarify whether opioid-sparing doses of dextromethorphan are able to decrease opioid-related side effects without causing hallucinations at similar rates to ketamine.

From King MR et al: Perioperative dextromethorphan as an adjunct for postoperative pain: a meta-analysis of randomized controlled trials, *Anesthesiology* 124(3):696–705, 2016.

BOX 10.3

Pain Assessment and Reassessment

Principles

- Pain is multidimensional. Patients experience its aspects in different, personal ways. Comprehensive pain assessment considers the physical, sensory, behavioral, sociocultural, cognitive, affective, and spiritual dimensions of pain.
- Patients who have difficulty communicating their pain require particular attention. This includes patients who are cognitively impaired, psychotic, or severely emotionally disturbed; children; the elderly; patients who do not speak English; and patients whose level of education or cultural background differs significantly from that of the healthcare team.
- Unexpectedly intense pain, particularly if sudden or associated with altered vital signs, such as hypotension, tachycardia, or fever, is reported and evaluated immediately; diagnoses, such as wound dehiscence, infection, or deep vein thrombosis should be considered.
- Family members should be involved when appropriate.

Pain Assessment Tools

- The most reliable indicator of the existence and intensity of pain and any resultant distress is the patient's self-report.
- Self-report measurement includes numeric or verbal descriptor ratings and visual analogue scales.
- Tools should be reliable, valid, and easy for the patient and nurse or physician to use. One may use these tools by showing a diagram to the patient to indicate the appropriate rating. One may also simply ask the patient for a verbal response: "On a scale of 0 to 10 with 0 as no pain and 10 as the worst pain possible, how would you rate your pain?" or "Please describe your pain for me, from no pain to mild, moderate, severe, or pain as bad as it could be."
- Tools must be appropriate for the patient's gender and age, developmental, physical, emotional, cognitive, and cultural status. In a cultural pain assessment, pose questions such as "What words would you use to describe your pain?" "Tell me about your beliefs about your pain." "How do you take your medication for pain?" "How can I help you with your pain?"

Preoperative Preparation

- Discuss the patient's previous experiences with pain and beliefs about and preferences for pain assessment and management.
- Give the patient information about pain management therapies and the rationale underlying their uses.
- Develop with the patient a plan for pain assessment and management.
- Select a pain assessment tool and teach the patient to use it.
- Provide the patient with education and information about pain control, including nonpharmacologic options, such as relaxation, distraction, imagery, and massage.
- Inform patients that it is easier to prevent pain than to attempt to reduce it after it is established, and that communication of unrelieved pain is essential for its relief. Emphasize the importance of a factual report of pain, avoiding stoicism or exaggeration.

Postoperative Assessment

- Assess the patient's perceptions, along with behavioral and psychologic responses. Observations of behavior and vital signs should not be used instead of a self-report, unless the patient is unable to communicate.
- Assess and reassess pain frequently during the immediate postoperative period. Determine frequency of assessment based on the procedure performed and severity of pain. Assess pain every 2 hours during the first postoperative day after major surgical procedures (assess for procedure-specific pain).
- Increase frequency of assessment and reassessment if pain is poorly managed.
- Record pain intensity and response to intervention in an easily visible and accessible place, such as a bedside flow sheet or in the electronic health record.
- Revise the management plan if pain is poorly controlled.
- Review with the patient before discharge the interventions used and their efficacy, and provide specific discharge instructions regarding pain and its management. Have patient "teach-back" or repeat instructions in his or her own words.

Modified from Booker SS, Herr KA: Pain management for older African Americans in the perianesthesia setting: the eight "I's," *JOPAN* 30(3):181–188, 2015; Sussex R: *How different cultures experience and talk about pain* (website), 2015. www.theconversation.com/how-different-cultures-experience-and-talk-about-pain-49046. (Accessed 16 January 2017); Tung W-C, Li Z: Pain beliefs and behavior among Chinese, *Home Health Care Manage Pract* 27(2):95–97, 2015; Wyatt R: Pain and ethnicity, *AMA J Ethics* 15(5):449–454; 2013.

---

as a bolus, while the nurse observes the patient's response. The patient should be able to open his or her eyes and talk to the nurse within 1 to 2 minutes of administration; naloxone is discontinued when the patient can take deep breaths on instruction and respond to physical stimulation.

Other techniques that have been shown to reduce pain for surgical patients include infiltration of the incision site with a local anesthetic in the OR before the initial incision and use of a long-acting local anesthetic at the incision site at the conclusion of the surgery. Local anesthetics as part of a multimodal approach to pain management can contribute to a considerable decrease in opioid dosage with minimal side effects (ASA, 2012; Chou et al., 2016). One option is perineural local anesthetic infusion, in which a catheter is threaded along or into the wound. A diluted concentration of a long-acting local anesthetic is delivered to the surrounding nerves by an infusion pump. Thorough patient education is imperative, including timing of removal of the catheter for patients who will be discharged home

with the pump. It also is important to know the type of anesthetic the patient received during surgery and the type of local anesthetic in the pump to prevent overdose. Multimodal analgesia allows a smaller dose of each component, helping to minimize adverse effects.

Nonpharmacologic interventions used to relieve pain include positioning for comfort, verbal reassurance, touch, applications of heat or cold, massage, TENS, distraction, and biofeedback. Cognitive modalities should also be considered as an adjunct to pharmacologic interventions for pain including guided imagery and other relaxation methods, hypnosis, intraoperative suggestions, and music (Chou et al., 2016). Nonpharmacologic interventions are designed to supplement, not substitute, pharmacologic interventions.

The physiologic effects of pain can be harmful to postoperative patients (Patient Safety). Such effects include decreased thoracic movement, increased splinting, reduced lung compliance and volume (leading to atelectasis), decreased mobility, increased risk of thromboembolism, exaggerated catecholamine response (which

SURGICAL PHARMACOLOGY

Dosing Data for Nonopioid Analgesics

Drug	Usual Adult Dose	Usual Pediatric Dose[a]	Comments
Oral			
Acetaminophen (Ofirmev)	Oral: 650–975 mg q4h IV per 15-min infusion: 1000 mg maximum single dose q6h to maximum total dose of 4000 mg/24 h	Oral: 10–15 mg/kg q4h IV per 15-min infusion: 15 mg/kg q6h to maximum total dose of 75 mg/kg per 24 h	Acetaminophen lacks peripheral antiinflammatory activity of NSAIDs Do not exceed the maximum daily dose of acetaminophen or hepatic injury may result, including risk of severe hepatotoxicity and death Available also in liquid and suppository
Aspirin	650–975 mg q4h	Not recommended for children	The standard against which other NSAIDs are compared Inhibits platelet aggregation; may cause postoperative bleeding
Choline magnesium trisalicylate (Trilisate)	1000–1500 mg bid	25 mg/kg q12h	May have minimal antiplatelet activity; also available as oral liquid
Diflunisal (Dolobid)	1000 mg initial dose followed by 500 mg q12h	—	—
Etodolac (Lodine)	200–400 mg q6h	—	—
Fenoprofen calcium (Nalfon)	200 mg q4–6h	—	—
Flurbiprofen	100 mg bid, tid, qid	—	—
Ibuprofen (Motrin, Caldolor, others)	Oral: 400 mg q4–6h IV: 400–800 mg q6h to maximum of 3200 mg; dilute in 100 mL normal saline or 5% dextrose and infuse over 30 min	Oral: 10 mg/kg q6–8h IV formulation for adults only	IV ibuprofen is contraindicated for the treatment of perioperative pain for CABG surgery
Ketoprofen (Orudis)	25–75 mg q6–8h	—	—
Magnesium salicylate	650 mg q4h	—	Many brands and generic forms available
Meclofenamate sodium (Meclomen)	50 mg q4–6h	—	—
Mefenamic acid (Ponstel)	250 mg q6h	—	—
Naproxen (Naprosyn)	500 mg initial dose followed by 250 mg q6–8h	5 mg/kg q12h	Also available as oral liquid
Naproxen sodium (Anaprox)	550 mg initial dose followed by 275 mg q6–8h	—	—
Oxaprozin	600 mg q24h	—	Long half-life, so can be given once daily
Salsalate (Disalcid, others)	500 mg q4h	—	May have minimal antiplatelet activity
Sodium salicylate	325–650 mg q3–4h	—	Available in generic form from several distributors
Selective COX-2 Inhibitor			
Celecoxib (Celebrex)	100–200 mg q12–24h; maximum of 400 mg	—	Reduces risk of GI side effects and renal toxicity No effects on platelet aggregation May have a higher risk of having heart attack or stroke
Parenteral NSAID			
Ketorolac	30 or 60 mg IM initial dose followed by 15 or 30 mg q6h Oral dose after IM dose: 10 mg q6–8h IV dose: 30 mg for healthy adults and 15 mg for adults >65 years	— — —	IM dose not to exceed 5 days; IV administration comparable to 10 mg IM morphine —

[a]Drug recommendations are limited to NSAIDs for which pediatric dosing experience is available.

NOTE: Only the above NSAIDs have FDA approval for use as simple analgesics, but clinical experience has been gained with other drugs as well.

bid, Twice daily; *CABG,* coronary artery bypass graft; *COX-2,* cyclooxygenase type 2; *GI,* gastrointestinal; *IM,* intramuscular; *IV,* intravenous; *NSAID,* nonsteroidal antiinflammatory drug; *qid,* four times daily; *tid,* three times daily.

Modified from Acute Pain Management Guideline Panel: *Acute pain management in adults: operative procedures. Quick reference guide for clinicians,* AHCPR pub. no. 92-0019, Rockville, MD, 1992; Agency for Health Care Policy and Research, US Public Health Service, US Department of Health and Human Services; Odom-Forren J: *Drain's perianesthesia nursing: a critical care approach,* ed 7, St Louis, 2017, Elsevier; Pasero C, McCaffery M: *Pain assessment and pharmacologic management,* St Louis, 2011, Mosby.

SURGICAL PHARMACOLOGY

Dosing Data for Opioid Analgesics

Drug	Approximate Equianalgesic Oral Dose	Approximate Equianalgesic Parenteral Dose	Recommended Starting Dose (Adults >50 kg Body Weight)		Recommended Starting Dose (Children and Adults <50 kg Body Weight)[a]	
			Oral	Parenteral	Oral	Parenteral
Opioid Agonist						
Morphine[b]	30 mg q3–4h (around-the-clock dosing)	10 mg q3–4h	30 mg q3–4h	10 mg q3–4h	0.3 mg/kg q3–4h	0.1 mg/kg q3–4h or 0.05–0.1 mg/kg IV q1–2h
	60 mg q3–4h (single dose or intermittent dosing)	—	—	—	—	—
Codeine[d]	130 mg q3–4h	75 mg q3–4h	60 mg q3–4h	60 mg q2h (IM/Sub-Q)	1 mg/kg q3–4h[e]	NR
Hydromorphone[b] (Dilaudid)	7.5 mg q3–4h	1.5 mg q3–4h	6 mg q3–4h	1.5 mg q3–4h	0.06 mg/kg q3–4h	0.015 mg/kg q3–4h
Hydrocodone (in Lorcet, available as Lortab, Vicodin, others)	30 mg q3–4h	NA	10 mg q3–4h	NA	0.2 mg/kg q3–4h[e]	NA
Levorphanol (Levo-Dromoran)	4 mg q6–8h	2 mg q6–8h	4 mg q6–8h	2 mg q6–8h	0.04 mg/kg q6–8h	0.02 mg/kg q6–8h
Meperidine (Demerol)[b] Not recommended for long-term pain management	300 mg q2–3h	100 mg q3h	NR	100 mg q3h	NR	0.75 mg/kg q2–3h
Methadone (Dolophine, others)	20 mg q6–8h	10 mg q6–8h	20 mg q6–8h	10 mg q6–8h	0.2 mg/kg q6–8h	0.1 mg/kg q6–8h
Oxycodone (Roxicodone, also in Percocet, Percodan, Tylox, others)	30 mg q3–4h	NA	10 mg q3–4h	NA	0.2 mg/kg q3–4h[e]	NA
Oxymorphone[c] (Numorphan)	NA	1 mg q3–4h	NA	1 mg q3–4h	NR	NR
Opioid Agonist-Antagonist and Partial Agonist						
Buprenorphine (Buprenex)	NA	0.3–0.4 mg q6–8h	NA	0.4 mg q6–8h	NA	0.004 mg/kg q6–8h
Butorphanol (Stadol)	NA	2 mg q3–4h	NA	2 mg q3–4h	NA	NR
Nalbuphine (Nubain)	NA	10 mg q3–4h	NA	10 mg q3–4h	NA	0.1 mg/kg q3–4h
Pentazocine (Talwin, others)	150 mg q3–4h	60 mg q3–4h	50 mg q4–6h	NR	NR	NR

[a]CAUTION: Dosages listed for patients with body weight <50 kg cannot be used as initial starting doses in infants <6 months of age. Consult the Agency for Healthcare Research and Quality *Clinical practice guideline for acute pain management: operative or medical procedures and trauma* for management of pain in neonates for recommendations.

[b]Meperidine is not typically used for long-term pain management because of breakdown into the neurologic stimulant normeperidine.

[c]For morphine, hydromorphone, and oxymorphone, rectal administration is an alternate route for patients unable to take oral medications, but equianalgesic doses may differ from oral and parenteral doses because of pharmacokinetic differences.

[d]CAUTION: Codeine doses >65 mg often are inappropriate because of diminishing incremental analgesia with increasing doses but continually increasing constipation and other side effects.

[e]CAUTION: Doses of aspirin and acetaminophen in combination opioid/nonsteroidal antiinflammatory drug preparations also must be adjusted to the patient's body weight.

NOTE: Published tables vary in the suggested dosages that are equianalgesic to morphine. Clinical response is the criterion that must be applied for each patient; titration to clinical response is necessary. Because there is not complete cross-tolerance among these drugs, it is usually necessary to use a lower equianalgesic dose when changing drugs and to retitrate to response.

CAUTION: Recommended dosages do not apply to patients with renal or hepatic insufficiency or other conditions affecting drug metabolism and kinetics.

IM, Intramuscular; *NA,* not available; *NR,* not recommended; *Sub-Q,* subcutaneous.

Modified from Acute Pain Management Guideline Panel: *Acute pain management in adults: operative procedures. Quick reference guide for clinicians,* AHCPR pub. no. 92-0019, Rockville, MD, 1992; Agency for Healthcare Research and Quality, US Public Health Service, US Department of Health and Human Services; Odom-Forren J: *Drain's perianesthesia nursing: a critical care approach,* ed 7, St Louis, 2017, Elsevier; Pasero C, McCaffery M: *Pain assessment and pharmacologic management,* St Louis, 2011, Mosby; Schick L, Windle P, editors: *PeriAnesthesia nursing core curriculum,* ed 3, St Louis, 2016, Mosby.

PATIENT SAFETY

Educating Patients About Medications for Pain Management

- Explain the purpose, dosage, schedule, and route of administration of any prescribed medications and side effects to report to the physician or nurse.
- Give the patient general guidelines for the use of pain medications.
- Explain that a variety of pain relief measures may be necessary for some types of pain.
- Instruct the patient to use pain relief measures before pain becomes severe. Determine the patient's ability or willingness to participate actively in the use of pain relief measures, and suggest measures the patient believes would be helpful.
- Encourage the patient to try a pain relief measure at least twice before abandoning it as ineffective. Instruct the patient to keep an open mind as to what may relieve pain.
- Discuss the use of nonopioid analgesics. Inform the patient that nonopioid analgesics include acetaminophen, aspirin, and nonsteroidal antiinflammatory drugs, such as ibuprofen, indomethacin, and naproxen.
- Explain the maximum amount of acetaminophen for 24 hours and how to calculate if on an opioid that includes acetaminophen—especially if the patient plans to augment the opioid with extra acetaminophen.
- Explain that nonopioid medications are generally well tolerated, but have the potential to cause GI ulceration, renal and hepatic toxic effects, and inhibition of platelet aggregation.
- Tell the patient that if the nonopioid drug does not have a therapeutic effect initially, the dosage should be increased before another type of drug is tried.
- Discuss the use of opioids, which are indicated for severe postoperative pain or intractable pain such as that associated with cancer. Opioids include morphine, hydromorphone, and methadone; these may be administered by oral route, IV, intrathecally, or epidurally.
- Explain that fixed dosage schedules with adequate doses for pain relief provide more constant blood levels and predictable pain relief. Discuss use of additional doses that may be needed for breakthrough pain.
- Discuss the side effects of opioid analgesics, including vomiting, respiratory and CNS depression, and constipation. For example, constipation requires the use of laxatives and stool softeners (e.g., senna [Senokot]).
- Review the use of opioid agonists and antagonists, including nalbuphine (Nubain), butorphanol (Stadol), pentazocine (Talwin), and buprenorphine (Buprenex).
- Explain the use of analgesic potentiators. Inform the patient that these potentiating drugs include hydroxyzine (Vistaril); diazepam (Valium); lorazepam (Ativan); diphenhydramine (Benadryl); and phenothiazine derivatives, such as promethazine (Phenergan), prochlorperazine (Compazine), and chlorpromazine (Thorazine).
- Discuss other types of drugs used in pain control, including tricyclic antidepressants, such as amitriptyline (Elavil), imipramine (Tofranil), and doxepin (Sinequan), and butyrophenones, such as droperidol (Inapsine) and haloperidol (Haldol).
- Discuss and demonstrate use of equipment for administering pain-relief medications: external and implantable pumps for IV, epidural, and intrathecal administration of opioid analgesics; PCA or PCEA, particularly for the management of acute postoperative pain; continuous wound infiltration with an ambulatory infusion pump; and TENS.
- Explain how to safely dispose of leftover medications.

CNS, Central nervous system; *GI*, gastrointestinal; *IV*, intravenous; *PCA*, patient-controlled analgesia; *PCEA*, patient-controlled epidural anesthesia; *TENS*, transcutaneous electrical nerve stimulation.

increases cardiac work and myocardial oxygen demand), increased risk for myocardial ischemia, impaired immune system, and delayed return of bowel and gastric function. Physiologic responses to acute pain include increased BP and heart rate, dilated pupils, perspiration, increased respiratory rate, and decreased respiratory excursion (Quinlan-Cowell, 2017).

Psychologically, patients in pain may display fear, helplessness, anxiety, anger, or frustration (Wilson et al., 2016). There is an association between poorly controlled postoperative pain and the risk of developing chronic pain, which emphasizes the importance of pain control in the perioperative period (Quinlan-Cowell, 2017). Patients of differing cultures respond to and communicate pain differently. A patient may believe that nonverbal communication expresses the pain to the nurse, but the nurse may not recognize the clues. Common misconceptions about pain also abound. These misconceptions must be recognized and corrected (Table 10.3).

Guidelines to address management of acute postoperative pain are available from specialty organizations such as the American Pain Society (APS), American Society of Pain Management Nurses (ASPMN), ASA, and ASPAN. Procedure-specific and evidence-based pain management guidelines are available through a web-based program called PROSPECT or Procedure Specific Postoperative Pain Management (Prospect, 2015). These clinical practice guidelines and recommendations were developed by consensus of an international group of surgeons and anesthesia care providers who reviewed pain research and graded the evidence (Fig. 10.11). These recommendations have been incorporated into many enhanced recovery after surgery (ERAS) protocols.

Unfortunately, patients who are managed with opioids as part of their analgesic program can have adverse events related to the medication. Two of the most serious opioid-related adverse events are unintended advancing sedation (which generally precedes respiratory depression) and respiratory depression. Education of the healthcare team and use of multimodal pain management are of utmost importance in decreasing these events (ASPAN US PR Strategic Work Team, 2014). Nursing care includes identifying patients who are at risk for unintended sedation and respiratory depression, assessing and monitoring patients who are using opioids for pain management, and intervening to prevent the deterioration of the patient's condition (Evidence for Practice). Pasero (2013) and Putnam (2016) offered detailed strategies to prevent opioid-related sentinel events after discharge from the PACU that include identifying at-risk patients, assessing for respiratory depression, changing the way pain is managed (from opioid only), and providing comprehensive education.

TABLE 10.3	
Misconceptions About Pain	
Misconception	**Correction**
Best judge of the existence and severity of patient pain is the physician or nurse caring for the patient	The patient is the authority about his or her pain; the patient's self-report is the most reliable indicator of the existence and intensity of pain; verbal patients should be able and willing to self-report pain
Clinician must believe what the patient says about pain	The clinician must accept and respect the patient's self-report of pain and proceed with an appropriate assessment and treatment; the clinician is entitled to a personal opinion but should not allow it to guide practice
Patients should not receive analgesics until the cause of pain is diagnosed	Symptomatic relief of pain should be provided while the investigation of cause proceeds; use a reliable and valid pain intensity scale
Visible signs, either physiologic or behavioral, accompany pain and can be used to verify its existence and severity	Even with severe pain, periods of physiologic and behavioral adaptation occur, leading to periods of minimal or no signs of pain; a mutually developed plan with comfort-function-mood goals yields meaningful reductions in pain
Pain never killed anyone	Unrelieved pain may be dangerous and is unacceptable; postoperative pain can delay healing and contribute to complications that can be life-threatening; acute pain warns of actual or potential tissue damage and resolves when healing has occurred; unrelieved postoperative pain is a complication or risk, not an acceptable consequence of surgery
If the patient requires higher doses of opioids than other patients, "he's hitting the PCA button too often"	There is no set dose of opioid that is effective for all patients; even an opioid-naive patient may require 6× more opioid than another patient; a patient who is opioid-tolerant may require 100× the opioid of an opioid-naive patient

PCA, Patient-controlled analgesia.

Modified from Booker SU, Haedtke C: Assessing pain in verbal patients, *Nursing* 4G(2):65 60, 2016; Edwards RR, Berde CB: Pain assessment. In Benzon H et al. editors: *Essentials of pain medicine*, ed 3, St Louis, 2011, Saunders; Pasero C, McCaffery M: *Pain assessment and pharmacologic management*, St Louis, 2011, Mosby.

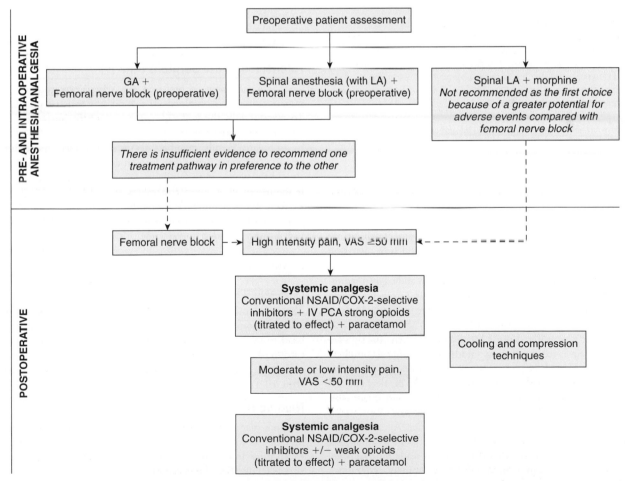

FIG. 10.11 Algorithm for the management of postoperative pain: total knee arthroplasty. *COX-2,* Cyclooxygenase type 2; *GA,* general anesthesia; *IV,* intravenous; *LA,* local anesthesia; *NSAID,* nonsteroidal antiinflammatory drug; *PCA,* patient-controlled analgesia; *VAS,* visual analogue scale.

The American Society of PeriAnesthesia Nurses Prevention of Unwanted Sedation in the Adult Patient: Evidence-Based Practice Recommendation

The purposes of this practice recommendation are to (1) promote the identification of patients at high risk for opioid-induced sedation and respiratory depression before administration of opioid analgesics and (2) enhance the assessment of sedation during opioid administration as a means of preventing life-threatening respiratory depression. The strategic work team made the following three overarching recommendations:

1. Assess and screen patients for individual and iatrogenic risk factors associated with the development of unwanted or advancing sedation and/or respiratory depression.
2. Assess for unwanted sedation in phase I and phase II PACU.
3. Perform an individualized discharge assessment of inpatients. Opioid analgesics are commonly prescribed for postoperative pain. An opioid-only approach to pain treatment has contributed to adverse events such as excessive sedation and life-threatening respiratory depression. Current accepted guidelines recommend multimodal analgesia, which is a more balanced approach to postoperative pain management than opioid-only treatment. Sedation can occur at any time during opioid therapy, but is most pronounced at the beginning of treatment and with subsequent increases in opioid dose. Sedation occurs before respiratory depression, which explains why increased sedation is the first sign that respiratory depression may occur. This evidence-based practice recommendation discusses risk factors of unwanted sedation in detail, discusses sedation scales that are available in the literature, and details the assessment that should occur before discharge including no transfer of the patient at the peak effect of the opioid and the importance of an accurate hand-off report.

Modified from American Society of PeriAnesthesia Nurses Recommendation Strategic Work Team: The ASPAN prevention of unwanted sedation in the adult patient evidence-based practice recommendation, *J Perianesth Nurs* 29(5):344–353, 2014.

Discharge From the Postanesthesia Care Unit

The PACU nurse completes a final assessment immediately before the patient's discharge and transfer to the surgical unit, assessing vital signs, level of consciousness, condition of the operative site, pain and comfort level, I&O, respiratory function and oxygen saturation, and mobility. If the patient requires ongoing oxygen therapy, a transport oxygen canister is provided, and an oxygen supply is prepared in the transfer surgical unit.

The patient is considered ready for discharge when vital sign are stable, the patient is recovered from anesthesia, no surgical complications are expected, and the patient meets medically approved criteria (ASA, 2017; O'Brien, 2017a). The patient should be alert enough to call for assistance. The dressings should be dry and intact with receptacles emptied. Discharge is usually by an anesthesia care provider, who may be present and write a discharge order. Alternatively, a numeric scoring system approved by the department of anesthesia may be used to determine whether the patient is ready for discharge. A common scoring system is the Aldrete score. Activity, respiration, circulation, consciousness, and oxygen saturation level are scored from 0 to 10; a total score of 8 to 10 is generally acceptable for PACU discharge, with exceptions made by physician order. A hand-off report is given to the nurse who will assume care for the patient on the surgical or other unit. This report may be given by telephone before the patient leaves the PACU or in person after the patient reaches the unit. The report includes a preoperative history, pertinent information regarding the patient's surgery and recovery, medications the patient was given, physician's orders, and all other appropriate information.

Admission to the Ambulatory Surgery Phase II Unit

When the patient has had an ambulatory surgery procedure, the next step after discharge from phase I PACU care is transfer to phase II PACU care (Ambulatory Surgery Considerations). The nursing role in phase II PACU typically focuses on preparation for care at home. The patient is transitioned to oral analgesics, and discharge instructions are provided to the patient and caregiver. The length of time required for phase II care is directly related to the type of procedure and readiness for discharge status of patient.

Fast-Tracking the Ambulatory Surgery Patient

In some instances the surgeon and anesthesia provider may determine that the patient is a candidate for "fast-tracking." In fast-tracking the patient bypasses PACU phase I and goes directly to PACU phase II care. The patient must meet phase I discharge criteria before leaving the OR. Each healthcare facility must have criteria in place to safely, appropriately, and effectively use fast-tracking. At the very least, discharge criteria from the OR should include awake or easily arousable, hemodynamically stable, breathing effectively on room air, minimal pain and nausea, and stable condition of surgical site (ASPAN, 2016).

Admission to the Surgical Unit

The patient's room is prepared for admission, and any necessary equipment is obtained. The patient is assisted into the bed. To prevent falls the bed rails are raised until the patient is fully awake. The patient is informed to call the nurse for assistance to ambulate. Family members also are instructed and enlisted to maintain safety for the patient. Equipment and the patient's condition should be explained to family members present. A special concern is the use of PCA. Family members should be instructed that the PCA is for the patient's use only and that pushing the PCA button for the patient can have a detrimental effect on the patient's well-being.

Postoperative Nursing Considerations

Assessment

The nurse in the receiving unit makes an immediate assessment as soon as the patient transfers to the bed. The nurse may choose a head-to-toe or systems assessment. Parameters include respiratory, cardiovascular, and neurologic status. The condition of the dressing and surgical site and patient comfort and safety also are assessed (Box 10.4).

Nursing Diagnosis

Nursing diagnoses related to the care of the postoperative patient include the following:
- Risk for Infection
- Ineffective Breathing Pattern
- Acute Pain
- Imbalanced Nutrition: Less than Body Requirements
- Impaired Physical Mobility

AMBULATORY SURGERY CONSIDERATIONS

Important Education and Information for Patients Who Are Discharged From Phase II Recovery to Home

Anesthesia
- Advise patient of common side effects: dizziness and drowsiness (have assistance if needed); sore throat; PDNV.
- For the next 24 hours the patient should not drive or operate machinery, drink alcohol, or sign important papers, and a responsible adult should stay with the patient.

Activity Limitations
- Advise patient to go home and rest for next 24 hours.
- Inform patient of any limits to activity because of procedure.

Diet
- Instruct patient how to progress to regular diet, or give instructions to patient detailing specific diet required because of procedure.

Safety Concerns
- Review preparation of home for patient return (e.g., removal of rugs that increase fall risk, sleeping area close to bathroom).

Reconciling Medication Information (TJC, 2016)
- Discuss new take-home medications or prescriptions. Document last dose of medication on patient's written instructions if given before discharge. Confirm that patient has prescription or that it has been electronically sent to patient pharmacy. Have patient repeat back.
- Discuss resumption of home medications. Physician should have noted which home medications the patient is to continue after discharge. Have patient repeat back.
- Instruct the patient to take the medication with food (unless contraindicated) to decrease stomach irritation.
- Discuss the use of acetaminophen or ibuprofen if the patient has no pain medication ordered (unless contraindicated). Have patient repeat back.
- Advise patient not to take acetaminophen if taking other pain medications that include acetaminophen as an ingredient. Have patient repeat back.

Surgical Procedure
- Discuss any information that pertains to specific procedure (e.g., when to remove dressing, when to resume showers or baths, ice at site, weight-bearing or activity restrictions). Confirm that patient can state correct name of procedure performed. Have patient repeat back.

Bowel Habits
- Increase dietary fiber and fluids.
- Use stool softener if needed.

When to Call the Healthcare Provider
- Fever greater than 101°F (38°C) orally
- Pain that becomes worse or is not relieved by pain medication
- Bleeding that is unexpected
- Warmth, redness, or swelling at the operative site
- Evidence of pus from the surgical incision
- Inability to eat or drink by day after discharge
- Persistent nausea and vomiting
- Inability to void

Follow Up Care
- Instruct patient about next appointment with physician or ascertain that appointment is already scheduled.
- Give patient telephone number for physician's office.
- If applicable, give patient telephone number of ambulatory surgery center.

Home Procedures
- If patient requires procedures at home such as dressing change or emptying drainage reservoir, ascertain that a responsible adult has received instructions and given a return demonstration of action.

Written Instructions
- All discharge instructions should be in writing and given to the patient, including all the pertinent information included previously, specific information about any new medications, and a list of home medications that physician requests be continued or discontinued.

PDNV, Postdischarge nausea and vomiting.

BOX 10.4

Patient Assessment on Admission to Postoperative Unit From the Postanesthesia Care Unit

- Respiratory status
- Patency of airway
- Respirations: depth, rate, character
- Breath sounds: presence, character
- Circulatory status
- Pulse, blood pressure
- Skin color, temperature
- Capillary filling
- Neurologic status
- Level of consciousness
- Ability to move extremities, peripheral pulses (as applicable)
- Dressing
- Presence of drainage
- Presence of tubes to be connected to drainage systems
- Comfort
- Presence of pain, nausea, vomiting

- Pain score
- Patient positioned for comfort and to facilitate ventilation
- Other comfort measures as determined by patient preference (e.g., warm blanket, music, massage)
- Safety
- Use of two patient identifiers
- Necessity for side rails
- Call cord within reach and instructions on operation reviewed
- Equipment
- Monitors connected and functioning
- IV fluids: location of insertion site, type and size of IV device, type of infusion, rate, amount in bag, patency of tubing, assessment of site
- Drainage systems (e.g., nasogastric, chest, urinary): type, patency of tubing, connection of appropriate container, character and amount of drainage

IV, Intravenous.

Outcome Identification

Outcomes identified for the selected nursing diagnoses could be stated as follows:

- The patient will be free from infection as indicated by normal vital signs; temperature within normal range; normal white blood cell count; clear breath sounds; clear, yellow urine; and warm, dry skin.
- The patient's respirations will be easy, unlabored, and adequate in rate and depth.
- The patient will verbalize subjective assertions of comfort: "I am in no pain." "My pain is under control and I can perform activities of daily living." The patient will have no objective signs of discomfort (e.g., grimaces, tachycardia).
- The patient will eat well from prescribed diet; weight loss will be minimal.
- The patient will ambulate at an appropriate level and perform other activities appropriate for condition.

Planning

Planning for the postoperative patient requires knowledge of surgical procedures and underlying medical conditions. Throughout the patient's stay, planning involves the patient, family, and caregiver or significant others (as appropriate and desired by the patient) with setting measurable goals to be achieved by discharge. A Sample Plan of Care for the postoperative patient follows.

Implementation

Wound Healing

Nursing care of the postoperative patient includes assessment of wound healing. Nursing interventions focus on preventing and monitoring wound complications. The nurse uses strict aseptic technique when placing a new dressing. Monitoring for signs and symptoms of infection includes noting any of the following: elevated body temperature; red, swollen, warm area surrounding the incision; elevated white blood cell count; tachycardia; or purulent drainage from the wound (Hoch, 2014). For a detailed discussion of wound healing, see Chapter 9.

Adequate Respirations

Postoperative patients are at risk for pulmonary complications because of increased respiratory secretions, decreased lung expansion, depression of the respiratory center, and the possibility of aspiration of gastric contents. These complications can be minimized by appropriate nursing management, including elevating the head of the bed whenever possible; encouraging coughing, turning, and deep breathing every 2 hours; ambulating the patient as soon as possible; and encouraging hydration (Hoch, 2014).

Circulation

Venous stasis in the postoperative patient can lead to thrombophlebitis, which is usually a preventable complication. Platelets adhere to the

---

SAMPLE PLAN OF CARE

Admission to the Postoperative Patient Care Unit

Nursing Diagnosis
Risk for Infection related to altered skin integrity, compromised aseptic technique, or malnutrition

Outcome
The patient will be free from infection, as indicated by normal vital signs; temperature within normal range; normal white blood cell count; clear breath sounds; clear, yellow urine; and warm, dry skin.

Interventions
- Monitor vital signs every 4 hours or as prescribed.
- Monitor temperature every 4 hours as needed; document and report increased temperature.
- Monitor laboratory values for evidence of infection; report variance from normal.
- Encourage patient to take deep breaths or sustained maximal inspiration or use respiratory aids.
- Preserve closed urinary system and provide catheter care. Remove catheter as soon as possible.
- Encourage patient to eat foods high in protein and vitamin C.
- Avoid antiinflammatory drugs such as steroids to facilitate healing.
- Use aseptic technique when changing dressings; change soiled dressings immediately.
- Monitor contents of wound drainage catheters.
- Teach patient, family members, and caregivers how to care for surgical site, what to expect, and when and who to call if drainage at incision or drain sites increases or if other

symptoms develop, such as fever, increased pain at site, and redness and swelling of incision.

Nursing Diagnosis
Ineffective Breathing Pattern related to postoperative pain, decreased energy, fatigue, decreased lung expansion, surgery

Outcome
The patient's respirations will be easy, unlabored, and adequate in rate and depth.

Interventions
- Monitor respirations and chest expansion frequently for 24 to 48 hours after the surgical intervention.
- Place the bed in high-Fowler position if possible.
- Auscultate lungs and evaluate productiveness of cough; document any adventitious breath sounds and nature and amount of sputum associated with cough (if present).
- Have patient cough and deep breathe at regular intervals; collaborate with patient to identify cues to remember to undertake these activities or recommend 10 deep breaths each hour.
- Encourage use of respiratory aids (e.g., incentive spirometry, as appropriate).
- Treat underlying conditions, such as pain.
- Demonstrate splinting incisional area with pillow before cough.
- Encourage patient to turn and change positions at least every 2 to 3 hours.
- Encourage early and regular ambulation and explain importance to patient, family, and caregivers.

venous wall and form a thrombus, with resultant potential for deep vein thromboembolism (DVT) or pulmonary embolus (PE).

Prevention may include administration of prophylactic heparin, aspirin, dextran, or warfarin. Application of an intermittent pneumatic compression device (IPCD) or graduated compression stockings may be ordered. Nursing measures that prevent DVT include applying the stockings whether the patient is in or out of bed, teaching the patient not to cross the legs, having the patient perform isometric leg exercises, and encouraging early ambulation.

If thrombophlebitis is suspected (pain or tenderness, erythema, localized area of warmth, swelling), the patient should return to bed and the physician notified. Treatment consists of rest, heat, graduated compression stockings, and anticoagulant therapy.

Urinary Function

One of the priorities during surgery and immediately afterward is to keep the patient well hydrated so that voiding occurs 6 to 8 hours after surgery. Usually intake is greater than output for 48 hours, as fluid and electrolyte balance returns to normal. Every effort is made to refrain from use of a catheter to avoid the risk of urinary tract infection. Measures to help the patient void include warming the bedpan, letting water run, applying warm water to the perineum, and allowing the patient to use the bathroom when possible. If discomfort is present and the bladder is palpable, catheterization becomes necessary. A portable bladder ultrasound may be used to assess the volume of urine in the bladder. A straight catheter is preferred, but in the event that several catheterizations are required, an indwelling catheter is inserted. Hydration of the patient becomes a priority. I&O is recorded accurately. A urine output of less than 0.5 mL/kg/hr is reported to the physician (Hoch, 2014).

Bowel Elimination

The postoperative patient who undergoes abdominal or pelvic surgery may have decreased peristalsis for at least 24 hours; this may persist

---

SAMPLE PLAN OF CARE

Admission to the Postoperative Patient Care Unit—cont'd

Nursing Diagnosis
Acute Pain

Outcome
The patient will verbalize subjective assertions of comfort: "I am in no pain." "My pain is under control and I can perform activities of daily living." The patient will have no objective signs of discomfort (e.g., grimaces, tachycardia).

Interventions
- Discuss the concept of pain and what it means for patient (e.g., throbbing, aching, stabbing, burning, feeling of "tightness").
- Educate patient, family members, and caregivers on the use of pain rating scale:
  - Show pain rating scale and explain its purpose.
  - Explain the components of the scale (if numeric scale used, explain what the numbers mean).
  - Set realistic comfort/function goals.
- Encourage patient to report pain, emphasizing that this is an important part of his or her care.
- Consider personal, cultural, spiritual, and ethnic components in developing a pain management plan with patient.
- Document assessment of pain (intensity, duration, location, and frequency) and response to pain management therapies.
  If patient has continuous local anesthetic infusion therapy, also known as *site-specific infusion therapy* (common with select orthopedic procedures, abdominal hysterectomy, mastectomy, or hernia repair):
- Assess site to ensure dressing is intact and catheter site is clean and dry.
- Query patient to determine whether symptoms of LAST are present (dizziness, ringing in the ears, metallic taste, tingling or numbness of lips, slowed speech); contact physician to initiate immediate treatment if assessment is positive.
- If patient is to be discharged with infusion therapy, provide verbal and written instructions.
- Support patient in the use of personally effective nonpharmacologic pain management strategies (e.g., relaxation techniques, distraction, massage, biofeedback, music, guided imagery, meditation).

Nursing Diagnosis
Imbalanced Nutrition: Less Than Body Requirements related to surgery

Outcome
The patient will exhibit adequate nutritional intake from prescribed diet; weight loss will be minimal.

Interventions
- Encourage patient to eat foods high in protein and vitamin C.
- Offer frequent, small amounts of food or high-protein liquids to patient with little or no appetite.
- Encourage ambulation (improves appetite)
- Schedule procedures not to conflict with mealtime.
- Administer pain medication as needed.
- Determine patient's previous history of PONV or PDNV; consult with physician regarding preventive measures for discharge if history is positive.
- Refer to nutritional support team if appropriate; dietary consultation may be important for patient with cultural or ethnic food preferences.

Nursing Diagnosis
Impaired Physical Mobility related to surgical procedure or pain

Outcome
The patient will ambulate at an appropriate level and carry out other activities appropriate for condition.

Interventions
- Encourage muscle-strengthening exercises before ambulation.
- Encourage ambulation or position changes and extremity exercises at least every 8 hours.
- Encourage leg exercises in bed.
- Before attempting to ambulate, have patient dangle legs over side of bed until pulse rate has stabilized and patient is not dizzy.
- Have two people help ambulate if patient is weak or obese.
- Encourage patient to walk further with each ambulation.
- Teach proper use of appropriate assistive devices (e.g., crutches, slings, walkers) and observe return demonstration.

LAST, Local anesthetic toxicity; *PDNV*, postdischarge nausea and vomiting; *PONV*, postoperative nausea and vomiting.

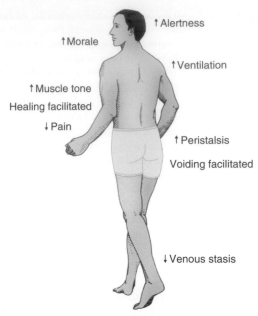

↑ Alertness

↑ Morale

↑ Ventilation

↑ Muscle tone

Healing facilitated

↓ Pain

↑ Peristalsis

Voiding facilitated

↓ Venous stasis

FIG. 10.12 Benefits from early postoperative ambulation.

PATIENT ENGAGEMENT EXEMPLAR

Planning Ahead

NAQC guiding principle number 5 states that the "nurse patient relationship is grounded in an appreciation of patient's rights and expands on the rights to include mutuality. Mutuality includes sharing of information, creation of consensus, and shared decision making."[a] Postoperative care and pain management need to be discussed before the patient's procedure. Perioperative nurses should share information with the patient letting them know what to expect, what the outcomes of surgery might be, patient limitations after surgery, and plan for any needed equipment or help at home. Postoperative pain expectations should be discussed to find out what pain means to the patient, what he or she can reasonably tolerate, what type of pain he or she has experienced in the past, and what actions were taken to alleviate the patient's pain. Patients can explain what they value and what is most important to them, and any decisions can be made together.

[a]Nursing Alliance for Quality Care (NAQC): *Fostering successful patient and family engagement: nursing's critical role* (website). www.naqc.org/WhitePaper-PatientEngagement. (Accessed 17 June 2016).

for several days for gastrointestinal (GI) surgery patients (Hoch, 2014). Increased fluid intake and early ambulation promote return of peristalsis. Bowel sounds are auscultated with a stethoscope to ensure that peristalsis has returned, and the abdomen assessed for distention. Constipation occurs frequently after surgery because of the effects of anesthetic agents and opioids, immobility, and decreased GI motility. Fluids, roughage, and bulk laxatives can relieve constipation; occasionally a suppository or an enema is needed.

Early Ambulation

Early ambulation expedites recovery and prevents complications by increasing muscle tone, improving GI and urinary tract function, stimulating circulation, and increasing vital capacity (Hoch, 2014) (Fig. 10.12). Ambulation usually is postponed if severe infection or thrombophlebitis is present.

Evaluation

Evaluation of the postoperative patient outcomes on the surgical unit might be stated as follows:

- The patient's vital signs, temperature, urinary output, breath sounds, and laboratory values were within normal limits; the surgical site showed no signs or symptoms of infection.
- The patient's breathing was easy and unlabored, at a normal rate and of adequate depth.
- The patient verbalized freedom from pain, was able to perform activities of daily living, and was free from facial grimaces, moaning, and other evidence of pain or discomfort.
- The patient was eating well; there was no weight loss or complaints of nausea or vomiting.
- The patient ambulated regularly and was assessed as capable of performing appropriate activities.

Patient, Family, and Caregiver Education and Discharge Planning

Ideally patient, family, and caregiver education and discharge planning begin before the patient's admission for surgery (Patient Engagement Exemplar). The patient, family, and caregiver are prepared to assume any care that may be needed after discharge. If needed, community resources are used. Home healthcare is a valuable resource for patients with treatment needs after discharge. The nurse responsible for the patient's care in the acute care setting collaborates and communicates with the home health team as soon as the need is identified so that the patient's care will be coordinated and consistent.

The patient, family members, and caregivers are instructed in the proper care of the wound or incision and signs and symptoms of a wound infection. They should know how to take a temperature and when the physician should be notified for elevated temperature. They should be knowledgeable about medication that the patient will be using at home, including analgesics. Appropriate nonpharmacologic methods of pain control, such as imagery, distraction, massage, music therapy, and relaxation, also can be taught. An appointment for a return visit with the surgeon should be scheduled. The patient is advised to resume normal activities gradually according to the physician recommendations.

The chapters on surgical interventions in Unit II have incorporated important elements for patient, family, and caregiver education and discharge planning. These elements assist the perioperative nurse in identifying and teaching what patients need to know and facilitate safe self-care during recovery from operative and other invasive procedures.

Key Points

- Immediate postoperative patient care includes the basic life-sustaining needs, airway, breathing, and circulation (ABCs), and are of the highest priority.
- Hand-off reports for postoperative patients are a critical time that require clear, focused communication. Perioperative risks for communication problems are transfer from OR to PACU, from PACU to phase II PACU, or from PACU to inpatient bed. Try to have no interruptions or distractions during handoffs and care transitions.
- Continuous assessment of postoperative patients in the PACU includes assessment of vital signs, including pulse oximetry and $ETCO_2$, wound, pain and comfort, and other appropriate parameters (these are often procedure specific).

- Complications can occur quickly in the PACU, including airway obstruction, laryngospasm, bronchospasm, aspiration, cardiac dysrhythmias, delirium, excessive pain, and nausea and vomiting.
- The function of phase II PACU is to assist the patient in discharge and home readiness.

Critical Thinking Questions

Your new patient in the PACU is a 35-year-old male who presented for bariatric surgery with extreme obesity (405 pounds; 5 feet 4 inches tall). He underwent general anesthesia for a laparoscopic roux-en-y gastric bypass. He was given morphine 6 mg, ondansetron 8 mg, dexamethasone 4 mg, and midazolam 4 mg during surgery. The nursing and anesthesia history include type 2 diabetes, hypertension, and gastric reflux. He previously stated that he has been told he snores at home on occasion. He is a single parent with one child 3 years of age. He has limited insurance and needs to go back to work as soon as possible. His only previous surgery was an appendectomy when he was 12 years old. He takes metformin, omeprazole, and metoprolol at home. His initial vital signs are 190/90, 120, 32, 88% oxygen saturation on room air, T 100.5°F. His pain level is self-reported as 8 (0–10 scale) and he reports mild to moderate nausea. What are your major concerns about this patient? What are his risk factors? List the components of your nursing assessment in priority order. Address each of the assessment findings and discuss your interventions for each finding.

℮volve *The answers to the Critical Thinking Questions can be found at http://evolve.elsevier.com/Rothrock/Alexander*

References

American Association of Nurse Anesthetists (AANA): *Postanesthesia care standards for certified registered nurse anesthetists* (website), 2013. www.aana.com/resources2/professionalpractice/Documents/PPM%20PACU%20Standards.pdf. (Accessed 14 January 2017).

American Society of Anesthesiologists (ASA): *Standards for postanesthesia care* (website), 2014. standards-for-postanesthesia-care%20(2).pdf. (Accessed 1 January 2017).

American Society of Anesthesiologists (ASA): *Practice guidelines for preoperative fasting and the use of pharmacologic agents to reduce the risk of pulmonary aspiration: application to healthy patients undergoing elective procedures: an updated report by the American Society of Anesthesiologists Task Force on Preoperative Fasting and the Use of Pharmacologic Agents to Reduce the Risk of Pulmonary Aspiration, Anesthesiology* 126(3):376–393, 2017.

American Society of Anesthesiologists (ASA): *Practice guidelines for acute pain management in the perioperative setting: an updated report by the American Society of Anesthesiologists Task Force on Acute Pain Management* (website), 2012. practice-guidelines-for-acute-pain-management-in-the-perioperative-setting%20(1).pdf. (Accessed 14 January 2017).

American Society of PeriAnesthesia Nurses (ASPAN): *2017-2018 perianesthesia nursing standards, practice recommendations and interpretive statements*, Cherry Hill, NJ, 2016, ASPAN.

ASPAN US PR Strategic Work Team: The ASPAN prevention of unwanted sedation in the adult patient evidence-based practice recommendation, *J Perianesth Nurs* 29(5):344–352, 2014.

Apfel C et al: Who is at risk for postdischarge nausea and vomiting after ambulatory surgery?, *Anesthesiol* 117:475–486, 2012.

Apfel CC: Postoperative nausea and vomiting. In Miller RD et al, editors: *Miller's anesthesia*, ed 8, Philadelphia, 2015, Saunders Elsevier.

Apfel CC et al: A simplified risk score for predicting postoperative nausea and vomiting, *Anesthesiol* 91:693–700, 1999.

Baker DW: *Joint Commission statement on pain management* (website), 2016. www.jointcommission.org/joint_commission_statement_on_pain_management/. (Accessed 14 January 2017).

Booker SQ, Haedtke C: Assessing pain in nonverbal adults, *Nursing* 46(6):66–69, 2016.

Carlisle H: Promoting use of capnography in acute care settings: an evidence-based project, *JOPAN* 30(3):201–208, 2015.

Chou R et al: Management of postoperative pain: a clinical practice guideline from the American Pain Society, the American Society of Regional Anesthesia and Pain Medicine, and the American Society of Anesthesiologists' Committee on Regional Anesthesia, Executive Committee, and Administrative Council, *J Pain* 17(2):131–157, 2016.

DeJohn P: Helping to avoid postdischarge nausea and vomiting, *OR Manager* 29(1):28–29, 2013.

Drain C: The respiratory system. In Odom-Forren J, editor: *Drain's perianesthesia nursing: a critical care approach*, ed 7, St Louis, 2017, Elsevier.

Fiszer D et al: Next-generation sequencing of RYR1 and CACNA1S in malignant hyperthermia and exertional heat illness, *Anesthesiology* 122:1033–1046, 2015.

Fowler MA, Spiess BD: Post anesthesia recovery. In Barash PG et al, editors: *Clinical anesthesia*, Philadelphia, 2013, Lippincott, pp 1555–1579.

Gan TJ et al: Consensus guidelines for the management of postoperative nausea and vomiting, *Anesth Analg* 118(1):85–113, 2014.

Garrett JH: Effective perioperative communication to enhance patient care, *AORN J* 104(2):112–117, 2016.

Golembiewski J: Pharmacological management of postoperative shivering, *JOPAN* 30(4):357–359, 2015.

Guenther U et al: Patients prone for postoperative delirium: preoperative assessment, perioperative prophylaxis, postoperative treatment, *Curr Opin Anesthesiol* 29(3):384–390, 2016.

Hall RJ et al: Delirium detection and monitoring outside the ICU, *Clin Anaesthesiol* 2(26):367–383, 2016.

Hoch CR: Nursing management: postoperative care. In Lewis SM et al, editors: *Medical-surgical nursing: assessment and management of clinical problems*, ed 9, St Louis, 2014, Elsevier.

Hooper VD: Care of the patient with thermal imbalance. In Odom-Forren J, editor: *Drain's perianesthesia nursing: a critical care approach*, ed 7, St Louis, 2017, Elsevier.

Hooper VD et al: Thermoregulation. In Schick L, Windle PE, editors: *PeriAnesthesia nursing core curriculum: preoperative, phase I and phase II PACU nursing*, ed 3, St Louis, 2016, Elsevier.

Koivuranta M et al: A survey of postoperative nausea and vomiting, *Anaesthesia* 52(5):443–449, 1997.

Langham GE et al: Noninvasive temperature monitoring in postanesthesia care units, *Anesthesiology* 111:90–96, 2009.

Makic MBF: Pain management in the non-verbal critically ill patient, *J Perianesth Nurs* 28(2):98–101, 2013.

Moola S, Lockwood C: Effectiveness of strategies for the management and/or prevention of hypothermia within the adult perioperative environment, *Int J Evid Based Health* 9(4):337–345, 2011.

Nicholau TK: The postanesthesia care unit. In Miller RD et al, editors: *Miller's anesthesia*, ed 8, Philadelphia, 2015, Saunders Elsevier.

Nightingale F: *Notes on hospitals*, ed 3, London, 1863, Longman, Green, Roberts, Longman & Green.

O'Brien D: Patient education and care of the perianesthesia patient. In Odom-Forren J, editor: *Drain's perianesthesia nursing: a critical care approach*, ed 7, St Louis, 2017a, Elsevier.

O'Brien D: Postanesthesia care complications. In Odom-Forren J, editor: *Drain's perianesthesia nursing: a critical care approach*, ed 7, St Louis, 2017b, Elsevier.

Odom-Forren J: Postanesthesia recovery. In Nagelhout JJ, Plaus KL, editors: *Nurse anesthesia*, ed 5, St Louis, 2014, Saunders.

Odom-Forren J et al: The relationship of pain and nausea in postoperative patients for 1 week after ambulatory surgery, *Clin J Pain* 31:845–851, 2015.

Odom-Forren J, Clifford TL: Evolution of periAnesthesia care. In Schick L, Windle P, editors: *Perianesthesia nursing core curriculum: preoperative, phase I and phase II PACU nursing*, ed 3, St Louis, 2016, Elsevier.

Pasero C: The perianesthesia nurse's role in the prevention of opioid-related sentinel events, *J Perianesth Nurs* 28(1):31–37, 2013.

Pasero C, McCaffery M: *Pain assessment and pharmacologic management*, St Louis, 2011, Mosby.

Pasero C, Stannard D: The role of IV acetaminophen in acute pain management, *Pain Manage Nurs* 13(2):107–124, 2012.

Prospect: *Procedure-specific postoperative pain management* (website), 2015. www.postoppain.org. (Accessed 14 January 2017).

Putnam K: Monitoring to prevent postoperative opioid-induced respiratory depression, *AORN J* 103(2):7-p, 2016.

Quinlan-Cowell A: Pain management. In Odom-Forren J, editor: *Drain's perianesthesia nursing: a critical care approach*, ed 7, St Louis, 2017, Elsevier.

Schick L: Perianesthesia complications. In Schick L, Windle PE, editors: *PeriAnesthesia nursing core curriculum*, ed 3, St Louis, 2016, Elsevier.

Seifert PC et al: Crisis management of malignant hyperthermia in the OR, *AORN J* 100(2):189–202, 2014.

Seifert PC, Wadlund DL: Hypotension in the OR, *AORN J* 102(1):64–73, 2015.

Sessler DI: Perioperative thermoregulation and heat balance, *Lancet* 387(10038): 2655–2664, 2016.

Spence DL et al: Obstructive sleep apnea and the adult perioperative patient, *J Perianesthes Nurs* 30(6):528–545, 2015.

Surgical Care Improvement Project (SCIP): *NQF-endorsed voluntary consensus standards for hospital care* (website), 2016. http://hospitalcoremeasures.com/pdf/scip/2t_SCIP-Card-2.pdf. (Accessed 2 January 2017).

The Joint Commission (TJC): *Hospital: 2017 national patient safety goals* (website), 2016. www.jointcommission.org/hap_2017_npsgs/. (Accessed 14 January 2017).

Viswanath O et al: *Emergence delirium: a narrative review* (website), 2015. www.hoajonline.com/journals/pdf/2049-9752-4-2.pdf. (Accessed 2 January 2017).

Weinger MB et al: A multimodal intervention improves postanesthesia care unit handovers, *Anesth Analg* 121(4):957–971, 2015.

Wilson L et al: Pain and comfort. In Schick L, Windle P, editors: *PeriAnesthesia nursing core curriculum: preoperative, phase I and phase II PACU nursing*, ed 3, St Louis, 2016, Elsevier.

CHAPTER **11**

Gastrointestinal Surgery

BRITTA E. DEVOLDER

Gastrointestinal (GI) surgery encompasses a large number of surgical and procedural interventions to diagnose, treat, and prevent spread of congenital and pathologic conditions. Curative procedures, coupled with palliative techniques, can assist with alleviating debilitating symptoms of disease, allowing for comfort and nutritive capabilities while promoting quality of life and death with dignity. Endoscopic and minimally invasive interventions decrease infections and complications. Clinical research uses patient outcomes to compare the effectiveness of new approaches and innovative methods to more traditional methods of GI procedures; such research continues to grow rapidly, providing new evidence for practice and decision making (Hopkins et al., 2015; Johnson and Hope, 2015; Thomas and Wyatt, 2015; Duke and Farrell, 2016).

GI surgery encompasses surgical management throughout the GI tract, which includes the esophagus, stomach, small and large intestines, and rectum. Gastroenterology is a medical specialty that uses endoscopy to locate, identify, mark, and sometimes treat intraluminal pathology in the GI tract (Hayman and Whiteford, 2016). Endoscopic procedures are a critical component of surgical diagnosis, staging of disease, and postoperative evaluation. Although general surgeons and endoscopists may specialize in laparoscopic or robotic approaches, surgical endoscopy, bariatrics, surgical oncology, or colorectal surgery, perioperative nurses and scrub personnel must be familiar with the fundamentals of GI surgery and common patient care requirements.

Surgical Anatomy

The GI tract, or alimentary canal, is a continuous, tubelike structure that spans the abdomen (Fig. 11.1). Beginning in the mouth, the GI tract includes the pharynx; esophagus; stomach; small intestine, consisting of the duodenum, jejunum, and ileum; and large intestine. The large intestine consists of the cecum, ascending colon, transverse colon, descending colon, sigmoid colon, rectum, and anus. The length of the GI tract totals about 6 meters (20 feet). Basic functions of the GI tract are ingestion, secretion, mixing, digestion, propulsion, absorption, and elimination by defecation. The GI tract creates a complex microbiologic ecosystem to support and maintain essential life-sustaining digestive and protective functions. Substantial populations of microorganisms, both obligate anaerobes and facultative bacterial spores, exist in the intestinal lumen. The organisms of the upper tract differ from those of the lower tract, with the highest concentration in the distal bowel. These organisms can and do contribute to contamination and disease processes within the intestinal tract and throughout the body.

The esophagus is a collapsible musculomembranous tube through which ingested material moves, by peristalsis, from the pharynx to the stomach. After exiting the pharynx, the esophagus passes through the neck, posterior to the trachea and anterior to the vertebral column. The mediastinal portion of the esophagus enters the thoracic cavity at the level of the first thoracic vertebra where it lies posterior to the heart. The esophagus enters the peritoneal cavity through the esophageal hiatus of the diaphragm, where it joins the cardia of the stomach. The lower esophageal sphincter (LES) is at the terminal end of the esophagus; its function is to prevent reflux of gastric contents. Blood supply to the esophagus originates from branches of the inferior thyroid arteries, bronchial arteries, the thoracic aorta, and branches of the left gastric and inferior phrenic arteries. The venous drainage from the esophagus empties into the subclavian veins, the azygos vein on the right, the hemiazygos vein on the left, and through the coronary vein in the portal circulation. The nerve supply is from branches of the vagus nerve and the sympathetic nervous system.

The stomach lies in the upper abdominal cavity, to the left of the midline, inferior to the diaphragm and anterior to the pancreas.

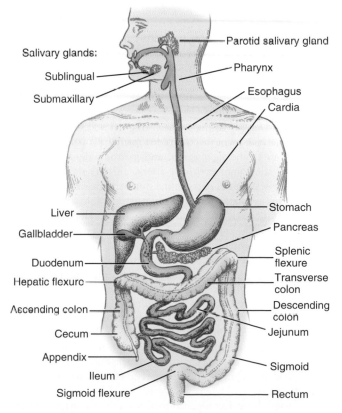

Salivary glands:
Sublingual
Submaxillary

Parotid salivary gland
Pharynx
Esophagus
Cardia

Liver
Gallbladder
Duodenum
Hepatic flexure
Ascending colon
Cecum
Appendix
Ileum
Sigmoid flexure

Stomach
Pancreas
Splenic flexure
Transverse colon
Descending colon
Jejunum
Sigmoid
Rectum

FIG. 11.1 Alimentary canal and its appendages.

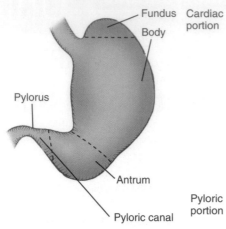

FIG. 11.2 Regional anatomy of stomach.

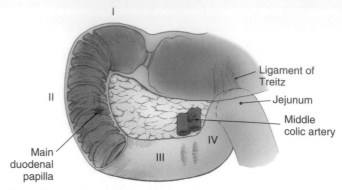

FIG. 11.3 Duodenum consists of four portions: *I,* superior duodenum; *II,* descending duodenum; *III,* horizontal duodenum; *IV,* ascending duodenum.

It is attached to the spleen on the left by the gastrosplenic ligament, the liver on the right by the hepatogastric ligament, the duodenum on the right by the gastroduodenal ligament, and the transverse colon inferiorly by the posterior layer of the greater omentum. Physiologically, cells in different regions of the stomach have unique functions related to digestion. Description of the stomach is by names related to each region, such as the cardia, fundus, body, antrum, and pyloric canal (Fig. 11.2). The fundus lies inferior to the left lobe of the liver and medially adjacent to the spleen. Inferior to the fundus, the body and antrum curve obliquely to the right, before terminating at the pylorus. The concave, or medial, margin of the stomach is referred to as the lesser curve and the convex, or lateral, margin of the stomach is known as the greater curve.

The omentum is a double layer of fatty peritoneum attached along the greater curve of the stomach. It drapes down loosely over the intestines and then folds posteriorly on itself before sweeping upward to attach along the transverse colon. The mesentery is also a double layer of peritoneum, but it differs from the omentum in that it connects the small bowel and parts of the colon to the posterior abdominal wall and contains the blood supply, nerves, and lymphatics of the intestines within its layers.

The blood supply to the stomach originates at the celiac trunk of the aorta, which branches into the left gastric, splenic, and common hepatic arteries. The right gastric and gastroduodenal arteries are branches of the common hepatic artery. The left and right gastric arteries supply the lesser curve of the stomach; the stomach's greater curve receives its supply from the right gastroepiploic artery, a branch of the gastroduodenal artery, and the left gastroepiploic artery, which originates from the splenic artery. Additional blood supply comes from the inferior phrenic arteries and the short gastric arteries located between the greater curve and the spleen. The gastric veins follow the same pathways as the arteries and drain into the portal vein. The right gastroepiploic vein drains into the superior mesenteric vein and the left gastroepiploic vein drains into the splenic vein. Regional lymph nodes are located at the gastroesophageal junction (GEJ), the splenic hilum, and the pylorus; they receive gastric lymphatic drainage, all of which empties into the celiac nodes and ultimately into the cisterna chyli and thoracic duct. The autonomic, sympathetic, parasympathetic, and enteric nervous systems regulate gastric function.

The stomach receives ingested food from the esophagus to begin the digestive process; it then propels partially digested food, or chyme, into the duodenum through the pylorus. In anticipation of receiving ingested material, the stomach prepares for its role in digestion by increasing motility, producing gastric acid, and releasing pepsinogen, intrinsic factor, gastric fluids, and mucus. Peptide hormones in the stomach (gastrin, somatostatin, and ghrelin) function directly and indirectly to regulate gastric secretions and motility. Gastrin causes enterochromaffin-like (ECL) cells in the body of the stomach to release histamine, stimulating gastric acid secretion from the parietal cells. Somatostatin inhibits gastrin, histamine, and acid secretion. Production of ghrelin occurs in the fundus. It stimulates gastric motility as well as the appetite, regulates hunger and satiety during meals, and plays a role in long-term body weight regulation (King and Hines, 2013). Research regarding ghrelin's role in obesity and potential medications for the treatment of obesity is ongoing (Anini and Shin, 2015).

The longest part of the GI tract is the small intestine, which begins at the pylorus and ends at the ileocecal valve. There is variation in length of the adult small intestine but typically it is about 3 meters long with a diameter of approximately 2.5 cm. The small intestine consists of three parts: the duodenum (20 cm), the jejunum (110 cm), and the ileum (155 cm). The duodenum begins with a 2-cm mobile intraperitoneal portion called the duodenal bulb. The remaining duodenum is retroperitoneal and fixed posteriorly by peritoneal attachments. The duodenal bulb dilates. Circular folds, known as plicae circulares of Kerckring, characteristic of the small intestinal mucosa, begin in the duodenum, continue through the jejunum, and become less prominent in the ileum. These plicae allow for greater mucosal surface area to absorb nutrients. The duodenum forms a C-shaped curve around the head of the pancreas; within this curve is the ampulla of Vater or main duodenal papilla, in which the common bile duct and the main pancreatic duct enter through the posteromedial wall (Fig. 11.3). The duodenum continues in a medial direction along the inferior border of the body of the pancreas before it ascends slightly to the duodenojejunal flexure, at which point it becomes the jejunum.

The blood supply to the duodenum comes from the gastroduodenal artery, located behind the duodenal bulb (Fig. 11.4). At the inferior margin of the bulb, the gastroduodenal artery divides into the right gastroepiploic and superior pancreaticoduodenal arteries to supply the proximal duodenum and head of the pancreas. The inferior pancreaticoduodenal artery, a branch of the superior mesenteric artery, supplies the transverse and ascending portions of the duodenum, as well as the head and body of the pancreas.

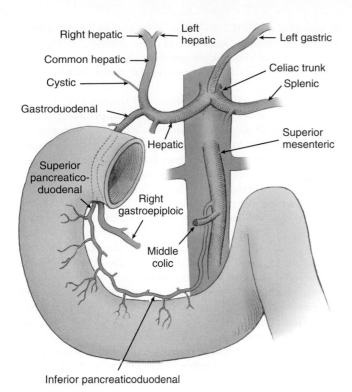

FIG. 11.4 Arterial blood supply of the duodenum.

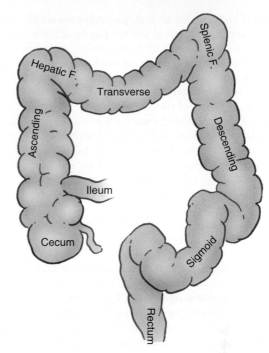

FIG. 11.5 Anatomic division of large intestine, showing locations of hepatic flexure and splenic flexure. *F,* Flexure.

In the left upper quadrant, the ligament of Treitz supports the duodenojejunal flexure and serves as a landmark to identify the beginning of the jejunum. The jejunum continues for about 2.5 meters (8 feet) before it transitions into the ileum in the right lower quadrant. The ileum continues for about another 3.5 meters (12 feet) before it ends at the ileocecal junction.

Blood supply to the jejunum and ileum comes entirely from their respective branches of the superior mesenteric artery. The mesentery of the jejunum and ileum is about 5.5 meters (18 feet) long, allowing for its mobility within the abdominal cavity. Peyer patches, a form of lymphatic tissue, generously litter the ileum mucosa on the antimesenteric boarder. The rich lymphatic drainage of the small bowel plays a major role in fat absorption. Lymphatic drainage from the mucosa proceeds through the wall of the small intestine to lymph nodes adjacent to the mesentery. It then proceeds to larger lymphatics that communicate with the retroperitoneal cisterna chyli and from there to the thoracic duct, where it terminates in the internal jugular vein. The lymphatics of the intestine play a major role, both in the body's immune defense and in the distribution of cells arising from intestinal neoplasms.

The large intestine (Fig. 11.5) consists of the cecum, colon, rectum, and anal canal (not illustrated). The cecum attaches to the lateral abdominal wall by peritoneal attachments called cecal folds. The terminal branch of the superior mesenteric artery, the ileocolic artery, supplies blood to the cecum.

The appendix is a 7- to 10-cm blind-ended tube of tissue that extends from the posteromedial wall of the cecum, below the ileocecal junction, and attaches to the cecum by the mesoappendix. The blood supply to the appendix comes from the appendicular artery, which is a branch of the terminal part of the ileocolic artery.

The ascending colon extends upward from the cecum to the hepatic flexure, where it lies behind the right lobe of the liver and

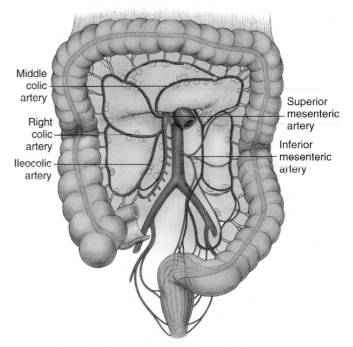

FIG. 11.6 Blood supply of the colon.

in front of the anterior surface of the right kidney. It receives its blood supply from the ileocolic and middle colic arteries (Fig. 11.6). The transverse colon begins at the hepatic flexure and ends at the splenic flexure. It lies below the stomach, suspended by the transverse mesocolon. The blood supply to the transverse colon is via the middle colic artery (see Fig. 11.6). The descending colon extends downward from the splenic flexure to become the sigmoid colon.

The sigmoid colon makes an S-shaped curve toward the midline, where it descends to transition into the rectum at the rectosigmoid junction. The arterial supply to the descending and sigmoid colon comes from the left colic and sigmoid arteries. The superior, middle, and inferior rectal arteries supply the rectum and anal canal. The marginal artery of Drummond forms an arcade of collateral circulation along the inner border of the colon.

Distinguishing physical characteristics of the colon are the teniae coli, epiploic appendices, and haustra. The teniae coli are three separate, longitudinal bands of muscle distributed along the length of the colon. The epiploic appendices are fatty appendages attached to the colon along the teniae and have no particular function. Haustra are sacculations of the colon wall along the contracted teniae, giving it a segmented appearance.

The rectum begins at the rectosigmoid junction, in which the teniae coli merge at the level of the sacral promontory. The absence of distinct teniae serves as a visual landmark for the upper margin of the rectum. The rectum has three characteristic lateral curves, or flexures, that coincide internally with transverse rectal folds called valves of Houston (Birnbaum, 2015). The rectum lies on the sacrum posteriorly. As it descends into the pelvis, the posterior rectum attaches to the anterior surface of the sacrum by the rectosacral fascia. It also attaches to the pelvis by fascia extending from the right and left pelvic sidewalls. In males, the rectovesical fascia, or Denonvilliers fascia, separates the anterior rectum from the seminal glands, prostate, bladder, ureters, and ductus deferens. In females, the rectovaginal fascia separates the anterior rectum from the vagina. The terminal rectum, or ampulla, dilates to receive and hold feces before passage into the anal canal. The GI tract terminates in the anal canal, which is a 3- to 5-cm funnel-shaped passage. The anal canal begins at the anorectal junction, which is separated from the anal verge by the internal and external anal sphincters.

The large intestine recovers water, electrolytes, and nutrients from succus entericus, which is a mixture of undigested fluids, starches, proteins, and bile salts received from the ileum. The remaining waste product descends toward the rectum, solidifies into feces, and stores in the rectal ampulla until its expulsion through the anal canal, or, commonly, defecation.

Perioperative Nursing Considerations

GI surgery and endoscopic procedures vary widely, depending on the patient's medical diagnosis and history, the purpose of the intended procedure, the surgical approach, and the involved anatomic structures. Other influencing factors include the patient's goals and desire for treatment, the surgeon's preferred approach based on training and experience, and the availability of advanced technologies in imaging, access, and instrumentation.

Assessment

Patient-centered care begins with an assessment that integrates information about the physiologic and psychosocial status of the patient into an individualized plan of care. Key sources of information that facilitate and guide the assessment process include medical history, physical examination, physician orders, and results from laboratory and other diagnostic studies. Laboratory studies might include a complete blood count, as well as a complete metabolic panel to measure serum glucose, serum electrolytes, kidney function, liver function, and serum proteins. Coagulation studies such as international normalized ratio (INR) and prothrombin time or partial

thromboplastin time (PT/PTT) may be appropriate if patients present with hepatic disease or long-term use of anticoagulants (Feeley et al., 2013). Abnormal values require specific notation and communication to the surgeon and anesthesia provider (lab values are presented in Appendix A).

Diagnostic procedures, determined by the patient's presenting signs and symptoms, the location of suspected pathology, and the potential sites of metastasis, may include esophageal manometry, pH monitoring, and motility studies. Additional tests may include radiologic studies, with or without contrast markers; endoscopic examinations; abdominal or endoscopic ultrasound (EUS); computed tomography (CT) imaging scans; magnetic resonance imaging (MRI); or positron emission tomography (PET). Endoscopic imaging has evolved to include chromoendoscopy, confocal laser endomicroscopy, endocystoscopy, optical coherence tomography magnification endoscopy, narrowband imaging, and wireless video capsule endoscopy, all recognized and utilized diagnostic options. These provide enhanced details of GI anatomy and are essential tools in identifying and staging GI malignancies to determine surgical options and other treatments (Ou et al., 2015; Lipka et al., 2015a; Micic and Semrad, 2016; Toomey et al., 2015).

Barriers to patient communication such as language, sensory deficits, and altered cognitive function, along with distractors, such as pain or emotional stress, require assessment during the preoperative interview. Acknowledge emotions as legitimate feelings. Encourage and allow the patient to express tearfulness or verbalize feelings of fear, anger, denial, depression, nervousness, or anxiety.

After confirming the patient's identity, ask the patient to verify, in his or her own words, the name of the scheduled procedure, the planned approach, and laterality if applicable. Because of the nature and unpredictability of GI surgery, if a minimally invasive approach is planned, the patient must understand the possibility of the need to convert to a laparotomy. If intestinal diversion via ileostomy or colostomy is a possibility, determine whether a wound ostomy continence nurse (WOCN) has marked the site of the stoma and assess the patient's understanding of this part of the procedure (Patient Engagement Exemplar). Individualized ostomy site selection by a WOCN helps prevent appliance leaks and peristomal skin complications (Salvadalena et al., 2015). The optimal ostomy site is located within the rectus muscle reducing the risk of peristomal hernias; avoids placement in or across a skin fold, crease, or at the belt line; and is visible and easily accessible to enable the patient to perform self-care postoperatively. A WOCN's preoperative counseling and education, aimed at assisting the patient, family, and caregiver to adapt to expected lifestyle changes, to accept altered body image, to address sexuality concerns, and to understand elements of ostomy self-care, demonstrate a positive effect on long-term outcomes. In emergent cases or when a WOCN is not available, the surgical team should be educated to identify the site and educate the patient appropriately (Salvadalena et al., 2015).

The perioperative nurse checks the review of systems (Table 11.1) in the medical record to identify and confirm patient conditions that can increase risks of perioperative complications. Current medications, including use of supplements, require review with the patient. Verify the last dose taken on all medications. GI conditions requiring procedural or surgical intervention are often accompanied by alterations in nutritional status, which can cause increased risk for infection, poor wound healing, pressure injuries, and overgrowth of bacteria in the GI tract (Birnbaum, 2015; Puplampu and Simpson, 2015). Assessment of the patient's nutritional status includes determining the patient's body mass index (BMI) (Box 11.1), history of

PATIENT ENGAGEMENT EXEMPLAR

What Patient Engagement Looks Like

NAQC guiding principle number 6 states "clinicians must recognize that the extent to which patients and family members are engaged or choose to engage may vary greatly based on individual circumstances, cultural beliefs and other factors."

Consider this scenario:

Mrs. Kipton is scheduled for a low anterior colon resection, possible end-to-end anastomosis, or a possible APR with a permanent colostomy. When Karla, the perioperative nurse, meets Mrs. Kipton in the preoperative holding area, patient-centered communication might sound like the following:

"Good morning, my name is Karla. I am a registered nurse and I will be taking care of you during your surgery." Mrs. Kipton introduces Karla to her daughter. Karla gets permission to continue the patient interview in the daughter's presence and then says, "Can you tell me what procedure you are having today?" Mrs. Kipton replies, "I would like for you to talk to my daughter." Karla says, "That is fine, Mrs. Kipton, I will be happy to talk to her." She then asks her daughter what the procedure is going to be. She says, "My mom has cancer near the end of her colon that has to be removed. The surgeon told us she might need to have a colostomy if the cancer is too big for him to put her back together." To confirm that Mrs. Kipton and her daughter understand the significance of having a colostomy and an APR, Karla says, "Yes, that is what it says here on your surgical consent form. The end of your colon is called the rectum. If the cancer is too low in your

rectum, making it unsafe for the surgeon to remove all of the cancer and still reconnect your healthy bowel to your remaining rectum, the entire rectum will be removed and a colostomy made. Your surgeon will bring the end of the healthy bowel up through a small hole in your abdominal wall, where it will be secured with stitches. The surgeon will then make another incision all of the way around the opening where your bowel movements come out and finish removing the rectum from the outside. If you do need to have a colostomy, instead of having bowel movements like you do now, your colon will empty into a small plastic bag that snaps onto a ring that is part of a pad that adheres to your skin. Unfortunately, we do not know exactly what the surgeon will find until he gets inside. If you do need a colostomy, the bag will be located there, on the left side of your abdomen, where Jan, the nurse who will teach you all about caring for your colostomy, put a mark yesterday. Is this what you both understand?" Mrs. Kipton glances at her daughter who nods yes and then replies, "Yes, we do understand and thank you for describing things so that we could understand what you were saying. We were having difficulty understanding all of this; it is very overwhelming." Throughout the perioperative process, patients' and families' levels of understanding are assessed and confirmed through dialog such as this. Respecting the patient's level of engagement and wishes for including family members is important to maintain a respectful and trustworthy nurse patient relationship.

APR, Abdominal perineal resection; *NAQC,* Nursing Alliance for Quality Care.
From Nursing Alliance for Quality Care (NAQC): *Fostering successful patient and family engagement: nursing's critical role* (website). http://www.naqc.org/WhitePaper-PatientEngagement. (Accessed 17 June 2016); Modified from Bertakis KD, Azari R: Patient-centered care is associated with decreased health care utilization, *J Am Board Fam Med* 24(3):229–239, 2011; Delbanco T, Gerteis M: A patient-centered view of the clinician-patient relationship. In Basow DS, editor: *UpToDate,* Waltham, MA, UpToDate, 2012; Mulsow JJ: Beyond consent—improving understanding in surgical patients, *Am J Surg* 203(1):112–120, 2012.

BOX 11.1

Calculating a Patient's Body Mass Index

A patient's body mass index (BMI) is an estimate of total body fat. BMI is a weight-to-height ratio that is used to determine if an individual is underweight, at a healthy weight, overweight, or obese. BMI is expressed as kilograms per square meter and calculated by the following formula:

$$BMI = (\text{weight in pounds} \div \text{height in inches}^2) \times 703$$

Calculated BMI (kg/m²)	Meaning
25–29.9	Overweight
30–34.9	Obese: class I
35–39.9	Moderately obese: class II
40–49.9	Severely or extremely obese: class III
≥50	Super obese: class IV

Modified from Bray GA, Perreault L: Obesity in adults: prevalence, screening, and evaluation. In Pi-Sunyer FX, editor: *UpToDate,* Waltham, MA, 2016, UpToDate; Ogden CL et al: *Prevalence of obesity among adults and youth: United States 2011-2014, NCHS data brief no. 219,* Hyattsville, MD, 2015, National Center for Health Statistics.

recent weight loss or gain, difficulty swallowing, nausea, vomiting, diarrhea, constipation, and NPO status.

Components of a nursing physical assessment include notation of general appearance and body mass distribution. Assessments of skin integrity, quality of peripheral pulses, presence of neuropathies, and physical limitations help determine baseline data for evaluation of outcomes related to positioning and hydration status. Focused examination of the patient's abdomen includes inspection for skin integrity, hair distribution, scars, and distention. Palpation to assess for rigidity; referral; and/or localization of pain, masses, and unusual pulsations may follow if indicated.

Relevant social assessment includes use of tobacco, alcohol, or recreational drugs. Inquiries about the patient's ability to perform activities of daily living; circumstances of the patient's home situation; and availability of family, friends, or other support systems during hospitalization and after discharge play an important part of discharge planning.

Nursing Diagnosis

Nursing diagnoses related to the care of patients undergoing GI surgery might include the following:

- Anxiety related to perioperative events
- Deficient Knowledge related to impending surgery
- Disturbed Body Image related to intestinal diversion (when diversion possible or planned)

TABLE 11.1

Preoperative Nursing Review of Systems

System	Condition	Increased Risk	Relevant Assessment Data
Cardiovascular	Ischemic heart disease	Cardiac death, nonfatal MI	Recent MI, cardiac surgery, cardiac stents, nitrate use for angina, abnormal ECG (pathologic Q waves)
	Heart failure	Respiratory complications, fluid and electrolyte imbalances, activity intolerance	Pulmonary edema-crackles, dyspnea at rest, tachycardia, hypertension or hypotension, reduced urinary output, PVCs and other dysrhythmias, restlessness, anxiety
	Hypertension BP 130–139/80–89	BP instability, arrhythmias, myocardial ischemia	Beta-blockers, ACEIs, ARBs, calcium channel blockers
Endocrine	Insulin-dependent diabetes, uncontrolled	Postoperative infections, cardiovascular complications	A1C >8% Fasting blood glucose ≥200
	Obesity	Cardiovascular (DVT) and respiratory complications (pneumonia), wound infection, delayed wound healing, obstructive sleep apnea	BMI >30
Immune	Malignancy, HIV, rheumatoid arthritis, SLE	Infection, difficult intubation and IV access, risk of aspiration, pulmonary embolism	Malnourished, recent treatment with chemotherapy, chronic use of glucocorticoids (prednisone), renal insufficiency
Pulmonary	COPD, asthma, respiratory infection	Postoperative respiratory complications	Abnormal chest x-ray, poor pulmonary function, inhaler use, cough, breathlessness, tobacco use
Renal	End-stage renal disease	Altered medication metabolism	Azotemia, abnormal serum potassium
Liver	Hepatitis, cirrhosis	Altered medication metabolism, bleeding	Malnutrition, vitamin K deficiency, ascites
GI	Malnutrition	Poor wound healing	Decreased albumin, transferrin, prealbumin
Anticoagulant therapy	Atrial fibrillation, coronary stents, recent DVT	Intraoperative and postoperative bleeding	Prolonged bleeding times, epistaxis, bruising Medication list includes aspirin, clopidogrel, dabigatran, warfarin, NSAIDs, COX-2 inhibitors, dipyridamole
Coagulopathy	von Willebrand disease		

ACE, Angiotensin-converting enzyme; *ACEI,* angiotensin-converting enzyme inhibitors; *ARBs,* angiotensin-receptor blockers; *BMI,* body mass index; *BP,* blood pressure; *COPD,* chronic obstructive pulmonary disease; *COX-2,* cyclooxygenase-2; *DVT,* deep vein thrombosis; *ECG,* electrocardiogram; *GI,* gastrointestinal; *HIV,* human immunodeficiency virus; *IV,* intravenous; *MI,* myocardial infarction; *NSAIDs,* nonsteroidal antiinflammatory drugs; *PVC,* premature ventricular contraction; *SLE,* systemic lupus erythematosus.

Modified from Hassilgren P et al: Perioperative management: practical principles, molecular basis of risk and future direction. In Fischer J, editor: *Fischer's mastery of surgery,* Philadelphia, 2012, Lippincott Williams & Wilkins; Ignatavicius DD, Workman LM, editors: *Medical-surgical nursing: patient-centered collaborative care,* St Louis, 2016, Elsevier.

- Risk for Perioperative Hypothermia
- Risk for Infection at the surgical site
- Risk for Perioperative Positioning Injury
- Risk for Impaired Tissue Integrity related to lasers, thermal devices, electrosurgery, radiation, or chemical solutions
- Risk for Injury from retained surgical items, wrong procedure, wrong site, or administration of wrong or incorrect medications
- Risk for Imbalanced Fluid Volume

Outcome Identification

Outcomes identified for selected nursing diagnoses could be stated as follows:
- The patient will demonstrate or verbalize decreased anxiety and ability to cope throughout the perioperative period.
- The patient will verbalize understanding of the surgical procedure, expected responses, and postoperative self-care requirements.
- The patient will demonstrate acceptance of expected changes in appearance.
- The patient will be at, or returning to, normothermia at the conclusion of the immediate postoperative period.
- The patient will be free from signs and symptoms of surgical site infection.

- The patient will be free from perioperative positioning injury.
- The patient will be free of evidence of impaired tissue integrity.
- The patient will be free from injury related to retained surgical items, wrong procedure, wrong site, and medication errors.
- The patient's fluid volume, electrolyte levels, and acid-base balance will be consistent with or improved from preoperative baseline levels.

Planning

Preoperative assessment provides the perioperative nurse with critical information to develop an individualized plan of care. Analysis of patient-specific physiologic and psychosocial data assists in identifying nursing interventions to comfort patients, mitigate risks for complications, prevent injury and infection, and help the patient to achieve the best possible outcomes. Planning for optimal patient care also includes ensuring that necessary instruments, supplies, and equipment are at hand for the planned procedure. A Sample Plan of Care for patients undergoing GI surgery can be found on p. 293. GI surgery also is one of the pioneering surgical services to focus on enhanced recovery after surgery (ERAS) pathways (Enhanced Recovery After Surgery).

ENHANCED RECOVERY AFTER SURGERY

Programs for Colorectal Surgery

Evidence-based strategies enhance recovery after elective colorectal surgery, accelerate a patient's return to preoperative levels of health and functional status, and facilitate early discharge. They reduce the surgical stress response and organ dysfunction that can occur after major abdominal surgery. Also known as fast-track programs or surgical care bundles, ERAS programs combine individual evidence-based strategies to create standardized preoperative, intraoperative, and postoperative pathways of care. These are implemented by multidisciplinary patient care teams to improve patient outcomes and reduce healthcare costs. Examples of a colorectal ERAS fast track program follow.

Preoperative Strategies
- Preadmission counseling including:
  - Extensive patient education about ostomy care
  - Expectation management for recovery milestones such as return to regular diet, driving, work, and other activities
  - Addressing self-care needs or challenges, and ensuring patients and their caregivers know what postoperative conditions require them to seek medical attention after discharge
- Preoperative assessment, risk evaluation, and optimization of comorbid conditions
- Eliminating or selective bowel preparation
- Fluid and carbohydrate loading
- Fasting: meat and fried and fatty food for 8 hours; light meals and unclear liquids for 6 hours; clear liquids for 2 hours

- Antibiotic prophylaxis
- Thromboprophylaxis
- No premedication

Intraoperative Strategies
- DVT prophylaxis
- Antibiotic prophylaxis
- High concentration of inspired oxygenation
- Mid-thoracic epidural analgesia
- Anesthesia using rapid-onset, short-acting anesthetic gases and medications
- Balanced fluid management: avoidance of salt and water overload
- Temperature regulation: maintain normothermia via warming devices and warm IV fluids
- Laparoscopic approach when possible
- Eliminate drain use

Postoperative Strategies
- Minimize use of opioid analgesia when possible
- Aggressively manage nausea
- Enteral nutrition on day 1
- Liquid diet within a few hours after surgery
- Early mobilization (on day of surgery)
- Early removal of urinary catheter
- Eliminate NG tube usage
- Avoid salt and water overload
- Stimulate gut motility
- Audit compliance and outcomes

DVT, Deep vein thrombosis; *ERAS,* enhanced recovery after surgery; *IV,* intravenous; *NG,* nasogastric.
Modified from Brady KM et al: Successful implementation of an enhanced recovery pathway: the nurse's role, *AORN J* 102(5):469–481, 2015; Hohenberger H, Delahanty K: Patient-centered care: enhanced recovery after surgery and population health management, *AORN J* 102(6):578–583, 2015; Scott MJ et al: Enhanced recovery after surgery (ERAS) for gastrointestinal surgery, part 1: pathophysiological considerations, *Acta Anaesthesiol Scand* 59(10):1212–1231, 2015.

SAMPLE PLAN OF CARE

Nursing Diagnosis
Anxiety related to perioperative events

Outcome
The patient will demonstrate or verbalize decreased anxiety and ability to cope throughout the perioperative period.

Interventions
- Explain preoperative activities and expectations (e.g., IV lines, skin preparation, positioning), sequence of sensory experiences and activities in the OR, and postoperative expectations (e.g., PACU, drains, catheters, dressings).
- Provide time for patient, family members, and caregiver to ask questions and express concerns.
- Determine effective coping strategies used by patient in the past; support these as appropriate.
- Minimize stimuli in the OR that can contribute to anxiety (e.g., high noise levels, excessive talking, music that is not the patient's preference).
- Remain with the patient during induction; convey caring behaviors (e.g., appropriate touch; a soft, reassuring voice; warm blankets for thermal comfort).

- Maintain the patient's dignity and privacy.
- Communicate unresolved or excessive anxiety to team members.

Nursing Diagnosis
Deficient Knowledge related to impending surgery

Outcome
The patient will verbalize understanding of the surgical procedure, expected responses, and postoperative self-care requirements.

Interventions
- Verify information the patient, family, and caregiver need and want to know. Determine current knowledge level and perceptions of surgery. Take into consideration language, culture, hearing or visual impairment, health literacy, cognitive impairments, and any relevant disability.
- Initiate preoperative education and discharge planning early in the perioperative process.
- Assess readiness to learn and patient's preferred learning style.
- Include family or patient's accompanying responsible adult in teaching. Use simple language. Present information in the

Continued

SAMPLE PLAN OF CARE—cont'd

patient's dominant language (use an interpreter if necessary). Note any sensory impairments and accommodate them. When possible, provide written information that replicates verbal education.

- Verify patient's understanding of material presented by having the patient repeat back, in his or her own words, information that has been presented. Correct misunderstandings.
- Communicate patient or family concerns to appropriate surgical team members or make appropriate referral.

Nursing Diagnosis
Disturbed Body Image related to intestinal diversion (when diversion possible or planned)

Outcome
The patient will demonstrate acceptance of expected changes in appearance and self-care.

Interventions
- Encourage verbalization of feelings about anticipated alterations in body function if diversion procedure planned.
- Elicit the patient's and family's (if appropriate) perceptions of planned surgical intervention.
- Identify effective sources of support.
- Encourage patient to implement cultural, religious, ethnic, or social customs associated with perceived loss.
- Provide accurate information relevant to patient's postoperative expectations (general principles of ostomy care and solutions to concerns that may worry patient).
- Refer patient to WOCN if this has not already been done.

Nursing Diagnosis
Risk for Perioperative Hypothermia

Outcome
The patient will be at or returning to normothermia at the conclusion of the immediate postoperative period.

Interventions
- Determine patient's risk to develop inadvertent hypothermia.
- Regulate ambient room temperature in range between 68°F and 78°F (20°C and 25.6°C) as appropriate.
- Monitor patient temperature during surgery.
- Minimize unnecessary patient exposure. Keep patient covered with warm blankets before induction. Ask patient if he or she is comfortable and warm enough.
- Use effective skin-surface warming methods (e.g., forced-air warming, circulating water garment, energy transfer pads) preoperatively, intraoperatively, and in PACU as needed.
- Use warmed irrigating solutions and fluid replacement therapy (e.g., IVs) as appropriate. Follow manufacturer's recommendations when using warming equipment.
- Cover patient with a warm blanket before transport to the PACU.

Nursing Diagnosis
Risk for Infection at the surgical site related to operative or other invasive procedure

Outcome
The patient will be free from signs and symptoms of surgical site infection.

Interventions
- Identify patient-specific risk factors for infection (e.g., altered nutritional status, chronic diseases, preoperative chemotherapy, radiation therapy).

- Follow institutional protocol for perioperative skin preparation (patient bath or shower preoperatively with prescribed antimicrobial agent; intraoperative skin preparation with antimicrobial agent).
- Initiate evidence-based practices to create and maintain a sterile field.
- Protect the patient from cross-contamination: use bowel/GI technique as appropriate.
- Designate appropriate wound classification (clean, clean-contaminated, contaminated, dirty/infected) at end of procedure.
- Initiate traffic control measures/protocols.
- Administer medication as prescribed (e.g., antibiotic prophylaxis), using safe medication practices. Label and document all medications on and off the sterile field.

Nursing Diagnosis
Risk for Perioperative Positioning Injury

Outcome
The patient will be free from signs of perioperative positioning injury.

Interventions
- Assess patient for physical alteration, prosthetics, or corrective devices requiring modifications to procedure-specific position.
- Position patient in body alignment with attention to possible modifications of surgical position, patient limitations, and safety.
- Use adequate body supports, restraints, and padding of pressure sites specific to planned position, patient body mass, and length of procedure. Reassess position status throughout procedure, especially after positional changes (as possible).
- Lift and transport patient carefully with sufficient assistance and lifting aids as needed.
- Reassess patient for signs and symptoms of positional injury at conclusion of procedure.

Nursing Diagnosis
Risk for Impaired Tissue Integrity related to lasers, thermal devices, electrosurgery, radiation, or chemical solutions

Outcome
The patient will be free of evidence of impaired tissue integrity.

Interventions
- Inspect skin condition and determine patient's risk factors related to skin injury.
- If hair must be removed from surgical site, select removal method most likely to preserve skin integrity.
- Protect patient from thermal, electrical, laser, and chemical injury by following institutional practice guidelines. Implement fire safety precautions with skin prep solution.
- Before applying dressings, clean and dry skin at incision site or sites.
- Prevent stretching of the skin when securing dressings with tape.
- Reassess patient for signs of skin injury at the conclusion of procedure and document findings.
- Remove blood/body fluids and apply clean gown and blankets before transfer to PACU.

Nursing Diagnosis
Risk for Injury from retained surgical items, wrong procedure, wrong site, or medication administration

SAMPLE PLAN OF CARE—cont'd

Outcome

The patient will be free from injury related to retained surgical items, wrong procedure, wrong site, or administration of wrong or incorrect medications.

Interventions

- Confirm patient identity, using two identifiers.
- Initiate preoperative verification process. Verify surgical procedure, and involve patient in marking surgical site.
- Identify any allergies to medications.
- Perform and document required counts. Take a "pause for the count" to avoid distractions.
- Administer medications and solutions as prescribed. Label all medications and solutions on and off the sterile field. Use safe medication practices. Document medications administered.
- Verify and record implants (as applicable).
- Follow protocols to contain, identify, label, preserve, transfer, and transport surgical specimens. Use safe specimen management practices.

Nursing Diagnosis
Risk for Imbalanced Fluid Volume

Outcome

The patient's fluid volume, electrolyte levels, and acid-base balance will be consistent with or improved from preoperative baseline levels.

Interventions

- Review baseline laboratory data; confer with surgeon or anesthesia provider regarding deviations from normal.
- Assess nutritional status, skin turgor, renal status, and other conditions or medications affecting fluid, acid-base, and electrolyte balance.
- Collaborate with surgeon and anesthesia provider in accurately estimating fluid and blood loss and maintaining or correcting losses (administration of fluid replacement therapies, blood products, electrolytes, or medications).
- Record all solutions administered from the surgical field.
- As appropriate, include EBL in hand-off report to receiving unit. In some institutions, calculation of a surgical Apgar score occurs at the end of the surgical procedure, based on the EBL, lowest mean arterial pressure (expressed in mm Hg), and the lowest heart rate rhythm recorded on the anesthesia record during the procedure. The score helps identify patients with a higher likelihood of developing complications after surgery.

EBL, Estimated blood loss; *GI*, gastrointestinal; *IV*, intravenous; *PACU*, postanesthesia care unit; *WOCN*, wound ostomy continence nurse.

Implementation

The perioperative nurse implements the plan of care throughout all phases of the patient's surgical experience. Communication and cooperation between all members of the surgical team by working together to help the patient achieve identified outcomes is essential. There is strong evidence that preoperative checklists prevent a number of surgical safety events as well as decrease postoperative complications (Mayer et al., 2016; Shekelle et al., 2013). Specialized checklists related to the GI ERAS have been developed and are used by the entire surgical team to promote standardization and compliance with identified bundles (Mayson et al., 2016; Wu et al., 2015).

Most patients undergoing open and laparoscopic GI surgery require general endotracheal anesthesia (anesthesia techniques appear in Chapter 5). A midthoracic epidural, placed preoperatively as an adjuvant to general anesthesia, can decrease postoperative pain, increase adherence to pulmonary exercises, and promote early ambulation. Intravenous (IV) moderate sedation is appropriate for outpatient endoscopic procedures, such as esophagogastroduodenoscopy (EGD) or colonoscopy.

Fluid management during significant blood loss may require arterial monitoring and frequent intraoperative sampling of hemoglobin and hematocrit (H&H), arterial blood gases (ABGs), electrolytes, and coagulation studies. A type and screen or type and crossmatch may be ordered preoperatively in anticipation of intraoperative blood/blood component transfusion. Replacement fluids include packed red blood cells (PRBCs), albumin, platelets, fresh frozen plasma (FFP), electrolytes, and colloids or crystalloids.

Before elective surgery, patients may choose to donate one or two units of autologous blood for use at surgery. Friends and family members may also donate donor-directed, compatible blood. Autotransfusion, or cell salvage, of the patient's blood during surgery may not be appropriate, given the potential contamination from bowel contents or from malignant GI tumors. A nasogastric (NG) tube, inserted to decompress the stomach, suctions gastric secretions in select procedures. Insertion of a temperature monitoring urinary catheter decompresses the bladder and provides accurate measurement of urinary output and renal function as well as body temperature.

Administration of IV antibiotics occurs before the incision and repeats as needed to maintain adequate levels throughout the procedure (Surgical Pharmacology). Antibiotic solutions may be used for irrigation during the procedure and before closure. Use of hemostatic agents, anticoagulants, steroid preparations, and local anesthetics is possible. The best guide for planning medications, therefore, is a comprehensive and frequently updated pick-list, or surgeon/procedure preference sheet. Extended antibiotic use, a weakened immune system, and poor hand hygiene can lead to *Clostridium difficile* infection. This infection is extremely hard to treat, and a new treatment is discussed in the Research Highlight box.

Chapter 6 thoroughly discusses safely positioning the patient for surgery. Common positions for patients undergoing GI procedures include supine position, low modified lithotomy position, and jackknife position. In supine or modified lithotomy position, the patient's arms are secured on armboards or tucked at the sides. When there are surgical reasons to tuck the arms at the side, pad the elbows to protect the ulnar nerve, turn the palms inward, and maintain the wrist in a neutral position (AORN, 2016). When the patient is in modified lithotomy position with arms secured on armboards, ensure there is adequate space between the base of the armboards and the stirrup holders for the surgeon and first assistant to stand. This can be challenging with patients of short stature. Ensure the hands and fingers are protected when raising or lowering the foot of the operating room (OR) bed. Exposure of key anatomy may require frequent intraoperative changes in the orientation of the OR bed. Common positions used to shift abdominal organs away from the operative site to optimize visualization include Trendelenburg, reverse Trendelenburg, and tilting of the OR bed from side to side into a lateral

SURGICAL PHARMACOLOGY

Commonly Administered Antibiotics in Gastrointestinal Surgery

Medication/Category	Dosage/Route	Purpose/Action	Adverse Reactions	Nursing Implications
Cefazolin (first-generation cephalosporin)	IV 1–2 g loading dose, up to 12 g in 24 h	Enteric gram-negative bacilli, gram-positive cocci	—	Administer loading dose within 1 h of incision; may repeat with 500 mg to 1 g after 2 h intraoperatively, followed by 500 mg to 1 g every 6–8 h for 24 h postoperatively
Cefoxitin (second-generation cephalosporin)	IV 2 g	Enteric gram-negative bacilli, enterococci, clostridia	Diarrhea	Administer within 1 h of incision; can redose with 2 g every 6 h for no more than 24 h after surgery
Ampicillin sulbactam (aminopenicillin and beta-lactamase inhibitor)	IV 2 g, loading dose with 1 g 6 h	*Enterococcus faecalis,* gram-negative bacilli	Diarrhea, nausea	Administer within 30 min of incision; routine use no longer recommended; reserve only for patients at highest risk of endocarditis
Clindamycin	<80 kg: IV 600 mg 81–160 kg: IV 900 mg >160 kg: IV 1200 mg	Aerobes, anaerobes, enteric gram-negative bacilli	Nausea, enhances susceptibility for *Clostridium difficile* infection	Dilute each 300 mg in 50 mL D_5W and give over 10–60 min; redose after 6 h
Ertapenem/carbapenem	IV 1 g	Enterobacter, *Escherichia coli*	Diarrhea	Adjust dose for renal impairment
Metronidazole hydrochloride	500 mg or 15 mg/kg with a redose 7.5 mg/kg after 6 and 12 h after initial dose	Anaerobes	Headache, nausea, vaginitis	Infuse over 1 h Do not give IV push Incompatible with aztreonam and possibly ceftriaxone
Vancomycin (glycopeptide)	IV 1000 mg or 10–15 mg/kg over 1 h	MRSA, *Staphylococcus aureus, Enterococcus*	Erythematous rash on face and upper body, hypotension	Infuse over 1 h, within 120 min of incision, adjust dose for renal impairment, incompatible with many other antibiotics, check y-site compatibility before hanging
Ciprofloxacin (fluoroquinolone)	IV 400 mg	Gram-negative bacilli, *Streptococcus pneumoniae,* gram-positive cocci, mycobacterial species	Rash, anorexia, nausea, vomiting, headache, dizziness, phototoxicity, long-term use increases risk for tendonitis or tendon rupture	Administer within 2 h of incision, incompatible with many other antibiotics and commonly used anesthetics, check y-site compatibility before hanging
Levofloxacin (fluoroquinolone)	IV 500 mg	Gram-negative bacilli, *S. pneumoniae,* gram-positive cocci, mycobacterial species	Long-term use increases risk for tendonitis or tendon rupture	Infuse over 1 h, within 120 min of incision
Aztreonam (miscellaneous)	IV 2 g	Gram-negative bacteria	—	Administer within 1 h of incision; redose at 4 h
Gentamicin	IV 5 mg/kg; use weight-based dosing for obese use: dosing weight = ideal body weight + 0.4 (actual weight − ideal body weight)	Gram-negative bacteria	—	Administer within 1 h of incision, limit to a single preoperative dose For patients 20% above ideal body weight use determining equation Use caution with patients with renal insufficiency

IV, Intravenous; *MRSA,* methicillin-resistant *Staphylococcus aureus.*

Modified from Bratzer DW et al: Clinical practice guidelines for antimicrobial prophylaxis in surgery, *Am J Health-Syst Pharm* 70(3):195–283, 2013; Mohabir PK, Gurney J: *Antibiotic prophylaxis for surgical procedures, Merck Manuals* (website). www.merckmanuals.com/professional/special-subjects/care-of-the-surgical-patient/antibiotic-prophylaxis-for-surgical-procedures. (Accessed 5 November 2016).

RESEARCH HIGHLIGHT

Fecal Microbiota Transplantation Therapy

Fecal transplant therapy is a procedure that is gaining in popularity to treat a number of conditions both acquired and congenital. One study focused on outcomes of fecal transplants on CDIs in immunocompromised and nonimmunocompromised patients. In this small retrospective study, a total of 107 patients' data were collected from the FMTs performed. Treatment results 12 weeks post-FMT were analyzed. Twelve patients were excluded from the study because of incomplete follow-up or death. Of the 95 patients in the final results, 58 were nonimmunocompromised and 35 were immunocompromised.

The procedures evaluated in the study consisted of donor stool prepared in a standardized manner introduced via an upper GI route or colonoscopy. The donor stool was from a number of sources including relatives, friends, and universal donors. To be deemed successful, the recipients needed to show a primary response, defined as relapse of diarrhea symptoms with a previous positive *Clostridium difficile*. A nonresponder of the first FMT was allowed to repeat up to three times before being considered a full nonresponder to FMT treatment.

Of the 95 patients studied, FMT had a 97.9% success rate in treating CDI in both immunocompromised and nonimmunocompromised patients. For SAEs, 101 patients were included in a retrospective review; 10.9% experienced SAE. Six of the eleven SAE patients died; none were attributed to the FMT. The remaining five SAE patients developed other infections or exacerbations of existing disease, possibly related to the FMT. This study did not address any adjunct therapies such as antibiotic use or other recommendations such as single rooms, hospitalization, or use of contact precautions. Overall the study concluded that FMT was equivalent in the immunocompromised and nonimmunocompromised populations and that it was a valid treatment for *C. difficile*.

CDIs, Clostridium difficile infections; *FMT,* fecal microbiota transplant; *SAE,* serious adverse event.

Modified from Mandalia A et al: Fecal transplant is as effective and safe in immunocompromised and non-immunocompromised patients for *Clostridium difficile, Int J Colorectal Dis* 31(5):1059–1060, 2016.

position. The surgical team collaboratively positions the patient and ensures that the patient is secured properly to the OR bed before draping. Special considerations to address unique challenges of positioning the obese patient appear in detail in Chapter 6. Measures for safe patient handling and lifting appear in Chapter 3.

GI surgery patients are at increased risk for venous thromboembolism (VTE) events such as DVT and pulmonary embolism (PE). Mechanical VTE prevention includes the use of graduated compression stockings and intermittent pneumatic compression devices (IPCDs) on the lower extremities. An IPCD has an electrically operated pump that intermittently inflates sleeves wrapped around the lower legs or the lower legs and thighs, compressing the veins and increasing venous blood flow toward the heart (Elpern et al., 2013). IPCDs are applied and turned on before induction of anesthesia. Wrap the sleeves around the legs smoothly to prevent folds when the legs are positioned in stirrups. Ensure that there are no pressure points from the hose connections. Hang the unit or place it on the floor under the OR bed in an area away from team members' feet and areas that may be wet. Place a blanket or mat under the unit to lessen vibration noise (AORN, 2016).

Patients having GI surgery are also at risk for perioperative hypothermia. Core body temperature is often measured throughout the procedure. The four most reliable sites for core monitoring of temperature are the tympanic membrane, distal esophagus, nasopharynx, and pulmonary artery. Risk factors for unplanned hypothermia include extremes of age, low body weight, open-cavity surgery, thyroid disorders, diabetic neuropathy, peripheral vascular disease, a cold OR, infusion of cold fluids, and irrigating the abdomen with cold normal saline or other solutions (AORN, 2016). Warming the patient before induction of anesthesia may help reduce redistribution of core body heat to the periphery (AORN, 2016) and contribute to normothermia in the PACU (Nicholson, 2013; Nieh and Su, 2016). Use all devices for warming patients and solutions according to the manufacturer's instructions (Wu, 2013).

Hair removal at the operative site, per surgeon order, occurs in the preoperative holding area as close as possible to the time of surgery. Hair removal is usually accomplished with clippers.

Antimicrobial skin preparation and draping receive extensive coverage in Chapter 4. Abdominal skin preparation follows general protocols for laparotomy, with generous borders should the surgeon extend the incision or need to accommodate the creation of stomas and drain placement. The perioperative nurse takes precautions to prevent accumulation or pooling of prep solutions under the patient or in the patient's hair to prevent chemical skin injury and surgical fires (risk management strategies for preventing surgical fire are discussed in Chapter 2). Sites within the prepped area with high concentrations of microorganisms, such as an existing stoma, draining fistula, or the rectum, are prepped last. Before surgical skin prep, cover and protect existing stomas with an occlusive sterile clear plastic dressing or a collection appliance or isolate them with a plastic drape secured with adhesive strips.

Draping the abdomen follows standard draping process as for laparotomy, discussed in Chapter 4. If the patient is in modified lithotomy position, extra drapes are needed under the buttocks and to cover the stirrups. Plan for additional drapes, towels, gowns, and gloves for the surgical team to implement proper techniques to keep clean and dirty items separate during open bowel procedures (often referred to as "bowel technique" or "GI technique").

The surgeon may request placement of ureteral catheters by a urologist before a GI procedure begins. The catheters may be lighted and inserted to enable the surgeon to see and palpate the ureters during the GI procedure. A basic cystoscopy setup includes sterile ureteral catheters, two of each size (see Chapter 15).

If transabdominal intraoperative endoscopic examination of the bowel lumen is necessary, endoscopes of an appropriate length should be sterile and set up on a separate sterile table. Consider this table contaminated after removal of the scope. Ensure availability of endoscopic accessories such as a light source, a mechanism to insufflate the bowel, and a suction device for intraluminal secretions. Team members who were involved in the endoscopic procedure change gown and gloves before proceeding with the remainder of the surgical intervention.

Additional accessory instruments or devices may include a sterile plastic drawstring intestinal bag to confine loops of normal bowel from the operative segment or sterile radiopaque surgical towels. If planning intraoperative ultrasound, ensure the components of a high-resolution ultrasound system are available, including necessary sterile probes or transducers.

GI linear and circular stapling devices streamline resection and approximation of GI viscera. Stapling devices typically accept multiple cartridge "reloads" for successive use and can be straight or curved and linear or circular; they can apply staples only, or they can apply staples and cut tissue between the staple lines. These instruments deliver double or triple rows of closely spaced, staggered inert staples, and are designed for use in open or laparoscopic procedures. The staples approximate tissue while preserving blood supply to tissue edges. Stapling devices for laparoscopic use have longer shafts, have articulating heads, use triple staple technology, provide for tissue compression before staples are fired, and accommodate larger bites of tissue. Personnel must be familiar with types of available stapling instruments, device operation, assembly if indicated, and proper loading of cartridges. A variety of staplers and reloads are available for GI procedures.

Common suture materials used in GI procedures include permanent silk sutures and absorbable polyglycolic acid and polydioxanone (PDS) sutures. Generally, surgeons use 3-0 and 4-0 sutures on a semicircular intestinal (tapered) needle on intestinal tissues. Ligatures for small vessels usually require a 3-0 or 4-0 suture, whereas larger vessels may require a size 0 or 2-0. For closure of enterotomies or hand-sewn anastomosis of the bowel, surgeons commonly use size 3-0 or 4-0 absorbable suture on the mucosa and seromuscular layers. Some surgeons may also want controlled-release 3-0 or 4-0 silk sutures available. For abdominal closure, the fascia and peritoneum are closed as one layer using a running suturing technique with a number 1 or 0 slow absorbing suture (e.g., PDS) on a large tapered needle. The surgeon's preference will dictate which skin staples or suture should be available for skin closure.

Bowel technique (also referred to as GI, contamination, or isolation technique) prevents cross-contamination of the wound or abdomen with bowel organisms. Surgeons also use this technique during cancer procedures to prevent mechanical metastasis, or "seeding" of malignant cells, throughout the abdomen. Bowel technique begins as soon as the GI tract is clamped and transected, and proceeds through wound irrigation, before wound closure. Instruments used for bowel resection and anastomosis are kept separate from the rest of the sterile back table. Contaminated GI tract instruments are handed off or left on a separate Mayo stand. After wound irrigation, the entire surgical team dons fresh gowns and gloves and switches to the closure setup of clean instruments. Additional towels or drapes may be placed on top of initial drapes. Planning during preoperative setup includes having the necessary extra instruments to accommodate bowel technique. Surgeon preference and institutional protocol determine the details of the bowel technique (AORN, 2016).

Surgical specimens may be contaminated with microorganisms or malignant cells. Careful handling of the specimen is important to prevent cross-contamination of instruments and the sterile field. The surgeon determines how the specimen is to be labeled and prepared for transfer to pathology. Accuracy is verified with the surgeon by reading back (referred to as "write down, read back, and verify") the label and pathology form before removing the specimen from the room or before the surgeon leaves the room, and documented according to institutional protocol. Specimens may be sent fresh, in saline, or in a preservative solution. Tissue may be sent for frozen-section examination to verify pathologic condition and to determine whether tissue margins are free of malignant cells. Specimens to be entered into research protocols may require further special handling, storage, transport, and documentation.

Closed suction drains evacuate fluids from the abdominal cavity. A variety of catheters (e.g., Malecot, Pezzer) are inserted into the stomach as a gastrostomy tube, decompressing the stomach until normal bowel peristalsis returns. A red rubber catheter may be used

as a jejunostomy tube to deliver postoperative enteral nutrition. Most drains and feeding tubes secure to the skin with a nonabsorbable suture. Gastrostomy tubes and jejunostomy tubes require appropriately sized catheter plugs or are connected to a drainage bag before patient transfer from the OR. All tubes and drains require labeling and documentation according to type and location.

Determination and documentation of wound classification occurs at the end of the procedure. Controlled entries into the GI tract without spillage of gastric or bowel contents are classified as "clean-contaminated." Gross contamination from the GI tract, major breaks in sterile technique, or visible presence of acute infection changes the classification to "contaminated." Further discussion of wound classifications can be found in Chapter 9.

Evaluation

Evaluation of patient care continues throughout the procedure and through patient transport to the PACU or surgical intensive care unit (SICU). Accounting for all sharps, instruments, and soft goods is mandatory in accordance with hospital policy and procedure.

Secure dressing(s), drains, and any pain management pump tubing to prevent dislodging or damage during transfer from the OR bed. Assess the skin for redness or bruising. Remove the electrosurgical unit (ESU) dispersive pad, inspect the site, and document skin condition. Clean the patient of any remaining blood or fluids. Ensure that the patient is covered with a clean gown and warm blanket before being transported to the PACU or SICU. Any variances require reporting to the surgeon, documentation in the patient's record, and inclusion in the hand-off report to the nurse in the PACU, SICU, or nursing unit. Patient outcomes, based on the perioperative nursing diagnoses, undergo review. Postoperative documentation reflects and measures how each outcome was met and notes significant variations from desired results. Outcomes for the plan of care for a patient undergoing GI surgery might be stated as follows:

- The patient verbalized decreased anxiety and ability to cope.
- The patient verbalized understanding of the surgical procedure, expected responses, and postoperative self-care requirements.
- The patient demonstrated acceptance of expected changes in appearance.
- The patient was at, or will return to, normothermia at the conclusion of the postoperative period.
- The patient will be free from signs and symptoms of surgical site infection.
- The patient was free from perioperative positioning injury.
- The patient was free of evidence of impaired tissue integrity.
- The patient was free from injury related to retained surgical items, wrong procedure, wrong site, and medication errors.
- The patient's fluid volume, electrolyte levels, and acid-base balance are consistent with or improved from preoperative baseline levels.

Patient, Family, and Caregiver Education and Discharge Planning

Patients undergoing surgical intervention for GI disorders vary greatly in length of time and complexity of recovery. Recovery and convalescence depend on the procedure, surgical approach, surgical site, anesthesia, pain management, and health of the patient. Teach patients that coughing and deep-breathing exercises will be necessary after surgery to prevent pneumonia by opening alveoli and removing pooled excretions. Coughing can be uncomfortable after abdominal surgery. Show the patient how to splint the incision by holding a small pillow or folded blanket firmly over the incision while coughing.

Incentive spirometry provides a visible measurement of inspiratory effort and is a helpful tool to encourage deep breathing. When possible, provide preoperative instructions for use with return demonstration and allow the patient to practice with the spirometer. Inform the patient that early ambulation helps regain overall muscle tone and strength, supports cardiac and pulmonary function, reduces or prevents the risk of DVT in lower extremities, and boosts a sense of well-being. Preventing pulmonary and vascular complications also helps reduce hospital readmission rates.

Pain management is critical for recovery. Explain the methods of pain control that might be available after surgery. For example, placing an epidural catheter immediately before surgery for postoperative pain control is possible, but can limit postoperative early ambulation. For most major GI procedures, patient-controlled analgesia (PCA) provides consistent pain control in the first 1 to 3 postoperative days (Hübner et al., 2015). Surgeons often order additional medication for breakthrough pain (Penprase et al., 2015).

Inform patients that narcotics may delay return of normal bowel peristalsis. Most patients experience a temporary decrease in bowel activity for about 3 days after GI surgery, which is called "postoperative ileus." Activity (or motility) of the small intestine usually returns to normal within a few hours after surgery. Stomach motility returns to normal within 24 to 48 hours, and the large intestine returns to normal within 48 to 72 hours (Birnbaum, 2015; Wolthuis et al., 2016). Prevention of postoperative ileus allows faster recovery and positive outcomes (Research Highlight).

Consider postoperative ileus prolonged when it lasts beyond the expected 3 days. Signs and symptoms are absence of bowel sounds, abdominal distention, diffuse abdominal pain, nausea, and vomiting (Wolthuis et al., 2016). Causes vary and can arise from neurogenic, inflammatory, hormonal, pharmacologic, or mechanical effects of surgery, including overmanipulation of the intestines. Identifying early bowel sounds through abdominal auscultation may signal the return of small intestine motility; only the passage of flatus or stool, however, indicates full return of bowel function and resolution of postoperative ileus (Wolthuis et al., 2016).

Many lifestyle changes occur for patients with a new ostomy. A WOCN helps patients learn how to care for their stoma and surrounding skin, about proper appliance selection and application, stoma irrigation, diet, and bowel training. A WOCN consultation assists the patient to consider quality-of-life strategies to deal with key issues such as clothing selection, self-esteem, body image, sex and intimacy, travel, public toileting, and odor control (Salvadalena et al., 2015). An excellent patient resource for learning about living with an ostomy is the United Ostomy Associations of America (www.ostomy.org).

After some GI surgeries, patients may require prolonged nutritional support with total parenteral nutrition (TPN) or enteral feedings. Obtaining referral and consultation for home care support and nursing care to administer TPN or enteral feedings is an essential part of discharge planning. General discharge instructions for the patient undergoing GI surgery include both verbal and written instructions (Patient, Family, and Caregiver Education).

Ambulatory surgery considerations and education are based on patient, procedure, and anesthesia selection. Patient instructions preoperatively and at discharge are critical to encourage positive outcomes, and depend on the patient's ability, self-efficacy, and family support for home care.

RESEARCH HIGHLIGHT

Use of Chewing Gum to Prevent Postoperative Ileus

Chewing gum is an accepted intervention for encouraging return of peristalsis and bowel function and prevention of prolonged postoperative ileus. Chewing gum after surgery stimulates the stomach and tricks the GI tract into thinking that the person is eating. Postoperative ileus is a common surgical complication with one out of three colorectal surgery patients experiencing ileus.

A comprehensive study summed the results of a total of 81 randomized control trials researching the use of chewing gum in returning postoperative bowel function. A total of 9072 patients were included in the review. The authors used a risk of bias assessment tool to independently review the studies and clinical trials, then they used a random-effects model with meta-analysis to further assess the data within subgroups of surgical site, time to bowel sounds, time to first flatus, time to bowel movement, and length of hospital stay.

The results of their analysis note that chewing gum was well tolerated and cost-effective. Studies using an ERAS pathway did not see as much benefit to chewing gum because of their other initiatives for reducing postoperative ileus. Overall, there was some evidence to support chewing gum on earlier returning bowel sounds and flatus and bowel movements than those who did not chew gum, but no effect on LOS. The authors recommend that further randomized clinical trials be completed to achieve higher quality data to fully evaluate the benefits of chewing gum for patients, especially within those institutions using an ERAS pathway.

ERAS, Enhanced recovery after surgery; *GI,* gastrointestinal; *LOS,* length of stay.
Modified from Short V et al: Chewing gum for postoperative recovery of gastrointestinal function, *Cochrane Database Syst Rev* 2:CD006506, 2015.

Surgical Interventions

Laparotomy

Laparotomy is surgical entrance into the abdominal cavity. The purpose of a laparotomy may be to explore the abdomen to make a diagnosis or as a means to perform a planned surgical procedure. Surgeons access the abdominal cavity by a variety of incisions, which are described next.

Open Abdominal Incisions

Various incisions to enter the abdominal cavity appear in Fig. 11.7. Key elements in planning the location and length of surgical incisions are access to the targeted pathology with sufficient visualization to complete the procedure without undue trauma to surrounding organs, preserving abdominal wall function, and ensuring secure wound closure. An optimally placed incision has many benefits, and many incision options are available. The incision must be able to be extended if unexpected findings require additional exposure to complete the procedure and be able to be closed securely with minimal risks for disruption. No one incision is able to cover all necessary access points (Verhaeghe, 2015). Other factors considered are the patient's condition and need for fast abdominal entry, uncertainty of diagnosis and need for flexibility, previous surgical scars, potential need for future abdominal surgery or ostomy, body habitus (physique), risk for bleeding, postoperative pain, and cosmetic results.

The layers of the abdominal wall appear in Fig. 11.8. In the midline, the abdominal wall consists of the skin, subcutaneous fat, the linea alba, preperitoneal fat, and peritoneum. At the midline, the anterior and posterior rectus sheaths fuse together to form the

PATIENT, FAMILY, AND CAREGIVER EDUCATION

General Discharge Instructions for Gastrointestinal Surgery Patients

Before discharge patients receive verbal and written information about postoperative activity, diet, wound care, when and with whom to make follow-up appointments, and what to do and who to call if they experience problems at home. All discharge medications are reviewed to ensure the patient understands the purpose of the medication, when to take it, and possible side effects.

Written instructions may include the following:

- Walking is good for you. Start with short walks. Gradually increase your physical activity as you grow stronger.
- Avoid lifting heavy items (greater than 10 pounds) until cleared to do so by your surgeon.
- Continue with deep-breathing exercises every 2 hours throughout the day.
- Avoid sitting for prolonged periods (greater than 1 hour) without getting up and walking around. This will help prevent blood clots from forming in your legs.
- Expect to get tired easily. Plan for several periods of rest throughout the day.
- Expect changes in appetite and alterations in how food tastes. You may find that you get full faster and eat less than you did before surgery. Eat four to six small meals throughout the day rather than three large meals. Follow all dietary restrictions your surgeon has prescribed. If there are no restrictions,

gradually work up to your preoperative dietary habits. If you are on a liquid diet, avoid caffeine, carbonated beverages, and drinks high in sugar content. It is important to drink plenty of water to stay hydrated.
- Keep your incision(s) clean and dry. A small amount of clear or pink drainage from your incision may occur for a few days after you go home. You can use a gauze pad to cover your incision to protect your clothes until the drainage stops.
- Take the pain medicine you have been prescribed if you need it.
- Do not drive or operate heavy equipment while taking pain medication.
- Take only the medications that are listed in your written discharge instructions as prescribed.
- Call your surgeon if you experience any of the following symptoms:
  - Temperature greater than 101°F (38.4°C)
  - Increasing abdominal pain
  - Persistent nausea or vomiting
  - Persistent diarrhea or absence of bowel movements
  - Sudden pain, swelling, or warmth in one or both of your legs
  - Shortness of breath or difficulty breathing
  - Redness, bright red bleeding, or yellow foul-smelling drainage at the incision site(s)

Modified from Hovsepian J et al: Postoperative instructions preoperatively—evaluating the effectiveness of a teaching model on patient satisfaction regarding instructions for home care, *J Perianesth Nurs* 32(3):231–237; 2016; Riccardi R, MacKay G: Fast-track protocols in colorectal surgery. In Weiser M, editor: *UpToDate,* Waltham, MA, 2016, UpToDate.

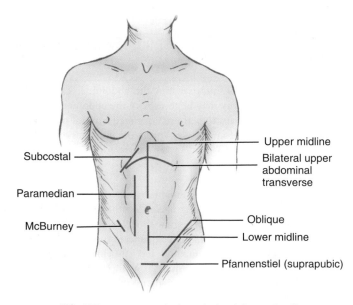

FIG. 11.7 Incisions made through the abdominal wall.

Subcostal
Paramedian
McBurney
Upper midline
Bilateral upper abdominal transverse
Oblique
Lower midline
Pfannenstiel (suprapubic)

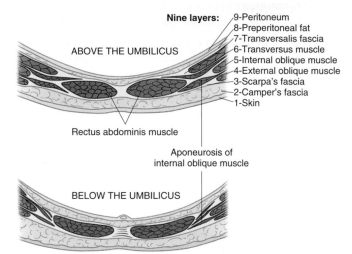

FIG. 11.8 Horizontal section of abdominal wall. Aponeurosis of internal oblique muscle splits into two sections, one lying anterior and the other posterior to rectus abdominis muscle, forming an encasing sheath around muscle above the umbilicus. Below the umbilicus, aponeuroses of all muscles pass anterior to rectus sheath.

Nine layers:
9-Peritoneum
8-Preperitoneal fat
7-Transversalis fascia
6-Transversus muscle
5-Internal oblique muscle
4-External oblique muscle
3-Scarpa's fascia
2-Camper's fascia
1-Skin

ABOVE THE UMBILICUS

Rectus abdominis muscle

Aponeurosis of internal oblique muscle

BELOW THE UMBILICUS

linea alba, an avascular, nerve-free structure that vertically divides the right and left rectus muscles from the xiphoid process to the symphysis pubis. Lateral to the linea alba, the anterior and posterior rectus sheaths cover the rectus muscles (Fig. 11.9). On the lower abdominal wall, the arcuate line is a landmark located about one-third of the distance between the umbilicus and the symphysis pubis. Above this imaginary line, the aponeurosis of the internal oblique muscle splits and joins the aponeuroses of the external oblique muscle

anteriorly and the transversalis fascia posteriorly to form the anterior and posterior rectus sheaths. Below the arcuate line there is no posterior rectus sheath.

Procedural Considerations: Open Laparotomy

A basic laparotomy set includes instruments for sharp and blunt dissection, clamping tissue, grasping tissue, suturing, cutting suture, and retracting tissue. An instrument list may include Metzenbaum

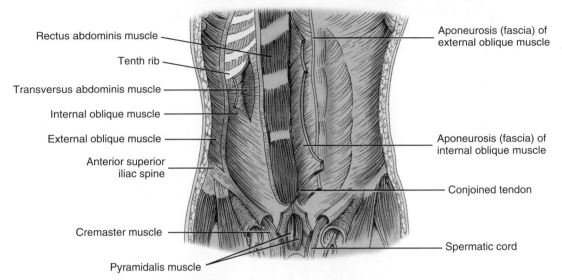

Rectus abdominis muscle

Tenth rib

Transversus abdominis muscle

Internal oblique muscle

External oblique muscle

Anterior superior
iliac spine

Cremaster muscle

Pyramidalis muscle

Aponeurosis (fascia) of
external oblique muscle

Aponeurosis (fascia) of
internal oblique muscle

Conjoined tendon

Spermatic cord

FIG. 11.9 Superior muscles of abdominal wall.

scissors, curved Mayo scissors, straight Mayo scissors (also called suture scissors), tissue forceps with teeth, Adson tissue forceps with teeth, Russian tissue forceps, DeBakey tissue forceps, Ferris Smith tissue forceps, Crile or Kelly hemostats, mosquito clamps, Péan clamps, Allis clamps, Babcock clamps, right-angle clamps, assorted needle holders, ringed forceps, and towel clips. The following retractors are usually included in various sizes: Deaver, Richardson, Harrington, Army Navy, malleable, and abdominal wall. Additional instruments to have available might include self-retaining retractors such as a Balfour, or Bookwalter set; atraumatic intestinal clamps; Yankauer and Poole suction tips; and longer versions of basic instruments for procedures in the pelvis, in obese patients, or in thoracoabdominal procedures. An ESU, smoke evacuator, and suction machine are basic to performing laparotomy.

Before any incision is made, but after surgical prepping and draping, all surgical team members pause for a time-out briefing that includes the components of The Joint Commission's (TJC) Universal Protocol for preventing wrong-site, wrong-procedure, wrong-person surgery. It is critical that time-out procedures are followed, that all team members are involved, and that everyone is in agreement in accordance to institutional policy.

Vertical Incisions

Midline Incision

A midline incision offers fast entry into the abdomen, provides excellent exposure to any part of the abdominal cavity, can be closed securely and rapidly, and is the standard incision for exploratory laparotomy (Verhaeghe, 2015). The incision starts above the umbilicus and is carried down through the subcutaneous layer to the linea alba. At the umbilicus the surgeon diverts the incision from the midline, around rather than through the umbilicus (Fig. 11.10A). Incision of the linea alba exposes the peritoneum (see Fig. 11.10B). To prevent injury to underlying structures, before incising the peritoneum surgical assistants use hemostats or smooth forceps to lift the peritoneum away from the intestines or other structures. The surgeon lifts the abdominal wall to protect underlying structures and extends the peritoneal incision in either direction as needed (see Fig. 11.10C), and can carry the extension of the incision cephalad to just below the xiphoid process. Taking culture samples may occur

at this point. If a more extensive exposure of the liver is needed, the surgeon can divide and ligate the falciform ligament between two clamps. The surgeon also can extend the incision caudad, down to just above the symphysis pubis, taking care not to injure the bladder. Use of laparotomy pads and suction is needed for exposure. The abdominal wall is often retracted with large Richardson retractors during initial exploration. Once the affected organs are identified, a self-retaining retractor, such as a Balfour or Bookwalter retractor system, is used to establish hands-free exposure. Wound protectors are often used to reduce surgical site infections and provide surgical site retraction, keeping the wound edges moist (Mihaljevic et al., 2015b).

Current literature notes that closure of midline incisions should incorporate all layers of the abdominal wall except the skin. The STITCH technique, also known as small bites, recommends that closure is done using interrupted sutures no more than 5 mm apart to close the wound and prevent abdominal incisional adhesions. Although this increases the time for closure, the longer-term benefits and reduction of postoperative complications counteract the extended surgical time (Deerenberg et al., 2015). Closure of the skin can also occur with skin staples, absorbable subcuticular sutures, adhesive skin tapes, dermal glue, or negative pressure devices (Mihaljevic et al., 2015a; Rajendran et al., 2016; Semsarzadeh et al., 2015). Surgeons seldom use internal or external retention sutures for primary abdominal closure. This is because there is little evidence to support their effectiveness in preventing wound disruption and there is an association between them and increased incisional pain and wound complications (Rajendran et al., 2016). In circumstances in which retention sutures are needed, #1 or #2 nonabsorbable suture material is appropriate, coupled with prepackaged retention bridges or flexible tubing bolsters to protect the incision site.

Paramedian Incision

Surgeons place paramedian incisions about 2 to 5 cm lateral to either side of the midline on the upper or lower abdomen. Incision of skin and subcutaneous tissue exposes the anterior rectus sheath, which in turn is incised vertically. Lateral retraction of the rectus muscle exposes the posterior rectus sheath, also then incised vertically. Entry into the peritoneum occurs in the same fashion as the midline incision.

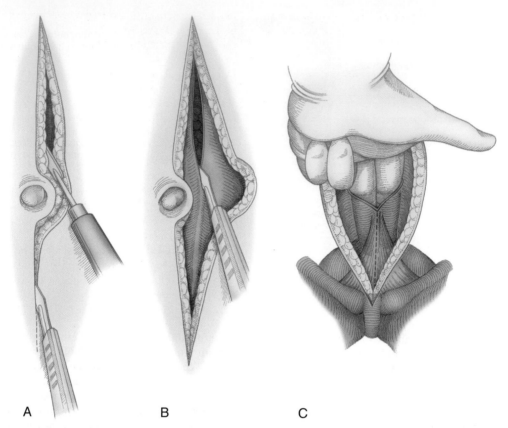

FIG. 11.10 (A) Midline laparotomy incision around the umbilicus. (B) External fascia is incised. (C) Entry into the peritoneal cavity.

A possible benefit of the paramedian incision is a potentially decreased risk for dehiscence or hernia; disadvantages include risk of injury to the epigastric vessels and risk of nerve injury resulting in paralysis of the rectus muscle. Closure is similar to the midline incision.

Oblique Incisions

The oblique inguinal incision is between the pubic tubercle toward the anterior iliac crest, slightly above and parallel to the inguinal ligament. It is the standard incision for open inguinal herniorrhaphy. The incision through the external oblique muscle provides access to the cremaster muscle, inguinal canal, and cord structures. This incision typically does not interrupt major abdominal arteries.

McBurney Incision

Use of the McBurney muscle-splitting incision is common for open appendectomy. In the lower right abdomen, the surgeon incises the skin along the skin tension lines at a point one-third of the distance between the anterior iliac spine and the umbilicus. Electrosurgical dissection of the subcutaneous layer and Scarpa fascia carries down to the external oblique fascia. The fascia is then sharply divided along its fibers. The internal oblique and transversus abdominis muscles are split in the direction of their fibers and retracted to expose the transversalis fascia and peritoneum. The fascia and peritoneum are incised together in the same direction as the incision (Rajendran et al., 2016). This incision is quick and easy to open, close, and extend medially or laterally if additional exposure is necessary. The surgeon can close the transversalis fascia and peritoneum together with absorbable suture and loosely approximate the muscles

with interrupted absorbable sutures. The external oblique fascia is closed with interrupted or continuous absorbable suture. In large patients with a subcutaneous layer less than 2 cm, Scarpa fascia may be approximated. Closure of the skin is according to surgeon preference. A transverse modification of a McBurney incision is the Rocky-Davis or Elliot modification.

Subcostal Incision

A subcostal (Kocher) incision begins approximately 3 cm below the xiphoid process and extends laterally, staying 2.5 to 3 cm below and parallel to the costal margin. The incision descends through the subcutaneous layer. The anterior fascia of the rectus muscle is identified and divided; division of the rectus, external oblique, internal oblique, and transversalis muscles follows. Electrocoagulation of the superior epigastric vessels in the rectus muscle may follow or they may undergo division between clamps and ligation. The surgeon lifts the peritoneum from the underlying viscera and sharply opens it. A right subcostal incision is appropriate for open procedures of the gallbladder, biliary system, and pancreas (Fig. 11.11), as is a left subcostal incision for open access to the spleen.

Joining of the right and left subcostal incisions in the midline is appropriate to make a "chevron" incision. Chevron incisions provide excellent exposure for gastric, duodenal, pancreatic, and portal system procedures. Closure of the subcostal incision is in layers. The falciform ligament is approximated if divided. Closure of the peritoneum, posterior rectus fascia, and anterior rectus fascia is with absorbable, running, or interrupted sutures. Skin closure is with absorbable subcuticular sutures or skin staples. Disadvantages of this incision include poor cosmesis and increased postoperative pain (Mizell et al., 2015; Muysoms et al., 2015).

Thoracoabdominal Incision

The thoracoabdominal incision joins the thoracic and abdominal cavities together. It provides exposure to the esophagus, cardia of the stomach, liver, spleen, kidneys, adrenal glands, lungs, aorta (left side), inferior vena cava (right side), and esophagus. The patient is

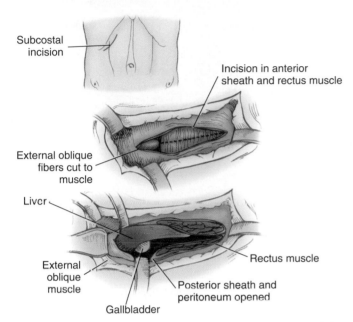

FIG. 11.11 Subcostal incision in upper right quadrant. Anterior sheath has been divided transversely, and muscle is exposed. Posterior sheath and peritoneum have been opened transversely.

in a semilateral position with the torso rotated 45 degrees and both hips on the OR bed (Fig. 11.12). Entry into the abdomen is first through a subcostal or midline incision. Entry into the thoracic cavity occurs by extending the incision in a posterolateral direction (Mizell, 2015). The thoracic incision is carried down through the latissimus dorsi, serratus anterior, and external oblique muscles. The intercostal muscles undergo division in the eighth intercostal space, and the pleural cavity is lifted to protect the lung and opened sharply. Removal of a short piece of costal cartilage can provide additional exposure before insertion of a self-retaining rib retractor, and slowly opened to expand the intercostal space. Division of the diaphragm is next, after which division of the phrenic vessels between clamps and ligation follows. Before closing, chest tubes are inserted into the pleural cavity through separate stab incisions. The diaphragm is closed using two layers of nonabsorbable suture via an interrupted vertical mattress technique, the divided ribs approximated with heavy sutures, and the chest wall and abdominal muscles closed in layers. Absorbable suture is appropriate to close the chest muscles, as is a delayed absorbing suture for closure of the abdomen. The skin edges are approximated and secured with suture, staples, skin-bonding adhesive, or skin tape strips (Rajendran et al., 2016).

Transverse Incisions

Pfannenstiel Incision

The Pfannenstiel incision is optimal for pelvic surgery. The surgeon makes a 10- to 15-cm skin incision transversely, about 3 to 5 cm above the symphysis pubis, usually within the pubic hairline (Fig. 11.13). Opening the anterior rectus fascia transversely occurs next. Elevation of the fascial edges with heavy clamps follows, as does blunt separation of the fascia from the underlying rectus muscle. The rectus muscles undergo separation at the midline raphe; the transversalis fascia, posterior rectus fascia, and peritoneum are divided vertically along the midline. This incision provides good exposure, secure closure, and acceptable cosmesis. Closure of the peritoneum

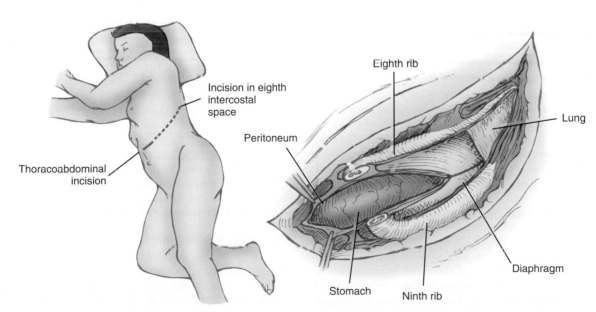

FIG. 11.12 Thoracoabdominal incision. Patient is placed on unaffected side. Incision is usually made from a point midway between the xiphoid process and the umbilicus to the costal margin at the site of the eighth costal cartilage. Dissection is carried down to the peritoneum and pleura. Costal cartilage and diaphragm are divided, and the stomach is exposed.

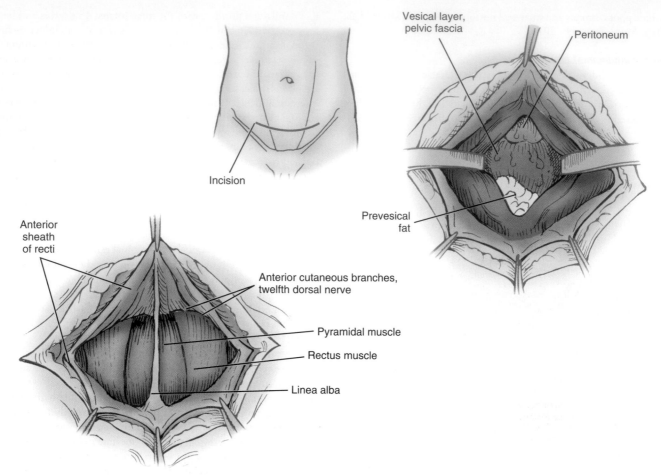

FIG. 11.13 Pfannenstiel incision (suprapubic).

is with continuous absorbable suture. Approximation of the rectus muscles is with interrupted absorbable suture. The anterior fascia is closed with slow-absorbing continuous suture.

Incision Complications

Dehiscence and Evisceration

Wound *dehiscence* is a risk of abdominal surgery and constitutes a disruption or separation of the wound edges that occurs when tension of the abdominal wall overcomes the tensile strength of the suture or integrity of the surgical knot. *Evisceration* occurs when bowel or other abdominal structures protrude through the open wound. Prolonged hypothermia with decreased tissue oxygenation, bleeding, devitalized or strangulated tissue, and excessive dead space in the subcutaneous layer can lead to seroma formation, wound infection, and disruption of a surgical wound.

Other risk factors for dehiscence include obesity, advanced age, male gender, chronic pulmonary disease, coughing, malignancy, previous radiation, trauma, poor nutritional status, and chronic steroid use (Mizell et al., 2015). Additional risk factors associated with and/or leading to wound dehiscence include excessive tension on the wound edges; incisions longer than 18 cm; improper surgical technique such as placing sutures too close to the wound edges; placing sutures too close to each other; strangulating tissue by pulling or tying sutures too tightly; or surgical knots that are insecure or cut too short, which can cause unraveling.

Nerve Injury

Injury to abdominal wall nerves can cause chronic pain, loss of sensation, or abdominal wall weakness. Nerve injuries occur when nerves are severed during incision, entrapped with suture during closure, or compressed or stretched with retractors or instruments. Nerve damage can be permanent or intermittent; if it persists longer than 3 months it should be surgically explored if detrimental to functioning (Antoniadis et al., 2014).

Minimally Invasive Surgery: Laparoscopy

From its origins in gynecologic surgery, laparoscopy has evolved from a minimally invasive technique used primarily for sterilization and diagnostic purposes into a surgical approach adopted by many surgical specialties to perform major resection, extraction, and repair of intra-abdominal organs (Box 11.2).

Procedural Considerations

Most laparoscopic procedures advance in similar fashion and require the same basic equipment, instruments, and supplies. Mentally organizing laparoscopic procedures into common components of progression facilitates the planning process. The general progression of a laparoscopic procedure includes (1) gaining abdominal access, (2) establishing pneumoperitoneum, (3) exposing the targeted organ, (4) completing the critical steps of the procedure, (5) extracting a specimen, (6) irrigating the wound, and (7) closing the incisions.

BOX 11.2

Minimally Invasive Approaches to Gastrointestinal Surgical Procedures

Robotic Gastrointestinal Procedures
- Nissen and Toupet fundoplication
- Gastric bypass
- Sleeve gastrectomy
- Colectomy
- Rectal resection
- Small bowel resection
- Gastrectomy
- Esophagectomy

Single-Incision Laparoscopic Surgery Gastrointestinal Procedures
- Appendectomy
- Right hemicolectomy
- Proctocolectomy

Natural Orifice Transluminal Endoscopic Surgery Gastrointestinal Procedures
- Transvaginal appendectomy
- Transgastric appendectomy
- Transgastric gastrojejunostomy (cadaver and animal studies only)
- PEG tube salvage
- Transrectal colectomy (currently in international human clinical trials)
- Transesophageal Heller myotomy

PEG, Percutaneous endoscopic gastrostomy.
Modified from Johnson H, Hope WW: Laparoscopic approaches in general surgery: is there anything new? In Latifi R et al, editors: *Technological advances in surgery, trauma and critical care,* ed 1, New York, 2015, Springer; Lopez NE et al: Single-incision laparoscopic surgery through an ostomy site: a natural approach by an unnatural orifice, *Surg Laparosc Endosc Percutan Tech* 25(1):74–78, 2015; Steinemann D: *Feasibility, safety and outcome of transrectal hybrid-NOTES anterior resection, ClinicalTrials.gov* (website). https://clinicaltrials.gov/ct2/show/NCT01992406. (Accessed 28 November 2016).

General equipment for laparoscopic procedures includes a variety of access port devices; visualization and insufflation equipment; energy-generating devices for coagulating, sealing, stapling, and dissecting tissue; and devices or equipment to evacuate surgical smoke. Instruments include laparoscopic dissectors, graspers, scissors, needle holders, knot pushers, suction/irrigator, and endoscopic staplers.

Any laparoscopic procedure may need conversion to an open procedure; it is always prudent to have a laparotomy instrument set readily available. If not specified by institutional policy or protocol, the decision to have laparotomy instruments opened and counted *before* the procedure begins depends on patient assessment, experience of the surgical team, and expected technical difficulty of the intended procedure. If anticipated, the possibility or probability of converting to an open procedure should be part of the preoperative team briefing. Sharps, soft goods, and other countable items opened on the field require counting before the procedure begins, regardless of approach or incision size. Reasons to convert to an open approach may include abdominal adhesions that prevent abdominal access (Evidence for Practice), significantly distorted anatomy that precludes safe dissection; gross fecal contamination or infection, uncontrollable bleeding; or pulmonary or cardiac changes related to the patient's inability to tolerate pneumoperitoneum or extreme positioning required for exposure (Jafari et al., 2015).

Operative Procedure

1. The surgical team positions, preps, and drapes the patient as appropriate for the intended procedure. Common patient positions for laparoscopic procedures are supine, lithotomy, and modified lithotomy.
2. Insufflation tubing, camera cord, light cord, and cords for energy-generating devices are secured to the sterile drapes with nonpenetrating clamps or a weighted magnetic drape; ends are passed off the sterile field for connection to the appropriate control units. Drape penetrating methods, such as towel clamps or staples, can lead to perforations in the drape potentially increasing the risk for infection. To lessen the risk of fire, complete all cable connections before activating fiberoptic light sources and ensure that the light cords do not rest on sterile drapes when activated.
3. The surgeon enters the abdomen by a variety of techniques. The three discussed here are common GI laparoscopy techniques.

Abdominal Access: Closed Technique

1. The surgeon makes an infraumbilical skin incision with a #11 or #15 blade. The length of the skin incision accommodates the size of the access port intended for this site.
2. One or two towel clips are used to elevate the abdominal wall before insertion of the Veress needle through the linea alba and peritoneum.
3. To verify correct positioning of the tip of the Veress needle, a 10-mL syringe, partially filled with normal saline, is attached to it. Gentle aspiration on the syringe will yield bloody fluid or intestinal content if the needle has entered a vessel or the intestine. No aspirate appears if the needle tip is clear. A "saline drop test," performed by injecting a small amount of saline into the clear chamber located just below the hub of the Veress needle, follows. If the Veress needle has entered the abdominal cavity, the saline in the chamber quickly drops into the abdomen.
4. Insufflation tubing, attached to the Veress needle, enables insufflation of the abdomen. Position the insufflator so the surgeon can visualize insufflation pressures and flow rate.
5. After establishing pneumoperitoneum, the surgeon removes the Veress needle and blindly inserts a 5-mm or 10-mm access port. Insufflation tubing is then transferred to the access port.

The size of the laparoscope typically determines the size of the access port at this site. An alternate site to gain initial access to the abdomen is in the upper right quadrant, about three fingerbreadths below the right costal margin in the midclavicular line. Surgeons often select this site when lower abdominal wall adhesions are suspected because of previous surgery.

Abdominal Access: Cutdown or Hasson Technique

1. The surgeon makes an infraumbilical skin incision as described previously for the closed technique. Blunt dissection of subcutaneous tissue with a tonsil clamp follows.
2. The linea alba is exposed using small and/or narrow handheld retractors.
3. The surgeon then places stay sutures (heavy absorbable suture on a small, heavy, curved needle) through the fascia on each side of the midline. Using two hemostats to elevate the abdominal wall, the loose ends of the sutures are clamped (referred to as "tagged") while the surgeon incises the fascia and peritoneum vertically to accommodate the access port.
4. Insufflation of the abdomen is with CO_2 as previously described.

EVIDENCE FOR PRACTICE

Preventing Abdominal Adhesions

The incidence of abdominal adhesions after GI surgery is high. Adhesions are fibrous bands of tissue between abdominal structures that are normally not connected. They can be very thin and avascular or they can be very thick and contain blood vessels and nerves. Injury or inflammation of the peritoneal surface triggers the body's natural healing process, which begins with an inflammatory response at the site of the injury. In the final stages of this process, fibrin deposits, degrades, and reabsorbs at the site of injury. Interruption or disturbance of this final phase of healing by the presence of foreign bodies, medications, blood, bacteria, or devitalized tissue can result in adhesion formation.

Adhesions can form between the peritoneal surfaces of the abdominal wall and its underlying abdominal structures, or they can form between adjacent structures within the abdomen such as the omentum, small bowel, and colon. They may be asymptomatic, but often result in complications that can occur in the early postoperative stage or years after an abdominal surgery. Complications include small bowel obstruction, abdominal/pelvic pain, and infertility.

Methods that have been used to prevent or minimize the formation of postoperative adhesions fall into one of the following categories: surgical technique, physical barriers, and pharmacologic agents. Recommended surgical techniques to prevent adhesions include gentle handling of tissue to minimize trauma, meticulous hemostasis, minimizing tissue ischemia, keeping tissues moist, and limiting the introduction of foreign materials such as talc from surgical gloves, lint from sponges, excess suture material, and char from electrocoagulated tissue. For long laparoscopic procedures, the use of heated and humidified CO_2 to insufflate the abdomen can decrease the incidence of peritoneal adhesions. Physical barriers may prevent or minimize the incidence of adhesions by keeping peritoneal surfaces separated during the healing process.

Examples and characteristics of solid physical barriers are as follows:

- Oxidized regenerated cellulose (Surgicel/ Interceed; Ethicon, Inc., Somerville, NJ).
  - Absorbable, flexible, knitted fabric.
  - Indicated for open and laparoscopic procedures.
  - Available in 1.5 × 2-inch or 3 × 4-inch sheets.
  - Excess fluid must be removed from injured tissue before placement.
  - Injured tissue must be completely covered by the product.
  - Moisten lightly with irrigation to keep in place after placement.
  - Will absorb in 2 weeks.
- Hyaluronic acid sheets with carboxymethylcellulose (Seprafilm; Genzyme Biosurgery, Cambridge, MA).
  - Transparent, brittle filmlike material that breaks easily when bent.
  - Indicated for open procedures that do not involve bowel anastomosis. It cannot be passed through a trocar without breaking into pieces.
  - Material readily adheres to moist surfaces, including surgical gloves and surgical instruments. Handle with dry gloves and instruments. When it comes into contact with wet surfaces, it forms a sticky gel that is difficult to reposition.
  - Product comes out of the sterile package positioned between two sheets of paper to facilitate handling and proper positioning the film. Do not remove the paper.
  - Available in 5 × 6-inch sheets.
  - Will absorb in 7 days.
- Expanded polytetrafluorethylene (Preclude Peritoneal Membrane, Gore-Tex Surgical Membrane; W.L. Gore & Associates, Newark, DE).
  - Flexible, nonabsorbable fabric sheet.
  - Can be cut to size. It should extend 1 cm beyond the injured tissue to facilitate anchoring in place with suture.
  - Nonabsorbable monofilament suture such as nylon or polypropylene used to suture in place.
- Polyethylene glycol (SprayGel; Confluent Surgical, Inc., Waltham, MA).
  - Comes in two syringes full of polyethylene glycol–based solutions that are simultaneously dispensed onto the injured tissue.
  - Spray forms an adherent gel-like barrier.
  - Components of the gel break down in 5 to 7 days and are absorbed by the kidneys.
- Liquid physical barriers include the following:
  - Hyaluronic acid (Sepracoat; Genzyme Corporation, Cambridge, MA).
  - Cross-linked hyaluronic acid (Intergel, Hyalobarrier gel; Baxter Healthcare Corporation, Deerfield, IL).
  - Icodextrin 4% (Adept; Baxter Healthcare Corporation).

Modified from Deas T, Sinsel L: Ensuring patient safety and optimizing efficiency during gastrointestinal endoscopy, *AORN J* 99(3):396–406, 2014; Glick JB et al: Achieving hemostasis in dermatology part II: topical hemostatic agents, *Indian Dermatol Online J* 4(3):172–176, 2013; Mais V: Peritoneal adhesions after laparoscopic gastrointestinal surgery, *World J Gastroenterol* 20(17):4917–4925, 2014; TenBroek RP et al: Benefits and harms of adhesion barriers for abdominal surgery: a systematic review and meta-analysis, *Lancet* 383(9911):48–59, 2014.

Abdominal Access: Direct Visual Entry

Another common technique for laparoscopic access to the abdomen uses an optical view access port to visualize layers of the abdominal wall as they are entered.

Insufflation of the abdomen may occur before or after insertion of the access port.

1. The surgeon makes the incision as previously described for open entry techniques.
2. A laparoscope inserts into the center of the access port's trocar. The trocar has a clear, nonbladed tip for visualization. The camera focuses on the inside tip of the trocar.
3. The trocar and port lock onto the shaft of the laparoscope; with a twisting motion, combined with controlled downward pressure, the access port, trocar, and laparoscope advance as one unit through the abdominal wall. The surgeon visualizes each layer of the abdominal wall as the trocar passes through.
4. With pneumoperitoneum established, the surgeon visually explores the abdomen to verify that the procedure can proceed laparoscopically as planned.
5. Additional access ports are inserted under direct laparoscope visualization. Size, number, and position of these ports are planned based on the surgical procedure and anticipated use of instruments, stapling devices, and size of the specimen to be extracted. For

example, certain instruments, such as endoscopic staplers, will pass only through 11-mm or 12-mm access ports. When expecting a large specimen, the surgeon may position access ports so that they can be joined together at the end of the procedure to accommodate extraction of the specimen. The laparoscope generally remains in the infraumbilical port. The surgeon uses at least two additional ports to perform the procedure and may insert additional ports, if needed, for instruments used by the first assistant.

6. At the end of the procedure, removal of access ports is done under direct visualization. Removal of the laparoscope from the umbilical port follows, as does evacuation of the pneumoperitoneum into a smoke evacuation system. Next is removal of the umbilical port. The midline fascial incision is closed with a size 0 absorbable suture on a taper needle if the incision is greater than 5 mm.

7. Skin incisions are closed according to surgeon preference and may include a subcuticular technique with 3-0 or 4-0 absorbable sutures. Dressings are then applied.

Single-Incision Laparoscopic Surgery

Procedural Considerations

Single-incision laparoscopic surgery (SILS) is a modification of the traditional laparoscopic approach in which abdominal access is achieved through multiple channels in a single-access port. The surgeon makes a single abdominal incision to accommodate the size of the access port; the laparoscope and all instruments enter via one port. Various single-access port systems with different numbers and sizes of channels are available. Location and orientation of the incision for the access port depend on patient anatomy and the procedure being performed. The umbilicus is a common site for port placement (Jafari et al., 2015).

Before development of modified laparoscopes and instruments, surgeons used standard rigid laparoscopes and laparoscopic instruments to perform single-incision procedures. The proximity and parallel orientation of these instruments often resulted in instrument "sword-fighting/collisions" within the abdomen and "clashing hands" conflicts outside the abdomen. In addition, the small working space of a single port inhibited the ability to place the laparoscope and instruments in the traditional and familiar laparoscopic "triangular" orientation. Visual perspective of the anatomy and working space significantly changed for the better as laparoscopes with flexible rotating tips developed to enhance visualization. Likewise, instruments with bendable rotating tips and curved flexible shafts have increased maneuverability. Advancements in robotic technology also allow utilization of single-port robotic surgery with Intuitive Surgical, Inc.'s (Sunnyvale, CA) own line of endowristed instrumentation.

Reported benefits of SILS are improved cosmesis (Di Saverio et al., 2016), reduced surgical trauma, less postoperative pain, and shorter hospital stays. SILS procedures that are GI specific include appendectomy, right hemicolectomy, extended right hemicolectomy, proctocolectomy, and ileostomy for ulcerative colitis (UC), high anterior colon resection, restorative proctocolectomy with ileoanal pouch, and utilizing stoma sites as entry for colorectal procedures (Johnson and Hope, 2015; Lopez et al., 2015).

Robotic-Assisted Laparoscopy

Robotic assistance enhances laparoscopic GI procedures such as Nissen fundoplication, bowel resection, Heller myotomy, gastric bypass, and gastrostomy (Goldner and Woo, 2015). The da Vinci surgical system (Intuitive Surgical, Inc.) is the most widely used robotic system for commercial use in the United States (Roy and Evans, 2016). Robotic instruments that provide haptic (tactile) and force feedback or are controlled by the surgeon's voice, eyes, or head movements, are being developed (Diana and Marescaux, 2015). Surgical robots that use endoscopic or bronchoscopic approaches have received US Food and Drug Administration (FDA) approval (Al Idrus, 2016). As healthcare systems consider starting a robotics program, advantages and disadvantages of owning and using a surgical robotic system require evaluation (Robotic-Assisted Surgery).

Procedural Considerations

Patient safety in robotic surgery is a collaborative effort involving the entire surgical team. Education and training are determined through needs assessment and training plans for the entire team to ensure patient safety, efficiency, and ability to respond in an adverse event (Gomez et al., 2015). The team must understand the physical configuration of system components (Cologne and Senagore, 2015; Gomez et al., 2015).

ROBOTIC-ASSISTED SURGERY

Advantages and Disadvantages

Advantages
- Binocular, three-dimensional (3-D) real-time visual feedback.
- High-definition technology.
- Hand controls at surgeon's console are ergonomically positioned.
- Scaled adjustment of movement allows for very fine precision dissection and suturing capabilities with no tremor.
- Articulating robotic arms mimic full rotation of wrists giving surgeon better range of motion, dexterity, and control.
- Stability of camera.
- Four operating arms: one for an instrument in each of the surgeon's hands, one for the scope, and one for an assistant's instrument.
- Surgeon sits at a console outside of the sterile field rather than stands.
- Assistant and scrub person are in the sterile field.
- Assistant may use an instrument to retract or provide suction, pass suture, pass clips as needed, or may exchange instruments.

Disadvantages
- Large bulky equipment.
- Limited field of view.
- Surgeon not at the field; depends on someone else to insert instruments.
- Increased distance from the field increases time delay in movement (more of a consideration for telesurgery across long distances).
- Initial cost of equipment.
- Cost of yearly maintenance of equipment and software upgrades.
- Increases the length of procedures.
- Setup time.
- Steep learning curve.
- Requires specialized training and a dedicated surgical team.
- Calibration of instruments.
- Care and handling of instruments.
- Emergent access to the abdomen takes more time because of the need to undock the robot.

The perioperative nurse and scrub person need to be competent in assembly, disassembly, and proper shutdown of all equipment. Additional responsibilities include calibration and configuration of the system; troubleshooting; draping robotic arms, endoscope, and other related equipment; docking the robot to the patient; disconnecting the arms from the trocars; removing instruments from the trocars; and undocking and disconnecting the system components (Kang et al., 2016).

Three mobile carts house the components of the da Vinci surgical system. These include the surgeon's console, where the surgeon sits to control the robotic arms; the patient cart, which holds four robotic arms and a touchscreen monitor; and the vision cart, which holds the camera control unit, light source, insufflator, ESU, and possibly other laparoscopic accessory items. Additional "resident" consoles can be used for teaching or dual-surgeon purposes.

Equipment used with the da Vinci system is specific to the system and includes a 0- and 3-degree high-definition endoscope system with 3-D technology; a camera, light cord, monopolar hook cautery, sterile drapes for the robotic arms; and special access ports designed to connect or dock with the robotic arms. Access ports come in three sizes: 8.5 mm for the endoscope, two 5-mm ports for the surgeon's instruments, and a 10-mm port for other instruments if needed. The "endowristed" da Vinci instruments are unique in that they are capable of a wide range of motion similar to that of the surgeon's wrist. An instrument set may include a Cadiere forceps, clip applier, curved dissecting scissors, Maryland dissector, various graspers, and needle holders for suturing.

Robotic-assisted laparoscopic procedures can last for several hours. Individual patient risk factors are assessed (Patient Safety) as attention is paid to increased risk for perioperative hypothermia, fluid management, DVT, surgical site infection, pressure ulcers, and position-related injuries or complications (Chang et al., 2014).

Operative Procedure

1. The surgeon places access cannulae into the abdomen, using one of the techniques previously described for laparoscopy.
2. To calibrate the system and prepare for docking the arms to the access ports, the cart with the robotic arms is positioned over the patient with guidance from the surgeon.
3. The surgeon attaches the robotic arms to the trocars and inserts the camera and instruments into the abdomen.
4. The surgeon leaves the sterile field to perform the procedure from the surgeon console.
5. A scrub person and a first assistant remain in the sterile field. The first assistant's role may include exchanging instruments for the surgeon, retracting tissues, instilling irrigation, suctioning, or cutting suture.

Natural Orifice Transluminal Endoscopic Surgery

Natural orifice transluminal endoscopic surgery (NOTES) continues to be a promising alternative approach for GI surgery. When compared with open and laparoscopic techniques, potential benefits of NOTES include no visible scars, possibly less pain, and potentially shorter LOS (Johnson and Hope, 2015). Disadvantages are that the surgeon must open a closed viscera to access the abdomen, complications related to failure of that opening to heal after closure can result in peritonitis, and male gender limits the vaginal approach.

Procedural Considerations

Surgeons perform NOTES procedures by entering the abdominal cavity through an incision created in the wall of a natural orifice

---

Ensuring Safe Patient Positioning for Colorectal Robotic Surgery: Utilizing a Second "Time-Out"

This study investigated if a second time-out for lengthy robotic procedures reduced positioning injuries and complications in robotic surgery patients. A surgical checklist was developed to address the most common complications and injuries present postrobotic procedures. The use of a checklist standardizes a proactive surgical team approach, which is necessary for enhancing communication within the team and promoting high standards of patient safety. Study recommendations for the second time-out are broken into general patient considerations, surgeon considerations, anesthesia considerations, and nursing considerations.

- General patient considerations:
  - Turn all room lights on.
  - Verify patient's head and eye placement and padding.
  - Check for pooling of preparation solutions at buttocks and lower back.
  - Check extremities for mottled appearance.
  - Verify sufficient padding at pressure points.
  - Verify safety strap security.
- Surgeon considerations:
  - Determine if the length of the procedure is usual for the operation.
  - Evaluate progression of surgery.
  - Identify cause(s) for prolonged operative time.
  - Evaluate need to convert to a different approach.
  - Evaluate need for another surgeon assistant.
  - Evaluate surgeon and surgical assistant fatigue.
  - Evaluate surgeon and surgical assistant break needs.
- Anesthesia considerations:
  - Check vital signs and report to team.
  - Evaluate extent of blood loss.
  - Evaluate patient's urine output and color.
  - Evaluate need for antibiotic redosing.
  - Evaluate need to draw labs.
- Nursing considerations:
  - Perform or review surgical counts.
  - Check equipment for proper functioning.
  - Check for placement and functional status of IPCDs.
  - Update administration on room time and discuss needs for additional or relief nursing and scrub personnel.

Conclusions from the implementation of the checklist were positive; the second time-out took less time than anticipated, and promoted team awareness of the patient's status and tolerance of the procedure. Future studies are needed for a greater analysis of effectiveness at additional facilities.

IPCD, Intermittent pneumatic compression devices.
Modified from Song JB et al: The second "time-out": a surgical safety checklist for lengthy robotic surgeries, *Patient Saf Surg* 7(19):1–6, 2013.

---

such as the stomach (peroral transgastric), rectum (transanal), or the vagina (transvaginal). Instruments are in development to overcome the challenges related to closing the defect created in the natural orifice.

Pure NOTES procedures are transluminal procedures performed using flexible endoscopes and instruments passed through the scopes' working channels. Many surgeons use a hybrid NOTES technique that combines laparoscopic visualization with natural orifice access.

Using a transvaginal hybrid NOTES technique, the surgeon inserts a 3-mm or 5-mm access port at the umbilicus to create a pneumoperitoneum. The surgeon next inserts a rigid laparoscope into the abdominal access port to visualize entry of the vaginal access port from inside the abdomen and then moves the laparoscope to the vaginal access port. It is possible to insert a grasper through the umbilical port to use as a retractor to facilitate the NOTES procedure. GI procedures modified for a NOTES or hybrid NOTES approach include transvaginal appendectomy, transgastric appendectomy, transvaginal and transgastric cholecystectomy, full-thickness resection of gastric cancer with laparoscopic lymph node dissection, percutaneous endoscopic gastrostomy (PEG) tube salvage, transesophageal Heller myotomy; and transanal minimally invasive surgery (TAMIS) (Nassif, 2015).

Gastrointestinal Endoscopy

GI endoscopy permits visual inspection of the mucosal lining of the esophagus, stomach, duodenum, colon, and rectum; it is performed for a wide range of screening, surveillance, diagnostic, and therapeutic procedures. Table 11.2 includes common therapeutic and diagnostic endoscopic procedures.

GI endoscopy takes place via flexible video endoscopes; most utilize 3-D technology. Endoscopy setup includes a light source, suction, irrigation, air source, ESU, video processor, camera for photo documentation of findings, and at least one monitor for visualization. Containers with saline for biopsy specimens and water-soluble lubricating jelly are available.

Flexible endoscopes are semicritical patient care devices that undergo high-level disinfection before each use (see Chapters 4 and 8). They are easily damaged by misuse and must be cleaned, disinfected, and stored according to the manufacturer's recommendations. They vary in length and diameter, depending on intended use. Using wheeled knobs and buttons on the handle of the scope, the endoscopist can deflect the tip of the scope up and down, left and right, instill air or water, and activate suction. Diagnostic endoscopes can be as small as 9 mm. For planned therapeutic procedures, the endoscope has a larger diameter to accommodate the working channel through which endoscopic instruments pass. Specialized endoscopes with overtubes and balloons enable examination of the small bowel. Because instrumentation for therapeutic endoscopic procedures may penetrate the intestinal mucosa, they are considered "critical" devices that must be sterilized before each use.

Endoscopy instruments and accessories include cytology brushes, snares, biopsy forceps, specimen retrieval nets, long-needle injection/aspiration catheters, and hydrostatic balloons. Instruments for hemostasis include appliers for clips, bands, and loops; monopolar or bipolar electrocoagulation probes; and argon plasma coagulation probes. Radiofrequency ablation (RFA) balloons, removable stents, and permanent stents may be necessary for therapeutic procedures.

Preprocedure preparation for EGD (sometimes called "upper GI endoscopy") includes limiting ingestion of solid foods and liquids for prescribed periods before the procedure. Preparation for colonoscopy, tailored to the patient's individual needs, includes preprocedure limitation of oral intake, as well as bowel cleansing preparations (Mathus-Vliegen et al., 2013).

Endoscopic procedures most commonly occur with moderate sedation/analgesia to ensure patient comfort, cooperation, and a safe and complete examination. Medications and safety measures for moderate sedation appear in Chapter 5. Monitoring the patient's airway, vital signs, oxygenation, level of consciousness, and comfort continues throughout the procedure and postprocedure recovery (Ambulatory Surgery Considerations).

Esophagogastroduodenoscopy

Procedural Considerations

EGD affords visualization of the oropharynx, esophagus, stomach, and proximal duodenum. It is the gold standard for diagnostics (Goldberg and Raufman, 2016). The procedure begins with the patient in left lateral decubitus position with neck flexed forward. To enhance passage of the endoscope for better visualization, the

TABLE 11.2

Endoscopic Procedures

Procedure	Indications (Diagnostic/Screening/Surveillance)	Indications (Therapeutic)
Esophagogastroduodenoscopy	• Abnormal upper GI x-ray • Upper GI bleeding • Dysphasia • Persistent heartburn • Persistent epigastric pain • Persistent vomiting • GERD • Odynophagia • Pyrosis • Ingestion of caustic substance • Gastric polyposis • Surveillance (Barrett esophagus, gastric ulcers)	• EMR • ESD • Foreign body retrieval • Sclerosing of esophageal varices • Stricture dilation • Ablation of tumors • Palliative stenting of tumors • Control of bleeding • Placement of PEG tube • Polypectomy • RFA • Endoscopic 270-degree fundoplication
Colonoscopy	• Screening (cancer) • Diagnosis (inflammatory colitis) • Surveillance (ulcerative colitis) • GI bleeding	• Polypectomy • Decompression • Hydrostatic balloon dilatation of strictures • Palliative dilation of obstructions with self-expanding metal stents • Detorsion of volvulus • Fecal microbiota transplant

EMR, Endoscopic mucosal resection; *ESD*, endoscopic submucosal dissection; *GERD*, gastroesophageal reflux disease; *GI*, gastrointestinal; *PEG*, percutaneous endoscopic gastrostomy; *RFA*, radiofrequency ablation.

AMBULATORY SURGERY CONSIDERATIONS

Increasing Efficiency and Safety for Gastrointestinal Endoscopy

GI endoscopy is often done in ASCs. Proper planning and preparation from the ASC perspective and good preoperative scheduling and preparation for patients enhance both efficiency and safety.

Perioperative staff in ASCs often fill multiple roles. These multiple roles can pose challenges for competency assessment and verification. Moderate sedation requires monitoring by an RN with the proper training and competencies or a CRNA. More complicated procedures need staffing to represent their acuity, along with an anesthesia provider for sedation greater than moderate sedation. A circulating nurse is mandatory for patient assessment. The ability for medical technicians or GI medical technicians to assist endoscopists when biopsies are taken is determined by external regulations.

Infection control protocols in ASC settings create environments less like procedure suites and more like ORs. Traffic control, attire, and terminal cleaning procedures are similar to that of an OR environment. Increased regulations and focus on stringent cleaning and disinfection of endoscopes may strain efficiency in ASCs with longer processing times. Scope manufacturers have updated IFUs to ensure that endoscopes are processed appropriately.

Policies and procedures assist with formulating a framework for standardization. Many organizations, including AORN, the American Society of Anesthesiologists, and the American Society for Gastrointestinal Endoscopy, provide guidelines and recommendations to assist with growing and often conflicting regulations. With proper planning, training, and implementing changing regulations, ASC staff can focus on maintaining patient safety, efficiency, and cost containment in the GI suite.

AORN, Association of periOperative Registered Nurses; *ASC*, ambulatory surgical center; *CRNA*, certified registered nurse anesthetist; *GI*, gastrointestinal; *IFU*, instructions for use; *RN*, registered nurse.
Modified from Deas T, Sinsel L: Ensuring patient safety and optimizing efficiency during gastrointestinal endoscopy, *AORN J* 99(3):396–406, 2014.

endoscopist may direct or use other positions such as supine, semi-Fowler, or sitting.

Procedure

1. The endoscopist or anesthesia provider may anesthetize the posterior pharynx with a topical agent such as benzocaine spray or gel.
2. A bite-block, positioned over the shaft of the endoscope and placed between the patient's upper and lower teeth, prevents the patient from accidentally biting down on the shaft of the endoscope during the procedure.
3. The endoscopist gently advances the tip of the lubricated gastroscope through the mouth and esophagus, and into the stomach and duodenum.
4. Visual inspection of the target organ follows.
5. Biopsies or brushings are obtained as needed; safe specimen handling practices are initiated.
6. Indicated therapeutic procedures follow.
7. While visualizing the mucosa, the endoscopist slowly withdraws the endoscope.
8. Once the patient's gag reflex returns, the patient is moved to a monitoring area and offered fluids.

Deep Small Bowel Enteroscopy

Procedural Considerations

The small bowel can be difficult to view endoscopically because of its length and contractility. Although video capsule endoscopy allows for visualization of the small bowel, therapeutic procedures cannot follow. All reports and images of capsule endoscopy results should be available at the time of any surgery (Ou et al., 2015). Double-balloon enteroscopy (DBE) is a technique that provides both visualization and the capability to perform therapeutic procedures in the small bowel (Micic and Semrad, 2016). Other techniques include single-balloon enteroscopy and spiral enteroscopy. Before the day of the procedure, patients receive instructions to fast after midnight and undergo a bowel prep to empty the colon. DBE commences from the mouth or the anus, or both, depending on the location of the suspected lesion. Because of longer procedure times, general anesthesia is frequently used for the oral approach (Lipka et al., 2015b).

Procedure: Double-Balloon Enteroscopy

1. The balloon-tipped endoscope inserts (back-loaded) through a soft overtube, which also has a balloon.
2. The endoscope inserts orally, through the esophagus and stomach, into the duodenum.
3. When the scope will not advance any more, the operator inflates the balloon on the endoscope.
4. The overtube advances over the endoscope to the first balloon, and the balloon on the overtube inflates.
5. With both balloons inflated, the operator withdraws the endoscope slightly to pleat the small bowel on the overtube, providing a straight pathway to advance the endoscope.
6. After deflating the endoscope balloon, the operator advances the scope.
7. The cycles of inflation and deflation, and advancement and withdrawal, repeat until the endoscope cannot advance farther.
8. The team marks the most distal location reached by the scope with a tattoo for later identification with capsule endoscopy.
9. The process reverses as the operator withdraws the scope.

Colonoscopy

Procedural Considerations

Colonoscopy provides endoscopic visualization of the colon from the rectum to the ileocecal valve. The clinician inspects the mucosa for abnormalities such as sites of bleeding, polyps, inflammation, ulceration, or tumors during both insertion and withdrawal of the colonoscope. Colonoscopy can be diagnostic and therapeutic (see Table 11.2). Performance of colonoscopy also is possible through an ostomy stoma to inspect an anastomosis site or identify recurrence of disease or bleeding. Likewise, reservoir pouches can undergo inspection postoperatively for anastomosis integrity, inflammation, bleeding, and other abnormalities. Tattooing lesions found during colonoscopy that will require surgical removal is common; this assists with localization of the lesion during a later operative procedure. Tattooing does not rule out the use of intraoperative colonoscopy to verify location of a colon lesion that is otherwise difficult to identify.

Procedure

The patient is positioned on the left side with knees bent. The operator passes a well-lubricated colonoscope slowly into the anal canal and advances it continually until it reaches the cecum. The endoscopist or surgeon may ask for a repositioning of the patient to prone position or may ask the perioperative or endoscopy nurse to apply gentle abdominal pressure or to lift the patient's left side to assist advancement of the scope. With sigmoidoscopy, examination extends only to the left colon. Flexible sigmoidoscopy is achievable without sedation with a cooperative patient. After endoscopic examination, the patient is observed for bleeding, pain, signs of perforation, or reaction to medications.

Endoscopic Ultrasound

EUS combines endoscopy and ultrasound, using sound waves to generate an image of the histologic layers of the esophageal, gastric, and intestinal walls. EUS is critically important in staging GI malignancies and determining surgical options and potential for therapeutic resection. The frequencies used, higher than those used in traditional ultrasound, provide highly accurate depths of any mucosal invasion. Endoscopic image-enhancement techniques include high-resolution endoscopes with narrowband imaging and magnification to identify mucosal surface details; narrowband filters to see capillary patterns, pits, and villi; and chromoendoscopy (staining techniques) and fluorescence to differentiate between normal and dysplastic tissue (Lim et al., 2013).

Endoscopic Procedures for Gastroesophageal Reflux Disease

Gastroesophageal reflux disease (GERD) is a condition in which the LES is incompetent and allows stomach contents to reflux into the esophagus. GERD symptoms include heartburn, regurgitation, and dysphagia. Less common GERD-related symptoms include chest pain, hypersalivation, and painful swallowing.

Complications of GERD are esophagitis and Barrett esophagus (BE) caused by repeated or prolonged exposure to gastric acid. Endoscopic procedures to treat GERD by improving the gastro-esophageal flap valve, improving function of the LES, or tightening the tissue at the GEJ are available for patients who are unresponsive to or cannot take GERD medications, or who do not wish to have a surgical procedure.

Endoscopic GERD procedures include RFA, intraluminal endoscopic sewing devices, transmural fasteners, and staplers. Two newer therapies, the Stretta (Mederi Therapeutics, Norwalk, CT) and EsophyX (EndoGastric Solutions, Inc., Redmond, WA), are gaining traction against the laparoscopic Nissen fundoplication (Hopkins et al., 2015). The Stretta procedure delivers controlled amounts of radiofrequency (RF) heat energy through a balloon catheter positioned endoscopically in the distal esophagus, creating thermal lesions that tighten the tissue at the LES. The EsophyX technique endoscopically creates a 200- to 300-degree internal plication of the gastric fundus to create a neogastroesophageal valve. The SRS endoscopic stapling system staples the gastric fundus to the esophagus to create a neogastroesophageal valve flap (Hopkins et al., 2015). The EndoCinch (C.R. Bard, Inc., New Providence, NJ) device endoscopically places sutures in mucosal folds at a location distal to the "Z"-line of the GEJ.

Endoscopic Procedures for Barrett Esophagus

BE is the presence of metaplastic changes to cells lining the esophagus as a result of chronic exposure to gastric acid. BE can progress to dysplasia, or precancerous changes, increasing the risk of the development of adenocarcinoma of the esophagus. BE treatment aims to prevent progression to dysplasia by minimizing or eliminating acid reflux through diet, lifestyle changes, and antireflux medications. When BE progresses to a high-grade dysplasia, endoscopic treatment

options include RFA, endoscopic mucosal resection (EMR), and photodynamic therapy (PDT).

Radiofrequency Ablation

RFA involves application of RF energy to the abnormal cells using the Barrx 360 system by Medtronic (Minneapolis, MN). The system consists of a generator, a guidewire, and a sizing catheter with a 4-cm long balloon used to measure the inner diameter of the esophagus. The ablation catheters are 165 cm long, with a balloon tip that contains a bipolar electrode with 60 tightly coiled electrode rings that wrap around the balloon. The clinician introduces the ablation catheter, inflates the balloon, applies RF energy, repositions the balloon and endoscope, and repeats the process along the length of abnormal tissue. The clinician then removes the ablation catheter, cleans the electrode, irrigates and cleans the esophagus, and repeats the process as necessary. After 12 weeks, if residual abnormal tissue remains, repetition of the original procedure is possible or small focal ablation can follow with the Barrx 90 electrode, which has a flat panel electrode to apply RF energy to smaller areas.

Endoscopic Mucosal Resection

EMR is excision of dysplastic lesions related to BE. Before EMR, EUS may help determine the depth of invasion into the esophageal wall. Saline is injected in the lesion or dysplastic tissue to separate the superficial mucosa from deeper submucosal and muscular layers. Separation of these tissue planes facilitates snare resection. Using suction attached to the endoscope, the clinician pulls the elevated lesion into a cap secured to the end of the scope and resects it with a rigid wire snare. The tissue specimen is then submitted for histologic examination (Hwang et al., 2015).

Photodynamic Therapy

PDT is a laser ablation technique. Dysplastic tissue uptakes a photosensitizer drug, Photofrin II (sodium porfimer), activated by the laser. IV administration of the drug occurs 48 hours before the procedure to allow for tissue uptake. Normal tissue excretes the drug sooner than abnormal or dysplastic tissues. The mucosal layer retains the drug, limiting the depth of the laser effect. After 48 hours the procedure commences. The clinician introduces the laser fiber through the endoscope channel and directs laser light toward the mucosa, causing tissue destruction and cell death in those areas identified by the uptake of the photosensitizer drug. The patient may continue to be light sensitive for 60 to 90 days after the injection and must take precautions to prevent cutaneous burns. Unlike EMR, PDT does not provide a tissue specimen. Clinicians often combine PDT with endoscopic resection.

Percutaneous Endoscopic Gastrostomy Tube Insertion

A PEG procedure involves percutaneous insertion of a uniquely designed gastrostomy tube into the stomach under endoscopic visualization. A PEG tube provides a means to provide enteral feedings to patients unable to ingest food orally, but who have a normally functioning GI tract. This procedure may occur in the endoscopy suite under IV sedation/analgesia or in the OR under general anesthesia in conjunction with another surgical procedure.

Procedural Considerations

Supplies include a prepackaged PEG tube kit. The contents of the kit vary depending on the technique used. Three techniques are the pull method (Ponsky technique), push method (Sacks-Vine technique), and the sheath method (Russell technique, which is rarely used and not described). Kits for the Ponsky and Sacks-Vine techniques contain a knife handle with a #11 blade, a 14- to 18-gauge trocar needle, a long silk suture, a guidewire, a gastrostomy tube, and a skin disk to secure the tube. A gastroscopy setup with a flexible scope, a wire snare, light source, air source, suction, and monitor is required. This procedure requires an endoscopist and an assistant. The patient is positioned supine. The monitor is positioned so that the physician (endoscopist or surgeon) and assistant can see it during tube insertion. The abdomen is prepped and preoperative antibiotics administered. If the patient is awake, a bite-block is inserted into the patient's mouth.

Procedure (Ponsky Technique)

1. The gastroscope is inserted and advanced into the fundus of the stomach. Insufflation of the stomach with air through the gastroscope follows. The flexible tip of the scope is angled anteriorly to provide transillumination through the anterior stomach and abdominal wall. Using transillumination, the physician confirms there are no abdominal viscera between the stomach and the anterior abdominal wall.
2. The physician injects local anesthetic at the site of the intended gastrostomy site if the patient is awake.
3. The physician then makes a small stab wound with a #11 blade.
4. As the 14- to 18-gauge trocar needle inserts through the abdominal wall and the anterior wall of the stomach, entry of the needle into the stomach is visualized with the gastroscope.
5. The long silk suture passes through the trocar needle into the stomach, in which a wire snare that has been passed through the working channel of the gastroscope entraps it.
6. After removal of the trocar needle, a hemostat is clamped to the end of the suture that remains outside the abdomen.
7. The gastroscope and snare are removed together, pulling the suture out of the patient's mouth.
8. The suture is attached to the tapered distal end of the gastrostomy tube, guided into the oral cavity, down the esophagus, into the stomach, and pulled out through the abdominal wall.
9. Reinsertion of the gastroscope follows to confirm correct positioning of the feeding tube.
10. The gastrostomy tube is secured in place against the abdominal wall using the disk.
11. The distal end of the tube is plugged, the stomach deflated, and the procedure ends.

Procedure (Sacks-Vine Technique)

Steps 1 through 4 are identical to the Ponsky technique (the pull method) just described. Instead of passing a long silk suture as mentioned in step 5, a guidewire is passed, ensnared, and pulled through the mouth in which a feeding tube threads over the guidewire and then is "pushed" through the mouth, into the stomach, and through the skin, where the assistant grabs the feeding tube as it exits. The remainder of the procedure is the same as the pull method.

Surgery of the Esophagus

Esophagectomy

Esophagectomy is indicated for cancer, dysplastic mucosal changes, and stricture of the esophagus caused by injury or benign disease. Most malignant tumors of the esophagus and GEJ are squamous cell carcinoma (SSC) or adenocarcinoma (Watanabe et al., 2013). Adenocarcinoma occurs at the GEJ and is associated with BE, GERD, obesity, and smoking (Hur et al., 2013).

Determination of the treatment and prognosis for patients with esophageal cancer is based on the cancer cell type, tumor location, depth of invasion, involvement of lymph nodes or spread to other structures, and overall physical condition of the patient. Preoperative evaluation involves many medical disciplines and often includes endoscopic examination and biopsy, EUS, and a PET scan with or without CT scan to assess for metastasis. Patients may also undergo diagnostic laparoscopy, thoracoscopy, mediastinoscopy, or bronchoscopy before proceeding with esophagectomy (Watanabe et al., 2013). Some patients receive chemotherapy and radiation before esophagectomy.

The approach depends on location and size of the tumor in the esophagus, the extent of planned lymph node dissection, the type of conduit used to replace the esophagus, and surgeon preference. Open approaches include transhiatal esophagectomy (THE), transthoracic esophagectomy (TTE or Ivor Lewis), and en bloc, or "tri-incisional" esophagectomy.

Reestablishing continuity of the GI tract after esophagectomy occurs by performing an anastomosis between the proximal esophagus and a variety of esophageal replacement conduits. The surgeon can create the anastomosis through a cervical incision or a chest incision; its location depends on location of the esophageal tumor and the approach used for esophagectomy. The anastomosis is either hand sewn or endostapled. A cervical anastomosis requires linear cutting staplers, whereas a thoracic anastomosis requires an end-to-end or circular stapling device. The most common conduit to replace the transected esophagus is the stomach. Other conduits include the jejunum and colon, both of which may require microvascular anastomosis. Additional supplies, such as microvascular instruments, a microscope, and related supplies, are then required.

Procedural Considerations

Instrumentation includes a thoracotomy set, laparotomy set, long and short vascular instruments, GI instruments, long versions of basic instruments, deep retractors, self-retaining abdominal and rib retractors, linear and circular stapling devices, and long vascular ligating clip appliers and clips in a variety of sizes. Additional supplies to have available include short and long silk sutures and ties in a variety of diameters according to surgeon preference; one or two long $\frac{1}{2}$- or 1-inch Penrose drains, one or two chest tubes (sized according to surgeon preference) with appropriate 5/1 connector(s), and a closed chest drainage system; and a closed suction drain(s) with suction bulb(s). If planning for resection of cervical esophageal cancer, instruments and supplies for pharyngectomy, laryngectomy, thyroidectomy, neck dissection, and tracheostomy should be available as well.

Minimally invasive esophagectomy (MIE) requires laparoscopic and thoracoscopic instruments, video and insufflation equipment, and energy-generating devices. If the surgeon plans to perform an EGD, a mediastinoscopy, or a bronchoscopy immediately before the procedure, additional equipment and/or staff is necessary. Postoperatively, patients are NPO (nothing by mouth) for an extended time while the esophagogastric anastomosis heals. Preoperative planning for insertion of a feeding jejunostomy ensures appropriate supplies are available in the OR.

Esophagectomy requires general anesthesia with endotracheal intubation. A double-lumen endotracheal tube provides the option for single-lung ventilation if thoracic exposure is needed. A radial artery catheter for blood pressure monitoring is inserted as is an indwelling urinary catheter. The patient's position on the OR bed depends on the planned surgical approach. Appropriate measures to prevent hypothermia and pressure injuries are initiated.

If needed, a pathologist renders intraoperative histologic confirmation of tumor-free margins. An intraoperative EGD may be done to confirm location of the tumor. A thoracic epidural or interscalene perineural blockade can augment postoperative pain management. Patients undergoing esophagectomy may transfer to the SICU after surgery.

Transhiatal Esophagectomy

The transhiatal approach requires an upper midline abdominal incision and an incision in the left neck. The preferred left-side-of-the-neck approach decreases risk of injury to the recurrent laryngeal nerve, because it descends and recurs lower (around the aortic arch rather than the subclavian artery) as it does on the right side (Namm and Posner, 2015).

Operative Procedure

1. The patient is supine. Skin prep includes the neck, chest, and abdomen.
2. The surgeon makes an upper midline incision, extends it cephalad to the xiphoid process, and explores the abdomen, after which a self-retaining retractor is positioned. Removal of the xiphoid process may achieve better access to the hiatus.
3. The liver is retracted to the right and the stomach mobilized to expose the esophageal hiatus. A Penrose drain encircles the esophagus for manipulation and retraction.
4. Performance of a pyloromyotomy facilitates postoperative gastric drainage into the duodenum.
5. The esophageal hiatus is enlarged, facilitating mobilization of the thoracic esophagus.
6. The surgeon makes a left neck incision just above the clavicle and exposes the cervical esophagus, taking care not to injure the recurrent laryngeal nerve with excessive lateral retraction.
7. A second Penrose drain is passed around the cervical esophagus, and mobilization of the cervical and upper thoracic esophagus using blunt finger dissection follows.
8. The cervical esophagus is divided with a linear stapler; it is then pulled through the mediastinum into the abdomen.
9. A linear cutting stapler is used to resect the esophagus, cardia, and part of the lesser curve of the stomach. This "tubularizes" the stomach, preparing it for the cervical esophagogastric anastomosis.
10. The stomach "tube" is pulled through the esophageal hiatus and posterior mediastinum into the neck.
11. Closure of the crura is with interrupted 2-0 nonabsorbable sutures; fixation of the stomach to the diaphragm is with a 3-0 silk suture.
12. A feeding jejunostomy tube is placed.
13. The anastomosis between the stomach and cervical esophagus is created through the neck incision.
14. Closure of the abdomen is with a running 0 PDS suture; skin closure is with staples.
15. A second stab incision is made and a closed suction drain (Jackson-Pratt) placed in the neck wound.
16. Closure of the neck incision in two layers follows, according to surgeon preference.
17. A chest x-ray taken in the OR ensures there is no pneumothorax or hemothorax.

Transthoracic Esophagectomy: Ivor Lewis

The TTE entails both an upper midline abdominal incision and a right thoracotomy incision. If the surgeon performs the procedure in one stage, the patient is in supine position with a roll under the torso on the side of the planned thoracotomy. Elevation of the arm on the side of the thoracotomy can be on an over armboard, draped out of the surgical field, or the arm may be prepped and draped into the surgical field. The neck, chest, and abdomen are prepped.

Alternatively, for a two-stage technique, patient placement position is supine for the abdominal portion of the procedure and then repositioned on the left side for the thoracic portion. Before repositioning, the abdomen is closed and dressed. Positioning aids (beanbag, over armboard, etc.) and supplies for reprepping and redraping are available.

Operative Procedure

1. The surgeon makes an upper midline abdominal incision, retractors are positioned, and mobilization of the stomach follows, as described previously for the transhiatal approach.
2. The surgeon next makes a separate thoracotomy incision in the sixth or seventh intercostal space on the intended side. The anesthesia provider may clamp the double-lumen endotracheal tube on the affected side to deflate the lung for better visualization. Gentle retraction of the lung with a handheld retractor exposes the pleura overlying the esophagus. The surgeon then lifts and incises the pleura.
3. A long Penrose drain encircles the esophagus for manipulation. Mobilization of the esophagus is circumferential, proximal, and distal to the tumor, ensuring tumor resection achieves clear margins.
4. Transection of the esophagus is proximal to the tumor, using a linear cutting stapling device.
5. The surgeon pulls the previously mobilized stomach into the chest through the esophageal hiatus of the diaphragm and fires a linear cutting stapling device across the proximal fundus and cardia of the stomach to complete the esophageal resection.
6. To reconnect the proximal esophagus to the stomach, placement of the anvil of a circular stapling device such as an EEA is in the proximal esophagus. The EEA stapler inserts into the stomach and connects to the anvil through an opening made in the stomach. Firing of the stapler follows and the anastomosis between the remaining esophagus and stomach is complete. Closure of the opening in the stomach is with nonabsorbable suture. Alternatively, the surgeon may hand sew the end to end anastomosis between the proximal esophagus and stomach in two layers, using interrupted 3-0 nonabsorbable sutures.
7. To decrease tension on the staple line of the anastomosis, the stomach can be tacked to the prevertebral fascia and to the esophageal hiatus with interrupted 3-0 nonabsorbable sutures.
8. A 36-French (F) chest tube is inserted through a separate stab wound and the thoracotomy incision closed in layers, according to surgeon preference.
9. Closure of the abdominal incision is as described previously for the transhiatal approach.

En Bloc (Tri-Incisional) Esophagectomy

This technique is the most radical approach to esophagectomy.

Operative Procedure

1. Through a right thoracotomy, the surgeon removes the esophagus and surrounding healthy tissues en bloc. The venous and lymphatic vessels are also ligated, divided, and removed with the specimen. Radical thoracic and mediastinum lymph node dissection follows.

2. Through an upper midline incision, stomach mobilization through the abdominal incision is as described in the transhiatal approach, and a radical upper abdominal lymph node dissection follows.
3. Preparation of the gastric conduit is as previously described; its delivery to the neck is through the posterior mediastinal space.
4. The surgeon creates a cervical esophagogastric anastomosis through the neck incision (Lee and Altorki, 2015).
5. The incision is closed and dressings applied.

Minimally Invasive Esophagectomy

Minimally invasive modifications to open esophagectomy are common (Watanabe et al., 2013). Any of these procedures may also occur with robotic assistance. Team communication regarding the intended approach for esophagectomy is an essential part of preoperative planning, should be properly annotated on the consent, and discussed during the briefing and/or time-out to ensure that all necessary equipment and supplies are readily available for the appropriate procedure or in case it requires conversion to an open procedure.

Laparoscopic Esophageal Myotomy (Modified Heller Myotomy)

Esophageal myotomy treats achalasia, a condition in which degeneration of the nerves to the lower esophagus results in inability of the LES to relax with swallowing. Normally the LES, a circular band of muscle encircling the esophagus, relaxes to allow ingested food and liquids to pass into the stomach. After swallowing, the LES contracts to prevent gastric reflux into the esophagus. Patients with achalasia have difficulty swallowing because the LES remains in a state of constant contraction. Over time, the peristaltic function of the esophagus may decrease and the proximal esophagus becomes dilated. Because of prolonged mucosal irritation of the esophagus, untreated achalasia increases the risk of esophageal cancer. Symptoms include difficulty swallowing, regurgitation of undigested food and liquids, heartburn, difficulty burping, hiccups, choking after meals, nighttime cough, and weight loss (Smith, 2015). Achalasia is not curable, but esophageal myotomy can alleviate its symptoms. The goal of myotomy is to relieve the obstruction caused by the contracted LES while preventing postoperative gastric reflux, scarring, and subsequent stricture. The most common approach to esophageal myotomy is the laparoscopic modified Heller myotomy combined with partial gastric fundoplication to prevent gastric reflux (Bhayani et al., 2014).

Procedural Considerations

The procedure requires general anesthesia with endotracheal intubation. The patient is in modified lithotomy or split-leg position. The OR bed will be in a steep reverse Trendelenburg position. Setup includes standard laparoscopy equipment, instruments, and supplies. The surgical team will use five access ports: two ports are for the surgeon, the third port is for the 30-degree laparoscope, the fourth is for a liver retractor, and the fifth is for the first assistant to use. Laparoscopic instruments include fine curved or right-angled dissectors, a hook dissector, clip appliers, liver retractor, atraumatic or Babcock graspers, ultrasonic shears, needle holders, and suture to close the crura and perform the antireflux procedure.

Use of intraoperative gastric endoscopy is common to confirm location of the Z-line at the GEJ and to inspect for unintended perforations of the mucosa. A flexible gastroscope, light source, video camera and monitor, suction, air source, and other related equipment are ready on a separate nonsterile table or cart.

Operative Procedure: Laparoscopic Technique

1. Abdominal access is obtained according to surgeon preference, and pneumoperitoneum then established.
2. Insertion of the liver retractor to retract the left lobe of the liver follows.
3. The surgeon identifies the right and left crura and opens the retroesophageal space.
4. A Penrose drain passes around the esophagus and its ends are secured together. The Penrose drain is used to manipulate the esophagus during mobilization.
5. Using blunt dissection, the distal esophagus is mobilized circumferentially.
6. A curved dissector is used to develop the plane between the esophageal mucosa and the inner muscular layer. A hook dissector can be used to divide the muscle. The myotomy begins about 2 cm proximal to the GEJ, extends proximally for about 8 cm, and then extends distally to a point approximately 2 to 3 cm below the GEJ on the anterior stomach.
7. Endoscopy is performed.
8. The antireflux procedure follows.
9. Instruments and access ports are removed and the incision closed according to surgeon preference.

Excision of Pharyngoesophageal (Zenker) Diverticulum

Pharyngoesophageal diverticula are the most common type of esophageal diverticula. Zenker diverticulum is considered "false diverticulum" because it involves only two layers of the esophageal wall, the mucosa and submucosa. Zenker diverticula herniate through the thyropharyngeus and cricopharyngeus muscles, forming a sac in which food can embed and infection can occur (Smith, 2015). As the diverticulum enlarges, symptoms develop such as a persistent cough, excessive salivation, regurgitation of undigested food, halitosis, voice changes, retrosternal pain, and intermittent dysphasia. Repair of Zenker diverticulum occurs through an incision in the neck or endoscopically.

Procedural Considerations

Instrumentation includes a thyroid set with fine dissecting hemostats, 5-inch Adson or other fine-toothed forceps, and lateral retractors. The procedure requires general anesthesia or a cervical block. Positioning of the patient is supine with a shoulder roll to extend the neck. The head may be turned away from the operative side. Skin prep extends from the mandible to the nipples and includes the neck and anterior chest. If using an alcohol-based prep solution, then team members assess fire risk and take appropriate action to prevent surgical fires. Results of a preoperative barium esophagram can confirm location of the diverticulum (or diverticula, if there is more than one).

Operative Procedure

1. The surgeon makes a vertical incision parallel to the inner border of the sternocleidomastoid muscle (SCM), between the level of the hyoid bone and a point 2 cm above the clavicle; an alternative is a transverse incision centered over the middle third of the SCM.
2. Handheld retractors are used to retract the SCM and carotid sheath laterally and the thyroid gland and larynx medially. Care is taken to not stretch the recurrent laryngeal nerve with excessive medial retraction. The surgeon may divide the omohyoid muscle with electrosurgery or retract it superiorly to expose the diverticulum.

3. The sac of the diverticulum is grasped with an Allis clamp and dissected from surrounding tissue. The anesthesia provider then may insert an esophageal dilator into the esophagus.

4. Performance of an 8- to 10-cm esophageal myotomy above and below the extruding diverticulum follows to expose its base.

5. If larger than 2 cm, resection of the diverticulum follows. Resection can be with a linear cutting and stapling device or with a scalpel, followed by closure of the mucosal defect with a running 4-0 absorbable suture.

6. Removal of the esophageal dilator is next and an NG tube replaces it. Saline is poured into the wound and a small amount of air instilled through the NG tube to test the staple line or suture closure for any leaks.

7. A closed suction drain is placed in the wound through a separate stab incision.

8. After removal of the retractors, closure of the platysma is done with interrupted stitches using a 4-0 absorbable suture.

9. Closure of the skin follows according to surgeon preference, and a nonabsorbable suture secures the drain to the skin. Dressings are applied.

Paraesophageal Hiatal Hernia Repair

The esophageal hiatus is the opening in the diaphragm through which the esophagus enters the abdominal cavity. Normally the phrenoesophageal membrane anchors the distal esophagus and the GEJ to the diaphragm. With a type I, or "sliding," hiatal hernia, widening of the esophageal hiatus and relaxation of the phrenoesophageal membrane allows the GEJ to migrate into the thoracic cavity, often resulting in the development of GERD. Types II, III, and IV hiatal hernias are "paraesophageal" hiatal hernias, which have a true hernia sac. In type II hernias, the GEJ remains fixed in its abdominal position while the fundus of the stomach migrates into the chest next to the esophagus through a localized defect in the phrenoesophageal membrane. As the defect enlarges, more of the stomach moves into the thoracic cavity, rotating around the fixed GEJ. Type II paraesophageal hernias progress to type III hernias as the hernia defect continues to enlarge and the GEJ itself begins to migrate into the chest along with the rest of the stomach. When other organs such as the colon, spleen, pancreas, and small bowel enter the hernia sac, the paraesophageal hiatal hernia becomes a type IV hiatal hernia.

Symptoms of hiatal hernia may include epigastric or chest pain, heartburn, chronic cough, regurgitation of undigested food, dysphagia, early satiety, vomiting, aspiration, and iron deficiency anemia. Possible complications of paraesophageal hiatal hernias include esophageal reflux gastritis; gastric ulceration; gastric volvulus with risk of strangulation, necrosis, and perforation; gastric outlet obstruction; hemorrhage; and pneumonia.

Surgical repair can be via laparotomy, thoracotomy, or laparoscopy. Some surgeons reserve an open approach for patients who have had previous abdominal surgeries and a thoracotomy approach when an open abdominal approach has failed (Smith, 2015).

Procedural Considerations

For an open abdominal approach, instrumentation and supplies include the following: a laparotomy set, long instruments, a self-retaining retractor, and a long ¼- to 1-inch Penrose drain. Thoracic instruments are available if an open thoracic approach is possible. The laparoscopic approach is the most common technique and is described in the next section.

Basic laparoscopy instruments and video equipment are needed. Additional laparoscopic instruments include a 30-degree laparoscope, two Babcock graspers, clip applier, ultrasonic shears, fan liver retractor, and a laparoscopic needle holder and knot pusher or other suturing device. Nonabsorbable suture is required to close the diaphragmatic defect and perform the fundoplication. Specialized long suture is needed for extracorporeal tying with a knot pusher, and standard 18-inch suture is used for intracorporeal tying techniques.

This procedure requires general anesthesia. Arrangement of Bougie or Maloney esophageal dilators in a variety of sizes (32F to 60F) is in ascending order on a nonsterile table for the anesthesia provider to insert during the procedure. Bougie and Maloney esophageal dilators do have expiration dates, so care is taken to track and replace ahead of anticipated use. Ensure water-soluble lubricant is on the nonsterile table to facilitate passage of the dilators. Stomach decompression with an NG tube may be needed as may insertion of a urinary bladder catheter. Patient placement is in supine or low modified lithotomy position, depending on surgeon preference. Arms may be padded and tucked at the patient's sides if necessary. The abdomen is prepped from nipple line to the pubic symphysis.

Operative Procedure: Laparoscopic Approach

1. Abdominal access and establishment of pneumoperitoneum depend on surgeon preference.

2. Retraction of the left lobe of the liver exposes the esophageal hiatus.

3. The surgeon gently reduces the hernia sac and stomach, opens the hernia sac, dissects it free, and excises it.

4. A Penrose drain passes behind and around the distal esophagus, enabling manipulation of the esophagus during dissection.

5. Using laparoscopic Babcock graspers or other nontraumatic graspers, the surgeon pulls the stomach and at least 2.5- to 3-cm of the distal esophagus into the abdominal cavity.

6. The anesthesia provider inserts the appropriately sized esophageal dilator (56F to 60F). Insertion of the dilators requires critical coordination with the surgeon to ensure the stomach's retraction at the appropriate angle to facilitate smooth passage and prevent perforation of the esophagus or stomach.

7. The surgeon approximates the crural fibers with interrupted size 0 nonabsorbable sutures to close the crura posterior to the esophagus. The esophageal dilator acts as a stent to ensure closure of the defect is not too tight around the esophagus. Note: If the hiatal defect is extremely large, use of a piece of biologic mesh to reinforce the repair is likely.

8. An antireflux procedure follows, using a 360-degree or a 270-degree posterior fundoplication. Fundoplication is described in the following section.

9. Removal of the esophageal dilator and Penrose drain is next.

10. The surgeon may suture the stomach to the anterior abdominal wall to keep it from sliding back into the chest.

11. Removal of the liver retractor, instruments, and trocars is under direct visualization, followed by removal of the laparoscope. After release of pneumoperitoneum, removal of the final access port follows.

12. Closure of all incisions ends the procedure.

Laparoscopic Nissen Fundoplication

Recurrent or persistent reflux of gastric contents, caused by defective or incompetent LES, into the esophagus or mouth constitutes GERD. In addition to an incompetent LES, patients simultaneously may have a hiatal hernia. In the presence of a hiatal hernia, the LES migrates into the thoracic cavity, altering the normal pressure gradient between the abdominal cavity and the thoracic cavity. The resulting increase in abdominal pressure can alter the LES's ability to adequately prevent reflux. If a hiatal hernia is present, it is repaired along with Nissen fundoplication.

Symptoms of GERD include heartburn, regurgitation of gastric contents, chest pain, and difficulty swallowing. Diagnostic studies include EGD, barium swallow, 24-hour esophageal pH monitoring, and esophageal manometry to rule out other causes of gastric reflux such as esophageal motility disorders. Complications of GERD include esophagitis, ulcers, stricture, aspiration pneumonia, BE, and esophageal cancer. Initial treatment for GERD includes dietary changes, weight loss, lifestyle changes, and medications such as antacids, histamine antagonists, and proton pump inhibitors. When these treatments fail to relieve symptoms, or if patients cannot tolerate or comply with prescribed medication regimens, consideration shifts to surgical intervention. A description of the most common surgical procedure performed for GERD, laparoscopic Nissen fundoplication, follows.

Procedural Considerations

Basic setup includes laparoscopy instruments and video equipment. Additional laparoscopic instruments include a 30-degree laparoscope, two Babcock graspers, clip appliers, ultrasonic shears, fan liver retractor, and a laparoscopic needle holder and knot pusher or other suturing device. Nonabsorbable suture is used to close the diaphragmatic defect and perform the fundoplication. Specialized long suture for extracorporeal tying with a knot pusher and standard 18-inch suture for intracorporeal tying techniques are available.

This procedure requires general anesthesia. Bougie or Maloney esophageal dilators in sizes 32F to 60F are arrayed in ascending order on a nonsterile table for the anesthesia provider to insert during the procedure. Ensure water-soluble lubricant is also on the table to facilitate passage of the dilators. If stomach decompression is needed, an NG tube is required. An indwelling urinary catheter is often required. Patient position is in supine or low modified lithotomy position per surgeon preference. The abdomen is prepped from nipple line to the pubic symphysis.

Operative Procedure

1. The surgeon gains abdominal access and pneumoperitoneum follows. The laparoscope is inserted in the umbilical access port.
2. Two trocars are placed under direct visualization to the right and left of the midline above the umbilicus and below the xiphoid process. These two ports are used for dissection and suturing. Additional ports are placed in the left and right lower abdomen.
3. A fan-shaped retractor, used to lift and retract the left lobe of the liver to expose the GEJ, inserts through the right lower port.
4. A Babcock grasper, inserted through the left lower port, is positioned on the fundus of the stomach, enabling the first assistant to provide lateral and downward traction.
5. The surgeon identifies the right and left crura and opens the retroesophageal space, creating a window through which the fundus will pass.
6. A Penrose drain is passed around the esophagus and its ends are secured together; the drain enables manipulation of the esophagus (Fig. 11.14).
7. The surgeon then mobilizes the cardia, fundus, and upper portion of the greater curve of the stomach. This may include ligation and division of the short gastric vessels between the fundus and

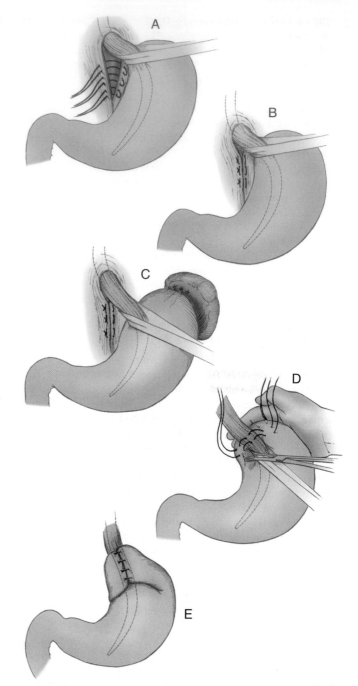

FIG. 11.14 Nissen fundoplication procedure begins with complete mobilization of the distal esophagus to create a posterior esophageal window for passage of the fundus of the stomach. (A) After the esophagus is mobilized, a Maloney or bougie esophageal dilator (40F to 48F) is passed orally into the stomach. (B) A Penrose drain around the esophagus retracts the esophagus laterally to expose the esophageal hiatus. (C) Heavy mattress sutures (0 braided nonabsorbable) are placed in the crura of the diaphragm to narrow the aperture of the hiatus but not so tight to constrict the esophagus, which is the purpose of stenting the esophagus with the Maloney dilator. (D) The fundus of the stomach is pulled through the posterior esophageal window and wrapped around the distal esophagus. (E) The 360-degree wrap is secured with nonabsorbable sutures to complete the procedure.

the spleen. Division of the short gastric vessels occurs either between clips or with ultrasonic shears.

8. The surgeon passes a Babcock from right to left behind the esophagus to grasp the fundus and pull it behind and around the esophagus, creating a 360-degree wrap. Noting any tension on the wrap, the surgeon may extend the stomach mobilization along the greater curve if needed.

9. Before closing the crura or suturing the wrap, the anesthesia provider inserts the appropriately sized esophageal dilator (56F to 60F). Insertion of the dilators requires critical coordination with the surgeon to ensure the stomach retracts at the appropriate angle to facilitate smooth passage and to prevent perforation of the esophagus or stomach.

10. The surgeon approximates the crural fibers with interrupted size 0 nonabsorbable sutures to close the hiatal defect, or crura, posterior to the esophagus. The esophageal dilator acts as a stent to ensure closure of the defect around the esophagus is not too tight.

11. If a hiatal hernia is present, it is repaired by approximating the crura posterior to the esophagus with nonabsorbable interrupted sutures.

12. With the esophageal dilator still in position, the gastric wrap is secured to itself with nonabsorbable interrupted sutures.

13. Removal of the esophageal dilator follows.

14. After release of pneumoperitoneum, the abdomen is inspected for hemostasis.

15. Instruments and ports are removed and incisions closed.

There are common variations of the Nissen fundoplication. The Rossetti-Nissen fundoplication also uses a 360-degree wrap; the procedure, however, does not entail ligation of the short gastric vessels. The Toupet fundoplication uses a partial 270-degree wrap, whereas the Dor fundoplication adopts a partial 180-degree fundal wrap anterior rather than posterior to the esophagus (DeHaan et al., 2016).

Surgery of the Stomach

Pyloroplasty

A pyloroplasty is a gastric drainage procedure that widens the pylorus to allow greater egress of stomach contents into the duodenum. The most commonly performed technique is the Heineke-Mikulicz pyloroplasty, described here (Shabino et al., 2016).

Procedural Considerations

Instrumentation and supplies include a laparotomy set and a self-retaining retractor. If closure of the pylorus is hand sewn, a long 3-0 absorbable suture on a tapered GI needle and several 3-0 silk sutures on the same type of needle are available. If the pyloric closure will be with a stapler, a linear stapler is available. The procedure requires general anesthesia with endotracheal intubation. Patient placement is supine. The abdomen is prepped. Unless gastric distention is present, there is no insertion of an NG tube. A urinary bladder catheter may not be needed because the time needed to complete this procedure is relatively short.

Operative Procedure

1. The surgeon makes a small midline laparotomy incision in the upper abdomen.

2. With the antrum of the stomach and duodenum exposed, the surgeon identifies the pylorus.

3. The surgeon next makes a full thickness 3-cm longitudinal incision between the stomach and the duodenum, parallel to the axis of the pylorus.

4. After placing sutures on the superior and inferior edges of the incision, a hemostat tags the sutures at the halfway point. A team member applies perpendicular traction to the sutures to facilitate horizontal closure of the incision.

5. The surgeon closes the pylorus incision in two layers, using a running 3-0 absorbable suture on the mucosa followed by interrupted seromuscular stitches with 3-0 nonabsorbable sutures.

6. Alternatively, the surgeon can use a linear stapler (TA 55) to close the pylorus.

7. Abdominal closure is in two layers and dressings are applied.

Repair of Perforated Peptic Ulcer

Repair of a perforated peptic ulcer may be performed via laparotomy or laparoscopically. The most common site of perforation is the anterior surface of the first portion of the duodenum (Shabino et al., 2016). The standard procedure for operative management of a perforated peptic ulcer is a Graham patch closure as described next (Shabino et al., 2016). Because the physical condition of the patient with a perforated peptic ulcer can deteriorate rapidly, the need for surgical intervention can become urgent.

Procedural Considerations

A standard laparotomy instrument set is needed for an open approach. The laparoscopic technique requires basic laparoscopy instruments and equipment including four trocars, laparoscopic needle holders, dissectors, graspers, and scissors. The technique for closure of the perforated ulcer is the same for laparotomy and laparoscopy with the exception of using intracorporeal suturing techniques for the laparoscopic approach.

Operative Procedure: Open Technique

1. The surgeon makes an upper midline laparotomy incision.

2. Exploration of the upper abdomen to locate the site of the perforation follows.

3. The surgeon performs a tissue biopsy of the ulcer to rule out malignancy.

4. To "close" the perforation, the surgeon places a small pedicle of omentum over the perforation and secures it to the stomach wall with interrupted 3-0 absorbable sutures; the omentum patch is called a Graham patch.

5. The abdomen is then irrigated with copious amounts of warm saline.

6. Closure of the abdomen is in two layers. Dressings are applied.

Gastrojejunostomy

A gastrojejunostomy establishes a permanent communication between the proximal jejunum and the stomach as a means to bypass an obstruction of the distal stomach or proximal duodenum resulting from an unresectable gastric tumor or severe pyloric stenosis (Shabino et al., 2016).

Procedural Considerations

Setup includes laparotomy and GI instrument sets. Circular and linear cutting stapling instruments are available in several sizes. Patient positioning is supine, after which induction of general anesthesia takes place. The anesthesia provider inserts an NG tube after intubation. Placement of an indwelling urinary catheter precedes abdominal skin prep.

Operative Procedure

1. The surgeon makes an upper midline abdominal incision, explores the abdomen, and directs placement of warm, moist packs and positioning of a self-retaining retractor.
2. After identifying the ligament of Treitz, the surgeon grasps a loop of proximal jejunum with a Babcock forceps and measures it (Fig. 11.15A). The surgeon determines the location of the anastomosis on the stomach and positions the jejunum against the stomach wall several centimeters posterior to the greater curve.
3. The surgeon next places nonabsorbable 2-0 or 3-0 traction sutures through the seromuscular layer at each corner of the intended anastomosis and then a row of interrupted 3-0 nonabsorbable sutures in the seromuscular layers of the jejunum and stomach to create the back wall of the anastomosis (see Fig. 11.15B).

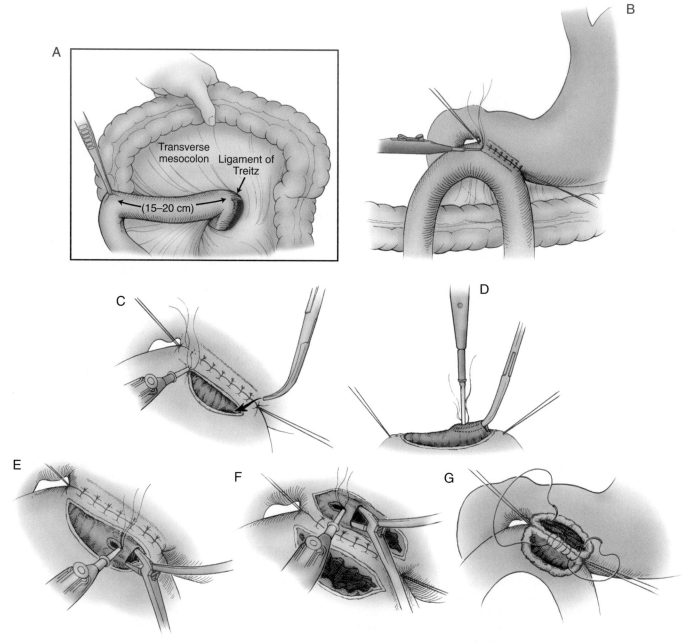

FIG. 11.15 Gastrojejunostomy. (A) Selection of a segment of jejunum that will be anastomosed to the stomach; the distance between the ligament of Treitz and the anastomosis should not be excessively long or under any tension. (B) Posterior row of interrupted sutures is placed between the gastric and jejunal serosae, and the sites of the gastric and jejunal stomas are scored with the electrosurgical pencil. (C) Jejunal stoma is created by dissecting through the serosa and muscularis with the electrosurgical pencil. An opening is made in the mucosa, and a right-angled clamp is inserted into the lumen. (D) Clamp is opened and elevated. (E) Electrosurgery is applied between the two jaws of the clamp. (F) Procedure is repeated to create the gastric stoma. (G) Full-thickness anastomosis is begun posteriorly.

4. The field is now draped for open anastomosis; bowel technique is initiated.
5. The surgeon opens the jejunum and stomach along the length of the back wall suture line (see Fig. 11.15C–F).
6. The surgeon closes the posterior and anterior mucosal layers with two 3-0 running absorbable sutures placed through the full thickness of the jejunum and stomach (see Fig. 11.15G).
7. The anastomosis is completed with a row of stitches placed in the anterior serosal layer, using interrupted 3-0 nonabsorbable sutures.
8. After removal of the traction sutures, team members discard contaminated instruments into a basin.
9. The wound is irrigated with warm saline
10. Sterile surgical team members don fresh gowns and gloves, switch to the clean closing instruments, close the abdominal wound in layers, and apply a dressing.

Partial Gastrectomy: Billroth I and Billroth II Reconstruction

Partial gastrectomy refers to resection of the distal stomach for treatment of malignant gastric tumors and complications of peptic ulcer disease such as bleeding, perforation, and obstruction. The extent of gastric resection depends on the type and location of the gastric lesion. The Billroth I procedure is a distal gastrectomy with GI reconstruction to connect the gastric remnant to the duodenum via an end-to-side or end-to-end anastomosis (gastroduodenostomy) (Fig. 11.16). Billroth I procedures entail resections at, or distal to, the antrum of the stomach. The Billroth II procedure is a distal gastrectomy combined with GI reconstruction to connect the gastric remnant to the jejunum via end-to-side or an end-to-end anastomosis (gastrojejunostomy). Billroth II procedures address gastric lesions extending proximal to the antrum.

Procedural Considerations

Setup requires basic laparotomy instruments, long instruments, and GI instruments. Also available are long, straight, and angled clip appliers and clips in assorted sizes; a self-retaining abdominal retractor; and a medium-length fine right-angle clamp. Linear cutting and end-to-end stapling instruments and cartridges are available in a variety of sizes. The patient is supine and general anesthesia induced. The anesthesia provider inserts an NG tube after endotracheal intubation. Insertion of an indwelling urinary catheter occurs before abdominal skin prep. Team members take appropriate precautions to prevent DVT, hypothermia, and pressure injuries.

Operative Procedure: Billroth I

1. The surgeon opens and explores the abdomen through an epigastric midline incision.
2. A self-retaining retractor is positioned to optimize exposure.
3. Mobilization of the greater curve of the stomach begins with sharp entry into the gastrocolic ligament, midway along the greater curve. Working toward the duodenum, the surgeon frees the stomach from the gastrocolic omentum by ligating and dividing the gastric branches of the gastroepiploic vessels close to the gastric wall. This occurs with clamps and ties, hemostatic clips, ultrasonic shears, or with a sealing bipolar instrument. For malignant tumors, the surgeon leaves the gastrocolic omentum attached to the stomach and resects closer to the transverse colon instead.
4. Mobilization of the greater curve continues, and clamping and division of the right gastroepiploic vessels follow.

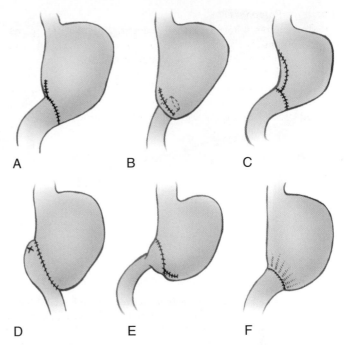

FIG. 11.16 Diagrams illustrating resections of stomach with anastomosis of stomach and duodenum (gastroduodenal anastomosis). All are modifications of the Billroth I technique, in which the stomach is moved to the duodenum. (A) Billroth I: after pylorus is removed, lesser curvature is partially closed and duodenum is sutured to the open end of stomach at its lower margin. (B) Kocher: distal end of stomach is closed, and duodenum is transferred up to the posterior margin of closed stomach. (C) Schoemaker: lesser curvature of stomach is sutured closed and brought down to the same size as the duodenum, and end-to-end anastomosis is done. (D) von Haberer-Finney: side of duodenum is transferred up to the end of stomach so that the entire end of the stomach is open for direct anastomosis. (E) Horsley: lesser curvature end of the stomach is used to suture to the duodenum and closes greater curvature end. (F) von Haberer: modification of operation shown in D. Stomach is narrowed or puckered so that it fits the end of the duodenum. Modification of this is done by some surgeons as follows: duodenum is split longitudinally and its ends are flared open so that the opening is large enough to fit the open end of the stomach.

5. The surgeon mobilizes the first and second portions of the duodenum to facilitate the gastroduodenostomy.
6. The surgeon next mobilizes the lesser curve of the stomach and divides and ligates the right gastric vessels between clamps, preserving the left gastric artery if possible.
7. The operative field undergoes preparation for open anastomosis (bowel technique).
8. The distal margin of the gastric resection includes the proximal duodenum. Its division is either between intestinal clamps or with a linear stapler. The surgeon divides the proximal stomach with a large GI stapling device.
9. The gastrectomy is complete. The staple line of the gastric remnant may be reinforced with a running 3-0 silk suture.
10. Next, the surgeon positions the duodenum adjacent to the gastric remnant at the planned anastomosis site and secures it at the corners with nonabsorbable 3-0 traction sutures placed through the serosa at each corner. A hemostat tags these sutures.
11. The surgeon places a row of interrupted 3-0 nonabsorbable sutures in the seromuscular layer of the duodenum and the stomach to create the back wall of the anastomosis.

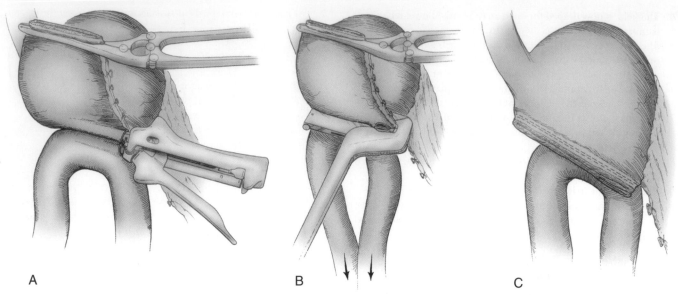

FIG. 11.17 Subtotal gastrectomy with stapled Billroth II anastomosis. (A) Distal stomach has been dissected free and resected just distal to the pylorus. A proximal limb of jejunum is transferred up to anastomose to the posterior wall of the stomach with a linear stapling instrument that transects between two parallel staple lines. (B) Stomach is elevated, and a 90-degree mechanical stapling device is placed across the distal stomach. (C) Completed subtotal gastrectomy with stapled antecolic gastrojejunostomy.

12. The surgeon makes matching enterotomies in the duodenum and stomach equidistant from the back wall suture line.

13. Anastomosis of the posterior and anterior mucosal layers of the enterotomies is with two 3-0 running absorbable sutures placed through the full thickness of the duodenum and stomach walls.

14. Closure of the front wall of the anastomosis is with a row of interrupted 3-0 nonabsorbable sutures placed in the seromuscular layer. The anastomosis is complete.

15. After removal of traction sutures, team members discard contaminated instruments into a basin.

16. Sterile surgical team members don fresh gowns and gloves, switch to clean closing instruments, close the abdominal wound in layers, and apply a dressing.

Operative Procedure: Billroth II

Instruments and supplies for Billroth II (gastrojejunostomy) (Fig. 11.17) are the same as described for Billroth I.

1. The surgeon opens and explores the abdomen through an epigastric midline incision.

2. A self-retaining retractor is positioned to optimize exposure.

3. Mobilization of the greater curve begins with sharp entry into the gastrocolic ligament, midway along the greater curve. Working toward the duodenum, the surgeon frees the stomach from the gastrocolic omentum by ligating and dividing the gastric branches of the gastroepiploic vessels close to the gastric wall, leaving the gastrocolic omentum. For malignant tumors, resection of the gastrocolic omentum follows.

4. Mobilization of the greater curve continues, after which clamping and division of the right gastroepiploic vessels occur.

5. The surgeon mobilizes the lesser curve of the stomach and divides the right gastric vessels between clamps. The vessels are ligated. The left gastric artery is preserved if possible.

6. Division of the duodenum just distal to the pylorus is with a GI linear stapling device.

7. The surgeon fires a large GI stapler across the stomach and directs removal of the gastric specimen. A bioabsorbable buttressing material can reinforce the staple line.

8. The surgeon mobilizes a loop of proximal jejunum, pulls it up in front of the colon, and positions it adjacent to the posterior wall of the remaining stomach.

9. Placement of a row of interrupted 3-0 nonabsorbable sutures in the seromuscular layer of the jejunum and the stomach creates the back wall of the anastomosis.

10. Creation of matching enterotomies in the jejunum and stomach equidistant from the back wall suture line follows.

11. The surgeon anastomoses the posterior and anterior mucosal layers of the enterotomies with two 3-0 running absorbable sutures placed through the full thickness of the duodenum and stomach walls.

12. Closure of the front wall of the anastomosis is with a row of interrupted 3-0 nonabsorbable sutures placed in the seromuscular layer. The anastomosis is complete.

Distal gastrectomy with laparoscopic Billroth I or II reconstruction is also possible. Standard laparoscopic instruments, equipment, and supplies are needed. Laparoscopic hemostatic energy-generating devices such as a bipolar vessel-sealing instrument or ultrasonic shears are available along with a wide variety of laparoscopic GI linear and circular stapling instruments. A subtotal gastrectomy, a more extensive gastric resection, removes at least four-fifths of the stomach (Smith, 2015).

Total Gastrectomy

As the name implies, total gastrectomy entails complete stomach resection. Reestablishment of GI continuity is with a Roux-en-Y anastomosis between the jejunum and esophagus (esophagojejunostomy) (Fig. 11.18). A Roux-en-Y anastomosis is a Y-shaped anastomosis that includes a Roux, or alimentary, limb and a "Y" limb.

Procedural Considerations

Basic laparotomy instruments, long instruments, and GI instruments are required. Also needed are straight and angled clip appliers and clips in assorted sizes, a self-retaining abdominal retractor, and a medium-length fine right-angle clamp. Linear cutting and end-to-end stapling instruments and cartridges are available. The patient is positioned supine and general anesthesia induced. The anesthesia provider inserts an NG tube after endotracheal intubation. After insertion of an indwelling urinary catheter, abdominal skin prep follows. Initiate precautions to prevent DVT, hypothermia, and pressure injuries according to hospital protocol.

Operative Procedure

1. The surgeon opens and explores the abdomen via a midline or bilateral subcostal incision. A self-retaining retractor is positioned to optimize exposure.

2. For malignant tumors, the gastrocolic omentum along the greater curve undergoes resection from the transverse colon and removal with the stomach.

3. Clamping and division of the right and left gastroepiploic vessels follow.

4. Mobilization of the fundus requires division of the short gastric vessels located between the spleen and fundus. Care is taken not to tear the splenic capsule with excessive retraction.

5. After mobilization of the lesser curve of the stomach, the left and right gastric vessels are individually clamped, divided, and ligated.

6. Using a GI linear stapler distal to the pylorus, the surgeon divides the first portion of the duodenum. Reinforcement of the staple line on the duodenal stump may be necessary with interrupted or running 3-0 absorbable sutures to prevent leakage or to control bleeding on the staple line.

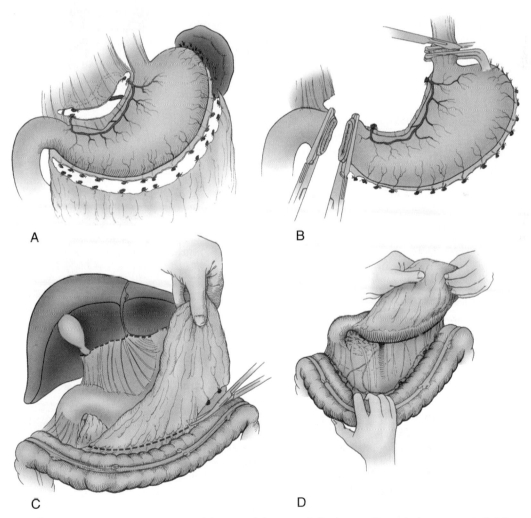

A   B

C   D

FIG. 11.18 Total gastrectomy. (A) Mobilization of the stomach for benign disease is demonstrated. Serial division of the vessels in the gastrocolic ligament and gastrohepatic ligament is performed to free the greater and lesser omentum. The short gastric vessels connecting the stomach to the spleen are divided, and the spleen is preserved. (B) Duodenum is divided distally to the pylorus, and the proximal line of division is at the distal intra-abdominal esophagus. (C) For malignancies the line of resection includes both the lesser and the greater omentum. (D) Retrogastric area is inspected for tumor involvement. The spleen and tail of the pancreas may be included in the resection.

Continued

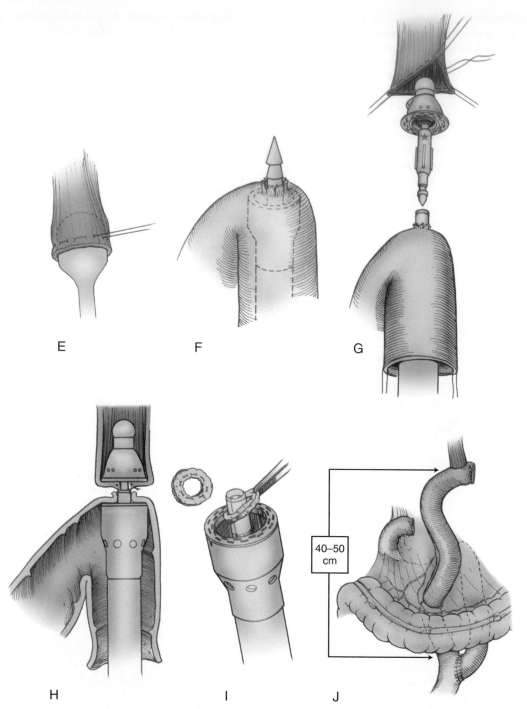

E   F   G

40–50 cm

H   I   J

FIG. 11.18, cont'd (E) Sizer is inserted into the lumen of the distal esophagus. (F) EEA or intraluminal anastomosis is inserted into the lumen of the jejunum to facilitate esophagojejunostomy. (G) Anvil is inserted into the distal esophagus in which purse-string sutures will be snugged around the protruding arm of the anvil. (H) Distal esophagus and the jejunum are united by the mechanism of the stapling device, and the intraluminal anastomosis will be performed. (I) "Donuts," distal esophagus, and jejunal tissues are examined for integrity and completeness. (J) Esophagojejunostomy completed.

7. The left lobe of the liver undergoes mobilization and retraction cephalad to expose the esophageal hiatus.
8. Mobilization and transection of the distal esophagus is with a GI linear stapling device.
9. Using a GI stapler the surgeon divides the jejunum about 40 cm from the ligament of Treitz and creates a Roux limb of approximately 50 cm to be brought up to the esophageal stump through a hole created in the mesentery of the colon. This is called a retrocolic technique.
10. The surgeon creates a side-to-side jejunojejunostomy between the proximal jejunum and a segment distal to the Roux loop to allow for biliary and pancreatic drainage.
11. Using an end-to-end circular stapling device, the surgeon creates the esophagojejunostomy.

12. The anvil of the stapler either passes down the esophagus through the mouth, or the surgeon makes an enterotomy to position the anvil directly in the esophagus (see Fig. 11.18G).
13. The stapler passes through an enterotomy made at the staple line of the Roux limb.
14. Once the anvil and the stapler join together (see Fig. 11.18H), the surgeon fires the stapler, achieving anastomosis between the esophagus and the Roux limb of the jejunum. The surgical team ensures that the remaining anvil and stapler pieces are all accounted for in the surgical counts. Closure of the enterotomies is with a small linear stapling device. After inspection of the donuts (see Fig. 11.18I), the anastomosis is complete (see Fig. 11.18J).
15. Using a flexible gastroscope, the surgeon inspects the anastomosis.
16. After irrigation of the abdomen with warm saline, closure in layers follows as previously described, and a dressing is applied.

Bariatric Surgery

Bariatric surgery, also termed "weight loss" or "weight reduction" surgery, is surgical treatment of obesity. According to the National Center for Health Statistics, obesity is a disease affecting more than 36.5% of US adults with highest prevalence in females and middle-aged people (Ogden et al., 2015). In 2013, 468,609 bariatric procedures were performed worldwide (Segal-Lieberman et al., 2016). Obesity is defined by BMI, which is an estimate of total body fat using a height-to-weight ratio. BMI does not fully represent all ethnic groups and because it does not directly measure body fat, it can be skewed by other factors (Ogden et al., 2015) (see Box 11.1).

Obese patients typically present with serious coexisting health conditions, such as diabetes, cardiopulmonary disease, obstructive sleep apnea (OSA), gallstone disease, hypertension, hyperlipidemia, and joint disease. Previous eligibility criteria for patients seeking bariatric surgery included a BMI of 40 kg/m² or greater without coexisting medical problems or those with a BMI of 35 kg/m² or greater with comorbidities such as type 2 diabetes (T2D), hypertension, hyperlipidemia, or OSA. In recent guidelines, patients with diabetes or metabolic syndrome and a BMI of 30 to 34.9 kg/m² may be offered a bariatric procedure (Segal-Lieberman et al., 2016). This underscores evidence that remission of diabetes is durable in a significant proportion of bariatric surgery patients, prompting emergence of the terminology "metabolic surgery" to treat T2D as well as to reduce cardiometabolic risk factors in obese patients (Fencl et al., 2015; Sudan et al., 2015). Patients must demonstrate psychologic stability and motivation to commit to postsurgical lifestyle changes. Formal mental health evaluations are necessary in patients who actively abuse alcohol or recreational drugs, or who have poorly controlled psychiatric disease; bariatric surgery may be contraindicated for these patients (Blackburn et al., 2016; Dawes et al., 2016).

There are three categories of bariatric procedures: restrictive (such as laparoscopic adjustable gastric banding [LAGB], described next, and laparoscopic sleeve gastrectomy [not described]), malabsorptive, or a combination of both. *Restrictive* procedures reduce the size of the stomach. When the patient eats, food is digested and absorbed normally, but the smaller capacity of the stomach gives the feeling of fullness, and the patient eats less. In *malabsorptive* procedures, surgery reduces the absorptive capacity of the small intestine with a bypass of a segment or segments of the proximal small bowel.

Adjustable Gastric Band

Adjustable gastric banding is a restrictive procedure using a silicone strip and adjustable elastic ring called an adjustable gastric band. The band is laparoscopically placed around the top of the stomach. The surgeon sutures a fold of stomach around the band to secure

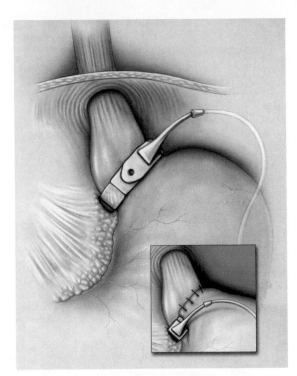

FIG. 11.19 Proper position of the Lap-Band. The silicone band around the fundus of the stomach creates a small gastric pouch. The inner lining of the band contains an inflatable balloon connected to a subcutaneous port on the patient's abdomen (not shown). The band can inflate or deflate to adjust stomach size as needed.

it in place (Fig. 11.19). The band has a port, which is inflated with saline 4 weeks postoperatively. The constriction created by the inflated band restricts the amount of ingested food that can enter the stomach, preventing overeating. This procedure is adjustable and reversible and has been shown to improve long-term health, including reducing risks of cardiovascular disease and T2D (Cobourn et al., 2013).

Laparoscopic Roux-en-Y Gastric Bypass

Roux-en-Y gastric bypass (RYGB) is a largely restrictive and mildly malabsorptive procedure that reroutes the passage of ingested food and fluid from a small pouch created with surgical staples or sutures in the proximal stomach to a segment of the proximal jejunum. Laparoscopic RYGB is relatively common in the United States.

Procedural Considerations

All patients undergoing bariatric surgery need special consideration because they usually have associated serious comorbidities that place them at heightened risk during the procedure. A special OR bed that can accommodate patients who weigh more than 350 pounds (159 kg) is required. In addition to laparoscopic instrumentation and accessory supplies, extra-large blood pressure cuffs and extra-long trocars are necessary. Positioning requires additional padded safety restraints, pressure-reduction devices to reduce the risk of pressure injury, and properly fitting IPCDs. The perioperative nurse anticipates the potential for anesthesia assistance during intubation and airway management.

Operative Procedure

1. This surgery requires placement of five trocars above the umbilicus (Fig. 11.20): two on the midline, two in the left upper quadrant,

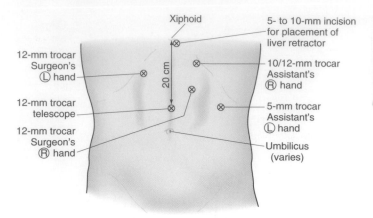

FIG. 11.20 Trocar configuration for laparoscopic Roux-en-Y gastric bypass.

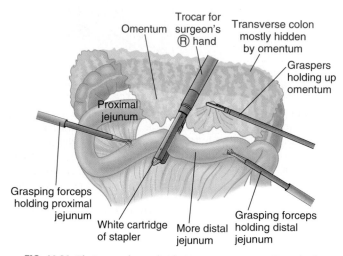

FIG. 11.21 Placing stapler to divide jejunum to create a Roux limb.

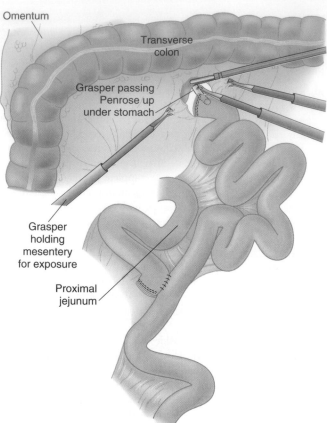

FIG. 11.22 Passing the Roux limb into a retrocolic and retrogastric position.

and one in the right upper quadrant (RUQ). The surgeon also makes an incision for the liver retractor.

2. The surgeon mobilizes the omentum and identifies the ligament of Treitz.
3. Using a vascular stapler the surgeon divides the jejunum 40 cm distal to the ligament of Treitz (Fig. 11.21).
4. While the proximal jejunum is left to lie in the patient's right side, the surgeon lifts the Roux limb superiorly and passes it through the transverse colon mesentery (Fig. 11.22).
5. With several loads of a linear stapler, the surgeon creates a gastric pouch.
6. The surgeon next anastomoses the Roux limb to the proximal gastric pouch. Methylene blue is instilled to check for leaks. The surgeon may perform the gastrojejunostomy with either traditional suturing techniques or a circular EEA stapler.
7. The surgeon closes any mesenteric defects, inspects the abdomen, and directs closure of the port sites.

With RYGB, avoidance of a critical segment of the calorie- and nutrition-absorbing mucosal surface occurs. The gastric pouch is generally less than 30 mL in volume. This procedure results in considerable weight loss for the patient. Serious complications, however, can arise, including hemorrhage, anastomotic leaks, PE, pneumonia, infection, small bowel obstructions or stenosis, and

incisional hernia (Table 11.3). Nutritional deficits, nausea, flatus, diarrhea, and dumping syndrome are other common complications.

Biliopancreatic diversion (BPD) (Fig. 11.23) and duodenal switch (Fig. 11.24) are largely malabsorptive and mildly restrictive procedures. In both, the Roux limb and the biliopancreatic limb are longer, leaving a shortened common channel for digestion and absorption of proteins, fats, and carbohydrates. These procedures present serious risks of complications, nutritional deficiencies, liver abnormalities, anemia, and lactose intolerance.

Surgery of the Small Bowel

Meckel Diverticulectomy

Meckel diverticulum forms when the vitelline duct fails to close completely by birth. The diverticulum includes all layers of the intestinal wall, and ileal, gastric, or pancreatic mucosa can line it. Meckel diverticulum is uncommon and in most cases does not cause symptoms. The most common complication is GI bleeding, followed by intussusception, obstruction, strangulation, diverticulitis, and volvulus (Steele and McGregor, 2016).

Procedural Considerations

Laparotomy and GI sets are required. Linear stapling devices are available. Patient positioning is supine, and general anesthesia is administered. The anesthesia provider may insert an NG tube after intubation. Insertion of an indwelling urinary catheter precedes abdominal skin prep.

TABLE 11.3
Complications of Bariatric Surgery

Procedure	Surgery-Related Complications
Adjustable gastric band	• Band erosion into the stomach • Slippage with gastric prolapse • Port infection • Tubing disconnection • Pouch dilation • Stomal obstruction • Gastric perforation • Delayed gastric emptying • Bleeding • Incisional hernia • Esophageal dilatation; esophagitis • Hiatal hernia
Vertical banded gastroplasty	• Staple line disruption • Anastomotic stenosis and obstruction • Erosion of mesh band • Gastroesophageal reflux • Vomiting
Sleeve gastrectomy	• Anastomotic leak • Gastric leaks • Stenosis of gastric outlet • Bleeding from mobilization of the greater curve of the stomach • Bleeding from short gastric vessels • Bleeding from staple line • Bleeding from splenic injury
Roux-en-Y gastric bypass	• Gastric remnant distention • Stricture of the gastrojejunal anastomosis • Marginal ulcers • Gallstones • Internal hernia in the mesentery • Ventral hernia • Dumping syndrome • Vitamin deficiency • Renal failure • Postoperative hypoglycemia
Biliopancreatic diversion with duodenal switch	• Anastomotic leak • Loose stools/diarrhea/frequent flatus • Protein calorie malnutrition • Anemia • Metabolic bone disease • Fat-soluble vitamin deficiency; vitamin B$_{12}$ deficiency
Non–procedure-specific complications	• DVT • PE • Cardiovascular complications • Pulmonary complications • Addiction transfer (drugs, alcohol) • Depression; suicide • Failure to lose weight or weight regain

DVT, Deep vein thrombosis; *PE,* pulmonary embolism.
Modified from Ellsmere JC: Late complications of bariatric surgical operations. In Jones D, editor: *UpToDate,* Waltham, MA, UpToDate, 2016; Puplampu T, Simpson S: Nursing care of the bariatric surgery patient. In Agrawal S, editor: *Obesity, bariatric and metabolic surgery,* ed 1, Switzerland, 2015, Springer International Publishing.

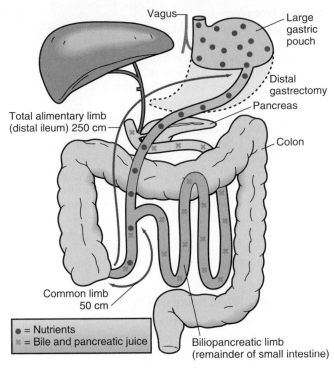

FIG. 11.23 Configuration of the biliopancreatic diversion, which is transection of the stomach with anastomosis of the duodenum to the distal ileum. In this malabsorptive procedure, the pancreatic enzymes and bile enter near the ileum, allowing nutrients to pass from the stomach to the distal ileum without being digested. Weight loss occurs because of the partial gastrectomy, which restricts intake, and because of the shortened alimentary canal, which causes malabsorption.

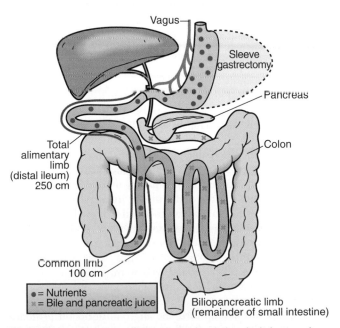

FIG. 11.24 Configuration of the duodenal switch, which leaves a larger portion of the stomach intact, including the pyloric valve. This alleviates dumping syndrome.

Operative Procedure

1. The surgeon opens the abdomen through a low midline or right lower quadrant incision and identifies the diverticulum.
2. If the diverticulum is long and narrow with a narrow base, it is double-clamped and divided at its base.
3. Closure of the bowel beneath the clamp is with full-thickness 3-0 absorbable sutures.
4. A row of inverting sutures using 3-0 or 4-0 nonabsorbable suture is used to close the outer layer.
5. Alternatively, a linear GI stapler may be used to resect the diverticulum.

If the base is broad, the surgeon may isolate the loop of bowel containing the diverticulum from the mesentery and perform a limited small bowel resection. Completion of an anastomosis of the divided ends is with an inner continuous layer of 3-0 synthetic absorbable sutures and an interrupted outer layer of 4-0 nonabsorbable sutures. Closure of the abdominal wound follows. This procedure can also be performed laparoscopically using an endoscopic GI linear stapling device.

Appendectomy (Open Approach)

Appendectomy is severance and removal of the appendix from its attachment to the cecum through a right lower quadrant, muscle-splitting incision (McBurney). This procedure removes an acutely inflamed appendix.

Procedural Considerations

Setup requires a basic laparotomy instrument set. Patient positioning is supine, and general anesthesia is administered. Culture tubes and specimen labels are available.

Operative Procedure

1. The surgeon usually makes a right lower quadrant muscle-splitting (McBurney) incision. Retraction of muscles with Richardson or Parker retractors exposes the peritoneum.
2. The peritoneum is lifted and entered. Peritoneal fluid is collected with aerobic and anaerobic culture swabs. Extension of the incision is then done with Metzenbaum scissors.
3. The distal appendix is grasped with Babcock forceps and gently lifted, exposing the mesoappendix containing the appendiceal artery.
4. The mesoappendix is dissected from the appendix and the artery ligated with a 2-0 nonabsorbable suture.
5. The appendix is elevated and a purse-string stitch placed in the cecum around the base of the appendix using an absorbable 2-0 suture.
6. A 3-0 synthetic absorbable suture ligature is tied around the base of the appendix, distal to the purse-string stitch.
7. Bowel technique commences by placing protective gauze sponges over the cecum to protect the wound from spillage. A basin is brought to the field for the specimen and the bowel-contaminated instruments.
8. The appendix is amputated with a scalpel. Soiled instruments are discarded into the basin.
9. After irrigation of the wound with warm saline, the wound is closed in layers with clean instrumentation and new surgical gowns and gloves.

If the appendix has ruptured, the surgeon irrigates the peritoneal cavity with copious warm fluids and inserts a closed suction drain in the appendiceal bed. Deeper layers of the site are closed; the subcutaneous tissue and skin may remain open. The wound is packed with moist fine-mesh gauze for healing by secondary intention. This healing method may apply in any case in which bowel contamination or abscess formation is present. It allows clean healing and protects against subcutaneous wound infection.

Appendectomy (Laparoscopic)

The laparoscopic approach to appendectomy is appropriate for uncomplicated appendicitis. In the presence of perforation, conversion to an open procedure will likely be necessary.

Procedural Considerations

Setup requires standard laparoscopic instrumentation, equipment, and supplies. The procedure requires placement of three trocars. The patient is positioned supine and general anesthesia induced. Insertion of an indwelling urinary catheter precedes abdominal skin prep.

Operative Procedure

1. Pneumoperitoneum is established. A 5-mm trocar is placed at the umbilicus for insertion of the laparoscope (if a 5-mm laparoscope is not available, use of a larger trocar is an alternative). A 5-mm (or larger) trocar placed in the RUQ serves as the working port. Another 5-mm trocar placed in the midline suprapubic site serves as the traction trocar.
2. A 5-mm laparoscopic Babcock forceps is inserted into the RUQ trocar for grasping and retracting the cecum toward the liver.
3. The surgeon grasps the appendix at its tip with a grasping forceps inserted through the suprapubic trocar and holds it in an upward position.
4. After removal of the Babcock forceps, insertion of a dissecting instrument through the RUQ trocar enables creation of a mesenteric window in the mesoappendix (the peritoneal fold connecting the appendix to the ileum).
5. Dissection, performed in proximity to the appendix, begins directly under the base and progresses 1 to 2 cm in length.
6. Depending on surgeon preference, the appendix may be transected in one of several ways: (1) with an endoscopic linear stapling instrument, (2) with a ligating loop instrument, or (3) with a suturing instrument.
7. In the endoscopic stapling technique, grasping forceps rotate the tip of the appendix so that the surgeon can snug the stapling device to the base of the appendix and close it. The stapling instrument is fired and withdrawn; inspection of the staple line follows. The remainder of the mesoappendix is dissected, hemostasis achieved, and the appendix removed through the RUQ port.
8. It is possible to use a specimen pouch to extract the appendix.
9. The abdomen is irrigated using a suction and irrigation device and pneumoperitoneum released.
10. Closure of trocar sites is with suture; a dressing or skin-bonding sealer is applied.

Resection of the Small Intestine

Small bowel resection removes a segment of diseased, obstructed, or necrotic small intestine. When possible, connecting the distal and proximal segments of the remaining small bowel restores continuity.

Procedural Considerations

Setup requires laparotomy and GI sets. GI linear stapling instruments should be available in a variety of sizes. Patient positioning is supine with general anesthesia. The anesthesia provider may insert an NG tube after intubation. Insertion of an indwelling urinary catheter precedes abdominal skin prep. If the planned procedure is laparoscopic, basic laparoscopic equipment, instrumentation, and stapling devices are available.

Operative Procedure

1. The surgeon incises the abdominal wall through a midline incision and explores the peritoneal cavity. Wound edges require protection with warm, moistened laparotomy pads or a wound protector. A wound protector keeps the wound edges moist and has shown a positive correlation with reducing surgical site infections (Mihaljevic et al., 2015b). Positioning of a self-retaining abdominal retractor optimizes exposure.
2. The surgeon identifies the diseased segment of small intestine.
3. Small mesenteric windows, created at the proximal and distal ends of the diseased small bowel segment, accommodate the arms of the linear staplers.
4. The surgeon positions the staplers across the small bowel and fires them.
5. Using clamps and suture ties with either a bipolar sealing device or ultrasonic shears, the surgeon mobilizes the transected small bowel from its mesentery.
6. Using a two-layer suturing technique or GI linear staplers, the surgeon reestablishes continuity of the GI tract with a functional end-to-end, end-to-side, or side-to-side anastomosis.

End Ileostomy

An end ileostomy entails bringing a transected portion of the ileum through the abdominal wall to divert small bowel content away from the GI tract distal to the ileostomy. An ileostomy can be temporary or permanent.

Procedural Considerations

Laparotomy and GI sets along with linear stapling instruments are required. Patient positioning is supine with general anesthesia. The anesthesia provider may insert an NG tube after intubation. Insertion of an indwelling urinary catheter precedes abdominal skin prep. An ostomy appliance is available for the stoma.

Operative Procedure

1. Through a midline incision the surgeon explores the peritoneal cavity and determines the pathologic condition.
2. Mobilization and resection of the ileum follow, as described in a small bowel resection.
3. The skin is incised at the predetermined site of the ileostomy.
4. Next the surgeon makes a cruciate (cross-shaped) incision in the fascia and peritoneum to accommodate two fingers.
5. The proximal end of the ileum is grasped with a Babcock clamp.
6. The surgeon pulls the ileum through the abdominal wall to the skin, ensuring that it does not stretch or twist, and that there is no compromise of its blood supply.
7. The ileum is secured to the parietal peritoneum on the abdominal wall with interrupted 3-0 nonabsorbable sutures.
8. Closure of the abdomen follows.
9. The stoma is sutured to the skin with everted absorbable sutures to protect the serosal surface against drainage from the stoma.
10. An ostomy appliance, cut to fit the diameter of the ileostomy, is placed over the stoma to collect small bowel contents.

An alternative to an end ileostomy is the Kock pouch. This involves creation of an ileal pouch with a nipple valve connected to a stoma on the skin. When working properly the stoma and pouch are continent and do not continually drain stool. A catheter, inserted into the stoma every 4 to 6 hours, evacuates contents, eliminating the need for an external appliance (Erickson et al., 2016).

Intestinal Transplantation

Intestinal failure occurs when there is an inadequate length of healthy small bowel necessary to absorb enough fluids, electrolytes, and other essential nutrients from ingested food to sustain life without the assistance of long-term use of TPN (O'Keefe, 2015). One cause of intestinal failure is short bowel syndrome (SBS). SBS arises as a result of multiple or extensive bowel resections to treat complications of Crohn disease, mesenteric infarction, trauma, or malignancies. Complications of long-term TPN include thrombosis of TPN access sites, catheter-related sepsis, and liver failure (Lacaille et al., 2015). Intestinal transplantation (ITx) is reserved to treat patients with intestinal failure who otherwise have failed medical management and are no longer candidates for TPN.

Procedural Considerations

ITx requires a specialized team with coordination between the organ procurement team and the recipient team to minimize the cold ischemia time of the donor organ. Instruments include a laparotomy set, vascular instruments, and any other transplant-related equipment necessary to prepare the graft. Patient positioning is supine with general endotracheal anesthesia. If central venous access is not attainable, the anesthesia provider may request transesophageal Doppler ultrasound to monitor cardiac status of the patient. Insertion of an NG tube and urinary catheter follows. Possible performance of a feeding jejunostomy or gastrostomy requires that those additional supplies are available (Lacaille et al., 2015).

Operative Procedure

1. The transplant surgeon completes the final visual inspection and assessment of the donor organ. The location of the recipient's incision depends on previous surgical incisions and the location of present or planned stomas.
2. The surgeon dissects the recipient inflow and outflow vessels.
3. An anastomosis is created from the superior mesenteric artery of the donor organ to the recipient's infrarenal aorta.
4. Connecting the donor superior mesenteric vein to the recipient portal vein or vena cava establishes venous drainage of the donor organ.
5. Reperfusion begins with release of venous flow as the clamps open.
6. Release of the arterial clamp follows.
7. Continuity of the intestine returns after establishing vascular supply. Proximal anastomosis joins the donor jejunum to the recipient stomach, duodenum, or proximal jejunum. A side-to-side anastomosis joins the distal ileum with the remaining colon.
8. The surgeon brings up the distal end of the graft as an end or loop ileostomy, which is usable for later endoscopic evaluation and intestinal biopsies.
9. The surgeon inspects the intact intestine, verifies hemostasis, and closes the abdomen.

Surgery of the Colon

Colostomy

Reestablishing continuity of the GI tract after colon resection sometimes is neither recommended nor feasible. Creation of a colostomy requires bringing the proximal end of the divided colon (or a loop of colon) through the anterior abdominal wall and suturing it to the skin to divert the fecal stream. A temporary colostomy, or fecal diversion, may be necessary to allow an abdominal infection to resolve, or to allow a distal anastomosis to heal. A permanent colostomy may be needed after colon resection when the remaining colon is of insufficient length to allow safe reconnection. Preoperative collaboration with a WOCN helps prepare patient transition after intraoperative determination of colostomy permanence (Salvadalena et al., 2015).

Procedural Considerations

Setup requires laparotomy instruments and GI instruments. The surgeon may use a GI linear stapler to transect the colon. Several 3-0 absorbable sutures on a controlled-release tapered GI needle are commonly used to sew the colostomy to the skin. A colostomy appliance covers the stoma. If a loop colostomy is planned, additional items may include a colostomy rod, red rubber tubing, or a loop ostomy bridge. Patient positioning is supine with general anesthesia. The anesthesia provider may insert an NG tube after intubation. Insertion of an indwelling urinary catheter precedes abdominal skin prep.

End Colostomy

Operative Procedure

1. The surgeon opens the abdomen, protects the wound edges, retracts the colon, and divides or resects it (Fig. 11.25).
2. Mobilization of the proximal end of the colon ensures that it will reach the anterior abdominal wall without excess tension.
3. A Kocher clamp is placed on the skin at the ostomy site (marked preoperatively). Lifting the Kocher puts traction on the skin while the surgeon uses a knife to cut the lifted skin.
4. Using electrosurgical dissection, the circular incision is carried down to the fascia. A cruciate incision is made in the fascia to accommodate the diameter of the colon. Army Navy retractors are placed.
5. A Babcock is inserted into the abdomen, and the surgeon grasps and pulls the colon through the skin.
6. The surgeon secures the colon internally to the peritoneum of the anterior abdominal wall to prevent it from slipping back into the abdomen during abdominal closure and to prevent future formation of a hernia around the stoma. A handheld retractor is used to lift the abdominal wall slightly during placement of these sutures.
7. After closure of the abdomen, the incision undergoes either dressing with sterile gauze or covering with a sterile towel while the colostomy matures.
8. To mature the colostomy, the surgeon sutures the colon to the skin at evenly spaced intervals around the circumference of the stoma. The colostomy appliance is cut to fit the diameter of the stoma and then secured to the skin. The skin around the stoma should be clean and dry before application of the ostomy appliance.

Loop Colostomy: First Stage. For a temporary loop colostomy, instead of transecting the bowel, the surgeon makes a small opening in the mesentery near the bowel with curved hemostats and Metzenbaum scissors. A Penrose drain is passed around the colon, and a Péan holds the two ends together. Mobilization of the loop of colon is as described for end colostomy. The surgeon uses the Penrose drain to pull the loop of colon through the abdominal wall (Fig. 11.26). Closure of the abdominal incision is next. A loop ostomy bridge or a 14F red rubber catheter is used to support and retain the loop of colon in position on the abdominal wall. The loop of intestine is left intact and a petrolatum gauze dressing applied.

Loop Colostomy: Second Stage. After 48 hours the surgeon opens 75% to 80% of the colon loop with the tip of an electrosurgical pencil. Absorbable sutures may secure the colostomy to the skin if the procedure is performed in the OR. If sutures are not used the surgeon can perform this procedure in the patient's room or in a treatment room. Application of an ostomy appliance completes the second stage of loop colostomy.

Closure of a Colostomy

Closure of a colostomy reestablishes GI continuity. Closure of the fascial defect at the ostomy site is with a heavy absorbable suture. The subcutaneous fat and skin may be left open to heal by secondary intention or closure may follow according to surgeon preference. The stoma site is considered contaminated.

Procedural Considerations

Setup requires laparotomy and GI sets. Linear stapling instruments are available. Patient positioning is supine with general anesthesia. Insertion of an indwelling urinary catheter precedes abdominal skin prep. Depending on what portion of the bowel is to undergo reconnection, the patient remains supine or is repositioned in low lithotomy. Low lithotomy is necessary if surgery involves the sigmoid colon or rectum, and access to the anus is required to insert a circular stapler to perform an end-to-end anastomosis. If the ileum is to be connected to the transverse or left colon, the patient remains supine.

Operative Procedure

1. A midline laparotomy incision begins the procedure as previously described.
2. The surgeon makes a circumferential incision around the colostomy to free it from the abdominal wall, allowing it to drop back into the abdomen.
3. Resection with a GI linear stapler (or between bowel clamps) of the distal portion of the colon that was attached to the skin follows.
4. Positioning the proximal and distal segments of bowel end to end, the surgeon makes an enterotomy in the proximal end, inserts the anvil of the circular stapler, and secures it with a purse-string stitch using a nonabsorbable suture.
5. An assistant moves between the legs to insert the cutting circular stapler through the anus into the rectum. A separate table for this portion of the procedure is set up for the assistant performing the "below part." The anvil and the stapler connect and tighten, and the stapler fires to connect the bowel to the rectum. Removal of the proximal and distal bowel donuts from the stapler follows, the donuts undergo inspection for completeness, and the surgeon checks the anastomosis for leaks. The surgical team ensures that the remaining anvil and stapler pieces are all accounted for in the surgical counts.
6. To check for leaks the proximal colon undergoes occlusion with a bowel clamp. Warm saline is instilled into the abdomen. The assistant instills air gently into the rectum from below while the surgeon observes the abdomen for bubbles. If present, bubbles indicate a leak that must be oversewn with suture. If there are no bubbles, the assistant dons a new gown and gloves before returning to the abdomen. New sterile drapes are placed over the legs.
7. The abdomen is closed in layers and a dressing applied.

Colon Resection

The purpose of colon resection is to remove malignant and nonmalignant lesions, to relieve an obstruction or a stricture, to repair a

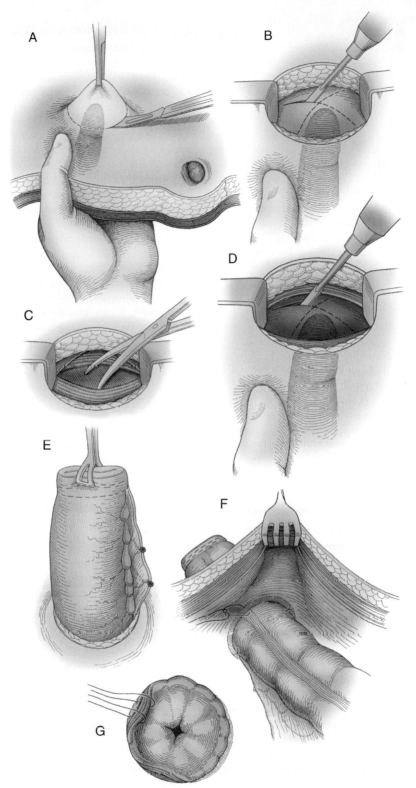

FIG. 11.25 Construction of a colostomy through the anterior abdominal wall. (A) Core of subcutaneous tissue is removed after making a circular skin incision with a #10 blade and using an electrosurgical pencil to dissect down to the anterior fascia. (B) Muscle fibers are split. (C) Tissues are dissected to the posterior layers, and the peritoneum is opened (D). (E) Colon is delivered through the abdominal wall so that it extends 2 to 3 cm beyond the skin surface. (F) Bowel is tacked internally to the peritoneal defect. (G) Four sutures are placed in each quadrant, incorporating the full-thickness cut end of the colon, the serosal surface approximately 1 to 2 cm below the open end of the colon, and up to the dermis. Additional sutures are used to mature the stoma, which refers to everting the mucosa to create a stable opening through which feces can evacuate.

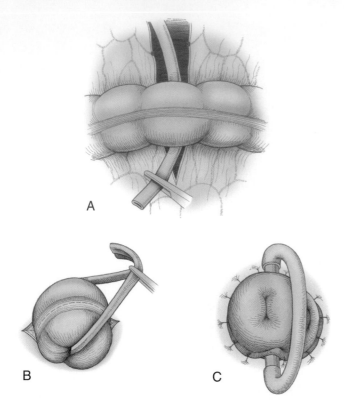

FIG. 11.26 Transverse loop colostomy. (A) Mesentery adjacent to the colon is taken down so that a Penrose drain may be passed beneath the colon. (B) Colon is pulled through the transverse incision and opened longitudinally along the teniae. (C) Apparatus or rod is placed underneath the stoma; sutures are used to mature the colostomy. The rod can be removed after the seventh postoperative day.

traumatic injury, or to treat inflammatory diseases of the bowel. The most common colon resections (Fig. 11.27) are right hemicolectomy, transverse colon resection, left hemicolectomy, low anterior colon resection (Fig. 11.28), and abdominal perineal colon resection (not illustrated). The extent of colon resected depends on the indication. Typically for malignant lesions, the resection includes the affected segment of colon and its regional lymph nodes, with the goal of removing as much tumor as possible at the time of surgery. Optimally the procedure also includes restoration of GI tract continuity, but when restoration is not possible, such as with abdominal perineal resection (APR) for low-lying rectal cancer, a permanent colostomy may be required.

Supplies and instruments are the same for all types of colon resection. Instrumentation required includes a laparotomy set, GI instruments, long instruments, a self-retaining abdominal retractor, and a variety of GI linear and circular stapling devices. EEA sizers should be available. A long electrosurgical pencil tip is often needed and is available. An extra Poole-type suction tip is kept clean for use when irrigating the abdomen with warm saline at the end of the procedure. Many surgeons perform an intraoperative colonoscopy, sigmoidoscopy, or ultrasound. Endoscopes and related equipment are readily available along with a sterile ultrasound probe. All bowel resection procedures require use of bowel technique as previously described to keep contaminated instruments separate from uncontaminated instruments and supplies. Replacement gowns and gloves for scrubbed personnel are required.

Open Right Hemicolectomy With Ileocolostomy

Procedural Considerations

Right hemicolectomy involves resection of the terminal ileum, the cecum, the ascending colon, and a portion of the transverse colon. It serves to remove disease of the cecum, ascending colon, or hepatic flexure. Extended right hemicolectomy removes lesions located in the transverse colon. A functional end-to-end, side-to-side, or end-to-side anastomosis creates a connection between the transverse colon and terminal ileum. These anastomosis techniques require one GI linear cutting stapler, three reloads, and one TA stapler. Alternately, the surgeon may hand sew the anastomosis in two layers using 3-0 absorbable and nonabsorbable suture on a tapered GI needle. Patient positioning is supine with general anesthesia. The anesthesia provider may insert an NG tube after intubation. Insertion of an indwelling urinary catheter precedes abdominal skin prep.

Operative Procedure

1. The surgeon opens through a midline incision and explores the peritoneal cavity. A self-retaining retractor is used to optimize exposure. Moist laparotomy sponges protect the wound edges or may pack the small bowel out of the immediate surgical field.
2. The surgeon identifies and confirms the lesion and then determines the extent of the resection.
3. The surgeon creates a mesenteric window for the GI linear stapler at the site of transection of the terminal ileum and then divides the ileum.
4. Next the terminal ileum is freed from its mesenteric attachment. The mesenteric vessels undergo clamping, division with Metzenbaum scissors, and ligation with silk ties.
5. Mobilization of the cecum and its retraction medially expose the right peritoneal reflection. The right ureter is identified and protected.
6. Lateral mobilization carries up and around the hepatic flexure, with care taken not to damage the second portion of the duodenum.
7. At the limit of the planned resection, the surgeon creates a window in the mesentery of the transverse colon to allow insertion of the GI linear stapler. The stomach is identified as it lies behind the transverse colon.
8. The surgeon scores the mesentery between the transected ends of bowel with the electrosurgery pencil. Next, the mesenteric vessels are isolated, clamped with Péan clamps, divided with Metzenbaum scissors, and ligated with 2-0 nonabsorbable or absorbable suture.
9. When the mesenteric resection is complete, the freed specimen passes off the field.
10. In preparation for the anastomosis, bowel technique commences.
11. With the stapled ends of the proximal and distal bowel facing the same direction, the transected ends of the bowel are in side-by-side position. The surgeon cuts a small corner of each segment diagonally across the staple line. Four mosquito clamps hold the two holes open to accept one leg each of a GI linear stapler. The stapler closes and fires, creating the anastomosis between the two segments of bowel. Three Allis clamps approximate the remaining enterotomy in a transverse direction, and a linear stapler fires along the clamps. Using heavy Mayo scissors or a knife, the surgeon excises the remnant of tissue held by the Allis clamps.

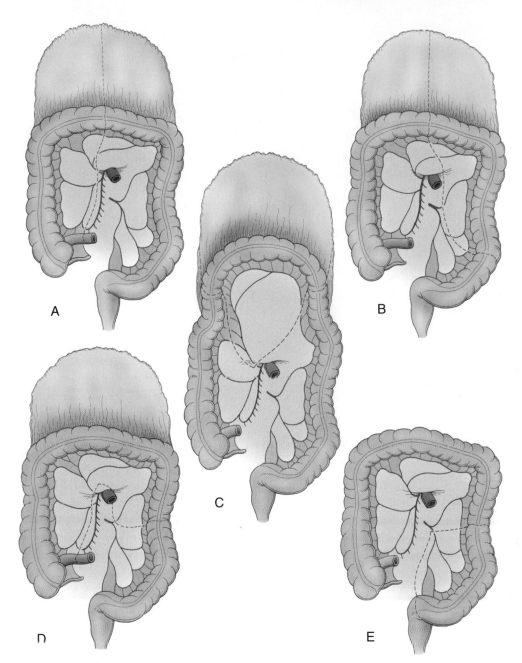

FIG. 11.27 Resection lines for various types of colon resection. (A) Right hemicolectomy and ileocolostomy. (B) Left hemicolectomy. (C and D) Transverse colectomy. (E) Anterior resection of sigmoid colon and rectosigmoidostomy.

12. The staple lines undergo inspection for hemostasis. Contaminated instruments are placed in a basin, and the surgical team changes gowns, gloves, and instruments.

13. The abdomen is irrigated with warm saline, closed in two layers using fresh sterile instruments, and dressings applied.

Laparoscopic Colon Resection

More and more colorectal surgical procedures use the laparoscopic approach. There is growing evidence that laparoscopic surgical outcomes are as good if not better than open approach surgical outcomes (Masoomi et al., 2015). Benefits of laparoscopic colon resection include less postoperative pain, potential for quicker return

of bowel function, shorter hospital stays, and faster return to normal activity after surgery. Multidisciplinary ERAS programs are becoming common for preoperative preparation and postoperative care of patients undergoing laparoscopic colorectal surgery (see Enhanced Recovery After Surgery box on page 293).

Procedural Considerations

Required instruments include a laparotomy set, laparoscopy instruments, and supplies, including a 30-degree laparoscope; a variety of laparoscopic GI linear and circular stapling devices; bipolar tissue sealing forceps; ultrasonic shears; atraumatic grasping forceps to manipulate the bowel; and laparoscopic suturing instruments

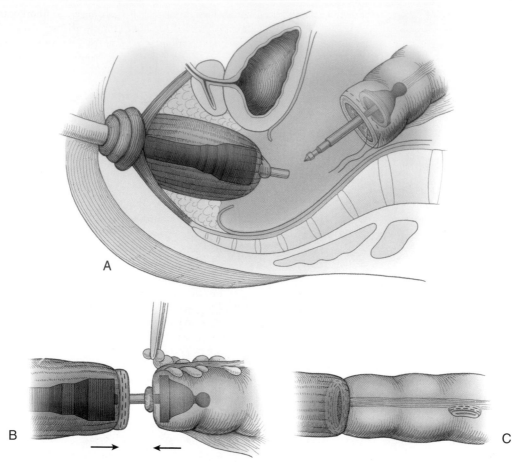

FIG. 11.28 EEA stapling device, used to perform low anterior anastomosis. (A) Stapler is introduced into the anus, and the anvil is placed into the proximal colon loop. (B) EEA is advanced to the level of the anvil, and the EEA is closed and fired. (C) Circular double-staggered row of staples joins the bowel; simultaneously, the circular blade in the instrument cuts the stoma. The instrument is gently removed. The resulting anastomosis is illustrated with bowel wall transparent to depict reconstruction.

or devices such as needle holders, knot pushers, and specialized suture.

Depending on the segment of bowel to be removed, patient positioning is supine or modified lithotomy position. Tucking the patient's arms allows for full access to all abdominal trocars by the surgeon and assistants. For sigmoid colectomy or low anterior colectomy, access to the rectum is necessary to perform an end-to-end anastomosis. The surgeon may stand on the patient's right, left, or between the patient's legs. Application of IPCDs minimizes the risk of DVT. Restraining straps or wide cloth tape secures the patient to the OR bed to prevent shifting during steep position changes. A beanbag device also may aid positioning. Insertion of an NG tube and urinary catheter precedes abdominal skin prep. A preoperative or intraoperative sigmoidoscopy or colonoscopy can verify the location of the lesion to be resected.

Operative Procedure (Laparoscopic Right Hemicolectomy)

1. Pneumoperitoneum is established, and the surgeon enters the abdomen as described in the section on laparoscopy.
2. Placement of additional access ports (usually 5 mm) depends on the segment of colon being resected.
3. Beginning at the level of the cecum, the surgeon mobilizes the colon from its lateral peritoneal attachments using ultrasonic

shears or bipolar vessel-sealing forceps. Some laparoscopic surgeons will mobilize the colon from a medial to lateral direction, taking the mesenteric blood vessels before mobilizing the lateral attachments. The description here is for the lateral to medial approach. Atraumatic graspers provide gentle medial traction on the colon. Patient positioning is as needed to optimize exposure.

4. The surgeon identifies the cecum and terminal ileum. The right ureter is also identified and protected. Mobilization of the cecum and ileum follows. The surgeon creates a small mesenteric window and places a GI stapler in the window across the terminal ileum. The stapler fires and transects the bowel.
5. The lateral peritoneal dissection carries up and around the hepatic flexure, as the surgeon takes care not to damage the second portion of the duodenum.
6. At the limit of the planned resection the surgeon creates a window in the mesentery of the transverse colon to allow insertion of the GI linear stapler.
7. Positioned across the transverse colon, the stapler fires, transecting the transverse colon.
8. Division of the mesentery between the transected ends of the bowel follows, using a GI linear stapler, ultrasonic shears, a bipolar vessel-sealing device, or hemostatic clips and laparoscopic

scissors. If the surgeon uses the stapler, several staple cartridges are necessary.

9. Bowel continuity is reestablished by intracorporeal or extracorporeal creation of a functional end-to-end or side-to-side anastomosis using GI linear stapling devices.

10. Closure of mesentery defects is with 3-0 nonabsorbable figure-of-eight sutures, according to surgeon preference.

11. The abdomen is irrigated and then inspected for hemostasis. Access ports are removed under direct visualization and port sites closed.

Transverse Colectomy

Transverse colectomy removes malignant lesions of the ascending, transverse, and left colon. The extent of resection depends on the pathology and location of the lesion to be removed (see Fig. 11.27C and D). A functional end-to-end anastomosis reestablishes bowel continuity.

Procedural Considerations

Patient positioning is supine with general anesthesia. The anesthesia provider may insert an NG tube after intubation. Insertion of an indwelling urinary catheter precedes abdominal skin prep.

Operative Procedure

1. The surgeon opens the abdomen through a midline incision and explores the peritoneal cavity. A self-retaining retractor is placed to optimize exposure. Moist laparotomy sponges protect the wound edges or may pack the small bowel out of the immediate field.

2. The surgeon identifies and confirms the lesion and determines the extent of the resection.

3. Incising the lateral peritoneal attachments mobilizes the hepatic flexure of the colon. Mobilization of the splenic flexure of the colon follows in a similar fashion.

4. A mesenteric window is created for the GI linear stapler at the proximal and distal site of transection. The linear stapler divides the bowel. A staple reload achieves the second resection.

5. The surgeon uses hemostats, Metzenbaum scissors, and 3-0 nonabsorbable ligatures on the middle and left colic vessels.

6. Bowel technique commences and creation of a functional end-to-end anastomosis takes place as described for right colectomy.

Low Anterior Resection of the Sigmoid Colon With End-to-End Rectosigmoidostomy

A low anterior resection removes malignant lesions in the sigmoid colon or proximal rectum or treats inflammatory bowel disease of the colon. This resection removes the distal portion of the sigmoid colon and rectosigmoid portion of the rectum (see Fig. 11.27E). Surgery can include reestablishment of continuity between the proximal sigmoid colon and the rectum if the distal rectal margin is cancer free and adequate length remains to create a tension-free well-vascularized anastomosis (Jafari et al., 2015).

Procedural Considerations

Laparotomy and GI sets are required. Linear stapling instruments as well as end-to-end curved mechanical stapling instruments (EEA) are necessary along with long instruments for pelvic dissection. A rigid sigmoidoscope may be required both before patient preparation and after anastomosis. A self-retaining retractor is required. A table with rectal instruments, the rigid sigmoidoscope, an end-to-end circular stapler, and suction tubing is readied for the portion of the procedure performed through the anus. Another table with instruments reserved for closure of the abdomen may also be prepared. If requested, a urologist places stents before abdominal prep; equipment and supplies for a cystoscopy and insertion of ureteral stents are needed. Lighted or unlighted ureteral stents help identify the ureters intraoperatively.

Operative Procedure

1. The surgeon opens the abdomen through a midline incision and explores the peritoneal cavity. A self-retaining retractor is placed to optimize exposure. Moist laparotomy sponges protect the wound edges or may pack the small bowel out of the immediate field.

2. The surgeon identifies and confirms the lesion and determines the extent and feasibility of the resection.

3. Lateral mobilization of the sigmoid colon begins along the avascular peritoneal reflection using sharp and blunt dissection, taking care to protect the left ureter and gonadal vessels as they enter the pelvis.

4. Medial mobilization follows, as the surgeon takes care to visualize and protect the right ureter.

5. The surgeon develops the presacral space and frees the rectum circumferentially from its anterior, posterior, medial, and lateral attachments with blunt and sharp dissection and bipolar vessel-sealing forceps.

6. Retraction of the uterus or bladder, if needed, is with a lighted retractor, Harrington, Deaver, or other long retractor.

7. The surgeon identifies the distal margin of resection and transects the rectum with a curved articulating GI linear stapler.

8. Resection of the proximal sigmoid colon is with a GI linear stapler.

9. Mobilization of the remaining sigmoid and left colon from their lateral attachments follows as needed to allow for a tension-free anastomosis to the rectum.

10. The proximal and distal segments of bowel are positioned end to end. The surgeon makes an enterotomy in the proximal end, inserts the anvil of the circular stapler, and secures it with a purse-string stitch using nonabsorbable suture.

11. An assistant moves between the legs to insert the cutting circular stapler anally into the rectum. The assistant performing the "below part" requires the previously set up table for this portion of the procedure. The anvil and the stapler connect and tighten; the stapler then fires to connect the bowel to the rectum (see Fig. 11.28). Removal of the proximal and distal bowel donuts from the stapler and inspection ensure they are complete circles. The donuts are included as part of the specimen. The surgical team ensures that the remaining anvil and stapler pieces are all accounted for in the surgical counts.

12. The anastomosis is checked for leaks. The proximal colon is occluded with a bowel clamp, and warm saline is instilled into the abdomen. The assistant then gently instills air into the rectum from below while the surgeon observes the abdomen for bubbles; bubbles indicate a leak that needs oversewing with suture. If there are no bubbles, the assistant dons a new gown and gloves before returning to the abdomen. A new sterile drape is placed over the legs.

13. The abdomen is closed and dressings applied.

Abdominoperineal Resection

APR (Fig. 11.29) is complete excision of the sigmoid colon, rectum, and anus for low rectal or anal cancers, complications of UC or Crohn disease, or fecal incontinence (Kwaan et al., 2015).

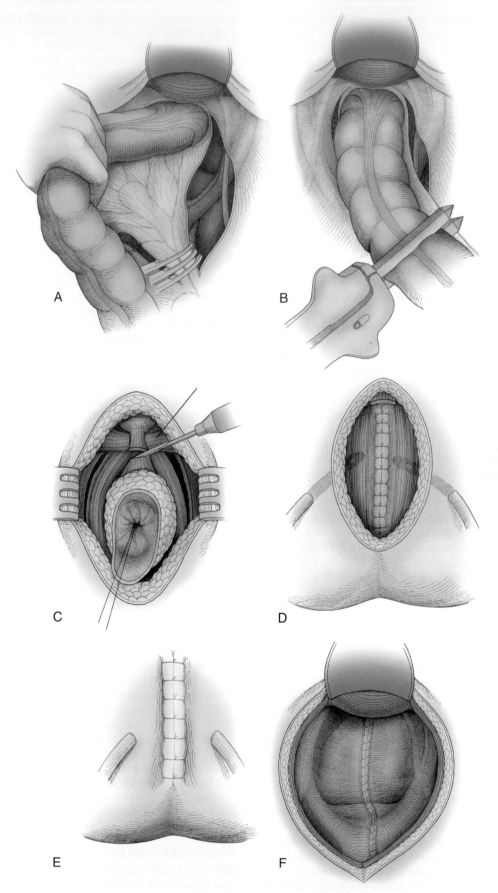

FIG. 11.29 Abdominoperineal resection for cancer of the rectum. (A) Sigmoid colon is deflected to the right to complete the rectosigmoid peritoneal detachment. (B) Distal sigmoid is transected to allow for better access to mobilize the rectum from the sacrum. (C) Rectal stump is excised from the perineal approach. (D) Drains are placed and moved through stab wounds; the levator tissues are reapproximated with 2-0 synthetic absorbable sutures. (E) Perineal skin is closed. (F) Pelvic peritoneal floor is closed from the abdominal approach.

Procedural Considerations

The abdominal portion of the procedure occurs with the patient in supine or lithotomy position. If the perineal portion of the procedure requires the jackknife position, the abdominal part will occur with the patient supine. After mobilization and transection of the rectum the abdomen undergoes closure and dressing, and patient positioning changes to jackknife position for perineal dissection. If two teams work simultaneously, patient positioning is modified lithotomy, and two setups are required. Insertion of an indwelling catheter into the urinary bladder occurs after induction of anesthesia. Before perineal prep, the rectum may be irrigated with povidone-iodine solution and then sewn closed with a purse-string stitch. A cystoscopy and placement of ureteral stents may follow. The anesthesia provider may insert an NG tube after intubation. A GI instrument set and a colostomy appliance are required for the abdominal portion of the procedure. A rectal set is required for the perineal portion of the procedure.

Operative Procedure

1. The surgeon opens the abdomen through a midline incision and explores the peritoneal cavity. A self-retaining retractor is used to optimize exposure. Moist laparotomy sponges protect the wound edges or may pack the small bowel out of the immediate surgical field.
2. The surgeon identifies and confirms the lesion and determines the extent and feasibility of the resection.
3. The abdominal portion of the procedure proceeds as described for a low anterior resection.
4. The surgeon mobilizes and resects the proximal colon for creation of a colostomy (completed after closure of the abdomen).
5. The surgeon makes an incision around the anus in an elliptic manner outside the sphincter muscles with a generous margin of perianal skin. A self-retaining rectal retractor is used for exposure.
6. Hemorrhoidal vessels are suture ligated and divided.
7. The surgeon divides the anococcygeal ligament and levator ani muscle to enter the pelvic fossa.
8. Mobilization and removal of the sigmoid and rectal stump are through the perineal incision.
9. Any bleeding points are clamped and tied.
10. Drains are placed and exteriorized through stab wounds in the buttocks.
11. If two teams are not available for synchronous excision of the perineum, the perineal portion of the operation follows completion of the abdominal resection.

Ileoanal Endorectal Pull-Through (Ileal Pouch–Anal Anastomosis)

Ileal endorectal pull-through, also called ileal pouch–anal anastomosis (IPAA), reestablishes GI continuity between the ileum and the rectum after proctocolectomy if the anal sphincter muscles are intact. Proctocolectomy with IPAA is the procedure of choice to treat UC or familial adenomatous polyposis (FAP), a heredity condition in which patients are at high risk to develop colon cancer at an early age (Rengifo-Cam et al., 2016). To decrease the frequent number of stools produced after a straight ileoanal anastomosis, the surgeon creates a pouch in the shape of a J, and then staples it to the remaining anus (Fig. 11.30). IPAA requires two surgical procedures. At the time of the proctocolectomy the surgeon creates the ileoanal J pouch, but to allow the pouch staple lines to heal properly, a diverting ileostomy is also created. At the second operation some 8 to 12 weeks later, closure of the ileostomy follows (Hayman and Whiteford, 2016; Salvadalena et al., 2015).

Procedural Considerations

Patient positioning is modified lithotomy. The anesthesia provider inserts an NG tube after intubation. Insertion of an indwelling urinary catheter precedes abdominal skin prep. Setup includes a laparotomy set, GI instrument set, perineal set, rectal instrumentation, and a self-retaining retractor system. Preparation of separate instrument tables accommodates the distinct rectal and abdominal approaches. A proctoscope is available for use at the conclusion of the procedure to check for anastomotic leaks. Application of an ileostomy appliance occurs at the end of the procedure.

Operative Procedure

1. The surgeon opens the abdomen through a midline incision and explores the peritoneal cavity. A self-retaining retractor is used to optimize exposure. Moist laparotomy sponges protect the wound edges or may pack the small bowel out of the immediate surgical field.
2. Using a GI linear stapler between the cecum and the distal ileum, the surgeon divides the bowel, taking care to preserve the ileocolic vessels.
3. The terminal ileum and an adjacent segment of ileum are placed side by side in the pelvis to create the pouch. A measuring device gauges the distance of the mesenteric pedicle to the apex of the pouch. Preservation of blood supply to the pouch occurs by taking care to prevent tension on the mesentery.
4. Sequential firings of a 75-mm GI stapler in the two limbs of the ileum create the J pouch, after which the surgeon makes an opening in the bottom of the pouch. One surgeon moves between the legs to perform the perineal portion of the procedure while the other surgeon stays "above."
5. A self-retaining rectal retractor (e.g., Lone Star) is placed to provide exposure of the anal canal. Injection of about 10 to 20 mL of 0.25% bupivacaine with 1:200,000 epinephrine into the submucosal plane of the anus lifts the anal mucosa off the longitudinal muscle. Next the anal canal mucosa is circumferentially excised.
6. The surgeon hand sews the opening at the bottom of the pouch to the dentate line (also called the pectinate line) in the anal canal with interrupted 2-0 absorbable sutures.
7. After the anastomosis is complete it is tested for leaks. The abdomen is filled with warm saline. The ileum is occluded with a bowel clamp proximal to the J pouch. Air instillation with a proctoscope follows. Bubbles in the abdomen indicate a leak, which is oversewn with nonabsorbable suture.
8. With the pouch complete, the surgical team dons new sterile gowns and gloves before closing the abdomen and creating a loop ileostomy on a previously designated site.
9. Dressings and an ileostomy appliance are applied.
   Alternatively, the surgeon may opt to create a Y pouch by aligning the distal ileum in an S configuration (Fig. 11.31) with each of the three limbs about 10 cm in length. The most distal 2 cm of the ileum are not incorporated into the pouch; instead it is preserved for anastomosis to the anus. The surgeon manually incises the three limbs and anastomoses them to create a pouch. Mucosal tissue is anastomosed with absorbable suture; nonabsorbable suture is used on the serosal layer. The surgeon pulls the preserved distal end of the ileum and the pouch through the rectal stump and anastomoses it to the anus. This completes the anal portion of the procedure.

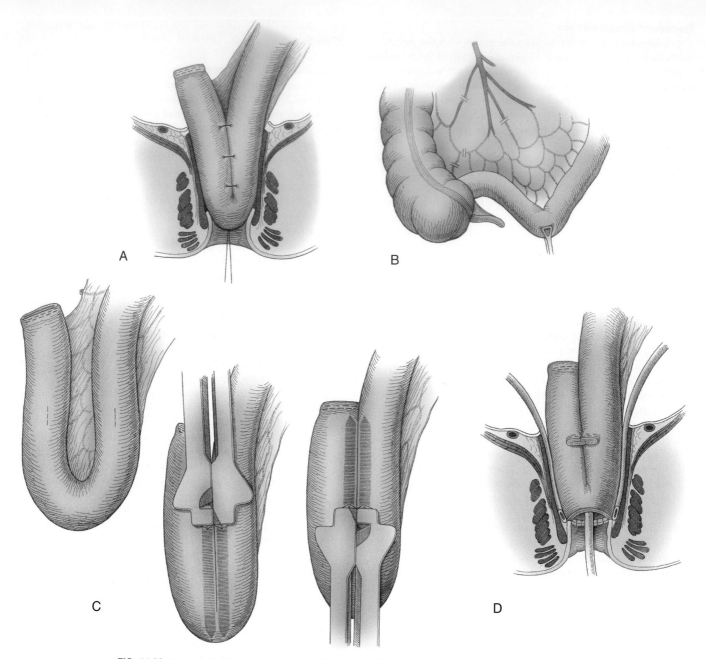

FIG. 11.30 J pouch for ileoanal endorectal pull-through. (A) The J pouch is created at the terminal ileum by folding two adjacent loops of small bowel, approximately 10 to 15 cm each, parallel to each other. (B) Mesenteric vascular arcades may need to be divided to provide adequate length for anal anastomosis. (C) Two loops are anastomosed using a mechanical cutting and stapling device (GIA). (D) Opening is made at the bottom of the pouch, and the pouch is pulled through rectal stump. Bottom of the pouch is anastomosed to anus.

Surgery of the Rectum

Hemorrhoidectomy

Hemorrhoidectomy, an ambulatory or office-based surgical procedure, is excision of internal and external hemorrhoids. Hemorrhoids can cause rectal bleeding, pain, and itching. When hemorrhoids do not respond to conservative medical treatment, surgical excision is appropriate (De la Garza and Counihan, 2013).

Procedural Considerations

Preoperative anal dilation helps expose the vessels and contributes to patient comfort in the immediate postoperative period. Many surgeons prefer to perform a rigid proctoscopy to rule out rectal disease before surgery. Spinal, caudal, epidural, and local anesthesia are options. Patient positioning usually is in lithotomy or jackknife with the buttocks taped apart. A rectal set is needed.

Operative Procedure

1. The surgeon inserts an anal retractor to expose the hemorrhoid(s).
2. The hemorrhoid is grasped with an Allis or Babcock clamp and traction applied.
3. The surgeon positions and ties a 2-0 absorbable suture around the apex of the hemorrhoid.
4. Excision of the hemorrhoid is with electrosurgery, a knife blade, or Metzenbaum scissors. Care is required to preserve the rectal sphincter.
5. The anal mucosa is closed with a 2-0 absorbable suture and a petrolatum gauze dressing placed over the wound in the anal canal.

Excision of Pilonidal Cyst and Sinus

Excision of a pilonidal cyst and sinus is removal of the cyst with sinus tracts from the gluteal fold overlying the sacrum (Fig. 11.32). Pilonidal cysts and sinuses result from ingrown hairs in the gluteal fold. Pilonidal cysts are more common in men. They rarely become symptomatic until the individual reaches adulthood. Symptoms vary from a mild, irritating, draining sinus tract to a painful, acute abscess that may recur frequently. Treatment consists of drainage in the acute stage and total surgical excision during remission. Complete excision of the cyst and sinus tracts prevents recurrence. The defect

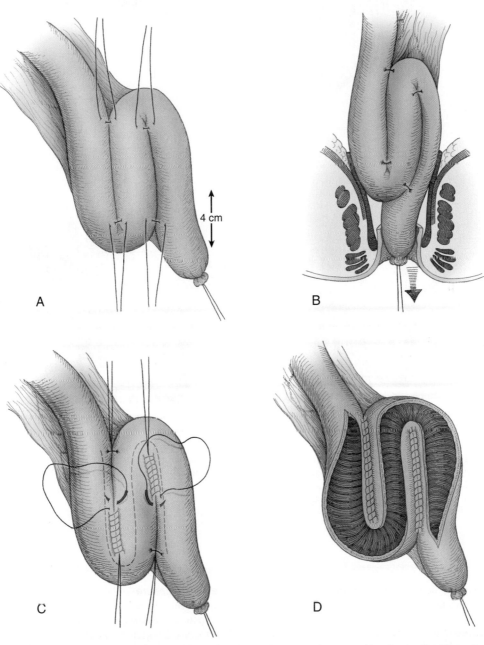

FIG. 11.31 The S pouch for ileoanal endorectal pull-through. (A) Pouch is created by aligning distal ileum in an S configuration with each limb (three in total) approximately 12 cm in length. (B) Length is measured before anastomosis begins. (C) Three limbs are incised and anastomosed to create the pouch. (D) Incision is made.

Continued

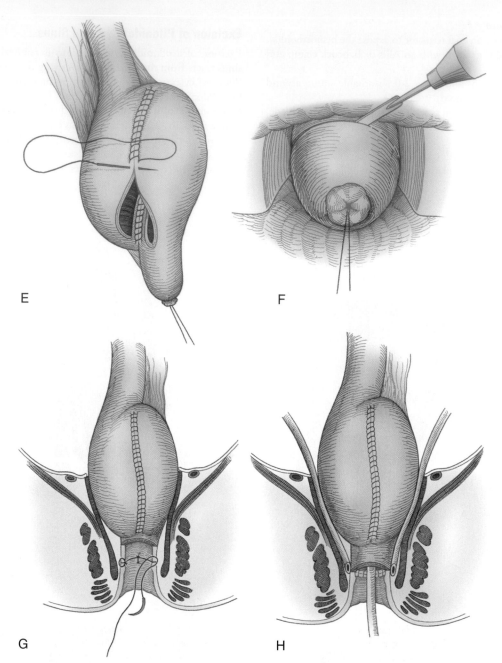

FIG. 11.31, cont'd (E) Pouch is closed using suture for the formation of the reservoir. (F) Distal ends of ileum and pouch are pulled through the rectal stump, and the lower outflow tract is trimmed. (G), With 3-0 absorbable sutures, the outflow tract is anastomosed to the anus at the dentate line. (H) Drain in place in the lumen of the newly created ileoanal-rectal canal.

resulting from recurrence may be too large for primary closure; if so, the wound is left open to heal by granulation.

Procedural Considerations
Setup includes a minor set and rectal instruments, as well as methylene blue, a 10-mL or 20-mL syringe, and a blunt-tipped needle. The patient is positioned in jackknife with the buttocks taped open laterally and secured to the sides of the OR bed.

Operative Procedure
1. The surgeon identifies the sinus tract(s) with a probe and makes an incision over the probe.
2. The tract(s) is injected with methylene blue using a blunt needle.
3. The surgeon makes an elliptic incision down to the fascia.
4. With a curette, granulation tissue is removed.
5. The surgeon completes excision of the cyst and sinus tract(s), and any bleeding is controlled.

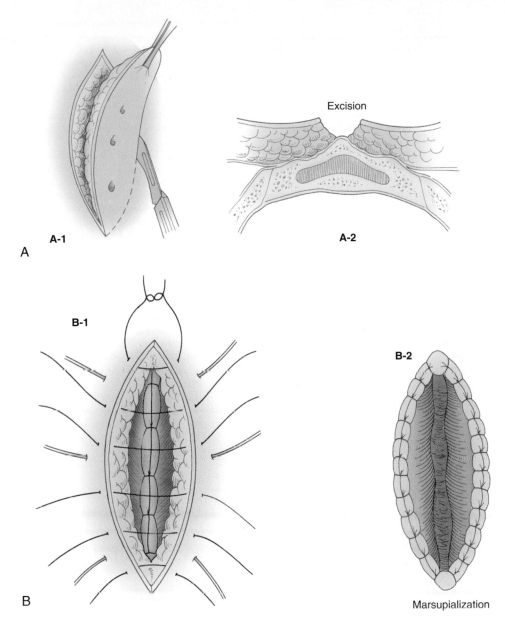

FIG. 11.32 Pilonidal cyst. The pilonidal sinus tract is identified with an injection of methylene blue into the tract. (A) Wide elliptic incision *(A-1)* is made to include all the subcutaneous tracts and tissue that are part of the fascia overlying the sacrum and coccyx *(A-2)*. (B) Closure of the wound can be primary *(B-1)* or secondary *(B-2)*.

6. If the surgeon plans to close the skin, extensive "undermining" of the skin may be needed to avoid excessive tension on wound edges.

Key Points

- GI surgery is a very broad field that encompasses surgical procedures of the esophagus, stomach, small intestine, large intestine, and rectum.
- Many GI surgical procedures have been adapted to accommodate minimally invasive and robotic approaches.
- A sound understanding of surgical anatomy and common approaches to the structures of the GI tract are critical to planning perioperative patient care.

- Planning care for patients undergoing GI surgery requires a team approach with clear communication among the entire surgical team.

Critical Thinking Question

Your next patient is scheduled for a robotic, bariatric Roux-en-Y procedure. Knowing that this is a complicated procedure, patient, and setup, what are some of the patient care factors you will consider in preparing for this patient?

⊖volve *The answer to the Critical Thinking Question can be found at http://evolve.elsevier.com/Rothrock/Alexander.*

References

Al Idrus A: *FDA clears Auris Surgical's robotic endoscopy system* (website), 2016. www.fiercebiotech.com/medical-devices/fda-clears-auris-surgical-s-robotic-endoscopy-system. (Accessed 8 November 2016).

Anini Y, Shin K: SAT-655: role of TNF-alpha in the altered ghrelin secretion in obesity, *Endocr Rev* 36(2):2015.

Antoniadis G et al: Iatrogenic nerve injuries, *Dtsch Aerztebl Int* 111(16):2014.

Association of periOperative Registered Nurses (AORN): *Guidelines for perioperative practice*, Denver, CO, 2016, The Association.

Bhayani NH et al: A comparative study on comprehensive, objective outcomes of laparoscopic Heller myotomy with per-oral endoscopic myotomy (POEM) for achalasia, *Ann Surg* 259(6):1098–1103, 2014.

Birnbaum E: Surgical anatomy of the colon, rectum and anus. In Ratto C et al, editors: *Coloproctology*, ed 1, Switzerland, 2015, Springer International Publishing.

Blackburn AN et al: The gut in the brain: the effects of bariatric surgery on alcohol consumption, *Addict Biol* 2016. [Epub ahead of print].

Chang C et al: Patient positioning and port placement for robot-assisted surgery, *J Endourol* 28(6):631–638, 2014.

Cobourn C et al: Five-year weight loss experience of outpatients receiving laparoscopic adjustable gastric band surgery, *Obes Surg* 23(7):903–910, 2013.

Cologne KG, Senagore AJ: Development of minimally invasive colorectal surgery: history, evidence, learning curve, and current adaptation. In Bardakcioglu O, editor: *Advanced techniques in minimally invasive and robotic colorectal surgery*, New York, 2015, Springer.

Dawes AJ et al: Mental health conditions among patients seeking and undergoing bariatric surgery: a meta-analysis, *JAMA* 315(2):150–163, 2016.

De la Garza M, Counihan TC: Complications of hemorrhoid surgery, *Semin Colon Rectal Surg* 24(2):96–102, 2013.

Deerenberg EB et al: Small bites versus large bites for closure of abdominal midline incisions (STITCH): a double-blind, multicentre, randomised controlled trial, *Lancet* 386(10000):1254–1260, 2015.

DeHaan RK et al: Esophagogastric junction distensibility is greater following Toupet compared to Nissen fundoplication, *Surg Endosc* 31(1):193–198, 2016.

Di Saverio S et al: Single-incision laparoscopic appendectomy with a low-cost technique and surgical-glove port: "how to do it" with comparison of the outcomes and costs in a consecutive single-operator series of 45 cases, *J Am Coll Surg* 222(3):e15–e30, 2016.

Diana M, Marescaux J: Robotic surgery, *Br J Surg* 102(2):e15–e28, 2015.

Duke MC, Farrell TM: Training and credentialing in new technologies. In Stain SC, et al, editors: *The SAGES manual ethics of surgical innovation*, Switzerland, 2016, Springer International, pp 147–157.

Elpern E et al: Original research: the application of intermittent pneumatic compression devices for thromboprophylaxis, *Am J Nurs* 113(4):30–36, 2013.

Erickson G et al: The road to recertification, *J Wound Ostomy Continence Nurs* 43(3):308–309, 2016.

Feeley MA et al: Preoperative testing before noncardiac surgery: guidelines and recommendations, *Am Fam Physician* 87(6):414–418, 2013.

Fencl JL et al: The bariatric patient: an overview of perioperative care, *AORN J* 102(2):116–131, 2015.

Goldberg E, Raufman JP: Stomach and duodenum: anatomy and structural anomalies. In Podolsky DK et al, editors: *Yamada's atlas of gastroenterology*, Oxford, UK, 2016, John Wiley & Sons, Ltd.

Goldner B, Woo Y: Robotic gastrectomy for gastric cancer: an American perspective, *Transl Gastrointest Cancer* 4(6):453–460, 2015.

Gomez PP et al: Development of a virtual reality robotic surgical curriculum using the da Vinci Si surgical system, *Surg Endosc* 29(8):2171–2179, 2015.

Hayman AV, Whiteford MH: Hybrid laparoscopic and endoscopic techniques: colon and rectum. In Kroh M, Reavis K, editors: *The SAGES manual operating through the endoscope*, ed 1, Switzerland, 2016, Springer International Publishing.

Hopkins J et al: Update on novel endoscopic therapies to treat gastroesophageal reflux disease: a review, *World J Gastrointest Endosc* 7(11):1039–1044, 2015.

Hübner M et al: Randomized clinical trial on epidural versus patient-controlled analgesia for laparoscopic colorectal surgery within an enhanced recovery pathway, *Ann Surg* 261(4):648–653, 2015.

Hur C et al: Trends in esophageal adenocarcinoma incidence and mortality, *Cancer* 119(6):1149–1158, 2013.

Hwang JH et al: Endoscopic mucosal resection, *Gastrointest Endosc* 82(2):215–226, 2015.

Jafari MD et al: Patient positioning, instrumentation, and trocar placement. In Ross H et al, editors: *Minimally invasive approaches to colon and rectal disease*, ed 1, New York, 2015, Springer.

Johnson TG, Hope WW: Laparoscopic approaches in general surgery: is there anything new? In Latifi R et al, editors: *Technological advances in surgery, trauma and critical care*, ed 1, New York, 2015, Springer.

Kang MJ et al: Perioperative nurses' work experience with robotic surgery: a focus group study, *Comput Inform Nurs* 34(4):152–158, 2016.

King J, Hines O: Anatomy and physiology of the stomach. In Yeo CJ, editor: *Shackelford's surgery of the alimentary tract*, ed 7, Philadelphia, 2013, Saunders.

Kwaan MR et al: Abdominoperineal resection, pelvic exenteration, and additional organ resection increase the risk of surgical site infection after elective colorectal surgery: an American College of Surgeons national surgical quality improvement program analysis, *Surg Infect (Larchmt)* 16(6):675–683, 2015.

Lacaille F et al: Intestinal failure–associated liver disease: a position paper of the ESPGHAN working group of intestinal failure and intestinal transplantation, *J Pediatr Gastroenterol Nutr* 60(2):272–283, 2015.

Lee PC, Altorki NK: Open radical en bloc esophagectomy. In Kim J, Garcia-Aguillar J, editors: *Surgery for cancers of the gastrointestinal tract*, ed 1, New York, 2015, Springer.

Lim LG et al: Comparison of probe-based confocal endomicroscopy with virtual chromoendoscopy and white-light endoscopy for diagnosis of gastric intestinal metaplasia, *Surg Endosc* 27(12):4649–4655, 2013.

Lipka S et al: No evidence for efficacy of radiofrequency ablation for treatment of gastroesophageal reflux disease: a systematic review and meta-analysis, *Clin Gastroenterol Hepatol* 13(6):1058–1067, 2015a.

Lipka S et al: Single versus double balloon enteroscopy for small bowel diagnostics: a systematic review and meta-analysis, *J Clin Gastroenterol* 49(3):177–184, 2015b.

Lopez NE et al: Single-incision laparoscopic surgery through an ostomy site: a natural approach by an unnatural orifice, *Surg Laparosc Endosc Percutan Tech* 25(1):74–78, 2015.

Masoomi H et al: Risk factors for conversion of laparoscopic colorectal surgery to open surgery: does conversion worsen outcome?, *World J Surg* 39(5):1240–1247, 2015.

Mathus-Vliegen E et al: Consensus guidelines for the use of bowel preparation prior to colonic diagnostic procedures: colonoscopy and small bowel video capsule endoscopy, *Curr Med Res Opin* 29(8):931–945, 2013.

Mayer EK et al: Surgical checklist implementation project: the impact of variable WHO checklist compliance on risk-adjusted clinical outcomes after national implementation: a longitudinal study, *Ann Surg* 263(1):58–63, 2016.

Mayson K et al: Adherence to components of an ERAS protocol for elective colorectal surgery after implementation, *Clin Nutr ESPEN* 12:e46–e47, 2016.

Micic D, Semrad CE: Small bowel endoscopy, *Curr Treat Options Gastroenterol* 14(2):220–235, 2016.

Mihaljevic AL et al: Postoperative negative-pressure incision therapy following open colorectal surgery (Poniy): study protocol for a randomized controlled trial, *Trials* 16(1):471, 2015a.

Mihaljevic AL et al: Wound edge protectors in open abdominal surgery to reduce surgical site infections: a systematic review and meta-analysis, *PLoS ONE* 10(3):e0121187, 2015b.

Mizell JS: Principles of abdominal wall incisions. In Sanfey H, editor: *UpToDate*, Waltham, MA, 2015, UpToDate.

Mizell JS et al: Principles of abdominal wall closure. In Sanfey H, editor: *UpToDate*, Waltham, MA, 2015, UpToDate.

Muysoms FE et al: European Hernia Society guidelines on the closure of abdominal wall incisions, *Hernia* 19(1):1–24, 2015.

Namm JP, Posner MC: Transhiatal esophagectomy. In Fisichella PM, Patti MG, editors: *Atlas of esophageal surgery*, ed 1, Switzerland, 2015, Springer International Publishing.

Nassif G: Transanal minimally invasive surgery, *Clin Colon Rectal Surg* 28(3): 176–180, 2015.

Nicholson M: A comparison of warming interventions on the temperatures of inpatients undergoing colorectal surgery, *AORN J* 97(3):310–322, 2013.

Nieh HC, Su SF: Meta-analysis: effectiveness of forced-air warming for prevention of perioperative hypothermia in surgical patients, *J Adv Nurs* 71(10):2294–2314, 2016.

Ogden CL et al: *Prevalence of obesity among adults and youth: United States 2011–2014, NCHS data brief no. 219*, Hyattsville, MD, 2015, National Center for Health Statistics.

O'Keefe SJ: Nutritional issues in the short bowel syndrome-total parenteral nutrition: enteral nutrition and the role of transplantation. In Meier RF, editor: *The importance of nutrition as an integral part of disease management*, vol 82, New Delhi, 2015, Karger Publishers.

Ou G et al: Effect of longer battery life on small bowel capsule endoscopy, *World J Gastroenterol* 21(9):2677–2682, 2015.

Penprase B et al: The efficacy of preemptive analgesia for postoperative pain control: a systematic review of the literature, *AORN J* 101(1):94–105, 2015.

Puplampu T, Simpson S: Nursing care of the bariatric surgery patient. In Agrawal S, editor: *Obesity, bariatric and metabolic surgery*, ed 1, Switzerland, 2015, Springer International Publishing.

Rajendran K, et al: Clinical study of abdominal closure and their related complications following midline laparotomy, *Glob J Res Anal* 5(1):25–27, 2016.

Rengifo-Cam W et al: Familial adenomatous polyposis. In Boardman L, editor: *Intestinal polyposis syndromes*, ed 1, Switzerland, 2016, Springer International Publishing.

Roy S, Evans C: Overview of robotic colorectal surgery: current and future practical developments, *World J Gastrointest Surg* 8(2):143–150, 2016.

Salvadalena G et al: WOCN Society and ASCRS position statement on preoperative stoma site marking for patients undergoing colostomy or ileostomy surgery, *J Wound Ostomy Continence Nurs* 42(3):249–252, 2015.

Segal-Lieberman G et al: Revisiting the role of BMI in the guidelines for bariatric surgery, *Diabetes Care* 39(Suppl 2):S268–S273, 2016.

Semsarzadeh NN et al: Closed incision negative-pressure therapy is associated with decreased surgical-site infections: a meta-analysis, *Plast Reconstr Surg* 136(3):592–602, 2015.

Shabino PJ et al: Gastric and duodenal surgery. In Chen H, editor: *Illustrative handbook of general surgery*, ed 2, Switzerland, 2016, Springer International Publishing.

Shekelle PG et al: *Making health care safer II: an updated critical analysis of the evidence for patient safety practices, Comparative Effectiveness Review No. 211 (prepared by the Southern California-RAND Evidence-based Practice Center under contract no. 290-2007-10062-I), AHRQ Publication No. 13-E001-EF* (website), 2013. www.ahrq.gov/research/findings/evidence-based-reports/ptsafetyuptp.html. (Accessed 28 September 2016).

Smith CD: Esophageal strictures and diverticula, *Surg Clin North Am* 95(3): 669–681, 2015.

Steele CW, McGregor JR: Inverted meckel diverticulum presenting as the lead point of small intestinal intussusception in adulthood, *J Hepatol Gastroint Dis* 2(132):2, 2016.

Sudan R et al: Morbidity, mortality, and weight loss outcomes after reoperative bariatric surgery in the USA, *J Gastrointest Surg* 19(1):171–179, 2015.

Thomas WE, Wyatt MG: *General surgery: key articles from the surgery journal*, London, 2015, Elsevier.

Toomey PG et al: The effect of product safety courses on the adoption and outcomes of LESS surgery, *JSLS* 19(2):e2015.00007, 2015.

Verhaeghe PJ: Abdominal incision: the gold standard has yet to be defined, *J Am Coll Surg* 220(3):375–376, 2015.

Watanabe M et al: Minimally invasive esophagectomy for esophageal cancer: an updated review, *Surg Today* 43(3):237–244, 2013.

Wolthuis AM et al: Incidence of prolonged postoperative ileus after colorectal surgery: a systematic review and meta-analysis, *Colorectal Dis* 18(1):O1–O9, 2016.

Wu CL et al: Initiating an enhanced recovery pathway program: an anesthesiology department's perspective, *Jt Comm J Qual Patient Saf* 41(10):447–456, 2015.

Wu X: The safe and efficient use of forced-air warming devices, *AORN J* 97(3): 302–308, 2013.

CHAPTER 12

Surgery of the Biliary Tract, Pancreas, Liver, and Spleen

JANICE A. NEIL

A pathologic condition in the liver, biliary tract, pancreas, or spleen often requires surgical intervention. These organs are highly vascular and control many of the body's metabolic and immune functions. Surgical intervention may be indicated for infection, cystic anomalies, congenital anomalies, metabolic diseases, trauma (see Chapter 28), or malignancy. Many new cases of malignancy of the gallbladder, pancreas, or extrahepatic biliary tract are diagnosed each year, and the prognosis for these is often poor (Jackson and Evans, 2017; Dudeja et al., 2017). Pancreatic cancer remains the fourth leading cause of death in the United States (Dudeja et al., 2017) and is widely recognized as one of the most aggressive solid tumors. Only a minority of patients presenting with pancreatic cancer are surgical candidates because of local tissue invasion or metastasis (Clancy, 2015). Surgeries of the liver and biliary tract have become more advanced as research and new technology permit more complete diagnoses of pathologic conditions. Resection of the liver for carcinoma has achieved a recognized role for cure or substantial palliation with safety and low morbidity.

Each year an estimated 700,000 cholecystectomies are performed to treat complications of gallstones (cholecystitis, biliary pancreatitis). Today laparoscopic cholecystectomy is considered the gold standard for treating gallbladder disease, but in some complicated cases the traditional "open" approach is still required. Those situations may include gallbladder cancer and patients with cirrhosis (American College of Surgeons, 2016). Compared with open-incision cholecystectomy, laparoscopic cholecystectomy results in reduced trauma to tissues as well as shorter postoperative recoveries, which are distinct advantages. Laparoscopic cholecystectomies were the precursor to numerous abdominal procedures now performed or assisted with the laparoscope.

New diagnostic technology and intraoperative use of ultrasonography, biliary endoscopy, and radiography enable surgeons to better treat diseases of the biliary tract. Solid organ transplantation, such as for the liver and pancreas, is a common way to treat primary hepatic tumors, end-stage liver disease, and insulin-deficient diabetes. Liver transplant procedures include entire organ transplants as well as living-related organ donations.

This chapter explores the most common open and minimally invasive procedures performed on the liver, biliary tract, pancreas, and spleen.

Surgical Anatomy

The liver is in the right upper quadrant of the abdominal cavity, beneath the dome of the diaphragm, and directly above the stomach, duodenum, and hepatic flexure of the colon. The external covering, known as *Glisson capsule,* is composed of dense connective tissue. The visceral peritoneum extends over the entire surface of the liver, except at its posterior attachment to the diaphragm. This connective tissue branches at the porta hepatis into a network of septa that extends into an intrahepatic network of support for the more than 1 million hepatic lobules. The porta hepatis is located on the inferior surface of the liver and provides entry and exit for the major vessels, ducts, and nerves. The hepatic artery maintains the arterial blood supply. Venous blood from the stomach, intestines, spleen, and pancreas travels to the liver by the portal vein and its branches (Fig. 12.1). The hepatic venous system then returns blood to the heart via the inferior vena cava.

Lobules are the functional units of the liver. Each lobule contains a portal triad that consists of a hepatic duct; a hepatic portal vein branch; and a branch of the hepatic artery, nerves, and lymphatics. A central vein is located in the center of each lobule and provides venous drainage into the hepatic veins.

Lobules also contain hepatic cords, hepatic sinusoids, and bile canaliculi. The hepatic cords consist of numerous columns of hepatocytes, which are the functional cells of the liver. The hepatic sinusoids are the blood channels that communicate among the columns of hepatocytes. The sinusoids have a thin epithelial lining composed primarily of Kupffer cells (phagocytic cells that engulf bacteria and toxins). The sinusoids drain into the central vein.

Bile is manufactured by the hepatocytes. The bile canaliculi are tiny bile capillary vessels that communicate among the columns of hepatocytes. The bile canaliculi collect and transport bile to the bile ducts in the portal triad of each lobule, from which bile then flows into the hepatic ducts at the porta hepatis. These ducts join immediately to form one common hepatic duct that merges with the cystic duct from the gallbladder to form the common bile duct (Fig. 12.2). The common bile duct opens into the duodenum in an area called the *ampulla,* or *papilla of Vater,* located about 7.5 cm below the pyloric opening from the stomach. Bile contains bile salts, which facilitate digestion and absorption, and various waste products.

The liver is essential in the metabolism of carbohydrates, proteins, and fats. It metabolizes nutrients into stores of glycogen, which are used for regulation of blood glucose levels and as energy sources for the brain and body functions.

The liver plays several important roles in the blood-clotting mechanism. It is the organ that synthesizes plasma proteins, excluding gamma globulins but including prothrombin and fibrinogen. Vitamin K, a cofactor to the synthesis of prothrombin, is absorbed by the metabolism of fats in the intestinal tract as a result of bile formation by the liver. Patients with liver disease may have altered blood-coagulation abilities.

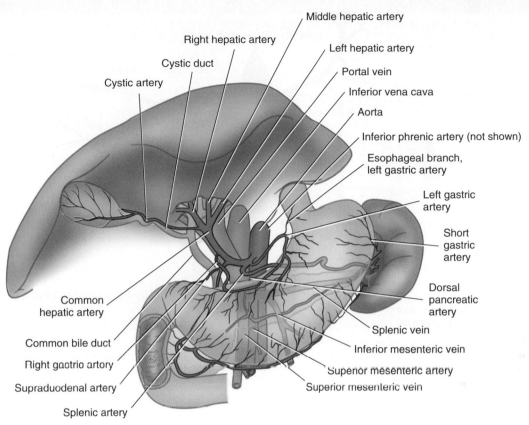

FIG. 12.1 Intricate relationships of the arterial and venous blood supply of the liver, gallbladder, pancreas, spleen, and the biliary ductal system.

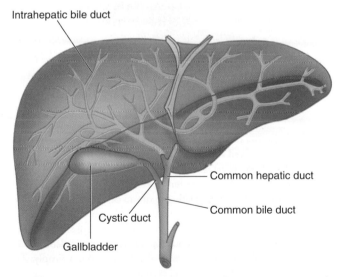

FIG. 12.2 Biliary system can be divided into three anatomic areas: the intrahepatic bile duct, the extrahepatic bile duct (common hepatic and common bile ducts), and the gallbladder and cystic duct.

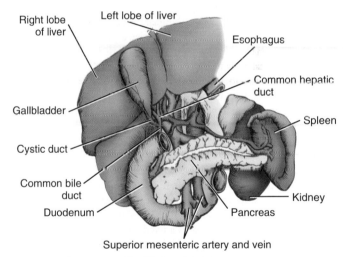

FIG. 12.3 Gallbladder and surrounding anatomy.

The liver also synthesizes lipoproteins and cholesterol. Cholesterol is an essential component of the blood plasma. It serves as a precursor for bile salts, steroid hormones, plasma membranes, and other specialized molecules. A diet high in cholesterol reduces the amount that must be synthesized by the liver. When the diet is deficient in cholesterol, the liver increases synthesis to maintain levels necessary for production of vital chemical molecules.

The liver also functions in the metabolic alteration of foreign molecules or biotransformation of chemicals. The microsomal enzyme system (MES) plays a major role in the body's response to foreign chemicals, such as pollutants, drugs, and alcohol. Patients with liver disease may have an altered response to chemical substances. This consideration is important in the induction and management of general anesthesia for patients with liver disorders.

The gallbladder, which lies in a sulcus on the undersurface of the right lobe of the liver, terminates in the cystic duct (Fig. 12.3).

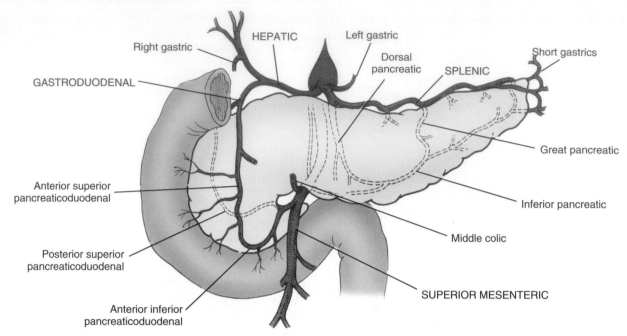

FIG. 12.4 Arterial supply to the pancreas arises from the celiac axis (hepatic and splenic arteries) and the superior mesenteric artery. The blood supply to the head of the gland is by way of the pancreaticoduodenal (anterior and posterior) arcades that arise from the gastroduodenal artery (superior) and superior mesenteric arteries (inferior).

This ductal system provides a channel for the flow of bile to the gallbladder, in which it becomes highly concentrated during storage. The liver produces about 600 to 1000 mL of bile each day. The gallbladder's average storage capacity is 40 to 70 mL. As foods, especially fats, are ingested, the duodenal cells release cholecystokinin. When the musculature of the gallbladder contracts, bile is forced into the cystic duct and through the common duct. As the sphincter of Oddi in the ampulla of Vater relaxes, bile is released, flowing into the duodenum to aid in digestion by emulsification of fats. The gallbladder receives its blood supply from the cystic artery, which is a branch of the hepatic artery. The triangle of Calot contains the cystic artery (and sometimes the right hepatic artery); it is an anatomic landmark in surgical removal of the gallbladder (Jackson and Evans, 2017). Its boundaries may be remembered as the "3 Cs": *c*ystic duct, *c*ommon hepatic duct, and *c*ystic artery. Innervation for the gallbladder and biliary tree is controlled by the autonomic nervous system. Parasympathetic innervation stimulates contraction, whereas sympathetic innervation inhibits contraction.

The pancreas (see Fig. 12.3) is a fixed structure lying transversely behind the stomach in the upper abdomen. The head of the pancreas is fixed to the curve of the duodenum. Blood is supplied to the pancreas and the duodenum from the celiac axis and superior mesenteric artery (Fig. 12.4). The body of the pancreas lies across the vertebrae and over the superior mesenteric artery and vein. The tail of the pancreas extends to the hilum of the spleen. In total, the pancreas extends about 25 cm. Pancreatic secretions containing digestive enzymes are collected in the pancreatic duct, or duct of Wirsung, which joins with the common bile duct to enter the duodenum about 7.5 cm below the pylorus. The dilated junction of the two ducts at the point of entry forms the ampulla of Vater.

The pancreas also contains groups of cells, called *islets,* or *islands, of Langerhans,* which secrete hormones into the blood capillaries

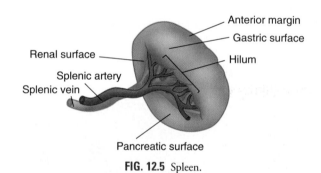

FIG. 12.5 Spleen.

instead of into the duct. These hormones are insulin and glucagon, and both are involved in carbohydrate metabolism.

The spleen (Fig. 12.5) is in the upper left abdominal cavity, with full protection provided by the tenth, eleventh, and twelfth ribs; its lateral surface is directly beneath the dome of the diaphragm. The anterior medial surface is in proximity to the cardiac end of the stomach and the splenic flexure of the colon. The spleen is covered with peritoneum that forms supporting ligaments. The splenic artery, a branch of the celiac axis, furnishes the arterial blood supply. The splenic vein drains into the portal system.

The spleen has many functions. Among them are defense of the body by phagocytosis of microorganisms, formation of nongranular leukocytes and plasma cells, and phagocytosis of damaged red blood cells. It also acts as a blood reservoir.

Perioperative Nursing Considerations

Assessment

The patient with hepatobiliary disease may have extreme jaundice, urticaria, petechiae, lethargy, and irritability. Depending on the extent of the disease, bleeding and coagulation times may increase and the platelet count decrease, contributing to intraoperative concerns with achieving hemostasis. A thorough nursing history is necessary for proper assessment of the health status of patients with dysfunctions of the hepatobiliary system, pancreas, or spleen. Assessment includes data about the patient's history of chronic disease, current medications, perceptions of his or her disease, comfort status, nutritional status, fluid and electrolyte balance, bowel and elimination patterns, energy level and independence, and exposure to toxins.

Establishing an objective database for a person with hepatobiliary or pancreatic dysfunction requires particular attention to characteristic signs of organ dysfunction (Evidence for Practice). Increased abdominal girth and distention, palmar erythema, distended periumbilical veins, hemorrhagic areas, spider nevi, muscle wasting, and dry mucous membranes are some characteristic signs and symptoms. Vascular volume is assessed by noting vital signs, including any orthostatic changes, skin turgor, temperature, and appearance, as well as weight gain or loss. Physical examination of the patient's abdomen includes palpation and percussion to evaluate tenderness, ascites, and organ enlargement.

Common laboratory tests to assess liver function are those that evaluate fat metabolism, protein metabolism, blood coagulation properties, bilirubin metabolism, and antigens and antibodies of hepatitis, as well as common tests of pancreatic function, can be found in Appendix A. Radiographic studies commonly used to evaluate function of the liver, pancreas, and spleen include abdominal examination, upper gastrointestinal (GI) series, transabdominal ultrasound studies, computed tomography (CT) scan, radioisotope scanning, nuclear magnetic resonance (NMR) imaging, angiography, cholecystography, and cholangiography. The hepatic iminodiacetic

acid (HIDA) scan can be used to evaluate the physiologic secretion of bile. State-of-the-art imaging includes contrast-enhanced magnetic resonance imaging (MRI), MR cholangiopancreatography (MRCP), endoscopic ultrasound (EUS), and high-resolution, thin-section spiral CT for imaging pancreatic and biliary structures. In addition, fluorodeoxyglucose positron emission tomography (FDG-PET) is a whole-body technique that can detect metastases, the recognition of which may change surgical management (Jackson and Evans, 2017).

Endoscopy and biopsy are more invasive diagnostic procedures. Endoscopic retrograde cholangiopancreatography (ERCP) (Fig. 12.6) allows direct visualization of the biliary tract, injection of radiographic dye into the ductal system, and biopsy when indicated. Percutaneous transhepatic cholangiography (PTC) uses percutaneous insertion of a long flexible needle into a bile duct of the liver. Contrast medium is injected, and serial x-ray examination is performed. Arteriography of the liver, biliary tree, pancreas, and spleen requires femoral arteriotomy and placement of a catheter into the celiac branch of the abdominal aorta under fluoroscopic visualization. Contrast medium is then injected, and serial x-ray examination allows the vessels to be visualized during the perfusion and drainage phases.

Nursing Diagnosis

After reviewing the nursing assessment, the perioperative nurse formulates nursing diagnoses. Nursing diagnoses related to the care of patients undergoing surgery of the liver, biliary tract, pancreas, or spleen might include the following:

- Anxiety related to impending surgical procedure, perioperative events, and surgical outcome
- Risk for Imbalanced Fluid Volume

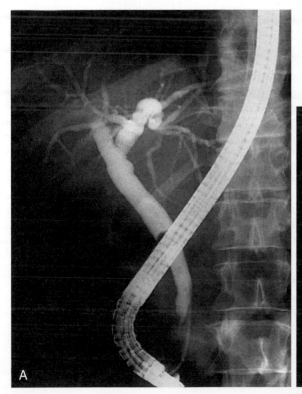
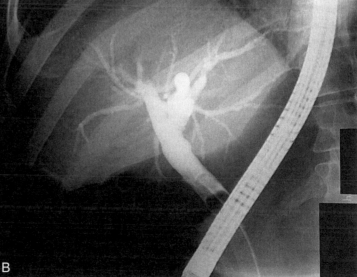

FIG. 12.6 (A) Endoscopic retrograde cholangiopancreatography demonstrates several calculi within the distal common bile duct. (B) Stone removal with a Fogarty catheter.

EVIDENCE FOR PRACTICE

National Surgical Quality Improvement Project: Hepatic, Pancreatic, and Complex Biliary Surgery

HPB surgery can be associated with major morbidity and significant mortality. For several years the ACS National Surgical Quality Improvement Program has gathered a large amount of data on patients undergoing many types of surgery. Improved outcomes result in fewer complications and decreased costs. Using standard reporting systems leads to decreases in morbidity and mortality by improved management. More than 400 academic and community hospitals nationwide participate in reporting to the NSQIP data set. Standardized reporting of surgeries, complications, and histopathology results are tracked. This tracking allows hospitals to achieve measurable improvements in quality care. An ACS-NSQIP "HPB risk calculator" was developed to help better risk stratify patients being considered for complex surgical procedures. Validations of the NSQIP findings related to hepatic surgery include the following:

- A retrospective review of liver resections captured by single-institution "standard" ACS-NSQIP data and a prospectively maintained database was performed.
- The ACS-NSQIP demonstrated high fidelity with the prospective database with respect to preoperative characteristics, median length of surgical stay, and 30-day mortality.
- The standard ACS-NSQIP overall complication rate was lower than the actual rate of complications (29.6% versus 43.2%; $P < .001$).
- More standards and rates need to be developed to capture liver-specific complications including biliary leak, liver failure, pleural effusion, postoperative ascites, and small bowel obstruction.
- A retrospective analysis of patients who underwent major and minor hepatic resection found the surgical risk calculator to have superior predictive power on mortality and morbidity.
- Institutions should further customize the morbidity risk to their own patient demographics.

ACS, American College of Surgeons; *HPB,* hepatic, pancreatic, and complex biliary; *NSQIP,* National Surgical Quality Improvement Program.
Modified from American College of Surgeons: *National Surgical and Quality Improvement Program (NSQIP)* (website). www.facs.org/quality-programs/acs-nsqip. (Accessed 3 November 2016); Kneuertz PJ et al: Risk of morbidity and mortality following hepato-pancreato-biliary surgery, *J Gastrointest Surg* 16(9):1727–1735, 2012; National Surgical and Quality Improvement Program (NSQIP): *Surgical risk calculator* 2016 (website). http://riskcalculator.facs.org/RiskCalculator/. (Accessed 3 November 2016); Daar DA et al: *Validation of the ACS-NSQIP liver module: a single-center experience* (website). www.avensonline.org/wp-content/uploads/JSUR-2332-4139-S2-0005.pdf. (Accessed 18 October 2016); Madhavan S et al: *A comparison, validation and improvisation of POSSUM and ACS-NSQIP surgical risk calculator in patients undergoing hepatic resection,* Abstract of the 12th World Congress of the International Hepato-Pancreato-Biliary Association, 20–23 April 2016, São Paulo, Brazil HPB 2016, 18(S1):e157 (website). www.hpbonline.org/article/S1365-182X(16)30388-4/fulltext. (Accessed 3 November 2016).

- Risk for Perioperative Hypothermia related to exposure of body surface or abdominal cavity and effects of anesthesia on thermoregulation
- Risk for Infection related to organ systems involved (portions of the GI tract)
- Risk for Perioperative Positioning Injury
- Risk for Impaired Skin Integrity related to invasion of body structures, disruption of skin surface
- Acute Pain related to surgical procedure

Outcome Identification

Statements about desired outcomes reflect nursing diagnoses identified for a patient population. Nursing diagnoses are also individualized according to cultural, ethnic, religious, and spiritual values, as well as an individual patient's status. From these are derived the outcomes the perioperative nurse wishes to achieve. The best outcome statement has specific criteria by which the perioperative nurse intends to measure whether the outcome has been met. These criteria are more meaningful when they are established in partnership with the patient. Not all outcomes will be planned with the patient, but ones relating to nursing diagnoses such as anxiety and coping can and should reflect patient participation. Outcomes identified for the selected nursing diagnoses might be stated as follows:

- The patient will verbalize management of anxiety and ability to cope, demonstrate knowledge of his or her psychologic responses to the planned procedure, and show an understanding of the planned sequence of perioperative events.
- The patient will maintain fluid volume equilibrium throughout the operative procedure.
- The patient will evidence an intraoperative core body temperature within the normal range (96°F to 99°F [35.5°C to 37.2°C]).
- The patient will be free of clinical signs and symptoms of surgical site infection (SSI).
- The patient will maintain baseline neuromuscular function and intact skin at positional pressure sites.
- The patient will demonstrate understanding of the plan to heal the incision site.
- The patient will report that the pain management regimen relieves pain to a satisfactory level (Ackley and Ladwig, 2014).

Planning

Planning the patient's care requires knowledge of the anatomy and subsequent physiologic complications that may occur with surgical interruption of tissues. Planning is driven by intended outcomes. The experienced perioperative nurse reflects on those intended outcomes and, using theory, science, and what has been learned through experience, identifies actions required for outcome achievement (Benner et al., 2009). Principles of safe surgical positioning, maintenance of asepsis, prevention of biologic and electrical hazards, and provision of proper instrumentation and equipment are a few constituents of the plan of care that are based on theory and science and augmented by nursing experience.

A review of the nursing assessment and a patient interview provides insights as to the specific needs of the patient. Reviewing the patient's medical and surgical history, as well as age, size, and nutritional status, assists the perioperative nurse in developing an effective plan of care. A Sample Plan of Care for a patient undergoing surgery of the liver, biliary tract, pancreas, or spleen follows.

Implementation

Patients having surgery of the liver, biliary tract, pancreas, or spleen are usually given a general anesthetic. The following pertinent factors should be considered in caring for these patients.

Universal Protocol

The Joint Commission (TJC) requires that the "wrong site, wrong procedure, wrong person" prevention protocol be carried out before each surgical procedure (TJC, 2016). This protocol was discussed in Chapter 2.

SAMPLE PLAN OF CARE

Nursing Diagnosis

Anxiety related to impending surgical procedure, perioperative events, and surgical outcome

Outcome

The patient will verbalize management of anxiety and ability to cope, demonstrate knowledge of his or her psychologic responses to the planned procedure, and indicate an understanding of the planned sequence of perioperative events.

Interventions

- Greet the patient positively; determine the name he or she prefers to be called.
- Introduce the patient to the OR team.
- Avoid hasty movements or gestures of indecision.
- Speak slowly and clearly when addressing the patient, and use terminology the patient can understand.
- Offer emotional reassurance by using touch, assisting the patient to a position of comfort on the OR bed, and offering warm blankets (thermal comfort).
- Classify the patient's level of anxiety (mild, moderate, or severe) by asking the patient and observing signs of anxiety (e.g., clenching/unclenching hands, crying, tremors).
- Determine the patient's personally effective coping mechanisms and facilitate use of these.
- Identify the patient's special concerns, values, and wishes concerning his or her care.
- Provide explanations of perioperative events, encourage questions.

Nursing Diagnosis

Risk for Imbalanced Fluid Volume

Outcome

The patient will maintain fluid volume equilibrium throughout the surgical procedure.

Interventions

- Review orders for blood/blood products; have products available in easily accessible, refrigerated storage for timely access.
- Communicate availability of blood/blood products during the preoperative briefing or time-out.
- Measure, communicate, and record estimated or real fluid volume loss throughout the surgical procedure.
- Anticipate and communicate to blood bank personnel the potential need for additional blood and blood products.
- Collaborate with anesthesia provider in fluid replacement therapies using safe blood administration practices.
- Check laboratory values intraoperatively; monitor and note deviations in study results; read back critical laboratory values; report to surgeon and anesthesia provider.

Nursing Diagnosis

Risk for Perioperative Hypothermia related to exposure of body surface or abdominal cavity and effects of anesthesia on thermoregulation

Outcome

The patient will maintain an intraoperative core body temperature of 96°F to 99°F (35.5°C to 37.2°C).

Interventions

- Determine thermal comfort: ask the patient if he or she is cold.
- Adjust room temperature and humidity to accommodate preservation of body temperature.

- Provide warm blankets on transfer to OR bed.
- Expose only that part of the body necessary for the surgical prep; cover all other body surfaces to maintain body heat.
- Provide warm irrigation solutions, first ensuring solution temperature is less than 105°F (40.5°C).
- Collaborate with anesthesia provider in warming intravenous (IV) fluids and blood/blood products before infusion.
- Use other active warming measures (such as forced-air warming system) for preventing hypothermia.
- Monitor body temperature to evaluate response to thermoregulation measures.

Nursing Diagnosis

Risk for Infection related to organ systems involved (portions of the gastrointestinal tract)

Outcome

The patient will be free of clinical signs and symptoms of surgical site infection.

Interventions

- Implement aseptic technique; communicate and correct breaks in asepsis.
- Ensure that preoperative antibiotics are administered as ordered; prophylactic antibiotics should be administered 1 hour before surgical incision is made. Follow guidelines for safe medication practices.
- Contain and confine contaminants appropriately.
- Ensure that all sterilization procedures have been performed properly.
- Ensure the integrity of sterile supply packaging is intact before dispensing items to the sterile field.
- As ordered, verify that patient has performed preoperative showers or baths.
- Perform intraoperative skin preparation with institutionally approved antimicrobial agent.
- Implement measures to prevent cross-contamination.
- Initiate traffic control and environmental measures that reduce risk for infection.
- Use aseptic technique in applying dressings to surgical sites.
- Correctly classify wound according to established wound classification system.
- Manage culture specimen collection according to institutional policy and safe practices for specimen management.

Nursing Diagnosis

Risk for Perioperative Positioning Injury

Outcome

The patient will maintain baseline neuromuscular function and intact skin at positional pressure sites.

Interventions

- Identify any physiologic alterations or mobility limitations that may affect procedure-specific positioning.
- Implement measures to prevent shearing forces during patient transfer to and from OR bed and during positional changes.
- Ensure that all positioning equipment is clean and functioning properly.
- Ensure patient is in optimal anatomic alignment after induction of anesthesia.
- Adequately pad all bony prominences and vulnerable neurovascular areas.
- Secure limbs to ensure position is maintained and to prevent limb from falling from positioning device (as appropriate to procedure-specific position).

Continued

SAMPLE PLAN OF CARE—cont'd

- Verify correct position during time-out.
- Ensure that no weight or stress is placed on body parts and structures during the surgical intervention.
- Check protective padding and safety restraints after all positional changes, as possible.

Nursing Diagnosis
Risk for Impaired Skin Integrity related to invasion of body structures, disruption of skin surface

Outcome
The patient will regain integrity of skin surface.

Interventions (Postoperative)
- Monitor incision site for color, redness, swelling, warmth, and pain.
- Avoid positioning patient on incision site.
- Individualize plan according to patient's skin condition, needs, and preferences.
- Monitor incision edges for intactness, bleeding, and drainage.
- Maintain a moist wound healing environment that is balanced with the need to absorb exudate.

Nursing Diagnosis
Acute Pain related to surgical procedure

Outcome
The patient will report that the pain management regimen relieves pain to a satisfactory level, using a pain assessment scale.

Interventions (Postoperative)
- Review use of a pain scale with the patient, family, and caregiver before surgery.
- Identify cultural and value components related to pain.
- Provide patient, family, and caregiver with information on pain management.
- Determine whether the patient is experiencing pain at the time of the initial postoperative assessment.
- Assess and document intensity and location of pain.
- Treat pain as ordered; document response to treatment.
- Use a preventive approach to keep pain at or below an acceptable level.

Positioning the Patient

For biliary surgery the patient is placed in supine position. Arms are placed on padded armboards with the palms up and fingers extended. Armboards are maintained at less than a 90-degree angle to prevent brachial plexus stretch. If there are surgical reasons to tuck the arms at the side, pad the elbows to protect the ulnar nerve, face the palms inward, and maintain the wrists in a neutral position (AORN, 2016). A drape, commonly referred to as a drawsheet, secures the arms. It should extend above the elbows and be tucked snugly, but not tightly, under the patient, not under the mattress. This prevents the arm from shifting downward intraoperatively and resting against the OR bed rail. A small positioning aid may be placed under the lower right side of the thorax to elevate the lower rib cage, providing better exposure and access to the viscera in the right upper quadrant of the abdomen. Alternatively, a lateral tilt of the OR bed may be used in combination with reverse Trendelenburg for procedures such as laparoscopic cholecystectomy.

Positioning for laparoscopic procedures requires exercising caution when applying safety straps. Given that the patient may be placed in a severe side tilt or reverse Trendelenburg position, safety or restraining straps must be placed securely, but not too tightly. Attention is given to proper alignment of the patient's body and extremities, and padded footboards are applied to prevent the patient from slipping. Areas of pressure in the selected surgical position (see Chapter 6) and bony prominences are padded well to prevent interruption of circulation and pressure injury to tissues and neurovascular structures. These precautions are especially important for diabetic, circulatory-impaired, immunocompromised, and elderly patients. Close monitoring of the patient is essential during positional changes, especially in laparoscopic procedures with decreased lighting in the room.

When anticipating an operative cholangiogram, the perioperative nurse ensures that the OR bed has been equipped and positioned so that C-arm image intensification can be accomplished efficiently. Radiation-protection devices for the surgical team and patient are made available and applied/worn as indicated.

Thermoregulation

The risks of intraoperative hypothermia have been well documented. When laparotomy is performed, patients are at further risk for perioperative hypothermia. To prevent unplanned hypothermia, the perioperative nurse takes affirmative measures to maintain body temperature in the OR. Proper environmental temperature and humidity prevent body heat loss caused by evaporation and convection. A forced-air warming blanket placed over the patient's upper body, head, and neck assists in maintaining body temperature. Minimizing body exposure to ambient air and using warm irrigating solutions also support thermoregulation. The temperature of irrigating fluids should be no higher than body temperature (98.6°F [37°C]) (AORN, 2016). A blood- and fluid-warming device may be used by the anesthesia provider to deliver intravenous (IV) fluids at a temperature higher than room air temperature (see Chapter 5). The anesthesia provider commonly monitors the patient's core temperature by use of an esophageal temperature probe when duration and complexity of the surgical procedure place the patient at risk for perioperative hypothermia. Additional comfort measures include using warm blankets before and after surgery.

Application of Intermittent Pneumatic Compression Device

Patients undergoing lengthy surgical procedures are at risk for venous dilation and blood pooling in the lower extremities. This may predispose the surgical patient to develop venous thromboembolism (VTE) in the postoperative period. Intermittent pneumatic compression devices (IPCDs), in conjunction with graduated compression stockings (referred to as mechanical prophylaxis), are applied in the OR before commencing lengthy surgical procedures to prevent or minimize VTE risks (AORN, 2016).

Draping the Patient

After the abdominal prep the surgical team allows time for the prep solution to dry and vapors to dissipate. This is an essential patient safety precaution when flammable prep solutions are used in conjunction with electrosurgery (or other energy-generating sources,

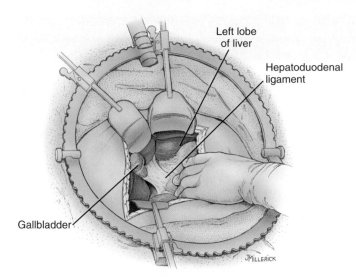

FIG. 12.7 Bookwalter self-retaining retractor in place to provide optimal exposure to the abdominal viscera.

such as a laser). Sterile towels are then arranged to accommodate the intended incision. A sterile drape sheet may be placed over the patient's lower torso and a laparotomy sheet then placed to provide a wide sterile field and to cover all exposed body surfaces except the incision site. Further information on draping can be found in Chapter 4.

Instrumentation

Instrumentation for open (i.e., performed via a laparotomy incision) surgeries of the liver, biliary tract, pancreas, and spleen includes a basic laparotomy set, biliary probes and forceps for dilating and exploring the ducts of the pancreas and biliary tract, vascular clamps, GI clamps, and ligating clips and appliers of all sizes. Linear stapling instruments also should be available. A self-retaining system such as the Bookwalter retractor set (Fig. 12.7) provides excellent exposure of the abdominal viscera. In addition, a flexible choledochoscope, Cavitron ultrasound suction aspirator (CUSA), intraoperative ultrasound, laser, argon beam coagulator, harmonic scalpel, LigaSure, and electrosurgical unit (ESU) may be required to perform certain procedures on the hepatobiliary system. Safe practices when using devices that generate surgical smoke require the use of a smoke evacuation system and accessories in both open and laparoscopic procedures (AORN, 2016). Chapter 8 discusses the safe use of energy-generating devices.

The basic equipment for minimally invasive surgery (MIS) procedures consists of two high-density monitors, an insufflation unit, ESU, light source, camera, and 0- and 30-degree telescopes in 10- and 5-mm sizes. A printer is optional. An ultrasonic dissecting unit is often used with MIS procedures. Trocars and sleeves are available in reusable, disposable, and reposable designs. Trocars and sleeves are commonly designed to accommodate 10- to 5-mm instruments and 12- to 5-mm accessories and instruments. MIS instruments include scissors and shears, dissecting forceps, atraumatic grasping forceps, hooks, Babcock clamps, retractors, needles, suturing devices, pouches, suction-irrigating devices, and mechanical stapling devices.

Thrombin, Gelfoam, Surgicel, Avitene, and other chemical hemostatic agents (Surgical Pharmacology) should be available in the operating room (OR) suite. Radiographic dye, supplies, and

radiation-protection devices are required if intraoperative radiography or angiography is planned as part of the procedure.

Drainage Materials

Tubes and catheters are selected for the areas to be drained. If a defective drain is used, a free fragment may remain in the wound on removal of the tube. The scrub person notes the condition of all drainage materials and tests them for patency before they are placed in the patient.

Soft rubber or latex tissue drains may be used after an open cholecystectomy or a choledochostomy. Verify that the patient has no latex allergy before using these devices and substitute nonlatex drains if necessary. The surgeon will prepare a latex rubber T-tube drain of suitable size after exploring the duct. The center of the crossbar is notched opposite the junction of the vertical limb so that its ends will bend more readily during removal. The ends are beveled and tailored to fit the duct.

Drains are usually exteriorized through separate stab wounds and anchored to skin edges to prevent their retraction. The perioperative nurse documents the types of drains and reservoirs inserted during the procedure. Depending on institutional protocol, these may be identified with an applied label. All drains and their locations should be included in the perioperative nurse's hand-off report to the nursing unit to which the patient is transferred postoperatively.

Aseptic Considerations

When the common duct is opened or an anastomosis is established between a duct and other parts of the alimentary tract, it may be the institution's policy or the surgeon's preference to isolate contaminated instruments and materials from the remainder of the operative field, as described for GI surgery (see Chapter 11). The wound is classified according to a standard system: any procedure in which the alimentary tract is entered under controlled conditions and without unusual contamination is considered a *clean-contaminated wound;* if there is gross spillage, however, the wound is classified as *contaminated.* Proper wound classification is considered an important predictor of postoperative SSI. (See Chapter 4 for a discussion of SSIs.)

Blood Products

During the preoperative verification process the perioperative nurse ascertains the type and amount of blood and blood products, both requested and available, and ensures the patient has a signed consent for transfusion. Constant, ongoing evaluation of blood loss is communicated to the anesthesia provider and surgical team during the procedure. When additional blood or blood products are required, the perioperative nurse communicates with blood bank personnel so that products are readily available and the required steps are carried out to verify blood/blood products with the anesthesia provider before transfusion.

Autologous blood or donor-directed blood products may be used in elective procedures involving the liver, biliary tract, pancreas, and spleen. Cell-saver devices may be used when potential contamination of the blood from bile or bowel does not exist.

Evaluation

Evaluation of the patient after surgery includes examination of all skin surfaces and comparison with preoperative assessment data. Abdominal drains, chest drainage systems, urinary drainage systems, and peripheral infusion lines are assessed for patency. Fluid volume use and loss are documented and communicated appropriately. A report of the patient's history, preoperative assessment, intraoperative

SURGICAL PHARMACOLOGY

Chemical Hemostatic Agents

Agent	Chemical Composition	Actions	Perioperative Precautions
Absorbable gelatin: powder or compressed forms (Gelfoam)	Purified porcine gelatin, beaten, dried, and heat sterilized	On areas of capillary bleeding, deposits fibrin, forming a clot. Absorbs 45 times its own weight.	Compressed form often dipped in warm saline or soaked in thrombin. Must be squeezed to remove air. Will absorb in body, but often removed to prevent compression on nearby structures.
Absorbable collagen (Collastat, Superstat, Helistat, Lyostypt)	Bovine collagen origin	Collagen activates coagulation mechanism, aggregation of platelets.	Must be kept dry and applied with dry gloves. Do not use in infected areas or in pooled blood. Excess material may be trimmed once hemostasis is achieved.
Microfibrillar collagen (Avitene, Surgiflow, Instat)	Hydrochloric acid salt of purified bovine corium collagen	Promotes adhesion of platelets and prompt fibrin deposition.	Applied dry. Use firm pressure against bleeding surface. Will absorb. Removed if used near optic nerve or spinal cord.
Oxidized cellulose (Surgicel, Surgicel Nu-Knit)	Absorbable oxidation product of cellulose	On contact with blood, clot forms. Increases in size and forms gel. Absorbs 10 times its own weight.	Applied dry. May be sutured in place.
Fibrin sealant (fibrin glue) (Tisseel, Beriplast, and Biocol)	Solution of concentrated fibrinogen and factor XIII are combined with a solution of thrombin and calcium	Mimics the final stage of the clotting cascade.	Apply fibrin sealant topical as a thin layer.
Phenol and alcohol	Chemical compounds used to electrocoagulate tissue across lumen of appendix	Phenol coagulates proteins, and 95% alcohol neutralizes phenol.	Phenol is caustic and may cause severe burns.
Epinephrine (Adrenalin)	Adrenal hormone	Powerful vasoconstrictor; prolongs action of local anesthetics to decrease bleeding.	Gelatin sponges may be soaked in 1:1000 epinephrine; especially useful in ear and microsurgical procedures.
Tannic acid	Powder from astringent plant	Used on nose and throat mucous membranes to stop capillary bleeding.	Also used in dental procedures.
Silver nitrate	Crystals of silver nitrate compound mixed with silver chloride and molded onto applicator sticks	Astringent and antimicrobial. Seals areas of surgical incisions.	May also be used in treatment of burns.
Thrombin	Enzyme extracted from bovine blood	Accelerates coagulation of blood. Unites rapidly with fibrin to form clot.	May be used topically as a dry powder or as a solution in which gelatin sponges are dipped. May also be sprayed onto site. Topical use only. Loses potency after 3 h.
Zeolite beads (QuikClot)	Derived from form of volcanic pumice	Beads cause hemostasis by absorbing water from blood.	Used for emergency hemostasis in uncontrollable bleeding or evisceration, especially in trauma. Causes an exothermic reaction. Must be removed; not biodegradable.
Kaolin-based product	Natural mineral form of hydrated aluminum silicate that is insoluble in water	QuikClot has been incorporated into a new product for hemostasis.	For uncontrolled emergency bleeding. American troops have been deployed for combat with this product.
Zinc chloride paste	Chemical compound	Causes coagulation over a denuded area.	Sometimes used after Mohs micrographic surgery.
Ferric subsulfate 20% (Monsel solution)	Chemical compound	Creates coagulation over denuded areas caused by shaved biopsies.	Applied with cotton swab causing vessels to occlude by denaturing protein.

Modified from Goodman T, Spry C: *Essentials of perioperative nursing*, ed 6, Burlington, MA, 2017, Jones & Bartlett; Phillips NF: *Berry and Kohn's operating room technique*, ed 12, St Louis, 2013, Mosby; Silvergleid AJ, Peralta E: *UpToDate: fibrin sealant* (website). www.uptodate.com/contents/fibrin-sealant. (Accessed 12 October 2016).

events, and postoperative evaluation is communicated to the post-anesthesia care unit (PACU) or surgical intensive care unit (SICU) nurse during the handoff.

Evaluation of patient status can be phrased as outcome statements such as the following:

- The patient verbalized management of anxiety and ability to cope, expressed awareness of his or her psychologic responses to the planned procedure, and indicated an understanding of the sequence of perioperative events.
- The patient maintained equilibrium in fluid volume; hematocrit remained in the expected range; vital signs were stable.
- The patient's intraoperative core body temperature remained consistently in the 96°F to 99°F (35.5°C to 37.2°C) range.
- The patient's surgical incision was dressed aseptically and was dry and intact. There will be no clinical signs or symptoms of infection.
- At the conclusion of the surgical procedure skin surfaces were clean, intact, and free of reddened areas; adequate capillary filling was noted after blanching of tissues. The patient had palpable pulses in all distal extremities and showed no evidence of diminished neuromuscular function.
- The patient will be able to perform activities of recovery with acceptable levels of pain.

Patient, Family, and Caregiver Education and Discharge Planning

The length of time and complexity of recovery vary greatly for patients undergoing surgical intervention for disorders of the liver, biliary tract, pancreas, or spleen. Laparoscopic cholecystectomy may be performed on an ambulatory surgery basis with extended recovery and observation of 6 to 8 hours (Ambulatory Surgery Considerations). In contrast, patients undergoing liver transplant or resection may require extensive recovery that includes a stay in the intensive care unit.

Patients undergoing laparotomy for surgical procedures on the liver, biliary tract, pancreas, or spleen may have varying degrees of postoperative edema, decreased GI peristalsis, and alterations in tissue oxygenation and lymphatic drainage, depending on the amount of manipulation, resection, and trauma to the normal anatomic structures of these viscera. General anesthesia is commonly administered. Smooth muscle relaxation is imperative for most major abdominal procedures. The patient usually experiences decreased peristalsis for 2 to 5 days after laparotomy. A nasogastric (NG) tube or gastrostomy tube may be inserted to evacuate large volumes of gastric juices. Diet is introduced only after bowel sounds return. The patient may experience nausea and vomiting if food or oral fluid is introduced too early for the GI system to function with normal absorption and motility.

Coughing and deep breathing are important for patients recovering from general anesthesia and abdominal surgery. Splinting of the abdominal muscles and use of an incentive spirometer assist the patient in postoperative coughing and deep breathing. Early ambulation assists the patient to regain overall muscle tone and prevents VTE in the lower extremities.

Pain management is very important in the patient's recovery and discharge planning. For most patients undergoing abdominal surgery, patient-controlled analgesia (PCA) or epidural analgesia may be used for better and more consistent control of pain and discomfort in the first 1 to 3 postoperative days. Narcotics may, however, add to the length of time for normal bowel peristalsis to return, and their use is monitored closely after the third postoperative day.

AMBULATORY SURGERY CONSIDERATIONS

Same-Day Surgery Versus Overnight Stay: Laparoscopic Gallbladder Surgery

Many patients have same-day surgery for elective laparoscopic cholecystectomy. As surgical stays for laparoscopic cholecystectomy become shorter, sometimes with a 4- to 8-hour observation before discharge, patient education and discharge planning become even more critical. In fact, single-site cholecystectomy is becoming more popular. The surgical site is at the top of the umbilicus, which results in a hidden incisional scar postoperatively (Svoboda et al., 2015). Control of postoperative pain, nausea, and vomiting is paramount for successful same-day discharge. Before the patient departs the ambulatory surgery center, the nurse verifies that the patient is hemodynamically stable, oriented, and alert; tolerates oral fluids; has voided; has dressings that are clean and dry; and has resolved or controlled PONV. Important discharge preparation includes information about early and continuing ambulation to decrease VTE risk, diet, changes in bowel patterns (feces may pass more quickly after cholecystectomy), steps to take if diarrhea is persistent, when to call the surgeon or other healthcare provider (for routine follow-up as well as problems with bleeding, fever, abdominal distention, persistent pain, jaundice, persistent cough, or shortness of breath), and medication management strategies (these are especially important if a bile acid binder has been prescribed). After reviewing this and other important discharge planning information, have the patient, family, and caregiver, if applicable, "teach-back" instructions in their own words and allow an opportunity to ask questions.

PONV, Postoperative nausea and vomiting; *VTE,* venous thromboembolism.
Modified from Society of American Gastrointestinal and Endoscopic Surgeons (SAGES): *Laparoscopic gallbladder removal (cholecystectomy) patient information from SAGES* (website). www.sages.org/publications/patient-information/patient-information-for-laparoscopic-gallbladder-removal-cholecystectomy-from-sages/. (Accessed 3 November 2016); Svoboda S et al: Robotic single-site cholecystectomy in the obese: outcomes from a single institution, *Surg Obes Relat Dis* 11(4), 882–887, 2015; Croghan A: Nursing management: liver, pancreas, and biliary tract problems. In Lewis SL et al, editors: *Medical-surgical nursing: assessment and management of clinical problems,* ed 9, St Louis, 2016, Mosby.

General discharge instructions for the patient undergoing surgery for disorders of the liver, biliary tract, pancreas, or spleen might include the recommendations found in the Patient, Family, and Caregiver Education box. In addition to such general instructions, surgical patients and their family or caregiver should receive surgery-specific instructions. The discharge nurse reviews medications the patient will be taking after discharge (medication reconciliation) along with purposes, dosages, schedules, and routes of administration for each, as well as any side effects to be reported. Both verbal and written instructions are provided, with phone numbers of those to call if questions arise and instructions for emergency situations. Patients should "teach-back," in their own words, all instructions and should be able to state the name of their surgical procedure. For most patients, a healthcare provider (such as the surgeon, nurse practitioner [NP] or physician assistant [PA]) should be notified if any of the following develop:

- Persistent fever (body temperature of 101°F [38.3°C] or higher)
- Bleeding
- Increased abdominal swelling or pain

- Chills
- Persistent cough or shortness of breath
- Persistent pain, redness, swelling, or purulent drainage from incision sites

Follow-up care may also require providing referrals for home care (or other) services.

PATIENT, FAMILY, AND CAREGIVER EDUCATION

General Discharge Instructions for Patients Undergoing Surgery for Disorders of the Biliary Tract, Pancreas, Liver, or Spleen

- Keep incision area(s) clean and dry.
- Swelling inside the gastrointestinal tract may produce a feeling of tightness; this should decrease in 6 to 8 weeks.
- Add solid foods to the diet gradually. Chew solid foods well, and avoid gulping; eating fast; or swallowing large, bulky portions.
- Avoid carbonated beverages for 3 to 4 weeks to help prevent gas bloating.
- Plan small, frequent meals because the feeling of fullness comes quickly.
- Increase exercise gradually to return to normal activities of daily living. Exercise regularly.
- Make an appointment for follow-up care with the surgeon.

Surgical Interventions

Surgery of the Biliary Tract

Laparoscopic Cholecystectomy

Cholecystectomy (removal of the gallbladder) is performed for the treatment of diseases such as acute or chronic inflammation (cholecystitis) or stones (cholelithiasis) (Box 12.1). About 90% of cholecystectomies are done laparoscopically, and it is the gold standard for the treatment of gallstone disease (Kamiński, 2014) and the surgical treatment of choice for patients who meet appropriate criteria for safe laparoscopic intervention. Preoperative evaluation of patients having laparoscopic cholecystectomy differs little from that for patients scheduled for open cholecystectomy. For patients with a history of peptic ulcer disease, a flexible esophagogastroduodenoscopy (EGD) may be performed to rule out existing disease. For patients with suspected ductal stones, a preliminary ERCP or other diagnostic evaluation is often done. A laparoscopic procedure always has the potential to be converted to a laparotomy, which is a potential the patient should be informed about before the surgical procedure. Laparotomy instrumentation and supplies should be available in the OR. Postoperative pain can be an issue after laparoscopic cholecystectomy (Research Highlight).

Procedural Considerations

Patients are generally admitted to the ambulatory surgery center (ASC) on the morning of surgery and commonly require less than

RESEARCH HIGHLIGHT

Postoperative Pain in Patients Who Have Undergone Laparoscopic Cholecystectomy: Medication Interventions

Although about 90% of all cholecystectomies done in the United States are done laparoscopically, postoperative (postop) pain may still be an issue necessitating delays in discharge or requiring overnight stays in ambulatory surgery centers. In some cases, the postop pain can be as severe as open cholecystectomy. Postop pain can come from several origins including the following (Sjövall et al., 2015):

- Distension-induced neuropraxia of the phrenic nerves (failure of nerve conduction caused by structural changes)
- Pain from insufflated gas (volume, type, and temperature of the gas)
- An acid-base imbalance (carbon dioxide-induced pneumoperitoneum)
- Size of wounds used for instrumentation
- Presence of drains
- Sociocultural factors individual to the patient

There are several techniques for treating postop pain including local analgesics, NSAIDs, opioids, and anticonvulsants. It is important to know which medication or combination of medications is the most effective and least harmful. Wound and port site local anesthetic injections decrease abdominal wall pain by 1 to 1.5 units on a 0 to 10 pain scale. Inflammatory pain and shoulder pain can be controlled by NSAIDs or corticosteroids (Sjövall et al., 2015).

The Cochrane Central Register of Controlled trials, MEDLINE, EMBASE, Science Citation Expanded, and the World Health Organization International Clinical Trial Registry Platform were searched to identify randomized clinical trials to enhance a review of the benefits and harms of different analgesics in treating

postop pain in patients who underwent laparoscopic cholecystectomy (Gurusamy et al., 2014). The review was based on 25 randomized trials that included 2505 patients (Brynelson, 2016). Interventions reviewed were NSAIDs, opioid analgesics, anticonvulsant analgesics, and comparisons of one of more of these agents. Analgesics were administered via oral, IV, rectal, subcutaneous, or sublingual routes.

Some of the highlights of the findings include the following:

- NSAIDs, opioids, and anticonvulsant analgesics led to significantly less (intervention group) pain compared with the control (or inactive) groups.
- There was no significant increase in length of stay when pain medications were administered.
- NSAIDs delivered during surgery were the most effective for postop pain reduction.
- When NSAIDs were compared with anticonvulsant analgesics, pain was significantly lower in the anticonvulsant medication-administered group. The comparison between anticonvulsant analgesics and opioids revealed that pain was less in the anticonvulsant analgesic group as well.

Nursing implications are as follows:

- The nurse should expect several types of pain-relieving medications ordered to treat postop pain in patients who have undergone laparoscopic cholecystectomy.
- Different classes of medications other than opioids may be more effective in reducing pain.
- A combination of opioids with nonopioid analgesics and local anesthetics may yield the best result.

IV, Intravenous; *NSAIDs,* nonsteroidal antiinflammatory drugs.

Modified from Brynelson S: Pharmacological interventions for prevention or treatment of postoperative pain in people undergoing laparoscopic cholecystectomy, *J Perianesth Nurs* 31(3):257–259, 2016; Gurusamy KS et al: Pharmacological interventions for prevention or treatment of postoperative pain in people undergoing laparoscopic cholecystectomy, *Cochrane Database Syst Rev* 3:CD008261, 2014; Sjövall S et al: Laparoscopic surgery: a narrative review of pharmacotherapy in pain management, *Drugs* 75(16):1867–1889, 2015.

BOX 12.1

Overview of Cholelithiasis and Cholecystitis

The two most common diseases of the biliary tree are *cholelithiasis* (stone formation in the gallbladder) and *cholecystitis* (inflammation of the gallbladder). These conditions may occur alone but usually occur simultaneously. Gallstones are becoming more common in the United States, affecting an estimated 8% to 10% of adults. Cholecystectomy is one of the most common surgeries performed. Gallstones are usually found in individuals older than 40 years, with a high incidence in people of Pima and Navajo Native American tribes, white women, and blacks.

Clinical conditions that may predispose one to gallstones include diabetes, obesity, cirrhosis, ileal disease or resection, cancer of the gallbladder, and pancreatitis. Cholecystitis usually results from obstruction of the cystic duct from gallstones (acute calculous cholecystitis); in a few patients, however, it results from stasis, bacteria, or sepsis (acute acalculous cholecystitis).

Pathophysiology

The pathophysiology of gallstones depends largely on the type of stone, the stone's location within the ductal system, and the nature of its occurrence (i.e., acute or chronic). Gallstones form as a result of the imbalance of cholesterol, bile salts, and calcium. The metabolism of cholesterol is often altered so that the bile is supersaturated, leading to precipitation and formation of stones. Cholesterol stones are the most common type and occur more often in women. Mixed stones are a combination of pigment and cholesterol stones. The exact cause of gallstone formation is unclear. Contributing factors include the following:

- *Supersaturation of bile with cholesterol.* Bile is composed mainly of water, with other components including cholesterol, bile salts, and pigments. Cholesterol alone is insoluble in water; it must be combined with other components (e.g., bile salts) to remain in solution. When bile salts are insufficient to maintain cholesterol in solution, cholesterol crystals form.
- *Bile stasis.* This occurs when the gallbladder has not contracted normally in response to a meal and the bile is stagnant and then becomes thick and concentrated. This occurs in patients receiving TPN for a prolonged period. Approximately 50% of these patients develop "sludge" (a mucus gel composed of calcium bilirubinate and cholesterol crystals) in the gallbladder by

week 6 of TPN therapy. Gallstones frequently occur during periods of fasting or dieting, during which there is a lack of stimulus for the gallbladder to contract.

- *Nucleation.* A nucleus (nidus) is formed of agents such as bacteria, bile, pigments, cellular debris, and calcium salts. Additional substances aggregate around this nucleus, forming a stone.
- *Genetics* may be a factor, as evidenced by increased prevalence in people of Pima and Navajo descent.

Some stones may form and pass through the ducts without causing clinical manifestations (asymptomatic cholelithiasis). Symptomatic cholelithiasis occurs when stones intermittently become lodged in the cystic duct, causing biliary colic (episodic pain in the right upper quadrant or epigastric area). The pain usually occurs after meals, especially high-fat meals, as a result of increased intraluminal pressure when the gallbladder attempts to contract to release bile (a normal response to food entering the duodenum) against the obstructing stone.

Cholecystitis develops as stones become impacted within the cystic duct, causing unyielding obstruction, edema, distention, and inflammation of the gallbladder. In chronic cholecystitis, gallstones remain, causing recurrent obstructions and producing changes in the gallbladder wall from recurrent edema and inflammation. The muscular coat becomes fibrous, and the gallbladder functions less effectively.

Complications

Edema and distention of the gallbladder walls decrease blood supply, resulting in patchy areas of necrosis and gangrene. Perforation of these areas can then occur. Bile leakage through these perforations into the peritoneum results in peritonitis. Abscess formation may occur if secretions from the ruptured gallbladder are confined by the omentum or other adjacent organs (e.g., colon, stomach, duodenum, or pancreas).

Stone migration from the gallbladder to the CBD may cause cholangitis (acute CBD inflammation). The presence of gallstones in the CBD is called choledocholithiasis. CBD stones are a major source of morbidity in patients with symptomatic gallstone disease. Stone migration to the ampulla of Vater can cause pancreatitis.

CBD, Common bile duct; *TPN,* total parenteral nutrition.
Modified from Croghan S. Nursing management liver, pancreas and biliary problems. In Lewis SL et al, editors: *Medical-surgical nursing: assessment and management of clinical problems,* ed 8, St Louis, 2016, Mosby.

---

a 24-hour stay or admission to an extended recovery unit (ERU). A general anesthetic is used, and antibiotic prophylaxis may be administered in the immediate preoperative period. The following instrumentation, supplies, and equipment are required for laparoscopic cholecystectomy: laparoscope, two 5-mm trocars and sheaths, two 10-mm or 11-mm trocars and sheaths (trocar size depends on surgeon preference and may vary), a #7 knife handle with a #11 blade, multiple clip appliers, blunt grasping forceps (an assortment of alligator, Babcock, and spatula), and laparoscopic scissors. A laparoscopic video unit and secondary "slave" monitor, laparoscopic camera and control unit, light source, CO_2 source and insufflation unit, ESU, suction-irrigator (disposable), filtered insufflation tubing (disposable), and a pressure bag for IV saline 0.9% are commonly used. Instrumentation and supplies for laparoscopic common bile duct exploration should be available in the room. This may include a balloon-tipped Fogarty catheter; wire baskets; dilators; a T-tube;

and a small, flexible choledochoscope. The patient is positioned supine with the usual comfort and safety measures observed. A Foley catheter (for bladder decompression) and an NG tube (for decompression of the stomach) may be inserted. Anesthesia is administered, the time-out completed, and the patient then placed in reverse Trendelenburg position of 10 to 20 degrees.

Pneumoperitoneum may be accomplished using the closed or open technique. In the closed technique, a special hollow insufflation needle (Veress) with a retractable cutting sheath is inserted into the peritoneal cavity through a supraumbilical incision and used for insufflation. In the open technique, sometimes termed the *Hasson technique,* a small incision is made above or below the umbilicus into the peritoneal cavity. A blunt-tipped cannula (Hasson cannula) with a gas-tight sleeve is inserted, and then insufflation takes place. This approach is used for patients who have had a prior abdominal incision near the umbilicus or for those who have the potential for intraperitoneal adhesions. The Hasson technique may also use sutures, placed on either side of the sleeve, to anchor and hold the sleeve in place.

The gas of choice for pneumoperitoneum is CO_2. Gas flow is initiated at 1 to 2 L/min. Elevated CO_2 levels and respiratory acidosis may occur because CO_2 diffuses into the patient's bloodstream during laparoscopy. Intra-abdominal pressure is normally between 8 and 10 mm Hg, and the surgeon commonly uses that range as an indicator for proper Veress needle placement. If the pressure gauge shows a higher pressure, the needle may be in a closed space (such as fat), be buried in omentum, or be in the lumen of the intestine. The perioperative nurse sets the insufflation unit to a maximum pressure of 15 mm Hg. When intra-abdominal pressure reaches 15 mm Hg, flow will stop. Pressure higher than 15 mm Hg may result in bradycardia or a change in blood pressure, or it may force a gas embolus into an exposed blood vessel during the operative procedure. Most insufflation units are equipped with an alarm to alert the operative team if the intra-abdominal pressure is exceeded. Alarm systems on clinical equipment should be activated and sufficiently audible with respect to competing noise in the OR. The surgeon and the anesthesia provider may frequently ask for the pressure reading.

Operative Procedure

1. A small skin incision is made in the folds of the umbilicus with a #11 blade on a #7 knife handle.
2. Pneumoperitoneum is created using either the open or closed technique.
3. An 11-mm trocar (trocar size depends on surgeon preference and may vary) is inserted through the supraumbilical incision; this becomes the umbilical port.
4. The laparoscope with attached video camera is inserted through the umbilical port, and the peritoneal cavity is examined. The surgeon usually stands on the left side of the patient, and the first assistant stands on the right. Video monitors are positioned at eye level at both the right and left sides of the operative field. The patient is then placed in a 30-degree reverse Trendelenburg position and tilted slightly to the left.
5. Three additional trocars are inserted into the peritoneal cavity under direct visualization of the laparoscopic view (Fig. 12.8).
6. Blunt grasping forceps are inserted through the medial 5-mm port to grasp the gallbladder.
7. The gallbladder is retracted laterally (Fig. 12.9A), exposing the triangle of Calot. The junction of the gallbladder and cystic

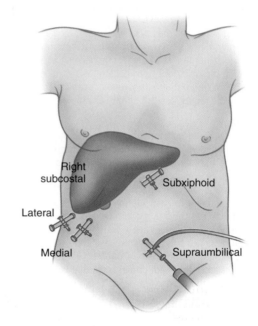

FIG. 12.8 Trocar placement for laparoscopic cholecystectomy.

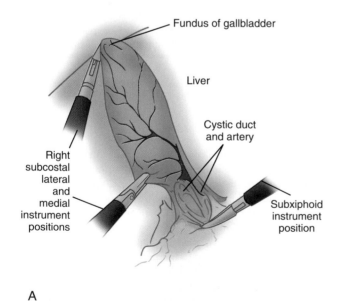

A

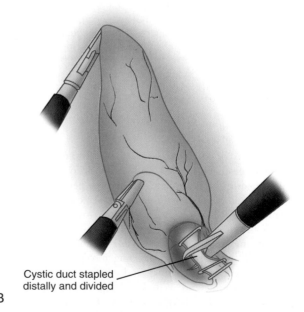

B

FIG. 12.9 (A) Gallbladder is retracted cephalad (using the grasper on the fundus) and laterally at the infundibulum. The peritoneum overlying the gallbladder infundibulum and neck and cystic duct is divided bluntly, exposing the cystic duct. (B) Once the gallbladder–cystic duct junction has been clearly identified, clips are placed proximally and distally on the duct and it is sharply divided.

duct are then identified. The endoscopic dissector, hook, and scissors are used to partially dissect the base of the gallbladder off the liver bed. Electrosurgery is also used. The electrosurgical instrument (active electrode) may have a channel through which suction can be applied to evacuate smoke plume. Some disposable instruments permit suction, electrocoagulation, and irrigation through the same instrument.

8. Hemoclips are placed proximally and distally on the cystic artery, and the artery is divided. The use of a disposable, preloaded, multiple-clip applier assists in the placement of ligating clips in a more efficient manner than a singly loaded, reusable applier.

9. An intraoperative cholangiogram may be performed by placing a hemoclip proximally on the cystic duct, incising its anterior surface, and passing the cholangiogram catheter into the duct. Once the cholangiogram is completed, two clips are placed distally on the cystic duct and it is divided (see Fig. 12.9B). A pre-tied loop ligature may be used if the duct is large.

10. Attention is then given to dissecting the gallbladder out of its fossa.

11. The surgical site is inspected for hemostasis. The gallbladder is dissected off the liver. Intraoperative bile spillage may necessitate additional irrigation and antibiotics.

12. The gallbladder is then removed through the umbilical port (Fig. 12.10). An endobag or similar specimen-retrieval accessory may be used to secure the gallbladder for extraction.

13. The peritoneal cavity is decompressed. The port sites are closed and dressed with Steri-Strips.

Laparoscopic Transcystic Duct Exploration of the Common Bile Duct

1. If the intraoperative cholangiogram indicates stones are present in the common bile duct, exploration can proceed using the same opening created for the cholangiogram.

2. A balloon catheter may be used to dilate the cystic duct enough for the stones to be removed.

3. A choledochoscope can be inserted through the cystic duct incision to visualize stones. The choledochoscope needs to have a working channel of at least 1.2 mm. Saline at body temperature is used to irrigate the common bile duct to aid in visualization.

4. A straight wire basket is threaded past the stone, and opened. When the stone is entrapped the basket is withdrawn. The choledochoscope and basket are removed together as a unit. The process is repeated until all stones are removed.

Laparoscopic cholangiography, choledochotomy, and common bile duct exploration are common procedures (Jackson and Evans, 2017). A single-port access approach is an alternative to the multiport technique in which one incision is made at the umbilicus with trocar insertion at different points of the single port. Generally this type of approach is used in optimal conditions such as when there is no acute inflammation or gallbladder pathology, because of a higher risk of bile duct injuries.

Single-Incision Laparoscopic Cholecystectomy (Single-Incision Laparoscopic Surgery)

The Robotic-Assisted Surgery box highlights information on robotic-assisted procedures of the gallbladder, pancreas, liver, and spleen.

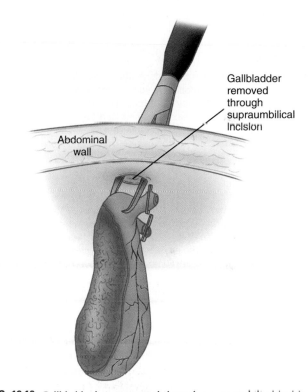

Gallbladder removed through supraumbilical incision

Abdominal wall

FIG. 12.10 Gallbladder being removed through a supraumbilical incision.

ROBOTIC-ASSISTED SURGERY ▋▋

Gallbladder, Pancreatic, Liver, and Spleen Surgeries

Robotic surgery enables surgeons to perform more advanced and complex procedures. The surgeon controls two robotic arms with laparoscopic instruments and cameras while sitting at a console. Surgical assistants are positioned at the field. The systems are not technically robots because they lack independent motion; instead, they are computer-assisted telemanipulators. The benefits of robotic technology include the following:

For surgeons:
- Three-dimensional magnified vision
- Enhanced ergonomics
- Hand tremor filtration
- Motion scaling

- Useful in confined spaces that are located in unfavorable anatomical locations
- Improved manual dexterity
- Increases the dexterity of endowrist instruments
  For patients:
- Reduced length of hospital stay
- Improved postoperative recovery time
- Decreased postoperative pain
- Decreased blood loss
- Reduced tissue trauma and inflammatory response to surgery
  However, robotic-assisted procedures such as the ones mentioned in this box often include steep learning curves as well

Continued

ROBOTIC-ASSISTED SURGERY

Gallbladder, Pancreatic, Liver, and Spleen Surgeries—cont'd

as increased costs associated with the purchase of the robot and training of personnel. Serious events from robotic surgery include unintended laceration/puncture, bleeding/hemorrhage, patient-positioning injuries, retained surgical items (also referred to as foreign bodies), and infection. Many facilities have training and credentialing processes to increase safe robotic surgery outcomes. It has been suggested by various authors that, in the majority of clinical settings, there is little or no advantage in using robotics systems versus traditional laparoscopic techniques as far as clinical outcomes are concerned. Unbiased clinical trials are needed to obtain high-quality data on robotic surgical procedures.[a]

Robotic-Assisted Laparoscopic Cholecystectomy[b]

Laparoscopic cholecystectomy was one of the first procedures to demonstrate the utility of surgical robots in general surgery. Highlights of robotic-assisted laparoscopic cholecystectomy include the following:

- Robotic operative times may be slightly longer because of equipment setup.
- Several studies have been done about the efficacy of robotic-assisted laparoscopic versus laparoscopic cholecystectomy. In terms of feasibility, safety, and reproducibility, robotic-assisted and laparoscopic cholecystectomy have comparable results.
- Robotic-assisted techniques can be useful in handling biliary injuries that may occur during laparoscopic cholecystectomy.
- The cost of robotic-assisted cholecystectomy remains higher compared with laparoscopic cholecystectomy.
- Injuries to the bile duct account for more than 80% of iatrogenic bile duct injuries. Technical skill has been noted to be a factor. The use of the robotic system helps decrease technical difficulties because of its three-dimensional magnified vision.
- Robotic single-site cholecystectomies are gaining acceptance as a safe alternative because of the improved ergonomics the robot provides.
- Single-site robotic cholecystectomies can be used in the obese patient with excellent short-term outcomes.

Robotic-Assisted Laparoscopic Pancreatic Procedures[c]

Pancreatic surgery still presents a difficult challenge for surgeons because of its technical complexity, extensive dissection, and restoration of bowel continuity (Memeo et al., 2016). However, robotic pancreatic surgery is rapidly expanding. Some of the procedures using robotic-assisted technology include the following:

- Pancreaticoduodenectomy: Selection criteria is carefully assessed; tumor size >10 cm, the need for vascular resection, and invasion of adjacent organ tissue are often contraindications. Laparoscopic approaches only allow two-dimensional views, whereas the robotic-assisted type can assist in the complex visceral dissection and reconstruction of digestive continuity.
- Hybrid laparoscopic and robotic: A minimally invasive technique that uses both laparoscopic and robotic approaches is often an effective technique that overcomes technical challenges, especially in pancreaticoduodenectomy.
- Distal pancreatectomy: The most frequent malignancies are ductal adenocarcinoma, neuroendocrine tumor, and pancreatic metastasis. Conversion rates to open cases range from 0% to 39%, and most were caused by difficulties in dissection or vascular invasion. Distal pancreatectomy with or without splenic preservation can be performed for lesions of the distal pancreas.
- Other robotic surgeries that have been done include total pancreatectomy, central pancreatectomy, and tumor enucleation.

Robotic-Assisted Liver Procedures[d]

- Surgeons using this approach must be highly skilled in open and advanced laparoscopic techniques because of the technical aspects as well as obtaining adequate tumor resection.
- Benign and malignant robotic-assisted wedge resections and right hepatectomy are the most commonly performed procedures.
- Blood loss is not significantly different from the laparoscopic approach.
- Sectoral, segmental, or subsegmental resections are possible as well as difficult-to-reach positions.
- Allows for more complex resections in the area of the hilar structures and major blood vessels; ergonomics are improved for nonanatomic wedge resections.
- Liver tumor microwave coagulation therapy is a promising entity for the robotic-assisted approach in the placement of the multiple needles required. This percutaneous technique is used as a method to treat inoperable liver tumors.

Robotic-Assisted Spleen Procedures[e]

- Partial splenectomy is a spleen-preserving technique that can be used in trauma, lesions, or hematologic conditions.
- The robotic system is especially useful in difficult splenectomies, splenectomy in liver cirrhosis, splenic tumors, and malignant hemopathies.

[a]Modified from Dubeck D: Robotic-assisted surgery: focus on training and credentialing, *Pennsylvania Patient Safety Advisory* 11(3), 93–101, 2014; Strickland E: DOC BOT preps for the OR, *IEEE Spectr* 63(6):32–37, 2016; Fernandes E, Giulianotti PC: Robot-assisted pancreatic surgery, *J Hepatobiliary Pancreat Sci* 20(6), 583–589, 2013; Mueller CL, Fried GM: Emerging technology in surgery: informatics, electronics, robotics. In Townsend CM et al, editors: *Sabiston textbook of surgery*, ed 20, Philadelphia, 2017, Saunders; Szold A et al: European Association of Endoscopic Surgeons (EAES) consensus statement on the use of robotics in general surgery, *Surg Endosc* 29(2):253–88, 2015; Tsuda S et al: SAGES TAVAC Safety and Effectiveness Analysis–DaVinci Surgical System (Intuitive Surgical, Sunnyvale, CA), *Surg Endosc* 29(10):2873–2884, 2015.

[b]Modified from Ayloo S et al: Laparoscopic versus robot-assisted cholecystectomy: a retrospective cohort study, *Int J Surg* 12(10):1077–1081, 2014; Bibi S et al: Single-site robotic cholecystectomy: the timeline of progress, *World J Surg* 39(10), 2386–2391, 2015; Kamiński JP et al: Robotic versus laparoscopic cholecystectomy inpatient analysis: does the end justify the means? *J Gastrointest Surg* 18(12):2116–2122, 2014; Lee SH et al: The first experiences of robotic single-site cholecystectomy in Asia: a potential way to expand minimally-invasive single-site surgery, *Yonsei Med J* 56(1): 189–195, 2015; Prasad A et al: Robotic assisted Roux-en-Y hepaticojejunostomy in a post-cholecystectomy type E2 bile duct injury, *World J Gastroenterol* 21(6):1703–1706, 2015; Svoboda S et al: Robotic single-site cholecystectomy in the obese: outcomes from a single institution. *Surg Obes Relat Dis* 11a(4):882–887, 2015; Vidovszky TF et al: Single-site robotic cholecystectomy in a broadly inclusive patient population: a prospective study, *Ann Surg* 260(1):134–141, 2014.

[c]Modified from Boggi U et al: Robotic-assisted pancreatic resections, *World J Surg* 40(10):2497–2506, 2016; Memeo R et al: Robotic pancreaticoduodenectomy and distal pancreatectomy: state of the art, *J Visc Surg* 15(3):353–359, 2016; Parisi A et al: Robotic pylorus-preserving pancreaticoduodenectomy: technical considerations, *Int J Surg* 21(Suppl 1):S59–S63, 2015; Walsh RM, Chalikonda S: How I do it: hybrid laparoscopic and robotic pancreaticoduodenectomy, *J Gastrointest Surg* 20(9):1650–1657, 2016; Suman P et al: Robotic distal pancreatectomy, *JSLS* 17(4):627–635, 2013.

[d]Modified from Liu S et al: Automatic multiple-needle surgical planning of robotic-assisted microwave coagulation in large liver tumor therapy. *PLOS/1, 2016* (website). http://journals.plos. org/plosone/article?id=10.1371/journal.pone.0149482. (Accessed 18 October 2016); Ocuin L, Tsung A: Robotic-liver resection for malignancy: current status, oncologic outcomes, comparison to laparoscopy, and future applications, *J Surg Oncol* 112(3): 295–301, 2015: Song, T: Recent advances in surgical treatment of hepatocellular carcinoma. *Drug Discov Ther* 9(5):319–330, 2015; Tsuda S et al: SAGES TAVAC Safety and Effectiveness Analysis–DaVinci Surgical System (Intuitive Surgical, Sunnyvale, CA), *Surg Endosc* 29(10):2873–2884, 2015.

[e]Balaphas A et al: Partial splenectomy in the era of minimally invasive surgery: the current laparoscopic and robotic experiences, *Surg Endosc* 29(12):3618–1327, 2015; Giza D et al: Robotic splenectomy: what is the real benefit?, *World J Surg* 38(12):3067–3073, 2014.

Cholecystectomy (Open Approach)

Because laparoscopic cholecystectomy has become the procedure of choice for the treatment of most gallbladder disease, experience with open cholecystectomy has drastically declined (Jackson and Evans, 2017). The few contraindications to the laparoscopic approach to cholecystectomy include patients with suspected or diagnosed cancer of the gallbladder, third trimester of pregnancy, cirrhosis with portal hypertension, generalized peritonitis, septic shock, previous surgery that prevents access, and poor pulmonary or cardiac reserve (Jackson and Evans, 2017). Such patients may not be able to tolerate the pneumoperitoneum required in laparoscopy. Further, if the surgeon is unable to identify all anatomic structures during a laparoscopic approach, conversion to an open procedure becomes necessary.

Procedural Considerations

A basic laparotomy set and biliary instruments are used when cholecystectomy is performed through an open abdominal incision. The patient is positioned supine and receives a general anesthetic. After the patient is intubated, the anesthesia provider may insert an NG tube. Antibiotic prophylaxis may be administered. When an operative cholangiogram is anticipated, the perioperative nurse ensures that the OR bed has been equipped and positioned so that C-arm image intensification can be efficiently accomplished. Radiation-protection devices for the surgical team and patient are used during image intensification.

Operative Procedure

1. The abdominal cavity is opened through a right subcostal or upper midline incision.
2. Hemostasis of capillary vessels is achieved with electrocoagulation. Larger vessels are clamped with hemostats and ligated with suture material.
3. Retractors and laparotomy packs are placed as the abdominal cavity is carefully examined.
4. The common duct is palpated for evidence of stones, and pathologic conditions are determined.
5. Harrington, Deaver, or self-retaining retractors, such as an upper-hand or Gomez retractor, are placed to provide exposure. Long tissue forceps and suction are used to manipulate tissues. The surrounding organs are isolated from the gallbladder region by moistened laparotomy packs and deep retractors.
6. To facilitate gentle traction, Péan forceps are usually placed on the body of the gallbladder (Fig. 12.11A).
7. The peritoneal fold overlying the junction of the cystic and common duct is incised with a #7 knife handle and a #15 blade, long Metzenbaum scissors, and forceps. Suction is available, and bleeding vessels are clamped and ligated or electrocoagulated.
8. Adhesions are separated by blunt dissection with small, round, dry dissector sponges; sponges on holders; and blunt right-angled clamps.
9. Dissection is continued to expose the neck of the gallbladder, the cystic artery, and the cystic duct. Lateral traction on the

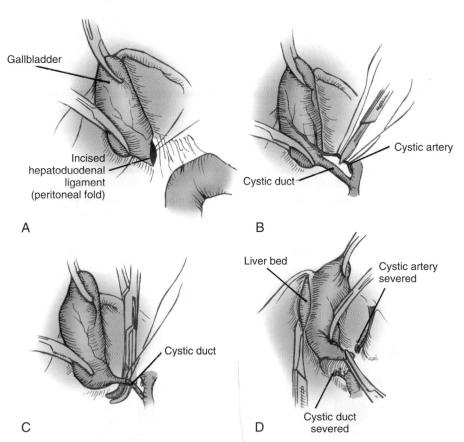

FIG. 12.11 Cholecystectomy. (A) With Péan forceps in place, gentle traction is maintained as peritoneum over the triangle of Calot is incised. (B) Cystic artery is clearly visualized, doubly ligated, and divided. (C) Cystic duct is carefully dissected and identified before forceps and ligatures are applied. (D) Dissection of gallbladder from liver bed is completed.

gallbladder neck allows incision of the peritoneum overlying the triangle of Calot.

10. Dissection is continued to expose the cystic artery as it enters the wall of the gallbladder.

11. On complete exposure and visualization of the branches, the cystic artery is doubly ligated with silk or clamped with ligating clips and divided (see Fig. 12.11B).

12. Occasionally a third ligature or clip may be used. If the cystic artery has more than one branch, each is ligated and divided separately.

13. Abnormalities of the arterial and ductal anatomy are common (Fig. 12.12), and the surgeon and assistant work with care to identify these structures.

14. The true junction of the cystic duct with the common bile duct is visualized.

15. The cystic duct is identified and carefully dissected down to its junction with the hepatic duct.

16. Any stones in the cystic duct are "milked" back into the gallbladder, and a tie is placed around the proximal part of the cystic duct.

17. If necessary, a cholangiogram is performed at this time (see the following section, Intraoperative Cholangiogram). If a cholangiogram is not done, the cystic duct is doubly ligated and divided (see Fig. 12.11C). A fine, absorbable transfixion suture may be used on the stump of the cystic duct near the common bile duct.

18. The gallbladder is then dissected from the liver bed and removed (see Fig. 12.11D).

19. All bleeding is controlled; reperitonealization of the liver bed, if indicated, is accomplished with interrupted or continuous fine absorbable intestinal sutures.

20. A closed suction drain may be inserted near the cystic duct stump. The free end of the drain is exteriorized through a stab wound in the lateral abdominal wall.

21. The wound is closed in layers and a dressing applied.

Intraoperative Cholangiogram

An intraoperative cholangiogram is usually performed with both open and laparoscopic cholecystectomy to visualize the common bile duct and the hepatic ductal branches, and to assess the patency of the common bile duct.

Procedural Considerations

An intraoperative cholangiogram requires fluoroscopy to visualize filling of the ducts. Before the patient's arrival in the OR, the perioperative nurse confirms that a radiolucent bed is available or prepares the OR bed with an image-intensification attachment. Ensure that the patient has not had previous allergic reactions to the x-ray medium before dispensing the pharmaceutic agent to the sterile field. Safe medication practices are followed for labeling and dispensing all medications on and off the sterile field. X-ray aprons or leaded shields are used for all members of the surgical team and the patient. Because the patient's abdomen remains open while the x-ray equipment is positioned directly over the operative site, appropriate draping to maintain asepsis is necessary. Radiopaque sponges and any unnecessary instruments are removed from the abdominal site to avoid obscuring the view of the contrast medium filling the ducts.

The scrub person prepares a cholangiocath by attaching a stopcock with a 20-mL syringe of saline and a 20-mL syringe of contrast medium to the Luer-Lok ports. All air bubbles are removed because they might be misinterpreted as gall duct stones on the x-ray film.

Intraoperative Procedure

1. The cholangiocath is irrigated with saline before and during its insertion into the cystic and common bile ducts.

2. The cholangiocath is inserted into the duct using atraumatic grasping forceps. Irrigation during insertion facilitates dilation and reduces trauma to the ductal lumen.

3. The cholangiocath is anchored in the lumen of the common bile duct by the surgeon's preferred method. Common methods are

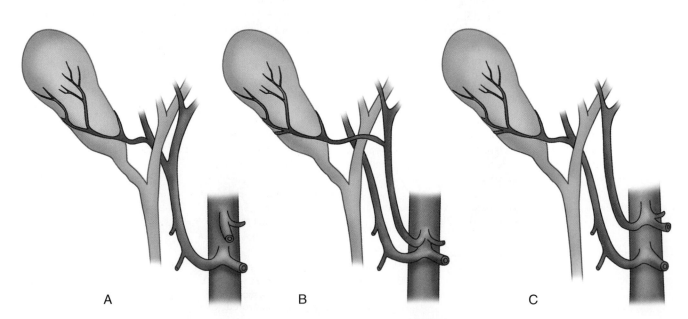

A   B   C

FIG. 12.12 Arterial blood supply of the liver and biliary system is variable. (A) The most common anatomic arrangement is a cystic artery arising from the right hepatic artery. (B) Dual hepatic blood supply is found in 15% to 20% of patients, with the right hepatic artery arising from the superior mesenteric artery in a significant number of patients, as in C.

applying a Ligaclip proximal to the insertion site; tying or suturing the catheter in place; or using a ring-jawed holding clamp, such as a Swenson clamp, which has been designed specifically for this purpose.

4. With placement of the cholangiocath confirmed and anchored, all radiopaque sponges, instruments, and obstructing equipment are removed from the field.

5. The surgical field is draped with a sterile drape sheet to maintain asepsis of the wound and field. The image-intensifier equipment (C-arm) is positioned as the surgeon redirects the stopcock to allow for injection of the contrast medium. If stones are found, the surgeon removes them under fluoroscopic guidance.

Cholecystostomy

Cholecystostomy establishes an opening into the gallbladder for drainage and removal of stones. The open approach is usually selected for patients with advanced medical problems who cannot tolerate general anesthesia or more extensive surgery. Ultrasound-guided percutaneous cholecystostomy has become an accepted procedure for patients who are not otherwise good candidates for surgery. Because of the high incidence of gangrene, perforation, and empyema, open cholecystostomy is often the preferred approach. Many patients are critically ill. If the diagnosis is uncertain, percutaneous cholecystostomy can be both diagnostic and therapeutic. About 90% of patients improve with percutaneous cholecystostomy (Jackson and Evans, 2017). In the rare situation when interventional radiology is not available, an open procedure may be done, as is described here.

Procedural Considerations

A large Toomey syringe (50 mL) or an Asepto syringe may be needed for irrigation purposes. If a local anesthetic is used, the anesthetic agent, syringes, and needles are assembled. Protocols for safe administration and labeling of all medications/solutions on and off the sterile field are followed. Specified drainage tubes or catheters should be available. The patient is positioned supine. Although many surgeons prefer a right subcostal incision, when cholecystostomy procedures are performed as emergencies, a quicker midline or transverse incision may be used. Instrumentation includes a basic laparotomy set plus a gallbladder set.

Operative Procedure

1. After incision into the abdominal cavity, the gallbladder is isolated by retraction of the surrounding viscera.
2. The fundus of the gallbladder is grasped with an Allis or Babcock forceps and, if needed, the proposed opening is encircled by means of an absorbable purse-string suture, leaving the ends long.
3. If the gallbladder is distended or tense, it may be isolated with moistened laparotomy packs to protect the abdominal cavity from contamination.
4. If decompression of the gallbladder is required, a large-bore needle (e.g., 18 gauge) may be inserted with suction attached. Gallbladder contents are aspirated and the site closed using surgical clips on a clip applier.
5. If a trocar is used within the purse-string suture, suction tubing is attached to the trocar sheath.
6. As the contents are aspirated, culture specimens may be taken. The contaminated trocar and sheath are removed and isolated in a discard basin.

7. The opening into the gallbladder can be enlarged with Metzenbaum scissors. Gallstones are removed with malleable scoops and stone forceps.
8. Irrigating the gallbladder with isotonic saline solution may be necessary to remove small stones, grit, or pastelike material. A syringe with a catheter or an Asepto syringe is sometimes used for irrigation.
9. Remaining contaminated instruments are placed in a discard basin.
10. A drainage tube is inserted into the gallbladder opening. The purse-string suture is tightened around the catheter, with care taken not to occlude it.
11. The free end of the catheter or tube is exteriorized through a stab wound and then anchored to the skin edges, as described for open cholecystectomy.
12. Drainage of the abdominal cavity is established with the exterior ends of each drain secured.
13. The wound is closed in layers, as described for laparotomy, and dressings applied at the incision and drain sites.

Common Bile Duct Exploration (Open Approach)

With the advent of endoscopic, percutaneous, and laparoscopic techniques (Fig. 12.13), open exploration of the common bile duct is rare. However, when these methods are not available, when they are not possible because of prior surgery, or when an open procedure is otherwise necessary, open common bile duct exploration is performed. Intraoperative ultrasound may be used to delineate relevant anatomy, detect bile stones, and decrease the risk of bile duct injury (Jackson and Evans, 2017).

Procedural Considerations

The patient is positioned supine after administration of a general anesthetic. The anesthesia provider may insert an NG tube after intubation. An indwelling urinary catheter may be inserted before the abdominal skin prep. Instrumentation includes a basic laparotomy set with the addition of gallbladder instruments. T-tubes of assorted sizes should be available. Intraoperative cholangiography is likely to be used to confirm that all stones have been removed; radiation-protection devices for the patient and surgical team are required. Culture tubes are needed. Soft rubber catheters for irrigation, balloon-tipped catheters such as the biliary Fogarty catheter, stone baskets, and the surgeon's preferred cholangiocath should be available, as well as both flexible and rigid choledochoscopes. A choledochoscope requires the following:

- Choledochoscope with accessories: biopsy forceps, stone-grasping forceps, and a sheath that can be used to direct other instruments into various portions of the biliary tract
- Video camera and viewing screen
- Light cord
- 0.9% normal saline (1000-mL bag)
- Sterile IV tubing
- Pressure bag
- Light source for the choledochoscope

Distending the common duct is necessary for better visualization and is accomplished by irrigating the duct with copious amounts of sterile saline. A pressure bag is placed around an IV bag of 0.9% saline, and pressure to 300 mm Hg is applied. Sterile tubing is then passed from the sterile field and attached to the saline bag. The scrub person attaches the distal end of the sterile IV tubing directly to the irrigating stopcock on the scope.

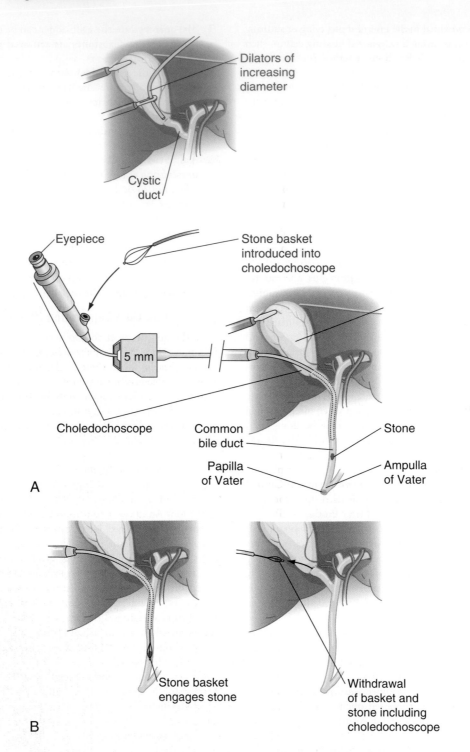

Dilators of increasing diameter

Cystic duct

Eyepiece

Stone basket introduced into choledochoscope

5 mm

Choledochoscope

Common bile duct

Stone

Papilla of Vater

Ampulla of Vater

A

Stone basket engages stone

Withdrawal of basket and stone including choledochoscope

B

FIG. 12.13 (A) Laparoscopic common bile duct exploration. After dilation of the cystic duct, the flexible choledochoscope is inserted into the abdomen through the small trocar and maneuvered into the distal common bile duct. (B) Stone basket is passed through the working channel of the choledochoscope and is used to snare a common duct stone. The stone basket and choledochoscope are then withdrawn together.

Operative Procedure

1. The abdomen is opened through a subcostal incision or midline incision.
2. If the gallbladder has not been previously removed, it is exposed and removed or retracted by means of laparotomy packs and retractors.
3. The common duct may be identified by means of an aspirating syringe and fine-gauge needle to make certain that the suspect duct is not a blood vessel. Culture specimens may be obtained.
4. The common duct region is isolated with moistened laparotomy packs and narrow-blade retractors. A discard basin for contaminated

instruments is placed at the lower end of the operative field, and suction is prepared for immediate use.

5. Two fine-traction sutures are placed in the wall of the duct, below the entrance of the cystic duct. A longitudinal incision is made in the common duct, between the traction sutures, with a long #3 knife handle and #15 or #11 blade, and enlarged with Potts angled or Metzenbaum scissors.

6. Visible stones are removed with gallstone forceps, after which exploration of the duct is begun with small, malleable scoops, proximal and then distal to the opening. Isotonic solution in an Asepto syringe and a soft, small-lumen catheter or a balloon-tipped catheter are used to facilitate the removal of small stones and debris as well as to demonstrate patency of the common bile duct in its entirety to the duodenum.

7. The choledochoscope may be used to identify additional stones. The scope is inserted into the common duct, which is then flushed with saline. After visualizing the duct to ensure that no stones remain, a T-tube is placed in the common bile duct and the choledochotomy is closed around the tube. A final cholangiogram is performed to be certain all stones have been removed. The wound is closed, the T-tube anchored to the skin, and dressings applied. Sterile tubing is used to connect the T-tube to a small drainage container or bag.

Anastomoses: Cholecystoduodenostomy, Cholecystojejunostomy, Choledochoduodenostomy, Choledochojejunostomy, and Transduodenal Sphincteroplasty

There are several types of anastomoses between the gallbladder and the small bowel. Many of these procedures can be done laparoscopically but exposure can be poor because of anatomic complexities (Lee and Hong, 2015). With more prevalent use of ERCP and laparoscopic common bile duct exploration, the need for these procedures has been drastically reduced (Priego et al., 2015).

• Cholecystoduodenostomy and cholecystojejunostomy create an anastomosis between the gallbladder and duodenum or the gallbladder and jejunum, respectively, to relieve an obstruction in the distal end of the common duct (tumor of the ducts involving the head of the pancreas or the ampulla of Vater, an inflammatory lesion, a stricture of the common duct, or the presence of stones).

• Choledochoduodenostomy is an anastomosis between the common duct and the duodenum, and choledochojejunostomy is an anastomosis between the duct and the jejunum. These procedures (referred to as choledochal drainage procedures) may be necessary in postcholecystectomy patients to circumvent an obstructive lesion and reestablish the flow of bile into the intestinal tract.

• Transduodenal sphincteroplasty achieves a choledochoduodenostomy between the distal end of the common duct and the side of the duodenum. The sphincters normally affecting the distal common and pancreatic ducts are rendered functionless because the stoma is noncontractile and therefore remains permanently open. An indication for transduodenal sphincteroplasty is sphincter of Oddi dysfunction, which is a poorly defined clinical syndrome characterized by pain characteristic of biliary colic and recurrent acute pancreatitis. Both endoscopic sphincterotomy and transduodenal sphincteroplasty with transampullary septectomy have been used with similar results. The procedure described in the following section has the advantage of including division of the transampullary septum, which promotes pancreatic duct drainage.

Procedural Considerations

Surgical approaches are similar for these anastomoses. Instrumentation for an open procedure includes a basic laparotomy set; gallbladder instruments with two curved Doyen intestinal forceps with guards, or similar atraumatic holding forceps; and a self-retaining retractor system. Linear stapling devices, and T-tubes and stents in varying sizes are available. Fluoroscopy is anticipated and radiation-protection devices for the patient and the surgical team are available. The patient is positioned supine after administration of a general anesthetic. The anesthesia provider inserts an NG tube after intubation. An indwelling urinary catheter is inserted before abdominal skin preparation.

Open Operative Procedure: Cholecystoduodenostomy and Cholecystojejunostomy

1. The abdomen is opened, the gallbladder exposed, the contents aspirated, and the pathologic condition confirmed.

2. The anastomosis site is prepared, posterior serosal silk sutures placed, and open anastomosis performed.

3. Anastomosis of the gallbladder to the duodenum or loop of the jejunum is usually performed as a two-layer anastomosis.

4. The serosa of the duodenum or loop of the jejunum is sutured to the full thickness of the fundus of the gallbladder.

5. A 1- to 1.5-cm opening is made into the small bowel and gallbladder in corresponding positions. GI technique (also referred to as bowel technique) (see Chapter 11) is instituted.

6. Interrupted fine monofilament (5-0 or 4-0) sutures are then placed around the entire circumference.

7. Contaminated instruments are placed in the discard basin, and the operative field is prepared for closure.

Surgery of the Pancreas

Drainage or Excision of Pancreatic Cysts (Open Method)

Pancreatic pseudocysts are localized collections of pancreatic secretions in a cystic structure. Surgical drainage is indicated for patients with pancreatic pseudocysts that cannot be treated with endoscopic techniques or for patients whose endoscopic treatment fails. There is increasing evidence that transgastric and transduodenal endoscopic drainage are safe and effective approaches (Dudeja et al., 2017).

The preferred operative therapy in patients with uncomplicated pseudocysts is internal drainage by one of three options: cystojejunostomy (use of a defunctionalized Roux-en-Y jejunal limb) (Fig. 12.14), cystogastrostomy (drainage into the stomach), or cystoduodenostomy (drainage into the duodenum) (Dudeja et al., 2017). Treatment depends on the location of the cyst. Cystogastrostomy is a faster and technically simpler procedure when the cyst adheres to the posterior wall of the stomach. Cystojejunostomy is the more versatile drainage procedure. Cystoduodenostomy is used in selected cases, depending on cyst location, but has limited utility.

Procedural Considerations

The patient is positioned supine after administration of a general anesthetic. The anesthesia provider may insert an NG tube after intubation. An indwelling urinary catheter may be inserted before abdominal skin preparation. Instrumentation and supplies include a basic laparotomy set, gallbladder instruments, a GI set, and a self-retaining retractor system.

Operative Procedure

1. A midline incision is made into the abdomen.
2. A self-retaining retractor system is used to expose the pancreatic area.

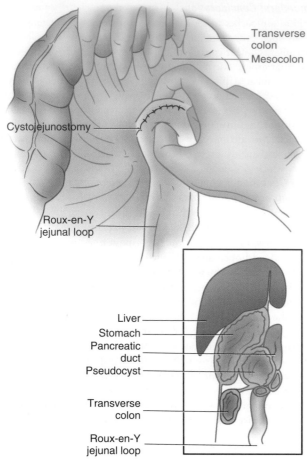

FIG. 12.14 Internal drainage of a pancreatic pseudocyst by Roux-en-Y cystojejunostomy through the base of the transverse mesocolon.

3. The pancreatic cyst is examined and the area isolated with moist packs.

4. Internal drainage may be accomplished by an incision into the anterior wall of the stomach, directly opposite the cyst if it adheres to the posterior wall, providing drainage through the GI tract.

5. A fistula is established between the anterior wall of the cyst and the posterior wall of the stomach. Many surgeons prefer an anastomosis between the cyst and a Roux-en-Y loop of jejunum (see Fig. 12.14) or into the duodenum directly, depending on the location of the cyst.

6. The anterior gastrostomy is closed and wound closure completed.

Laparoscopic Pancreatic Cyst–Gastrostomy

Laparoscopic techniques may be used for internal drainage procedures for pancreatic pseudocysts. CT imaging is used to diagnose the pancreatic pseudocyst. An EUS may provide additional information. The location, size, and thickness of the wall of the pseudocyst are assessed to determine the more appropriate procedure for drainage, either a laparoscopic pancreatic cyst–gastrostomy or a Roux-en-Y pancreatic cystojejunostomy. Endoscopic drainage of pseudocysts may also be done in centers where endoscopists are experienced in percutaneous drainage techniques. Laparoscopic treatment of pancreatic pseudocysts enables definitive drainage with faster recovery (Galketiya et al., 2015).

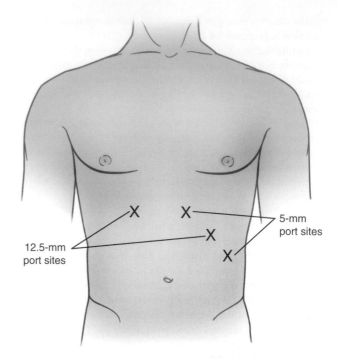

FIG. 12.15 Port sites for trocar placement in laparoscopic pancreatic cyst–gastrostomy.

Procedural Considerations

General anesthesia is induced. An NG tube is usually inserted. The patient is positioned supine. Equipment and instrumentation are a 30-degree telescope (10 mm or 5 mm); a video camera; two high-density video monitors; a high-flow insufflator with CO_2 tank; an ESU; two 12.5-mm trocar ports; two 5-mm trocar ports (trocar size depends on surgeon preference and may vary); an endodissecting instrument (5 mm) or atraumatic grasping forceps (5 mm); endoshears/scissors (5 mm) with electrocoagulation connection; an endo-Babcock instrument; a mechanical stapling device; a 10-mm endoclip applier; a 10-mm endosuturing instrument (optional); 2-0 suture material, 7-inch length (optional); an electrocoagulation hook; a long 5-mm laparoscopic needle; and an endoretractor.

Operative Procedure

1. Pneumoperitoneum is created and the trocars inserted via port sites as illustrated in Fig. 12.15.

2. The pancreatic pseudocyst is located by entering the lesser sac at the greater curvature. Hemostasis is achieved by using the endoclip applier. An endostapling device (gastrointestinal anastomosis [GIA] type) with vascular cartridges is used to dissect the greater curvature.

3. The surgeon assesses the site for entry into the stomach. An endoretractor may be used to retract the left hepatic lobe.

4. Using electrodissection, an incision centered between the lesser and greater curvatures is made on the anterior wall of the stomach and then extended.

5. A long laparoscopic aspiration needle is inserted into the intra-abdominal and gastric cavity. The camera is advanced to visualize the posterior wall of the stomach.

6. The needle is inserted into the cyst and its presence is confirmed by aspiration.

7. A small incision is made into the cyst and the pancreatic fluid aspirated.

8. The endostapling device is inserted into the gastric cavity. The smaller jaw of this instrument is inserted into the pseudocyst. The stapling device is closed. It is important that the anastomosis not be under tension. The stapling device is fired and the anastomosis checked for integrity. An endosuturing instrument is used to close any defects in the anastomotic line.

9. An NG tube is directed into the pseudocyst.

10. The two edges of the anterior wall gastrostomy are approximated using endograsping forceps (atraumatic) or an endodissecting instrument. The gastrostomy is then closed using an endostapling device (TA type).

11. A drain is placed, the abdomen deflated, trocar ports removed, and trocar sites closed and dressed.

Other Laparoscopic Pancreatic Procedures

Laparoscopic pancreatic surgery is an emerging approach that has not yet gained wide acceptance because of the complexity of the procedures, the accuracy needed to perform the operation, and the typically steep learning curve required to master the procedures (Dubeck, 2014). Laparoscopic resection of lesions in the body and tail of the pancreas is done in specialized centers. Pancreatic exploration and resections of peri-pancreatic tissue, endocrine tumors, pancreatic carcinomas, and cystic tumors have all been achieved laparoscopically (Rosok et al., 2010). Laparoscopic surgery may be used as an initial step to rule out metastatic disease before resection.

Severe attacks of acute pancreatitis can result in pancreatic necrosis that may require debridement and drainage by surgical or radiologic methods. Minimal access techniques include laparoscopy with necrosectomy (resection of necrotic tissue) (Gomatos et al., 2016).

Pancreaticoduodenectomy (Whipple Procedure)

Pancreatic cancer is treated using a multidisciplinary approach that often includes surgeons, gastroenterologists, oncologists, radiologists, nurses, and nutritionists. Tumors arise from the exocrine glands (95%) and endocrine glands (5%) in the pancreas. Ductal adenocarcinoma constitutes 80% of all pancreatic tumors. Most tumors begin in the head of the exocrine gland; obstruct the bile duct; and extend to the duodenum, intestines, and spine. Metastasis occurs to regional lymph nodes, and common metastatic sites include the liver and lungs. Because symptoms most often occur late in the disease, the prognosis is usually poor. A Whipple procedure involves removal of the head of the pancreas, the entire duodenum, a portion of the jejunum, the distal third of the stomach, and the lower half of the common bile duct, with reestablishment of continuity of the biliary, pancreatic, and GI tract systems. For patients who have cancer of the ampulla of Vater, newer less invasive pancreatic-sparing duodenectomy techniques are used as an alternative to pancreaticoduodenectomy (Dudeja et al., 2017).

Procedural Considerations

A basic laparotomy set, a GI instrument set, a self-retaining retractor system, linear stapling devices, and appropriate drains and catheters are required. The perioperative nurse ensures that ordered blood and blood products are available. Pancreaticoduodenectomy may take 5 to 6 hours and require the transfusion of many units of blood or blood products. The patient is positioned supine after administration of a general anesthetic. Attention is paid to padding positional pressure points with gel pads or using a pressure-reducing OR bed mattress. IPCDs are applied as well as a forced-air warming device and other active warming measures to prevent hypothermia. The anesthesia provider inserts an NG tube after intubation. An indwelling urinary catheter is inserted before abdominal preparation. The abdomen is prepped from nipple line to midthigh.

Operative Procedure

1. The abdomen is entered through either an upper transverse, a bilateral subcostal, or a long paramedian incision. Resectability is assessed, exploring for hepatic metastases, serosal implants of tumor, and lymph node metastases. If these are outside the zone of resection, the disease is unresectable.

2. Laparotomy packs and retractors are used to expose the operative site and protect vital structures.

3. The duodenum is mobilized using the Kocher maneuver (incision of peritoneal reflection lateral to the second portion of the duodenum) with Metzenbaum scissors and subsequent blunt dissection of loose areolar tissue.

4. Mobilization of the duodenum continues and bleeding vessels are ligated, often with silk.

5. The gastrocolic ligament and the gastrohepatic omentum are divided between curved forceps and ligated or transfixed.

6. The gastroduodenal and right gastric arteries are clamped, divided, and ligated.

7. The prepyloric area of the stomach is mobilized.

8. The operative field is prepared for open anastomosis by isolating the area with laparotomy sponges.

9. By placing two long Allen or Payr clamps near the midportion of the stomach, the transection is completed.

10. The duodenum is reflected, the common duct is divided, and the hepatic end is marked or tagged for later anastomosis.

11. The jejunum is clamped with two Allen forceps and the duodenojejunal flexure divided.

12. The pancreas is divided and the duct carefully identified.

13. Further mobilization of the duodenum and division of the inferior pancreaticoduodenal artery are done to permit complete removal of the specimen.

14. The most common reconstructive technique is anastomosis of the pancreas to the jejunum first, followed by the bile duct and then the duodenum (Fig. 12.16).

15. Drains may be placed, the abdomen closed, and an abdominal dressing applied.

Laparoscopic Whipple Resection

Laparoscopic Whipple resection is challenging. It is performed with increased frequency at high-volume centers. It has short-term outcomes similar to the open approach. Dissection of the pancreatic head from the portal vein and superior mesenteric artery is very challenging. Given the complexity of the procedure and the fact that the major morbidities after pancreaticoduodenectomy are not related to the size of the incision, the laparoscopic Whipple procedure has not yet become widely adopted (Dudeja et al., 2017). However, Rosok and colleagues (2010) described the following method for the laparoscopic Whipple procedure.

Operative Procedure

The patient is placed in supine position. In addition to trocars used for distal resection, two additional trocars are placed lateral to the right rectus sheath in the medioclavicular line. All dissection is done with a vessel-sealing device in accordance with standard oncologic surgical principles. Anastomosis is done with a 4-cm incision with a minimally invasive laparotomy retractor ring used with specially designed instruments. Hepaticojejunostomy is achieved with an end-to-side anastomosis using monofilament sutures. In addition,

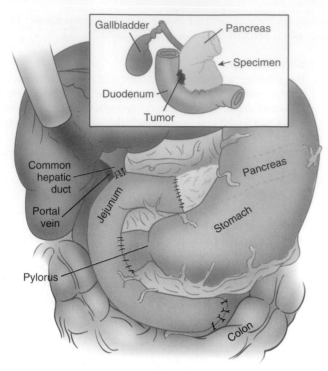

FIG. 12.16 Pylorus-preserving pancreaticoduodenectomy and the subsequent reconstruction. Inset at the top depicts the resected specimen. The jejunal limb is passed through and sutured to the transverse mesocolon.

the pancreatic anastomosis is made as an end-to-side pancreatico-gastrostomy. The gastroenterostomy is stapled as a side-to-side anastomosis using an endoscopic stapling device.

Pancreatic Transplantation

Pancreatic transplantation is the implantation of a pancreas from a donor into a recipient for patients with type 1 (formerly known as juvenile-onset) diabetes. Options for pancreatic transplant include a pancreas transplant alone (PTA), an option chosen for patients with functioning kidneys; a simultaneous pancreas-kidney transplant (SPK), because severe diabetes is often associated with chronic renal failure; or a pancreas after kidney (PAK) transplant, in which the pancreas is transplanted sometime after the kidney transplant. Pancreatic transplantation differs from other organ transplants in that it does not have immediate lifesaving results. It is done in the hope of preventing debilitating side effects of diabetes, such as cardiovascular, retinal, and renal disease. If a patient with insulin-dependent diabetes undergoes a successful pancreatic transplant, it may eliminate the need for frequent glucose monitoring, decrease the need for rigid dietary restrictions, and reduce the need to closely monitor for hypoglycemic events (Becker and Witkowski, 2017). Transplant is most effective in people with few or no secondary diabetic complications because it may reverse or stop the progression of these complications. A new option on the horizon for persons with diabetes is an implanted microelectromechanical system (MEMS). It includes an implantable insulin pump that delivers insulin in response to blood glucose levels (Jivani et al., 2016), which could replace injectable insulin and glucose meters.

Procedural Considerations

Communication among team members is essential in all transplant surgeries. The verification process for organ transplant, established

BOX 12.2

Cultural Considerations in Organ Transplantation

The following are some of the policies set forth by the HRSA to ensure organs for transplant are distributed fairly.

Organ Offers

Nondiscrimination in Organ Allocation

A candidate's citizenship or residency status in the United States must not be considered when allocating deceased donor organs to candidates for transplantation. Allocation of deceased donor organs must not be influenced positively or negatively by political influence, national origin, ethnicity, sex, religion, or financial status.

Order of Allocation

The process of allocating deceased donor organs occurs with these steps:

1. The match system eliminates candidates who cannot accept the deceased donor based on size or blood type.
2. The match system ranks candidates according to the allocation sequences in the organ allocation policies.
3. The OPO must first offer organs to potential recipients in the order that the potential recipients appear on a match run.
4. If no transplant program on the initial match run accepts the organ, the host OPO may give transplant programs the opportunity to update their candidates' data with the OPTN contractor. The host OPO may do an updated match run and allocate the organ according to the updated candidate data.
5. If no transplant program within the Donation Service Area or through an approved regional sharing arrangement accepts the organ, the Organ Center will allocate an abdominal organ first regionally and then nationally, according to allocation policies. The Organ Center will allocate thoracic organs according to *Policy 6: Allocation of Hearts and Heart-Lungs* and *Policy 10: Allocation of Lungs.*
6. Members may export deceased donor organs to hospitals in foreign countries only after offering these organs to all potential recipients on the match run. Members must submit the *Organ Export Verification Form* to the OPTN contractor before exporting deceased donor organs.

HRSA, Health Resources and Services Administration; *OPO*, Organ Procurement Organization; *OPTN*, Organ Procurement and Transplant Network.
Modified from Organ and Transplantation Network: *Policies* (website). https://optn.transplant.hrsa.gov/media/1200/optn_policies.pdf#nameddest=Policy_05. (Accessed 3 November 2016).

by the United Network for Organ Sharing (UNOS), must be followed to ensure that the organs of the donor and the recipient are compatible (Patient Safety) (Box 12.2). Prevention of technical failure is the main objective for pancreatic transplant. Many variables are associated with the procedure and no single technique is universally used. The majority of pancreas transplants performed in the United States are SPK procedures (Fig. 12.17). Instrumentation includes a transplant set as described for kidney transplantation in Chapter 15. In addition, vascular instruments and instruments for resection of the duodenal segment and management of the pancreatic duct are required. A linear stapling device may be used.

The patient is positioned supine after administration of a general anesthetic. The anesthesia provider may insert an NG tube after intubation. An indwelling urinary catheter is inserted before the abdominal skin prep and is attached to a urometer. Like other transplant procedures, these procedures are lengthy, lasting 5 to 7 hours. Positional pressure sites must be padded and a pressure-reducing

PATIENT SAFETY

Transplant of Donor Organs/Tissues: Example of Procedure for Establishing Identity and Matching Donor With Recipient

Before transplant surgery, several checkpoints are implemented to ensure identity and matching between the organs/tissues of the donor and the recipient.

Before the patient enters the OR, the following must occur:

Verification (Presurgical)

1. Verification is done of donor ID, donor blood type and subtype (if used for allocation), and organ type (with laterality if applicable), for all deceased donors before incision. Verification is completed by a qualified healthcare professional who is an OPO employee and the surgeon recovering the donor organ(s).
2. When the intended recipient is known, verification is made of the unique intended recipient identifier and intended recipient blood type. Verification is done, if the donor and intended recipient are blood type compatible or intended incompatible, by two qualified healthcare professionals, one of which must be an OPO staff member.
3. Verification of specified data elements on all living donors, not just those within the same facility, is done. Verification must occur *before administration of general anesthesia* on the day of organ recovery. The elements to be verified are the living donor ID, organ type and laterality (if applicable), donor blood type and subtype (if used for ensuring transplant compatibility or allocation), intended recipient unique identifier, intended recipient blood type, that the donor and intended recipient are blood type compatible or intended incompatible, and that the correct donor organ has been identified for the correct intended recipient. Verification is done by the recovery surgeon and another licensed healthcare provider.
4. An organ check-in process must occur for all organs received from facilities outside the transplanting facility.
5. An additional pretransplant verification protocol starts before organ arrival at a facility. The elements to be verified include the expected donor ID, expected organ (and laterality if applicable), expected donor blood type and subtype (if used for allocation), recipient unique identifier, recipient blood type, and that the expected donor and recipient are blood type compatible (or intended incompatible).

For all verifications, the policy specifies acceptable sources that can be used to verify each required data element.

A transplant hospital may specify whether a candidate is willing to accept an organ from a donor known to have certain infectious diseases, according to the following:

Donor Infectious Disease Screening Options if the Donor Tests Positive for:	Then Candidates May Choose Not to Receive Offers on the Following Match Runs:
• Cytomegalovirus (CMV)	• Intestine
• Hepatitis B core antibody (HBcAb)	• Heart, intestine, kidney, liver, lung, pancreas, heart-lung, kidney-pancreas
• Hepatitis B nucleic acid test (NAT)	• Heart, intestine, kidney, liver, lung, pancreas, heart-lung, kidney-pancreas

Donor Infectious Disease Screening Options if the Donor Tests Positive for:	Then Candidates May Choose Not to Receive Offers on the Following Match Runs:
• Hepatitis C (HCV) antibody	• Heart, intestine, kidney, liver, lung, pancreas, heart-lung, kidney-pancreas
• Hepatitis C nucleic acid test (NAT)	• Heart, intestine, kidney, liver, lung, pancreas, heart-lung, kidney-pancreas
• HIV; organs from HIV-positive donors may only be recovered and transplanted according to the requirements in the Final Rule	• Kidney, liver; use of HIV-positive donor organs is only permissible for kidney and liver transplantation at this time

Modified from Organ Procurement and Transplantation Network: *Policies* (website). https://optn.transplant.hrsa.gov/governance/policies. (Accessed 15 October 2016).

1. Once a transplant has been posted, PTCRs are faxed from the HLA laboratory to the OR where the transplant is to occur. The blood bank will fax ABO reports.
2. The OR charge nurse verifies the posted recipient's PTCR and the ABO report.
3. The organ arrives at the OR.
4. The circulating nurse applies an Addressograph label to the box with the organ.
5. The circulating nurse and another registered nurse together do the following:
   a. Verify the tag on the organ with the PTCR to ensure the following matches:
      i. Recorded ABO type of the recipient is the same or is compatible with the recorded ABO type of the donor
      ii. The UNOS number on the organ is the same as the UNOS number on the PTCR.
   b. Identify the patient using the usual hospital policy.
   c. Sign the transplant verification form.
   In the OR, the following must occur:
6. Preliminary anatomic checks are done by the transplant surgeon. The transplant surgeon verifies
   a. that the UNOS number on the PTCR is the same as the UNOS number on either the organ container or the paperwork provided; and
   b. the compatibility of the organ and the patient by ABO blood type.
   The transplant surgeon then signs the transplant verification form.
7. Once the patient is taken into the OR, the OR team takes a time-out.
8. The transplant verification form and PTCR are a permanent part of the patient's medical record.
9. The transplant verification form (deceased donor) is attached to the record.

HLA, Human leukocyte antigen; *OPO,* Organ Procurement Organization; *PTCR,* preliminary transplant crossmatch reports; *UNOS,* United Network for Organ Sharing.

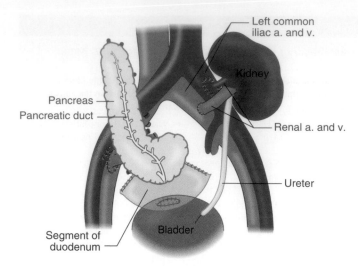

FIG. 12.17 Transplantation of the pancreas with drainage of the bladder through a pancreaticoduodenocystostomy. A renal transplant is also shown with the common iliac vessels used for vascular anastomoses. *a*, Artery; *v*, vein.

mattress placed on the OR bed. Given the patient's diabetes mellitus, maintaining skin and tissue integrity is paramount. IPCDs will likely be used. The anesthesia provider carefully monitors blood glucose levels throughout the procedure. Blood and blood products are ordered, and their availability verified. Blood-warming devices, a forced-air warming device, warmed irrigating solution (105°F [<40.5°C]), and other measures are used to maintain normothermia. The patient is usually transferred to the SICU on completion of the procedure.

Measures to address and reduce patient and family anxiety are part of all transplant programs. At-home rehabilitation is a gradual process, and social services and other resources are part of the transplant team. The patient must take immunosuppressive drugs indefinitely.

Operative Procedure (Whole-Organ Pancreatic Transplantation)

1. The whole-organ pancreatic transplantation procedure is performed through an oblique incision opposite the side of the renal transplant in the lower abdominal quadrant. A midline incision may also be used for pancreatic transplant.
2. The external iliac artery and vein are skeletonized and lymphatics are tied off with 4-0 nonabsorbable ligatures.
3. The external iliac vein is clamped with noncrushing vascular clamps and a #11 blade is used to make a venotomy.
4. The venotomy incision is extended with Potts scissors.
5. An end-to-side anastomosis of the donor portal vein to the recipient's external iliac vein is performed with four double-armed 5-0 polypropylene sutures.
6. The external iliac artery is then clamped and an aortic punch is used to make an arteriotomy.
7. An end-to-side anastomosis of the recipient's external iliac artery with the donor aortic patch containing the origin of the superior mesenteric artery and the celiac axis is performed with four double-armed 6-0 polypropylene sutures.
8. Management of the pancreatic duct is then performed, according to the type of en bloc procedure performed.
9. Various enteric procedures for drainage of pancreatic duct secretions have been performed with whole-organ transplants en bloc with

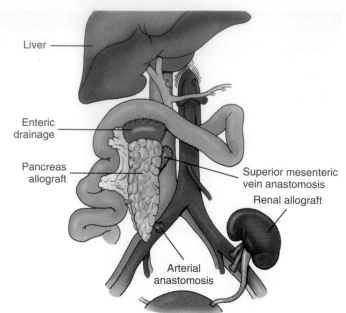

FIG. 12.18 Pancreas and kidney transplants (pancreas after kidney or simultaneous pancreas-kidney transplant) with the donor pancreas vascularized to facilitate enteric exocrine drainage to a proximal portion of the jejunum (enteric drainage technique). The donor kidney is implanted in the left iliac fossa, anastomosed to the femoral vessels and a ureteroneocystostomy is performed.

a segment of duodenum and the spleen. They include cutaneous jejunostomy, drainage into an ileal loop, and duodenojejunostomy with end-to-end or side-to-side anastomosis. Direct grafting of the pancreatic duct into the enteric or urinary system is also performed for management of exocrine secretions. Surgical procedures include pancreaticojejunostomy with an established Roux-en-Y loop of jejunum (Fig. 12.18), pancreaticoductoureterostomy, and pancreaticocystostomy. The whole-organ pancreas transplant may also be performed as a pancreaticoduodenal transplantation or a pancreaticoduodenal-splenic transplantation (Research Highlight).

Surgery of the Liver

Drainage of Abscess

Abscesses of the liver occur primarily by spread of bacteria or other organisms through the portal system (a direct route after trauma), the biliary tract, or the hepatic artery (in generalized septicemia). In addition, direct extension from a subdiaphragmatic or subhepatic abscess can lead to a liver abscess. Broad-spectrum antibiotics are started that cover gram-positive, gram-negative, and anaerobic bacterial strains. In most instances percutaneous drainage is effective and safe for hepatic abscesses. Laparoscopic drainage procedures have been reported with some success and are a reasonable option for select patients (Dudeja and Fong, 2017). However, open procedures (described in the following sections) may be required, often via the transperitoneal route. This approach permits inspection of the abdominal cavity for the underlying source of the abscess.

Procedural Considerations

A basic laparotomy set is used. Biliary instrumentation, drainage materials, and aerobic and anaerobic culture tubes are needed. Safe

RESEARCH HIGHLIGHT ‖

Islet Cell Transplantation: Pancreatic Islet Cell Transplantation

The pancreatic islets, responsible for insulin production (also called islets of Langerhans), are scattered throughout the pancreas. Destruction of these cells by an autoimmune process leads to type 1 diabetes. A procedure to replace these cells is the pancreatic islet transplantation. In 2000, islet transplantation was first developed by Shapiro in Canada (Clinical Islet Transplant Consortium, 2017).

The main goal of pancreatic transplantation is to replace the islet cells (insulin-producing cells) of the pancreas. Islet transplantation is a minimally invasive procedure that avoids an abdominal procedure and its possible surgical complications.

There are several indications for islet transplantation, including persons with hard to control blood glucose, frequent hypoglycemia, and occurrence of microvascular and macrovascular changes.

For this type of transplantation, one or more pancreases are procured from deceased donors. Special attention is given to proper cooling of the organ and taking care to not injure the capsule (Becker and Witkowski, 2017; Lazear, 2016).

The method of preparation is as follows:

1. The pancreas(es) is dissociated during enzymatic digestion with collagenase.
2. The islets are separated from acinar tissue during gradient purification.
3. Islets can be cultured for up to 72 hours, which allows an elective procedure and preparation of the patient.

The islets are then infused via a catheter through the upper abdomen into the portal vein of the liver by an interventional radiologist. It can be done with local anesthesia. With only the islets transplanted, pain and recovery time are diminished compared with whole-pancreas transplantations. Currently this procedure is experimental in the United States. Research continues to investigate the best ways to implant the islet cells and to prevent their rejection. Widespread acceptability has not occurred because of the following reasons:

1. The necessity of several donors in some cases to provide enough islet cells
2. Enough islet cells transplanted to decrease the need for outside sources of insulin
3. Graft failure because of continued autoimmunity and alloimmunity
4. The high amount of immunosuppressive drugs required after transplantation
5. Oxidative stress caused by hypoxia or inflammation
6. Loss of function caused by poor revascularization

Pancreatic Islet Cell Development and Regeneration

Stem-cell based treatment has been used to stimulate islet graft cells in preclinical and clinical settings in which special attention is given to engraftment-enhancing treatment to various types of stem cells. As stem-cell research and development broadens, there may be potential to create pancreatic beta cells in the laboratory that can be used for transplant.

Modified from Cunha JP et al: Stem-cell-based therapies for improving islet transplantation outcomes in type 1 diabetes, *Curr Diabetes Rev* June 28, 2016 [Epub ahead of print]; Clinical Islet Transplantation Consortium: *What is islet transplantation?* (website). www.citisletstudy.org/islet.html. (Accessed 28 June 2017); Hajizadeh-Saffar E et al: Inducible VEGF expression by human embryonic stem cell-derived mesenchymal stromal cells reduces the minimal islet mass required to reverse diabetes, *Sci Rep* 5:9322, 2015; Romer AI, Sussel L: Pancreatic islet cell development and regeneration, *Curr Opin Endocrinol Diabetes Obes* 2(4):255–264, 2015; Becker Y, Witkowski P: Kidney and pancreas transplantation. In Townsend CM et al, editors: *Sabiston textbook of surgery*, ed 20, Philadelphia, 2017, Saunders; Lazear J: Nursing management, diabetes mellitus. In Lewis S et al, editors: *Medical-surgical nursing: assessment and management of clinical problems*, ed 9, St Louis, 2016, Mosby.

practices for handling specimens such as cultures are initiated. The patient is positioned supine after administration of a general anesthetic. The anesthesia provider may insert an NG tube after intubation. An indwelling urinary catheter may be inserted before the abdominal skin prep.

Operative Procedure

1. The incision preferred by many surgeons is the transperitoneal route; the surgical approach may be modified, however, according to the location of the abscess (e.g., in a high posterior abscess, the transpleural approach may be selected).
2. The abdomen is opened as described for laparotomy and abdominal inspection carried out.
3. The abscess is mobilized and evacuated, and cultures obtained.
4. Surgical drains are placed and the wound closed.

Hepatic Resection

Anatomically the liver is divided into left and right lobes, with the caudate lobe lying in the dorsal segment. Resection of the liver is undertaken for primary tumors, benign conditions (e.g., hepatolithiasis), and metastatic tumors. Hepatic resection is usually approached in one of three ways. The *anatomic* approach is based on the premise that malignant cells distribute along the portal venous segmental supply. In the *enucleation* approach specific benign lesions with limited chance of local invasion are removed. The third approach *(nonanatomic)* includes resections appropriate for a pathologic process in which a limited margin is acceptable, such as in tumor debulking (Dudeja and Fong, 2017).

Many advances have improved the outcomes for patients undergoing hepatic surgery. One of these is an improved understanding of the segmental anatomy of the liver, making intrahepatic dissection safer and more precise. There are many ways to transect liver tissue and many methods to coagulate and control vessels, and these vary according to the disease requiring resection. Removal of normal liver should be kept to a minimum in these cases, and techniques such as enucleation are appropriate, although a major resection is occasionally necessary. For malignant disease, a margin of normal tissue is important, and formal anatomic resections yield the best results. Techniques such as wedge resection often result in higher rates of margin involvement and disease recurrence. They are, therefore, used carefully and sparingly (Dudeja and Fong, 2017).

The liver is divided into eight segments. The common surgeries for liver segments include the following (Dudeja and Fong, 2017):

- Right hepatectomy: Segments V through VIII (right *hepatectomy* and right hemihepatectomy); this can be extended further to include segment IV (right-left trisectionectomy)

- Left hepatectomy: Segments II through IV compose the left liver (left *hepatectomy* and left hemihepatectomy). This can be extended further to the right to include segments V and VIII.
- Trisegmentectomy: Removal of segments IV, V, VI, VII, and VIII.
- Left lateral segmentectomy or left lateral sectionectomy: Resection of segments II and III.
- Right posterior sectorectomy-sectionectomy and right anterior sectorectomy-sectionectomy: Segments VI and VII or the right anterior sector (segments V and VIII).

For patients with liver carcinoma, there are also other treatment options. These include the following (Dudeja and Fong, 2017):

- Ablation: Cryotherapy, radiofrequency ablation, and microwave use heat or cold to destroy tumors. This may be done at the time of laparotomy or laparoscopy.
- Transarterial embolization and chemoembolization: Usually done percutaneously, this therapy induces ischemic necrosis. Chemotherapeutic agents may also be added.
- Radiotherapy: A combination of ablation and transarterial external beam radiation.
- Systemic treatment with chemotherapy.
- Hormonal and immunotherapy: These new therapies are on the horizon and have been used in a limited number of patients.

Procedural Considerations

Instruments used are a laparotomy set, biliary instruments, vascular instruments, noncrushing liver clamps, a self-retaining retractor, and a surgical stapler. Supplies and equipment should be available for thermoregulation, electrosurgery, measurement of portal pressure, and replacement of blood loss. For major liver procedures, intraoperative ultrasound (to guide vessel isolation and minimize vascular occlusion), the argon beam coagulator, and the CUSA are used. Special blunt needles for suturing liver tissue are also necessary.

The patient is placed in supine position. Mild Trendelenburg position may be requested by the surgeon. The anesthesia provider may insert an NG tube after induction of general anesthesia and intubation. An indwelling urinary catheter is inserted before abdominal skin preparation. The abdomen is prepped from nipple line to midthigh. Surgeons often use a right subcostal incision, with the ability to extend with a left subcostal if necessary. In some instances a median sternotomy or right thoracotomy incision is required, and chest instruments are then necessary. Liver sutures, absorbable or nonabsorbable (according to surgeon preference), vessel loops, and umbilical tapes are available on the sterile field.

Hemostatic material, such as Gelfoam, Surgicel, or Avitene, and absorbable collagen sheets are readily available when the resection begins. The potential for bleeding exists both intraoperatively and postoperatively because of the high vascularity of the liver. If postoperative bleeding and subsequent hypovolemia occur, it may become necessary to call a rapid response team.

Surgeons use various methods to remove liver tissue. A CUSA allows the surgeon to dissect tissue using ultrasonic waves incorporated with fluid and suction. The ultrasonic waves cut through liver tissue, emulsifying it and diluting the tissue with fluid so that it can be suctioned. The ESU active electrode (pencil or handpiece) uses electrical current to cut through and desiccate liver tissue. Finger-fracture of liver tissue is performed by digital pressure against the parenchyma.

Operative Procedure

1. Through a right subcostal incision, the abdominal cavity is opened and examined.

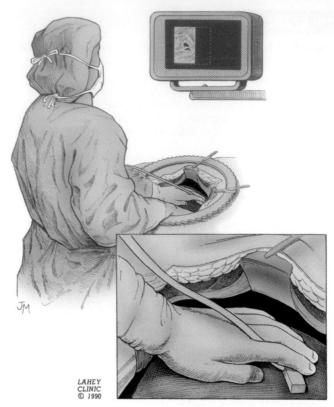

FIG. 12.19 Use of intraoperative ultrasound using a 7-MHz T-probe to permit assessment of the liver.

2. Pathologic condition is determined and resectability evaluated.
3. Moist laparotomy packs are inserted and a self-retaining retractor placed.
4. Intraoperative ultrasonography (US) is performed to assess all segments of the liver (Fig. 12.19). Ultrasound-guided digital intraparenchymal isolation of vessels is used during resection.
5. Lymph nodes in the porta hepatis and along the gastrohepatic ligament are then assessed by palpation to determine extrahepatic metastasis.
6. The intended resection line is scored with the blade tip of the ESU pencil, and coagulation is set at the surgeon's selected setting (Fig. 12.20).
7. The liver parenchyma is then delicately resected using the CUSA handpiece (Fig. 12.21).
8. Once the portion of the liver is resected, the remaining liver resection margins are assessed for bleeding and bile leakage.
9. A laparotomy sponge may be placed against the transected surface for several minutes. The laparotomy sponge is gently rolled from the surface, which is then examined for bile leakage.
10. Areas may then be oversewn with 2-0 or 3-0 absorbable suture, or an intended layer of eschar is applied using electrocoagulation or the argon beam coagulator.
11. Abdominal drains may be placed along the liver bed and exteriorized through the abdominal wall through separate stab wounds.
12. The abdominal wound is then closed and dressings applied.

Laparoscopic Hepatic Surgery

Procedural Considerations

Laparoscopy for liver resection is a highly specialized field. It can present severe technical difficulties such as bleeding control. Other

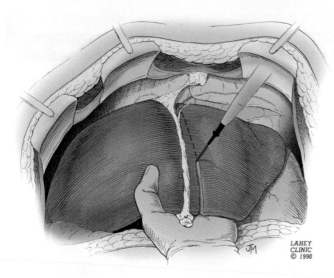

FIG. 12.20 Use of electrosurgical pencil with blade tip to score the line of resection on the surface of the liver.

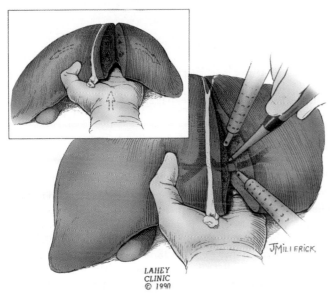

FIG. 12.21 Use of the Cavitron ultrasonic surgical aspirator handpiece to dissect through the hepatic parenchyma.

limitations relate to inadequate retraction, the inability to assess safe margins of resection with the loss of tactile sense, difficulty with safe parenchymal transection, and the potential for injury of adjacent structures (Song, 2015). However, laparoscopic liver surgery has become a safe and effective approach in many institutions (Boggs, 2015).

Minimally invasive hepatic resection approaches include pure laparoscopic, hand-assisted laparoscopic, and a hybrid approach in which the procedure is begun laparoscopically to mobilize the liver and start dissection, followed by a small laparotomy to complete the parenchymal transection. Single-incision approaches have also been developed in an attempt to minimize abdominal wall trauma (Claude et al., 2014).

Laparoscopic ultrasound navigation is often an important element in laparoscopic hepatic surgery. It enables determination of tumor location and its relationship to adjacent vascular and biliary structures.

At low power it causes no tissue damage and is used mainly for diagnostic purposes. With a high-frequency setting, ultrasound can be used to dissect, cut, and coagulate (Eisele, 2016).

Liver Transplantation

Liver transplantation is implantation of a liver from a donor into a recipient. The procedure includes retrieving or procuring the liver from a donor, transporting the donor liver to the recipient's hospital, performing a hepatectomy on the recipient, and then implanting the donor liver. Reanastomoses are then undertaken of the suprahepatic vena cava, infrahepatic vena cava, portal vein, and hepatic artery; biliary reconstruction with end-to-end anastomosis of donor and recipient common bile ducts; or Roux-en-Y anastomosis if the recipient's bile duct is absent as a result of biliary atresia.

Liver transplantation is indicated for patients with chronic hepatocellular disease, chronic cholestatic disease, metabolic liver disease, primary hepatic cancer, acute fulminant liver disease, and inborn errors of metabolism. When malignancies are the cause of end-stage liver disease, the right upper quadrant may be radiated intraoperatively—after hepatectomy and before transplantation.

Patients undergo extensive physiologic and psychologic assessment and evaluation by physicians and transplant coordinators before being placed on a national-network waiting list. The potential for postoperative complications (Table 12.1) requires ongoing evaluation.

Procedural Considerations

Successful transplantation requires the cooperative efforts of the organ procurement agency and the staff of the donor and recipient hospitals. Usually two members of the surgical team from the recipient's hospital travel to the donor's hospital to procure the donated liver. Multiple transplant teams may arrive at the donor hospital to procure various organs for transplantation. UNOS policies dictate a detailed system for checking and rechecking organs for transplantation to ensure that organs of the donor and recipient are compatible (see Patient Safety box). These policies are strictly followed before any transplantation can take place. Safe practice further requires that hospital policies are consistent with applicable law and organ donation regulations, address patient and family preferences for organ donation, and specify the roles and desired outcomes for every stage of the donation process.

Preparing the Operating Room for the Donor. The donor OR is set up for a major laparotomy procedure. Basic instrumentation and equipment include a basic laparotomy set, cardiovascular instruments, power sternal saw, and nephrectomy instruments. A sterile, draped, medium-size instrument table is needed for preparation of the liver away from the main sterile field and instrument tables. The procurement team provides special Collins solution for flushing the organs, sterile plastic containers and ice chests for organs, and in situ flush tubing. The liver is generally placed in two Lahey bags immediately after procurement.

Preparing the Operating Room for the Recipient. Each transplant surgeon has preferred instruments, supplies, and sutures. Generally the following are needed in the recipient's OR: a basic laparotomy set, a cardiovascular instrument set, an assortment of T-tubes, a slush unit or means of providing iced lactated Ringer's solution, two ESUs, a forced-air warming device, a temperature probe, IV volumetric pumps on stands, two blood warmers or water baths, an indwelling urinary catheter, an insertion tray, and a urometer. An argon beam coagulator may be used and should be available. A defibrillator is located in the room with sterile external paddles available.

TABLE 12.1

Assessment and Prevention of Common Postoperative Complications Associated With Liver Transplants

Assessment	Prevention
Acute Graft Rejection	
Occurs from fourth to tenth postoperative day	Expect prophylaxis with immunosuppressant agents, such as cyclosporine
Manifested by tachycardia, fever, RUQ or flank pain, diminished bile drainage or change in bile color, or increased jaundice	Diagnose early to treat with more potent antirejection drugs
Laboratory changes include increased levels of serum bilirubin, transaminases, and alkaline phosphatase, and prolonged prothrombin time	Use antibiotic prophylaxis
Infection	
Can occur at any time during recovery	Diagnose early and treat with organism-specific antiinfective agents
Manifested by fever or excessive, foul-smelling drainage (urine, wound, or bile); other indicators depend on location and type of infection	Perform frequent cultures of tubes, lines, and drainage
	Remove invasive line as early as possible
	Use good hand hygiene
Hepatic Complications (Bile Leakage, Abscess Formation, Hepatic Thrombosis)	
Manifested by decreased bile drainage, increased RUQ abdominal pain with distention and guarding, nausea or vomiting, increased jaundice, and clay-colored stools	Keep T-tube in dependent position and secure to patient; empty frequently, recording quality and quantity of drainage
Laboratory changes include increased levels of serum bilirubin and transaminases	Report manifestations to physician immediately
	May necessitate surgical intervention
Acute Renal Failure	
Caused by hypotension, antibiotics, cyclosporine, acute liver failure, or hypothermia	Monitor all drug levels with nephrotoxic side effects
Indicators of hypothermia include shivering, hyperventilation, increased cardiac output, vasoconstriction, and alkalemia	Prevent hypotension
	Observe for early signs of renal failure and report them immediately to physician
Early indicators of renal failure include changes in urinary output, increased BUN and creatinine levels, and electrolyte imbalance	Report manifestations to physician immediately

BUN, Blood urea nitrogen; *RUQ,* right upper quadrant.
Modified from Ignatavicius DD, Workman ML: *Medical-surgical nursing: patient-centered collaborative care,* ed 8, Philadelphia, 2016, Saunders.

Large-bore cannulae for IV monitoring and fluid or blood replacement lines are placed in addition to an arterial line and a central venous line.

Two surgeon headlights and light sources will be necessary to augment visualization of the abdominal site. A venovenous bypass system may be used to support peripheral blood flow. To support the many steps of the transplant procedure, these additional supplies should be available: extra drape sheets, table covers, gowns, towels, gloves, surgical soft goods such as sponges, gauze dissectors, and laparotomy pads; cold IV Ringer's solution; sterile IV administration set for flushing the new liver; umbilical tape; booties; hemostatic agents; and vessel loops.

A cart containing sutures and the numerous other small items should be arranged and placed in the room for each procedure. This minimizes the need for the circulating nurse to leave the patient and surgical team to obtain extra supplies.

Liver transplantation is a lengthy procedure that takes many hours. The following aspects of implementing a plan of care deserve special attention.

Patient Positioning. The patient is placed supine with knees slightly flexed and padded. An indwelling urinary catheter is inserted after induction of anesthesia. Accurate body alignment is essential. A gel pad that is the length of the OR bed or a pressure-reducing OR bed mattress is used, with attention to all potential pressure areas. Heel protectors are applied and IPCDs are placed on the patient's legs. The safety strap is placed over the lower part of the thighs and secured. A forced-air warming device is applied over the upper body, neck, and head to assist in maintaining normothermia. Fluid warmers are used to warm blood products and IV solutions.

Skin Preparation. The patient is prepped from the neck to midthigh, bedline to bedline. Prep solution should not pool at the bedline or wet the sheets on the OR bed. Fire safety precautions for prep solutions are followed.

Blood Loss and Replacement. Blood loss may be extensive and replacement must be timely. The perioperative nurse confirms that blood products are available at the beginning of the procedure (this may be incorporated into the time-out). These include 10 units each of packed red blood cells (RBCs) and fresh frozen plasma (FFP) and 1 unit of pooled donor platelets. The perioperative nurse remains available to assist the anesthesia provider during the insertion of peripheral and arterial lines. An autologous cell-saver device may be used to assist in blood replacement by way of autotransfusion.

Intraoperative Laboratory Testing. It is possible that as many as 50 blood specimens will be drawn for analysis during the procedure. Safe specimen collection practices are implemented. These specimens must be recorded on the blood-loss record and calculated into replacement needs. Specimens are delivered to the laboratory immediately. A telephone in the OR is useful for receiving and reading back critical test results/reports directly from the laboratory. Safe practices for reporting critical test results require the perioperative nurse to verify the critical test results such as these by "reading back" the result (AORN, 2016; Potter et al., 2013). Standard Precautions in collection of specimens are observed.

Length of Procedure. Procedures may last from 6 to 20 hours. Special attention is paid to maintaining the integrity of the sterile environment, given the length of surgery and number of people entering and exiting the OR.

Communication With Family. Frequent reports to the family are important. Family members often are knowledgeable about liver function tests and laboratory values and want this information in addition to reports on the condition of their loved one. One person should be assigned in advance to make regular contacts with family and support persons (Patient Engagement Exemplar). The UNOS team also works closely in communicating with the donor's and recipient's families.

Communication Among Teams. The perioperative nurse ensures that communication occurs among teams. Coordination among the procurement team, anesthesia team, and surgical teams is essential for a successful transplant procedure. Perioperative nursing responsibilities also include monitoring and communicating blood-loss volume in suction canisters and on sponges, the availability of blood and blood products, laboratory results, time of organ arrival, ischemic time, and other events as they unfold in preparation for and during the transplant procedure.

Operative Procedure

1. Bilateral subcostal incisions are made with a midline incision extended toward the umbilicus. If necessary, the xiphoid is removed. The right side of the chest is entered if additional exposure is needed.
2. Initial dissection of the underlying tissues is achieved with electrosurgery and suture ligatures.

PATIENT ENGAGEMENT EXEMPLAR

Partnerships and Communication

Patient-centered care is a guiding principle of excellence in perioperative nursing care. Patients and families are increasingly asking to partner with healthcare providers in making decisions that affect their own health or the health of a family member. Making a decision to have a liver transplant is often an emotional one; it is a lifesaving surgery that involves the death of another person who has donated a liver and this can cause many different feelings for patients and families. Perioperative nurses as partners with the patient/family should understand this and be present to discuss concerns and feelings. As partnerships are formed, perioperative nurses communicate with words that can easily be comprehended and understand the anxiety they may be feeling about the procedure. When speaking with the family of a liver transplant patient, the nurse might say:

> I understand that your family member is having a liver transplant today. The procedure involves getting the liver from a donor, transporting it to this hospital, and putting it in the patient. This requires the cooperative efforts of the organ procurement agency and the staff of the donor and recipient hospitals. Members of the surgical team from our hospital are traveling to the donor's hospital now to get the donated liver. We will be using a detailed system for checking and rechecking to make sure that the liver of the donor and recipient match. Since this is an effort of many people, we will be keeping you informed at each step and give you regular updates as the surgery progresses.

3. Isolation of all hilar structures and dissection to mobilize the lobes of the native liver are performed.
4. The retrohepatic vena cava is skeletonized, as are the hepatic artery, portal vein, common bile duct, and inferior vena cava.
5. The donor liver is examined.
6. Preparations may be made at this time for venovenous bypass using an extracorporeal assist device if the patient is unstable.
7. The infrahepatic vena cava and the suprahepatic vena cava are clamped, as are the portal vein, the hepatic artery, and the common bile duct.
8. Native hepatectomy is then performed.
9. The donor liver is placed in the right upper abdomen, and revascularization of the donor organ begins with end-to-end anastomoses in the vena cava and portal vein, with double-armed fine vascular suture.
10. At this point the clamps on the portal vein, suprahepatic vena cava, and infrahepatic vena cava are released slowly, and blood flow through the vena cava and portal vein is restored.
11. The anastomosis sites are checked for leaks.
12. If it was used, venovenous bypass is discontinued, and the cannulation sites are closed.
13. The postrevascularization phase focuses on achieving hemostasis. Complete hemostasis may require extensive time at this point. Bleeding may be exacerbated by a fibrinolytic episode associated with the reperfusion of the donor organ. The liver is monitored for a change in color from dusky to pink. An intraoperative Doppler may be used to confirm patency of the blood supply.
14. The anastomosis of the hepatic artery is then commenced, followed by bile duct reconstruction. This varies with the status of the recipient's biliary tract. If biliary atresia is the cause of the patient's end-stage liver disease, choledochoenterostomy into a Roux-en-Y loop of jejunum is performed (Fig. 12.22).
15. The anastomoses are checked for leaks.
16. Drains are placed behind and in front of the liver and exteriorized. The abdomen is then closed.

Donor Hepatectomy

Donor hepatectomy is performed for procurement of a healthy liver for transplantation into a patient who has end-stage liver failure. This procedure occurs only after the donor patient has been determined to be brain dead and family consent for organ donation has been obtained. Donor hepatectomy can be performed at any hospital. Organ procurement agencies arrange contact with transplant centers when a viable organ donor has been identified.

Procedural Considerations

Once the liver transplant candidate has been identified, the procurement team from that transplant center travels to the institution in which the organ donor is hospitalized. If multiple organs are being donated, surgeons from several transplant centers may arrive to procure the organs they will be transplanting at their respective centers.

The procedure for procurement of multiple organs differs according to the transplant centers represented. Most commonly, the systemic cooling of the donor's body temperature is started before the procurement of the heart. Cannulation sites also vary according to which organs are procured.

Perioperative nurses at the donor hospital are responsible for supplying a basic laparotomy setup with instrumentation to open the sternum. Basic vascular clamps are also required to clamp the major vascular structures. Cold lactated Ringer's solution for parenteral

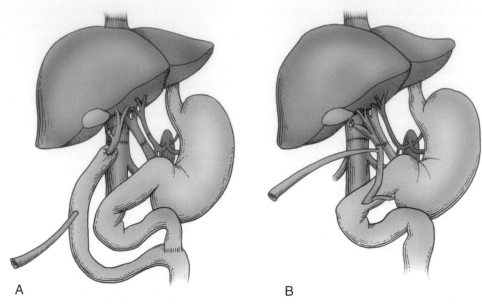

FIG. 12.22 Completed orthotopic liver transplant with Roux-en-Y biliary reconstruction (A) and end-to-end anastomosis of the donor-to-recipient common bile ducts (B).

infusion and cold Ringer's solution for irrigation are usually used in large amounts.

Operative Procedure

1. The donor patient is positioned supine on the OR bed. The skin area from neck to midthigh is prepped and draped.
2. A midline incision is made from the suprasternal notch to the pubis.
3. A subcostal incision is performed bilaterally on the abdomen for better exposure of the abdominal viscera.
4. Retractors are placed to provide optimal exposure of the organs that will be procured.
5. The aorta and vena cava, superior and inferior to the liver and kidneys, are skeletonized by dissection and ligation of the lymphatics and smaller vasculatures.
6. The porta hepatis is dissected; the superior mesenteric artery and celiac trunk are then dissected and delicately exposed as close to the aorta as is convenient.
7. The superior mesenteric vein is dissected and prepared for cannulation. The donor is heparinized and systemically cooled.
8. If the heart is to be procured, removal takes place at this time.
9. Further cooling and flushing of the pancreas, liver, and kidneys are achieved by cannulation and infusion of cold lactated Ringer's solution through the inferior vena cava just superior to the bifurcation.
10. The liver, pancreas, spleen, and a segment of the duodenum harboring the pancreatic duct are procured en bloc by placing clamps on the suprahepatic and infrahepatic venae cavae.
11. The suprahepatic vena cava is transected with a surrounding cuff of diaphragm intact.
12. The infrahepatic vena cava is transected above the level of the renal veins.
13. The celiac axis is detached from the aorta as an aortic patch or taken with a full aortic circumference.

14. The duodenal segment is procured, using a linear stapling device at opposite ends of the segment.
15. The en bloc organs are taken to a back table for further dissection and ligation to separate the liver from the en bloc pancreas, spleen, and duodenal segment graft. Meanwhile, other members of the procurement team continue working to free the kidneys and ureters if they are to be taken.
16. The liver is placed in a basin of cold Ringer's solution, double-bagged in sterile Lahey bags, and placed in an ice chest for transport to the recipient's hospital.
17. The kidneys are placed in sterile cassettes and mechanically perfused.
18. The pancreatic en bloc graft is also placed in a basin of cold Ringer's solution, bagged, and transported in a thermal chest of ice.
19. The abdomen is closed with a single layer of size 1 or 0 nonabsorbable suture.
20. Drapes are removed, and the donor patient is cleaned and washed. Tubes and infusion lines are tied off or clamped. Sometimes family members of the donor patient request to view the body after organ donation. This factor may be important in helping them face their loss. Before family viewing, cover the donor's body with a warm blanket. The perioperative nurse assists the family in their grieving process by providing a quiet and private environment in which to say good-bye to their family member. The nurse should stay with family members to support them.
21. The donor patient is then transported by stretcher to the morgue.

Living-Related Liver Transplantation

Just as kidney transplantation has evolved into living-related donor possibilities, so too has liver transplantation. The capacity of the liver to regenerate provided the scientific basis for development of the living-related donor transplantation procedure. Reduced-size and split-liver transplantations have been performed successfully. Reduced-size liver transplantation has been performed for infants, children, or very small adults with results comparable to those obtained with whole-organ transplantation. Safety issues are of the highest priority for a living donor. Careful selection of the candidate, combined with fastidious surgical technique, minimizes potential complications (Ascher, 2017). Minimally invasive techniques (laparoscopic approaches) are used in some institutions. Recipients may have an increased risk for postoperative complications such as pulmonary emboli, portal vein thrombosis, bile duct injury, and liver insufficiency secondary to a resection that is too extensive (Ascher, 2017). Prospective living donors are thoroughly evaluated with a protocol that includes blood group compatibility, a comprehensive history and physical examination, laboratory studies, psychosocial evaluation, independent advocate opinion, anatomic compatibility, review of candidacy with the donor, and presentation to a selection committee (Goldaracena et al., 2015). As cloning, biogenetic engineering, and other technologic advances increase the possibilities for organ transplants, society will need to address ongoing debates of ethical dilemmas surrounding transplantation (Research Highlight).

RESEARCH HIGHLIGHT ||

Liver Transplant and Hepatitis C in the New Era of Direct-Acting Antiviral Agents

The impact of new anti-viral drugs for HCV has the potential for improving the lives of patients who need liver transplants. Until recently, effective treatment for HCV was often not well tolerated and/or effective.

Cirrhosis and liver carcinoma caused by HCV are the most common indications for liver transplant in the United States. In patients with HCV infection, all patients have recurrence of HCV after transplantation. In addition, patients with HIV and HCV have an increased risk of mortality from liver failure. Transplants on immunocompromised patients were previously considered a contraindication.

The approval of the new drug sofosbuvir in 2013 had a huge effect on persons with HCV and liver disease. It targets the RNA within the HCV cell and prevents replication of the virus. This drug combined with ribavirin and/or ledipasvir is now the recommended treatment and cure for HCV. In addition, these direct-acting antiviral agents have minimal side effects and have been approved for the treatment of preliver and postliver transplant patients.

Use of the new drugs has the following advantages:

- Decreasing the incidence of liver failure caused by HCV and the need for liver transplants.
- Persons on the wait list for liver transplant can achieve a pretransplant virologic cure.
- In persons who have had a liver transplantation with an HCV occurrence, the drug regimen can be simplified with fewer side effects as well as cure HCV.
- Patients with HIV and HCV can have fewer drug interactions and simplified regimens.

Such advantages present the potential for changing the need for liver transplantations and/or greatly improving outcomes.

HCV, Hepatitis C virus.

Modified from Righi E et al: Impact of new treatment options for hepatitis C virus infection in liver transplantation, *World J Gastroenterol* 21(38):10760–10775, 2015; Audrey C, Raffael B: Liver transplantation for hepatitis C virus in the era of direct-acting antiviral agents, *Curr Opin HIV AIDS* 10(5): 361–368, 2015; Harvoni: *I am hepatitis cured, I let go* (website). www.harvoni.com. (Accessed 18 October 2016); Mah'moud MA: Current management of hepatitis C virus, *N C Med J* 77(3):188–193, 2016.

Surgery of the Spleen

Splenectomy (Open Approach)

Splenectomy is removal of the spleen. It is performed for multiple reasons: trauma to the spleen; specific malignant conditions (Hodgkin disease and non-Hodgkin lymphomas; hairy cell, chronic lymphocytic, and chronic myelogenous leukemias); hemolytic jaundice or splenic anemia; idiopathic thrombocytopenic purpura (ITP); tumors, cysts, or splenomegaly; or accidental injury during vagotomy or other procedures involving mobilization of the splenic flexure of the colon. If accessory spleens are present, they are also removed because they are capable of perpetuating hypersplenic function. In most instances patients evaluated for elective splenectomy are considered candidates for laparoscopic splenectomy; contraindications include severe portal hypertension, uncorrectable coagulopathy, severe ascites, extreme splenomegaly, extensive adhesions, and most traumatic injuries to the spleen. For these patients an open approach is indicated. If splenectomy is required because of trauma and there is massive hemorrhage, a surgical-crisis checklist may be implemented; Arriaga and colleagues (2013) found checklist use was associated with significant improvement in managing OR emergencies.

Procedural Considerations

Instrumentation is as described for a basic laparotomy, plus two large right-angled pedicle clamps, long instruments, and hemostatic materials and devices. Abdominal suction apparatus is available, and a cell-saver may be requested. The patient is positioned supine. After induction of general anesthesia and intubation, the anesthesia provider may insert an NG tube. An indwelling urinary catheter may be inserted before the abdominal prep. The abdomen is prepped from nipple line to midthigh. The OR bed is moved to reverse Trendelenburg position with a slight tilt to the right. A midline abdominal incision provides access to the spleen and allows maximal exposure of all abdominal organs. Occasionally a subcostal approach is used for a patient without traumatic injury. Rarely, a thoracoabdominal approach is used.

Operative Procedure

1. The abdomen is opened through the selected incision.
2. Retractors are placed over moistened laparotomy packs and exploration is carried out.
3. The costal margin is retracted upward.
4. The splenorenal, splenocolic, and gastrosplenic ligaments are clamped and divided with long dressing forceps, long hemostats, sponges on holders, and long Metzenbaum or Nelson scissors.
5. Adhesions posterior to the spleen are freed.
6. The spleen is delivered into the wound.
7. The short gastric vessels are now easily identified, clamped, divided, and ligated.
8. The cavity formerly occupied by the spleen is packed with moist laparotomy pads, if necessary.
9. The splenic artery and vein are dissected free with fine dissecting scissors and forceps.
10. The artery is clamped and doubly ligated. The artery is ligated first to permit disengorgement of blood from the spleen and facilitate return of venous blood to the circulatory system.
11. The splenic vein is then clamped, divided, and ligated.
12. The specimen is removed, bleeding vessels controlled, and the wound closed in layers, as described for laparotomy. Dressings are applied.

13. Drainage is usually required only if extensive adhesions to the diaphragm were divided or if significant clotting abnormalities exist.

Laparoscopic Splenectomy

Laparoscopic splenectomy is standard procedure for surgical treatment of benign hematologic disorders; its benefits include less postoperative pain, decreased intraoperative bleeding, and decreased length of stay (Balaphas et al., 2015; Poulose and Holzman, 2017). Indications are the same as with open procedures, with the exception of the contraindications noted previously. The laparoscopic technique has been successfully used in blunt trauma as well.

Procedural Considerations

After induction of general anesthesia, an NG tube and indwelling urinary catheter are inserted, and IPCDs are applied to the lower extremities. The patient is positioned in right lateral position, with the OR bed flexed and kidney rest raised to increase the distance between the lower rib and iliac crest. The anterior abdomen is brought close to the edge of the OR bed. A beanbag positioning device may be used. Safety restraints are placed, especially in anticipation of a possible slight backward patient tilt. Alternatively, supine or modified lithotomy position may be used. The surgeon stands on the patient's right side, as does the scrub person, and assistants stand to the left.

Instrumentation and equipment include a 30-degree telescope (10 mm or 5 mm), a camera (triple-chip or single-chip), a high-flow insufflator with tank, a high-resolution monitor (second monitor optional for assistant), a printer (optional), a Surgineedle or Veress needle, four 12-mm trocars (trocar size depends on surgeon preference; some surgeons substitute one or two of the 12-mm trocars with 5-mm trocars or even 3-mm trocars), endoshears/scissors, ultrasonic endoshears, an endodissecting forceps or endograsper (atraumatic), an endoretractor, an endoclip applier, a linear stapling device (GIA type) with vascular cartridges, an endoretrieval pouch, and a suction-irrigation system. As with other laparoscopic procedures, instruments and supplies are available if it becomes necessary to convert to an open approach.

Operative Procedure

1. Pneumoperitoneum is created and the first trocar placed under direct visualization. Three to five 2- to 12-mm operating ports are used, with the camera port at the umbilicus.
2. The laparoscope is inserted through the port and the camera placed.
3. The stomach is retracted to expose the spleen and a search made for any accessory spleens.
4. Initial dissection is begun by mobilizing the splenic flexure of the colon.
5. The splenocolic ligament is divided using sharp dissection, mobilizing the inferior pole of the spleen. The spleen is now retracted cephalad, taking care not to rupture the splenic capsule during retraction.
6. The lateral peritoneal attachments of the spleen are then incised using either sharp dissection or ultrasonic endoshears.
7. The lesser sac is entered along the medial border of the spleen.
8. With the spleen elevated, the short gastric vessels and main vascular pedicle are visualized. The tail of the pancreas is also visualized and avoided.
9. The short gastric vessels are divided by means of an ultrasonic dissector, endoclips, or an endovascular stapling device.

10. After the short gastric vessels have been divided, the splenic pedicle is carefully dissected from both the medial and lateral aspects.
11. After the artery and vein are dissected, the vessels are divided by application of the endovascular stapler. Multiple vascular branches may be encountered and each is taken individually.
12. The spleen is now devascularized and ready for removal.
13. An endoretrieval pouch is introduced through one of the trocar sites, usually the left lateral site.
14. The pouch is opened and the spleen placed into it. The drawstring is grasped and the pouch closed, leaving only the superior pole attachments, which are now divided.
15. The open end of the pouch is exteriorized from the abdomen through the supraumbilical port or epigastric trocar site. The spleen is then morcellated and removed in fragments.
16. The laparoscope is reinserted and the splenic bed is assessed for hemostasis.
17. If necessary a drain is placed in the intra-abdominal cavity, the abdomen deflated, and the trocars removed.
18. The trocar sites are then closed.

A single-port access approach is an alternative to multiport techniques. One incision is made at the umbilicus. Each trocar is inserted through a separate fascial location within the single umbilical incision. A slight extension of the incision may be necessary for the spleen removal from the abdominal cavity. The benefits of this approach include a concealed scar, decreased adhesion formation, less parietal trauma, and faster recovery (Corcione et al., 2014).

Key Points

- A pathologic condition in the liver, biliary tract, pancreas, or spleen often requires surgical intervention. Surgeries of the liver and biliary tract have become more advanced as research and technology permit more complete diagnoses of pathologic conditions.
- The nursing process of assessment, outcome identification, planning, implementation, and evaluation is used in every phase of perioperative patient care. Planning for such care requires knowledge of the anatomy and subsequent physiologic complications that may occur with surgical interruption of tissues.
- Cholecystectomy is the most common, nonemergency abdominal operation performed in the United States. Laparoscopic cholecystectomy has become the gold standard surgical intervention for the treatment of cholecystitis.
- The patient with hepatobiliary disease may have extreme jaundice, urticaria, petechiae, lethargy, and irritability. Depending on the extent of the disease, bleeding and coagulation times may be increased and the platelet count decreased, contributing to intraoperative concerns with achieving hemostasis.
- Laparoscopic pancreatic surgery is an emerging approach that is gaining acceptance. Pancreatic cancer is treated using a multidisciplinary team that often includes surgeons, gastroenterologists, oncologists, radiologists, nurses, and nutritionists.
- Pancreaticoduodenectomy (Whipple procedure) is the removal of the head of the pancreas, the entire duodenum, a portion of the jejunum, the distal third of the stomach, and the lower half of the common bile duct, with reestablishment of continuity of the biliary, pancreatic, and GI tract systems.
- Anatomically the liver is divided into left and right lobes with the caudate lobe lying in the dorsal segment. This translates into eight segments. Resection of the liver is undertaken for primary

tumors, benign conditions (e.g., hepatolithiasis), and metastatic tumors.

- Liver transplantation is the implantation of a liver from a donor into a recipient. The total procedure involves retrieving or procuring the liver from a donor, transporting the donor liver to the recipient's hospital, performing a hepatectomy on the recipient, and then implanting the donor liver. Successful transplantation requires the cooperative efforts of the organ procurement agency and the staff of the donor and recipient hospitals.
- Splenectomy is removal of the spleen. It is performed for multiple reasons: trauma to the spleen; specific malignant conditions (Hodgkin disease and non-Hodgkin lymphomas; hairy cell, chronic lymphocytic, and chronic myelogenous leukemias); hemolytic jaundice or splenic anemia; ITP; tumors, cysts, or splenomegaly; or accidental injury during vagotomy or other procedures involving mobilization of the splenic flexure of the colon.

Critical Thinking Question

A 45-year-old man is scheduled for a living related liver transplant. He will be donating part of his liver to his son who has liver failure. When you greet him in preop holding to start your assessment, you note that he is concerned about what the consequences will be for him. He asks you if his liver will return to normal functioning. What factors would you incorporate into your plan of care for this patient?

℮volve *The answer to the Critical Thinking Question can be found at http://evolve.elsevier.com/Rothrock/Alexander.*

References

Ackley BJ, Ladwig GB: *Nursing diagnosis handbook: an evidence-based guide to planning care*, ed 10, St Louis, 2014, Mosby.

American College of Surgeons: *Open operation rates for gallbladder removal drop 90 percent at one Texas institution over the course of 30 years. News from the American College of Surgeons* (website), 2016. www.facs.org/media/press-releases/jacs/gallbladder040716. (Accessed 3 November 2016).

Arriaga AF et al: Simulation-based trial of surgical-crisis checklists, *N Engl J Med* 368(3):246–253, 2013.

Ascher N: Liver transplantation. In Townsend CM et al, editors: *Sabiston textbook of surgery*, ed 20, Philadelphia, 2017, Saunders.

Association of periOperative Registered Nurses (AORN): *Guidelines for perioperative practice*, Denver, CO, 2016, The Association.

Balaphas A et al: Partial splenectomy in the era of minimally invasive surgery: the current laparoscopic and robotic experiences, *Surg Endosc* 29(12):3618–3627, 2015.

Becker Y, Witkowski P: Kidney and pancreas transplantation. In Townsend CM et al, editors: *Sabiston textbook of surgery*, ed 20, Philadelphia, 2017, Saunders.

Benner P et al: *Expertise in nursing practice: caring, clinical judgment, and ethics*, ed 2, New York, 2009, Springer.

Boggs W: *Short-term outcomes favor laparoscopic over open liver resection* (website), 2015. www.chronicliverdisease.org/reuters/article.cfm?article=20151216Scie 1837308750. (Accessed 18 October 2016).

Brynelson S: Pharmacological interventions for prevention or treatment of postoperative pain in people undergoing laparoscopic cholecystectomy, *J Perianesth Nurs* 31(3):257–259, 2016.

Clancy TE: Surgery for pancreatic cancer, *Hematol Oncol Clin North Am* 29(4):701–716, 2015.

Claude T et al: Single incision laparoscopic hepatectomy: advances in laparoscopic liver surgery, *J Minim Access Surg* 10(1):14–17, 2014.

Clinical Islet Transplantation Consortium: *What is islet transplantation?* (website), 2017. www.citisletstudy.org/islet.html. (Accessed 28 June 2017).

Corcione F et al: Robotic single-access splenectomy using the Da Vinci Single-Site® platform. A case report, *Int J Med Robot* 10(1):103–106, 2014.

Dubeck D: Robotic-assisted surgery: focus on training and credentialing, *Pennsylvania Patient Safety Advisory* 11(3):93–101, 2014.

Dudeja V, Fong Y: The liver. In Townsend CM et al, editors: *Sabiston textbook of surgery*, ed 20, Philadelphia, 2017, Saunders.

Dudeja V et al: Exocrine pancreas. In Townsend CM et al, editors: *Sabiston textbook of surgery*, ed 20, Philadelphia, 2017, Saunders.

Eisele RM: Advances in local ablation of malignant liver lesions, *World J Gastroenterol* 22(15):3885–3891, 2016.

Galketiya K et al: Management of pancreatic pseudocyst: where do we stand?, *AMJ* 9(1):9–11, 2015.

Goldaracena N et al: Live donor liver transplantation: a valid alternative for critically ill patients suffering from acute liver failure, *Am J Transplant* 15(6):1591–1597, 2015.

Gomatos IP et al: Outcomes from minimal access retroperitoneal and open pancreatic necrosectomy in 394 patients with necrotizing pancreatitis, *Ann Surg* 263(5):992–1001, 2016.

Gurusamy KS et al: Pharmacological interventions for prevention or treatment of postoperative pain in people undergoing laparoscopic cholecystectomy, *Cochrane Database Syst Rev* (3):CD008261, 2014.

Jackson PG, Evans SRT: Biliary system. In Townsend CM et al, editors: *Sabiston textbook of surgery*, ed 20, Philadelphia, 2017, Saunders.

Jivani RR et al: Biomedical microelectromechanical systems (BioMEMS): revolution in drug delivery and analytical techniques, *Saudi Pharm J* 24(1):1–20, 2016.

Kamiński JP et al: Robotic versus laparoscopic cholecystectomy inpatient analysis: does the end justify the means?, *J Gastrointest Surg* 18(12):2116–2122, 2014.

Lazear J: Nursing management, diabetes mellitus. In Lewis S et al, editors: *Medical-surgical nursing: assessment and management of clinical problems*, ed 9, St Louis, 2016, Mosby.

Lee JS, Hong TH: Laparoscopic choledochojejunostomy in various hepatobiliary and pancreatic surgeries: a single surgeon's experience, *J Laparoendosc Adv Surg Tech A* 25(4):305–310, 2015.

Memeo R et al: Robotic pancreaticoduodenectomy and distal pancreatectomy: state of the art, *J Visc Surg* 153(5):353–359, 2016.

Potter P et al: *Documentation and informatics. Fundamentals of nursing*, ed 8, St Louis, 2013, Mosby.

Poulose BK, Holzman MD: The spleen. In Townsend CM et al, editors: *Sabiston textbook of surgery*, ed 20, Philadelphia, 2017, Saunders.

Priego P et al: Laparoscopic choledochoduodenostomy: an option in cases of obstructive biliary tract, *Am Surg* 81(5):E195–E197, 2015.

Rosok BI et al: Single-centre experience of laparoscopic pancreatic surgery, *Br J Surg* 97(6):902–907, 2010.

Sjövall S et al: Laparoscopic surgery: a narrative review of pharmacotherapy in pain management, *Drugs* 75(16):1867, 2015.

Song T: Recent advances in surgical treatment of hepatocellular carcinoma, *Drug Discov Ther* 9(5):319–330, 2015.

Svoboda S et al: Robotic single-site cholecystectomy in the obese: outcomes from a single institution, *Surg Obes Relat Dis* 11(4):882–887, 2015.

The Joint Commission (TJC): *Universal protocol for preventing wrong site, wrong procedure and wrong person surgery* (website), 2016. www.jointcommission.org/standards_information/up.aspx. (Accessed 28 June 2016).

CHAPTER 13
Hernia Repair

JAMES D. SMITH, JR.

A hernia is a condition in which an organ or tissue protrudes through the wall of the cavity normally containing it. Hernias can be congenital in origin, or they may be the result of prolonged weakness or traumatic injury, including weakness at previous surgical sites. They can occur in any body cavity, and include intracranial hernias, spinal disk hernias, and internal hernias of the abdominal cavity. The most common form of hernias, however, and the ones most people associate with the word "hernia," are those of the abdominal wall.

Abdominal wall hernias are categorized according to their location (Fig. 13.1) and primarily consist of inguinal, femoral, umbilical, epigastric, and spigelian hernias. Ventral hernias occur along the abdominal midline and encompass both umbilical and epigastric hernias. Inguinal hernias are further classified as either direct or indirect, based on the location of the herniation within the inguinal region. Traumatic hernias, including surgical site hernias, can occur anywhere, and they are not further classified by location.

Abdominal wall hernias affect 4% of the population over 45 years of age, with inguinal hernias accounting for 75% of all abdominal wall hernias. There are approximately 20 million inguinal hernia repairs performed annually in the world, making them one of the most common surgical procedures. Men have a much higher risk of acquiring inguinal hernias than women, at 27% compared with 3%. Women have a higher incidence of femoral hernias than men, although they still have more inguinal hernias than femoral (Broadhurst and Wakefield, 2015).

Currently, there are multiple techniques available for the treatment of each type of abdominal wall hernia. These techniques include open, laparoscopic, and robotic-assisted procedures, with or without mesh or biologic grafts. Each of these techniques, and its variants, carries specific benefits and risks that must be addressed to provide a safe and effective herniorrhaphy.

Surgical Anatomy

The surgical presentation of a hernia is a bulge at the hernia site. This bulge is primarily made up of abdominal contents contained within a pouch of peritoneum called a "hernia sac," but it may contain preperitoneal fat as well. When the presence of the bulge is intermittent, the tissues involved move in and out of the defect, and the hernia is said to be reducible. When the bulge cannot be reduced, the hernia is considered incarcerated. An incarcerated hernia may be chronic or acute. In the case of a chronic incarceration, the hernia contents or sac develop adhesions preventing reduction of the hernia. In the case of an acute incarceration, reduction may be prevented by malrotation or swelling of hernia contents, or by narrowing of the fascial defect related to patient tension and pain. Patients with incarcerated hernias may present with signs of intestinal obstruction, such as vomiting, abdominal pain, and distention. The greatest danger of an incarcerated hernia is that it may become strangulated. In the event of a strangulated hernia, the blood supply of the trapped sac contents becomes compromised, causing tissue death. A strangulated hernia is a surgical emergency, requiring prompt surgical intervention to prevent necrosis of the bowel and other trapped tissues.

Inguinal Hernias

The inguinal region, also called the groin, is the inferolateral portion of the abdomen bordered by the anterior superior iliac spine superolaterally, the pubic tubercle medially, and the thigh inferiorly. The abdominal wall in the inguinal region is composed of multiple layers of supporting muscle and fascia. Moving from superficial to

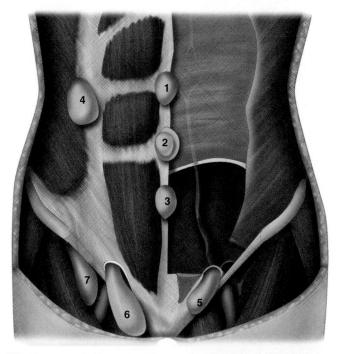

FIG. 13.1 Types of abdominal wall hernias. Diagram of the anterior abdominal wall, depicting site of abdominal wall hernias: *1*, supraumbilical hernia; *2*, umbilical hernia; *3*, infraumbilical hernia; *4*, spigelian hernia; *5*, direct inguinal hernia; *6*, indirect inguinal hernia; *7*, femoral hernia.

deep, they consist of the external oblique muscle, the internal oblique muscle, the transversus abdominis muscle, the transversalis fascia, and the peritoneum (Fig. 13.2). Each of the muscles is covered by a thin, fascial aponeurosis. A pathway, known as the inguinal canal, travels inferiorly and medially through the groin and allows the passage of structures from the abdominal wall to the external genitalia. The inguinal canal is approximately 4 cm long and contains the spermatic cord and associated structures in males and the round ligament in females. An inguinal hernia occurs when abdominal contents enter the inguinal canal.

The inguinal canal consists of anterior, posterior, superior, and inferior walls, as well as two openings known as rings. The anterior wall consists of the aponeurosis of the external oblique, reinforced by the internal oblique muscle laterally. The posterior wall is formed by the transversalis fascia. The superior wall, called the roof, is formed by the transversalis fascia, internal oblique, and transversus abdominis. The inferior wall, or floor, is composed of a "rolled-up" portion of the external oblique aponeurosis (EOA) called the inguinal ligament, or Poupart ligament. The opening into the inguinal canal from the abdomen is called the deep, or internal, ring. It is located above the midpoint of the inguinal ligament, lateral to the epigastric vessels. At the other end of the canal, the superficial, or external, ring opens superiorly to the pubic tubercle (Fig. 13.3).

If the EOA is opened and the cord or round ligament is mobilized, then the posterior wall and floor of the inguinal canal are exposed. The transversalis fascia of the posterior inguinal wall is the structure that becomes defective and is susceptible to indirect, direct, or femoral hernias. When a weakening or a tear in the aponeurosis of the transversus abdominis and the transversalis fascia occurs, the potential for development of a direct inguinal hernia is established (Fig. 13.4).

The posterior inguinal floor can be divided into two areas. The superior lateral portion contains the internal ring, and the inferior medial area contains the attachment of the transversalis aponeurosis and fascia to the Cooper ligament (iliopectineal line). The Cooper ligament is the site of insertion of the transversalis aponeurosis along the superior ramus from the symphysis pubis laterally to the femoral sheath. The inguinal portion of the transversalis fascia arises from the iliopsoas fascia and not from the inguinal ligament.

Direct and Indirect Inguinal Hernias

There are two types of inguinal hernias, direct and indirect. They are identified by their location in relation to the inferior (deep) epigastric blood vessels. The inferior epigastric vessels arise from the external iliac vessels and enter the inguinal canal just proximal to the internal ring. The triangle formed by the epigastric vessels laterally, the inguinal ligament inferiorly, and the rectus abdominis muscles

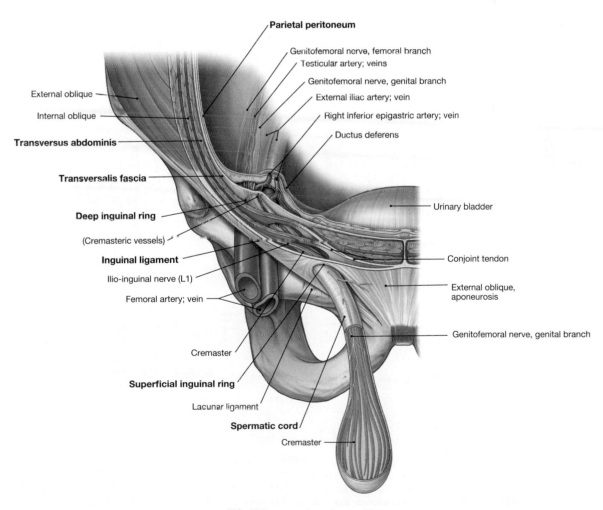

FIG. 13.2 Inguinal canal anatomy.

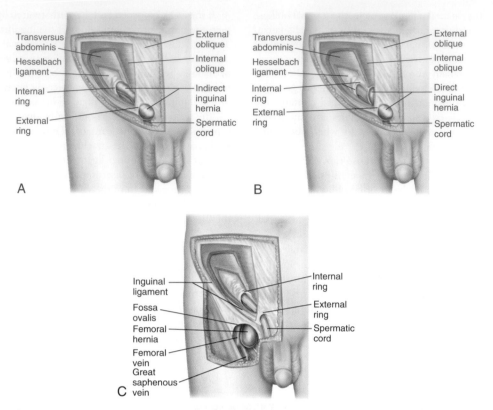

FIG. 13.3 Anatomy of region of common pelvic hernias. (A) Indirect inguinal hernia. (B) Direct inguinal hernia. (C) Femoral hernia.

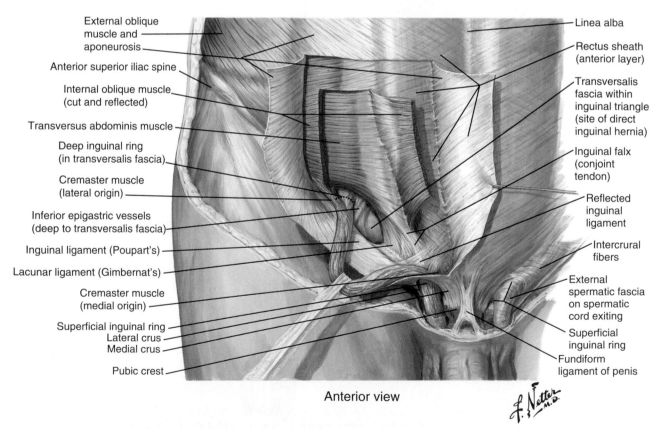

Anterior view

FIG. 13.4 Muscular planes of the lower abdomen. The right spermatic cord is retracted inferiorly to show the floor of the inguinal canal and the location of a potential direct inguinal hernia.

medially is referred to as the Hesselbach triangle (Fig. 13.5). Hernias that occur within the Hesselbach triangle are called direct inguinal hernias. Indirect inguinal hernias occur laterally to the deep epigastric vessels (Fig. 13.6).

An indirect hernia enters the inguinal canal via the deep inguinal ring. Indirect hernias may be either congenital, representing a persistence of the processus vaginalis, or acquired. A congenital hernia sac has a small neck, is thin-walled, and is closely bound to the cord structures. With an acquired indirect hernia the neck is wide and the sac is both short and thick-walled. Because it follows the course

of the cord structures, the indirect hernia sac may extend into the scrotum or labia. Indirect hernias are far more common than direct hernias, particularly in males and children.

Direct hernias enter the inguinal canal though the posterior wall of the inguinal canal, medial to the epigastric vessels. Because they protrude into the inguinal canal but not into the cord, they typically do not involve the scrotum. Being an acquired rather than congenital hernia, direct inguinal hernias result from weakening of the abdominal musculature. When both direct and indirect hernias are present, the defect is called a *pantaloon hernia*, from the French word for "pants."

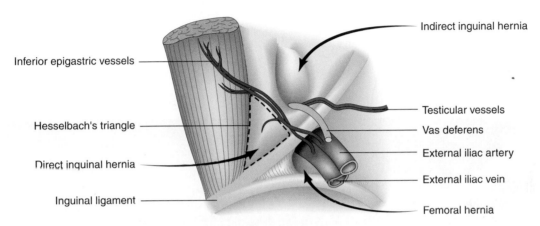

FIG. 13.5 Hesselbach triangle. The boundaries of the Hesselbach triangle are the deep epigastric vessels laterally, inguinal ligament inferiorly, and rectus abdominis muscle medially.

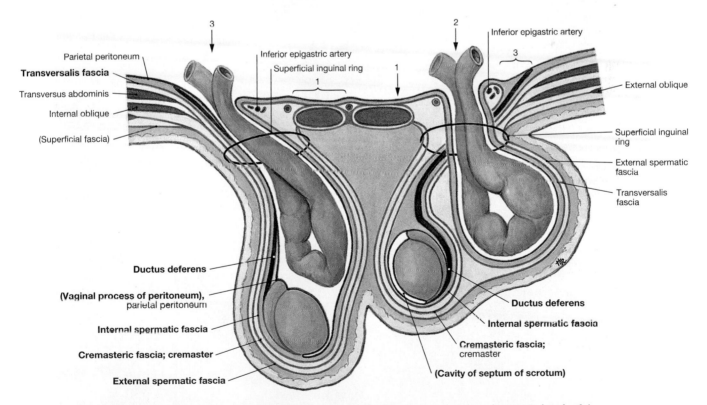

FIG. 13.6 Indirect versus direct inguinal hernias. *Left side of image:* Lateral, indirect hernia. *Right side of the image:* Medial, direct hernia. Indirect hernia shown passing through the deep inguinal ring, lateral to the inferior epigastric vessels. Direct hernia shown entering the inguinal canal medial to the inferior epigastric vessels.

Femoral Hernias

The femoral vessels pass from the groin into the thigh by way of the femoral sheath. Femoral hernias occur in the smallest, most medial compartment of the femoral sheath, which is called the femoral canal. This canal is roughly rectangular and is bordered by the femoral vein laterally, the lacunar ligament medially, the inguinal ligament anteriorly, and the pectineal ligament and pectineus muscle posteriorly (Fig. 13.7). The canal allows for passage of lymphatic vessels through an opening at the superior border known as the femoral ring, which is where femoral herniations also occur.

Femoral hernias are far less common than inguinal hernias, accounting for about 5% of groin hernias. They are also far less likely to occur in children and are more common in women than men. In elderly women they can occur almost as frequently as inguinal hernias.

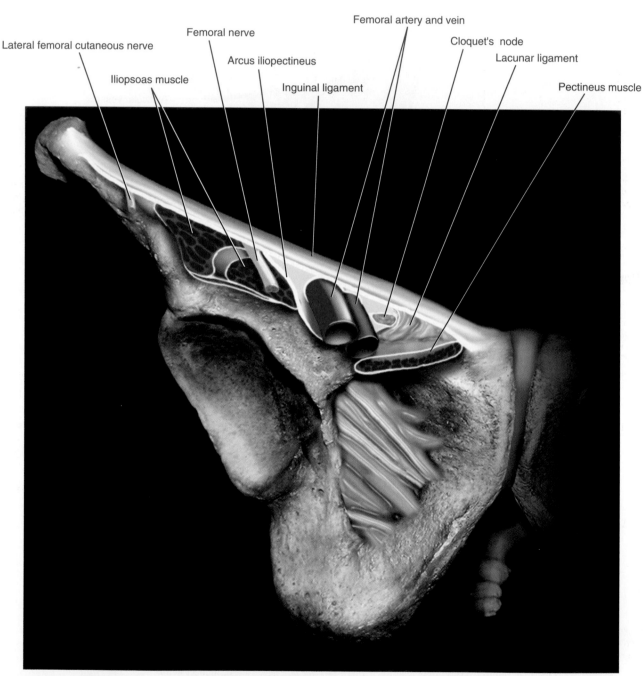

FIG. 13.7 This frontal view of the right hemi-pelvis shows, from medial to lateral, the femoral canal, Cloquet's lymph node, the femoral vein, the femoral artery, the femoral nerve, and lateral femoral cutaneous nerve. These major structures lie on the pectineus and iliopsoas muscles.

Obturator Hernias

The obturator foramen is an opening at the base of the pelvis, which allows for passage of vessels and nerves from the pelvis into the medial thigh. The foramen contains a fibrous membrane, called the obturator membrane, which almost completely closes the foramen. The remaining opening, through which the structures pass, is called the obturator canal. Although rare, hernias can occur through the obturator canal. They occur most frequently in emaciated elderly women. There is no obvious bulge associated with these hernias, and diagnosis is often made when a computed tomography (CT)

scan is performed related to symptoms of intestinal obstruction. The patient may also present with a palpable mass in the medial thigh, or pain on the medial aspect of the thigh with internal hip rotation, which is called the Howship-Romberg sign. Although rare, this hernia has a high incidence of morbidity and mortality related to strangulation of entrapped tissues, including bowel, omentum, and urinary bladder.

Ventral Hernias

The anterior abdominal wall is composed of five muscles (Fig. 13.8). Laterally, three muscles are layered with their fibers running in

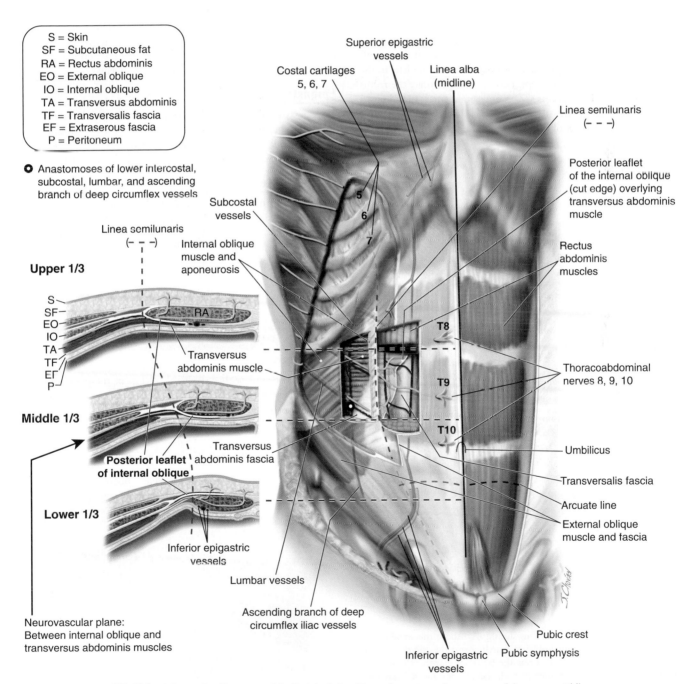

FIG. 13.8 Abdominal wall anatomy: Myofascial relationships and neurovascular anatomy of the upper, middle, and lower thirds of the abdominal wall.

different directions, providing added strength, and preventing hernias. The most superficial of these muscles is the external oblique, followed by the internal oblique, and finally by the transversus abdominis, under which lies the transversalis fascia. Bilaterally, the aponeuroses of the three muscles intertwine at the midline, forming a fibrous structure called the linea alba, which runs from the xiphoid process superiorly to the symphysis pubis inferiorly. Medial to these muscles lies the rectus abdominis, with the pyramidalis lying superficially to it at the inferior edge, and attaching to the pubis bone. These muscles are encased in a fibrous case called the rectus sheath, which is made up of the aponeuroses of the three lateral muscles lateral to where they fuse and form the linea alba. The lateral edge of the rectus sheath forms a curved line along the border between the lateral muscles and the rectus abdominis called the semilunar line, or spigelian line. From the upper limit of the rectus abdominis to below the umbilicus, the rectus sheath is composed of an anterior sheath superficial to the rectus muscle, and a posterior sheath deep to it. At approximately one-third the distance from the umbilicus to the pubic crest, where the inferior epigastric vessels perforate the rectus abdominis, the posterior rectus sheath ends at a demarcation known as the arcuate line, or line of Douglas (Fig. 13.9). Inferior to this line, the posterior border of the rectus abdominis is the transversalis fascia.

The weakest points of the abdominal musculature, and the most common sites for hernias to occur, lie along the linea alba, and secondarily, the semilunar line. These include epigastric hernias, umbilical and paraumbilical hernias, and spigelian hernias.

Umbilical Hernias

The umbilicus, or belly button, is the scar formed by the sloughing of the umbilical cord shortly after birth. It lies along the linea alba and is used as a landmark for dividing the abdomen into quadrants. Normally the layers of the abdominal wall fuse at the site of the umbilicus by the age of 2, closing the umbilical ring through which the umbilical cord passed. A true umbilical hernia occurs when the umbilical ring fails to close, allowing abdominal contents to protrude through. These hernias are seen almost exclusively in younger children. A paraumbilical hernia occurs at the weakened area near the closed umbilical ring, typically along the midline above or below the umbilicus. Most people simply refer to these as umbilical hernias. They are the most common of the ventral hernias.

Epigastric Hernias

The epigastrium is the area between the sternum and the umbilicus. Epigastric hernias occur along the linea alba above the umbilicus and are similar to umbilical hernias. They are more common in young children and tend to be small, particularly in adult patients.

Spigelian Hernias

Hernias occurring along the semilunar line (spigelian line) are called spigelian hernias (Fig. 13.10). They are rare and often difficult to diagnose. The most common location is below the arcuate line, where the posterior rectus sheath becomes deficient. The spigelian hernia sac often passes through the transversus and internal oblique aponeuroses and then spreads out under the intact EOA, creating an unusual presentation and complicating diagnosis.

Perioperative Nursing Considerations

Assessment

Assessment begins with a thorough review of the patient's history, which includes previous surgeries related to the herniated area. Information relating to a familial history of hernias, the patient's

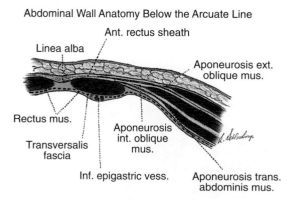

FIG. 13.9 Cross-sections of the rectus sheath. (A) Above the arcuate line, the aponeurosis of the external oblique muscle forms the anterior sheath, and the transversus aponeurosis forms the posterior sheath. The internal oblique muscle splits to contribute to both the anterior and the posterior sheaths. (B) Below the arcuate line, all aponeuroses pass anterior to the rectus.

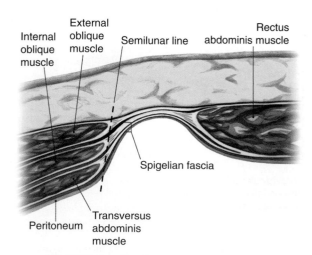

FIG. 13.10 Spigelian fascia and location of hernias.

nutritional status, duration of the symptoms, a history of or current obesity, increased intra-abdominal pressure, chronic cough, constipation, benign prostatic hypertrophy, intestinal obstruction, colon malignancy, or pregnancy is noted. A list of the patient's current medications is reviewed, along with any history of chronic illness and allergies, including latex allergies. The patient's occupation and physical activities are listed. If part of institutional protocol, verification of preoperative showering or bathing with an antiseptic agent is done during assessment.

Pain is often a notable symptom for the patient, and it may be described as a burning sensation. An accurate description of the type and degree of pain is included in the assessment; review general information about onset, duration, severity, and quality of pain, and about exacerbating and remitting factors. Patients often describe the feeling of a foreign body, or mass, at the hernia site. This may appear on arising in the morning and disappear while sleeping.

The diagnosis of hernia is accompanied by clinical physical examination. Palpation of the herniated area may suggest the contents of the hernia sac. Fingertip palpation allows the examiner to feel the edges of the external ring or abdominal wall. Having the patient stand and cough during the examination also helps in the evaluation of the herniated area. If a definitive diagnosis is not confirmed, ultrasonic scanning and imaging techniques (e.g., CT) may be used.

In some patients a hernia may cause no symptoms; the only sign may be a swelling or protrusion in an area of the abdominal wall. If the hernia is unilateral, the patient may note the lack of a protrusion on the other side in comparison. The area may be visible when the patient stands or coughs and may disappear on reclining. Femoral hernias can be difficult to diagnose and may resemble an enlarged lymph node.

During the last few decades the practice of obtaining routine preoperative studies (e.g., complete blood count [CBC], chest x-ray, and electrocardiogram [ECG]) has been a subject of much controversy. It has been somewhat established that performing routine screening tests in patients who are otherwise healthy is of little value in detecting diseases and in changing the anesthetic management or outcome. For this reason, current emphasis has shifted toward enacting preemptive, multimodal pathways designed to promote improved surgical outcomes. This approach, called enhanced recovery after surgery (ERAS), relies on a thorough history and physical examination of the patient, accompanied by preoperative nutritional enhancement and a preemptive approach to postoperative pain control (Enhanced Recovery After Surgery). Thus an otherwise healthy patient presenting for hernia repair will have, in some institutions, only selective testing, which reduces cost without sacrificing safety or quality of surgical care.

Nursing Diagnosis

Nursing diagnoses related to the care of the patient undergoing hernia surgery might include the following:

- Anxiety related to impending surgical procedure, perioperative events, and surgical outcome
- Risk for Perioperative Positioning Injury
- Risk for Thermal Injury
- Risk for Surgical Site Infection

Outcome Identification

Outcome measurement and management are important parts of perioperative nursing care. Outcomes identified for the selected nursing diagnoses could be stated as follows:

- The patient will verbalize management of anxiety and will exhibit relaxed facial expressions and body movements.
- The patient will be free of injuries related to surgical positioning.

ENHANCED RECOVERY AFTER SURGERY

Use of Enhanced Recovery After Surgery Pathways Related to Ventral Hernia Repair

ERAS pathways represent a standardized, multimodal approach to managing patients after surgical procedures. Most of the early ERAS research focused on gastrointestinal surgery, with significant improvements in LOS, postoperative complications, and readmission rates. Consequently, pathways for other surgical procedures are being developed and studied, such as this one for VHR.

Although ERAS pathways are designed to improve a patient's recovery after surgery, they involve changes to care throughout the perioperative period. The VHR pathway includes guidelines for care in preoperative, intraoperative, and postoperative periods. In the preoperative period, new emphasis is on nutrition, with the administration of supplement shakes for 5 days before surgery. On the day of surgery, the pathway includes administration of two medications previously not used for VHR. The first is gabapentin, which is used to reduce the need for anesthetics as well as the need for narcotic pain control both during and after surgery. It also provides antianxietal effects. The second medication is alvimopan, a peripherally acting μ-opioid antagonist, which helps prevent constipation effects of opioids without reducing their analgesic efficacy. The use of these two medications allows intraoperative narcotic and anesthetic usage to be minimized. Intraoperatively a TAP block is performed using liposomal bupivacaine for long-acting postoperative pain relief. Postoperatively strong emphasis is placed on intestinal recovery. Gabapentin and alvimopan are continued, narcotic use is minimized, and nasogastric tubes are not routinely used. Diet advancement is also changed under the ERAS pathway. Patients are no longer kept NPO until passing flatus. Instead, they are given limited clear liquids on the first postoperative day, including a nutritional supplement drink, ad lib clear liquids on day two, and a regular diet on day three.

The use of ERAS pathways for the management of surgical patients represents a dramatic shift away from care based primarily on the preferences and training of the surgeon and anesthesia provider. It is a standardization of the spectrum of care with the goal of returning the patient to normal function as quickly as possible. Use of this pathway for VHR resulted in quicker transition to oral narcotics, quicker return of bowel function, shorter hospital stays, fewer postoperative complications, and reduced readmission rates. The success of studies such as this one will certainly lead to the development and refinement of ERAS pathways for multiple surgical procedures.

ERAS, Enhanced recovery after surgery; *LOS,* length of stay; *NPO,* nothing by mouth; *TAP,* transversus abdominis plane; *VHR,* ventral hernia repair.
Modified from Majumder A et al: Benefits of multimodal enhanced recovery pathway in patients undergoing open ventral hernia repair, *J Am Coll Surg* 222(6):1106–1115, 2016.

- The patient will be free of both internal and external thermal injuries.
- The patient will remain free of surgical site infection throughout the postoperative period.

Planning

The perioperative nurse formulates a plan of care for the patient undergoing herniorrhaphy by assimilating knowledge pertaining to the anatomy involved, principles of asepsis, the planned surgical procedure, and requisite information provided/gained during planning specific to the surgical patient (Patient Engagement Exemplar). Instrumentation, draping, and positioning for the procedure depend on the type of hernia and repair to be performed and will differ for open versus laparoscopic repairs.

A Sample Plan of Care for a patient having surgery for hernia repair is shown on p. 385.

Implementation

Although it is important to customize the plan of care by procedure, the use of safety checklists has reduced complication rates (Gillespie et al., 2014) and become the recognized standard of care (Patient Safety). For this reason the Association of periOperative Registered Nurses (AORN) has combined the surgical checklists of the World Health Organization (WHO), and The Joint Commission (TJC) to produce a comprehensive surgical checklist (AORN, 2016). The following procedures represent one application of the checklist to the performance of hernia surgery.

Preprocedure Check-In

The patient is identified using multiple identifiers, including full name, date of birth, and medical record number. These should match the ID band. The patient verbally confirms that the surgical procedure/procedural consent matches the planned procedure, site, and side for which the team is preparing. The presence of a current history and physical; preanesthesia assessment; nursing assessment; relevant diagnostic and radiologic test results; blood products; or any special equipment, devices, or mesh implants is confirmed. An intravenous (IV) line is inserted. Monitors, such as a three-lead or five-lead ECG, pulse oximeter, and blood pressure cuff, are attached per institutional protocol. The surgeon marks the location of the surgery. A transversus abdominis plane (TAP) block may be performed to help with postoperative pain control of certain hernias (Fayezizadeh et al., 2016) (Research Highlight). If ordered, prophylactic antibiotics are administered within 1 hour of incision. This usually takes place just before leaving the preoperative area or on arrival in the operating room (OR).

Operating Room

Before the patient arrives in the OR, the sterile field is established. Sterility and completeness of all instrument sets is confirmed. All

PATIENT ENGAGEMENT EXEMPLAR

It Takes a Team

Regardless of the type of planned hernia repair, the entire perioperative team is involved. Discussions among the patient and anesthesia provider, perioperative nurse, surgical assistant, and surgeon cover specific topics to ensure that the patient knows what to expect and what is expected of the patient.

Topics for Discussion With the Perioperative Team
- Preoperative dietary recommendations
- Targeted nutritional and dietary advice for obese patients in the weeks before surgery; weight loss may improve anesthetic management and postoperative rehabilitation

- Immediate preoperative preparation
- Continuation, alteration, or cessation of normal medications
- Need for fasting (nothing by mouth [NPO])
- Choice of anesthetic technique
- Informed consent
- Information on pain management (begin pain management education preoperatively)
  Postoperatively, patients need to know what to expect.

This information is presented in the Patient, Family, and Caregiver Education box on p. 389.

Modified from Hobbs JL: A dimensional analysis of patient-centered care, *Nurs Res* 58(1):52–60, 2009; PROSPECT (procedure specific postoperative pain management): *Herniorrhaphy* (website). www.postoppain.org/sections/?root_id=28415&section=6. (Accessed 2 November 2016).

PATIENT SAFETY

Comprehensive Surgical Checklist

In 2004 TJC instituted Universal Protocols for the prevention of wrong-site, wrong-procedure, or wrong-person surgery. These now standard protocols include both written and verbal confirmation that the correct procedure is being done on the correct side of the correct patient. In 2008 WHO created a surgical safety checklist, expanding on TJC's Universal Protocols. Since that time, studies show that use of a surgical checklist combined with a structured training program consistently reduces adverse events. Despite this sentinel event data show that wrong-patient, wrong-site, or wrong-procedure surgery remains a frequently reported event. Root cause analysis of this sentinel event is often determined as "human factors." One way to improve care is through adherence to comprehensive, properly applied surgical checklists. The AORN comprehensive surgical checklist engages the entire surgical team in ensuring the patient's safety from the preoperative area until they leave the OR. The checklist is separated into four sections, by the specific verifications to be performed at given times, as follows: preprocedure check-in, sign-in, time-out, and check-out, which are used in this chapter.

AORN, Association of periOperative Registered Nurses; *TJC,* The Joint Commission; *WHO,* World Health Organization.
Modified from Stratton M: The power of checklists, *AORN J* 103(6):549–551, 2016.

SAMPLE PLAN OF CARE

Nursing Diagnosis
Anxiety related to impending surgical procedure, perioperative events, and surgical outcome

Outcome
The patient will verbalize management of anxiety, and will exhibit relaxed facial expressions and body movements.

Interventions
- Assess the patient's level of anxiety by asking questions and observing for signs of anxiety (e.g., clenched hands, tense movements, displays of emotion).
- Greet the patient positively and ask how they prefer to be addressed.
- Introduce the patient to the OR team, maintaining a calm, supportive manner.
- Offer emotional reassurance by using touch (as appropriate), helping the patient to a position of comfort on the OR bed, and providing warm blankets (thermal comfort).
- Determine the patient's personally effective coping mechanisms and facilitate use of them.
- Identify the patient's special concerns, values, and any cultural or spiritual wishes concerning his or her care.
- Provide explanations of perioperative events; encourage questions.

Nursing Diagnosis
Risk for Perioperative Positioning Injury

Outcome
The patient will be free of injuries related to surgical positioning.

Interventions
- Determine procedure-specific positioning needs (e.g., open repair versus laparoscopic versus robotic repair). Provide appropriate positioning and padding accessories.
- Note the patient's height, weight, age, and skin integrity. Make adjustments to the OR bed to maintain proper body alignment and support.
- Aid the patient to a comfortable position on the OR bed. Apply safety straps as appropriate to the procedure, explaining their necessity to the patient.
- For procedures performed in other than the supine position (e.g., laparoscopic or robotic), place the patient on a stabilization device (e.g., beanbag, gel pad, foam pad).
- Pad and secure all limbs and bony prominences, placing them in anatomic alignment, with no hyperextension of the joints.
- Assess all equipment brought to the surgical field after draping and throughout the surgery to ensure no undue pressure is applied to the patient.

Nursing Diagnosis
Risk for Thermal Injury

Outcome
The patient will be free of both internal and external thermal injuries.

Interventions
- Check the ESU and all energy-generating devices for proper function.
- Apply the ESU dispersive electrode (grounding pad) to clean, dry skin over a large muscle mass; avoid scar tissue, orthopedic hardware, hairy surfaces, joint surfaces, and bony prominences.
- Avoid pooling of prep solutions, and allow prep solutions to completely dry before draping.
- Visually inspect all energy-generating instruments for insulation integrity.
- Separate energy-generating cords from each other and from light cords to avoid capacitive coupling.
- Place the ESU active electrode (handpiece, pencil) and other energy-generating sources in a protected location (such as a sterile holster) when not in use.

Nursing Diagnosis
Risk for Surgical Site Infection

Outcome
The patient will remain free of infection throughout the postoperative period.

Interventions
- Review patient history for increased risk of infection; perform any special precautions indicated.
- Verify sterility of all items introduced to the sterile field.
- Verify room temperature between 68°F and 75°F, and humidity between 20% and 60%.
- Verify administration of prophylactic antibiotics (if ordered) within 1 hour of incision, or in accordance with your institution's policy.
- Remove any hair at the operative site (only if ordered) using clippers as opposed to a razor.
- Maintain patient normothermia through the use of warmed IV fluids, warmed forced-air blankets, warming blankets, and so forth.
- Use proper hand hygiene and sterile technique for all patient procedures (e.g., IV line starts, indwelling urinary catheter insertion).

ESU, Electrosurgical unit; *IV*, intravenous.

---

soft goods, such as sponges, sharps, and instruments, are counted and recorded according to institution protocols. Any planned or potentially necessary grafts/meshes are verified as available, and expiration dates checked. Electrical and specialty equipment (e.g., electrosurgical unit [ESU], laparoscopes, robot) is tested for proper function as applicable.

Sign-In
The patient is transferred to the OR bed. Appropriate safety straps are applied. Monitors (pulse oximeter, blood pressure cuff, and ECG leads) are reattached. Arms are padded for safety and comfort.

Intermittent pneumatic compression devices (IPCDs) are applied per institution protocol. Before induction of anesthesia, the patient's identity, procedure, and procedure site are again confirmed verbally and by site marking. A discussion among all members of the surgical and anesthesia teams verifies patient allergies, airway risks, expected blood loss, and the plan of care. The patient then receives a general anesthetic, an inguinal nerve block, a field block, a spinal or epidural block, a regional anesthetic with sedation, or a local anesthetic (Surgical Pharmacology) with moderate sedation/analgesia. An indwelling urinary catheter is placed, if appropriate, for the scheduled procedure. Any needed changes to the position are made securing

RESEARCH HIGHLIGHT ‖

Use of Transversus Abdominis Plane Blocks With Liposomal Bupivacaine for Postoperative Pain Control After Open Ventral Hernia Repair

A primary concern associated with open VHR is postoperative pain control. Open VHR is an invasive procedure, often involving large upper abdominal incisions, extensive dissection, and the fixation of mesh, frequently resulting in an increased need for narcotic pain control (both IV and oral) and extended LOS. In this study, researchers examined the efficacy of TAPb, utilizing LB, to improve postoperative pain control. Effectiveness was gauged by postoperative utilization of narcotics, numerical rating scale pain scores, time to oral narcotics, and LOS.

One hundred patients undergoing open VHR were enrolled, with 50 receiving TAPb and the remaining 50 in the control group. The TAPb consisted of 20 mL of LB with volume expanded with 150 mL of normal saline to a total volume of 170 mL, to which was added 50 mL of 0.25% bupivacaine, for a total volume of 220 mL. The TAP was accessed via the cut edge of the transversus muscle, and 20 mL of the solution was injected into the TAP under direct visualization at five vertical levels (subcostal, upper-abdominal, midabdominal [×2], and pelvic side wall) bilaterally.

Postoperatively, patients were evaluated for pain on the day of surgery and on postoperative days (PODs) 1 to 3. Patients receiving TAPb with LB had significantly less pain and required significantly fewer narcotics from the day of surgery through the second POD, with the greatest differences on the day of surgery. This was attributed to the 48- to 72-hour duration of LB, which was combined with standard bupivacaine for maximum effect on the day of surgery, with decreasing effect over the next two PODs. The TAPb patients also made a quicker transition to oral narcotics and experienced a 24% decrease in their LOS. The study authors believe these results advocate for the use of TAPb with LB in open VHR.

IV, Intravenous; *LB*, liposomal bupivacaine; *LOS*, length of stay; *POD*, postoperative day; *TAPb*, transversus abdominis plane block; *VHR*, ventral hernia repair.
Modified from Fayezizadeh M et al: Efficacy of transversus abdominis plane block with liposomal bupivacaine during open abdominal wall reconstruction, *Am J Surg* 212(3):399–405, 2016.

SURGICAL PHARMACOLOGY

Common Medications Used in Hernia Surgery

Medication/Category	Dosage/Route	Purpose/Action	Adverse Reactions	Nursing Implications
Lidocaine (Xylocaine)/ amide local anesthetic	With epi: 7 mg/kg max Without epi: 4.5 mg/kg max Local injection	Provide local anesthesia	For both lidocaine and bupivacaine: lightheadedness; nervousness; apprehension; euphoria; confusion; dizziness; drowsiness; tinnitus; blurred or double vision; vomiting; sensations of heat, cold, or numbness; twitching; tremors; convulsions; unconsciousness; respiratory depression; and arrest	For both lidocaine and bupivacaine: Patients should be informed of the effects of local anesthetics in advance Most adverse reactions are caused by overdose or inadvertent intravascular injection Administered medication amounts should be closely monitored and documented
Bupivacaine (Marcaine, Sensorcaine)/ amide local anesthetic	With epi: 3.2 mg/kg Without epi: 2.5 mg/kg Local injection	Provide local anesthesia		
Epinephrine/ sympathomimetic vasoconstrictor (Epi)	1:100,000 or 1:200,000 added to local anesthetic	Used to reduce toxicity, prolong duration of anesthesia, and control bleeding	Anxiety, restlessness, tremor, weakness, dizziness, sweating, palpitations, pallor, local ischemia, nausea and vomiting, headache, and respiratory difficulties	Epi cannot be used on digital blocks or penile blocks because of risk of ischemia and necrosis For hernia repair, monitor vital signs

the arms and padding all prominences to prevent nerve or pressure injuries. The surgical site is exposed and prepped with an institution-approved antiseptic solution. Prep solutions, especially when alcohol based, are allowed to fully dry before draping to prevent the accumulation of flammable vapors under the drapes. When the prep solution is fully dried, the patient is sterilely draped by the scrub person, the surgical assistant, and/or the surgeon.

Time-Out

Before the skin incision is made, the circulating nurse calls a "time-out," during which all nonessential activity stops. During the time-out team members are introduced, and the identity of the patient, the procedure, operative side, incision site, correct and completed consent, and visible site marking are all confirmed. A fire risk assessment is discussed. Any relevant images are displayed. The surgeon states the anticipated duration of the procedure, the expected blood loss, and any critical or nonroutine steps to be performed. The anesthesia provider states the type of prophylactic antibiotic, and time given, along with any additional anesthesia concerns. The scrub person and circulating nurse verify the presence of all needed equipment and supplies, the sterility of instruments and implants, and add any additional concerns they may have.

Intraoperative

Performance of the surgical procedure involves each member of the surgical team acting in concert. The surgeon performs the procedure while coordinating actions of the other team members. The surgical assistant provides exposure/visualization utilizing retractors, clamps, scissors, ties, or other instruments as needed to enhance the performance of the surgery. The surgical assistant may control the camera in laparoscopy, or be the direct care provider at the OR bed while the surgeon works from a robotic console (Robotic-Assisted Surgery). Scrub persons maintain the sterile field and provide the surgeon with instruments, medications, mesh, or other needed items. The circulating nurse maintains all equipment, opens needed items onto the sterile field, and documents all aspects of the procedure. The anesthesia provider monitors and documents the patient's vital signs and anesthetic status, adjusting medications and fluids as needed.

Sign-Out

After the procedure, but before the patient leaves the OR, the surgical team performs and documents a debriefing. This usually includes the name of the procedure performed, noting any differences from the originally planned procedure; completion and correctness of all counts; any specimens, which are identified and labeled; and the determined wound classification. The team discusses key concerns for the patient, team performance, and the events of the procedure, documenting any significant events or needed changes for future surgeries.

Evaluation

At the end of the procedure, examine all skin surfaces to assess variances with preoperative data. Extubation is timely to avoid stress on the repaired hernia site. If the patient coughs or strains while waking, pressure is applied to the site of the repair as a support measure. Any palpation of a disruption of the repair is reported to the surgeon immediately.

Evaluation can be phrased in outcome statements, such as the following:
- The patient verbalized management of anxiety; facial expression and body movements were relaxed.
- The patient was free of injuries related to surgical positioning.
- The patient was free from any internal or external thermal injuries.
- The patient will remain free of surgical site infection throughout the postoperative period.

When the patient's care is transferred to the postanesthesia care unit (PACU) nurse, the perioperative nurse gives a hand-off report pertaining to relevant events and patient status during the operative procedure. This report includes the procedure performed; the location, status, and dressings on all incisions; the location of any drains; the presence of an indwelling urinary catheter, if applicable; and a brief synopsis of the patient's history and physical as it pertains to his or her surgical care.

Patient, Family, and Caregiver Education and Discharge Planning

Greater involvement of patients in their care increases the likelihood of achieving the best outcomes. For the hernia patient to assume such responsibilities, plans for patient, family, and caregiver education along with plans for discharge and home recovery need to be designed. Preferably, discharge planning is begun before admission. This is important because hernia repair is frequently performed as an ambulatory procedure (Ambulatory Surgery Considerations). Issues such as recovery times, analgesic requirements, complication rates, and times for return to full activity are inherent to patient education and discharge planning. These issues are also pertinent to ERAS pathways, particularly for large ventral hernias, and the Enhanced Recovery After Surgery box on p. 383 discusses them further. Anticipated postoperative care, including incision care, incisional splinting as appropriate to the repair approach, and the importance of early ambulation and deep breathing is reviewed. The Patient,

ROBOTIC-ASSISTED SURGERY ▌▌

Key Points in Hernia Surgery

- Robotic hernia surgery currently refers to use of the da Vinci surgical system (robot) to perform hernia repair.
- Robotic surgery is a variant of laparoscopic surgery. Setup and instruments for the procedure may be different, but patient considerations for robotic surgery are essentially the same as with their laparoscopic counterparts.
- Use of the robot for hernia repair is still new. Although the number of procedures is increasing, studies have yet to be completed to support or refute robotic-assisted hernia repair.
- Each of the laparoscopic hernia repairs described in this chapter can be performed robotically.
- Robotic instruments provide far greater articulation and dexterity than standard laparoscopic instruments. This allows the surgeon to more easily suture both tissue and mesh, and it reduces the need to rely on tacks for securing mesh.
- A binocular robotic camera provides the surgeon with true three-dimensional laparoscopic vision. This improved vision combined with improved instrument dexterity allows for finer dissection of the hernia sac and defect as well as safer

identification and manipulation of blood vessels and other structures.

- Adequate training for the entire surgical team is essential. After placement of the robotic ports, the surgeon leaves the surgical field and sits at the console. The scrub person and surgical assistant need to be competent with docking/undocking procedures and instrument insertion and removal, and the entire perioperative team must be proficient with emergency shut down procedures.
- Care is taken to ensure that the robotic arms do not apply pressure to the patient, either during docking or with movement of the arms. Evaluation of both patient and robot positioning is ongoing to prevent patient injury.
- When the robot is docked, the position of the OR bed cannot change, and the position of the patient on the OR bed cannot change. (Note: There is currently one OR bed that will integrate bed movement with the position of the robotic arms.) Always make sure the bed is locked and the patient fully secured. If the patient is in a Trendelenburg/reverse Trendelenburg or tilted position at the time of docking, patient sliding/shifting could cause severe injury.

AMBULATORY SURGERY CONSIDERATIONS

Use of Transversus Abdominis Plane Block With Ambulatory Totally Extraperitoneal Herniorrhaphy

TAP block is a peripheral nerve block used for postoperative pain control in a wide variety of abdominal surgical procedures, including colon resection, cesarean section, and prostatectomy. It has also been shown to be effective for ventral hernia repair (see Research Highlight: Use of Transversus Abdominis Plane Blocks With Liposomal Bupivacaine for Postoperative Pain Control After Open Ventral Hernia Repair). TEP inguinal herniorrhaphy is a laparoscopic technique for the repair of inguinal hernia that does not invade the peritoneal space. This approach allows for a tension-free preperitoneal repair without the level of postoperative pain associated with open repair, and without the risks associated with entering the peritoneum. TEP procedures are increasingly performed on an ambulatory surgery basis. In this study, use of TAP blocks was reviewed with patients undergoing ambulatory TEP hernia repair without neuromuscular block (curarization).

Anesthesia

General anesthesia was administered to all patients using propofol and sufentanil, without neuromuscular block. Airways were maintained with an LMA during anesthesia. Anesthesia was maintained using sevoflurane, with additional sufentanil as needed.

Ultrasound-Guided Transversus Abdominal Plane Block

TAP blocks provide blockade of the sensory nerves downward from the T12-L1 level. This reduces parietal and peritoneal pain, making postoperative recovery easier. Current use of ultrasound guidance to identify the proper plane for injection allows the provider to visualize the correct space, making the block more effective and easier to perform.

Efficacy

The duration of analgesia with TAP blocks is from 24 to 48 hours. TAP blocks are associated with reduction in postoperative narcotic use and postoperative nausea and vomiting. There are no contraindications for use, other than an allergy to the local anesthetic used for the block. The technique is considered appropriate for all patients undergoing ambulatory hernia repair.

LMA, Laryngeal mask airway; *TAP,* transversus abdominis plane; *TEP,* totally extraperitoneal.

Modified from Meyer A et al: Totally extraperitoneal (TEP) endoscopic inguinal hernia repair with TAP (transversus abdominis plane) block as a day-case: a prospective cohort study, *J Visc Surg* 152(3):155–159, 2015.

Family, and Caregiver Education box presents specific home care requirements. Pain management is important as a part of discharge planning; surgical patients frequently report inadequate pain management during their postoperative recovery and convalescence.

Surgical Interventions

Surgery for Repair of Groin Hernias

Repair of Inguinal Hernias

Operative procedures for repair of inguinal hernias include open, laparoscopic, and robotic approaches. The open, nonprosthetic approach seeks to reestablish the integrity of the transversalis fascia and simultaneously reestablish and strengthen the posterior inguinal floor. There are several techniques to accomplish this, two of which are described. The more common practice at this time, however, is to perform a stress-free repair using mesh to supplement tissue strength and prevent recurrence. There are a variety of mesh systems available for both open and laparoscopic repairs, including onlay, mesh plug, and bilayer systems (Research Highlight).

Procedural Considerations

The patient is in the supine position for all groin hernia repairs but may be modified to Trendelenburg to facilitate laparoscopic or robotic procedures. Arms are secured on padded armboards with the palms up and fingers extended. Armboards are maintained at less than a 90-degree angle to prevent brachial plexus stretch. If there are procedural reasons to tuck the arms at the side, as may occur in laparoscopic hernia repair, pad the elbows to protect the ulnar nerve, face the palms inward, and maintain the wrist in a neutral position. A drawsheet may be used to secure the arms. It is tucked snugly, but not tightly, under the patient, and not under the mattress. This prevents the arm from shifting downward intraoperatively and resting against the OR bed rail. Padded arm sleds may also be used for this purpose.

The patient's skin from above the umbilicus to midthigh is exposed, prepped with antimicrobial solution, and draped with sterile drapes. Care is taken to avoid pooling of prep solution in the perineal area. Allow 3 minutes of drying time with alcohol-based prep solutions before applying drapes to avoid trapping flammable fumes. A sterile drape is placed under the scrotum because it may become necessary to enter the scrotum.

Operative Procedure

Native Tissue Repairs. The initial steps of an open inguinal repair are identical, regardless of the type of repair performed. These steps are presented here, and the individual repairs described later proceed from the point of the step 5.

1. A skin incision is made obliquely between the anterior superior iliac spine and the pubic tubercle, or in a natural skin line within that area for better cosmesis. Dissection is carried through Scarpa fascia and subcutaneous tissue, exposing the EOA.

2. The EOA is opened by way of a small incision over the inguinal canal, lateral to the inguinal ring and in the direction of its fibers, to the external ring. The aponeurotic flaps are reflected back along the iliohypogastric and ilioinguinal nerves, which are identified and preserved from injury (Fig. 13.11). The ilioinguinal nerve is a sensory nerve that innervates the medial thigh and the scrotum.

3. The spermatic cord and surrounding structures are bluntly dissected and freed circumferentially from the canal. A moistened Penrose drain is often used to gently retract the vessels and vas deferens.

4. The cremaster muscle is incised longitudinally to expose the cord structures (and hernia sac with indirect hernias). The muscle may be completely divided for better visualization if needed. This does, however, increase the risk of cord damage and testicular descent.

5. If an indirect sac is identified, it is carefully dissected away from the cord until the neck of the hernia is clearly delineated. The sac is then reduced into the preperitoneal space. If the sac is opened, intentionally or inadvertently, the hernia contents are reduced, and the sac is ligated and excised. For an indirect hernia

Patients rely on information given to them at discharge to properly care for themselves. These instructions need to be clear, consistent, and as comprehensive as possible. They are provided both verbally and in writing to the patient and/or their primary caregiver. Many facilities follow up by phone call with the patient within 24 to 48 hours of their surgery, which has been shown to increase patient satisfaction and reduce postoperative concerns (Daniels et al., 2016).

Discharge instruction sheets address basic patient needs and concerns. This information is fully discussed with the patient and/or caregiver, utilizing a teach-back technique to ensure that all of the information has been received and understood. Encourage questions, and provide both verbal and written answers using easy to understand, nontechnical language.

Things to Be Addressed in a Postoperative Instruction Sheet for Hernia Repair
What to Expect
The effects of anesthesia and surgery can easily be mistaken for problems. It is important to let the patient know what is normal and what is not normal. This may be done as a separate section of the instruction sheet or incorporated into an individual section. Either way the following items should be discussed:
- *Pain:* There will be pain at the incision site(s) and in the deeper tissues. This will vary depending on the procedure, the use and type of local blocks, or pain pumps. Pain should improve over the course of recovery, as with any injury.
- *Swelling:* This occurs more routinely with inguinal hernia repair, but can occur with other hernias as well. Men will have scrotal swelling with inguinal hernia repair, which can be pronounced enough to convince them the hernia has recurred or that an injury occurred in surgery. Also, the accumulation of fluid at the surgical site (seroma) can have the appearance of recurring hernia. These effects should resolve over several weeks.
- *Bowel changes:* Depending on the type of anesthesia and pain medication, and the effects of antibiotics or stress, patients may experience transient constipation or diarrhea for several days. A stool softener may be recommended in their postoperative instructions.
- *Fatigue:* It is normal to tire more easily throughout the recovery period, and fatigue should not be considered abnormal.

What to Do
Instructions explain any actions to be taken or avoided to promote healing. This section varies by hernia procedure, facility, and physician. It is individualized to the needs of the patient. In some form, the following issues are addressed:
- *Pain relief:* Ice packs to control swelling, and consequently reduce pain, are especially helpful for inguinal hernia repair, both at the incision site and on the scrotum. Safety measures

and length of application are reviewed. Pain medications range from over-the-counter analgesics to prescribed narcotics. Instructions for use, and any associated risks, are included in both written and verbal form. Emphasis is placed on the danger of driving while under the influence of narcotics.
- *Antibiotics:* If antibiotics are prescribed, the need to take them as directed and complete the prescribed course is emphasized.
- *Wound care:* Incisions may be covered by Steri-Strips, surgical glue, or gauze dressings. Care of dressings is reviewed. Bathing instructions vary but generally bathing is avoided until there is physician approval. Patients are instructed on how to examine their incision(s), looking for erythema, abnormal swelling, bleeding, drainage, and signs of infection.
- *Diet:* Most patients are able to return to a normal diet after discharge; some loss of appetite may occur for several days. Caution against a heavy meal on the day of surgery to avoid anesthesia-associated nausea. Fluids are encouraged. Foods high in fiber, along with extra fluid intake, may prevent or alleviate constipation.
- *Activity:* Quicker return to normal activity is increasingly being promoted as beneficial to healing. One general guideline stipulates that if it hurts, then do not do it. Depending on the procedure, guidelines on increasing activity often include time restrictions on heavy lifting (e.g. over 10 pounds), involvement in sports, or sexual activity. Whatever the restrictions, make certain the patient understands them, and fully discuss the difference between normal postoperative discomfort and abnormal pain.

When to Seek Medical Care
There are several complications that can occur after hernia repair. Patients are taught to recognize them and get prompt medical care when they occur. The patient should contact their physician or go to the emergency room for any of the following conditions:
- *Failure of the repair:* If a popping or a tearing sensation occurs along with pain at the surgical site, failure of the repair may have occurred. This occurs most often at times of strong abdominal tension, such as coughing, sneezing, or straining with defecation.
- *Dehiscence:* Part or all of an incision may reopen after surgery. A small skin-level dehiscence may not require reclosure, but it should be examined.
- *Infection:* Signs and symptoms of an infection include fever, increased pain, erythema (redness and warmth at the incision site), a swollen or hard incision, or purulent drainage, which is often thick; foul smelling; and white, yellow, or green in color.
- *Allergic reaction:* Reactions to antibiotics or pain medication can include rash, hives, itching, nausea/vomiting, weakness, or difficulty breathing. If any of these things occur, patients should cease taking medications and contact their physician. For cases of difficult breathing, they should call 911 immediately.

Modified from Care after adult hernia repair: Elsevier Interactive Patient Education ©2016 Elsevier Inc. Last revised: June 24, 2016.

in which the sac extends into the scrotum, the sac is usually opened and reduced, possibly leaving the distal end of the sac open to prevent the formation of a hydrocele.

Shouldice Repair. In the Shouldice repair a multilayer imbricated repair of the posterior wall of the inguinal canal using nonabsorbable continuous running sutures is performed. A running stitch is believed to evenly distribute tension and prevent recurrence. The posterior wall

of the inguinal canal is reconstructed by superimposing suture lines, progressing from deep to more superficial layers. First, the transversus abdominis aponeurotic arch is secured to the iliopubic tract with a stitch running laterally from the pubic tubercle to the medial flap made up of the transversalis fascia, the internal oblique muscle, and the transversus abdominis. Next, the internal oblique and transversus abdominis muscles and aponeuroses are sutured to the inguinal ligament using

RESEARCH HIGHLIGHT ‖

Biosynthetic Coated Meshes Using Extracellular Matrix-Based Biomaterial Scaffolds

The use of PP mesh, known for its strength and durability, is well established for hernia repair. It is also associated with a chronic inflammatory response at the site of the repair and the production of fibrous local scar tissue. The use of biosynthetic meshes woven from ECM materials has the advantage of providing a biologic scaffold for improved tissue remodeling with reduced amounts of fibrosis. Unfortunately, their more rapid rate of in vivo degradation, and subsequent loss of strength, leads to higher recurrence rates. In this study, researchers evaluated the efficacy of PP mesh subjected to a hydrogel coating of ECM. They compared the fibrotic response and mechanical strength of various types of coated and uncoated PP meshes implanted in rats and explanted at 14 and 180 days.

Porcine dermal ECM was prepared, powdered, and placed in solution. Both lightweight and heavyweight PP meshes were individually added to this solution, allowing the ECM to form a hydrogel coating around the mesh and between the mesh fibers. The prepared mesh was then sterilized and implanted along a surgically created defect in the ventral abdomen of the test animals. At 14 days, some samples of the mesh were explanted and examined for inflammatory response and fibrous connective tissue deposition. At 180 days, the remaining samples were explanted and examined for the same characteristics. Eight of the samples were tested for mechanical strength at the 180-day point.

The researchers determined that the ECM coating resulted in a decrease in proinflammatory macrophages (M1) at the 14-day point. They associated this early reduction in the foreign body response of the host to the 180-day finding of decreased mature collagen deposition. Mechanical strength at 180 days was not statistically affected by the ECM coating. These combined findings conclude that the application of ECM coating to PP mesh results in a decreased early inflammatory response, leading to a long-term decrease in collagen deposition. This reduction in scar tissue over the course of 6 months (180 days) led to the deposition of more constructive tissue, without affecting the long-term strength of the synthetic PP mesh.

ECM, Extracellular matrix; *PP*, polypropylene.
Modified from Faulk DM et al: ECM hydrogel coating mitigates the chronic inflammatory response to polypropylene mesh, *Biomaterials* 35(30):8585–8595, 2014.

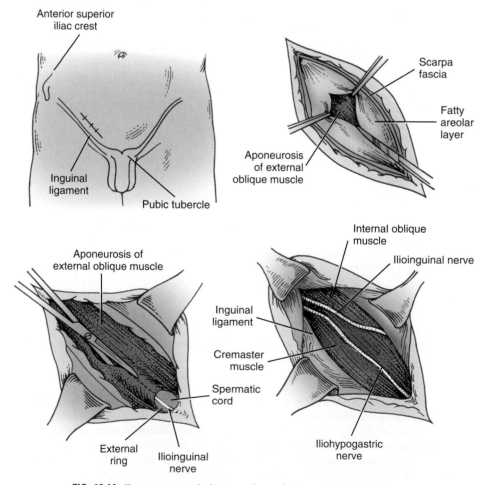

FIG. 13.11 Skin incision with division of superficial muscle and fascial layers.

a stitch that begins with the stump of the divided cremaster muscle and runs medially back to the pubic tubercle. The Shouldice repair is associated with a low recurrence rate and a high degree of patient satisfaction.

Desarda Repair. The Desarda repair uses a 1- to 2-cm flap of the EOA as a native tissue patch, which functions similarly to the synthetic patch in a Lichtenstein repair (see later section). In this technique the underside of the EOA is bluntly dissected approximately 2 inches superiorly, and then the adhesive attachments of the inferior EOA are dissected. This frees up the EOA for creation of the tissue flap and low-tension closure after the repair. After the cord structures have been isolated and the hernia reduced, the lateral edge of the medial flap of the EOA (the upper flap) is sutured to the inguinal ligament, deep to the spermatic cord. This is carried out beginning at the fusion of the EOA and the rectus sheath (the medial corner), and continued until the internal ring is narrowed, but without cord constriction. The stitches pick up the inguinal ligament and transversalis fascia and attach them to the EOA. The medial flap of the EOA is then incised from the symphysis pubis to 1 to 2 cm past the internal ring, at a width equal to the gap between the inguinal ligament and the muscle arch (approximately 1–2 cm). The upper edge of this flap is then sutured to the internal oblique aponeurosis (or conjoined muscle). The inguinal canal is then closed by suturing the new edge of the medial (upper) flap to the lateral (lower) flap (Youssef et al., 2015). Desarda described the technique, using running absorbable (PDS) sutures, whereas other descriptions use interrupted, nonabsorbable sutures. This hernia repair has a low recurrence rate, comparable to a Lichtenstein repair, while reducing the cost and foreign-body complications associated with synthetic hernia repairs (Youssef et al., 2015).

Mesh

The use of implanted prosthetics in hernia repair has grown steadily as more and better prosthetic materials are developed. There are implant options for all abdominal wall hernia repairs, whether performed open, laparoscopically, or robotically.

Prosthetics can be made of synthetic, biosynthetic, or biologic material. They may also be used in combination as composite meshes. Synthetic mesh materials are nonabsorbable and include polypropylene, polyester, polytetrafluoroethylene (PTFE), and expanded polytetrafluoroethylene (ePTFE). They are intended for long-term support and promote either tissue ingrowth or encapsulation. Because these are permanent foreign bodies, they are at risk of bacterial colonization, which may require explantation. They are, therefore, an increased infection risk for cases with wound classes II to IV (see Chapter 9 for a discussion of wound classification).

Biosynthetics, which are synthesized biodegradable polymers woven into monofilament or multifilament meshes, are intended to provide short-term strength, along with a scaffold, which allows for tissue ingrowth. Ideally tissue ingrowth increases in strength as the mesh strength decreases, providing a permanent hernia repair. Being biodegradable, they are less subject to colonization and do not require explantation. There is, however, a risk of recurrence related to absorption of the mesh without adequate tissue ingrowth.

Biologic meshes are made of collagen, which has been processed to remove all cellular material. These meshes may be human, porcine, or bovine in origin. They also provide strength for the hernia repair, along with a matrix for permanent incorporation into natural tissues. Being natural tissue, they can be used in all wound classes, with less risk of infection than synthetic materials. A process called collagen crosslinking adds to the strength of the mesh, but reduces the ability to undergo cellular infiltration and be fully incorporated by the native tissues. Biologic meshes are processed several different ways, both with and without crosslinking, providing multiple options for various surgical needs. The main drawback to biologic mesh is the cost, which can run into the tens of thousands of dollars. For this reason synthetic and biosynthetic meshes are often chosen for procedures at a lower risk of infection.

Composite meshes are intended for intraperitoneal use and are designed to provide strength and ingrowth to the abdominal wall while preventing visceral adhesions. To facilitate this, two types of material are combined; they must be properly oriented to the abdominal wall and the viscera. Although the side attached to the wall is primarily nonabsorbable polypropylene, the visceral element may be either absorbable or permanent. Absorbable composite components are intended to allow neoepithelialization of the permanent mesh to occur before being absorbed. Permanent composite components provide an ongoing barrier, with a microporous mesh, or promote parietal tissue growth as a protective barrier, using a macroporous mesh.

Having such a large number of options for the use of mesh in hernia repairs necessitates close coordination between the surgical staff and the surgeon on a patient-by-patient basis. The best option for a healthy patient with an umbilical hernia may not be appropriate for a diabetic patient with poor wound healing and a history of infections. Having the appropriate mesh, or an assortment of probable meshes, available and date-checked is part of the surgical time-out.

One additional form of mesh for hernia repair is currently in the development stage, but it has strong potential for future use. Researchers have produced an injectable viscous biomaterial capable of conversion to a solid, elastic implant through exposure to ultraviolet light (Skrobot et al., 2016). The material used is derived from fatty acids, and once available, it could provide new options for minimally invasive hernia repair.

Mesh Repairs

Lichtenstein Repair. The Lichtenstein repair uses a single sheet of polypropylene mesh to provide stress-free support of the floor of the inguinal canal. The initial steps of this repair are the same as those for native tissue repair, and are described in steps 1–5 listed in the previous section, Native Tissue Repairs. The sheet of polypropylene mesh, trimmed to lie flat on the floor of the inguinal canal, is sutured in place, beginning with the apex of the mesh 2 cm medial to the pubic tubercle, where the anterior rectus sheath inserts into the pubic bone (Fig. 13.12). Sutures into the pubic tubercle or periosteum are avoided because they can cause chronic postoperative pain. The mesh is slit at the lateral end to accommodate the spermatic cord. A continuous nonabsorbable suture secures the lower edge of the mesh to the inguinal ligament, beginning at the medial apex, and extending laterally to beyond the internal ring. The two cut edges of the mesh are sutured together, forming a snug but non-constricting mesh ring around the spermatic cord. Keeping the mesh lax, the upper edge is sutured to the internal oblique aponeurosis and rectus sheath with interrupted nonabsorbable sutures. The iliohypogastric nerve should be identified and avoided, splitting the mesh to do so, if necessary. The two tails of the split end of the mesh are trimmed at about 5 cm past the internal ring and laid flat under the EOA. It is unnecessary to suture them in place, and doing so may cause injury to the femoral nerve. The inguinal canal and superficial tissues are then closed in standard fashion. This technique is uncomplicated and associated with low recurrence rates

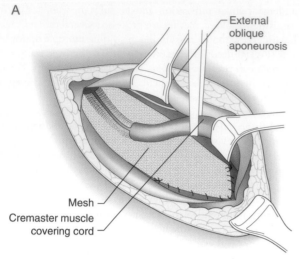

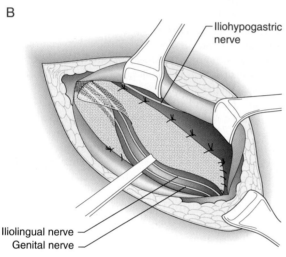

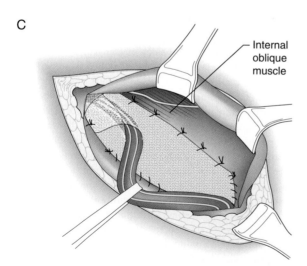

FIG. 13.12 Tension free inguinal hernia repair using overlay mesh with a Lichtenstein technique right-sided hernia. (A) The lower border of the mesh is secured in place with a continuous suture to the inguinal ligament. (B) Interrupted sutures are placed between the upper edge of the mesh and the underlying aponeurosis. (C) A suture is placed laterally to close the two tails around the internal ring.

and low postoperative pain. It can be performed using multiple anesthetic modalities, including local and regional blocks. For these reasons, it is the most common mesh technique used.

Mesh-Plug Repair. The mesh-plug repair is a tension-free, preperitoneal repair, using a cone-shaped mesh plug inserted into the hernia defect to prevent extrusion of abdominal contents through the defect. This plug is frequently, although not always, covered by an onlay mesh similar to that used in a Lichtenstein repair, but with few, if any, sutures needed to hold it in place. Such an approach is known as a "plug and patch" repair (Fig. 13.13). As with other open herniorrhaphies, the initial dissection is performed as previously listed in steps 1–5 in the Native Tissue Repairs section. At this point, the preperitoneal plane, into which the plug is placed, is exposed. For an indirect hernia, the sac is dissected away from the cord structures, allowing visualization of the preperitoneal fat pad. The sac may then be reduced. If the hernia is direct, the attenuated fascia is circumferentially dissected at the hernia opening, creating an opening into the preperitoneal plane. The plug is then inserted into the defect, for both direct and indirect hernias, and secured flush with the hernia opening using interrupted nonabsorbable sutures. These sutures do not provide structural strength, which is not needed with a stress-free repair. They are simply to prevent movement of the mesh before adhesion of the tissues to the mesh has occurred. Prefabricated plugs often have multiple mesh petals that may be retained or removed to accommodate hernia defects of various sizes. After insertion of the plug, the onlay mesh is applied, if it is used. The inguinal canal and superficial tissues are then closed in standard fashion. The mesh-plug technique has been recommended for the treatment of primary and recurrent direct and indirect inguinal hernias, as well as femoral hernias. It is associated with low recurrence rates and low postoperative complications. The technique requires little dissection, can be performed quickly, and is cost-effective.

Bilayer Repair. The bilayer repair uses a three-dimensional mesh to create a triple repair. The mesh has a round preperitoneal underlay component and an oval overlay component, connected by a tubular stem, which acts as a mesh plug. It may be used for any inguinal hernia repair, but in the case of a pantaloon hernia, the epigastric vessels are ligated, and the defects are connected to form a single defect. To perform this repair, the initial dissection is carried out after steps 1–5 listed in the Native Tissue Repairs section. As with the mesh-plug repair, the sac is dissected away from the cord structures and reduced for indirect hernia. The defect is fully circumscribed for both indirect and direct hernias. The preperitoneal space is then bluntly dissected with a sponge to create a flat surface for the underlay portion of the mesh. This portion of the mesh is inserted through the defect and unfurled with a finger to lie smoothly on the underside of the transversalis fascia. This extends laterally to the Cooper ligament, protecting the femoral canal. This portion of mesh requires no suturing and is held in place by intra-abdominal pressure, which prevents recurrence. The connecting tube fills the defect at this point, effectively plugging it. The onlay portion of the mesh is then laid smoothly on the floor of the inguinal canal and minimally secured with interrupted sutures medial to the pubic tubercle, at the midportion of the inguinal ligament, and at the midportion of the transversus muscle arch. A slit is made in the mesh to allow passage of the spermatic cord and secured with a stitch to form a ring around the cord. The inguinal canal and superficial layers are then closed. This technique is associated with low recurrence and few complications. Although it requires blunt dissection of the preperitoneal space, it provides comprehensive coverage, protecting the entire myopectineal orifice, which includes both the inguinal and femoral canals.

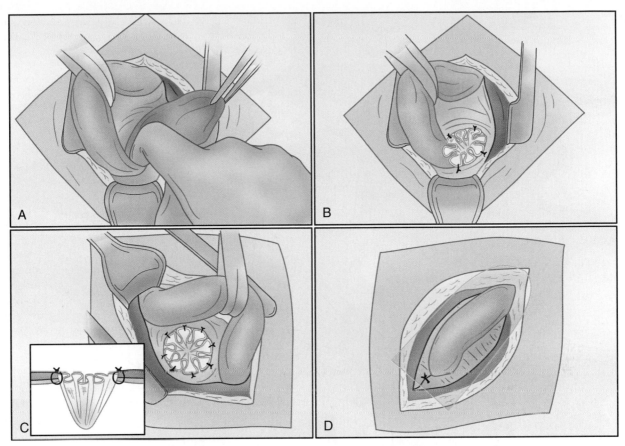

FIG. 13.13 Mesh-plug repair using the PerFix plug. (A) Hernia sac is dissected free of the cord structure to the level of the internal ring. (B) Typically, a large plug is used. Some of the internal petals may be removed if the plug is too bulky. (C) Large or extra-large PerFix plug is inserted. The plug should not be stretched to fill the defect. Typically, 8 to 10 sutures are used. (D) Sutureless onlay patch. The tails of the onlay patch are taken around the cord and sutured together. The onlay patch is not sutured to the floor of the inguinal canal.

Repair of Femoral Hernias. Although femoral hernias occur less frequently than inguinal hernias, they are far more likely to become incarcerated or strangulated. Therefore surgical repair is always recommended. Femoral hernias can be repaired using any of the methods for repairing inguinal hernias. Although open repairs are performed using both natural tissue and stress-free repairs, just as with inguinal hernias, differences in the anatomy require adjustments in techniques. For this reason one stress-free surgical technique specific to femoral hernia repair is described in the following section.

Operative Procedure

Mini-Mesh Repair for Femoral Hernia. The mini-mesh technique (Kulacoglu, 2014) uses a small piece of polypropylene mesh, cut to accommodate the size of the femoral canal, in a stress-free overlay technique. This technique uses a traditional inguinal approach as described in steps 1–5 listed in the Native Tissue Repairs section. Dissection is then carried out in an infrainguinal approach. The hernia sac is dissected free and reduced into the abdomen. The femoral canal is then fully exposed, clearly delineating the hernia defect. The patch is trimmed to cover the defect and sutured to the Cooper ligament with interrupted nonabsorbable sutures. Sutures are placed inferior and superomedial to the femoral vein, at the inferior and the medial aspects of the canal, and at the caudal flap of the transversalis fascia (Fig. 13.14) (Kulacoglu, 2014). The inguinal

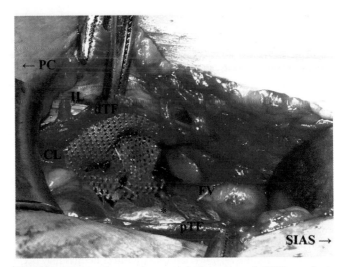

FIG. 13.14 Mini-mesh secured to cover the femoral canal. *FV,* Femoral vein; *CL,* Cooper ligament; *IL,* inguinal ligament; *dTF,* distal flap of transversalis fascia; *pTF,* proximal flap of transversalis fascia; *PC,* pubic corner; *SIAS,* spina iliaca anterior superior. *Preperitoneal fat tissues are retracted with a sponge.

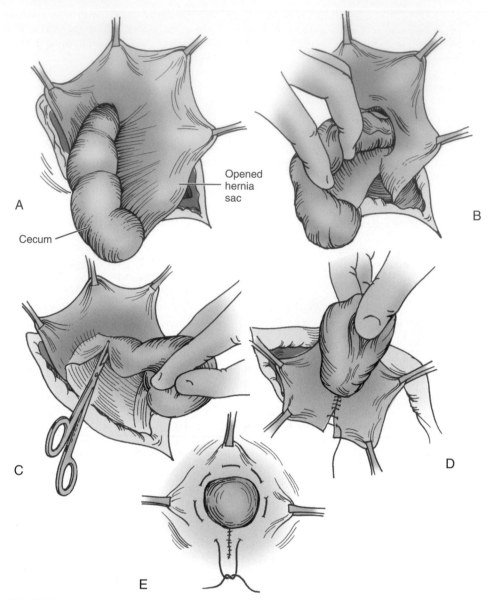

FIG. 13.15 Right sliding hernia. (A) Cecum forms posterior wall of hernia sac. (B) Peritoneum is excised medially (C) and laterally (D) to allow mobilization of cecum for subsequent reduction to peritoneal cavity. Lateral and medial margins are approximated. (E) After reduction, high ligation is accomplished using a purse-string suture.

floor is then closed using running nonabsorbable sutures as in the Shouldice technique described in the Native Tissue Repairs section. The inguinal canal and superficial layers are then closed. This technique provides an uncomplicated approach to repairing femoral hernias in the absence of concurrent inguinal hernia.

Repair of Sliding Hernias. Direct or indirect hernias may occur as sliding hernias. A sliding inguinal hernia occurs when the wall of a viscus forms a portion of the wall of the hernia. The most common sliding hernias involve the bladder in direct hernias, the sigmoid colon in left indirect hernias, and the cecum in right indirect inguinal hernias. This hernia must be recognized early in the repair because attempts at surgical removal of the entire sac will injure the sliding viscus.

Operative Procedure

All operations designed to repair sliding hernias adhere to the basic principle of repairing the defect in the transversalis fascia. To free the bowel from the sac, the following steps are taken:

1. The sac is opened in an area in which no bowel is present and is excised medially and laterally to a point at which the bowel can be mobilized (Fig. 13.15).
2. The lateral and medial peritoneal margins are approximated.
3. The bowel is reduced to the peritoneal cavity, and high ligation of the sac is performed.
4. Repair of the transversalis fascia is done by one of the methods previously described.

Laparoscopic Inguinal Hernia Repairs. Techniques used for laparoscopic herniorrhaphy primarily consist of the transabdominal preperitoneal patch (TAPP) repair and the totally extraperitoneal patch (TEP) repair. The difference between TAPP and TEP repairs is the manner in which the preperitoneal space is entered. The TAPP uses intraperitoneal trocars and the creation of a peritoneal flap over the posterior inguinal region. TEP provides access to the preperitoneal space without entering the peritoneal cavity. Both techniques use a mesh patch to create the repair. They are also both excellent options for repairing bilateral hernias when there are no contraindications, such as an inability to tolerate general anesthesia, a history of surgery involving the preperitoneal space, or a large scrotal or incarcerated hernia.

Laparoscopic hernia repairs have the advantage of a quicker return to normal activity and less postoperative pain than open repairs. Laparoscopic approaches, especially the TEP approach, have a higher incidence of recurrence. Open approaches have a higher occurrence of chronic postoperative pain, but a lower incidence of complications, including damage to epigastric vessels.

Procedural Considerations

After induction of general anesthesia the patient is placed in supine position with the arms tucked at the sides and padded. An indwelling urinary catheter is used by some surgeons to maximize the preperitoneal space and decompress the bladder, preventing injury and increasing the field of view. If the patient has voided preoperatively, urinary catheterization may not be used. The skin is prepped and draped to include the lower abdomen, genital area (manipulation of the scrotal sac may be necessary), and upper thighs. After introduction of the laparoscope, the patient is placed in a 20- to 30-degree Trendelenburg (see Chapter 6 for positioning precautions) so that viscera fall away from the inguinal area. The following items are needed: appropriately sized trocars and scopes (a 30-degree laparoscope is most commonly used), an appropriate selection of meshes, ESU and appropriate smoke evacuation system, blunt graspers, a tacking device (absorbable or nonabsorbable tacks, per surgeon choice) or fibrin glue applicator system, laparoscopic clip applier, suction irrigator, balloon dissector for TEP repair (used to create the preperitoneal space), the primary monitor, and a video cart.

Operative Procedure: Totally Extraperitoneal Patch Approach

The TEP technique laparoscopically develops and insufflates the preperitoneal space, allowing the surgeon to reduce and patch inguinal hernias without making an open incision, or entering the peritoneum. This is accomplished by inserting an inflatable dissecting balloon into the preperitoneal space under laparoscopic visualization. This port is used primarily for visualization, with two additional working ports placed.

1. An infraumbilical incision is made. The anterior rectus sheath is incised, and the ipsilateral rectus abdominis muscle is retracted laterally.
2. With blunt dissection, a space is created beneath the rectus.
3. A dissecting balloon (preperitoneal distention balloon [PDB]) is inserted superficial to the posterior rectus sheath, tunneled past the arcuate line into the preperitoneal space, advanced to the pubic symphysis, and then inflated under direct laparoscopic vision (Fig. 13.16).
4. The space is opened and the PDB removed and replaced with a blunt-tip trocar. The preperitoneal space is insufflated to a pressure of approximately 12 mm Hg.

5. Two additional trocars are then placed in the midline. A 5-mm or 11-mm port is placed approximately 2 inches below the camera port, and a 5-mm port is placed the same distance below that.
6. Using a 30-degree laparoscope, the inferior epigastric vessels and lower portion of the rectus sheath are identified and retracted anteriorly.
7. The Cooper ligament is cleared from the pubic symphysis to the level of the external iliac vein.
8. The iliopubic tract is identified. Care is taken to avoid injury to the femoral branch of the genitofemoral nerve and the lateral femoral cutaneous nerve.
9. Lateral dissection is carried out to the anterior superior iliac spine.
10. The spermatic cord is skeletonized.
11. A direct hernia sac is gently reduced by retraction if it has not already been reduced by balloon expansion of the peritoneal space. A small indirect sac is mobilized from the spermatic cord and reduced into the peritoneal cavity. A large or irreducible sac may be divided proximally, near the internal ring. The proximal peritoneal sac is closed with a loop ligature or clip to prevent pneumoperitoneum from occurring.
12. A piece of polypropylene mesh is inserted and unfolded to cover the direct, indirect, and femoral spaces and rest over the cord structures. The mesh is carefully secured with a tacking stapler, beginning near the pubic tubercle, extending down the Cooper ligament, going up the midline, and along the upper border of the mesh. Care is taken to avoid any nerves or blood vessels. Mesh may also be secured using fibrin glue, which prevents nerve or vascular injury. Both methods are equally effective in preventing migration of mesh.
13. The preperitoneal space is then desufflated under laparoscopic visualization, and the ports closed, making sure to close the fascial defect on any port larger than 8 mm to prevent creation of an incisional hernia.

Surgery for Repair of Hernias of the Anterior Abdominal Wall

Ventral or Incisional Hernias

Ventral hernias can appear spontaneously or any time after abdominal surgery. Spontaneously occurring ventral hernias include epigastric and umbilical hernias. Incisional hernias occur at the site of previous abdominal surgery, which becomes a weak spot in the presence of any condition that prevents proper healing of the incision site, or which causes weakening of the abdominal wall. Operations that involve wound contamination, or wounds that become infected, are more prone to developing subsequent ventral hernias. Patients taking steroids, those diagnosed with chronic obstructive pulmonary disease (COPD), and patients with a poor nutritional state and resulting hypoproteinemia are also predisposed to ventral hernia formation.

Ventral/incisional hernia repairs can be done using open, laparoscopic, or robotic techniques; they include natural-tissue and stress-free repairs. If all layers of the abdominal wall are easily identified, anatomic layer-by-layer repair may be done. A type of overlap method for repair is also sometimes used. Vertical and transverse overlap procedures are referred to as *vest-over-pants repairs.* For large defects, in which approximation of tissue would result in closure with excessive tension or would cause either circulatory or respiratory compromise, synthetic or biologic materials such as surgical mesh or patches are often used to bridge the gap.

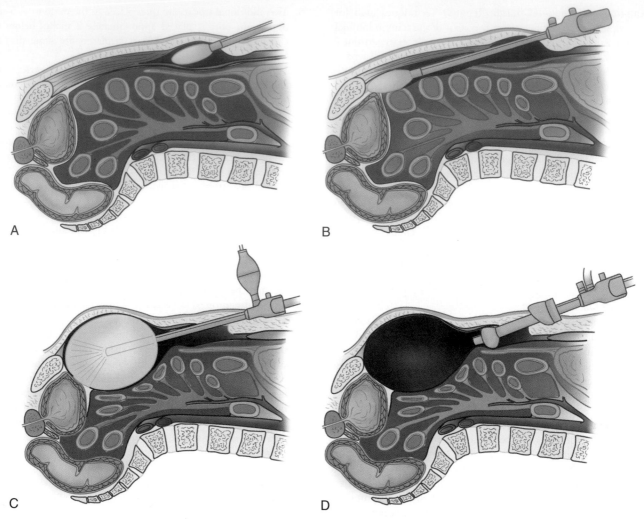

FIG. 13.16 Totally extraperitoneal patch (TEP) laparoscopic hernia repair. (A) TEP approach for laparoscopic hernia repair is demonstrated. Access to the posterior rectus sheath is gained in the periumbilical region. A balloon dissector is placed on the anterior surface of the posterior rectus sheath. (B) Balloon dissector is advanced to the posterior surface of the pubis in the preperitoneal space. (C) Balloon is inflated, creating an optical cavity. (D) The optical cavity is insufflated by carbon dioxide, and the posterior surface of the inguinal floor is dissected.

Umbilical Hernias

True umbilical hernias occur primarily in young children and frequently disappear spontaneously by 2 years of age. If the defect persists, a simple approximation of the overlying fascia is all that is necessary for repair (see Chapter 26 for a description of umbilical hernia repair in children). In adults, umbilical hernias are actually paraumbilical and represent a defect in the linea alba just above or below the umbilicus. This is also a common location for incisional hernias because it is a routinely used port site for laparoscopic procedures. These hernias tend to occur more frequently in obese people (Evidence for Practice), making diagnosis more difficult. Umbilical hernias are potentially dangerous because they often have small necks and frequently become incarcerated. Surgical repair is indicated for all adults with both symptomatic and asymptomatic umbilical hernias. Because umbilical hernias tend to have small defects, they are more likely to be repaired using

native tissue than other hernias, although they may also be repaired using any of the techniques applicable to all ventral/incisional hernias.

Epigastric Hernias

Epigastric hernias are defects in the midline of the abdominal wall between the xiphoid process and the umbilicus. Patients with epigastric hernias can have nausea, abdominal pain, or epigastric pain similar to that observed with cholecystitis or duodenal ulcers. When these hernias are small and acute, they may be closed primarily, with or without mesh. For larger hernias, especially those accompanied by loss of abdominal domain (when more of the viscera is outside the abdominal cavity than inside), primary closure of the fascia creates a much higher risk of recurrence and the potential for increased intra-abdominal pressure (IAP). This increase in IAP can result in a potentially life-threatening condition called abdominal compartment syndrome (ACS). ACS is defined as "the presence of organ dysfunction

EVIDENCE FOR PRACTICE

Perioperative Nursing Care of the Obese Patient

Obesity is defined as having a BMI of at least 30. Further delineations list a BMI of 35 to 39.9 as severely obese, and a BMI of 40 or greater as morbidly obese. Current estimates show 30% of the population of the United States falls into one of these categories. This is four times greater than it was in the 1980s (Leonard et al., 2015). Obesity is associated with multiple comorbidities, including heart disease, hypertension, sleep apnea, vascular compromise, and diabetes. Each of these conditions is exacerbated as BMI increases. Care of this patient population in the surgical setting presents unique challenges and requires increased coordination between all members of the surgical team participating in the hernia repair.

Preoperatively, even routine surgical procedures require additional testing, which may include ECG, chest x-ray, glucose/HbA1c, CBC, and a metabolic panel. The history and physical is carefully reviewed for current respiratory, circulatory, and skin status. Comorbidities and their implications are discussed with the surgeon and anesthesia provider. Obese patients have an increased risk of SSI, DVT, and PE. Prophylactic antibiotic compliance, with a weight-adjusted dosage, is essential, and prophylactic anticoagulant medications are frequently given.

There are significant challenges to safely providing anesthesia to the obese patient. Nursing interventions may include obtaining a difficult airway cart, assisting with intubation, providing cricoid pressure as directed, or elevating the patient's head and chest with a wedge. They may also need to be placed in reverse Trendelenburg position for both intubation and extubation.

The obese patient undergoing hernia repair requires special considerations for positioning, staffing, and surgical supplies. The OR bed must be rated to safely hold the weight of the patient. Extensions and longer safety straps may be needed. To transfer and position the patient without injury to the patient or staff, additional staff members or a lifting device may be needed. Appropriately sized IPCD sleeves should be applied. Because of an increased risk for pressure and nerve injuries, special care is taken to pad bony prominences and maintain tension-free positioning of extremities. Because obese patients have an increased risk of inferior vena cava compression in the supine position, the patient may require a wedge under the right flank, or need to be maintained in a left lateral tilt. If the planned hernia procedure requires the patient to be in Trendelenburg, the patient's tolerance of the position should be tested before the incision is made. Larger surgical instruments and longer laparoscopic trocars are available as needed. When prepping, additional care should be taken to ensure skin folds are fully cleaned, prepped, and allowed to dry to avoid inadequate prepping, unwanted pooling, and possible chemical burns.

BMI, Body mass index; CBC, complete blood count; DVT, deep vein thrombosis; ECG, electrocardiogram; IPCD, intermittent pneumatic compression device; PE, pulmonary embolism; SSI, surgical sight infections.

Modified from Fencl JL et al: The bariatric patient: an overview of perioperative care, AORN J 102(2):116–131, 2015.

---

as a result of increased abdominal pressure or intraabdominal hypertension" (Ferreira and Pressman, 2017). ACS reduces blood flow to abdominal organs, which can result in fatal organ failure. The primary surgical causes of ACS are reduction and primary closure of a long-standing hernia. For this reason large and/or chronic ventral hernias are repaired using stress-free techniques. One laparoscopic and one open option are presented here.

Laparoscopic Ventral Hernia Repair

The technique described here uses a transabdominal approach, with a mesh that includes an antiadhesion surface on the visceral side. The defect is covered without being reapproximated, preventing loss of abdominal space. Because the defect is covered from the inside, abdominal straining pushes the patch against the defect, helping to prevent recurrence.

Procedural Considerations

After induction of general anesthesia the patient is placed in supine position with the arms tucked at the sides and padded. An indwelling urinary catheter is used by some surgeons to decompress the bladder, especially if they anticipate a surgical time greater than 2 hours. IPCDs are placed on the legs to prevent DVT. Subcutaneous heparin may be given for the same reason. The skin is prepped and draped to include the entire abdomen, from the nipples to the pubic symphysis. The following items are needed: appropriately sized trocars and scopes (a 30-degree laparoscope is most commonly used), an appropriate selection of meshes and nonabsorbable sutures, ESU and appropriate smoke evacuation system, blunt graspers, a tacking device (absorbable or nonabsorbable tacks, per surgeon choice) or

fibrin glue applicator system, laparoscopic clip applier, suction irrigator, the primary monitor, and a video cart.

Operative Procedure: Laparoscopic Ventral Hernia Repair

1. Laparoscopic ports are placed based on the location of the hernia. Typically, three or four will be used, and they are placed as laterally as possible for midline hernia repair. After placement of the first port, additional ports are placed under visualization with a 30-degree scope. At least one port must be 10 to 12 mm to allow introduction of the mesh into the abdomen. Adhesiolysis may need to be carried out in the placement of ports or for visualization of the hernia. This should be done with "cold" scissors if possible to prevent thermal injuries, which could go undiagnosed during the procedure.

2. The hernia sac is then reduced using blunt dissection with atraumatic graspers. The sac is not normally excised unless the bowel is closely adherent to it.

3. In addition to clearing any adhesions from the abdominal wall, any excessive tissue in the vicinity of the defect must be taken down. This may include the falciform ligament or any excessive fat. The cleared area should allow for fixation of the mesh with an overlap of 4 to 5 cm in all directions. For incisional hernias, the surgeon may choose to cover the entire previously incised area, regarding it as a weakened area that is prone to additional herniation.

4. The size of the defect is measured to determine the appropriate size of the mesh. It is important to lower the pneumoperitoneum pressure to 5 to 8 mm Hg while measuring to reduce tissue distortion. The defect is then measured using a ruler introduced

into the abdomen. A diagram of the hernia and anticipated mesh coverage may be drawn on the skin to aid in suturing the mesh at the proper location.

5. The appropriately sized mesh is opened onto the field, and sutures are placed at the superior, inferior, and bilateral edges. The tails of the sutures are left long because they will be used to suture the mesh to the abdominal fascia.

6. The mesh is rolled up and introduced into the abdomen, in which it is oriented to fully cover the defect with 4 to 5 cm of overlap, with the antiadhesive surface facing the viscera.

7. Stab incisions are made in the skin at the location of the sutures in the mesh. A transfascial retrieval device is used to pull each of the tails of the sutures through the fascia and stab incisions. These tails are then tied, securing that point of mesh to the fascia. The order of suturing is usually superior, inferior, and then bilateral, making sure to adjust incision sites to draw the mesh taut against the abdominal wall. The skin of each stab incision is elevated with a hemostat to prevent dimpling of the skin.

8. The remainder of the mesh is secured to the abdominal wall circumferentially. This may be done with tacks or sutures. Tack fixation is more common with standard laparoscopy, whereas suturing is greatly facilitated when using a robotic approach.

9. The abdomen is then evaluated for bleeding or injury, the ports are removed, the pneumoperitoneum is released, and port sites are closed.

Open Ventral Hernia Repair Using Component Separation Technique

This technique is used for the repair of large, complex midline hernias. It is an increasingly common method for restoring the integrity and function of the abdominal wall. Component separation refers to separating the overlapping layers of the external and internal oblique muscles, which allows greater mobilization of the rectus sheath toward the midline (Fig. 13.17). Although this technique can be used with and without mesh, natural tissue-only repairs have a higher incidence of recurrence. Variants of the procedure include mesh underlay, overlay, and bridging with synthetic or biologic grafts. The following technique describes an underlay with closure of the rectus sheath over the mesh.

Operative Procedure: Component Separation Hernia Repair

1. A midline incision is carried down to the hernia defect. Any infected tissue, existing mesh, and hernia sacs are excised.

2. The subcutaneous fat is dissected off the rectus sheath bilaterally to the junction of the rectus abdominis and the external oblique muscle. Care is taken to preserve the perforating vessels of the periumbilical rectus abdominis, which decreases the risk of infection and dehiscence.

3. A longitudinal incision is made in the EOA along the semilunar line from the costal margin to the arcuate line.

4. The avascular plane between the external and internal oblique muscles is bluntly dissected, allowing advancement of the rectus sheath to the midline.

5. An underlay patch, containing an antiadhesive visceral surface and providing a 4- to 5-cm fascial overlap, is placed deep to the rectus sheath and sutured in place with nonabsorbable sutures. Initial sutures are placed at the upper and lower apices to provide appropriate tension and a smooth distribution of the mesh.

6. The rectus sheath is then closed over the mesh.

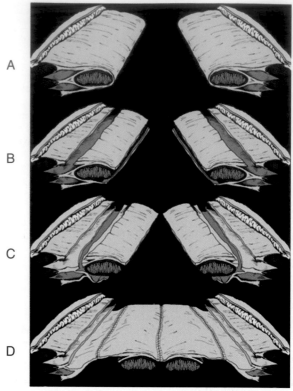

FIG. 13.17 Components separation technique for abdominal wall reconstruction. (A) Normal anatomy above the arcuate line. (B) The posterior rectus sheath is mobilized from the rectus muscle, and the external oblique fascia is divided. (C) The internal oblique component of the anterior rectus sheath is divided down to the arcuate line. (D) Completed repair, suturing the medial border of the posterior sheath to the lateral border of the anterior sheath, with approximation of the medial portion of the anterior sheath in the midline.

7. One or two large bulb suction drains are placed in the subcutaneous space.

8. The skin is then closed, excising any redundant skin caused by the repair, and dressings applied.

Spigelian Hernias. The semilunar line, or linea spigeli, marks the transition from muscle to aponeurosis in the lateral rectus abdominis muscle. The area of aponeurosis that lies between the semilunar line and the lateral edge of the rectus muscle is referred to as the *spigelian zone*. A defect in this area is called a spigelian hernia. The hernia sac frequently passes through the transversus and internal oblique aponeuroses and then spreads out under the intact EOA. Spigelian hernias are uncommon and are generally difficult to diagnose because of their unusual presentation. Ultrasound imaging improves the diagnosis of such hernias. When ultrasound is not conclusive, CT can better visualize the hernia orifice. When the hernia spontaneously reduces, even a CT might not provide sufficient diagnosis. In such a case, diagnostic laparoscopy may be required for confirmation; laparoscopic repair would be indicated at the time of diagnosis.

Surgical repair of a Spigelian hernia is recommended because of a high incidence of incarceration. Defects are typically small and can be repaired using an open primary closure with or without mesh, stress-free repairs using preperitoneal or bilayer mesh, or laparoscopically using an intraperitoneal onlay technique.

Key Points

- A hernia is an abnormal protrusion of an organ or tissue through a defect in its surrounding walls.
- Although hernias can occur at various sites of the body, they most commonly involve the abdominal wall, particularly in the inguinal region.
- Hernias may be inguinal (direct or indirect), femoral, ventral, umbilical, or incisional (occur at previous sites of surgical incisions). Indirect inguinal hernia is the most common hernia and occurs more commonly in males.
- Options for hernia repair (herniorrhaphy) include open surgical approaches, laparoscopic techniques, and robotic-assisted procedures, using native tissue repairs, multiple types of synthetic and biosynthetic mesh, or biologic grafts.
- More than 1 million hernia repairs are performed in the United States each year.
- Hernias can be reducible or incarcerated. Incarcerated hernias require prompt surgical evaluation.
- When blood supply to contents of an incarcerated hernia becomes compromised, the hernia is said to be strangulated. A strangulated hernia is a surgical emergency.
- The type and anatomic structures of the hernia guide procedural considerations and surgical approach.
- Tension-free repairs using a mesh patch with an open surgical technique are the dominant methods for inguinal hernia repair.
- Laparoscopic inguinal hernia repairs also use tension-free mesh repairs, with several repair options. The most common techniques are the TEP and TAPP approaches.
- Most hernia repairs are performed on an ambulatory surgical basis.
- The perioperative plan of care includes a thorough review of discharge instructions for care at home.

Critical Thinking Questions

A 78-year-old male patient presents to the emergency department with complaints of a 3-month history of right inguinal swelling and tenderness. The patient is married, smokes ½ a pack of cigarettes per day, is retired, and has a history of cardiac stent placement 2 years ago. He states his pain has increased in the last 24 hours, but denies nausea and vomiting. CT scan confirms the diagnosis of incarcerated right inguinal hernia, and the patient is transferred to the preoperative area for surgery later in the day. What change in the patient's condition makes this a surgical emergency? Which factors in the patient's history are considered most relevant to his convalescence? What are the patient, family, and caregiver education priorities for this patient after an inguinal hernia repair?

evolve *The answers to the Critical Thinking Questions can be found at http://evolve.elsevier.com/Rothrock/Alexander.*

References

Association of periOperative Registered Nurses (AORN): *AORN comprehensive surgical checklist* (website), 2016. www.aorn.org/surgicalchecklist. (Accessed 6 December 2016).

Broadhurst JF, Wakefield C: Adult groin hernias: acute and elective, *Surgery* 33(5):214–219, 2015.

Daniels S et al: Call to care: the impact of 24-hour postdischarge telephone follow-up in the treatment of surgical day care patients, *Am J Surg* 211(5):963–967, 2016.

Fayezizadeh M et al: Efficacy of transversus abdominis plane block with liposomal bupivacaine during open abdominal wall reconstruction, *Am J Surg* 212(3):399–405, 2016.

Ferreira J, Pressman A: Abdominal compartment syndrome. In Ferri FF, editor: *Ferri's clinical advisor 2017*, ed 1, 2017, Elsevier.

Gillespie BM et al: Effect of using a safety checklist on patient complications after surgery: a systematic review and meta-analysis, *Anesthesiology* 120(6):1380–1389, 2014.

Kulacoglu H: Mini-mesh repair for femoral hernia, *Int J Surg Case Rep* 5(9):574–576, 2014.

Leonard KL et al: Perioperative management of obese patients, *Surg Clin North Am* 95(2):379–390, 2015.

Skrobot J et al: New injectable elastomeric biomaterials for hernia repair and their biocompatibility, *Biomaterials* 75:182–192, 2016.

Youssef T et al: Randomized clinical trial of Desarda versus Lichtenstein repair for treatment of primary inguinal hernia, *Int J Surg* 20:28–34, 2015.

CHAPTER 14
Gynecologic and Obstetric Surgery

SUSAN A. CARZO

At some point, many women face undergoing gynecologic surgery. Surgical procedures on the female reproductive system occur for diagnostic, therapeutic, or cosmetic reasons. Conditions such as abnormal bleeding, typically from the uterus, cervix, or vagina; benign or suspected malignant neoplasms; infertility; or the need to remove or repair weakened structures require surgery. More US inpatient hospital stays for surgical procedures are performed on women than men (Weiss and Elixhauser, 2014). An essential component of perioperative nursing care for women focuses on a holistic approach with sensitivity to their special needs.

Surgical Anatomy

Female reproductive organs and their relationships are shown in Figs. 14.1 and 14.2. Adult female structures associated with reproduction are the external organs (vulva), associated ligaments and muscles, soft tissues and contents of the pelvic cavity, and bony pelvis.

Female External Genital Organs (Vulva)

The external organs, called collectively the *vulva,* include the mons pubis, the labia majora and labia minora, the clitoris, the vestibular glands, the vaginal vestibule, the vaginal opening, and the urethral opening (Fig. 14.3).

The mons pubis is a mound of adipose tissue covered by skin and, after puberty, by hair. It is situated over the anterior surface of the symphysis pubis.

The labia majora are two folds of adipose tissue, covered with skin, that extend downward and backward from the mons pubis. Varying in appearance according to the amount of adipose tissue, they unite below and behind the mons pubis to form the posterior fourchette and in front of the mons pubis to form the anterior fourchette. The labia minora are the two hairless, flat, delicate folds of skin that lie within the labia majora. Each labium splits into lateral and medial parts. The lateral part forms the prepuce or hood of the clitoris and the medial part forms the frenulum. The posterior folds of the labia are united by a delicate fold extending between them, forming the fossa navicularis.

The clitoris is the homolog of the penis in the male. It hangs freely and terminates in a rounded glans (small, sensitive vascular body). Unlike the penis, the clitoris does not contain the urethra. The vaginal vestibule is a smooth area surrounded by the labia minora, with the clitoris at its apex and the fossa navicularis at its base. It contains openings for the urethra and the vagina.

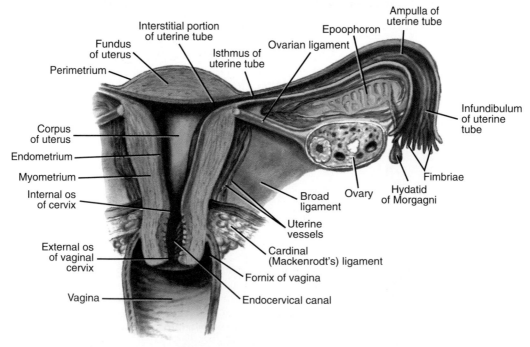

FIG. 14.1 Female reproductive organs.

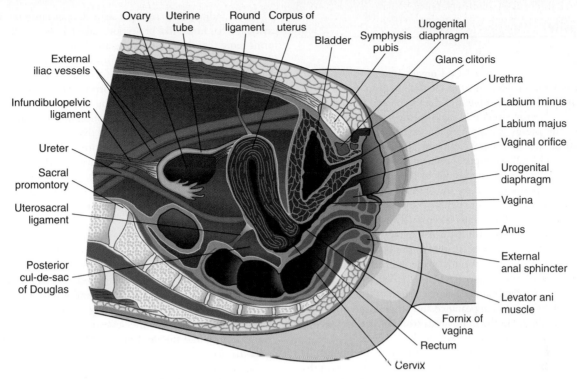

FIG. 14.2 Female pelvic organs as viewed in midsagittal section.

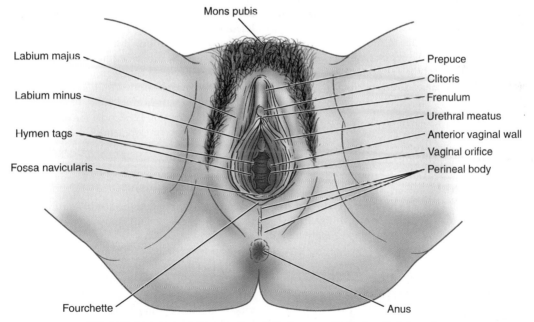

FIG. 14.3 Structures of the external genitalia that are collectively called the *vulva*.

The urethra, which is about 4 cm long in premenopausal women, is close to the anterior vaginal wall and connects the bladder with the urethral meatus. Two small paraurethral ducts, which are commonly known as *Skene ducts,* lie on either side of the urethral meatus and drain the *Skene glands.*

The vaginal opening lies posterior to the urethral meatus. The hymen surrounds the virginal vaginal opening and may be circular, crescentic, or fimbriated. Its remnants after vaginal intercourse are the carunculae hymenales or hymenal tags.

Bartholin glands and ducts are located on each side of the lower end of the vagina at the 5 and 7 o'clock positions. The narrow ducts open into the vaginal orifice on the inner aspects of the labia minora. The glands secrete mucus and can become infected or inflamed.

Pelvic Cavity

Uterus

The uterus is an inverted pear-shaped organ situated in the pelvic cavity between the bladder and the rectum. It gains much of its support from its direct attachment to the vagina and from indirect attachments to nearby structures, such as the rectum and pelvic diaphragm. The uterus is supported on each side by the broad, round, cardinal, and uterosacral ligaments and levator ani muscles (see Figs. 14.1 and 14.2). The upper lateral points, the uterine cornua, receive the fallopian tubes. The fundus of the uterus is the upper, rounded portion positioned above the level of the tubal openings and just below the pelvic brim. Below, the body (corpus) of the uterus joins the cervix. The corpus is separated from the cervix by a slight constriction in the internal canal called the *isthmus*. The cervix lies at the level of the ischial spines. The body of the uterus communicates with the cervical canal at the internal orifice, called the *internal os*. The constriction (endocervical canal) ends at the vaginal portion of the cervix at the external orifice, called the *external os*. The external os varies in appearance and is typically round and 2 to 3 mm in diameter in the nulliparous woman; after delivery, it may become oval, round, or wide and slitlike.

The uterine body has three layers: (1) the outer peritoneal, or serous, layer, which is a reflection of the pelvic peritoneum; (2) the myometrium, or muscular layer, which houses smooth muscle, nerves, blood vessels, and lymphatics; and (3) the endometrium, or mucosal layer, which lines the cavity of the uterus.

The ureters descend into the pelvis posteriorly at the level of the ovaries, after which they pass under the uterine arteries and run laterally along the base of the paracervical ligament, where they connect to the posterior bladder, anterior to the vagina. Given the proximity of the ureters to the female reproductive organs, it is important to identify and understand their anatomic relationship to other structures within the pelvic cavity during gynecologic surgical procedures.

Fallopian Tubes (Oviducts)

The Greek word *salpinx,* meaning "trumpet" or "tube," is used to refer to the fallopian tubes (Fig. 14.4). The tubes are paired and consist of a musculomembranous channel about 10 to 13 cm long, forming the canals through which the ova are conveyed to the uterus from the ovaries. The outer surfaces of the tubes are covered by peritoneum. The inner layers are composed of muscular tissue lined with ciliated epithelium. Each tube receives its blood supply from the branches of the uterine and ovarian arteries and has four parts:

(1) the infundibulum is trumpet shaped, opens into the abdominal cavity, and has finger-like projections called *fimbriae;* (2) the ampulla forms more than half of the tube and is thin walled and tortuous; (3) the isthmus is cylindric and forms approximately one-third of the tube; and (4) the remainder of the fallopian tube is known as both the intramural or interstitial portion. Measuring approximately 1 cm in length, it passes through the wall of the uterus.

It has been theorized that after conception, transfer of fertilized ovum into the uterus is accomplished through vascular changes that occur during contraction of the smooth muscle fibers of the tube. The peristaltic action of the muscular layer and the ciliary movement propel the ovum toward the uterus.

The right tube and ovary are in close proximity to the cecum and appendix; the left tube and ovary are situated near the sigmoid flexure.

Ovaries

The ovaries are located on each side of the uterus. The ovaries and tubes are collectively known as the *adnexa*. Each ovary lies within a depression (ovarian fossa) on the lateral wall of the pelvic cavity and above the broad ligament (see Fig. 14.1). The anterior border of each ovary is attached to the posterior layer of the broad ligament by a peritoneal fold (mesovarium) and is suspended by the ovarian ligament.

The ovaries are small almond-shaped organs composed of an outer layer, known as the *cortex,* and an inner vascular layer, known as the *medulla.* The medulla consists of connective tissue containing nerves, blood vessels, and lymph vessels. The ovary is covered by epithelium, not peritoneum. The cortex contains ovarian (graafian) follicles in different stages of maturity. After ovulation, the corpus luteum arises from the graafian follicle that expelled the ovum.

The ovaries produce ova after puberty and also function as endocrine glands, producing hormones such as estrogen, secreted by the ovarian follicles. Estrogen controls the development of secondary sexual characteristics and initiates growth of the lining of the uterus during the menstrual cycle. Progesterone, which is secreted by the corpus luteum, is essential for implantation of the fertilized ovum and for the development of the embryo. Testosterone is also secreted in much smaller amounts than in the male and is responsible for libido in the female.

Ligaments of the Uterus

The uterus has numerous ligaments to support its structure such as the broad, round, cardinal, and uterosacral ligaments (see Figs. 14.1 and 14.2).

The pelvic peritoneum extends laterally, downward, and posteriorly from each side of the uterus. A double fold of pelvic peritoneum forms the layers of the broad ligament, enclosing the uterus. These layers separate, covering the floor and sides of the pelvis. The fallopian tube is situated within the free border of the broad ligament. The free margin of the upper division of the broad ligament, lying immediately below the fallopian tube, is termed the *mesosalpinx.* Each ovary lies behind its respective broad ligament.

Round ligaments are fibromuscular bands attached to the uterus. Each round ligament passes forward and laterally between the layers of the broad ligament to enter the deep inguinal ring.

Cardinal ligaments (also known as paracervical or Mackenrodt ligaments) are composed of connective tissue with smooth muscle fibers and provide strong support for the uterus. They are found at the base of each of the broad ligaments and contain or house the uterine artery and vein.

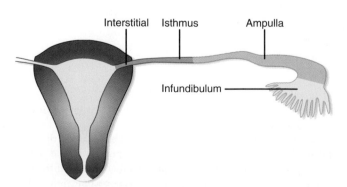

FIG. 14.4 Anatomic segments of the fallopian tube.

Uterosacral ligaments are a posterior continuation of the peritoneal tissue. The ligaments pass posteriorly to the sacrum on either side of the rectum.

Vagina

The vagina is a rugated musculomembranous tube. It carries the menstrual blood from the uterus, serves as the organ for sexual intercourse, and is the terminal portion of the birth canal. The anterior wall measures 6 to 8 cm in length and the posterior wall 7 to 10 cm (see Figs. 14.1 and 14.2). The anterior wall of the vagina is in proximity to the bladder and urethra. The lower posterior wall is anteriorly adjacent to the rectum. The upper portion of the vagina lies above the pelvic floor and is surrounded by visceral pelvic fascia. The lower half is surrounded by the levator ani muscles.

Cervix

The cervix consists of a supravaginal portion, closely associated with the bladder and the ureters, and a vaginal portion, which projects downward and backward into the vaginal vault. The projection of the cervix into the vaginal vault divides the vault into four regions—anterior, posterior, right lateral, and left lateral—called *fornices*.

The posterior fornix is in contact with the peritoneum of the pouch or cul-de-sac of Douglas. The rectovaginal septum lies between the vagina and rectum. The dense connective tissue separating the anterior wall of the vagina from the distal urethra is termed the *urethrovaginal septum*.

Bony Pelvis

The pelvis is the portion of the trunk below and behind the abdomen. The bony pelvis is composed of the ilium, symphysis pubis, ischium, sacrum, and coccyx. The so-called *pelvic brim* divides the abdominal false portion, located above the arcuate line, from the true portion of the pelvis, located below this line. The bony pelvis accommodates the growing fetus during pregnancy and the birth process.

The true pelvis is considered to have three parts: inlet, cavity, and outlet. The muscles lining the pelvis facilitate movement of the thighs, give form to the pelvic cavity, and provide a firm elastic lining to the bony pelvic framework. All organs located in the pelvis are covered by endopelvic fascia, which is important in maintaining the normal strength within the pelvic floor.

The fascia covering the muscles is usually dense and firm, whereas the fascia covering organs is often thin and elastic. The nerves, blood vessels, and ureters coursing through the anatomic structures of the pelvis are closely associated with muscular and fascial structures.

Pelvic Floor

The pelvic floor acts as a supportive sling for the pelvic contents (Fig. 14.5). The pelvic fascia may be divided into three general groups: parietal, diaphragmatic, and visceral. The parietal pelvic fascia covers the muscles of the true pelvic wall and perineum. The diaphragmatic fascia covers both sides of the pelvic diaphragm, which is made up of the levator ani and coccygeal muscles. The visceral fascia is thin and flexible and covers the pelvic organs. The floor of the pelvis, known as the *pelvic diaphragm*, gives support to the abdominal pelvic viscera in this region. It consists of the levator ani and coccygeal muscles with their respective fascial coverings, separating the pelvic cavity from the perineum.

The levator ani muscles, varying in thickness and strength, may be divided into three parts: the iliococcygeal, the pubococcygeal, and the puborectal muscles. The fibers of the levator ani muscles blend with the muscle fibers of the rectum and vagina. The pubovaginal fibers of the pubococcygeal portion of the levator ani muscles, lying directly below the urinary bladder, help to control micturition (urination). The pubococcygeal fibers of the levator ani muscles control and pull the coccyx forward and assist in the closure of the pelvic outlet. The fibers pull the rectum, vagina, and bladder neck upward toward the symphysis pubis to close the pelvic outlet and

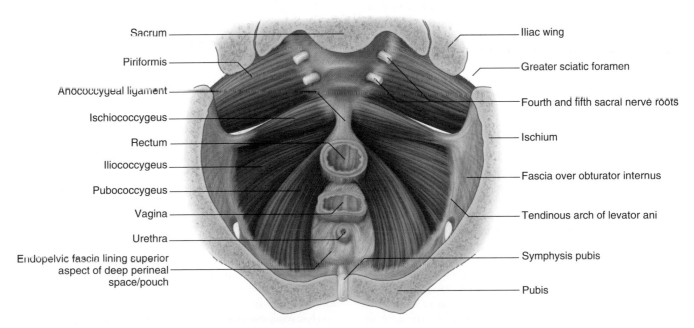

FIG. 14.5 Muscles of the female pelvis viewed from above. The sacral nerve roots have been divided close to the sacral foramina. The anorectal junction, vagina, and urethra have been divided at the level of the pelvic floor.

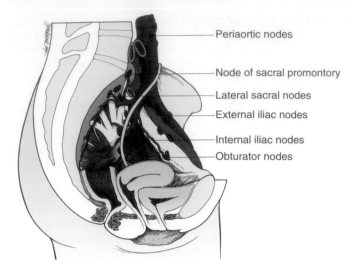

- Periaortic nodes
- Node of sacral promontory
- Lateral sacral nodes
- External iliac nodes
- Internal iliac nodes
- Obturator nodes

FIG. 14.6 Major lymphatics of the pelvis. The major lymph nodes of the pelvis follow the major vessels. Each group of nodes receives contributions from multiple organs. The groupings are somewhat arbitrary because there is no distinct separation of individual node groups.

are responsible for the flexure at the anorectal junction. Relaxation of the fibers during defecation permits a straightening at this junction. During childbirth, the action of the levator ani muscles directs the fetal head into the lower part of the passageway.

Vascular, Nerve, and Lymphatic Supply of the Reproductive System

The blood supply of the female pelvis derives from the internal iliac branches of the common iliac artery, supplemented by the ovarian, superior rectal, and median sacral arteries, which are branches of the aorta. The nerve supply of the female pelvis comes from the autonomic nerves that enter the pelvis in the superior hypogastric plexus (presacral nerve). The lymphatics of the female pelvis either follow the course of the vessels to the iliac and preaortic nodes or empty into the inguinal glands (Fig. 14.6).

Perioperative Nursing Considerations

Assessment

Perioperative patient care depends on thorough nursing assessment and planning skills. Gynecologic patient information is gathered through nursing and physician interviews, evaluation of the patient's systems, physical examination, collection of medical and surgical histories, and diagnostic testing. Family history of gynecologic disease, hypertension, diabetes, and heart disease are key elements to consider when assessing and planning patient care.

Skillful communication is an essential component of any nursing assessment. Patient interviews occur in ambulatory surgical centers, preoperative holding rooms, and on hospital patient care units. During the preoperative interview, the perioperative nurse offers support and patient education and obtains information for the surgical procedure and nursing plan of care (Goodman and Spry, 2017). The nurse also ensures privacy during the patient interview whenever possible, providing a safe environment for sharing sensitive

information. Questions about reproduction and gynecologic history may embarrass or be distressful for the patient. Personal values, native language, and cultural beliefs are all considered and respected during the interview process.

Throughout the assessment, the perioperative nurse remains open, nonbiased, compassionate, and supportive to assist in establishing a trusting therapeutic relationship. Creating such a relationship facilitates the nurse's assessment for intimate partner violence (IPV). IPV is a major health concern worldwide with a reported global prevalence of 30% (Esposito, 2016; WHO, 2016). The perioperative nurse must identify and understand the warning signs of IPV. Any patient concerns about her own safety during the perioperative period and beyond are addressed (Patient Safety).

The gynecologic patient's history contains a complete obstetric history including a chronologic listing of each pregnancy, length of gestation, type of delivery, complications during pregnancy, duration of labor, and fetal weight. Her menstrual cycle and its data should include age at onset, length of cycle, amount of flow, duration of bleeding, abnormal bleeding, and any pain or discomfort during menses. The amount of flow is noted in relation to the number of pads and tampons used during her menstrual cycle; onset of menopause is also noted. Additional elements of gynecologic assessment are prior Papanicolaou (Pap) test results, gynecologic surgical procedures, vaginal discharge or infections, pain, and sexual and infertility history. See the laboratory values in Appendix A for common studies in the reproductive assessment of gynecologic patients.

Gynecologic disorders may be associated with urinary problems. The perioperative nurse asks about stress incontinence or loss of urine while coughing, sneezing, exercising, or laughing. Getting up at night to urinate may reflect irritative changes in the bladder, shifting of extravascular fluids in the recumbent position, or decreased bladder capacity. Any urgency, pain, or burning sensations during urination are also queried. Frequent urination may reflect compression of the bladder by an ovarian or uterine mass, particularly if this has been progressive.

A medication history includes the use of all prescription and nonprescription medications. These include analgesics, oral contraceptives, estrogen therapy, diuretics, antihypertensives, cardiac medications, and use of herbal supplements or nutraceuticals. Herbal supplements can interfere with the patient's ability to clot effectively during surgery (e.g., vitamins C and E and St. John's wort) (see Chapter 30 for a discussion of integrative therapies). It is essential to note the name, frequency, dose, and duration of all medications in the patient's record during the perioperative assessment. The nurse continues the assessment by reviewing the physician's history and physical examination, laboratory results, and results of diagnostic studies. This review helps in planning intraoperative care.

The gynecologic patient may undergo numerous preoperative diagnostic studies, depending on the gynecologic problem or disease. Studies performed as part of preoperative assessment include ultrasonography, computed tomography (CT) scanning, and magnetic resonance imaging (MRI). These studies contribute to evaluation of patients suspected of having a malignancy and/or possible disease involvement of other surrounding organs. The vaginal and pelvic ultrasound assists with diagnosing adnexal disease, endometrial hyperplasia, and uterine fibroids, as well as detecting blood or fluid within the pelvis.

Hysterosalpingograms (HSGs) or sonohysterograms are commonly performed in the radiology department; they identify abnormalities in the uterine cavity or possible occlusions within the tubal folds. These diagnostic tools are most useful in detecting causes of infertility

PATIENT SAFETY

Assessment Techniques for Intimate Partner Violence

IPV is actual or threatened physical or sexual violence, psychologic aggression (including coercive tactics), or emotional abuse by a spouse, ex-spouse, boyfriend, girlfriend, ex-boyfriend, ex-girlfriend, or date. The partner need not cohabit with the victim. IPV may also include rape and stalking; it crosses all ages and segments of society and is not limited to certain economic groups or educational levels.

Nurses and other healthcare providers may represent the first and only contact that an isolated woman seeks outside an abusive relationship and are a primary source of relief. Therefore screening for IPV should be an important part of the perioperative assessment. The CDC publication, *Intimate Partner Violence and Sexual Violence Victimization Assessment Instruments for Use in Healthcare Settings,* presents and summarizes a variety of screening tools. Characteristics common to the tools include trying to normalize the conversation with neutral opening statements, such as, "In this health service, we are concerned about your health and safety, so we ask all women about violence and safety at home. Are you safe at home? Are you ever afraid of your partner?" In addition, healthcare providers should use direct questions when violence is suspected, such as, "Have you ever been hit, kicked, or punched by someone close to you?"

Cues to abuse include delay in seeking medical assistance (hours or days), vague explanations of injuries, nonspecific complaints, a partner who seems reluctant to leave the woman alone with the healthcare provider, and substance abuse. Physical signs include new and old injuries to the face, breasts, abdomen, and buttocks; fractures that have a suspicious etiology; injuries at various stages of healing; and patterns that indicate injuries made by biting or fist/hand patterns. Pregnant women have an increased risk for IPV and therefore should be thoroughly assessed by the perioperative nurse.

If the nurse suspects IPV, he or she is mandated in most states to report the abuse. Domestic violence is considered a crime in all states, but the category (e.g., misdemeanor or felony) varies by state definition. Nurses must be aware and knowledgeable of the reporting requirements for the state in which they reside. In addition to reporting the abuse or suspected abuse, the nurse must document the findings in the medical record. If appropriate to the situation, photographs can be taken and included in the record.

Nurses in ambulatory surgery must assess the patient's safety before she is discharged and provide her with written information about her legal options, shelters, crisis intervention services, and counseling. The National Domestic Violence Hotline (1-800-799-SAFE) is available 24 hours a day, 7 days a week. Nurses also facilitate patient safety by providing education to women and empowering their understanding that abuse is a violation of their basic human rights, promoting assertiveness, and recommending resources that enhance their independence.

CDC, Centers for Disease Control and Prevention; *IPV,* intimate partner violence.
Modified from Basile KC et al: *Intimate partner violence and sexual violence victimization assessment instruments for use in healthcare settings: version 1.0* (website), 2007. www.cdc.gov/violenceprevention/pdf/ipv/ipvandsvscreening.pdf. (Accessed 16 January 2017); Breiding MJ et al: *Intimate partner violence surveillance uniform definitions and recommended data elements, version 2.0* (website), 2015. www.cdc.gov/violenceprevention/pdf/intimatepartnerviolence.pdf. (Accessed 16 January 2017); World Health Organization (WHO): *Violence against women fact sheet* (website), 2016. www.who.int/mediacentre/factsheets/fs239/en/. (Accessed 16 January 2017).

and identifying intrauterine masses that appear as endometrial thickening on routine ultrasonography.

Colposcopy with binocular magnification often happens in the surgeon's office. Patients who have an abnormal Pap test suggestive of dysplasia undergo this examination. Colposcopy identifies cellular abnormalities involving the vulva, vagina, or cervix and helps identify localized areas of dysplasia and carcinoma in situ (CIS). Exocervical biopsies or endocervical curettage samples can be obtained during the colposcopic procedure to rule out invasive carcinoma or to detect early adenocarcinoma of the cervix.

Gynecologic Carcinoma

Gynecologic cancers commonly occur in the cervix, ovaries, vagina, and endometrial layer of the uterus. Less common sites for gynecologic carcinomas are the vulva and fallopian tubes. Risk factors associated with gynecologic cancers are human papillomavirus (HPV) infection; inherited familial predisposition to cancer, such as Lynch syndrome (hereditary nonpolyposis colorectal cancer [HNPCC]); and *BRCA* gene mutations. Other risk factors linked with these cancers are obesity, high-fat diets, sexually transmitted diseases (STDs), diabetes, race, and age.

Endometrial cancer (Fig. 14.7) is the most common gynecologic cancer in women in the United States. An estimated 60,050 new cases were predicted for 2016 (National Cancer Institute, 2016). Uterine sarcomas are less common and account for up to 8% of uterine cancers. It is estimated 1 in 36 women will be diagnosed with endometrial cancer during their lifetime. Patients with this type of cancer may be asymptomatic or they may experience postmenopausal bleeding as their primary symptom. The average age of women diagnosed with endometrial cancer is 60 years of age; it is unusual to be diagnosed in women younger than 45 years of age.

It is estimated that invasive cervical cancers were diagnosed in over 12,500 women in 2016 (ACS, 2016b). HPV is one of the main causes of cervical cancer. Pap test screening provides early detection, aids in cancer treatment, and lowers mortality rates by detecting early changes in cervical cells and enabling prompt treatment (Table 14.1). In its early invasive stage, cervical cancer may be asymptomatic or associated with painless vaginal spotting, postcoital bleeding, or irregular intermenstrual bleeding. During the early preinvasive stage, the disease may be described as dysplasia. From moderate or severe dysplasia, the disease progresses to CIS. Preinvasive cancers may also be designated as cervical intraepithelial neoplasia (CIN) and classed according to severity of histologic abnormalities (ACS, 2016h; Jhingran et al., 2014):
CIN1: Mild
CIN2: Moderate
CIN3: Severe, to CIS (Fig. 14.8)

Ovarian cancer is the leading cause of death from gynecologic malignancies in the United States. The majority occur in postmenopausal women; half of the women who are diagnosed are 63 or older (ACS, 2016e). It is frequently diagnosed in later disease stages because of the absence of early symptoms. Signs and symptoms

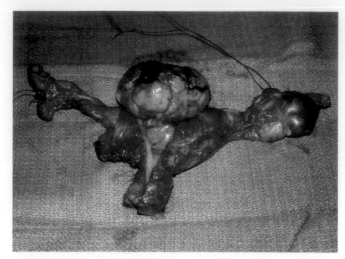

FIG. 14.7 Total abdominal hysterectomy and bilateral salpingo-oophorectomy showing large polypoid adenocarcinoma of the endometrium with deep myometrial invasion.

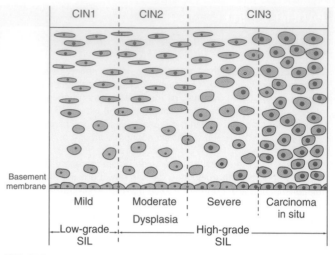

FIG. 14.8 Diagram of cervical epithelium showing progressive changes and various terms used. *CIN,* Cervical intraepithelial neoplasm; *SIL,* squamous intraepithelial lesion.

TABLE 14.1

Screening Methods for Cervical Cancer: Joint Recommendations of the American Cancer Society and the American Congress of Obstetricians and Gynecologists

Population	Recommended Screening Method	Comment
Women younger than 21 years	No screening	Women should begin cervical cancer screening by age 21
Women ages 21–29 years	Pap test every 3 years	HPV testing as follow-up if abnormal Pap test
Women ages 30–65 years	HPV and Pap test (co-testing) every 5 years	HPV testing beginning at age 30 until age 65 is optional
	Pap test alone is acceptable every 3 years	—
Women older than 65 years	If regular screening in previous 10 years has been negative, and no history of previous serious preinvasive cancers (CIN2 or CIN3) in the last 20 years, screening may stop	Women with a history of CIN2 or CIN3 should continue screening for at least 20 years after the abnormality was found
Women who underwent total hysterectomy	No screening is necessary. If cervical cancer or moderate to severe cervical cell changes, screening should be done for 20 years after surgery.	Applies to women without a cervix and without a history of CIN2, CIN3, or cancer in the past 20 years
Women who underwent a supracervical hysterectomy (cervix was not removed)	Continue cervical cancer screening guidelines as above	—
Women vaccinated against HPV	Follow age-specific recommendations (same as unvaccinated women)	—
Women who should have more frequent screening	—	Women with a history of cervical cancer, women who have HIV, or who have been exposed to DES before birth, and women with a weakened immune system

CIN, Cervical intraepithelial neoplasia; *DES,* diethylstilbestrol; *HIV,* human immunodeficiency virus; *HPV,* human papillomavirus.
Modified from American Cancer Society (ACS): *The American Cancer Society guidelines for the prevention and early detection of cervical cancer* (website), 2016. www.cancer.org/cancer/cervicalcancer/moreinformation/cervicalcancerpreventionandearlydetection/cervical-cancer-prevention-and-early-detection-cervical-cancer-screening-guidelines. (Accessed 21 January 2017); American Congress of Obstetricians and Gynecologists (ACOG): *Cervical cancer screening* (website), 2016. www.acog.org/Patients/FAQs/Cervical-Cancer-Screening. (Accessed 19 January 2017).

can be vague and are often accompanied by indicators typically attributable to common gastrointestinal (GI) diseases such as hiatal hernia, diverticular disease, or gallbladder disease. Tumors (Fig. 14.9) that are epithelial account for about 85% to 90% of ovarian cancers. Germ cell tumors account for less than 2%, and gonadal stromal cell tumors of the ovary account for about 1%. More than

half of stromal cancer is found in women over 50 years of age (ACS, 2016g).

Ovarian tumors spread to the peritoneal surfaces of the abdominal and pelvic cavities by intraperitoneal dissemination, local extension, lymphatic invasion, and transdiaphragmatic passage. Common sites for invasion and metastasis occur where there is stasis of peritoneal

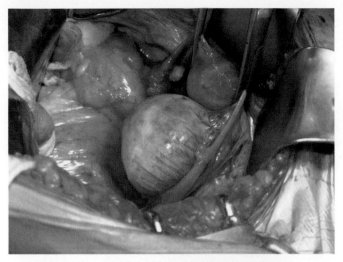

FIG. 14.9 Gross stage IA ovarian cancer. The right ovarian mass is free of adhesions and visible adjacent to a normal fallopian tube and uterine corpus.

fluid circulation such as the omentum, uterus, cul-de-sac, bladder, underside of the diaphragm, paracolic gutter, mesentery and serosa of large and small bowel, and the surface of the liver (Green, 2016).

Vulvar cancer (Fig. 14.10) represents about 4% of gynecologic cancers (ACS, 2016d) and is typically slow growing. Noninvasive vulvar cancer appears most often in women younger than 50, whereas invasive vulvar cancer appears in women 70 or older. In younger women, the incidence is often linked to genital warts (condylomata acuminata) caused by HPV. Symptoms include irritation and pruritus or nonhealing lesions in the perineal area. In women over 70 there is an association with lichen sclerosus and squamous hyperplasia (ACS, 2016f; Jhingran et al., 2014).

Vaginal cancer is rare and may be associated with a prior diagnosis and treatment of cervical cancer or precancer. Approximately 1 of every 1100 women will develop vaginal cancer. There are fewer than 1000 deaths per year (ACS, 2016c) associated with this disease. Approximately 90% of vaginal cancers are metastatic. Sources of metastases include cancers of the endometrium, cervix, vulva, breast, colon, rectum, and kidney (Jhingran et al., 2014). Vaginal cancer, generally asymptomatic in the early stages, may present as painless spontaneous or postcoital bleeding and dyspareunia; urinary symptoms develop in the later stages with anterior tumors; constipation is associated with posterior tumors (Jhingran et al., 2014).

Fallopian tube cancer is very rare, with an incidence of less than 1%. Most women are asymptomatic. Depending on the degree of tubal obstruction, symptoms may include vaginal bleeding, vaginal discharge, and lower abdominal pain (Schmeler and Gersheson, 2017). Research has shown that there may be a correlation between high-grade ovarian and peritoneal serous carcinomas and the distal portion of the fallopian tube (Evidence for Practice). Fallopian tube cancers are also more likely to be associated with a predisposing genetic mutation, such as BRCA1 or BRCA2. Preinvasive lesions are thought to arise in the fimbriated end of the fallopian tube (Siraj and Chern, 2015).

Nursing Diagnosis

Perioperative nursing care is a planned process that is implemented to ensure safe, effective, and efficient patient outcomes. Nursing diagnoses are formulated after reviewing the patient's record and conducting a patient assessment. All significant collected data are

---

EVIDENCE FOR PRACTICE

The Role of Salpingectomy in the Prevention of Ovarian Cancer

ACOG released a *Committee Opinion* in January 2015 on the role of salpingectomy for the prevention of OC. The opinion notes that evidence has shown that epithelial ovarian cancers, such as serous, endometrioid, and clear cell, may begin in the distal portion of the fallopian tube and endometrium and not on the surface of the ovary as once thought. Women with the *BRCA* gene mutation who had risk-reducing surgery (BSO) were found to have 1% to 5% early tubal malignancy in the fimbriated end of the tube.

Further supporting the role of BSO in preventing OC was a meta-analysis of 77 studies, of which three were included: one cohort study and two population-based case-control studies. In these three studies, 3509 patients underwent BSO and 5,655,702 controls did not. Over the combined study period, 29 of the 3509 BSO patients developed OC compared with 44,006 of the 5,655,702 without BSO. A fixed effects model revealed a significant decrease in the risk of OC occurrence in the patients who underwent BSO relative to the controls (OR = 0.51, 95% CI 0.35–0.75, I^2 = 0%). The authors concluded that BSO reduces the risk of OC by 49%.

ACOG encourages physicians to initiate discussions on the benefits of BSO with or without oophorectomy when the patient is scheduled to have a benign hysterectomy, pelvic surgery, or tubal ligation. Low-risk women who have BSO and preserve their ovarian function (BSOR) could also reduce their risk for ovarian cancer while protecting their quality of life. Premenopausal women who have ovarian function have a protective effect on decreasing their risk of cardiovascular disease, osteoporosis, and even cognitive impairment from early surgical menopause. If they are of childbearing age and wish to have children, they may have the option of in vitro fertilization.

The ACOG committee recommends further investigation with randomized clinical trials to verify the role of BSO in the prevention of ovarian cancer.

ACOG, American Congress of Obstetricians and Gynecologists; *BSO*, bilateral salpingo-oophorectomy; *BSOR*, bilateral salpingectomy with ovarian retention; *CI*, confidence interval; *OC*, ovarian cancer; *OR*, odds ratio.
Modified from American Congress of Obstetricians and Gynecologists (ACOG): *Salpingectomy for ovarian cancer prevention* (website), 2015. www.acog.org/Resources-And-Publications/Committee-Opinions/Committee-on-Gynecologic-Practice/Salpingectomy-for-Ovarian-Cancer-Prevention. (Accessed 16 January 2017); Yoon SH et al: Bilateral salpingectomy can reduce the risk of ovarian cancer in the general population: a meta-analysis, *Eur J Cancer* 55:38–46, 2016.

---

reviewed, prioritized, and incorporated into the perioperative plan of care. The gynecologic patient may have multiple nursing diagnoses that warrant perioperative nursing interventions including the following:

- Anxiety and Disturbed Body Image related to planned surgical intervention
- Urinary Retention related to edema, anesthesia, opioids, or pain
- Risk for Infection at the surgical site related to operative or other invasive procedures
- Risk for Perioperative Hypothermia
- Risk for Perioperative Positioning Injury

Outcome Identification

Outcomes identified for the selected nursing diagnoses could be stated as the following:

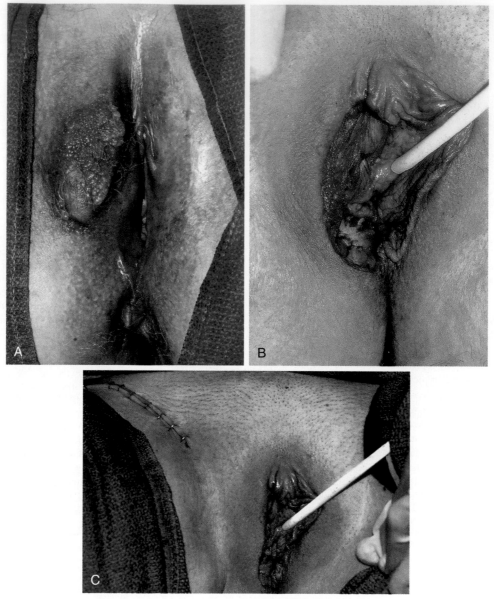

FIG. 14.10 Cancer of the vulva. (A) T1 lesion on the right side of the vulva. (B) Defect after excision of the primary lesion. (C) Postoperative results after closure and node dissection via separate incisions.

- The patient will verbalize reduced or controlled anxiety and acknowledge feelings regarding her body image.
- The patient will maintain or regain normal patterns of urinary elimination.
- The patient will remain free from a surgical site infection (SSI).
- The patient will remain normothermic.
- The patient will be free from injury related to surgical positioning.

Planning

Planning enables the perioperative nurse to provide patient care in an organized and individualized manner. Planning involves preparation for both psychosocial and physiologic needs. Part of planning efficient and effective patient care is gathering necessary equipment and supplies, positioning accessories, surgical devices, and adjuncts requisite to the specific gynecologic surgical procedure. For example, if the gynecologic patient is undergoing a lengthy surgical procedure,

the perioperative nurse has available a forced-air warming device, pressure-reducing positioning devices, graduated compression stockings, and intermittent pneumatic compression devices (IPCDs). Undertaking these actions assists with maintaining the patient's body temperature, promoting skin integrity, and preventing venous stasis, which aids in the prevention of thrombus or emboli formation (Research Highlight). Nursing interventions that will help the gynecologic patient reach desired outcomes are identified for each patient. A typical Sample Plan of Care for the gynecologic patient follows.

Implementation

During implementation of the plan of care, the perioperative nurse performs the identified nursing interventions. Implementation includes gathering the appropriate instruments and patient care supplies, positioning the patient on the operating room (OR) bed,

Venous Thromboembolism Rates in Women Undergoing Minimally Invasive Surgery for Endometrial Cancer With Different Modes of Thromboprophylaxis

VTE is a well-documented, preventable hospital-related surgical complication in the United States. Compared with laparotomy surgical procedures, VTE occurrence after MIS is rare. Risk factors associated with VTE for women include age, weight, prior history of VTE, malignancy, varicose veins, and the type of surgery performed.

A retrospective cohort study of 1413 women was conducted in a community-based healthcare system in northern California from January 2009 to 2014. Patients underwent MIS for endometrial cancer or complex hyperplasia with atypia; 739 (52.3%) underwent a robotic-assisted procedure, whereas 674 (47.7%) underwent a laparoscopic procedure. They all received mechanical or sequential compression devices (SCDs) as part of VTE prophylaxis per individual hospital policy. Sixty-one percent additionally received pharmacologic prophylaxis. A clinical diagnosis of a VTE was determined within 30 postoperative days and confirmed by one of three diagnostic studies: Doppler ultrasound, computed tomography, or ventilated-perfusion scan.

The study identified a total of 5 of 1413 (0.35%) women with a VTE event, robotic-assisted surgical procedures identified 4 of 739 patients (0.54%), and laparoscopic procedures identified 1 of 674 (0.15%) patients. Patients who received mechanical prophylaxis and additional pharmacologic prophylaxis had a VTE rate of 0.23%, whereas patients who received mechanical prophylaxis alone had a rate of 0.55%. The rate of VTE did not differ statistically between the two different modes of thromboprophylaxis. The study authors concluded that women undergoing MIS should not be included in the high-risk group for VTE. Pharmacologic prophylaxis may not be warranted for women undergoing MIS for endometrial cancer.

MIS, Minimally invasive surgery; *VTE*, venous thromboembolism.
Modified from Freeman AH et al: Venous thromboembolism following minimally invasive surgery among women with endometrial cancer, *Gynecol Oncol* 142(2):267–272, 2016.

ensuring IPCDs are functioning, maintaining normothermia, performing antimicrobial skin preparation, inserting urinary catheters, draping the patient, creating and maintaining a sterile field, initiating safety measures, and monitoring the patient. The nurse ensures all medications are given as ordered, that is, preoperative antibiotic and deep vein thrombosis (DVT) prophylaxis, when applicable. Throughout the patient's perioperative experience, the nurse continues to collect data, adjusts the plan of care, and updates documentation. Hand-off reports are given to relief personnel, ensuring continuity during care transitions.

Instrumentation

The planned gynecologic surgical procedure and any anticipated intraoperative surgical interventions determine what instrumentation is needed. A basic vaginal instrument tray (also called a "kit" or "set") is required for vaginal and vulvar surgery. A basic open abdominal gynecologic instrument tray is required for open abdominal gynecologic surgery. Laparoscopic, hysteroscopic, or specialized robotic instruments are used during minimally invasive surgery (MIS). Surgeon's instrument preferences as well as each facility's instrument tray components vary. The instrumentation described in this chapter is not meant to be all inclusive. For most abdominal gynecologic procedures, a dilation and curettage (D&C) tray is also available.

Positioning

Patient-positioning principles, methods, and safety measures for different surgical positions are described in Chapter 6. Stirrups for lithotomy position may support only the patient's feet (canvas, fabric, or gel-pad ankle straps) or may cradle and support the thighs, popliteal spaces, and lower legs. Padded cradle stirrups promote maintenance of skin integrity and aid in preventing nerve injury (such as peroneal neuropathy). The nurse anticipates that the patient's position may be modified based on the surgical procedure and surgeon's preference. The patient is placed in the lithotomy position for most vaginal and vulvar surgeries. Careful attention is focused on preventing injury

Nursing Diagnosis
Anxiety and Disturbed Body Image related to planned surgical intervention

Outcome
The patient will verbalize reduced or controlled anxiety and acknowledge feelings regarding her body image.

Interventions
- Determine the patient's previous experience and expectations with surgery as well as her level of knowledge related to the planned surgical intervention.
- Assess the patient's level of anxiety and physical reactions to anxiety (e.g., tachycardia, tachypnea, blood pressure elevation, and nonverbal expressions of anxiety); classify her anxiety as low, moderate, or high.
- Use a calming presence and nonthreatening touch (if welcome) to communicate comfort and caring. Acknowledge denial, anger, or depression as normal feelings when adjusting to change in body image or function. Determine and respect her personal space.

- Provide time for and encourage expression of concerns or needs. Clarify and correct any misconceptions she may express about her diagnosis and the effect it will have on her body image.
- Explore coping skills previously used by the patient to relieve anxiety (e.g., relaxation, deep breathing, imagery, listening to music); reinforce these and facilitate their use.
- Explain the sequence of perioperative nursing activities and procedures by using nonmedical terms and clear, concise language that the patient can understand. Encourage questions and expression of concerns. Reinforce information provided by other healthcare team members.
- Minimize environmental stimuli and noise while maintaining patient's privacy.

Nursing Diagnosis
Urinary Retention related to edema, anesthesia, opioids, or pain

Outcome
The patient will maintain or regain normal patterns of urinary elimination.

Continued

SAMPLE PLAN OF CARE—cont'd

Interventions

- Before surgery, explain that an indwelling or temporary (straight) catheter will be inserted (if applicable).
- Verify the presence of any latex allergy; a latex-free catheter is required for latex-allergic patients.
- Insert indwelling or straight catheter using aseptic technique.
- Secure tubing to prevent inadvertent stretching or stress on indwelling catheter.
- Document size of catheter inserted and who inserted it.
- Keep drainage bag below the level of the bladder.
- Observe and document the color and amount of urine on insertion; report abnormalities preoperatively or postoperatively to the surgeon and document any changes.
- Check patency of catheter and drainage system whenever patient is repositioned.
- Discuss with the patient the importance of adequate postoperative fluid intake and early ambulation.
- Clarify any patient misconceptions.
- Encourage the patient to verbalize feelings and concerns regarding inability to void postoperatively and discomfort or pain associated with the presence of an indwelling catheter.

Nursing Diagnosis

Risk for Infection at the surgical site related to operative or other invasive procedures

Outcome

The patient will remain free from SSI.

Interventions

- Administer and document antibiotic prophylaxis as prescribed. Follow safe practices for all medications administered. Label all medications on and off the sterile field.
- Initiate measures to warm patient and maintain normothermia.
- Prepare surgical site with an antiseptic solution; document skin condition at surgical site and solution used.
- Apply dressing to surgical site before sterile drapes are removed to prevent contamination of incision.
- Use infection prevention and control practices.
- Maintain aseptic technique and monitor members of the surgical team for breaks in technique.
- Correctly classify surgical wound at end of procedure.
- Document presence, location, and type of any drains inserted during surgical intervention.

- Review with patient signs and symptoms of infection at surgical site: redness, swelling, warmth, tenderness, pain.
- Discuss the importance of proper handwashing techniques, especially when changing surgical wound dressings, as applicable.

Nursing Diagnosis

Risk for Perioperative Hypothermia

Outcome

The patient will be free from perioperative hypothermia.

Interventions

- Initiate measures to warm patient and maintain normothermia. Begin with preoperative warming and continue intraoperatively.
- Prevent unnecessary skin exposure when prepping, positioning, or moving the patient.
- Place an active warming device (e.g., forced-air warming blanket) on patient after transfer to OR bed.
- Use warm IV and irrigating fluids (as applicable).

Nursing Diagnosis

Risk for Perioperative Positioning Injury

Outcome

The patient will be free from injury related to surgical positioning.

Interventions

- Document any preexisting patient considerations (e.g., nutritional status, weight, preoperative chemotherapy, limitations in mobility or range of motion, neurovascular impairments) that place the patient at risk for positioning injury.
- Use adequate numbers of personnel, or a transfer device, to transfer and position the patient.
- Place safety belts and straps on the patient and secure to the OR bed without friction or undue pressure.
- Assess and document condition of dependent skin areas.
- Use pressure-reducing positioning devices.
- Pad and protect bony prominences and dependent pressure sites.
- Maintain proper body alignment.
- Apply graduated compression stockings and IPCDs as indicated.
- Reassess padding and protection during any positional changes when this does not compromise the integrity of the sterile field.

IPCD, Intermittent pneumatic compression device; *IV,* intravenous; *SSI,* surgical site infection.

and vascular compression. A minimum of two caregivers must position the patient's legs. They are supported above and below the knee joint while positioning to prevent hyperextension of the knee. The legs are raised and placed in the stirrups simultaneously. When lowering the patient's legs, legs are brought together simultaneously and lowered to the bed one at a time to maintain the patient's hemodynamic status (AORN, 2017).

For abdominal gynecologic surgery, Trendelenburg (low or standard) position is usual. This position facilitates access to omentum as well as to the pelvic and paraaortic lymph nodes. It further allows access to the sigmoid colon if a sigmoid resection is required because of metastatic disease.

Steep Trendelenburg position is used during robotic-assisted surgery for exposure of the pelvic organs. This position allows gravity to assist the bowel in falling back into the abdominal cavity and out

of the pelvis, providing optimal exposure. Using steep Trendelenburg position for prolonged procedures may increase cardiovascular risk because of decreased pulmonary compliance and functional residual capacity (FRC) and increase central venous, intraocular, and intracranial pressures (Cassorla and Lee, 2015). Steep Trendelenburg for long periods of time may result in edema of the face, eyes, tongue, and larynx. Anesthesia providers assess for airway edema and obstruction before extubation (Cassorla and Lee, 2015).

For Trendelenburg position, always protect from integumentary, musculoskeletal, and nerve injury while ensuring adequate circulatory, renal, and respiratory functions. Cassorla and Lee (2015) recommended:

- Position the patient's arms on padded armboards with the palms up and fingers extended to prevent ulnar nerve injury whenever possible.

- Maintain armboards at less than a 90-degree angle to prevent stretching the brachial plexus.
- If there are surgical reasons to tuck the arms at the patient's side, pad the patient's elbows to protect the ulnar nerve, face the palms inward toward the hip, and maintain the wrists in a neutral position.
- Secure the arms with a folded drawsheet.
- Wrap the drawsheet over the patient's arms and then snuggly tuck directly under the patient, not under the mattress, to prevent the arm from shifting downward intraoperatively and resting against the OR bed rail, where fingers could be inadvertently compressed and injured.

The bladder is often decompressed at the beginning of the procedure by placing a straight (in and out) or indwelling urinary catheter to monitor urinary output. This practice can also aid in the prevention of bladder injury. The surgeon may request the perioperative nurse to "back fill" the bladder in a retrograde manner intraoperatively with sterile normal saline to assist in determining bladder margins for safe tissue dissection.

The sizes of sutures, needles, and drains depend on the surgical procedure, surgeon preference, and patient needs. The perioperative nurse consults with the surgeon before the procedure to ensure all essential items are readily available.

Prepping

Skin preparation and routine draping procedures are described in Chapter 4. Care is taken to prevent cross-contamination and to avoid pooling under the patient when prepping multiple areas, as in an abdominal hysterectomy. Prep the abdomen before beginning the vaginal prep using the clean to dirty principle (AORN, 2017) and avoid splashing vaginal prep solution onto the already prepped abdomen. Two separate prepping setups are used and kept separate. The perioperative nurse takes care when performing vaginal preps on patients who had vaginal bleeding and may have clots in the vaginal vault. The clots and any gross blood on the thighs or vulva must be removed before beginning the prep. This practice ensures the prepping solution will come into contact with the skin and all mucous membranes of the perineum and vaginal area. All soiled prepping drapes are removed before draping to prevent fire risk and chemical burns caused by pooling (AORN, 2017). Women who have undergone radiation of the pelvis, as well as younger and older female patients, may have narrow or foreshortened vaginal vaults. Take extra care when prepping these patients; it may be best to prep the stenotic vagina with irrigation using a bulb syringe.

Examination Under Anesthesia

Many physicians perform a pelvic examination after the patient is anesthetized and positioned, but before the operative site is prepped. The perioperative nurse anticipates this examination and ensures that nonsterile gloves and an appropriate lubricant are available. Culture specimens (e.g., gonococcal, chlamydial, trichomonal) and a Pap test may be obtained during the examination. Verify with the surgeon that the lubricants used are compatible with cytologic evaluation. Safe specimen practices are initiated.

Dressings, Drains, and Packing

Various dressings are used in gynecologic surgery and may range from simple (e.g., wound closure tapes and surgical skin glue) to complex (i.e., multilayer gauze, ostomy appliances, and abdominal binders). Perineal pads and mesh pants are often used in combination after hysterectomy and vaginal surgeries.

Closed or open drains may be used with or without a reservoir. Indwelling catheters are also commonly used in gynecologic surgery and may be removed postoperatively. All drains and catheters are secured for patient comfort and to avoid dislodgement. Verify in advance that the patient does not have a latex allergy because many of these drains contain latex.

Packing may be used in fistulas or other abnormally created cavities to support and stent the vagina, absorb postoperative drainage, or aid in hemostasis. Products used for vaginal packing include narrow or large fine-mesh gauze available in various yardages. Vaginal packing is usually moistened with saline or coated with antibiotic, antifungal, or an estrogen cream before insertion. Packing is inserted with care to avoid distention of the vaginal vault and compression of its vascular structures. If more than one pack is required or if the length of packing needs to be cut, it is documented in the patient's record and communicated during the patient hand-off report. This ensures all vaginal packing is accounted for when removed postoperatively.

Evaluation

During evaluation, the perioperative nurse determines whether the patient met the previously established outcomes. Some outcomes can be reached during the preoperative and intraoperative phases of care; they are evaluated before the patient's discharge from the OR. Others require ongoing monitoring and measurement in the postoperative phase, and these are denoted by the word "will" to indicate their ongoing nature. Part of the perioperative nursing hand-off report to the postanesthesia care unit (PACU) includes the outcomes of the nursing plan of care. They can be phrased as follows:

- The patient will effectively cope with her anxiety and disturbance in body image; questions will continue to be answered and misconceptions clarified. Her anxiety was reduced; she verbalized concerns and used personally effective coping strategies during her procedure.
- Urinary elimination patterns and patency were maintained; urinary output was adequate. Color and amount of urine were monitored for any changes, documented in the patient record, and communicated to the surgeon and anesthesia provider.
- The patient's skin integrity and surgical asepsis were maintained. There will be no signs of SSI.
- Perioperative normothermia was maintained.
- There was no apparent evidence of injury related to surgical positioning; range-of-motion and neurovascular status will be consistent with preoperative levels.

In addition, the perioperative nurse evaluates and reports the patient's alertness and orientation status, pain level, presence of drains and catheters, and respiratory status in the hand-off report to the PACU nurse.

Patient, Family, and Caregiver Education and Discharge Planning

Patient, family, and caregiver education, along with discharge planning, are critical perioperative nursing activities. Many gynecologic surgical procedures happen on an ambulatory basis, both in hospitals and ambulatory surgical centers. Hospital stays for patients requiring admission after their surgical procedure continue to shorten. Therefore patient education and discharge planning begin before admission during preadmission testing. Regardless of the procedure to be performed, the perioperative nurse begins patient, family, and caregiver education with vital postoperative care information (Enhanced Recovery After Surgery).

ENHANCED RECOVERY AFTER SURGERY

Enhanced Recovery Pathway in Gynecologic Surgery

ERAS pathways in gynecologic surgery use a multimodal clinical evidence-based approach to perioperative care. ERAS promotes early return of GI function and is associated with both shorter hospital stays and reduced hospital costs without increasing complications or readmission rates. Its main goal is to optimize patient outcomes by decreasing the body's response to stress associated with surgery. Pathway interventions focus on three main surgical phases: preoperative, intraoperative, and postoperative.

Preoperative

- Patient counseling and education: implement these as early as possible and provide educational materials.
- Preoperative diet: carbohydrate-loading drinks are often used to mitigate preoperative caloric restriction, improve insulin resistance, and lead to shorter hospital stays.
- Avoid mechanical bowel preparation: there are more negative effects from bowel preparation than benefits. These negative effects may include patient discomfort, dehydration, electrolyte disturbances, need for prolonged fasting, and delay of postop bowel function. Bowel preparation does not benefit intraoperative visualization or bowel handling.
- Preemptive analgesia: the theory is that pain medications block the pain receptors before they are stimulated, which promotes better pain control and less postop use of pain medications.

Intraoperative

- Anesthesia: advances in anesthetic medications, availability of short-acting volatile anesthetics, and the use of continuous propofol decrease PONV, assist with rapid awakening, and decrease systemic opioid requirements.
- Maintain normothermia: core body temperatures below 36°C have been associated with increased risk of bleeding, impaired drug metabolism and oxygen transportation, cardiac morbidity, and increase in infection. It is important to monitor intraoperatively for both hypothermia and hyperthermia.
- Avoid intraoperative fluid overload: fluid overload may lead to electrolyte abnormalities, peripheral soft tissue and small

bowel edema (leading to delay in bowel function), and pulmonary congestion.

- Prevent PONV: female gender and gynecologic and MIS surgery are recognized as contributors to PONV. Women who are at high risk for PONV may benefit from a transdermal scopolamine patch applied within 2 hours before anesthesia and surgery.
- Avoid NGTs: routine use of NGTs has been associated with increased rates of postoperative pneumonia, atelectasis, and fever. The ERAS Society recommends against routine use of NGTs in both benign and oncologic gynecologic surgery.
- Limit prophylactic peritoneal drains: peritoneal drains should be considered when there is a concern for postoperative bleeding or when a very low anterior bowel resection has been performed without a temporary bowel diversion.

Postoperative

- Early postoperative feeding: encourage patient consumption of liquid and solid intake within 24 hours postoperatively. Studies show early return of bowel function and shorter hospital stays with no change in postoperative complications.
- Early mobilization: helps protect against muscle loss as well as pulmonary and VTE complications.
- Early urinary catheter removal: within 24 hours after surgery. This practice has shown less frequent urinary tract infections, early ambulation, and shorter hospital stays.
- Perioperative pain management: one of the most central goals of ERAS is pain control while minimizing opioid use.
- Multimodal pharmacologic analgesia: using two or more medications to act synergistically for pain control.
- Regional analgesia: i.e., TEA, TAP blocks, and IPLA.
- Postoperative fluid management: patients are encouraged to drink immediately after surgery and IVs are discontinued once patients can maintain hydration.
- Laxative use and prevention of postoperative ileus: the goal is to hasten return of GI function. Chewing gum early postoperatively has also shown to improve GI function.

ERAS, Enhanced recovery after surgery; *GI,* gastrointestinal; *IPLA,* intraperitoneal local anesthetic; *IV,* intravenous; *MIS,* minimally invasive surgery; *NGT,* nasogastric tube; *PONV,* postoperative nausea and vomiting; *TAP,* transverse abdominis plane; *TEA,* thoracic epidural analgesia; *VTE,* venous thromboembolic.
Modified from Kalogera E, Dowdy SC: Enhanced recovery pathway in gynecologic surgery, *Obstet Gynecol Clin North Am* 43(3); 551–573, 2016.

The main goal is to restore normal body function, which may include early ambulation, prevention of respiratory complications, wound care, drain care, catheter care, anticipated postoperative discomfort, managing postoperative pain, restrictions in activity, diet, and any other patient concerns. Other topics, such as progression of activities, returning to work, lifting limitations, emotional and physical issues, sexual activity, general nutritional needs, and health maintenance are also part of the educational process.

Gynecologic patients are provided with specific information regarding postoperative signs and symptoms to report, especially in relation to vaginal bleeding and the surgical wound, along with restrictions related to douching and vaginal penetration (tampons or sexual intercourse). Today, patients may go home on the same day as their surgical procedure or be admitted for a 23-hour stay (Ambulatory Surgery Considerations). Simple, clear information

and instructions such as those presented in the Patient, Family, and Caregiver Education box enhance patient learning.

Lasers in Gynecologic Surgery

Carbon dioxide and argon lasers are used in gynecology to treat extrauterine disease such as pelvic endometriosis, cervical dysplasia, condylomata acuminata, pelvic adhesive disease, and premalignant diseases of the vulva and vagina. Lasers are generally used in conjunction with the colposcope and operating microscope, or the laparoscope. A laser plume evacuator or suction system is used to remove surgical smoke and fumes from the operative field in both open and MIS procedures (AORN, 2017). Surgical personnel in the room wear a high-filtration laser mask to prevent exposure from the laser plume and implement laser safety precautions (see Chapter 8 for a discussion of lasers and laser safety).

AMBULATORY SURGERY CONSIDERATIONS

Minimally Invasive and Robotic Gynecologic Surgery

Many gynecologic procedures are performed using minimally invasive techniques. An advantage of MIS is that patients can be discharged on the day of surgery or within 23 hours of admission. Other advantages of MIS are fewer incision-related complications and less postoperative pain, better cosmesis, lower intraoperative blood loss, and faster postoperative recovery. Perioperative nurses involved in gynecologic ambulatory procedures should consider the following factors when planning and implementing perioperative patient care.

Preoperative Care

Preoperative care of patients undergoing MIS focuses on early patient teaching. Provide patients with written and verbal instructions, review preadmission procedures, and alleviate concerns or confusion. Teaching focuses on the following:

- Specifics of the particular surgical procedure: provide educational pamphlets or informative websites such as for robotic-assisted procedures. Be sure websites show an HON code of conduct seal.
- Anxiety: ensure that the patient understands the surgeon controls the robot and the robot is only a surgical tool to aid the surgeon to be more efficient and effective.
- Levels of postoperative pain and any activity limitations: remember that patients and their families will provide much of the postoperative care at home after surgery.
- Complications: review signs and symptoms to watch for and ensure the patient knows when to contact her healthcare provider about problems (e.g., infection, uncontrolled pain, sudden change in vaginal discharge).
- Care of the operative site: provide written instructions when teaching because preoperative anxiety may distract the patient's attention and her comprehension or retention of teaching material. These instructions are reviewed again postoperatively, before discharge.
- Preprocedural screening of patients: aimed at identifying risks for infection, clotting disorders, hypertension, heart or lung disease, and numerous other diseases that may interfere with the patient's care. The patient's general health is assessed to ensure that she can tolerate the procedure and the anesthesia plan of care. MIS procedures use CO_2 gas to create visual space in the peritoneum (which is called a *pneumoperitoneum*). Insufflation with

CO_2 can cause cardiopulmonary and hemodynamic complications.

The following are possible complications associated with CO_2 insufflation:

- Hyperkalemia
- Pulmonary complications
- Cardiovascular and vascular complications
- Subcutaneous emphysema
- Metabolic inflammatory responses
- Gas embolism (rare)

Intraoperative Care

Intraoperative care is specific to the planned procedure. In robotic-assisted procedures, the nursing team must know how to set up, calibrate, and operate the robotic system. During surgery, monitoring cues and messages from the robotic system are important. Troubleshooting is critical to ensure patient safety and to avoid prolonging the procedure. Knowing emergency protocols is vital in MIS and robotic-assisted procedures. The surgical team may find that developing a checklist for surgical emergencies, such as converting to an open procedure, assists in efficient care and positive surgical outcomes rather than relying on memory alone.

Postoperative Care

Postoperative care of the MIS patient is provided according to the same standards as those of traditional surgery. Early care focuses on stabilizing the patient, maintaining pain control, carefully monitoring the operative site, carefully monitoring vital signs and level of consciousness, and following specific care requisites for the particular procedure.

As length of stay for these patients is generally short, keen assessment skills are important to handle issues before discharge. Teaching within the shortened time frame may be impeded by patients and family who are not ready to learn because of postoperative pain or the effects of anesthesia. The nurse provides verbal and written discharge instructions, has the patient or family member teach-back key points in their own words, and, when possible, follows up with the patient and her family after discharge to ensure that complications do not arise and patients are having no problems following instructions. Before discharge, complete (or review) medication reconciliation and discuss new medication with the patient and her family.

HON, Health on the Net; MIS, minimally invasive surgery.
Modified from Arriaga AF et al: Simulation-based trial of surgical-crisis checklists, *N Engl J Med* 368:246–253, 2013; The Joint Commission (TJC): *Ambulatory health care: 2017 national patient safety goals* (website). www.jointcommission.org/ahc_2017_npsgs/. (Accessed 17 January 2017); Uccella S et al: Laparoscopic versus open hysterectomy for benign disease in women with giant uteri (≥1500 g): feasibility and outcomes, *J Minim Invasive Gynecol* 23(6):922–927, 2016; Unger CA et al: Risk factors for robotic gynecologic procedures requiring conversion to other surgical procedures, *Obstet Gynecol Int J* 135(3):229–303, 2016.

PATIENT, FAMILY, AND CAREGIVER EDUCATION

Gynecologic Surgery

When possible, provide the patient and her caregiver with verbal and written instructions. Provide them with the phone number of the physician, nurse practitioner, or physician assistant to call if questions arise. Use visual aids to enhance instruction. Encourage the patient to verbalize any concerns she may have regarding her condition and surgery. Misconceptions about the outcome of gynecologic surgery are common. Patients may believe that undergoing a hysterectomy will cause depression, nervousness, mental instability, weight gain, wrinkles, masculinity, and hirsutism. Provide education to correct misconceptions and discuss other concerns, such as fear of death, cancer, loss of femininity and childbearing ability, pain management, and changes in sexuality. Education points for common gynecologic procedures are as follows.

Continued

PATIENT, FAMILY, AND CAREGIVER EDUCATION

Gynecologic Surgery—cont'd

Dilation and Curettage of the Uterus
- Notify physician if an elevated temperature or foul-smelling vaginal discharge develops.
- Clean the perineum after elimination and change perineal pads often.
- Eat foods high in iron and protein to promote tissue repair and red blood cell replacement.
- Avoid sexual intercourse, tub baths, and the use of tampons for 2 weeks to allow healing and prevent infection.
- Slight bleeding is normal. However, if bleeding is as heavy as during your normal menstrual period or if it lasts longer than 2 weeks, call your physician.

If a procedure was performed for miscarriage, add the following:
- Mood swings and depression are common after pregnancy loss because of hormonal changes as well as with the emotional consequences of the loss. It can be helpful to talk to friends, family, or clergy about your loss.
- Support groups may be helpful while you recover.
- Allow yourself (and your partner) to grieve the loss before becoming pregnant again.
- Attempts at a subsequent pregnancy should be postponed until you check with your physician.

Endometrial Ablation
- Vaginal discharge is expected for 4 to 6 weeks.
- Your next menstrual period may be irregular.
- You may find analgesics or NSAIDs helpful for pain relief (if not contraindicated).
- You can return to your normal activities within several days.
- Call your physician if you have heavy bleeding or signs of infection.
- Avoid sexual intercourse and the use of tampons for 2 weeks to allow healing and prevent infection.

Vulvectomy
- Avoid sexual activity for 4 to 6 weeks or as long as directed by your healthcare provider.
- Rest frequently.

- Avoid crossing your legs and sitting or standing for long periods.
- Avoid tight, constricting clothing, and wear cotton underwear.
- Keep your perineal area clean and dry. Rinse perineum after each elimination with warm water, and pat dry. Avoid sitting on the toilet for prolonged periods of time, particularly if you are constipated and strain to defecate.
- Report any temperature greater than 102.2°F (39°C).
- Report any swelling, redness, unusual tenderness, drainage, or foul odor of the incision site to your healthcare provider.
- Eat a well-balanced diet to promote healing.
- Elevate legs periodically.

Myomectomy or Hysterectomy
- You will no longer have a period, although you may have some vaginal discharge after you go home.
- Eat foods high in protein, iron, and vitamin C to aid tissue healing; include foods with high fiber content, and drink six to eight glasses of water daily.
- Rest when tired; resume activities as your comfort level permits. Avoid vigorous exercise, vacuuming, and heavy lifting for 6 weeks. Avoid sitting for long periods. Resume driving when your comfort allows or when your healthcare provider approves.
- Avoid tub baths, intercourse, and douching until after your follow-up examination.
- When vaginal intercourse is resumed, use water-soluble lubricants to decrease discomfort.
- Report the following symptoms to your healthcare provider: vaginal bleeding, GI changes, persistent postoperative symptoms (e.g., cramping, distention, change in bowel habits), and signs of wound infection (e.g., redness, swelling, heat, or pain at the incision site).
- If your ovaries were removed you may experience symptoms of menopause, including hot flashes, night sweats, and vaginal dryness. Other symptoms may include sleep disturbance, fatigue, anxiety, and depression.
- Hormone replacement therapy may be prescribed.

GI, Gastrointestinal; NSAIDs, nonsteroidal antiinflammatory drugs.
Modified from Lowdermilk DL: Structural disorders and neoplasms of the reproductive system. In Lowdermilk DL, Perry SE, editors: *Maternity and women's health care*, ed 11, St Louis, 2016, Mosby; Cashion K: Hemorrhagic disorders. In Lowdermilk DL, Perry SE, editors: *Maternity and women's health care*, ed 11, St Louis, 2016, Mosby.

Surgical Interventions

Vulvar Surgery

A variety of malignant and nonmalignant conditions affect the vulva. Benign lesions are generally excised. The treatment of early malignant disease of the vulva is accomplished by a local wide excision, or, for more multicentric or extensive lesions, by simple or radical vulvectomy with possible inguinofemoral lymph node dissection depending on the extent of invasion.

Excision of Condylomata Acuminata

Vulvar/perineal condyloma is caused by HPV (Fig. 14.11), most commonly the low-risk HPV subtypes (6 and 11), which are transmitted sexually. These warty lesions may extend into the vaginal vault or the anus and may be aggravated by hormonal changes during pregnancy. Depending on the viral strain, the condition may be benign or associated with high-risk subtypes of HPV, often leading to moderate or severe dysplasia and malignancy. Surgical treatment ranges from desiccation of the lesions with a monopolar electrosurgical unit (ESU) to sharp excision or eradication through use of the laser. Surgical personnel in the room wear high-filtration laser masks to prevent exposure and possible viral contamination from airborne contaminants caused by the ESU or laser plume (AORN, 2017). Surgical intervention is based on the type and extent of the lesions.

Superficial Vulvectomy

Superficial vulvectomy is the removal of the external skin from the affected area, which has been previously identified after applying 3% to 5% acetic acid. The purpose of this procedure is to preserve

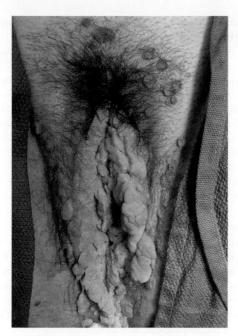

FIG. 14.11 Condylomata acuminata.

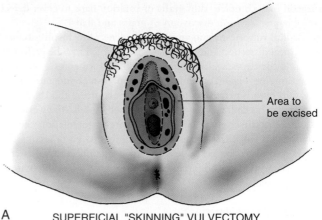

A   SUPERFICIAL "SKINNING" VULVECTOMY

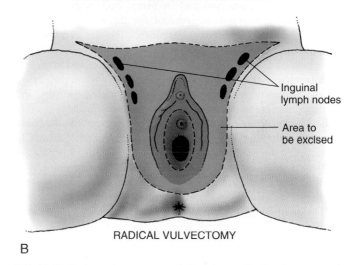

B   RADICAL VULVECTOMY

FIG. 14.12 Outline of incisions used for (A) superficial vulvectomy and (B) radical vulvectomy.

the underlying structures of the external genitalia. This procedure treats not only dysplasia, but also leukoplakia, intractable pruritus, or other types of skin lesions and chronic venereal granulomas.

Procedural Considerations

The basic vaginal instrument tray is required, plus an ESU, if desired. The nurse assists with placing the patient in lithotomy position (see Chapter 6 for positioning considerations) and then performs a perineal and vaginal prep.

Operative Procedure

The external skin is excised from the affected area (Fig. 14.12A).

Simple Vulvectomy

Simple vulvectomy is removal of the labia majora and labia minora, possibly but not preferably the glans clitoris, and occasionally tissue from the perianal area. A simple vulvectomy is usually done to treat CIS of the vulva when it is multicentric. Rarely, a simple vulvectomy is necessary for the treatment of either leukoplakia or intractable pruritus.

Procedural Considerations

The instruments required and patient positioning are as described for superficial vulvectomy.

Operative Procedure

1. The surgeon incises the affected skin, usually starting anteriorly above the clitoris. The incision is continued laterally to the labia majora, to the midline of the perineum, and around the anus if involved. A knife, hemostats, radiopaque gauze sponges on sponge-holding forceps, tissue forceps, and Allis forceps are required. Bleeding vessels are clamped, ligated, or electrocoagulated with the ESU.
2. Periurethral and perivaginal incisions are made. Bleeding of this vascular area can be controlled by means of Kelly or Crile hemostats and electrocoagulation with the ESU. Ligation of blood

vessels should be minimal. Allis-Adair forceps are used for holding diseased tissues.
3. Using curved dissecting scissors, tissue forceps, Allis forceps, and sponges on holding forceps, the surgeon undermines and mobilizes the skin and subcutaneous tissues.
4. The wound is closed, usually by simple bilateral Z-plasty. In some cases, the surgeon excises the skin around the anus to accomplish a sliding skin flap.
5. Closed-wound drainage catheters may be placed in dependent areas; an indwelling urinary catheter is inserted and its tubing secured. Vaginal gauze packing may be placed in the vagina. Dressings are applied.

Radical Vulvectomy and Groin Lymphadenectomy

Radical vulvectomy and groin lymphadenectomy involve dissection of the following structures: the labia majora; the labia minora; the clitoris; the mons veneris; involved terminal portions of the urethra, vagina, and other vulvar organs; and the superficial and deep inguinofemoral nodes, portions of the round ligaments, portions of the saphenous veins, and the lesion itself. In the past, dissection was carried out en bloc; however, now the procedure is discontinuous, and minimal skin, if any, in the groin is sacrificed. It also may involve reconstruction of the vaginal walls and pelvic floor and closure of the abdominal wounds if a segment of vagina is resected. A plastic surgeon may complete skin grafts or rotation flaps to cover defects (see Chapter 22 for a discussion of grafts and flaps).

Radical vulvectomy and groin lymphadenectomy involve abdominoperineal dissection and groin dissection, which may be performed as a one- or two-stage operation. When performed as a one-stage operation, it is optimally done by a four-person perioperative team. The skin prep is extensive, including the abdomen and thighs; if a skin graft is needed, the donor site is prepped as well. Many extensive lesions alternatively may be treated with chemoradiation therapy, avoiding loss of intestinal or bladder function. Early lesions may also be treated by sentinel node biopsy to avoid unnecessary dissection of negative nodes and attendant morbidity, including chronic lymphedema.

Procedural Considerations

The patient lies supine and may be placed in Trendelenburg and low lithotomy positions, as required for the various stages (see Chapter 6 for positioning considerations). The skin prep includes the abdomen, perineum, vagina, and thighs. An indwelling urinary catheter is often inserted to act as a urethral marker and to prevent postoperative urethral trauma. The perioperative nurse prepares to receive numerous specimens during lymph node dissection, and safe specimen management practices are implemented. As in other radical surgeries, the perioperative nurse prepares to measure blood loss and anticipates measures to assist the anesthesia provider in maintaining normovolemia.

For radical vulvectomy, the basic vaginal instrument tray is required, along with assorted sizes of Richardson retractors, Volkmann rake retractors, skin hooks, and closed wound drainage systems.

For groin lymphadenectomy, the basic abdominal gynecologic instrument tray is required, along with Schnidt tonsil forceps, Kantrowitz right-angle thoracic clamps, ligating clips and appliers, suture ties, an ESU, and closed wound drainage systems.

Operative Procedure

Radical Vulvectomy

1. The skin incisions of the abdomen and thigh join with those for vulvectomy. The incisions in the vulva encircle the urethra.
2. In the vulvar dissection, the surgeon removes the terminal portions of the urethra and vagina, the mons veneris, the clitoris, the frenulum, the prepuce of the clitoris, Bartholin and Skene glands, and fascial coverings of the vulva with the specimen (see Fig. 14.12B).
3. Reconstruction of the vaginal walls and the pelvic floor is completed.
4. An indwelling urinary catheter is inserted and its tubing secured; a closed wound drainage system is placed in the denuded area; and pressure dressings are applied.

Groin Lymphadenectomy

1. The surgeon makes the first skin incision on the side of the primary lesion. If nodes on the same side of a lateralized lesion are negative on histologic section, it will not be necessary to perform the contralateral node dissection. The end of the incised skin is grasped with Allis forceps. The incision is extended to the aponeurosis of the external oblique muscle.
2. The fascia over the inguinal ligament and the fascia lata of the upper thigh are exposed, separated, and freed with retractors, blade, scissors, hemostats, and radiopaque soft gauze sponges.
3. Bleeding vessels, including the superficial iliac artery and vein, the epigastric artery and vein, and the superficial external pudendal artery and vein, are preserved when possible; otherwise, they are

clamped and ligated. Smaller bleeding vessels are controlled with the ESU.
4. Using Metzenbaum scissors, tissue forceps without teeth, and retractors, the surgeon excises the nodes most commonly involved with metastatic disease. These nodes are those superficial to the cribriform fascia and medial to the femoral vein. The surgeon pays particular attention to the resection of these nodes and, if suspicious, they are likely to be submitted for frozen-section examination. Involvement of these nodes is indicative of a need for postoperative groin irradiation, and then only grossly involved nodes need be removed.
5. The lymphatic node beds may be identified in the future by placing metal clips in the area during the procedure. Fine, long, sharp tissue dissection scissors are needed.
6. The node-bearing regions are exposed for complete dissection by means of retractors and are protected by warm, moist radiopaque laparotomy pads. The saphenous vein is preserved, if possible, to reduce risk of postoperative lymphedema. If not possible, ligation is performed using scissors, forceps, and hemostats and then doubly tied.
7. The surgeon clears the femoral canal of its lymphatics; the round ligament is clamped, cut, and ligated.
8. The wound is closed using the surgeon's preferred suture material, drains are inserted and secured, and dressings are applied.
9. An indwelling urethral catheter is inserted and its tubing secured before the patient is transferred to the PACU.

Gynecologic Surgery Using Vaginal Approach

Plastic Reconstructive Repair of the Vagina (Anterior and Posterior Repair; Colporrhaphy)

A vaginal repair is done to correct a cystocele, rectocele, enterocele, or to reestablish the support of the anterior and posterior vaginal walls and restore the bladder and rectum to their normal positions.

A cystocele is a herniation of the bladder that causes the anterior vaginal wall to bulge downward (Fig. 14.13). A defect in the anterior vaginal wall is usually caused by obstetric or surgical trauma, advanced age, or an inherent weakness. A large protrusion may cause a sensation of pressure in the vagina or present as a mass at or through the introitus; it may also cause voiding difficulties.

A rectocele occurs when the anterior rectal wall (posterior vaginal wall) protrudes into the vagina. Generally the anterior rectal wall forms a bulging mass beneath the posterior vaginal mucosa (Fig. 14.14). As the mass pushes downward into the lower vaginal canal, the rectum may be separated from the fascial and muscular attachments of the urogenital diaphragm and the pelvic wall. The levator ani muscles become stretched or separated. The patient may present with a mass protruding into the vagina, difficulty in evacuating the lower bowel, hemorrhoids, and a feeling of pressure.

An enterocele is a herniation of the peritoneum through the central portion of the vaginal vault in women who have undergone prior hysterectomy. If a woman has a uterus, the herniation is between the uterosacral ligaments. An enterocele can contain a loop of the small intestine.

Procedural Considerations

The procedure is done with the patient in lithotomy position (see Chapter 6 for positioning considerations). The basic vaginal instrument tray is required. Vaginal retractors are used for exposure. The labia may be sutured to the medial thigh on each side to expose the vaginal introitus. A D&C tray should be available.

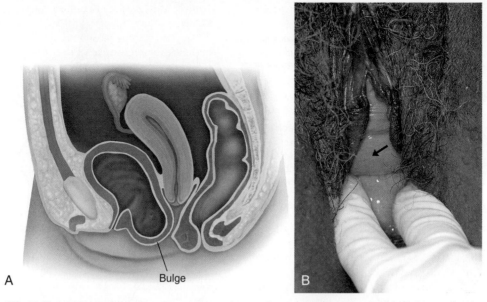

FIG. 14.13 (A) Cystocele resulting from unrepaired tears of muscles of the pelvic floor and those under the bladder, usually resulting from childbirth, surgical trauma, advanced age, or inherent weakness. (B) Cystocele *(arrow).*

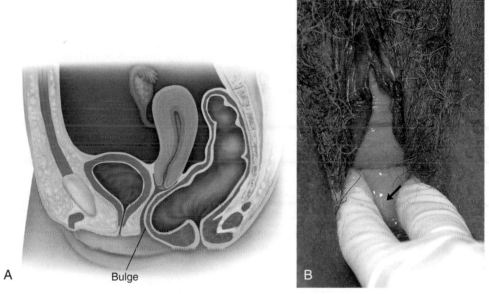

FIG. 14.14 (A) Rectocele resulting from unrepaired tears of the muscles of the pelvic floor and those under the bladder, usually resulting from childbirth, surgical trauma, advanced age, or inherent weakness. (B) Rectocele *(arrow).*

Operative Procedure

Cystocele Repair

1. The bladder is drained by straight catheterization or insertion of an indwelling urinary catheter (surgeon's preference). Areolar tissue between the bladder and vagina at the bladder reflection is exposed. A mixture of IV normal saline and vasopressin or local anesthetic with epinephrine may be injected into the tissue for hemostasis and to facilitate tissue plane dissection. Full-thickness dissection of the vaginal wall is done up to the bladder neck with a blade, curved scissors, tissue forceps, Allis-Adair or Allis forceps, and radiopaque gauze sponges. Bleeding vessels are clamped and tied with ligatures or controlled with a bipolar or monopolar ESU.

2. The surgeon mobilizes the urethra and bladder neck with a knife blade, radiopaque gauze sponges, and curved scissors.

3. Sutures are placed adjacent to the urethra and bladder neck in such a manner that, after they have been tied, the bladder neck and the posterior urethrovesical angle are narrowed (Fig. 14.15A).

4. The surgeon sutures the connective tissue on the lateral aspects of the cervix into the cervix to shorten the cardinal ligaments.

5. Allis-Adair forceps are applied to the edges of the incision, and the left flap of the vaginal wall is drawn across the midline. Edges

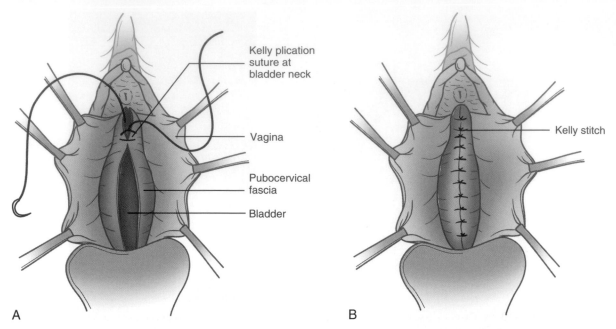

FIG. 14.15 Cystocele repair. (A) Placement of a Kelly stitch in the pubocervical fascia at the junction of the urethra with the bladder neck. (B) Repair of the cystocele as the pubocervical fascia is sutured; thus the cystocele is plicated.

are trimmed according to the size of the cystocele. The surgeon repeats the process on the right flap of the vaginal incision.

6. The anterior vaginal wall is closed in a manner resulting in reconstruction of an anterior vaginal fornix (see Fig. 14.15B). Cystoscopy instrumentation may be required to evaluate the integrity of the urethra and ureteral orifices. A perineal pad may be applied.

Rectocele Repair

1. The surgeon places Allis forceps posteriorly at the mucocutaneous junction on each side, at the hymenal ring, and just above the anus (Fig. 14.16A). A mixture of IV normal saline and vasopressin or local anesthetic with epinephrine may be injected into the tissue for hemostasis and to facilitate tissue plane dissection. Skin and mucosa are incised and dissected from the muscles beneath with a knife blade, tissue forceps, curved scissors, and radiopaque gauze sponges.

2. Allis-Adair forceps are placed on the posterior vaginal wall, scar tissue (from obstetric trauma) is removed, and the surgeon continues the dissection to the posterior vaginal fornix and laterally, depending on the size of the rectocele (see Fig. 14.16A–B).

3. The perineum is denuded by sharp dissection, and trimming of the posterior vaginal wall is carried out with Allis forceps and curved scissors (see Fig. 14.16C).

4. The rectal wall proximal to the puborectal muscle is strengthened by placement of sutures.

5. Bleeding is controlled, and the surgeon closes the vaginal wall from above, downward to the anterior edge of the puborectal muscle. The rectocele is repaired from the posterior fornix to the perineal body. Remains of the transverse perineal and bulbocavernosus muscles are used to augment the perineum. The anterior edge of the levator ani muscle may be approximated (see Fig. 14.16D).

6. The mucosa and skin are trimmed, and the remaining closure is performed with interrupted sutures.

7. The vagina may be packed with 2-inch vaginal gauze packing with an added antibiotic, antifungal, or an estrogen cream. An indwelling urinary catheter is inserted and the tubing is secured. A perineal pad may be applied.

8. The surgeon will require an additional pair of sterile gloves if a rectal digital examination is performed to prevent cross-contamination of the vaginal, rectal, and anal tissue flora.

Enterocele Repair. Enterocele repair is illustrated in Fig. 14.17. The peritoneal sac is carefully dissected from the underlying rectum, the overlying bladder, or both, so that the peritoneal tissues are completely freed from the surrounding structures. The sac is opened to establish true identification and is then closed as high as possible by permanent purse-string sutures. The portion of peritoneal tissue distal to the purse-string ties is then excised, and the area is reinforced locally by transverse suture closure using any available supportive tissues. This technique is used to prevent recurrence.

Perineal Repair. Perineal repair is illustrated in Fig. 14.18.

Vesicovaginal Fistula Repair. A vesicovaginal fistula (a communication between the urinary bladder and the vagina) is repaired by free dissection of the mucosal tissue of the anterior vaginal wall, closing of the fistula tract, and repair of the fascial attachments between the bladder and vagina, with establishment of urinary drainage. Fistulas vary in size from a small opening that permits only slight leakage of urine into the vagina to a large opening that permits all urine to pass into the vagina (Fig. 14.19). They may result from radiation therapy, radical surgery for the management of pelvic cancer, chronic ulceration of the vaginal structures, penetrating wounds, or obstetric trauma. Vesicovaginal fistulas are repaired either through the vaginal or transperitoneal approach (see Chapter 15 for a description of the transperitoneal approach).

Urethrovaginal Fistula Repair (Vaginal Approach). A urethrovaginal fistula (a communication between the urethra and the vagina) (see Fig. 14.19) usually causes constant incontinence or difficulty

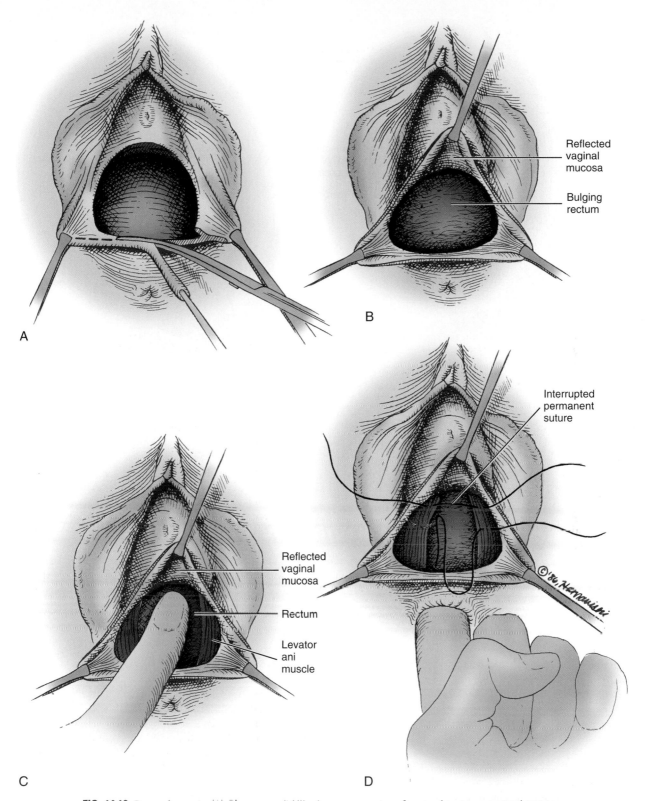

FIG. 14.16 Rectocele repair. (A) Placement of Allis clamps at margins of perineal incision; perineal incision is being made. (B) Reflected vaginal mucosa with rectum bulging. (C) Depression of rectum identifying margins of levator ani muscle. (D) Placement of sutures in perirectal tissue and levator ani bundles.

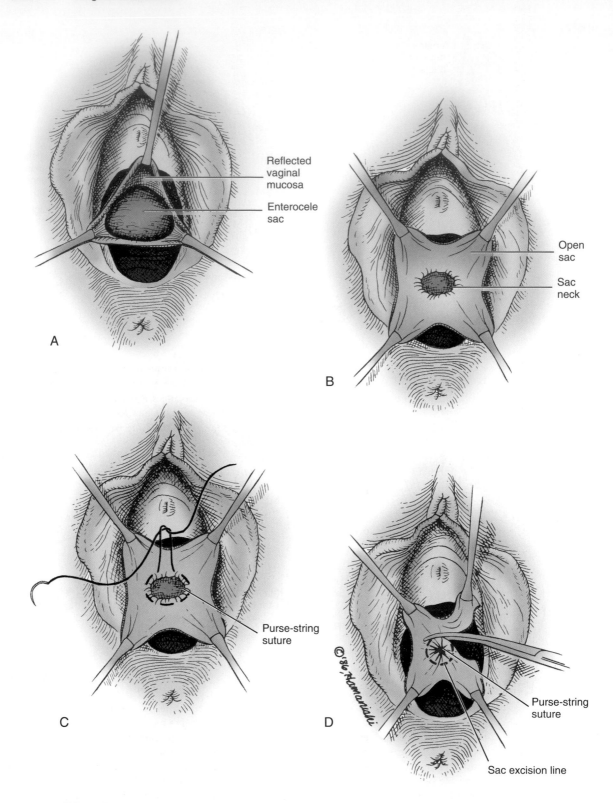

FIG. 14.17 Enterocele repair. (A) Appearance of enterocele sac with vaginal wall reflected. (B) Appearance of open enterocele sac with sac neck identified. (C) Placement of purse-string suture at neck of enterocele sac. (D) Excision of enterocele sac.

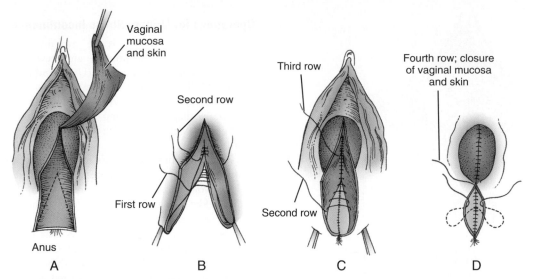

FIG. 14.18 Repair of complete lacerations of the perineum. (A) Lower margins of incision. (B) Placement of first and second rows of sutures. (C) Second and third rows of sutures. (D) Fourth row of sutures.

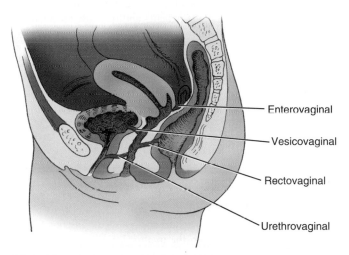

FIG. 14.19 Genital fistulas may present as communications between the urethra, bladder, one of the ureters, or the bowel and some part of the genital tract. Two of the most common types are urethrovaginal and vesicovaginal, both of which empty into the vaginal canal.

in retaining urine. This condition occurs after damage to the anterior wall and bladder, radiation therapy, or parturition.

Procedural Considerations. The basic vaginal instrument tray is required, with the addition of Kelly fistula or Metzenbaum scissors, dressing forceps, probes, skin hooks, Frazier suction tips, urethral catheters, and sterile saline to distend the bladder intraoperatively to check for leaks. The patient is placed in lithotomy position (see Chapter 6 for positioning considerations).

Operative Procedure

1. After traction sutures are placed around the fistulous tract, the surgeon grasps the tissues with Allis-Adair forceps and plain tissue forceps.
2. The surgeon excises scar tissue around the fistula, locates the cleavage between the bladder and vagina, and mobilizes the flaps using scissors, forceps, and radiopaque gauze sponges.

3. The bladder mucosa is inverted toward the interior of the bladder with interrupted sutures. The sutures are passed through the muscularis of the bladder down to the mucosa.
4. A second layer of inverting sutures is placed in the bladder and tied, completely inverting the bladder mucosa toward the interior.
5. The surgeon closes the vaginal wall in multiple layers, approximating the anterior and posterior vaginal walls distal to the closure of the bladder with interrupted sutures in a direction opposite the closure of the bladder wall.
6. The bladder is distended with sterile saline to detect any leaks. An indwelling urinary catheter is inserted and the tubing is secured. A perineal pad may be applied.

Ureterovaginal Fistula

A ureterovaginal fistula (a communication between the distal ureter and the vagina) develops as a result of injury to the ureter. In some cases, reimplantation of the ureter into the bladder or ureterostomy may be done (see Chapter 15 for a description of these procedures).

Rectovaginal Fistula Repair (Vaginal Approach)

A rectovaginal fistula is an abnormal communication between the rectum and vagina (see Fig. 14.19). Surgical repair is via the vaginal approach. It includes repair of the perineum, fascia, and muscle-supporting structures between the rectum and vagina, closing the fistula (Fig. 14.20). In the presence of a large rectovaginal fistula, as in patients who have had radiation therapy or incurable cancer, a colostomy may be performed (see Chapter 11 for a description of the procedure for colostomy). The surgeon requires an additional pair of sterile gloves if a rectal digital examination is performed during the procedure to prevent cross-contamination.

Procedural Considerations. The basic vaginal instrument tray is required. The patient is placed in lithotomy position (see Chapter 6 for positioning considerations)

Operative Procedure

1. The surgeon excises the scar tissue and tract between the rectum and vagina (Fig. 14.21); edges of fresh tissue are approximated with absorbable sutures (surgeon's preference).

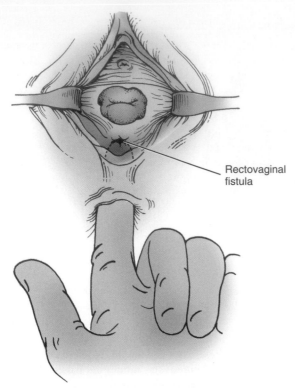

FIG. 14.20 Rectovaginal fistula. Examiner's finger puts tension on rectovaginal septum.

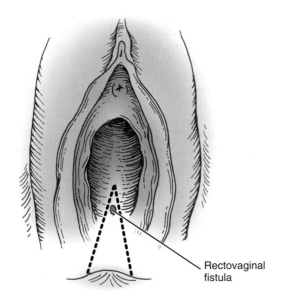

FIG. 14.21 Repair of rectovaginal fistulas of all types is essentially the same as shown here. Portion of scar tissue to be excised is included within dotted lines; repair is as described for complete lacerations of perineum (see Fig. 14.18).

2. The rectum and vaginal walls are mobilized; the rectum is closed with inversion of the mucosa into the rectal canal. Occasionally, a myocutaneous flap is used in reconstruction to augment closure.
3. The vagina is closed transversely or in a sagittal plane different from that of the rectal canal. The vaginal mucosal layer is inverted into the vaginal wall; an indwelling urinary catheter is inserted and the tubing is secured. A perineal pad is applied.

Operations for Urinary Stress Incontinence

Urinary incontinence (UI) is the involuntary loss of urine. The three main types of incontinence are stress urinary incontinence (SUI); urge urinary incontinence (UUI); and mixed urinary incontinence (MUI), which describes the simultaneous presence of both types of UI (Lemack and Anger, 2016). The patient may have preoperative diagnostic voiding or urodynamic testing in the physician's office to determine which type of UI is present (Dmochowski et al., 2016).

Normal micturition depends on a finely coordinated group of voluntary and involuntary movements. As a result of volitional impulses, voiding may be inhibited or stopped by the intrinsic muscles of the bladder neck and proximal urethra and the puborectalis division of the levator ani muscle (see Chapter 15).

Previous pelvic procedures sometimes cause scarring and distortion, with displacement of the bladder neck. Conditions such as uterine prolapse, cystocele, urethrocele, cystourethrocele, or urogenital fistulas after radiation therapy may be associated with SUI. Women who have had vaginal births are more likely to suffer SUI because of direct injury to ligamentous and fascial support as well as pelvic floor nerves and tissues (Lemack and Anger, 2016).

The procedure selected depends on the severity of SUI, the extent of the condition causing it, the patient's ability to use the anatomic mechanism for voluntary inhibition of urination, and any previous procedures. States of SUI are classified in relation to frequency and degree of incontinence, the presence of other diseases, and the function of the pubococcygeal muscle (levator ani). Surgery for SUI entails repair of the fascial supports and the pubococcygeal muscle surrounding the urethra and the bladder neck. Surgeons perform this repair through either a vaginal or an abdominal approach. Synthetic and biologic prosthetic materials as well as autologous fascia are used for SUI repairs (Dmochowski et al., 2016). Another available treatment option is the tension-free vaginal tape (TVT) sling (see Chapter 15 for a discussion of the TVT sling procedure).

The desired outcome of surgery for SUI is to improve the performance of a dislodged or dysfunctional vesical neck, to restore normal urethral length, and to tighten and restore the anterior urethral vesical angle. In this manner, the urethrovesical junction remains above the levator musculature of the pelvic floor and continence is preserved under the stress of coughing or sneezing. Surgery is performed by gynecologists, urologists, and by a subspecialty of surgeons trained in gynecology and urology known as urogynecologists. Procedures for a vesicourethral suspension (Marshall-Marchetti-Krantz procedure) and pubovaginal sling (PVS) using autologous fascia are described in Chapter 15.

Construction of a Vagina

Repairing or overcoming a congenital or surgical defect of the vagina is accomplished by (1) obtaining a skin graft, which is applied to a mold and placed in the area of vaginal reconstruction, or (2) making a simple opening in the area of vaginal reconstruction and placing a mold to permit spontaneous epithelialization of the area.

Procedural Considerations

For a skin graft, the plastic surgery instrument tray is required, with the addition of a dermatome, marking pen, and nonadherent gauze dressing. For vaginal construction, the basic vaginal instrument tray is required, with the addition of iris scissors, skin hooks, a vaginal mold, Halsted mosquito hemostats, and a ruler.

Operative Procedure

1. The skin graft is taken most commonly from the buttock because it provides a better cosmetic result in young women than the former approaches of harvesting skin from the abdomen or anterior area of the thigh. The donor site is dressed in the routine manner with nonadherent gauze and a pressure dressing.

2. The skin graft is kept in a moist radiopaque gauze sponge in a closed container until it is ready to be used. Communication of where the graft is on the back table occurs between scrub persons when there is a change of personnel to prevent the graft from being thrown off the field inadvertently. The graft is clearly marked on the back table.

3. The surgeon uses sharp dissection to create a vaginal orifice, taking care to prevent damage to the rectum and bladder. A mold is used to apply the donor skin or simply to hold the dissected area open to permit spontaneous epithelialization (Fig. 14.22).

Trachelorrhaphy (Cervical Repair)

Trachelorrhaphy is removal of separated or torn surfaces of the anterior and posterior cervical lips and reconstruction of the cervical canal. It is performed to treat deep lacerations of a cervix that is relatively free from infection.

Procedural Considerations

The basic vaginal instrument tray is required, along with an ESU and a conization loop electrode, if desired. An indwelling or straight urinary catheter may be inserted into the bladder, depending on the surgeon's preference. The patient is in lithotomy position (see Chapter 6 for positioning considerations).

Operative Procedure

1. The labia may be retracted with Allis-Adair tissue forceps or sutures. The surgeon grasps the cervix with a tenaculum.

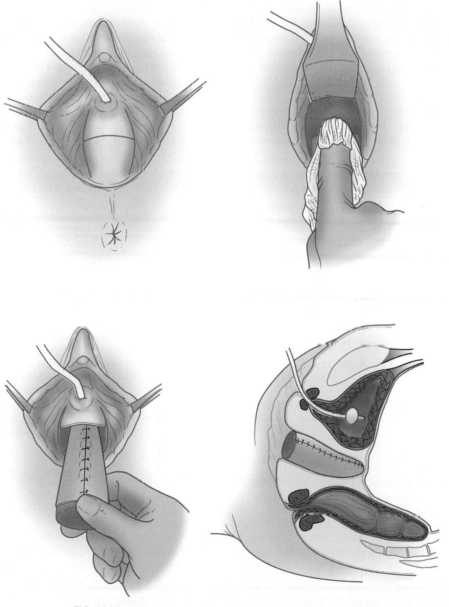

FIG. 14.22 Vaginal reconstruction using split-thickness skin graft.

2. The tissue of the exocervix is denuded with a blade. Using sharp dissection, the surgeon undermines the flaps. Bleeding vessels are clamped and ligated or controlled by a monopolar ESU throughout the procedure. The mucosa is dissected from the cervix.
3. A small distal portion of the cervical canal is coned with a blade or a loop electrode to remove tissue.
4. The denuded and coned areas are covered by transversely suturing the mucosal flaps of the exocervix, using interrupted sutures. Tissue forceps, hemostats, and radiopaque gauze sponges are needed. The sutures are placed in such a manner that the fibromuscular tissue of the cervix is included, eliminating dead space where a hematoma may form, and providing a complete reconstructed cervical canal.
5. The indwelling urinary catheter is removed (surgeon's preference).
6. A vaginal pack may be inserted. A perineal pad is applied.

Dilation of the Cervix and Curettage

D&C is done for diagnostic purposes for a variety of pelvic conditions, such as abnormal uterine bleeding. D&C is also performed to obtain tissue for diagnosis when carcinoma of the endometrium is suspected, in the study of infertility, or for removal of uterine polyps. A common indication for D&C is incomplete abortion (e.g., miscarriage) or therapeutic abortion. The perioperative nurse is sensitive to the emotional needs of a patient experiencing a recent miscarriage (Box 14.1).

Procedural Considerations

In a D&C procedure, instruments are introduced through the vagina for the purpose of dilating the cervix. Numerous cervical dilators are available. The patient is in lithotomy position (see Chapter 6 for positioning considerations).

Operative Procedure

1. The surgeon places a Jackson or Auvard weighted speculum in the posterior vagina. A Sims or Deaver retractor is placed anteriorly to expose the cervix. The anterior lip of the cervix is grasped with a tenaculum (Fig. 14.23).
2. The direction of the cervical canal and the depth of the uterine cavity are determined by means of a blunt probe or graduated uterine sound.
3. The surgeon dilates the cervix using graduated Hegar or Hanks dilators and/or a Goodell uterine dilator. Lacrimal probes may be needed if severe cervical stenosis is present, such as in patients who are nulligravida, are postmenopausal, have had scarring from previous cervical procedures (loop electrosurgical excision procedure [LEEP]), or have undergone radiation therapy in the past.
4. Exploration for pedunculated polyps or myomas may be done with a polyp forceps.
5. Using a sharp curette the surgeon scrapes the interior of the cervical canal to obtain an endocervical tissue specimen. To obtain an endometrial specimen, the surgeon scrapes the endometrial lining of the uterus. For specific identification and the site of specimens, the endocervical specimen is scraped with the curette first, and then a separate specimen is curetted from the uterine endometrium. As with any specimen, a confirmation of its identity is obtained from the surgeon and sent to pathology for diagnosis (see Chapter 2 for a discussion of safe specimen practices).

BOX 14.1

Supporting Patients Through Miscarriage or Stillbirth

A diagnosis of pregnancy is often a joyous occasion. Many women, however, can experience perinatal loss, which is defined as ectopic pregnancy, miscarriage, or fetal death. Miscarriage occurs in about 10% to 15% of all pregnancies occurring before 20 weeks of gestation. Stillbirths occur in 1 in 160 pregnancies after 20 weeks of gestation. Causes of many miscarriages and infant deaths are not always known. The known causes generally fall into three broad categories: birth defects; problems with the umbilical cord or placenta; and certain conditions of the mother (obesity, high blood pressure, or uncontrolled diabetes). Perinatal loss may occur with little or no advance warning for the mother, and surgical procedures at this time increase the woman's sense of vulnerability. The perioperative nurse can play a sensitive and supportive role when providing care for patients who present to the OR with miscarriage or cesarean birth for fetal demise.

By definition, a miscarriage is a pregnancy loss that occurs before 20 weeks of gestation. In the United States, state laws may stipulate that, in addition, the weight of the fetus is less than 350 g and signs of life are absent. Abortion is the medical term used for both spontaneous and elective pregnancy termination occurring before 20 weeks of gestation. Terms used to identify the diagnosis should also be chosen carefully. Many women find the term abortion harsh and unkind when referring to spontaneous events. Some may feel insulted or misunderstood, believing that abortion refers only to an elective procedure. The term miscarriage is more neutral and should be used consistently for early loss. Infant death is better referred to as "has died" or "there is no heart beat" rather than "lost," "gone," or "passed." Also, avoid using clinical terminology because this may convey a perceived lack of sincerity and respect. The nurse must be sensitive to the cultural and religious needs of both the patient and family during this time.

When discussing perinatal loss with a woman, initiate the conversation by referring to the pregnancy and listen for the patient's use of such terms as pregnancy, baby, or my son or daughter when referring to the loss. Such neutrality encourages the woman to express her feelings. Additional suggestions for communicating with parents include the use of phrases and open-ended questions such as the following:
• "I am sad for you."
• "How are you doing with all of this?"
• "This must be hard for you."
• "What can I do for you?"
• "I am here, and I want to listen."
• "I am sorry."
Avoid the following phrases:
• "Be thankful you have another child."
• "I know how you feel."
• "You have to keep going for her sake."
• "You're young and you can have others."
• "Better for this to happen now, before you knew the baby."
• "There was something wrong with the baby anyway."

Modified from Black BP: Perinatal loss, bereavement, and grief. In Lowdermilk DL, Perry SE, editors: Maternity and women's health care, ed 11, St Louis, 2016, Mosby; Centers for Disease Control and Prevention (CDC): Facts about stillbirth (website), 2016. www.cdc.gov/ncbddd/stillbirth/facts.html. (Accessed 19 January 2017); March of Dimes: Loss and grief (website). www.marchofdimes.org/complications/loss-and-grief.aspx. (Accessed 19 January 2017).

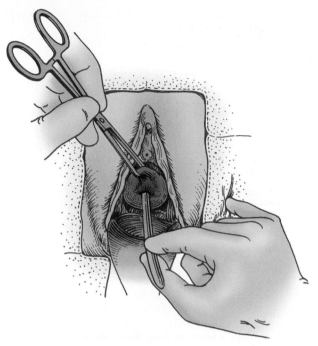

FIG. 14.23 Dilation of cervix and curettage. Vaginal wall retracted; cervix held by tenaculum; cervix dilated with dilator. Uterine cavity curetted with sharp curettes.

6. Fragments of endometrium or other dislodged tissues may be removed with warm, moist radiopaque gauze sponges on sponge-holding forceps.
7. The surgeon may take multiple punch biopsies of the suspected cervical lesions with a cervical biopsy forceps to supplement the diagnostic studies.
8. Retractors are withdrawn, the tenaculum is removed from the cervix, and hemostasis is evaluated at the site of the tenaculum and biopsy sites (if taken). A vaginal pack may be inserted. A perineal pad is applied.

Suction Curettage

Suction curettage is vacuum aspiration of the uterine contents. Aspiration has proved to be a safe and effective method for early termination of pregnancy and for use in missed and incomplete spontaneous abortions. Advantages include less dilation of the cervix, less damage to the uterus, less blood loss, less chance of uterine perforation, and reduced danger of infection. Suction curettage is the treatment of choice for benign gestational trophoblastic neoplasia, more commonly known as hydatidiform mole (molar pregnancy). Hydatidiform mole is a condition that arises from growth of embryonic tissue containing only paternal genetic material possibly arising from fertilization by the sperm in a defective egg that has no nucleus or from fertilization of the egg by two sperm. This results in the synthesis of material, which is termed a mole and consists of multiple fluid-filled vesicles resembling a cluster of grapes (Fig. 14.24). Preoperative and postoperative laboratory blood and imaging studies are performed for diagnosis and patient follow-up (Roth, 2017).

Procedural Consideration

The D&C tray is required, plus one tray of Pratt, Hawkin, or Hank uterine dilators, placenta forceps, urethral catheter, sterile suction cannulae (various sizes), aspirator tubing, a vacuum aspirator unit,

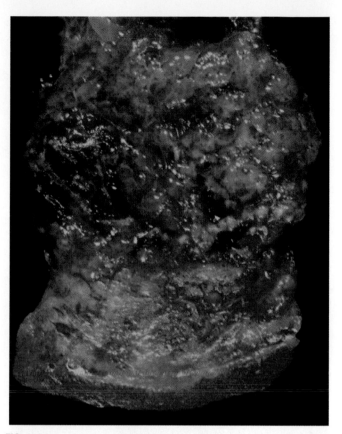

FIG. 14.24 Complete hydatidiform mole. Enlarged, transparent, and cystically dilated villi fill the uterine cavity. Note vesicles have the appearance of grapelike clusters.

and oxytocic drugs. The patient is in lithotomy position (see Chapter 6 for positioning considerations).

Operative Procedure

1. The surgeon exposes the cervix with an Auvard weighted speculum and an anterior retractor, grasps it with a sharp tenaculum, and draws it toward the introitus.
2. The cervix is dilated enough to be able to insert a 10- to 14-mm curette, depending on the uterus size.
3. The appropriate-size cannula is inserted into the uterus until the sac is encountered. The suction is turned on with immediate disruption and aspiration of the contents. Continued gentle motion of the cannula removes the uterine contents (Fig. 14.25). Use of uterine curettes may supplement suction in removing the entire uterine contents, but this must be done judiciously because it carries the risk of Asherman syndrome (intrauterine adhesions or scarring) from removal of the basal layer of the endometrium.
4. Retractors and the tenaculum are removed and a perineal pad is applied.

Removal of Pedunculated Cervical Myomas (Cervical Polyps) or Submucosal Leiomyomas (Fibroids)

Cervical polyps (small pedunculated lesions) stem from the endocervical canal and consist almost entirely of columnar epithelium with or without squamous metaplasia (Fig. 14.26). They vary in size and are soft, red, and friable. Bleeding may result from the slightest trauma. Submucosal fibroids are located underneath the endometrium and can protrude into the vagina or out of the cervical canal. Pedunculated lesions are removed from the cervical canal by dissection

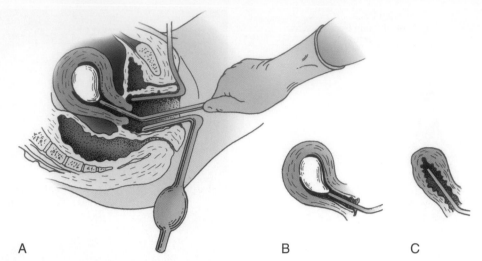

FIG. 14.25 Suction curettage. (A) Insertion of cannula. (B) Gentle suction motion to aspirate contents. (C) Uterine contents evacuated.

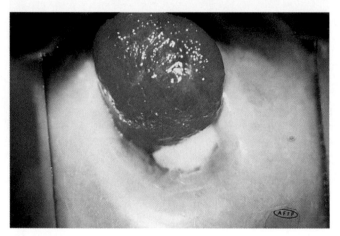

FIG. 14.26 Cervical polyp. A large polyp protrudes from the external cervical os.

with a blade electrode or resectoscope. Usually, the surgeon also performs endometrial and endocervical curettage, and a cytologic slide may be taken because some of these may represent early primary adenocarcinomas.

Procedural Considerations

A D&C tray, the ESU, and a blade electrode or resectoscope are required. The patient is in lithotomy position (see Chapter 6 for positioning considerations).

Operative Procedure

1. The surgeon grasps the anterior lip of the cervix with a tenaculum. The canal is sounded and dilated either to visualize or to palpate the base of the polyp pedicle.
2. The base of the polyp or submucosal fibroid is dissected out with a blade or monopolar ESU. An endoloop may be used as a lasso around the base of the polyp or submucosal fibroid to excise it. Bleeding is controlled with a monopolar ESU or manual pressure using a radiopaque gauze sponge. A resectoscope with the use of a monopolar or bipolar ESU may also be used for dissection.

3. The tenaculum is removed from the cervix, hemostasis is established, and the retractors are withdrawn.
4. A vaginal pack may be inserted for hemostasis if needed. A perineal pad is applied.

Conization Biopsy of the Cervix

Conization biopsy of the cervix is generally performed for the diagnosis or treatment of cervical dysplasia. Lugol's solution or 3% to 5% acetic acid is available to stain cervical tissue to differentiate between healthy and diseased tissue. The procedure may be initiated with colposcopy and punch biopsy, followed by the use of a monopolar ESU, and a cone biopsy with either a blade or LEEP. Hemostasis is controlled with a ball electrode and a monopolar ESU.

Procedural Considerations

Instruments required include a D&C tray along with an ESU, a conization electrical loop, and/or a ball-tipped electrode. The patient is in lithotomy position (see Chapter 6 for positioning considerations).

Operative Procedure

1. The surgeon retracts the posterior vaginal wall with a speculum and the anterior vaginal wall with lateral retractors. The outer portions of the cervix are grasped with a tenaculum, and the cervix is drawn toward the introitus. Cystic areas of the cervix may be treated with a monopolar needle electrode and ESU or laser. An endometrial biopsy may be done (Fig. 14.27A). The cervical stroma deep to the site of resection is infiltrated with a local anesthetic with epinephrine to provide mechanical and pharmacologic vasoconstriction before the procedure; typically 20 mL is used to provide hemostasis. Safe medication practices are initiated. Label all solutions on the sterile field. Bleeding points are coagulated with an ESU or laser.
2. The surgeon uses the electrical loop or a blade (see Fig. 14.27B–C) to remove the diseased tissue and obtain a histologic specimen for pathologic diagnosis. The surgeon may place a tagging suture at 12 o'clock to determine the position of the specimen for diagnostic purposes. Safe specimen management practices are implemented. The 3-mm ball-tipped electrode and a monopolar ESU may be used for hemostasis.

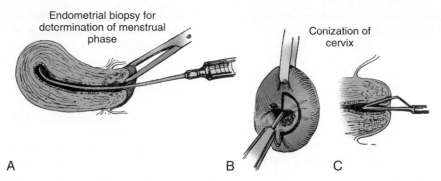

Endometrial biopsy for determination of menstrual phase

Conization of cervix

A   B   C

FIG. 14.27 (A) Endometrial biopsy technique. (B and C) Conization loop used to treat cervical conditions or obtain specimens for diagnostic tests.

3. If a wide conization is performed, the cervix rarely requires suturing. Vaginal packing may be used. An indwelling urinary catheter may be inserted and the tubing is secured. A perineal pad is applied.

Internal Radiation Therapy (Brachytherapy) for Cervical and Endometrial Malignancy

Internal radiation therapy (brachytherapy) is used to treat certain cervical and endometrial malignancies, either on its own or in conjunction with external beam radiation treatment (EBRT) and/ or chemotherapy. Radiation is either delivered at a low-dose rate (LDR) or at a high-dose rate (HDR) into or near the diseased tissue using several different applicator modes (e.g., Fletcher-Suit applicator for internal radiation). LDR brachytherapy requires the patient's admission to the hospital, whereas HDR brachytherapy is on an ambulatory basis. For LDR in women who have had a hysterectomy for endometrial cancer, a cylinder containing radioactive material is placed into the vagina (intracavity). If a uterus is still present, as would be the case with primary cervical cancer, a rod (tandem) is placed in the vagina along with small metal holders (ovoids) close to the cervix (tandem and ovoid brachytherapy). Tandem and ovoids are placed in either the OR under general anesthesia or in the interventional radiology department using moderate sedation/ analgesia. The radioactive material (LDR) is often loaded into the devices when the patient returns to a shielded hospital room. Patients may remain in the hospital for 1 to 3 days with the radioactive material in place, on bed rest, under the supervised care of medical personnel, and have limited contact with family. Cesium has generally replaced radium insertions for treatment of malignancy of the cervix and endometrium. Although LDR brachytherapy, typically used with cesium-137 (Cs-137), has been the traditional approach, the use of HDR therapy, used with iridium-192 (Ir-192), is rapidly increasing (Smith and Jhingran, 2017).

Procedural Considerations

The patient is in lithotomy position. The bladder is drained with an indwelling urinary catheter and the tubing is secured. The catheter balloon is inflated with a radiopaque medium for radiographic visualization after insertion of the cesium. An indwelling rectal marker is also placed by the surgeon for radiographic visualization. Various types of cesium applicators may be used according to the surgeon's preference and the area of malignancy. The cesium is loaded into the applicators later in the radiation department or in the patient's room under controlled conditions, in which all personnel are monitored by use of dosimeters.

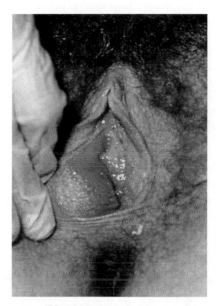

FIG. 14.28 Bartholin abscess.

Interstitial Therapy

Afterloading cesium needles are available in various lengths with small diameters for insertion into the tissue surrounding the cervix. They are inserted vaginally with a needle applicator and are used as a supplement to intravaginal or intrauterine sources. As with LDR therapy, radioactive material (Ir-192 usually) is only loaded in the radiotherapy suite or in the patient's shielded room. To facilitate removal, the needles have wires or threads attached to their distal ends.

Marsupialization of Bartholin Duct Cyst or Abscess

A cyst in a Bartholin gland usually results from retention of glandular secretions caused by blockage in the duct system (Fig. 14.28). This causes infection and resultant scarring of the Bartholin duct. Marsupialization of a Bartholin duct cyst or abscess involves removal or incision of the cyst through the vaginal outlet and drainage of the area. In true marsupialization, the cyst is surgically exteriorized by resecting the anterior wall and suturing the cut edges of the remaining cyst to the adjacent edges of the skin.

Procedural Considerations

The basic vaginal instrument tray is required, plus a 15-gauge needle, a syringe, and culture tubes (aerobic and anaerobic) to obtain a culture of the cyst if infection is suspected, iodoform or plain gauze packing, and a drain, if desired by the surgeon.

Operative Procedure

1. The labia minora may be sutured to the perineal skin on the medial side of the thigh to expose the vaginal introitus.
2. A stellate (starlike) incision is then made into the mucosa, which is distended over the cyst.
3. The surgeon dissects the cyst wall. The tissue may be marsupialized, everted with sutures, and left open.
4. A drain or packing may be inserted and a perineal pad applied.

Vaginal Hysterectomy

Vaginal hysterectomy is removal of the uterus through an incision made in the vaginal wall and the pelvic cavity. Contraindications to a vaginal approach are a large uterine tumor (either benign or malignant) or pelvic malignancy extending beyond the uterus.

Procedural Considerations

Instruments include the basic vaginal instrument tray. An abdominal gynecologic instrument tray should be available in case laparotomy is indicated. To facilitate dissection and decrease bleeding, the vaginal walls may be infiltrated with a local anesthetic (vasoconstrictors are optional). The patient is in lithotomy position (see Chapter 6 for positioning considerations).

Operative Procedure

1. The labia minora may be sutured to the medial thigh to expose the vaginal introitus. The surgeon places a weighted vaginal retractor to retract the posterior vaginal wall.
2. A tenaculum or suture ligature is placed on the cervix to permit traction on the cervix.
3. The surgeon incises the anterior vaginal wall with a blade through the full thickness of the wall (Fig. 14.29A). A circumferential mixture of IV normal saline and vasopressin or local anesthetic with epinephrine may be injected before incision into the submucosa tissue for hemostasis and to facilitate tissue plane dissection. The bladder is freed from the anterior surface of the cervix by sharp and blunt dissection. The bladder is then elevated to expose the peritoneum of the anterior cul-de-sac, which is entered by sharp dissection (see Fig. 14.29B).
4. The peritoneum of the posterior cul-de-sac is identified and incised.
5. The surgeon clamps, cuts, ligates, or uses a handheld vessel sealing and dividing device on the uterosacral ligaments (see Fig. 14.29C–D). If sutures are used, the ends of the ligatures are left long and are tagged with a clamp.
6. The uterus is drawn downward, and the bladder is held aside with retractors and moist radiopaque laparotomy pads.
7. The surgeon clamps, cuts, and ligates, or uses a handheld vessel sealing and dividing device on the cardinal ligaments on each side. The uterine arteries are doubly clamped, cut, and ligated or controlled with a handheld vessel sealing and dividing device.
8. The fundus is delivered with the aid of a uterine tenaculum.
9. When the ovaries are preserved, the surgeon clamps and cuts the round ligament or uses a handheld vessel sealing and dividing device bilaterally on the uteroovarian ligament and the fallopian tube (see Fig. 14.29E) and then removes the uterus. The pedicles are ligated if the surgeon uses the clamp and cut technique.

10. The surgeon reapproximates the peritoneum between the rectum and vagina with a continuous or interrupted suture. Retroperitoneal obliteration of the cul-de-sac is accomplished by passing sutures from the vaginal wall through the infundibulopelvic and round ligament, through the cardinal ligament, and out the vaginal wall. Sutures are tied on the vaginal aspect of the new vault (see Fig. 14.29F–G). The round, cardinal, and uterosacral ligaments may be individually approximated for additional support.
11. Any existing cystocele and rectocele and the perineum are repaired. In the presence of prolapse, reconstruction of the pelvic floor may be required.
12. An indwelling urethral catheter is inserted and the tubing is secured. The vagina may be packed and a drain inserted. A perineal pad is applied.

Gynecologic Surgery Using Minimally Invasive Techniques

Hysteroscopy

Hysteroscopy is the endoscopic visualization of the uterine cavity, intracavity, and tubal orifices. Both assessment and operative procedures can be completed during a hysteroscopy procedure. The common indications for hysteroscopy include evaluation of abnormal uterine bleeding (with possible endometrial ablation), location and removal of "lost" intrauterine devices (IUDs), evaluation of infertility, diagnosis and surgical treatment of intrauterine adhesions, verification and excision of submucous leiomyomas or endometrial polyps, resection of uterine septa or submucous leiomyomas, and tubal sterilization. A diagnostic laparoscopy may be done in association with hysteroscopy to assess the patient intra-abdominally. Contraindications for diagnostic or operative hysteroscopy include pregnancy; pelvic infection; cervical malignancy; and, in some instances, heavy bleeding.

A major potential complication of hysteroscopy is perforation of the uterus and/or injury to surrounding intestine, urinary tract structures, or the great vessels of the uterus. A diagnostic laparoscopic intraperitoneal examination is then needed to assess and evaluate the extent of the perforation, provide hemostasis, and repair any injured structures (Baggish, 2016a; Carlson et al., 2017).

A significant potential complication of hysteroscopy is the intravasation of the fluid used to distend the uterine cavity. Intravasation with systemic absorption can lead to hyponatremia. Signs and symptoms of hyponatremia include bradycardia, hypertension followed by hypotension, nausea, vomiting, headache, visual disturbances, agitation, confusion, and lethargy. The perioperative nurse is responsible for monitoring hysteroscopy fluid intake and output accurately during the procedure. Monitoring may be manual (i.e., calculating the difference between inflow and outflow) or automatically calculated on commercially available hysteroscopy pumps, which decrease the chance of human error. If a discrepancy of 1 to 1.5 L (nonelectrolyte medium; e.g., 1.5% glycine) or 2.5 L (electrolyte medium, e.g., Ringer's lactate or normal saline) or more occurs (less for patients depending on age, comorbidities, cardiovascular disease, and body mass index [BMI]), the surgeon and anesthesia provider are alerted and consideration is given to terminating the procedure (Carlson et al., 2017). At the end of the procedure, the hysteroscopy deficit should be communicated to the surgeon, anesthesia provider, and the PACU nurse during handoff, and documented in the patient's perioperative record. In contrast, intravasation of normotonic solution, although safer, can still lead to congestive heart failure in susceptible individuals.

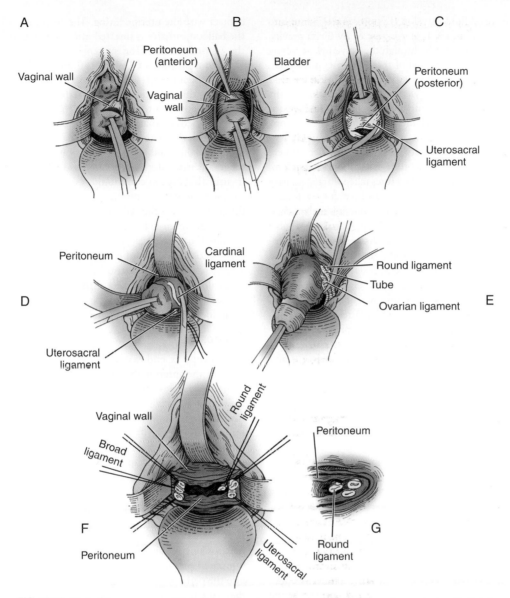

FIG. 14.29 Vaginal hysterectomy. (A) Incision of vaginal wall around cervix. Anterior vaginal wall slightly elevated. (B) Deaver retractor on each side; one Deaver retractor under bladder. Peritoneum opened. (C) Posterior cul-de-sac opened. Heaney clamp applied to left uterosacral ligament. (D) Left uterosacral ligament cut and tied. Clamp applied to left cardinal ligament. (E) Clamp applied to ovarian ligament, round ligament, and fallopian tube. (F) Uterosacral ligament, broad ligament, and round ligament shown in their respective normal positions. (G) Peritoneum closed and cardinal ligament, broad ligament, and uterosacral ligament reattached to angle of vagina. Left uterosacral and broad ligaments anchored.

Procedural Considerations

Instruments include a D&C tray, a hysteroscopy tray, polyethylene tubing or pump tubing, fiberoptic light source, the ESU, pressure-infusion pump, and a video camera and monitor. Other instrumentation includes a resectoscope, instrumentation needed for resection of uterine polyps or submucous leiomyomas, and an endometrial ablation device (if applicable). The patient is in lithotomy position (see Chapter 6 for positioning considerations).

Operative Procedure

1. The surgeon places an Auvard weighted speculum and an anterior retractor to expose the cervix; the anterior lip of the cervix is grasped with a tenaculum and is drawn toward the introitus.

2. The direction of the cervical canal and the depth of the uterine cavity are determined by means of a graduated uterine sound.

3. The surgeon dilates the endocervical canal with graduated Hegar or Hank uterine dilators to 6 mm, 7 mm, or 8 mm, depending on the size of the hysteroscope or resectoscope (if applicable).

4. The hysteroscope pump tubing is primed using the surgeon's choice of fluid and according to manufacturer's directions.

5. The surgeon introduces the hysteroscope to the level of the internal cervical os.

6. To achieve satisfactory visualization and sustained intrauterine pressure, the uterine cavity is distended with saline (normal saline solution [NSS]), Ringer's lactate, or 1.5% glycine. Fluids may be under continuous pressure when delivered by means of

a pressure-controlled fluid-infusion (hysteroscopic) pump into the irrigating channel of the hysteroscope or by direct gravity. The outflow fluid can run freely through the polyethylene tubing connected to the outflow channel of the hysteroscope or drain freely into an under buttocks drainage drape. If an under buttocks drainage drape is used, polyethylene tubing is attached to the bottom of the drainage drape and then to the suction canister, where it can be measured and monitored for a hysteroscopy deficit.

7. Exploration of the uterine cavity is begun. A video camera monitor is used to enhance visibility for the operative team. Procedures may be videotaped and pictures taken intraoperatively for recordkeeping, future reevaluation, and patient teaching.

8. The surgeon may introduce ancillary instruments, such as rigid and flexible biopsy forceps, scissors, grasping forceps, or a tubal occlusive device through the operating channel of the hysteroscope. Insulated coagulation electrodes and an ESU are used with a resectoscope; a "rollerball" electrode is used for both monopolar and bipolar electrode devices.

9. If submucosal leiomyomas or large uterine endometrial polyps are present, a tissue-removing device (MyoSure; Hologic, Inc., Marlborough, MA) may be inserted through the hysteroscope. This device removes submucosal smooth muscle tissue by suctioning and drawing the tissue into the device to safely cut and remove it.

10. On completion, the hysteroscope and any remaining instruments and retractors are withdrawn, the fluid deficit reported and recorded, and a perineal pad applied.

Endometrial Ablation

Endometrial ablation is performed to treat abnormal uterine bleeding. A pregnancy test (if applicable) will be done before ablation. A D&C may be performed before ablation to diagnose abnormal bleeding (Ryntz and Lobo, 2017).

The overall goal of endometrial ablation is to create amenorrhea or reduce menstrual bleeding to a normal or tolerable flow for the patient. It may be an alternative to hysterectomy in some patients with chronic menorrhagia. The procedure uses an ESU, thermal energy, or radiofrequency (RF). Patients who wish to have children are offered other alternative treatments for their abnormal uterine bleeding. Women who have suspected abnormal pathology or large uteri represent contraindications for this procedure (Ryntz and Lobo, 2017).

An adapted urologic resectoscope delivers electrical energy using continuous-flow irrigation to either coagulate or resect the endometrium. Endometrial ablation can also be carried out with a resectoscope and an ESU with either a loop or a rollerball electrode attachment. When using the resectoscope, 1.5% glycine is chosen as the distending medium because it is electrolyte free and compatible with the use of an ESU.

Reported complications associated with endometrial ablation using an ESU include hemorrhage, fluid intravasation, uterine perforation, recurrent bleeding, uterine perforation with associated injury to bowel and bladder, cervical lacerations, and rupture of a fallopian tube. One of the main disadvantages of using an ESU for endometrial ablation is that it must be done in conjunction with a hysteroscopy.

Endometrial ablation using thermal energy can be performed with a uterine balloon catheter. This catheter conforms to the internal uterine contour and contains a heating element. The surgeon performs suction curettage before ablation therapy to provide maximal balloon contact with the uterine lining. The cervix is dilated to 5 mm, and the balloon catheter is inserted into the uterus until the tip touches the uterine fundus. The surgeon inflates the balloon with sterile D₅W to a pressure of 160 to 180 mm Hg. The solution is heated to a temperature of 188°F (86.6°C) and maintained for 8 to 10 minutes. This procedure may be performed on an ambulatory basis and does not require hysteroscopy (Ryntz and Lobo, 2017).

Endometrial ablation using RF energy is accomplished with a wandlike device with a retractable triangular mesh end. The surgeon introduces the wand into the uterine cavity, then extends the triangular mesh. The triangular mesh conforms to the uterine cavity and measures its size. The surgeon communicates the uterine cavity measurements to the perioperative nurse, who confirms the measurements and inputs them into the RF controller. The surgeon then activates the RF wand, which delivers energy to the uterine cavity for about 90 seconds. Once the cycle is completed the surgeon retracts the triangular mesh into the wand and removes the wand from the uterine cavity.

A general anesthetic is usually administered, although a paracervical block along with IV conscious sedation/analgesia can be used. Either of these procedures can also be performed in the physician's office using local anesthesia or a paracervical block.

Laparoscopy

Laparoscopy is endoscopic visualization of the peritoneal cavity through the anterior abdominal wall after establishment of a pneumoperitoneum. It is used to investigate and diagnose causes of abdominal or pelvic pain, infertility, and to evaluate pelvic masses. Ancillary procedures such as adhesiolysis, fulguration of endometriotic implants (Fig. 14.30), aspiration of cysts or peritoneal fluid for cytologic study, ovarian or tissue biopsy, ovarian cystectomy, oophorectomy, removal of an ectopic pregnancy, tuboplasty, or tubal sterilization may be performed via laparoscopy. Lasers, tissue-sealing devices, or an ESU with either a bipolar or monopolar active electrode are often used during laparoscopy.

Procedural Considerations

Laparoscopy requires general anesthesia. Trocar port sites are often infiltrated or injected with local anesthetic before trocar insertion into the peritoneal cavity. The perioperative nurse assists with placing the patient in modified lithotomy position (see Chapter 6 for

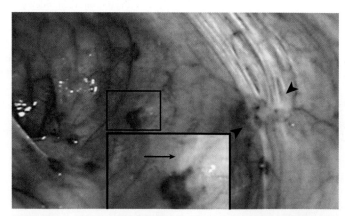

FIG. 14.30 A hemorrhagic area of the right cul-de-sac *(small box)* is seen on magnification to lie adjacent to a clear macule of endometriosis *(large box)* and may contain a gland/stroma complex of endometriosis obscured beneath the hemorrhage. The base of the right uterosacral ligament demonstrates thickening of whitish fibrosis and entrapment of old dark blood between the *arrowheads.*

positioning considerations). The abdomen, perineum, and vagina are prepped and draped for a combined procedure. Specially designed drapes with openings for both abdominal and perineal areas may be used. The bladder is emptied, with straight catheterization or through insertion of an indwelling urinary catheter, to prevent injury during trocar port placement.

The surgeon may perform a D&C in conjunction with laparoscopic procedures when indicated. After exposing the cervix and confirming the position and depth of the uterus, the surgeon introduces a uterine manipulator into the cervix to manipulate the uterus during the laparoscopy for better visibility. Most uterine manipulators have an intrauterine cannula port used for intraoperative chromopertubation. Chromopertubation tests for tubal patency by injecting a diluted mixture of methylene blue or sterile NSS through the intrauterine cannula into the cervical canal. If the fallopian tubes are patent, dye or fluid can be seen exiting at the tube's fimbriated ends.

The usual instruments for the vaginal portion of the procedure include a D&C tray, with the addition of a uterine manipulator, intrauterine cannula, diluted methylene blue or sterile normal solution, and a 60-mL syringe with extension tubing for chromopertubation.

An abdominal gynecologic instrument tray should be readily available in the event a laparotomy is necessary.

Operative Procedure

1. The surgeon may inject local anesthetic before making a small vertical percutaneous incision (0.7–1.2 cm) at or within the inferior margin of the umbilicus.

2. Elevating the skin with a towel clamp on either side of the umbilicus or grasping below the umbilicus with a radiopaque gauze sponge for traction, the surgeon inserts an insufflation (Veress) needle through the layers of the abdominal wall into the peritoneal cavity. Some surgeons prefer a direct optical access trocar insertion technique or the open laparoscopic Hasson technique to establish pneumoperitoneum, insufflating through the valve of the trocar sleeve rather than through a Veress needle (see Chapter 11 for a description of these two access approaches).

3. Once the Veress needle is inserted into the peritoneal cavity, a 10-mL syringe partially filled with sterile saline may be attached to the needle and used for aspiration. If the needle has entered a blood vessel, blood is aspirated. If a loop of intestine or the stomach has been entered, bowel contents or malodorous gas is aspirated. If the needle is free in the peritoneal cavity, nothing is aspirated.

4. The surgeon attaches Silastic, one-way filtration tubing to the Veress needle where it is then connected to a CO_2 gas insufflator. The perioperative nurse confirms settings for CO_2 insufflation rate and maximum pneumoperitoneum pressure with the surgeon before insufflation begins. Approximately 3 to 4 L of CO_2 is delivered into the peritoneal cavity to achieve pneumoperitoneum. CO_2 is commonly used as the insufflation medium because it is nontoxic, highly soluble in blood, and rapidly absorbed from the peritoneal cavity. The intra-abdominal pressure is usually set between 12 and 15 mm Hg and is closely monitored to prevent overdistension of the abdomen and to ensure free passage of gas into the peritoneal cavity. Veress needles or trocar stopcocks are inspected for leaks and to confirm they are in the open position to allow for the free flow of CO_2 into the insufflation tubing. Opening or initial pressures are in the 2- to 8-mm range and slowly rise with insufflation. The abdominal cavity should symmetrically distend with early loss of dullness to palpation over the liver in the right upper quadrant.

5. After insufflation is complete, the Veress needle is withdrawn and replaced with a 5-mm or 10-mm trocar, covered by a trocar sleeve (port). This is inserted through the abdominal wall and into the peritoneal cavity. The angle of the trocar is approximately 45 degrees toward the concavity of the pelvis. The Silastic, one-way filtration tubing is attached to the trocar sleeve and insufflation resumes. With the trocar sleeve in place, the surgeon withdraws the trocar and introduces the laparoscope.

6. The surgeon visualizes the pelvis, lower abdomen, and visceral contents. If the lens of the laparoscope fogs, application of a commercially available defogger solution may control the problem. The laparoscope may also be prewarmed or warmed intraoperatively in a metal scope warmer filled with warm sterile water. Alternatively, the surgeon may touch the lens to a loop of intestine to clear it. There are commercial insufflation units that warm the CO_2 either by a separate warming attachment connected to one-way infiltration tubing or incorporated into the insufflation tubing itself.

7. The anesthesia provider places the patient in Trendelenburg position.

8. The video camera is attached to the laparoscope to aid the surgical team's visualization, as well as to record the procedure for future reference, medical teaching, or patient education. If ancillary instruments such as biopsy forceps, a tissue-sealing device, or bipolar forceps are needed, the surgeon inserts a second trocar under direct visualization at the suprapubic region or at the right or left lower lateral oblique region of the abdomen. If needed, a third port is also introduced.

9. The surgeon may test for tubal patency (if applicable) using chromopertubation.

10. After the planned intra-abdominal procedure, the surgeon withdraws the laparoscope, allows the insufflated gas to escape from the trocar port or by suction, and removes any remaining trocar ports. Some surgeons remove the trocar ports under direct vision before removing the laparoscope.

11. The trocar incisions are closed (fascia, if necessary, followed by a subcuticular stitch), and wound closure strips, small dressings, or skin glue is applied.

12. The surgeon removes the uterine manipulator (if used) and checks the cervix for bleeding. If bleeding is present, pressure may be applied with a radiopaque sponge on a sponge-holding forceps.

13. A perineal pad is applied.

Laparoscopic Salpingostomy for Ectopic Tubal Pregnancy

Ectopic pregnancy is gestation developing outside of the endometrial cavity. Risk factors for developing an ectopic pregnancy include use of IUDs for contraception, pelvic inflammatory disease, tubal ligation, tubal dysfunction (as with endometriosis), in vitro fertilization, smoking, salpingitis, hormonal imbalance, and previous ectopic pregnancy. Although the fallopian tube is the most common site for ectopic pregnancies (occurring in up to 90% of all cases), ectopic pregnancies can also develop on the cervix, on the ovary, or within the peritoneal cavity (Kho and Lobo, 2017; Cashion, 2016). Women who experience ectopic pregnancy generally present with abdominal pain, abnormal vaginal bleeding, and a palpable adnexal mass. Diagnosis is confirmed through measurement of human chorionic gonadotropin (hCG) levels and the use of ultrasound to determine the absence of a gestational sac within the endometrial cavity. A serious complication of ectopic pregnancy is tubal rupture and

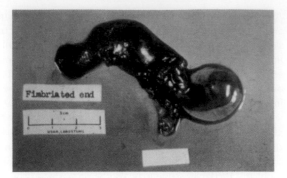

FIG. 14.31 Ruptured ectopic pregnancy with fetus in sac.

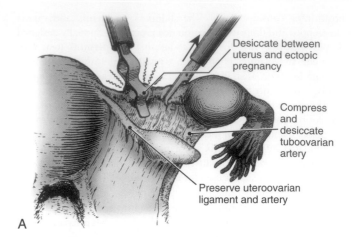

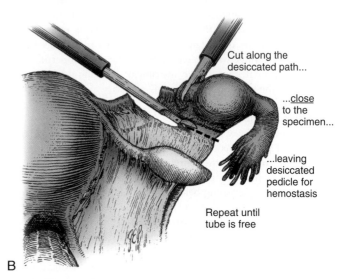

FIG. 14.32 (A) Electrodesiccation of the proximal fallopian tube during salpingectomy. (B) Excision of the fallopian tube.

hemorrhage (Fig. 14.31). Ultrasound is also useful in identifying free fluid in the peritoneal cavity, which could be blood or cystic fluid. Ruptured ectopic pregnancy is considered a surgical emergency and is associated with severe abdominal pain, tachycardia, and hypotension. The patient may also experience shoulder pain because of irritation of the diaphragm from the hemoperitoneum.

Ectopic pregnancy may be treated medically with methotrexate (if unruptured) or surgically through salpingostomy, segmental resection, fimbrial expression, or salpingectomy (Fig. 14.32). Methotrexate destroys rapidly dividing cells by blocking folic acid uptake in embryonic cells and is often administered in conjunction with surgery (Cashion, 2016). Laparoscopic and/or ultrasound-guided application of methotrexate directly into the fallopian tube may also be used. This approach decreases the toxicity of systemic administration of methotrexate (Kho and Lobo, 2017). Women who have had an ectopic pregnancy are at an increased risk for another one (Kho and Lobo, 2017).

Procedural Considerations

Procedural considerations for laparoscopic salpingostomy are identical to those for any laparoscopic procedure, with the addition of methotrexate. The surgical team may find that developing a checklist for surgical emergencies such as ruptured ectopic pregnancy assists in efficient care rather than relying on memory (Arriaga et al., 2013).

Operative Procedure

The operative procedure begins as described in steps 1 through 8 of the laparoscopy.

1. Immediate evacuation of blood or fluid is done to enhance visibility and to assess the pelvic organs and structures.
2. The surgeon mobilizes the distal end of the fallopian tube to perform an adhesiolysis. Grasping forceps are placed on either side of the fallopian tube, and gentle traction is applied.
3. Before making an incision into the tube, coagulation of the serial vessels on both sides of the anticipated incision may be performed. A dilute solution of IV saline and vasopressin may be injected into the mesenteric margin to avoid excessive bleeding (Fig. 14.33).
4. The surgeon makes a single incision with scissors from the mesenteric to the antimesenteric side of the fallopian tube, in which the products of conception are exposed.
5. The tissue is removed gently with forceps while constant irrigation (hydrodissection) is maintained with an isotonic solution (Fig. 14.34). Vigorous evacuation is avoided so that the highly vascular, underlying interstitial layer is not disturbed.
6. Small bleeding vessels can be ligated with a fine, nonreactive suture or with a monopolar ESU laparoscopic instrument. Simple

traumatic compression of bleeding margins will also promote hemostasis. Mesosalpingeal vessel ligation may be performed.
7. The tubal incision may be allowed to close by secondary intention or, as in the instance of salpingostomy, the incision may be closed in one or two layers, with 6-0 interrupted sutures.
8. The procedure ends as described in steps 10 through 13 of the laparoscopy.

Laparoscopic Ovarian Cystectomy

Ovarian cystectomy is frequently performed via the laparoscopic approach.

Operative Procedure

The operative procedure begins as described in steps 1 through 8 of the laparoscopy.

1. After successful laparoscopic entry, adhesiolysis is achieved (if applicable).
2. On entry, peritoneal washings for cytology are obtained, if indicated. Safe specimen practices are initiated.
3. The ovarian cyst is mobilized and the cortex grasped with a biopsy instrument.
4. The surgeon incises the cortex to expose the cyst wall with scissors, a monopolar ESU laparoscopic instrument, or the CO_2 laser.

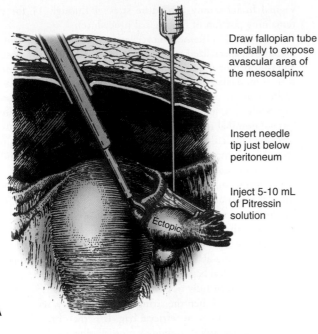

Draw fallopian tube medially to expose avascular area of the mesosalpinx

Insert needle tip just below peritoneum

Inject 5-10 mL of Pitressin solution

Ectopic

A

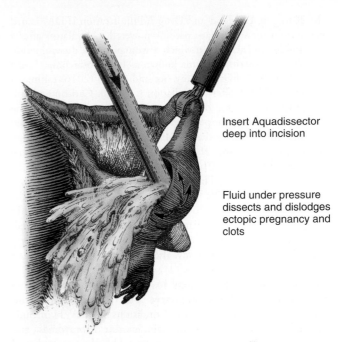

Insert Aquadissector deep into incision

Fluid under pressure dissects and dislodges ectopic pregnancy and clots

FIG. 14.34 Hydrodissection (Aquadissector) used to separate ectopic pregnancy from fallopian tube during salpingostomy.

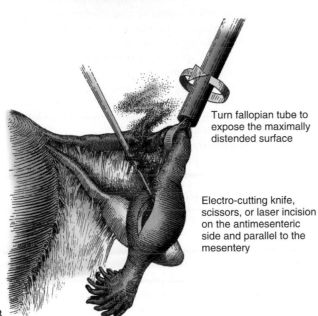

Turn fallopian tube to expose the maximally distended surface

Electro-cutting knife, scissors, or laser incision on the antimesenteric side and parallel to the mesentery

B

FIG. 14.33 Salpingostomy. (A) Injection of vasopressin into mesosalpinx. (B) Incision made into fallopian tube.

5. The incision is enlarged using scissors, and pressurized hydrodissection is used to separate the cyst from the ovarian stroma.
6. The cyst is dissected, placed in a laparoscopic retrieval bag, and removed intact through a trocar port.
7. Alternatively, the cyst may be opened, evacuated, thoroughly cleaned by lavage with the hydrodissector, and then removed. The patient is usually changed to supine from Trendelenburg while the fluid is removed and the pelvic cavity cleaned by lavage. Supine position assists in preventing fluid entry into the upper abdominal cavity.
8. Hemostasis is controlled using a laparoscopic monopolar ESU instrument.

9. The ovary usually does not require suturing; however, if the edges gape widely, the surgeon may approximate them loosely with interrupted 4-0 synthetic absorbable suture.
10. The procedure ends as described in steps 10 through 13 of the laparoscopy.

Laparoscopic-Assisted Vaginal Hysterectomy

Laparoscopic-assisted vaginal hysterectomy (LAVH) offers an alternative to total abdominal hysterectomy (TAH) and vaginal hysterectomy. The patient avoids having a large abdominal incision, extended hospital stay, and a long recovery period, all of which occur with TAH. LAVH is associated with less postoperative pain than TAH. Patients who are not candidates for a traditional TAH (e.g., those with numerous comorbidities) may be candidates for LAVH. This procedure also allows for contained extracorporeal, either intravaginally or intra-abdominally, morcellation (contained manual coring) of large benign uterine fibroids that can then be removed by extending the incision (mini-laparotomy) of one of the trocar sleeve ports or through the vagina.

Contained intra-abdominal or intravaginal morcellation uses a specimen retrieval bag. Once the uterus is in the laparoscopic retrieval bag, CO_2 is insufflated into the bag, ensuring safe distance between the morcellator and the bag, as well as between the bag and any intra-abdominal structures. The surgeon then cores the fibroid or benign enlarged uterus into narrow strips. This is done with a power or electrical instrument with a rapid circular cutting blade at its tip or a knife blade. A laparoscopic tenaculum inserted through the port of the morcellator is used to control and remove the tissue. The cored narrow strips can be easily evacuated through the port of the morcellator device with each pass of the morcellator. The assistant or surgeon continues to morcellate the uterus until it is small enough to extract through the vagina, a trocar port, or mini-laparotomy. The surgeon uses a knife and tenaculum for intravaginal contained morcellation. Vaginal hysterectomy does not commonly allow for morcellation of large uterine fibroids.

In 2014, the US Food and Drug Administration (FDA) issued a warning on the use of laparoscopic-powered morcellators after a highly published incident in which a woman had a dissemination of unsuspected uterine sarcoma known as leiomyosarcoma (LMS) after a laparoscopic hysterectomy. See and Chern (2016) estimated the chances of LMS after morcellation is 1:350. Carlson and colleagues (2017) estimated the chances as 1:350 to 1:1000. Placing the uterus in a contained specimen retrieval bag specifically designed for morcellation reduces the risk of dissemination of both benign and malignant cells from fragmented tissue within the abdominal cavity (See and Chern, 2016).

Although not described here, in laparoscopic-assisted supracervical hysterectomy (LASH), the body of the uterus is removed and the uterine cervix is left intact. To remove the benign uterus in a LASH procedure, contained morcellation or mini-laparotomy is required. If pain and bleeding persist, the uterine cervix is removed laparoscopically (laparoscopic trachelectomy, also known as cervicectomy) at a later date.

The surgeon uses laparoscopy to visualize the pelvis and can determine whether disease is present. This is not possible with traditional vaginal hysterectomy. Conditions for LAVH include postmenopausal bleeding, pelvic pain, uterine leiomyomas, and adnexal masses. Patients with postmenopausal bleeding are evaluated for the presence of endometrial cancer or atypical endometrial hyperplasia to select the appropriate procedure. Contraindications for LAVH may include a history of abdominopelvic surgery, salpingitis or endometriosis, lymphadenectomy, and some types of endometrial cancer or large uterine leiomyomas.

Procedural Considerations

Procedural considerations, accessory instrumentation, and approach are similar to those used in other laparoscopic surgical procedures. The patient is placed in low lithotomy position with attention to positioning interventions to protect the patient from injury (see Chapter 6 for positioning considerations). A two-procedure table setup is used to prevent cross-contamination. One setup is used for the laparoscopic portion of the procedure and the other for the vaginal portion.

Operative Procedure

The operative procedure begins as described in steps 1 through 8 of the laparoscopy and may include the following:

1. The broad ligament is dissected with a blunt or sharp laparoscopic instrument or a laparoscopic monopolar ESU instrument.
2. Dissection of the round and infundibulopelvic ligaments is completed using a bipolar coagulation device or with a 5-mm or 10-mm laparoscopic vessel sealing and dividing device.
3. Continued dissection of the broad ligaments is performed up to the bladder and posterior uterine borders.
4. Dissection continues by freeing the urinary bladder from the lower uterine segment, thus creating a bladder flap.
5. The uterine vessels are sealed bilaterally and divided with a vessel sealing and dividing device or a monopolar ESU laparoscopic instrument using cutting current. The ESU is used to divide the upper paracervical ligament and devascularize the uterus.
6. The laparoscope and instruments are then removed. The light source is turned off for fire prevention safety. The surgeon, assistant, and scrub person now turn their attention to the vaginal portion of the procedure.
7. The surgeon may inject the vaginal submucosa circumferentially with a diluted sterile IV saline and vasopressin mixture (see

vaginal hysterectomy procedure steps 4 through 11 for the remaining portion of the vaginal procedure).

8. If intravaginal contained morcellation is done, the uterus is placed in a specialized retrieval bag before vaginal cuff closure and the opening brought out through the vagina. The specimen is then morcellated in the bag using a tenaculum, knife blade, and/or curved mayo scissors. The vaginal cuff is then closed (see vaginal hysterectomy procedure step 10). If contained intra-abdominal morcellation is done (see below) the uterus is placed in the cul-de-sac and an occluder is inserted into the vagina to maintain CO_2 pneumoperitoneum for the remainder of the procedure.
9. The surgeon, surgical assistant, and scrub person change their surgical gown and gloves and return to the laparoscopy. The laparoscope is reintroduced to verify hemostasis and to confirm integrity of the vaginal cuff closure. Irrigation is carried out and any clots are suctioned and removed.
10. If contained intra-abdominal morcellation is done, a laparoscopic specimen retrieval bag is inserted through a trocar port, the bag is deployed until fully open, the detached uterus is deposited into the bag, and then the string is pulled tightly, securing the uterus in the specimen retrieval bag. It is then brought up to the abdominal wall. Contained morcellation of the uterus is performed following the manufacturer's safety instructions and hospital policy relating to morcellation. The remaining tissue is extracted in the specimen retrieval bag through a mini-laparotomy; contained manual coring and specimen extraction is similarly done through the mini-laparotomy site.
11. The end of the procedure is as described in steps 10 through 11 of the laparoscopy with additional sutures needed for closure of the mini-laparotomy site.
12. An indwelling urinary catheter is inserted and the tubing secured. A perineal pad is applied.

Robotic-Assisted Procedures for Gynecologic Procedures

Robotic-assisted laparoscopic surgery represents the newest available technology for minimally invasive gynecologic procedures. It has transformed modern surgery. The only available robotic system currently used in hospitals within the United States is the da Vinci surgical system (Intuitive Surgical, Inc., Sunnyvale, CA) (Carlson et al., 2017). The system consists of three separate components:

1. The *surgeon's console* has a three-dimensional high-definition viewer, hand manipulators (master controls), and foot controls. Once docked, the surgeon is seated at the console away from the surgical field and able to manipulate the robotic arms, camera, and magnification of the surgical field.
2. The *vision system* provides a three-dimensional image through an endoscope equipped with a stereoscopic camera and dual optics. There is also a viewing monitor for the assistant and team to visualize the surgical procedure.
3. The *patient side cart* has four robotic arms with fixed pivotal points, three of which can be used with robotic 360-degree wristed (i.e., jointed) instruments in 7 degrees of freedom, and the other is for holding and stabilizing the endoscope and camera.

Robotic technology in gynecologic surgery is used for hysterectomies, pelvic reconstructive surgery, and gynecologic oncology procedures (Carlson et al., 2017; Magrina, 2016). Surgical advantages include three-dimensional visualization and magnification of the surgical field, elimination of surgeon hand tremors, ergonomic advantages for the surgeon, and enhanced dexterity with precise and defined

ROBOTIC-ASSISTED SURGERY ▍▍

Procedural and Positioning Considerations in Robotic-Assisted Surgery: Steep Trendelenburg

Robotic-assisted surgery presents special procedural and surgical positioning considerations and challenges. In gynecologic surgery, steep Trendelenburg position is used for gravity and to keep bowels in the upper abdomen and away from the surgical area. The surgical team must understand these special considerations and challenges, and integrate optimal techniques in their plan of care to maintain safe patient care.

- The perioperative nurse and surgical team must be educated and familiar with the specialized equipment used for robotic-assisted surgery to facilitate a smooth and safe experience for the patient.
- Lithotomy positioning is used for robotic-assisted pelvic surgery; general safety position guidelines for the lithotomy position are assessed, planned, implemented, and evaluated (see Chapter 6 for general positioning considerations).
- For the most part, once any of the robotic arms are docked, the patient OR bed cannot be moved unless the robot is fully undocked. There is only one available system (TruSystem 7000dV OR Table; Trumpf Medical, Charleston, SC), designed to work with the da Vinci Xi Surgical System from Intuitive Surgical that allows dynamic patient positioning while the surgeon operates during robotic-assisted procedures.
- Because steep Trendelenburg position is used, meticulous positioning considerations are used. Face, eye, breast, arm, and hand pads are used to prevent positioning injury.

- A steep Trendelenburg position test may be done before incision to ensure patients with high BMIs can tolerate (e.g., respiratory and circulatory systems) the intraoperative position.
- To assist in preventing patient nerve and dermal injury caused from the patient sliding to the head of the bed because of steep Trendelenburg, the perioperative team uses specialized memory foam or beanbag positioning aids.
- The perioperative team monitors the patient's position at intervals intraoperatively.
- Likewise, the team monitors the patient's arm position to ensure robotic arms are not resting on the patient. For procedural reasons, arms are tucked by the patient sides, and padded with foam or gel pads; arm sleds may be used.
- Shoulder braces are not recommended because they may cause a compression injury to the brachial plexus.
- Intraocular pressure (IOP) increases in steep Trendelenburg; procedural time should be monitored and repositioning should be considered during prolonged surgical procedures ("supine rest"). Increased IOP can lead to blindness.
- IV fluids may be kept to a minimum to prevent paralaryngeal and facial edema until the patient returns to supine position.
- Instruments to convert to an open abdominal procedure are always readily available.
- Emergent safety checklists are established for conversion from a robotic-assisted procedure to a laparotomy.

Modified from Cassorla L, Lee JW: Patient positioning and associated risks. In Miller RD, editor: *Miller's anesthesia*, ed 8, Philadelphia, 2015, Churchill Livingstone; Hortman C, Chung S: Positioning considerations in robotic surgery, *AORN J*, 102(4):434–440, 2015.

---

microscopic tissue dissection capabilities (Carlson et al., 2017; Magrina, 2016). Direct patient advantages compared with traditional open procedures include smaller incisions, reduced blood loss and infection rate, shorter hospital stays, and fewer postoperative complications (Ulm et al., 2016). Robotic-assisted procedures can also be used in extremely obese patients for whom conventional laparoscopy would be ineffective or difficult.

Procedural Considerations

Robotic-assisted laparoscopic procedures are performed under general anesthesia. Procedural considerations applicable to laparoscopic surgery are appropriate for robotic-assisted surgery including both prepping and draping practices. Some special procedural and positioning considerations are noted in the Robotic-Assisted Surgery box.

Operative Procedure

1. The surgeon places a uterine manipulator (surgeon's preference) into the cervix along with a vaginal balloon occluder. This device is used to manipulate the uterus intraoperatively and to prevent CO_2 from escaping through the vagina during dissection of the uterus and cervix.
2. A Veress needle is placed, and the surgeon establishes an adequate pneumoperitoneum. Alternately, the open Hasson technique may be used (see Chapter 11).
3. The surgeon incises the skin at or above the umbilicus and inserts a disposable 12-mm trocar port for the camera. Some surgeons place this port either slightly to the right or left of the umbilicus, especially when lymph node dissection is contemplated. The robotic laparoscopic telescope with the attached camera is then introduced into the pelvic cavity. Fire safety

practices require that the light source shutter is only opened when the robotic laparoscopic camera is being monitored.

4. Two or three additional robotic 8-mm trocar ports are created for the robotic instrument arms. A supplementary trocar port (placed on the patient's right or left lateral abdominal area) is created for the assistant to use for any additional instrumentation, removal of specimens, retraction, insertion and removal of sutures, and for irrigation and suctioning purposes. Once all the trocar ports are placed, the robotic laparoscopic camera is removed and the light source shutter closed for fire safety.
5. The anesthesia provider positions the patient in steep Trendelenburg, and the bed is positioned to the lowest height.
6. The perioperative nurse drives the patient cart up to and between the patient's legs, or to the right or left side of the OR bed (lateral docking), while observing and maintaining integrity of the sterile field. Patient safety is closely monitored. All team members are attentive when the patient cart is being driven into position and again at the end when the cart is driven away from the patient and parked.
7. Both the surgeon and the surgical assistant attach the robotic camera and instrument arms to their respective trocar ports. The cart is now considered docked. The cart must be in the "drive (D)" position and the brakes set.
8. The robotic laparoscopic camera is reintroduced into the abdominal cavity and then, under direct visualization, the robotic instruments are inserted into the pelvic cavity. The monopolar and bipolar cords of the ESU are attached to the robotic instrument scissors and robotic bipolar instrument, respectively.
9. The surgical assistant remains at the sterile field to assist the surgeon and monitor the patient and surgical field throughout

the procedure. The surgeon moves to the console to perform the laparoscopic robotic-assisted portion of the procedure.

10. The surgeon begins by bilaterally skeletonizing tissue using the robotic laparoscopic monopolar and bipolar ESU instruments around the infundibulopelvic, round, and broad ligaments as well as the uterine artery pedicles. Once coagulated and dissected completely, the tissue is divided using the robotic laparoscopic scissor instrument.

11. Additional dissection is performed to divide the cardinal and uterosacral ligament complex bilaterally.

12. Either the scrub person or the surgical assistant provides cephalad pressure on the uterus by means of the uterine manipulator while the surgeon performs a circumferential colpotomy. This elevates the cervix up and away from the location of the ureters and protects them from injury.

13. Once the uterus and cervix are detached, they are delivered into the patient's vagina and positioned to maintain CO_2 pneumoperitoneum by the surgical assistant. If there is suspicion of uterine malignancy that may warrant lymph node dissection for tumor staging, the specimen is removed by the surgical assistant and sent to pathology for a frozen diagnosis as ordered by the surgeon. An occluder is inserted into the vagina to maintain CO_2 pneumoperitoneum. If appropriate, pelvic and paraaortic lymph node dissection is now carried out. Specimens can be withdrawn in a retrieval bag through the vagina or trocar port.

14. The surgeon closes the vaginal cuff using a running absorbable barbed suture.

15. Hemostasis is established and robotic instruments are removed under direct visualization. The robotic laparoscopic camera is then removed along with the trocar ports. The light shutter is closed for fire safety.

16. The perioperative nurse safely backs the cart away from the patient and parks it away from the surgical field. The cart is now considered undocked.

17. The surgeon returns to the sterile field and, along with the surgical assistant, completes the procedure as in steps 10, 11, and 13 of the laparoscopy. The occluder (if used) is removed from the vagina at the end of the procedure.

Laparoendoscopic Single-Site Surgery

Laparoendoscopic single-site surgery (LESS) is an evolving surgical approach that has recently become a more available option for women undergoing minimally invasive gynecologic surgical procedures. Other names for this common technical approach are single-site laparoscopy (SSL), single-port laparoscopy (SPL), and single-incision laparoscopic surgery (SILS) (LaMattina and Barth, 2014). The LESS procedure uses an open Hassan technique, a single-site incision at the umbilicus, with standard and specially designed instruments and endoscopes. Most incisions range from approximately 2 to 7 cm in length; up to five instruments can be inserted and manipulated through a single port at one time (LaMattina and Barth, 2014). LESS access port systems are either gel-based or have multichanneled ports.

Most laparoscopic gynecologic surgical procedures such as an LAVH, salpingo-oophorectomy, and laparoscopic tubal ligation (LTL) can be accomplished with the LESS approach. Patient advantages with an LESS procedure include less postoperative pain; better cosmesis; and elimination of potential injury to the inferior epigastric vessels, as well as the iliohypogastric or the ilioinguinal nerves. These injuries may occur when lateral ports are placed in the traditional laparoscopic surgical approach.

Procedural Considerations

Procedural considerations are the same as with laparoscopic surgery with the addition of one of the many available LESS ports (surgeon's preference), laparoscopic articulating instruments, and a flexible endoscope. As with all laparoscopic procedures, an open abdominal instrument and gynecologic tray is readily available. General anesthesia is administered, a urinary catheter is inserted, and skin prep and draping are carried out as described in the laparoscopy procedure.

Operative Procedure

1. The surgeon places a uterine manipulator (surgeon's preference) into the cervix, usually along with a vaginal balloon occluder.

2. The surgeon may inject local anesthetic before incising the skin for the open Hasson technique (see Chapter 11).

3. The surgeon inserts the LESS port.

4. A laparoscopic endoscope is placed, followed by the surgeon's choice of laparoscopic instruments.

5. Visualization of the pelvis, lower abdomen, and the visceral contents is begun.

6. The anesthesia provider positions the patient in steep or modified Trendelenburg.

7. The surgical procedure is carried out as described in the similar laparoscopic surgical procedures.

8. The procedure is completed as described in steps 10 through 13 of the laparoscopy.

Gynecologic Surgery Using the Abdominal Approach

Total Abdominal Hysterectomy

TAH is the removal of the entire uterus, including the corpus and the cervix. TAH may be performed for symptomatic pelvic relaxation or prolapse, chronic pain associated with pelvic congestion, pelvic inflammatory disease, endometriosis, recurrent ovarian cysts, uterine leiomyomas (fibroids), dysfunctional uterine bleeding (DUB) in perimenopausal women, or adenomyosis. TAH procedures are the most common surgical procedure performed on women in the United States unrelated to pregnancy (Gor and Rivlin, 2015) with or without BSO (Patient Engagement Exemplar).

In a study reported by Shah and colleagues (2015), the authors concluded that operative time for all three approaches to hysterectomy (TAH and vaginal and laparoscopic) increased with BMI. Increased BMI was also associated with more surgical risks, with abdominal hysterectomies resulting in the highest surgical risks for events such as wound infection and wound dehiscence when compared with vaginal or laparoscopic hysterectomy.

Procedural Considerations

The abdominal prep (lower area of contamination) may be completed before vaginal and perineal prep, which includes the cervix. When the abdominal prep is completed first, the perioperative nurse uses caution when prepping the already prepped abdomen. There is insufficient evidence to support whether the abdomen or perineal area should be prepped first; caution is used in either instance (AORN, 2017). An indwelling urinary drainage catheter is inserted to provide continual bladder drainage. The patient begins in supine position and is then repositioned to Trendelenburg position. A basic abdominal gynecologic instrument tray and a self-retaining retractor are required. Provisions are made to remove instruments that come into contact with the cervix and vagina from the surgical field, avoiding vaginal contamination of the abdominal incision (isolation technique).

Operative Procedure

1. In an obese patient or for exploration of the upper abdominal cavity, a left rectus (paramedian) or vertical midline incision is usual. For simple hysterectomy in a woman of normal size and with a normal size uterus, a Pfannenstiel incision is often used. The surgeon opens the abdominal layers and peritoneum as described for a laparotomy (see Chapter 11).

2. Once the peritoneal cavity is opened, the anesthesia provider puts the patient in Trendelenburg position to provide better visualization of the pelvic organs.

3. A self-retaining retractor is used for exposure and moist radiopaque laparotomy pads are used to pack the intestines into the upper abdomen. The round ligament is grasped with forceps, clamped, cut, and ligated. A handheld vessel sealing and dividing device can be used throughout the procedure during which ligaments and vessels are clamped, cut, and ligated. If the surgeon cuts the pedicles, a #10 blade or Metzenbaum scissors is used; sutures may be tagged with a hemostat for traction. This procedure is done on both sides (Fig. 14.35A).

4. Using blunt dissection, the surgeon separates the anterior layer of the broad ligament close to the uterus on each side. Bleeding vessels are clamped and ligated. The fallopian tube and the uteroovarian ligaments are doubly clamped together, incised, and doubly tied with suture ligatures (see Fig. 14.35B).

5. The surgeon pulls the uterus forward to expose the posterior sheath of the broad ligament and incises the ligament with Metzenbaum scissors. Ureters are identified. The uterine vessels and uterosacral ligaments are doubly clamped, divided by sharp dissection at the level of the internal os, and ligated with suture ligatures (see Fig. 14.35C).

6. The severed uterine vessels are clamped at the paracervical ligament, cut, and suture ligated, or bluntly dissected away from the cervix on each side with the aid of radiopaque gauze sponges on sponge-holding forceps, scissors, and tissue forceps.

7. The bladder is separated from the cervix and upper vagina with sharp and blunt dissection assisted by radiopaque gauze sponges on sponge-holding forceps. The bladder may be retracted with a moist radiopaque laparotomy pad and an angular blade retractor. The vaginal vault is incised close to the cervix with a blade or scissors (see Fig. 14.35D).

8. The surgeon grasps the anterior lip of the cervix with an Allis or Kocher clamp. Using scissors, the surgeon dissects the cervix and amputates it from the vagina. The uterus is removed. The scrub person places any potentially contaminated instruments used on the cervix and vagina into a discard basin and passes them from the field (including sponge-holding forceps and suction). Bleeding is controlled with hemostats and sutures or a monopolar ESU.

9. The vaginal vault is closed as one layer with interrupted figure-of-eight sutures to ensure the vault of the vagina is closed completely and to prevent any risk for prolapse. Angle sutures anchor all three connective tissue ligaments to the vaginal vault. The pedicles, fallopian tubes, and ovarian ligaments are left free of the vault.

10. The surgeon may close the peritoneum over the bladder, vaginal vault, and rectum (see Fig. 14.35E). The packed radiopaque laparotomy pads are removed, and the omentum is drawn over the bowel.

11. The abdominal wound is closed as described for laparotomy closure (see Chapter 11).

12. An abdominal dressing and perineal pad are applied. The indwelling urinary catheter tubing is secured.

Salpingo-Oophorectomy

Salpingo-oophorectomy is removal of a fallopian tube and all or part of the associated ovary. Unilateral salpingo-oophorectomy may be done to treat chronic salpingo-oophoritis, for ectopic tubal gestation, or for certain disease conditions of the adnexa or large adnexal cysts. Some indications for BSO are malignancy, premalignant states, and as a risk-reducing procedure for patients at high risk for malignancy (*BRCA1* or *BRCA2* gene and Lynch syndrome). In most cases, this procedure is done laparoscopically unless a large adnexal mass is present.

Procedural Considerations

The basic abdominal gynecologic instrument tray is required.

Operative Procedure

1. The skin is incised, and the abdominal layers are opened, as described for laparotomy (see Chapter 11).

2. The affected tube is grasped with Allis or Babcock forceps. The ureter is first identified and then the infundibulopelvic ligament is clamped with hemostats, cut, and ligated. A laparoscopic vessel sealing and dividing device can be used throughout the procedure during which ligaments and vessels are clamped, cut, and/or ligated.

3. The mesosalpinx is grasped with hemostats and divided with the suspensory ligament of the ovary.

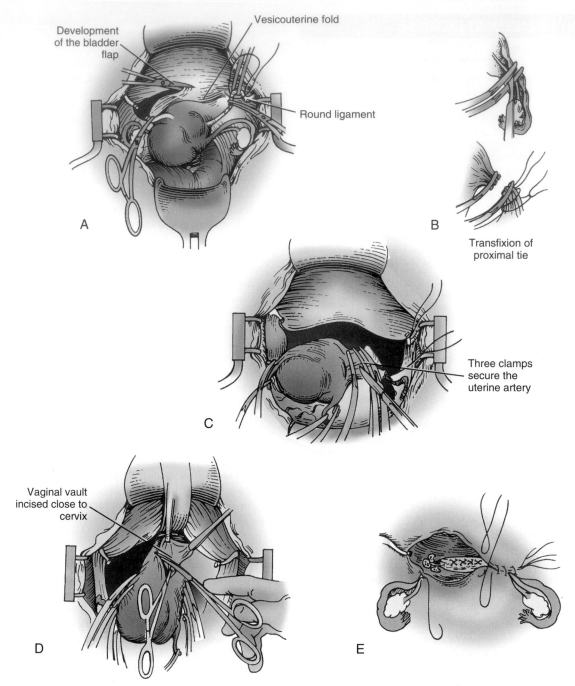

FIG. 14.35 Abdominal hysterectomy for single fibroid uterus. (A) Peritoneum retracted with self-retaining retractors; organs are protected with laparotomy packs saturated in warm normal saline solution. Transverse incision made through uterine peritoneum and extended to each side of uterine attachments of round ligaments. Bleeding vessels clamped and ligated. Round ligament grasped, ligated, and cut. (B) Tube and ovarian ligaments clamped, cut, and sutured. (C) Uterus pulled forward, posterior sheath of broad ligaments divided, and uterine artery and veins secured by three heavy curved clamps. Pedicle divided, leaving two hemostats on proximal pedicle. (D) Bladder separated from cervix and upper vagina. Vaginal vault opened and grasped with Allis forceps. Allis forceps placed on anterior lip of cervix, and dissection of cervix carried out to complete its amputation from vagina. (E) Three connective tissue thickenings anchored to vaginal vault, vaginal mucosa approximated, and vault closed. As shown, peritoneum is closed with continuous suture.

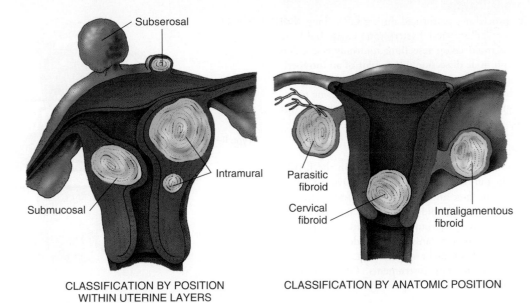

Subserosal

Intramural

Submucosal

Parasitic
fibroid

Cervical
fibroid

Intraligamentous
fibroid

CLASSIFICATION BY POSITION
WITHIN UTERINE LAYERS

CLASSIFICATION BY ANATOMIC POSITION

FIG. 14.36 Classification of uterine leiomyomas.

4. The cornual attachment of the tube is excised with a blade or curved scissors. Bleeding vessels are clamped and ligated.
5. The edges of the broad ligament are peritonealized from the uterine horn to the infundibulopelvic ligament as described for TAH.
6. If both tubes and ovaries are to be removed, steps 2 through 5 are completed on the opposite side.
7. The abdominal wound is closed as described for laparotomy (see Chapter 11).
8. An abdominal dressing is applied. The indwelling urinary catheter tubing is secured.

Abdominal Myomectomy

Uterine fibroids (Fig. 14.36) are the most common benign tumors. They contain fibrous tissue and arise from the muscular wall of the uterus. African American women have a higher incidence of uterine fibroids than do white women (Dolan et al., 2017). Another term for uterine fibroids is *uterine leiomyomas*. They may also be located in the submucosal area or the subserosal surface of the uterus. On occasion, they may become pedunculated and extend into the cervical canal. Rarely, a subserosal fibroid may pedunculate and migrate to become a parasitic fibroid attached to the omentum or mesentery. Abdominal myomectomy is removal of fibroid tumors by carefully separating each one from the uterine wall and its blood supply. Myomectomy is usually done in young women who have symptoms indicating the presence of uterine fibroids who wish to preserve their potential fertility. Submucosal fibroids may decrease the chances of conception and increase miscarriage (Dolan et al., 2017).

Uterine fibroids often cause pelvic pain and pressure or may accentuate the severity of bleeding associated with DUB. Myomectomy may be performed as a prophylactic measure with other abdomino-pelvic surgery. Preoperative preparation may include preoperative injections of leuprolide acetate (Lupron), a synthetic version of the naturally occurring gonadotropin-releasing hormone (GnRH) over several months' time, to reduce the volume of the fibroid and decrease its blood supply. This intervention mimics the postmenopausal state for women who receive it because it reduces the amount of estrogen the body synthesizes, reducing the size of the fibroid.

Procedural Considerations

The basic abdominal gynecologic instrument tray and an ESU are required. A laser may also be used. The patient is prepped as described for abdominal hysterectomy.

Operative Procedure

The procedure begins as in steps 1 and 2 of the TAH.
1. To contract the musculature of the uterine wall, a drug such as vasopressin and sterile IV 0.9% sodium chloride (NaCl) mixture may be injected into the fundus.
2. The surgeon grasps the fibroid tumor with a towel clip or tenaculum. The broad ligament may be opened with curved hemostats and Metzenbaum scissors to determine the course of the ureter and/or to free the bladder.
3. Each tumor is shelled out of its bed, using blunt and sharp instruments, a monopolar ESU, or the laser. Bleeding vessels are clamped and ligated or a monopolar ESU is used.
4. The uterus is reconstructed with interrupted or continuous sutures.
5. The peritoneum is closed, and then the abdominal wound is closed as described for laparotomy (see Chapter 11).
6. An abdominal dressing and perineal pad are applied. The indwelling urinary catheter tubing is secured.

Cytoreductive Surgery for Ovarian Cancer

Cytoreductive surgery (CRS) is when surgeons attempt optimal surgical tumor debulking for ovarian cancer. Evidence has shown that there is an inverse relationship between the amount of tumor left behind at the time of surgery and the patient's overall length of survival. The goal of CRS is to leave behind as little tumor as possible; less than 1 cm is adequate to improve survival. No residual gross disease is optimal. Ovarian cancer is the leading cause of gynecologic cancer death in women in the United States (ACS, 2016e). Most women who present at the time of diagnosis already have intra-abdominal spread with metastatic disease (stage III or IV) using staging criteria from the International Federation of Gynecology and Obstetrics (FIGO). The death rate for ovarian cancer is high for two main reasons: (1) the disease spreads early, and (2) the signs and symptoms of ovarian cancer are vague (Coleman et al., 2017).

Other operative procedures performed during CRS along with a TAH with BSO or supracervical hysterectomy with BSO are omentectomy; rectosigmoid colon resection; midtransverse colon resection; pelvic lymph node dissection; placement of an intraperitoneal chemotherapy catheter; and fulguration of macroscopic tumor on the diaphragm, bladder, pelvic side walls, and liver using either an argon beam coagulator (see Chapter 8 for a discussion of this energy-delivering device) or an ESU.

Procedural Considerations

The patient is positioned and prepped as described in the LAVH procedure. An indwelling urinary catheter is inserted. Ovarian cancer patients may present with large amounts of ascites and metastatic spread to the omentum, rectosigmoid colon, midtransverse colon, peritoneum, paracolic gutter, liver, and diaphragm. The perioperative nurse arranges the suction canisters in tandem to manage large amounts of ascites. Instrument requirements are the same as with TAH in addition to long instruments, GI instruments (as indicated), intestinal staplers, and possibly an argon beam coagulator.

Operative Procedure

1. The skin is incised, and the abdominal layers are opened, as described for laparotomy (see Chapter 11). If ascites is present, a small incision is made into the peritoneum and suction is used to drain the ascites.
2. The surgeon and surgical assistant do a thorough exploration and assessment of the pelvic and abdominal cavity and plan the surgical approach.
3. If omental involvement is visible, an omentectomy will be performed. If no omental involvement is visible, an omental biopsy may be taken. Safe specimen practices are initiated.
4. A TAH with BSO then follows as described in the TAH and salpingo-oophorectomy procedures.
5. Depending on the extent and involvement of the disease process with other organs, a rectosigmoid resection or other bowel resection (see Chapter 11) may be performed.
6. Fulguration of macroscopic surface tumor sites with a monopolar or bipolar ESU instrument or argon beam coagulator may be performed. Resection of enlarged lymph nodes may also be carried out at this time.
7. An intraperitoneal chemotherapy catheter may be placed into the peritoneal cavity at the end of the procedure. The port for the catheter is inserted and positioned under the skin above a bony area such as a rib or pelvic bone (ACS, 2016a).
8. The abdominal wound is closed as described in laparotomy (see Chapter 11). Drains may be used.
9. An abdominal dressing and perineal pad are applied. The indwelling urinary catheter tubing is secured.

Radical Hysterectomy (Wertheim)

Radical hysterectomy is en bloc dissection and wide removal of the uterus, tubes, ovaries, entire uterosacral and uterovesical ligaments, and upper vagina; this is often also undertaken with careful removal of all recognizable lymph nodes in the pelvis (Fig. 14.37). Complex and extensive dissection of tissue surrounding the ureters, bladder, bowel, and greater vessels of the pelvis is also undertaken (Jhingran and Meyer, 2017). There are many variations of radical hysterectomy procedures; the procedure performed depends on the diagnosis and extent of the disease process. Radical hysterectomy is performed for malignancy of the cervix.

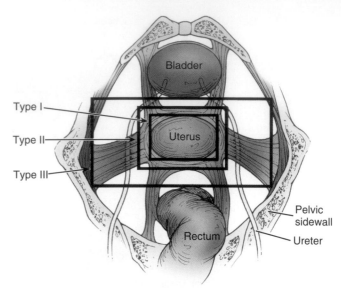

FIG. 14.37 Different types of hysterectomy: *Type I,* simple hysterectomy; *Type II,* modified radical hysterectomy; *Type III,* radical hysterectomy.

Procedural Considerations

As with any complex surgical procedure, blood loss and urinary output are closely monitored. The patient is prepped and draped as described for TAH. An indwelling urinary catheter is inserted. The basic abdominal gynecologic instrument tray is required, with the addition of long instruments and a self-retaining retractor.

Operative Procedure

1. The skin is incised, and the abdominal layers are opened, as described for laparotomy (see Chapter 11).
2. The surgeon cuts the peritoneum at its reflection on the anterior surface of the uterus between the round ligaments (Fig. 14.38A). Using blunt dissection, the surgeon frees the bladder surface from the cervix and vagina.
3. The right round and infundibulopelvic ligaments are clamped, cut with Metzenbaum scissors, and ligated with sutures or a monopolar ESU to expose the external iliac artery. A handheld vessel sealing and dividing device can be used throughout the procedure where ligaments and vessels need to be clamped, cut, and ligated. The ureter is identified and retracted with a vein retractor (see Fig. 14.38B).
4. The lymph and areolar tissues are dissected from the iliac artery, obturator fossa, and ureter with Lahey forceps, small gauze dissectors (also called "Kitners," "peanuts," or "pushers"), and Metzenbaum scissors. A complete lymph node dissection removes tissue from the femoral canal to the bifurcation of the iliac arteries bilaterally. The uterine artery and vein are clamped, cut, and doubly ligated.
5. The surgeon elevates the uterus and opens the cul-de-sac (see Fig. 14.38C); the uterosacral and cardinal ligaments are clamped, cut with scissors at some distance from the cervix, and doubly ligated with suture ligatures. Pararectal and paravesical areolar tissues are dissected free to skeletonize the upper vagina, and tissues are removed as near to the pelvic walls as possible.
6. If there is an exocervical lesion, the proximal vagina is cross-clamped with Heaney forceps leaving an adequate margin around the cervical lesion (see Fig. 14.38D) and divided using a blade on a long knife handle. The uterus and surrounding tissues are

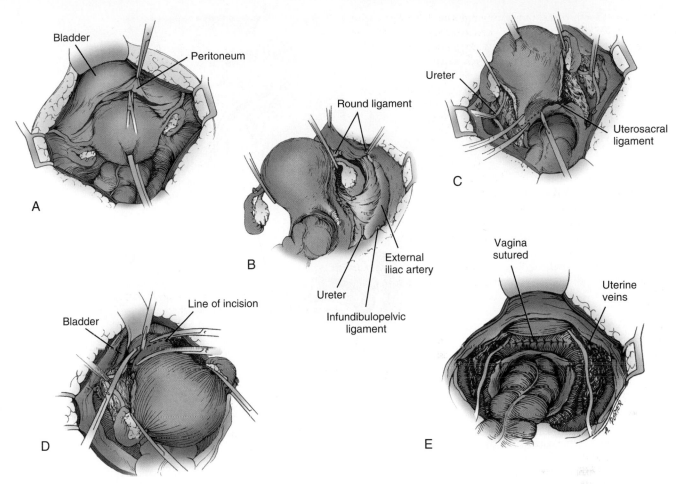

FIG. 14.38 Wertheim radical hysterectomy. (A) With upward traction applied on uterus, peritoneum is incised from round ligament to round ligament. (B) Right round and infundibulopelvic ligaments are ligated and cut, exposing right external iliac artery. (C) Uterus is held upward and forward, exposing cul-de-sac, which is incised as shown by dotted line. (D) After dissection is completed, vagina is doubly clamped preparatory to transection, after which the entire specimen is lifted out en bloc. (E) Vagina is closed. Peritoneum remains to be reperitonealized.

removed. A monopolar ESU is used to minimize venous oozing from small venules and capillaries. Lowering the head of the OR bed 15 degrees is also helpful in reducing oozing of blood and serum.

7. The surgeon sutures the vagina with an interrupted or running locked stitch, and may insert closed suction drains from above (see Fig. 14.38E). The peritoneum may be closed with a continuous running suture or left open.

8. The abdominal wound is closed as described for laparotomy (see Chapter 11). Vaginal packing and drains may be used. A suprapubic indwelling catheter may be placed to assist in managing postoperative bladder atony and for bladder drainage.

9. An abdominal dressing and perineal pad are applied. The indwelling urinary catheter tubing is secured.

Pelvic Exenteration

Pelvic exenteration is en bloc removal of the rectum, the distal sigmoid colon, the urinary bladder and distal ureters, all pelvic reproductive organs, and lymph nodes. In some patients, a perineal phase may also be required to excise all pelvic cancer with a negative margin. In this case, the entire pelvic floor with the accompanying pelvic peritoneum, levator muscles, and perineum may be excised. A partial exenteration, either anterior and/or posterior, may be performed, depending on the origin of the carcinoma and the extent of local tissue invasion (Fig. 14.39).

Pelvic exenteration is the surgical treatment for advanced or recurrent carcinoma of the cervix after radiation therapy. Exenteration is considered only after a thorough investigation of the patient and disease status to determine if the disease is isolated to the central pelvis and there is a reasonable chance of a cure (Jhingran and Meyer, 2017). The need to create urinary and bowel diversions is also considered, together with the patient's ability to cope with these diversions postoperatively.

Plastic surgery may be required for creation of a neovagina. Psychologic preparation and support of the patient and family by the perioperative nurse and physician are prime requisites.

Procedural Considerations

Utmost care is taken in positioning the patient because of the duration of surgery (see Chapter 6 for positioning considerations). The patient is in supine position with legs abducted in the modified lithotomy position (i.e., lower extremities resting on a well-padded plantar

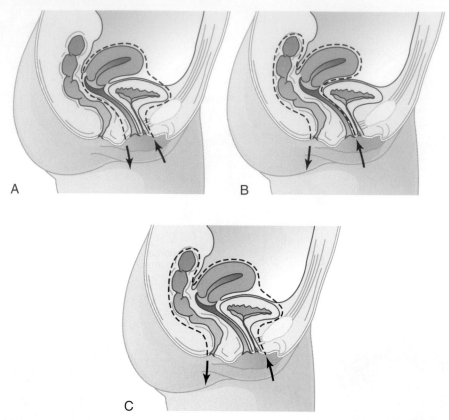

FIG. 14.39 Organs removed in pelvic exenteration. (A) Anterior exenteration. (B) Posterior exenteration. (C) Total pelvic exenteration.

surface rather than on the heel or popliteal area) or slightly elevated in that position to allow access to the perineum without disruptive position changes. Skin prepping includes the abdomen, thighs, perineum, and vaginal vault.

The perioperative team is alert to fluid and blood loss throughout the procedure. Irrigation solutions are accurately measured, and radiopaque laparotomy pads weighed, to more accurately assess blood volume loss, and the anesthesia provider and surgical team are apprised of these measurements.

When the colon is transected or ureteral drainage is diverted into a segment of the ileum, GI technique (bowel technique) should be followed as described in Chapter 11.

Separate instrument trays are required for the abdominal and perineal approaches. Extra drapes, gowns, and gloves are readily available.

For the abdominal approach, the basic abdominal gynecologic instrument tray and instruments for abdominoperineal resection (see Chapter 11) are required.

For the perineal approach, the basic vaginal instrument tray is required. To prevent contamination, the anus may be closed with a purse-string suture.

Operative Procedure

1. A long vertical midline incision from the symphysis pubis to the umbilicus is made, and the abdomen is opened as described for laparotomy (see Chapter 11). If a perineal phase is to be performed (in contrast to a supralevator exenteration), a second incision within the perineum encircling the vestibule and anus is also made.

2. The surgeon explores the peritoneal cavity for metastasis to the liver, the lymph nodes of the celiac axis, the superior mesenteric artery, and the paraaortic tissues.

3. The pelvis is explored, and the peritoneum along the brim of the pelvis is examined for lymph node involvement. Frozen sections may be indicated to be certain that there will be negative margins. The obturator fossa and the region of the uterosacral ligaments are explored. When findings at exploration are negative, retractors are placed and the small bowel is isolated with moist radiopaque laparotomy pads (Fig. 14.40).

4. The surgeon frees the sigmoid mesocolon and sections it with intestinal clamps and a blade or a stapling device. The proximal end is exteriorized through an opening in the left side of the abdomen; an intestinal clamp is left across the lumen until later when the permanent colostomy will be secured to the skin (see Chapter 11).

5. The remaining sigmoid mesentery is clamped with curved hemostatic or Kelly clamps, cut, and ligated down to and including the superior hemorrhoidal vessels. Long instruments and sutures are used to reach the deep pelvic structures.

6. The distal sigmoid colon is closed with an inverting suture. The sigmoid colon and rectum are freed from the sacrococcygeal area by blunt and sharp dissection.

7. The lateral pelvic peritoneum is cut along the iliac vessels; the ovarian vessels and round ligaments on each side are clamped with a curved hemostatic or Kelly clamp, cut, and doubly ligated. The surgeon can use a handheld vessel sealing and dividing device throughout the procedure where ligaments and vessels need to be clamped, cut, and ligated.

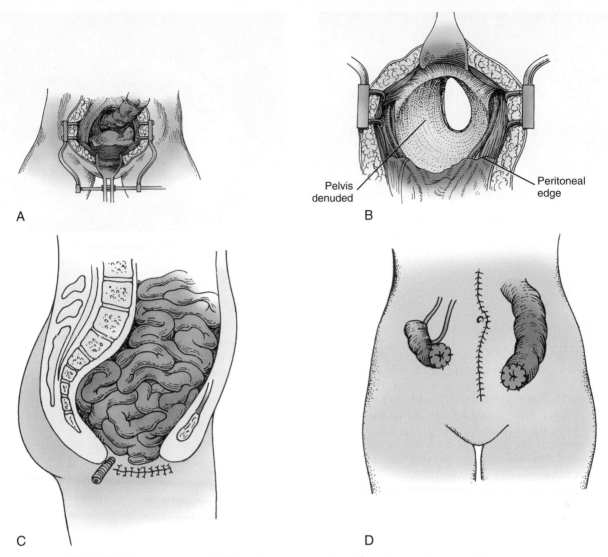

FIG. 14.40 Pelvic exenteration. (A) Pelvic viscera in situ as viewed from the operating surgeon's vantage point after retractors are placed and small bowel is isolated with moist laparotomy packs. (B) Empty pelvis after dissection of paravesical and paravaginal tissues and removal of specimen en bloc. (C) Sagittal view of small bowel above pelvic defect. Perineal packing or drain may be used. (D) After closure of abdominal wall, colostomy and urostomy stomas are sutured to skin edges.

8. The surgeon incises the peritoneum over the dome of the bladder with a long knife handle and blade or Metzenbaum scissors, and separates the bladder from the symphysis pubis down to the urethra.

9. The ureters are identified and divided 2 to 3 cm below the brim of the pelvis. The proximal end is left open to allow urinary drainage, whereas the distal end is ligated.

10. The external iliac vein is retracted to allow evacuation of the contents of the obturator fossa, leaving the obturator nerve intact. Care must be taken in dissection not to damage the sacral plexus and sciatic nerve. Occasionally, some component of the hypogastric (internal iliac) vessels may also be excised.

11. In the perineal phase, the surgeon isolates the internal pudendal vessels, ligates them with transfixion sutures, and cuts them. The remaining soft tissue attachments of the pelvis are clamped and cut. Steps 10 and 11 are then performed on the opposite side.

12. The perineum is incised by an elliptic incision that includes the clitoris and anus. The ischiorectal fat is incised up to the area of the levator muscle.

13. The coccygeal attachment of the rectum is severed. The levator muscles are severed at their lateral attachments by using a long knife handle with a blade; hemostasis is maintained by pressure and traction.

14. The paravesical and paravaginal tissues are resected by means of a knife from the periosteum of the symphysis pubis and superior pubic rami. The specimen is completely freed and removed from the pelvis (Fig. 14.41).

15. After residual bleeding vessels are identified and controlled by transfixing ligatures or the ESU, the surgeon closes the subcutaneous tissue with interrupted sutures. A drain is placed in the wound, and the skin is closed.

16. The ileal or colonic segment for the conduit is fashioned next, and the ureters are anastomosed to it. The external stoma is placed on the right side of the abdomen.

17. A jejunostomy catheter occasionally may be inserted into the proximal jejunum to aid in postoperative bowel decompression. It is connected to the bowel with a purse-string suture and exteriorized to the skin, where it is sutured in place.

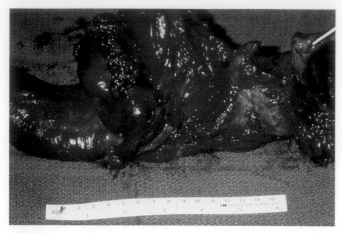

FIG. 14.41 Total pelvic exenteration specimen: bladder, uterus, cervix, and rectum.

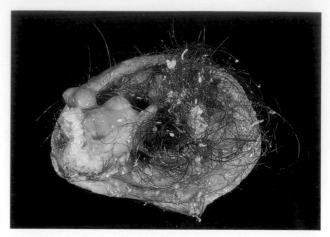

FIG. 14.42 Gross appearance of a cut-open dermoid cyst. Note the presence of hair-bearing skin.

18. A gastrostomy tube may be placed into the stomach in the same manner.

19. Hemostasis is assessed and controlled. The small intestine is carefully repositioned into the pelvis. Packs and retractors are removed.

20. The peritoneum, rectus muscles, and fascial sheaths are closed with interrupted figure-of-eight sutures. The skin is closed with interrupted sutures or staples.

21. The colostomy stoma is prepared by removing the intestinal clamp from the sigmoid colon, opening the colon, and suturing the stoma to the skin edges (see Chapter 11).

22. Dressings are applied to the abdominal wound, drain, and secured tube sites. Drainage devices are applied to the colostomy and urostomy stomas.

Surgery for Conditions Affecting Fertility

Oophorectomy and Oophorocystectomy

Oophorectomy is removal of an ovary. Oophorocystectomy is removal of an ovarian cyst. Functional cysts constitute the majority of ovarian enlargements, with follicular cysts being the most common. Functional cysts develop in the corpus luteum. Benign cystic teratomas, also known as dermoid cysts, are very common and are composed of ectodermal tissues (sweat glands, hair follicles, and teeth) (Fig. 14.42). Other tissues found in dermoid cysts include skin and skin appendages, cartilage, bone, and respiratory and GI tract epithelium (Dolan et al., 2017). Ovarian epithelial tumors, serous cystadenomas, and mucinous cystadenomas are prone to malignant change.

The choice of operation depends on the patient's age and symptoms, findings during physical examination, and direct examination of the adnexa during surgical exploration. If the ovarian tumor is recognized as benign, only the visibly diseased portions of the adnexa are removed. In the presence of dermoid, follicular, and corpus luteum cysts, the cyst is usually enucleated and most of the ovarian parenchyma is preserved. In a tubal pregnancy, the ectopic pregnancy may be removed from the tube or the entire ectopic fallopian tube may be removed concomitant with, in some instances, the ovary. In most cases, this procedure is done laparoscopically unless there is a large adnexal mass present.

Procedural Considerations

The basic abdominal gynecologic instrument tray is required. An 18-gauge needle and 30-mL or 60-mL syringe is likely to be needed to aspirate ovarian cyst fluid.

Operative Procedure

1. The skin is incised and the abdominal layers are opened as described for laparotomy (see Chapter 11).

2. After the abdominal cavity is opened, the surgeon has several options:

   a. For removal of a large ovarian cyst, an 18-gauge needle with a 30-mL or 60-mL syringe attached may be used to aspirate the cyst. Suction is readily available. All normal ovarian tissue is preserved when possible.

   b. For removal of a smaller ovarian cyst, a clamp is placed at the base of the cyst, and the cyst is excised. The wound in the ovary is closed with absorbable suture (depending on hemostasis and surgeon's preference) (Fig. 14.43).

   c. For removal of a dermoid cyst, the field is protected with radiopaque laparotomy pads because cystic contents cause irritation if they are spilled into the peritoneal cavity. An incision is made along the base of the cyst between the wall and normal ovarian tissue. The cystic wall is dissected away. The ovary is closed with interrupted or continuous sutures.

   d. For decortication of an enlarged ovary and wedge resection, a large segment of the ovarian cortex opposite the hilum is removed. The cysts are punctured with a needle and collapsed. A wedge of ovarian stroma, extending deep into the hilum, is resected with a #15 blade; the cortex of the ovary is closed with interrupted or continuous sutures.

3. To prevent prolapse of the tube into the cul-de-sac, the tube may be sutured to the pelvic side wall.

4. The abdominal wound is closed as described for laparotomy (see Chapter 11).

5. An abdominal dressing is applied.

Microscopic Reconstructive Surgery of the Fallopian Tube

Reconstructive surgery of the fallopian tube is done to restore patency and function of the fallopian tube, promoting the possibility of

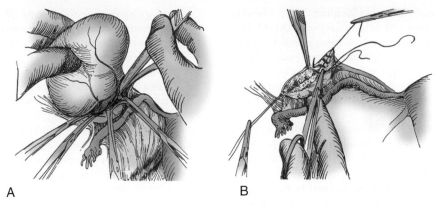

FIG. 14.43 Resection of small cyst from ovary. (A) Incision made around ovary near junction of cyst wall and normal ovarian tissue. Knife handle is convenient instrument for removal of cyst contents. (B) Wound in ovary closed.

fertilization. Fallopian tubal obstruction can occur in the distal (more common) or proximal portion of the tube, and sometimes in both. Fertility outcomes after surgery depend on the location of the tubal obstruction and the amount of disease (Lobo, 2017). Reconstructive surgery of the tube, broadly called *tuboplasty,* includes reanastomosis (after a tubal ligation), salpingoneostomy, fimbrioplasty, and lysis of adhesions. An HSG and laparotomy can assist in determining the extent and area of obstruction before reconstructive tubal surgery.

Microsurgical techniques are used with a mini-laparotomy and/or laparoscopy. Microsurgical tubal anastomosis permits atraumatic, accurate alignment of fallopian tube segments. The CO_2 laser may be adapted to the operating microscope, or the freehand approach may be used in tubal reconstructive surgery. These procedures may be performed in fertility clinics by fertility specialists.

Procedural Considerations

The patient is in supine position. The surgeon may place a Kahn, Calvin, Rubin, Hui, or HUMI cannula or a pediatric Foley catheter into the uterine cavity for intraoperative chromopertubation with diluted methylene blue. Intraoperative chromopertubation can also be achieved by applying a Buxton uterine clamp around the lower segment of the uterus and inserting an Angiocath catheter through the fundus into the cavity. A radiopaque vaginal pack may be inserted to help elevate the uterus.

The basic abdominal gynecologic instrument tray is required, with the addition of iris scissors (one curved and one straight), Adson forceps without teeth, Halsted mosquito hemostats, a tray of Bowman lacrimal probes, Webster needle holders, Frazier suction tip, Kirschner retractor (if desired), and a Buxton uterine clamp (if desired).

Basic microsurgical instruments include microscissors (one curved and one straight), bayonet microscissors, jeweler's forceps, microforceps, fallopian tube forceps, petit-point mosquito hemostats, micro–needle holders (one curved and one straight), ball-tipped nerve hook, and glass or Teflon rods.

Accessory items include micro–needle electrodes for the ESU; an ESU pencil; bipolar forceps with cord, irrigator, syringes, and blunt needles for irrigation of the tissues; plastic or Silastic tubing and connectors; diluted methylene blue or indigo carmine solution; diluted heparinized lactated Ringer's solution; microscope; microscope drape or operative loupes; and a video monitoring system (if desired).

Operative Procedure

Operative procedures for correction of postsurgical tubal occlusion are usually performed under the operating microscope. Other reconstructive procedures vary according to the nature of the pathologic condition of the tube and may be performed under the operating microscope or by use of operative loupes.

In microsurgery, the surgeon minimizes tissue injury to prevent postoperative adhesions and promote positive outcomes. Microsurgical instruments are specialized and delicate. To prevent damage, they are used only for the microsurgery portion of the procedure. Each of these instruments is designed to permit gentle, atraumatic handling of tissues and to avoid abrasions, lacerations, and vascular damage.

The tissues are continually irrigated to prevent drying of the serosal surfaces. Lactated Ringer's solution alone or with heparin added may be used for this purpose. Meticulous hemostasis is required. Irrigation is also used to identify bleeding vessels. Hemostasis is achieved by an ESU with a micro–needle monopolar electrode or very fine bipolar forceps. When a CO_2 laser is used, smoke from laser vaporization is evacuated to prevent carbon deposits on the tissue.

Tubal Ligation

Tubal ligation is the interruption of fallopian tube continuity, resulting in sterilization of the patient. Generally the indication for sterilization depends entirely on the desire of the patient. Certain medical indications and concern for the psychosocial needs of the patient are factors, and occasionally an obstetric indication exists, such as genetic abnormality. In the United States sterilization is a voluntary procedure. Thorough presurgical counseling is needed for the patient and her husband or significant other because this procedure is not predictably reversible. Patients may elect to have the procedure performed laparoscopically at an ambulatory surgery center.

Tubal ligation can be performed immediately postpartum after vaginal delivery or at the time of cesarean birth (Baggish, 2016b). This timing does not delay patient discharge time. There is emerging opinion for a change in practice arising from multiple clinical trials to opt for a risk-reducing bilateral salpingectomy, instead of a simple tubal ligation, to decrease the risk of ovarian cancer (Rivlin and Westhoff, 2017).

Operative Procedure

Many surgical methods and techniques are available for tubal ligation such as laparoscopic clips, Silastic bands, and thermal coagulation (i.e., bipolar ESU instrument) (Rivlin and Westhoff, 2017). Materials that do not create artifacts on x-rays or interfere with MRI are often used. The objective of each method is to achieve complete closure of the fallopian tube to prevent conception. General surgical considerations are directed to excising a section of each fallopian tube, ligating the severed ends, achieving hemostasis, and incorporating the proximal stump within layers of the mesosalpinx. Excised segments are sent for pathologic examination.

Laparoscopic Tubal Occlusion. The operative procedure begins as described in steps 1 through 8 of laparoscopy.

1. An accessory trocar port is inserted at the suprapubic region for the occluding instrument.
2. Once the tube has been identified and isolated in the grasping forceps sterilization is completed by using a laparoscopic bipolar ESU instrument, or by placing a spring clip or Silastic band.
   a. *Bipolar ESU coagulation* occurs when electrical current passes only through the tube from prong to prong. At least 3 cm of the tube is destroyed to prevent spontaneous recanalization. It is recommended that the tube be grasped at least 2 to 3 cm away from the uterocornual junction. This technique leaves a stump of isthmus to absorb the intrauterine fluid under pressure and minimize fistula formation, aiding in the prevention of a future ectopic pregnancy.
   b. The *spring clip* occludes the isthmus of the tube by two plastic jaws (Fig. 14.44A–B). The tube is compressed by a stainless

steel spring that presses the jaws together. Spring clip application requires careful surgical technique to ensure the clip is completely across the isthmus of the tube (see Fig. 14.44C). Some surgeons apply two spring clips positioned close together on each tube when using this approach.
   c. With a *Silastic band*, the tube is drawn 1.5 cm into a 0.5-cm–diameter metal cylinder, which destroys approximately 3 cm of the tube (Fig. 14.45A). A Silastic ring stretched on the outside of the cylinder is released to form an occlusion (see Fig. 14.45B). Over time, about 3 cm of the constricted tube necrose and the tubes separate (see Fig. 14.45C).
3. Trocar site closure is completed as described for laparoscopy.

Mini-Laparotomy Approach

1. The surgeon creates a 2- to 5-cm transverse incision approximately 6 cm above the pubic hairline. The surgeon may infiltrate the incision with local anesthesia before incision or at the end of the procedure.
2. A self-retaining or small handheld retractor is placed through the incision and into the peritoneal cavity. The fallopian tube is grasped with a Babcock clamp and gently pulled up. Spring clips or Silastic bands can be applied, or the original Pomeroy method of ligation can be carried out. The Pomeroy technique (Baggish, 2016b) provides a tissue segment specimen from each tube. The tube is pulled up with an Allis clamp or mosquito hemostat. A Kelly clamp is then placed across the base of the pulled up knuckle

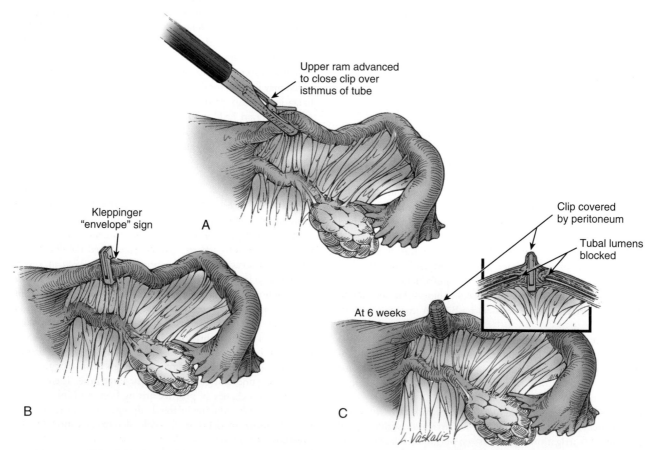

FIG. 14.44 Spring clip. (A) Isthmic portion (first 2–3 cm of tube) is maneuvered into the open jaws of the clip until it is snug against the hinge. (B) Closing the clip will create the Kleppinger envelope sign, which is a fold of tubal peritoneum in the hinge of the clip. (C) Failure to get the clip completely across the isthmus may result in pregnancy. Some surgeons routinely use two clips close together on each tube.

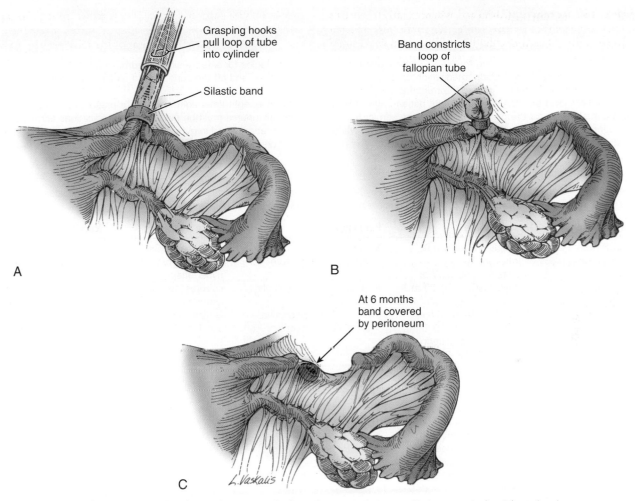

FIG. 14.45 Silastic band. (A) About 3 cm of tube is drawn into a 5-mm cylinder over which a Silastic band has been stretched. (B) Releasing the band constricts the knuckle of tube with eventual necrosis. (C) As with the Pomeroy technique, 6 months later the stumps are about 3 cm apart.

portion of the tube, excised superior to the Kelly clamp, and then ligated. Hemostasis is confirmed.

3. Closure of the incision (fascia, if necessary, followed by a subcuticular running suture) is followed by placement of wound closure strips, small dressings, or skin glue.

Obstetric Surgery

Providing safe, quality nursing care for the perioperative patient is the goal of every surgical team. The interventions necessary to reach this goal intensify with the pregnant woman who presents for surgery. The team is now faced with the challenge of caring for at least two patients, the mother and her child. Maternal changes in pregnancy increase as gestation progresses and include hormonal fluctuations, mechanical changes to the viscera related to the enlarging uterus, increased metabolic and oxygen demands, and hemodynamic changes. The fetus also has unique metabolic and hemodynamic needs that must be considered. Hazards of performing surgery on the pregnant patient include fetal loss, fetal asphyxia, premature labor, premature rupture of the membranes, and thromboembolic events, which can be increased because of the physiologic changes of pregnancy. Physiologic changes affect cardiovascular and hemodynamic, respiratory, GI, coagulation, and renal systems (Flood and

Rollins, 2015). Many local and inhaled anesthetic medications used in the perioperative setting can cross into the placental circulation (Flood and Rollins, 2015).

Special considerations for the obstetric surgical patient include continuous monitoring of the fetal heart rate, rapid induction for general anesthesia to prevent aspiration, and preparation for the possible use of tocolytics (e.g., medications to decrease uterine activity) to prevent labor (Surgical Pharmacology). Neonatal resuscitative drugs and equipment are readily available when performing surgery on pregnant women in the second trimester and beyond. If the surgical approach allows, the pregnant woman is positioned with a lateral tilt or with a wedge or pillow under her right hip to provide uterine displacement and relieve pressure on the maternal vena cava. This position promotes blood flow to the placenta.

Cervical Cerclage

Cervical incompetence is a condition characterized by habitual midtrimester spontaneous abortions. The condition is characterized by a shortening of the length of the cervix (observed on ultrasound) and funneling of the cervix. Surgical intervention is designed to prevent cervical dilation and shortening. This procedure gives better support by means of suture or surgical tape to the cervix. Introduced

Medications Used in Gynecology and Obstetrics

Part of safe perioperative patient care focuses on safe medication practices. Strategies for safe medication administration include standardizing labeling of medication, medication containers, and other solutions on and off the surgical field, separating sound-alike and look-alike medications, and minimizing interruptions and distractions.

In addition to practicing the "eight rights" (right patient, right medication, right dose, right time, right route, right reason, right response, and right documentation) for the medications he or she administers, the perioperative nurse must be familiar with medications administered to the patient by others (e.g., anesthesia providers, surgeons). Many of the medications used in gynecologic and obstetric surgery are unique to the specialty or have unique uses within the specialty. The perioperative nurse must be familiar with how these medications work, dosage ranges, adverse reactions, and nursing implications.

Oxytocics

Medications that increase motor activity within the uterus by hormonal stimulation, or direct stimulation on the smooth muscles, usually resulting in uterine contractions. Oxytocic medications are used intraoperatively and postoperatively.

Medication/Category	Dosage/Route	Purpose/Action	Adverse Reactions	Nursing Implications
Oxytocin (Pitocin) Functional class: Hormone Chemical class: Oxytocic, uterine-active agent	Incomplete abortion: IV Infusion: 10 units/500 mL D$_5$W or 0.9% NaCl at 10–20 mU/min, max 30 units/12 h Postpartum hemorrhage: IV: 10–40 units in 1000 mL nonhydrating diluent infused at 20–40 mU/min IM: 3–10 units after delivery of placenta Control of postpartum bleeding: Dilute 10–40 units/1000 mL of solution; run at 10–20 mU/min; adjust rate as needed Have crash cart available on unit (magnesium sulfate at bedside)	Missed or incomplete abortion; postpartum bleeding Acts directly on myofibrils, producing uterine contraction; vasoactive antidiuretic effect	Bradycardia, PVCs, hypotension/ hypertension, seizures, tetanic contractions, N/V, constipation, anaphylaxis	Monitor VS and I&O Assess for hemorrhage Monitor uterine contractions Teach patient to report adverse reactions (bleeding, blurred vision, difficulty speaking, wheezing, itching, swelling)
Methylergonovine Maleate (Methergine) Functional class: Oxytocic Chemical class: Ergot alkaloid	PO: 200 mcg tid to qid × ≤7 days IM/IV: 200 mcg q2–4h × 1–5 doses	Stimulates uterine, vascular, and smooth muscle, causing contractions; decreases bleeding; arterial vasoconstriction Prevention, treatment of hemorrhage postpartum or postabortion, uterine contractions	N/V, cramping, headache, hypotension/ hypertension, dysrhythmias, tinnitus, dizziness, seizures, dyspnea, leg cramps, allergic reactions	Monitor VS, bleeding; watch for indication of hemorrhage. Ergot toxicity: tinnitus, hypertension, palpitations, chest pain, nausea, vomiting, weakness; cold, numb extremities

Tocolytics

Medications that decrease uterine contractility. Most commonly used in the perioperative setting during fetal surgery or in surgical procedures on pregnant females. Tocolytics may also be used in the PACU.

Medication/Category	Dosage/Route	Purpose/Action	Adverse Reactions	Nursing Implications
Magnesium sulfate Functional class: anticonvulsive, electrolyte	IV 4–5 g IV infusion; with 5 g IM in each gluteus, then 5 g q4h *or* 4 g IV infusion, then 1–3 g/h continuous infusion, maximum dose in patients with severe renal disease is 40 g/d or 20 g/48 h	To treat and prevent seizures and eclampsia	N/V, muscle weakness, sweating, confusion, respiratory depression, depressed reflexes, vasodilation, hypotension	Seizure precautions. Monitor VS Maintain accurate I&O Monitor renal function Ensure IV calcium gluconate is available to reverse magnesium sulfate toxicity

Antimetabolites

Medications that interrupt cell division. Antimetabolite medications may be administered intraoperatively or postoperatively.

Medication/Category	Dosage/Route	Purpose/Action	Adverse Reactions	Nursing Implications
Methotrexate (Rheumatrex, Trexall) Functional class: Antineoplastic-antimetabolite Chemical class: Folic acid antagonist	IM: 50 mg/m^2	Ectopic pregnancies Inhibits an enzyme that reduces folic acid, which is needed for nucleic acid synthesis in all cells	N/V, dizziness, seizures, headache, confusion, dizziness, blurred vision, hepatotoxicity, nephrotoxicity	Discuss need for weekly repeated hCG levels Monitor WBC counts Encourage patient to report symptoms of infection

SURGICAL PHARMACOLOGY

Medications Used in Gynecology and Obstetrics—cont'd

Medication/Category	Dosage/Route	Purpose/Action	Adverse Reactions	Nursing Implications
Miscellaneous Agents				
Estradiol cream (Estrace cream) *Functional class:* Estrogen, progestins	Topical cream given intravaginally, 0.1 mg/g	Lubricant for vaginal packing for treatment of moderate to severe vasomotor symptoms associated with menopause and vaginal atrophy	N/V, dizziness, headache, local irritation, vaginal discharge	Assess preoperatively for any sensitivity to topical estrogens
Vasopressin (Pressyn) *Functional class:* Pituitary hormone	Given as a local injection Available in 20 units/mL (is diluted in sterile IV saline per direction of surgeon)	To help control bleeding; causes vasoconstriction	Dysrhythmias, bradycardia, hypertension, chest pain, headache, uterine cramping, N/V	Monitor VS Verify dilution with surgeon
Methylene blue (Urolene Blue), methylthioninium chloride Description: Water soluble dye	May be given IV or during chromopertubation IV: 1% injection 10 mg/mL During chromopertubation diluted in saline per direction of surgeon	To test patency of fallopian tubes or ureters Converts ferrous iron to ferric iron producing methemoglobin	Abdominal pain, dizziness, headache, urine and fecal discoloration, hypertension, N/V, diaphoresis, mental confusion	Warn patient about urine and stool discoloration Check VS and assess for mental confusion Monitor VS Verify dilution with surgeon

hCG, Human chorionic gonadotropin; *I&O,* intake and output; *IM,* intramuscular; *IV,* intravenous; *N/V,* nausea or vomiting; *PACU,* postanesthesia care unit; *PO,* by mouth; *PVC,* premature ventricular contractions; *tid,* three times daily; *qid,* four times daily; *VS,* vital signs; *WBC,* white blood cell.

Modified from Gold Standard: *Methylene blue* (website), 2016. www.clinicalkey.com/#!/content/drug_monograph/6-s2.0-390. (Accessed 21 January 2017); Skidmore-Roth L: *Mosby's 2017 nursing drug reference,* ed 30, St Louis, 2017, Elsevier; Wolters K: *Nursing 2017 drug handbook,* ed 37, Philadelphia, 2017, Lippincott.

by Shirodkar in 1951, cervical cerclage provides a mechanical closure to the cervix. Cerclage is accomplished via a vaginal approach (Shirodkar and McDonald approaches). The McDonald cerclage is the more common approach (Cashion, 2016) and uses a suture to secure and close the cervix by passing a suture through four points on the cervix (i.e., at the 12, 3, 6, and 9 o'clock positions). The cervical cerclage is generally removed in an office procedure when the woman reaches the 36th week of gestation (Cashion, 2016), or when spontaneous labor begins, or the child is delivered by cesarean birth.

Procedural Considerations: Vaginal Approach

A gentle vaginal surgical prep is carried out. Instruments include the basic vaginal instrument tray, with the addition of right and left Deschamps ligature carriers, trocar needles, nonabsorbable sutures for the internal os, and the surgeon's preference for closure of the mucosal incisions.

Operative Procedure: Shirodkar/McDonald

1. Anterior and posterior vaginal retractors are placed, and the cervix is pulled down with smooth ovum or sponge-holding forceps. With smooth tissue forceps and dissecting scissors, the mucosa over the anterior cervix is opened to permit the bladder to be pushed back (Fig. 14.46).
2. The surgeon lifts the cervix and incises the posterior vaginal mucosa at the level of the peritoneal reflection. The corners of the anterior and posterior incisions are bilaterally approximated in the area of the lateral mucosa with curved tonsil or Allis forceps.
3. The prepared ligature is placed at the desired level by passage of the material through the approximated tissue and then drawn tight posteriorly to close the cervix; it is then tied. It is not

necessary to suture the ligature to the underlying tissues. The suture material used for this ligation is 5-mm Dacron or Mersilene tape. The anterior and posterior mucosal incisions are usually closed with 2-0 absorbable suture to complete the procedure.

4. The McDonald cerclage is performed in a similar manner, using the same instruments, supplies, and preparation. The suture is not buried in the submucosa in the McDonald technique (Fig. 14.47).

Abdominal Surgery During Pregnancy

The incidence of immediate need for abdominal surgery occurs as frequently among pregnant women as among nonpregnant women of childbearing age. Diagnosis of abdominal problems in the pregnant woman is challenging because of the enlarged uterus and displaced organs. Mild leukocytosis and increased levels of alkaline phosphatase and amylase are normal during pregnancy; abnormally high or rising laboratory values should be noted. Ultrasound is the safest and most commonly used diagnostic study during pregnancy, avoiding any ionizing radiation exposure to the fetus. MRI also can be used as a diagnostic tool (Montgomery, 2016; Schwartz and Ludmir, 2017).

Laparotomy or laparoscopy may be required for conditions such as appendicitis, acute cholelithiasis, ovarian masses, and intestinal obstruction. Appendicitis is the most common nonobstetric surgical condition that complicates pregnancy and occurs in about 1 in 1000 pregnancies (Montgomery, 2016).

Fetal Surgery

Developments in prenatal diagnosis have progressed so far that clinicians may consider the fetus to be the patient. Serious congenital anomaly is diagnosable by ultrasonography, alpha-fetoprotein specimen, amniocentesis, chorionic villi sampling, or percutaneous umbilical blood sampling. When an anomaly is identified, a

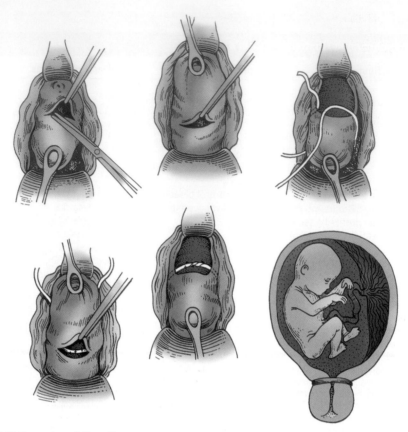

FIG. 14.46 Principles of Shirodkar operation for treatment of incompetent internal cervical os during pregnancy.

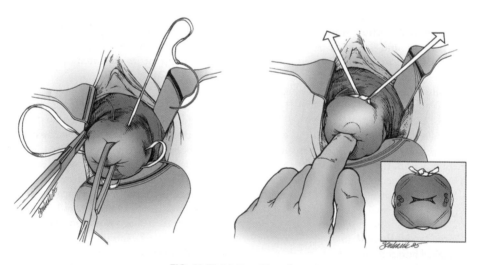

FIG. 14.47 McDonald cerclage.

multidisciplinary team reviews the mother's complete medical history and prenatal ultrasonograms. (For more information on fetal surgery, see Chapter 26.)

Cesarean Birth

Cesarean birth, also referred to as *cesarean section* or *C-section*, is delivery of the fetus or fetuses through abdominal (laparotomy) and uterine (hysterotomy) incisions. Generally cesarean birth is used whenever further delay in delivery may seriously compromise the fetus, the mother, or both, or when vaginal delivery cannot be accomplished safely. In recent years, cesarean birth has increased because of fetal monitoring, fetal scalp blood sampling for pH determination, and a widespread emphasis on recognition of actual or suspected impairment of fetal well-being if delivery is delayed. Reasons for cesarean birth include failure to progress, malposition and malpresentation, cephalopelvic disproportion, abruptio placentae, toxemia, fetal distress, uterine dysfunction, placenta previa, prolapsed cord, previous pelvic surgery, cervical dystocia, active herpes genitalis, extensive condylomatous disease, and diabetes. Multiple pregnancies also may be an indication for cesarean birth. In certain situations and after appropriate counseling, elective cesarean delivery may be a medically acceptable option. Cesarean births may be classified as primary (woman's first cesarean), repeat (indicates a previous cesarean birth), elective (a scheduled procedure in either of the previous categories or at maternal request), or emergency (there is an immediate need for intervention). The surgical team may find that developing a checklist for surgical emergencies, such as emergency cesarean birth, assists in efficient care rather than relying on memory alone (Arriaga et al., 2013).

Cesarean birth is ranked as the most commonly performed major surgical procedure in the United States. In 2013, nearly a third of births were performed by cesarean section (Mistry et al., 2016).

Cesarean birth may take place in an OR in the obstetric labor suite or in the main OR. Patients about to undergo cesarean birth need careful assessment and emotional support. Because cesarean birth may involve emergency situations, the mother may express grave concern for her infant's well-being. If the mother has participated in childbirth classes, she may believe she has failed in some way. The perioperative nurse remains aware of the psychologic as well as physiologic needs of mothers. Mothers may choose to remain awake after administration of a regional anesthetic; the mother's birthing partner may be permitted to accompany and support her in the OR and witness the birth (based on hospital policy). The birthing partner will need the perioperative nurse's assistance in preparing for the delivery by washing hands and donning scrub attire or a protective gown. The perioperative nurse reassures and encourages the birthing partner to coach and lend support to the mother during this intensely stressful time. The birthing partner is included in the bonding process that is initiated at birth. The mother, if awake and stable, is shown and encouraged to hold her infant. The perioperative nurse promotes a positive, family-centered experience.

If the cesarean birth is performed as an emergency, the family-centered approach may not be feasible. In emergency situations the mother's support person or persons need to be directed to the surgical waiting area, where information will be communicated regarding the condition of the mother and infant. The support person or persons may then accompany the infant as he or she is transferred to the nursery. In an emergency cesarean birth, certain perioperative procedures may be omitted, such as initial surgical counts. When this occurs, institutional protocol for waived counts governs.

Procedural Considerations

The patient is supine with elevation of the right side to displace the uterus and prevent vena cava compression. Bony prominences are padded, and the patient is positioned in good body alignment with a safety strap above the knees. Antibiotics are administered by the anesthesia provider if not previously given. The perioperative nurse assists the anesthesia provider with the administration of a regional anesthetic before placing the patient in the supine position. Throughout this process maternal vital signs and fetal heart tones are monitored and recorded per institutional protocol.

If a general anesthetic is used, all preparations, including skin prep (Research Highlight), bladder drainage, draping, suction connection, counts, and gowning and gloving of scrubbed personnel, are done before induction. In many hospitals, healthcare providers qualified to deliver newborn care and resuscitation are in attendance for the delivery. A radiant warmer and resuscitative equipment for immediate postdelivery care of the infant are available. These infants

RESEARCH HIGHLIGHT

A Comparison of Two Skin Antiseptic Agents at Cesarean Delivery

SSIs occur in 5% to 12% of cesarean deliveries, whereas 2% to 5% occur in all surgical procedures. Cesarean deliveries are the most common surgical procedure among women in the United States; about 32.7% (1.3 million) of the 3.9 million births in 2013 were by cesarean delivery. Associated SSIs are estimated to cost $3,529 per occurrence. This unplanned incidence can place an extra burden on the new mother, interfering with breastfeeding and therefore the development of the mother-infant bonding relationship.

Researchers conducted a pragmatic, randomized controlled trial of 1147 women who underwent cesarean delivery at Washington University Center in St. Louis, Missouri, between September 2011 and June 2015. They were randomized to receive either 2% chlorhexidine gluconate with 70% isopropyl alcohol ($n = 572$) or 8.3% povidone-iodine with 72.5% isopropyl alcohol ($n = 575$) as a skin preparation (1 : 1 ratio).

It is known that the skin can harbor numerous pathogens that can contribute to SSIs. Effective and diligent preoperative skin asepsis decreases the chances of SSIs. Twenty-three patients (4.0%) in the chlorhexidine-alcohol group developed SSI compared with 42 patients (7.3%) in the iodine-alcohol group.

This study found that using a preoperative skin antisepsis combination of chlorhexidine-alcohol at cesarean delivery significantly lowered the patient risk for SSI compared with use of the iodine-alcohol preparation. The AORN scored this study with a rate of I A using the AORN Research Evidence Appraisal Tool. This score is representative of the best research available for evidence-based perioperative practice. Perioperative nurses should consider using the evidence from this study to guide their practice during future cesarean deliveries.

AORN, Association of periOperative Registered Nurses; *SSI,* surgical site infection.
Modified from Tuuli MG et al: A randomized trial comparing skin antiseptic agents at cesarean delivery, *N Engl J Med* 374(7):647–655, 2016; Evidence appraisal of Tuuli MG et al: A randomized trial comparing skin antiseptic agents at cesarean delivery, *AORN J* 103(5):537-542, 2016.

are considered to be at risk until there is evidence of physiologic stability.

The skin is prepped and draped as for abdominal surgery. The vagina is not prepped. An indwelling urinary catheter is inserted and secured. Instruments include the basic abdominal gynecologic tray, with the addition of Lister bandage scissors, Foerster sponge-holding (ring) forceps, Pennington forceps, cord clamps, a DeLee retractor, delivery forceps, a head extractor (if desired), laboratory tubes for cord blood, a drain (optional), and a bulb syringe.

Operative Procedure

1. The surgeon makes an infraumbilical midline vertical incision or lower transverse Pfannenstiel incision that is long enough to allow the infant to be delivered without difficulty; the length of the incision varies with the estimated size of the fetus.
2. The abdomen is opened in layers as described in laparotomy (see Chapter 11). The rectus and pyramidalis muscles are separated in the midline by sharp and blunt dissection to expose the underlying transversalis fascia and peritoneum.
3. The peritoneum is elevated with two Crile hemostats about 2 cm apart, and the peritoneum is palpated to rule out the inclusion of bowel, omentum, or bladder. The surgeon opens the peritoneum and enters the abdominal cavity.

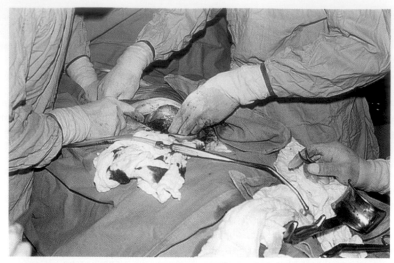

FIG. 14.48 Fundal pressure applied. Infant's head emerging from hysterotomy.

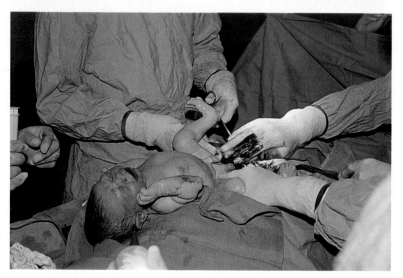

FIG. 14.49 Cord clamped in preparation for passing infant off field.

4. Bleeding sites within the abdominal incision may be clamped but not ligated until later, unless they obstruct the field of vision. If the patient has a general anesthetic, speed is used to prevent an anesthetized infant. An ESU is used for hemostasis.

5. The surgeon quickly palpates the uterus to determine the size and presenting part of the fetus as well as the direction and degree of rotation of the uterus.

6. The reflection of the visceral peritoneum above the upper margin of the bladder and overlying the anterior lower uterine segment is gently separated by sharp and blunt dissection.

7. The developed bladder flap is held downward beneath the symphysis with a bladder retractor such as the DeLee.

8. The uterus is opened with a blade through the lower uterine segment about 2 cm above the bladder flap. Once the uterus is opened, the incision can be extended by cutting laterally with large bandage scissors or by simply spreading the incision by means of lateral pressure applied with each index finger when the lower uterine segment is thin.

9. The presenting membranes are incised. Suction is imperative here, and many surgeons prefer no suction tip (only the large, open end of the suction tubing) during the expulsion and suctioning of amniotic fluid.

10. All retractors are removed. The fetal head is gently elevated manually, by use of obstetric forceps, or with the use of a vacuum apparatus through the incision. Once the fetal head is delivered, the surgical assistant provides transabdominal fundal pressure (Fig. 14.48) to aid in the delivery of the shoulders and extremities.

11. As soon as the head is delivered, a bulb syringe or aspirator tip is used to aspirate the exposed nares and mouth to minimize aspiration of amniotic fluid and its contents.

12. Oxytocin (20 units per liter of fluid or as directed by the surgeon) may be administered IV by the anesthesia provider as soon as the shoulders are delivered (or after delivery of the infant), so that the uterus contracts. Some surgeons inject 10 units of oxytocin directly into the muscular layer of the uterus either before or after the delivery of the placenta. Use of oxytocin minimizes blood loss.

13. On delivery of the entire infant, the cord is clamped and cut (Fig. 14.49), and the infant is given to the member of the team

who is responsible for any resuscitation efforts. A sterile gown or sheet is provided to the individual receiving the infant.

14. The edges of the uterine incision are promptly clamped with Péan forceps, ring forceps, Allis clamps, or Pennington clamps.

15. The placenta is delivered and placed in a large receptacle from the back table. Fundal massage or manual removal may be used to hasten delivery of the placenta and reduce bleeding.

16. One or two separate layers of suture may be used to close the uterine incision. The surgical team conducts a count to verify that no surgical items have been retained in the uterine cavity.

17. After closure of the uterine incision, hemostasis is established. The cut edges of the visceral peritoneum overlying the uterus and bladder may or may not be approximated. If the surgeon elects to close this layer, it is completed with a continuous running suture.

18. Any blood, blood clots, vernix, and amniotic fluid in the pelvis and peritoneal cavity are removed. The pelvic cavity may be lavaged until clear. The fallopian tubes and ovaries are also inspected. If scheduled, tubal ligation is carried out at this point.

19. The peritoneum and each abdominal layer are closed.

20. After the wound is closed, the perioperative nurse massages the patient's fundus and cleans any clots expressed from the vagina.

21. An abdominal dressing and perineal pad are applied.

Key Points

- Surgical procedures on structures of the female reproductive system are performed for diagnostic, therapeutic, or cosmetic purposes.
- A holistic approach with sensitivity to the special needs of women's health, their cultural beliefs and practices, as well as their sense of vulnerability, are essential components of perioperative patient care.
- Adult female structures associated with the process of reproduction are the external organs (vulva), the associated ligaments and muscles, the soft tissues and contents of the pelvic cavity, and the bony pelvis.
- The gynecologic patient's history includes a chronologic listing of each pregnancy, length of gestation, type of delivery, complications during pregnancy, duration of labor, and fetal weight; data on menstrual patterns are also collected.
- Lasers are frequently used in gynecologic procedures in conjunction with the colposcope and operating microscope, or the laparoscope.
- MIS and laparoscopic robotic-assisted surgery have specific advantages in approaching and treating gynecologic conditions.
- The incidence of immediate need for abdominal surgery occurs as frequently among pregnant women as among nonpregnant women of childbearing age.
- Cesarean birth is ranked as the most commonly performed major surgical procedure in the United States.

Critical Thinking Questions

A 45-year-old patient is scheduled for a laparoscopic robotic-assisted hysterectomy with possible BSO at 7:30 this morning. You are her perioperative nurse. After you have introduced yourself and properly identified her, you start reviewing her medical record for key factors to incorporate in your plan of care. You note she is morbidly obese and has medically controlled hypertension. This morning in the preoperative holding room, her blood pressure was 150/86 mm Hg and her fasting blood glucose taken 1 hour ago was 230 mg/dL. She has been fasting for 8 hours and did not take her insulin this morning as she usually does. She did, however, take her blood pressure medication with a sip of water around 5 a.m.

What additional perioperative nursing and positioning considerations are you planning for this patient? Will you anticipate monitoring her blood glucose level intraoperatively? If so, how often? Will you add this information to the time-out data you share with the surgical team? When reviewing the patient's medical record, you also note she has had several previous laparoscopic and open abdominal procedures. What additional instrumentation will you have available? What concerns do you have about her metabolic syndrome and the role it will play in her postoperative recovery?

⊖volve *The answers to the Critical Thinking Questions can be found at http://evolve.elsevier.com/Rothrock/Alexander.*

References

American Cancer Society (ACS): *Chemotherapy for ovarian cancer* (website), 2016a. www.cancer.org/cancer/ovariancancer/detailedguide/ovarian-cancer-treating-chemotherapy. (Accessed 19 January 2017).

American Cancer Society (ACS): *What are the key statistics about cervical cancer?* (website), 2016b. www.cancer.org/cancer/cervicalcancer/detailedguide/cervical-cancer-key-statistics. (Accessed 19 January 2017).

American Cancer Society (ACS): *What are the key statistics about vaginal cancer?* (website), 2016c. www.cancer.org/cancer/vaginalcancer/detailedguide/vaginal-cancer-key-statistics. (Accessed 19 January 2017).

American Cancer Society (ACS): *What are the key statistics about vulvar cancer?* (website), 2016d. www.cancer.org/cancer/vulvarcancer/detailedguide/vulvar-cancer-key-statistics. (Accessed 19 January 2017).

American Cancer Society (ACS): *What are the key statistics of ovarian cancer?* (website), 2016e. www.cancer.org/cancer/ovariancancer/detailedguide/ovarian-cancer-key-statistics. (Accessed 19 January 2017).

American Cancer Society (ACS): *What are the risk factors for vulvar cancer?* (website), 2016f. www.cancer.org/cancer/vulvarcancer/detailedguide/vulvar-cancer-risk-factors. (Accessed 19 January 2017).

American Cancer Society (ACS): *What is ovarian cancer?* (website), 2016g. www.cancer.org/cancer/ovariancancer/detailedguide/ovarian-cancer-what-is-ovarian-cancer. (Accessed 19 January 2017).

American Cancer Society (ACS): *Work-up of abnormal pap test results* (website), 2016h. www.cancer.org/cancer/cervicalcancer/moreinformation/cervicalcancer preventionandearlydetection/cervical-cancer-prevention-and-early-detection-abn-pap-work-up. (Accessed 19 January 2017).

Arriaga AF et al: Simulation-based trial of surgical-crisis checklists, *N Engl J Med* 368(3):246–253, 2013.

Association of periOperative Registered Nurses (AORN): *Guidelines for perioperative practice*, Denver, 2017, The Association.

Baggish MS: Complications of hysteroscopy. In Baggish MS, Karram MM, editors: *Atlas of pelvic anatomy and gynecologic surgery*, ed 4, Philadelphia, 2016a, Elsevier.

Baggish MS: Tubal sterilization. In Baggish MS, Karram MM, editors: *Atlas of pelvic anatomy and gynecologic surgery*, ed 4, Philadelphia, 2016b, Elsevier.

Carlson SM et al: Endoscopy: hysteroscopy and laparoscopy. In Lobo RA et al, editors: *Comprehensive gynecology*, ed 7, Philadelphia, 2017, Elsevier.

Cashion K: Hemorrhagic disorders. In Lowdermilk DL, Perry SE, editors: *Maternity & women's health care*, ed 11, St Louis, 2016, Elsevier.

Cassorla L, Lee JW: Patient positioning and associated risks. In Miller RD, editor: *Miller's anesthesia*, ed 8, Philadelphia, 2015, Saunders.

Coleman RL et al: Neoplastic diseases of the ovary. In Lobo RA et al, editors: *Comprehensive gynecology*, ed 7, Philadelphia, 2017, Elsevier.

Dmochowski RR et al: Slings. In Wein AJ et al, editors: *Campbell-Walsh urology*, ed 11, Philadelphia, 2016, Elsevier.

Dolan M et al: Benign gynecologic lesions. In Lobo RA et al, editors: *Comprehensive gynecology*, ed 7, Philadelphia, 2017, Elsevier.

Esposito N: Violence against women. In Lowdermilk DL, Perry SE, editors: *Maternity and women's health care*, ed 11, St Louis, 2016, Mosby.

Flood P, Rollins MD: Anesthesia for obstetrics. In Miller RD, editor: *Miller's anesthesia*, ed 8, Philadelphia, 2015, Elsevier.

Goodman T, Spry C: *Essentials of perioperative nursing*, ed 6, Burlington, MA, 2017, Jones & Bartlett Learning.

Gor HB, Rivlin ME: *Hysterectomy* (website), 2015. http://emedicine.medscape.com/article/267273-overview. (Accessed 19 January 2017).

Green AE: *Ovarian cancer* (website), 2016. http://emedicine.medscape.com/article/255771-overview#a1. (Accessed 19 January 2017).

Jhingran A et al: Cancers of the cervix, vulva, and vagina. In Neiderhuber JE et al, editors: *Abeloff's clinical oncology*, ed 5, Philadelphia, 2014, Saunders.

Jhingran A, Meyer LA: Malignant diseases of the cervix. In Lobo RA et al, editors: *Comprehensive gynecology*, ed 7, Philadelphia, 2017, Elsevier.

Kho RM, Lobo RA: Ectopic pregnancy. In Lobo RA et al, editors: *Comprehensive gynecology*, ed 7, Philadelphia, 2017, Elsevier.

LaMattina JC, Barth RN: Laparoendoscopic single-site surgery an evolving surgical approach. In Cameron JL, Cameron AM, editors: *Current surgical therapy*, ed 11, Philadelphia, 2014, Elsevier.

Lemack GE, Anger JT: Urinary incontinence and pelvic prolapse. In Wein AJ et al, editors: *Campbell-Walsh urology*, ed 11, Philadelphia, 2016, Elsevier.

Lobo RA: Infertility. In Lobo RA et al, editors: *Comprehensive gynecology*, ed 7, Philadelphia, 2017, Elsevier.

Magrina JF: Robotic surgery in gynecology. In Baggish MS, Karram MM, editors: *Atlas of pelvic anatomy and gynecologic surgery*, ed 4, Philadelphia, 2016, Elsevier.

Mistry K et al: *HCUP statistical brief #211: variation in the rate of cesarean section across U.S. hospitals, 2013* (website), 2016. www.hcup-us.ahrq.gov/reports/statbriefs/sb211-Hospital-Variation-C-sections-2013.pdf. (Accessed 19 January 2017).

Montgomery KS: Medical-surgical disorders. In Lowdermilk DL, Perry SE, editors: *Maternity and women's health care*, ed 11, St Louis, 2016, Elsevier.

National Cancer Institute: *Cancer stat facts: endometrial cancer* (website), 2016. https://seer.cancer.gov/statfacts/html/corp.html. (Accessed 18 January 2017).

Rivlin K, Westhoff C: Family planning. In Lobo RA et al, editors: *Comprehensive gynecology*, ed 7, Philadelphia, 2017, Elsevier.

Roth L: Molar pregnancy. In Ferri FF, editor: *Ferri's clinical advisor 2017 edition*, Philadelphia, 2017, Elsevier.

Ryntz T, Lobo RA: Abnormal uterine bleeding. In Lobo RA et al, editors: *Comprehensive gynecology*, ed 7, Philadelphia, 2017, Elsevier.

Schmeler KM, Gersheson DM: Fallopian tube and peritoneal carcinoma. In Lobo RA et al, editors: *Comprehensive gynecology*, ed 7, Philadelphia, 2017, Elsevier.

Schwartz N, Ludmir J: Surgery during pregnancy. In Gabbe SG et al, editors: *Obstetrics: normal and problem pregnancies*, ed 7, Philadelphia, 2017, Elsevier.

See A, Chern B: Contained intra-abdominal morcellation: is it the way forward? *Gynecology and Minimally Invasive Therapy* 5(3):99–101, 2016.

Shah DK et al: Association of body mass index and morbidity after abdominal, vaginal, and laparoscopic hysterectomy, *Obstet Gynecol* 125(3):589–598, 2015.

Siraj SHM, Chern B: Salpingectomy and prevention of ovarian carcinoma, *Gynecology and Minimally Invasive Therapy* 5(3):102–105, 2015.

Smith JA, Jhingran A: Principles of radiation therapy and chemotherapy in gynecologic cancer. In Lobo RA et al, editors: *Comprehensive gynecology*, ed 7, Philadelphia, 2017, Elsevier.

Ulm MA et al: A comparison of outcomes following robotic-assisted staging and laparotomy in patients with early stage endometriod adenocarcinoma of the uterus with uterine weight under 480g, *Gynecology and Minimally Invasive Therapy* 5(1):24–29, 2016.

Weiss AJ, Elixhauser A: *HCUP statistical brief #180: overview of hospital stays in the United States, 2012* (website), 2014. www.hcup-us.ahrq.gov/reports/statbriefs/sb180-Hospitalizations-United-States-2012.pdf. (Accessed 19 January 2017).

World Health Organization (WHO): *Violence against women fact sheet* (website), 2016. www.who.int/mediacentre/factsheets/fs239/en/. (Accessed 19 January 2017).

CHAPTER 15

Genitourinary Surgery

HELENE P. KOREY MARLEY

Advances in genitourinary (GU) surgery, with the use of robotics, laparoscopic techniques, cryotherapy, brachytherapy, lasers, ultrasonography, lithotripters, innovative diagnostic measures, and minimally invasive surgical approaches, have expanded treatment options. As urologic surgery becomes more complex and far more precise, the perioperative nurse is challenged to maintain up-to-date knowledge, documented competence, and new technical skills. More procedures are performed on an ambulatory or short-stay basis, allowing limited time for patient, family, and caregiver education and discharge planning. The success of surgical intervention and patient outcomes depends greatly on the nurse's ability and knowledge in designing, developing, and implementing an effective perioperative plan of care.

Surgical Anatomy

The normal GU system includes one pair of kidneys, two ureters, the urinary bladder, the urethra, and the prostate gland in the male.

Also considered essential to the GU system are the adrenal glands, male reproductive organs, and the female urogynecologic system.

Urine is excreted by the kidneys and conveyed to the bladder through the ureters. Urine is stored in the bladder, which serves as a reservoir until its full capacity (350–700 mL) is reached, and is eliminated from the body by way of the urethra. Normal urinary output ranges from 0.5 to 1 mL/kg of body weight per hour for the average adult.

Kidneys

The kidneys are located in the retroperitoneal space along the lateral borders of the psoas muscle, one on each side of the vertebral column at the level of the twelfth thoracic to the third lumbar vertebrae. Usually the right kidney is several centimeters lower than the left because the liver rests superior and anterior to the right kidney (Fig. 15.1).

Each kidney is surrounded by a mass of fatty and loose areolar tissue known as *pararenal fat.* A capsule enclosing the renal space is known as the *fascia renalis.* This is composed of *Gerota fascia* (anterior

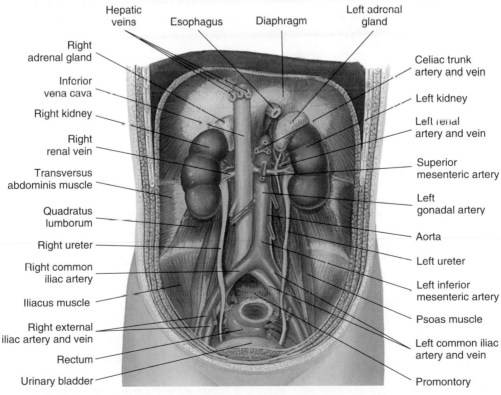

FIG. 15.1 Location of urinary system organs.

renal fascia) and *Zuckerkandl fascia* (posterior renal fascia). These structures help keep the kidneys in their normal anatomic position. The anterior and posterior relationships of the kidneys are shown in Fig. 15.2.

On the medial side of each kidney is a concave area known as the *hilum,* through which the renal artery and vein enter and exit. The renal pelvis, a funnel-shaped structure that lies within the kidney and posterior to the renal vascular pedicle, divides into several branches called *calyces* (Fig. 15.3). When surgery is indicated in these structures, a posterior flank approach is preferred. When surgery for the removal

of a mass is anticipated, a transabdominal or thoracoabdominal incision may be chosen.

The kidneys are highly vascular organs that process approximately one-fifth of the body's entire volume of blood at any one time. The blood supply to the kidney is conveyed through the renal artery (a large branch of the aorta) and leaves through the renal vein. On entering the kidney, the renal artery divides into anterior and posterior sections. These undergo further division into interlobular arteries from which smaller afferent branches pass to the glomeruli. Efferent arterioles in the glomeruli then pass to the tubules of the nephron.

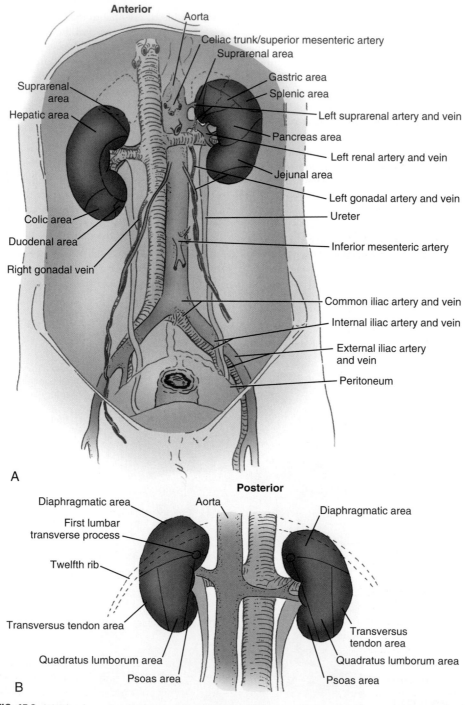

FIG. 15.2 (A) Blood supply of kidneys and relationship of kidneys and ureters to the main arteries and veins and the intraperitoneal organs. (B) Relationship of the kidneys and ureters to the spinal column.

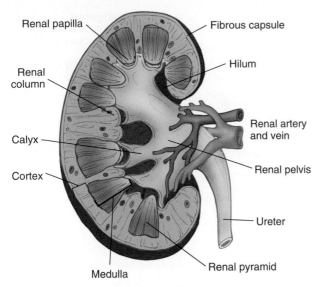

FIG. 15.3 Normal kidney.

The renal lymphatic supply originates beneath the capsule of the kidney and empties into the lumbar lymph nodes at the junction of the renal vascular pedicle and aorta. The nerves of the autonomic (involuntary) nervous system originate from the lumbar sympathetic trunk and from the vagus nerve. Removal of the nerve pathways does not impair renal function. The renal artery and vein with their accompanying nerves and lymphatics are referred to as the *pedicle* of the kidney.

Adrenal Glands

The adrenal glands lie retroperitoneally beneath the diaphragm, capping the medial aspects of the superior pole of each kidney. On the right side the gland is triangular and adjacent to the inferior vena cava; on the left side it is a rounded, crescent-shaped gland posterior to the stomach and pancreas. Each adrenal gland has a medulla, which secretes epinephrine (adrenaline), and a cortex, which secretes steroids and hormones. Secretions from the adrenal cortex are influenced by the activity of the pituitary gland. The adrenal glands are liberally supplied with arterial branches from the inferior phrenic and renal arteries and from the aorta. Venous drainage is accomplished on the right side by the inferior vena cava and on the left by the left renal vein. The lymphatic system accompanies the suprarenal vein and drains into the lumbar lymph nodes.

Ureters

Each ureter is a continuation of the renal pelvis. The ureter extends in a smooth S curve from the renal pelvis to the base of the bladder (Fig. 15.4). It is approximately 25 to 30 cm long and 4 to 5 mm in diameter in the adult. This fibromuscular cylindric tube is lined by transitional epithelium (urothelium) and lies on the psoas muscle, passing medially to the sacroiliac joints and laterally to the ischial spines. As urine accumulates in the renal pelvis, slight distention initiates a wave of muscular contractions. This peristaltic activity continues down the ureter, propelling urine into the bladder.

Urinary Bladder

The adult urinary bladder is a hollow, muscular viscus that acts as a reservoir for urine until micturition (voiding) occurs. It has an outer adventitial layer and inner urothelial layer. The trigone, a

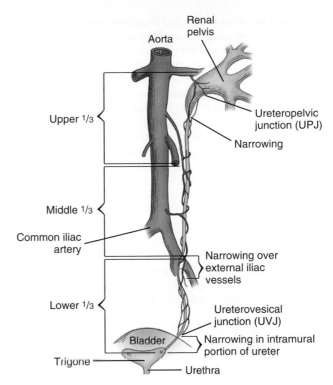

FIG. 15.4 Anatomy of ureter.

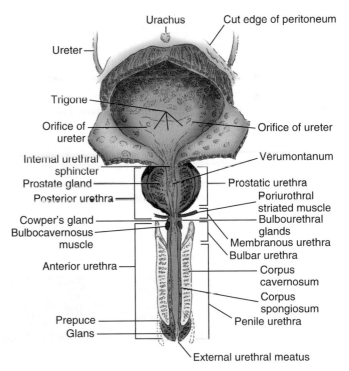

FIG. 15.5 Anatomy of male urinary bladder, prostate gland, and urethra.

triangular area, forms the base of the bladder. The three corners of the trigone correspond to the orifices of the ureters and the bladder neck (opening of the urethra) (Fig. 15.5). The ureteral orifices, on the proximal trigone at the interureteric ridge, are approximately 2.5 cm apart. The bladder neck (internal sphincter) is formed from converging detrusor muscle fibers of the bladder wall that pass distally to form the smooth musculature of the urethra. Physiologically the bladder fills with urine and expands into the abdominal cavity. The extraperitoneal location is advantageous because a suprapubic (above the pubic arch) incision may be performed without violating the peritoneum and potentially causing intraperitoneal complications.

The main arterial supply of the bladder comprises the superior, middle, and inferior vesical arteries. These vessels are derived from the internal iliac (hypogastric) artery, the obturator and inferior gluteal arteries, and in females the uterine and vaginal arteries. The bladder has a rich venous supply that drains into the internal iliac (hypogastric) vein. The lymphatic system is served by the vesical, external, and internal iliac and common iliac lymph nodes.

The bladder's size, position, and relationship to the bowel, rectum, and reproductive organs vary according to the bladder's distention. In the female the vagina lies dorsal to the base of the bladder and parallel to the urethra (Fig. 15.6). In the male the prostate gland is interposed between the bladder neck and the urethra (Fig. 15.7). These anatomic relationships influence the symptoms that a patient experiences preoperatively and are important landmarks during pelvic surgery.

The process of bladder evacuation appears to be initiated by nerve cells from the sacral division of the autonomic nervous system. These sacral reflex centers are controlled by higher voluntary centers in the brain. Stimulation of the sacral centers results in contraction of the bladder muscles and relaxation of the bladder outlet sphincters.

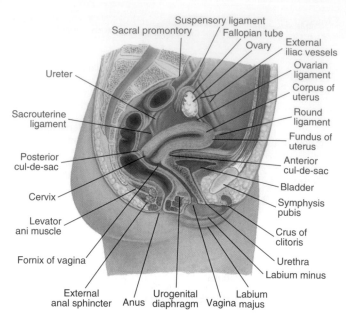

FIG. 15.6 Female genitourinary and reproductive anatomy.

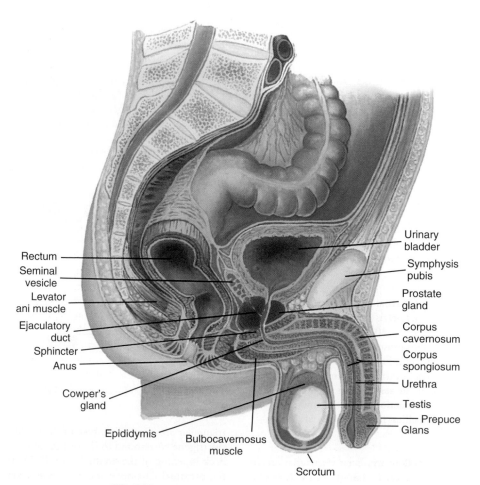

FIG. 15.7 Male genitourinary and reproductive anatomy.

Muscles inside and adjacent to the urethral wall and from the pelvic floor maintain closure of the sphincters of the bladder, thus enabling continence.

Urethra

The male urethra, normally 20 to 25 cm long, extends from the bladder neck to the tip of the penis and varies in diameter from 7 to 10 mm. It is divided into two portions: the proximal (sphincteric) urethra and the distal (conduit or anterior) urethra, both of which undergo further subdivision. The proximal urethra is commonly referred to as the *posterior urethra,* where it is elevated by the verumontanum, extending from the bladder neck through the prostate and the membranous portion. Within the posterior urethra lie the prostatic and membranous portions (see Fig. 15.5). As the urethra exits the prostate and crosses the pelvic (urogenital) diaphragm, it is called the *membranous urethra.* The distal urethra, commonly called the *anterior urethra,* is subdivided into the bulbar, pendulous (penile), and glandular urethras. The bulbar urethra is the area most prone to urethral strictures in the male. The prostatic urethra is approximately 3 cm long and is the widest portion of the urethra. On the floor of the prostatic urethra is the verumontanum, which contains the openings of the ejaculatory ducts. The membranous urethra is the shortest portion, measuring approximately 2.5 cm and extending from the external sphincter to the apex of the prostate. The penile, or pendulous, urethra lies within the corpus spongiosum. The urothelium of the urethra is continuous with that of the bladder.

The female urethra is a narrow membranous tube about 3 to 5 cm long and 6 to 8 mm in diameter. Slightly curved, it lies behind and beneath the symphysis pubis, anterior to the vagina. It passes through the internal and external sphincters and the urogenital diaphragm. The periurethral glands of Skene open on the floor of the urethra just inside the meatus. Because the female urethra is so short and in proximity to the anal and vaginal areas, microorganisms find easy access to the bladder and can cause urinary tract infections (UTIs).

Prostate Gland

The prostate gland is a walnut-shaped organ composed of fibromuscular and glandular components. It is located at the base of the bladder neck and completely surrounds the urethra. The gland is about 4 cm at the base, is about 2 cm in depth, and normally weighs 20 to 30 g (see Figs. 15.5 and 15.7).

The four glandular regions within the prostate have two major zones (the peripheral zone and the central zone) and two minor zones (the transitional zone and the periurethral zone). Many clinicians still refer to prostate lobes as intraurethral lobes (right and left lateral) and extraurethral lobes (posterior and median). The posterior lobe is readily palpable during rectal examination and prone to cancerous degeneration. Benign prostatic hyperplasia (BPH, often referred to as hypertrophy) generally occurs in the transitional zone (intraurethral lobe).

Behind the prostatic capsule is a fibrous sheath known as the *true prostatic capsule,* which separates the prostate gland and the seminal vesicles from the rectum. This fascia is an important landmark during perineal prostatectomy.

The lobes of the prostate gland secrete highly alkaline fluid that dilutes the testicular secretion as it is excreted from the ejaculatory ducts. These secretions are believed to be essential to the passage of spermatozoa and helpful in keeping them alive. The arterial supply to the prostate is derived from the pudendal, inferior vesical, and hemorrhoidal arteries.

Male Reproductive Organs

The male reproductive organs include several paired structures: the testes, epididymides, seminal ducts (vasa deferens), seminal vesicles, ejaculatory ducts, and bulbourethral glands. Other organs of the reproductive tract are the penis, prostate gland, and urethra.

The *scrotum* is located behind and below the base of the penis and in front of the anus. Within the scrotum are two cavities, or sacs, that are lined with smooth, glistening tissue (the tunica vaginalis). Normally a small amount of clear fluid is contained in the tunica vaginalis. Each loose sac contains and supports a testis, an epididymis, and some of the spermatic cord. The two sides of the scrotum are separated from each other by a median raphe (septum).

The *testes* manufacture the spermatozoa and also contain specialized Leydig cells that produce the male hormone *testosterone.* Each testis consists of many tubules in which the sperm are formed, surrounded by dense capsules of connective tissue. The tubules coalesce and continue into the adjacent epididymis, in which the sperm mature and are stored. At the upper pole of the testis is the appendix testis, a small body that may be pedunculated (stalked) or sessile (flat).

The *epididymis* is a long, convoluted duct located along the posterolateral surface of the testis. It is closely attached to the testicle by fibrous tissue and secretes seminal fluid, which gives the sperm a liquid medium in which to migrate. The vas deferens (ductus deferens, seminal duct) is a distal continuation of the epididymis as it enters the prostate gland and conveys the sperm to the seminal vesicle.

The *vas deferens* extends from the epididymis into the abdomen and lies within the spermatic cord in the inguinal region. The spermatic cord also contains veins, arteries, lymphatics, nerves, and surrounding connective tissue (cremaster muscle), which give support to the testes. The terminal portion of each vas deferens is called the *ejaculatory duct;* it passes between the lobes of the prostate gland and opens into the posterior urethra.

The *accessory reproductive glands* include the seminal vesicles, prostate gland, and bulbourethral gland. The seminal vesicles unite with the vas deferens on either side, are situated behind the bladder, and produce protein and fructose for the nutrition of the sperm cell. Sperm and prostatic fluid are discharged at the time of ejaculation.

The *Cowper glands* (bulbourethral glands) are located on each side at the juncture of the membranous and bulbar urethras. Each gland, by way of its duct, empties mucous secretions into the urethra.

The *penis* is suspended from the pubic symphysis by the suspensory ligaments. The penis contains three distinct vascular, spongelike bodies surrounding the urethra: two outer bodies called the *right corpus cavernosum* and *left corpus cavernosum* and an inner body, the *corpus spongiosum urethrae.* These tissues contain a network of vascular channels that fill with blood during erection (see Fig. 15.7). At the distal end of the penis the skin is doubly folded to form the prepuce, or foreskin, which serves as a covering for the glans penis. The glans penis contains the urethral orifice.

Perioperative Nursing Considerations

Assessment

Patients entering a hospital or ambulatory surgery unit for GU surgery may exhibit many emotions and reactions, including fear, embarrassment, helplessness, hostility, anger, and grief. The urology patient population varies from infants with congenital anomalies to elderly people with physiologic impairments. Because many procedures are performed on an ambulatory basis, the nursing staff must prepare to quickly meet patients' specific needs, from preoperative teaching to postoperative home care. The patients' families need to be involved in this preparation process. Patient education begins in the surgeon's office. Communication between the office and perioperative nursing staff allows continuity of care and increases the efficiency and effectiveness of surgical procedures.

In addition to routine admission information, the perioperative nurse will review the patient's urologic and cardiac histories. This information includes but is not limited to vital signs, allergies (including latex), the patient's primary problem, history of the present illness, nature of symptoms, and limitations imposed by the disease condition. In some cases patients may be seen who are not having a primary urologic procedure but instead are scheduled for an ancillary urologic procedure (e.g., insertion of ureteral catheters or stents to facilitate positive identification of the ureters and reduce the potential for severing or ligating them during pelvic or abdominal procedures). The nurse reviews all data pertinent to the proposed operative procedure. Nursing observation should include the patient's general physical appearance as well as nonverbal behaviors, such as restlessness, which may indicate discomfort or anxiety. Any limitations in mobility or sensory deficits should be noted. Urologic procedures frequently require positions that create unusual stress for the patient, both anatomic and physiologic, such as compression of the vena cava and dependent lung during lateral positioning. Also large amounts of irrigating fluids are frequently used intraoperatively in urologic procedures, which may affect the patient's electrolyte status. Assessment provides the perioperative nurse with data adequate to support preoperative planning, intraoperative implementation, and postoperative evaluation (Patient Safety).

The patient may undergo several studies preoperatively, including measurement of levels of serum and urine electrolytes, blood glucose, and blood urea nitrogen (BUN); urinalysis and urine cultures; cardiac enzymes; complete blood count (CBC); prothrombin time (PT) and partial thromboplastin time (PTT); blood chemistry profiles (see the laboratory values in Appendix A); electrocardiogram (ECG); and chest x-ray examination. The nurse reviews the patient's medical history, focusing on medication use (including the use of over-the-counter medications and herbal supplements), any infectious processes, or chronic diseases. Specific GU studies can be found in the patient's medical record. They may encompass all or some of the following: computed tomography (CT) scans, magnetic resonance imaging (MRI), bone and dual energy x-ray absorptiometry (DEXA) scans, positron emission tomography (PET), ProstaScint scans, intravenous (IV) pyelograms or urograms (IVPs or IVUs, respectively), GU flat plate (KUB [kidney, ureter, bladder]), urodynamic studies (UDS), fluoroscopic examinations (angiography, cavernosography), prostate-specific antigen (PSA), and ultrasonography. After the nurse reviews the medical record, assessment information is compiled, perioperative nursing diagnoses are identified, and the perioperative plan of care is formulated.

Nursing Diagnosis

Nursing diagnoses related to the care of patients undergoing GU surgery might include the following:
- Anxiety
- Risk for Perioperative Positioning Injury
- Impaired Urinary Elimination
- Risk for Deficient Fluid Volume

PATIENT SAFETY

Geriatric Syndromes and Urology

A large number of urology patients are in the geriatric population. Geriatric syndromes occur more commonly among older adults, and can have a direct effect on urologic health. Examples of geriatric syndrome include frailty, falls, pressure ulcers, polypharmacy, delirium, and UI. These are described in Chapter 27.

Geriatric syndromes and how they pertain to patient safety in urologic patients are as follows:

- *Frailty* can be predictive of both morbidity and mortality outcomes in urologic patient wound healing. Preoperative assessment is essential in predicting and providing safe measures, including increased nutritional status preoperatively.

- *Falls*, potentially injurious, are an increased risk in the patient with UI and use of indwelling urinary catheters. Catheters have been referred to as a single point restraint making it difficult for the patient to mobilize. Patients often forget they have a catheter. Efforts at reducing the use of indwelling catheters as well as following falls prevention guidelines are essential to reducing falls.

- *Pressure ulcer* formation is increased in UI patients from chronic moisture leading to tissue loss. Positioning and transfers during surgery, padding pressure points, and proper positioning during dorsal lithotomy position are especially important in the prevention of ulcer formation. Positioning patients while awake can provide a comfortable position and prevent injury.

- *Polypharmacy* in adult patients can cause potential risk postoperatively. Demerol is a common pain medication given postoperatively, causing potential risk for delirium and adverse events, and should be avoided in the elderly patient. When Demerol is used, lower doses should be prescribed and closely monitored to determine patient response.

- *Delirium* can increase the risk of readmission rates, reoperation, caregiver requirements, and mortality within the first year after surgery. Prevention of delirium is key, and PCA is used to avoid overdosage. Maintaining proper sleep cycle and making sure patient's hearing aids and glasses and mobility devices are at the bedside support delirium prevention as well.

- *UI* is inclusive in the falls and pressure ulcer categories.

PCA, Patient-controlled analgesia; *UI,* urinary incontinence.
Modified from Griebling TL: Aging and geriatric urology. In Wein AJ et al, editors: *Campbell-Walsh urology,* ed 11, Philadelphia, 2015, Elsevier.

- Impaired Gas Exchange
- Sexual Dysfunction

Outcome Identification

Outcomes identified for the selected nursing diagnoses could be stated as follows:
- The patient will verbalize an acceptable anxiety level to the perioperative nurse.
- The patient will be free from injury related to the surgical position.
- The patient will demonstrate or regain a normal pattern of urinary elimination.
- The patient will maintain adequate fluid volume and electrolyte balance.

- The patient will maintain adequate oxygen supply and alveolar ventilation.
- The patient will discuss fears and concerns regarding sexual function.

Planning

Plans of care are the organizing framework for perioperative nursing activities, in which nursing interventions are clinical processes in a quality health outcome model. Frequently the urology patient presents a complex medical picture. Any alterations in the patient's physical, mental, or emotional status may greatly influence both the surgical and the postoperative course. A review of the patient's record; communication with the patient or family; recognition of specific psychosocial, cultural, ethnic, and spiritual needs of the patient and family; and knowledge gained from other members of the patient care team are all used to formulate the nursing database (Sample Plan of Care).

Implementation

The perioperative nurse begins implementation of the patient care plan during the patient interview. Information that is concise and simply presented enhances the final surgical outcome. Meeting the patient's emotional needs is a nursing priority. A calm patient retains more information and is cognitively and emotionally more receptive to perioperative teaching. The nurse provides explanations of what to expect throughout the operative period to allay the patient's fears and nurture confidence in the nursing care provided. Establishment of this relationship is key to assisting patients to minimize the effect of the surgical experience on their coping ability and to be emotionally comfortable. Perioperative nursing care requires not only the collection of pertinent patient data but also the coordination of numerous supplies and equipment to support the smooth implementation of the plan of care.

Patient Safety

The perioperative nurse considers several factors in advocating for the patient during the intraoperative period. Institutions have various protocols and processes in place to support patient safety. A critical safety protocol that the nurse is responsible to follow is to ensure the correct patient, correct procedure, and correct site surgery. Such a protocol includes proper patient identification, proper operative site identification, proper procedure identification, and proper medication identification. All wrong-site, wrong-procedure, and wrong-patient surgery occurrences are considered sentinel events by The Joint Commission (TJC). In addition, the Association of periOperative Registered Nurses (AORN) has established guidelines for patient safety (AORN, 2016).

To fulfill these requirements, preoperative verification, surgical site marking, and time-out processes must occur for every surgical procedure. What the patient expresses as the intended surgical procedure is compared with what is documented on the operative permit and other items, such as the (OR) schedule. Patient identification is achieved by also asking the patient to state his or her full name and birth date. This information is compared with the patient identification bracelet. Documentation of the processes implemented is completed on the designated institutional form or forms.

The surgeon marks the surgical site with a permanent nontoxic marking pen. The patient should be involved in this process. A standard policy needs to be developed within the particular facility as to how marking will be accomplished for urologic, endoscopic, and abdominal procedures, particularly when they involve laterality. This mark should be clearly visible after prepping and draping.

Time-out is a pause in the activity that occurs before the start or incision on all procedures. The entire team stops to verbally confirm the patient's identity, verify the patient's position, state and agree on the procedure and surgical site, and review that all implants and necessary equipment are available and ready. The nurse documents this process according to hospital policy.

When medications are used intraoperatively, the containers should always be marked with the medication and dose (refer to Chapter 2 for a full discussion of medication safety). The scrub person, who may be a registered nurse or surgical technologist, verifies the medication and dosage verbally when passing the drug in its administration device to the surgeon. Local anesthetics that contain epinephrine should be used with caution in urology. Many urologic interventions involve "end-organs," for example, the scrotum, testicles, and penis. The use of epinephrine in these areas can result in an ischemic situation and should be avoided.

Positioning

Thorough understanding of the urologic OR bed and its functions is essential for optimum patient positioning. The position in which the patient is placed for surgery is determined by the particular operation to be performed. For urologic operative procedures the patient may be placed in the lateral, supine, prone, or lithotomy position. Any of these positions may be exaggerated to give optimum access to the organ involved, particularly in radical surgery of the prostate and bladder. When the patient is supine, his or her arms are placed on padded armboards with the palms up and fingers extended. Armboards are maintained at less than a 90-degree angle to prevent brachial plexus stretch. If there are surgical reasons to tuck the arms at the side or rest on a specially designed sled, all bony prominences in contact with the OR bed must be padded to protect the ulnar nerve, the palms face inward, and the wrist is maintained in a neutral position. A drape secures the arms. It should be tucked snugly under the patient, not under the mattress. This prevents the arm from shifting downward intraoperatively and resting against the OR bed rail. Acting as the patient's advocate, the nurse takes considerable care to ensure that the surgical position does not interfere with respiration or circulation. It is essential to avoid displacement of the joints and undue tension on neurovascular bundles or ligaments. A patient positioned laterally (flank position) for renal surgery has the spine extended for greater access to the retroperitoneal space. Padding and stabilized support with gel pads, pillows, sandbags, and straps should be available for precise anatomic positioning and safety (see Chapter 6). When an electrosurgical unit (ESU) is to be used, care must be taken that the patient does not contact metal parts of the OR bed. In some procedures involving stones of the kidneys or ureters, intraoperative fluoroscopy may be required. When fluoroscopy (C-arm) is to be used, the patient must be placed on an OR bed compatible with its use. Whenever possible, the perioperative nurse takes measures to protect the patient from undue radiation exposure to the thyroid and chest areas by using small leaded shields. In urologic procedures it generally is not feasible to shield the reproductive organs during fluoroscopy.

Aseptic Techniques and Safety Measures

Prevention of infection is an important nursing goal in the care of the GU patient. It is, however, seldom possible to confirm freedom from infection intraoperatively or immediately postoperatively. Aseptic techniques must be carefully maintained and monitored. Skin

SAMPLE PLAN OF CARE

Nursing Diagnosis
Anxiety

Outcome
The patient will verbalize an acceptable anxiety level to the perioperative nurse.

Interventions
- Provide an accepting and supportive environment.
- Use touch (as appropriate) to convey caring and support.
- Encourage expression of feelings.
- Promote feelings of self-worth.
- Provide comfort measures (e.g., warm blankets, pillow).
- Facilitate or assist patient in using personally effective coping strategies (e.g., relaxation, deep breathing, music, imagery).
- Maintain patient privacy.
- Encourage participation of patient, family, and caregiver in plan of care.

Nursing Diagnosis
Risk for Perioperative Positioning Injury

Outcome
The patient will be free from injury related to the surgical position.

Interventions
- Maintain proper body alignment.
- Assess range of motion and musculoskeletal, peripheral vascular, and cardiovascular status preoperatively.
- Pad all bony prominences.
- Avoid compression of vulnerable nerves and neurovascular bundles.
- Secure patient to operating room (OR) bed without friction or pressure.
- Provide support stockings or intermittent pneumatic compression sleeves as indicated.
- Initiate measures to warm patient and maintain normothermia.

Nursing Diagnosis
Impaired Urinary Elimination

Outcome
The patient will demonstrate or regain a normal pattern of urinary elimination.

Interventions
- Assess bladder for distention.
- Instruct patient in importance of any postoperative antibiotic or anticholinergic therapy.
- Follow aseptic technique during catheter insertion and connection to drainage device.
- Maintain closed urinary drainage system.
- Note amount, color, and character of urine; report abnormalities.
- Keep drainage tubing and collection device below the level of the patient's bladder.
- Keep urine draining freely; avoid kinks in tubing.
- Check patency of catheter after all position changes.
- Secure drainage tubing to patient to prevent pulling or retraction during transfer.

- Include catheter care and measures to facilitate voiding after catheter removal as part of preoperative patient, family, and caregiver education and discharge planning.
- Provide patient with information/referral on preventing recurrent UTI.

Nursing Diagnosis
Risk for Deficient Fluid Volume

Outcome
The patient will maintain adequate fluid volume and electrolyte balance.

Interventions
- Provide appropriate IV solutions, volumetric pumps, and fluid warmers.
- Monitor patency of all IV lines.
- Record volume of IV and irrigating fluids instilled.
- Monitor ECG, vital signs, and cardiopulmonary status as appropriate.
- Monitor blood loss and volume replacement.
- Monitor urinary output, and note color; report output less than 30 mL/hr and changes in color or clarity.
- Collaborate with anesthesia provider in monitoring serum electrolyte status.
- Monitor pH and specific gravity of urine as appropriate.

Nursing Diagnosis
Impaired Gas Exchange

Outcome
The patient will maintain adequate oxygen supply and alveolar ventilation.

Interventions
- Review breathing exercises and use of incentive spirometer with patient preoperatively.
- Position patient to provide maximum lung perfusion; have positioning devices available; check that these are clean and functioning properly.
- Assist anesthesia provider in applying cardiac monitor leads, blood pressure cuff, and pulse oximeter.
- Collaborate with anesthesia provider in monitoring ventilation or perfusion.
- Administer oxygen as required; assist with intubation and maintenance of airway during positioning.

Nursing Diagnosis
Sexual Dysfunction

Outcome
The patient will discuss fears and concerns regarding sexual function.

Interventions
- Clarify patient's understanding of risks and benefits of surgical procedure.
- Provide an open, accepting environment for the patient to discuss potentially embarrassing issues.
- Maintain patient privacy and dignity.
- Consider making a referral for patient to discuss options available to achieve sexual function postoperatively.

preparation and draping procedures (see Chapter 4) vary, depending on the surgery to be performed and institutional protocols. Special care must be taken when cleansing the female perineal area to avoid contamination from the rectum to the urethra. Prepping solutions should be applied with downward strokes and the sponge discarded once it has contacted the inner vaginal or anal areas (Spruce, 2016). Transurethral passage of instruments and catheters requires meticulous technique to prevent retrograde infections of the urinary tract, and single doses of antimicrobial agents reduced infections to between 1% and 5% (Schaeffer et al., 2015).

Visualization of the bladder during transurethral procedures is often enhanced by darkening the room. Provision should be made for proper adjustments to lighting. ESUs and fiberoptic light systems are common adjuncts in urologic surgery. The nurse and scrub person must be familiar with the manufacturer's safety precautions and recommendations during their use.

Use of Irrigating Fluids

When the bladder is entered, sterile distilled irrigating fluid is administered to distend it for effective visualization. Commercially prepared sterile irrigation solutions with appropriate closed administration sets are highly recommended. Such closed systems prevent the inherent risks of cross-contamination. Large volumes of irrigating solutions are frequently used, particularly during more extensive endoscopic procedures. When these solutions are at the room temperature of the OR, they are cold compared with the patient's internal body temperature and can cause hypothermia. Solution-warming units are available commercially and are a useful tool to help decrease this risk. The drawback to these units may be that the warmth delays clotting, increasing the risk of blood loss.

Commercially prepared sterile irrigation solutions are available in collapsible bags and rigid plastic containers, both of which have the same advantages: neither depends on air, and each may be hung in series, providing continuous irrigation without interruption. Air bubbles, a problem that distorts visibility during the procedure, are eliminated with these systems.

For simple observation cystoscopy, retrograde pyelography, and simple bladder tumor fulgurations, sterile distilled water may be used without complication. However, during transurethral resection of the prostate (TURP), venous sinuses may be opened and varying amounts of irrigant are invariably absorbed into the bloodstream. Studies indicate that the use of distilled water during TURP may result in hemolysis of erythrocytes and possible renal failure. Other important complications include dilutional hyponatremia and cardiac decompensation.

Therefore a clear, nonelectrolytic, and iso-osmotic solution should be used. The most widely used urologic irrigating fluids are 3% sorbitol, an isomer of mannitol, and 1.5% glycine, an aminoacetic acid solution. In dilute solutions, sorbitol and glycine have many properties that make them particularly useful for irrigation during transurethral prostatectomy. At slightly hypotonic concentrations they do not produce hemolysis. However, if too much intravasation occurs with glycine, an encephalitic state can result from the ammonia produced (Surgical Pharmacology). Because the solutions are non-electrolytic, they do not cause dispersion of high-frequency current with consequent loss of electrosurgical cutting capacity, as occurs with normal saline.

During ureteropyeloscopy, sterile normal saline is the irrigant of choice unless electrosurgery is to be used. This solution most closely approximates a physiologic solution, which is an important factor if perforation and extravasation of fluid into the retroperitoneum occur. If electrosurgery is required, as with a TURP, 3% sorbitol or 1.5% glycine should be used.

Thorough knowledge of the potential hazards encountered intraoperatively during transurethral surgery is extremely important. Although complications are more prevalent in the postoperative stage, close observation during the intraoperative period is essential. Signs and symptoms such as sudden restlessness, apprehension, irritability, confusion, nausea, slow pulse rate, seizures, dysrhythmias, and rising blood pressure may be suggestive of TURP syndrome, which is a severe hyponatremia caused by systemic absorption of irrigating fluid used during surgery (Collins and Terris, 2014). Minimal amounts of fluids should be given and urine output carefully monitored. Irrigation fluid should be under as little pressure as possible and the bladder emptied before it reaches full capacity to prevent intravesical pressure. During ureteropyeloscopy it is frequently necessary to use a pressure bag to ensure adequate visualization of the upper urinary tract. Serum electrolyte values should be obtained, and if a low serum sodium value is reported, hypertonic sodium chloride is administered by means of a slow IV drip, often on a volumetric pump. IV diuretics such as furosemide (Lasix) may be required to prevent possible pulmonary edema associated with the administration of hypertonic saline. If the patient's reaction is severe, surgery may have to be terminated.

Endoscopic and Ancillary Equipment

Cystoscopic and ancillary equipment often varies from one institution to another. Therefore it is valuable to have a reference manual or standard setup cards that illustrate and describe in detail the required instrumentation for each specific procedure.

The basic cystoscopy tray should include instruments and accessory items that are routinely used for all cystoscopy procedures. If ureteral catheterization is planned, catheterizing telescopes or an Albarrán bridge, which can be packaged and sterilized separately, may be easily added to the basic cystoscopy setup. Instruments for transurethral surgery and other special procedures may be wrapped, sterilized, and placed on separate trays so that they are available on request. This concept minimizes handling of the delicate lensed instruments and ultimately reduces costly repairs.

Cystoscopic procedures frequently require additional instrumentation. Instruments of various types and sizes, such as a visual obturator, biopsy forceps, urethral sounds, Phillips filiforms and followers, and Ellik evacuators are available as prepackaged, sterile, disposable items. The reusable products may also be packaged separately and sterilized.

Ureteral and Urethral Catheters

A variety of ureteral and urethral catheters are designed for specific procedures. Ureteral catheters are manufactured of polyurethane material and are graduated so that the surgeon may determine the exact distance the catheter has been inserted into the ureter (Fig. 15.8). Most manufacturers provide sterile disposable catheters wrapped in peel-open packages to allow aseptic handling during ureteral insertion. Some indications for the use of ureteral catheters are to (1) perform retrograde pyelography, (2) identify the ureters during pelvic or intestinal surgery, and (3) bypass partial or complete obstruction that may be present as a result of ureteral tumors, calculi, or strictures. Not uncommonly, it is necessary to insert a ureteral stent in a pregnant female because of hydronephrosis or obstructing calculi.

The most commonly used catheters include the open-ended, whistle tip, cone tip, and olive tip. When a retrograde ureterogram

SURGICAL PHARMACOLOGY

Agents Used in Urologic Surgery

Category	Dose/Route	Purpose/Action	Adverse Reactions	Nursing Implications
Bulking Agents				
Coaptite Macroplastique	Transurethral, periurethral One or more 1-mL syringes	Correct UH, ISD, SUI	Swelling, urinary retention Local tissue infarction/ necrosis, vascular occlusion, embolus	Avoid injection into blood vessels. Do not use bulking agents in presence of acute cystitis, urethritis, or other genitourinary infection.
Neurotransmitter Inhibitors				
Botulinum toxin	100–300 units intravesically	Correct overactive bladder, SUI	Bladder pain, UI, urinary retention	Patient education in CIC
Irrigants				
Glycine (monocarboxylic amino acid)	1.5%, 3–5 L, intravesically	No hemolysis or dispersion of electrocurrent Used for all monopolar ESU cases: TURP, bladder tumor resection	Increased ammonia production Encephalitic reaction Biosynthesis of heme Blurred vision CNS disturbances TURP syndrome if absorbed	Contraindicated with clozapine usage Use with caution in diabetic patients, patients with liver disease; inhibitory neurotransmitter
Sorbitol (nonelectrolytic, iso-osmotic, hypotonic aminoacetic acid)	3%, 3–5 L, intravesically	Isomer of mannitol, no hemolysis or dispersion of electrocurrent	TURP syndrome if absorbed	Hyperglycemia may occur in patients with diabetes mellitus Use with caution in patients with renal or cardiac compromise
Water	Distilled, 3–5 L, intravesically	Irrigant, lyse cancer cells	Hyponatremia, hemolysis of erythrocytes	Avoid with TURP Intravasation can lead to dilutional hyponatremia, cardiac decompensation, and renal failure
Normal saline	0.9%, 3–5 L, intravesically	Physiologic irrigant used with all laser procedures	Hypernatremia	Not for use with electrosurgery Disperses electrocurrent
Injectables				
Indigo carmine	40 mg, IV or local	Colorize urine, vessels	Hypertension	Moderately reduces oxygen saturation
Phenylephrine (Neo-Synephrine)	0.05% (5 mg), SubQ	Vasoconstriction for priapism	Hypertension, reflex bradycardia	May decrease renal blood flow Contraindicated in patients with hypertension
Papaverine	30 mg/mL, 2 mL in solution, intercavernosally	Vasodilation, antispasmodic Artificial erection	Dizziness, dysrhythmia, hypotension, flushing, hypothermia	Contraindicated in AV block, pregnancy Depressed AV or intraventricular conduction, physiologic antagonist
Vasopressin (Pitressin)	20 units/mL: 2 mL (40 units) in solution, local	Vasoconstriction	Water intoxication, dizziness, headache, pallor	May cause tenesmus, tremors, cramps, abdominal pain, hyponatremia; retards absorption of local anesthetics Contraindicated in patients with uremia, coronary artery disease, hypertension
Topical				
Methylene blue	1 mL/100 mL NS, topical	Colorize tissues, vessels	Hypertension, dizziness, headache, anemia, diaphoresis	Do not use in patients with severe renal disease, hemolytic anemia Destroys erythrocytes; may cause methemoglobinuria
Other				
B&O suppository (belladonna/ opium)	16.2 mg/30 mg, rectal	Prevent/decrease bladder/ureteral spasm/pain relief	Constipation, decreased sweating	Use with precaution in patients who take MAOIs, agents that affect GI motility, select narcotics May cause cardiovascular instability, paralytic ileus, respiratory depression, toxin-mediated diarrhea, pseudomembranous enterocolitis

AV, Atrioventricular; *CIC,* clean intermittent catheterization; *CNS,* central nervous system; *ESU,* electrosurgical unit; *GI,* gastrointestinal; *ISD,* intrinsic sphincter dysfunction; *IV,* intravenous; *MAOIs,* monoamine oxidase inhibitors; *NS,* normal saline; *SubQ,* subcutaneous; *SUI,* stress urinary incontinence; *TURP,* transurethral resection of the prostate; *UH,* urethral hypermobility; *UI,* urinary incontinence.

Modified from DailyMed: *Current Medication Information* (website) http://dailymed.nlm.nih.gov/dailymed/about.cfm. (Accessed 6 September 2016); Hodgson BB, Kizior RJ: *Saunders nursing drug handbook 2016,* St Louis, 2016, Elsevier; NCBI PubChem Project: http://pubchem.ncbi.nlm.nih.gov. (Accessed 6 September 2016).

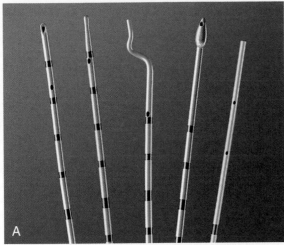

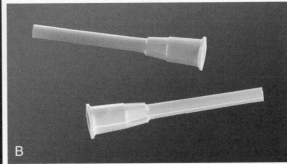

FIG. 15.8 (A) Ureteral catheters. (B) Adapters.

is indicated, a cone-tipped ureteral catheter may be helpful in occluding the ureteral orifice to accomplish the x-ray study effectively. When a ureteral catheter is left indwelling, a special adapter (see Fig. 15.8B) may be connected to the end of the ureteral catheter to facilitate connection to a closed urinary drainage system. A small slit may also be created in the Foley catheter, and the distal end of the ureteral catheter can be slipped into it and taped in place.

Indwelling double-pigtail or double-J stents are available and are passed cystoscopically to reside within the ureter. When the guidewire is removed from the core of the stent, a proximal and distal J or "pigtail" forms in the tubing to retain the stents. Many of these stents have a nonabsorbable suture attached to the distal end, which extends through the urethral meatus. A suture may be easily tied to the distal end of those that do not. The surgeon can then remove the stent in the office setting postoperatively without needing to perform a cystoscopy.

Urethral catheters have a multitude of functions as stents, as drainage tubes, and in diagnostic studies in the OR. They are generally divided into two categories—plain and indwelling (retention)—and range in different French (F) sizes, most commonly 10F through 30F. The Foley catheter is the most frequently used retention catheter and is manufactured with a variety of balloon sizes, tip styles, lengths, and eye arrangements.

After transurethral prostatic surgery a three-way Foley catheter with a 30-mL balloon capacity may be left indwelling. This type of catheter is preferred because it facilitates continuous bladder irrigation (CBI), and the large balloon aids in achieving hemostasis in the prostatic bed. The surgeon may apply light traction on the Foley catheter with a leg strap, adhesive catheter anchor, or tape. This traction causes pressure against the bladder neck and aids in hemostasis. The goal is to prevent traumatic catheter removal in men.

A hematuria catheter, a three-way Foley specifically for patients with excessive clot formation, is also available. This catheter is reinforced with a stretch spiral wire within the catheter lining that permits vigorous aspiration without fear of lumen collapse.

Diagnostic studies performed in the cystoscopy suite may require special catheters for specific studies. A Davis or Trattner triple-lumen double-balloon urethrographic catheter or any of a variety of urodynamic catheters may be used to diagnose lesions of the female urethra, such as urethral strictures, diverticula, and fistulas. To accomplish female urethrography, the catheter is inserted through

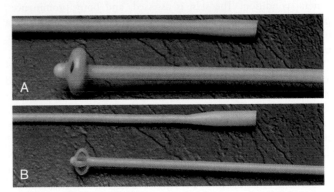

FIG. 15.9 (A) Pezzer (mushroom) catheter. (B) Malecot (bat-winged) four-winged catheter.

the urethra into the bladder; the two balloons on the catheter are inflated, one in the bladder and one at the external urethral orifice, effectively isolating the urethra. Contrast medium is injected to visualize the entire urethra.

Another type of self-retaining catheter frequently used in the OR is the Pezzer catheter, which is also known as a *mushroom* catheter (Fig. 15.9A). It may be straight or angulated with a large single channel and a preformed tip in the shape of a mushroom. The flexible mushroom tip helps keep the catheter in place. This catheter is used primarily for suprapubic bladder drainage, often for poor-risk patients who have uremia, neurogenic bladder syndrome, or possibly long-standing urinary retention. The catheter is inserted into the bladder through a midline or small transverse abdominal wall incision and secured to the abdomen with suture or tape. The Malecot four-winged catheter, often used as a nephrostomy tube to provide temporary or permanent diversion of urine after kidney surgery and when renal tissue needs to be restored, may also be used for suprapubic drainage (see Fig. 15.9B). A Foley catheter of preferred size is frequently chosen for either purpose. Nephrostomy tube replacement is accomplished by introducing the catheter into the surgical tract with a straight catheter guide and securing it in place with a suture or a nephrostomy retention disk that is one size smaller than the nephrostomy tube being used. The flanges of the disk are taped or sutured to the skin. The use of other variations of urethral catheters is described throughout the chapter.

Photography in Urology

The use of photographic and video imaging equipment in urologic surgery serves to document the patient's disease, the progress of a disease process, and long-term follow-up study. It is also an important teaching resource. Video equipment adapts to endoscopic instrumentation and has the capability of projecting an enhanced image on a television monitor, permitting members of the surgical team to observe and learn during the actual surgical procedure. Other visual aids, such as slides and photographs, are used in teaching, as visual references in publication, and as documentation in patient records.

When any form of photography or video imaging is used, the patient's privacy must be ensured, and an informed consent should be obtained. Special release forms should also be signed preoperatively by the patient for any videotapes or photographs to be used in teaching or publications.

Evaluation

Before the patient is taken to the postanesthesia care unit (PACU) or observation unit, the perioperative nurse evaluates the patient's general condition. The skin is assessed, and bony prominences, prepped and draped areas, and areas contacted by the attachment of ancillary equipment are observed for signs of pressure, irritation, or other changes from the preoperative status.

Many urology patients are discharged to the PACU with catheters and drains inserted, including urethral, ureteral, suprapubic, and wound drains. A local anesthetic may have been used for either primary analgesia or postoperative pain management (preemptive analgesia); preoperative or intraoperative infiltration of the surgical site blocks sensory input, resulting in postoperative analgesia. A hand-off report to the PACU nurse should include intraoperative position, problems encountered specific to the patient, and the patient's preoperative physical status as well as comprehension and anxiety levels. Documentation of medications administered from the sterile field or by the perioperative nurse intraoperatively should include time of administration, name of medication, dosage, site and route of administration, and the name of the person who performed the application or injection. Drains should be documented as to size and type, insertion site, time and date of insertion, type of collection device, name of the person who performed the insertion, and character of drainage. When several drains are in place, additional labeling on the collection devices is beneficial. Any postoperative observations before or during transport should be recorded. Evaluation should also address whether the patient met the identified outcomes related to specific nursing diagnoses in the perioperative nursing plan of care. Attainment of identified desired outcomes, included in the documentation and report to the PACU, may be phrased as follows:

- The patient verbalized an acceptable anxiety level to the perioperative nurse.
- The patient had no evidence of positional injury; neurovascular status was consistent with preoperative level, and skin integrity was intact.
- The patient maintained patency of the urinary catheter with no signs of blockage or urinary retention. Urinary output remained within normal limits. The patient will void without difficulty after catheter removal.
- The patient had no evidence or signs of fluid volume or electrolyte imbalance; vital signs were stable, arterial blood gases were within normal limits, and urinary output was maintained at acceptable levels.
- The patient maintained adequate gas exchange; lung expansion and O_2 saturation were satisfactory.
- The patient discussed fears and concerns regarding sexual function.

Patient, Family, and Caregiver Education and Discharge Planning

Patient, family, and caregiver education and preparation for discharge allow perioperative nurses to plan for the urologic surgery patient's care across a continuum. Information is tailored according to the procedure and the patient's status (Ambulatory Surgery Considerations). Information provided should be presented in language the patient can understand (lay terms) and clarified with the patient by having the patient repeat back in his or her own words the information provided. When possible and with the patient's approval, family members or others who will serve as caregivers should be included in the educational process at the outset. Institutions may find it helpful to inventory the patient education materials available for select surgical procedures. An example of patient education for home care after nephrectomy is presented in the Patient, Family, and Caregiver Education box.

AMBULATORY SURGERY CONSIDERATIONS

Cystoscopy, Transrectal-Guided Ultrasound Biopsy of the Prostate

A commonly performed ambulatory urologic procedure is a cystoscopy, transrectal ultrasound guided biopsy of the prostate (cysto/TRUS). To minimize complications, patient selection is determined by the healthcare team. Patients classified as physical status 1 or 2, as per the American Society of Anesthesiologists, generally pose no great risk for procedures performed with general, IV moderate sedation and local anesthetics. The majority of cysto/TRUS patients have this procedure performed with IV sedation/local. To decrease pain during and immediately after the procedure, a viscous local anesthetic is injected into the rectum and the urethra after IV sedation is initiated.

Preoperative and postoperative teaching of the patient and his family is essential because the family will be the primary caregiver on discharge. Teaching begins in the surgeon's office. The office staff provides patients with a prescription for antibiotics with instructions to begin the medication 24 hours before the procedure and to continue oral antibiotics postoperatively until the prescription is completed. The office staff also advises the patient to take a cleansing enema 2 to 3 hours before the procedure. Both the antibiotics and the enema decrease the chances of postoperative infection.

Patient and family anxiety levels will be high pending the postoperative diagnosis. The patient may also be anxious because of the nature of the procedure and anesthetic used. The perioperative nurse plays a key role in supporting the patient and his family throughout the ambulatory surgical experience.

Discharge assessment after anesthesia includes the following:
- Airway patency, respiratory function, and oxygen saturation
- Stable vital signs
- Hypothermia resolved
- Level of consciousness and muscular strength
- Adequate pain control

AMBULATORY SURGERY CONSIDERATIONS

Cystoscopy, Transrectal-Guided Ultrasound Biopsy of the Prostate—cont'd

- Mobility
- Skin color and condition
- Condition of the surgical site
- Intake and output
- Comfort
- Anxiety
- Significant other interaction
- Numeric score if used

Before discharge the nurse instructs the patient to increase his clear liquid intake and monitor urine output. Postoperative burning on urination and blood in the urine as well as blood draining from the rectum are common. Patients are instructed to keep the perineum clean. The nurse ensures that the patient has a prescription for pain medication, clarifies the instructions for dosage and frequency, and instructs the patient to call the surgeon for any temperature higher than 101°F (38°C). The nurse provides all instructions verbally and gives the patient and his family a written copy of the instructions. The patient calls the physician as directed for results of the biopsy.

A postdischarge phone call to the patient is recommended. This allows the nurse to review the patient's postoperative status, provide reassurance if necessary, and reinforce any teaching. The call also provides the patient and his family with an opportunity to ask additional questions.

IV, Intravenous.

PATIENT, FAMILY, AND CAREGIVER EDUCATION

Home Care Education for the Nephrectomy Patient

Give the patient and the caregiver both verbal and written instructions. Provide them with the name and telephone number of a physician or nurse to call if questions arise. At the end of reviewing home care instructions, have the patient or family member repeat back, in his or her own words, information provided.

General Instructions After Discharge

- Continue walking when you return home. The walking will help you build strength. Gradually increase the amount of walking you do each day. It is very important that you continue walking when you are discharged from the hospital. Not only will this build strength but will also aid in preventing blood clots from the legs.
- Take planned rest periods during the day. The best gauge is your own body and how you feel.
- Avoid bending. If you must pick something up, bend with your knees, not your waist; stoop to pick up the item.
- Avoid heavy lifting (greater than 5 pounds). Anything you need to brace yourself to pick up is too heavy. Also avoid strenuous activity.
- Climb stairs as necessary, taking them slowly at first. You may wish to group your activities, so that you do not have to make many trips up and down stairs during the first week you are home.
- Shower as directed by your surgeon. Gently wash the incision with soap and water, rinse well, and pat dry. Avoid tub baths until the incision is completely healed. If you had an open nephrectomy you will have tape strips on the incision. They will fall off in about a week.
- Do not drive any motorized vehicle, or sign any legal documents while you are taking pain medications. The medications may alter visual perception and impair judgment.
- Avoid driving for at least 4 weeks after surgery or until you are not taking pain medications or are pain free. Take breaks every couple of hours if you are on extended trips. Get out of your car and walk around a bit.

Diet

- Eat a well-balanced diet to promote healing and good bowel function. Return to your normal fluid intake unless otherwise directed by the surgeon.
- Avoid constipation. If you become constipated, there are alternatives to consider. Increase the roughage in your diet. Drink prune juice or orange juice. You can take an over-the-counter laxative of your choice. Drink 6 to 8 glasses of water per day.

Reasons to Call the Physician

- Your incision becomes red or swollen
- The skin around your incision is warmer than elsewhere and is slightly red
- There is drainage from your incision
- There is an opening in your incision
- You are having difficulty passing urine or your urine output becomes less than it normally has been
- You have chills or fever of 101°F or more
- Your pain is severe and is not relieved by pain medication

Follow-Up Care

When providing patient education, stress the importance of regular follow-up visits. Make sure the patient has the necessary names and telephone numbers to reach his or her surgeon as needed.

Modified from Tower Urology at Cedars-Sinai Office Tower: *Robotic laparoscopic partial or radical nephrectomy* (website). https://www.towerurology.com/services/nephrectomy/2016. (Accessed 9 August 2017).

Discharge instructions should be printed and include community resources and support groups as appropriate for the surgical intervention and the patient's diagnosis. These too should be presented in easily understood terms, reviewed, and confirmed by having the patient repeat back in his or her own words the information provided.

Any requisite skills that the patient or family will require should be demonstrated, with return demonstrations as time permits. Perioperative nurses may find it helpful to involve institutional resource persons or departments such as the social services department in developing information related to home care services, durable medical equipment, and transfers to aftercare facilities other than home (skilled nursing center, rehabilitation facility, other long-term care facility). Patients and their families need preparation for mastering information and tasks that need to be performed. The goal of such interdisciplinary discharge planning is to provide information for the patient that is comprehensive and easy to use. This is part of perioperative nursing's ethical and professional responsibility to patients; it also meets TJC's requirements of providing consistent patient, family, and caregiver education.

Surgical Interventions

Diagnostic and Endoscopic Procedures

Cystoscopy

Cystoscopy is an endoscopic examination of the lower urinary tract, including visual inspection of the interior of the urethra, the bladder, and the ureteral orifices. In a male patient special attention is given to the examination of the verumontanum (which contains the ejaculatory duct), the bladder neck, and the median and lateral lobes of the prostate. In a female patient the urethra, bladder neck, and bladder are examined.

Cystoscopy is an important diagnostic tool that provides the surgeon with valuable information concerning the patient's urologic condition. Traditional white light cystoscopy is the standard. A new blue light cystoscopy was recently introduced for diagnosing non–muscle-invaded bladder tumors that are otherwise undetected with the standard cystoscopy. An imaging agent, hexaminolevulinate HCl, and a photodynamic light source are required. At this time, there are a limited number of facilities using this system (Calvaresi et al., 2014). More indications for cystoscopy include hematuria, urinary retention, UTI, cystitis, tumors, fistulas, vesical calculus disease, and urinary incontinence. Urinary incontinence in postmenopausal women may be related to estrogen deprivation.

Procedural Considerations

On arrival to the preoperative area all patients should be greeted by name and identified by their identification bracelet and number. The perioperative nurse should review the chart for operative consent and pertinent laboratory reports; IVPs and any other diagnostic x-ray studies ordered preoperatively should also be available for review. Customarily the patient voids immediately before transport to the OR. The time of urination and the output volume should be documented for ruling out residual urine in the bladder.

After the patient is placed on the cystoscopy bed, correct positioning requires optimum relaxation of muscles of the legs and perineum. Proper positioning is a vital consideration for patient safety and comfort. Lithotomy is the position most often used. Allen and Yellofin stirrups are boot-style stirrups that support the foot and calf. These have thick gel padding within the stirrup and provide optimum patient comfort and protection, relieving pressure on the popliteal space. They are especially beneficial for the patient who has limited hip mobility and altered peripheral circulatory status. The nurse should assess the patient's bilateral pedal pulses preoperatively and postoperatively when using any stirrups. Stirrups should be adjusted carefully to avoid undue pressure on the calf. If knee crutches are used, the curve of the yoke suspension should flow outward from the perineum, in the same manner as the patient's legs. Padding the knee crutches reduces pressure on the popliteal areas. If sling stirrups that support only the feet are used, the post should be padded and

positioned to prevent pressure on the peroneal nerve. Special pads are designed for use with both of these stirrups.

After the patient is properly positioned, the anesthesia provider may tilt the OR bed so that the patient's head is slightly higher than the buttocks to allow the prep solution to drain into the collecting pan. Pooling of solutions beneath the patient may cause skin reaction and chemical irritation, as well as the potential for burns if an ESU is used. If the cystoscopic procedure requires the use of an ESU, the nurse ensures that the dispersive pad is placed on the patient in direct contact with the skin as close to the operative site as is practical. When placing the ESU pad, the nurse avoids hairy areas, bony prominences, scar tissue, and proximity to prosthetic metal implants or pacemakers.

Next, the nurse or surgeon dons gloves and preps the entire pubic area, including the perineum, with an antimicrobial solution. A disposable drape sheet with a sterile screen material incorporated into it is a standard part of the cystoscopy drape pack. The surgeon and scrub person drape the patient in a manner that ensures aseptic technique is maintained during the urologic procedure. If a general or spinal anesthetic is required, the anesthesia provider administers it before prepping and draping. If a local anesthetic is preferred, the surgeon instills it into the urethra of the male patient after prepping and draping but before instrumentation. For a female patient, the surgeon places a cotton applicator that has been dipped into the anesthetic solution in the urethral meatus. Usually, viscous lidocaine (Xylocaine), 1% or 2%, is used. If the patient is allergic to lidocaine, instillation of 50 to 60 mL of lubricant accompanied by anesthesia-monitored sedation is often adequate to afford the surgeon painless access to the urethra and bladder. The patient should be informed that a sensation of pressure is to be expected.

The basic cystoscopy setup requires a cystoscopy pack, a sterile gown or apron, sterile gloves, a fiberoptic light source, a prep cup and solution, gauze sponges, the cystourethroscope (Fig. 15.10), a short bridge and fiberoptic light cord, lateral and foroblique telescopes, a Luer-Lok stopcock, irrigation tubing and sterile water irrigant, and water-soluble lubricant. Additional items that should be sterile and available include a calibrated container to measure residual urine,

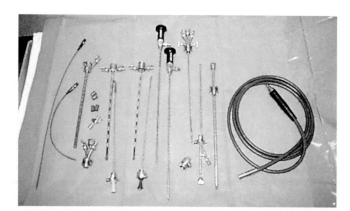

FIG. 15.10 Basic instruments for cystoscopy, catheterization, electrosurgery, and retrograde ureteral pyelography (add ureteral catheter of choice). *Left to right,* Bugbee electrodes, single-horn Albarrán deflecting bridge, nipple adapters, stopcock, short double-horn bridge, 23F and 17F foroblique cystourethroscopes and sheaths, 30- and 70-degree telescopes, double-horn Albarrán deflecting bridge, single-horn examining bridge, visual obturator, and fiberoptic cable.

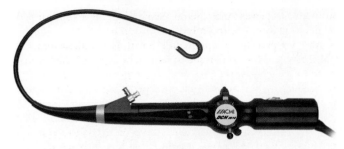

FIG. 15.11 Flexible cystoscope.

test tubes with screw tops for urine specimens, an Albarrán bridge and rubber catheter nipples or adapters, a medicine glass for dye, anesthetic solution, disposable 10- and 20-mL syringes, medication labels and a marking pen, a penile clamp (to occlude the male urethra after local anesthetic is instilled), contrast material, an ESU and dispersive pad, and a Bugbee electrode.

The flexible cystoscope (Fig. 15.11) is used for patients with obstructive symptoms resulting from prostatic hyperplasia and rigid prostatic urethra. In addition, the flexible cystoscope can be used for patients who cannot assume a lithotomy position, such as those with spinal cord injuries or severe arthritis. Flexible cystoscopy may be accomplished with the use of a local anesthetic. It affords the patient a higher degree of comfort, is less traumatic to the urethra, and can be performed in the patient's bed on the nursing unit.

Cleaning, sterilization, disinfection, and maintenance of endoscopic equipment are important procedures in the care of fiberoptic lensed instruments. Ultimately this process reduces costly repairs and ensures the availability of properly functioning instruments. See Chapter 8 for the procedure to correctly process endoscopic equipment.

Endoscopy of the GU tract is considered a class II (clean-contaminated) procedure and, according to the Centers for Disease Control and Prevention (CDC) and the Association for Professionals in Infection Control and Epidemiology (APIC) guidelines, presently requires disinfection rather than sterilization. High-level disinfection with an agent, such as activated glutaraldehyde or dialdehyde, which can destroy vegetative microorganisms, most fungal spores, tubercle bacilli, and small nonlipid viruses, is recommended. In most situations the routine of meticulous cleaning of endoscopic instruments and making sure that all channels are accessed, followed by appropriate high-level disinfection, provides reasonable assurance that the items are safe to use. The level of disinfection is based on the contact time, temperature, and concentration of the active ingredients of the disinfectant, as well as the nature of microbial contamination.

Many institutions are, however, treating endoscopic interventions as sterile procedures because the sterilization of instruments provides the greatest assurance that the risk of infections transmitted by contaminated instruments has been eliminated (see Chapter 4). Some options available include glutaraldehyde solution, hydrogen peroxide solution, an automated peracetic acid unit, an ethylene oxide (ETO) "gas" sterilizer, a hydrogen peroxide and plasma sterilizing unit, and high-vacuum or gravity steam autoclaving for those components that may be sterilized in this manner. The manufacturer's recommendations should always be followed. If soaking is chosen the lid should remain on the soaking container when not in use, and personnel should wear masks when in direct contact with the fumes. It is also imperative that the instrumentation be thoroughly rinsed in sterile distilled water after removal from the soaking solution and

before use. Glutaraldehyde residue remaining in the channels or on the lens can result in chemical burns for the patient and the surgeon.

Stone removal, bladder biopsy, and bladder fulguration may be accomplished by using special cystoscopic accessories. This procedure is called a *litholapaxy.* Lowsley forceps, Wappler rigid cup forceps, and flexible foreign body forceps may also be used. Bladder fulguration requires the use of flexible-stem electrodes available in various French sizes and tip configurations such as the ball, cone, dome, and bayonet.

Operative Procedure

1. The surgeon lubricates the cystourethroscope and introduces it into the urethra, withdraws the obturator, and drains the bladder. Residual urine may be measured at this time if the patient voided before the examination. The specimen may be saved for cultures or cytologic studies.

2. The surgeon connects the cystourethroscope to the irrigating system and inserts and locks the telescope in place. If the patient is awake, telling the patient to try to urinate also helps facilitate passage of the scope. The surgeon controls the rate of flow and volume of fluid by adjusting the stopcock on the scope. If difficulty is encountered during insertion, the visual obturator may be used to introduce the scope under direct vision. This accessory is constructed to smooth the fenestrated edges of the cystourethroscope. It requires the use of the telescope for direct vision and permits irrigation during introduction.

3. For retrograde ureteral catheterization and pyelography, the surgeon passes ureteral catheters through the cystoscope sheath and then through the ureteral orifice and into the ureter via the Albarrán bridge. A radiopaque substance (e.g., nonionic, low-osmolar agents Omnipaque 300 and Optiray 320; or ionic high-osmolar Renografin-60 and Hypaque 50) is injected. Fluoroscopic imaging is used to outline the entire upper urinary collecting system.

Periurethral-Transurethral Injection of Bulking Agents

Coaptite injection is an ambulatory surgery procedure achievable with the patient administered a local anesthetic with or without sedation. Coaptite (calcium hydroxylapatite; Boston Scientific, Marlborough, MA) is a synthetic injectable composed of spherical particles and is prepackaged in a sterile 1-mL syringe containing the coaptite material. Injection needles available are 14.6-inch, 21-gauge, noncoring needles for transurethral use or for periurethral insertion. Female patients with intrinsic sphincter deficiency (ISD) demonstrated by urodynamic evaluation and male patients (usually after prostatectomy) with incontinence lasting more than 1 year may benefit from this procedure. Other indications for coaptite injection include urethral hypermobility (UH), stress urinary incontinence (SUI) secondary to previous stricture treatment, trauma, or myelodysplasia (Herschorn, 2015).

Macroplastique (Uroplasty Inc., Hopkins, MN) is a bulking product composed of polydimethylsiloxane (a silicone elastomer) particles suspended in a polyvinylpyrrolidone carrier gel and is packaged in a sterile 3-mL syringe containing 2.5 mL of product. Instillation of the bulking agent is achieved by attaching the rigid transurethral needle to the 3-mL syringe containing the agent. The 3-mL syringe is then placed in a manual plunger device and injected. It is designed to treat women with SUI secondary to documented ISD. Macroplastique is a nondegradable and nonresorbable permanent implant that provides a durable effect. Macroplastique is currently approved by the US Food and Drug Administration (FDA) for use in women only (Herschorn, 2015).

Botox (onabotulinum toxin A) is FDA approved for neurogenic detrusor overactivity (also called overactive bladder in patients with a neurologic condition) and used off label for idiopathic overactive bladder. Rarely it is also used off label for interstitial cystitis and very rarely for BPH. Doses between 100 and 300 units are used depending on surgeon preference and patient preference. Higher doses are more likely to cause urinary retention or incomplete bladder emptying, requiring intermittent catheterization, than lower doses. Patients with neurogenic bladder who already perform intermittent catheterization usually receive higher (300 units) doses, whereas those who do not perform catheterization receive 100 to 200 units. This treatment is covered by insurance for the neurogenic overactive bladder patients. Repeat injections are generally needed between 12 and 15 months and can be repeated indefinitely (Anderson et al., 2015).

Procedural Considerations

Coaptite and Macroplastique require no refrigeration. Patient skin testing is not required for either product. Botox is stored in the refrigerator. A urine culture and sensitivity is done approximately 10 days preoperatively. It is optimal to use a video system for the procedure. A basic cystoscopy set is required. The patient is usually positioned in the lithotomy position (Herschorn, 2015).

Operative Procedure

1. The surgeon instills urethral anesthetic and may supplement the anesthesia with a perineal block of 1% or 2% lidocaine. Cystoscopic examination is performed before the bulking agent is injected to rule out any associated findings. It is recommended that the irrigation be instilled by use of a pressure bag to minimize extravasation of the material by increasing the intraurethral pressure.
2. The surgeon introduces the injection needle provided by the manufacturer through the cystoscope and places the tip transurethrally, below the urethral mucosa, just distal to the bladder neck. Positioning of the needle tip is accomplished when the surgeon sees the indentation of the urethra by the tip while manipulating the needle.
3. Coaptite and Macroplastique are injected until the urothelium enlarges and meets in the midline, approximating the appearance of lateral lobe enlargement of the prostate. Botox is injected into 10 to 30 locations in the bladder including the trigone.

Transurethral Ureteropyeloscopy

Transurethral ureteropyeloscopy is an endoscopic examination of the ureters and renal pelvis. The use of rigid or flexible ureteroscopes or ureteropyeloscopes provides the opportunity to diagnose filling defects in the ureter and renal pelvis, congenital anomalies, hematuria, ureteral obstruction, and damage from trauma. Manipulation, fragmentation, basketing of ureteral and renal calculi, and retrieval of foreign bodies are possible with transurethral ureteropyeloscopy. Extracorporeal shock-wave lithotripsy (ESWL), electrohydraulic lithotripsy (EHL), sonic lithotripsy, or laser lithotripsy may accompany the procedure. It may also be used to manage residual sludge after these treatments.

Ureteral strictures may be treated transurethrally, and biopsies of tumors of the ureter and renal pelvis are performed under direct visualization. Internal ureteral stents may also be inserted for ureteral patency. These range in size from 3F to 8.5F and are available in single-J, double-J, and pigtail configurations.

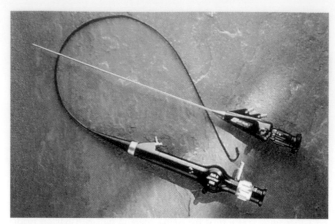

FIG. 15.12 Flexible ureteropyeloscope and rigid ureteropyeloscope.

Procedural Considerations

The setup is similar to that for a cystoscopy with the addition of a rigid or flexible ureteroscope system (Fig. 15.12). A critical factor in this procedure is allowing enough time for careful dilation of the ureter under C-arm fluoroscopy. The flexible ureteroscope has gained popularity because of its inherent tip mobility, which provides a more panoramic view of the entire circumference of the ureter. The perioperative nurse must be prepared to tilt the radiolucent operative bed at head and foot and laterally, as well as raise the bed.

In addition to the standard cystoscopy setup, the following items should be available: a rigid or flexible ureteroscope, ureteral dilators of graduated sizes and styles, size 3F to 5F ureteral stone baskets of various styles, a ureteral grasping forceps, biopsy forceps, snare, scissors, catheters of various styles and sizes, stents, guidewires, balloon dilators, and radiographic contrast material. Patient allergies should be checked before the use of radiographic contrast material.

Operative Procedure

1. The surgeon inserts the ureteropyeloscope and accesses the ureter with a guidewire under fluoroscopic control. The ureter is irrigated as the guidewire is advanced. The scrub person assists by maintaining slight tension on the wire.
2. An additional working guidewire is placed by the surgeon to be used as a safety wire.
3. The surgeon passes the ureteroscope over the working guidewire, biopsies any suspicious lesions, and performs diagnostic pyeloscopy and ureteroscopy. The characteristics of calculi are observed to determine the best treatment approach. Urine may be obtained for cytologic and microbiologic examination. If a calculus is small enough to be delivered through the ureter, the surgeon engages it in a retrieval basket and removes it under visual as well as fluoroscopic control. If, after ureteral dilation, the calculus does not appear to be small enough for delivery, lithotripsy (fragmentation) is performed through the ureteroscope, or ESWL may be performed later. Lithotripsy may be performed with ultrasonic (through a rigid ureteroscope) or electrohydraulic lithotripters or with the tunable pulse-dyed or holmium:yttrium-aluminum-garnet (Ho:YAG) lasers. Appropriate laser precautions must be enforced. Chapter 8 discusses laser safety issues in more depth.
4. The surgeon assesses the ureter for integrity (perforation or laceration) with retrograde pyelography.
5. A ureteral stent is placed over the remaining safety guidewire, and the guidewire is removed.

Surgery of the Penis and the Urethra

Laser Ablation of Condylomata and Penile Carcinoma

Laser ablation of condylomata or penile cancer is the eradication of diseased tissue by means of a laser beam. Laser therapy has been determined to be effective for condylomata and penile cancers that are refractory to other treatments. One of the major advantages of the laser is that heat is distributed evenly to the tissue underlying the lesion. When any laser is being used, precautions appropriate to that system must be initiated (see Chapter 8).

Procedural Considerations

Laser treatment may be performed successfully with local infiltration of an anesthetic. A U-shaped, crater-like lesion of predetermined depth with a 2-mm radius can be created. A power setting ranging from 2 to 20 watts on continuous or super-pulse mode is commonly used. With laser ablation, less edema and necrosis occur, fibrosis is minimized, and rapid healing is facilitated. The argon, CO_2, potassium-titanyl-phosphate (KTP), and neodymium (Nd):YAG lasers are all suitable for this therapeutic application.

Operative Procedure

1. The surgeon moves the beam transversely across the tissue and then in a crosshatch matrix, treating all perimeters of the lesion. Throughout the procedure the surgeon wipes the area with acetic acid (5% vinegar), which results in greater visualization of the diseased tissue and allows therapy to deeper layers.
2. At the end of the procedure the wound is coated with an antibiotic ointment and left uncovered.

Circumcision

Circumcision is the excision of the foreskin (prepuce) of the glans penis. Circumcision in adult males is performed for the relief of phimosis, a condition in which the orifice of the prepuce is stenosed or too narrow to permit easy retraction behind the glans. Another condition that may require circumcision is balanoposthitis, which is an inflamed glans and mucous membrane with purulent discharge. Circumcision may also be performed to prevent recurrent paraphimosis (a condition in which the prepuce cannot be reduced easily from a retracted position). (See Chapter 26 for pediatric considerations during circumcision.)

Procedural Considerations

The perioperative nurse assists in positioning the patient in the supine position. A plastic or minor instrument set and a local anesthetic with IV sedation are sufficient. An ESU should be available.

Operative Procedure

1. The surgeon clamps the prepuce in the dorsal midline and incises it toward the coronal margin (Fig. 15.13A), leaving about 5 cm of coronal mucosa intact. If the prepuce is adherent, a probe or hemostat may be used to break up adhesions.
2. A similar procedure is performed ventrally. The two incisions are then joined circumferentially. Alternatively, a superficial circumferential incision is made in the skin with a scalpel at the level of the coronal sulcus and the mucosa at the base of the glans.
3. The surgeon undermines redundant skin between the circumferential incisions and removes it as a complete cuff (see Fig. 15.13B).

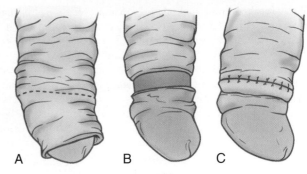

FIG. 15.13 Circumcision.

4. Bleeding vessels are coagulated or clamped with mosquito hemostats and ligated with fine absorbable ligatures.
5. The surgeon approximates the raw edges of the skin incision to a coronal cuff of mucosal prepuce, generally with 4-0 or 5-0 absorbable sutures on atraumatic, plastic cutting, or fine gastrointestinal (GI) needles (see Fig. 15.13C).
6. The wound is dressed with petrolatum gauze.

Excision of Urethral Caruncle

A urethral caruncle is a benign lesion or inflammatory prolapse of the external urinary meatus in the female. Excision entails the removal of these papillary or sessile tumors from the urethra.

Procedural Considerations

The perioperative nurse assists with placing the patient in the lithotomy position. A minor or plastic set, an ESU, and a local anesthetic are used. A urethral catheter of an appropriate size may be required if the distal urethral prolapse is severe.

Operative Procedure

1. The surgeon uses a small, fine-tipped Metzenbaum or plastic scissors to expose the tumor and excise it within a wedge of ventral urethral tissue.
2. Figure-of-eight 4-0 absorbable sutures are placed at the edge of the incision to achieve hemostasis.

Urethral Meatotomy

Urethral meatotomy is an incisional enlargement of the external urethral meatus to relieve congenital or acquired stenosis or stricture at the external meatus.

Procedural Considerations

The perioperative team places male patients in the supine position and female patients in the lithotomy position for this procedure. Prepping and draping are as described for urethral catheterization. The surgeon administers local anesthesia. A plastic instrument set is required.

Operative Procedure

1. The surgeon places a straight hemostat on the ventral surface of the meatus.
2. An incision is made along the frenulum to enlarge the opening and overcome the stricture.
3. Hemostasis is obtained by clamping the bleeding vessels and ligating them with fine absorbable sutures.

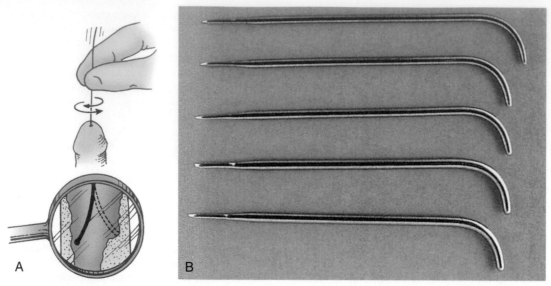

FIG. 15.14 (A) Method of using coudé-tipped bougie for passing stricture. (B) Variety of urethral sounds (dilators).

4. The surgeon sutures the mucosal layer to the skin with fine absorbable sutures.
5. A dressing of petrolatum gauze is applied.

Urethral Dilation and Internal Urethrotomy

Urethral dilation and internal urethrotomy are performed to provide relief of distal lower urinary tract obstruction. Urethral strictures or narrowing of the urethra may be caused by a congenital malformation that is usually found at the external urinary meatus. Infection or trauma may also contribute to stricture of the membranous and pendulous urethra. Urethral stricture disease may be treated by periodic and gradual dilation or internal urethrotomy.

Procedural Considerations

The perioperative nurse assists with placing the male patient in the supine position for routine urethral dilation and in the lithotomy position for other procedures. The female patient is placed in the lithotomy position. Prepping and draping are conducted as appropriate to the patient's position and gender. The surgeon administers a local anesthetic either (1) by placing cotton-tipped applicators, which have been dipped into viscous 2% lidocaine (Xylocaine), into the urethral opening or (2) by using a urethral syringe to instill the lidocaine. Female urethral dilation is performed with short, straight metal dilators or with hollow McCarthy dilators. The latter allows a urine specimen to be obtained.

In addition to a cystoscopy setup, required instrumentation includes urethrotomes; the resectoscope working element with sheath, obturator, and cold knives; urethral dilators; Phillips filiforms and followers; Van Buren sounds; and a silicone Foley catheter. Before use, the filiforms and followers should be carefully inspected for damaged or weak points, particularly around the scored-threaded end.

Operative Procedure

Gradual Dilation

1. In a male patient the surgeon lubricates and anesthetizes the urethra with a viscous anesthetic that is instilled into the urethra with a urethral or Uro-Jet syringe. A penile clamp occludes the penile urethra at the coronal sulcus and keeps the anesthetic within the urethra.
2. Phillips filiforms of various tips and sizes are introduced first in an attempt to pass an instrument beyond the urethral stricture. Followers of increasing size are connected to the filiforms and passed through the strictured portion of the urethra, stretching the scarred area (Fig. 15.14A).
3. Slow dilation is also achieved with a small catheter or follower left in the urethra. It leads to softening of the stricture over the course of several days.

Internal Urethrotomy

1. The surgeon inserts the assembled visualizing urethrotome into the urethra.
2. When necessary, the surgeon feeds a filiform or ureteral catheter into the catheterizing channel to help identify the patent portion of the urethra.
3. The surgeon advances the urethrotome to the desired position, and incises the urethral scar with the blade. The normal urethra is incised 1 cm proximally and distally beyond the stricture to achieve optimum results.
4. A silicone Foley catheter is inserted and left in place for 3 to 5 days after surgery.

Urethroplasty

Urethroplasty is reconstructive surgery of the urethra for strictures, urethral fractures, or narrowed segments of the urethral lumen that are congenital, inflammatory, or traumatic in origin. Urethral grafts are generally required and may include free skin grafts and mobilized vascular flaps. There are many combinations of these procedures, and in all of them some type of temporary urinary diversion may be used, depending on the location and severity of the condition.

Typically the patient complains of obstructive symptoms, frequently associated with a UTI. Techniques used to determine diagnosis include urodynamics (voiding pressures above and below the site of obstruction), urinary flow cytometry, IVU to rule out an upper tract lesion, cystoscopy, and urethrography. The length and density of the diseased urethra are determined to plan the appropriate reconstructive procedure. Any associated UTI must be treated and eradicated before surgical intervention. Definitive repair should not be done for 10 to 12 weeks after use of diagnostic instrumentation to allow the inflammatory reaction to subside.

Procedural Considerations

The patient is placed in the exaggerated lithotomy position by the perioperative nurse and one other person. Routine prepping and draping procedures are used with precautions for isolating the anus (e.g., the use of an impervious plastic adherent drape). The setup includes a minor instrument set with fine plastic instruments for dissection and plastic repair. Strictures may be located deep, requiring fiberoptic lighting. An ESU may be required.

Operative Procedure

Johanson Urethroplasty. The Johanson urethroplasty is a two-stage procedure to repair and reconstruct the male urethra for severe urethral stricture disease. Approximately 3 months after completion of the first stage, if the operative site is healing and the patient is voiding adequately, a second-stage procedure is performed. Vascularized flaps of preputial or penile skin may be mobilized to the ventrum by leaving them attached to the outer surface of the prepuce or as an island flap. One modification is the transverse preputial island flap neourethra with glans channel positioning for the meatus. Preputial skin is preferred because of its rich reliable blood supply and non–hair-bearing characteristics.

First Stage

1. The surgeon makes an inverted U incision in the perineum from the inner borders of the ischial tuberosities up to and including the base of the scrotum.
2. A Van Buren sound is passed into the urethra up to the stricture (see Fig. 15.14B). The bulbocavernosus muscle is dissected and retracted laterally.
3. The surgeon makes an incision in the urethra over the strictured area and extends it in each direction at least 1 cm beyond the diseased area. The abnormal scar tissue is excised or simply incised, because scrotal skin ultimately increases the lumen.
4. A 28F sound is passed through both the proximal and the distal urethral lumens to rule out further stricture.
5. The surgeon sutures the remaining urethral mucosa to the scrotal skin with 4-0 absorbable sutures.
6. A cystotomy tube to divert the urinary stream may be left indwelling and removed in 5 to 7 days.

Second Stage (Mobilized Vascular Flap)

1. A red rubber catheter is temporarily inserted into the bladder through the proximal urethral stoma.
2. The surgeon incises the penoscrotal skin longitudinally, adjacent to the urethra.
3. A new urethra is constructed by developing the ventral preputial skin that is dissected free and fanned out. The rectangle of skin is rolled into the neourethra and measured.
4. A channel is sharply created on the ventral aspect of the glans, in a plane just above the corpora.
5. The surgeon removes the glans tissue, forming a groove approximately 14F in diameter.
6. Layers of subcutaneous tissue are dissected free from the dorsal penile skin to create an island flap that is spiraled to the ventrum. The surgeon brings the flaps together in the midline and closes with a continuous or interrupted 4-0 absorbable suture.
7. The neourethra is anastomosed proximally to the urethra and carried to the tip of the glans.

8. The dorsal penile flaps are transposed laterally to the midline, and the surgeon excises the excess skin.
9. The surgeon closes with 4-0 absorbable interrupted mattress sutures around the glans and down the penile shaft. A bulky pressure dressing is applied.
10. Suprapubic cystostomy drainage is an option, but a urethral catheter usually suffices.

Horton-Devine Urethroplasty (Urethral Patch Graft). Urethral patch graft is a one-stage operative procedure that incorporates a free skin graft to correct a urethral stricture. Free skin grafts should be at full thickness. Because the free graft must be revascularized, it is important that it have a perfect skin cover of well-vascularized dorsal, preputial, penile skin.

1. The surgeon passes a 17F panendoscope into the posterior urethra, and then passes a 20F urethral dilator into the posterior urethra.
2. A perineal vertical midline incision is made into the urethral lumen. The surgeon reinserts the panendoscope and examines the incision to determine whether it crosses the stricture.
3. The defect is measured, and the surgeon makes a circumferential incision on the posterior penile shaft to harvest an oval piece of skin the size of the defect.
4. The epidermal side of the graft is defatted, and 4-0 absorbable sutures are placed at the apex and base.
5. The surgeon sutures the apex into position at the proximal and distal ends of the stricture with the epidermal side toward the urethral lumen.
6. The graft is anastomosed proximally to the urethra with the suture line of the graft next to the corpus. The middle glans dart is fixed to the corpus. The graft is formed into a neourethra over a Silastic stenting catheter.
7. The surgeon reinserts the panendoscope and irrigates the urethra to check for suture-line leaks.
8. A Foley or fenestrated catheter is inserted to serve as a stent.
9. The surgeon approximates and closes the corpus spongiosum over the patched area as a separate layer with interrupted 3-0 absorbable sutures. Subcutaneous 4-0 absorbable sutures are placed.
10. The skin and the graft site are closed with interrupted 4-0 sutures.
11. A suprapubic catheter is inserted to divert urine for healing. Petrolatum gauze is wrapped around the penis and covered with gauze sponges and fluffed dressings. A scrotal support is applied to provide support and pressure.

Penectomy

Penectomy is the partial or total removal of a cancerous penis. The procedure selected depends on the extent of involvement and disease stage. Invasive penile cancer not suited for irradiation because of its size, depth, or location is best dealt with by penectomy. Excision of a 2-cm gross tumor margin is adequate for local management. Partial penectomy may afford a sufficient length for directable and upright urination. At least 3 cm of viable proximal shaft is necessary for consideration of a partial penectomy. If the residual stump is inadequate in length, detachment and mobilization of the suspensory ligaments may be an option in selected patients. A total penectomy is generally required when tumor margins are beyond a 2-cm retrievable length from the penoscrotal junction.

Options are available to limit the extent of the disfiguring surgery used in the past for penile cancer. Chemotherapy agents, often combined with irradiation, are proving effective in shrinking penile carcinomas that would have previously mandated radical penectomy.

Reconstruction is possible after penectomy. Evaluation must take into account sexual, urinary, and cosmetic factors. Extensive or proximally invasive lesions that include the scrotum, perineum, abdominal wall, and pubis necessitate emasculation as well as expanded resection of involved tissues.

Procedural Considerations

The setup necessary is similar to that for any inguinal surgery, with the addition of a medium Penrose drain for use as a tourniquet.

Operative Procedure
Partial Penectomy

1. The lesion is excluded by a towel attached to the planned amputation line. The surgeon applies a Penrose drain to act as a tourniquet at the base of the penis (Fig. 15.15A).
2. After circumferential skin incision, the surgeon divides the cavernous bodies to the urethra with a 2-cm gross margin (see Fig. 15.15B).
3. Dorsal vessels are ligated, margins of the tunica albuginea are approximated, and the urethra is dissected proximally and distally (spatulated) to obtain a 1-cm redundant flap (see Fig. 15.15C).
4. Without sacrificing the tumor margin, the surgeon divides the urethra. Interrupted sutures are placed on the opposite margins of the tunica albuginea to secure the corpora. The tourniquet is removed, and hemostasis is achieved.
5. After the dorsal urethrotomy, a skin-to-urethra anastomosis is performed. The redundant skin flap is then dorsally approximated (see Fig. 15.15D).
6. A small urinary catheter is inserted, and a nonadherent dressing is applied.

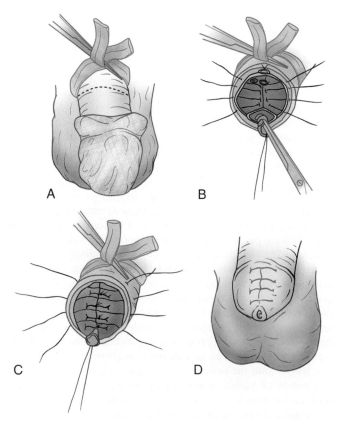

FIG. 15.15 Partial penectomy.

Total Penectomy

1. A vertical elliptic incision is made around the penile base (Fig. 15.16A).
2. The distal urethra and its ventral traction are divided through an incision in Buck fascia, mobilizing the urethra and aiding its dissection, which extends from the corpora to the bulbar region.
3. The surgeon separates and ligates the corpora (see Fig. 15.16B). The suspensory ligaments and dorsal vessels are divided as corporal dissection is performed.
4. The urethra is transected from the corpora (see Fig. 15.16C).
5. An ellipse of skin approximately 1 cm in size is taken from the perineal area. A tunnel is fashioned in the perineal subcutaneous layer of tissue. A traction suture through the tunnel, at the penile base, aids dissection for transposition of the urethra to the perineum (see Fig. 15.16D).
6. The surgeon grasps the urethra with forceps and transfers it to the perineum. The urethra is spatulated, and a skin-to-urethra anastomosis is performed through a buttonhole incision in the perineum (see Fig. 15.16E).
7. The primary incision is closed horizontally, elevating the scrotum away from the urethral opening (see Fig. 15.16F).
8. An indwelling urinary catheter is inserted, and the wound is covered with a nonadherent dressing.

Surgical Management of Priapism

Priapism is defined as an abnormal persistent erection of the penis. Priapism is a true urologic emergency that may lead to permanent erectile dysfunction and penile necrosis if left untreated. Surgical management (shunt surgery) is indicated after repeated penile aspirations and injections of sympathomimetics have failed or if such an attempt has resulted in a significant cardiovascular effect. The object of shunt surgery is reoxygenation of the cavernous smooth muscle. Shunt procedures reestablish corporal inflow by relieving venous outflow obstruction. Open shunting will require general anesthesia and an OR suite. After shunting, follow-up with the patient regarding erectile function is required. A penile implant is considered if (1) aspiration and sympathomimetics have failed, (2) distal and proximal shunting procedures have failed, and (3) ischemia has been present for longer than 36 hours.

Procedural Considerations

The setup for shunting is as described for penile implant including instrumentation.

Operative Procedure
Unilateral Shunt Procedure

1. A transscrotal or transperineal incision is made.
2. The surgeon incises the proximal corpus cavernosum as well as the corpus spongiosum at the base of the penis.
3. This newly formed fistula is joined together medially and laterally using 3-0 absorbable suture.
4. The surgeon closes the incision with 4-0 absorbable suture in a running subcuticular stitch, and a dressing is applied.
5. The penis is placed flush with the lower abdomen for patient comfort. Mesh underpants are useful as a nonadherent support dressing. An ice pack may be applied to reduce swelling.

Penile Implant

A penile prosthesis is implanted for treatment of organic sexual impotence. Sexual impotence may be caused by (1) diabetes mellitus, (2) priapism, (3) Peyronie disease, (4) penile trauma, (5) pelvic

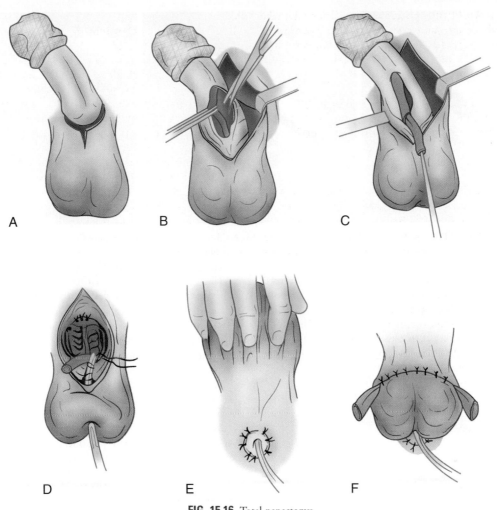

FIG. 15.16 Total penectomy.

surgery, (6) neurologic disease (in selected cases), (7) vascular disease, (8) hypertension, and (9) idiopathic impotence. The penile implant serves as a stent to enable vaginal penetration for sexual intercourse. Penile implants are available as malleable one-piece devices, self-contained inflatable devices, and two- and three-piece devices. The procedure described for the inflatable penile implant is the same for the three-piece device.

Procedural Considerations

The anesthesia provider administers either a spinal or a general anesthetic. The perioperative nurse assists with positioning the patient in either the supine or the lithotomy position, as directed by the surgeon. A 5- to 10-minute skin prep is usually performed before draping is performed. To prevent urethral injury and potential urinary retention, the surgeon may insert a 14F or 16F Foley catheter to identify the urethra intraoperatively. The ESU may be required. The surgeon may inject a local anesthetic of 0.5% plain bupivacaine (Marcaine) or 1% etidocaine (Duranest) at the beginning of the procedure into the incisional sites. Often a penile block, composed of 0.9% saline (150 mL), 1% plain lidocaine (50 mL), and 30 mg/mL papaverine (2 mL), is instilled intraoperatively before the incision into the corpus cavernosum. This enables the surgeon to evaluate erectile size and provides some postoperative pain management.

The scrub person sets up a separate sterile Mayo stand or small table covered with a plastic drape for the implants. It is recommended

that the implants not be in contact with paper or cloth that may shed fiber particles.

The instrument setup includes a minor set with fine instruments, plus Hegar dilators, the penile prosthesis of choice (Fig. 15.17), the Furlow Inserter, the closing tool, the assembly tool for clamping connectors (Fig. 15.18A), and the connectors of choice (see Fig. 15.18B). Medications needed in the operative field include 50 mL of 1% lidocaine, 150 mL of injectable 0.9% normal saline, 1 mL of methylene blue (optional by surgeon preference), 2 mL of papaverine, 50 mL of 0.5% bupivacaine or 1% etidocaine, 50,000 units of bacitracin, and 80 mg of kanamycin. Medication safety practices must be implemented for all medications on the sterile field.

A serious risk with a penile implant is infection. Infection rates for first-time implantation are low at 1%, but the rate can rise to as high as 18% with reimplantation procedures. Within the past decade with the introduction of models that have been irradiated and embedded with minocycline hydrochloride and rifampin (Inhibizone), the incidence of infection has decreased by 50% to 70% even after 11 years of follow-up (Francois-Eid, 2015). The sterile team should be double-gloved throughout the procedure. A 5-minute antimicrobial prep of the operative area is critical in reducing skin flora. The anus should be isolated in the perineal approach. Intraoperatively and before insertion of the implant components, a prophylactic antibiotic irrigant of bacitracin and kanamycin in normal

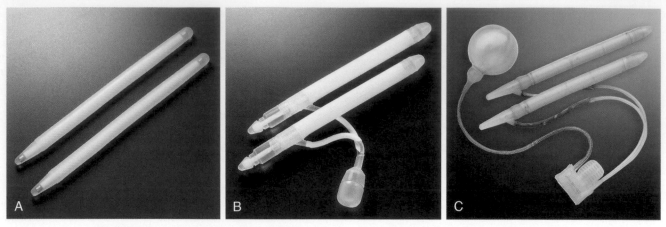

FIG. 15.17 (A) AMS malleable 650 penile prosthesis. (B) AMS Ambicor inflatable two-piece penile prosthesis. (C) AMS tactile inflatable penile prosthesis, three-piece with rifampin (Inhibizone).

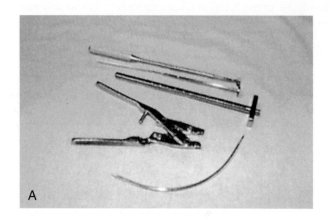

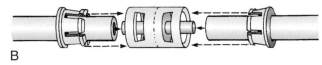

FIG. 15.18 (A) *Top to bottom,* Closing tool, Furlow inserter, assembly tool, and tubing passer. (B) Quik-connectors.

saline is used on the implants without rifampin and in the insertion sites. Systemic antibiotics may also be required. As with any implant procedure, it is vital to maintain an environment conducive to infection prevention. The perioperative nurse ensures that traffic in and out of the OR is minimized.

It is recommended that the implants with rifampin not be soaked in any solution before implantation because this may cause the antibiotic component to disintegrate. The area to be implanted may be irrigated with antibiotic solution, and the implant itself may be dipped in a sterile solution of 0.9% normal saline to assist with insertion if desired. Prophylactic antibiotic protocols remain the same.

Operative Procedure

Implantation of Noninflatable (Semirigid) Prosthesis

1. The surgeon inserts a 14F or 16F Foley catheter and attaches it to a drainage collection device to be maintained within the sterile field. The amount and color of urine are noted. The catheter is left in place intraoperatively to assist in identifying the urethra.
2. A midline incision is made from the base of the penis into the scrotum for approximately 3 cm. Some surgeons may choose a suprapubic or dorsal penile approach.
3. The surgeon incises the tunica albuginea over the most proximal portion of the corpora in a longitudinal manner, and places stay sutures.
4. The corpora are dilated proximally and distally with 7- to 14-mm Hegar dilators, depending on the diameter of the implant chosen. The corpora are dilated to 1 mm more than the implant size. Care is taken to not perforate the urethra.
5. The surgeon measures the corporal length with a Furlow inserter or sizing instrument.
6. After placement of the closure sutures, the surgeon inserts the prosthesis into the corpora. Proper placement is evident immediately by a change in the configuration of the penis with no buckling of the glans.
7. The surgeon closes the tunica albuginea using the previously placed 2-0 absorbable continuous suture; 3-0 or 4-0 absorbable interrupted sutures are used for skin closure.
8. Petrolatum gauze or 2-inch tube gauze may be used for the dressing.

Implantation of Inflatable Prosthesis

1. The surgeon inserts a 14F or 16F Foley catheter and attaches it to a drainage collection device to be maintained within the sterile field. The amount and color of urine are noted. The catheter is left in place intraoperatively to assist in identifying the urethra.
2. A 3-cm long suprapubic incision is made.
3. The surgeon incises the tunica albuginea of each corpus in the most proximal portion, and places stay sutures.
4. The corpora are dilated distally and proximally with 7- to 14-mm Hegar dilators. Dilation should be 1 mm more than the diameter of the chosen implant. The 700CX implant is 12 mm at its widest point. When this is used, the dilation at the distal end should be 13 mm. The proximal end, however, should be 14 mm to accommodate the input tubing.
5. The surgeon measures the corporal length with the Furlow inserter.

6. Corporal sutures of 2-0 absorbable material are placed along the tunica incision and tagged. Some surgeons prefer to place these sutures last and use the closing tool to prevent puncture of the cylinders.

7. The cylinders are packaged with attached traction sutures of 4-0 braided polyester at the distal end. The surgeon places the suture through the eye of a 2½-inch Keith needle, and slides the needle into the groove of the Furlow inserter.

8. The surgeon guides the Furlow inserter along the corporal tunnel, and pushes the plunger to release the Keith needle, which punctures the glans.

9. The Keith needle is grasped with a heavy hemostat and pulled through the glans, allowing the cylinders to slide to the channel opening. The surgeon removes the Furlow inserter, inserts the cylinder, and guides it to its proper position beneath the glans penis.

10. If necessary, rear tip extenders are added to the proximal end of the cylinder. The proximal end is positioned in the crus.

11. The procedure is repeated on the other side.

12. The surgeon palpates the external inguinal ring and uses blunt dissection to create a path. Dissecting scissors are used to separate the transversalis fascia on the inguinal floor. If the Ambicor implant with self-contained reservoir is being placed, steps 12 through 14 are eliminated.

13. The perivesical space is enlarged to allow palpation of the Cooper ligament. The reservoir is then positioned into the perivesical space.

14. The surgeon fills the reservoir with 65 or 100 mL of saline solution (depending on the reservoir size selected) and pulls it against the floor of Hesselbach triangle.

15. The pump is then placed into the most dependent portion of the scrotum. It is generally positioned on the patient's dominant side. The space is created by blunt dissection lateral to the testicle.

16. The rods and reservoir tubings are connected to the pump with the connectors of choice, using the assembly tool to clamp them in place, and tested for inflation and deflation.

17. The surgeon closes the tunica of the scrotum over the pump with a running stitch of 3-0 absorbable suture.

18. The prosthetic device is left in a partially inflated position to reduce bleeding and promote healing for 24 hours postoperatively (Figs. 15.19 and 15.20). (After 24 hours the implants are deflated for the remainder of the "healing phase" so the reservoir pocket heals with the reservoir in "full position" to prevent autoinflation.)

19. The surgeon closes the incision with 4-0 absorbable suture in a running subcuticular stitch, and a dressing is applied.

20. The penis is positioned flush with the lower abdomen for patient comfort. Mesh underpants are useful as a nonadherent support dressing. An ice pack may be applied to reduce swelling.

21. The Foley catheter is left in place during the immediate 24-hour postoperative period and then usually removed.

Deep Dorsal and Emissary Vein Ligation

Undertaken for vascular compromise–related impotence, this procedure entails the ligation or elimination of the penile deep dorsal vein and its tributaries. Care is taken to avoid damage to the arteries and nerves lying alongside the deep dorsal vein. A common cause of erectile dysfunction in patients with organic impotence is vascular compromise. Before surgical intervention is undertaken, a definitive diagnosis of a corporal leak is made through dynamic infusion cavernosometry and cavernosography. Diagnostic results may indicate failure-to-store or failure-to-fill impotence. Patients with vascular compromise in a given anatomic region tend to be compromised elsewhere as well. Many have diabetes or hypertension. Because of this the perioperative nurse must exercise great care in positioning the patient to prevent further damage to the patient's altered tissue perfusion. The cavernous and crural veins are suture ligated. All circumflex and emissary branches are ligated or coagulated. The suspensory ligament is detached, and the entire deep and accessory dorsal vein is removed.

Revascularization of the Penile Arteries

The relationship of focal arterial occlusive disease to sexual dysfunction has prompted efforts to rectify the resulting impotence. Reconstructive surgery has been attempted in patients who demonstrate correctable vascular disease in the large arteries. The most widely attempted repairs are end-to-end and end-to-side microscopic anastomoses of the distal inferior epigastric artery to the proximal deep dorsal artery near the pubic level, below the rectus muscle and Buck fascia. The surgeon makes paramedian and infrapubic incisions and frees and tunnels the arteries. This procedure requires both urologic and vascular surgeons.

Surgery of the Scrotum and Testicles

Hydrocelectomy

A hydrocele is an abnormal accumulation of fluid within the scrotum. The fluid is contained within the tunica vaginalis. Excessive secretion or accumulation of hydrocele fluid may be the result of infection or trauma. A hydrocelectomy is the excision of the tunica vaginalis of the testis to remove the enlarged, fluid-filled sac.

Procedural Considerations

The team places the patient in the supine position. Prepping and draping of the patient include routine cleansing of the external genitalia and draping with a fenestrated sheet. A minor instrument set is required, plus a small drain; a 30-mL syringe with a 20-gauge, 2-inch aspirating needle; and a suspensory dressing.

Operative Procedure

1. The surgeon administers a local anesthetic into the cord at the base of the scrotum with 10 to 15 mL of plain 1% lidocaine.

2. An anterolateral incision is made in the stretched skin of the scrotum over the hydrocele mass with a #10 or #15 blade.

3. Bleeding is controlled with Crile hemostats, the ESU, or vessel ligation with 3-0 absorbable ligatures. Stretching the skin of the scrotum compresses the scrotal vessels.

4. An incision is then made between the blood vessels. The fascial layers are incised to expose the tunica vaginalis.

5. The surgeon uses sharp and blunt dissection to free the hydrocele.

6. The sac is opened, and clamps are placed on each side incorporating the tissue adjacent to the tunica vaginalis and the skin.

7. Using Martius clamps, the surgeon everts the incised edges. The tension placed by the Martius clamp compresses the incised edge, controls bleeding, and prevents dissection between the tissue layers.

8. A pouch is created by dissecting between the tunica vaginalis and the dartos layer. Scrotal pressure is released. This pouch will hold the testis after the repair.

9. The surgeon opens the tunica vaginalis and evacuates the fluid contents.

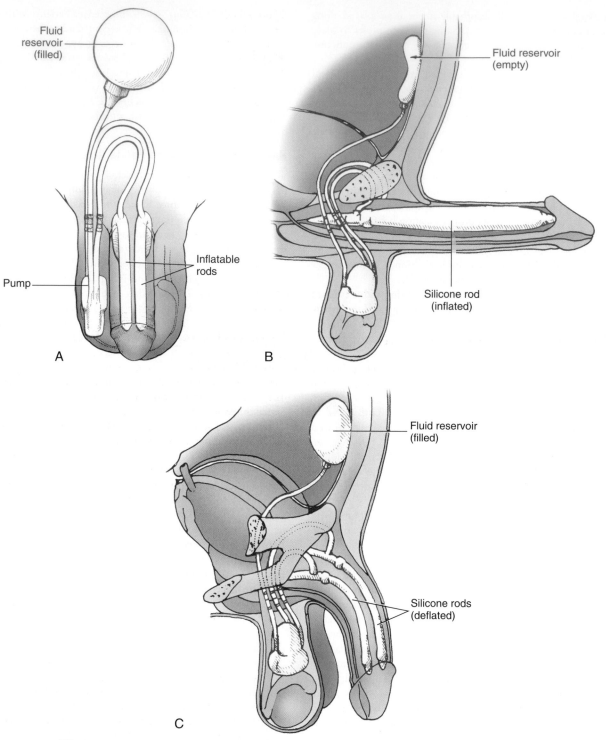

FIG. 15.19 AMS inflatable 700CX penile prosthesis. (A) Frontal view. (B) Sagittal view, penis in the erect position. (C) Sagittal view, penis in the flaccid position.

10. The testis is lifted, and the sac is inverted so that it surrounds the testicular attachments and epididymis.
11. Excess tunica vaginalis may be excised. The surgeon sutures the tunica edges along the peritoneal surface with 3-0 absorbable suture in an interrupted fashion to the juncture of the testis. Six to eight sutures are placed around the circumference of the testis (Fig. 15.21). Some surgeons elect to sew the sac behind

the spermatic cord in an interrupted fashion, and others may choose a continuous radial stitch around the posterior testis and epididymis.
12. The testis is replaced into the scrotum.
13. A drain may be placed into the scrotum and exteriorized through a stab wound in its most dependent portion. The drain is loosely sutured to the external scrotal wall to prevent migration.

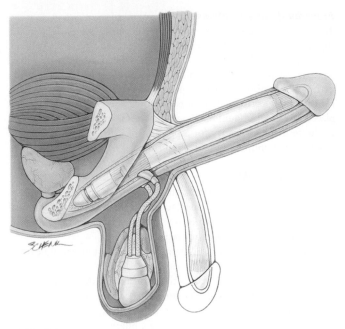

FIG. 15.20 AMS Ambicor inflatable two-piece implant, sagittal view.

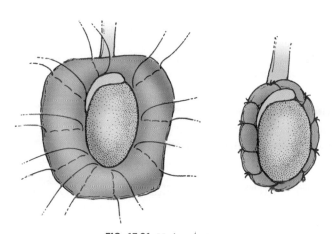

FIG. 15.21 Hydrocelectomy.

14. The surgeon closes the scrotal incision with 3-0 absorbable sutures in a full-thickness continuous manner or in layers with 3-0 and 4-0 continuous absorbable sutures.
15. A fluff compression dressing contained in a scrotal support or mesh underpants aids in reducing postoperative scrotal edema.

Vasectomy

A vasectomy is the excision of a section of the vas deferens. The operation is usually performed selectively as a permanent method of sterilization. Because of the serious implications of permanent sterilization, particular attention must be paid to acquiring informed consent.

The patient having elective sterilization for birth control is encouraged to return to the office setting for sperm-count analysis. Generally two successive negative counts are sufficient to indicate that sterility has been achieved. Elective vasectomies are frequently performed in the office setting.

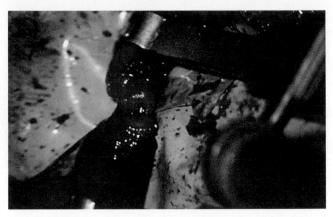

FIG. 15.22 Two portions of the vas in approximator clip with background material as the proximal end is sutured through the serosa to the mucosa with 10-0 nylon.

Vasovasostomy

Vasovasostomy is the surgical reanastomosis of the vas deferens, generally with the goal of restoring male fertility after vasectomy. Reanastomosis may often alleviate chronic testicular pain, a not infrequent complication after vasectomy. A precise reconnection can be performed with the use of a microscope and a modified two-layer anastomosis. Success rates vary, but in general, patency can be demonstrated by the presence of sperm in the semen within 4 weeks after vasovasostomy (Sabanegh et al., 2015). When there are no longer two viable segments of vas deferens, a similar procedure, the epididymovasostomy, may be performed. This involves anastomosis of a vas deferens to a segment of the epididymis. Postoperative precautions include no lifting or ejaculation for a minimum of 2 weeks. The sperm count and viability of sperm are rechecked at 3- and 15-month intervals. If sperm are not present by 6 months, the operation is considered a failure (Sabanegh et al., 2015).

Procedural Considerations

A minor instrument set is required, with the addition of selected microsurgical instruments and sutures. The procedure is frequently done under monitored anesthesia care with local injection of 0.5% plain bupivacaine (Marcaine) and 1% lidocaine (Xylocaine) in a 50:50 ratio.

Operative Procedure

1. After the vas deferens has been located by external manipulation, the surgeon makes a vertical scrotal incision.
2. The testicle, epididymis, and vas are displaced from the scrotum. The vasectomy site is identified, and the scarred area is excised.
3. The surgeon trims the proximal end of the vas deferens until fluid is expressed. Fluid is collected on a glass slide and examined for the presence of live sperm. Surgery continues even if results for sperm are negative unless an epididymal obstruction exists.
4. The distal end of the vas is resected until a normal lumen is visible.
5. The distal and proximal lumens are then dilated.
6. The surgeon places the two portions of the vas in an approximator clip and inserts a piece of background material underneath to provide contrast and improve visibility. Six stitches of 10-0 nonabsorbable microsuture are placed in the inner layer. The proximal end is sutured through the serosa to the mucosa, and the distal end is sutured through the mucosa to the serosa (Fig. 15.22).

7. A second layer of 8 to 10 stitches of 9-0 nonabsorbable suture is placed without penetrating the lumen of the vas.
8. The surgeon closes the incision in two layers with interrupted 3-0 and 4-0 absorbable sutures.
9. Gauze sponges and a scrotal support are placed on the patient to provide a pressure dressing.

Spermatocelectomy

Spermatocelectomy is removal of a spermatocele, which is a lobulated intrascrotal cystic mass attached to the superior head of the epididymis. Spermatocele is usually caused by an obstruction of the tubular system that conveys the sperm and may be a late complication after vasectomy.

Procedural Considerations

The setup for a spermatocelectomy is as described for a hydrocelectomy, plus a microscope and slides, if desired.

Operative Procedure

1. The mass is approached through a scrotal incision as described for hydrocelectomy.
2. The surgeon identifies the structures of the testis and spermatic cord and dissects the cystic structure free.
3. Bleeding is controlled with the ESU.
4. The wound is closed and dressed as described for hydrocelectomy.

Varicocelectomy

A varicocelectomy is the high ligation of the gonadal veins of the testes. Varicocelectomy is done to reduce venous backflow of blood into the venous plexus around the testes and to improve spermatogenesis.

Varicoceles occur more frequently on the left side because the gonadal vein of the left testis unites retroperitoneally with the renal vein at a 90-degree angle and is consequently under greater backpressure. As a result of this unusual backpressure, the pampiniform plexus of the spermatic cord becomes tortuous and engorged, resembling a bag of worms.

Procedural Considerations

The setup for inguinal varicocelectomy is as described for an inguinal hernia repair (see Chapter 13). A microscope may be used to better visualize the vessels involved.

Operative Procedure

The incision may be through a suprainguinal approach or an oblique inguinal approach over the external inguinal ring.

1. The surgeon identifies the structures of the spermatic cord and dissects the vessels free from the vas deferens.
2. The abnormal dilated veins in the inguinal canal are clamped and ligated. The redundant portions are excised. A drain may be placed.
3. The incision is closed in layers.

Testicular Biopsy

A biopsy of the testicle involves a wedge excision of suspicious tissue for diagnostic confirmation. Men experiencing infertility who are azoospermatic or oligospermatic with a normal or minimally elevated level of follicle-stimulating hormone may be evaluated through this means. Biopsy may also be performed to obtain sperm cells for in vitro fertilization techniques.

Procedural Considerations

The perioperative nurse assists with positioning the patient in the supine position, and the anesthesia provider administers a general, regional, or spinal anesthetic. A minor instrument set is used. Special fixatives, such as Bouin or Zenker solution, must be available when pathologic confirmation is required. If retrieval of sperm cells is planned, the perioperative nurse ensures the biopsy specimen is placed in a small amount of saline, kept warm, and taken immediately to the fertility laboratory for aspiration of cells. Formalin destroys the germinal epithelium and should not be used.

Operative Procedure

1. The scrotum is held firmly on its posterior aspect. This causes the skin on the anterior aspect to stretch tightly over the incisional site, forcing the epididymis to remain posterior and allowing the scrotal skin to part without retraction.
2. The surgeon makes a 1- to 2-cm vertical incision, taking care to avoid injury to the epididymis.
3. The incision is continued to the tunica vaginalis. As the tunica is incised, there should be a normal efflux of clear fluid.
4. Absorbable 4-0 stay sutures are placed in the tunica vaginalis. Two more are placed in the tunica albuginea.
5. Using the scalpel in a shaving action, no-touch technique, the surgeon resects a small ellipse of tunica with its tubules. The tissue is placed in the fixative or sent to the histology department as a fresh specimen.
6. The wound is closed in three layers with 3-0 and 4-0 absorbable suture.
7. Gauze sponges and fluffed dressings are placed over and around the scrotum. A scrotal support is applied to provide pressure and support.

Orchiectomy

An orchiectomy is the removal of the testis or testes. Removal of both testes is castration and renders the patient sterile and deficient in the hormone *testosterone,* which is responsible for development of secondary sexual characteristics and potency. This operation, like vasectomy, has legal implications that require attention to acquiring informed consent for surgery. Bilateral orchiectomy is usually performed to control symptomatic metastatic carcinoma of the prostate gland. A unilateral orchiectomy is indicated because of testicular cancer, trauma, or infection. Testicular cancer is the most common solid malignancy affecting males between the ages of 15 and 35. Germ cell tumors account for 95% of testicular tumors. Testicular tumors usually present as a nodule or painless swelling of one testicle. Approximately 30% to 40% of patients complain of a dull ache or heavy sensation in the lower abdomen, perianal area, or scrotum, whereas acute pain is the presenting symptom in 10%. Gynecomastia presents as a symptom caused by metastases. Evaluation of the patient includes physical examination, ultrasound, CT, or MRI as well as serum beta human chorionic gonadotropin (hCG) and alpha-fetoprotein (AFP) (Light, 2015). Testicular implants are available for cosmetic purposes. These must be ordered preoperatively based on preoperative measurements for size. This procedure has recently been approached through endoscopic techniques, usually in conjunction with laparoscopic herniorrhaphy.

Procedural Considerations

The perioperative nurse assists with positioning the patient supine, and the anesthesia provider administers a general, spinal, or regional anesthetic. A minor instrument setup is required.

Operative Procedure
Scrotal Approach

1. For benign conditions the incision is made over the anterolateral surface of the midportion of the scrotum.
2. The surgeon carries the skin incision through the subcutaneous and fascial layers through the tunica vaginalis, exposing the testicle.
3. Retractors are placed, and bleeding vessels are clamped and ligated.
4. The spermatic cord is divided into two or three vascular bundles. Each vascular bundle is doubly clamped, cut, and ligated, first with 0 absorbable suture ligature and then with a proximal free 0 absorbable tie.
5. The vas is separately ligated with a 0 absorbable tie. The testis is removed.
6. The procedure is repeated on the opposite side if bilateral excision is planned.

Inguinal Approach

1. For malignant conditions the incision is begun just above the internal ring, extending downward and inward over the inguinal canal to the external inguinal ring.
2. The surgeon exposes the inguinal canal and dissects the spermatic cord free, cross-clamps it, and divides it into vascular bundles at the internal ring.
3. Gentle forward traction is applied to the cord, which is dissected from its bed.
4. The testis is everted into the wound from the scrotum and excised.
5. The procedure is repeated on the opposite side if bilateral excision is planned.
6. Bleeding is controlled with the ESU. A small drain may be placed in the empty hemiscrotum if desired.
7. The surgeon reapproximates the external oblique fascia with 2-0 absorbable interrupted sutures.
8. Subcutaneous tissue, including Scarpa fascia, is closed with 4-0 absorbable sutures.
9. The skin is reapproximated with surgical staples or 4-0 subcuticular sutures.

Radical Lymphadenectomy (Retroperitoneal Lymph Node Dissection)

Radical lymphadenectomy is a bilateral resection of retroperitoneal lymph nodes. Lymph node dissection is performed for treatment of nonseminomatous testicular tumors or in conjunction with an open prostatectomy for prostate cancer. Dissection usually includes lymph nodes, channels, and fat around both renal pedicles; the vena cava; and the aorta, including the bifurcation of the aorta.

Procedural Considerations

The perioperative nurse assists with placing the patient in the supine position. The anesthesia provider administers a general anesthetic. If the dissection is unilateral, the patient is supine with the operative side tilted upward. Long, fine dissection instruments along with basic laparotomy instruments are required.

Although this procedure may be performed laparoscopically, this approach has not yet become the standard of practice because of its technical difficulty.

Operative Procedure

1. The surgeon makes a midline abdominal incision from the xiphoid process to the symphysis pubis.
2. The abdominal contents are explored to determine the degree of gross nodal involvement. The colon is either packed within the abdominal cavity or mobilized and kept moist outside the abdomen.
3. The surgeon opens the posterior peritoneum between the aorta and the vena cava.
4. Using blunt and sharp dissection, the surgeon removes the lymphatic structures and fat en bloc from around both renal pedicles, the vena cava, and the aorta from above the renal hilum to beyond the bifurcation of the iliac vessels on the side of the original testicular neoplasm.
5. The spermatic vessels of the affected side are removed down to and including the stump of the previous orchiectomy.
6. The inferior mesenteric artery may be sacrificed if technically necessary, but the superior mesenteric artery is not disturbed.
7. The ureter on the affected side is skeletonized to remove any perilymphatic tissue.
8. If reperitonealization is desired, the posterior peritoneum is closed with a 2-0 absorbable continuous suture.
9. The surgeon repositions the viscera into the abdominal cavity, and closes the wound in layers, usually without placement of a drain.

Surgery of the Prostate Gland

Glandular hyperplasia of the prostatic urethra usually manifests itself after 50 years of age. Prostatic enlargement may be benign or malignant and may occur in one or more lobes of the prostate but most frequently occurs in the lateral or median lobes. Progressive growth of the hyperplastic gland compresses the remaining normal prostatic tissue, forming what is called a *surgical capsule*. The growth of adenomatous tissue slowly encroaches on the prostatic urethral lumen, causing obstruction of urinary outflow. The surgeon and patient must consider several factors when determining the best route for removal of the prostatic obstruction: the age and medical condition of the patient, the size of the gland and location of the pathologic condition, and the presence of associated medical disease (Patient Engagement Exemplar).

Prostate cancer is the most frequently diagnosed cancer in men, and is the second leading cause of cancer death in American men, behind only lung cancer (ACS, 2016a, 2016b). Because of the prevalence of prostate cancer and the similarity of symptoms to BPH, the American Urological Association (AUA) recommends that starting at age 40 the PSA test and digital rectal examination (DRE) should be offered to men at average risk (Evidence for Practice).

A blood sample is drawn to determine the PSA level, followed by a DRE. The blood is often drawn first because manipulation of the gland has been known to alter the efficacy of the PSA test. The PSA test is considered a valuable tool for early detection of carcinoma of the prostate, but if used alone, it will miss 20% to 30% of all prostate cancers. If the test value is elevated, the patient is at risk for carcinoma of the prostate; a PSA value greater than 10 ng/mL is highly suggestive of prostatic carcinoma. PSA tests cut metastatic prostate cancer rates by 50% (Castellino, 2015). Clinical evaluation and an elevated PSA usually indicate the need for a transrectal ultrasound needle biopsy to confirm the diagnosis. When the results of the biopsy are positive for malignancy, additional diagnostic studies are indicated including measurement of free and total serum PSA II levels, bone scans, and CT and MRI scans of the pelvis (Jemal et al., 2015).

The most commonly used system to grade prostate cancer is the Gleason score. To calculate the Gleason score, the pathologist evaluates

PATIENT ENGAGEMENT EXEMPLAR

Centered Care: Use of a Questionnaire

The AHRQ notes that in a patient-centered model, patients become active participants in their own care and receive services designed to focus on their individual needs and preferences, in addition to advice and counsel from health professionals.

One method that can be useful to engage the patient is a symptom severity questionnaire. An example of a patient-centered care questionnaire is the AUA severity index for ranking BPH symptoms. Because BPH is rarely life-threatening but can have a considerable effect on a patient's quality of life, treatments are more preference driven than for conditions such as cancer, so patients must be involved more fully in treatment decisions.

Each of the seven questions included asks the patient to rank a particular symptom on a scale of 0 to 5, with 5 being the most severe. The symptoms are incomplete emptying, frequency, intermittency, urgency, weak urinary stream, hesitancy, and nocturia. On completion of the test, the numbers are added up to determine the overall severity of BPH-related symptoms. Based on these totals, the patient's symptoms are classified as mild, moderate, or severe.

Measures of symptoms and BPH-specific health status provide the most detailed and sensitive measures of treatment

effectiveness from the patient's perspective, according to AHRQ-funded researchers.

The AUA severity index is described below:

1. Over the past month or so, how often have you had a sensation of not emptying your bladder completely after you finished urinating?
2. Over the past month or so, how often have you had to urinate again less than 2 hours after you finished urinating?
3. Over the past month or so, how often have you found you stopped and started again several times when you urinated?
4. Over the past month or so, how often have you found it difficult to postpone urination?
5. Over the past month or so, how often have you had a weak urinary stream?
6. Over the past month or so, how often have you had to push or strain to begin urination?
7. Over the last month, how many times did you usually get up to urinate from the time you went to bed at night until the time you got up in the morning?

For questions 1–6, there is a choice of six possible answers: never; less than one time in five; less than half the time; about half the time; more than half the time; almost always. Question 7 has six possible answers, ranging from 0 to 5 or more.

AHRQ, Agency for Healthcare Research and Quality; *AUA*, American Urological Association; *BPH*, benign prostatic hyperplasia.
Modified from Agency for Healthcare Research and Quality (AHRQ): *Expanding patient-centered care to empower patients and assist providers* (website), 2002. https://archive.ahrq.gov/research/findings/factsheets/patient-centered/ria-issue5/ria-issue5.html. (Accessed 3 December 2016); American Urological Association (AUA): *BPH symptom score index* (website). http://www.dupagemedicalgroup.com/userfiles/file/patientForms/symptom-score-sheet-bph%20copy.pdf. (Accessed 3 December 2016).

the prostatic tissue to determine which type of cell is the most common and which type is the second most common and gives each of the two cell types a score from 1 to 5. The two scores are combined to determine the total score. Higher numbers are an indication of more abnormal, aggressive cancer cells. Men with a Gleason score of 2 to 4 are generally cured by surgery; scores from 5 to 6 indicate mildly aggressive cancer cells; a score of 7 indicates the cancer is moderately aggressive. Scores between 8 and 10 indicate highly aggressive tumors and are associated with a poor prognosis after surgery (Barocas et al., 2015). Additional prostate cancer-staging tools are the tumor, node, metastasis (TNM) system and the AUA system (Box 15.1).

If the prostate gland is cancerous, a radical retropubic or radical perineal prostatectomy, in conjunction with open or laparoscopic pelvic lymph node dissection, is usually performed. TURP may also be used in men who cannot have a radical prostatectomy, or to relieve symptoms caused by prostate cancer before other treatments begin. Select patients with well-differentiated or moderately differentiated lesions may be candidates for transperineal, ultrasonically guided implantation of radium seeds (brachytherapy) or cryoablation of the prostate (cryotherapy). Newer therapies for detection and treatment of prostate cancer are being developed (Research Highlight). Many patients desire to retain sexual function. The surgeon may attempt to save the neurovascular bundles in what is termed a nerve-sparing approach. The site and size of the prostatic lesion, however, often determine whether this can be achieved successfully and without undue risk to the patient.

BOX 15.1

American Urological Association Prostate Cancer Stages

Stage A: Clinically Unsuspected Disease
A1   Focal carcinoma, well differentiated
A2   Diffuse carcinoma, usually poorly differentiated

Stage B: Tumor Confined to Prostate Gland
B1   Small, discrete nodule of one lobe of the gland
B2   Large or multiple nodules or areas of involvement

Stage C: Tumor Localized to Periprostatic Area
C1   Tumor outside prostate capsule, estimated weight ≤70 g, seminal vesicles uninvolved
C2   Tumor outside prostate capsule, estimated weight >70 g, seminal vesicles involved

Stage D: Metastatic Prostate Cancer
D1   Pelvic lymph node metastases or ureteral obstruction causing hydronephrosis, or both
D2   Bone, soft tissue, organ, or distant lymph node metastases

Modified from Nelson WG et al: Prostate cancer. In Abeloff MD et al, editors: *Abeloff's clinical oncology*, ed 5, Philadelphia, 2014, Churchill Livingstone.

EVIDENCE FOR PRACTICE

Diagnosing and Managing Prostate Cancer

Early detection is important in diagnosing and managing prostate cancer. Information relating to a patient's profile in initiating the algorithm includes the following:

Risk Factors

1. *Age:* After 50 years old, the risk increases rapidly; about 64% of all prostate cancer cases are diagnosed in men ages 65 and older. Although the lifetime risk for prostate cancer is 3%, prostate cancer is the most common noncutaneous cancer in men in the United States, and the second leading cause of male cancer mortality.
2. *Race:* African American men and Jamaican men of African descent have the highest prostate cancer incidence rates in the world.

3. *Diet:* High dietary fat is associated with a greater risk for developing cancer.
4. *Family history:* Risk is increased for men who have first-degree relatives with prostate cancer.

Candidates for Early Detection (USPSTF)

1. Screening of asymptomatic men ages 55 to 69 years

Diagnostic Measures Used in Combination for Early Detection (USPSTF)

1. DRE
2. Ultrasonography may be included.

Screening for Prostate Cancer: Clinical Summary of USPSTF Recommendation

Population	Adult males
Recommendation	**Do not use PSA-based screening for prostate cancer. Grade: D**
Screening tests	Contemporary recommendations for prostate cancer screening all incorporate the measurement of serum PSA levels; other methods of detection, such as digital rectal examination or ultrasonography, may be included. There is convincing evidence that PSA-based screening programs result in the detection of many cases of asymptomatic prostate cancer, and that a substantial percentage of men who have asymptomatic cancer detected by PSA screening have a tumor that either will not progress or will progress so slowly that it would have remained asymptomatic for the man's lifetime (i.e., PSA-based screening results in considerable overdiagnosis).
Interventions	Management strategies for localized prostate cancer include watchful waiting, active surveillance, surgery, and radiation therapy. There is no consensus regarding optimal treatment.
Balance of harms and benefits	• The reduction in prostate cancer mortality 10 to 14 years after PSA-based screening is, at most, very small, even for men in the optimal age range of 55 to 69 years. • The harms of screening include pain, fever, bleeding, infection, and transient urinary difficulties associated with prostate biopsy, psychological harm of false-positive test results, and overdiagnosis. • Harms of treatment include erectile dysfunction, urinary incontinence, bowel dysfunction, and a small risk for premature death. • Because of the current inability to reliably distinguish tumors that will remain indolent from those destined to be lethal, many men are being subjected to the harms of treatment for prostate cancer that will never become symptomatic. • The benefits of PSA-based screening for prostate cancer do not outweigh the harms.
Relevant USPSTF recommendations	Recommendations on screening for other types of cancer can be found at https://www.uspreventiveservicestaskforce.org/.

For a summary of the evidence systematically reviewed in making these recommendations, the full recommendation statement, and supporting documents, please go to https://www.uspreventiveservicestaskforce.org/.

Disclaimer: Recommendations made by the USPSTF are independent of the US government. They should not be construed as an official position of the Agency for Healthcare Research and Quality or the US Department of Health and Human Services.

DRE, Digital rectal exam, *PSA,* prostatic-specific antigen; *USPSTF,* US Preventive Services Task Force.
From US Preventive Services Task Force (USPSTF): *Clinical summary: prostate cancer: screening* (website), March 2017. https://www.uspreventiveservicestaskforce.org/Page/Document/ClinicalSummaryFinal/prostate-cancer-screening. (Accessed 1 December 2017).

Surgery for prostate enlargement may be preceded with a biopsy procedure. Depending on the results of the biopsy, a variety of procedures are available to address the benign or malignant condition.

Prostatic Core Needle Biopsy

Needle biopsy of the prostate is indicated for patients in whom prostatic cancer is clinically suspected. It may be accomplished transrectally with a needle designed for this purpose or transperineally.

Procedural Considerations

Needle biopsy of the prostate has the risk of both intraoperative and postoperative bleeding. A cystoscopic examination may accompany a needle biopsy. Most needle biopsies are performed in the surgeon's office or ultrasound department.

The most significant potential complication of a biopsy is systemic infection. This risk can be decreased with antibiotic administration before and after the procedure and bowel cleansing before the

---

RESEARCH HIGHLIGHT

Promising Biopsy Technique Transrectal Ultrasound/ Magnetic Resonance Imaging Fusion

One of the most promising newer biopsy techniques is TRUS/ MRI fusion. It combines the familiarity of real-time TRUS guidance with detailed information from an MRI. A prebiopsy MRI identifies target lesions suspicious for cancer based on imaging characteristics. TRUS of the prostate is performed with MRI, and real-time images are combined creating a 3D prostate reconstruction which allows rapid identification of the MRI target lesions for biopsy in minutes. Two TRUS/MRI fusion systems approved by the FDA are available in the United States. The UroNav platform (Phillips/Invivo, Gainesville, FL) has the largest collection of published data to date and has been under study at the National Cancer Institute since 2004. The other is the Artemis Platform with ProFuse (Eigen, Grass Valle, CA), which uses a mechanical arm to direct the biopsy. Several other manufacturers are developing systems in the United States and abroad.

FDA, US Food and Drug Administration; *MRI,* magnetic resonance imaging; *TRUS,* transrectal ultrasound.
From Raskolnikov D et al: Current ability of multiparametric prostate magnetic resonance imaging and targeted biopsy to improve the detection of prostate cancer, *Urol Pract* 1(1):13–21, 2014.

examination. The patient takes antibiotics 24 hours before the procedure and is advised to use a sodium phosphate enema 2 to 3 hours before the test is performed. Before the examination, an antiseptic solution mixed with a viscous local anesthetic often is instilled into the rectum and allowed to coat the tissues for 5 to 15 minutes. The surgeon may also inject local anesthetic into the prostate and seminal vesicles transrectally with a 22-gauge, 22-cm injection needle through the needle guide on the transducer.

Operative Procedure

Transrectal, Ultrasonically Guided Biopsy. Transrectal, ultrasonically guided biopsy is commonly performed in the surgeon's office using a high-frequency transrectal ultrasound transducer to assess the prostate gland. The technique allows the surgeon to assess the size, volume, and shape of the prostate and the likelihood of the presence of a malignancy. Biopsy specimens of suspicious areas or lesions may be obtained with a needle passed across the rectal wall, with the aid of ultrasound guidance. The needle penetrates the rectal mucosa with a core biopsy system. Color-flow imaging may also be used to help identify areas that are likely invaded with prostatic carcinoma or have acute and chronic inflammation. Highly vascular areas carry a greater probability of harboring a carcinoma. A full bladder helps delineate the base of the prostate.

The surgeon visualizes the prostate in three dimensions, allowing more accurate localization of abnormalities and extent of disease. For the axial view, the transrectal transducer is placed deeply into the rectum, just proximal to the seminal vesicles, to about 10 cm above the anal verge. Here the vas deferens may be distinguished. The transducer is slowly withdrawn to the level of the base of the gland, enabling visualization of the inner gland. Seminal vesicles are seen in cross section. To evaluate the prostate in the sagittal planes, the surgeon rotates the probe clockwise or counterclockwise (Fig. 15.23). A series of 12 biopsy specimens is generally taken with a disposable "core biopsy" needle. These are taken from the right and left medial and lateral apices, the right and left midline, and the right and left medial and lateral bases. Lesions as small as 2 to 3 mm are visible with this procedure.

Transperineal Biopsy. The perioperative nurse assists with placing the patient in the lithotomy or lateral position. The procedure may be performed with the patient receiving a general, regional, or local anesthetic. The surgeon performs a rectal examination to identify the induration. The needle is inserted through the perineal skin and guided ahead until the tip is against the lesion. The biopsy specimen

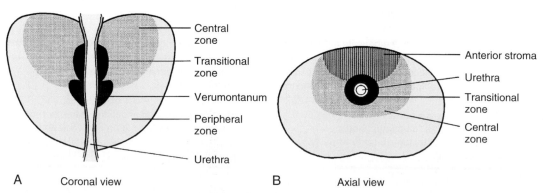

A   Coronal view   B   Axial view

FIG. 15.23 Schematic drawing of zonal anatomy of the prostate (*nonshaded area* is peripheral zone). (A) Coronal view. (B) Axial view.

is taken in the same fashion as described for the transrectal approach. Some surgeons may incise the site with the #11 or #15 blade and place a 4-0 absorbable closing suture.

The surgeon may also use the transperineal approach to perform template biopsies with ultrasound guidance, using the brachytherapy (seed implant) template. The perioperative nurse assists with placing the patient in the lithotomy position, and secures his scrotum toward the abdomen with a transparent adhesive dressing. The surgeon positions the brachytherapy grid, template fixation device, and probe with cradle adjacent to the patient's perineum. Using the ultrasonic transrectal transducer the surgeon measures the prostate and calculates its total volume. Biopsies are then obtained transperineally through the template grid.

Transurethral Resection of the Prostate Gland

During a TURP, the surgeon passes a resectoscope into the bladder through the urethra and resects successive pieces of tissue from around the bladder neck and the lobes of the prostate gland, leaving the capsule intact. The resectoscope has a stabilized cutting loop that is used to resect tissue and coagulate blood vessels by means of electric current. The electric current that powers the electrode is supplied by a high-frequency ESU. The current settings are specified by the surgeon, who activates the cutting or coagulating current with a foot pedal during the course of the procedure.

TURP is one surgical method of treating benign obstructive enlargement of the prostate gland. Several factors influence the surgical approach: size of the gland and location of the pathologic condition, age and condition of the patient, and presence of associated diseases.

Procedural Considerations

The instrument setup for TURP is as described for cystoscopy with additional necessary instruments. The four principal types of resectoscopes are McCarthy, Nesbit, Iglesias, and Baumrucker. Adult resectoscopes range in size from 24F to 28F and have the following components: foroblique telescope, operating element, cutting loops, and postresectoscope sheaths and obturators. A TURP requires a resectoscope (multiple working elements); a foroblique telescope as well as a backup telescope; stabilized or unstabilized cutting loops; a postresectoscope sheath with its corresponding articulated obturator; a high-frequency cord; a short bridge; a Toomey syringe or the Ellik or Urovac evacuator; van Buren sounds; a 22F or 24F, 30 mL, three-way Foley catheter; a disposable urologic drape with rectal sheath; and a system for CBI and urinary drainage. Supplementary instruments include a resectoscope adapter and a lateral telescope.

The continuous-flow resectoscope (CFR) has unique components that include an outlet stopcock to which a suction tube is attached, an inflow tube on the inner sheath, and outflow holes on the outer sheath. These features enable the surgeon to resect tissue without interruption to empty the bladder, which also must be done with the standard resectoscope. In addition to the CFR, which replaces the standard resectoscope, the setup includes thick-walled Silastic suction tubing and a continuous-flow pump. The continuous-flow technique decreases intravesical pressure on the bladder during the procedure, provides a clearer field of vision because of the constant inflow and outflow of irrigant, and reduces the operating time because the resection process does not need to be interrupted to evacuate the bladder. It also provides a "still" bladder for the resection of bladder tumors.

A continuous flow of isotonic and nonelectrolytic irrigating fluid is necessary to ensure transmission of electric current and clear visualization throughout surgery. Irrigating solution such as 3% sorbitol or 1.5% glycine, 3 to 5 L, may be connected in tandem to provide a constant flow. Warming units, available for these solutions, help eliminate the hypothermia often experienced when large amounts of cold irrigants are used. On the other hand, when solutions are warm, the patient may show a tendency to bleed more. The perioperative nurse must remain alert to the status of the irrigation solution and replace it as required.

During transurethral prostatic surgery, the return of irrigation fluid must be monitored because intravasation and absorption of fluid into open prostatic venous sinuses or bladder perforation may occur. The perioperative nurse should be aware of the early signs and symptoms and measures used to remedy these complications (Collins and Terris, 2014). The patient usually experiences significant respiratory changes and abdominal discomfort. Continued extravasation and absorption can lead to hypovolemia and hyponatremia. Other important observations are rigidity and swelling of the lower abdomen, coupled with changes in sensorium. If extravasation of irrigating fluid is evident, the surgical procedure is discontinued and a cystogram is obtained immediately to determine whether bladder perforation has occurred. Insertion of a Foley catheter is generally all that is necessary to control the situation. In the rare instance of a major perforation, surgical closure may be accomplished through a cystotomy incision.

Operative Procedure

1. The surgeon dilates the urethra with sounds sized from 20F to 30F.
2. Cystourethroscopy is performed to assess the degree of prostatic obstruction and to inspect the bladder. Some surgeons perform this diagnostic procedure several days before surgery, whereas others perform the examination in the OR immediately before surgery.
3. The surgeon passes a well-lubricated postresectoscope sheath with its fitted Timberlake obturator into the urethra.
4. The Timberlake obturator is removed, and the working element (resectoscope), assembled with the foroblique telescope and cutting loop, is inserted through the sheath.
5. The irrigation tubing, light cord, and high-frequency cord are appropriately connected, and the surgeon opens the stopcock to allow the irrigation fluid to fill the bladder.
6. With the bladder distended, the surgeon inspects the prostatic urethra and bladder trigone.
7. After determining the location of the ureteral orifice, the surgeon begins electrodissection, alternating cutting and coagulating currents as required (Fig. 15.24).
8. The bladder is drained, washing out prostatic tissue and small blood clots. At times the surgeon may use the Ellik evacuator to remove resected prostatic tissue. The Ellik is used by removing the working element of the resectoscope, fitting the nozzle of the evacuator onto the resectoscope sheath, and removing the bladder contents by manual pulsatile pressure. The scrub person ensures an Ellik or Urovac evacuator or a Toomey syringe is readily available for manual irrigation. Fluid may be drawn from the irrigant directly into the resectoscope sheath through the already attached tubing.
9. When the resection is completed, the surgeon inspects the prostatic fossa to ensure that all bleeding points have been coagulated.

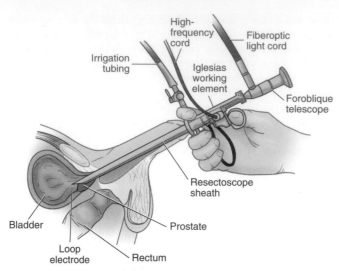

FIG. 15.24 Sectional view illustrating removal of portion of hypertrophied middle lobe of prostate gland with Iglesias resectoscope.

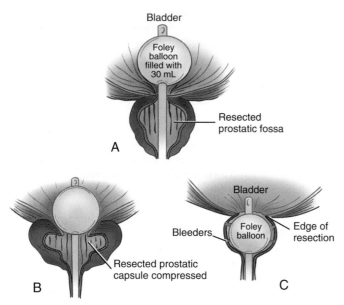

FIG. 15.25 (A and B) Proper position for Foley catheter with inflated balloon beyond prostatic capsule. (C) Improper position.

10. The resectoscope is then removed, and a Foley catheter (22F or 24F, two-way or three-way, 30-mL balloon) is inserted into the bladder for urinary drainage. The balloon is inflated (Fig. 15.25A), pulled gently in traction against the bladder neck, and secured, to help control venous bleeding (see Fig. 15.25B). The Foley balloon must not be inflated within the prostatic fossa (see Fig. 15.25C), in which it may cause excessive bleeding from the resected prostatic capsule. If desired, continuous irrigation with gravity drainage is initiated, with normal saline as the bladder irrigant instead of sorbitol or glycine. A 3- to 4-L urinary drainage system is suggested to avoid frequent emptying of the drainage bag.

Transurethral Incision of the Prostate

Transurethral incision of the prostate (TUIP) is a procedure in which the prostate is incised at the 5 and 7 o'clock positions to provide relief of obstruction, with results similar to those provided by a complete transurethral resection but with a lower incidence of bladder neck contracture and retrograde ejaculation. The shorter operative time inherent with the procedure minimizes fluid absorption and may decrease postoperative pulmonary and cardiovascular complications. The procedure may be performed with cold or hot knives as well as the standard resectoscope, or laser fiber (TULIP). This procedure is appropriate for sexually active patients with moderate to small obstructive prostates without a significant middle-lobe component. One major disadvantage is the potential for missing occult prostatic cancer. Despite this, some clinicians view this as an underused, feasible form of treatment.

Transurethral Incision of the Ejaculatory Ducts

Transurethral incision of the ejaculatory ducts is performed for the relief of obstructed ejaculatory ducts, a common condition in men with chronic prostatitis and prostatic calculi. Symptoms closely mimic prostatodynia and include aching in the perineal and genital areas with no lasting or significant improvement from conservative therapy (antibiotics and analgesics). The resectoscope loop is guided with transrectal ultrasound imaging to the dilated ejaculatory ducts, and the obstructed ducts are resected. Calculi may be fragmented if necessary and removed. A catheter generally is not needed.

Photoselective Vaporization of the Prostate

The KTP laser is now used to treat BPH or prostatic enlargement. *Green-light photoselective vaporization of the prostate (PVP)* is a new minimally invasive approach performed on an ambulatory basis. The approach is the same as with other endoscopic techniques. A noncontact laser fiber is used to heat the prostate tissue and rapidly vaporize it to a penetration depth of 0.8 mm with minimal to no blood loss. Vaporization occurs from within the tissues, in which the collagen matrix eventually bursts as a result of the vapor buildup. The laser is operated in a continuous wave mode and induces a coagulation zone of only 1 to 2 mm in thickness. This prevents the excessive sloughing of necrotic tissue. The patient may not always need a Foley catheter after the procedure.

Interstitial Laser Coagulation of the Prostate

Interstitial laser coagulation (ILC) with the Indigo laser is a minimally invasive procedure for treatment of urinary outflow obstruction secondary to BPH. It is indicated for men older than 50 years with a median or lateral prostatic lobe volume of 20 to 85 mL. Designed for those men who wish to minimize the risk for incontinence and impotence found with conventional TURP, this procedure is now performed in the office setting about 80% of the time.

The procedure is contraindicated for the treatment of prostate cancer and for those patients who had previous brachytherapy with radioactive seeds. However, some physicians may elect to perform ILC before brachytherapy (or cryotherapy) in the hopes of minimizing, if not relieving, the postoperative voiding symptoms associated with these more definitive treatments.

Procedural Considerations

The patient is placed in the lithotomy position and prepped as for cystoscopy. An optional local anesthetic with oral or monitored IV sedation is generally adequate. Oral sedation is used more commonly with the office-based procedure; if the surgery takes place in the hospital or ambulatory center, monitored IV sedation may be used. An ultrasound machine with transrectal capability is often used to measure the size of the prostate gland and determine the appropriate

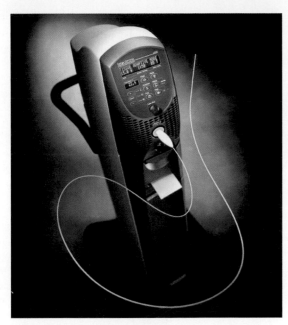

FIG. 15.26 Indigo Optima laser unit with diffuser-tip fiber.

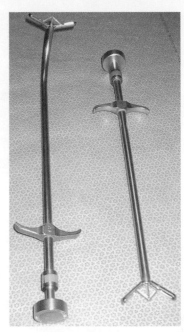

FIG. 15.27 Curved and straight Lowsley tractors in open position.

number of laser applications (sticks). Some surgeons choose to measure by cystoscopy alone.

The setup includes a 17F or 23F panendoscope and 30-degree fiberoptic lens, ultrasound and transrectal transducer, and the Indigo laser machine with laser fiber (Fig. 15.26). The fiber has graduated black depth markings used to guide placement into the prostate gland. The laser machine automatically times each "stick" for 2 minutes, 30 seconds. The perioperative nurse ensures that all laser safety precautions are observed (see Chapter 8).

Operative Procedure

1. The surgeon inserts the transrectal transducer and measures the prostatic volume. (This may have been performed as an office procedure preoperatively.) Local anesthetic may be injected through the transducer guide pin with an 8-inch spinal needle or with the 8-inch collagen injection needle if ultrasound is not used.
2. Cystoscopy is performed, and the prostatic urethra is evaluated.
3. The surgeon introduces the laser fiber through the panendoscope and passes it into the lateral lobe of the prostate gland through the urethral wall to the desired depth.
4. This is repeated one to three times on each side, depending on the measured prostatic volume.
5. A TUIP may be performed using the bare-tip fiber.
6. A 16F or 18F urethral catheter is inserted and connected to straight drainage. A 16F suprapubic Foley catheter may also be used and attached to irrigation or drainage.

Transurethral Microwave Therapy/Transurethral Needle Ablation

Transurethral microwave therapy (TUMT) is a minimally invasive method of applying heat to the prostate gland for the relief of the symptoms associated with BPH and bladder-outlet obstruction. TUMT maintains temperatures in the urethra, sphincter, and rectum at a level that is physiologically safe while heating the tissue deep within the transitional zone of the prostate. A water-cooled catheter is combined with microwave radiation to the lobes of the prostate. This treatment is an office-based procedure.

Transurethral needle ablation (TUNA) is also a minimally invasive office procedure for the treatment of BPH of the median and lateral lobes. This technique delivers radiofrequency (RF) energy through two electrodes that are embedded in a special urethral catheter. Specific target areas of the prostate are thermally ablated by the RF energy and combined inductive heating of water molecules, leaving the urethra and the remainder of the prostate intact.

Simple Retropubic Prostatectomy

Simple retropubic prostatectomy is the enucleation of hypertrophic prostatic tissue through an incision in the anterior prostatic capsule by an extravesical approach. The retropubic approach offers excellent exposure of the prostate bed and vesical neck and readily controllable intraoperative and postoperative bleeding.

A preoperative bowel prep and antibiotic therapy are the standards of care for all open prostatectomies.

Procedural Considerations

The perioperative nurse assists with positioning the patient in a slight Trendelenburg position with the pelvis elevated and the legs slightly abducted. Although the draping procedure must conform to individual OR policies, the following procedure is suggested for draping the patient:

1. The first towel, with a cuff, is placed under the scrotum.
2. The next three towels are placed around the lower abdominal incision site, followed by a sterile laparotomy sheet.
3. A fifth towel, folded in half, is placed over the penis and scrotum below the retropubic incision site and secured with two nonperforating towel clamps.

The instrument setup includes a basic laparotomy set and bladder and prostatic instruments (Figs. 15.27 and 15.28). The following supplies should be readily available: Jackson-Pratt drains; water-soluble lubricant; Toomey and Asepto syringes; urinary drainage system; 20F, 5-mL Foley catheter; 22F or 24F, 30-mL Foley catheter; 10- and 30-mL syringes; and a self-retaining retractor (Fig. 15.29).

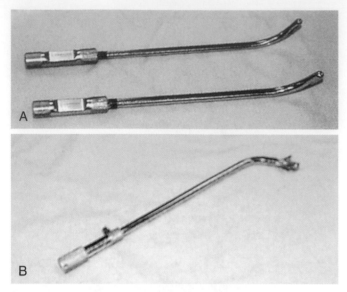

FIG. 15.28 (A) Urethral suture guides. (B) Roth grip-tip urethral suture guide.

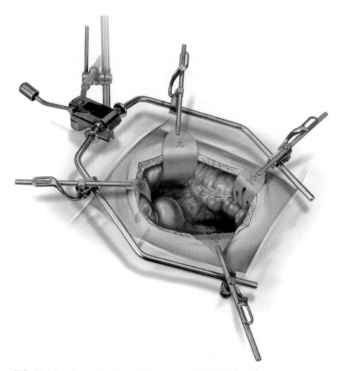

FIG. 15.29 Adjustable Omni-Tract surgical UO400 urology retractor system.

Operative Procedure

1. The surgeon inserts a 20F or 22F Foley catheter with 30-mL balloon into the urethra and through the bladder neck and inflates it. This is clamped and maintained within the sterile field. Frequently a three-way catheter is used for CBI.
2. Through a Pfannenstiel or low vertical midline incision, the surgeon incises the anterior rectus sheath along with portions of the internal and external oblique muscles.
3. The rectus abdominis muscles are retracted laterally to expose the space of Retzius.

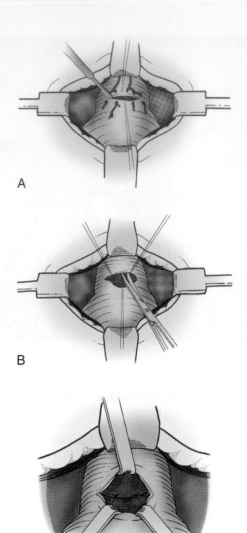

FIG. 15.30 Retropubic prostatectomy.

4. After placement of traction sutures, the anterior portion of the prostatic capsule is incised transversely (Fig. 15.30A).
5. The prostatic adenoma may be dissected or finger enucleated from the surgical capsule (see Fig. 15.30B).
6. The surgeon places hemostatic sutures at the 5 and 7 o'clock positions, encompassing the vesical neck and prostatic capsule, to ligate the primary blood supply to the prostate. Other bleeding points within the capsule may be suture ligated with 2-0 absorbable sutures.
7. The prostatic capsule incision is closed with either a continuous or an interrupted 0 absorbable suture (see Fig. 15.30C).
8. A drain is placed in the space of Retzius and exteriorized through the fascia and skin via a separate stab incision.
9. The abdominal incision is then closed in layers, and the wound is dressed.
10. If CBI is to be used, normal saline solution irrigation is initiated through a 3-L closed irrigation system.

Suprapubic Prostatectomy

Suprapubic prostatectomy is the removal, through a transvesical approach, of periurethral glandular tissue obstructing the outlet of the urinary tract. A low midline, or Pfannenstiel, incision may be used. One advantage of the suprapubic approach is that it allows access for surgical correction of any existing bladder condition such as vesical calculi or vesical diverticula. Control of bleeding is a major consideration in any prostatectomy and is one disadvantage of the suprapubic approach. Because the prostate is located beneath the symphysis pubis, ligation of bleeding capsular vessels is difficult. However, control of hemorrhage and replacement of blood loss, coupled with skilled perioperative nursing care and early mobilization of the patient, have greatly minimized complications.

Procedural Considerations

Spinal, epidural, or general anesthesia may be selected for patients having a suprapubic prostatectomy, depending on their medical condition. The patient is placed in a slight Trendelenburg position with the umbilicus elevated and the legs slightly abducted. Draping and instrumentation are as described for retropubic prostatectomy.

Operative Procedure

1. The surgeon inserts a 20F or 22F Foley catheter with 30-mL balloon into the urethra and through the bladder neck and inflates it. This is clamped and maintained within the sterile field. This maneuver facilitates identification of the bladder.
2. A transverse or midline lower abdominal incision is made through the skin and the two layers of superficial fascia (Fig. 15.31A).
3. The external and internal oblique muscles are cut along the lines of the original incision.
4. The surgeon clamps, electrocoagulates, or ligates any bleeding vessels.
5. The rectus muscles are separated in the midline and retracted laterally.
6. After the placement of traction sutures, the surgeon opens the bladder at the dome with a scalpel. Liquid contents are aspirated, and the bladder incision is enlarged.
7. The bladder is visually and manually explored for calculi, a tumor, or diverticula.
8. The surgeon manually enucleates the adenomatous tissue using the tip of the index finger inserted through the vesical neck into the prostatic urethra (see Fig. 15.31B). If difficulty is experienced with the enucleation, the surgical assistant may place a finger into the rectum to elevate the prostate gland. Aseptic technique is maintained during enucleation with the use of a sterile second glove on the hand used in the rectum.
9. After enucleation is completed, attention is directed to maintaining good hemostasis by suture ligation of the vesical neck at the 5 and 7 o'clock positions. Other significant bleeding points may also be ligated.
10. A suprapubic catheter is placed into the bladder lumen through a small stab incision.
11. A 22F or 24F, two-way or three-way Foley catheter with a 30-mL balloon is inserted into the urethra in place of the original one, and the balloon is inflated to a size that prevents the catheter from falling or being pulled into the prostatic fossa (see Fig. 15.31C).
12. The surgeon closes the cystotomy incision with interrupted 2-0 absorbable sutures.
13. A drain is left along the cystotomy incision, exteriorized through a separate stab wound, and secured to the skin with a silk suture.
14. The muscles, fascia, and subcutaneous tissues are closed in layers, and a dressing is applied.
15. To reduce clot formation and maintain catheter patency, normal saline irrigation solution may be connected to the Foley catheter

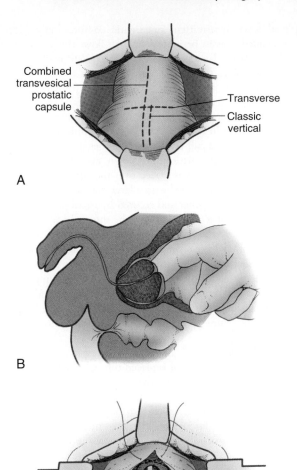

FIG. 15.31 Suprapubic prostatectomy.

to provide continuous irrigation to the bladder. Continuous irrigation may be initiated during closure.

Simple Perineal Prostatectomy

Simple perineal prostatectomy is the removal of the prostate gland through a perineal approach. A perineal approach is most suitable when an open prostatic biopsy is desired and, after receipt of pathologic confirmation, radical excision is to follow. Other advantages include preservation of the bladder neck, improved urethrovesical anastomosis, and easier control of bleeding. Some surgical disadvantages are (1) inability to perform biopsy of the iliac and obturator nodes for determining extension of disease and (2) possible formation of urethrorectal fistulas.

Procedural Considerations

The patient is placed in an exaggerated lithotomy position with the legs above the level of the pelvis. The perioperative nurse places a bolster beneath the sacrum to allow the perineum to be as parallel to the OR bed as possible, with the buttocks extending several inches over the bed edge. Stirrups should be well padded to protect the popliteal fossa. Intermittent pneumatic compression devices are recommended to assist peripheral vascular flow. The patient is often placed in a steep Trendelenburg position. Well-padded shoulder braces, placed over the acromial processes in a manner to prevent stretch or pressure injury, may be required to prevent the patient from sliding upward on the bed. Routine skin preparation is performed and includes an interior rectal prep. Special draping is as follows:

1. A towel folded in half is placed over the pubic area.
2. Two towels with a cuff are placed on either side of the perineum.
3. Two legging drapes, with points down, are placed over the legs.
4. One impervious drape is placed over the anus.
5. A large sheet fully opened with a large cuff is placed across from one stirrup to the other and secured by towel clamps.
6. A laparotomy sheet follows, with the short end to the floor.

The instrument setup is as described for suprapubic prostatectomy, omitting abdominal self-retaining retractors and adding straight and curved Lowsley tractors, Roux retractors, Jackson retractors with short and long blades, Doyen vaginal retractors, Young retractor, perineal prostatic retractors, Sauerbruch retractors, and a narrow and wide self-retaining perineal retractor, such as the Thompson retractor or the Omni-Tract surgical UO100 pelvic retractor system.

Operative Procedure

1. A curved Lowsley tractor is placed through the urethra into the bladder and held back by the surgical assistant, causing the prostate to be pushed down toward the perineum.
2. An inverted U-shaped incision is made from one ischial tuberosity to another, curving just anteriorly to the anus (Fig. 15.32A).
3. Three Martius or Allis clamps are secured to the posterior edge of the incision and retracted downward, over the anal drape.
4. The surgeon clamps any subcutaneous bleeders with straight mosquito hemostats and electrocoagulates or ties them with 3-0 absorbable ligatures.
5. The central tendon is isolated, clamped, and cut distally to the external anal sphincter (see Fig. 15.32B).
6. The rectourethral muscle is incised and pushed downward from the central tendon.
7. The levator ani muscle is exposed and retracted laterally (see Fig. 15.32C).
8. The prostate gland is exposed. The surgeon may send biopsies of the prostate for pathologic confirmation. If the results are negative, the prostatic adenoma is removed. If the frozen section reveals malignancy, a radical prostatectomy may be done at this time.
9. If simple enucleation is to be performed, the prostatic capsule is incised and the Lowsley tractor is removed (see Fig. 15.32D).
10. The urethra is divided, and the Young prostatic retractor is inserted.
11. The blades are opened, drawing the prostate down, and the adenoma is manually enucleated from the surgical capsule.
12. A 22F Foley catheter with 30-mL balloon is inserted through the urethra into the bladder.
13. Bleeding is controlled at the 5 and 7 o'clock positions.
14. The capsulotomy incision is repaired with a continuous 2-0 absorbable suture (see Fig. 15.32E).
15. A drain is left in place at the level of the capsulotomy incision.
16. The surgeon reapproximates the subcutaneous tissue with 3-0 absorbable suture.
17. The skin incision is reapproximated with 4-0 absorbable subcutaneous sutures.
18. The wound is dressed according to the surgeon's preference and taped or held with a supportive device, such as mesh underpants.

Transrectal Seed Implantation (Interstitial Radiotherapy With Brachytherapy)

Brachytherapy of the prostate gland is a procedure that requires a collaborative, multidisciplinary approach to patient care. The radiation oncologist and medical physicist, in addition to the surgeon, are vital to an optimum outcome from the initial planning stage throughout the postoperative surveillance. Preplanning is required to determine the size of the prostate, dose of each seed, the spacing necessary between each seed, and the number of seeds required. A template plan is developed preoperatively by using the ultrasound and the probe-anchoring equipment to measure and map the appropriate seed sites within the prostate. This may be accomplished in the surgeon's office, radiology department, or oncology clinic. The implant plan is finalized at the time of surgery.

The facility that offers this treatment must be licensed for "Group 6" with the radioactive materials licensing department of their respective state. If seed implantation is indicated as an adjunct to radiation therapy, it should be performed 3 to 4 weeks after the radiation treatment.

During percutaneous implantation of iodine-125 or palladium-103 seeds, the patient is positioned in the lithotomy position. The surgeon visualizes the prostate with transrectal ultrasonic imaging, and locates the midportion of the prostate on a transverse image. This location becomes an index for positioning the axial ultrasound plane at the base of the prostate. Approximately 2 to 3 hours should be allowed from start to completion. The procedure is amenable to outpatient management using a regional or general anesthetic.

Iodine seeds are commercially available in titanium-encased rods called magazines, which absorb the electrons. The rods have to be secured by the attending radiologist, who brings them to the procedure and monitors their handling. They cannot go to central processing for sterilization unless a radiologist or radiology technician accompanies them through the process, so the perioperative nurse ensures that the recommended practices for immediate use sterilization are followed (AORN, 2016). These seeds may also be embedded in an absorbable suture that allows them to remain positioned appropriately in relation to themselves and their location within the prostate and minimizes the risk of seed migration. Palladium seeds, which are not presently available prethreaded, are plated onto a graphite pellet. The pellets are loaded into titanium tubes with a lead marker. The half-life of iodine-125 (60 days) is longer than that of palladium-103 (17 days) and allows the therapy to be delivered over the duration of tumor cell replication, altering the ability of the tumor cells to multiply. Compared with iodine-125, palladium-103 affords a larger dose of radiation in a shorter time interval to more rapidly growing tumors.

Procedural Considerations

Percutaneous implantation of radioactive seeds allows the delivery of significantly higher doses of radiotherapy to the prostate than provided by external beam therapy. The radius of penetration around each seed is only 5 mm, thus sparing adjacent organs. The typical radiation dose that can be delivered by external beam may be 6500 centigrays (cGy), whereas the dose that can be delivered with implantation of seeds alone is in the range of 12,000 to 16,000 cGy. Some patients may receive hormone therapy to shrink the prostate gland for 3 months before implantation, and some will undergo radiation therapy before implantation. Patients with stage A or stage B prostate cancer are appropriate candidates, and selection is not

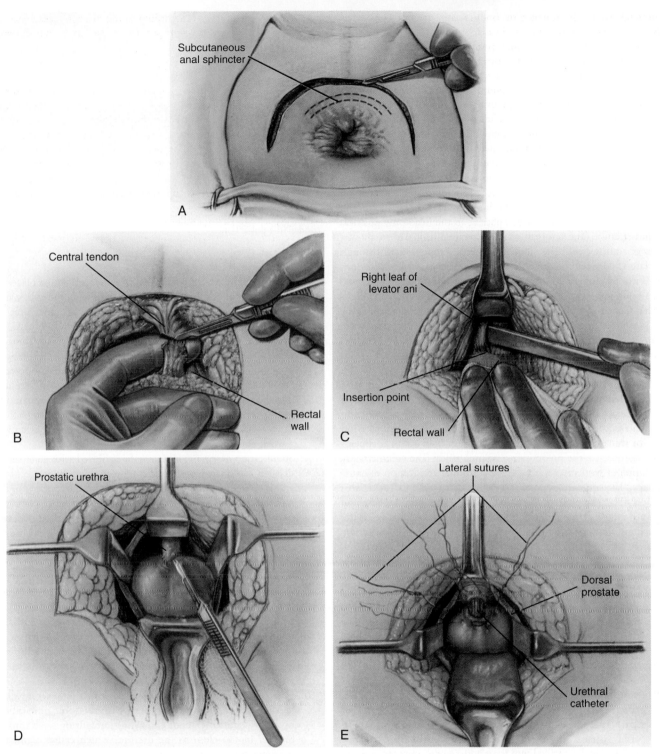

FIG. 15.32 Simple perineal prostatectomy.

influenced by a rise in the PSA level, biopsy specimens indicative of further involvement, or age. Ideal patients for brachytherapy treatment as monotherapy are those with low-risk parameters (PSA ≤10, Gleason score 6 or less, and low-volume disease on biopsy).

Possible complications include the risk of intraoperative seed displacement into the bladder; implantation too close to the urethra, resulting in postoperative urethral stricture or prolonged dysuria;

and implantation into the perineum if the needles are withdrawn too quickly. There is also the chance of migration of seeds, placed just outside the periphery of the gland and in the periprostatic plexus, to the lung. The nurse instructs the patient to avoid extended contact with children and pregnant females and to keep a 15-foot distance from this population group for 6 to 8 weeks. The patient must strain his urine, and any seeds expelled should be retrieved and returned to the oncologist. Body wastes are not considered hazardous, however.

Bleeding from the percutaneous sites is minimal, but postoperative ecchymosis of the perineum is to be expected. Other postoperative complications that may occur in the first 12 months include acute cystitis, prostatitis, and urinary retention. Late complications may include chronic prostatitis with cystitis, urethral stricture with contracture, stress with urge or total incontinence, proctitis, and impotence. Some patients may require posttreatment TURP, bladder-neck incision, suprapubic catheter insertion, or urethral dilation to alleviate the previously mentioned conditions. Much less commonly, rectovesical or rectoprostatic fistula can occur, requiring interventions such as laparotomy, colostomy, and urinary diversion. Patients are generally able to void 24 to 48 hours after implantation. The perioperative nurse positions the patient in the lithotomy position with assistance. The scrotum must be secured cephalad to allow a clear operating field. The surgeon places a traction stitch through the lateral edges of the scrotum and anchors it to the groin region.

With an experienced team, seeding is done with real-time ultrasound imaging. Throughout the procedure, random room checks with a Geiger counter are performed to determine radiation levels. All personnel, surgical equipment, and trash (including disposable drapes) are scanned before leaving the room at the end of the procedure.

Operative Procedure

Before seeding is begun, the surgeon positions the ultrasound transducer so that the posterior margin of the prostate is parallel to the axis of the ultrasound transducer. The direction of seed insertion and the transverse images of the prostate must have a similar appearance to those on the preoperative volume study. The volume study and implant worksheet are used for continual verification of coordinates. The surgeon attaches a stabilizer bar to the OR bed. This secures the "stepping unit," which allows a 5-mm incremental forward-and-backward motion of the probe. The sled that holds the transducer is attached to the stepping unit. The probe must be securely anchored so that the position of the prostate relative to the needles used to implant the seeds remains unaltered throughout the procedure. For the needles to be positioned appropriately, the template with labeled grid is attached to the transrectal transducer so that the needles placed through the probe grid match the grid locations on the plan. The grid is labeled alphabetically Aa, Bb, Cc, and so on, with the center of the prostate corresponding to D on the grid. The plan is designed to avoid the urethra, bladder neck, and rectum to prevent urethrorectal fistula formation, irradiation of the bladder, and scarring at the bladder neck level.

1. At the beginning of the procedure the surgeon inserts a urethral catheter, drains the bladder, and then refills it with 150 mL of sterile water. The bladder then provides an "acoustic void" to better visualize the prostate. If fluoroscopy is used, contrast medium can be instilled into the bladder to delineate the position of the bladder neck.

2. The surgeon removes the urethral catheter during implantation of seeds to avoid placement of seeds close to the urethra. The catheter causes the tissue surrounding the urethra to be compressed, and if attempts are made to implant seeds into this compressed tissue, penetration of the catheter and urethra may occur. The catheter also causes an acoustic shadow that prevents visualization of the anterior prostate gland.

3. The scrub person covers the ultrasound probe with a sterile probe cover filled with 15 mL of sterile water to remove the

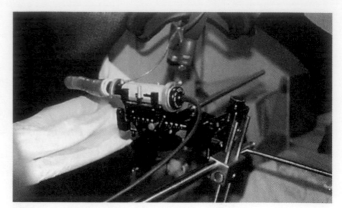

FIG. 15.33 Transducer on stepping unit and slide, angled upward to "get under" the pubic bone.

artifact. Alternatively, a gel-filled probe cover can be placed on the end of the ultrasound probe. Filling with too much fluid will change the configuration of the prostate and alter the anatomic presentation. The transducer is aimed with the tip upward at a 10- to 20-degree angle (Fig. 15.33). The posterior wall of the prostate must be far enough away from the probe so that the posterior row of seeds is placed just inside the posterior capsule. Seeds are implanted by means of loaded needles placed into the prostate according to the template plan, with the midline seeds placed slightly off center to avoid the urethra. Alternatively, individual seeds can be placed through the hollow needles with a Mick applicator that uses a long plunger.

4. Stabilization of the prostate may be achieved with stabilization needles placed laterally to the center into the right and left lobes and then removed once the anterior seeds are in place. Another method is to use a Foley catheter as a retractor for implantation of the periphery and until implantation near the urethra occurs. The best method may be to overcompensate for the rotation of the prostate by angling or turning the needle slightly opposite to the direction desired.

5. The most anterior seeds are placed first so that imaging of the anterior portion of the gland is not obscured by the ultrasonic shadows created by seeds placed posteriorly. If strands are used, hydrocortisone (Anusol-HC) is used to seal the bevel before implantation. Strands should be cut cleanly with electrosurgery to seal the ends and avoid frayed ends, which may be split further when the stylet is inserted into the needle, adversely affecting seed placement.

6. Contrary to normal needle insertion with the bevel up, these needles are placed into the prostate with the solid, or back, side up. Every effort is extended to avoid implanting seeds into the bladder or too close to the urethra, which causes significant postoperative irritative symptoms.

7. When placing the anterior needles, passage of the needle may be prevented by the inferior arch of the pubic bone. The needle tip is visualized as a bright echo, and the angle may be altered to compensate for the bone. Alternatively, the placement of the anterior seeds may be postponed until the end when the template may be dropped down, the probe positioned parallel to the pubic arch, and the needles inserted past the anterior portion into the prostate. Rarely, the template may need to be removed from the ultrasound probe at the conclusion of the procedure to allow "freehand" placement of anterior needles.

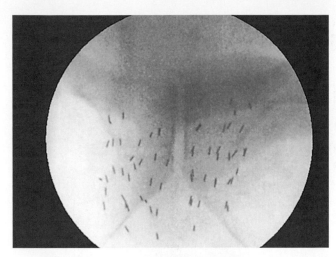

FIG. 15.34 Fluoroscopic view of completed seed implant.

8. The needle is inserted beyond the desired site and then retracted. The first seed determines where the balance will lie because the seeds fall into a plane that follows the first seed in a specific needle. The target volume is greater than the actual volume of the prostate so the capsular edge of the prostate and just beyond are also subjected to seed penetration (Fig. 15.34). These peripherally placed seeds have a higher energy and may have a greater tendency for migration if the tissue is not dense enough to hold the seed in place.

9. The distribution of seeds is generally 80% peripheral and 20% central.

10. The surgeon performs a cystoscopy at the end of the treatment so that seeds protruding into the urethra or left in the bladder may be removed.

11. A Foley catheter is placed and left for 24 to 48 hours.

Nerve-Sparing Radical Retropubic Prostatectomy With Pelvic Lymphadenectomy

Radical prostatectomy is the treatment preferred for patients with organ-confined carcinoma of the prostate. This procedure involves removal of the entire gland, its capsule, and the seminal vesicles. Important anatomic structures that affect erectile function are within the surgical field. Whenever possible, the surgeon attempts to spare the posterolateral neurovascular bundles, supplying the corpora cavernosa, to preserve potency. Those with tumors confined in the prostatic capsule are the best candidates for nerve-sparing procedures. In the presence of more advanced tumor extension, the surgeon attempts to spare one of the bundles, allowing the chance for potency.

Procedural Considerations

Patient preparation and basic surgical instrumentation are as for the simple retropubic approach. Additional supplies include long-tipped, right-angled clamps; urethral suture guides; a Bookwalter or Wishbone (UO400) self-retaining retractor; long Martius clamps; straight and right-angled clip appliers and clips; and right-angled scissors.

Operative Procedure

1. The surgeon creates a vertical midline lower abdominal extra-peritoneal incision.

2. A bilateral pelvic lymphadenectomy is performed, removing the external iliac, obturator, and hypogastric nodes en bloc. Lymphadenectomy is done primarily for tumor staging.

3. The surgeon exposes the puboprostatic ligaments, and incises the endopelvic fascia on each side of the gland to the puboprostatic ligaments (Fig. 15.35A). Right-angled scissors are used to divide the puboprostatic ligaments. The dorsal vein complex is easily subject to injury, and excessive venous bleeding may occur during this phase of the procedure. The scrub person and the perioperative nurse need to be alert to this potential complication.

4. A plane is developed between the lateral prostatic border and the levator ani muscles with sharp and blunt dissection. Once visualized, the muscle is dissected laterally to the urogenital diaphragm.

5. The surgeon ligates and divides the collateral veins originating from the levator ani muscle and running laterally to the pubo-prostatic ligaments to free the apex of the prostate.

6. The dorsal venous complex, supplying the penis, is carefully retracted medially. Once a plane is developed, the venous complex is separated from the urethra with a long-tipped, right-angled clamp. The venous complex is ligated with 0 or 2-0 absorbable ligatures. Some surgeons opt to use a stapler designed for this purpose. The complex is then transected with a #15 blade. Backbleeding, from the vessels onto the anterior surface of the prostate, is suture ligated.

7. The surgeon uses a right-angled clamp to mobilize the urethra from the rectourethralis muscle between the two neurovascular bundles, avoiding damage to them.

8. A Penrose drain or vessel loop is passed around the urethra. The surgeon elevates and divides the urethra with a long-handled scissors or scalpel (see Fig. 15.35B). The catheter is clamped proximally and pulled upward through the urethral incision, where it is cut and held cephalad.

9. The posterior urethra is transected (see Fig. 15.35B).

10. The surgeon dissects the rectourethralis fibers free from and medial to the neurovascular bundles (see Fig. 15.35C–D).

11. Next the surgeon enucleates the prostate, divides the bladder neck, and clip-ligates the seminal vesicles (see Fig. 15.35E–F).

12. Once bleeding is controlled, the urethral suture guide is inserted in place of the Foley and six 2-0 absorbable sutures on a 5/8-inch curved needle are placed inside to outside on the distal urethral segment. These are tagged and left uncut to be anastomosed to the bladder neck (see Fig. 15.35G).

13. The surgeon trims and everts the bladder neck and creates a rosebud stoma. The sutures are placed from the urethra to a corresponding position on the bladder neck. When all are placed, they are brought together in single fashion and tied.

14. Closure is as for simple retropubic prostatectomy. Continuous postoperative irrigation is rarely used. A 22F, 30-mL Foley catheter is inserted and placed to gentle traction, and dressings are applied.

Radical (Total) Perineal Prostatectomy

Patient preparation and instrumentation are the same as for simple perineal prostatectomy. The radical approach is accompanied by laparoscopic or low abdominal lymph node dissection, if not previously performed as a separate procedure. Currently, laparoscopy is performed more frequently than the standard incisional approach. Supplies needed for laparoscopy include standard laparoscopic instrumentation, three 10-mm trocars, one 5-mm trocar, an insufflation needle, a video camera unit, and CO_2 insufflation supplies.

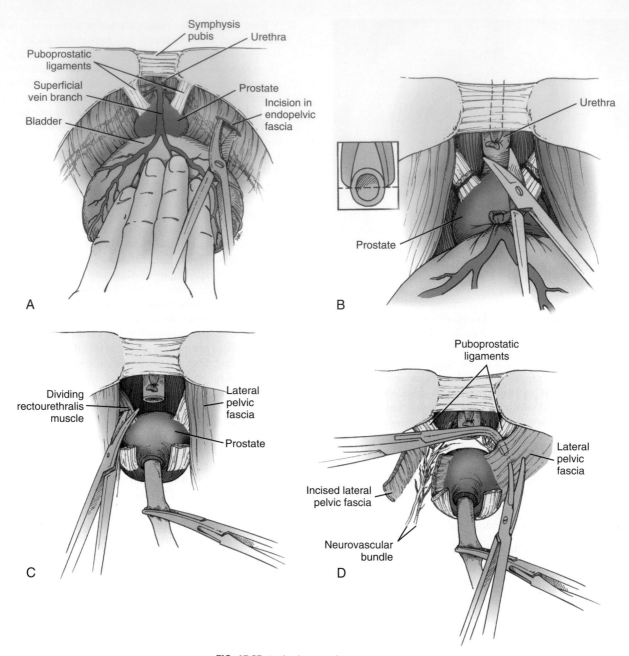

FIG. 15.35 Radical retropubic prostatectomy.

Procedural Considerations

Two operative setups are necessary. Most commonly, laparoscopy precedes prostatectomy. The patient is in the supine position for the laparoscopy, with the area of the umbilicus slightly elevated. Intermittent pneumatic compression devices and preoperative Foley catheterization are necessary. Instruments should be available in the OR to convert to an open procedure if necessary. Lymph nodes may be sent for frozen section, primarily for tumor staging.

Operative Procedure

Laparoscopic Lymph Node Dissection

1. The surgeon inserts the Veress needle and insufflates the abdomen.
2. Trocars are placed as follows: 10-mm trocars at the 12 o'clock (umbilicus), 3 o'clock, and 9 o'clock positions; a 5-mm trocar at the 6 o'clock position.
3. The surgeon grasps the peritoneum over the vas deferens, and incises it with scissors. The vas is identified, clipped or electrocoagulated, and divided.
4. The peritoneal dissection is continued laterally and cephalad to the sigmoid colon on the left and the ascending colon on the right.
5. After identification of the spermatic cord structures, iliac vessels, ureters, and psoas muscle, the surgeon extends the incision to the pubic ramus.
6. The Cloquet node is identified and freed from under the external iliac vein.
7. Dissection continues until the obturator nerve is isolated.
8. At the level of the bifurcation of the common iliac vein, the large lymph channel is located and removed. Endo Clips or scissors coagulation may be used. Clips offer a lower risk of postoperative lymphocele.

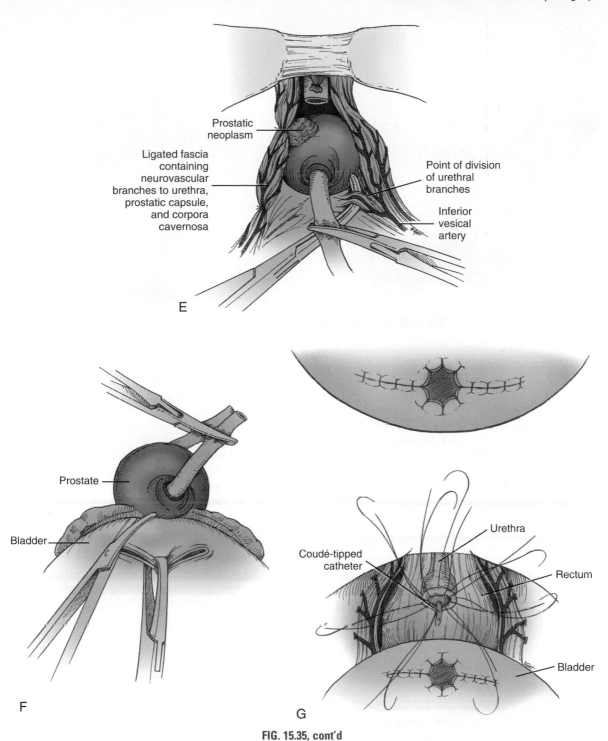

Prostatic neoplasm

Ligated fascia containing neurovascular branches to urethra, prostatic capsule, and corpora cavernosa

Point of division of urethral branches

Inferior vesical artery

E

Prostate

Bladder

F

Coudé-tipped catheter

Urethra

Rectum

Bladder

G

FIG. 15.35, cont'd

9. In a similar fashion the tissue overlying the external iliac artery is removed.
10. The procedure is repeated on the opposite side.
11. Hemostasis is achieved and the trocars are removed. Each trocar is removed under direct observation with the laparoscope to allow for identification of inner abdominal wall bleeding sites.
12. After evacuation of the CO_2 from the abdomen, the fascia layers are closed at the 12, 3, and 9 o'clock positions.
13. The surgeon closes the skin with 4-0 absorbable subcuticular sutures and dresses the wound.

14. The patient is then repositioned and prepared for radical perineal prostatectomy.

Radical Perineal Prostatectomy. Surgical approach is as for simple perineal prostatectomy (Fig. 15.36).
1. The surgeon incises a layer of subcutaneous fascia and uses blunt dissection to create a space within the ischial rectal fossa (Fig. 15.37A).
2. The central tendon is incised, permitting dissection to be performed beneath the triangle formed by the superficial external anal sphincter (see Fig. 15.37B).

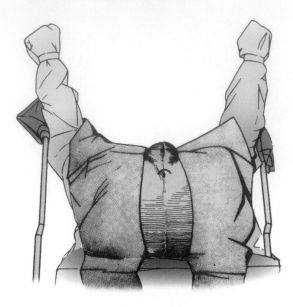
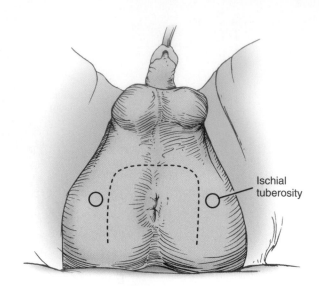

Ischial tuberosity

FIG. 15.36 Radical perineal prostatectomy, draping and incision.

3. The assistant retracts the sphincter to provide visualization of the rectourethralis (see Fig. 15.37C).
4. The true prostatic capsule is exposed by incision of the overlying fascia (see Fig. 15.37D).
5. After dissection of the periprostatic fascia unilaterally, the surgeon passes a right-angled clamp around the membranous urethra and incises it (see Fig. 15.37E).
6. Using a knife the surgeon severs the posterior bladder neck and retracts the bladder superiorly (see Fig. 15.37F).
7. Blunt dissection is used to develop a plane between the anterior bladder and the posterior prostate and seminal vesicles (see Fig. 15.37G).
8. The surgeon identifies the vascular pedicles at the 5 and 7 o'clock positions, and incises and divides them (see Fig. 15.37H).
9. Before closure of the bladder neck, the surgeon may place vest sutures of 0 or 2-0 absorbable material in a mattress fashion in the open bladder neck at the 2 and 10 o'clock positions and left long for later lateral perineal placement (see Fig. 15.37I).
10. Once the reanastomosis is accomplished, the vest sutures are crossed, passed through the perineal body laterally and parallel to the urethra (anterior to the incision), and secured either just beneath the skin or to the skin with suture buttons.
11. After placement of the Foley catheter, the urethra is then reanastomosed to the bladder neck with four to six 2-0 absorbable sutures placed at the 2, 4, 8, and 10 o'clock positions. Some surgeons opt to place sutures at the 6 and 12 o'clock positions as well.
12. A drain is placed anteriorly to the rectal surface and exteriorized through the incision line or through a separate stab wound.
13. The wound is closed as described in the simple procedure.

Laparoscopic Radical Prostatectomy

Laparoscopic radical prostatectomy (LRP) is a minimally invasive approach that may be offered to some patients in centers where practitioners are skilled in the technique. Patient selection is the same as that for radical retropubic or perineal prostatectomy. Those patients who have undergone androgen deprivation, radiation, or perineal surgery may not be good candidates for the procedure,

however. Advantages to an LRP over an open procedure are decreased intraoperative blood loss (attributable to the tamponade effect of the pneumoperitoneum on the venous sinuses, and improved access to and visualization of vascular structures), shorter hospital stays, and decreased postoperative pain. The return to continence and sexual potency is reported to be comparable with other approaches. Some practitioners suggest that retaining sexual potency is more likely because the neurovascular bundles may be visualized under magnification and are more readily preserved (Fulmer et al., 2015). Because of the high cost of the numerous disposable items needed, many institutions may opt to not offer this approach to their patients.

Procedural Considerations

Generally no bowel prep is performed preoperatively. IV administration of a third-generation cephalosporin and 2500 units of low-molecular-weight subcutaneous heparin on the morning of surgery is standard treatment.

With the assistance of at least one additional person, the perioperative nurse positions the patient in low lithotomy position with his arms at his sides. The abdomen, entire perineal area, and the upper and inner thigh region are prepped. This entire area is draped open, and separate leggings are used. The anesthesia provider places the patient in the Trendelenburg position. The perioperative nurse positions the video monitor between the patient's legs. A Foley catheter is inserted into the urethra and attached to drainage. After the procedure, heparin is given once daily for 2 weeks postoperatively. The drain and Foley catheter are generally removed on the third postoperative day, and the patient is discharged.

Operative Procedure

1. The surgeon inserts the Veress needle and insufflates the abdomen. Once an internal pressure of 15 mm Hg of CO_2 is achieved, the needle is removed and replaced with a 10-mm trocar.
2. The laparoscope is used to inspect the interior of the abdominal wall. A second incision is then created at McBurney point, a 10-mm trocar is inserted, and the CO_2 line is moved and reattached to this port to prevent fogging of the lens.

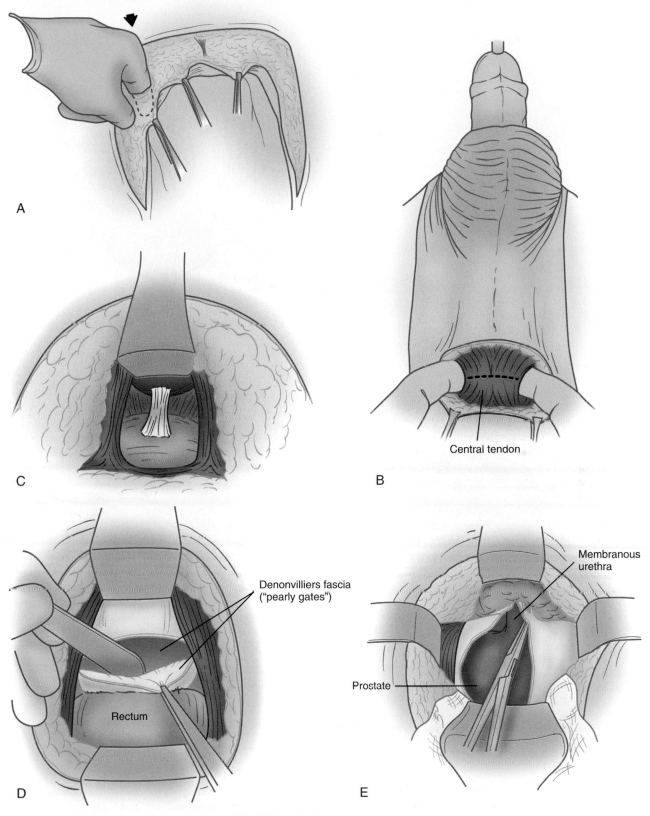

FIG. 15.37 Radical perineal prostatectomy.

Continued

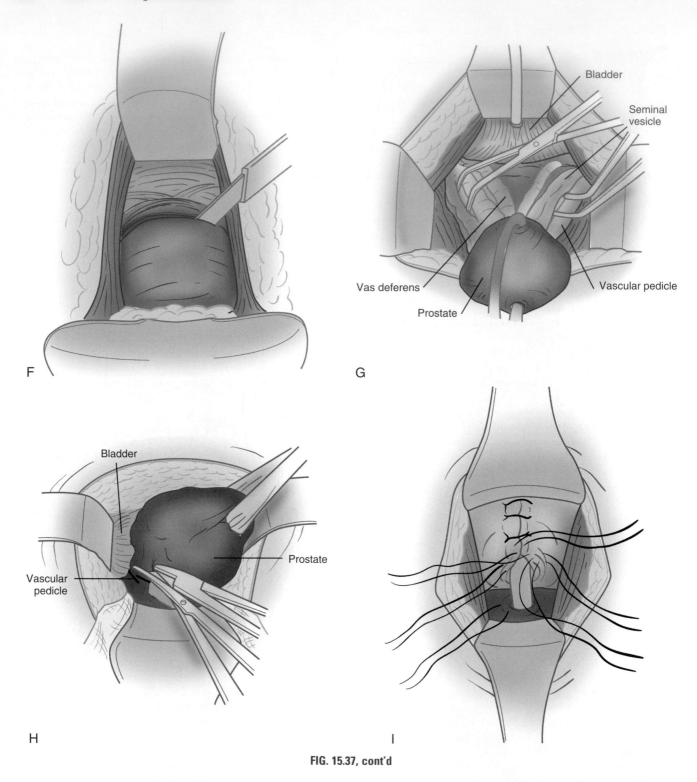

F

G

Bladder

Seminal vesicle

Vas deferens

Prostate

Vascular pedicle

H

Bladder

Vascular pedicle

Prostate

I

FIG. 15.37, cont'd

3. Three small incisions are made for 5-mm trocar placement: one inferolateral to McBurney point, one in the left iliac fossa, and the third midline between the umbilicus and pubis.
4. If a lymph node dissection is to be performed, this is accomplished first as described in laparoscopic lymph node dissection.
5. The surgeon incises the peritoneal reflection to expose the vas deferens and seminal vesicles. The vasal artery is coagulated, and the vas is transected bilaterally. The seminal vesicles are transected bilaterally and well mobilized.
6. Denonvilliers fascia is incised longitudinally close to the ampulla of the vas and seminal vesicles and placed on mild traction. Once the prerectal fat is visible, the surgeon begins inferior blunt dissection to the posterior surface of the prostate. Dissection is carried to the rectourethralis muscle.

7. The bladder is filled through the Foley catheter with approximately 120 mL of sterile saline to pull it posteriorly and help identify the bladder contours.

8. An incision is made medial to the medial umbilical ligament for the initiation of bladder dissection. This is carried to the vas and up the abdominal wall anteriorly and caudally until contact is made with the pubic ramus.

9. The urachus is divided in the midline and dissected to the level of the symphysis pubis, across the space of Retzius. A bipolar or monopolar dissector is often used for this purpose.

10. After the bladder is freed anteriorly and laterally, the surgeon manually empties it with a suction or syringe device.

11. The surgeon coagulates and incises the dorsal vein. The fascia of Zuckerkandl (fat) covering the prostate is resected or pushed laterally cephalad. The periprostatic space is entered, and the endopelvic fascia is incised on its line of reflection.

12. The puboprostatic ligaments are incised to allow dissection of the dorsal venous complex. This is accomplished with a curved monopolar or bipolar scissors. The vessels surrounding the dorsal venous complex are electrocoagulated with bipolar forceps and then ligated with 2-0 absorbable ligature passed from one side to the other.

13. Using sharp and blunt dissection, the surgeon develops a plane between the bladder neck and prostate. The anterior wall of the urethra is incised, and the Foley catheter is deflated and pulled into the operative field. The lateral and posterior urethral walls are then incised.

14. The posterior bladder neck is finally incised and the retrovesical space entered. The prostatic pedicles are bilaterally electrocoagulated with bipolar forceps.

15. A lateral incision is made to expose and preserve the neurovascular bundles on each side. They are dissected free of the prostatic base to the entrance of the pelvic floor and posterolateral to the urethra.

16. The surgeon transects the dorsal vein complex and retracts it anteriorly to expose the anterior urethral wall. A knife is used to cut across the anterior urethra, and a urethral suture guide is pushed through the urethrotomy into the pelvis. The posterior wall is then transected.

17. The prostate is retracted superiorly and the remaining attachments freed.

18. The surgeon creates the urethrovesical anastomosis with interrupted 3-0 absorbable sutures using two needle holders. Once all sutures are placed and tied, the Foley is reinserted and the bladder filled to check the patency of the anastomosis.

19. A specimen collection bag is passed through the second port at McBurney point and opened. The prostate is placed in the sac, the sac is closed, and the string is cut. The port is removed and the string to the sac is placed on the abdomen outside the port, a mosquito clamp is attached to the end, and the port is reinserted.

20. Abdominal pressure is lowered to 5 mm Hg, and peritoneal incisions are left open. The surgeon places a drain in the pelvis through the lower left port and sutures it to the skin. The abdominal muscles are split, and the specimen is extracted after removal of the trocar. All trocars are then removed and the incisions closed in a routine manner.

Robotic-Assisted Laparoscopic Radical Prostatectomy

An overview of robotic-assisted surgery and its benefits for the patient are featured in Chapter 8. Specific information relating to urologic procedures is noted in the Robotic-Assisted Surgery box.

Surgery of the Bladder

Operations on the urinary bladder may be performed through an open abdominal incision or a transurethral route. Diagnostic procedures are often undertaken via the transurethral route. Bladder tumors, diverticula, congenital defects, or trauma may necessitate an open abdominal approach. A thorough diagnostic workup and endoscopic examination help to determine the appropriate surgical approach to be used. Radical procedures, such as total cystectomy, are performed for the treatment of invasive carcinoma of the bladder and require permanent urinary diversion.

For most open bladder surgery the patient is placed in the supine position with a bolster under the pelvis. The Trendelenburg position may be desired because this position tilts the head down and allows the viscera to fall cephalad. This allows excellent exposure of the pelvic organs, including the bladder. The patient is draped as described for routine suprapubic prostatectomy, using a disposable impermeable drape that is placed immediately below the bladder incision. A catheter may be inserted into the urethra and the bladder distended with sterile saline at the start of surgery for easy identification. An ESU is required. The instrument setup for open bladder operations requires a basic laparotomy set, plus Mason-Judd bladder retractors; long and short thyroid traction forceps; retropubic needle holders (or other long needle holders); one trocar; vessel loops; a catheter stylet; a closed-wound suction system; and assorted Foley, Pezzer, and Malecot catheters.

Suprapubic Cystostomy

Cystotomy is an opening made into the urinary bladder through a low abdominal incision. When a drainage tube is inserted into the bladder through an abdominal incision, the procedure is a cystostomy.

Procedural Considerations

The patient is in the supine position. Anesthesia may be general, spinal, or local with sedation. A basic laparotomy set is generally sufficient for the procedure. Foley catheters ranging from 22F to 30F should be available, as well as Malecot suprapubic catheters and a drainage bag. Frequently a flexible cystoscopy is incorporated as part of the procedure.

Operative Procedure

1. After making a vertical or Pfannenstiel incision the surgeon divides the rectus fascia along the midline (Fig. 15.38A).

2. The bladder is distended with saline solution that is instilled with an Asepto syringe through a catheter.

3. The surgeon uses sharp and blunt dissection to dissect free the dome of the bladder (see Fig. 15.38B).

4. Using a pair of Martius forceps, the surgeon grasps the walls of the bladder on either side of the midline (see Fig. 15.38C).

5. Two traction sutures may be placed through the bladder wall and held with straight hemostats.

6. The surgeon incises the bladder downward with a scalpel. Bleeding vessels in the bladder wall are clamped and ligated.

7. The bladder contents are aspirated with a suction device.

8. The bladder opening may be extended if the bladder is to be explored for diverticula or calculi.

9. The surgeon inserts a large-size Malecot or Pezzer catheter into the bladder (see Fig. 15.38D).

10. The incision is closed snugly about the catheter with absorbable sutures to render the closure watertight around the cystostomy tube.

ROBOTIC-ASSISTED SURGERY ▌▌

Laparoscopic Radical Prostatectomy

Robotic-assisted laparoscopic radical prostatectomy is a procedure gaining popularity in urology.

Procedural Considerations

Before the patient's arrival to the OR the perioperative nurse and scrub person collaborate to ensure that all the necessary instrumentation and equipment are available for the procedure. Depending on the robotic system used, a standard laparoscopic setup is used with the addition of the robotic instrumentation and equipment, as described in Chapter 8.

Patients undergoing robotic prostatectomy receive a general anesthetic. The perioperative nurse assists with positioning the patient in the supine position with his legs in Allen stirrups. After the procedure begins, the anesthesia provider places the patient in the Trendelenburg position to displace the viscera from the pelvis into the upper abdomen to improve visualization. When the patient is positioned and draped, the patient instrument cart is docked, and the surgeon inserts the trocars into the patient. Surgeons may use a transperitoneal or extraperitoneal approach to the prostatectomy. The transperitoneal approach is used more frequently because it typically provides better access to the gland and surrounding structures. The surgical dissection for robotic-assisted prostatectomy is similar to that performed in the laparoscopic approach, but it us performed under the control of the surgeon at the robotic console.

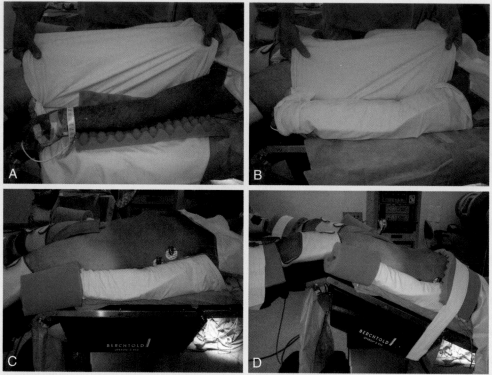

(A–C) Patient positioning for robotic-assisted radical prostatectomy. During positioning on the OR bed, the drawsheet and egg-crate padding are used to help secure the patient's hands and arms to the side in the neutral position, taking great care to protect from injury to the median and ulnar nerves. (D) To prevent the patient from sliding when in the steep Trendelenburg position, heavy cloth tape and egg-crate padding are placed across the patient's chest. (From Wein AM, Kavoussi LR, Partin AW et al: *Campbell-Walsh urology*, ed 11, St Louis, 2016, Elsevier.)

11. The muscle, fascia, and subcutaneous tissue are closed with absorbable suture.
12. The surgeon closes the skin with staples or suture.
13. The cystostomy tube is secured to the skin with a 0 or 2-0 nonabsorbable suture to prevent it from being inadvertently dislodged from the bladder. A drain such as a Jackson-Pratt may be left in the prevesical space.
14. The wound is dressed, and the cystostomy tube is connected to a straight urinary drainage system.

Transurethral Resection of Bladder Tumors

Bladder lesions may be removed using a standard resectoscope, working element, loop, and a foroblique telescope, which is passed through the urethra into the bladder. A 24F cystoscope sheath with a catheterizing bridge and biopsy forceps may be used to remove bladder tumors located at the very top or dome of the bladder (Fig. 15.39). Transitional cell carcinoma of the bladder is one of the most difficult lesions to track because it can occur wherever there is

ROBOTIC-ASSISTED SURGERY

Laparoscopic Radical Prostatectomy—cont'd

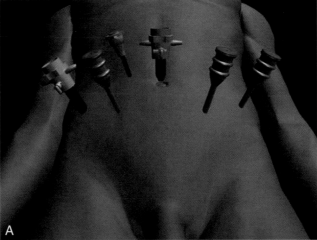

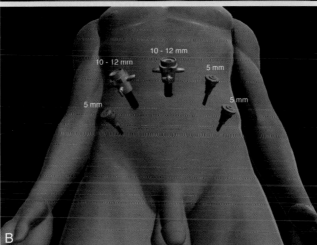

(A) Trocar configuration for robotic-assisted laparoscopic prostatectomy and (B) laparoscopic radical prostatectomy. (From Wein AM, Kavoussi LR, Partin AW et al: *Campbell-Walsh urology*, ed 11, St Louis, 2016, Elsevier.)

transitional cell lining of the urinary tract. Bladder cancer has a tendency to recur in other areas of the bladder, even after complete resection of the original lesion.

Usually the surgeon removes not only the bladder lesion but also a portion of the bladder muscle underlying the lesion so that the pathologist can determine whether any tumor has invaded the muscle. Random biopsy specimens of the normal bladder lining are also taken to ascertain if microscopic transitional cell carcinoma in situ (CIS) is present. Lesions that deeply invade the muscle must be treated with an open surgical procedure, such as a partial cystectomy or total cystectomy.

The resection technique, setup, and preparation of the patient are virtually the same as those for TURP. The anesthesia provider administers a general, spinal, or regional anesthetic. A retrograde pyelogram may be done to check for lesions in the upper urinary tract.

Sterile water is recommended as an irrigating solution in transurethral resection of bladder tumors. Because few vessels are uncovered during this short resection procedure, water absorption with hemolysis and systemic complications such as hyponatremia do not occur. In addition, cancer cells released during the procedure tend to absorb water, causing them to rupture and lyse rather than remain viable and capable of implanting themselves into the raw surface of the bladder created by the surgery. When the procedure is completed, the surgeon passes a large catheter, usually a 24F, into the bladder and connects it to drainage.

Transurethral Laser Ablation of Bladder Tumors

The Nd:YAG or Ho:YAG laser may be used to destroy small recurrent bladder tumors and to coagulate the tumor bed of larger bladder tumors resected with an electrosurgical loop. A powerful, highly focused beam of light in the near-infrared range is transmitted to the tumor site through a flexible glass fiber. This laser fiber is passed through the catheter channel of a cystoscope, and the fiber is directed by a deflecting laser bridge (Fig. 15.40). The advantages of a laser in the eradication of bladder tumors are as follows: (1) bleeding is minimized, (2) only sedation is required, (3) the operating time is shortened, (4) there is minimal damage to healthy tissue, and (5)

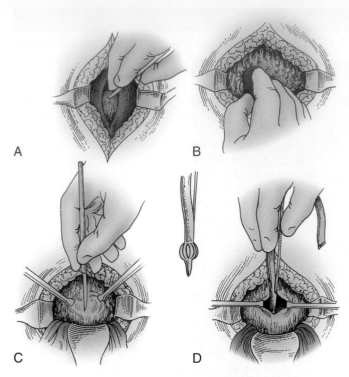

FIG. 15.38 Suprapubic cystostomy.

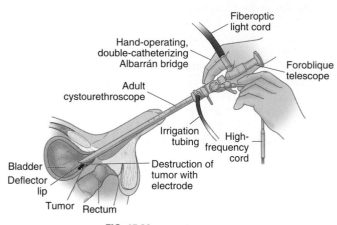

FIG. 15.39 Laser fulguration.

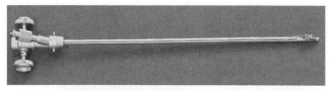

FIG. 15.40 Resectoscope with bridge.

postoperative drainage of the bladder by a urethral catheter is not needed.

Alternatives to Surgery for Superficial Bladder Cancer

Patients with various types of cancer may be treated in the urology office setting with various therapeutic modalities including the instillation of chemotherapeutic solutions. These measures may be initiated instead of surgery or as an adjunct to surgery. Instillations

are aimed at eradicating existing disease, reducing tumor recurrence and progression, and improving overall patient survival (Chang et al., 2016).

Patients with bladder cancer that has been staged as Ta, CIS, and T1 may be treated with intravesical, antineoplastic chemotherapy agents such as *thiotepa* (Thioplex), *mitomycin C* (Mutamycin), *doxorubicin* (Adriamycin), and *ethoglucid* (Epodyl). Chemotherapy has become the treatment of choice for low-risk patients.

Immunotherapy with *bacille Calmette-Guérin (BCG)* (TheraCys or Tice) is used to treat patients considered to have high-risk tumors. BCG, through an unknown mechanism, strengthens the body's immune reaction to cancer and is considered the most effective therapy for recurrent and residual bladder cancer.

Combination chemotherapy and immunotherapy have become standard treatment for patients with metastatic transitional cell carcinoma. BCG has been combined with *mitomycin C* and with *interferon alfa-2b*. The latter combination has been highly effective, rescuing approximately 60% of those who failed with BCG alone (Chang et al., 2016).

Trocar Cystostomy

Trocar cystostomy consists of draining the bladder by puncture with a needle or trocar and inserting a catheter.

Procedural Considerations

A minor instrument set along with a metal probe and grooved director, an Anthony suction tube and tubing, and trocar catheters or a prepackaged cystostomy kit is required. A local anesthetic may be used.

Operative Procedure

1. The surgeon nicks the skin at the site of the puncture with a scalpel and inserts the trocar into the bladder.
2. The trocar obturator is withdrawn, the bladder is drained through the trocar by suction, and a catheter is passed through the trocar cannula into the bladder.
3. The surgeon removes the cannula and sutures the catheter to the wound edges. The wound is dressed.

Suprapubic Cystolithotomy

Suprapubic cystolithotomy is the removal of calculi from the bladder. Obstructions, such as prostatic enlargement or foreign bodies, are common causes of bladder calculi and may be corrected at the time of surgery. In the past, special transurethral instruments such as the lithotrite were commonly used to crush vesical calculi manually. Bladder stones are often eradicated via the electrohydraulic lithotripter, which fragments the stone within the bladder by using an electric current to initiate shock waves (Fig. 15.41A), or by ultrasonic lithotripsy.

During ultrasonic lithotripsy ultrasound waves are transmitted through a hollow metal probe, which creates vibration at the tip. When applied to the surface of a calculus, the vibrating tip drills and fragments the calculus. This mechanical disintegration is continued until the stone is reduced to small fragments that are evacuated by suction through the hollow center of the probe (see Fig. 15.41B). The Ho:YAG laser may also be used for fragmentation of bladder calculi.

Procedural Considerations

Instruments for open bladder operations along with Millin T-shaped stone forceps, Millin capsule forceps, and Lewkowitz lithotomy forceps are required.

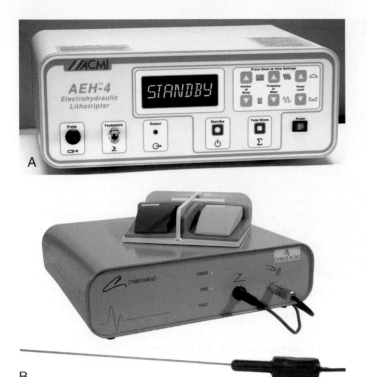

FIG. 15.41 (A) Electrohydraulic lithotripter. (B) Ultrasonic lithotripter.

Operative Procedure

The surgical approach is similar to that described for suprapubic cystotomy. When the bladder is opened, calculi are identified and extracted. If indicated, bladder outlet obstruction is repaired.

Repair of Vesical Fistulas

Vesical fistulas occurring between the bladder and the intestines or vagina may be repaired surgically. *Vesicointestinal fistulas* may be caused by ulcerative colitis, diverticulitis, or neoplasms of the colon or rectum. *Vesicovaginal fistulas* may be a complication of radiotherapy for cervical cancer, endoscopic procedures involving surgery of the trigone or vesical neck, obstetric injuries, and hysterectomies.

Procedural Considerations

The instrument setup is as described for open bladder operations. Intestinal instruments (see Chapter 11) are necessary for vesicointestinal fistulas. For vesicovaginal fistulas, vaginal preparation and a colporrhaphy set (see Chapter 14) with colostomy or ileostomy instruments are used.

Vesicointestinal fistulas are more common than vesicovaginal fistulas. Of the intestinal fistulas, the sigmoid colon is most often involved. A colostomy proximal to the fistula may be performed to protect the repaired segment of bowel. The communicating area of bladder and bowel is totally resected. Generally, an end-to-end bowel resection is performed after excision of the involved intestinal segment. The bladder is then repaired in three layers.

If the fistula is at the dome of the bladder, the approach will be transperitoneal, transvesical, or a combination of the two. If the fistula is in the trigone of the bladder, a vaginal approach may be used. A suprapubic tube is usually left in the bladder.

Operative Procedure

Vesicovaginal Fistula Repair: Vaginal Approach

1. Before placing the patient in the hyperflexed lithotomy or Kraske position (jackknife), the surgeon inserts a suprapubic catheter, clamps it, and connects it to closed drainage. If the intended position is Kraske, separate draping material and instrumentation are set up for the suprapubic catheter insertion with the patient supine. The catheter is secured, and the patient is turned for the procedure.
2. The area is draped with a lithotomy or laparotomy sheet as indicated per the patient's position.
3. The surgeon sutures the labia to the outer groin or inner thigh for retraction and visualization.
4. A weighted vaginal retractor is placed posteriorly, and the defect is examined. A relaxing vaginal incision may be necessary at the 5 or 7 o'clock position.
5. The surgeon inserts a 4F ureteral catheter through the fistula, and dilates the tract to admit an 8F balloon catheter. The balloon is inflated, and the catheter is used as a retractor.
6. The area is infiltrated with vasopressin (Pitressin) solution.
7. The surgeon incises the vaginal mucosa and perivesical fascia around the defect outside of the scarred tissue.
8. Two planes are developed (one between the mucosa and fascia and one between the fascia and the bladder wall) with fine scissors, forceps, and gauze (Kitner) dissectors.
9. The bladder wall is freed from the vaginal wall.
10. The vesical defect is grasped with Martius clamps, the scarred edges are everted, and the defect is closed vertically with interrupted 3-0 absorbable sutures after removal of the catheter previously placed. In some instances, a labial pedicle or full-thickness flap (Martius flap) may be placed between the vesical closure and the vaginal closure (Fig. 15.42). This prevents suture-line stress and overlay and removes the need for a relaxing incision. Larger fistulas that do not adequately reapproximate may necessitate a vascularized muscle flap to reinforce closure.
11. The surgeon approximates the perivesical fascia and vaginal mucosa separately with transverse interrupted 3-0 absorbable sutures. A one-sided ellipse of vaginal mucosa may be excised to offset the closure.
12. Alternatively, an inverted U incision may provide more exposure than other incisions and result in a posterior flap that completely covers the site of the defect.
13. The surgeon unclamps the suprapubic catheter, removes the labial stitches, and loosely packs the vagina.

Vesicovaginal Fistula Repair: Transperitoneal (Transvesical) Approach

1. The patient is placed in the low lithotomy and moderate Trendelenburg position. Both the perineum and the abdomen are prepped and draped appropriately. A laparoscopy pack works well for this approach.
2. The surgeon inserts ureteral catheters and places a 16F Foley catheter in the bladder and clamps it.
3. Tight gauze packing is placed into the vagina.
4. The surgeon makes a vertical midline or Pfannenstiel incision.
5. The peritoneum is incised and bluntly dissected from the dome of the bladder.
6. The small bowel is packed cephalad.
7. Stay sutures of 2-0 absorbable material are placed in the bladder dome, and the bladder is opened.

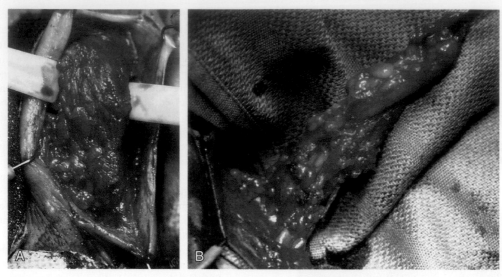

FIG. 15.42 Creation of Martius flap.

8. The surgeon divides the bladder wall and overlying peritoneum down to the fistula. Stay sutures are placed periodically to serve as retractors for bladder elevation.
9. The peritoneum is incised transversely at the level of the fistula, forming a pedicle flap.
10. The vagina and bladder are separated widely on each side of the fistula. An assistant places upward pressure on the packing to facilitate dissection.
11. As the fistula is exposed, the surgeon excises it until it is completely removed. A probe may be used to localize it, if small, or an 8F balloon catheter may be inserted and used for traction during dissection.
12. The bladder and vagina are freed from each other until there is enough mobility for separate closures.
13. The surgeon closes the vagina, without tension, with inverting 2-0 or 3-0 interrupted sutures in two layers.
14. The peritoneal flap is swung into the defect and sutured in place for reperitonealization. A long, attached peritoneal or free peritoneal pedicle flap may be needed for reperitonealization. Alternatively, the omentum may be manipulated from behind the right side of the colon for an omental graft. A vascularized muscle flap may be placed for fistulas resulting from radiation necrosis.
15. A 22F Malecot catheter and a wound drain are inserted and pulled through separate stab wounds in the abdomen.
16. The ureteral catheters are removed, and the bladder mucosa and submucosa are closed in separate layers with 2-0 or 3-0 absorbable suture in a running fashion.
17. The muscularis and adventitia are externally approximated with interrupted 3-0 sutures.
18. The wound is closed in layers.
19. Dressings are applied, the Foley is unclamped, the packing is removed, and the vagina is loosely repacked.

Vesicosigmoid Fistula Repair: Abdominal Approach

1. With the patient in the Trendelenburg position, a 20F or 22F, 5-mL Foley catheter is inserted and the bladder filled with 100 mL of sterile water. After the patient is prepped and draped as described for laparotomy, midline, or paramedian, and transperitoneal incisions are made.

2. The surgeon explores the abdomen.
3. The descending colon and sigmoid colon are mobilized by incising along the fascia fusion line of Toldt.
4. The involved loop of colon is identified. If a walled-off inflammatory mass is found, a transverse colostomy may be performed and a two-stage intervention considered.
5. Using blunt dissection, the surgeon separates the fistulous tract.
6. A probe is inserted to determine the extent of involvement.
7. The defects in the bladder and bowel are debrided to obtain healthy tissue. Large inflammatory masses require a colon resection.
8. The surgeon closes the bladder in two layers with a 3-0 absorbable submucosal running stitch and a 2-0 absorbable interrupted muscularis and adventitial stitch.
9. The edges of the bowel defect are trimmed to reach normal tissue, and stay sutures are placed on each side.
10. The cavity is pulled transversely, and the mucosa and submucosa are closed in one pass with a Connell stitch of 3-0 chromic catgut.
11. The surgeon approximates and closes the muscularis and serosa in one pass with 4-0 silk Lembert sutures.
12. The abdomen is irrigated with 2000 mL of sterile saline with an attempt to reach all areas.
13. A sump-style drain is placed intraperitoneally, and a Penrose or small Jackson-Pratt drain is placed suprapubically, exiting through separate stab wounds.
14. The surgeon closes the abdomen in layers in the conventional manner. If a colostomy was performed, it is opened for fecal diversion and the appropriate appliance applied.
15. Gauze and bulky absorbable dressings are applied and secured; Montgomery straps may be used.

Vesicourethral (Marshall-Marchetti-Krantz and Burch) Suspension

There is lack of a clear consensus as to which surgical procedure for stress incontinence is most effective, but contemporary practice is shifting to the urethral sling being the most widely used and having largely replaced the colposuspension (Marshall-Marchetti-Krantz [MMK] and Burch procedures).

Pubovaginal Sling With Autograft

Urethral slings are currently the procedure of choice for the surgical correction of female SUI. A variety of materials (autologous, allograft, xenograft, and synthetic) are used. Pubovaginal sling (PVS) placed at the bladder neck is able to improve SUI by providing a layer of tissue that compresses the urethra during times of increased intra-abdominal pressure.

The autologous fascial PVS remains the gold standard treatment for SUI with efficacious and durable outcomes. Rectus fascia is the most commonly used autologous material.

The incidence of PVS perforation and exposure is partially dependent on the composition of sling material. Synthetic slings perforate 15 times more often into the urethra and are exposed 14 times more often in the vagina than autologous, allograft, and xenograft slings. Urinary tract perforation by an autologous PVS is rare.

Procedural Considerations

The procedure is performed using either general or spinal anesthesia. After anesthesia is administered, the team places the patient in the dorsal lithotomy, moderate Trendelenburg position, and preps the abdomen (from umbilicus down) and vagina. Povidone-iodine is used for vaginal preparation, and chlorhexidine is used for abdominal prep. Sterile drapes are placed.

Operative Procedure

1. The surgeon places a weighted speculum in the vagina.
2. An 18F Foley catheter is inserted into the urethra. The patient should be placed in moderate Trendelenburg position.
3. A vaginal ring retractor is used initially for retracting the labia majora and later to retract the incision to further improve visualization and ease of dissection.
4. A 6- to 7-cm Pfannenstiel incision is made approximately 2 cm above the pubic symphysis and carried down to the rectus fascia.
5. The graft is harvested out of the rectus fascia using a scalpel or electrosurgery.
6. The fascia is closed with a running #1 polydioxanone suture (left long).
7. The graft is placed in 0.9% normal saline until needed.
8. Then 0.9% sterile normal saline is injected into the vaginal epithelium to aid in tissue dissection.
9. An inverted U-shaped incision is made using a #15 blade to expose the urethra and it is carried down through the vaginal epithelium.
10. An Allis clamp is placed below the meatus.
11. With an Allis clamp and Metzenbaum scissors, the surgeon creates lateral flaps and retracts them with the help of the vaginal ring retractor. The bladder is drained to avoid inadvertent injury.
12. The surgeon perforates the endopelvic fascia in a superolateral direction and spreads the Metzenbaum scissors widely. Using blunt finger dissection, the surgeon dissects the retropubic space. The infrapubic and retropubic planes are connected. Hemostasis is achieved with bipolar electrocoagulation.
13. Stamey needles are passed from above through the abdominal incision (tonsil clamps may be used instead of Stamey needles). The needles are in contact with the pubis until they are brought out lateral to the bladder into the vaginal incision.
14. A cystoscopy should be performed using a 70-degree lens to confirm bladder integrity.
15. After the extravesical passage is confirmed, the surgeon replaces the Foley catheter and an ampule of indigo carmine is injected to confirm ureteral efflux during final cystoscopy for sling tensioning.
16. The ends of the graft suture are passed through the Stamey needle eyelets. After marking the center of the graft with a clamp, the surgeon removes the Stamey needles and brings the ends of the suture out through the abdominal incision and tags them with hemostats.
17. The distal aspect of the graft is sutured to the periurethral tissue with two simple 4-0 polyglactin 910 sutures.
18. After adequate hemostasis is achieved, the vaginal incision is closed with a watertight, running 2-0 polyglactin 910 suture. Before final tensioning of the sling, the vagina should be closed and the weighted speculum removed to eliminate distortion that affects the final tension.
19. The polydioxanone sutures are tied down above the rectus fascia while cystoscopy with a 30-degree lens is performed to visualize adequate coaptation of the proximal urethra.
20. The abdominal incision is closed with a subcuticular 4-0 polyglactin 910 suture. The Foley catheter is left to straight drainage and a conjugated estrogen–covered vaginal packing is placed (Dmochowski, 2015).

Tension-Free Vaginal Tape Sling

A tension-free vaginal tape (TVT) sling is indicated for women diagnosed with UH, ISD, and pure stress incontinence caused by pelvic floor relaxation. It will not correct urge incontinence, although it may be used in women with combination stress and urge incontinence. This patient will need to have her urge incontinence controlled in another manner. It appears to be a viable option for the overweight and older female and for women who have had previous corrective measures that failed. It is not recommended for younger women who are pregnant or intend to become pregnant. Other contraindications include patients with intrinsic bleeding problems or who are receiving anticoagulant therapy. Risks include bladder perforation, perforation of pelvic viscera adherent to the pubis, retropubic hemorrhage and hematoma formation, infection, and urinary retention.

The tape is composed of polypropylene mesh encased in a plastic sleeve that has a center slit and is secured to a large, curved trocar needle at each end. A T-shaped introducer is attached to these needles for passage of the sling material. The mesh is passed through the pelvic tissue and positioned under the urethra, creating a supportive sling. Unlike other corrective procedures for incontinence, no screws, anchors, or internal sutures are required.

Procedural Considerations

The procedure may be performed using a local anesthetic with moderate sedation. After the sedation is administered, the perioperative nurse places the patient in the lithotomy position.

Operative Procedure

1. A 16F or 18F Foley catheter is inserted to drain the bladder.
2. The surgeon injects local anesthetic through the skin and into the muscle and fascia lateral to the midline and just above the symphysis pubis, bilaterally. Vasopressin (Pitressin) is commonly added to the anesthetic to help control bleeding.
3. Additional local anesthetic is injected suburethrally into the anterior vaginal mucosa to the retropubic space, bilaterally.

4. The surgeon performs a cystoscopy to confirm integrity of the bladder wall, urethral patency and length, and location of the ureters.

5. Two incisions, 0.5 to 1 cm in length, are made in the abdominal skin over each injection site.

6. The surgeon places a weighted speculum into the vagina and grasps the anterior vaginal mucosa with two Allis clamps.

7. Using a #10 or #15 blade, the surgeon makes a 1.5-cm incision into the anterior vaginal mucosa, 1 cm to the right of the external meatus.

8. Blunt Metzenbaum scissors are used to dissect suburethrally and periurethrally to the level of the endopelvic fascia.

9. The surgeon inserts a rigid stylet into the Foley catheter, and inserts the catheter into the bladder.

10. The bladder neck and urethra are deflected away to allow passage of the first needle by holding the Foley with its stylet against the inner ipsilateral thigh. An Allis clamp or hemostat may be placed in the center of the sling material to prevent twisting of the mesh or its sleeve.

11. After attaching the introducer, the first needle is passed 1 cm lateral to the urethra with the curve of the needle in the palm of the surgeon's hand. The needle penetrates the urogenital diaphragm behind the symphysis pubis.

12. Two fingers of the other hand are placed over the skin incision, the needle is pushed through the retropubic space, and the introducer is removed. The needle is guided up to partially protrude through the abdominal wall.

13. Before the trocar needle is extracted and removed, the surgeon removes the Foley and performs a cystoscopy. When bladder integrity has been confirmed, the first needle may be brought out through the abdominal wall and cut from the sling material, and a hemostat is attached to the mesh and sleeve.

14. The procedure is then repeated on the other side with the Foley directed toward the ipsilateral inner thigh during insertion and passage of the needle.

15. Once the tape is in place, the surgeon positions an 8F Hegar dilator between the tape and the urethra for tension testing. The patient is asked to cough, and the tape is adjusted until there is no leak or only a few drops of fluid are lost during coughing. The plastic sleeves are then removed by pulling them up through the abdominal incisions. The excess mesh that protrudes is cut at the skin surface.

16. The surgeon closes the vaginal mucosa with a running stitch of 2-0 chromic suture. Wound closure strips or skin sutures are used to close the abdominal incisions.

17. A perineal pad may be placed to absorb any vaginal bleeding. Abdominal dressings are applied at the surgeon's discretion. Vaginal packing and a postoperative Foley catheter are usually not necessary.

Transvaginal Sling With Bone Anchor

Indications and contraindications for this procedure are the same as those for the TVT sling procedure. The patient with severe osteoporosis may not be a good candidate for this technique because the bone anchors may not integrate into the pubic bone properly.

Risks with this technique include bladder perforation, inadequate fixation of the bone anchor (this generally requires abandoning the method and using a different type of sling approach), urinary retention, pain, osteitis pubis or osteomyelitis of the pubic bone, and recurrent incontinence.

Procedural Considerations

The procedure may be performed using a local anesthetic with moderate sedation. After the sedation is administered, the perioperative nurse places the patient in the lithotomy position. A formal incision may not be necessary for this procedure.

Operative Procedure

1. Before the procedure the scrub person loads a bone screw with preloaded #1 polypropylene suture onto the bone drill. A plastic cover fits over the screw, protecting the patient during insertion.

2. A Foley catheter is inserted, the bladder drained, and the catheter clamped.

3. The surgeon places Allis clamps on the mucosa and pulls gently upward to expose the anterior vaginal wall.

4. Tension is put on the polypropylene stitch that protrudes through the handle of the bone drill. The surgeon inserts the drill into the vagina in a line parallel to the plane of the symphysis pubis, and holds the drill head against the pubic bone (Fig. 15.43).

5. Insertion is complete when the polypropylene stitch stops rotating. Fixation of the screw is tested with a gentle downward tug on the suture. The bone screws should lie lateral to the symphysis pubis in the posterior mid-third of the pubic bone.

6. The Foley is opened and drained. If the urine is bloody a cystoscopy is performed. Some surgeons choose to routinely perform cystoscopy after each screw insertion to evaluate bladder patency.

7. A right-angle clamp is used to follow the tunnel of the polypropylene suture upward. A small puncture is created in the urethropelvic ligament to allow passage of the sling material into the retropubic space. The sling material may be cadaveric fascia or polypropylene mesh.

8. The surgeon creates a 2-cm tunnel between the midurethra and bladder neck, behind the vaginal wall.

9. The sling material is perforated with a Keith needle, and the polypropylene suture is passed through the eye of the needle. The suture is then transferred to the sling material. This is done twice on each end of the material.

10. The material is passed through the tunnel (Fig. 15.44).

11. Following cystoscopy, steps 4 through 6 are repeated on the contralateral vaginal wall. The polypropylene sutures are tied individually so that the material lies close to the pubic bone.

12. The vagina is sutured on each side with a single stitch of absorbable 2-0 suture.

13. A vaginal pack soaked in antibiotic or estrogen cream is inserted. The Foley catheter is drained and attached to a closed drainage system.

Implantation of InterStim Sacral Nerve Stimulator (Neuromodulator)

The InterStim system is indicated for the treatment of urinary urge incontinence, urinary retention, and significant urgency-frequency in patients who have failed traditional conservative measures or could not tolerate more invasive surgical procedures (Vasavada et al., 2015). The procedure is performed in two stages. During the first stage a lead is implanted and connected to an external stimulator. The patient is discharged and undergoes a trial period that lasts from 2 to 4 weeks to determine whether the device will be effective. During this trial period the patient maintains a diary to track symptoms and postvoid residuals. If the trial is successful, the patient will return for the subcutaneous implantation of a pulse generator.

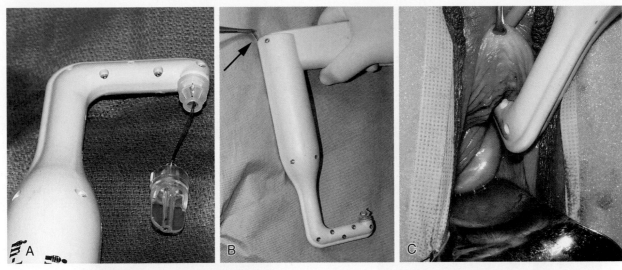

FIG. 15.43 (A) Bone anchor on bone drill with #1 polypropylene. (B) Bone drill ready; polypropylene extends out handle *(arrow)*. (C) Bone drill in place.

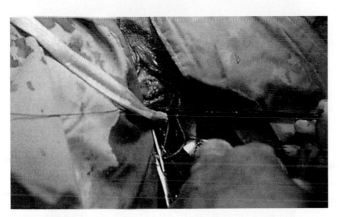

FIG. 15.44 Fascia lata graft being placed for suburethral sling procedure.

Some precautions must be taken by the patient who has had this device implanted. MRI studies are not recommended. Caution should be taken and the device turned off if the ESU will be used during any future surgery the patient might undergo. Female patients should be instructed to carry their purses on the opposite side of the implant.

Procedural Considerations

The perioperative nurse assists with positioning the patient in the prone position with a 30-degree flexion at the hips. Pillows may be placed under the patient's abdomen to support the lumbar area and decrease lordosis. Pillows are also placed under the ankles to elevate the feet and prevent pressure on the toes.

C-arm fluoroscopy is used to visualize sacral landmarks and verify lead position intraoperatively. Although general anesthesia may be used, monitored anesthesia care with a local anesthetic is preferable so that the patient may verbally respond to nerve stimuli during the procedure. It is suggested that no IV muscle relaxants be administered because this will affect the physiologic response to the stimulator. If electrocoagulation is needed, a bipolar system should be used, because unipolar current could travel into the sacral foramen. The patient is typically discharged from the hospital on the same day.

The nurse preps the patient's sacral area, buttocks, and perineum and applies the test stimulation ground pad to the patient's heel. An alternative to this placement is the calf or skin below the rib cage or iliac crest. The pad is approximately 5 to 8 cm in size and is attached by a test stimulation cable to the external stimulator. The patient is draped to expose the entire buttock area so that responses to nerve stimulation may be assessed. The feet and lower legs are also exposed to allow visualization of muscle response.

The surgeon locates and marks the sacral outline, S3 foramen, posterior iliac spine, coccygeal tip, and midline. To locate these landmarks, the surgeon palpates the upper border of the greater sciatic notch. The S3 sacral foramen is approximately one fingerbreadth from the midline, whereas the S2 and S4 foramina are one fingerbreadth above and below S3. The sacral crest corresponds to S4, and the S3 foramen is 9 cm above the coccygeal tip and 2 cm from the midline.

Operative Procedure

1. The surgeon inserts the needle into the S3 foramen. The external stimulator is activated to confirm correct placement of the needle. A bellows response (flattening of the perineum) and flexion of the great toe indicate the needle is in the S3 foramen.
2. The guidewire is inserted into the foramen needle.
3. A 5-mm stab wound is created for the lead introducer.
4. The surgeon slides the lead introducer, consisting of dilator and sheath, over the guidewire and advances it into the foramen. The depth marker on the directional guide is aligned with the top of the dilator.
5. The dilator is then removed, and the sheath remains in place.
6. The surgeon inserts the tined lead, with its stylet (Fig. 15.45), and passes it through the sheath until the second white marker is aligned with the back of the sheath. The four electrodes on the lead are now exposed and visible on fluoroscopy.
7. Nerve responses are again assessed at this time by connecting the mini J hook on the patient cable to the uninsulated section of the foramen needle. The electrodes are numbered 0 to 3, and the connector contacts on the needle correspond to these numbers. Beginning at the distal tip of the needle, all four electrodes are tested. The lead is repositioned according to the

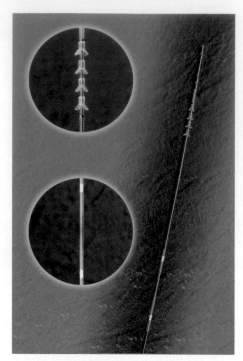

FIG. 15.45 InterStim tined lead.

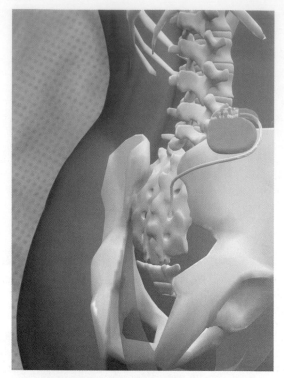

FIG. 15.46 Graphic placement of InterStim.

verbalized and visualized responses of the patient. The foramen producing the best results is chosen.

8. After the electrodes are in optimal position, the lead body proximal to the sheath is held in place and the sheath is slowly backed out of the wound. This is often accomplished under fluoroscopy.

9. As the sheath is withdrawn, the tines on the lead open, anchoring it in place.

10. The surgeon creates a tunnel for the subcutaneous neurostimulator generator pocket by means of the same incision. Placement is in the upper buttock below the beltline.

11. A pocket is created with the bipolar ESU. The pocket depth should not be greater than 4 cm to avoid interference with programming and shifting of the neurostimulator. The ideal pocket is 3 to 5 cm below the superior iliac crest and lateral to the outer sacral edge.

12. The surgeon uses the tunneling tool with its metal tip and plastic tube to develop the tunnel from the lead to the intended pocket. Once tunneling is achieved the metal tip is removed and the tool is withdrawn, leaving the plastic tubing in place. The proximal lead end is then fed through the tubing to the pocket, and the tubing is removed. The protective boot is placed over the end of the lead. Leads may be placed bilaterally at the surgeon's discretion.

13. The percutaneous extension is then tunneled from the eventual generator site to the opposite posterior iliac side, and exits the skin. This is then attached to the external device.

14. The incisions at all wound sites are closed. The wounds are dressed with small gauze and an occlusive dressing.

If the patient has a good response (50% or greater decrease in symptoms), then the area of generator site is extended in a second stage and the generator is connected to the lead (Figs. 15.46 and 15.47). The percutaneous extension is pulled out through the other side and taken away from the field.

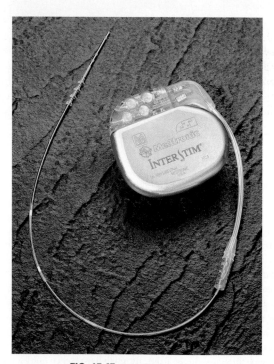

FIG. 15.47 InterStim implant.

Male Perineal Sling

The male perineal sling is designed to improve male incontinence by increasing outlet resistance. Using cadaveric dermis, fascia lata, or pericardium, the surgeon places a triangular sling under the bulbous urethra and anchors it with six screws that are placed into the inner portion of the descending ramus just below the symphysis pubis.

Other treatments for incontinence, including the use of botulinum A toxin, are being investigated.

Bladder Augmentation

Augmentation enterocystoplasty is a procedure performed to surgically enlarge the bladder capacity. A wide range of conditions that were previously treated with urinary diversion may now be successfully managed with this technique. Indications include reflex incontinence unresponsive to medical management, detrusor hyperactivity with compromised bladder function, chronically contracted bladder resulting from radiation or repeated infections, and neuropathic bladder combined with recurrent UTIs or compromised renal function. A segment of bowel is used to augment the bladder. The bowel is re-formed into a semispheric shape to decrease peristaltic contractions and anastomosed to the opened bladder dome. The result is a low-pressure reservoir that provides improved bladder capacity and urinary compliance. Almost all segments of bowel as well as the stomach have been used for bladder augmentation. Selection depends on anatomic factors, functional characteristics, and the surgeon's preference. In some cases, ureteral reimplantation or associated bladder-outlet procedures are incorporated in a one-stage procedure.

Postoperatively, intermittent catheterization and bladder irrigations may be necessary. The patient must be able and willing to learn and perform these procedures and must be accepting of this alteration in lifestyle.

Procedural Considerations

The nurse assists with positioning the patient in the supine position after the anesthesia provider administers a general or regional anesthetic. The female patient may be in a frog leg or lithotomy position, particularly if access to the perineum is necessary. The entire abdomen and genitalia are prepped and draped. The surgeon inserts a Foley catheter after the patient has been prepped and draped so that the bladder can be filled to capacity for visualization during the procedure. Basic laparotomy and intestinal instruments are required.

Operative Procedure

1. The surgeon makes a supraumbilical to symphysis midline abdominal incision.
2. The peritoneal cavity is exposed using a Bookwalter or similar retractor.
3. The surgeon examines the intestines and stomach, and chooses the appropriate segment for reconstruction (Fig. 15.48A).
4. A sagittal bladder incision is made from 2 cm cephalad to the bladder neck anteriorly across the anterior bladder wall, the peritonealized dome surface, and the posterior bladder wall to 2 cm above the posterior interureteric ridge. This causes the bladder to be bivalved in a clam-shaped design.
5. The surgeon places bilateral traction sutures along the bladder incision.
6. The length of the incision is measured to correlate with the corresponding segment of bowel or stomach. Average length required is 25 cm.
7. The surgeon mobilizes the segment of bowel and closes the mesentery cephalad so that the segment is on the retroperitoneum. The segment is left attached to its mesentery to maintain blood supply (see Fig. 15.48B).
8. The isolated segment is opened, trimmed, and detubularized. The surgeon then folds it double and sutures it to form a cup patch (see Fig. 15.48C).
9. Anastomosis is accomplished with a running, intermittent locking, absorbable suture, beginning at the posterior apex and running up each side.
10. With one-third of the attachment complete, the surgeon places sutures at the anterior apex and runs them bilaterally to meet cephalad (see Fig. 15.48D).
11. The surgeon fills the bladder to check the integrity of the anastomosis.
12. Abdominal closure is performed, and dressings are applied. The Foley catheter will remain for 7 to 14 days. Some surgeons may choose to place a suprapubic catheter instead of a Foley.

Implantation of Prosthetic Urethral Sphincter

Implantation of a prosthetic urethral sphincter is usually done as a last measure for patients with stress incontinence when other modalities have failed. Problems with the device have included foreign-body reaction, persistent urethral pressure causing urethral erosion, and fluid hydraulic failure. The artificial sphincter unit has an abdominally placed, pressure-regulated reservoir that maintains a constant predetermined pressure on the periurethral cuff. Because of the connection between the reservoir and cuff, any increase in intra-abdominal pressure transmits more fluid into the cuff. This connection allows for a compensatory increase in urethral resistance during coughing or straining.

The scrotal or labial pump shifts the fluid into the cuff to the reservoir to allow bladder emptying. The fluid reenters the cuff through a resistor in about 60 to 120 seconds. The locking button in the AMS 800 artificial sphincter unit traps fluid in the reservoir to allow activation of the cuff. The sphincter is available in a single-cuff and double-cuff model.

Procedural Considerations

Standard laparotomy and lithotomy positioning accessories are required, as well as the sphincter components, contrast material diluted according to the manufacturer's recommendations, and an antibiotic solution. The patient is placed in a modified lithotomy position.

Stricture disease is more commonly found in the male population, and the most common cuff placement is around the bulbous urethra. Bladder neck placement of the cuff is generally reserved only for females.

Operative Procedure
Bulbous Urethral Cuff

1. Perineal and transverse suprapubic incisions are made.
2. The surgeon mobilizes the bulbous urethra through a midline perineal incision (Fig. 15.49A).
3. A 2-cm space is created beneath the bulbocavernosus muscle and around the bulbous urethra.
4. The surgeon places the cuff, tab end first, around the bulbous urethra (see Fig. 15.49B).
5. The reservoir is placed beneath the rectus muscle through the suprapubic incision (see Fig. 15.49C).
6. The surgeon attaches the pump to the tubing passer, introduces it through the suprapubic incision, and transfers it to the scrotum through a subcutaneous tunnel created between the two incisions. The reservoir, cuff, and pump are connected and filled with contrast material or injectable saline to the appropriate volume (Fig. 15.50).
7. The wound is closed and dressed with gauze sponges. A urethral catheter is usually not inserted.

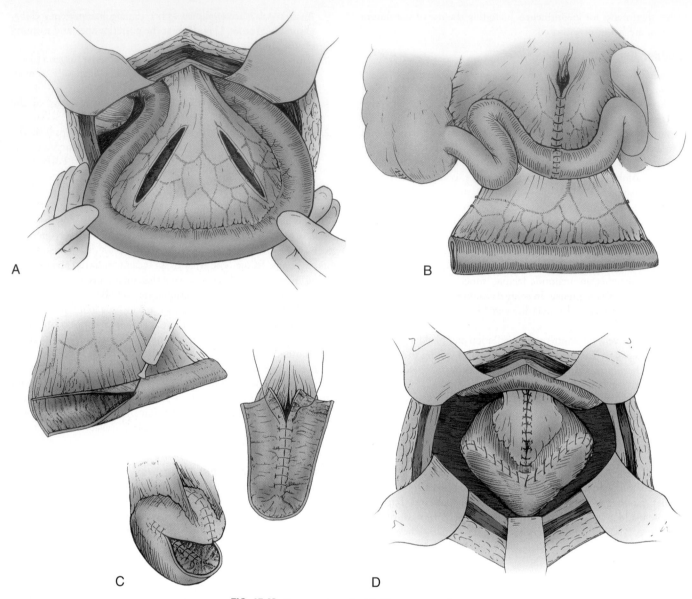

FIG. 15.48 Ileocystoplasty for bladder augmentation.

Radical Cystectomy With Pelvic Lymphadenectomy

Cystectomy is the total excision of the urinary bladder and adjacent structures along with pelvic lymph nodes. Cystectomy is a surgical consideration when a vesical malignancy has invaded the muscular wall of the bladder or when frequent recurrences of widespread papillary tumors do not respond to endoscopic or chemotherapeutic management. The patient should be medically able to withstand surgery with the expectation of reasonable longevity. Total cystectomy necessitates permanent urinary diversion into an ileal or colonic conduit. In a male patient, the prostate gland, seminal vesicles, and distal ureters are removed with the bladder and its peritoneal surface. In a female patient, the bladder, urethra, distal ureters, uterus, cervix, and proximal third of the vagina are removed. Radical cystectomy is one of the growing number of surgical procedures for which implementation of an enhanced recovery after surgery (Enhanced Recovery After Surgery) protocol may be indicated.

Procedural Considerations

The perioperative nurse places the patient in the supine position. Instruments are as described for major abdominal procedures. For a male patient, if the prostate and seminal vesicles are to be removed, prostatectomy instruments should be added. For a female patient, vaginal and abdominal hysterectomy as well as plastic surgery instruments should be added (see Chapters 14 and 22).

Operative Procedure

A midline incision from the epigastrium to the symphysis pubis, curving to the left of the umbilicus, is generally used.

1. The surgeon enters the peritoneal cavity above the umbilicus. The entire urachal remnant is clamped, divided, and ligated with heavy silk ligatures (Fig. 15.51A). It will be removed en bloc with the bladder.
2. The bladder dome is lifted at its peritoneal surface, and dissection proceeds laterally on either side with ligation of the major vesical

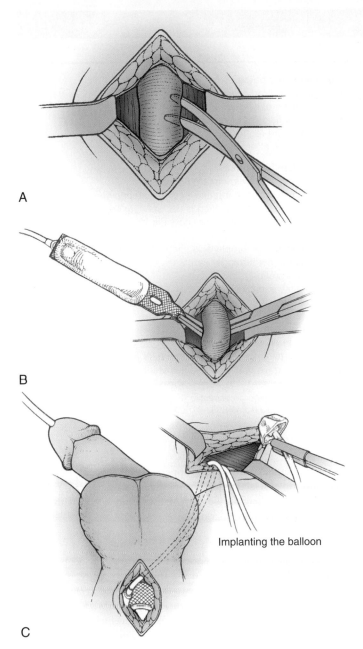

A

B

C

Implanting the balloon

FIG. 15.49 Implantation of artificial urinary sphincter.

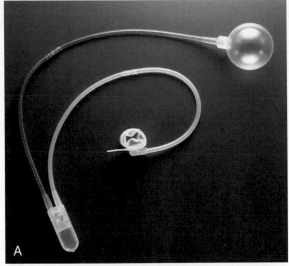

A

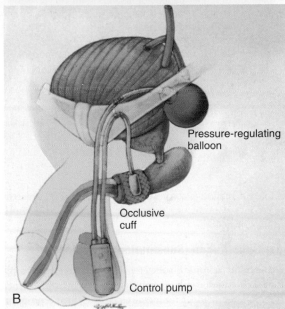

Pressure-regulating balloon

Occlusive cuff

Control pump

B

FIG. 15.50 (A) AMS 800 single-cuff artificial urinary sphincter. (B) Final placement of artificial urinary sphincter.

arteries to the level of the vas deferens or round ligament (see Fig. 15.51B).

3. The surgeon divides the vas deferens (in male patients) and cuts the urethra at the level of the pelvic diaphragm.

4. The ureters are identified and traced to the bladder. Care is taken to preserve the adventitial tissue (see Fig. 15.51C).

5. Abdominal exploration and pelvic lymphadenectomy with frozen sections are performed to rule out metastatic disease.

6. In the male patient the bladder is then retracted to expose the endopelvic fascia and puboprostatic ligaments. The prostate, dorsal venous complex, and seminal vesicles are dissected free, as described for a radical retropubic prostatectomy (see Fig. 15.51D). These will be removed in continuity with the bladder.

7. In the female patient the broad ligament is bilaterally incised posterior to the fallopian tube and ovary to the level of the posterior vagina to be removed en bloc with the bladder (see Fig. 15.51E). The endopelvic fascia is incised at the bladder neck to expose the proximal urethra. The vagina is then incised along the lateral walls to the level of the proximal urethra and bladder neck. The anterior vaginal wall is incised in a U fashion to circumscribe the urethra (see Fig. 15.51F). The vagina is reconstructed.

8. The surgical specimen consists of the bladder, distal ureters, prostate, seminal vesicles, and distal vas in the male and the bladder, uterus, fallopian tubes, and ovaries in the female and is removed en bloc.

9. The surgeon ligates the urethra with absorbable suture. If urethrectomy is indicated, this is done en bloc with the bladder.

10. Radiopaque soft goods are placed in the denuded pelvis, and pressure is applied to reduce blood loss from oozing.

ENHANCED RECOVERY AFTER SURGERY

Programs for Genitourinary Surgery

Evidenced-based strategies to enhance recovery after radical cystectomy surgery accelerate a patient's return to preoperative levels of health and functional status and facilitate early discharge by reducing surgical stress response and organ dysfunction that can occur after major genitourinary cancer surgery. Also known as fast track programs, enhanced recovery programs combine individual evidence-based strategies to create standardized preoperative, intraoperative, and postoperative pathways of care that are implemented by multidisciplinary patient care teams to improve patient outcomes and reduce healthcare costs. Examples of a genitourinary fast track program follow.

Preoperative Strategies
- Nutritional risk screening before surgery
- Preoperative oral nutrition supplementation
- Avoidance of longer periods of fasting
- Preoperative carbohydrate loading 24 hours before surgery if risk of undernutrition is present
- Avoidance of bowel prep
- Administration of opioid receptor antagonist, alvimopan, 30 to 60 minutes before surgery to promote bowel recovery
- Marking of ostomy site with patient in seated position

Intraoperative Strategies
- Deep vein thrombosis prophylaxis
- Antibiotic prophylaxis
- Balanced fluid management
- Temperature regulation
- Limited use of nasogastric tubes

Postoperative Strategies
- Fluid dynamics are monitored
- Initial observation in intensive care or stepdown units
- Routine nasogastric suction is not needed; considered in compromised mentation or known issues with airway protection
- Thromboembolic prophylaxis should be continued in the absence of hemorrhage
- Early ambulation
- Pulmonary exercise
- Early return of bowel function, use of recommended medications if needed
- Antiemetics for nausea
- Early enteral feeding
- Minimize narcotic pain medication (use ketorolac and acetaminophen unless contraindicated)

Modified from Jensen BT et al: Preoperative nutritional status and the impact on radical cystectomy recovery: an international comparative study, *Urol Nurs* 36(3):133–140, 2016; Persson B et al: Initial experiences with the enhanced recovery after surgery (ERAS) protocol in open radical cystectomy, *Scan J Urol* 49(4):302–307, 2015.

11. Urinary diversion is accomplished by means of an isolated ileal or colonic conduit, an orthotopic diversion, or a continent urinary diversion.

Bladder Substitution (Substitution Cystoplasty)

The ideal candidate for a bladder replacement after cystectomy for carcinoma is a patient with a normal urethra; a proximally located, well-differentiated bladder tumor; absence of CIS; and proof, in the male patient, that the prostatic urethra is free of disease. High-dose radiation offers appreciable risks for postoperative complications and is contraindicated with enterourethral anastomosis. A discussion of techniques to create a neobladder follows.

Right Colocystoplasty

Depending on the extent of involvement, the right side of the colon may be used to replace the bladder, the bladder and prostatic urethra, or the bladder and prostate with a direct enteric-to-proximal bulbar urethral anastomosis. This procedure has become more functionally effective with the use of intermittent self-catheterization and selective implantation of a prosthetic urinary sphincter.

Ileocecal Bladder Substitution

The ileum has been used as a reservoir to restore urinary continuity because it possesses a low intraluminal pressure. However, the short mesentery does not always permit the bowel to reach the urethra and results are not consistently successful. There have been significant incidences of recurrent carcinoma, renal damage, incontinence, strictures, fistula, hypokalemia, anemia, suture-line breakdown, and stone formation after the procedure. Although most patients attain daytime urinary control, a small percentage still have problems with enuresis. Deterioration of the upper urinary tract as a result of infection and obstruction has historically been a significant risk with this procedure; therefore ileocecal substitution is met with mixed reactions and recommendations.

Sigmoidocystoplasty

Because of the sigmoid colon's ease of construction, bladder proximity, decreased obstruction from mucus, and large capacity, it has been more appealing as a tissue source to many surgeons in their attempt to create a new bladder. More efficient emptying with a larger reservoir capacity seems to occur with a sigmoid replacement. Results yield higher intraluminal pressures, more effective urinary flow rates, and less nocturnal incontinence than with ileal segments.

Ileoascending Bladder Substitution

In an effort to improve the intestinal reservoir's capacity and antirefluxing effectiveness, the use of the ascending colon as a continent reservoir was introduced. This technique has several anatomic advantages over other methods of bladder replacement. The segment used can include the hepatic flexure and proximal transverse colon. A large-capacity reservoir is obtained, and colonic incision or tailoring is not required to achieve an appropriate shape. It easily reaches any site within the pelvis and can be anastomosed directly to the urethra without tension.

Orthotopic Ileocolic Neobladder (Le Bag)

The Le Bag continent diversion technique uses the right colon and ileum as an orthotopic bladder replacement. Bladder substitution relies on meticulous dissection of the prostatic apex with preservation of the urinary sphincter and neurovascular bundles, as well as a

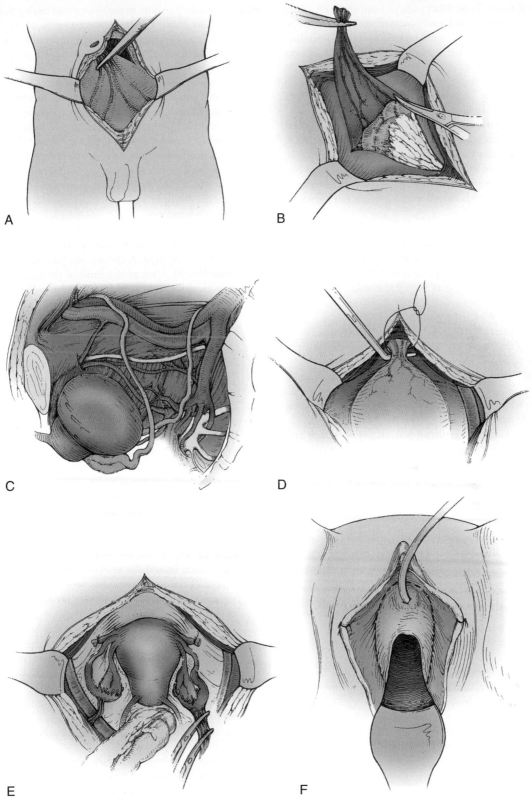

FIG. 15.51 Radical cystectomy.

watertight urethral anastomosis. Most patients have achieved a high degree of daytime continence and a minimum of nocturnal enuresis. Short-term complications encountered include bleeding, infection, urinary extravasation, bladder perforation, urethral stricture, fistula formation, urinoma, and small-bowel obstruction. Long-term problems include chronic constipation or diarrhea, compromised enterohepatic circulation, vitamin B_{12} deficiency, and urinary incontinence in a small percentage of patients.

Considerations influencing patient selection include age, general health, and fitness for extensive, complicated surgery. Contraindications include previous radiation therapy, bowel disease (diverticulosis, Crohn disease, colitis), and other major medical problems. Preoperative urethral biopsy specimens are frequently taken to rule out tumor or cellular atypia in the urethra, which would prevent this particular intervention.

Procedural Considerations. The patient is placed in the supine position. Intermittent pneumatic compression devices are applied before the induction of anesthesia. A cystectomy and prostatectomy or hysterectomy are performed. Major deep intestinal, bladder, and prostate or hysterectomy instruments, as well as a large self-retaining retractor, are needed.

Operative Procedure

1. After cystoprostatectomy, the right side of the colon is reflected medially along the mesentery to the hepatic flexure. The distal ileum that is to be used in the neobladder is inspected.
2. The surgeon divides the small bowel, positions it into an S shape, and places stay sutures of 2-0 or 3-0 absorbable material.
3. The posterior walls are sewn from inside to outside with running 3-0 absorbable suture.
4. A seromuscular wedge of the dependent cecum is excised, and the mucosa is everted with 4-0 absorbable sutures to form a bladder neck.
5. The left ureter is brought retroperitoneally under the sigmoid mesentery, a submucosal tunnel is created, and the ureters are reimplanted through the colonic wall. Anastomosis is done from the interior of the pouch.
6. The surgeon places anchor sutures of 3-0 or 4-0 silk at the outer entry point. The wall of the colon is anchored to the psoas muscle with 3-0 or 4-0 silk to prevent migration of the neobladder.
7. Ureteral stents are placed and exteriorized through the colonic segment and a separate abdominal stab wound, along with a catheter, to serve as a suprapubic tube.
8. Sutures of 2-0 absorbable material are placed around the urethral stump and tagged.
9. The surgeon inserts a Foley catheter into the urethra in a retrograde manner, and the urethra is anastomosed to the neobladder at the point of the new bladder neck.
10. The neobladder is closed in an intestinal fashion or with a GI stapler in a side-to-side anastomosis. The surgeon places drains, tests the bladder filled for leaks, and closes the wound.

Cutaneous Urinary Diversions

Ileal Conduit

The ileal conduit is the classic method by which the urine flow is diverted to an isolated loop of bowel. One end of the isolated loop is exteriorized through the skin so that the urine can be collected in a drainage bag, which is intermittently emptied. The surgeon consults with the enterostomal therapist preoperatively to determine the stoma site. The selected site, usually in the right lower quadrant of the abdomen, above the beltline, is marked with a fine needle

dipped in methylene blue to prevent erasure during skin preparation. The goal is to create a round, protruding stoma without wrinkles in the skin, to prevent urine leakage under the collecting device. The candidate for ileal diversion must have a retrievable ureter at least 1 cm in diameter with a thick, well-vascularized wall. The patient must be able to care for the appliance. Conditions amenable to diversion include neurogenic bladder, interstitial cystitis, and bladder carcinoma. Cystectomy may be performed before or after this procedure, depending on the patient's diagnosis. In cases that do not involve bladder cancer, the surgeon may choose to leave the bladder in situ rather than subject a debilitated patient to further surgery. In certain cases of extensive bladder carcinoma, the surgeon may elect to treat the patient with radiation in an attempt to decrease the size of the tumor and neutralize the regional lymph nodes before performing cystectomy.

Procedural Considerations. The perioperative nurse assists with positioning the patient in the supine position. Abdominal and GI instruments are required. A cystectomy, prostatectomy, or hysterectomy may also be done at the time of the surgery. Endostapling devices, with absorbable staples, should be available.

Operative Procedure

1. The bladder is decompressed with a catheter.
2. The surgeon enters the abdomen through a midline abdominal incision and places a self-retaining abdominal retractor to exclude the viscera from the region of dissection.
3. The ureters are identified and severed approximately 2.5 cm from the bladder.
4. The surgeon creates a retroperitoneal tunnel so that the left ureter lies close to the right ureter.
5. The distal ileum and mesentery are inspected to identify the bowel's blood supply.
6. A drain is passed through the mesentery, midway between the two main arterial arcades adjacent to the ileum at the proximal and distal ends of the selected segment. This segment usually makes up 15 to 20 cm of the terminal ileum, a few centimeters from the ileocecal valve. The ileocecal artery is preserved to maintain adequate circulation to the isolated ileal segment.
7. The surgeon incises the peritoneum over the proposed line of division of the mesentery.
8. Intestinal clamps are placed across the ileum, and the bowel is divided flush with the clamps.
9. Using GI technique (also referred to as bowel technique; see Chapter 11), the surgeon closes the proximal end of the isolated ileal segment first with a layer of absorbable sutures and then with a second layer of interrupted 2-0 nonabsorbable sutures.
10. The proximal and distal segments of ileum are reanastomosed end-to-end in two layers.
11. The surgeon closes the mesenteric incision with interrupted nonabsorbable sutures.
12. The closed proximal end of the conduit segment is fixed to the posterior peritoneum.
13. The ureters are implanted in the ileal segment, using fine instruments and 4-0 absorbable ureteral sutures on atraumatic needles.
14. The surgeon separates the peritoneum and muscle of the abdominal wall lateral to the original incision with blunt dissection.
15. The abdominal opening for the stoma is made, and the distal opening of the ileal conduit is then drawn through a fenestration in the muscle, fascia, and skin.

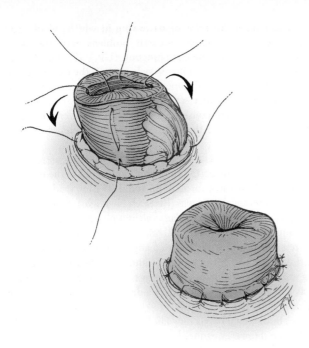

FIG. 15.52 Rosebud suture technique for stoma.

16. The ileum is fixed to the fascia with 2-0 sutures. A rosebud stoma is constructed as the ileum is sutured to the skin using subcuticular stitches (Fig. 15.52).
17. Ureteral stents are usually left in the stoma, and a urinary collecting pouch is placed over the rosebud stoma to collect urine.
18. The surgeon inserts closed-suction wound drains and closes the abdominal incision. The skin is reapproximated.

Continent Urinary Diversions

The Kock pouch, the right colocystoplasty, and the Camey version of the ileocystoplasty have been modified for anastomosis to a urethral stump or the prostatic capsule, resulting in effective continent bladder replacement. All continent urinary diversions create an easily catheterized stoma and a nonrefluxing ureteral anastomosis. Different parts of the bowel and the stomach have been used as continent reservoirs. The choice of the antireflux mechanism depends on the implantation site. The stoma does not require an appliance; therefore the site may be placed below the beltline or bikini line, permitting it to be catheterized when the patient is sitting. It may be anastomosed to the proximal urethra, thus forming an orthotopic bladder.

Ileal Reservoir (Kock Pouch)

Procedural Considerations. A continent reservoir formed into a U configuration is constructed from a section of ileum proximal to the ileocecal valve. The legs of the U are sewn together at the antimesenteric border. The intestine is opened adjacent to the antimesenteric border, and the back wall of the pouch is reinforced with absorbable suture.

Continence is achieved by the valve mechanism with the nipple valve attached to the skin. Nipple valves are created proximally and distally by intussusception of the bowel into the reservoir cavity.

Once the nipples are fixed to the sidewall of the reservoir with absorbable suture or polyglycolic staples, the anterior wall is closed. The ureters are anastomosed to the afferent limb of the pouch, preventing reflux. The efferent limb is drawn through the stoma site and anchored to the abdominal wall fascia.

Operative Procedure
1. The mesentery is divided and suture ligated or staple ligated along the avascular plane between the superior mesenteric artery and the ileocolic artery.
2. The surgeon divides the bowel, and four segments are measured and marked with silk suture tags. These segments will serve as the efferent conduit, the pouch, and the afferent limb.
3. A portion of the proximal ileum is resected and discarded along with a wedge of mesentery. Suction is passed down the lumen to clear any fecal material or mucus.
4. The surgeon closes the proximal end of the bowel with suture or staples.
5. The segment to be used is spread out in a U shape. The sides are sewn together with 3-0 absorbable suture in a running stitch or connected using a GI endostapler.
6. The surgeon uses the ESU to incise the bowel laterally to the suture in the two loops. The medial edges are oversewn with 3-0 or 4-0 silk.
7. The mesentery is cleared on the limb segments, and the lumens are intussuscepted into the open pouch.
8. Synthetic mesh is used to serve as a strut to prevent peristomal herniation and to fix the base of the efferent nipple to the abdominal wall, facilitating catheterization. The thoracoabdominal (TA) or similar endostapler is used to form each nipple and to attach the nipples to the back wall of the pouch.
9. An 8F stenting catheter is placed inside the nipple of the efferent conduit to prevent the formation of a collar that is too tight.
10. The surgeon secures the limbs with 3-0 or 4-0 silk suture.
11. The pouch is closed with sutures or the endostapler.
12. The ureters are anastomosed, as described previously in the Ileal Conduit section, to the afferent limb.
13. A small stoma site is prepared, as described previously in the Ileal Conduit section. A catheter of choice is placed in the stoma for postoperative care. Stents may be placed in the ureters for the immediate postoperative period. This necessitates initial placement of an ileostomy appliance until all systems are functioning.
14. A drain is placed, which exits through a separate stab wound.
15. The surgeon closes the wound. Retention sutures may be used. Bulky absorbent dressings are applied; Montgomery straps may be used.

Indiana Pouch

Procedural Considerations. The Indiana pouch technique is a modification of the original ileocecal diversion. The surgeon constructs a continent reservoir from the right side of the colon, which may include the ileum and cecum, the ileocecal valve, and ascending colon. Surgery proceeds as for any diversionary procedure. The ileocecal valve is reinforced with nonabsorbable suture. Two rows of nonabsorbable suture are used to then imbricate the ileal segment, which serves as a limb that can be catheterized once it is exteriorized to the skin level as a stoma. The cecal segment is detubularized by incising along the taenia and anastomosing the distal edge horizontally to the proximal portion. Intussusception of the ileocecal valve into the cecum and narrowing of the ileal segment attached to the skin allow for continence.

Operative Procedure

1. The large bowel is split down the antimesenteric border for approximately three-quarters of its length.
2. The U-shaped defect is closed.
3. The surgeon sutures the terminal ileum along its length over a small Robinson catheter using the intestinal technique.
4. The pouch is filled with 400 mL of saline, and a larger catheter is placed to determine its ability to be catheterized.
5. The ureters are tunneled into the cecum through its taenia and then tacked to the outer bowel wall. The cecum is secured to the pelvic wall. Ureteral stents may be placed.
6. The pouch is secured to the abdominal wall.
7. The surgeon prepares the stomal site as described previously in the Ileal Conduit section.
8. A 22F Malecot drain is placed in the reservoir to drain the cecostomy, exiting through a separate stab wound.

Surgery of the Ureters and Kidneys

Stones, infections, and tumors are the most common causes of urinary tract obstruction, necessitating surgery to prevent renal obstruction and subsequent renal failure. Obstruction may also result from congenital malformations or previous operations on the urinary tract (Fig. 15.53).

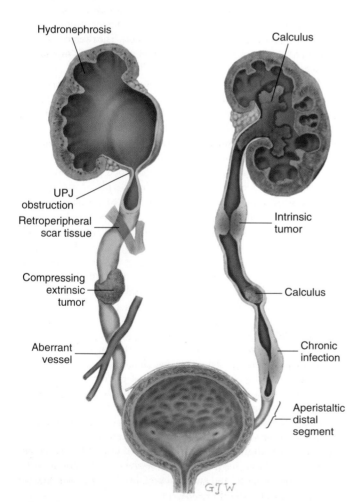

FIG. 15.53 Some common causes of urinary tract obstruction. *UPJ,* Ureteropelvic junction.

The ureter has three areas of narrowing in which calculi may become lodged and pose a potential problem with pain and obstruction: (1) the ureteropelvic junction (UPJ), (2) the crossing of the ureter over the external iliac vessels, and (3) the ureterovesical junction (UVJ). Urine may sometimes cause calculi to be washed down the ureter to produce severe ureteral colic. The majority of renal calculi are spontaneously passed into the bladder. However, if they become lodged in the ureter, surgical intervention may be indicated.

Although the causes of many kidney stones are obscure, certain conditions, such as obstruction, stasis, and imbalance of the metabolism, predispose to their formation. There is some evidence that statins may protect against stones (Research Highlight). Stones consist of various elements: calcium oxalate, calcium phosphate, magnesium ammonium phosphate, uric acid, calcium carbonate, and cystine. An increase in the concentration of any of these compounds can cause tiny crystals to form; as these clump together, they begin to form a stone. Stones removed during surgery are subjected to chemical analysis and should be submitted in a dry jar. Fixative agents such as formalin should not be used.

Stones in the renal pelvis may fall into the UPJ and obstruct the flow of urine. However, stones less than 3 cm in diameter may also pass down the ureter and lodge at a more distal location. A stone may remain in a renal calyx and continue to enlarge, eventually filling the entire renal collecting system (staghorn calculus). Diverticula may form and harbor stones that can be difficult to reach and treat. Hydroureteronephrosis, infection, and destruction of renal parenchyma frequently result from unrelieved obstruction.

Hypothermia may be used as an adjunct to renal stone surgery as a means of prolonging the safe period of renal ischemia. Several

RESEARCH HIGHLIGHT

Statins May Protect Against Kidney Stones

The prevalence of nephrolithiasis in the United States has increased substantially. In patients with hyperlipidemia statins might reduce the risk for kidney stone formation, according to one retrospective study.

The relationship between levels of lipids in the blood, the intake of statins, chronic kidney disease, and kidney stones is currently being researched and debated. At this time, the study results are not enough to prompt the prophylactic use of lipid-lowering drugs in patients at risk for nephrolithiasis. Elevated lipid levels have previously been associated with kidney stones. A study of 57,000 patients newly diagnosed with hyperlipidemia showed, for the first time, that the risk for stone development was lower in statin users than nonusers. Previous research on this subject lacked the analysis of laboratory values, and these supplementary laboratory data added a high degree of credibility to study findings.

The study's conclusion shows that statins have a protective effect against the formation of kidney stones in adults with hyperlipidemia. The findings are not enough to prompt a prophylactic use of statins and will remain an academic matter until there is more research.

From Sur RL et al: Impact of statins on nephrolithiasis in hyperlipidemic patients: a 10-year review of an equal access health care system, *Clin Nephrol* 79(5):351–355, 2013; Tasian GE et al: Annual incidence of nephrolithiasis among children and adults in South Carolina from 1997 to 2012, *Clin J Am Soc Nephrol* 7(3):488–496, 2016.

methods enable renal cooling: ice slush or cold saline solution, surface cooling coils, perfusion of cold solutions through the renal artery, or a variation of these basic techniques, such as perfusion of the renal pelvis with saline that has been cooled by a coil immersed in ice slush.

A refrigeration unit "slush machine" that produces sterile slush provides a cost-effective, time-saving alternative to the other methods of slush preparation. Commercially synthesized ultrafiltrate of sterile plasma in liter bottles is also available for use as the slush. Alternatively, a rigid plastic container of 1000 mL of normal saline or lactated Ringer's solution may be placed on its side in a freezer several hours before surgery. To prevent the solution from solidifying, the container should be rotated one-half turn every 20 to 30 minutes. Sterile slush may then be poured directly into a sterile basin as required.

The surgical approach in renal surgery depends on the patient's condition, the amount of exposure needed, and the surgical procedure to be performed. There are three principal surgical approaches to the kidney. The simple *flank,* or *transabdominal,* incision is most frequently used and may include removal of the eleventh or twelfth rib. The incision begins at the posterior axillary line and parallels the course of the twelfth rib. It extends forward and slightly downward between the iliac crest and the thorax. For the *lumbar* incision, the patient may be initially positioned supine and then rotated to lateral and slightly forward over protective bolsters with the operative side up. This effectively places the flank in an oblique position, causing the abdominal viscera to fall away from the operative incision, and affords an excellent approach to the renal pedicle. Alternatively, the patient may be placed prone with bolsters under the affected side to provide elevation. The *thoracoabdominal* exposure is used primarily for large upper pole renal neoplasms. The tenth and eleventh ribs are usually removed, and the chest cavity is opened, collapsing the lung. The leaves of the diaphragm are separated to expose the kidney.

Ureteral Surgery

Ureterostomy (ureterotomy) is opening the ureter for continued drainage from it into another body part. Cutaneous ureterostomy is diversion of the flow of urine from the kidney, through the ureter, away from the bladder, and onto the skin of the lower abdomen. A suitable urinary-collecting device is then placed over the ureteral stoma.

Ureterectomy is complete removal of the ureter. This procedure is generally used in collecting system tumors and includes nephrectomy and the excision of a cuff of bladder.

Ureteroureterostomy is segmental resection of a diseased portion of the ureter and reconstruction in continuity of the two normal segments.

Ureteroenterostomy is diversion of the ureter into a segment of the ileum (ureteroileostomy, or more commonly, ileal urinary conduit) or into the sigmoid colon (ureterosigmoidostomy). Ureteroneocystostomy (ureterovesical anastomosis) is division of the distal ureter from the bladder and reimplantation of the ureter into the bladder with a submucosal tunnel.

Reconstructive operations may be indicated because of a pathologic condition of the bladder or lower ureter that interferes with normal drainage. Conditions requiring urinary diversion or reconstruction of the urinary tract include malignancy, cystitis, stricture, trauma, and congenital ureterovesical reflux. Invasive vesical malignancy requiring surgical removal of the bladder necessitates urinary diversion.

Ureterocutaneous transplant, ureterosigmoid anastomosis, and ileal conduit are urinary diversionary procedures performed when the bladder is no longer functioning as a proper urine reservoir.

Etiologic factors causing irreparable vesical dysfunction are chronic inflammation, interstitial cystitis, neurogenic bladder, exstrophy, trauma, tumor, and infiltrative disease (amyloidosis). Ureterolithotomy is incision into the ureter and removal of an obstructing calculus.

Procedural Considerations

The site of the incision and position of the patient depend on the nature of the proposed surgery. The patient may be placed in the supine position for abdominal surgery, in the modified Trendelenburg position for low abdominal or pelvic surgery, or in the lateral position for high or midureteral obstructing calculi. The perioperative nurse ensures that the patient's arms are supinated when on armboards; in lateral position the upper arm is placed on an overbed armboard, such as the Allen lateral arm support, and the lower arm is supinated on a padded armboard. The kidney rest should lie just under the dependent iliac crest.

Instruments include a nephrectomy set, plus plastic instrumentation for pyeloplasty. Additional instruments may be required, depending on the type of operation and the surgical approach used.

Operative Procedure
Ureteral Reimplantation

1. The surgeon exposes the ureter through an incision determined by the location of the pathologic condition. A ureteral catheter, passed retrograde, may be used to facilitate identification and isolation of the ureter.
2. The ureter is dissected free with long forceps and scissors, picked up with fine traction sutures, freed from the surrounding tissues, and severed at the desired level.
3. The surgeon ligates the distal end of the ureter and transfers the proximal stoma to the site of anastomosis. The anastomosis is accomplished with fine dissection instruments and fine atraumatic sutures.
4. A soft splinting stent is usually left in place until healing has taken place and free drainage is ensured. The wound is closed in layers and dressings applied.

Ureterocutaneous Transplant (Anastomosis). The surgical approach is the same as that for a low ureterolithotomy.

1. The ureter is divided as far distally as possible.
2. The surgeon passes the severed ureter retroperitoneally through the lower abdominal wall and sutures it to the skin with an absorbable everting suture of 4-0 on an atraumatic needle to form a stoma. The ureter is handled gently with plastic instruments, fixation forceps, and iris scissors.
3. A small Silastic stenting catheter is passed up into the ureter and left in place for 48 to 72 hours, as ureteral edema subsides. The patient requires a urine-collecting device after surgery.

Ureterosigmoid Anastomosis

1. The surgeon enters the peritoneal cavity through a lower left paramedian incision.
2. The major portion of the large bowel is protected with moist laparotomy packs.
3. Deep retractors are placed, and the surgeon uses long forceps and scissors to incise the posterior peritoneum.
4. The ureters are identified, divided close to the bladder, mobilized, and brought through the posterior peritoneal incision to lie near the sigmoid. Traction sutures and smooth tissue forceps are used to handle the ureters.
5. The sigmoid colon is mobilized to prevent tension on the ureteroenteric anastomosis.

6. Using 3-0 nonabsorbable suture material, the surgeon sutures the sigmoid colon to the pelvic peritoneum at a point where the ureter falls easily on the bowel.

7. Using a scalpel with a #15 blade, the surgeon makes an incision into the taenia of the sigmoid down to the mucosal layer. The edges of the taenia are undermined to create two parallel flaps.

8. The ureter is laid on the bowel mucosa, and a small slit is made through the mucosa into the lumen of the colon.

9. With fixation forceps and iris scissors, the surgeon bevels the ureter to lie flat in the tunica incision.

10. The distal ureter is anchored to the bowel mucosa with 4-0 absorbable ureteral sutures on atraumatic needles. The other ureter is anastomosed in the same manner in a position slightly above the first.

11. The tunicae are then loosely reapproximated over the ureter with 4-0 absorbable sutures, creating an antireflux anastomosis.

12. The surgeon closes the posterior peritoneum with absorbable sutures. Drains are exteriorized retroperitoneally. The incision is closed and dressings applied.

Ureterolithotomy

Procedural Considerations. A KUB x-ray examination should be done immediately before surgery to determine the exact location of the stone. The surgeon may also schedule a cystoscopic examination preoperatively and may attempt to remove the stone endoscopically. The location of the stone determines the surgical approach. A stone high in the ureter requires a flank incision with possible removal of the twelfth rib; a more distal ureteral stone requires a lower abdominal incision.

Operative Procedure

1. After exposure of the ureter, the stone may be kept stationary with Babcock clamps or vessel loops applied above and below it.

2. With a #15 blade, the surgeon makes an incision in the ureter directly over the stone, which may be easily removed with Randall stone forceps.

3. A 10F catheter is passed proximally up and distally down the ureter while irrigating with saline to check for ureteral patency and to dislodge any remaining stone fragments.

4. The surgeon closes the ureter with 4-0 or 5-0 absorbable sutures. All stones should be placed in dry receptacles and sent to the chemistry laboratory for analysis.

Kidney Surgery

This section provides information about surgical procedures performed on the kidney for restoration of function or treatment of renal conditions.

Procedural Considerations

Patient preparation and instrument setup are as described for ureteral surgery.

Operative Procedure

Pyelotomy and Pyelostomy

1. The surgeon incises the pelvis of the kidney with a small scalpel blade. Fine traction sutures may be placed at the edges of the incision for gentle retraction while the pelvis and calyces are explored.

2. In pyelostomy, a small Malecot or Foley catheter is placed through the incision into the renal pelvis. Pyelotomy is used only for very short periods of renal drainage because tubes tend to be dislodged easily from the renal pelvis.

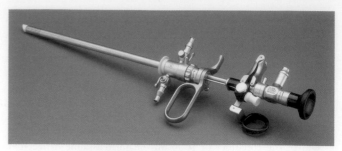

FIG. 15.54 Kuntz laser working element.

Percutaneous Nephrolithotomy

Percutaneous nephrolithotomy facilitates the removal or disintegration of renal stones using a rigid or flexible nephroscope (Fig. 15.54) passed through a percutaneous nephrostomy tract. Accessory instrumentation, such as the ultrasound wand, electrohydraulic lithotripter probe, laser fiber, stone basket, and stone grasper, is passed through the lumen of the nephroscope.

Ideally the patient is in good health and not obese and the calculus is 1 cm or less in diameter, free-floating, radiopaque, and solitary. However, there is a high population of obese patients who undergo percutaneous nephrolithotomy. Advances in technology complemented by the experience gained by the uroradiology team have allowed patients with more complex problems to be managed in this manner. Patients who have undergone previous renal surgery, have stone recurrence, or have an established nephrostomy tract may also benefit from this procedure.

Creation of the nephrostomy tract and removal of the stone can be accomplished by three different methods. Proper placement of the nephrostomy wire can decrease the operating time significantly. In the *one-step procedure*, creation of the nephrostomy tract, tract dilation, and stone removal are completed in a single session. This method is generally preferred unless there are contraindications. In the *immediate two-step procedure*, the radiologist places the nephrostomy tube under radiographic guidance and the surgeon removes the stone later the same day or the next morning. The second step is usually done in the OR with the patient administered a general anesthetic. In the *delayed two-step procedure*, the nephrostomy tract is established after the patient has been administered a local anesthetic. The patient is discharged the following day with a 22F or 24F nephrostomy tube connected to drainage. The patient is readmitted to the hospital 5 to 7 days later for the percutaneous removal of the stone after the patient has been administered a general anesthetic.

Of basic concern during the operative phase are the patient's position and body temperature, the potential for sudden and rapid blood loss, the type of anesthesia, medications required during surgery, and catheter management during and after the procedure. The patient's position, which may be prone or up to 30 degrees prone-oblique, and the draping procedure depend on whether the surgery is performed in the radiology department or the OR and the type of x-ray equipment that will be used.

Endopyelotomy

Endopyelotomy is currently considered the first-line therapy for primary and secondary UPJ obstruction in adults and secondary UPJ obstruction in children.

Procedural Considerations. Acucise endopyelotomy is the simultaneous dilation and incision of a ureteral stricture under fluoroscopic guidance. Only basic cystoscopic equipment and C-arm fluoroscopy are needed for this procedure. The Acucise balloon catheter will pass through a standard 25F cystoscope sheath.

Operative Procedure

1. The surgeon places an open-ended ureteral catheter into the distal ureter, and a retrograde pyelogram is performed to define the area of stenosis. A guidewire is then advanced into the renal collection system.
2. The Acucise catheter is placed over the guidewire and passed through the cystoscope. The Acucise catheter should be rotated under direct cystoscopic vision so the cutting wire is in correct lateral orientation.
3. The surgeon advances the cutting balloon catheter over the super stiff guidewire until the UPJ stenosis is visualized. The surgeon positions the cutting wire laterally at the UPJ and in the proximal and midureter.
4. After visualizing the wire in the lateral position, the surgeon gently inflates the balloon with dilute contrast media to ensure correct positioning across the UPJ.
5. After ensuring proper grounding of the patient, the cutting wire is activated at 75 to 100 watts (pure cut) for 5 seconds, and simultaneously dilute contrast is again instilled into the dilating balloon under continuous, fluoroscopic guidance. As the balloon inflates, the stricture is incised.
6. The incision is completed and a retrograde pyelogram is performed through the Acucise catheter to confirm extravasation at the incision site.

The surgeon removes the internal stent at 6 weeks postoperatively using a flexible cystoscope in males or a rigid cystoscope in females. Patients typically return 12 weeks after stent removal for postoperative IVP or differential renal scan with furosemide wash-out to confirm efficacy of the endopyelotomy.

Extracorporeal Shock-Wave Lithotripsy

ESWL units use water-filled cushions adjacent to the kidney area. An x-ray image intensifier with two monitors is used to visualize the kidney stone at the focal point of the shock wave. After every 100 shocks, fluoroscopy is used to locate remaining stone particles. Adjustments are made, and the patient is repositioned before further treatments. ESWL is often used with percutaneous nephrolithotomy and transurethral ureteropyeloscopy if the patient does not pass the gravel.

Stones that are treated with ESWL are fragmented by the energy focused on the stone with the lithotripter. The shock waves are administered from 30 minutes to 2 hours. Shock waves reverberate inside the stone, causing fragmentation with ultimate complete or partial destruction of the calculus. The amount of destruction depends on the number and energy of the shock waves delivered and the stone's hardness. This technique is effective because shock waves can be transmitted and focused through tissue without loss of energy. A loud, reverberating, popping sound occurs each time a wave pulse is activated. It is advisable that earplugs be worn.

The requirement for anesthesia is determined by the power of the shock wave, the area of shock-wave entry at the skin level, and the size of the shock-wave focal point. The summation of shock waves used during the procedure can cause pain at the skin level. Typically a general, spinal, or local anesthetic is used with the older lithotripters. Modern versions allow for lithotripsy with only IV sedation, oral sedation, or a transcutaneous electrical nerve stimulation (TENS) unit.

The use of a stent before ESWL depends on the patient and the character of the stone or stones. The patient should have a negative urine culture before stent placement. Studies show that complication rates decrease if a stent is used with a stone larger than 1.5 cm. A stent placed before ESWL tends to decrease the need for ancillary interventions, reduces overall complications, and assists in proper positioning for ESWL by delineating the ureteral anatomy and the precise stone location. On the other hand, those patients who tend to readily form stones may demonstrate calcification of the ureteral stent in a relatively short time. Without a stent the risk of silent renal obstruction resulting in loss of kidney function, obstruction of the ureter, nephritis, and sepsis is increased.

Complications related to ESWL are attributable to the cavitation effects of treatment and are proportional to the number of shocks. The ability of the kidney's tubular cells to survive shock waves is related to the number of shock waves to which the kidney is exposed and not to the energy level. Gross hematuria is seen almost universally, resolves in 12 to 48 hours, and is believed to be attributable to parenchymal edema that spontaneously heals within 1 week. Subcapsular or perirenal hematoma caused by perinephric fluid collections may occur and appears to be higher in the hypertensive patient. Subcapsular hematoma may resolve in 6 weeks or may take up to 6 months, whereas perirenal hematoma is relieved usually in a matter of days. Impairment of renal function may be seen in patients with solitary kidneys. Iliac artery and vein thromboses have been reported with lithotripsy for ureteral stones. The majority of lithotripsy patients demonstrate little or no long-term morbidity.

Laser Lithotripsy

Laser lithotripsy has become an exciting alternative to ESWL and EHL. The Ho:YAG, tunable pulse-dyed (coumarin), Er:YAG (erbium:yttrium-aluminum-garnet), the tunable Alexandrite (a chromium-doped mineral), or the Q-switched Nd:YAG laser systems have the ability to disintegrate stones without damaging soft tissue. The technique may be used during a ureteropyeloscopy or nephroscopy or to manage ureteral stones instead of performing a ureterolithotomy. When the laser probe is discharged in direct contact with the calculus, plasma (ionized gas) coats the stone's surface. This plasma expands with repeated firings, creating a shock wave that fractures the stone. Normal saline is used for continuous irrigation throughout the procedure. It is not necessary to immobilize the calculus. Everyone in the room must wear laser goggles, and all laser precautions apply (see Chapter 8).

Dismembered Pyeloplasty

Pyeloplasty is revision or plastic reconstruction of the renal pelvis. Pyeloplasty is performed to create a better anatomic relationship between the renal pelvis and the proximal ureter and to allow proper urinary drainage from the kidney to the bladder. A temporary nephrostomy is often included to protect the plastic reconstruction of the UPJ. Tissue healing usually occurs in 10 to 12 days, and the nephrostomy tube is removed once ureteral patency is demonstrated. *Ureteroplasty* is reconstruction of the ureter distal to the UPJ. A *dismembered pyeloplasty* is the combined correction of the redundant renal pelvis and resection of a stenotic portion of the UPJ.

Procedural Considerations. The instrument setup is as described for nephrectomy, plus fine plastic and vascular instrumentation and Randall stone forceps. A ureteral stent and red rubber catheters also are used. The perioperative nurse assists with positioning the patient in the lateral position.

Operative Procedure

Open Approach

1. The surgeon exposes the kidney and upper ureter through a supracostal flank incision.
2. Gerota fascia is entered, and the renal pelvis and ureter are freed while the kidney is rotated medially.
3. The surgeon frees the ureter and stabilizes it with a vessel loop below the level of the UPJ.
4. A 4-0 stay suture is placed in the tip of the ureter, and the ureter is incised, trimmed, and shaped to the desired contour with fine forceps and scissors.
5. Anchoring sutures of 4-0 material are placed for traction during reconstruction of the renal pelvis. A diamond-shaped incision is made into the renal pelvis, and the tissue is removed. The Y-V-plasty technique may be followed. It converts a Y-shaped surgical incision of the renal pelvis into a V by drawing the apex of the arms of the Y to the foot of the Y with absorbable sutures.
6. Sutures are placed at each end of the refashioned renal pelvis, passed to the ureteral stoma, and tagged. The pelvis is irrigated free of clots. The sutures are run in a continuous manner, creating the anastomosis.
7. A Silastic tubing may be used to stent the repaired pelvis until adequate healing has occurred. A nephrostomy tube is also placed within the pelvis to divert urine safely while the edema in the area of the repair resolves.
8. The surgeon closes Gerota fascia over the repair.
9. A drain is placed where the pelvis was reconstructed, and the surgical incision is closed in layers.

Laparoscopic Approach. UPJ obstruction has joined the rank of conditions that may be treated laparoscopically. Generally a standard transperitoneal approach is used. The patient may be placed supine with a lateral tilt or in lateral decubitus and the bed rotated to access the ports.

After placement of four trocars as in laparoscopic nephrectomy, the surgeon frees the proximal ureters and renal pelvis. The obstruction at the UPJ is excised, and a spatulated anastomosis is performed using running or interrupted sutures. A ureteral stent is usually left in place.

Decreased postoperative pain and shorter hospitalization make this approach appealing. A higher degree of skill is required for this technique, however, making it an option that has not become standard treatment as yet.

Nephroureterectomy: Open Approach

Nephroureterectomy is removal of a kidney and its entire ureter. This procedure is indicated for hydroureteronephrosis of such a degree that reconstructive repair is impossible. It is also used for collecting system tumors of the kidney and ureter.

Procedural Considerations. Open nephroureterectomy requires an extension of the incision anteriorly with the patient positioned semilaterally and fully prepped and draped for the surgeon to access the flank and lower abdomen. Only one instrument set is required, but a second skin-prep setup and set of sterile drapes may be necessary. An alternative to open nephroureterectomy is laparoscopic nephroureterectomy.

Operative Procedure

1. The surgeon exposes the kidney and upper ureter and performs a nephrectomy as described in the following procedure. The kidney may be placed in a plastic bag to prevent possible spillage of tumor cells.

2. The ureter is mobilized as far distally as possible. The OR bed is adjusted so that surgery on the lower ureter may proceed. The lower ureter and bladder are identified and mobilized.
3. The ureter and a small cuff of the bladder are removed in continuity, and the bladder is repaired with a single layer of 2-0 absorbable interrupted sutures. The ureter and cuff of bladder are pulled superiorly, and the intact kidney and ureter are removed.
4. An 18F or 20F Foley catheter is left in the bladder, and a drain is placed behind the bladder. The incision is closed in layers.

Nephrectomy: Open Approach

Nephrectomy is the surgical removal of a kidney. It is performed as a means of definitive therapy for many renal problems, such as congenital UPJ obstruction with severe hydronephrosis, renal tumor, renal trauma, calculus disease with infection, cortical abscess, pyelonephrosis, and renovascular hypertension.

In routine renal surgery the patient is placed in the lateral position with the dependent iliac crest over the kidney rest. The operative flank is uppermost, with the patient's back brought to the edge of the OR bed. The upper arm is supported on an overhead arm support, and the lower arm is supinated on a padded armboard. It may be flexed slightly at the elbow and angled cephalad to promote better access to the flank. The patient's legs are positioned by placing a pillow between them and flexing the lower leg at the knee. The upper leg remains extended. The kidney rest is then raised, and when the desired bed flexion is achieved, 3-inch adhesive tape is used to stabilize the patient throughout surgery. Routine skin preparation and draping procedures are performed.

Procedural Considerations. The nephrectomy setup includes a routine laparotomy setup; kidney instruments; a variety of red rubber, Malecot, or Pezzer catheters; a wound drainage system; and vessel loops. In certain nephrectomies the chest or the GI tract may be opened. If the chest is opened, appropriate instruments and postoperative chest drains are needed. Rib resection requires the addition of a Finochietto rib retractor, a large Matson costal periosteotome, an Alexander costal periosteotome, right and left Doyen rib raspatories, a Bethune rib cutter, a double-action duckbill rongeur, a Bailey rib approximator, and a Langenbeck periosteal elevator. When the GI tract is opened, GI technique is used for the anastomosis.

Operative Procedure

1. The incision is carried through the skin, fat, and fascia. Bleeding vessels are clamped and ligated.
2. The surgeon exposes and incises the external oblique, internal oblique, and transversalis muscles in the direction of the initial skin incision.
3. If necessary, a rib or ribs (eleventh and/or twelfth) may be resected to provide better access to the kidney. The surgeon strips the periosteum with an Alexander costal periosteotome and Doyen rib raspatory. A scalpel and heavy scissors are used to cut through the lumbocostal ligaments. The rib is grasped with an Ochsner clamp and cut with rib shears, removing the portion necessary to expose the kidney. Gerota fascia is identified and incised with Metzenbaum scissors.
4. The surgeon extends the incision and uses blunt and sharp dissection to expose the kidney and perirenal fat. The scrub person should save all perirenal fat that is removed during surgery, placing it in a small basin of normal saline for possible use as a bolster to stop bleeding.
5. The ureter is identified, separated from its adjacent structures, doubly clamped, divided, and ligated with absorbable 0 suture.

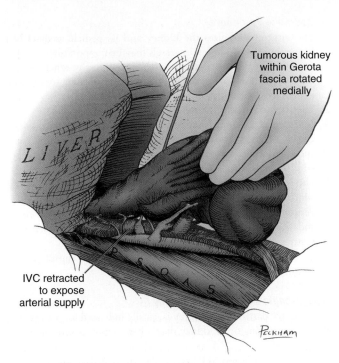

IVC retracted
to expose
arterial supply

Tumorous kidney
within Gerota
fascia rotated
medially

LIVER

PSOAS

PECKHAM

FIG. 15.55 Nephrectomy. *IVC,* Inferior vena cava.

6. The kidney pedicle containing the major blood vessels is isolated and doubly clamped; each vessel is triply ligated with heavy nonabsorbable ties. Each vessel is then severed, leaving two ligatures on the pedicle, and the kidney is removed (Fig. 15.55).
7. The renal fossa is explored for bleeding, and necessary hemostasis is achieved. The fossa is then irrigated with normal saline, and the irrigant is removed by suction.
8. The surgeon closes the fascia and muscle in layers with interrupted absorbable sutures. Retention sutures may be used in obese or chronically ill patients in whom wound healing may be delayed.
9. The skin edges are approximated with sutures or skin staples, and the dressing is applied.

Laparoscopic Nephrectomy

The approach for laparoscopic nephrectomy may be transabdominal (transperitoneal), extraperitoneal (retroperitoneal), or intraperitoneal. Transabdominal is the most common approach. Indications for laparoscopy are generally for benign disease, although more radical surgeries have been accomplished in this manner. A full mechanical antibiotic bowel prep is prescribed. Although surgery time may be longer than typical for an open procedure, postoperative recovery time, analgesia requirements, and total hospital stay are lessened. The procedure always includes cystoscopy with placement of a renal balloon catheter, a ureteral catheter, and a Foley urethral catheter under C-arm fluoroscopy. Indigo carmine may be injected into the skin overlying the renal pelvis.

The patient is initially placed on a beanbag in the supine position. A standard laparoscopy instrument and equipment setup that includes three 5-mm trocars, an insufflation needle, and two 10- to 12-mm trocars is used. Cystoscopic and ureteroscopic supplies are needed, as well as a 0.035-gauge Bentson guidewire, an occlusion balloon catheter, a 0.035-gauge Amplatz stiff guidewire, a 16F Foley catheter and drainage bag, indigo carmine, an irrigator-aspirator, a 1-L bag of saline, a 1-L pressure bag (to pressurize the irrigant to 250 mm Hg),

a #12 or #11 blade, 10-mm clip appliers, the entrapment sack, and tissue morcellator. An open setup should always be available in the event laparoscopy is unsuccessful.

Procedural Considerations. The patient is prepped and draped as for laparotomy. Use of a draping pack with four large adherent drape sheets, instead of a standard laparotomy sheet, affords better access for the port sites.

The patient may be placed in lateral decubitus position on a deflated beanbag positioner at the outset or turned after endoscopic intervention. Ensuring that the patient is adequately secured to the OR bed is critical. Before prepping the patient, the bed is tilted laterally to afford a central abdominal access. The patient is prepped and draped, and access of the first three ports is achieved. Before the surgeon inserts the remaining trocars, the anesthesia provider returns the bed to its normal configuration so that the patient is again in lateral decubitus position. The kidney rest is then elevated, and the operation continues.

Some surgeons begin the procedure with the patient supine. The patient's contralateral arm is padded with thick foam from the shoulder to the fingertips. The patient is prepped and draped for thoracoabdominal surgery. Extra draping materials are used when the patient is repositioned.

Operative Procedure

1. The surgeon accesses the peritoneal cavity through a 1-cm transverse, subumbilical stab-wound incision. After elevation of the anterior abdominal wall with towel clips, the Veress needle is inserted with the stopcock valve control in the closed position.
2. After the Veress needle is in place, sterile saline is dropped into the lumen of the needle and the valve of the needle is opened. If the saline enters freely (a successful test), the abdominal cavity is inflated with CO_2 until a pressure of 15 to 20 mm Hg is obtained. If saline does not enter freely, it indicates improper placement of the needle.
3. The surgeon nicks the rectus fascia with the knife blade, and replaces the Veress needle with the 10-mm trocar. Towel clips are again used on each side of the incision to stabilize the abdominal wall during insertion.
4. The 10-mm laparoscope is inserted.
5. A second incision is made immediately below the costal margin in the midclavicular line, and a 10- to 12-mm trocar is inserted.
6. The surgeon inserts the first of three 5-mm trocars through a small incision 2 cm below the umbilicus in the midclavicular line.
7. The last two 5-mm trocars are placed, one in the anterior axillary line level with the umbilicus and one subcostal in the anterior axillary line. All trocars are then withdrawn until 2 to 3 cm of each sheath protrudes into the abdomen. The surgeon may use polypropylene suture to secure the side arm ports to the patient's skin. Each trocar site is laparoscopically inspected after trocar insertion to identify any bleeding or perforation. On occasion it may be necessary to extend the incision for trocar insertion.
8. The surgeon mobilizes the ascending or descending colon with electrosurgical scissors and deflects it medially. The retroperitoneum is opened.
9. Using gentle motion on the ureteral catheter, the surgeon identifies and dissects the ureter. A Babcock forceps is clamped around the dissected ureter for retraction.
10. The ureter is dissected until the lower pole of the kidney is visualized (Fig. 15.56). Any veins encountered are clipped twice proximally and twice distally. The kidney is cleared of surrounding

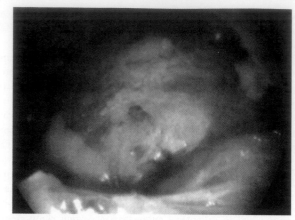

FIG. 15.56 Interior view of exposing right kidney laparoscopically.

tissue and freed laterally and superiorly. Gerota fascia is entered to free the adrenal gland and exclude it from the dissection.

11. The renal artery and vein are identified and cleared to create a 360-degree window around each vessel. The clip applier is inserted through the 10- to 12-mm port. Two clips are placed on the specimen side, and three clips are placed on the stump side of both the artery and the vein, which are then sharply incised.

12. Two pairs of clips are placed proximally and distally on the ureter, which is sharply incised. The specimen end is grasped, and the kidney is moved into the upper abdominal quadrant.

13. The surgeon introduces the entrapment sac through the 10- to 12-mm port. The bottom of the sac is pulled into the abdomen with graspers until the neck of the sac clears the end of the port and is then unfurled.

14. The sac is opened, and the ureteral stump with attached kidney is placed inside. The drawstrings are pulled tight, closing the mouth of the sac.

15. The anesthesia provider returns the patient to the supine position by tilting the OR bed, and the sac strings are extracted through the umbilical port. Under laparoscopic observation, the surgeon removes the port, and the neck of the sac is brought to lie on the abdominal surface. The tissue morcellator is inserted into the sac, and the kidney is morcellated under suction in a clockwise fashion.

16. The surgeon removes the instrumentation from the abdominal cavity, observing each trocar site, during and after removal, to ensure that hemostasis has been achieved. Fascial layers at the 12-mm trocar sites are closed with 2-0 or 3-0 absorbable suture in a figure-of-eight pattern.

17. Using a 4-0 absorbable suture, the surgeon performs a subcuticular closure of all port sites.

Heminephrectomy

Heminephrectomy is removal of a portion of the kidney. It is usually indicated for conditions involving the lower or upper pole of the kidney, such as calculus disease, or trauma limited to one pole of a kidney. In rare instances in which a patient has only one kidney, such surgery may be used for renal neoplasms to avoid the need for dialysis and subsequent renal transplantation.

Procedural Considerations. The setup is as described for nephrectomy with the addition of vascular and bulldog clamps.

Operative Procedure
1. The surgeon mobilizes the kidney and its pedicle as described for nephrectomy. The main vessels may be temporarily occluded for only 20 to 30 minutes, after which progressive renal damage may occur. Local hypothermia may be indicated to prolong ischemic operating time.

2. The renal capsule is incised and stripped back.

3. A wedge of kidney tissue containing the diseased or damaged cortex is excised. The surgeon clamps the interlobar fat or arcuate and interlobular arteries with Hopkins clamps and ligates them with 4-0 absorbable suture on urologic needles.

4. The surgeon reapproximates the open collecting system with a continuous 4-0 suture.

5. Perirenal fat is placed in the area in which tissue was excised, and the renal parenchyma is reapproximated with horizontal mattress sutures.

6. If possible, the surgeon reapproximates the renal capsule with a continuous 2-0 suture.

Laparoscopic Partial Nephrectomy

Laparoscopic partial nephrectomy is usually indicated for the removal of a tumor, leaving more kidney than a heminephrectomy (Schwartz et al., 2015).

Procedural Considerations. The setup is as described for laparoscopic nephrectomy.

Operative Procedure
1. Steps 1 to 8 of the laparoscopic nephrectomy procedure are completed.

2. The surgeon locates the tumor and then clears the fat around it. The surgeon tries to keep the fat directly above the tumor intact so the pathologists can confirm no advancement into the fat.

3. A 0.5- to 1-cm margin around the tumor is marked with the ESU. Some surgeons may use laparoscopic ultrasound to see the depth of the tumor.

4. The anesthesia provider administers IV mannitol and the surgeon clamps the hilum to prevent blood loss. Clamp time needs to be minimized to 30 minutes or else icing of the kidney is needed.

5. The surgeon uses scissors to sharply excise the tumor. If the collecting system of the kidney is entered, this needs to be closed separately. It can be checked for watertight closure with IV indigo carmine. Surgical bolsters and hemostatic matrix (e.g., FLOSEAL) are generally used for hemostasis.

6. After the sutures are placed, the surgeon removes the hilar clamp and monitors for bleeding. A closed-wound drain system may be placed.

7. The surgeon removes the instrumentation from the abdominal cavity, observing each trocar site, during and after removal, to ensure that hemostasis has been achieved. Fascial layers at the 12-mm trocar sites are closed with 2-0 or 3-0 absorbable suture in a figure-of-eight pattern.

8. Using a 4-0 absorbable suture, the surgeon performs a subcuticular closure of all port sites.

Radical Nephrectomy

Radical nephrectomy is excision of the kidney, perirenal fat, adrenal gland, Gerota capsule (fascia), and contiguous periaortic lymph nodes. This procedure is performed for parenchymal renal neoplasms. In the open approach, a lumbar, transthoracic, or transabdominal approach to the kidney is used, depending on the size and location of the lesion. The transthoracic or transabdominal approach is preferred because the blood vessels of the kidney can be more easily reached and ligated before the tumor is mobilized, decreasing the possibility of tumor embolization into the bloodstream. For the laparoscopic approach a retroperitoneal or transperitoneal approach may be used.

Procedural Considerations. The setups are as described for open nephrectomy and laparoscopic nephrectomy.

Operative Procedure. Generally the procedure is as described for nephrectomy with two exceptions: (1) the renal pedicle is ligated before the kidney is mobilized, and (2) Gerota capsule is not incised but is removed en bloc with the kidney. Involved lymph nodes surrounding the renal pedicle are excised. A chest tube is inserted if the transthoracic approach is used.

Kidney Transplant

Kidney transplant entails transplantation of a living-related or cadaveric donor kidney into the recipient's iliac fossa (Fig. 15.57). It is performed in an effort to restore renal function and thus maintain life in a patient who has end-stage renal disease.

Transplant From a Living Donor

The kidney donor must be in good health. ABO (blood typing) and histocompatibility (human leukocyte antigen [HLA] tissue typing) along with a negative white cell (lymphocyte) crossmatch determine donor-recipient compatibility. It is not necessary to match the Rh factor. After the donor has been chosen, a complete workup that includes history, physical examination, chest x-ray examination, ECG, CBC, BUN and creatinine values, blood chemistry profiles, coagulation studies, viral titers, and serologic testing is performed. Renal function is assessed by monitoring three creatinine clearances, urinalysis, and blood and urine cultures if hospitalized 72 hours or longer, followed by IVP and excretory urography. A flush aortogram assesses the vascular anatomy, and renal angiography pinpoints the kidney of choice while ruling out the presence of renal lesions. A kidney with a single renal artery is preferred, but kidneys with double and triple arteries may be used if necessary. If there is a family history of diabetes, a 5-hour glucose tolerance test is also performed (UNOS, 2016).

The ideal living donor is an identical twin, although a family member, friend, or altruistic donor may donate an organ. The living donor and the kidney recipient arrive in the preoperative registration area the morning of surgery. The patients are then brought to the preop holding area to be prepared for surgery.

Procedural Considerations. Two adjacent ORs are prepared for the procedures because surgery on the donor and surgery on the recipient proceed simultaneously.

Usually the left kidney is chosen for removal because the left renal vein is longer than the right renal vein. Two IV lines and a Foley catheter are required. The patient is placed on a beanbag positioning device and moved into a modified flank position with the torso in a 30-degree lateral decubitus position with the right side down after endotracheal intubation. The lower arm is positioned extended outward on a well-padded armboard at a right angle to the torso; the upper arm is positioned on an elevated lateral armboard. The patient's hips are rolled slightly posteriorly to allow exposure of the lower abdominal midline. Three pillows are placed between the patient's legs, and the ankles and feet are appropriately padded. An axillary roll is also placed and the radial pulse is confirmed in the right wrist. The bed is flexed to 30 degrees, and the upper portion is angled downward to approximately 140 degrees. The skin is prepped from midchest to pubis and draped to expose the flank area.

Required instruments and equipment are identical to those for a nephrectomy plus an IV pole and supplies for the sterile perfusion table. These include electrolyte solution (placed in an iced basin until needed), cystoscopy tubing, a large kidney basin with iced saline solution, an olive tip, a 30-mL syringe, Gerald forceps, tenotomy scissors, a smooth Christmas tree tip, mosquitos, and Kelly hemostats.

An electrolyte solution of histidine-tryptophan-ketoglutarate (HTK) or University of Wisconsin (UW) solution that contains 10,000 units of heparin is used to flush the harvested kidney (Olumi et al., 2015).

Operative Procedure

Open Approach

1. The donor nephrectomy procedure is as described for nephrectomy; however, the ureter and renal vein and artery require meticulous dissection.

2. Maximum length of the ureter is achieved by dividing it at or below the pelvic rim if possible. To preserve adequate ureteral vascularization, the surgeon is cautious not to skeletonize the ureter.

3. Particular care is taken to remove the maximum length of the renal vein and artery. Obtaining the maximum length of the left renal vein sometimes requires partial occlusion of the inferior vena cava with a Satinsky clamp and dissection of a portion of the inferior vena cava. This is done after the ureter has been freed.

4. Repair of the inferior vena cava is made with a continuous 4-0 or 5-0 vascular suture.

5. Five minutes before the surgeon clamps the renal vessels, 5000 units of heparin sodium and 12.5 g of mannitol are systemically administered to the patient to prevent intravascular clotting and maximize diuresis.

6. Furosemide, mannitol, and IV fluids are administered to the donor to maintain adequate urinary output from the donor's remaining kidney.

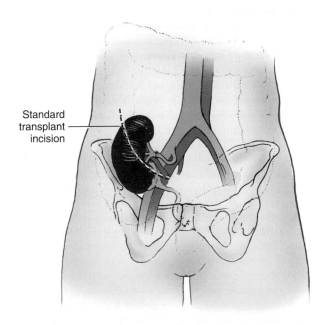

Standard transplant incision

FIG. 15.57 Transplanted kidney in recipient's iliac fossa.

7. Gentle handling of the kidney is essential. Team members must prevent undue traction on the vascular pedicle, which may induce vasospasm and reduce perfusion of the kidney.

8. To reduce warm ischemia time the surgeon double-clamps the vein and the artery, excises the kidney, and immediately places it in iced saline solution on a sterile back table, where the kidney is flushed with the designated electrolyte solution. Warm ischemia time (from the clamping of renal vessels to a point at which the kidney is perfused with cold electrolyte solution) should be kept to a minimum to prevent acute tubular necrosis and to maintain maximum renal function after transplantation.

9. Gerald forceps are used to expose the renal artery to permit insertion of an olive tip or smooth Christmas tree cannula. The cold electrolyte solution passes through the IV tubing and the needle catheter, flushing any remaining donor's blood from the kidney. This also decreases the kidney's metabolic rate by lowering its temperature. Flushing time is usually 2 to 5 minutes.

10. After flushing the surgeon may trim the vessels of adventitia to facilitate the vascular anastomosis to the recipient's iliac vessels.

11. The kidney, in iced saline solution and HTK or UW solution, is covered with sterile drapes and taken by the surgeon to the room in which the recipient's iliac vessels have been exposed.

12. Wound closure for the donor is as described for nephrectomy.

Hand-Assisted Laparoscopic Approach. The hand-assisted laparoscopic (HAL) approach allows surgeons direct hand contact with the operative field, maximizing tactile feedback and minimizing surgical injury to the patient. HAL differs from standard laparoscopy because surgeons are also able to introduce their hand into the operative field.

Procedural Considerations. A gel-port hand-port and three or four trocars are used. Generally, the hand-port and a 5-mm trocar are the working ports; a 10-mm trocar is used for the laparoscope, and an additional 5-mm trocar may be used if extra retraction is needed. Instruments required include the following: two 5-mm atraumatic graspers, 5-mm curved dissecting scissors, a coagulating hook, a bipolar grasper, two needle holders, a clip applier, a vascular stapler, and an atraumatic retrieval bag without a system for opening and closing it and a minimal opening of 15 cm. In addition, the standard open setup needs to be ready with open vascular instrumentation, a smooth Christmas tree adapter, sterile cystoscopy tubing, and sterile iced saline for ex vivo perfusion.

Operative Procedure

1. The surgeon creates a supraumbilical incision for the hand-port. After the hand-port is placed, a 10-mm trocar is placed through the hand-port to introduce pneumoperitoneum. A camera is introduced through the trocar to directly visualize the placement of the 5-mm working port, approximately two fingerbreadths cephalad to the hand-port. The 10-mm camera port is placed three fingerbreadths inferior to the xiphoid. An additional 5-mm trocar may be placed in the flank at the convex border of the kidney if extra retraction is necessary.

2. A bipolar ESU is used to incise the left lateral peritoneal reflection.

3. The descending colon is reflected medially from the beginning of the splenic flexure down to the level of the sigmoid colon, incising the phrenocolic ligaments completely. Care is taken to ensure no bowel injury or mesenteric defect occurs.

4. The surgeon divides the lienorenal and splenocolic ligaments at the inferior border of the spleen, allowing the spleen to be retracted superiorly and to mobilize the splenic flexure medially.

5. Gerota fascia is exposed by mobilizing the descending colon medially.

6. The plane is developed between Gerota fascia and the mesentery, adjacent to the lower pole of the kidney.

7. The plane medial to the gonadal vein and the ureter is developed and the structures are dissected off the psoas muscle, taking care not to devascularize the ureter.

8. The surgeon continues to dissect the medial aspect of the upper pole of the kidney, which is mobilized until the upper pole is completely free.

9. The left renal vein is then freed from its adventitial attachments and the adrenal and lumbar veins are identified, doubly clipped on both sides, and divided between clips.

10. After elevating the kidney, the surgeon performs additional dissection, usually posteriorly to the renal vein to identify and isolate the renal artery and after dividing the fibro-fatty and lymphatic tissue around the vessels.

11. The renal artery is dissected out, taking care to ensure there is space to pass the endovascular gastrointestinal anastomosis (GIA) stapler around the artery and vein.

12. The entire kidney is then freed of all its adventitial attachments.

13. The anesthesia provider administers 40 mg of furosemide (Lasix) and 12.5 mg of mannitol and 3000 units of heparin via the patient's IV.

14. Next the gonadal vein is double clipped and divided and the ureter is triple clipped and divided at the level of the iliac vessels.

15. After 3 minutes of systemic heparinization, the renal artery and vein are transected individually and sequentially with the endovascular GIA stapler.

16. The kidney is placed in the large basin with iced saline and flushed on the back table with 1 L of cold HTK or UW solution.

17. After the kidney is flushed, as described in the open donor nephrectomy, the kidney basin is covered with a drape and taken to the recipient OR.

18. The surgeon irrigates the peritoneum and achieves hemostasis. A drain may be inserted into the peritoneal space for a short time postoperatively.

19. The wounds are sutured and dressings applied.

Transplant From a Cadaveric Donor

The ideal cadaveric donor is young, free from infection and cancer, normotensive until a short time before death, and under hospital observation several hours before death. Permission to harvest the donor kidney must be obtained from the family and the medical examiner after brain death has been unequivocally established. Awareness of existing state legislation in this complex area is advisable.

The donor is completely evaluated. The medical history is reviewed for any possible contraindications, such as chronic disease, ongoing systemic infection, IV drug abuse, malignancy, heart or lung disease, trauma to the donor organ, and the presence of human immunodeficiency virus (HIV). Laboratory studies include blood typing, urinalysis, urine and blood cultures, BUN, serum creatinine, CBC, hepatitis B antigen evaluation, Venereal Disease Research Laboratory (VDRL) for the presence of venereal disease, and p24 antigen capture assay for the presence of HIV antigen. Evaluation of arterial blood gases, electrolyte values, and liver enzymes is also necessary. Because of improvements in medical therapy, the only absolute contraindications to organ donation are HIV and metastasis.

Preoperative management of the cadaver donor is vital to the success of the transplant. Organ perfusion, oxygenation, and hydration must be maintained. Arterial blood gas evaluation determines ventilatory support, and dopamine may be administered if fluids alone are not able to maintain an adequate systolic blood pressure. Urine output is monitored, and antibiotics may be administered to combat or prevent infection.

Procedural Considerations. After brain death has been established, the donor is taken to the OR with respiratory and cardiac function maintained mechanically. The donor is placed in the supine position and is prepared for a laparotomy. Anticoagulant and α-adrenergic receptor–blocking agents are administered systemically during the procedure. Adequate renal perfusion and function are maintained with IV fluids and diuretics.

Instruments and equipment are the same as those for nephrectomy, with the addition of Metzenbaum scissors, suture scissors, vascular forceps, DeBakey forceps, Dean hemostatic forceps, mosquito hemostats, DeBakey clamps, angled clip appliers with medium and large clips, bulldog clamps, vascular clamps, Deaver retractors, Harrington splanchnic retractors, vascular needle holders, a sternal saw or Lebsche knife and mallet, umbilical tapes, electrolyte solution (lactated Ringer's, Sachs, or Collins), cold packing in an iced basin until needed, an IV pole, IV extension tubes, a kidney basin with cold (4°C [39.2°F]) IV saline solution, a three-way stopcock, an 18-gauge needle catheter, a centimeter ruler, the perfusion machine or kidney transplantation equipment, and ice.

Operative Procedure

1. The surgeon makes a midline incision from the xiphoid process to the symphysis pubis with bilateral supraumbilical transverse extensions through the skin, subcutaneous layer, fascia, and muscle.
2. Hemostasis is obtained with clamps, ties, suture ligatures, and the ESU.
3. The kidney, renal vessels, and ureter are carefully dissected with Metzenbaum scissors, DeBakey forceps, and Dean hemostatic forceps.
4. The anesthesia provider administers 15,000 units of heparin sodium IV 5 to 10 minutes before the renal vessels are clamped.
5. The usual method of resection is en bloc resection (harvesting of donor kidneys) (Fig. 15.58), which involves the removal of sections of the inferior vena cava and aorta with both kidneys in continuity.
6. The surgeon makes an incision along the route of the small bowel mesentery up to the esophageal hiatus.
7. Next, the surgeon mobilizes the entire GI tract, spleen, and inferior portion of the pancreas dividing the celiac axis and the superior mesenteric artery, exposing the entire retroperitoneal region.
8. Using vascular clamps, the surgeon clamps and divides the inferior vena cava and aorta below the renal vessels.
9. The surgeon secures the lumbar tributaries with metal clips and divides them.
10. The kidneys and ureters are freed from their surrounding soft tissues.
11. The ureters are divided distally at the pelvic brim.
12. The surgeon clamps and divides the suprarenal aorta and inferior vena cava at the level of the diaphragm, close to the bifurcation.
13. The surgeon severs the vessels and kidney and ligates the aorta and vena cava.
14. After removal of the kidneys, immediate perfusion with cold (4°C [29.2°F]) UW or electrolyte solution is performed. The

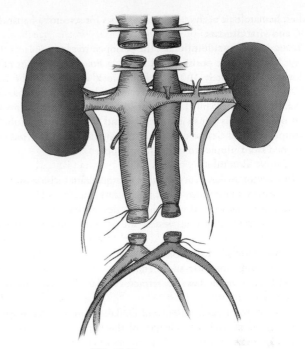

FIG. 15.58 En bloc resection.

kidneys are placed in a container of cold saline solution and surrounded by saline slush in an insulated carrier or placed on a hypothermic pulsatile perfusion machine for transport. While kidney perfusion is begun, the abdominal lymph nodes and spleen are removed for use in tissue typing.

15. The incision is closed with interrupted sutures, and the patient's artificial life-support systems are terminated. The perioperative nurse cares for the patient's body, preserving privacy and dignity at the patient's death.

Transplant Recipient

Each potential recipient is judged individually regarding kidney transplantation. Recipient ages range from <1 year to 75 years of age. Older patients are less tolerant of postoperative complications. Contraindications for renal transplantation include (1) systemic disease that precludes major surgery, (2) oxalosis (a metabolic disorder), (3) a positive HLA cytotoxic antibody screen, (4) untreatable cardiovascular disease, (5) active cancer, and (6) noncompliance (Collins, 2015). If required, a patient may need to undergo bilateral nephrectomy before renal transplantation for uncontrollable hypertension, for kidney infections, or for reflux when there is a significant history of infections. Occasionally a large polycystic kidney may need to be removed to create a space for the new kidney. Splenectomy may be performed at this time to improve leukopenia and enhance the effects of myelosuppressive and immunosuppressive drugs.

The transplant recipient requires optimal nutritional support and adequate dialysis. All potential sources of infection must be treated. Most commonly these include teeth, bladder, nasal sinuses, and skin. The patient may need a short course of hemodialysis to control fluid overload or electrolyte imbalances. A repeat cytotoxic crossmatch with fresh serum specimens should follow hemodialysis. Preoperative antibiotics are commonly administered. Other important diagnostic tools for preoperative evaluation are chest x-ray examination, abdominal ultrasonography, voiding cystourethrography, liver function studies, hematologic assays, and serum values for screening hepatitis, HIV, and viral diseases.

Procedural Considerations. The perioperative nurse places the patient in the supine position and inserts a Foley catheter into the bladder. Approximately 100 mL of antibiotic mixed in an IV bag of 0.9% normal saline is instilled into the bladder through cystoscopy tubing. The bladder is filled and drained four times. The fifth instillation of 100 mL is left in the bladder and the cystoscopy tubing is clamped until the time of the ureteral anastomosis. The patient is prepped from nipples to groin and draped.

Operative Procedure

1. The surgeon makes a curved right lower quadrant incision through the skin, subcutaneous layer, fascia, and muscle.
2. Bleeding is controlled with clamps, ties, and an ESU.
3. The inferior epigastric vessels are divided between suture ligatures.
4. Retroperitoneal dissection is performed by mobilizing the peritoneum superiorly and medially.
5. A self-retaining Bookwalter retractor is placed once exposure is attained.
6. Using Metzenbaum scissors and DeBakey forceps, the surgeon dissects along the entire length of the hypogastric artery and the external and common iliac arteries to the bifurcation of the aorta, continuing down the internal iliac artery.
7. The internal iliac artery is ligated distally and divided, with proximal control maintained by a vascular clamp.
8. The iliac vein may be dissected free by ligating and dividing the internal iliac venous branches with 3-0 nonabsorbable sutures or ligating clips. More commonly, only the hypogastric artery and that portion of iliac vein to be anastomosed are dissected free.
9. The donor kidney is brought into the operative field in a large basin of iced saline and HTK or UW solution.
10. The surgeon uses mosquito hemostats, 4-inch DeBakey forceps, and curved and straight fine scissors to make the necessary alterations on the donor kidney vessels to facilitate the anastomoses.
11. A Lambert Kay clamp is placed on the internal iliac vein.
12. A #11 blade is used to make a 1-cm incision in the iliac vein between the clamps.
13. The vessel is rinsed with heparin sodium solution (10 units/mL) in a 30-mL syringe with an olive tip.
14. Angled Potts scissors are used to extend the incision to accommodate the donor renal vein.
15. The surgeon performs the anastomosis of the donor kidney renal vein to the side of the recipient's iliac vein with 5-0 double armed vascular sutures.
16. In like manner the renal artery is anastomosed end-to-end with the proximal portion of the internal iliac artery using 5-0 vascular sutures.
17. Before placing the final sutures, the vessels are irrigated proximally and distally with heparin sodium solution with a 30-mL syringe with an olive tip.
18. The Lambert Kay clamps are removed from the venous vessels, and the anastomosis is checked for leakage.
19. The clamp on the internal iliac artery is then released, and the anastomosis is checked.
20. Meticulous inspection is made of the hilum and surface of the kidney for bleeding and infarction.
21. The anesthesia provider administers diuretics intravenously as needed.
22. Attention is then directed to the ureter and bladder.
23. Two Gerald forceps are used to grasp the anterior bladder wall.
24. Using a scalpel with a #10 blade, the surgeon makes a 4-cm anterior incision.
25. The ureter is passed through the bladder wall and tunneled suburothelially for 2 to 2.5 cm.
26. The surgeon sutures the spatulated end of the ureter into the bladder urothelium with four to six 5-0 atraumatic absorbable sutures, creating a ureteroneocystostomy.
27. A 6F ureteral stent is passed through the ureteroneocystostomy, up to the renal pelvis, and out through the urethra with the Foley catheter. This stenting catheter will remain in place for 36 to 48 hours to ensure ureteral patency during a period in which ureteral edema may occur.
28. Retractors are removed, and the bladder is closed with 5-0 atraumatic absorbable suture.
29. The renal anastomoses are again checked for bleeding.
30. The cystoscopy tubing is disconnected from the Foley catheter and a urometer is attached to the Foley catheter to monitor postoperative urine output.
31. The surgeon inserts closed-wound suction drains into the wound, exteriorizes them through the skin laterally, and secures the tubing with 2-0 nonabsorbable suture on a cutting needle.
32. Muscle and fascial layers are closed with a single layer of 0 nonabsorbable sutures on a large atraumatic needle.
33. The subcutaneous layer is closed with 3-0 absorbable sutures on an atraumatic needle.
34. Skin closure is accomplished with skin staples, and dressings are applied.

Adrenalectomy

Adrenalectomy is partial or total excision of one or both adrenal glands. It may be performed for several reasons: hypersecretion of adrenal hormones; neoplasms of the adrenal gland; or for secondary treatment of neoplasms elsewhere in the body that depend on adrenal hormonal secretions, such as carcinoma of the prostate and breast; and pheochromocytoma.

Care of the patient with pheochromocytoma carries with it particular concerns for the perioperative nurse. These patients are subject to extreme elevations in blood pressure, often accompanied by tachycardia, and hypovolemic states that can induce vascular collapse. If an adrenal tumor is being excised, early ligation of the adrenal vein is crucial in avoiding a sudden blood pressure elevation from the manipulation of the gland. After tumor removal there will be a rapid drop in blood pressure that can be minimized by maintenance of blood volume and administration of norepinephrine. With bilateral adrenalectomy, cortisone replacement is instituted.

Procedural Considerations

Adrenalectomy may be approached as a laparoscopic or an open procedure. The laparoscopic approach is generally associated with less morbidity and shorter hospital stays. For unilateral adrenalectomy the patient may be placed in the lateral or supine position, depending on the intended approach. If both glands are to be removed the supine or prone position is selected. The prone position is especially useful for a known disorder, such as aldosteronism, localized benign lesions and solitary adenomas of Cushing disease, and for debilitated patients with an advanced neoplasm.

The setup for a lateral approach is as described for nephrectomy, including rib resection instruments, vascular instruments, and vessel clips and appliers. The setup for an abdominal approach is as described for laparotomy, including vascular instruments, extra-long scissors, tissue forceps, Rochester-Péan forceps, Mixter forceps, and needle holders. Penrose tubing is needed for retraction. Vessel clips and appliers also may be needed, as well as various sizes of nonabsorbable braided sutures.

The setup for the posterior approach is as described for the lateral approach. The patient is placed prone in a 35-degree jackknife position with the kidney rest under the inferior margin of the anterior rib cage. Both arms should be carefully extended cephalad with adequate support under each shoulder.

Operative Procedure

Laparoscopic Approach

1. The surgeon makes a 1.5-cm incision at the tip of the twelfth rib. The thoracolumbar fascia is entered by blunt dissection, and the 12-mm balloon dissector is placed behind Gerota fascia and along the anterior axillary line. The balloon is inflated with 800 mL of saline, and the laparoscope is used to confirm balloon placement.
2. The operating balloon trocar is then placed in this position.
3. The surgeon inserts two 10-mm trocars on each side of the initial trocar, along the costal margin, in the anterior and posterior axillary line.
4. The fourth trocar is placed along the posterior costal margin.
5. Dissection begins near the renal hilum, incising into Gerota fascia.
6. The surgeon identifies, clips, and divides the adrenal arteries.
7. The anterior, lateral aspect of the gland is freed from the upper pole of the kidney.
8. The adrenal vein is clipped and divided.
9. The surgeon mobilizes the posterior, superior, and anterior surfaces of the adrenal gland. A fan retractor is used to retract the pancreas and spleen, or pancreas and liver, depending on which side the gland is being excised.
10. The adrenal branches of the inferior phrenic vessels and any accessory vessels are clipped and divided. The gland is removed through the original port using a retrieval sac. Hemostasis is achieved. The trocars are then sequentially removed, the incisions closed, and dressings applied.

Lateral Approach: Open

1. A flank, thoracolumbar, or transthoracic incision is performed as described for nephrectomy.
2. The rib underlying the chosen approach is resected or deflected for optimum exposure of the upper pole of the kidney.
3. The surgeon enters between the eleventh and twelfth ribs in a flank approach, the tenth and eleventh ribs in a thoracolumbar approach, and the ninth and tenth ribs in a transthoracic approach.
4. Using scissors, the surgeon makes an opening through the transverse fascia.
5. The pleura and diaphragm are protected with moist laparotomy packs, and Gerota fascia is incised to expose the kidney and adrenal gland.
6. The surgeon identifies the gland and dissects it free from the upper pole of the kidney with scissors and Babcock forceps.
7. The blood supply of the gland is identified, clamped or clipped, and divided. Bleeding vessels are ligated.
8. To release the gland the left adrenal vein, a branch of the left renal vein, is separated by clamping and cutting. The right adrenal vein, a tributary of the vena cava, is also divided. Fine vascular sutures may be required to repair inadvertent injury to the vena cava.
9. When hemostasis has been ensured, the surgeon closes the wound in sequential layers: muscle, fascia, subcutaneous tissue, and skin. Dressings are then applied.

Abdominal Approach

1. The surgeon incises the abdominal wall with an upper abdominal incision, and the peritoneal cavity is opened and explored. Hemostasis is established.
2. The abdominal wound is retracted, and the surrounding organs are protected with moist laparotomy packs.
3. The surgeon opens the retroperitoneal area near the diaphragm on the left side, exposing the renal fascia.
4. The renal fascia is opened to reveal the left kidney and adrenal gland.
5. Using blunt and sharp dissection, the surgeon frees the adrenal gland from the kidney, clamps all bleeding vessels, and ligates them with 3-0 nonabsorbable sutures.
6. After all bleeding is controlled, the surgeon replaces the kidney in the renal fascia, and closes it with interrupted 0 absorbable sutures.
7. The peritoneum is closed over the left kidney and renal fascia.
8. The abdominal retractors are rearranged to provide access to the peritoneum over the right kidney and adrenal gland. Care must be taken to prevent trauma to the liver.
9. The surgeon repeats the procedure on the right side, taking care to clamp and ligate the short adrenal vein.
10. The abdomen is inspected for bleeding vessels, which are clamped and ligated.
11. The wound is closed and dressings applied.

Posterior Approach

1. The surgeon makes an incision over the eleventh or twelfth rib.
2. The periosteum is elevated, avoiding the nerves and vessels on the inferior margin.
3. The diaphragm and pleura are displaced superiorly, the appropriate rib is resected, and hemostasis is achieved.
4. Gerota fascia is incised, and through sharp and blunt dissection the surgeon exposes the posterior aspect of the upper pole of the kidney.
5. The surgeon mobilizes the upper pole and places a padded retractor to deflect the kidney downward for the approach to the adrenal gland.
6. The suprarenal fat is meticulously dissected.
7. Vessel clips are used for control of smaller vessels.
8. Dissection continues superiorly, laterally, and inferiorly while the integrity of the hilum of the adrenal gland is maintained.
9. Using right-angled clamps, the surgeon frees, divides, and ligates the adrenal vein and artery.
10. Babcock clamps are used for manipulation and removal of the adrenal gland.
11. Bleeding is controlled, and the wound is inspected for injury to renal structures.
12. The surgeon closes Gerota fascia with interrupted absorbable sutures.
13. The wound is closed and dressings applied.

Key Points

- GU surgery encompasses a variety of procedures involving the adrenal glands, kidneys, ureters, lymphatic system, small intestine, bladder, prostate, urethra, penis, testicles, vaginal vault, rectum and inguinal region.

- Many GU procedures have adapted to robotic-assisted minimally invasive procedures, the most common being the robotic-assisted laparoscopic prostatectomy and robotic-assisted laparoscopic nephrectomy.
- Urologic procedures on men are more common because of the prevalence of benign and malignant prostatic conditions. BPH is one of the most common diseases of aging men, ranking in the top 10 most commonly diagnosed conditions in men older than age 50. Prostate cancer is the most frequently diagnosed cancer in men and is the second leading cause of cancer death in men.
- Key factors to consider in planning patient care include positioning and attention to fluid and electrolyte balance. Many procedures require lithotomy positioning, which has a high potential for patient injury. The use of various solutions to aid in visualization and electrosurgery during TURP (or laser TURP) procedures may contribute to hyponatremia.

Critical Thinking Questions

You are assigned as the perioperative nurse for a 62-year-old man who will undergo a robotic radical prostatectomy. The patient states he has a history of hypertension and inguinal hernia repair but denies any other history. However, while positioning the patient you note that he has bilateral incisional scars consistent with hip arthroplasty. His range of motion is severely inhibited in both joints. What risk factors must you take into consideration concerning positioning? How can traditional lithotomy positioning place the patient in further danger? What alternative position(s) would be safer for the patient?

e**volve** *The answers to the Critical Thinking Questions can be found at http://evolve.elsevier.com/Rothrock/Alexander.*

References

American Cancer Society (ACS): *Can prostate cancer be found early?* (website), 2016a. www.cancer.org/cancer/prostatecancer/detailedguide/prostate-cancer-detection. (Accessed 31 October 2016).

American Cancer Society (ACS): *Key statistics about prostate cancer?* (website), 2016b. www.cancer.org/cancer/prostatecancer/detailedguide/prostate-cancer-key-statistics. (Accessed 31 October 2016).

Anderson KE, Wein AJ: Pharmacologic management of lower urinary tract storage and emptying failure. In Wein AJ et al, editors: *Campbell-Walsh urology*, ed 11, Philadelphia, 2015, Elsevier.

Association of periOperative Registered Nurses (AORN): *Guidelines for perioperative practice*, Denver, 2016, The Association.

Barocas DA et al: Effect of the USPSTF Grade D Recommendation against screening for prostate cancer on incident prostate cancer diagnoses in the United States, *J Urol* 194(6):1587–1593, 2015.

Calvaresi AE et al: Implementing hexaminolevulinate HCl blue light cystoscopy: a nursing perspective, *AORN J* 100(5):490–496, 2014.

Castellino AM: *PSA tests cut metastatic prostate cancer rate by 50%* (website), 2015. www.medscape.com/viewarticle/853298. (Accessed 31 October 2016).

Chang SS et al: *Diagnosis and treatment of non-muscle invasive bladder cancer: AUA/SUO joint guideline* (website), 2016. www.auanet.org/education/guidelines/non-muscle-invasive-bladder-cancer.cfm. (Accessed 31 October 2016).

Collins BH: *Renal transplantation* (website), 2015. emedicine.medscape.com/article/430128-overview#a3. (Accessed 31 October 2016).

Collins MA, Terris MK: *Transurethral resection of the prostate* (website), 2014. http://emedicine.medscape.com/article/449781-overview. Accessed 31 October 2016).

Dmochowski R: Slings. In Wein AJ et al, editors: *Campbell-Walsh urology*, ed 11, Philadelphia, 2015, Elsevier.

Francois-Eid J: Surgery for erectile dysfunction. In Wein AJ et al, editors: *Campbell-Walsh urology*, ed 11, Philadelphia, 2015, Elsevier.

Fulmer BR et al: *Laparoscopic and robotic radical prostatectomy* (website), 2015. http://emedicine.medscape.com/article/458677-overview. (Accessed 31 October 2016).

Herschorn S: Injection therapy for urinary incontinence. In Wein AJ et al, editors: *Campbell-Walsh urology*, ed 11, Philadelphia, 2015, Elsevier.

Jemal A et al: Prostate cancer incidence and PSA testing patterns in relation to USPSTF screening recommendations, *JAMA* 314(19):2054–2061, 2015.

Light D: *Malignant testicular tumor imaging* (website), 2015. http://emedicine.medscape.com/article/381007-overview. (Accessed 1 November 2016).

Olumi AF et al: Open surgery of the kidney. In Wein AJ et al, editors: *Campbell-Walsh urology*, ed 11, Philadelphia, 2015, Elsevier.

Sabanegh E et al: *Vasovasectomy and vasoepididymostomy treatment & management* (website), 2015. http://emedicine.medscape.com/article/452831-treatment. (Accessed 1 November 2016).

Schaeffer AJ et al: Infections of the urinary tract. In Wein AJ et al, editors: *Campbell-Walsh urology*, ed 11, Philadelphia., 2015, Elsevier.

Schwartz MJ et al: Laparoscopic and robotic surgery of the kidney. In Wein AJ et al, editors: *Campbell-Walsh urology*, ed 11, Philadelphia, 2015, Elsevier.

Spruce L: Back to basics: surgical skin antisepsis, *AORN J* 103(1):96–100, 2016.

United Network for Organ Sharing (UNOS): *Living donation: information you need to know* (website), 2016. www.unos.org/wp-content/uploads/unos/Living_Donation.pdf. (Accessed 1 November 2016).

Vasavada SP, Rackley RR: Electrical stimulation and neuromodulation in storage and emptying failure. In Wein AJ et al, editors: *Campbell-Walsh urology*, ed 11, Philadelphia, 2015, Elsevier.

CHAPTER 16

Thyroid and Parathyroid Surgery

CARMENCITA DUFFY

Thyroid glandular diseases include goiter, benign and malignant nodules, hyperthyroidism, hypothyroidism, and inflammatory conditions. Goiters have been described since 2700 BCE, before the thyroid gland was even identified. During the Italian Renaissance, around 1500, Leonardo da Vinci depicted two glands located on either side of the larynx. In 1543 Vesalius labeled the tissue "laryngeal glands." However, Thomas Wharton, in a 1656 publication titled *Adenograpahia*, replaced the term with the "thyroid gland," from the Greek word *thyreoeides*, meaning "shield shaped."

Surgeons perform surgical procedures on the thyroid gland for various underlying causes. Surgery ranges from lobectomy with or without isthmusectomy, to subtotal or total thyroidectomy. Surgical approaches to thyroid and parathyroid surgery include open, minimally invasive surgery (MIS) and robotic techniques.

Surgical Anatomy

Thyroid Gland

The thyroid gland (Fig. 16.1) is a highly vascular organ that lies in the anterior portion of the neck, deep to the paired strap muscles, resting on the midline of the trachea. It attaches to the cricoid and trachea by the ligament of Berry. The inferior border of the thyroid varies and may rest above or below the sternal notch. The gland, weighing about 20 g, consists of right and left lobes united by a middle portion called the *isthmus* (Fig. 16.2). The isthmus sits near the base of the neck, between the second and fourth tracheal rings,

and the lobes lie beside the larynx, trachea, and esophagus. The pyramidal lobe, a long, thin projection of thyroid tissue protruding cephalad from the isthmus, is found in about 30% of patients at surgery; it is a vestige of the embryonic thyroglossal duct and migrates from the foramen cecum at the base of the tongue.

Blood supply to the thyroid is from the superior thyroid artery, which originates from the external carotid artery, and from the inferior thyroid artery, which originates from the thyrocervical trunk of the subclavian artery. The points at which these two arteries enter the thyroid gland are referred to as "poles" of the thyroid and are important anatomic landmarks during surgery. The thyroid gland drains via three pairs of veins (superior, middle, and inferior thyroid veins). Occasionally, a single thyroid artery (thyroidea ima) forms directly from the arch of the aorta or the innominate artery and rises in front of the trachea to enter the midline of the gland inferiorly.

The recurrent laryngeal nerve (RLN), a branch of the vagus nerve, innervates the intrinsic muscles of the larynx. The right RLN loops under the subclavian artery and ascends in an oblique direction lateral to the tracheoesophageal groove. The RLN contains both motor and sensory fibers. The motor component innervates intrinsic muscles of the larynx, with the exception of the cricothyroid muscle, which is innervated by the external branch of the superior laryngeal nerve (EBSLN). The sensory component supplies sensation to the larynx below the vocal cords. During surgery, surgeons take care to identify and protect this nerve. Immediate hoarseness occurs if the nerve is divided on one side. Bilateral RLN injury can result in acute airway obstruction postoperatively as the vocal folds occupy a paramedian position. An emergency tracheotomy may be necessary to relieve the obstruction. Injury to the EBSLN, which innervates the cricothyroid muscle, results in difficulty in shouting or singing high notes.

The thyroid gland produces three hormones: thyroxine (T_4) and triiodothyronine (T_3) (together known as the *thyroid hormones*) and calcitonin. T_3 and T_4 cannot be synthesized without iodine; together they regulate energy metabolism and growth and development. Calcitonin inhibits calcium resorption from bone and increases calcium storage in the bone. In addition, calcitonin increases renal excretion of calcium and phosphorus and decreases serum calcium levels. Calcitonin may be used as a tumor marker in medullary thyroid carcinoma. The anterior pituitary synthesizes thyroid-stimulating hormone (TSH) and stimulates the production and release of thyroid hormones and iodine uptake.

The most common cause of hyperthyroidism is Graves disease. Appropriate pharmacologic measures used in treatment of hyperthyroidism include antithyroid drugs, radioiodine therapy, and β-adrenergic blockers. Medications are considered useful in treating symptoms during thyrotoxic states and in returning the thyroid

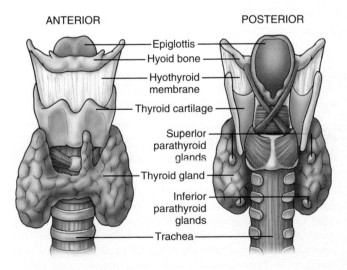

ANTERIOR   POSTERIOR

- Epiglottis
- Hyoid bone
- Hyothyroid membrane
- Thyroid cartilage
- Superior parathyroid glands
- Thyroid gland
- Inferior parathyroid glands
- Trachea

FIG. 16.1 Thyroid gland.

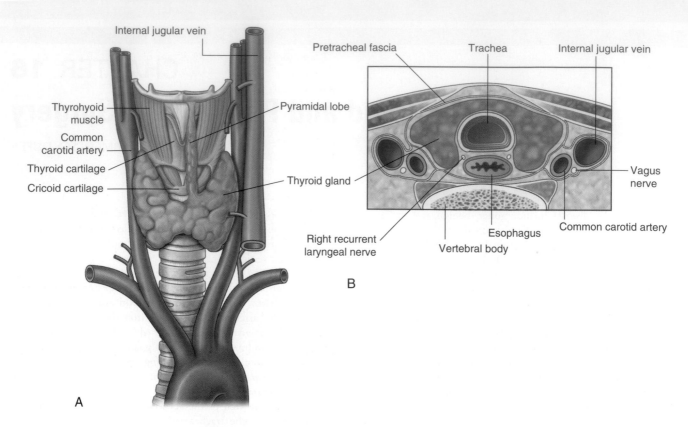

FIG. 16.2 (A and B) Thyroid in relation to surrounding structures.

hormone levels and metabolism to a normal state. Radiation therapy or surgery is ultimately necessary because the medication regimen is not considered a "cure."

In 2015 the American Thyroid Association (ATA) established revised guidelines for the management of thyroid nodules to include recommendations regarding initial evaluation, clinical and ultrasound criteria for fine-needle aspiration (FNA) biopsy, interpretation of FNA biopsy results, use of molecular markers, and management of benign thyroid nodules (Haugen et al., 2016).

Parathyroid Gland

The parathyroid glands are small ovoid masses, usually four in number, located behind the thyroid lobes. Normal parathyroid glands are generally small, lobular, and yellow, but their color may vary from yellow to mahogany. They are usually found bilaterally, in pairs, and are about the size of a lentil bean. It may be challenging to differentiate the glands from a lobule of fat, a thyroid nodule, or lymph node. Thyroid adenomas generally, although not always, tend to be larger, asymmetric, and more red-brown than normal parathyroids (Fig. 16.3). The upper pair of glands lies close to the posterior portion of the superior pole of the thyroid; the lower pair usually (about 60% of the time) lies near the posterior lateral aspect of the lower pole of the thyroid. Ectopic parathyroid glands, more common in the inferior parathyroid glands, may be found in various places throughout the neck and the superior mediastinum (Shivani and Goldenberg, 2016). To allow for interdisciplinary communication between pathologists, radiologists, surgeons, endocrinologists, and anesthesia providers, a classification system is used to determine the most commonly located positions for enlarged parathyroid glands. Each parathyroid gland measures approximately $3 \times 3 \times 3$ mm and

generally weighs less than 50 mg; the upper glands are generally smaller than the lower ones. Both upper and lower parathyroid glands receive their blood supply from the inferior thyroid artery (Fig. 16.4).

The parathyroid glands secrete parathyroid hormone (PTH), an antagonist to calcitonin. Both PTH and calcitonin work together to maintain calcium homeostasis (Fig. 16.5) by increasing calcium removal from storage in bone and increasing absorption of calcium by the intestines. When the parathyroid glands do not secrete sufficient amounts of PTH, hypocalcemia may develop. When there is an insufficient amount of PTH, calcium does not metabolize and is excreted from the body. Hypocalcemia varies from an asymptomatic biochemical abnormality to a life-threatening disorder, depending on the duration, severity, and rapidity of development. Hypoparathyroidism often develops because of advanced thyroid cancer requiring radical resection surgery involving the central neck (Seong et al., 2016). Hypocalcemia also develops in 1% to 2% of patients after total thyroidectomy (TT) (Skugor, 2014).

Perioperative Nursing Considerations

Assessment

Patients with hyperthyroidism most likely have had appropriate drug therapy that has returned thyroid hormone levels and metabolic states to normal (euthyroid). Perioperative nurses assess for any symptoms that relate to accelerated metabolism (Box 16.1). The patient's baseline vital signs are noted for an abnormally elevated resting pulse rate, elevated systolic blood pressure, and cardiac symptoms such as palpitations or atrial fibrillation. Patients with

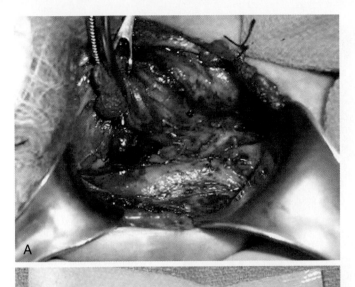

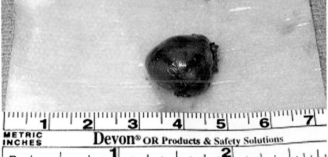

FIG. 16.3 (A) A right upper parathyroid adenoma in situ. The thyroid gland is retracted to the midline. The recurrent laryngeal nerve enters the operative field inferiorly and tracks superiorly in the tracheoesophageal groove. The carotid sheath lies lateral to the nerve. The adenoma is the lobular mahogany mass located at the superior pole of the thyroid. (B) Parathyroid adenoma after removal.

BOX 16.1

Common Symptoms and Signs of Thyroid Dysfunction

Hypothyroidism

- Fatigue, lethargy, weakness
- Weight gain, puffy face
- Cold intolerance, decreased sweating
- Dry, sparse, coarse hair; dry skin
- Anemia, pallor
- Hoarse voice, decreased hearing
- Poor concentration, depression
- Muscle stiffness and pain
- Generalized interstitial edema, inelastic cold skin
- Bradycardia, cardiac hypertrophy
- Constipation, decreased libido
- Menstrual irregularity (especially heavy menses; infertility)

Hyperthyroidism

- Vision changes: myopathy, ophthalmopathy, and exophthalmos
- Emotional lability, restlessness
- Irritability, nervousness
- Exercise intolerance, fatigue
- Dependent edema
- Weight loss (but perhaps weight gain), thirst, increased appetite (appetite may also be decreased)
- Heat intolerance and flushing
- Hyperactivity, especially children
- Cardiac palpitations; bounding, rapid pulse
- Increased sweating
- Insomnia, exhaustion
- Muscle weakness, tremor
- Dyspnea on mild exertion
- Frequent bowel movements
- Menstrual irregularity (oligomenorrhea; infertility)

Modified from Milas K: *Hyperthyroidism symptoms* (website). www.endocrineweb.com/conditions/hyperthyroidism/hyperthyroidism-symptoms. (Accessed 9 December 2016); Workman LM: Care of patients with problems of the thyroid and parathyroid glands. In Ignatavicius DD, Workman ML, editors: *Medical-surgical nursing: patient-centered collaborative care*, ed 8, St Louis, 2016, Elsevier.

---

overactive thyroid conditions have an increased risk of heart problems (Kramer, 2016), particularly atrial fibrillation, which may lead to premature death. The perioperative nurse's assessment includes whether anticoagulant and thyroid medications are being taken by the patient. Review the patient's cardiac and respiratory rates, muscle strength, elimination patterns, history of weight loss, heat intolerance, and emotional status.

Patients, especially if young, may be anxious about the disease and the success of surgery, and may express concerns about the cosmetic results of neck surgery. Patients concerned about body image should be able to discuss these issues with the perioperative nurse. Vocalists will likely be worried whether surgery will adversely affect their voice. The anesthesia provider, therefore, may use an endotracheal tube with a smaller diameter than usual to minimize trauma to the vocal cords. Assess skin integrity; patients with hyperthyroidism may have finely textured skin and edema in the lower extremities, placing them at higher risk for skin breakdown. The most typical complications of thyroid surgery, although infrequent, are hypoparathyroidism and injury to the RLN (Kaplan et al., 2016). Preoperative assessment of the patient's voice tone and quality is therefore noted.

Large thyroid nodules may cause a tracheal shift and present a challenge to the anesthesia provider for intubation and airway

management. The size of thyroid enlargement should be noted preoperatively and steps taken to prepare the operating room (OR) in anticipation of a difficult intubation. The "difficult airway" anesthesia cart should be in the room along with, preferably, two anesthesia providers and the circulating nurse standing by to assist with induction. The anesthesia provider will not extubate a patient who has been difficult to intubate until anesthetic gases have dissipated and level of consciousness is such that the patient can protect his or her own airway and maintain oxygen saturation with spontaneous breathing. If there is concern about postoperative edema and ensuing airway obstruction from a difficult induction, the anesthesia provider may administer steroids intraoperatively and choose to leave the endotracheal tube in postoperatively.

A grossly enlarged thyroid is also more difficult to excise, and intraoperative bleeding is more common and profuse. Hematoma development may rarely occur on emergence from anesthesia and require reexploration and ligation of the offending blood vessel. Hemorrhage may cause tracheal compression and airway compromise. Generally, patients who have larger glands excised require a drain postoperatively (Byrne, 2013). They are closely monitored during emergence from anesthesia and postoperatively. Excessive swelling at the operative site, with or without poor air exchange, is treated

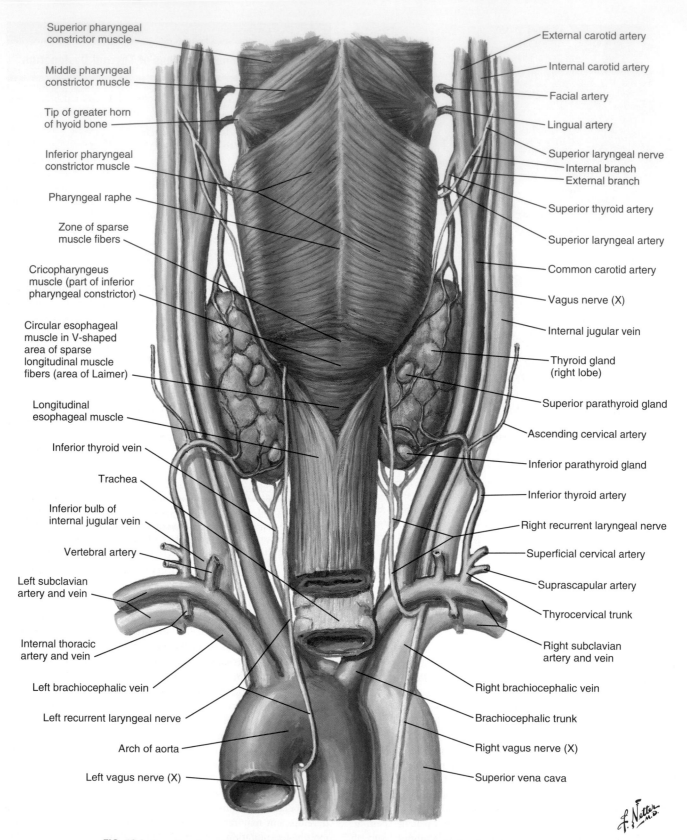

FIG. 16.4 Posterior view of thyroid and parathyroids. Note relation to carotid sheath and esophagus. Note pathway of recurrent laryngeal nerves.

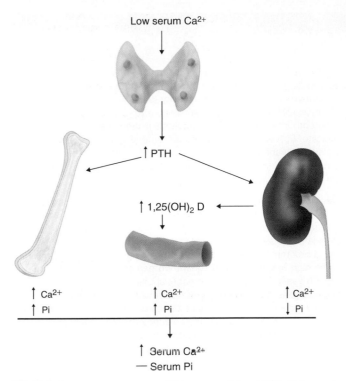

Low serum Ca²⁺

↑ PTH

↑ 1,25(OH)₂ D

| ↑ Ca²⁺ | ↑ Ca²⁺ | ↑ Ca²⁺ |
| ↑ Pi | ↑ Pi | ↓ Pi |

↑ Serum Ca²⁺
— Serum Pi

FIG. 16.5 Homeostatic response to a fall in serum calcium (Ca^{2+}). *Pi,* Inorganic phosphate; *PTH,* parathyroid hormone; *1,25(OH)₂D,* biologically active form of vitamin D.

as a potentially life-threatening emergency. The instrument table is kept sterile until the patient is extubated and has left the OR. A tracheotomy tray with tubes is readily available should an emergency tracheotomy be necessary.

In addition to clinical signs and symptoms, results of diagnostic tests are reviewed (Appendix A) (Evidence for Practice). Tests performed most commonly before thyroid surgery include measurements of TSH, T_3, and T_4 levels; radioisotope or ultrasonic scans; and an electrocardiogram (ECG).

Thyroid Assessment

In addition to palpation of the thyroid gland for size, contour, consistency, lymph nodes, fixation, tenderness, and bruits, computed tomography (CT) and magnetic resonance imaging (MRI) scans are used to assess a thyroid with suspected malignancy for encroachment of the tumor outside the thyroid capsule into the adjacent tissue of the neck (Hoang et al., 2015). Such scans are an effective means to confirm and evaluate invasion into surrounding tissue.

Ultrasound and autopsy studies show more than 50% of healthy adults have thyroid nodules, yet only 3% to 5% are palpable. Although most nodules are benign, 7% to 29% are cancerous. In the United States it was estimated that in 2016 there were about 62,450 new cases of thyroid cancer and about 1980 deaths (National Cancer Institute, 2016). Thyroid cancer is commonly diagnosed at a younger age than most other adult cancers. Nearly three of four cases are found in women. About 2% of thyroid cancers occur in children and teens. The chance of a thyroid cancer diagnosis has risen in recent years and is the most rapidly increasing cancer in the United States, tripling in the last three decades. Much of this increase appears to result from increased use of thyroid ultrasound, which can detect small thyroid nodules that might not otherwise have been found (ACS, 2016).

Preoperative Testing

Thyroid Isotope Scan (Thyroid Scintigraphy). Thyroid nodules, the most common endocrine problem in the United States, are any abnormal growth of thyroid cells. Most nodules are discovered during routine physical examination because they rarely are symptomatic. Imaging of the normal thyroid with radionuclide agents shows normal size, shape, position, and function of the thyroid, with no areas of decreased or increased uptake. When nodules are detected, they may be classified as *hot,* demonstrating increased uptake of radionuclide agent; this may indicate benign adenoma or localized toxic goiter. *Cold nodules* are hypofunctioning or nonfunctioning and may indicate cyst, nonfunctioning adenoma or goiter, lymphoma, localized area of thyroiditis, or carcinoma. Two commonly used agents in thyroid imaging are radioactive iodine and technetium 99m-pertechnetate ($^{99m}TcO_4^-$).

Ultrasound Scan. Ultrasound scans, also called *ultrasound imaging* or *sonography,* are noninvasive tests that use sound waves to create an image; they do not use ionizing radiation as in x-ray. Scans help determine whether a neck lump originates from the thyroid or adjacent anatomy. Thyroid scan with survey of the cervical lymph nodes is usually performed in all patients with known or suspected thyroid nodules (Haugen et al., 2016). Involvement of the vessels in the neck or mediastinum, although rare, can occur; it is critical that the surgeon and OR team know if this is the case before surgery, because it dictates the extent of the surgery.

New ultrasonic techniques have been applied to the thyroid. Three-dimensional (3-D) ultrasound has proven to be more accurate. Tissue harmonic imaging (THI) uses the first harmonic of the transmitted frequency for image formation and results in images with less "noise." These techniques improve image clarity but do not improve lesion characterization.

Fine-Needle Aspiration. Ultrasonography also helps facilitate accurate needle placement and sampling of the target nodule during FNA. When a tissue sample for pathologic examination is required, FNA of a palpable nodule is considered one of the most effective methods for identifying malignancy. FNA has high accuracy, low risk, and is cost-effective. A suspicious nodule usually implies a follicular neoplasm, which can be benign or malignant, and requires removal and evaluation by the histology department. The procedure is usually performed under ultrasound guidance, but may be performed in the surgeon's office. Several samples are usually taken from various parts of the nodule and are rated on a 1 to 6 scale ranging from benign to clearly malignant. When metastatic disease is found on preoperative imaging, an altered operative and disease management plan will be established for the patient. Patient preparation for FNA includes the following information:

- You will be lying down for the procedure and may expect coldness on your neck from the prepping solution.
- Local anesthesia may or may not be used.
- Once the prick of the needle is felt, no talking, swallowing, or moving is allowed.

FNA may be an emotionally stressful procedure for the patient. Vials of ammonia should be kept in the room in case the patient feels faint. Lowering the head (Trendelenburg position or sitting with the head down) is also important to treat vasovagal syncope. Postprocedure education should include (1) the necessity of refraining from using aspirin or aspirin-containing medications or nonsteroidal antiinflammatory drugs (NSAIDs) for the next 24 hours, and (2) the expectation of seeing a half-dollar–size bruise at the FNA site (Patient Engagement Exemplar). There are no restrictions on food or activity.

EVIDENCE FOR PRACTICE

Screening for Thyroid Dysfunction

The symptoms and signs of thyroid dysfunction are well established (see Box 16.1). A thorough history and physical are required. A history of exposure to neck or whole-body radiation or growing up in iodine-poor areas may lead to thyroid cancer. A rapidly expanding neck mass, new onset of hoarseness, neck or ear pain, or cough are symptoms of concern. Patients with symptoms suggestive of metastasis (e.g., a fixed, immobile mass and/or hoarseness, dysphagia, or respiratory symptoms) may undergo CT or MRI. Although calcifications were formerly considered a benign finding, some thyroid cancers demonstrate eggshell calcifications.

The AACE practice guidelines for diagnostic evaluation of hyperthyroidism and hypothyroidism recommend TSH assay as the single best screening test. Hyperthyroidism results in a lower than normal TSH level (suppressed TSH secretion). To diagnose hyperthyroidism accurately, TSH assay sensitivity, the lowest reliably measured TSH concentration, is 0.02 mIU/L or less.

An elevated serum TSH concentration is present in both overt and mild (subclinical) hypothyroidism. In the latter, the free thyroid hormone (fT_3 and fT_4) levels are, by definition, normal.

Hypothyroidism results from undersecretion of thyroid hormone. In the United States hypothyroidism affects nearly 11 million people each year. The most common cause of primary hypothyroidism is chronic autoimmune thyroiditis (Hashimoto disease). The most valuable laboratory test is measurement of TSH and free T_4 levels. Clinical hypothyroidism is treated with levothyroxine (L-thyroxine) replacement therapy. The AACE supports treating subclinical hypothyroidism if TSH levels are greater than 10 mcU/mL or if TSH levels are between 5 and 10 mcU/mL in conjunction with goiter or positive antibodies, or both. TPOAb measurements are also considered when evaluating patients with subclinical hypothyroidism.

Serum TSH measurement is the single most reliable test to diagnose all common forms of hypothyroidism and hyperthyroidism, with high sensitivity (98%) and specificity (92%). Periodic TSH measurements are done after 3 to 6 months and at 12-month intervals, or more frequently if the patient's symptoms indicate. Follow-up testing of serum T_4 levels in persons with persistently abnormal TSH levels can differentiate between subclinical (normal T_4 levels) and "overt" (abnormal T_4 levels) thyroid dysfunction.

Recommendations of Other Groups

In 2002 a consensus panel sponsored by the AACE, ATA, and the Endocrine Society found insufficient evidence to support population-based screening for thyroid dysfunction, although the panel recommended aggressive case-finding in those considered to be high risk, including pregnant women and women older than age 60 years. Later, a second panel appointed by the three organizations reviewed the same evidence. Although the panel acknowledged that the evidence does not support population-wide screening, it concluded that the evidence did not equate to lack of a benefit. It therefore issued a separate dissenting consensus statement that recommended routine population-wide screening for subclinical hypothyroidism and hyperthyroidism in adults. The ATA also recommends such screening in adults beginning at age 35 years and every 5 years thereafter.

The American Academy of Family Physicians adopted the USPSTF recommendation, which suggests that current evidence is insufficient to assess the balance of benefits and harms of screening for thyroid dysfunction in nonpregnant, asymptomatic adults (LeFevre, 2015).

AACE, American Association of Clinical Endocrinologists; *ATA,* American Thyroid Association; *CT,* computed tomography; *fT₃,* free triiodothyronine; *fT₄,* free thyroxine; *mcU,* microunits; *mIU/L,* milli-international unit; *MRI,* magnetic resonance imaging; *TPOAb,* antithyroid peroxidase antibody; *TSH,* thyroid-stimulating hormone; *USPSTF,* US Preventive Services Task Force. Modified from Gharib H et al: American Association of Clinical Endocrinologists, American College of Endocrinology, and Associazioine Medici Endocrinologi Medical Guidelines for Clinical Practice for the Diagnosis and Management of Thyroid Nodules—2016 update, *Endocr Pract* 22(5):622–639, 2016; USPSTF: *Thyroid dysfunction: screening* (website), 2015. www.uspreventiveservicestaskforce.org/Page/Document/UpdateSummaryFinal/thyroid-dysfunction-screening. (Accessed 5 January 2017).

PATIENT ENGAGEMENT EXEMPLAR

Patient-Centered Communication

Patient-centered care emphasizes recognition of the patient, the patient's family, or other designee as full partners in care delivery. When perioperative nurses provide patient education, either verbally or through written materials, they should be tailored to the patient's individual situation and be easily understood. Here are some suggestions for patient-centered communication when providing patient education for patients undergoing a thyroid aspiration:

- Be concise. ("You had a fine-needle aspiration of your thyroid gland today.")
- Focus on need-to-know information. ("Here are some important things to know.")
- Use words of one or two syllables.
- Avoid use of medical terms; use words laymen would use. ("An 'aspiration' means getting a small piece out through a needle.")
- Speak or write material in the first person. ("You will have a bruise about the size of a half-dollar.")
- Do not use fancy fonts or bold fonts; use bold only for items that are of critical importance. ("Call 911 if you have a hard time swallowing.")
- Ask the patient to "teach-back" the material to you rather than ask if the patient understood you. ("Please tell me in your own words what you can eat or drink this afternoon.")
- Be sure the patient can state the name of the surgical procedure. ("What is the name of the operation you had today?")
- Treat patients, their family, or designee with courtesy and respect. ("What else can I help you with?")

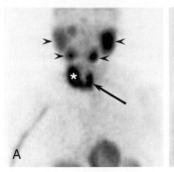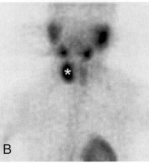

FIG. 16.6 (A) Early three-dimensional sestamibi image shows uptake in mass *(asterisk)*, in salivary glands *(arrowheads)*, and in thyroid gland *(arrow)*. (B) Late three-dimensional sestamibi image shows retention of radiotracer in the adenoma *(asterisk)*, with absence of radiotracer in the thyroid gland. Salivary glands normally retain radiotracer on late images.

Perioperative Patient Education. A patient's knowledge deficit about thyroid surgery can be alleviated with proper preoperative education. Invite the patient to verbalize questions and concerns. Alleviate anxiety; reassure the patient that you will be his or her nurse throughout the surgical procedure. Discuss perioperative events such as positioning on the OR bed, the incision site and type of dressing to be used, and any drains. Note that intermittent pneumatic compression devices (IPCDs) will be applied to be used for deep vein thrombosis (DVT) prophylaxis. Advise the patient that there are various ways of protecting their eyes during surgery, and if lacrilube is used, they can expect temporary blurred vision when they first open their eyes.

Postoperative education begins preoperatively. Include a time line for neck muscle recovery (expect 3–6 months), the importance of early neck flexion and extension to the patient's tolerance, diligent thyroid and/or calcium medication intake, regular postoperative follow up, the potential for body temperature changes, and how to access support management. Review pain assessment and management therapies.

Parathyroid Assessment

Elevation of serum PTH levels in association with hypercalcemia suggests hyperparathyroidism (HPT) in most cases (Velez et al., 2016). Normal PTH levels, serum calcium levels, and bone density T-scores may be found in Appendix A. Causes of primary HPT are single adenoma (80%–85%), four-gland hyperplasia (10%–15%), and rarely parathyroid carcinoma (<1%).

Nuclear Medicine. Preoperative localization studies with a parathyroid sestamibi scan (Fig. 16.6) or high-resolution ultrasonography can identify parathyroid adenomas with high sensitivity (70%–80%). Sensitivity decreases significantly for hyperplasia (<50%).

Improvements in anatomic detail may be achieved by using the single-photon emission computed tomography (SPECT)/CT. This system uses software that depicts 6 to 16 slices of tissue and produces 3-D images that help identify parathyroid adenomas (Wong et al., 2016).

Four-Dimensional Computed Tomography. This system uses a multiphase multidetector CT that provides rapid volumetric acquisition and in-plane spatial resolution of 1 mm or better. It provides a road map for the operating surgeon. There is improved sensitivity and specificity with this type of CT scan (Wong et al., 2016).

HPT causes an increase in the level of serum calcium and a decrease in the level of serum phosphate. Nursing diagnoses and plans of care are based on these imbalances and the severity of

---

BOX 16.2

Parathyroid Dysfunction

Hyperparathyroidism
Signs and Symptoms
- Polyuria, polydipsia, kidney stones
- Abdominal pain, constipation, nausea, anorexia
- Fracture risk (decreasing bone mineral density [BMD])
- Joint or back pain
- Depression, paranoia, mood swings
- Muscle weakness and atrophy

Hypoparathyroidism
Signs and Symptoms
- Personality disturbances: anxiety, depression, irritability
- Tetany: muscle cramps, spasms (hands, face, feet); paresthesia: numbness and tingling (around mouth, lips, and tongue [perioral])
- Dry, scaly skin; brittle nails; thin, patchy hair
- Weak tooth enamel/dental caries
- Cataracts

Modified from Kaplan EL et al: Surgery of the thyroid. In Jameson JL et al, editor: *Endocrinology: adult and pediatric*, ed 7, St Louis, 2016, Elsevier; Velez RP et al: Simplifying the complexity of primary hyperparathyroidism, *J Nurse Pract* 12(5):346–352, 2016.

associated symptoms. Some patients are asymptomatic, whereas others have symptoms that manifest themselves as disturbances in the central nervous system or cardiovascular, renal, gastrointestinal, or musculoskeletal system (Box 16.2).

Assessment includes determining whether the patient is apathetic or emotionally irritable; whether there is muscle weakness and atrophy, back or joint pain, nausea, vomiting, constipation, peptic ulcer disease, or cardiac dysrhythmia; and whether there is renal damage, stones, or disease. If any of these are present, the plan of care is adjusted. Otherwise, perioperative patient education and nursing management of the patient undergoing parathyroidectomy are essentially the same as those for thyroidectomy. In the early postoperative period for both TT and parathyroidectomy, the patient is closely observed for any signs of hypocalcemia. The serum calcium level reaches its lowest level in 48 to 72 hours after surgery and returns to normal within the following 2 to 3 days. Symptoms include numbness and tingling of extremities and around the lips. Hyperactive tendon reflexes and a positive Chvostek sign (tapping on the facial nerve elicits contraction of facial muscles) can be demonstrated on physical examination. Tetany may develop and is exhibited by carpopedal spasms, tonic-clonic convulsions, and laryngeal stridor, which can be fatal.

Nursing Diagnosis

Nursing diagnoses related to the care of patients undergoing thyroid and parathyroid surgery might include the following:
- Impaired Swallowing related to mechanical obstruction (enlarged thyroid preoperatively; edema or hematoma postoperatively)
- Risk for Ineffective thermoregulation related to altered metabolic rate and surgical environment
- Disturbed Body Image related to surgical scar in prominent location
- Ineffective Airway Clearance related to obstruction (enlarged thyroid preoperatively; edema or hematoma postoperatively) or bilateral RLN injury
- Impaired Gas Exchange related to postoperative bleeding or swelling or inability to move secretions

Outcome Identification

Outcomes identified for the selected nursing diagnoses may be stated as follows:

- The patient will maintain normal swallowing.
- The patient will maintain normal body temperature.
- The patient will verbalize decreased disturbance in feelings related to body image.
- The patient will maintain a patent airway.
- The patient will maintain effective gas exchange.

Planning

The inherent risks associated with surgery are reduced through careful planning, assessment, and tailoring the plan of care to your specific patient. As the patient's advocate, you are equipped with critical thinking and competency skill sets that provide a safe perioperative experience for the patient undergoing thyroid or parathyroid surgery. Consider a patient who is not at optimal weight at high risk for pressure injury (Scott, 2016); pad pressure areas to prevent skin, tissue, and nerve damage. Limit skin exposure, provide warm saline intraoperatively for irrigation, and use a patient-warming device (e.g., forced-air or underbody mat) (Rightmyer and Singbartl, 2016) to prevent perioperative hypothermia.

Although rare, a potentially fatal complication for patients with hyperthyroidism is thyroid storm (thyrotoxic crisis) (Hooley and Reagan, 2016). The perioperative staff must recognize and differentiate between uncomplicated thyrotoxicosis and thyroid storm (Table 16.1) and be prepared to act quickly. Thyroid storm can occur in patients whose hyperthyroidism has been partially controlled or has been untreated. Thyrotoxic crisis can be precipitated by a stressful event, such as surgery. Planning a quiet, calm atmosphere and helping the patient relax can reduce the risk of thyroid storm. Plan for appropriate interventions to assist in reducing body temperature and heart rate, provide oxygen and intravenous (IV) solutions, and administer medications as prescribed in the event thyrotoxic crisis occurs (Surgical Pharmacology).

See the following Sample Plan of Care for a patient undergoing thyroid and parathyroid surgery.

TABLE 16.1

Thyroid Storm

Thyroid storm may be difficult to differentiate from signs of uncomplicated thyrotoxicosis. The following table compares symptoms of uncomplicated thyrotoxicosis and thyroid storm.

Uncomplicated Thyrotoxicosis	Thyroid Storm: Severe Exacerbation of Thyrotoxicosis
Heat intolerance, diaphoresis	Hyperpyrexia, temperature in excess of 106°F (41.1°C), dehydration
Sinus tachycardia, heart rate 100–140 beats/min	Severe tachycardia (heart rate faster than 140 beats/min), hypotension, cardiac dysrhythmias, congestive heart failure
Diarrhea, increased appetite with weight loss	Nausea, vomiting, severe diarrhea, abdominal pain, hepatocellular dysfunction with jaundice
Anxiety, restlessness	Confusion, disorientation, agitation, delirium, psychosis, seizures, stupor, or coma

Implementation

Positioning

Proper positioning on the OR bed is crucial for optimal exposure of the thyroid gland. The patient is positioned supine. Some surgeons prefer a beach chair position or a wedge under the back. Moderate extension of the neck is required for maximal exposure; extension optimizes the space between the clavicles and the jaw (Byrne, 2013). A headrest provides proper support, keeps the head straight, and prevents aggravation of prior neck problems. Alternatively, a shoulder roll may be used. The arms are tucked at the side, the elbows are padded to protect the ulnar nerve, the palms faced inward, and the wrist maintained in a neutral position (AORN, 2017). A drape secures the arms. It should be tucked snugly, but not tightly, under the patient, not under the mattress. This prevents the arm from shifting downward intraoperatively and resting against the OR bed rail. All pressure points are padded, especially for patients not at optimal weight. Should the patient be too large to tuck the arms safely at the sides, arm sleds or side extensions for the OR bed may be used to accommodate the arms. Reduction of venous congestion can be accomplished by a 30-degree reverse-Trendelenburg tilt of the OR bed.

Skin Preparation

The operative area (chin and anterior neck region, lateral surfaces of the neck from the earlobes down to the outer aspects of the shoulder, and upper anterior chest region to the nipples) is prepped with an antimicrobial solution (prep solution). Appropriate precautions are taken to prevent pooling of solution under the neck or in the axillary area. When using an alcohol-based prep solution around the head and neck, there is an increased risk for a surgical fire. Follow the manufacturer's directions for the prep solution carefully; the patient's skin should be totally dry and all fumes from the prep solution dissipated before draping in accord with fire safety precautions. Bed sheets or towels that become soaked with a flammable prep solution should be removed from the OR. After the skin prep, the patient is draped with sterile towels and a fenestrated sheet. A sterile towel, lap sponge, or self-adherent tape strips may be placed on each side of the neck to prevent blood from pooling under the neck during surgery. Self-adherent tape strips or drapes also promote maintenance of the integrity of the sterile field and reduce the risk of intraoperative fire hazard by sealing off the operative site from anesthetic vapors that may have leaked and become trapped under the drapes. If lap sponges are used on each side of the neck during draping, communicate their placement and record them on the count sheet to avoid confusion when accounting for all items used throughout the procedure. After draping is complete and before the incision, a time-out is taken. All personnel suspend activity, and stop and listen closely during the time-out (TJC, 2016). The following are verified: correct patient identity, correct site (include laterality of applicable), and correct procedure to be performed; special patient considerations, positioning, drying time of antimicrobial skin prep solutions, proper equipment (e.g., laryngeal nerve monitors, IPCDs, energy-generating devices such as electrosurgical units [ESUs], warming devices); and availability of needed supplies. All antibiotics given to the patient are verbalized; include the dose, time, and amount given. The time-out is documented. The surgeon may then mark the incision site with the pressure of a full-length fine silk tie to help ensure a wound line that blends with the patient's neck creases and skin lines.

SURGICAL PHARMACOLOGY

Thyroid Storm: A Life-Threatening Condition Characterized by an Exaggeration of the Usual Physiologic Response Seen in Hyperthyroidism

Preoperative Prophylactic Care for Thyroid Storm

Use KI preoperatively in thyrotoxicosis to decrease thyroid blood flow.

Emergency Care During Thyroid Storm

- Maintain a patent airway and adequate ventilation.
- Administer supplemental oxygen.
- Establish vascular access for fluid resuscitation or medication administration.
- Monitor intake and output.
- Give antithyroid drugs as prescribed: propylthiouracil (PTU, Propyl-Thyracil), 300–900 mg/d; MMI (Tapazole), up to 60 mg/d.
- Administer KI solution IV, as prescribed.
- Initiate continuous cardiac monitoring.
- Prepare the patient for insertion of a central venous pressure line.
- Give β-adrenergic blockers such as propranolol (Inderal), IV as prescribed; administer slowly, over 3 minutes.
- Esmolol (Brevibloc), 500 mcg/kg IV followed by 50–200 mcg/kg, minimum maintenance dose, is useful in patients at risk for complications from beta-blockade and cardiovascular collapse.
- One hour after administration of PTU or MMI, hormone release can be inhibited by large doses of iodine, which reduce thyroidal iodine uptake. Lugol solution, 30 gtt/d orally in four divided doses, or a saturated solution of KI, 5 gtt orally or via an NG tube q6h, can be used.
- Ipodate sodium, 0.5–3 g/d PO, can be administered instead of iodine.
- Patients unable to take PTU or MMI also can be treated with lithium 300 mg PO q6h in conjunction with iodine. Adjust lithium dose to maintain levels at about 1 mEq/L.
- Plasmapheresis, plasma exchange, peritoneal dialysis exchange transfusion, and charcoal plasma perfusion are other techniques to remove excess circulating hormone for patients who do not respond to the initial line of management.
- Monitor vital signs every 30 minutes or more frequently as patient's condition dictates.
- Provide comfort measures.
- Control hyperthermia with application of ice packs and a cooling blanket.
- Give nonsalicylate antipyretics such as acetaminophen (normally 650 mg PO q4h).
- Aggressive fluid and electrolyte therapy, 3–5 L/d, is needed for dehydration and hypotension.
- Provide multivitamins, especially vitamin B_1, to prevent Wernicke encephalopathy.
- Glucocorticoids reduce iodine uptake and must be used with caution because they have significant adverse effects.
- Dexamethasone (Decadron, Dexone), 2 mg IV q6h, or hydrocortisone (Cortef, Solu-Cortef), 100 mg IV q8h, may be given.
- Control hypertension with agents such as guanethidine (Ismelin), 1–2 mg/kg/d orally, or reserpine, 2.5–5 mg IM q4-6h.
- Treat heart failure if present.
- Educate the patient, family, and caregiver about symptoms of thyroid storm and that they should call 911 for racing heart rate (tachycardia) that exceeds 140 beats per minute, atrial fibrillation, high fever, persistent sweating, shaking, agitation, restlessness, confusion, diarrhea, and unconsciousness.

CHF, Congestive heart failure; *d,* day; *IM,* intramuscular; *IV,* intravenous; *KI,* potassium iodide; *MMI,* methimazole; *NG,* nasogastric; *PO,* orally.
Modified from Davis CP: *Thyroid storm symptoms, causes, and treatment* (website), 2016. www.medicinenet.com/thyroid_storm_symptoms_causes_and_treatment/views.htm. (Accessed 5 January 2017); Misra M et al: *Thyroid storm* (website), 2015. http://emedicine.medscape.com/article/925147-overview. (Accessed 5 January 2017); Moore K: *Thyroid storm* (website). www.healthline.com/health/thyroid storm#Overview1. (Accessed 5 January 2017)

SAMPLE PLAN OF CARE

Nursing Diagnosis
Impaired Swallowing related to mechanical obstruction (enlarged thyroid preoperatively; edema postoperatively)

Outcome
The patient will maintain normal swallowing.

Interventions
- Keep suction line and suction catheter connected and active until patient is discharged from OR.
- Monitor for and report difficulty swallowing during emergence from anesthesia or transport to PACU.
- Gently suction oropharyngeal secretions as required.
- Keep vein open postoperatively until patient can swallow without difficulty.

Nursing Diagnosis
Risk for Ineffective Thermoregulation related to altered metabolic rate

Outcome
The patient's body temperature will be maintained within normal range.

Interventions
- Monitor patient's temperature; report abnormalities.
- Provide light covers if temperature is elevated or patient states that he or she is too warm.
- Use active warming (e.g., forced-air warming device) both preoperatively and intraoperatively to prevent perioperative hypothermia.

Continued

SAMPLE PLAN OF CARE—cont'd

- Use fluid warmer for IV fluids as needed to maintain body temperature.
- Limit skin exposure: expose only skin at the operative site.
- Maintain ambient room temperature between 68°F and 77°F to prevent perioperative hypothermia.

Nursing Diagnosis

Disturbed Body Image related to surgical scar

Outcome

The patient will verbalize decreased disturbance in feelings related to body image.

Interventions

- Describe incision location in natural fold of skin.
- Explain that techniques used for surgical closure minimize scarring.
- Educate patient in postoperative turning measures to decrease strain on suture line.
- Suggest that jewelry, scarves, and certain necklines can be used to cover scar until normal fading occurs.
- Advise patient to refrain from prolonged exposure to direct sunlight or tanning salons while incision is healing.

Nursing Diagnosis

Ineffective Airway Clearance related to obstruction secondary to enlarged thyroid (preoperatively), edema (postoperatively), or recurrent laryngeal nerve injury

Outcome

The patient's airway will remain patent.

Interventions

- Position patient so that enlarged gland does not obstruct airway. Head of transport vehicle may need to be elevated preoperatively. Postoperatively the head of the bed may need elevation to 30 to 45 degrees to ease air exchange and minimize edema.
- Assist anesthesia provider during induction and extubation. Have oxygen and suction available.

- Monitor respiratory rate and signs of respiratory distress (stridor, wheezing, dyspnea, labored respirations).
- If distress occurs because of recurrent laryngeal nerve injury, a tracheotomy may be required. Have oxygen, suctioning equipment, and a tracheotomy tray available.
- Observe neck dressing and back of neck for signs of postoperative edema or bleeding.
  - Hemorrhage at the incision site or respiratory distress from tracheal compression may require urgent reintubation for airway protection and a return to the OR for wound reexploration.

Nursing Diagnosis

Impaired Gas Exchange related to postoperative bleeding or swelling, bilateral recurrent laryngeal nerve surgical injury, or inability to move secretions

Outcome

The patient's gas exchange will remain effective.

Interventions

- Monitor respiratory status and results of pulse oximetry.
- If patient is extubated in the OR, be prepared to assist anesthesia provider; closely observe for respiratory stridor or respiratory obstruction (recurrent laryngeal nerve malfunction). Tracheotomy may be required; oxygen, suctioning equipment, and a tracheotomy tray should be available. A trach tube with a high-volume, low-pressure cuff is often indicated postoperatively for patients with head and neck cancer.
- Assess and document color of nailbeds (postoperative).
- Monitor surgical site for swelling and bleeding (postoperative).
- Suction patient's secretions as needed (postoperative).
- Monitor patency of surgical drain and amount/nature of drainage in collection device, as applicable (postoperative).
- Instruct patient in coughing and deep breathing: support the neck by placing both hands behind the neck when coughing to reduce strain on the suture line (postoperative).

IV, Intravenous; *PACU,* postanesthesia care unit.

Evaluation

Evaluation of intraoperative interventions determines the effectiveness of the plan of care. The hand-off report to the postanesthesia care unit (PACU) or the ambulatory recovery unit includes the surgical procedure, type of anesthesia used, any local anesthetics administered, location of drain (if any), dressing used, condition of skin postoperatively, and any other information specific to the patient's care. Documentation, using facility protocol, reflects achievement of patient outcomes related to planned interventions; include these in the hand-off nursing report to PACU personnel. Outcomes identified for the selected nursing diagnoses may be stated as follows:

- The patient will maintain normal swallowing.
- The patient maintained body temperature within a normal range.
- The patient verbalized decreased disturbance in feelings related to body image.
- The patient maintained a patent airway; there was no edema or hematoma at the surgical site or signs of respiratory distress.
- The patient maintained adequate gas exchange; O₂ saturation remained normal. The patient was extubated without incident.

Patient, Family, and Caregiver Education and Discharge Planning

Patient education and discharge planning include any family members, significant others, or even friends who will help the patient at home (Patient, Family, and Caregiver Education). Written discharge instructions are provided and orally reviewed, with clarification of information and correction of misperceptions. The name and telephone number of the physician or nurse to call with questions is provided, as is information regarding a follow-up office appointment, if available. General information, such as the name of the thyroid or parathyroid procedure and any changes that will occur as a result of the surgery, is explained. Signs and symptoms to report include those of hypocalcemia; the patient should report any numbness or tingling around the lips or extremities, twitching, or spasms. Explore the patient's concerns, anxieties, thoughts, and feelings. The advent of thyroidectomies and parathyroidectomies performed in ambulatory surgery centers has introduced a new set of needs and challenges for the patient, family, and perioperative staff (Ambulatory Surgery Considerations).

PATIENT, FAMILY, AND CAREGIVER EDUCATION

Home Care After a Thyroidectomy

- Give both patient and caregiver *verbal* and *written* instructions. Provide the name and telephone number of a physician or nurse to call if questions or problems arise. Have patient and/or caregiver repeat back instructions in his or her own words. Allow time for questions.
- Explain and discuss surgical procedure performed. The patient should be able to state the name of the surgical procedure performed.
- Wound/incision care:
  - Teach patient to keep the surgical site clean and dry.
  - Review methods to conceal surgical site without affecting healing. Suggest loosely buttoned collars, high-neck blouses, jewelry, or scarves.
  - Explain that paper strip(s) over wound will peel off in 7 to 10 days; when ends curl, strip may be removed.
  - Advise patient that incisions approximated with surgical glue may have glue peeled off at a prescribed postoperative day.
  - Inform patient that lotion may soften healing scar and improve its appearance (if approved by physician).
- Warning signs: review signs and symptoms that should be reported to physician or nurse.
  - *General:* respiratory distress, bleeding.
  - *Wound infection:* redness, warmth, swelling, persistent drainage from site, unrelieved tenderness.
  - *Total thyroidectomy:* review signs and symptoms of hypothyroidism.
  - *Parathyroid damage:* review signs of hypocalcemia: numbness, tingling, twitching, spasm, tetany.

- Medication management:
  - Explain purpose, dosage, schedule, and route of administration of any prescribed drugs, as well as side effects to report to physician or nurse. Have patient "teach-back."
  - Provide list of all medications patient is to take (including those that are not newly prescribed; this is part of discharge medication reconciliation and safety).
  - Discuss importance of not taking over-the-counter medications without first checking with physician or nurse.
  - If patient had total thyroidectomy, explain the importance of taking thyroid replacement medication regularly.
- Activity to tolerance. Do not overexert; balance activity with rest. Encourage patient to discuss allowances and limitations with respect to occupation, recreation, and activities.
- If patient has parathyroid damage, explain need for calcium supplements.
- Teach prescribed head and neck exercises and ways to support the neck when coughing or moving to prevent incisional strain.
- Discuss need to maintain balanced diet.

Follow-Up Care
- Stress importance of regular follow-up visits to monitor thyroid levels. Make sure patient has necessary names and telephone numbers.

Modified from Drugs.com. *Total thyroidectomy care notes* (website). www.drugs.com/cg/total-thyroidectomy-discharge-care.html. (Accessed 5 January 2017); Workman LM: Care of patients with problems of the thyroid and parathyroid glands. In Ignatavicius DD, Workman ML, editors: *Medical-surgical nursing: patient-centered collaborative care,* ed 8, St Louis, 2016, Elsevier.

AMBULATORY SURGERY CONSIDERATIONS

Patient Teaching, Preparation, and Screening: An Emphasis on Health Literacy

Thorough patient teaching and preparation with written instructions are critical for ambulatory surgery patients and their families. Limited health literacy has been related to problems understanding discharge information. Nurses require strong critical thinking, clinical reasoning, and assessment skills to screen patients for problems that may preclude discharge to home. Safe and successful ambulatory surgery depends in part on recognizing which patients can be sent home and which patients should be admitted.

Verify that patients have arranged for someone to drive them home and for a caregiver (family/friend) to assist during the first 24 hours at home. Surgery cannot be done on an ambulatory basis if these arrangements have not been made.

Patients are thoroughly and carefully screened as to eligibility for ambulatory thyroidectomy or parathyroidectomy. Ambulatory surgery is contraindicated in patients with grossly enlarged thyroids or comorbid medical conditions, such as cardiac disease, uncontrolled hypertension, brittle diabetes, and sleep apnea. Patients who had a difficult intubation or who bled excessively

during surgery are usually excluded from discharge on the same day as surgery.

Ascertain the patient's ability to understand and cooperate with discharge instructions. Part of health literacy is ensuring that the patient can process and understand health information. Use health literacy "universal precautions" by simplifying your communications.

The patient is sent home with prescriptions for pain management, calcium supplements, thyroid hormone (if indicated), and other medications specific to preexisting conditions. All medications should be reviewed (discharge medication reconciliation) and a list provided. Lower health literacy and a high number of medications may result in less understanding of medication regimens.

Patients must meet discharge criteria from ambulatory surgery: they must be fully awake; alert; and oriented and able to void, swallow, and drink fluids without nausea or vomiting.

Deep breathing, early mobility at home, and hydration are emphasized.

Continued

AMBULATORY SURGERY CONSIDERATIONS

Patient Teaching, Preparation, and Screening: An Emphasis on Health Literacy—cont'd

Patients are cautioned not to drive or drink alcohol for at least 24 hours.

Patients and families are under physical and emotional stress; they may find discharge information overwhelming. Standardized, printed discharge instructions from the surgeon, specific to the surgery performed, with space available to customize information for the patient, provide a valuable tool and reference resource for the patient and family/caregiver to use at home. This is an important part of health literacy for ambulatory surgery patients.

Verify that the patient and caregiver understand symptoms indicating a significant problem that needs immediate attention, as

well as actions to take and people to contact in case of an emergency. These include signs and symptoms of dyspnea, hemorrhage, thyroid storm (a dangerously elevated heart rate, blood pressure, and temperature), and hypocalcemia. Speak in plain language when describing signs and symptoms. Validate that the patient has no language, hearing, or vision barriers to understanding discharge instructions. Ask the patient and caregiver to repeat back instructions in their own words.

Instruct the patient to call the physician's office for a follow-up visit if this has not been done.

Modified from Agency for Healthcare Research and Quality (AHRQ): *Health literacy universal precautions toolkit* (website) . www.ahrq.gov/professionals/quality-patient-safety/quality-resources/tools/literacy-toolkit/index.html. (Accessed 5 January 2017); Rapporteur JA: *Health literacy: past, present, and future: workshop summary*, Washington DC, 2015, National Academy of Sciences.

Surgical Interventions

Unilateral Thyroid Lobectomy, Subtotal Lobectomy, Bilateral Subtotal Lobectomy, Near-Total Thyroidectomy, and Total Thyroidectomy

Unilateral thyroid lobectomy (or *hemithyroidectomy*) is the removal of one thyroid lobe with excision of the isthmus. The isthmus is completely removed to prevent postoperative hypertrophy in response to the lobectomy with subsequent airway impingement.

Subtotal lobectomy is a lobectomy that spares the posterior capsule and a portion of adjacent thyroid tissue. *Bilateral subtotal lobectomy* is removal of both lobes of the thyroid in the fashion stated for subtotal lobectomy. *Near-total thyroidectomy* is a total lobectomy with contralateral subtotal lobectomy.

Total thyroidectomy is the removal of both lobes of the thyroid and all thyroid tissue present. For patients with cancer of the thyroid, total or near-total thyroidectomy is the desired treatment. After surgery, the thyroid cancer patient may be treated with radioactive ablation therapy for residual or metastatic disease and thyroid hormone suppression therapy. The patient is then monitored by physical examination, laboratory studies (serum thyroid function and thyroglobulin levels), and radioactive scans.

The purpose of the surgical intervention relates to the patient's medical diagnosis. *Goiter* refers to any enlargement of the thyroid gland. It includes both benign and malignant nodules; enlargement is visible over the anterior neck. *Benign adenomas* are encased in a fibrous capsule, distinct from surrounding thyroid tissue.

Malignancies occur most commonly in patients younger than 20 or older than 60 years. Excising lymph nodes with suspected or known cancer of the thyroid remains a standard therapy. Radiologic studies aid in determining nodal metastasis and which levels of the neck to dissect. Contralateral metastasis is generally associated with large tumors. Young patients tend to respond favorably to treatment and have a better prognosis than older patients. Older patients are at greater risk for postoperative complications.

Graves disease, the most common cause of hyperthyroidism, is associated with diffuse, bilateral enlargement of the thyroid gland. Surgery is reserved for patients who fail medical therapy (antithyroid drugs and radioactive iodine) or have a contraindication to medical therapy.

Hashimoto thyroiditis is believed to be an autoimmune disease in which nontender enlargement of the gland occurs. Surgery is performed to relieve compression symptoms.

Nontoxic nodular goiter involves production of insufficient hormones and is noninflammatory; in such cases thyroid tissue proliferates in an apparent attempt to produce the minimal hormonal requirement. Surgery may be indicated to relieve tracheal or esophageal obstruction or to rule out a malignant nodule of the thyroid.

Total thyroidectomy may be done for malignant tumors (Box 16.3). An intraoperative frozen section may be indicated to confirm the diagnosis. If the diagnosis is not definitive by frozen section, a hemithyroidectomy may be the treatment of choice. If the permanent histologic report is benign, the patient's unaffected thyroid lobe is preserved. If, however, pathologic analysis demonstrates that the thyroid mass is malignant, a TT is often recommended.

Minimally invasive approaches to thyroid surgery include minimally invasive open thyroidectomy (MIT) and minimally invasive video-assisted thyroidectomy (MIVAT). Minimally invasive thyroid surgery is performed for both partial and TTs. Although more expensive than open procedures, robotic-assisted surgeries for thyroidectomy are done (Research Highlight: Using Robotics in Thyroid and Neck Dissection Surgeries) (Research Highlight: Robotic-Assisted Thyroidectomy in Differentiated Thyroid Carcinoma) (Robotic-Assisted Surgery). Researchers continue to conduct studies on natural orifice transendoscopic surgery (NOTES); in the future, skin incisions may become obsolete for some surgeries.

Thyroidectomy

Minimally invasive thyroidectomies reduce postoperative pain, decrease hospital lengths of stay, and improve cosmetic results. Minimizing dissection and resultant dead space eliminates the need for external drains in most cases. Smaller incisions, minimal use of surgical drains, and prophylactic calcium supplementation have enabled thyroid surgery to be performed safely with better surgical and cosmetic outcomes.

MIVAT is generally reserved for thyroid nodules within specific size limits as well as for low-stage papillary thyroid carcinomas. As MIVAT has evolved and surgeons have become more proficient with the technique, the only absolute contraindications for its use are (1) thyroid malignancies beyond low-stage papillary carcinoma and (2) preoperative evidence of lymph node metastasis. Relative

BOX 16.3

Malignant Thyroid Nodules

Papillary Carcinoma
- Most common form (70%–80%)
- Poorly encapsulated
- Calcifications present, which is uncommon in other carcinomas

Follicular Carcinoma
- Second most common form (about 10%)
- Well differentiated
- Associated with iodine deficiency

Hürthle Cell Tumor (Oncocytic Carcinoma)
- Derived from follicular epithelium
- Accounts for about 3% of thyroid malignancies
- Associated with regional nodal metastasis

Medullary Carcinoma
- Undifferentiated tumor
- Accounts for 5% to 8% of thyroid malignancies
- Higher death rate than differentiated

Anaplastic (Undifferentiated) Carcinoma
- Almost always advanced when the diagnosis is made
- Highly aggressive, metastasizes quickly
- Rapidly fatal; survival is measured in months (1-year survival is about 20%)

Other Thyroid Cancers
- Thyroid lymphoma
- Thyroid sarcoma

Modified from American Cancer Society: *What is thyroid cancer?* (website), 2016. www.cancer.org/cancer/thyroidcancer/detailedguide/thyroid-cancer-what-is-thyroid-cancer. (Accessed 5 January 2017); Kaplan EL et al: Surgery of the thyroid. In Jameson JL et al, editor: *Endocrinology: adult and pediatric,* ed 7, St Louis, 2016, Elsevier.

RESEARCH HIGHLIGHT

Using Robotics in Thyroid and Neck Dissection Surgeries

In this study, researchers compared the efficacy of robotic thyroidectomy via a gasless, axillary approach with conventional cervical and endoscopic techniques. Using a meta-analysis of 87 publications in which nine studies met inclusion criteria (totaling 2881 patients; 1122 underwent robotic thyroidectomy), their analysis showed that those undergoing robotic surgery had greater cosmetic satisfaction, with a pooled net outcome difference of −1.35 (95% CI: −1.69, −1.09). Robotic surgery had a longer operative time than a conventional technique (95% CI: 29.23, 54.87), although robotic surgery showed a trend to be shorter than an endoscopic approach. Analysis also showed that robotic, open, and endoscopic surgeries had similar risks. The authors concluded that robotic thyroidectomy surgery is as feasible, safe, and efficacious as endoscopic approaches and has superior cosmetic results compared with the conventional open approach.

CI, Confidence interval.
Modified from Jackson NR et al: Safety of robotic thyroidectomy approaches: meta-analysis and systematic review, *Head Neck* 36(1):137–143, 2014.

RESEARCH HIGHLIGHT

Robotic-Assisted Thyroidectomy in Differentiated Thyroid Carcinoma

This systematic review and meta-analysis evaluated the completeness and outcomes of robotic thyroidectomy, noting that a robotic-assisted thyroidectomy approach remains controversial in DTC. The meta-analysis compared oncologic outcomes and/or the surgical completeness between OT and RT in low-risk DTC. Ten studies met criteria and included 2205 DTC patients (752 [34.1%] had RT, whereas 1453 [65.9%] had conventional OT). The authors found that robotic surgery had significantly fewer central lymph nodes retrieved during central neck dissection (4.7 ± 3.2 versus 5.5 ± 3.8, SMD = −0.240, 95% CI: −0.364 to −0.116, $P < .001$) and higher preablation sTg levels (3.6 ± 6.7 ng/mL versus 2.0 ± 5.0 ng/mL, SMD = 0.272, 95% CI: 0.022 to 0.522, $P = .033$). Interestingly, these variations were more evident in the RTAA than the robotic bilateral axillo-breast approach. The analysis concludes that although there are differences in lymph nodes retrieved and a less complete thyroid resection performed, using a robotic transaxillary approach is unlikely to compromise the outcomes of low-risk DTC because of its inherently good prognosis.

CI, Confidence interval; *DTC,* differentiated thyroid carcinoma; *OT,* open thyroidectomy; *RT,* robotic thyroidectomy; *RTAA,* robotic transaxillary approach; *SMD,* standardized mean difference; *sTg,* stimulated thyroglobulin.
Modified from Lang BH et al: A systematic review and meta-analysis evaluating completeness and outcomes of robotic thyroidectomy, *Laryngoscope* 125(2):509–518, 2015.

ROBOTIC-ASSISTED SURGERY

Robotic Thyroidectomy: Key Points

These key points are considered regarding the decision to use a robotic thyroidectomy approach:
- Robotic surgery is ideal for patients with likely benign lesions less than 3 cm and a corresponding body mass index less than 35 kg/m².
- Careful attention must be given to the position of the patient's arms, and proper padding must be completed before the procedure to achieve optimal exposure and working space from the axilla to the thyroid.
- Working space should be developed without robotic assistance to establish thyroid bed exposure from a 5-cm incision in the axilla.
- Three robotic instruments along with a stereoscopic endoscope are likely sufficient to provide excellent visualization.

Modified from Holsinger FC, Chung WY: Robotic thyroidectomy, *Otolaryngol Clin North Am* 47(3):373–378, 2014.

contraindications include (1) prior conventional thyroidectomy, (2) nodules with a diameter larger than 30 mm and volume greater than 25 mL, and (3) a history of thyroiditis. When these criteria were met, Viani and colleagues (2015) found enhanced cosmetic results, lower postoperative pain, and similar oncologic results.

Procedural Considerations

The patient is positioned supine. A drape pack with a fenestrated sheet is required along with a basic instrument set and thyroid instruments. An energy-generating device such as an ESU, a surgical smoke evacuator (Chavis et al., 2016), gauze dissectors, and a small

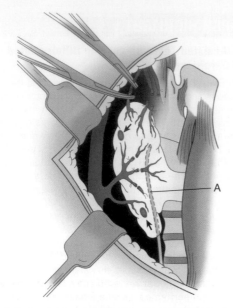

FIG. 16.7 Safe thyroid principles emphasize the following: division of all branch vessels on the capsule of the thyroid with fine mosquito hemostats to prevent injury to the superior laryngeal nerve while detaching the superior thyroid artery and to prevent injury to the parathyroid glands while detaching the inferior thyroid artery; mobilization of parathyroid glands *(arrows)* by medial-to-lateral dissection to preserve their vascular pedicle; and constant awareness of the location of the recurrent laryngeal nerve *(A)*, especially near its penetration into the larynx.

drain (optional) are commonly used. A headlight for the surgeon and assistant may be required. A nerve monitor used during surgery protects the RLNs. The patient is prepped from chin to the upper chest, using fire safety precautions. Surgeons may also use a harmonic scalpel or tissue fusion device. The harmonic scalpel blade retains its heat longer than an ESU blade. Appropriate precautions must therefore be used with the harmonic scalpel to avoid inadvertent injury to adjacent tissue. Thyroidectomies are done through a small incision, and visualization is critical for successful extraction. Bleeding can obscure the view and hinder progress of the surgery; therefore surgeons may opt to use hemostatic agents intraoperatively to maintain hemostasis.

Operative Procedure: Open Thyroidectomy

Fig. 16.7 provides an overview of safe thyroidectomy principles.

1. Setup for a nerve-monitoring system is strategically positioned during or after intubation. The device significantly reduces nerve location time while improving patient safety and decreasing surgeon stress during difficult dissections.
2. A transverse incision (slightly curved and symmetric) is made parallel to the normal skin line crease of the neck, through the skin and first layers of the cervical fascia and platysma muscle, about 2 cm above the sternoclavicular junction.
3. An upper skin flap is undermined to the level of the thyroid notch of the thyroid cartilage; double skin hooks or Allis clamps are placed on the dermis and retracted anteriorly and superiorly to facilitate dissection. A lower flap is then undermined to the sternoclavicular joint. A knife, fine curved scissors, tissue forceps, and gauze sponges are used to undermine the flaps. Bleeding vessels are clamped with hemostats and ligated with fine nonabsorbable sutures. Energy-generating or ultrasonic energy

devices help facilitate dissection with minimal vessel and tissue injury. Retraction with a vein retractor or Army-Navy retractor, or with a self-retaining neck retractor, helps identify the plane for dissection.

4. Flaps are held away from the wound with stay sutures inserted through the cervical fascia and platysma muscle.
5. The fascia in the midline is incised between the strap (sternohyoid and sternothyroid) muscles with a cold or hot knife or energy-generating device(s). Care is taken to preserve the anterior jugular veins. The fascia may be lifted on either side with forceps during the dissection to help define the plane of dissection and protect the jugular vessels. The sternocleidomastoid muscle may be retracted with a loop retractor. Ordinarily, it is not necessary to divide the strap muscles. If additional exposure is required, however, such as with a very large gland, they may be divided between clamps using Mastin muscle clamps, Kocher clamps, or hemostats. The divided muscles are retracted from the operative site to expose the target lobe.
6. The inferior and middle thyroid veins are ligated with fine nonabsorbable sutures or hemoclips and divided with Metzenbaum scissors or energy-generating devices.
7. The lobe is first rotated medially, and loose areolar tissue is then divided posteriorly and medially toward the tracheoesophageal sulcus with hemostats and Metzenbaum scissors. Small gauze sponges are used for blunt dissection. Bleeding is controlled with hemostats, hemoclips, and ligatures, as well as with the ESU (monopolar or bipolar), or other energy-generating devices.
8. The RLN, which enters the larynx immediately posterior to the cricothyroid articulation, is identified and carefully preserved. Electrocoagulation is not used in the vicinity of the recurrent or superior laryngeal nerves because the spread of current can damage these nerves. Nerve monitoring is used during dissection to identify proximity to the laryngeal nerves, thus preventing injury. Nerve-monitoring systems are a helpful adjunct in identifying and preserving the RLNs, but they are not a substitute for visualization. The monitoring device is located in the endotracheal tube inserted by the anesthesia provider during anesthesia induction. Vigorous suction and dissection may cause injury to the nerve and parathyroid glands. Bilateral injury to each EBSLN may result in paralysis of the cricothyroid muscles and make it impossible to produce high-pitched sounds. Although surgeons maintain visual identification of the RLN, significant improvement in identifying the nerve results and decreased risk of early phonation changes after thyroidectomy occurs when a nerve-monitoring device is used (Kim et al., 2015). The scrub person prepares a radiopaque 4 × 8-inch sponge on the end of a forceps for the surgeon or assistant to use in gently blotting the area.
9. The thyroid lobe is pulled downward, a Lahey goiter or polar retractor inserted as necessary, and the avascular tissue between the trachea and upper pole of the thyroid dissected with Metzenbaum scissors or energy-generating device.
10. The superior thyroid artery is defined by blunt dissection with a small gauze sponge (peanut) on a clamp; it is then isolated with a right-angle clamp. The artery is ligated with nonabsorbable suture or clamped and divided. Care is taken here to avoid injury to the superior laryngeal nerve. The upper parathyroid gland is often identified at this time.
11. The inferior thyroid artery is identified and preserved as is the inferior parathyroid. Only branches of the inferior thyroid artery that do not supply the parathyroid glands are ligated, using fine

forceps, sutures, and scissors or energy-generating device. The thyroid lobe is then dissected away from the RLN with hemostats and Metzenbaum scissors, or energy-generating device. Bleeding vessels are clamped with hemostats or hemoclips and ligated with fine nonabsorbable sutures.

12. The lobe is elevated with Babcock clamps and freed from the trachea with fine scissors, forceps, knife, and hemostats, or with cautious electrodissection. The fibrous bands attached to the trachea and cricoid cartilage are divided.

13. The isthmus of the gland is elevated with fine forceps and divided between hemostats with scissors, removing the lobe and isthmus. The cut edge of the remaining thyroid may be oversewn to maintain hemostasis. If a pyramidal lobe is present, it is removed, along with the lobe to which it is attached, to its termination in the neck, which may reach the hyoid bone. If it is necessary to transect the hyoid bone, hyoid scissors or a small bone cutter is used.

14. The cut surface of the opposite lobe requires careful hemostasis. Interrupted sutures may be used for this purpose as well as for reapproximation to the pretracheal fascia.

15. The excised thyroid is examined for inadvertent parathyroid inclusion. If a parathyroid is present, it is removed and reimplanted.

16. The strap muscles, if severed, are reapproximated with fine interrupted absorbable or nonabsorbable sutures. If necessary, a drain is inserted into the thyroid bed and exteriorized through the midline. Some surgeons prefer to drain the wound laterally through the sternocleidomastoid muscle and the lateral aspect of the incision, believing that this produces better healing and cosmetic results. A hemostatic agent may be placed in the lateral gutter to facilitate hemostasis.

17. The edges of the platysma muscle are reapproximated. The skin edges are then reapproximated with subcuticular fine absorbable sutures.

18. Wound closure tapes or surgical glue is applied to the wound edges, and gauze dressings, if required, are placed on the wound with minimal tape.

Substernal or Intrathoracic Thyroidectomy

Extensions of goiters enlarging into the substernal and intrathoracic regions may occur. If they cause tracheal and esophageal obstruction, they are usually excised surgically. Longer instruments are sometimes required. Splitting the sternum is rarely necessary because access to the substernal part of the gland is usually satisfactory through the standard thyroid incision.

Minimally Invasive Thyroidectomy

Minimally Invasive Open Thyroidectomy

The length of the incision is the major difference between minimally invasive and traditional thyroidectomy. Given its smaller size, the site of the minimally invasive incision is critical for optimum access and visualization. After the incision is made, the remaining procedure is the same as that for conventional thyroidectomy.

Minimally Invasive Video-Assisted Thyroidectomy

Procedural Considerations

The possibility of conversion to open thyroidectomy should be included on the operative consent form and discussed with the patient (Dhingra, 2015). Instruments and supplies for a possible open procedure are available and ready. The patient is positioned supine with slight neck extension. Surgical skin preparation is done as in an open procedure in the event conversion is necessary. Draping is as for thyroidectomy. A set of long Miccoli instruments is added to the standard thyroid or neck dissection setup. A 30-degree endoscope and harmonic scalpel with scissors are used to ligate and divide vessels. Fire safety precautions are implemented for illuminated light cords, endoscopes, light sources, and cable connections.

Operative Procedure

1. A horizontal incision of 3 cm or less is marked and then carefully made between the sternal notch and cricoid cartilage, usually less than 1 to 2 cm inferior to the cricoid (Fig. 16.8).

2. Subcutaneous tissue is electrodissected and the raphe of strap muscle is then separated superiorly and inferiorly for about 3 cm. The anterior jugular veins are preserved.

3. Gentle, blunt dissection is used to separate the strap muscle from the thyroid.

4. The middle thyroid vein is clipped and divided.

5. Miccoli retractors are used to retract the strap muscles and soft tissue, exposing the superior lobe and vascular bundle.

6. The endoscope is introduced to visualize the upper pole.

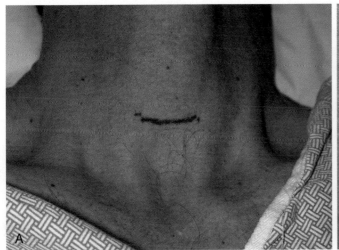
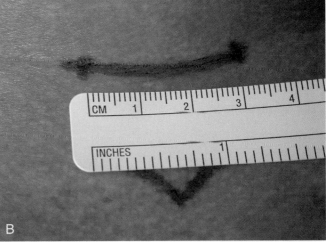

FIG. 16.8 (A) Minimally invasive video-assisted thyroidectomy incision location. (B) MIVAT incision length.

7. Miccoli spatula-shaped and aspirator dissectors are used to dissect the superior pole and vascular bundle (Fig. 16.9). Care is taken to identify and preserve the EBSLN.

8. The thyroid lobe is then retracted medially, and its lateral and posterior attachments are dissected. The RLN and parathyroids are protected and preserved (Fig. 16.10).

9. After sufficient mobilization of the lobe, the remainder of the procedure is accomplished under direct visualization. The isthmus is transected to complete the lobectomy.

10. The same procedure is repeated on the other side for complete thyroidectomy.

11. Hemostasis is achieved, the wound is irrigated, strap muscles are reapproximated, and the skin is closed (Fig. 16.11).

Thyroglossal Duct Cystectomy

Thyroglossal duct cysts (TDCs) are the most common congenital cyst found in the neck. These cysts are the second most common type of pediatric neck mass. Although this cyst may be found in patients of any age, most are noted during childhood; 50% usually are seen before 20 years of age and about 70% by 30 years of age. The thyroglossal duct is an embryonic structure arising from the descent of the thyroid gland into the anterior portion of the neck. Usually the cyst presents as an asymptomatic midline swelling and is painless. Occasionally the cyst may become infected because of its proximity to the oral cavity. When present in an adult, it exists as a pretracheal cystic pouch attached to the hyoid bone, with or without a sinus tract to the base of the tongue at the foramen cecum (Fig. 16.12). Thyroglossal duct cystectomy, often referred to as the Sistrunk procedure, requires complete excision of the cyst in continuity with its tract, the central portion of the hyoid bone, and the tissue above the hyoid bone extending to the base of the tongue to avoid recurrent cystic formation and to prevent infection. Only 1% of TDCs are malignant on histology, and the prognosis for treating this malignancy is good.

Procedural Considerations

The perioperative nursing assessment should be appropriate to the patient's age. Reassurance and age-appropriate information about

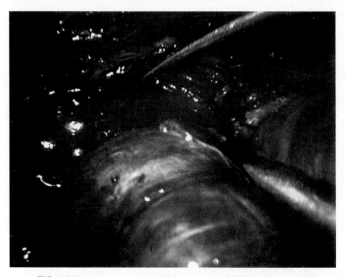

FIG. 16.9 Video-assisted dissection of the right superior pole.

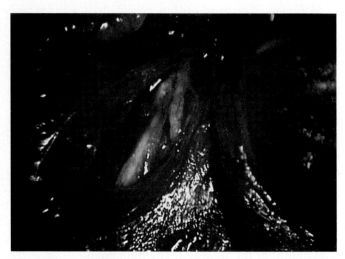

FIG. 16.10 Identification of the recurrent laryngeal nerve during video-assisted right thyroid lobectomy. A parathyroid gland is also identified.

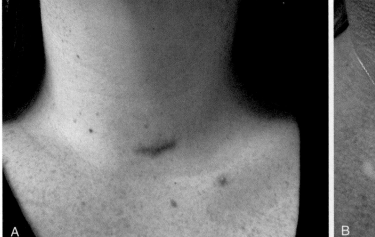

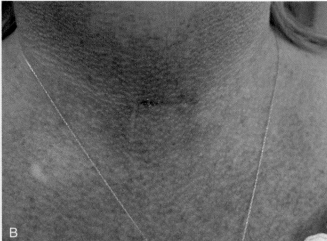

FIG. 16.11 (A) Surgical scar at 2 weeks. (B) Surgical scar at 6 weeks.

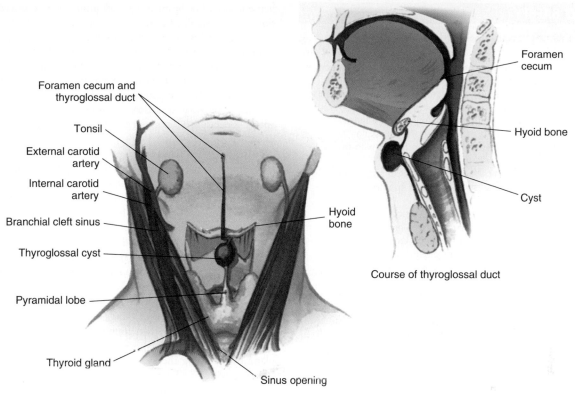

FIG. 16.12 Thyroglossal cyst showing both anterior and lateral views.

the procedure are given. The patient is positioned supine, with the neck supported in extension; the chin is elevated. Bone instruments are needed in addition to the basic instrument set.

Operative Procedure

1. The surgeon makes a transverse incision between the hyoid bone and thyroid cartilage through the subcutaneous tissue.
2. The platysma muscle is incised and flaps are raised as described for thyroidectomy.
3. The strap (sternohyoid and sternothyroid) muscles are separated in the midline.
4. Sharp and blunt dissection is used to mobilize the cyst and duct, up to the attachment to the hyoid bone. The hyoid bone is transected twice, removing the center section with bone-cutting forceps. The segment of bone and the cyst are freed from adjacent structures.
5. The duct is traced superiorly through or near the hyoid up to the musculature of the tongue and removed completely. Methylene blue dye injection is used occasionally to visualize the whole tract.
6. The cyst is removed and the strap muscles closed with interrupted fine nonabsorbable sutures. A drain may be placed. The skin is then closed with subcuticular fine absorbable sutures and dressings applied.

Parathyroidectomy

Parathyroidectomy is excision of one or more parathyroid glands. Normal or atrophic glands are generally not removed. The presence of adenomas (hypersecreting neoplasms), hyperplasia, or carcinoma requires surgical excision. For carcinomas, resection of the ipsilateral thyroid lobe and lymph nodes is essential, although metastasis may still occur. Any residual parathyroid cancer may secrete PTH, causing hypercalcemia and its attendant problems.

Previously, the gold standard for parathyroidectomy was bilateral neck exploration with biopsy of all four glands to confirm the presence of adenoma or hyperplasia. New technologies, however, offer less invasive surgical options that pinpoint the affected gland and obviate the need to biopsy, and potentially damage, healthy parathyroid glands. The four-gland exploration for single-gland involvement is being replaced by radio-guided, minimally invasive ambulatory procedures using intraoperative PTH levels and/or the gamma probe. Patients with a negative sestamibi scan are excluded from minimally invasive parathyroidectomy (MIP) protocols, although intraoperative PTH levels are still helpful in identifying multiple adenomas. Often the diagnosis of an adenoma can be made by gross inspection of the glands by the surgeon, but such diagnoses must be confirmed histologically by the pathologist.

Minimally invasive techniques cannot be used for hyperplasia. Hyperplasia requires removal of three and one-half glands through a bilateral neck exploration. A portion of a gland must remain to prevent hypocalcemia and its complications.

Procedural Considerations

During bilateral neck exploration, multiple biopsies may help to determine the presence or absence of parathyroid tissue. Numerous specimen containers should be available (Patient Safety). When parathyroidectomy using a minimally invasive approach with intraoperative PTH assays is planned, verify that a pathologist is alerted and ready to analyze blood samples and tissue specimens. If the surgeon is performing a focused parathyroidectomy (FP) (as described under the later section Minimally Invasive, Focused Parathyroid Surgery), several blood tubes are required to measure

Handling Multiple Specimens

The perioperative nurse is accountable for specimen collection, identification, and handling. Standardized specimen collection procedures should be used by all members of the surgical team. During parathyroidectomy, multiple specimens are often collected. To accurately identify and safely manage these specimens, the perioperative nurse does the following:

- Verify specimen collection and handling needs with the surgeon before beginning the procedure.
- Ensure availability of an adequate number of specimen containers, labels, laboratory forms, and appropriate preservative.
- Take an additional time-out when the specimen is collected, in which the surgeon, scrub person, and nurse agree on the name of the specimen, its type, source location, and preservative solution required for maintaining specimen integrity; minimize any distractions during this specimen verification process.
- Label the specimen with a patient label and provide the name of the contents on the container.
- Indicate the order of specimen harvesting when multiple specimens are collected (they may be labeled A, B, C, etc.).
- Communicate to the pathology department the nature of the procedure and anticipated specimens.
- Plan for direct communication about specimens between the surgeon and pathologist or perform a read-back or repeat-back of pathology findings verbally reported to you. Music is turned down and conversation kept to a minimum during read back/repeat back.
- Use Standard Precautions and Transmission-Based Precautions; label all specimens as biohazards.
- Log specimens according to institutional protocol for chain of custody.
- Arrange for timely transport of specimens to the pathology department.
- Include specimen management and status in your hand-off report if you are relieved during the procedure.
- Document specimen collection in the intraoperative nursing record according to institutional protocol. Electronic medical record (EMR) documentation facilitates ease in charting of time-stamped specimen labeling.
- Announce all specimens collected during the debriefing at the conclusion of the surgical procedure.
- Avoid surgical item counts during care and handling of specimens

Modified from AORN: Guidelines for the care and handling of specimens in the perioperative environment. In *Guidelines for perioperative practice,* Denver, 2017, The Association.

PTH levels intraoperatively. The circulating nurse notes excision time and collaborates with the anesthesia provider to anticipate and handle postexcision blood samples. Mediastinotomy instruments should be available (see Chapter 23). The patient is positioned, prepped, and draped as described for thyroidectomy. Hemoclips should be available.

Operative Procedure: Open Approach

In the classic open approach with the thyroid gland visible, the surgeon conducts a bilateral neck exploration of the "normal" locations of the four parathyroid glands. Meticulous hemostasis with mosquito hemostats and fine ligatures is a prerequisite to location and identification of these small glands.

The thyroid gland is gently rotated anteriorly to provide access to the posterior thyroid sulcus, which is where the parathyroid glands are almost always found. Identification of the parathyroid vascular pedicle, as it leaves either the superior thyroid artery or the inferior thyroid artery, is a means of locating both the inferior and superior glands. Metzenbaum scissors, mosquito hemostats, hemoclips, energy-generating devices, and gauze dissector sponges are used during dissection.

Attention then turns to the posterolateral surface of the thyroid lobe or just beneath the lower thyroid pole, where the inferior parathyroid glands are frequently found. Finding the vascular pedicle from the inferior thyroid artery may aid identification (see Fig. 16.4). Occasionally the lower pair is found in the thymic capsule or tissue, in which case a portion of the thymus is resected. A mediastinotomy is indicated for a small percentage of patients. Thoracoscopy (see Chapter 23) is a successful, minimally invasive technique that may be used to remove parathyroid tumors that are deep in the mediastinum.

If one of the parathyroid glands shows evidence of disease, an effort is made to find other glands on the same side to ensure that they are disease free. When found, biopsy is performed, and the area is marked with a hemoclip. The surgeon resects the diseased gland by clamping the vascular pedicle with mosquito hemostats, dividing with small scissors or a knife, and ligating with a fine nonabsorbable suture or hemoclip. The amount of parathyroid tissue that should be removed remains controversial and relates to whether single or multiple glands are involved. As noted, a portion of a gland must remain to prevent hypocalcemia and its complications.

An alternative for multiple gland involvement is to excise all four glands and to transplant a portion of one in an accessible site, such as the neck or forearm, for later removal if hypercalcemia recurs. The amount of remaining parathyroid tissue can then be adjusted to regulate PTH to the desired level. This eliminates reexploration and potential injury to the RLNs. The parathyroid is morcellized and divided into several segments. An incision is made in the forearm or neck, and four separate grooves with purse-string sutures are made in the muscle. Some parathyroid tissue is placed and secured in each groove. The sites are then marked with one, two, three, and four hemoclips, respectively. If PTH levels remain high, the sites can be easily identified by the clips and more parathyroid tissue excised.

The neck region is then explored for aberrant parathyroid tissue, which is also resected. The remainder of the procedure is as described for the thyroid gland.

Minimally Invasive, Focused Parathyroid Surgery

Although a variety of minimally invasive techniques have evolved, a widely used procedure is the focused minimally invasive open approach (FP), in which imaging has identified a single parathyroid lesion. A localization study with sestamibi scan or ultrasound is used to identify the offending adenoma and to determine an optimum incision site.

PTH-Guided Parathyroidectomy

Another approach is the intraoperative intact, rapid assessment PTH approach. Blood samples are drawn before, during, and after the procedure to measure PTH levels. A venous blood sample is obtained before IV insertion and sent for baseline preoperative measurement of PTH.

A 2-cm incision is made in the neck based on the localization studies. Once the suspect parathyroid gland is exposed, a preexcision blood sample is taken. As a result of manipulation, the preexcision blood level may test higher than the baseline level. The preexcision level becomes the marker for measuring the postexcision drop in PTH level.

The excised gland is placed in sterile saline and kept on the instrument table until the pathologist confirms a sufficient drop in PTH blood levels. A drop of 50% or more is considered verification that the parathyroid adenoma was excised (Kim and Krause, 2016). Blood levels may also be drawn at 5, 10, and 20 minutes post excision. When the adenoma is excised, a dramatic drop in PTH level is frequently achieved by the 10-minute postexcision PTH sample. If the 10-minute drop is significant, the surgeon may opt not to have the pathologist run a 20-minute postexcision blood sample. If the hormone level fails to drop sufficiently, the ipsilateral parathyroid is explored as the next most likely adenoma. False-positives have been reported in patients who have slow metabolic rates, are renal insufficient, or have large adenomas (3 g or greater).

Any normal parathyroid that was excised and placed in saline is then morcellized with a #15 blade to increase surface area and then reimplanted. After the fascia is reapproximated, a clamp or scissors is used to create a groove in the strap muscle. A purse-string stitch of fine nonabsorbable suture is placed around the groove. The morcellized parathyroid tissue is placed inside the groove and the purse-string tightened and tied. Parathyroid tissue responds well to reimplantation.

Sestamibi-Guided Parathyroidectomy

Another minimally invasive technique is the sestamibi-guided, or radio-guided, parathyroidectomy. MIP is considered the treatment of choice for HPT when a singular adenoma is present (Burke et al., 2013). Technetium-99m sestamibi is the imaging method of choice for localization of the parathyroid for patients with primary HPT. Sestamibi is administered preoperatively and a gamma probe used intraoperatively to pinpoint the adenoma. MIP is usually an ambulatory surgery procedure that has a 95% success rate using sestamibi imaging techniques. A higher success rate is also noted when an experienced endocrine surgeon consults in the radiology study interpretation.

Key Points

- The thyroid gland is situated in the ventral aspect of the neck and is composed of right and left lobes anterolateral to the trachea and connected by an isthmus. It secretes the thyroid hormones T_3, T_4, and calcitonin.
- Hyperthyroidism occurs when tissues are exposed to high levels of circulating thyroid hormone.
- Diagnosis and management of hyperthyroidism are based on patient history, clinical presentation, and blood work results (T_3, T_4, and TSH). TSH is synthesized by the anterior pituitary and stimulates the production and release of thyroid hormones and uptake of iodine.
- Treatment for hyperthyroidism includes antithyroid medication, radioiodine, β-adrenergic medications, and surgery (TT or subtotal thyroidectomy [STT]).
- Thyroid storm is an acute manifestation of hyperthyroidism.
- Hypothyroidism is a deficiency in thyroid hormone. It may be overt or subclinical. It is a common chronic condition and more common in women than men.

- The four parathyroid glands are small and located behind the thyroid gland. They monitor and control calcium by secreting PTH to closely control serum calcium levels.
- In HPT, calcium builds up, potentially leading to atherosclerosis, hypertension, and increased risk for atrial fibrillation, palpitations, osteopenia, osteoporosis, and formation of kidney stones. A serum calcium level greater than 13.5 mg/dL can produce life-threatening cardiac dysrhythmias.
- Head and neck irradiation in childhood and long-term lithium therapy are associated with a higher prevalence of primary HPT.
- Parathyroidectomy may be completed on an ambulatory surgery basis.

Critical Thinking Questions

Your patient, Ms. J., is a 30-year-old who has just undergone a thyroidectomy in OR #6. The surgeon has left the OR and you are the circulating nurse in the room. It is lunchtime, and a new perioperative nurse (J.R.) comes into the room to give lunch relief to the scrub person (A.S.), who is cleaning up her instruments and preparing to take them to the decontamination area. J.R. says that she will take the instruments to the decontamination area, and that A.S. needs to go to lunch now; she has many lunch reliefs to do today. The hospital policy requires that the scrub person remain in the room until the patient has been transferred to the PACU, but J.R. is unaware of this policy. As a novice perioperative nurse, she is concerned with the tasks of preparing for the next surgery. You are finishing the documentation at the computer station and turn around to see the anesthesia provider is having difficulty with the patient's airway. He has just extubated the patient, and his assistant has left the OR. You are alone in the room with this patient in distress. What would your priority nursing actions be at this time? What needs to be established for patient safety? What is the most probable cause for the patient's respiratory distress, and what actions will you need to perform to provide this patient with a positive patient outcome?

evolve *The answers to the Critical Thinking Questions can be found at http://evolve.elsevier.com/Rothrock/Alexander.*

References

American Cancer Society (ACS): *Key statistics for thyroid cancer* (website), 2016. www.cancer.org/cancer/thyroidcancer/detailedguide/thyroid-cancer-key-statistics. (Accessed 5 January 2017).

Association of PeriOperative Registered Nurses (AORN): *Guidelines for perioperative practice*, Denver, 2017, The Association.

Burke JF et al: Early-phase technetium-99m sestamibi scintigraphy can improve preoperative localization in primary hyperparathyroidism, *J Surg* 205(3): 268–273, 2013.

Byrne MD: Little gland, big problems, *OR Nurse* 7(1):23–28, 2013.

Chavis S et al: Clearing the air about surgical smoke: an education program, *AORN J* 103(3):289–296, 2016.

Dhingra JK: *Minimally invasive surgery of the thyroid treatment & management* (website), 2015. http://emedicine.medscape.com/article/1298816-treatment #d11. (Accessed 5 January 2017).

Haugen BR et al: 2015 American Thyroid Association Management Guidelines for Adult Patients with Thyroid Nodules and Differentiated Thyroid Cancer: The American Thyroid Association Guidelines Task Force on Thyroid Nodules and Differentiated Thyroid Cancer, *Thyroid* 26(1):1–133, 2016.

Hoang JK et al: Imaging thyroid disease: updates, imaging approach, and management pearls, *Radiol Clin North Am* 53(1):145–161, 2015.

Hooley J, Reagan S: *Hyperthyroidism: a storm brewing* (website), 2016. www.americannursetoday.com/hyperthyroidism-a-storm-brewing/. (Accessed 5 January 2017).

Kaplan EL et al: Surgery of the thyroid. In Jameson JL et al, editors: *Endocrinology: adult and pediatric*, ed 7, St Louis, 2016, Elsevier.

Kim L, Krause MW: *Hyperparathyroidism* (website), 2016. http://emedicine.medscape.com/article/127351-overview#a3. (Accessed 5 January 2017).

Kim S et al: Intraoperative neuromonitoring of the external branch of the superior laryngeal nerve during robotic thyroid surgery: a preliminary prospective study, *Ann Surg Treat Res* 89(5):233–239, 2015.

Kramer A: *How too much thyroid hormone affects your heart* (website), 2016. www.everydayhealth.com/atrial-fibrillation/living-with/how-much-thyroid-hormone-affects-your-heart/. (Accessed 5 January 2017).

LeFevre ML: *Clinical guideline, screening for thyroid dysfunction: U.S. Preventive Services Task Force Recommendation Statement. Annals of Internal Medicine,* 162(9) (website), 2015. http://annals.org/aim/article/2208599/screening-thyroid-dysfunction-u-s-preventive-services-task-force-recommendation. (Accessed 5 January 2017).

National Cancer Institute (NCI): *Thyroid cancer treatment (PDQ)—health professional version,* (website), 2016. www.cancer.gov/cancertopics/pdq/treatment/thyroid/HealthProfessional/page1. (Accessed 5 January, 2017).

Rightmyer J, Singbartl K: Preventing perioperative hypothermia, *Nursing 2016* 46(9):57–60, 2016.

Scott SM: Perioperative pressure injuries: protocols and evidence-based programs for reducing risk, *Patient Safety and Quality Healthcare* 13(4):21–28, 2016.

Seong JL et al: Risk factors of postoperative hypocalcemia after total thyroidectomy of papillary thyroid carcinoma patients, *Korean Journal of Endocrine Surgery* 16:70–78, 2016.

Shivani S-B, Goldenberg D: Surgical exploration for hyperparathyroidism, *Operative Techniques in Otorhinolaryngology* 27(3):126–135, 2016.

Skugor M: *Hypocalcemia,* Cleveland Clinic Center for Continuing Education. (website), 2014. www.clevelandclinicmeded.com/medicalpubs/diseasemanagement/endocrinology/hypocalcemia/. (Accessed 5 January 2017).

The Joint Commission (TJC): *2017 national patient safety goals, hospital accreditation program* (website), 2016. www.jointcommission.org/hap_2017_npsgs/. (Accessed 5 January 2017).

Velez RP et al: Simplifying the complexity of primary hyperparathyroidism, *The Journal for Nurse Practitioners* 12(5):346–352, 2016.

Viani L et al: Minimally invasive video assisted thyroidectomy (MIVAT) and papillary thyroid carcinoma, *Eur J Surg Oncol* 41(1):S6, 2015.

Wong K et al: Endocrine radionuclide scintigraphy with fusion single photon emission computed tomography/computed tomography, *World J Radiol* 8(6): 635–655, 2016.

CHAPTER **17**
Breast Surgery

KATHRYN J. TROTTER AND JANICE A. NEIL

Most surgical procedures of the breast aim to establish a definitive diagnosis or to treat breast cancer. Changing hormone levels from puberty throughout the remainder of life affect breast tissue in its physical and microscopic characteristics. With these inevitable changes, numerous aberrations and tumors can occur.

Breast changes, benign or malignant, are some of the most emotionally upsetting health problems to confront women. Breast cancer is likely the most common cancer in American women (Wolff et al., 2014). The most significant risk factors for developing breast cancer are female gender and aging (Breastcancer.org, 2015). Estimates are that one in eight women in the United States will develop breast cancer. If detected early, there is a 98.8%, 5-year survival rate (National Cancer Institute, 2016). Breast cancer risk doubles if a woman's mother, sister, or daughter had breast cancer. Early menarche (before 12 years of age) and a late natural menopause (after 55 years of age) are associated with a slightly increased risk to develop breast cancer. Five to ten percent of breast cancer cases are believed to be hereditary gene mutations passed on from a parent (ACS, 2016). Further, a woman who has cancer in one breast is at risk for cancer in the other breast (ACS, 2016). Earlier detection, improved treatments, and possibly decreased incidence as a result of declining use of postmenopausal hormonal treatment have slowed the annual increase in breast cancer mortality, most notably with larger decreases in women under age 50 (Breastcancer.org, 2015).

Surgical Anatomy

The breasts are bilateral mammary glands. They are surrounded by a layer of fat and are encased in an envelope of skin. Each breast extends vertically from the second to the sixth ribs and horizontally from the lateral edge of the sternum to the anterior axillary line. The largest part of each mammary gland rests on the connective tissue of the pectoralis major muscle and laterally on the serratus anterior (upper outer quadrant of each breast), with a normal globular contour occurring as a result of fascia support (Cooper ligaments) (Fig. 17.1). An elongation of mammary tissue normally extends laterally on the pectoralis major toward the axilla and is known as the *tail of Spence* (Fig. 17.2).

The breast consists of 12 to 20 glandular lobes separated by connective tissue. Each lobe drains by a single lactiferous duct that opens on the nipple. The nipple, located at about the fourth intercostal space, forms a conical projection into which the ducts open. A pigmented circular area called the *areola* surrounds the nipple. Smooth muscle fibers of the areola contract to allow for nipple projection.

Three major arterial systems (Fig. 17.3) supply the mammary glands with blood. The major supply of blood comes from the perforating branches of the internal mammary arteries, derived from the internal thoracic artery. The breast is additionally supplied by the lateral thoracic and thoracoacromial arteries as well as posterior intercostal arteries. Veins that mainly drain the breasts are the axillary, along with the subclavian, intercostals, and internal thoracic veins.

Lymph drainage generally follows the course of the vessels. Greater than 75% of lymph drainage, chiefly from the lateral quadrants, drains to the axillary lymph nodes. The remainder drains to either the parasternal nodes, the opposite breast (medial quadrants), or the inferior phrenic nodes' lower quadrants (Fig. 17.4). The internal thoracic nodes are few, but they are responsible for most lymph drainage from the inner half of the breast. Thus the lymph system

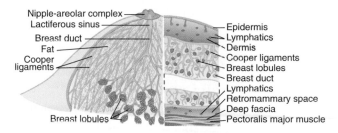

FIG. 17.1 Normal mature resting breast.

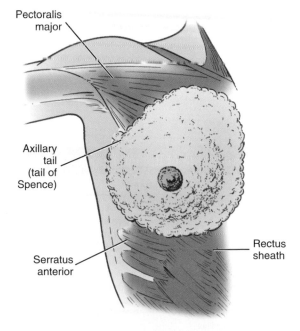

FIG. 17.2 Normal distribution of mammary tissue of adult female.

can be a channel for the spread of malignant disease from either breast to associated areas of the chest wall or to the axilla.

The sensory nerve supply is primarily threefold: the anterior lateral intercostal nerves, the medial intercostal nerves, and the cervical plexus. The anterior rami of the lateral cutaneous nerves of the intercostal nerves provide sensation to the lateral portion of the breast and nipple-areolar complex (NAC). The cervical plexus provides the superior medial innervation (de la Torre and Davis, 2013).

The mammary glands are present at birth in males and females. They are affected by three types of physiologic changes: (1) those related to growth and development, (2) those related to the menstrual cycle, and (3) those related to pregnancy and lactation. Hormonal stimulation, however, produces the development and function of these glands in females. Estrogen promotes growth of the ductal structures, whereas progesterone promotes lobular development. Occasionally, developmental errors of the breast occur. Additional nipples or extramammary tissue in the axilla or over the upper abdomen may be present. Absence of one or both nipples may also occur and may be associated with absence of the underlying pectoral muscle and chest wall.

Benign Lesions of the Breast

"Fibrocystic change in the breast" is an all-encompassing term used to describe many different breast changes. Examples of benign lesions that are generally considered when discussing fibrocystic changes are multiple lesions of fibrous disease, intraductal papilloma, cysts, and solid masses such as fibroadenoma (Table 17.1). These changes

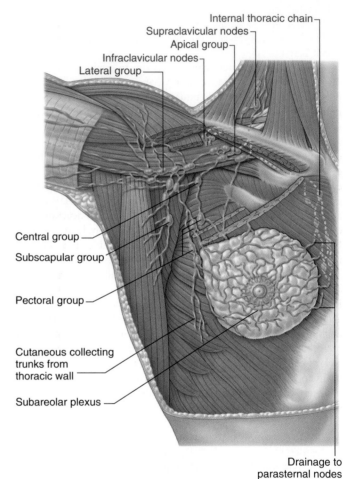

FIG. 17.4 Axillary lymph node groups.

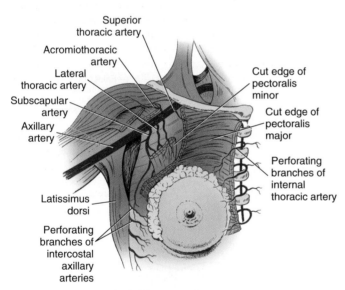

FIG. 17.3 Normal arterial blood supply of the breast.

TABLE 17.1		
Typical Presentation of Benign Breast Disorders		
Breast Disorder	**Description**	**Incidence**
Fibroadenoma	Most common benign lesion; solid mass of connective tissue that is unattached to surrounding tissue	Teenage years into 30s
FBC	Discrete, tender, mobile, and often bilateral; size may fluctuate with the menstrual cycle	Late teens and 20s
Ductal ectasia	Often associated with nipple discharge, dilation of the ducts with surrounding inflammation and fibrosis, may be accompanied by an intraductal mass	Women 40–50s, perimenopausal
Intraductal papilloma	Mass in duct that results in nipple discharge; mass is usually not palpable, typically bloody discharge is unilateral and uniductal	Women 40–55 years of age

FBC, Fibrocystic breast condition.
Modified from Collins LC, Schnitt SJ: Pathology of benign breast disorders. In Harris JR et al, editors: *Diseases of the breast,* ed 5, Philadelphia, 2014, Wolters Kluwer Health.

affect most women at some time in their lives. About two-thirds of women experience breast pain. Tenderness, fluctuations in size, and multiple lesions are common features that help differentiate these generally benign lesions from cancer.

Nipple discharge is more commonly physiologic. A postmenopausal woman who has some duct ectasia or who has borne children can sometimes express nipple discharge. The most common cause of serous or serosanguineous nipple discharge is a benign intraductal papilloma, along with medications such as tricyclines and antidepressants. Discharge is usually significant only if it is spontaneous, bloody, and persistent (Hunt and Mittendorf, 2017). Chronic unilateral nipple discharge, especially if bloody, prompts an investigation for occult carcinoma.

Breast Cancer in Men

Breast cancer in men is rare; less than 1% of breast carcinomas arise in men. Most male breast cancer is found between ages 60 and 70. Lifetime risk of developing breast cancer is 1 in 1000. Risk factors include increased age, radiation exposure, estrogen treatment, Klinefelter syndrome, cirrhosis of the liver, obesity, female relatives with a breast cancer diagnosis, and families in which the breast cancer susceptibility gene 2 *(BRCA2)* mutation has been identified (Hardin and Tsangaris, 2014). The most common type of tumor is infiltrating ductal carcinoma. Paget disease of the nipple, inflammatory carcinoma, and intraductal cancer have also been reported in men. Similar to women, symptoms include breast lumps, nipple inversion, nipple discharge, pain or pulling feelings, and skin or nipple changes such as dimpling, puckering, redness, or scaling. Staging of male breast cancer is identical to staging for female breast cancer. Treatment may include surgery, radiation therapy, chemotherapy, hormone therapy, and targeted therapy. A hormone receptor test precedes hormone therapy to determine whether estrogen and progesterone receptors are present. Adjuvant therapy of radiation, chemotherapy, or hormone treatment is appropriate after surgery to destroy cancer cells that cannot be detected. The prognosis for early-stage breast cancer in men is favorable. Five-year survival rates reach 100% for stage 0 and stage I tumors (MedicineNet.com, 2016).

Breast Cancer in Women

Breast cancer affects women primarily. Until it can be prevented, early detection is the best hope for cure. In the past, widespread medical wisdom suggested that all women practice monthly self-examination to detect palpable lesions. There is, however, now a growing debate over how valuable breast self-examination (BSE) is in detecting early breast cancer and increasing survival rates (Breastcancer.org, 2015). The US Preventive Services Task Force (USPSTF) does not recommend BSE, but encourages women to tell their physician/provider about lumps or changes in their breast (Crawford, 2015). The ACS advises women that BSE is optional (Oeffinger et al., 2015).

The most common form of breast cancer is invasive ductal carcinoma (Research Highlight). Eighty percent of newly diagnosed breast cancers are infiltrating (also referred to as invasive) ductal carcinoma (Breastcancer.org, 2015) (Table 17.2). Invasive breast cancers smaller than 1 cm may be treated with cryoablation by using a "cryoprobe" (a thin wandlike device inserted through the skin to the targeted lesion using ultrasound guidance). When inside the lesion core, the probe, which is filled with nitrogen gas, creates a "freeze ball" in the surrounding tumor tissue, which destroys it (Simmons et al., 2016). Cryoablation is being studied to evaluate its role as a nonsurgical treatment of early-stage breast cancer.

The cause of breast cancer remains unknown. Many factors, including environmental, dietary, and familial influences (ACS, 2016) may contribute to its development (Table 17.3). Long-term survival is optimized when detected early, reducing axillary lymph node involvement.

Less radical surgery is the treatment of choice today. Most small, noninvasive, and invasive breast cancers are treated by breast-conserving surgery (BCS). Surgical excision of the tumor, often with sentinel lymph node biopsy (SLNB) is the primary treatment. The use of radiation therapy alone or a combination of surgery, chemotherapy, targeted therapies, and radiation therapy are further treatment options. Adjuvant chemotherapy is particularly recommended for premenopausal women with axillary node involvement. Targeted

---

TABLE 17.2

Types of Breast Cancer

Breast Cancer Type	Percent of Breast Cancers	Specific Features
DCIS	20	Can appear as microcalcifications, can vary widely in appearance, and can have features of other histologic subtypes of breast cancer; if untreated, 60%–100% of cases advance to invasive carcinoma
LCIS	10	A marker for future breast cancer risk; begins in milk (lobules) glands of breast, may become invasive, grows as single file of malignant cells around ducts and lobules and presents most often as a poorly defined mass
Intraductal carcinoma	80	Cancer has grown through the ductal walls; is invasive
Medullary carcinoma	5	Forms distinct boundary between tumor tissue and normal tissue, well circumscribed, frequent phenotype of *BRCA1* hereditary breast cancer, contains lymphocytes
Tubular	2	Infrequently metastasizes to lymph nodes, slow growing, long-term survival approaches 100%
Inflammatory carcinoma	1–5	Rapidly growing, often with metastasis present at diagnosis, first manifestations are breast skin edema and redness and warmth with dimples or ridges; can be confused with mastitis; more common in African American women

DCIS, Ductal carcinoma in situ; *LCIS,* lobular carcinoma in situ.
Modified from American Cancer Society: *Types of breast cancer* (website). www.cancer.org/cancer/breastcancer/detailedguide/breast-cancer-breast-cancer-types. (Accessed 1 November 2016); Townsend CM et al: *Sabiston textbook of surgery: the biological basis of modern surgical practice,* ed 20, Philadelphia, 2017, Elsevier; Niederhuber JE et al: *Abeloff's clinical oncology,* ed 5, Philadelphia, 2014, Elsevier.

RESEARCH HIGHLIGHT

Advances in the Treatment of Ductal Carcinoma in Situ

DCIS is characterized by malignant epithelial cells confined to the ductal system of the breast and accounts for almost 30% of breast cancers each year. It is most commonly detected on screening mammography, and with increased screening rates there has been a significant rise in the incidence of DCIS. Traditionally, it has been managed through a combination of surgery, radiation therapy, and endocrine therapy. However, DCIS is now known to vary from a quiescent lesion with minimal clinical significance to a more aggressive disease that may become invasive cancer. Research in the last decade has altered treatment decisions, because individual prognostic indications now direct the plan of care.

Much of the current discussion on DCIS surrounds the question of overtreatment and possible elimination of surgery in selected cases. This is because the pathology shows different nuclear grades (how much the cellular nucleus resembles normal cells) from low to high within DCIS, just as with invasive cancer. Multigene assays are being developed such as the Oncotype DX DCIS Score, which is a 12-gene expression assay that estimates the 10-year risk of any local recurrence (DCIS or invasive). The test measures a group of cancer genes in the tissue sample to see how active they are. There are ongoing clinical trials that aim to evaluate both oncologic outcomes and the patient's quality of life with observation alone. This implies no surgery, but medications such as tamoxifen or the AIs may or may not be used. The future goal of developing a personalized therapy based on risk assessment should help to reduce morbidity, psychologic effects, and the disease's healthcare burden.

AI, Aromatase inhibitors; *DCIS*, ductal carcinoma in situ.
Modified from Margolese RG et al: Anastrozole versus tamoxifen in postmenopausal women with ductal carcinoma in situ undergoing lumpectomy plus radiotherapy (NSABP B-35): a randomized, double-blind, phase 3 clinical trial, *Lancet* 387(10021):849–856, 2016; Park TS, Hwang ES: Current trends in the management of ductal carcinoma in situ, *Oncology* 30(9):823–823, 2016; Solin LJ et al: A multigene expression assay to predict local recurrence risk for ductal carcinoma in situ of the breast, *J Natl Cancer Inst* 105(10):701–710, 2013.

TABLE 17.3

Risk Factors for Breast Cancer

Factors	Comments
High Increased Risk	
Female gender	99% of all breast cancers occur in women
Age >60 years	Median age at diagnosis is 61; risk increases until age 80
Genetic factors	Inherited mutations of *BRCA1* and/or *BRCA2* increase risk
History of previous breast cancer and familial breast cancer	Personal history of early onset (<40 years) breast cancer
	Two or more first-degree relatives with breast cancer
Noninvasive carcinoma	DCIS and LCIS
Moderate Increased Risk	
Family history	One first-degree relative with breast cancer
Age	Diagnosed with breast cancer at an early age
Radiation	High-dose radiation to the chest
Dense breasts	Mammographically extremely dense (>50%) breasts compared with less dense (11%–25%)
Low Increased Risk	
Reproductive history (nulliparity or first child born after age 30)	Childless women have an increased risk, as do women who bear their first child near or after age 30
Menstrual history (early menstruation or late menopause or both)	Risk for breast cancer rises as interval between menarche and menopause increases
Oral contraceptives	There is a slight increase in breast cancer risk in women taking oral contraceptives
HRT	Use of estrogen and progesterone for greater than 5 years increases risk
Obesity	Postmenopausal and adult weight gain
Personal history of breast cancer	>40 years old
Height	<5 feet 3 inches
Jewish heritage	Women of Jewish Ashkenazi heritage have higher incidences of *BRCA1* and *BRCA2* genetic mutations

DCIS, Ductal carcinoma in situ; *HRT*, hormone replacement therapy; *LCIS*, lobular carcinoma in situ.
Modified from American Cancer Society (ACS): *Breast cancer facts and figures 2015-2016*, Atlanta, 2016, ACS; Ignatavicius DD et al: *Medical-surgical nursing: patient-centered collaborative care*, ed 8, St Louis, 2016, Elsevier; Townsend CM et al: *Sabiston textbook of surgery: the biological basis of modern surgical practice*, ed 20, Philadelphia, 2017, Elsevier.

therapies are drugs or other substances that interfere with cancer growth and spread by inhibiting specific molecules involved in tumor growth and progression (Marriott et al., 2014). New studies and new therapeutic options are continually being developed and tested.

Conventional breast radiation, given once a day over 5 to 6 weeks to the entire breast, is called conventionally fractionated (CF) radiation therapy. A newer method, called hypofractionated (HF) radiation, delivers about the same dose as CF over 3 to 4 weeks. The American Society for Radiation Oncology (ASTRO) encourages using HF in people diagnosed at age 50 or older who have early-stage, hormone-positive, node-negative breast cancer who have not had chemotherapy. Fatigue and skin reactions are comparable to the longer course treatment. Accelerated partial breast irradiation (APBI) delivers radiation after a lumpectomy, reducing treatment time and excluding radiation to healthy tissue, but may miss some cancer cells that have migrated away from the tumor (Warshaw, 2015/2016). APBI is being studied in clinical trials.

Brachytherapy, also known as internal radiation, is another delivery method of radiation. Radioactive seeds are placed precisely into the adjacent cancerous breast tissue. There are two kinds of brachytherapy: interstitial and intracavitary. In *interstitial brachytherapy*, which is rarely used, many small, hollow catheters are inserted into the breast around the lumpectomy area and are left in place for several days. Radioactive pellets are inserted into the catheters for short periods each day and then removed. *Intercavitary brachytherapy* is the more common type of brachytherapy. A device is put into the space left from BCS, remaining in place until treatment is complete (usually 5 days). One end of the device extends out of the breast and the source of radiation, often pellets, is placed down through the tube for the proper time and then is removed. This is done twice a day on an ambulatory basis (ACS, 2016).

Screening Technologies

Imaging methodologies, such as mammography, ultrasonography (US), and breast magnetic resonance imaging (MRI), help to detect breast masses too small for clinical detection. The American Cancer Society (ACS) recommends mammograms for women ages 45 to 54, transitioning to biennial screening at 55 with an option to continue annual screening (Table 17.4). Women at high risk should have an MRI and, if 30 years or older, a mammogram every year. High-risk women include those who have a known breast cancer susceptibility gene 1 *(BRCA1)* or the breast cancer susceptibility gene 2 *(BRCA2)* mutation; those who have a first-degree relative with a *BRCA1, BRCA2,* or other gene mutation; and those who have a history of ductal breast cancer (DC), lobular carcinoma in situ (LCIS), atypical ductal hyperplasia, or atypical lobular hyperplasia

(ACS, 2016). The USPSTF advises women ages 50 years and older to have a biennial mammogram screening (CDC, 2016; Osterweil, 2016). The National Comprehensive Cancer Network (NCCN) and the American College of Obstetricians and Gynecologists (ACOG) recommend annual mammogram screening at age 40 (The Training Center, 2016).

Mammography and Imaging

The most common screening mechanism for asymptomatic women is mammography (Fig. 17.5). In mammography the entire breast is

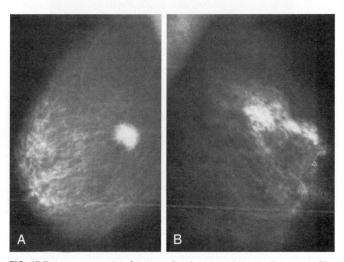

FIG. 17.5 Mammographic features of malignancy. (A) A stellate mass. The combination of density, surrounding spicules, and distortion of the breast architecture strongly suggests a malignancy in this mammogram. (B) Clustered microcalcifications. Fine, irregular, and branching forms suggest malignancy in this mammogram. Fine calcifications, less than 0.5 mm in size, are more often associated with cancer than are larger, coarse calcifications.

TABLE 17.4

Comparison of Screening Recommendations for Average-Risk Women

Guidelines	Recommendation
USPSTF, 2016	
40–49 years	Individualized decision making based on a woman's values, preferences, and health history (C recommendation)
50–74 years	Mammography every 2 years (B recommendation)
≥75 years	More research needed; indefinite evidence of benefit (I statement)
ACS, 2016	
40–44 years	Women should have the choice to start annual breast cancer screening with mammograms
45–54 years	Mammography every year
≥55 years	Mammography ever 2 years or annually according to personal preference; screening can continue if the woman is in good health and is expected to live at least 10 more years
NCCN, 2016	
≥40 years	Annual clinical breast examination and annual mammography; upper age limit for screening not established; screening can continue if the woman is in good health and is expected to live at least 10 more years

Key to USPSTF recommendations for practice: *A* (not shown), Offer or provide this service; there is high certainty that the net benefit is substantial. *B,* The USPSTF recommends the service. There is high certainty that the net benefit is moderate or there is moderate certainty that the net benefit is moderate to substantial. *C,* Offer or provide this service for selected patients depending on individual circumstances. *I statement,* read the clinical considerations section of USPSTF Recommendation Statement. If the service is offered, patients should understand the uncertainty about the balance of benefits and harms.

Adapted from American Cancer Society: *Breast cancer prevention and early detection, 2015–2016* (website), 2015. www.cancer.org/content/dam/cancer-org/research/cancer-facts-and-statistics/cancer-prevention-and-early-detection-facts-and-figures/cancer-prevention-and-early-detection-facts-and-figures-2015-2016.pdf. (Accessed 22 December 2016); National Comprehensive Cancer Network (NCCN): *NCCN clinical practice guidelines in oncology: breast cancer screening and diagnosis, version 1.2016 (free registration required)* (website). www.nccn.org/patients/guidelines/cancers.aspx. (Accessed 22 December 2016); Osterweil N: *USPSTF guidelines: biennial breast cancer screening from 50* (website). www.medscape.com/viewarticle/857027#vp_2. (Accessed 22 December 2016).

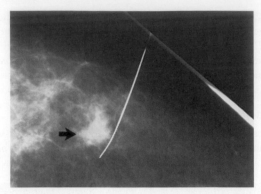

FIG. 17.6 Mammogram section. Craniocaudal view of breast. *Arrow* indicates breast lesion localized by wire before surgical excision.

BOX 17.1

Breast Imaging Reporting and Data System Assessment Scores

Category 0: The screening mammogram indicates additional screening is necessary. Prior mammograms, if available, are used for comparison. Additional imaging may include spot compression, magnification, special mammographic views, or ultrasound.
Category 1: The results are negative.
Category 2: The findings are benign.
Category 3: The findings are probably benign. Short-term follow-up is advised.
Category 4: The findings are suspicious. Biopsy is considered.
Category 5: The findings are highly suggestive of malignancy. Preliminary biopsy is needed; surgical treatment likely required.
Category 6: Known biopsy-proven malignancy. This category may be used for a second opinion before excisional biopsy, radiation therapy, chemotherapy, or mastectomy or for following tumor response during chemotherapy.

Modified from Hunt KK, Mittendorf EA: Diseases of the breast. In Townsend CM et al, editors: *Sabiston textbook of surgery*, ed 20, Philadelphia, 2017, Saunders.

visualized as x-ray beams are directed in several planes through it. Mammograms detect abnormal-appearing densities, irregular or spiculated margins, microcalcifications, and clusters of calcium deposits that are clinically nonpalpable. Screening mammography is most helpful in early detection because it can discover cancer several years before physical symptoms, such as a lump, develop. Often previous mammograms are used for comparison. The accuracy of mammography depends on careful x-ray technique and breast size, structure, and density. Radiation dosage varies with individuals and techniques. As a result of improved radiologic techniques, radiation exposure in a mammogram is very low. The benefits far outweigh the minute risks of radiation exposure. Advances in computer-assisted detection allow the computer to analyze the mammogram, placing asterisks and triangles on small potential problem areas, which a radiologist then reviews. If screening mammography reveals a suspicious area, the patient is asked to return for diagnostic mammography. When a lesion previously detected in a mammogram is too small to palpate, mammograms are repeated immediately before surgery. The lesion is localized by the insertion of a needle or a wire within a needle (often referred to as "needle" or "wire" localization) (Fig. 17.6).

Digital mammography, also known as full-field digital mammogram (FFDM), is similar to a standard mammogram in that an x-ray is used to take images of the breast. The mammogram is recorded and viewed on a computer where the image size, brightness, or contrast in certain areas of the film can be adjusted and seen more plainly. Digital images can be sent electronically to other sites for viewing and consulting with breast specialists. Radiologists also can use software to interpret digital mammograms. Digital screening mammograms are more accurate than film screening mammograms, with a 70% detection rate compared with 55% for film screens. Women most likely to benefit from digital screening are those younger than 50 with dense breast tissue and who are premenopausal or perimenopausal. More recently, to improve breast cancer detection, breast tomosynthesis (pseudo-three-dimensional [3-D] mammography) imaging has been added to two-dimensional (2-D) mammography during screening (Bernardi et al., 2016).

When a palpable mass or other abnormality is identified on screening mammography, additional diagnostic mammographic views are obtained, and the radiologist assigns a Breast Imaging Reporting and Data System (BI-RADS) score (Box 17.1). US may then be ordered.

US differentiates between solid and cystic lesions. A cyst is a fluid-filled sac and is considered a benign finding. A solid mass may

suggest malignancy and requires further evaluation. As a screening methodology alone, its sensitivity and specificity are less definitive than mammography. US can be useful with dense or dysplastic breasts and in pregnant or lactating women. Women 30 to 39 years of age benefit most from US after screening mammography. US has a sensitivity of 95.7% and discovers more cancerous lesions than mammography.

MRI is used as an adjunct to mammography in the detection of breast lesions. MRI uses a strong magnet to produce a complete image of the breast. There is no radiation. Breast MRI can image dense breast tissue. The ACS recommends that MRI be used for women at high risk. Such women include those who have known breast cancer–associated *BRCA1* or *BRCA2* gene mutations, have a first-degree relative with a *BRCA1* or *BRCA2* gene mutation, have a lifetime risk of breast cancer of 20% to 25% or greater according to risk-assessment tools, and had radiation therapy to the chest between 10 and 30 years of age. MRI also better determines definite size of the cancer and is useful in women with breast augmentation.

Molecular breast imaging (MBI) refers to a number of modalities that use a radiopharmaceutical agent in scanning, including breast-specific gamma imaging (BSGI) and positron emission mammography (PEM). It involves injection of a short-lived radiotracer, which is absorbed by breast tissue and preferentially so by breast tumors. MBI is useful in detecting breast cancer in women with dense breasts, those who present with a palpable abnormality not found on mammogram or US, and those who cannot tolerate MRI or who have metallic implants.

DNA-based genetic testing for *BRCA1* and *BRCA2* is recommended for women with family histories that suggest risk for these gene mutations and for women who are diagnosed with cancer premenopausally and have a hormone receptor negative cancer. These mutations may lead to the development of hereditary breast and/or ovarian cancer. Individuals with a harmful *BRCA* mutation have a lifelong chance of 50% to 80% risk of developing breast cancer and are more likely to be diagnosed before menopause (Breastcancer.

org, 2015). To test for *BRCA1* and *BRCA2*, a blood DNA sample is needed for full-length gene sequencing; a saliva sample can be sufficient, depending on need for panel testing. For breast cancer tumors, there are genomic profiling tools that are designed to spare patients side effects of unnecessary treatment when they do not need additional treatment (adjuvant therapy). One of the test results is a recurrence score, which correlates the chance of a specific tumor returning in the next 10 years. Genetic counseling is suggested before and after the workup (Arpino et al., 2013).

Diagnostic Techniques

Once a mass is identified, there are multiple techniques to establish a diagnosis. During a fine-needle aspiration biopsy (FNAB), a small area of the breast may be anesthetized with lidocaine. FNAB is mainly used for differentiation of solid from cystic masses but may also be performed when a new, dominant, unexplained mass is found. A 22-gauge needle with a 10-mL syringe is inserted into the mass, and a small amount of the contents is aspirated. The contents are then prepared on a slide for cytologic examination. If the content is fluid, the cyst should be emptied. Cyst fluid is usually clear or cloudy and green or amber. If the mass is solid, the needle is repetitively inserted into the mass while steady negative pressure is applied to the syringe; suction is released and the needle withdrawn. FNAB may be performed with ultrasound-guided insertion. The sample may be injected into a Pap cytology solution or slides fixed and submitted to pathology. The diagnostic accuracy depends on obtaining a proper amount of aspirate and also on the skill of the cytopathologist (Stahl et al., 2016).

A core needle biopsy is similar to an FNAB but a larger needle is used because actual breast tissue is removed rather than a sampling of cells. Core needle biopsy is preferred over excisional biopsy because it is minimally invasive and less expensive (Mayo Clinic, 2016). Types of core biopsies include US-guided core biopsy, stereotactic core biopsy, and MRI-guided core needle biopsy. A *US-guided core biopsy* does not require surgery. A large biopsy needle is placed into the breast tissue and the US aids in confirming the proper needle placement for biopsy. Tissue samples are then obtained through the needle. In *stereotactic core biopsy,* a large biopsy needle is inserted into the breast tissue; computerized mammographic pictures facilitate needle placement using digital imaging so the precise location of breast tissue is biopsied. Tissue samples are then withdrawn through the needle (Mayo Clinic, 2016). A small titanium clip is placed to mark the biopsy location. *MRI-guided core needle biopsy* provides an image that determines the exact location of the tumor using 3-D pictures and the computer (Mayo Clinic, 2016).

Surgical Treatment Considerations

Surgical treatment ranges from minimally invasive breast biopsy, BCS, wide excision of the tumor mass, or modified radical mastectomy involving the breast and axillary lymph nodes (Mayo Clinic, 2016). BCS is alternately called segmental mastectomy, lumpectomy, partial mastectomy, wide local excision, and tylectomy (Hunt and Mittendorf, 2017). The surgical goal is removal of the cancerous mass with a margin of normal tissue and a good cosmetic result. When a specimen of breast tissue is sent to the laboratory, it is inked to mark the relationship between the tumor and the surgical margins of the excision. The pathologist evaluates the margins on all sides of the tumor for malignant cells. No ink is the standard for adequate margins in invasive breast cancer (Hunt and Mittendorf, 2017). If a margin is positive, it indicates that malignant cells may remain in the breast. Reexcision to remove more tissue from the

operative tumor site is done to achieve clear margins (Hunt and Mittendorf, 2017).

The choice of procedure depends on the size and site of the mass, the characteristics of the cells, the stage of the disease, and the patient's choice. English literacy, health literacy, and cultural considerations are all components of evaluating and supporting a patient's choice in determining procedure options (Patient Engagement Exemplar). A breast cancer diagnosis is usually staged to measure the extent of the disease and to classify patients for possible treatment modalities (Fig. 17.7 and Table 17.5). The TNM (T = tumor; N = node; M = metastasis) classification has been adopted as a mechanism to clinically stage this disease. Staging results are used in designing a specific treatment plan. Radiation therapy, chemotherapy, or hormonal therapy may be used with surgery or as alternative treatment methods (Ambulatory Surgery Considerations).

Excised tumors or core needle biopsies are evaluated for their estrogen-binding and progesterone-binding abilities. Techniques have been developed to assess the ability of breast cancer to bind with estrogen and progesterone. This positive binding capability identifies the patient with a hormone-dependent tumor (Fig. 17.8). It is estimated that about two-thirds of all breast cancers are positive for estrogen binding, a majority of which are also positive for progesterone binding. The presence of these receptor sites is favorable to hormone manipulation, with the goal of preventing breast cancer cells from receiving estrogen stimulation. In these patients, and those who have negative axillary nodes, it is decidedly preferable to obtain a genomic assay of the primary cancer to find out the risk for recurrence

---

PATIENT ENGAGEMENT EXEMPLAR

Understanding Cultural Differences

Guiding principle number 8 states: "Acknowledgment and appreciation of culturally, racially or ethnically diverse backgrounds is an essential part of the engagement process."[a] Often, women going through a breast surgery are doing so because of a breast cancer diagnosis. Cultural differences among women vary greatly, and perioperative nurses need to understand cultural barriers to help women understand their diagnosis and treatment options. In some cultures, breast disease, cancer, and mastectomy are taboo topics and often are not discussed even among family members.[b] Nurses may be the first person to be able to cross that cultural barrier and discuss what is happening with the patient.[b] Women who do not speak or understand English may not trust the healthcare system. Having an interpreter present for women with low English literacy is imperative. Some women may feel embarrassment or guilt when diagnosed and may thus delay treatment or surgery.[b] Perioperative nurses who establish a relationship with the patient and family can discuss these feelings and honor any beliefs or wishes the patient may have. It is important to communicate those feelings and beliefs to other caregivers across the perioperative continuum. The American Cancer Society has information for patients in many languages and is a good resource for perioperative nurses to share with their patients.

---

[a]Nursing Alliance for Quality Care: *NAQC guiding principles: fostering successful patient and family engagement: nursing's critical role* (website), 2013. www.naqc.org/WhitePaper-PatientEngagement. (Accessed 17 June 2016).
[b]Steligo K: *Breast cancer differences in ethnic populations* (website), 2013. www.thebreastcaresite.com/after-surgery/breast-cancer-differences-ethnic-populations-2/. (Accessed 22 December 2016).

TABLE 17.5

Staging of Breast Cancer

Stage 0	Carcinoma in situ LCIS: abnormal cells in lining of a lobule DCIS: intraductal carcinoma; abnormal cells that are in lining of a duct
Stage Ia	Tumor <2 cm with no axillary lymph node involvement; cancer has not spread outside the breast; no lymph nodes are involved
Stage Ib	There is no tumor in the breast or the tumor is <2 cm; small groups of cancer cells larger than 0.2 mm but not larger than 2 mm are found in the lymph nodes (micrometastases)
Stage IIa	Cancer cells found in axillary lymph nodes, or tumor is <2 cm with metastasis to axillary lymph nodes, or tumor >2 cm but not >5 cm with no metastasis to axillary lymph nodes
Stage IIb	Tumor >2 cm but not >5 cm with positive axillary lymph nodes or tumor >5 cm with negative axillary lymph node involvement
Stage IIIa	Tumor ≤5 cm with metastases to axillary lymph nodes that are attached to each other or to other structures or has spread to lymph nodes behind the breast bone; or tumor ≥5 cm with spread to axillary lymph nodes that are alone or attached to each other or to other structures or has spread to lymph nodes behind the breast bone
Stage IIIb	Tumor of any size that has grown into the chest wall or skin of the breast causing swelling of the breast or nodules in breast skin and may have spread to axillary lymph nodes that are attached to each other and to other structures and may have spread to lymph nodes behind the breast bone
Stage IIIc	Tumor of any size that has spread either to the lymph nodes behind the breast bone and axillary lymph nodes or to the lymph nodes above or below the collarbone
Stage IV	Invasive breast cancer that has spread beyond the breast and nearby lymph nodes to other organs of the body, such as the lungs, distant lymph nodes, skin, bones, liver, or brain

DCIS, Ductal carcinoma in situ; *LCIS*, lobular carcinoma in situ.
Modified from Breastcancer.org: *Stages of breast cancer* (website). www.breastcancer.org/symptoms/diagnosis/staging. (Accessed 22 December 2016); National Breast Cancer Foundation, Inc.: *Breast cancer stages* (website). www.nationalbreastcancer.org/breast-cancer-stages. (Accessed 22 December 2016).

AMBULATORY SURGERY CONSIDERATIONS

Port Insertion for Breast Cancer Treatment

A breast cancer patient who needs further medical treatment may opt to have a port (implantable venous access system) placed under the skin in the chest, abdomen, or upper arm. This access port is used for frequent or continuous infusions of chemotherapeutic agents, solutions, other medications, pain management medication, or blood products as well as for repeated blood draws. Port insertion is commonly done in an ambulatory surgery setting by a surgeon or in the IR department by a radiologist. The port has a soft, pliable plastic catheter that is threaded into a large central vein such as the internal jugular vein, subclavian vein, or a vein in the upper or lower arm under x-ray guidance. The catheter is then attached to the port chamber (a metal or plastic base with a rubber dome), which is placed under the skin.

The patient is instructed to refrain from consuming solid foods or full liquids for at least 6 hours before the procedure. Clear liquids may be taken 2 hours before the procedure. Regular medications may be taken the morning of the insertion unless instructed otherwise. Aspirin, clopidogrel (Plavix), or warfarin should be discontinued before surgery. Ask the physician when these medications need to be stopped; usually they can be resumed the next day. Medication allergies are noted. The protocol for correct person, procedure, and side/site is observed. Conscious sedation or monitored anesthesia care is often used (see Chapter 5). After the procedure the patient will be observed for approximately 1 hour before discharge. Discharge instructions are given.

IR, Interventional radiology.
Modified from CancerNet.com: *Catheters and ports in cancer treatment* (website), 2015. www.cancer.net/navigating-cancer-care/how-cancer-treated/chemotherapy/catheters-and-ports-cancer-treatment. (Accessed 5 December 2016); Liang E: *Portacath* (website), 2015. www.sir.net.au/portacath_pi.html. (Accessed 5 December 2016); LaRoy JR et al: Cost and morbidity analysis of chest port insertion: interventional radiology suite versus operating room, *J. Am Coll Radiol* 12(6):563–571, 2015.

after treatment and the plan of care (Breastcancer.org, 2015). Use of selective estrogen receptor modulators (SERMs) and estrogen receptor downregulators (ERDs) after surgery and chemotherapy increase disease-free survival in premenopausal women with positive binding for estrogen. Postmenopausal women benefit from aromatase inhibitors (AIs). They appear to work better than estrogen receptor modulators on certain breast cancers, with fewer side effects.

Some of the most promising data reported for advanced breast cancer involve human epidermal growth factor receptor 2 (HER-2), a cellular protooncogene coding for a transmembrane receptor. Agents such as trastuzumab (Herceptin), used to target HER-2, were first approved for treatment of metastatic HER-2–positive breast cancer

in 1998. In 2012 pertuzumab was approved for use in combination with trastuzumab and with the chemotherapy agent docetaxel (Stenger, 2015). It is indicated for use in patients with metastatic HER-2–positive breast cancer who have not received previous treatment with either chemotherapy or HER-2–targeted therapy. Research and understanding of the immune system, development of methods to evaluate aspects of the immune response, and ongoing development of monoclonal antibodies continue to transform the field of immunotherapy and breast cancer treatment.

Clinical trials continue to explore clinical effectiveness of poly ADP-ribose polymerase (PARP) enzyme inhibitors in triple-negative breast cancer (TNBC) patients. These tumors are estrogen and

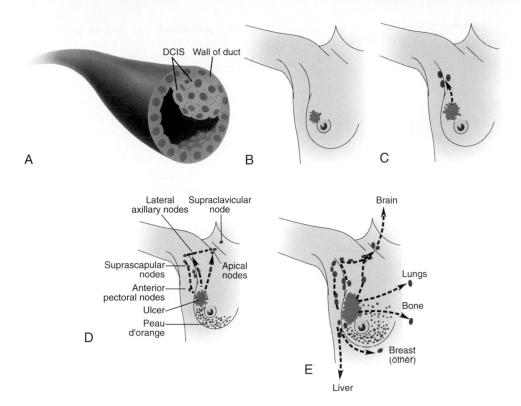

FIG. 17.7 Anatomic staging of breast cancer. (A) Stage 0 is carcinoma in situ. Lobular carcinoma in situ (LCIS) is defined as abnormal cells that are in the lining of a lobule. LCIS seldom becomes invasive cancer. However, having LCIS in one breast increases the risk of cancer for both breasts. Ductal carcinoma in situ *(DCIS)* is defined as abnormal cells that are in the lining of a duct. DCIS is also called intraductal carcinoma. The abnormal cells have not spread outside the duct and have not invaded the nearby breast tissue. DCIS sometimes becomes invasive cancer if not treated. (B) Stage I: tumor <2 cm with no axillary lymph node involvement. (C) Stage IIa: cancer cells found in axillary lymph nodes, or tumor ≤2 cm with metastasis to axillary lymph nodes, or tumor >2 cm but not >5 cm with no metastasis to axillary lymph nodes. Stage IIb: tumor >2 cm but not >5 cm with positive axillary lymph node involvement, or tumor >5 cm with negative axillary lymph node involvement. (D) Stage IIIa: tumor ≤5 cm with metastasis to axillary lymph nodes that are attached to each other or to other structures, or has spread to lymph nodes behind breast bone; or tumor >5 cm and has spread to axillary lymph nodes that are alone or attached to each other or to other structures, or has spread to lymph nodes behind the breast bone. Stage IIIb: tumor of any size that has grown into the chest wall or skin of the breast, causing swelling of the breast or nodules in breast skin; may have spread to axillary lymph nodes that are attached to each other and to other structures and may have spread to lymph nodes behind the breast bone. Inflammatory breast cancer: breast is red, swollen (at least stage IIIb). Stage IIIc: tumor of any size that has spread either to the lymph nodes behind the breast bone and axillary lymph nodes or to the lymph nodes above or below the collarbone. (E) Stage IV: distant metastatic cancer.

progesterone hormone receptor negative and HER-2/neu negative. TNBC is found in younger women, women of African American or Hispanic descent, and individuals with *BRCA1* mutations. It also is associated with a worse prognosis than other breast cancer subtypes (Bethea et al., 2015; Hunt and Mittendorf, 2017).

Breast cancer patients are increasingly seeking and using integrative therapies to enhance their surgical and medical treatment or recover from the side effects of treatment (see Chapter 30 for a discussion of integrative therapies). Along with using products such as green tea, botanicals, vitamins E and C, and flaxseed, breast cancer patients are incorporating massage therapy and meditation and enlisting the help of dietitians and nutritionists.

Perioperative Nursing Considerations

Assessment

Patients undergoing breast surgery will likely be extremely apprehensive about the possibilities of having a malignancy, losing a body part, facing a negative reaction from a partner and family, and experiencing a negative change in self-image. For this reason patients may have nurse navigators guide them through the maze of breast cancer treatment options and requirements. During a preoperative interview the perioperative nurse continues to assess the patient's level of anxiety and possible causes. Identification of fears and concerns

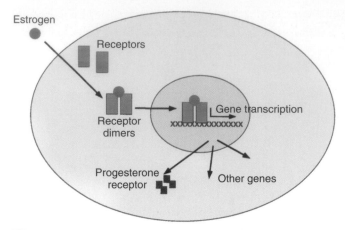

FIG. 17.8 Physiology of estrogen and the estrogen receptor, shown schematically. Estrogen binds to estrogen receptors, translocates to the nucleus of the cell, and interacts with cellular DNA. This interaction results in the transcription of estrogen-responsive genes, such as the receptor for progesterone. In addition, other genes are induced by the estrogen receptors that influence cell growth and differentiation.

helps in planning appropriate nursing interventions. The patient should identify the breast (and, if possible, the quadrant of the breast) in which the mass is located and participate in surgical site marking. The perioperative nurse may reinforce the patient's understanding of the proposed surgical procedure, verify that the patient can correctly state its name, and correct misunderstandings (as appropriate). Identifying the patient's support systems and coping mechanisms helps manage anxiety and enhances the discharge planning process. If the patient has lost a relative or close friend to breast cancer, her coping mechanisms may be affected because of memories of that loss.

Nursing Diagnosis

Based on nursing assessment, a perioperative nurse uses nursing diagnoses to develop a plan of care. Nursing diagnoses related to the care of patients undergoing breast surgery might include the following:

- Anxiety related to fear of cancer, the surgical intervention, or biopsy results
- Disturbed Body Image related to loss of body part
- Risk for Injury related to use of energy-generating devices (e.g., electrosurgery)
- Deficient Knowledge related to unfamiliarity with perioperative routines

Outcome Identification

Outcomes are derived from nursing diagnoses. They direct the perioperative nurse in selecting nursing interventions that will prevent, or intervene in, the actual or high-risk areas identified in the nursing diagnoses. Outcomes identified for the selected nursing diagnoses could be stated as follows:

- The patient will verbalize a level of anxiety that is personally acceptable.
- The patient will discuss feelings regarding body image changes resulting from the surgical procedure.
- The patient will experience no untoward injury from energy-generating devices (e.g., electrosurgery).

- The patient will verbalize an understanding of perioperative routines.

Planning

Using nursing diagnoses and desired outcomes, the perioperative nurse individualizes a plan of care for each patient and communicates with other colleagues on the patient care team. The plan of care for a patient undergoing breast surgery includes nursing interventions that allow the patient freedom to express concerns, have specific questions answered, and discuss breast reconstruction options, as appropriate. As part of planning patient care, priorities are established and a method of ensuring continuity of care established (Sample Plan of Care).

Implementation

Before surgery the perioperative nurse procures the necessary supplies, instruments, and equipment for the planned operation. The patient's operative site is marked by the surgeon outside of the operating room (OR) before any medications are given. Mammogram digital images or other imaging studies are available in the OR for the surgeon's review; their presence may be confirmed during the preoperative briefing. The facility protocol for identifying the correct surgical site and side is followed. Often this consists of a checklist that is initiated during the time-out and includes verbal communication among surgical team members, review of the medical record and informed consent, confirmation of imaging studies, and direct observation of the marked surgical site. Other preparation may include Foley catheter placement, axillary hair trim, and intermittent pneumatic compression devices (IPCDs). Intravenous (IV) antibiotics, started within 1 hour before the incision is made, may be administered (Patient Safety). A breast biopsy, performed after the patient has received a local anesthetic, requires adjunct sedation and monitoring equipment (e.g., electrocardiogram [ECG], pulse oximeter, blood pressure apparatus). Patient allergies are reviewed to avoid allergic or toxic reactions to local anesthetics, antibiotics, or pain medications. For a mastectomy, extra sponges and instruments are often needed. An electrosurgical unit (ESU) or surgical laser is used to provide both hemostasis and tissue dissection. Safe practices when using devices that generate surgical smoke require the use of a smoke evacuation system and accessories (AORN, 2016) (see Chapter 8 for a discussion of the ESU and surgical smoke evacuation). The incision site may be drained postoperatively with a closed wound suction device. Ensuring availability of supplies before the procedure allows the nurse to maintain a comforting presence while supporting, monitoring, and caring for the surgical patient.

After transfer to the OR bed, the patient is placed supine with the operative side near the edge of the bed. The arm on the involved side, with the palms up and fingers extended, is carefully placed on a padded armboard at no greater than 90 degrees to prevent brachial plexus stretch. If there are surgical reasons to tuck the arms at the side, pad the elbows to protect the ulnar nerve, turn the palms inward, and maintain the wrist in a neutral position (AORN, 2016). Depending on the location of the lesion and the planned surgery, a small pad can be placed under the operative side to facilitate exposure of the incision area. Positioning the OR bed in slight Fowler position with a lateral tilt away from the surgeon can also facilitate exposure. IPCDs are applied to prevent deep vein thrombosis (DVT). The anesthesia provider or circulating nurse places a forced-air warming device on the patient away from the surgical site (Evidence for Practice).

SAMPLE PLAN OF CARE

Nursing Diagnosis
Anxiety related to fear of cancer, the surgical intervention, or obtaining biopsy results

Outcome
The patient will verbalize a level of anxiety that is personally acceptable.

Interventions
- Encourage questions and allow time for verbalization of fear, distress, and anxiety. Use active listening and reflective questions.
- Review the surgeon's explanation of the planned procedure and the reason for it (as appropriate).
- Assess verbal and nonverbal signs of anxiety.
- Provide emotional support and comfort measures (warm blankets, touch as appropriate).
- Maintain quiet, calm environment.
- Demonstrate warmth and acceptance of the patient's anxiety.
- Determine the patient's personally effective coping techniques (or recommend some), such as relaxation, rhythmic breathing, or guided imagery. Support the patient in using these.
- Record patient reactions.

Nursing Diagnosis
Disturbed Body Image related to loss of body part

Outcome
The patient will discuss feelings regarding body image changes resulting from the surgical procedure.

Interventions
- Allow patient to discuss concerns about her sexual attractiveness, loss of confidence, or perceived loss of femininity.
- Promote an environment of support, respect, and comfort.
- Discuss available resources and options (external prosthesis, alternatives in garments and dress, reconstructive surgery, as appropriate). Make referrals to nurse on discharge unit or community agency as indicated.
- Maintain patient's privacy.
- Encourage a visit by a Reach to Recovery volunteer (as applicable).

Nursing Diagnosis
Risk for Thermal Injury related to use of energy-generating devices (e.g., electrosurgery)

Outcome
The patient will experience no untoward injury from energy-generating devices.

Interventions
- Position ESU dispersive pad as close to operative site as possible.
- Note any metal implants patient may have and do not place dispersive pad over these sites.
- Select a dispersive pad site that is clean and dry, with good muscle mass; note and document the condition of the skin at the selected site.
- Protect dispersive pad from fluids and contact with metal objects.
- Initiate fire safety precautions; ensure all prep solutions have dried before draping.
- Activate the ESU after dispersive pad and active electrode are connected.
- Set power setting as low as possible to achieve desired effect. Document power settings.
- Use holster for ESU active electrode on the sterile field.
- Provide supplies to remove excess char buildup from ESU active electrode (as applicable).
- Check dispersive pad contact and all connections after changes in position or requests to increase power.
- Evaluate and document skin condition on removal of the ESU dispersive pad.

Nursing Diagnosis
Deficient Knowledge related to unfamiliarity with perioperative routines

Outcome
The patient will verbalize understanding of perioperative routines.

Interventions
- Assess the patient's experience with previous surgical procedures.
- Review surgical team use of correct site surgery verification protocols.
- Explain that skin will be cleansed with antiseptic solution at the surgical site and that solution may feel cold.
- Provide clear and concise explanations of all nursing interventions.
- Explain roles and introduce healthcare team members present in the OR.
- Encourage questions.
- Describe types of dressings and equipment that may be used postoperatively. If lymph node dissection is performed, describe use of incisional closed wound drainage systems.
- Ask the patient to explain in her own words what type of surgery will be performed ("teach-back").

ESU, Electrosurgical unit.
Modified from Ackley BJ, Ladwig G: *Nursing diagnosis handbook: an evidence-based guide to planning care,* ed 11, Philadelphia, 2016, Mosby.

Skin preparation ("prep") depends on the location of the lesion and the surgery intended. Antimicrobial skin prep solutions vary. For a breast biopsy, the area prepped is usually the affected breast and the immediate surrounding skin. For a mastectomy, the area prepped can extend from above the clavicle to the umbilicus and from the opposite nipple to the bedline of the operative side, including the axilla, and possibly the upper arm on the operative side (Fig. 17.9). Some surgeons caution against vigorous scrubbing of the surgical site to prevent possible seeding of cancer cells from the main mass. Appropriate precautions to prevent pooling of solution under

the patient and to reduce the risk of surgical fire are taken during skin prep procedures.

Surgical drapes expose the affected breast and the preoperative site mark. For mastectomy, the arm on the operative side is draped free, using a stockinette and drapes that allow free movement of the arm to facilitate access to the axilla. A final time-out is performed before the incision.

During implementation of the plan of care, the perioperative nurse continues to collect data, continually reassesses the patient's needs and the needs of the surgical team, initiates nursing interventions, and

PATIENT SAFETY

Surgical Site Infections After Breast Cancer Surgery

The CDC wound classification system considers breast surgery as "clean." The definition of SSI is one that occurs within 30 days postoperatively with median time for an infection around 16 days postop. The SSI rate for clean surgical procedures is projected to be less than 2%. Risk factors for surgical site infection after breast cancer surgery include comorbid conditions such as

diabetes mellitus, hypertension, BMI >30, pulmonary disease, and smoking. A higher ASA classification is also a risk (Chung et al., 2015; Al-Hilli et al., 2015) (see Chapter 5 for a discussion of ASA classification).

Research about SSI after breast surgery is highlighted in several studies:

Study Information	Author
Higher risk of SSI with breast reconstruction with free flap	Al-Hilli et al., 2015; Chung et al., 2015
There were 18,696 mastectomies performed in 2004–2011 SSI rate: 8.1% Of those included are mastectomy, 5%; mastectomy with implants, 10.3%; mastectomy with flap, 10.7%; mastectomy with flap and implant, 10.3%	Olsen et al., 2015a
• For women who have mastectomy or lumpectomy, SSI follows bleeding as the second most common complication; SSI rate is higher in mastectomy versus conservative surgeries • SSI rate higher in incisions that had drains (Jackson-Pratt and Hemovac). Patients with seromas (collection of fluid) and hematomas (collection of blood) were more likely to develop SSI	Gil-Londoño et al., 2016
Bilateral versus unilateral mastectomies have similar infection rates	Silva et al., 2015
Most common organism of SSIs post breast cancer surgery is the *Staphylococcus* species despite preoperative antimicrobial prophylaxis	Rolston et al., 2014
Risk of SSI is significantly higher with reexcision	Olsen et al., 2015b

Perioperative nurses are constantly aware of factors that may cause SSIs and continuously monitor and implement measures to prevent them (see Chapter 4 for a thorough discussion of essential elements of sterile technique). Infections can increase costs, cause psychologic and emotional trauma, result in poor

cosmetic results, and delay adjuvant therapies. The findings of the previously mentioned studies remind the perioperative team that SSI after breast cancer surgery is higher than the expected clean classification.

ASA, American Society of Anesthesiologists; *BMI*, body mass index; *CDC*, Centers for Disease Control and Prevention; *SSI*, surgical site infection.
Modified from Chung CU et al: Surgical site infections after free flap breast reconstruction: an analysis of 2899 patients from the ACS-NSQIP datasets, *J Reconstr Microsurg* 31(6):434–441, 2015; Gil-Londoño J-C et al: Surgical site infection after breast cancer surgery at 30 days and associated factors, *Infectio*, 2016, doi: 10.1016/j.infect.2016.04.003; Olsen MA et al: Incidence of surgical site infection following mastectomy with and without immediate reconstruction using private insurer claims data, *Infect Control Hosp Epidemiol* 36(8):907–914, 2015; Olsen MA et al: Increased risk of surgical site infection among breast-conserving surgery re-excisions, *Ann Surg Oncol* 22(6):2003–2009, 2015; Rolston KV et al: Current microbiology of surgical site infections in patients with cancer: a retrospective review, *Infect Dis Ther* 3(2):245–256, 2014; Silva AK et al: The effect of contralateral prophylactic mastectomy and perioperative complications in women undergoing immediate breast reconstruction: a NSQIP analysis, *Ann Surg Oncol* 22(11):3474–3480, 2015; Al-Hilli Z et al: Reoperation for complications after lumpectomy and mastectomy for breast cancer from the 2012 National Surgical Quality Improvement Program (ACS-NSQIP). *Ann Surg Oncol* 22:S459–S469, 2015.

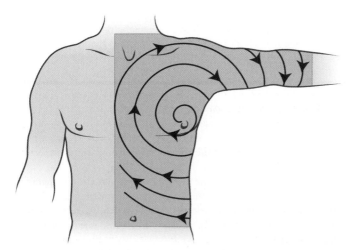

FIG. 17.9 Diagram of skin surgical preparation.

documents all care delivered. Formats for documenting perioperative patient care vary. However, documentation of patient problems and nursing interventions addressing these problems is essential. For the patient undergoing breast surgery, consideration should be given to document the patient's level of anxiety, the surgical position and accessory positioning devices used, the time-out, the location of the ESU dispersive pad, unit settings and identification number, results of perioperative monitoring, medications administered by the perioperative nurse or from the sterile field, specimens collected, and any closed wound drainage systems inserted into the surgical wound.

Evaluation

Evaluation of the patient before discharge from the OR includes both general observation parameters important for every surgical patient and specific evaluation of the goals of the plan of care. The patient's skin at dependent pressure sites, skin prep sites, and the dispersive pad placement site is assessed and any change in skin integrity is documented. The hand-off report to the nurse in the postanesthesia care unit (PACU) includes any unusual events or

EVIDENCE FOR PRACTICE

Preventing Unintended Perioperative Hypothermia

Hypothermia, a core body temperature less than 97°F (36°C), is a common occurrence in surgical patients. Heat loss from patient radiation (thermal loss) and convection are the two most significant sources in the OR. A slight drop in perioperative normothermia can be associated with considerable morbidity and mortality. Room temperature is the single most critical factor influencing actual heat loss. Up to 20% of patients experience unintended perioperative hypothermia. General, regional, and epidural anesthesia can also alter thermoregulatory mechanisms. Temperature management is a challenge for perioperative personnel. SSI is the most serious complication from hypothermia associated with administration of anesthetics. Myocardial ischemia, prolongation of medication effects, increased surgical bleeding, shivering, breaks in skin integrity, increased length of stay, and patient dissatisfaction with care are other untoward processes associated with hypothermia.

The AORN *Guidelines for Perioperative Practice* (AORN, 2016) outline steps for the prevention of unplanned hypothermia. Begin with an assessment of the factors associated with hypothermia. Monitor patients closely and develop evidence-based practices for maintaining normothermia. Use prewarming for 35 minutes, but at least 10 minutes, for preventing perioperative hypothermia. Two common types of prewarmers are forced-air warmers and warm cotton blankets. A review to determine the best method for prewarming found forced-air warming the most effective. Many ambulatory surgery centers do not routinely use forced-air warmers, especially for shorter surgeries such as lumpectomy. To investigate this practice, a RCT of patients having lumpectomies was undertaken; two groups received prewarming interventions at an ambulatory surgery center. Group 1 had forced-air warming and Group 2 had warm cotton blankets. Both groups had warmed IV fluids; their temperature was monitored every 15 minutes using infrared ear thermometers and digital hygrometers. Results showed no significant difference between the two groups' temperature changes. This suggests that warm blankets may be just as effective in prewarming patients who are having short procedures, such as lumpectomy, when warmed IV fluids are also given.

Perioperative nurses implement steps to maintain normothermia such as the following:
- Determine patient temperature on admission
- Assess for signs and symptoms of hypothermia
- Implement presurgical warming methods (forced-air or warm blankets) for at least 10 minutes
- Maintain room temperature at or above 75°F (24°C)
- Institute active warming for patients who are hypothermic
- Perform frequent intraoperative temperature monitoring, limit skin exposure, warm IV fluids
- Reassess temperature on arrival and discharge to the PACU.

IV, Intravenous; *PACU*, postanesthesia care unit; *RCT*, randomized controlled trial; *SSI*, surgical site infection.
Modified from Connelly L et al: The optimal time and method for surgical prewarming: a comprehensive review of the literature, *J Perianesth Nurs* 32(3):199–209, 2016; AORN: *Guidelines for perioperative practice*, Denver, 2016, The Association; Menzel M et al: Implementation of a thermal management concept to prevent perioperative hypothermia: results of a 6-month period in clinical practice, *Der Anaesthesist* 65(6):423–429, 2016; Nadia HI, Raha AR: Routine intraoperative forced-air warmer usage in prevention of perioperative hypothermia: to use or not to use in daycare breast lumpectomy?, *J Surg Acad* 5(1):34–43, 2015.

patient problems during surgery, use of any closed wound drainage systems in the wound, and achievement of identified patient outcomes. Outcomes, based on the nursing diagnoses selected, should be part of the documentation as well as the hand-off report. Outcomes identified for the selected nursing diagnoses could be stated as follows:
- The patient verbalized an acceptable level of anxiety; she communicated her specific anxieties, her facial expression and body structures were relaxed, and her vital signs remained within her normal range.
- The patient discussed feelings regarding possible body image changes resulting from the surgical procedure; her preferred coping strategies were reviewed and supported during the procedure.
- The patient experienced no untoward injury from energy-generating devices; there were no skin changes at the site of the ESU dispersive pad.
- The patient verbalized an understanding of perioperative routines; she cooperated with requests and was provided with ongoing explanations.

Patient, Family, and Caregiver Education and Discharge Planning

Discharge planning begins as soon as the patient is informed of the necessity for surgery or when the nurse first meets the patient. According to the extent of the anticipated surgery, information about appropriate exercises to enhance recovery, prosthetic devices, reconstruction options, and available community support groups are explained. The perioperative nurse provides or reinforces information based on the patient's desire for information, readiness to learn, and anxiety level.

The patient is often discharged within hours of or on the day after surgery. Instruct the patient and other caregivers regarding aseptic wound care, care for closed wound drainage systems (if present), and pain management. Include possible signs of complications, along with instructions regarding when and how to notify the physician. Teach postoperative exercises to the patient to facilitate her return to normal activities. Coordinate home care (if necessary) with the physician and the patient. A follow-up telephone call to the patient helps the nurse assess the patient's ability to cope with her diagnosis and surgery. The Patient, Family, and Caregiver Education box provides sample discharge information.

Surgical Interventions

Biopsy of Breast Tissue

The diagnosis of breast lesions using a minimally invasive procedure, as discussed previously in the section Diagnostic Techniques, is preferred. In an *incisional biopsy*, a portion of the mass is surgically excised using a curved incision line. The tissue is sent for pathologic examination. In an *excisional biopsy*, the entire tumor mass is excised along with a small margin of normal tissue for examination as with incisional biopsy.

Procedural Considerations

Biopsy is usually performed after the patient receives a local anesthetic, a local anesthetic with IV moderate sedation/analgesia, a laryngeal mask airway (LMA), or a general anesthetic with intubation, depending on the patient's condition and medical history. An active warming device and IPCDs are placed on the patient. The short delay between biopsy and further treatment has not been shown to adversely affect survival. However, when an extensive surgical procedure is anticipated in conjunction with the biopsy or when multiple lesions are to be excised and the amount of local anesthetic would exceed the maximum safe dose, general anesthesia is used. A minor instrument set is used for biopsy; the ESU is often requested. Separate instruments are used for each biopsy site when there are multiple lesions. Perioperative staff are sensitive to the fact that the patient may be alert during the procedure; use caution with oral pathology reports called over a speaker phone. Pathology reports, especially if the report confirms malignancy, should be discussed when the patient is fully awake and has a support system available.

Operative Procedure: Open Breast Biopsy

1. An incision in the direction of the skin lines (curvilinear) or along the border of the areola is made over the tumor mass; the circumareolar incision gives the best cosmetic result. If the lesion is located in an extremely lateral or medial site, a radial incision may be used.
2. Gentle traction is applied to the mass. If the lesion is small, the entire mass and an edge of normal tissue are removed by sharp dissection. If a large lesion is present, a small incisional biopsy of the main mass is done. The specimen should not be

PATIENT, FAMILY, AND CAREGIVER EDUCATION

Discharge Instructions and Home Care for Breast Surgery Patients

Give both the patient and the caregiver *verbal* and *written* instructions. Provide them with the name and telephone number of a physician or nurse to call if questions arise. Use visual aids to assist in instruction.

General Information
- Review explanation of the disease, the surgical procedure performed, and adjuvant therapy to be carried out.
- Explain that if the axillary nodes were removed, the affected arm may swell and is less able to fight infection. Discuss measures to prevent lymphedema:
  - Exercise arm daily (provide specific exercises).
  - Report loss of shoulder or joint mobility.
  - When healing is complete, begin strengthening and stretching exercises.

Wound/Incision Care (Select Applicable Education Based on Surgical Procedure Performed)
- Encourage the patient to look at her incisions so she can see what is normal. Teach her how to care for the skin at the site of surgery.
- Advise her that there may be a dry gauze dressing over the incision site and the drain site.
- Provide information regarding dressing changes, amount of fluid leakage at closed wound drainage system site that is normal, when to change soiled drain-site dressing (including emptying and measuring drain reservoir), and what to report to a physician or nurse.
- Discuss numbness in the area of surgery and typical sensations (heaviness, tingling, and "pins and needles"). These are likely to resolve by 1 year after surgery.

For modified radical mastectomy:
- Teach the patient to change the dressing, assess the appearance of her incision and closed wound drainage system site, milk or strip clots through the drainage tubing to maintain patency, empty the drainage container, and record the amount and character of drainage.
- Caution her not to abduct the affected arm or elbow above the shoulder until closed wound drainage systems are removed.
- Instruct her to report any redness or drainage around the closed wound drainage system.
- Instruct her to avoid use of deodorants or antiperspirants until stitches and drains have been removed from the axilla and the wound has healed. If no closed wound drainage system is present, she may shower.
- Caution her not to allow injections, placing of IV lines, drawing of blood, or taking of blood pressure in her affected arm if axillary dissection was done.

- Instruct her to avoid wearing constricting clothing or jewelry on her affected arm and to carry her handbag on the unaffected arm if axillary dissection was done.
- Discuss types of temporary and permanent prostheses available; assist with referral as needed.
- Advise her not to use an external prosthesis or bra pad until swelling has subsided and incisional healing is complete. Tell her to check with a physician or nurse before getting fitted for a breast prosthesis. This usually occurs about 6 weeks after surgery as long as wounds are healing and any postoperative edema has resolved.
- Discuss types of reconstruction available (as appropriate).
- Stress importance of noticing changes in her remaining breast and adhering to prescribed regimen for mammography of her unaffected breast.

Warning Signs
Review signs and symptoms that should be reported to a physician or nurse:
- Swelling of arm.
- Drainage from incision, excessive drainage or blood in drainage unit, difficulty keeping unit flat.
- Infection: redness, purulent drainage, pain, incision warm to touch.

Medications
- Explain purpose, dosage, schedule, and route of administration of any prescribed medications, as well as side effects to report to a physician or nurse. Have her repeat these back or review them with you (medication reconciliation). If she is taking an opioid analgesic, initiate a bowel protocol (including a laxative and stool softener) to prevent constipation.
- Discuss alternative methods of postoperative pain management: visualization, guided imagery, meditation, relaxation, biofeedback, music, and other personally effective techniques.

Activity
- Encourage discussion of allowances and limitations with respect to occupation, recreational sports, activities, and postdischarge therapies.
- Encourage resumption of self-care activities (feeding, combing hair) and activities of daily living as tolerated.
- Remind her that fatigue related to breast cancer treatment often increases during adjuvant breast cancer treatments such as chemotherapy and radiation therapy.
- Explain that sexual activity may be resumed when desired. The partner should use a position that does not place pressure on her chest wall.

PATIENT, FAMILY, AND CAREGIVER EDUCATION

Discharge Instructions and Home Care for Breast Surgery Patients—cont'd

- Discuss the need to continue postmastectomy exercises to regain full range of motion (as applicable).

Follow-Up Care
- Stress the importance of regular follow-up visits. Make sure she has the necessary names and telephone numbers.
- Prepare her for adjuvant therapies: hormone therapy, chemotherapy, and radiation therapy.

Psychosocial Care
- Encourage verbalization about feelings and fears regarding diagnosis, adjunctive therapy, and actual and perceived changes in body image and sexuality.
- Encourage patient and family to seek individual or group counseling to reduce emotional stress and help with effective coping.

Referrals
- Provide referrals to the breast care navigator (if available); if not, refer to a home health service and social services as indicated.
- Assist the patient to obtain referral services to breast cancer survivorship programs and contact support groups, such as the American Cancer Society's Reach to Recovery program, to cope with alterations in body image and other concerns.
- Encourage follow-up care with the patient's primary care provider for ongoing healthcare needs.
- If chemotherapy or radiation therapy is prescribed postdischarge, ensure that the patient and family have specific instructions about appointments, anticipated side effects, and self-management at home.
- Provide reliable printed and online resources for patient, family, and caregiver education.

IV, Intravenous.

Modified from Justice M: Care of patients with breast disorders. In Ignatavicius DD, Workman ML, editors: *Medical-surgical nursing–patient-centered collaborative care,* ed 8, St Louis, 2016, Elsevier; MedlinePlus: *Mastectomy—discharge* (website), 2015. https://medlineplus.gov/ency/patientinstructions/000244.htm. (Accessed 22 December 2016); UCSF Medical Center: *Mastectomy: instructions after surgery* (website). www.ucsfhealth.org/education/mastectomy_instructions_after_surgery/. (Accessed 13 December 2016).

placed into a formalin solution if a frozen section or further studies are to be done on the tissue to determine cancer treatment for the patient. Formalin immersion prevents frozen-section examination. For diagnostic biopsies, the surgeon orients the specimen and the pathologist inks all margins. This assists the surgeon in reexcision if the pathologist finds positive margins on the specimen. The tissue can be examined by frozen section to determine immediate diagnosis if desired. If a 48-hour permanent section is required for definitive diagnosis, the patient is scheduled at a later time for any further surgery that may be necessary.

3. If the lesion is benign, hemostasis is ensured and subcutaneous breast tissue approximated with absorbable suture. A cosmetic subcuticular skin closure is used when possible.

Operative Procedure: Open Breast Biopsy With Needle (Wire) Localization or Radioactive Seed

In some instances, such as when a lesion previously detected on mammogram is too small to palpate or the lesion is not amenable to stereotactic core biopsy, a localization procedure may be necessary before surgery. This can be achieved with placement of a wire or radioactive seed. The needle (wire)-localization breast biopsy (NLBB) localizes the lesion by the insertion of a needle or a wire within a needle. The wire is placed within the suspected area, and the distal end is left on the outside of the skin. The needle may be left in place or removed after insertion of the wire (see Fig. 17.6). The needle or wire is then protected by a dressing or cup taped over the wire for protection during transport, and the patient is sent to the OR for surgical biopsy. Mammograms are repeated immediately before surgery. Care is taken during transfer to the OR bed and gown removal not to dislodge or bump the wire. Similar care is taken during positioning, prepping, and draping. Digital images are sent to the OR with the wire entry visible on the image, or are available on the computer system in the OR suite.

1. The skin incision is placed precisely over the expected location of the mammographically determined lesion to minimize tunneling through the breast tissue.
2. Dissection is carried out using the wire as a guide.
3. Tissue around the wire is removed en bloc with the wire and sent for specimen mammography in the radiology department. Radiography can also be done intraoperatively.
4. The patient is kept on the OR bed with the sterile field maintained until confirmation that the lesion has been excised. It is then sent from radiology or the OR to the pathology department.
5. Needles and portions of needle/wire are counted to prevent a retained surgical item.

Operative Procedure: Radioactive Seed Placement

Radioactive seeds can also be used to localize nonpalpable breast lesions intraoperatively (radioactive seed localization [RSL]) (Pouw et al., 2015). They can be placed up to 5 days before surgery, which is an advantage over needle (wire) localization, which must be done the day of surgery. They require the use of a probe to identify the seed intraoperatively, which can often be the same probe used to perform the sentinel lymph node (SLN) procedure. The seeds are placed in the radiology department, usually under US or mammographic guidance. A needle is inserted into the breast and is used as a guide to place a radioactive seed in the area of concern. The radioactive seeds are slightly larger than the clips placed during a breast biopsy, and they are removed at the time of surgery. The surgical procedure is similar to a breast biopsy with needle localization, except dissection is carried out using the probe and seed as a guide. Tissue around the seed is removed en bloc with the seeds and sent for specimen mammography.

Incision and Drainage for Abscess

Incision of an inflamed and suppurative area of the breast is performed to drain an abscess. Breast abscesses are very painful. They occur most frequently during the first 4 weeks of breastfeeding. Staphylococcal or streptococcal organisms enter the breast through abraded or lacerated nipple surfaces or through the lactiferous ducts. Chronic abscesses are rare. Drainage is required when the breast abscess is apparent. Biopsies may be done for additional diagnosis along with cultures for appropriate antibiotics.

Procedural Considerations

Breast abscess drainage may require a general anesthetic. Initially, percutaneous drainage or aspiration may alleviate the pressure. If not, surgery may be necessary. Instruments are the same as those for biopsy.

Operative Procedure

1. Generally a radial incision extending outward from the nipple or a circumareolar incision is preferred. A short incision into the thoracomammary fold may be used for deep breast abscesses in the lower or outer quadrant.
2. After skin incision, the wound is deepened until pus is encountered.
3. A curved hemostat is directed into the cavity to determine the extent of the abscess. Specimens for aerobic and anaerobic organisms are usually taken for culture.
4. Exploring the cavity with the index finger breaks up loculations.
5. The opening is enlarged to ensure adequate drainage, the cavity is irrigated with warm saline solution with or without antibiotics, and bleeding vessels are ligated with absorbable sutures or coagulated.
6. The wound is drained or loosely packed with medicated gauze. Healing occurs by second intention.

Breast-Conserving Surgery

Lumpectomy, also known as partial mastectomy or wide local excision, is a procedure that conserves the breast. It is removal of a tumor mass with a margin of 1 to 1.5 mm of normal tissue. The MarginProbe system, which emits an electric field and senses the returning signal from tissue under evaluation, may be used to examine specimen margins. Many surgeons, however, perform cavity shave margins (CSMs). Performing routine CSM has been shown to decrease rates of positive margins and thus reexcision rates. It is also helpful for pathologists in defining margins more precisely (Chagpar et al., 2015).

1. The initial steps are the same as for open breast biopsy.
2. After the main specimen is removed, 1- to 2-mm margins are sharply excised ("shaved") from each cavity margin (superior, lateral, inferior, medial, anterior, and posterior) and are sent to pathology separately from the main specimen with proper labeling.
3. Clips are applied to mark the excisional cavity walls.
4. The incision is closed and dressings applied.

Surgical clips left in the operative site assist the radiation oncologist. Alternatively, a bioabsorbable marker may be placed in the breast that contains marker clips (Fig. 17.10) (Research Highlight). BCS, with subsequent radiation therapy, is often the treatment of choice for small tumors. BCS is not usually an option for patients with (1) two or more cancer sites in separate quadrants of the breast; (2) persistent positive margins after reasonable surgical attempt; (3) diffuse, malignant-appearing microcalcifications; or (4) those who have undergone previous radiation to the affected breast. BCS, when combined with sentinel node or axillary node dissection (Fig. 17.11) and irradiation in stage I and stage II breast cancers, yields long-term survival rates equivalent to those for mastectomy and axillary staging. If one or more axillary nodes are involved, then chemotherapy is recommended.

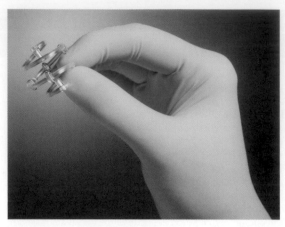

FIG. 17.10 BioZorb is an absorbable marker placed in the breast that contains marker clips that can be seen on x-ray.

RESEARCH HIGHLIGHT

BioZorb: A Bioabsorbable Marker That Aids in Targeted Therapies

BioZorb is an absorbable helix tissue marker that is placed in the breast intraoperatively. It contains marker clips that can be seen on x-ray and identifies the area in the breast for radiation therapy. It is slowly absorbed by the body over time, allowing for more targeted radiation therapy and reduced treatment times.

The following are features of BioZorb:
- Quickly and easily implanted in the breast during lumpectomy.
- Reliably identifies the 3-D region in which the tumor was removed.
- Readily visible with all breast imaging modalities.
- Facilitates TBRT, providing more accurate delineation of post-lumpectomy margins; decreases treatment time.
- Significantly reduces PTVs.
- Excellent cosmetic outcomes; absorbs within a year.

PTV, Planned treatment volumes; *TBRT,* targeted beam radiotherapy.
Modified from Cross MJ et al: Impact of a novel bioabsorbable implant on radiation treatment planning for breast cancer, *World J Surg* 41(2):464–471, 2016; Focal Therapeutics: *BioZorb: the difference is easy to visualize* (website). www.focalrx.com. (Accessed 23 December 2016).

Procedural Considerations

In patients with large breasts, increased bleeding may occur, requiring the ESU, a smoke evacuation system, and additional hemostatic clamps. The procedure is as described for open breast biopsy.

Focused ultrasound offers a potentially noninvasive alternative to surgical lumpectomy. Instead of surgical lumpectomy, the physician uses MRI or US guidance to identify the breast tumor, and then directs a focused beam of acoustic energy through the skin into the tumor. The beam heats and destroys the tumor without damaging nearby structures or tissues. Follow-up MRI determines whether the entire tumor has been destroyed. If required, focused US can be repeated (Focused Ultrasound Foundation, 2016).

Lymph Node Biopsy

Identification and microscopic examination of the SLNs, the first lymph nodes along the lymphatic channel from the primary tumor

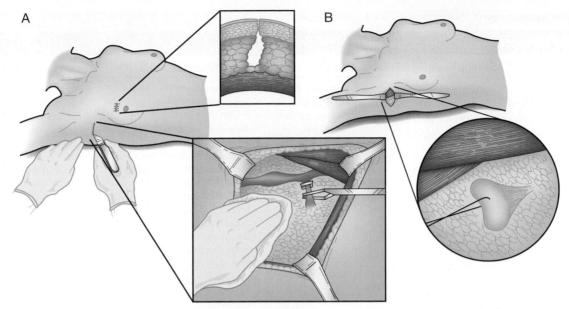

FIG. 17.11 Breast-conserving surgery. (A) Incisions are placed directly over the mass to be removed. A transverse incision in the low axillary region is used for sentinel node biopsy or axillary dissection. *Inset,* Excision cavity of breast-conserving surgery. (B) In sentinel node biopsy, a similar transverse incision is made that may be located by percutaneous mapping with the gamma probe if radiolabeled colloid is used. The sentinel node is located by its staining with dye, radioactivity, or both, and dissected free as a single specimen.

site, help to determine the need for additional or more extensive surgeries and treatments of early-stage invasive breast cancer for patients thought to have low to moderate risk for involvement of lymph nodes. Focus on SLNs is premised on the belief that if cancer cells have traveled through the lymph nodes, then the cells will lodge in the first nodes. SLNs are not located in the same site in every patient. If SLNs are negative, no other nodes in the lymph node channel are likely to be involved. Evidence of a positive node may require an axillary lymph node dissection (ALND) and adjunct therapy (Camp and Smith, 2014). ALND may not be recommended for patients with positive SLNs who will be treated with adjuvant systemic therapies and whole-breast radiotherapy (Camp and Smith, 2014). ALND is also inappropriate for patients with palpable nodal disease, those who have received preoperative chemotherapy, and those who have undergone mastectomies or who do not receive postoperative radiotherapy or partial-breast radiotherapy. Complications of SLNB include risk of allergic reactions to the blue dye or radioisotope use, rare instances of sensory or motor nerve damage, and pain.

Procedural Considerations

The procedure for SLNB is similar to that for breast biopsy. The sentinel node is identified by injection of either isosulfan blue dye, methylene blue dye, or the radioisotope technetium-99m sulfur colloid, which is a gamma-emitting material. Isosulfan blue and methylene blue dyes are contraindicated in patients with known hypersensitivity (Surgical Pharmacology). Careful patient monitoring is mandatory. A crash cart is available in case of severe anaphylactic reaction. The surgical staff coordinates the procedure with the nuclear medicine department. If technetium is used, a sterile handheld detector is required. In addition to a minor instrument set, if blue dye is used, a 5-mL syringe, a 25-gauge needle, an alcohol wipe, and the dye are required. For technetium, the gamma-tracer probe, counter, and sterile sleeve for the probe are required. Multiple

specimen containers are on hand along with pathology request forms. The surgeon may request that each specimen be numbered on the specimen container and the pathology request form. Safe practices for handling surgical specimens are implemented. A number of studies have shown that using a combination of isosulfan blue dye and technetium results in the lowest false-negative results (Hunt and Mittendorf, 2017). SLNB is replacing levels I and II ALND as the standard procedure for staging axillary lymph nodes.

Operative Procedure: Using Isosulfan Blue Dye or Methylene Blue Dye

1. Blue dye is injected around or near the tumor, or dye may be injected into the area of the breast mass that has been exposed as part of a breast biopsy (Hunt and Mittendorf, 2017).
2. This may be followed by a lymphatic massage (Hunt and Mittendorf, 2017).
3. The sentinel nodes stained with the blue dye are identified and excised.
4. The nodes are sent to the pathology department for examination.
5. Based on the results, the surgeon may or may not proceed with further ALND or the planned surgery, and may elect BCS (see Fig. 17.11).

Operative Procedure: Using Technetium

1. The tumor or previous biopsy site is injected with a small amount of radioactive tracer 20 minutes to 8 hours before surgery. It can also be injected after anesthesia is induced and the time-out completed.
2. This is followed by massage.
3. A handheld detector is passed over the top of the patient's chest to identify the area of the sentinel node (a positive reading). The probe may also be used with the addition of a sterile sleeve during excisional biopsy. Isosulfan blue dye may be used in conjunction with technetium during a procedure to enhance visibility of nodes.

SURGICAL PHARMACOLOGY

Drugs Used Intraoperatively in Breast Surgery

Medication Category	Dosage/Route	Purpose/Action	Adverse Reactions	Nursing Implications
Methylene blue: indicator dye, sentinel node mapping	Locally injected	Injected in periphery of an area exposed as part of a breast biopsy; sentinel nodes stained are identified and excised	Hypersensitivity reactions in some patients (hives; difficulty breathing; swelling of the face, lips, tongue, or throat)	Sentinel lymph node mapping, can be used alone or in combination with radiocolloid technetium-99m sulfur colloid
Isosulfan blue injection 1% aqueous solution: indicator dye, sentinel node mapping	Locally injected subcutaneously	Delineates lymphatic vessels draining the region of injection	Hypersensitivity reactions in some patients (urticaria, blue hives, a generalized rash, or pruritus); bronchospasm and respiratory compromise unusual; patients with a sulfa allergy do not display a cross-sensitivity to isosulfan blue dye; contraindicated in those individuals with known hypersensitivity to triphenylmethane or related compounds	Adjunct to lymphography; can be used alone or in combination with radiocolloid technetium-99m sulfur colloid

Modified from Hunt KK, Mittendorf EA: Diseases of the breast. In Townsend CM et al, editors: *Sabiston textbook of surgery*, ed 20, Philadelphia, 2017, Saunders; *Methylene blue. Gold standard drug monograph*, Elsevier, 2016; Drugs.com: *Isosulfan blue injection* (website). www.drugs.com/pro/isosulfan-blue-injection.html. (Accessed 21 December 2016).

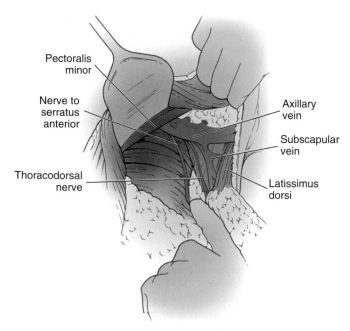

FIG. 17.12 Axillary dissection.

4. The surgeon marks the skin with a marking pen to indicate the reactive area.
5. The area is prepped and excisional biopsy of the SLN proceeds.

Axillary Lymph Node Dissection

ALND (Fig. 17.12) is removal of axillary nodes through an incision in the axilla after determining that the sentinel node is malignant. Removal and examination of the axillary nodes allow staging of the disease. Adjunct treatment can be more accurately planned when the pathologic stage is determined.

Procedural Considerations

The patient is placed supine on the OR bed with the operative side near the bed edge. The arm on the operative side is extended to less than 90 degrees on an armboard. The skin is prepped and draped as previously described.

Operative Procedure

1. An incision is made slightly posterior and parallel to the upper lateral border of the pectoralis major muscle or transversely across the axilla, below the hair line.
2. The fascia is incised over the pectoralis muscle, and the pectoralis minor muscle is exposed. Major blood and lymphatic vessels are clamped and ligated. Use of the ESU is avoided around the axillary vessels and nerves to reduce the risk of inadvertent injury and subsequent impaired muscle function.
3. The tissue over the axillary vein is incised.
4. The surgeon removes lymph nodes between the pectoralis major and pectoralis minor muscles, taking care not to injure the medial and lateral nerves of the pectoralis major.
5. Axillary fat and lymph nodes are freed from the chest wall and axillary vein carefully to avoid skeletonization. The long thoracic nerve along the chest wall near the axillary vein is identified, and the thoracodorsal nerve posteriorly is dissected free from the specimen.
6. The fat and nodes are removed.
7. A closed wound drainage system is usually placed through a separate stab incision to allow for lymphatic drainage, and the wound is closed.

Subcutaneous Mastectomy

Subcutaneous mastectomy uses both skin-sparing and nipple-sparing techniques. These are similar except the incision for skin sparing

ROBOTIC-ASSISTED SURGERY

Robotic Nipple-Sparing Mastectomy for Treatment of Breast Cancer and Immediate Robotic Breast Reconstruction With Implant

Surgeons at the European Institute of Oncology in Milan, Italy, in late 2016 reported that they had completed the first 29 surgeries consecutively, using single port RNSM and IRBR with implants successfully in a preliminary assessment of feasibility, reproducibility, and surgical and oncologic safety. Their purpose was to develop a new technique for mastectomy that used the da Vinci Xi (Intuitive Surgical, Sunnyvale, CA) through a single portal incision at the axillary fold that leaves no visible scarring and preserves the breast-skin envelope and nipple-areola complex. The surgeon-reporters noted the robot offered advantages such as robotic optical 3-D vision with a tenfold image magnification, better light intensity viewing the proper surgical dissection plane, and a minimally invasive approach with a greater anatomically sparing mastectomy. Future studies will include whether this minimally invasive approach offers a solution for complete excision of mammary tissue, including all ducts in the nipple, with a good result aesthetically (i.e., whether preservation of the skin envelope including the nipple-areola complex does or does not amplify oncologic recurrence rates), as well as cost analyses, length of operative times and learning curves, and patient satisfaction.

IRBR, Immediate robotic breast reconstruction; *RNSM*, robotic nipple-sparing mastectomy.
Modified from Toesca A et al: Robotic nipple-sparing mastectomy for treatment of breast cancer: feasibility and safety study, *Breast* 31:51–56, 2017.

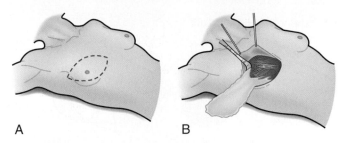

FIG. 17.13 Simple mastectomy. (A) Skin incisions are generally transverse and surround the central breast and nipple-areolar complex. (B) Skin flaps are raised sharply to separate the gland from the overlying skin and then the gland from the underlying muscle. Simple mastectomy divides the breast from the axillary contents and stops at the clavipectoral fascia.

includes the NAC, whereas the nipple-sparing incision does not. This mastectomy removes all breast tissue with the overlying skin. Sometimes, the nipple is left intact (nipple-sparing mastectomy [NSM]). This procedure is recommended for patients who have central tumors of noninvasive origin, chronic cystic mastitis, hyperplastic duct changes, multiple fibroadenomas, or a history of previous biopsies. Women with a higher body mass index and larger breasts are no longer excluded automatically because of presumed increased nipple loss from ischemia (Coopey et al., 2013). Robotic-assisted NSM is also possible (Robotic-Assisted Surgery).

Procedural Considerations

The patient is positioned as for biopsy. If reconstruction is planned at the time of mastectomy, appropriate equipment and supplies (see Chapter 22) are required.

Operative Procedure

1. An incision is usually begun in the inframammary crease and made on the medial or lateral aspect of the breast. Some surgeons initially remove and preserve the NAC by using lateral extensions of wide circumareolar incisions.
2. Blunt dissection follows to elevate the breast from the pectoral fascia.
3. The breast tissue is separated from the skin, attempting to remain in a plane between subcutaneous tissue and the breast. Dissection carries out toward the axilla. With care, 90% or more of the breast tissue, including the tail of Spence, can be removed. Some lymph nodes in the axillary area also may be removed. Bleeding vessels are clamped and ligated.
4. To assess the NAC base for tumor on permanent histologic evaluation, the NAC is inverted through the incision, and a thin

slice of tissue is removed from the base to establish a true margin. This ensures viability of the NAC while obtaining an adequate tissue sample.
5. Insertion of a closed wound suction catheter typically follows. The wound is closed, and a light pressure dressing applied.

Simple Mastectomy

Simple mastectomy is removal of the entire involved breast without lymph node dissection (Fig. 17.13). A simple mastectomy serves to remove extensive benign disease, a malignancy believed to be confined to the breast tissue, or as a palliative measure to remove an ulcerated advanced malignancy.

Procedural Considerations

The patient is positioned as for biopsy.

Operative Procedure

1. A transverse elliptic incision (see Fig. 17.13A), using a knife, curved scissors, and the ESU, frees the skin edges from the fascia. Bleeding vessels are clamped with hemostats and ligated with sutures or electrocoagulated.
2. Warm, moist laparotomy pads protect the skin edges of the wound; the breast tissue is grasped with Allis forceps and dissected free from the underlying pectoral fascia with curved scissors, a knife, or an ESU.
3. The tumor and all breast tissue are removed, but the axillary fat pad is not entered unless the procedure includes SLNB. Bleeding vessels are clamped and ligated or electrocoagulated.
4. A closed wound drainage catheter is inserted and anchored to the skin with a fine suture. The wound is closed with fine sutures or staples and a dressing applied.

Modified Radical Mastectomy

Modified radical mastectomy follows a tissue biopsy with positive diagnosis of malignancy; it removes the involved breast and all or partial axillary contents (Fig. 17.14). This surgery is only considered after careful discussion among the patient, family, and surgeon. A modified radical mastectomy removes the entire involved area with the aim of decreasing the spread of malignancy. This surgery's elliptic incision encompasses the NAC, a biopsy scar if an open biopsy has been performed, and excess skin of the breast. The underlying pectoral muscles are not removed. Patients who meet criteria for mastectomies may be considered for immediate reconstruction (see Chapter 22). Reconstruction is based on the patient's cosmetic and physiologic needs (Hunt and Mittendorf, 2017).

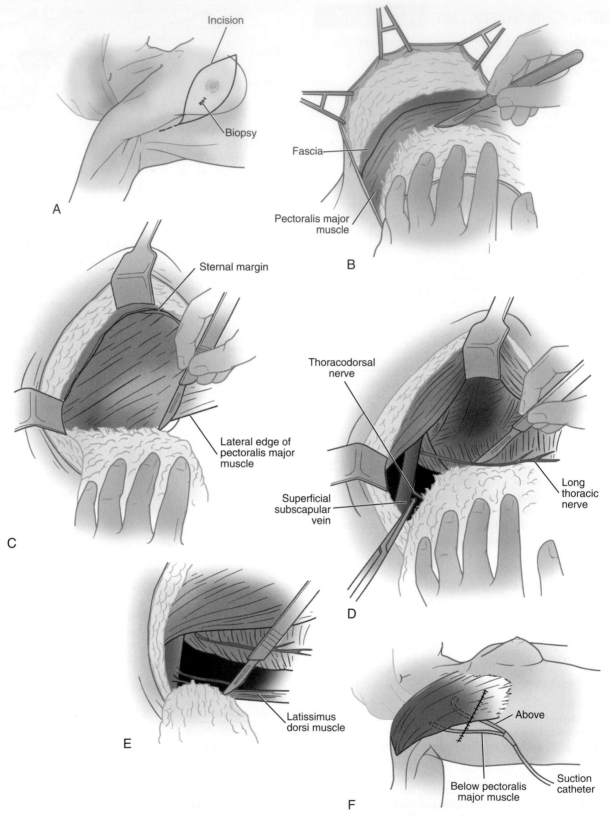

FIG. 17.14 Modified radical mastectomy. (A) Lines of incision. (B) Resection of breast from lateral edge of pectoralis major muscle. (C) Dissection of breast from lateral edge of pectoralis major muscle. (D) Thoracodorsal and long thoracic nerves identified. (E) Resection from latissimus dorsi muscle. (F) Incision is closed, and closed wound drainage systems are placed.

Procedural Considerations

The patient is placed supine on the OR bed with the operative side near the bed edge. The arm on the operative side is extended to less than 90 degrees on a padded armboard. The skin is prepped and draped. Tissue removed during surgery undergoes microscopic analysis to further classify it (type, tumor size, grade, invasion, lymphocytic response, and clean margin size). Additional analyses such as hormone receptor status (estrogen and progesterone positive or negative) and HER-2/neu expression may also be performed. This information assists the oncologist in planning subsequent adjuvant therapies.

Operative Procedure

1. An oblique elliptic incision with lateral extension toward the axilla is made through the subcutaneous tissue (see Fig. 17.14A). Hemostats and ligatures or electrocoagulation control bleeding points.
2. The skin is undercut in all directions to the limits of the dissection with a #3 knife handle with a #10 blade, curved scissors, or the ESU. Knife blades require frequent change to ensure precise dissection.
3. The margins of the skin flaps are covered with warm, moist laparotomy pads and retracted. Resection of fascia and breast from the pectoralis major muscle follow (see Fig. 17.14B), starting near the clavicle and extending down to the midsternum; the pectoralis muscle remains intact.
4. The intercostal arteries and veins are clamped and ligated.
5. Retraction of the axillary flap allows for dissection of the axilla. Careful attention is directed to preventing injury to the axillary vein and to the medial and lateral nerves of the pectoralis major muscle.
6. Dissection of the fascia from the lateral edge of the pectoralis muscle follows (see Fig. 17.14C). Vessels are ligated in the axilla and adjacent to the sternum. The fascia is then dissected from the serratus anterior muscle. The thoracic and thoracodorsal nerves are preserved (see Fig. 17.14D).
7. The breast and axillary fascia are freed from the latissimus dorsi muscle and suspensory ligaments (see Fig. 17.14E). The specimen is then passed off the field.
8. The surgical area is inspected for bleeding sites, which are ligated and electrocoagulated. The wound is irrigated with normal saline. Closed wound suction catheters are inserted into the wound through stab wounds and secured to the skin with a nonabsorbable suture on a cutting needle (see Fig. 17.14F).
9. A few absorbable sutures may be used in the subcutaneous tissue to approximate the skin edges. The incision is closed with suture material of choice, staples, or a running subcuticular stitch.
10. Wound closure tapes, antibiotic ointment, and a nonadherent wound dressing such as Adaptic may be applied.
11. The dressing consists of either a simple gauze dressing or a bulky absorbent dressing held in place by a surgical bra or ACE bandage.

Key Points

- Each breast has 15 to 20 lobes; each lobe has many smaller lobules, which end in dozens of tiny bulbs that can produce milk. These all link by ducts, which in turn lead to the nipple in the center of the areola.
- There are many benign breast conditions such as breast tumors and solitary lumps, fibrocystic changes, nipple problems and discharge, and infections or inflammation.
- Fibroadenomas in the breast consist of both glandular and connective tissue. They usually occur in women between 20 and 30 years of age and are benign breast tumors.
- A woman has about a one in eight chance of being diagnosed with breast cancer at some time during her life. Breast cancer is the most frequently diagnosed cancer in women in the United States.
- Breast cancer in men is rare; less than 1% of all breast cancers occur in men.
- Aside from gender, the strongest risk factor for breast cancer is age; other risk factors include a personal or family history of breast cancer, menstruation before age 12, menopause starting after age 55, a first full-term pregnancy after age 30, never having been pregnant, dense breasts, obesity after menopause, excessive alcohol use, and inherited changes in certain genes.
- *BRCA1* and *BRCA2* are genes that belong to a class of genes known as tumor suppressors. Mutation of these genes has been linked to both hereditary breast and ovarian cancers.
- After breast cancer has been diagnosed, ensuing tests determine whether cancer cells have spread within the breast or to other parts of the body.
- A biopsy is performed to determine the type of breast cancer, hormone receptor (estrogen, progesterone, or both), and HER-2–positive type. This, as well as tumor markers, aids in developing treatment plans.
- Lumpectomy is a surgical procedure that involves removing a suspected malignant tumor or lump and a small margin of surrounding tissue from the breast.
- Simple or total mastectomy involves removing the entire breast tissue but not the muscle tissue under the breast. This mastectomy can be combined with an SLNB.
- In a traditional mastectomy the surgeon removes an ellipse of skin that includes the skin of the NAC.
- In an NSM, a periareolar incision (nipple and areola intact) may be made, but the inframammary incision is more commonly used.
- The first node that lymphatic fluid passes through in a group of lymph nodes is called the SLN.
- SLNB is done by removing one to five SLNs from an underarm. The nodes are then examined by a pathologist to determine whether they are positive for cancer cells.
- After breast cancer surgery, patients should have a physical examination and a review of symptoms every 3 to 6 months for the first 2 to 3 years, then every 6 months until year 5, and annually thereafter. They should continue to have mammograms as prescribed.

Critical Thinking Question

Your patient, a 48-year-old Latin female, is undergoing a left breast lumpectomy with SLN dissection. In the preoperative area, you greet her to begin your assessment and establish baseline information necessary for her perioperative experience. You feel that she is having a hard time stating the name of her procedure and understanding it; she is not sure what the procedure entails, particularly the sentinel node biopsies. What steps would you take to facilitate a smooth transition to the intraoperative phase?

evolve *The answer to the Critical Thinking Question can be found at http://evolve.elsevier.com/Rothrock/Alexander.*

References

Al-Hilli Z et al: Reoperation for complications after lumpectomy and mastectomy for breast cancer from the 2012 National Surgical Quality Improvement Program (ACS-NSQIP), *Ann Surg Oncol* 22:S459–S469, 2015.

American Cancer Society (ACS): *Types of breast cancers* (website), 2016. www.cancer.org/cancer/breastcancer/detailedguide/breast-cancer-breast-cancer-types. (Accessed 13 December 2016).

Arpino G et al: Gene expression profiling in breast cancer: a clinical perspective, *Breast* 22(2):109–120, 2013.

Association of periOperative Registered Nurses (AORN): *Guidelines for perioperative practice*, Denver, 2016, The Association.

Bernardi D et al: Breast cancer screening with tomosynthesis (3D mammography) with acquired or synthetic 2D mammography compared with 2D mammography alone (STORM-2): a population-based prospective study, *Lancet Oncol* 17(8):1105–1113, 2016.

Bethea TN et al: *Abstract C49: relation of family history of cancer to risk of ER+, ER–, and triple-negative breast cancer in African American women* (website), 2015. http://cebp.aacrjournals.org/content/25/3_Supplement/C49.short. (Accessed 13 December 2016).

Breastcancer.org: *Symptoms and diagnosis* (website), 2015. www.breastcancer.org/symptoms. (Accessed 13 December 2016).

Camp MS, Smith BL: Lymphatic mapping and sentinel lymphadenectomy. In Cameron LJ, editor: *Current surgical therapy*, ed 11, St Louis, 2014, Elsevier.

Centers for Disease Control and Prevention (CDC): *What is breast cancer screening?* (website), 2016. www.cdc.gov/cancer/breast/basic_info/screening.htm. (Accessed 13 December 2016).

Chagpar AB et al: A randomized, controlled trial of cavity shave margins in breast cancer, *N Engl J Med* 373(6):503–510, 2015.

Chung CU et al: Surgical site infections after free flap breast reconstruction: an analysis of 2899 patients from the ACS-NSQIP datasets, *J Reconstr Microsurg* 31(6):434–441, 2015.

Coopey SB et al: Increasing eligibility for nipple-sparing mastectomy, *Ann Surg Oncol* 20(10):3218–3222, 2013.

Crawford C: *USPSTF still recommends mammography for women 50-74* (website), 2015. www.aafp.org/news/health-of-the-public/20150424mammograms.html. (Accessed 13 December 2016).

de la Torre J, Davis MR: Anatomy for plastic surgery of the breast. In Neligan PC, editor: *Plastic surgery*, ed 3, Philadelphia, 2013, Saunders.

Focused Ultrasound Foundation: *Breast cancer* (website), 2016. www.fusfoundation.org/diseases-and-conditions/women-s-health/breast-cancer. (Accessed 23 December 2016).

Gil-Londoño J-C et al: Surgical site infection after breast cancer surgery at 30 days and associated factors, *Infectio* 2016. doi: 10.1016/j.infect.2016.04.003.

Hardin R, Tsangaris T: Male breast cancer. In Cameron JL, editor: *Current surgical therapy*, ed 11, Philadelphia, 2014, Saunders.

Hunt KK, Mittendorf EA: Diseases of the breast. In Townsend CM et al, editors: *Sabiston textbook of surgery*, ed 20, Philadelphia, 2017, Saunders.

Marriott J et al: *Breast cancer care gets personal* (website), 2014. www.americannursetoday.com/breast-cancer-care-gets-personal/. (Accessed 14 December 2016).

Mayo Clinic: *Breast biopsy: what you can expect* (website), 2016. www.mayoclinic.org/tests-procedures/breast-biopsy/details/what-you-can-expect/rec-20236113. (Accessed 13 December 2016).

MedicineNet.com: *Male breast cancer* (website), 2016. www.medicinenet.com/male_breast_cancer/article.htm. (Accessed 14 December 2016).

National Cancer Institute Surveillance, Epidemiology, and End Results Program: *Cancer stat facts: female breast cancer* (website), 2016. https://seer.cancer.gov/statfacts/html/breast.html. (Accessed 13 December 2016).

National Comprehensive Cancer Network (NCCN): *NCCN clinical practice guidelines in oncology: breast cancer screening and diagnosis, version 1.2016* (website; free registration required), 2016. www.nccn.org/patients/guidelines/cancers.aspx. (Accessed 22 December 2016).

Oeffinger KC, Fontham ETH et al: Breast cancer screening for women at average risk: 2015 guideline update from the American Cancer Society, *JAMA* 314(15):1599–1614, 2015.

Olsen MA et al: Incidence of surgical site infection following mastectomy with and without immediate reconstruction using private insurer claims data, *Infect Control Hosp Epidemiol* 36(8 Suppl):907–914, 2015a.

Olsen MA et al: Increased risk of surgical site infection among breast-conserving surgery re-excisions, *Ann Surg Oncol* 22:2003–2009, 2015b.

Osterweil N: *USPSTF guidelines: biennial breast cancer screening from 50* (website), 2016. http://www.medscape.com/viewarticle/857027. (Accessed 22 December 2016).

Pouw B et al: Heading toward radioactive seed localization in non-palpable breast cancer surgery? A meta-analysis, *J Surg Oncol* 111:185–191, 2015.

Rolston KV et al: Current microbiology of surgical site infections in patients with cancer: a retrospective study, *Infect Dis Ther* 3:245–256, 2014.

Silva AK et al: The effect of contralateral prophylactic mastectomy and perioperative complications in women undergoing immediate breast reconstruction: a NSQIP analysis, *Ann Surg Oncol* 22(11):3474–3480, 2015.

Simmons RM et al: A phase II trial exploring the success of cryoablation therapy in the treatment of invasive breast carcinoma: results from ACOSOG (Alliance) Z1072, *Ann Surg Oncol* 23(8):2438–2445, 2016.

Stahl DL et al: The breast. In Baggish MH, Karram MM, editors: *Atlas of pelvic anatomy and gynecologic surgery*, ed 4, Philadelphia, 2016, Elsevier.

Stenger M: *CLEOPATRA Overall survival analysis: significant benefit for pertuzumab plus trastuzumab/docetaxel in HER2-positive metastatic breast cancer* (website), 2015. www.ascopost.com/issues/may-25-2015/cleopatra-overall-survival-analysis-significant-benefit-for-pertuzumab-plus-trastuzumabdocetaxel-in-her2-positive-metastatic-breast-cancer. (Accessed 13 December 2016).

The Training Center: *Breast cancer facts and stats* (website), 2016. https://qap.sdsu.edu/screening/breastcancer/facts.html. (Accessed 13 December 2016).

U.S. Preventive Services Task Force (USPSTF): *Breast cancer: screening* (website), 2016. https://www.uspreventiveservicestaskforce.org/Page/Document/UpdateSummaryFinal/breast-cancer-screening. (Accessed 24 July 2017).

Warshaw R: *Understanding radiation therapy* (website), 2015/2016. www.lbbc.org/sites/default/files/InsightWinter2015%20FINAL_General.pdf. (Accessed 13 December 2016).

Wolff AC et al: Cancer of the breast. In Niederhuber JE, editor: *Abeloff's clinical oncology*, ed 5, Philadelphia, 2014, Saunders.

CHAPTER 18

Ophthalmic Surgery

EILEEN DICKSON MIELCAREK

Eyesight is not essential to life, but quality of vision enables us to have a higher quality of life. Much of what we learn throughout our lifetime and how we understand and navigate our world is through our vision. According to the latest available data, a survey of more than 11,000 people in 11 countries to gauge eye care habits and perceptions, the Barometer of Global Eye Health respondents said they would rather lose a limb, lose 10 years of their life, or receive a 50% cut in income than lose 50% of their vision (Bausch + Lomb, 2012). Early detection of eye disease through regular eye examinations can provide the most effective treatment when needed and ultimately preserve vision.

There is a disconnect between Americans' fear of losing their vision and not taking the necessary steps to preserve and enhance their eyesight. The previously mentioned survey revealed that more than two-thirds of respondents did not have a recent eye examination, which is the most basic step necessary to preserve eyesight. In addition, 7 in 10 respondents said they were somewhat or very knowledgeable about their eye healthcare, yet 97% of eye doctors say the public does not sufficiently understand proper eye healthcare. Part of the disconnect may be attributed to the fact that sick or diseased eyes often look normal, and certain diseases exhibit no warning signs or evolve slowly over time. Because vision impairment increases the risk of mortality and morbidity from other chronic conditions and is often associated with a reduced quality of life, eye and vision health should be a population health priority (National Academies of Sciences, Engineering, and Medicine, 2016).

The ocular surgical interventions discussed in this chapter are delicate, microscopic, and demand careful planning and execution by both the surgeon and the perioperative staff. As technology advances in eye care, surgical interventions become more detailed and require advanced instrumentation as well as more planning and team participation. The perioperative nurse must keep abreast of changes in technology, procedural techniques, safety issues, efficiency, communication, and patient education resources to provide optimal care to ophthalmic surgery patients.

Surgical Anatomy

The eyes are one of the more complex organs of the human body. Vision begins with a focal point of light, which travels through the cornea, lens, and vitreous fluid, and lands on the retina to be sent to and interpreted by the brain. Clear vision requires all of the following: healthy, functioning eye structures; adequate light; intact neurovascular communication with the brain; and the brain's effective interpretation of the images relayed. The following cycle, if completed in the full sequence, leads to accurate visual images:

1. Light rays emanate from an object in the field of vision and transmit to the eye. These light rays pass through the clear cornea, which accounts for approximately 65% of the refractive power of the eye.
2. Iris muscles control the size of the pupil to allow the appropriate amount of light into the eyes.
3. The rays pass through the crystalline lens, which changes shape to accommodate the refraction and focus between distant and near images. The lens accounts for 35% of the refractive power of the eye.
4. The rays travel through the clear vitreous fluid and land directly on the macula, the central part of the retina, and the area of highest sensitivity for details. The nerve endings of the retina pass the images as nerve impulses through the optic nerve to the brain, where the occipital area interprets the images (Fig. 18.1).

The American Academy of Ophthalmology (AAO) recommends that healthy adults receive an eye examination every 2 years, even if vision is normal and unchanged. Children should receive a baseline

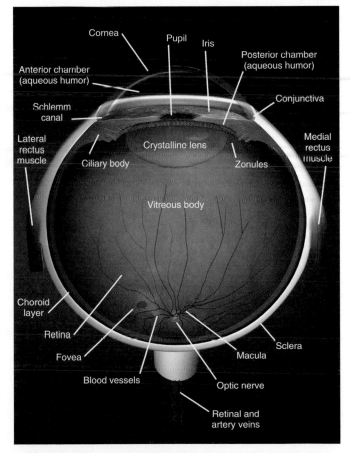

FIG. 18.1 Anatomy of the eye. Horizontal section through left globe.

eye examination by an ophthalmologist before starting school, even if no signs of impairment or complications are present. Diabetic individuals of any age should see an ophthalmologist every year because they are at higher risk for eye diseases (AAO, 2014).

Refractive Apparatus

As light rays pass through the eye, there are opportunities for the light not to land directly on the macula. Refractive errors occur when images do not focus and fall directly on the retina, but these can be corrected with eyeglasses or contact lenses. *Myopia* (nearsightedness) occurs when the focal point of the light rays is behind the retina. *Hyperopia* (farsightedness) occurs when the light rays focus in front of the retina. *Astigmatism* occurs when the cornea is cylindrically shaped instead of spherical, and the light rays diverge as they reach the retina. *Presbyopia* is the natural aging of the eye in which the lens cannot change shape and accommodate for the focusing needed to see close objects. Myopia, hyperopia, and astigmatism are considered lower order aberrations that account for the majority of refractive errors (Fig. 18.2). Higher order aberrations are complex microscopic irregularities present on the surface of the cornea, lens, and retina that can affect the quality of visual acuity.

Eyeglasses that minimize images are prescribed to refocus light rays in myopic patients; eyeglasses that magnify images are prescribed for hyperopic patients; and magnifying bifocals or reading glasses are prescribed for presbyopic patients. Presbyopia occurs in everyone older than age 45, even if they have perfect distance vision. The unit of measure in refraction is called a diopter. The more diopters required to correct vision, the worse unaided vision one has.

Cornea

The cornea is the transparent, avascular window through which light passes to the retina; it joins the white sclera at a transitional zone called the limbus. The cornea is composed of five layers: the epithelium, Bowman membrane, the stroma, Descemet membrane, and the endothelium (Fig. 18.3). The epithelium consists of constantly renewing cell layers with many nerve endings, accounting for the cornea's great sensitivity to foreign bodies and abrasions. Bowman membrane is a connective tissue thickening that forms a barrier to trauma and infection under the epithelium. If damaged, Bowman membrane does not regenerate and a permanent scar is formed. The stroma accounts for 90% of the corneal thickness and is composed of precisely layered fibers. If this layering is disrupted (e.g., by edema), corneal clarity decreases. Descemet membrane is a thin layer between the endothelial layer of the cornea and the stroma. The corneal endothelium is a single layer of hexagonal cells that acts as a fluid pump to keep the cornea clear by maintaining the proper level of stromal dehydration for clarity. Because corneal endothelial cells do not regenerate, damage to this layer may cause persistent corneal edema and loss of transparency.

The *sclera* is the opaque "white" part of the strong external layer, and it is made up of collagenous fibers loosely connected with fascia. The sclera receives the attachments of the extraocular muscle tendons, and it is pierced by the ciliary arteries and nerves posteriorly by the optic nerve. The sclera provides the eye with form and shape and encompasses the entire side and back of the eye.

Conjunctiva

The conjunctiva is a thin, transparent mucous membrane divided into a palpebral portion (lining the inside of the eyelids) and a bulbar portion (lining the surface of the globe). The junction between the palpebral and bulbar conjunctivae forms a forniceal sac.

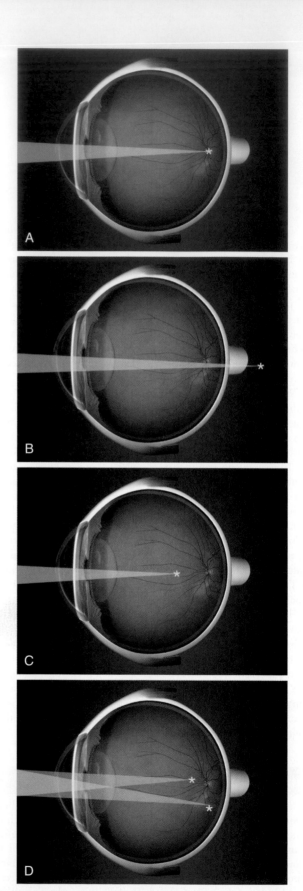

FIG. 18.2 (A) Emmetropia (perfect vision). (B) Myopia (nearsightedness). (C) Hyperopia (farsightedness). (D) Astigmatism can present with hyperopia or myopia.

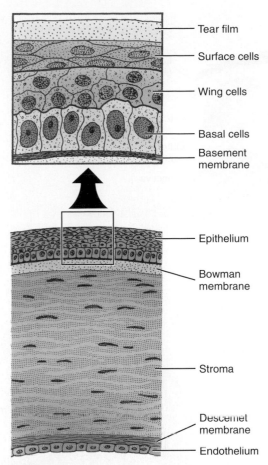

FIG. 18.3 Five layers of cornea. *Inset,* Layers of epithelium.

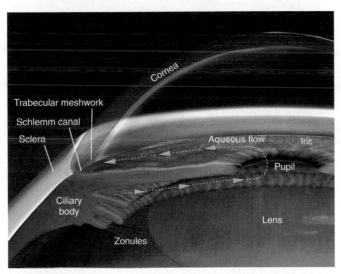

FIG. 18.4 Anterior chamber, ciliary body, and aqueous circulation.

Crystalline Lens

The biconvex lens is suspended behind the iris and connected to the ciliary body by delicate collagenous strings called *zonules* (Fig. 18.4). The lens changes shape and focus (accommodation) by either relaxation or tightening of the zonular fibers. Over time (particularly

after age 40), the lens and zonules become progressively less elastic, resulting in presbyopia.

Vitreous Humor

The vitreous body is a transparent, gelatinous mass composed of 99% water and 1% collagen and hyaluronic acid. It fills the posterior four-fifths of the eyeball and is adherent to the retina at the vitreous base. The vitreous supports the shape of the eye internally and gives the eye its shape.

Retina

The retina is an extension and modification of the brain designed to perceive light and relay visual signals through the optic nerve back to the occipital brain. The central portion of the retina is called the macula and is responsible for central detailed vision (20/20), whereas the peripheral retina is responsible for spatial orientation, night vision, and peripheral vision. The visual sensory nerve endings of the retina pass the images as nerve impulses through nerve fibers of the optic nerve to the brain, in which the occipital area interprets the images.

Supporting Structures

Nerve and Blood Supply

The optic nerve (second cranial nerve) extends between the posterior eyeball and the optic chiasm. This cranial nerve carries visual impulses as well as the sensations of pain, touch, and temperature from the eye and its surrounding structures to the brain, in which they are interpreted. The ophthalmic artery, the main arterial supply to the orbit and globe, is a branch of the internal carotid artery. It divides into branches supplying the globe, muscles, and eyelids. The central retinal artery and central retinal vein travel through the optic nerve and provide a separate blood supply for the retina.

Lacrimal Apparatus

The lacrimal gland produces aqueous tears and secretes them through a series of ducts onto the anterior ocular surface, keeping the cornea moist and washing away any debris. The tears then flow inward to the puncta, from which they are conducted by the canaliculi to the lacrimal sac and finally pass into the nasolacrimal duct. The lacrimal apparatus effectively functions like a sink, with a faucet (main and accessory lacrimal glands) and drain (lacrimal puncta, canaliculi, sac, and nasolacrimal duct) (Fig. 18.5).

Eyelid

Eyelids provide protection to the eye from debris and foreign bodies and continuous tear moisture to the cornea (blinking). The anterior eyelid layers contain the eyelid skin; ocular adnexa (eyelashes and associated glands); and subcutaneous tissue, lymphatics, and muscles. The tarsus is a plate of dense fibrous tissue that forms the main scaffolding of the eyelids. Within the tarsus are the meibomian glands, which secrete the oily component (sebum) of the tear film. The orifices of these sebaceous glands are found at the eyelid margin just posterior to the eyelashes.

The palpebral fissure refers to the space between the margins of the two eyelids. When the eye is closed, the fissure becomes a mere slit and the cornea is completely covered by the upper eyelid. The upper eyelid is more mobile and larger than the lower. The eyelids are closed by the orbicularis oculi muscle, and the upper lid is opened by the levator muscle.

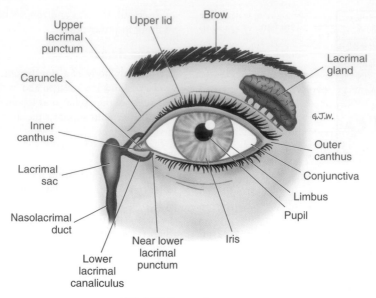

FIG. 18.5 Lacrimal apparatus.

Tears

Tears are essential for keeping the cornea lubricated to maintain clarity and optical performance. Tears have three layers: the mucous layer that sits closest to the cornea, the aqueous water layer, and the oily lipid layer. Aqueous tears are created by the lacrimal glands located within the upper temporal eyelid, the mucous layer by conjunctival cells, and an oily layer by meibomian glands in the eyelid. The cornea does not have blood vessels or blood flow, so tears provide antibodies and nutrition to the cornea, as well as flush out irritants and debris.

Muscles

Seven separate eye muscles control the movement of the eyeball. The muscles work in yoked pairs, with ocular movements generated by an increase in the tone of one set of muscles and a decrease in the tone of the antagonistic muscles. Named according to their relative position on the eyeball, the extraocular muscles of the eyeball include the four recti (the *superior, inferior, medial,* and *lateral*) and two oblique muscles (the *superior* and *inferior*). Except for the inferior oblique muscle, these muscles originate from the back of the orbit. The extraocular muscles are supplied by cranial nerves III (oculomotor, supplying the superior, inferior, and medial recti), IV (trochlear, supplying the superior oblique), and VI (abducens, supplying the lateral rectus) (Fig. 18.6).

Perioperative Nursing Considerations

Assessment

Patients undergoing eye surgery range from premature infants with retinopathy of prematurity or congenital conditions to elderly patients whose conditions result from the aging process. These patients need assessment of both their vision and general health status. A preoperative visit to the eye clinic or surgeon's office typically completes diagnostic testing and physical examination pertinent to the presenting eye condition requiring surgery. Communication with the physician's office staff to coordinate patient preparation and teaching and to collate preoperative test results increases the efficiency and effectiveness

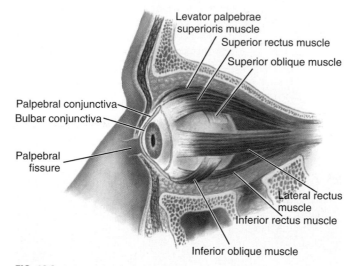

FIG. 18.6 Orbit and muscles. Medial rectus is located on the nasal side of the globe.

of preoperative procedures. Perioperative nurses often contact patients preoperatively by phone to provide needed information concerning the day of surgery and to obtain initial preoperative assessment information.

The perioperative nursing staff must be prepared to meet the specific needs of each patient and family, collaborate and communicate effectively for continuity of patient care, and prepare the patient for home care. On admission, a staff member should fully orient the patient to the physical surroundings. Constant description and reinforcement are important to visually impaired patients. Approaching the patient from the unaffected side increases the patient's independence and decreases the possibility of startling the patient.

Assessment is designed to collect and disseminate pertinent information and is carried out in a comprehensive, yet efficient, manner. A standard set of parameters should provide enough information to facilitate appropriate care in the event of an emergency. Physiologic information (e.g., height, weight, vital signs), psychosocial factors (e.g., support systems, fears, anxiety, cultural considerations), and environmental, education, and self-care needs are assessed. The general health history includes a comprehensive list of current medication therapy (often the patient is asked to bring currently prescribed medications to the appointment). The medical history is very important in cueing the nurse to evaluate for ocular manifestations of systemic disease. For example, the patient may present for retinal surgery as a consequence of retinopathy related to diabetes mellitus.

Data may be collected from family or significant others or directly from physicians or their office staff. Throughout this process the nurse encourages the patient to assume an active role in his or her healthcare needs. All information is documented so that it is readily available to others.

An ocular history, which includes the patient's primary problem, history of the present condition, symptoms, and visual limitations, is reviewed from the patient's initial visit to the eye care provider's office, and the nurse confirms these findings. Some common forms of ocular examination are shown in Fig. 18.7.

An external examination of the eye, including lids, lashes, conjunctivae, and lacrimal apparatus, should have been performed to detect any deviations from normal. The corneal reflex should have been tested and the cornea inspected for superficial irregularities. Pupil size and contour, as well as pupillary reaction, both direct and consensual, should be noted. Shallow anterior chamber depth alerts staff members to the potential for high pressures resulting from angle closure with dilation of the pupil.

The function of the extraocular muscles should have been determined. Movement should be synchronous, and visual lines should meet on a fixed object. Documentation of this examination must be descriptive, accurate, and concise. It is of value later in assessing the outcome of the procedure. The following observations are also important:

- General appearance of the eye (edema, asymmetry, redness, condition of conjunctiva, sclera, and skin around the eyes)
- Symptoms of irritation (itching, burning)
- Position of eyelids (opened and closed), condition of upper and lower lid surfaces, eyelid spasm
- Visual acuity, pupillary dilation (note if pupils are equal, round, reactive to light, and accommodative), visual fields
- Extraocular muscle movement
- Drainage from eye
- Current and significant past medical problems (eye disease, diabetes, cardiovascular disease, hypertension, allergies)
- Current medication history, including anticoagulants, analgesics, herbs, and nutritional supplements
- General: vital signs; restlessness, discomfort, anxiety; limitations in mobility; presence of prosthesis

After the assessment information has been compiled, nursing diagnoses are identified and the plan of care for the entire perioperative period is developed.

Nursing Diagnosis

Nursing diagnoses related to the care of patients undergoing ophthalmic surgery might include the following:
- Deficient Knowledge or Readiness for Enhanced Knowledge related to diagnosis, surgical intervention, medication management, and home care management
- Anxiety related to vision loss, surgical intervention, awake status during surgical intervention, fear of the unknown and surgical outcome
- Acute and/or Chronic Pain related to increased intraocular pressure (IOP) and surgical intervention
- Risk for Injury related to altered visual sensory perception

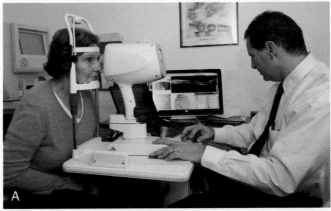

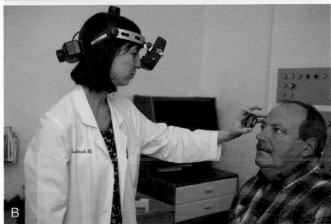

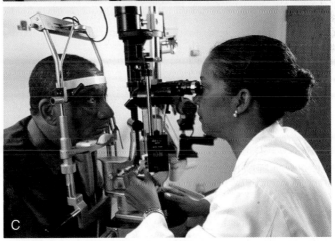

FIG. 18.7 (A) Optical coherence tomography (OCT) machine takes cross-section images of the retina, cornea, and anterior segment. It is used to diagnose glaucoma, retina issues, and cornea abnormalities. The femtosecond laser machine has a live OCT incorporated for real-time viewing. (B) After the eyes are dilated, an indirect ophthalmoscope provides the eye care professional with a wider view of the retina. (C) A slit lamp, with its high magnification, allows the eye care professional to examine the front of the eye.

Outcome Identification

Outcomes identified for the selected nursing diagnoses could be stated as follows:
- The patient, family, or significant others will verbalize knowledge of the diagnosis, planned surgical intervention, medication management, and requirements for home care maintenance before discharge.

- The patient will verbalize an acceptable level of anxiety and use personally effective coping mechanisms.
- The patient will express adequate comfort during and after the surgical intervention as determined by response on a verbal pain scale.
- The patient will be free from injury related to altered visual sensory perception.

Planning

Plans of care are the framework for organizing activities during perioperative patient care. Although ophthalmic surgery is often perceived as minor because of the small incision site and relatively short surgery period, the perioperative team must be fully prepared for potential complications or emergencies. Patients who are admitted for ophthalmic surgery often have complex medical histories. After a review of the patient's record, supplemented by a patient or family interview, collected data are incorporated into an individualized perioperative plan of care. A Sample Plan of Care for a patient undergoing ophthalmic surgery follows.

Implementation

Managing and Monitoring Patient Safety Needs

A key aspect of the perioperative nurse's role is patient safety. Because many ophthalmic procedures are performed with local anesthesia, the circulating nurse or an additional perioperative nurse must be prepared to monitor the patient and provide supportive care.

SAMPLE PLAN OF CARE

Nursing Diagnosis
Deficient Knowledge or **Readiness for Enhanced Knowledge** related to diagnosis, surgical intervention, medication management, and home care management

Outcome
The patient, family, or significant others will verbalize knowledge of the diagnosis, planned surgical intervention, medication management, and requirements for home care maintenance before discharge.

Interventions
- Determine knowledge level; address knowledge deficits or make appropriate referrals.
- Identify any barriers to communication (e.g., vision, hearing, speech, language spoken).
- Assess readiness to learn.
- Identify psychosocial status, noting anxiety or manifestations of stress.
- Assess coping mechanisms; support those that have been personally effective for the patient.
- Implement measures to provide psychologic support.
- Elicit perception of surgery; consider any cultural implications.
- Encourage patient participation in decision making and planning for postoperative care.
- Reinforce physician's explanations and clarify any misconceptions.
- Provide instructions based on age, health literacy status, culture, and other identified needs.
- Begin discharge education and planning during the preoperative period.
- Evaluate response to instructions; have patient teach-back in their own words.
- Evaluate environment and expectations for home care; make referrals as appropriate.

Nursing Diagnosis
Anxiety related to vision loss, surgical intervention, awake status during surgical intervention, and fear of the unknown and surgical outcome

Outcome
The patient will verbalize an acceptable level of anxiety and use personally effective coping mechanisms.

Interventions
- Allow the patient time to verbalize concerns.
- Help the patient identify sources of anxiety; classify anxiety as low, moderate, or high.
- Assist the patient to identify personal strengths and external resources; reinforce personally effective coping mechanisms.
- Observe for increased anxiety demonstrated through behavior (e.g., hand tremor, shakiness, restlessness, facial tension, voice quivering, increased perspiration, tearfulness).
- Provide information and answer questions concisely.
- Use touch (as appropriate) to communicate reassurance.
- Control environmental stimuli in the OR.

Nursing Diagnosis
Acute Pain and/or Chronic Pain related to increased IOP and/or surgical intervention

Outcome
The patient will remain comfortable during surgical intervention and postoperatively as determined by response on a verbal pain scale.

Interventions
- Identify cultural and value components related to pain.
- Instruct patient to verbalize pain during procedure performed using local anesthetic or sedation; use a validated pain rating scale.
- Observe for physical signs of pain, such as facial grimacing, groaning, muscle tightening, or changes in vital signs.
- Alert surgeon to any patient reports of significant pain from the injection or signs of local anesthesia toxicity (LAST) (e.g., tinnitus, tingling around the mouth) (if using local anesthesia).
- Ensure patient understands what is happening during the procedure (e.g., stinging or pressure from local anesthetic injection) and how long it will last.
- Monitor the presence of, or an increase in, eye pain, pain around orbit, blurred vision, reddened eye, abdominal pain, nausea, vomiting, neurologic changes, and changes in visual fields; initiate appropriate action.
- Implement measures to provide psychologic support.
- Implement pain guidelines; administer medications as prescribed.
- Instruct the patient to refrain from excessive exertion, such as crying, coughing, straining, lifting, bending, rubbing the eyes, and blowing the nose postoperatively.
- Discuss methods to promote patient comfort, such as music, guided imagery, and relaxation.

Nursing Diagnosis
Risk for Injury related to altered visual sensory perception

Outcome
The patient will be free from injury related to altered visual sensory perception.

SAMPLE PLAN OF CARE—cont'd

Interventions

- Review presenting medical condition and results of eye exams.
- Announce and introduce yourself to all patients with reduced vision; use a normal tone of voice unless the patient also has hearing problems.
- Explain perioperative events; seek patient cooperation in events such as transfer to OR bed, achieving position of comfort, remaining still during procedure, local anesthesia, sounds in the OR environment, etc.
- Demonstrate how to apply eyedrops; evaluate the patient (or family's) ability to self-administer (return demonstration).

- Teach the patient about common side effects of eye medications
- Teach principles of infection prevention (e.g., hand hygiene).
- Instruct the patient, family, and caregiver to watch for signs and symptoms of infection including redness, pain, swelling, drainage, and changes in visual acuity postoperatively and to report these problems promptly to the physician.
- Encourage the patient, family, and caregiver to discuss concerns about reduced or impaired vision.
- Review strategies with the patient, family, and caregiver related to how to alter home environment for patient safety, self-confidence, and independent living.
- Encourage patient to keep follow-up appointments.

Reassurance is especially important for patients who are awake because they can usually see and hear the surgery progressing. Ophthalmic patients, like other surgical patients, have increased sensitivity to noise and activities within the OR. The OR should be kept quiet and peaceful to decrease anxiety and increase cooperation, reducing the need for deep sedation.

Both the scrub person, who may be a registered nurse or surgical technologist, and the perioperative nurse manage additional patient safety needs. Foreign substances must not be introduced intraocularly. Lint-free drapes should be used to create the sterile field. Gloved hands should not touch the portion of an instrument used in an intraocular wound, and debris should be cleansed from instruments with cellulose sponges. All gloves should be powder free (FDA, 2016).

Members of the perioperative team have several important responsibilities in preparing the OR room and the equipment. Technologic advances in ophthalmic surgery require that perioperative nurses be familiar with equipment and check each piece carefully before the patient arrives in the OR. Organization and grouping of outlet cords must be checked to ensure clear walking areas. The availability of specially ordered intraocular lens (IOL) implants or prostheses needs to be checked to prevent delay or cancellation of the procedure. Scrupulous attention to aseptic technique is essential in preventing endophthalmitis (infection within the eye) and possible blindness. Safety-focused communication within the perioperative team includes the following:

- *Identification:* The perioperative nurse asks the patient to state his or her name and compares the name on the wristband with the name on the chart and surgical schedule while verbally confirming it with the patient or a family member. Two or more identifiers, such as birth date or medical record number, are required (TJC, 2017).
- *Verifications:* The patient or family member should state which eye is the operative site and which procedure is being performed. The nurse reviews the surgical consent, surgeon's preoperative orders, and operating room (OR) schedule to determine whether the correct operative eye has been prepared (including verification of operative eye using the word "right" or "left" [abbreviations are not accepted], marking of the operative site, and dilation, if appropriate) and other protocols have been carried out according to facility policies on correct-site surgery. If there is any discrepancy among the patient's response, the informed consent, the physician's orders, ophthalmic history, and exam, the discrepancy is corrected during the preoperative verification process. Immediately before the incision, this information, along with any implants or special

needs, is reconfirmed during the time-out (Patient Safety). Facility protocols may also require performance of a separate time-out before blocking the eye (Betsy Lehman Center, 2017).

Preventing Infection

As in any practice of nursing the primary way to prevent infection within ophthalmic surgery is handwashing. The Association of periOperative Registered Nurses (AORN) recommends hands should be washed before and after every patient contact, before performing a clean or sterile task, when hands are visibly soiled, after contact with the patient's surroundings, any time there is risk for contact with blood or other body fluids, before and after eating, and after using the restroom (AORN, 2017).

To prevent endophthalmitis, patients receive an antibiotic before surgery. The physician may also use a topical antibiotic such as vancomycin given intracamerally (within a chamber, such as the anterior or posterior chamber of the eye) for gram-positive coverage; gram-positive organisms are responsible for more than 90% of endophthalmitis (Shorstein et al., 2013) (Evidence for Practice). Symptoms of endophthalmitis are usually noticed 24 hours to 7 days after surgery (Jabbarvand et al., 2016). Toxic anterior segment syndrome (TASS) is a sterile postoperative inflammatory reaction caused by a noninfectious substance that enters the anterior segment, resulting in toxic damage to intraocular tissues. The process typically starts as early as 4 hours after the procedure and up to 48 hours after cataract surgery, especially those considered difficult surgery cases. TASS is limited to the anterior segment of the eye, is Gram stain and culture negative, and usually improves with steroid treatment. The primary differential diagnosis is infectious endophthalmitis. Possible causes of TASS include intraocular solutions with inappropriate chemical composition or concentration, pH, osmolarity, preservative, denatured ophthalmic viscosurgical devices, enzymatic detergents, bacterial endotoxin, oxidized metal deposits and residues, and factors related to IOLs such as residues from polishing or sterilizing compounds. An outbreak of TASS is an environmental and toxic control issue that requires complete analysis of all medications and fluids used during surgery, as well as complete review of instrument cleaning and sterilization protocols.

Safety Measures in Administering Medications

Medications used in the perioperative period are extremely important to the procedure's outcome and the patient's safety. Drugs for diagnosing and treating eye disorders are potent; one error could result in total, irreversible blindness.

PATIENT SAFETY

Using an Ophthalmic-Specific Checklist

Failure to embrace a safety culture can lead to serious adverse events. Using checklists to ensure critical information is shared among team members is one strategy to promote a safe environment of care and enhance communication. An example of a comprehensive ophthalmic-specific checklist is provided below.

The original checklist was developed by a task force comprised of members from the AAO, the ASORN, and other key ophthalmic societies, and divides surgical care into three main phases: before anesthesia sign-in, time-out before incision, and the postoperative sign-out before transferring the patient to the recovery area.

Before Anesthesia Sign-In	Before Incision Time-Out	Before Leaving OR Sign-Out

□ Patient has confirmed:
  • Allergies
  • Consent
  • Identity
  • Procedure
  • Site (which eye is to be operated on)
□ Site is marked
□ History and physical have been reviewed
□ Presurgical assessment complete
□ Anesthesia safety check done
 	
Does patient have difficult airway/aspiration risk?
□ Not applicable
□ No
□ Yes: equipment checked and available
	□ All team members have introduced themselves by name and role
	□ Surgeon, anesthesia provider, and nurse orally confirm:
	  • Patient
	  • Site
	  • Procedure
	□ Surgeon and nurse orally confirm:
	  • Antibiotic
	  • Devices
	  • Dyes
	  • Gas
	  • Implant style and power (may also be written on OR white board so all can see)
	  • Mitomycin-C/antineoplastics
	  • Tissue
	
	Anticipated critical events:
	□ Surgeon reviews:
	  • Critical steps
	    □ None anticipated
	    □ Reviewed
	  • Surgery duration
	    □ Anesthesia provider reviews any patient-specific concerns
	□ Nursing team reviews:
	  • Sterility (including indicator results)
	  • Equipment issues
	  • Concerns
		□ Nurse orally confirms with team the name of procedure recorded:
		  • Instrument, sponge, sharps count correct:
		    □ Not applicable
		    □ Yes
		  • Specimen labeled (including patient name):
		    □ Not applicable
		    □ Yes
		□ Nurse orally confirms with team whether there are any equipment issues to be addressed
		□ Surgeon, anesthesia provider, and nurse review key concerns for recovery and management of this patient
		
		Patient Label
		Date of Surgery: _____

Signature/Time	Signature/Time	Signature/Time

AAO, American Academy of Ophthalmology; *ASORN,* American Society of Ophthalmic Registered Nurses.
Modified from American Society of Cataract and Refractive Surgery (ASCRS): *ASC surgical safety checklist for ophthalmology* (website), 2012. www.ascrs.org/resources/asc-surgical-safety-checklist-ophthalmology. (Accessed 27 January 2017); American Academy of Ophthalmology's 2014 Wrong Site Task Force: *Wrong-site, wrong-IOL checklist* (website; free download required). www.betsylehmancenterma.gov/resources/tools-for-safe-cataract-surgery-1. (Accessed 30 January 2017).

The patient's medical and ocular histories determine the selection of appropriate ophthalmic agents. The perioperative nurse should be knowledgeable about the specific medications ordered, including purpose, strength, action, duration, adverse reactions, route of administration, and contraindications. This information should be included in the patient's initial assessment. For example, mydriatic and cycloplegic eyedrops may be contraindicated in narrow-angle glaucoma.

The nurse checks the medication label for name, strength, and expiration date during preparation and before administration. This precaution is especially important because many ophthalmic drugs are distributed in single-dose units that closely resemble each other. The patient must be positively identified, and the site of the administration must be clearly translated from the physician's orders.

Handwashing between patients when administering eyedrops is imperative. The nurse ensures that intraocular solutions are separated from those not used intraocularly.

All solutions on and off the sterile field must be clearly labeled. To meet The Joint Commission (TJC) 2017 National Patient Safety Goals, medications in a procedural setting must have labels that include drug name, strength/concentration, and amount. Medication errors are among the most common medical errors (TJC, 2017). Preprinted labels and sterile waterproof pens and labels are commercially available to avoid smearing from liquids.

Instillation of Eyedrops

Most medications prescribed for the eye are administered in the form of eyedrops. Perioperative nurses should have a firm grasp of

EVIDENCE FOR PRACTICE

Decreasing Postoperative Endophthalmitis With Intracameral Antibiotics

Postoperative endophthalmitis, defined as an inflammatory condition of the aqueous and/or vitreous humor, is a serious complication that can occur after any ocular surgery that disrupts the integrity of the globe. In the United States, reports of postoperative endophthalmitis after cataract surgery range from 0.04% to 0.41%. Postoperative endophthalmitis is generally the result of the perioperative introduction of bacteria to the patient's eye either from the patient's skin, lashes, or conjunctiva, or from contaminated instruments. Patients usually present within 6 weeks after surgery with symptoms of moderate to severe eye pain, decreased vision, photophobia, conjunctival hyperemia, discharge, chemosis (conjunctival edema), ocular and periocular inflammation, and hypopyon (pus in the anterior chamber). Endophthalmitis can result in decreased or permanent loss of vision; one-third of surgery patients who develop endophthalmitis do not gain vision better than light perception and counting fingers, and 50% never gain visual acuity better than 20/40.

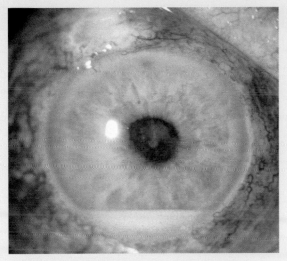

Eye with endophthalmitis, illustrating a hypopyon.

The practice of using antibiotic prophylaxis to prevent endophthalmitis after cataract surgery is well established; however, there is no consensus on the most appropriate agent or route to use. In European studies the use of intracameral cefuroxime was found to be effective in preventing endophthalmitis. An advantage of using the intracameral route is that the dose achieved in the anterior chamber is much higher than that achieved with topical administration.

Shorstein and partners (2013) undertook a study to determine postcataract surgery endophthalmitis in relation to practices for administering antibiotic prophylaxis using intracameral injections of cefuroxime, moxifloxacin, or vancomycin. Cefuroxime was the primary medication used for injection; moxifloxacin or vancomycin was used for patients with medication allergies.

In a more recent study, findings revealed that the average period between surgery and initial diagnosis of endophthalmitis was 8 days, with only 11% of cases developing more than 6 weeks after surgery. Diabetics were at a higher risk of developing endophthalmitis than their nondiabetic counterparts. Vitreous loss during surgery and extracapsular cataract extraction were also key factors that increased the risk of developing endophthalmitis. During the study, cultures were taken of each patient that developed endophthalmitis, and it was discovered that 36% of cases had positive culture results and 63% were negative. Eyes that tested positive for coagulase-negative staphylococci had better final visual acuity results than cases with enterococci and *Pseudomonas* species. Patients who lived in more rural locations had a significantly higher occurrence of endophthalmitis compared with urban patients. No follow-up study has yet been done to examine why patient locale had an effect on endophthalmitis patients, even though they were all treated at the same hospital facility. Interestingly, the rate of the disease was higher in left-eye surgeries than right-eye, even though there was a higher rate of surgeries performed on the right eye.

The authors concluded that an increase in the use of intracameral injection coincided with a large decline in the risk for endophthalmitis. There was a slight advantage to combining topical antibiotics with intracameral injection, and this warrants further study.

Modified from Hashemian H et al: Post cataract surgery endophthalmitis; brief literature review, *J Curr Ophthalmol* 28(3): 101–105, 2016; Jabbarvand M et al: Endophthalmitis occurring after cataract surgery, *Ophthalmology* 123(2):295–301, 2016; Shorstein NH et al: Decreased postoperative endophthalmitis rate after institution of intracameral antibiotics in a Northern California eye department, *J Cataract Refract Surg* 39(1):8–14, 2013.

---

instilling eyedrops and confirm that patients know how to properly instill drops for their postoperative care. Certain diseases such as arthritis can impede a patient's ability to instill his or her own eyedrops. The perioperative nurse should confirm that a caregiver is able to instill drops on behalf of the patient, as required, before discharge.

Before administering eyedrops, the perioperative nurse performs hand hygiene and checks the orders to verify which eye is to receive the drops. Check strength of the drug; if necessary, verify that it is for ophthalmic use. Put on gloves if there are secretions in or around the eye. The patient may be supine or sitting, with the head tilted back slightly. The nurse instructs the patient to look upward and then gently pulls the lower eyelid open to expose the lower conjunctival sac (Fig. 18.8). The prescribed number of drops is then administered without touching the tip of the dropper to the eye or fingers. Natural blinking distributes the drug evenly onto the eye surface.

To minimize systemic absorption of certain eyedrops, such as atropine, or maximize the absorption of the drop within the eye, the nurse may instruct the patient to immediately keep the eyelid closed and gently press on the nasolacrimal duct for 1 minute to prevent absorption into the circulatory system. When a toxic drug is instilled, the nurse uses a tissue or clean cotton ball to dry the inner corners of the patient's eyelids after each drop to minimize systemic absorption. When multiple eyedrop prescriptions are required, each drop of medication should be allowed to fully absorb within the eye before proceeding to the next. The nurse should wait at least 1 minute between applications of multiple eyedrops.

The nurse provides education about the expected effect of each medication so the patient is able to evaluate its effectiveness, detect signs and symptoms of adverse reactions, and know when to notify perioperative personnel concerning problems. The patient should also be well informed of any special considerations associated with specific medications so that appropriate safety precautions are taken.

Ophthalmic Pharmacology

Numerous medications are used during ophthalmic surgery (Surgical Pharmacology). They can be delivered as eyedrops, ointments, gels, or injected, or mixed in irrigations (Workman and LaCharity, 2016).

Text continued on p. 585

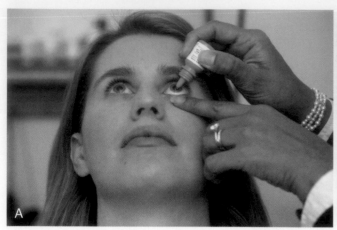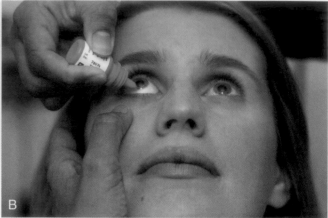

FIG. 18.8 Eye care professional applies eyedrops to dilate a patient's pupils. Positioning of the patient may require applying eyedrops from the left (A) or right side (B).

SURGICAL PHARMACOLOGY

Medications for Ophthalmic Surgery

Medication/Category	Dosage/Route	Purpose/Action	Adverse Reactions	Nursing Implications
Mydriatics (Dilation)				
Phenylephrine (Neo-Synephrine, Mydfrin)	Topical: 2.5%, 10% (occasionally used) Dosage per surgeon's order	Dilates pupil but permits focusing; causes vasoconstriction of conjunctiva and anterior vessels; used for objective examination of retina, testing of refraction, easier removal of lens; used alone or with a cycloplegic	Corneal microdeposits noted in almost all patients treated for more than 6 months (can lead to blurry vision) Hypertension, nausea, fever, narrow-angle glaucoma; interacts with tricyclic antidepressants	Standard red cap; use preoperatively; check for effect on cardiac and respiratory conditions; can stimulate sympathetic receptors; lasts 4–6 h
Cycloplegics (Dilation)				
Tropicamide (Mydriacyl)	Topical: 0.25%, 0.5%; mostly 1% is used Dosage per surgeon's order	Dilates pupil by paralyzing iris sphincter and accommodation muscles; anticholinergic, used for examination of fundus, refraction, uveitis, and relief of pain from ciliary spasm	Interacts with tricyclic antidepressants; cardiovascular effects in higher doses; use may cause delusions	Standard red cap; use preoperatively; may precipitate attack of narrow-angle glaucoma; lasts 4–6 h
Atropine	Topical: 0.5%, 1% Dosage per surgeon's order	Anticholinergic; dilates pupil; potent	Mydriasis, blurred vision, photophobia, decreased visual acuity, tearing, dry eyes or dry conjunctiva, eye irritation, crusting of eyelid	Standard red cap; used preoperatively; patient may be sensitive to light; may use slight pressure on lacrimal punctum to prevent systematic absorption; lasts 7–14 days
Cyclopentolate (Cyclogyl)	Topical: 0.5%, 1%, 2% Dosage per surgeon's order	Anticholinergic; dilates pupil; inhibits focusing	Extremely narrow anterior chamber angles Use with caution in Down syndrome patients Not used in younger than 1 year of age Tachycardia Hypertension May occasionally cause the full spectrum of systemic atropinic toxicity	Standard red cap; used preoperatively; duration up to 24 h

SURGICAL PHARMACOLOGY

Medications for Ophthalmic Surgery—cont'd

Medication/Category	Dosage/Route	Purpose/Action	Adverse Reactions	Nursing Implications
Epinephrine PF mixture	Intracameral or topical: (1:500)/0.3–0.5 mL Dosage per surgeon's order	Dilates pupil; added to BSS for irrigation to maintain pupil dilation; constricts blood vessels to prevent bleeding	—	Red cap; syringes should be well marked to measure 0.3 mL; comes in 1-amp vial
Combination Dilation Eyedrops				
Hydroxyamphetamine (Paredrine, Paremyd), tropicamide (Mydriacyl)	Topical: hydroxyamphetamine 1%; tropicamide 0.25% Dosage per surgeon's order	Combination of parasympathetic antagonist and sympathetic agonist; simplifies process of dilation	Tachycardia Hypertension Contraindicated for closed-angle glaucoma	Red cap; onset 15 min; Duration 45–60 min
Intracameral Injections				
Epi-Shugarcaine	9 mL BSS Plus 3 mL 4% lidocaine/4 mL epinephrine 1:1000 PF (bisulfate free)	Used to dilate pupil; helps maintain dilation intraoperatively; used for floppy iris syndrome and patients with small pupils	Inflammation or foreign body sensation Contraindicated if allergic to any of the ingredients	Caution: Must be precisely mixed by perioperative nurse according to surgeon's order Different strengths and mixtures possible Use blunt-tip 25- to 30-gauge cannula, 2-mL syringe
Miotics (Parasympathetic Constriction)				
Carbachol (Miostat)	Intracameral: 0.01% in 1.5-mL vial Dosage per surgeon's order	Potent cholinergic; constricts pupil; used intracamerally during anterior segment surgery	Ciliary or accommodative spasm, blurred vision, reduced night vision, diaphoresis, increased salivation, urinary frequency, nausea, diarrhea, bronchial asthma Use with caution with Parkinson disease	Green packaging; use blunt-tip anterior chamber needle; used intraoperatively
Acetylcholine chloride (Miochol-E)	Intracameral: 1% 1:100 solution in 2-mL dual-chamber univial Dosage per surgeon's order	Cholinergic; rapidly constricts pupil by activating parasympathetic nervous system; used intraocularly during anterior segment surgery to constrict a dilated pupil	Iris spasm that may be painful, flushing of face, corneal edema, decompensation, allergies to any ingredients	Onset 15–30 s; comes from medication-dispensing system; preset vials with green lettering
Pilocarpine hydrochloride	Topical: 1%, 4% Dosage per surgeon's order	Cholinergic; constricts pupil; used topically for lowering IOP in glaucoma	Acute uveitis, headaches, decreased night vision	Green top; used preoperatively and postoperatively; lasts 4–6 h
Topical Anesthetics				
Tetracaine hydrochloride (Pontocaine)	Topical: 0.5% Dosage per surgeon's order	Anesthetic and pain reliever	Can compromise cornea epithelium Category C pregnancy and lactation	Clear or white cap bottle; used preoperatively and postoperatively; onset 5–20 s; duration of action 10–20 min; if pain persists contact surgeon
Proparacaine hydrochloride (Ophthaine)	Topical: 0.5% Dosage per surgeon's order	Anesthetic and pain reliever	Known hypersensitivity to any component of the solution Softening and erosion of corneal epithelium have been reported	White cap bottles; used preoperatively; onset 5–20 s; duration of action 10–20 min; if pain persists contact surgeon

Continued

SURGICAL PHARMACOLOGY

Medications for Ophthalmic Surgery—cont'd

Medication/Category	Dosage/Route	Purpose/Action	Adverse Reactions	Nursing Implications
Lidocaine hydrochloride gel (Akten)	Topical: 3.5% Most often used 10 min before surgery Dosage per surgeon's order	Anesthetic and pain reliever	Known hypersensitivity to any component of the solution	Used preoperatively; apply to the surface of the eyeball under the upper and lower lids; can desensitize corneal nerves and may lead to neurotrophic corneal ulcers and melting
Injectable Anesthetics				
Lidocaine (Xylocaine), lidocaine-MPF (preservative free)	1%, 2%, 4% Dosage per surgeon's order; available for injection, as a gel for topical application	Anesthetic and pain reliever; local skin injection, retrobulbar and peribulbar blocks; gel (jelly) applied topically	Known hypersensitivity to any component of the solution; monitor cardiac and CNS symptoms; watch for LAST	Injected preoperatively and intraoperatively; onset 4–6 min; duration of action 40–60 min; 120 min with epinephrine
Bupivacaine (Marcaine, Sensorcaine), bupivicane-MPF (preservative free), hyaluronidase (Hydase) (enzyme)	0.25%, 0.50%, 0.75%; hyaluronidase: 1 mL Dosage per surgeon's order	Anesthetic and pain reliever; local skin injection facial nerve block; hyaluronidase is occasionally added to bupivacaine to enhance diffusion of the anesthetic	Watch dosage in patients with hepatic or renal disease	Preoperatively and intraoperatively; onset 5–11 min; duration of action 8–12 h with epinephrine; often used in 0.75% combination with lidocaine for blocks
Mepivacaine (Carbocaine)	1%, 2% Dosage per surgeon's order	Local anesthetic and pain reliever; injection: used for blocks	Long acting, can affect cardiac and CNS (LAST)	Onset 3–5 min; duration of action 120 min, greater with epinephrine
Viscoelastics/Adherents				
Sodium hyaluronate chondroitin sulfate (Healon, GV5, Amvisc, Provisc, Viscoat, DuoVisc)	Intracameral: Prepared syringes; dose labeled on syringe to surgeon's order	Coats and protects corneal endothelium, intraocular structure, and tissue; helps increase volume to push structures away such as filling capsular bag	Increased IOP, punctate keratitis, cystoid macular edema, postcapsular opacity No known contraindications if used according to manufacturer's instructions	Some brands require refrigeration; allow 30 min to warm to room temperature; check manufacturer's inserts for single-use syringe; GV5 requires surgeon certification
Irrigants				
BSS (Endosol)	Topical and intracamerally	Used to keep cornea moist during surgery; also used as internal irrigant into anterior or posterior segments	Corneal edema has occurred Use with caution with diabetic patients during vitrectomy	Solution most used in eye surgery; used preoperatively and intraoperatively; preservative free; do not use for more than one patient
BSS enriched with bicarbonate, dextrose, and glutathione (BSS Plus, Endosol Extra)	Intracameral; not for injection or IV infusion	Used as internal irrigant into anterior or posterior segment; provides better metabolic support for ocular tissues during long procedures	When corneal endothelium is abnormal, irrigation, trauma can cause bullous keratopathy	Used intraoperatively; need to reconstitute immediately before use by addition of part 1 to part 2 with transfer device; never use part 1 or part 2 alone; may result in damage to the eye
Steroid Antiinflammatory Agents				
Betamethasone sodium phosphate and betamethasone acetate suspension (Celestone)	Injection; comes in single-use local infiltration	Injected and used to treat severe allergic and inflammatory ocular conditions; also used with blocks	Foreign body sensation	Stored in medication-dispensing system; used preoperatively and intraoperatively

SURGICAL PHARMACOLOGY

Medications for Ophthalmic Surgery—cont'd

Medication/Category	Dosage/Route	Purpose/Action	Adverse Reactions	Nursing Implications
Dexamethasone (Decadron)	Injection: 4 mg/mL injected into conjunctiva	Adrenocortical; injected subconjunctivally postoperatively for inflammation prophylaxis and used to treat severe allergic and inflammatory conditions	Fungus infection, increased IOP	Stored in medication-dispensing system; used intraoperatively
Prednisolone (Pred Forte, Econopred, Inflamase)	Topical drops suspension: 1% Dosage per surgeon's order	For reducing inflammation and severe allergic conditions	Elevated IOP and cataract formation	Pink cap; shake bottle before use; preoperative and postoperative use
Fluoromethalone (FML, Flarex)	Topical eyedrops, suspension, or ointment: 0.1%, 0.25% Dosage per surgeon's order	For reducing inflammation and severe allergic conditions	Elevated IOP and subcapsular cataract formation	Pink cap; shake bottle before applying to cornea postoperatively; use ointment form for longer lasting dose
NSAIDs				
Nepafanec (Nevanac), flurbiprofen (Ocufen), ketorolac (Acular), diclofenac (Voltaren), bromofenac (Xibrom)	Topical eyedrops: 2–4 times daily	Topical treatment of inflammation	Adverse effect is corneal melting	Gray cap; used preoperatively and postoperatively
Antiinfectives				
Aminoglycosides: gentamicin (Genoptic, Gentak), besifloxacin (Besivance, Moxeza), tobramycin (Aktob, Tobrex), norfloxacin (Chibroxin) ophthalmic	Topical drops: 2–4 times daily Dosage per surgeon's order and manufacturer's instructions	Topical treatment of bacterial superficial ocular infections	Allergic reaction to ingredients, itching, redness	Brown or tan cap; used preoperatively and postoperatively
Quinolones: gatifloxacin (Zymaxid), ofloxacin (Ocuflox), ciprofloxacin (Ciloxan), levofloxacin (Iquix, Quixin), moxifloxacin (Vigamox) ophthalmic	Topical drops: 2–4 times daily Dosage per surgeon's order and manufacturer's instructions	Topical treatment of superficial bacterial ocular infections at time of surgery	Allergic reaction to ingredients, itching, redness	Brown or tan cap; used preoperatively and postoperatively
Injectable Antiinfectives				
Cefazolin (Ancef, Kefzol)	1 g mixed with 4.8 mL sterile water; use 0.5 mL for subconjunctival injections Dosage per surgeon's order	Prophylactically injected subconjunctivally/intracamerally for endophthalmitis	Hypersensitivity to any component	Perioperative nurse mixes medication; careful calculation and validation that dosage is correct; stability and sterility must be maintained; syringes must measure low concentrations, no air bubbles left in syringes; 6–24 h expiration
Vancomycin	1 g mixed with 20 mL sterile water Dosage per surgeon's order	Prophylactic for eye infections	Hypersensitivity to any component	Perioperative nurse reconstitutes drug according to manufacturer's instructions; careful calculation and validation of dosage; syringes must measure low concentrations, no air bubbles left in syringe
Tobramycin	Dosage per surgeon's order	Intravitreal injections for active endophthalmitis	Lid itching; hypersensitivity to any component	Careful calculation and validation that dosage is correct; syringes must measure low concentrations, no air bubbles left in syringe

Continued

SURGICAL PHARMACOLOGY

Medications for Ophthalmic Surgery—cont'd

Medication/Category	Dosage/Route	Purpose/Action	Adverse Reactions	Nursing Implications
Miscellaneous				
Cocaine	Topical: 1%–4%	Used on cornea to loosen epithelium before debridement and on nasal packing to reduce congestion of mucosa; topically used for packing for dacryocystorhinostomy Afrin spray (oxymetazoline) may be used topically instead of 4% cocaine	Damage or soften corneal epithelium Sloughing of tissue with too much vasoconstriction	Never injected; must be kept with controlled substances
Hyperosmotic agent, mannitol (Osmitrol)	IV dosage per surgeon's order	IV osmotic diuretic to reduce IOP	Use with caution in renal disease, dehydration, diuresis	Administered IV by anesthesia provider
Trypan (VisionBlue)	Intracameral: 0.6%	For capsule staining and identification in complex cataract surgery	Can stain IOL implant up to 1 wk if not irrigated out of the eye	Precaution: Confirm label for ophthalmic use; follow manufacturer's instructions
Tissue plasminogen activator (TPA) (Activase)	6.25–25 mcg per 0.1 mL Loaded into syringe after defrosted	Used to treat fibrin formation in postvitrectomy patients; lysis of clots on retina	Bleeding	Drug is stored in frozen single-dose aliquots; must be defrosted at least 30 min to reach room temperature
Corneal fibrin glue (Tisseel, Evicel, Artiss)	Corneal glue	Biologically derived tissue sealant; used for controlling bleeding and to secure tissue to the surface of the eye (e.g., securing conjunctival tissue during pterygium surgery or ocular surgery where amniotic membrane is used to cover an abnormality or conjunctival defect)	—	Begins to polymerize in about 30 s to 1 min; totally secure in 10 min
Acetazolamide sodium (Diamox)	IV 500 mg or 125–500 mg orally; frequency depends on dosage	Carbonic anhydrase inhibitor; IOP lowering by suppressing the secretion of aqueous humor	Swelling of lens, myopia, gastrointestinal intolerance, drowsiness, lethargy, depression, renal sulfa hypersensitivity	Orange packaging; administered IV by anesthesia provider; communicate about sulfa allergies and report to surgeon if there is a reaction; receive order from surgeon to discontinue use
Antimetabolite				
Mitomycin (MMC), fluorouracil (5-FU)	Topical: 0.2–0.4 mg/mL for 90 s or longer per surgeon's orders; application is done with several Weck-Cel sponges	Antimetabolite used topically to inhibit scar formation in glaucoma-filtering procedures and pterygium excision	Known reaction to any components; MMC is toxic and potentially hazardous; avoid exposure to unintended tissue	Chemotherapeutic drug; handle and discard in compliance with OSHA and facility policies for safe use of antineoplastics

BSS, Balanced salt solution; *CNS*, central nervous system; *IOL*, intraocular lens; *IOP*, intraocular pressure; *IV*, intravenous; *LAST*, local anesthetic systemic toxicity; *MPF*, Methylparaben free; *NSAIDs*, nonsteroidal antiinflammatory drugs; *OSHA*, Occupational Safety and Health Administration; *PF*, preservative free; *s*, seconds.

NOTE: Color codes for topical ocular medication caps are based on the American Academy of Ophthalmology recommendations to the Food and Drug Administration to aid patients in distinguishing among drops, minimizing the chance of using an incorrect medication.

Modified from Review of Ophthalmology: *Ocular sealants and glues in review* (website), 2014. www.reviewofophthalmology.com/article/ocular-sealants-and-glues-in-review. (Accessed 16 February 2017); *Ophthalmic drug fact sheet*, St Louis, 2011, Wolters Kluwer Health; Brodie SE, Francis JH: Aging and disorders of the eye. In Fillit HM, editor: *Brocklehurst's textbook of geriatric medicine and gerontology*, ed 2, St Louis, 2017, Elsevier; Gault JA, Vander JF: *Ophthalmology secrets in color*, ed 4, Philadelphia, 2016, Elsevier; Gyang KO: *Ocular drugs handbook: an easy reference guide to eye medications*, Bloomington, IN, 2008, AuthorHouse; Workman ML: Care of patients with eye and vison problems. In Ignatavicius DD, Workman LL: *Medical-surgical nursing: patient-centered collaborative care*, ed 8, St Louis, 2017, Elsevier.

Anesthesia

Local Anesthesia. The three types of ocular blocks are retrobulbar, peribulbar, and subtenon (parabulbar). The typical anesthetic agents used in the blocks are 2% lidocaine, 0.75% bupivacaine, and hyaluronidase (enzyme). The total volume mixed is generally 10 mL; however, the usual volume given is much less and depends on the technique chosen by the surgeon. Ocular blocks are performed by the surgeon because of the proximity to major nerve endings and muscles.

Ocular Blocks. The *retrobulbar block* has the highest risk of all the ocular blocks (Fig. 18.9). This block uses a 3-L syringe armed with a retrobulbar needle; the needle's tip is specially designed not to lacerate blood vessels. The surgeon places the needle inferior to the globe, in the outer one-third of the orbital rim. After the needle is past the equator of the globe, it is directed toward the orbital apex while the patient is looking upward and inward. This block is given retro, or behind the eye (muscle cone). The advantages of this widely used block are the relatively small volume of solution required, excellent anesthesia, and loss of voluntary eye muscle control. Its risks include perforation of the globe, hemorrhage, damage to the optic nerve, and injection of the muscle; a major risk is brainstem anesthesia.

The *peribulbar block* carries a moderate risk and is given outside of the muscle cone (Fig. 18.10). The surgeon begins with the needle in the inferior lateral orbital rim. It is then directed under and away from the globe. The peribulbar block uses a larger volume of local anesthetic and diffuses into the retro space. The advantages of this block include increased safety because there is less chance of hitting

the optic nerve or causing brainstem anesthesia. Associated risks are perforation (smaller risk than the retrobulbar block), hemorrhage, unpredictable akinesia, conjunctival chemosis, and extended lead time for effects to set up.

A *subtenon block* is administered after facial skin preparation (prep). The surgeon makes a small inferior nasal incision with dissection past the equator of the globe using blunt scissors. The injection is given inferior nasal to the globe using a blunt cannula. The advantages of this block include increased safety because the surgeon is unlikely to perforate the globe, relatively quick onset, and smaller volumes than the peribulbar block. Disadvantages are chemosis, inconsistent akinesia, and the time for the block to take effect.

Topical Anesthesia. The most common ophthalmic anesthetic agents are proparacaine and tetracaine. These topical anesthetics are useful to check IOP and temporarily relieve pain for diagnostic purposes. Topical anesthetics are given in the OR before the facial prep. Each medication is applied in the superior and inferior conjunctival fornices with the patient in supine position. The cornea becomes numb with the first drop, but the conjunctiva is more difficult to numb and may require another application. The process is finished with the application of lidocaine gel to the upper and lower conjunctival surface. Advantages of topical anesthesia include no risk of perforation or retrobulbar hemorrhage and quick onset. Disadvantages include no akinesia and no block of the seventh nerve to prevent the patient from squeezing the eye.

Positioning

Positioning the patient for ophthalmic surgery generally requires additional devices for stabilizing the head, protecting bony prominences, and providing appropriate alignment to prevent peripheral neurovascular injury. The ophthalmology stretcher, which is a combination transport device and OR bed, is often used for convenience and comfort. This stretcher, with a tapered head end, allows for closer access to the patient's face and eliminates transfers for the patient. The perioperative nurse positions the patient with a foam donut or headrest under the head and a pillow under the back of the knees. For procedural reasons, the nurse often tucks the patient's arms at the side, pads the elbows to protect the ulnar nerve, faces the palms inward, and maintains the wrists in a neutral position; a drape, tucked snuggly under the patient, not under the mattress, prevents the arm from shifting downward intraoperatively and resting against the OR bed rail (AORN, 2017).

If patients are to be sedated, the nurse asks if they are comfortable. Some elderly patients prefer not to discuss their discomfort for fear

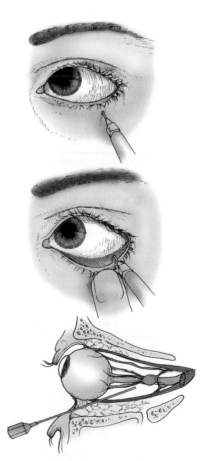

FIG. 18.9 Retrobulbar block.

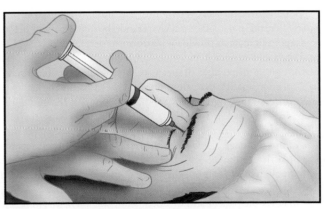

FIG. 18.10 Peribulbar block.

of being bothersome, so it is important to pay attention to their body language and cues.

Intraocular surgery is usually carried out with the use of a microscope. A special wrist rest may be used to stabilize the surgeon's hands and may include perforated tubing or a bar to provide oxygen under the drapes. The nurse should attach the tube to the bed and secure it approximately 2.5 cm below the patient's lateral canthus before draping. The wrist rest may be placed unilaterally or may encircle the head. A strip of tape is sometimes placed over the patient's forehead (avoiding the eyebrows) and secured to the OR bed to provide head stabilization.

Prepping

The operative site is prepped under aseptic conditions, usually after the anesthetic is administered. A sterile prep tray commonly contains sterile normal saline solution, irrigation bulb, basins, gauze sponges, cotton-tipped applicators, towels, and antimicrobial skin disinfectant.

Some surgeons order one or two drops of 5% povidone-iodine solution administered to the eye surface before prep of the face and eyelids to reduce rates of conjunctival bacterial load and risk of endophthalmitis (AORN, 2017). Unless the patient has been administered a general anesthetic, a topical anesthetic drop is placed to minimize the stinging sensation. Povidone-iodine may be contraindicated in patients with allergic reactions to *topical* iodine. For these patients a mixture of baby shampoo and balanced salt solution (BSS) can be used as the agent for the facial prep instead of povidone-iodine.

The nurse cleans the patient's lid margins by inverting the lids and cleaning with cotton-tipped applicators moistened with antimicrobial skin disinfectant, taking care to prevent the solution from entering the patient's ears. The eye may then be irrigated with normal saline solution using an irrigating bulb. When toxic chemicals or small particles of foreign matter must be removed, the eye surface and conjunctival sac are thoroughly flushed with tepid sterile normal saline solution using an irrigation bulb or an Asepto syringe. The nurse pats dry the prep area so the drape with adherent backs will hold. The surgical prep is completed before draping and starting the procedure so the solution has adequate time to dry.

Draping

Special concerns for eye surgery draping include repelling water, eliminating lint and fiber particles, and providing adequate air exchange for patients receiving local anesthetics. A cardboard bridge that adheres to the sides of the patient's face may be used to support the drape above the patient's mouth and nose. The surgeon may request that the nurse place a Mayo stand above the patient before the draping process to provide a platform to decrease the weight of the drapes and surgical handpieces/tubing on the patient. The use of a one-piece disposable drape, with a self-adherent, fenestrated plastic section for the eye, eliminates the need to lift the patient's head during draping and facilitates drape removal at the end of the procedure. The eyelids may be separated when applying the self-adherent plastic eye drape to keep the eyelashes out of the operative eye. A fluid drainage bag with a wicking strip may also be adhered to the plastic eye drape.

In an alternative method, the surgeon may drape the head with a half-sheet and two towels, use a large sheet or U-drape or split sheet to cover the patient and OR bed, and place a fenestrated plastic eye drape over the operative site (Fig. 18.11).

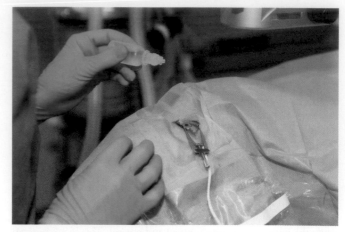

FIG. 18.11 Draped patient. The scrub person keeps the cornea moist with saline solution during eye surgery.

Instrumentation

Additional instruments, depending on the type of procedure, can be added to the basic instrument set. Special surface finishes are used to reduce light reflection. Instruments are designed with round handles for smoother motion and rotation under the microscope. Instruments are placed on the Mayo stand; the order of their use can be listed on the surgeon's preference card or computerized pick list.

A variety of ophthalmic forceps are designed for specific use with different tissues of the eye. Fixation forceps, used to hold tissue firmly in place or provide traction before incision, have an angled tooth that overlaps for secure fixation. Suturing forceps, used to pick up wound edges for dissection or suturing, are single-toothed forceps with the tooth at a right angle to the shank of the forceps. Tying forceps have a flat platform for holding suture as it is tied.

Care and Handling. To maintain the quality and precision of all ophthalmic instruments, including microsurgical instruments, strict criteria for care and handling must be followed. Storage cases protect instrument tips and cutting surfaces. Instruments should be inspected under magnification when purchased and before and after each use, observing for burrs on tips, nicks on cutting surfaces, and alignment of jaws. The scrub person should clean eye instruments used during the procedure with nonfibrous sponges to avoid damaging delicate instrument tips. Personnel handling instruments should know the name and purpose of each instrument. Tissue can be damaged by the use of an inappropriate instrument, and instruments can be damaged by inappropriate use. After use, instruments should be cleaned, thoroughly dried, and terminally sterilized before storage in protective containers.

It is recommended that microsurgical instruments are cleaned according to manufacturer's instructions for use (IFU). If permissible, they may undergo ultrasonic cleaning with distilled water and an appropriate enzymatic cleansing agent. Enzymatic detergents may elevate the risk for TASS; instruments must be thoroughly rinsed and IFU carefully followed (Mamalis, 2016). They can be individually handheld or immersed together in the ultrasonic cleaner as long as they are not touching each other. These instruments have small lumens, which must be thoroughly cleaned to remove debris that may cause TASS (Goodman and Spry, 2017). Instruments should be rinsed with distilled water and thoroughly dried. A hot-air blower (never a towel) should be used for drying instruments. Instrument lubricant should not be used on an irrigating cannula because residue can be introduced into the eye and cause damage.

In addition to basic care and handling, a routine preventive maintenance program should be established for sharpening, realigning, and adjusting precision eye instruments. Keeping an instrument in good repair is much less expensive than buying a new one. Disposable instruments offer accessibility and quality assurance; for example, forceps are properly aligned for each use because they have not been used on other procedures. Benefits for the institution include elimination of costs related to repairs. Knives are available with retractable blades to minimize occupational exposure to bloodborne pathogens from accidental sharps injuries.

Equipment Used. A wide range of equipment is used in ophthalmic surgery. The perioperative team's knowledge of proper functioning and troubleshooting should be confirmed through inservice education and training specific to new equipment. For safety, all items must be used according to the IFU and tested for proper performance before the patient enters the OR. Although products and manufacturers may vary, the following are some of the typical pieces of equipment and accessories used in ophthalmic surgeries:

- *Phacoemulsification machines (phaco):* These machines produce ultrasound frequency vibrations, which in a fluid medium emulsify and break up the cataract. Irrigation and aspiration (I/A) handpieces are used. Phaco tips and handpieces can be chosen with different diameters and straight or curved tips. Ultra-chopper tips are available for torsional handpieces. The scrub person must be aware of the high speed in which ultra-chopper tips function; the slightest wrong movement may shatter the cataract. Bipolar electrosurgical unit (ESU) and anterior vitrectomy handpieces may also be attached when needed. The surgeon controls the foot pedal and chooses one of the following modes by depressing the pedal to a certain position: irrigation alone; irrigation and aspiration; and irrigation, aspiration, and phacoemulsification combined. Some machines also have an anterior vitrector. As the surgeon manipulates the handpiece and operates the foot pedal to emulsify the lens nucleus, the perioperative nurse monitors the function of the instrument and operates the console controls to change settings such as irrigation bottle height. The irrigation used is BSS. Tubing attached to the handpiece has low compliance and helps reduce the intraoperative fluid surge that may occur after an occlusion blockage suddenly releases. It is important to ensure that all parts of the phaco machine are functioning properly before the procedure. Improperly used phaco units can cause corneal burns.
- *Posterior vitrectomy machines:* Functions on these machines may include vitrectomy with cutter handpieces for removal of vitreous; extrusion for gentle aspiration near sensitive retina and macula; oil infusion; bipolar electrosurgery or diathermy; and motorized cutting with electric scissors attachment. Foot pedal or manual controls can set eye pressure and cut and suction rates.
- *Cryotherapy machine:* The cryotherapy machine is generally used to cause an inflammatory reaction in the retinal tissue that seals a break or tear. The unit uses nitrous oxide as the freezing agent. Adequate pressure settings are needed for acceptable levels of freeze. External and intraocular handpieces are available.
- *Lasers:* Lasers are used for various applications in eye procedures, whether for clearing an opacified posterior capsule after cataract surgery, for reshaping or creating a flap of the cornea, or for direct use inside the eye during posterior vitrectomy. Settings must be confirmed with the surgeon. When the laser is in use,

everyone in the OR must wear appropriate protective eyewear according to the laser's wavelength. Warning signs are posted on doors, and windows are covered to avoid scatter outside the room (Chapter 8 further discusses laser safety measures).
- *ESU units:* Bipolar or monopolar ESUs may be used. Fire precautions are observed, especially in the presence of oxygen (Chapter 8 further discusses ESU safety measures).
- *Operating microscope:* Most ophthalmic procedures are performed using a surgical microscope. Proper care and maintenance of the operating microscope are essential to ensure optimal functioning and durability of this sophisticated, expensive piece of equipment.

It is the perioperative nurse's responsibility to adjust the microscope's oculars (eyepieces) before surgery to obtain the clearest view of the operating field. The perioperative nurse must be familiar with how to adjust pupillary distance (e.g., the distance between pupils of the user's eyes) and diopter settings on the oculars for operator vision correction to work without eyeglasses comfortably. The angle of the ocular should also be adjusted for appropriate viewing and personal comfort without scrunching or stretching. Users who have significant astigmatism should wear their eyeglasses and set the oculars at zero because uncorrected astigmatisms cannot be entered into the microscope's ocular setting. If there is an uncorrected refractive error, the minus (myopia) or plus (hyperopia) error should be entered on the ocular dial, each hash mark indicting a diopter of correction. Users should be aware of their own refractive errors because they can cause decreased visual acuity during surgery. For safety, the microscope should be tested and adjusted for proper performance before the patient enters the room. The centering buttons on the microscope for the vertical and horizontal planes should be set before the procedure begins by pushing each button once. The microscope spotlight should be in gross focus, obtained by manually raising or lowering the microscope head or the OR bed height. Some microscopes used for other applications such as plastic surgery may use light sources that are so bright they can damage the retina. The nurse must ensure that the microscope used in ophthalmic surgery is specifically intended and safe for eye surgery. Other responsibilities include full command of how the scope needs to be focused and all the movements of the arms of the scope. Microscopes are adjusted for right eye and left eye procedures (Fig. 18.12).

Ophthalmic Sutures

Sutures used in ophthalmic surgery are very fine and range in size from 4-0 to 10-0. Handling and arming these sutures can be a challenge for the scrub person with uncorrected presbyopia. Fine eye sutures produce minimum reaction and discomfort for the patient. They should be handled as little as possible to avoid weakening and fraying. Ophthalmic needles also are very delicate and must be handled with extreme care and inspected for evidence of burrs before use. During ophthalmic microscopic procedures, a modified neutral zone is used. The scrub person should place the sharp in the surgeon's hand. The surgeon should then return the sharp to the designated neutral zone (AORN, 2017).

Ophthalmic Dressings

At the completion of the operation, the operative eye area is cleansed with saline sponges. After plastic surgery procedures on the lids or lacrimal ducts, antibiotic ophthalmic ointment may be thinly spread over the skin and eyelashes to prevent adhesion of the bandage.

folded eyepatch covered with a second single-layer eyepatch, may be used when compression is desired.

Application of Corneal Shields. Contact lenses, applied directly onto the cornea, are used by patients to correct refractive errors instead of eyeglasses. It is important for the perioperative nurse to confirm that patients have removed all contact lenses before surgery and understand they must abstain from contact lens use until the ophthalmologist permits. Collagen corneal shields look like contact lenses and are used postoperatively to distribute postoperative medication and protect the eye after surgery.

Perioperative nurses should be able to apply corneal shields to the patient's eye with comfort. The nurse applies a glove to the dominant hand and places the corneal shield on the index finger. Using the nondominant hand, the upper eyelid is gently lifted while pulling down the lower lid with the middle finger of the dominant hand. The nurse instructs the patient to slightly look up and then gently places the corneal shield on the cornea and instructs the patient to blink the shield into place. The corneal shield may naturally fall out of the eye during the postoperative period, usually within 4 to 12 hours. The nurse discusses this with the patient and reinforces that it is a normal process and the shield should be reapplied.

Evaluation

The nurse evaluates the patient's general condition before transport to the postanesthesia care unit (PACU) or observation unit. The general appearance of the skin is assessed, with areas around the face and bony prominences noted for redness or other changes from the preoperative condition.

A hand-off report to the receiving nurse in the PACU or observation area includes postoperative positioning requirements, potential problems specific to the patient, and preoperative anxiety level and use of coping mechanisms.

Evaluation should address whether the patient met the desired perioperative nursing outcomes; the patient's responses may be documented as outcome statements. The following examples are based on the nursing diagnoses identified in the plan of care:

- The patient, family, or significant others verbalized knowledge regarding the diagnosis, planned intervention, medication management, and requirements for home care maintenance.
- The patient verbalized an acceptable level of anxiety and used effective coping mechanisms.
- The patient remained comfortable during the intervention as determined by pain scale response.
- The patient will remain free from injury related to altered visual sensory perception.

Patient, Family, and Caregiver Education and Discharge Planning

Patient education is one of the nurse's greatest contributions. Some facilities have programs with group teaching for patients; in other settings, education is provided individually. Depending on the setting, the nursing role in patient education may include review of preoperative expectations, individual patient needs, surgeon's instructions, procedure, IOL choices (if applicable), and overview of the surgery experience.

Implementation of the plan of care actually begins during the patient interview. Planning to meet the patient's educational needs should play an equal role with meeting other needs. Verbal review and reinforcement of information initially provided in the physician's office ensures consistency in teaching. Written material and audiovisual media (closed circuit television, DVDs, tablet computers, photos,

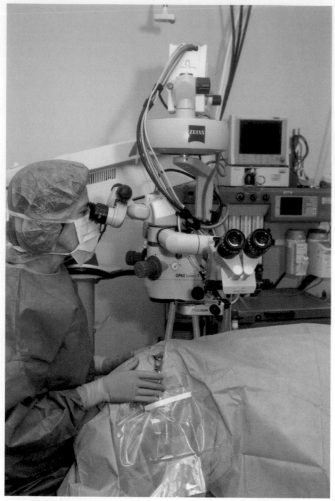

FIG. 18.12 When the patient is in position, the perioperative nurse sets the microscope into focus. Head is positioned properly for surgery.

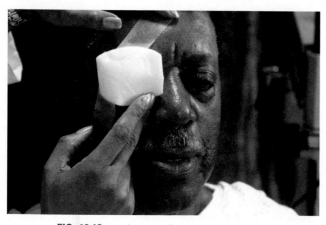

FIG. 18.13 Application of a protective eyepatch.

The initial dressing is a sterile eye pad secured with nonallergenic tape (Fig. 18.13). After intraocular operations, when external pressure on the eyes might be harmful, the initial dressing is covered with a protecting, perforated aluminum plate or plastic eye shield. Postcataract dressings range from traditional eye pads to collagen corneal shields rehydrated in an antiinfective-antiinflammatory solution to no dressing at all. A pressure bandage, consisting of a

PATIENT ENGAGEMENT EXEMPLAR

Patient-Centered Care in Ophthalmic Surgery

Patient-centered care recognizes the obligation to understand and meet patients' expectations, and partnerships between nurses and patients are a cornerstone of patient-centered care. It is especially important to fulfill that obligation in providing care to ophthalmology patients who may be experiencing challenges with visual acuity. Providing patient-centered care is further challenged by the ambulatory nature of most ophthalmic procedures. In 1992 the Institute for Family-Centered Care was established. It has nine principles, among which are respect for patient's values, preferences, and expressed needs and involvement of family and friends.

In the scenario that follows the nurse practices patient-centered care by considering the effect of communication and relationships on the outcomes of the patient's care.

Mr. B. is an energetic 76-year-old African American male with glaucoma in both eyes and a dense cataract in the left eye. Glaucoma has left him blind in the right eye, with some peripheral loss in the left eye. Mr. B. has been married for 45 years and goes to church every Sunday with his wife. She is the main caregiver.

In providing patient-centered communication for Mr. B., the nurse notes, "I see on your consent for today's surgery that you are having a trabeculectomy on the left eye combined with cataract removal and implementation of a lens. Can you tell me in your own words what that means?" She then listens carefully to

determine that Mr. B. understands the procedure. An indication that Mr. B. understands might include the following response:

"The doctor tells me that the pressure in my good eye is too high, like a basketball that has too much air in it. She wants to make a release valve so that fluids can drain and stop the high pressure. The doctor also said I have a cataract and she will remove that and put a new lens in at the same time. I might have to keep taking my pressure drops, but I may have to take them less often if the surgery works."

Before discharge, Mr. B.'s patch will be removed. The perioperative nurse should work with his wife to orient him to the room and those around him. Even with the patch removed his visual acuity will be greatly diminished the first 24 hours and he will continue to require constant care. Mr. B. should have light perception and can count fingers and see blurry images until further healing occurs. The nurse partners with the patient and his wife to ensure they both understand to continue the eyedrop regimen and make sure labels can be seen by the patient. They may need to use a magnifying glass or write larger letters on forms and medicine bottles. The nurse reinforces that Mr. B. will be required to wear the shield while sleeping, so he will not be able to navigate by himself. The nurse may also explore community assistance as part of patient-centered care to assist Mr. B. and his wife through the initial recovery period and challenges associated with partial blindness.

Modified from Frampton SB, Guastello S: Patient-centered care: more than the sum of its parts—Planetree's patient-centered hospital designation programme, *World Hosp Health Serv* 46(4):13–16, 2010; Rawson JV, Moretz J: Patient- and family centered care: a primer, *J Am Coll Radiol* 13(12 Pt B):1544–1549, 2016.

and patient information websites) may be used to enhance patient education programs but do not eliminate the need for direct interchange with patients and feedback from them.

Family members or friends should be included to add support and increase understanding of the planned surgery. The loss of sight produces the same staged coping behaviors of grieving that move the individual from denial to acceptance. Thorough preoperative preparation of the patient and those who will assist with care at home in the postoperative period plays a vital role in the successful outcome of the surgical procedure (Patient Engagement Exemplar). General guidelines for patient, family, and caregiver education for the patient undergoing ophthalmic surgery include the following:

- Purpose and desired results of preoperative eyedrops and sedation
- Explanation of what to expect from the anesthetic
- Activities and routines of the intraoperative period
- What to expect immediately after surgery, including pain and visual acuity
- Designated driver after procedures
- Verbal and written IFUs of eyedrops and other medications
- Any limitations on activities (bending, lifting, eye rubbing, special positioning)
- Wound care, protective sunglasses
- Signs and symptoms of complications
- Follow-up postoperative phone calls from the ambulatory surgery center, as applicable
- Who to call with questions or concerns
- Follow-up appointments

The Patient, Family, and Caregiver Education box has additional examples of instructions specific to cataract surgery.

Surgical Interventions

Surgery of the Lens

Cataract Extraction

Cataract surgery is the leading diagnosis for ambulatory surgery visits, with more than 3 million lens extractions performed yearly in the United States (Ambulatory Surgery Considerations). It is estimated that more than 24 million Americans older than age 40 have a cataract, and this number is expected to increase as baby boomers continue to age (NEI, 2016a).

Normally, light passing through a clear lens projects a sharp image onto the retina. The lens is made of mostly water and protein and over time some of the protein may clump together, leading to clouding of the lens (cataract). Exposure to ultraviolet light has been linked to acceleration of cataract development. Vision gradually gets worse as the lens changes from clear to a yellow or brown (Fig. 18.14). The cataract eventually makes it difficult to differentiate certain colors, to read, or to perform routine activities. Other symptoms include blurred vision, difficulty using current eyeglasses, having poor night vision, noticing glare from headlights or lamps, perceiving that sunlight is too bright, and double vision. In addition to age related cataracts, the following other types of cataracts exist:

- *Congenital:* Children may be born with cataracts or develop them throughout their youth.
- *Traumatic:* After eye injury or electric shock; cataracts may develop even years later.
- *Secondary:* After eye surgery for other conditions, cataracts may develop, or they may be associated with other health problems

PATIENT, FAMILY, AND CAREGIVER EDUCATION

Discharge Instructions and Home Care After Cataract Surgery

- Give both the patient and the caregiver verbal and written instructions. Provide them with the name and telephone number of the surgeon or nurse to call if questions arise. Stress handwashing for patient and caregiver.
- Advise the patient to avoid squeezing the eyelids shut or touching the eyes postoperatively.
- Encourage the patient to wear eyeglasses during the day to avoid rubbing the eye and provide protection from environmental hazards.
- Review the signs and symptoms that should be reported to the surgeon or nurse such as sudden onset of eye pain or pressure, photophobia, sudden decrease in vision, sudden and severe headaches, excessive redness or watering of eyes, swelling, nausea, or vomiting. Discuss the need to wear an eye shield while sleeping the first week postoperatively. Tape may be used to hold the shield in place. The patient should avoid sleeping on the stomach or operated side for the first week after surgery.
- Discuss that vision may not be clear for the first few days postoperatively.
- Instruct that sunglasses must be worn at all times while outside after cataract surgery to avoid ultraviolet light damage and reduce glare and photophobia.
- Reinforce that if the patient is receiving a standard IOL implant he or she will still need to wear eyeglasses; however, the prescription may not be as strong. Approximately 3 to 6 weeks after surgery, the new prescription will be given. Vision may feel unbalanced until the new prescription is ordered and the trained optician delivers new eyeglasses.
- Discuss that if a multifocal IOL is implanted, it may take time for visual acuity to adjust completely (up to 3 months), especially until after the second eye is operated on.
- Remind the patient not to use eyedrops from previous surgeries because this may promote infections. An eyedrop checklist should be given to the patient to keep track of the eyedrop schedule. Make sure the patient/caregiver can read the instructions; have them read back.
- Review the proper instillation of eyedrops with patient and caregiver. (Note: If the surgery on the second eye was just performed, the patient may still be taking drops for the first eye. Review the specific drops for each eye and provide a checklist for each eye. Instruct the patient to follow the surgeon's directions for tapering drops for the first eye.)
- Instruct the patient not to use handkerchiefs to wipe the eyes if eyedrops spill over; instead use disposable single-use tissues.
- Advise the patient to avoid constipation by drinking plenty of water and eating a diet high in fiber.
- Explain the need to avoid strenuous exercise for 2 to 3 weeks. Check with the physician before resuming heavy occupational or recreational activities. Note that sexual relations can usually resume after 1 week.
- Discuss limiting the amount of computer and close reading during the first few days after surgery because this may dry out the eyes and prevent the new IOL from stabilizing.
- Review that pets carry dander and germs that can irritate the surgery site. Discuss precautions with the patient and caregiver such as not sleeping in the same bed as pets and to be conscious of contacting pet saliva.
- Stress the importance of regular follow-up care with the physician.

Modified from surgery instructions from Mielcarek Eye Lifetime Vision Center in Media, PA, under the guidance of Medical Director Leon Mielcarek, MD, FACS.

AMBULATORY SURGERY CONSIDERATIONS

Empathic, Patient-Centered Communication

Most eye surgeries are performed in ambulatory surgery centers that limit personal patient interaction with nurses compared with inpatient surgeries. Efficiency, increased flow, and work management concerns also reduce the time for perioperative nurses to bond with and care for the surgery patient. Patients still desire and require a hands-on approach to their eye care, so finding an appropriate balance between comforting care and efficiency in the surgery center can be challenging.

Perioperative nurses often observe anxious behavior in surgery patients, yet little acknowledgment or intervention may be taken to document or respond to the anxiety. A patient-centered care approach to nursing may be lost to fast-paced efficiency approaches to patient care.

A 2016 study explored the relationship between empathic patient-centered communication and both psychologic and clinical outcomes. Based on the premise that empathic communication appreciates the patient's emotions; expresses that awareness to the patient; and leads to the patient feeling he or she is understood, respected, and validated, 104 ambulatory surgery patients were randomly assigned to an IG or CG. The CG received

standardized information regarding hospital norms and descriptions of surgical preparation procedures. The information delivery to the CG lasted about 15 minutes and was conducted in individual patient sessions. The IG also had about a 15-minute individual discussion, but this was conducted by nurses trained in empathic, patient-centered communication.

The STAI-Y was used to assess anxiety. Sociodemographic data were collected from patient clinical records. Both groups were similar in sociodemographic data. STAI-Y and clinical data were collected immediately before and immediately after the preoperative surgical interview, which took place about a month before surgery. Follow-up assessment was conducted 24 hours after surgery and again 1 month after surgery. Postoperative data collection included clinical outcomes such as wound healing, surgery recovery, return to normal activities of daily living, pain, and patient satisfaction. Study findings confirmed that anxiety levels decreased, information satisfaction increased, recovery was faster, and wound healing improved in the IG. The study authors concluded that empathic, patient-centered communication was effective in reducing preoperative anxiety and increasing surgical recovery, patient satisfaction, and wound healing.

CG, Control group; *IG,* intervention group; *STAI-Y,* State-Trait Anxiety Inventory Form Y.
Modified from Pereria L et al: Preoperative anxiety in ambulatory surgery: the impact of an empathic patient-centered approach on psychological and clinical outcomes, *Patient Educ Couns* 99(5):733–738, 2016.

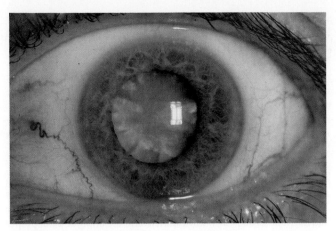

FIG. 18.14 Hypermature age-related corticonuclear cataract with a brunescent (brown) nucleus.

such as diabetes, steroid use, smoking, and prolonged exposure to sunlight.

Cataract removal is warranted when the cataract interferes with everyday activities such as driving, reading, and watching television. Presence of a cataract may also create difficulties for the ophthalmologist to assess vitreous and retina issues. Potential complications, although rare, are discussed as part of informed consent before surgery. Potential problems include vision-threatening infections, bleeding, inflammation, vision loss, double vision, and high or low eye pressure. In patients with vision in only one eye, risks and benefits of surgery are carefully evaluated.

Certain medications and diseases may prevent the pupil from properly dilating or may cause unexpected iris contractions during surgery. Intraoperative floppy iris syndrome (IFIS) may cause complications during cataract surgery, but those complications are partially reduced when proper precautions are taken in at-risk patients. Patients who are under long-term treatment for glaucoma therapy, who use alpha-blockers such as tamsulosin (Flomax), or who have diabetes are more prone to IFIS.

Patients who have had previous refractive surgery such as laser-assisted in situ keratomileusis (LASIK) or photorefractive keratectomy (PRK) have a compromised cornea, and postoperative refractions are less predictable. Optiwave refractive analysis (ORA) can be used intraoperatively to analyze the reflected wave of light exiting the eye, give the surgeon an accurate measure of the eye's focusing capabilities, and better predict postcataract results for visual acuity. ORA measurement is completed after the cataract nucleus has been removed but before the IOL is inserted.

Patients expect to see well without glasses as early as the day after surgery. It is important to manage postoperative vision expectations of patients so they understand proper healing times and fluctuations. If patients are scheduled for surgery in both eyes a few weeks apart, they may experience some imbalances because one eye has postoperative refraction and the other eye has preoperative vision. This imbalance is not an indication of the final visual acuity outcome of cataract surgery. The stronger the presurgery eyeglass prescription the more likely imbalances may occur and the more the perioperative nurse must communicate the imbalances so patients are prepared and avoid premature disappointment. Patients with cataracts in both eyes generally have their procedures performed at separate times, usually 4 to 8 weeks apart.

Months or years after cataract surgery, residual epithelial cells may grow back on the capsular bag causing opacification of the posterior capsule and a haze in vision. A YAG laser may be indicated for capsulotomy, creating a hole in the center of the capsule to allow light to pass through and restore clear vision.

There are two separate types of cataract surgery: the removal of the cataractous lens with extracapsular cataract excision (ECCE) via a phaco method, or an intracapsular cataract extraction (ICCE) method with insertion of an artificial IOL to restore visual acuity. The femtosecond laser is used by some surgeons to perform capsulorrhexis before an ECCE or ICCE procedure (Fig. 18.15).

In the ECCE procedure the anterior portion of the capsule is opened in a controlled manner using a 25-gauge needle or a capsule forceps. Phaco uses high-frequency ultrasonic energy to break the hardened lens material into fragments that can then be aspirated from the eye with saline. The surgeon removes only the lens nucleus from the eye, leaving the posterior capsule behind to hold the IOL implant. The ICCE method of cataract removal consists of removing the entire lens within its capsule with a cryoprobe. It is rarely performed except in the event of a dislocated lens. If an ICCE is scheduled, alpha-chymotrypsin (Catarase, Chymar), an enzyme that acts to weaken the zonules of the lens, is used; a cataract cryoprobe needs to be available.

Intraocular Lens

Extraction of the cataractous lens removes one of the major refractive components of the eye. Four options for replacing this lost refractive power include (1) IOL implantation; (2) astigmatism IOL implantation; (3) advanced technology bifocal (multifocal) IOL implantation; or (4) aphakia (no implant), which requires the use of thick eyeglasses postoperatively. IOLs offer many advantages to patients, including reduced dependence on eyeglasses and reduced thickness of any eyeglass correction needed.

The adoption of the IOL has allowed cataract surgery to become a procedure of choice with increased visual freedom. The redefinition of aging in the baby-boomer generation has spurred research for improved performance of IOLs. Active adults understand cataract surgery has also become refractive surgery and can significantly reduce their dependence on eyeglasses and contact lenses. The expectations of vision after cataract surgery have increased, and patients are demanding better outcomes. The perioperative nurse holds a crucial job on the ophthalmic surgical team to provide detailed, educated, and accurate assistance to help achieve the patient's heightened expectations.

IOLs are made of silicone or acrylic resin and are available in various diopter powers. The necessary diopter power, customized for each patient, is determined by measuring the curvature of the patient's cornea (keratometry) and the axial length (length from cornea to retina). A complex mathematic formula is then used to calculate the correct lens power needed for the desired results. This work is performed in the surgeon's office, and desired IOL orders are transmitted to the hospital a week before the surgery date.

The standard IOL implant reimbursed by insurance can reduce the prescription for hyperopia or myopia, but it does not correct for astigmatism or presbyopia. After cataract surgery the patient's distance prescription can be significantly reduced, but he or she will most likely need to wear some form of bifocal glasses for most activities.

Advanced technology multifocal IOLs provide both distance and near focus at the same time (AAO, 2016). When this option is chosen, the patient's expectations of visual acuity after surgery are heightened. The astigmatism and multifocal IOLs require an extra out-of-pocket expense for patients, furthering their high expectations of performance and visual acuity.

Toric IOLs are designed to reduce hyperopia or myopia as well as astigmatism to reduce a patient's dependence on eyeglasses for distance as much as possible. Toric IOLs have different optical power and focal length in two orientations perpendicular to each other. A small degree of astigmatism can be corrected during femtosecond laser-assisted cataract surgery (FLACS). The patient will still need eyeglasses for close reading and computer work, but will gain freedom from eyeglasses for activities such as driving and watching television. Advanced technology bifocal or accommodating IOLs give the patient the most freedom from eyeglasses because they correct for distance as well as reading. Patients have reported excellent visual acuity results with bifocal IOLs. Advanced technology IOLs also require more preparation, precision, and detailed work on the surgeon's behalf, which requires extra attention by the perioperative nurse.

Over the past few years numerous microsurgical techniques have been developed for IOL insertion through a smaller self-sealing incision and through a clear corneal incision. With the advent of the smaller 2.8-mm or less incision diameter, IOLs have evolved to become foldable. The scrub person must understand the importance of proper folding techniques (Fig. 18.16). IOLs that are folded incorrectly into the injector can be inserted upside down or backward, negatively affecting postsurgical refractions. The more the surgeon has to manipulate the incorrectly folded IOL, the higher the risk of inflammation. Astigmatism and multifocal IOLs require particular attention while folding into the injector because they have a smaller room for error and require more precise insertion. IOL manufacturers supply IOLs in a preloaded injector to reduce the risk of misloading.

Perioperative personnel must be familiar with specific institutional policies pertaining to IOLs and their use. The AAO developed

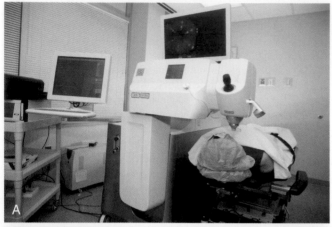

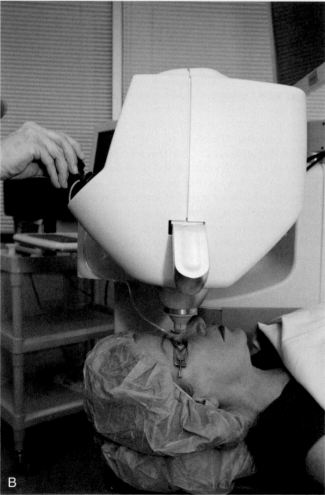

FIG. 18.15 (A) Femtosecond laser is used in cataract surgery to perform the capsulorrhexis. The room is nonsterile and adjacent to the OR. (B) The patient is positioned under the femtosecond laser with a speculum in place and docking cone in position for the surgeon.

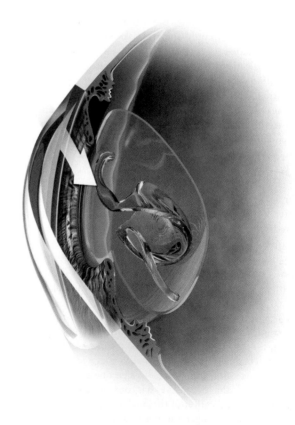

FIG. 18.16 Intraocular lens (IOL) is folded into the injector by the scrub person, handed to the surgeon, and the surgeon places the folded IOL into the capsular bag. In some instances the haptics need to be adjusted with a Sinskey hook to line up the refraction.

recommendations to minimize the occurrence of preventable errors such as wrong IOL implant, damaged IOL implantation, or upside down IOL loading and implantation. The recommendations emphasize the importance of heightened communication and verifications of preoperative calculations of lens style and power ordered and documentation as a written order. Ophthalmic surgery presents high risks for errors, partly because of the high volume of procedures (Custer et al., 2016). It is recommended that the surgeon have some form of written documentation regarding the case specifics and IOL specifications (white board or copy of operative plan taped to microscope) available to view when scrubbed, gowned, and seated at the surgical microscope (Custer et al., 2016). Advanced IOL implants are customized and are ordered from the manufacturer at least 7 to 10 days before the date of cataract surgery. Many surgery centers have one designated nurse that is in charge of ordering the advanced technology IOLs for all surgery patients. It is important for the perioperative nurse to use a standardized protocol for communicating and double checking the availability of these implants before the surgery day so there are no unnecessary delays or surgery cancellations.

Posterior chamber lenses (PCLs) can be implanted only when the cataract is removed by ECCE. Placement behind the iris in the bag or in the sulcus is the most physiologic position for an artificial lens (PCL) and is the most common method. Anterior chamber lenses (ACLs), placed in front of the iris, are used in the absence of capsular support, including after vitreous loss or ICCE and for secondary lens implantation (when the cataract was previously removed without lens replacement).

Femtosecond Laser-Assisted Cataract Surgery

FLACS emerged much faster than phacoemulsification technology. Femtosecond (femto) refers to the speed of the optical pulse of the laser, which is one quadrillionth of a second (10^{-15}). This short pulse duration allows less tissue damage during surgery as well as more precisely focused ablation in the cornea or anterior chamber. The laser can be set to different depths to reach different levels within the anterior chamber, all without generating heat during the ablation process. The use of the Femto laser during cataract surgery can create more accurate initial incisions, yielding more predictable and standardized capsulorrhexis. These findings are significant because a fraction of a millimeter in eye surgery can alter the desired postoperative results. The femtosecond laser can precut the cataractous nucleus for the surgeon so less ultrasound energy is needed for nucleus removal. The more dense and "hard" the cataract, the more benefit there is to using the femtosecond laser to precut the cataract (Olson, 2016).

Femtosecond is a continuation of the LASIK model of providing refractive improvements to patients to enhance their lifestyle, as well as increase the reproducibility and consistency of cataract surgery. LASIK surgery created a desire in patients for better visual acuity without glasses, as well as an acceptance to pay out of pocket to improve their vision, and ultimately a higher expectation of vision after cataract surgery. FLACS helps the surgeon increase precision on eyes that have previously undergone LASIK surgery or refractive keratotomy (RK), because the cornea has been compromised and more variations in postcataract surgery refractive outcomes are possible (Alio et al., 2016).

Complication rates are comparable to rates for manual cataract surgery. Continuing surgeon experience, modification of techniques, and improved technology will determine the effect of lasers on the quality of cataract surgery and patient outcomes. One notable physical difference for the femtosecond laser patient is the possible increase in subconjunctival hemorrhages as the result of having to dock the laser on the eye. The patient may experience a "bloodshot" eye for 3 to 5 days after the procedure.

Procedural Considerations

Preoperative dilating drops, both sympathetic agonists (phenylephrine) and parasyfmpathetic antagonists (tropicamide, cyclopentolate, atropine, and homatropine), are instilled at prescribed intervals in the preoperative area. The nurse administers a drop of topical preservative-free tetracaine 0.5% numbing agent into the operative eye before the patient enters the OR. The patient is instructed to keep this eye closed to prevent the cornea from drying. As the patient is being positioned on the OR bed, the nurse administers another drop of tetracaine. During the procedure an intraocular anesthetic solution is usually injected and can be combined with intracameral epinephrine, lidocaine, and BSS (Epi-Shugarcaine) to help with poorly dilating pupils.

An armrest is positioned on the operative side, and the patient's head and the microscope are adjusted. The patient is instructed to look at the light of the microscope and is told where to fixate. If the patient cannot open the eye, a facial nerve block may be considered. If the patient cannot fixate on the light at all, the surgeon may administer a retrobulbar block.

Instrumentation varies with the surgeon's preference but usually includes a phaco handpiece and tip, I/A handpiece and tips, BSS, phaco blades (surgeon preference), capsule forceps, lens manipulators, hydrodissection cannula, pupil expander (iris retractor or Malyugin ring), IOL forceps, lens positioner hook, and the IOL and IOL injector. The nurse also ensures the following are available for unexpected procedures: anterior vitrectomy handpiece, Beehler forceps to dilate the pupil, 10-0 nylon or 10-0 Vicryl (polyglactin) suture, and a secondary IOL.

Machine settings are specific for each brand of phaco machine and are not interchangeable. Power and vacuum settings, irrigation bottle height, and foot pedal positions must be adjusted for each machine and for each surgeon. Perioperative nurses should consult instruction manuals for the machines and review required settings to avoid complications or delays. Through teamwork and adequate training and monitoring for competency, the surgical team can optimize technology for safety and efficiency in cataract surgery regardless of the equipment used.

Pressures in the anterior and posterior chambers are generally equal. After the surgeon makes the incision into the anterior chamber, aqueous fluid leaks out. Pressure in the anterior chamber falls below that in the posterior chamber, and vitreous from the back of the eye tries to push forward and could carry other structures with it. To minimize the risk from these pressure gradients, the surgeon injects thick viscoelastics early in the procedure, which do not leak.

The surgeon may choose to make the incision on two different points of the eye. An incision near the limbus, where the cornea meets the sclera, should not have an effect on the postsurgical refraction, whereas an incision point in clear cornea can purposefully adjust the postsurgical astigmatic refraction.

Combined Cataract Procedures With iStent Glaucoma Implant

A small implant, the iStent, can be implanted at the end of cataract surgery, after the IOL has been implanted. The iStent is implanted into the trabecular meshwork to reduce the block of fluid flow to Schlemm canal. The device improves the natural flow of fluid in the eye that is compromised in patients with open-angle glaucoma.

The device uses the same incision that was created to insert the IOL and is minimally invasive, so no additional anesthesia or surgical instruments are required. The iStent comes preloaded on a handle for the surgeon to implant. The surgeon turns the patient's head at a 30-degree angle and holds a gonio prism in one hand (usually the nondominant hand) while inserting the iStent through the cataract incision.

Operative Procedure
Cataract Extraction

1. The surgeon places an eyelid speculum after draping.
2. A 1-mm stab incision (paracentesis, tiny incision in cornea opposite the main incision) is made at 5 o'clock in the left eye or at 11 o'clock in the right eye into the anterior chamber.
3. Intercameral anesthesia may be administered: 1 mL of unpreserved lidocaine 1.0% is slowly injected into the anterior chamber through a 27- to 30-gauge cannula using a tuberculin syringe.
4. The surgeon injects viscoelastic material into the anterior chamber to deepen the chamber and widen the pupil.
5. The temporal or superior corneal incision is made with a keratome (diamond gem or single-use blade). Some surgeons may use a caliper to mark the incision width, and may use a second knife to make a vertical cut before the horizontal pass with the keratome (Fig. 18.17A).
6. BSS is continuously sprayed onto the eye to keep the cornea moistened and reduce the risk of dryness during surgery.
7. Capsulotomy and capsulorrhexis are performed with a capsulorrhexis forceps or other surgeon-preferred instrument. This step of tearing the capsule in a controlled manner is critical in creating a round, stable opening into the capsular bag (e.g., the saclike structure remaining within the eye after the phaco process) (see Fig. 18.17B).
8. Using a 30-gauge cannula and BSS solution, the surgeon performs hydrodissection (and sometimes hydrodelineation) to separate the center/nucleus from the capsule and maneuver the lens within the capsule (see Fig. 18.17C).
9. The surgeon uses a phaco tip to sculpt the nucleus with ultrasound vibration.
10. A second supporting instrument is inserted through the left-handed paracentesis incision to help rotate and divide the cataractous nucleus into quadrants (see Fig. 18.17D).
11. Cataractous nucleus removal usually proceeds in two phases: nuclear sculpting, in which the nucleus is cracked or sculpted into smaller fragments, and quadrantic emulsification of those fragments. If the cataract is too hard to emulsify, the surgeon can express the nucleus of the lens manually. This is known as non-phaco ECCE.
12. After removing the lens nucleus, the surgeon places an I/A tip into the eye and uses it to remove the remaining cortical material (see Fig. 18.17E). This combination of irrigation and aspiration is intended to maintain equilibrium within the eye. Removing the cortex minimizes postoperative inflammation.
13. The surgeon may polish the posterior capsule or aspirate anterior lens epithelial cells with a burred instrument.
14. The surgeon injects viscoelastic material to inflate the anterior chamber and capsular bag.
15. A posterior chamber IOL is carefully folded into the injector by the scrub person (following manufacturer's loading guidelines), passed to the surgeon, and placed into the eye by unfolding the capsular bag (see Fig. 18.17F–G). The IOL is centrally positioned with a Sinskey hook or the I/A tip. The surgeon may need to widen the corneal incision before placing the IOL.

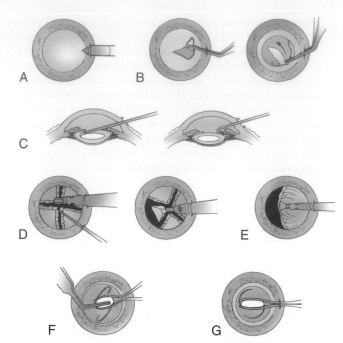

FIG. 18.17 Clear cornea cataract extraction. (A) A 2.6-mm or smaller incision is made into the cornea. (B) Manual capsulorrhexis is performed on anterior capsule of lens. (C) Nucleus of lens is loosened by hydrodissection. (D) Nucleus of lens is "cracked" into four quadrants and removed with phacoemulsification. (E) Irrigation and aspiration handpiece is used to strip the remaining cortex from the capsule. (F) Intraocular lens (IOL) is folded. (G) IOL is placed into the capsular bag.

16. The surgeon uses the I/A tip to remove any remaining viscoelastic material to let the eye pressures stabilize. Leaking of the wound may be controlled or prevented by hydrating the wound edges. Occasionally, a 10-0 nylon suture is necessary for diabetic, elderly, or extremely active patients or dense cataract removals.
17. Topical antibiotics or combination antibiotic-corticosteroid ointment or drops are placed on the eye. A shield is applied to prevent dust and debris from entering the surgery site and to prevent the patient from touching the eye.

Anterior Segment Vitrectomy

The main indications for vitrectomy in the anterior segment are as follows: vitreous loss during cataract extraction; opacities in the anterior segment; complications associated with vitreous in the anterior chamber; and miscellaneous causes, such as hyphema, pupillary membranes, and residual soft lens material.

Procedural Considerations

The procedure varies according to surgeon preference. A pathologic condition in the anterior segment can be approached through a limbal incision, as in lens extraction with vitreous loss, or through an open sky approach, after trephine incision for penetrating keratoplasty. Most phaco equipment has a vitrector that can be quickly attached if needed.

Operative Procedure
Anterior Vitrectomy for Vitreous Loss During Cataract Extraction

1. The surgeon introduces the vitreous cutter into the eye through the cataract wound. Saline infusion may be through the handpiece or a separate cannula with an infusion line.

2. The cutter is placed in the middle of the pupil, posterior to the iris, and enough vitreous is removed to ensure that no vitreous remains in the anterior chamber and that the iris has fallen back into its normal position.

3. The pupil is constricted with acetylcholine chloride intraocular solution. The anterior chamber may be re-formed with BSS.

4. The procedure is completed as for a lens extraction.

Anterior Vitrectomy for Anterior Segment Opacities, Hyphema, Pupillary Membranes, and Residual Soft Lens Material

1. Appropriate fixation sutures or a lid speculum is placed.

2. The surgeon makes an incision at the limbus either through clear cornea or under a conjunctival flap. One to three incisions are made, depending on the vitreous cutter chosen and the technique.

3. If a multifunction probe is not used, the surgeon places an infusion cannula into one incision and the vitreous cutter into another incision. A third incision may be used for an accessory instrument. The vitreous, blood, or other material is removed.

4. The surgeon closes the incisions and patches the eye.

Surgery of the Retina

Vitreoretinal Surgery

Vitreous fluid fills about two-thirds of the eye, helps keep the round shape of the eyeball, and is originally attached to the retina. The vitreous slowly liquefies, atrophies, and shrinks as we age. The vitreous then can become stringy, and shadows can be cast onto the retina, causing "floaters" ("cobwebs" or specks that float in the field of vision). They may look like spots, threadlike strands, or squiggly lines. Floaters are more noticeable when looking at bright objects, such as a white piece of paper. Floaters are more common in patients who have diabetes, have undergone cataract surgery, or are nearsighted. Over time the floaters usually settle below the line of sight but do not completely disappear. Floaters in and of themselves generally do not require treatment. However, if a patient experiences a sudden increase in the number of floaters, retinal examination is warranted to rule out a retinal tear, break, or hole (NEI, 2016b).

The retina, the light-sensitive layer of tissue lining the eye, sends visual signals via the optic nerve to the brain. Attached to the retina are millions of fine fibers intertwined with the vitreous. The shrinking vitreous in an aging eye causes the fine fibers to pull on the retinal surface. When the fibers break the vitreous separates and shrinks from the retina, causing traction on the retina. Normally the vitreous detaches from the retina (a posterior vitreous detachment [PVD]). However, sometimes the vitreous can create traction on the retina and pull a piece of the retina with it, creating a retinal tear. Fluid can then leak under the retina into the subretinal space, leading to a retinal detachment (RD); symptomatic breaks (manifested as new floating objects or flashing lights) are likely to progress to RD (Patient, Family, and Caregiver Education).

PVDs are usually not sight-threatening and, like floaters, typically do not require treatment. Patients at risk for the development of PVD are those who are nearsighted and more than 50 years of age, although the condition is very common after age 80. Again, it may not be noticeable but will simply be annoying because of an increase in floaters. A small but sudden increase in new floaters is a symptom of vitreous detachment. Flashes of light in side vision may also occur (NEI, 2016b).

Occasionally some of the vitreous fibers pull so hard on the retina that it causes RD (the sensory retina [neural layer] is separated from the underlying retinal pigment epithelium [RPE] layer). A sudden increase in floaters or flashing lights (a result of traction on the

RD, Retinal detachment.

retina) is a cardinal symptom of RD and an indication for evaluation by a retina specialist as soon as possible. The dilated eye examination is the only way to diagnose the exact cause of the vision problem; permanent loss of vision can occur without timely treatment (NEI, 2016c).

An additional symptom of RD is the appearance of a "curtain" in the field of vision, from above, below, or the side. RD generally occurs because of retinal tears or holes associated with injury, degeneration, or vitreous contraction. Other much less common causes include inflammation, retinal vascular problems, or even tumors of the retina and choroid. Patients who have previously had cataract surgery are at higher risk for RD. Males are more likely to develop RD than females, and the condition is more common in people older than 40 years (NEI, 2016c). Other risk factors include history of nearsightedness or RD in the other eye, family history of RD, presence of lattice degeneration (thinning of the retina in nearsighted people), and occurrence of an eye injury.

Other retinal diseases (Research Highlight) can produce changes that require vitreoretinal surgery. These generally include conditions that impair the ability of light to reach the retina (i.e., obstruction of the visual axis), or cause traction on the retina, produce fluid accumulation (i.e., exudation), leading to swelling within or under the retina. Occasionally surgery is performed for diagnostic reasons, to deliver medication in a targeted fashion, or to relieve intractable inflammation.

Microvascular disease is related to the eye's vulnerability as a result of its dense network of capillary vessels. Diabetes leads to retinal changes (diabetic retinopathy). The presence of diabetes for more than 15 years significantly increases the likelihood of developing some form of retinopathy, typically bilaterally. However, the severity

Gene and Stem Cell Therapy in Retinal Disease

The diagnosis and progression of diseases of the retina, most specifically AMD and RP, unfortunately often lead to vision loss. Although retinal disease is manageable, there are little to no treatments to reverse the disease process and accompanying vision loss. Research investigating gene and cell therapies shows promise in helping retina disease patients possibly keep their vision.

Both AMD and RP have strong genetic components. Scientists have successfully delivered cloned genes to specific retinal cells in humans. Studies have shown an increase in visual function over extended periods of time. The ultimate goal of this treatment is to regain some visual function. Clinical trials have used obstacle courses in dim light to measure the speed and accuracy of navigation before and after gene therapy. Before the therapy, study patients typically collided with obstacles and repeatedly veered off the course. Three years after gene therapy, patients completed the course without going off course, avoided obstacles, and stepped over obstacles in their direct path. This development is important to regain confidence and independence, as well as decrease the healthcare cost associated with daily support from blindness.

Compromise and total loss of the photoreceptors of the retina is the most common cause of end-stage irreversible blindness in the developed world. The two paths of affecting photoreceptors are by genetic correction by introducing modifier genes or by augmenting or replacing the cells entirely. The ideal approach is to replace the photoreceptors early in disease progression before the onset of photoreceptor loss and subsequent replacement. A key requirement for gene therapy is the safe delivery of the modifier genes to the layers of the retina. Clinical trials are starting to evidence safe, effective gene and cell transfers. Demonstration of clinical effectiveness of such eye procedures is prompting additional genetic research. New investigative strategies are enrolling subjects, and initial results are showing signs of efficacy. Clinically significant therapies are still years away, but initial gene and cell therapies have shown promising results to help recover vision from previously irreversible vision loss from retinal diseases.

AMD, Age-related macular generation; *RP,* retinitis pigmentosa.
From Maclaren R et al: Gene therapy and stem cell transplantation in retinal disease: the new frontier, *Ophthalmology* 123(10):S98–S106, 2016.

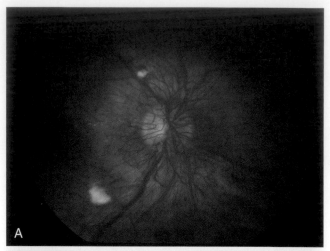
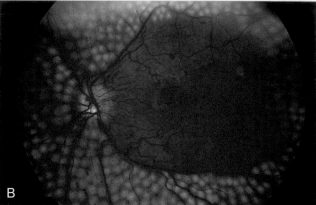

FIG. 18.18 (A) Proliferative retinopathy, an advanced form of diabetic retinopathy, occurs when abnormal new blood vessels and scar tissue form on the surface of the retina. (B) Fundus photo showing scatter laser surgery for diabetic retinopathy.

may be different between eyes. Retinopathy is classified in either of the following ways:

- *Background, or nonproliferative:* Disease is confined to the retinal surface. Retinal capillary walls develop microaneurysms (bulges) that can lead to leakage and development of exudates within the retina. Hemorrhages occur within the retina and are reabsorbed. Capillary membrane changes result in blocked capillaries and retinal ischemia. Eventually deterioration progresses to the next stage.
- *Proliferative:* Neovascularization, or the formation of new retinal blood vessels, can develop within the retina in an attempt to relieve ischemic anoxia secondary to microvascular damage caused by diabetes (Fig. 18.18). These new vessels are fragile and can rupture spontaneously, causing bleeding, and they are very permeable, causing leakage. Hemorrhage into the retina or vitreous can consequently ensue, leading to severe visual loss.

Neovascularization can develop into scar tissue that can produce traction, which may distort or even detach the retina. In RD, pigment

or blood cells are freed in the vitreous, causing flashes and floaters. Fluid from the vitreous cavity can seep through the retinal tears into the subretinal space and progressively detach the retina. The part of the retina that has separated from its nutritional source becomes damaged and relatively nonfunctional. On occasion inflammatory or scar tissue can develop on the retinal surface, leading to an epiretinal membrane that can distort vision. As the inflammatory or scar tissue, which is firmly attached to the retina, contracts, the retina can wrinkle or "pucker." When the wrinkle is over the area of the macula, the central vision becomes blurred and distorted.

In the same manner, as the shrinking vitreous pulls the retina, peripherally causing tears and RD, vitreous traction centrally can produce problems. When the macula is affected, it is more serious because of the effect on central vision, which is called a macular hole. Both macular pucker and macular hole have the same symptoms, distorted, blurred vision (NEI, 2016d). Additionally, a macular hole may present with distortion of straight lines and difficulty reading. Vision ranges from 20/25 to 20/400 (the latter for untreated macular hole). Fifty percent of very early macular holes close on their own.

Various types of RD are as follows:

- *Rhegmatogenous:* This is the most common type. Fluid exudate from a tear or break in the retina leaks under the retina, separating it from the RPE.
- *Tractional:* This form of RD is often secondary to diabetic retinopathy, especially if untreated. The retina also separates from

the RPE, which is caused by contraction of scar tissue on the retina's surface.

- *Exudative or serous:* In inflammatory retinal disease or trauma, fluid exudate leaks under the retina. In this RD type, however, there are no breaks or tears in the retina.

Location of the pathology on the retina affects visual symptoms. Macular pucker, for example (also called epiretinal membrane, preretinal membrane, retina wrinkle, or internal limiting membrane disease), generally affects the macula, located in the center of the retina. The macula normally provides sharp, central vision needed for reading, driving, and fine detail work, and when puckered can cause blurred, distorted central vision.

Various modalities for surgical treatment include laser treatments, scleral buckling, vitrectomy, and retinopexy. In addition to any of these therapies, freeze treatment (cryopexy) may be performed in the surgeon's office for small holes and tears to help "weld" and reattach the retina (NEI, 2016d).

Laser Treatment in Diabetic Retinopathy

Laser energy is used to apply burns to peripheral retinal tissue to help neovascularization regress. The pathophysiologic mechanism for regression of neovascularization is not completely understood, but is thought to occur as a result of the reduced retinal oxygen requirement as a result of the scarred retinal tissue. This method of eliminating abnormal vascularization is called panretinal photo coagulation (PRP). Again, in principle, early diagnosis and control of blood glucose levels are paramount, because laser treatment does indeed partially destroy the retina to help arrest neovascularization. Thus surgeons use the laser before excess damage occurs, electrocoagulating minute hypoxic areas to prevent the new vessels from forming. Laser treatments may begin in an office setting or later in the OR in conjunction with surgery. The laser may be applied through the slit lamp, with the indirect ophthalmoscope, or directly during vitrectomy surgery using an intraocular endolaser probe (see Fig. 18.18).

Vitrectomy

Vitrectomy is narrowly defined as removal of all or part of the vitreous gel (body). In the broader clinical sense, vitrectomy surgery can also include the excision and removal of fibrotic membranes, removal of epiretinal membranes, and electrocoagulation of bleeding vessels. In its normal state the vitreous gel of the eye is transparent. In certain disease states, bleeding from damaged or newly formed vessels may cause the vitreous to become opaque, which may then severely decrease vision. In addition to the patient's inability to see, the surgeon is unable to visualize the retina and therefore treat the underlying pathologic condition before permanent damage can occur. In these cases vitrectomy surgery is indicated to restore the patient's vision and to allow the surgeon to institute treatment if indicated.

Formation of membranes may block the visual axis and cause decreased vision. Contraction of these membranes may produce traction-type or rhegmatogenous RD. In these cases vitrectomy surgery is indicated to relieve the underlying pathologic processes leading to decreased vision.

Posterior Segment Vitrectomy

A pathologic condition in the posterior segment is usually approached through the pars plana, which is tissue that is anterior to the anterior attachment of the retina, typically located 3 to 4 mm from the limbus (corneoscleral junction). Because the pars plana has no retinal tissue, entry at this site poses little risk for RD. The main indications for posterior segment vitrectomy through the pars plana are as follows: long-standing vitreous opacities, advanced diabetic eye disease, severe intraocular trauma, retained foreign bodies; proliferative vitreoretinopathy, RD from giant tears, endophthalmitis, and diagnostic vitreous biopsy.

Essentially, vitrectomy vacuums any pooled blood to enhance clarity. Complications of vitrectomy include RD, retinal tears, cataract, and infection. The risk of no treatment can be total loss of vision.

Procedural Considerations. Vitrectomy of the posterior segment is a microsurgical procedure requiring a viewing system (e.g., operating microscope with an X-Y coupling, zoom lens, and fine focus), contact lens system or noncontact wide-angle viewing system (e.g., Biom), an illumination system, a cutting-suction-infusion system, and accessory instruments (Fig. 18.19).

The surgeon can hold the contact lens in place by hand or can suture it for stabilization. Another option for a sew-on lens is the use of a noncontact panoramic wide-angle viewing system. This system allows a wide, noncontact view of the macula and is mounted on the microscope and swings out of the way for extraocular phases of the vitrectomy. Other advantages are that it provides a good view under air, eliminates the time needed to sew on a lens, and does not require an assistant to hold the lens. The eye may be rotated freely to view the extreme periphery. The image is inverted by a manual knob, foot pedal, or hand control.

The infusion system consists of a 500-mL bottle of buffered BSS (such as BSS Plus or Endosol Extra), a standard intravenous (IV) administration set, and an infusion needle or sleeve. The level of IOP can be varied by elevating or lowering the infusion bottle in relation to the patient's eye and by adjusting the digital readout of the nitrogen gas–forced infusion.

Cutting and suction systems vary in sophistication and technology. All cutters engage tissue into a port and then cut it by the shearing action between the edges of a moving and a nonmoving part. Guillotine cutters have a linear back-and-forth action, whereas reciprocating or oscillating cutters rotate in a clockwise-counterclockwise fashion. The cutter may be part of a single-use multifunction handpiece. Suction is operated with a pump controlled by a foot switch to maintain the level of aspiration.

An endolaser or indirect laser delivery system is usually available for photocoagulation. Illumination for vitrectomy is *external,* using the operating microscope for anterior segment vitrectomy, and *internal,* using a fiberoptic light pipe (endoilluminator) for posterior segment vitrectomy. A special light pipe (cannonball) that illuminates a wider area is needed if a wide-angle viewing system is used on the microscope.

Replacement of the vitreous with air is facilitated with a special air-exchange unit that may be incorporated into the multifunction vitrectomy machine. Other substances for intraocular tamponade are liquid perfluorocarbons, silicone oil, perfluoropropane gas (C_3F_8), and sulfur hexafluoride gas (SF_6).

Several accessory instruments may be used for pars plana vitrectomy, depending on the extent of the procedure. Microhooks, picks, and subretinal forceps and scissors are used for dissection, peeling, and removing membranes (Fig. 18.20). These instruments can be manually operated with a thumb control or run with compressed air from the automated vitrectomy console. Even smaller 23- and 25-gauge trocars allow for finer instrumentation without the need for suturing the trocar sites. Foreign-body microforceps and various magnetic devices are used to retrieve foreign objects such as glass, metal, or other substances. An intraocular cryoprobe for cryocoagulation directly on the retina surface can be attached

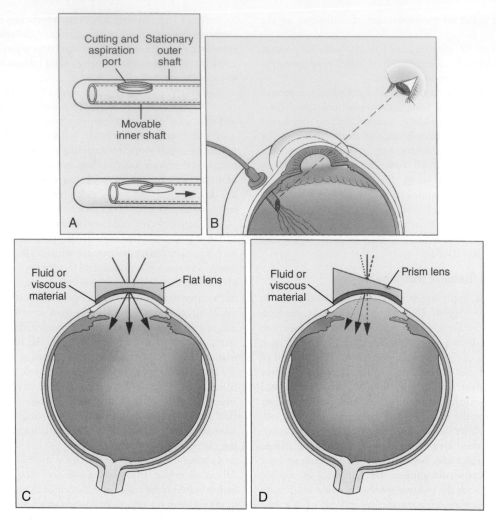

FIG. 18.19 Essential components for vitrectomy. (A) Vitrector probe with its cutting/aspirating port close to the tip of the intraocular portion of the handpiece. (B) Infusion cannula, placed in pars plana, is viewed for correct position. (C) Flat contact lens, resting on cushion of fluid or viscoelastic material on the cornea, is used for viewing posterior half of the vitreous cavity and retina. (D) Prism contact lens used for viewing anterior structures in the vitreous cavity.

to the cryotherapy device. Flute needles or disposable soft-tipped cannulae are handheld or attached to an extrusion or aspiration line for evacuating pools of blood or for fluid-gas exchange. The soft silicone tips can come close to the retina without scratching or damaging the tissue.

To prepare for a vitrectomy procedure, the perioperative nurse must know the location of the ocular problem, the surgeon's plan to address the problem, the instrumentation to be used, and the anticipated extent and length of the procedure. Instrument and equipment function should be thoroughly checked before the patient is transferred into the OR. When preparing for pars plana vitrectomy in the posterior segment, the perioperative nurse must be aware that a combined scleral buckling procedure may be necessary. Clear communication with surgeons paves the way for effective preparations.

In the case of retinal tears, C_3F_8, SF_6, liquid perfluorocarbons, and silicone oil can be used to provide retinal tamponade. Intraocular expansible gases (C_3F_8 and SF_6) can be used to provide retinal tamponade, but may require the patient to be positioned facedown for several weeks to help reattach the retina. The expansible gas is

slowly absorbed by the body (over a period up to 3 months) as aqueous humor produced by the ciliary body slowly displaces it. Silicone oil can be used for complicated cases and when positioning is difficult for patients. The disadvantage of silicone oil is that the patient will require another procedure to remove the silicone oil because the index of refraction of silicone oil is significantly different from that of vitreous, giving patients the impression that they are "looking through a crystal ball."

Liquid perfluorocarbons such as perfluorooctane (PFO; Perfluoron), being heavier than BSS, allow the retina to be pushed posteriorly and are used as a tamponade to help repair a giant retinal tear. The liquid is then removed from the posterior segment. Silicone oil is a highly viscous oil with a high surface tension that mechanically limits fibrovascular proliferation. The oil may be left in place, but it is recommended that it be removed within 1 year if the retina is reattached and stable. Silicone oil may cause increased IOP and secondary glaucoma. A National Eye Institute (NEI)-supported nationwide clinical trial comparing treatment of proliferative vitreoretinopathy with silicone oil or long-acting intraocular gas indicated

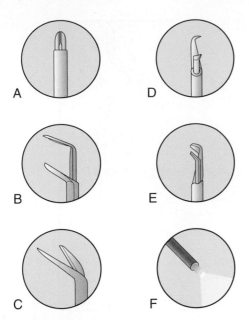

FIG. 18.20 Tips of microinstruments used in vitrectomy procedures. (A and B) Peeling forceps. (C) Horizontal scissors. (D) Vertical scissors. (E) Membrane peeler and cutter. (F) Lighted pick.

that either treatment was effective; thus surgeons have options in treating such cases (NEI, 2016d).

Vitrectomy procedures vary from less than 1 hour to more than 3 hours (Fig. 18.21). When a long procedure is anticipated, care must be taken to protect the patient's skin and reduce perioperative positioning pressure areas. A foam mattress pad, heel and elbow protectors, and elasticized stockings may be used. A wrist support may be placed around the patient's head to support the surgeon's wrist during manipulation of the intraocular instruments.

Because of the amount of fluid used in the operative field during this procedure, draping is done to allow for removal of infusion fluid from the field and the electric foot pedals are protected from fluid damage.

Operative Procedure
1. The surgeon places a lid speculum and incises the conjunctiva.
2. The surgeon sutures the infusion line in place with a purse-string suture (for 20-gauge surgeries) and checks it for proper placement.
3. Generally, three incisions are made through the pars plana: one for infusion, one for endoillumination, and one for a vitreous cutter or other instrument (e.g., pick, forceps, scissors, laser probe, extrusion needle). In the right eye these incisions are placed at 8, 10, and 2 o'clock; for the left eye, this corresponds to 2, 4, and 10. An illuminating chandelier can also be placed for bimanual surgery, typically at the 6 o'clock position.
4. The operating microscope is aligned. A wide-angle viewing system is swung into position, or a fundus lens is fixed on the anterior surface of the cornea.
5. If a dense cataract or retained lens material blocks the view of the retina, a lensectomy may be performed with a fragmatome or other ultrasonic handpiece at this time.
6. The surgeon removes the vitreous under direct visualization. Once the medium has been removed and the retinal condition visualized, the necessary injections or treatments (endolaser photocoagulation, repair of macular pucker, insertion of silicone oil, gas-fluid

exchange) are completed. A scleral buckling procedure may also be performed.
7. The trocars are removed from the pars plana incisions. Cultures from the vitreous washings are taken if necessary.
8. Subconjunctival injections of steroids or antibiotics are given. An eye pad and shield may be applied for protection of the eye.

Scleral Buckling

Procedural Considerations
In treating RD, the aim is to return the retina to its normal anatomic position. With scleral buckling, repair is done from outside the globe. The procedure's purpose is to cause an intrusion or push into the eye at the site of the pathologic source. Treatment by diathermy or cryotherapy causes an inflammatory reaction that leads to a permanent adhesion between the detached retina and underlying structures. The surgery also involves sealing off the area in which the tear or hole is located and may include drainage of the subretinal fluid.

The procedure may be performed using general anesthesia or monitored anesthesia care (MAC) with local blocks. The scleral buckling may be done using an episcleral (working outside of the sclera) technique or by scleral dissection (making a partial-thickness incision into the sclera and creating flaps to expose the underlying tissue). Both techniques may include drainage of subretinal fluid, encircling bands, diathermy, light coagulation, or cryotherapy. Cryosurgery or light coagulation may be used alone or in combination with a buckling procedure. A detailed drawing of the retina may be made before surgery and displayed in the OR. On the basis of this drawing, the surgeon opens the conjunctiva to a previously determined extent, for example, 90 degrees for a simple horseshoe tear or 360 degrees for an aphakic detachment.

Operative Procedure
1. The inferior, superior, lateral, and medial rectus muscles are isolated using 0 silk ties as traction sutures (Fig. 18.22).
2. Using the indirect ophthalmoscope, the surgeon locates the detachment and tear and marks the site with nonpenetrating diathermy by indentation or with a methylene blue marking pen.
3. Under direct visualization the surgeon applies the retinal cryoprobe to the external surface of the globe in the area of the pathologic condition and treats the area. An ice ball forms in the proper areas until the entire lesion has been treated.
4. The buckling component of the procedure secures silicone bands, sponges, plates, or tires to the sclera. The surgeon places nonabsorbable sutures (4-0 or 5-0) into the sclera surrounding the lesion and ties them over the silicone sponge, causing the outer shell of the eye to be pushed toward the elevated retina.
5. If an encircling band is to be used, the surgeon places mattress sutures into the sclera in four quadrants. A silicone band is passed 360 degrees around the eye under the sutures and the rectus muscles. The sutures are tied, and a self-holding Watzke sleeve is applied to the band to maintain a predetermined circumference. This causes a 360-degree constriction of the outer coats into the eye.
6. If drainage of subretinal fluid is desired, the surgeon chooses an area under direct visualization in which a significant fluid level exists under the retina, and places a diathermy mark on the sclera. The sclera is split to the choroid, and a small amount of diathermy is applied to the choroid bed. A 27-gauge ½-inch needle is then used to puncture the choroid into the subretinal space to permit fluid drainage.

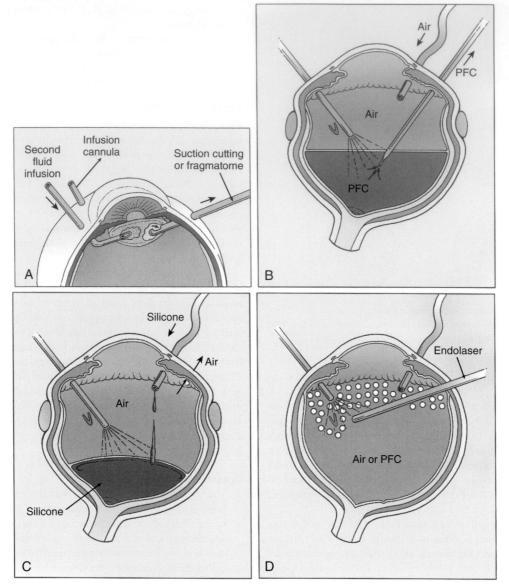

FIG. 18.21 Procedures done with vitrectomy. (A) Pars plana lensectomy performed with a second infusion line. (B) Air/perfluorocarbon *(PFC)* exchange. PFC has been placed in the vitreous cavity for removal of subretinal fluid and anatomic reattachment of the retina. Air under positive pressure is then placed through the infusion cannula as the PFC is simultaneously extruded through the tapered needle. (C) Silicone/air exchange. Silicone is inserted through the infusion cannula as a temporary intraocular tamponade. Silicone is heavier than air and fills the globe from the bottom up, and the air escapes through the sclerotomy site. In silicone/fluid exchange, the silicone floats on the fluid and the fluid is removed with an extrusion needle. (D) Endolaser photocoagulation is performed after the retina is returned to its normal position.

7. Air or replacement fluids may be introduced into the eye after draining the subretinal fluid. This is usually done through the pars plana under direct visualization.
8. The surgeon removes the traction sutures from around the muscles and closes the conjunctiva with 7-0 absorbable suture. A subconjunctival injection of an antibiotic, steroid, or both may be given, and an eye pad is applied.

Retinopexy

In pneumatic retinopexy an intraocular injection of an air bubble or therapeutic gases provides pressure against retinal breaks, allowing them to approximate the pigment epithelium. Retinopexy may be used in combination with scleral buckling and posterior vitrectomy; it may be performed as part of an ambulatory procedure for treatment of certain RDs, using laser photocoagulation with injection of the gas bubble followed by specific postoperative positioning. The gases are drawn through a Millipore 0.22-μm filter and may be mixed with filtered air so that concentrations may be varied. The gas bubble is a ratio mixture of gas and air. The higher the concentration of gas to air, the longer the bubble remains in the eye before being "absorbed." Patient positioning after retinopexy is often facedown for several days to weeks but may include tilting

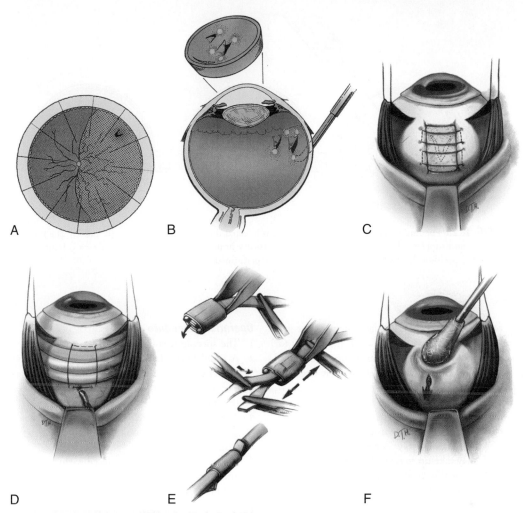

FIG. 18.22 Scleral buckling operation for treatment of retinal detachment. (A) Diagram of retina showing detachment of retina of temporal half of left eye, with retinal tear at equator of globe at 1 : 30 o'clock position. (B) Examination of fundus by means of ophthalmoscope and handheld lens and depression of sclera with diathermy electrode. Surgeon visualizes the field and places an electrode beneath retinal tear; burn mark is made on sclera at the site of retinal tear with diathermy electrode. (C) A sponge is sutured in place over the treated site of retinal tear. (D) Band and tire are used to encircle the eye. (E) Placement of Watzke silicone sleeve is one method to secure edges of encircling band. (F) Small incision is made through sclera, and choroid is finely incised to allow subretinal fluid to drain.

the head to one side or the other as well. The head position is determined by the location of the retinal tear or hole. For example, if the retinal tear or hole is located superior temporal in the right eye, the patient would be instructed to tilt the head down and to the left, so the bubble will float upward and to the right where the tear or hole is located. The larger the tear or hole, the longer the bubble needs to be in contact with the area to be reattached (Fig. 18.23).

SF_6 is a colorless, odorless, and nontoxic gas. It increases 2.5 times in volume within 48 hours after injection by drawing other gases, specifically nitrogen and oxygen, from the surrounding tissues. SF_6 bubbles remain for at least 10 days.

C_3F_8 is a colorless, odorless, and nontoxic gas. It quadruples its volume within 48 hours after injection. A 1-mm bubble can remain up to 30 to 50 days.

Because SF_6 and C_3F_8 are expansible gases, certain precautions are required. Patients are given a wristband to wear that states what kind of gas bubble is in their eye and when it was instilled. If they require surgery, they need to alert the anesthesia provider of the presence of the gas bubble. The intent of instilling a gas bubble is to sustain its size and hold the retina in place. SF_6 and C_3F_8 are inert, insoluble in water, and poorly diffusible. Because nitrous oxide (N_2O) is 117 times more diffusible than SF_6, it rapidly enters the gas bubble. With continued administration of N_2O, the injected gas bubble can increase to three times its original size. IOP can increase from 14 to 30 mm Hg; 18 minutes after discontinuation of N_2O, IOP decreases along with the smaller bubble size. Such quick and wide variations in bubble size can negatively affect the surgical outcome. Therefore N_2O should be discontinued at least 20 minutes before an intravitreal gas injection to ensure stable bubble size and IOP. Some anesthesia providers avoid using N_2O for any case in which intravitreal gas injection is anticipated. Patients are instructed to avoid air travel until the gas bubble is completely resolved or decreased to a level of 5% of the vitreous volume. Cabin

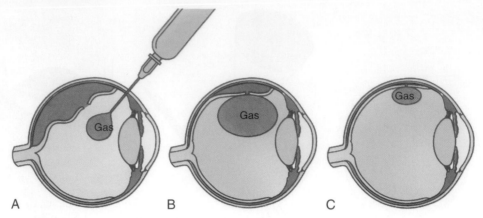

FIG. 18.23 Pneumatic retinopexy. (A) Gas bubble is injected through the pars plana. (B and C) The bubble closes and supports the retinal break. After a 7- to 10-day healing period and when the retina is returned to normal position, laser surgery or cryotherapy can be performed to seal the break.

pressurization in air travel will cause severe enlargement of the gas bubble with an increase in IOP and eye pain. Car or train travel to high elevations should also be avoided unless the change in altitude is done gradually. N_2O should be avoided so long as there is gas in the eye.

The majority of patients with RD can be successfully treated. Visual outcomes, however, are not always predictable, and additional treatment may be necessary. A successful anatomic result of retinal reattachment unfortunately does not always correlate with improvement in visual function. It may take up to several months to evaluate the final visual result. Occasionally, even with the best efforts and multiple attempts at repair, treatment may fail; sight may not be able to be restored. This discussion is part of informed consent. Repairing a detachment before the macula detaches provides the best visual results.

Surgery for Glaucoma

Glaucoma is a group of diseases that include optic neuropathy and associated visual field loss; elevated IOP is a primary risk factor (Mayo Clinic Health Letter, 2015). Glaucoma is caused from a build up of fluid in the eye, which causes pressure on the optic nerve. This pressure gradually begins to damage a person's peripheral vision with few warning signs, and if left untreated may cause permanent blindness (Fig. 18.24). Generally once the loss of peripheral vision occurs from glaucoma it cannot be restored.

Glaucoma can be treated with pressure-reducing drops and medications, with laser treatments such as argon laser trabeculectomy (ALT) or selective laser trabeculectomy (SLT), or with surgery.

Iridectomy

Peripheral iridectomy is removal of a section of iris tissue (Fig. 18.25); it is usually performed as part of a trabeculectomy procedure or when laser iridotomy is not feasible because of cloudy cornea or uveitis. Peripheral iridectomy is used to treat acute, subacute, or chronic angle-closure glaucoma when extensive peripheral anterior synechiae have not formed. This procedure is performed to reestablish communication between the posterior and anterior chambers, relieving pupillary block and permitting the iris root to drop away from the trabecular meshwork to reestablish the outflow of aqueous fluid through the Schlemm canal.

Operative Procedure

1. The speculum is introduced.
2. A small beveled incision is made at the superior limbus, or a perpendicular incision is made in the clear cornea.
3. The surgeon grasps the peripheral iris with forceps, pulls it through the incision, and excises it with a scissors.
4. The iris is repositioned by gently stroking the cornea with a blunt spatula or muscle hook. The iris can also be repositioned by irrigating with BSS.
5. A clear corneal incision is closed with 10-0 nonabsorbable suture, and a limbal incision is closed with an absorbable suture. Intracameral antibiotics may be injected, and an eye pad is applied.

Trabeculectomy (Filtration Surgery)

Trabeculectomy is a filtering procedure accomplished by incising a conjunctival flap and a scleral flap, creating a fistula, performing an iridectomy, and creating the filtering bleb (Fig. 18.26). Trabeculectomy is often combined with cataract removal and insertion of an IOL.

Procedural Considerations

Adjunctive medical therapy to decrease postoperative fibrosis includes application of an antimetabolite-soaked sponge (5-fluorouracil [5-FU] or mitomycin C) placed under the conjunctival flap. Multiple sponges are used to create diffuse blebs. Because 5-FU and mitomycin C are antimetabolites, nursing precautions for handling hazardous waste are followed. The perioperative nurse wears gloves while drawing up the antimetabolite from the vial to transfer to the operative field. All items used with the medication are disposed as hazardous waste. Instruments that contact antimetabolites should be washed separately.

Operative Procedure

1. Incisions are made into the conjunctiva and Tenon capsule, dissection is done, and a conjunctival Tenon capsule flap is created. Hemostasis is obtained with bipolar coagulation.
2. If antimetabolite is to be used, the surgeon applies it for 90 seconds to the sclera using multiple sponges before making any incision into the sclera. A small piece of sponge is saturated in the antimetabolite (5-FU or mitomycin C) and placed between the conjunctival Tenon capsule flap and the sclera. The sponge

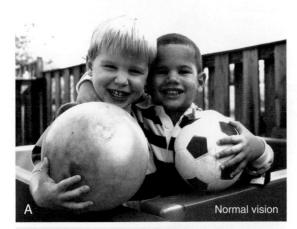

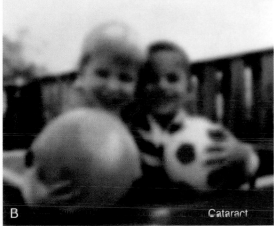

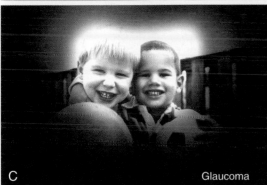

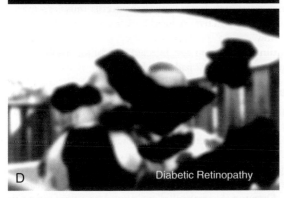

FIG. 18.24 Comparative views with (A) normal vision. A scene as it might be viewed by a person with cataract (B), as it might be viewed by a person with glaucoma (C), and as it might be viewed by a person with diabetic retinopathy (D).

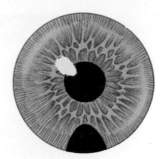

FIG. 18.25 Peripheral iridectomy.

is left in place for 3 to 5 minutes, then the site is irrigated vigorously with copious amounts of BSS.

3. The surgeon creates a square or triangular partial-thickness scleral flap (300 μm).
4. The scleral flap is retracted, and the surgeon makes an incision into and through the limbus into the anterior chamber with the tip of the blade. The limbal incision is extended to a rectangular flap of deep limbal tissue, which is then excised to create the fistula.
5. An iridectomy is performed.
6. The surgeon replaces the scleral flap and closes it with interrupted 10-0 nonabsorbable sutures. The conjunctival Tenon capsule flap is closed with a running suture, and the conjunctiva is closed.
7. BSS is injected through a cannula into the anterior chamber to deepen the anterior chamber and elevate the conjunctival bleb.
8. An eye pad and shield are applied.

Glaucoma Drainage Devices

Several types of drainage devices have been implanted into the posterior subconjunctival space with varying success when filtering procedures have been unsuccessful. These include the Molteno implant, Krupin valve, Ahmed device, Baerveldt device, and Schocket implant. Complications have been reduced through modifications in design and technique (Fig. 18.27).

Procedural Considerations

The glaucoma drainage device (GDD) and the pericardium or donor patch may be soaked in an antibiotic solution. The surgical technique for implanting GDDs is similar, regardless of the type of implant used. The drainage device and graft are documented as implants per facility protocol. The procedure is usually performed under local anesthesia with a retrobulbar or peribulbar block.

Operative Procedure

1. The surgeon incises the conjunctiva and exposes the sclera.
2. Measurements are taken for placement of the plate of the device. The plate is then sutured to the sclera.
3. After the patency of the device is checked, an occluding suture is inserted into the drainage tube.
4. With a needle, a tunnel is created into the anterior chamber for the tube and paracentesis tract.
5. The tube is trimmed and inserted into the anterior chamber. The tube is sutured to the sclera with 9-0 nonabsorbable suture.
6. The tube is covered with a patch graft of donor sclera or pericardium.
7. The occluding suture is passed through the Tenon capsule and the conjunctiva into the inferior cul-de-sac, secured with absorbable suture, and trimmed.

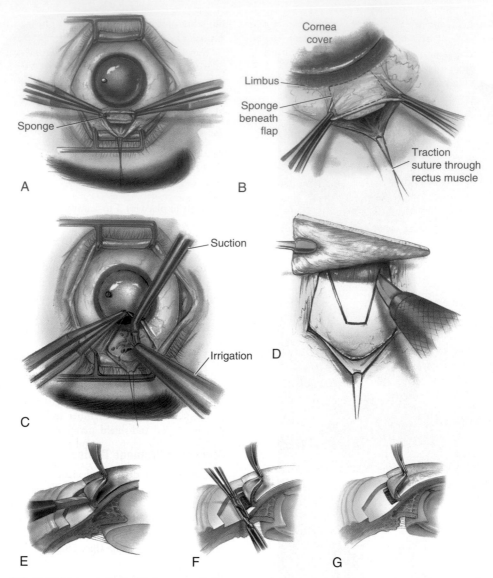

FIG. 18.26 Trabeculectomy. (A) Sponge soaked in antimetabolite is placed on sclera and (B) held in place for 90 seconds. (C) Area is thoroughly irrigated. (D) Scleral flap is formed. (E) Incision is made into anterior chamber. (F and G) Fistula is created by removing a flap of limbal tissue.

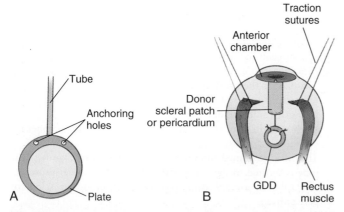

FIG. 18.27 Glaucoma drainage devices (*GDD*s). (A) Components of GDD. (B) GDD in place. Tip of drainage tube in anterior chamber. Donor scleral patch or pericardium covering tube from plate to edge of cornea.

8. Traction sutures from around the rectus muscles are removed, and the conjunctiva is closed with a continuous 7-0 absorbable suture.
9. Antiinfective agents are injected subconjunctivally. The eye is dressed with an eye pad and shield.

Canaloplasty

Canaloplasty is a surgical procedure performed when a small microcatheter is inserted into the eye around the trabecular meshwork. A viscoelastic is injected into the catheter to dilate it; this enlarges the main drainage channel (Schlemm canal). After the channel is enlarged the catheter is removed and a suture is placed within the channel. The suture is tightened to make sure the channel stays open. Opening the channel allows aqueous to flow out of the eye, reducing the IOP.

During this procedure a microscope, often requiring the capability to tilt at a 45-degree angle to enhance visualization, and bipolar

ESU are used. Instruments include an anterior segment tray, curved Stevens iris scissors, #15 blades, and lamellar or crescent blades. Medications used during the procedure are anesthetic eyedrops or injections (per surgeon's or anesthesia provider's preference), BSS, viscoelastic, antibiotic and steroid injections, antibiotic eye ointment, and cycloplegic drops. The surgeon makes a small limbal incision into the anterior chamber, injects a viscoelastic, and passes a small catheter around the trabecular meshwork around Schlemm canal. Ophthalmic ointment is applied followed by a patch and shield.

Surgery of the Conjunctiva

The conjunctiva is a transparent and elastic membrane that lines the inner surface of the eyelids and covers the sclera. Lacerations caused by injury as well as deficits resulting from excision of tumors, cysts, nevi, or pterygia can usually be repaired by simple undermining and suturing.

Pterygium Excision

A pterygium is a fleshy, triangular encroachment of conjunctiva onto the peripheral area of the cornea. Pterygia occurrence has been linked to increased exposure to ultraviolet light, so it is important to wear polarized sunglasses while outside during the day. Because pterygia tend to recur, surgery is delayed until vision is affected by encroachment on the visual axis, high astigmatism, or irritation.

Operative Procedure

Pterygia surgery can be done under topical; peribulbar; or, less commonly, retrobulbar anesthesia. A pterygium can also be excised totally and the limbus treated with an eye cautery or bipolar ESU. The sclera is typically covered using a conjunctival autograft or amniotic membrane graft, or, less commonly, left bare (Fig. 18.28).

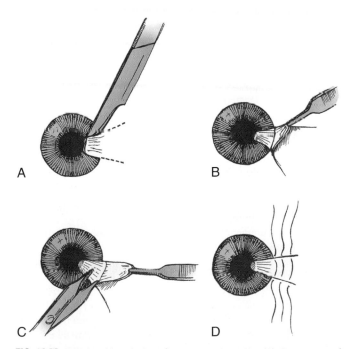

FIG. 18.28 McReynolds technique for pterygium excision. (A) Cornea around head of pterygium is incised. (B) Pterygium flap is dissected upward, leaving clear cornea. (C) Lower margin of pterygium is dissected, and the entire pterygium is freed from sclera. (D) Sutures are placed for closure of conjunctiva.

Surgeons have also adopted use of fibrin tissue adhesive in place of sutures for conjunctival grafts or amniotic membranes.

Surgery may be combined with application of the chemotherapeutic agent mitomycin C (typically 0.02 mg/mL for 3 minutes) for recurrent cases. In addition, a diamond burr drill may be used to smooth the corneal and limbal surfaces after the removal of tissue.

Excisional Biopsy

Any suspect lesion of the conjunctiva can be removed by a simple elliptic excision and sent for pathologic examination. The conjunctiva may or may not be closed, depending on the surgeon's particular technique.

Surgery of the Cornea

Surgery of the cornea is indicated for a variety of conditions in which cosmetic, therapeutic, restorative, or refractive outcomes are desired.

Repair of Lacerations

Corneal lacerations may be closed with direct appositional suturing with 10-0 suture viewed through an operating microscope or with a tissue adhesive, such as cyanoacrylate monomers. The sterile tissue adhesive is applied to well-dried tissue that has been properly oriented anatomically. It polymerizes and seals the wound on contact with the tissue. Culture specimens are usually obtained at the time of surgery. Antibiotics are injected subconjunctivally before the dressing is applied.

Refractive Corneal Procedures

Keratorefractive procedures are corneal procedures designed to correct myopia, hyperopia, and astigmatism. These procedures require reshaping the cornea to change the refractive power of the eye to reduce or eliminate the need for eyeglasses and contact lenses. The types of corneal refractive surgeries include PRK, LASIK, and wavefront-guided custom LASIK. Although most refractive procedures are truly surgical, few are performed in traditional hospital or ambulatory surgical facilities. However, refractive surgery has been performed for so many years that these same patients who are aging will present themselves for cataract surgery. It is recommended that the perioperative nurse be familiar with this branch of eye surgery.

LASIK Surgery

With the LASIK procedure the curvature of the corneal stroma is reshaped using an excimer laser to ablate certain areas. For nearsighted patients the central curvature of the cornea is flattened by removing stromal tissue from the center of the cornea. For farsighted patients the central curvature of the cornea is steepened by removing stromal tissue from the periphery of the cornea, leaving the center untreated.

Advances in LASIK have allowed surgeons to improve its overall results. Wavefront-guided LASIK surgery corrects for the lower order aberrations (refractions) as well as the patient's individual higher order aberrations. Custom-guided LASIK (Intralase), a US Food and Drug Administration (FDA)–approved femtosecond laser, is used to create the corneal flap. It can perform the cutting more accurately, quicker, and without using a mechanically moving metal keratome. This technology is more precise because the laser reads the patient's eye and uses these findings for calculations. During this precise process, stable eye positioning is paramount for the best results.

Photorefractive Keratectomy

PRK is a surface ablation technique that involves manual scraping to remove the corneal epithelium and to shape the surface of the cornea with the cool light of the excimer laser. Surface ablation avoids the complications of flap formation in LASIK and provides excellent visual results. A major drawback, however, is delayed visual rehabilitation and pain from the regrowth of corneal epithelium, although it can be controlled with topical and oral therapy. PRK is performed if a patient has thin corneas, previous corneal scarring, or other corneal diseases.

LASEK Surgery

Laser epithelial keratomileusis (LASEK) is similar to PRK because the procedure is performed on the surface of the cornea. After numbing the eye with topical anesthetic drops, the surgeon loosens the epithelium with a diluted alcohol solution and mechanically pushes it aside. A laser is then used to treat the corneal surface, similar to PRK and LASIK procedures. The epithelial flap is then returned to its original position, and a bandage contact lens is placed for the duration of the healing process, which may take several days.

Corneal Transplantation (Keratoplasty)

A corneal transplantation (keratoplasty) is performed when the patient's cornea is thickened or opacified by disease and degeneration. Corneal transparency may be impaired by scars, infection (bacterial, fungal, or viral), thermal or chemical burns, corneal dystrophies, edema after intraocular surgery, or keratoconus (abnormal steepening). Corneal transplantation, in which corneal tissue from one human eye is grafted to another, is done to improve vision when the retina and optic nerve are functioning properly. Because the cornea lacks blood vessels, it can be transplanted with less rejection and at a 90% success rate. Corneal transplant is one of the most frequently performed human transplant procedures. Eye Bank Association of America (EBAA) member eye banks in the United States provided 79,304 corneas for transplant in 2015 (EBAA, 2015). Lamellar grafts can be used to treat a pathology that is not of full thickness. One type of lamellar surgery, called deep anterior lamellar keratoplasty, is commonly used for patients who have keratoconus or partial-thickness corneal scars. If successful, the corneal stroma and epithelium are able to be replaced while keeping the host endothelium, which decreases the risk of transplant rejection and improves graft stability. Because of the technical difficulty of this procedure, it is common to convert to a full-thickness penetrating procedure. Another technique used for posterior corneal pathology is Descemet stripping endothelial keratoplasty (DSEK). This is used for patients who have Fuchs dystrophy, corneal edema caused by intraocular surgery, or failed corneal transplants. It consists of replacing the endothelium without transplanting the entire cornea. It offers improved corneal clarity with less astigmatism, shorter healing times, and less chance of wound dehiscence and rejection. Deep lamellar endothelial keratoplasty (DLEK) is another technique. It consists of replacing the endothelium without transplanting the full cornea to restore vision. This technique offers the potential for highly predictable corneal power for extended periods without the astigmatism that often occurs with penetrating keratoplasty. The transplanted endothelium is inserted into the host through a small incision, greatly reducing the risk of infection.

Phototherapeutic keratectomy (PTK) procedures use excimer laser ablation to remove superficial corneal lesions and smooth the corneal surface. PTK can be used for conditions that would require corneal transplant and may delay or replace the occurrence of penetrating keratoplasty in some cases.

Procurement of Corneas

Education on eye donation and transplantation is important for all surgical staff so that they understand that ocular tissue is a donated gift. Corneas and scleral grafts are gifts that were given by families as they were grieving the loss of their loved ones and should be treated as such.

The eye bank may be a central community agency or may be owned and operated by a hospital. Eye banks help coordinate the procurement of eyes from recently deceased persons under the EBAA guidelines. People of any age can be eye donors, and poor eyesight or cataracts does not influence eye viability (EBAA, 2015). The donor's family, medical, and social histories are reviewed. It is not necessary to perform antigen matching as with other tissue or organ transplants, but blood serum tests for human immunodeficiency virus (HIV) and hepatitis B and C virus are performed on the donor. The procurement team removes donor eyes within 6 hours of death in accordance with legal regulations. Tissue, such as a cornea, must be recovered, processed, and transplanted in controlled surgical environments. If the donor eye is unsuitable for the cornea to be transplanted, the eye can be used for research or education.

Many individuals have signed donor cards or eye-donor designation on their drivers' licenses. A special consent form is required and should be signed by the authorized next of kin and by a hospital representative designated by the institution. Federal regulations require hospitals to report all deaths and imminent deaths to organ procurement organizations. With the collaboration of hospitals, organ procurement organizations, and eye and tissue banks, the family of each potential donor is informed about the option to donate organs or tissues.

Enucleations may be done in the hospital morgue or emergency department under aseptic conditions. The procured cornea is placed in Optisol GS sterile buffered tissue culture medium within 12 hours of death and transplanted within 3 to 7 days. Optisol GS sterile buffered tissue culture medium contains polypeptides, dextran, and antibiotics (gentamicin and streptomycin) and can preserve a donor cornea for 14 days under refrigeration. It is best if corneal transplantation is performed in 2 or 3 days because the cornea may become boggy from constant exposure to the tissue culture solution.

Donor Tissue Procurement

Procedural Considerations. Postmortem preparation includes elevating the donor's head with a pillow to minimize edema in the face or near the eye. The eyes are irrigated and lightly taped closed to avoid pressure on the eye. A small ice pack may be applied to the forehead or over the eyes if the donor is not in a refrigerated morgue within 1 hour of death.

For the procurement procedure, the eyes are washed and irrigated in the routine manner of preparation for eye surgery. The sterile field, drapes, and instruments are essentially the same as those for an enucleation on a living patient (see page 614).

Operative Procedure

1. Eye specimen jars are labeled for right and left eyes.
2. The speculum is inserted, and after routine enucleation the donated eye is placed with the cornea up and secured in a metal eye cage or on gauze in the sterile specimen jar.
3. The eye sockets are packed with cotton, and the lids are closed.
4. Specimen jars are sealed with tape and labeled with the donor's name or identification number, time of death, time of enucleation, and date. The jars are placed on crushed ice in an insulated carrier

and transported to the eye bank. The entire cornea with a scleral rim is placed in Optisol GS before transplant.

Corneal Transplant

Procedural Considerations. For the transplant procedure the nurse positions and preps the patient in the same fashion as for a cataract procedure. Corneal transplant is typically done under local or general anesthesia. For local anesthesia, most surgeons use a retrobulbar or peribulbar block in addition to a facial block to obviate procedural pain. It is very important to have adequate akinesia and anesthesia so the patient cannot squeeze the eyelids after removal of the host corneal button. It is also important for the anesthesia provider to keep the patient comfortable during this crucial step in transplantation. Any posterior pressure during this time can lead to suprachoroidal hemorrhage or expulsion of the intraocular contents. For this reason, many surgeons give mannitol to lower IOP pressure before surgery.

Operative Procedures

Penetrating Keratoplasty

1. After insertion of a wire lid speculum, the surgeon may place a Flieringa ring or bridle sutures to support the structure of the eye. If a ring is used, the surgeon secures it in place with four 5-0 Dacron sutures (Fig. 18.29).
2. A corneoscleral button that has been refrigerated and stored in Optisol GS is removed from its container.
3. The surgeon places the donor corneoscleral button on a sterile Teflon block with the epithelial (outside) surface down. Using the corneal trephine as a punch, the surgeon presses out the

button. A drop of Optisol GS may be used to cover the donor button until it is implanted.

4. Using a handheld trephine or a disposable suction trephine, a corneoscleral button is excised from the recipient's cornea. The diameter of the cornea removed from the recipient's eye is usually 0.25 mm smaller than the graft taken from the donor's eye.
5. Peripheral iridectomies or iridotomies may be performed at this time at the surgeon's discretion; a cataract extraction with IOL implantation may also be performed if the lens is opaque.
6. The surgeon places the graft into the opening of the recipient's eye and anchors it in place with four single-armed sutures placed at the four cardinal meridians, viewed through an operating microscope. Some surgeons preplace sutures in the graft. The surgeon sutures the graft to the host with either continuous or interrupted 10-0 nonabsorbable sutures.
7. Air or sodium hyaluronate may be injected into the anterior chamber of the recipient's eye to keep the iris from adhering to the suture line. Mydriatic or miotic solutions are used at the surgeon's discretion.
8. A subconjunctival injection of antibiotic solution or a topical application of antibiotic drops may be used at the completion of the procedure. Antibiotic ointment is applied, followed by an eye pad and a protective shield.

Lamellar Keratoplasty

1. The surgeon inserts the eye speculum, then places the superior rectus and inferior rectus bridle sutures (if needed).
2. The perioperative nurse presents the donor eye from the eye bank to the sterile field; the scrub person washes it in BSS.
3. If the lamellar graft has not already been cut by the eye bank, the surgeon will make a groove to the desired depth in the cornea using a trephine. The lamellar graft is completed using either a keratome or sharp dissection with a blade, and the graft is placed in Optisol solution or BSS.
4. The recipient cornea is trephined to the appropriate depth. A lamellar resection can then be performed, removing the anterior part of the cornea. If a deep anterior lamellar keratoplasty is being performed, the surgeon may insert a needle or cannula into the deep corneal stroma after placing the groove. Air is then injected to find a plane for dissection between the corneal stroma and the inner layer of the cornea (Descemet membrane). This is called the "big bubble technique."
5. The donor tissue is sutured in place with an interrupted or continuous 10-0 nonabsorbable suture.
6. A mydriatic agent and subconjunctival or topical antibiotics may be used and the eyepatch applied.

Descemet Stripping Endothelial Keratoplasty

1. The surgeon inserts a lid speculum and uses a trephine to mark the corneal epithelium for the size of endothelial graft that will be placed. Multiple paracentesis incisions are made, and a viscoelastic agent is injected to maintain a formed anterior chamber. A temporal corneal incision is made.
2. Using a reverse Sinskey hook the surgeon scores and strips the Descemet membrane. Venting incisions may be placed full thickness through the remaining host cornea using a sharp point blade. Aspiration is then used to remove the viscoelastic from the anterior chamber, and an anterior chamber maintainer is typically placed to facilitate graft placement.
3. Attention is directed to the donor corneal button. The button may be cut by the eye bank, or may need to be cut to the appropriate thickness using a microkeratome and artificial anterior chamber system.

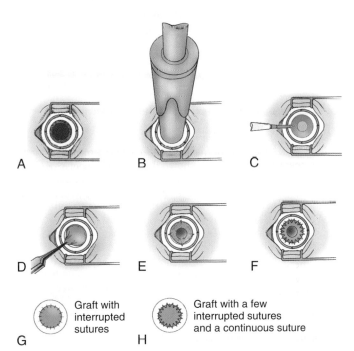

FIG. 18.29 Corneal transplantation. (A) Eye of patient who will undergo corneal transplantation. Flieringa fixation ring is sutured in place with 5-0 nonabsorbable sutures. (B) Corneal trephine is placed on recipient cornea, and partial penetration is made approximately three-quarters through stroma. (C) Anterior chamber is entered through groove, and the remainder of button is excised with right and left corneal microscissors. (D) Corneal button is removed. (E) Donor cornea graft is sutured in place with four sutures. (F) Donor cornea graft is sutured in place with interrupted or continuous 10-0 nonabsorbable suture (G and H).

Graft with interrupted sutures

Graft with a few interrupted sutures and a continuous suture

4. The endothelial graft can be inserted into the anterior chamber by several different methods. Many graft inserters are available that attach to the irrigation on a phaco unit. Other common methods of insertion include the use of a Busin glide or folding, using forceps.

5. After the graft is in the anterior chamber, a 10-0 nonabsorbable suture is placed at the wound and the graft is unfolded so the endothelial surface is facing down. When the graft is in good position, a cannula is used to inject an air bubble under the graft, displacing it up against the corneal stroma and increasing the IOP so the graft will adhere to the posterior cornea. The air is typically left in position for 30 minutes to 1 hour after which part of it is released to prevent pupillary block. Some surgeons perform an iridectomy and leave a full air bubble in the eye. The surgeon may remove the air in the OR or at a slit lamp.

6. Antibiotic and mydriatic drops are then placed on the eye and the eye may be patched.

Surgery of the Lacrimal Gland and Apparatus

Surgery of the lacrimal gland is usually performed for treatment or diagnosis of tumors of the lacrimal fossa or to correct epiphora, which is abnormal overflow of tears related to a congenital or acquired obstruction of the lacrimal drainage system.

Surgery of the Lacrimal Fossa

Surgery of the lacrimal fossa is performed for biopsy of any structure in the lacrimal fossa.

Operative Procedure

The lacrimal fossa, which is in the upper temporal quadrant of the orbit, may be approached directly through the lid or through the conjunctiva by everting the upper lid. The lacrimal gland is divided into a palpebral and an orbital part by the orbital septum. Surgery on the palpebral portion may produce a dry eye.

Nasolacrimal Duct Procedures

Operative Procedure

Simple Probing

1. Using a punctual dilator, the surgeon widens the tear duct opening along the medial aspect of the upper and lower eyelids.

2. A lacrimal probe (sizes vary from 00 to 4) is passed through the punctum, canaliculus, lacrimal sac, and nasolacrimal duct into the nasal cavity (under the middle meatus).

3. Adequacy of the duct opening is confirmed via metal-on-metal contact with the probe within the nasal cavity or via irrigation of fluorescein-tinged saline through the tear duct, aspirated in the nose.

Probing With Intubation. After opening the duct as described in the previous procedure, the surgeon may place a Silastic tube or stent in one or both canaliculi to reduce the chance of postoperative obstruction.

The surgeon threads the polyglactin leader on the stent through a stylet inserted into the punctum and retrieves it from the nasal cavity in the nose with a hook. Bicanalicular stents may use a pliable metal rod attached to the Silastic tube.

Dacryocystorhinostomy

Dacryocystitis (Fig. 18.30) is an infection in the lacrimal sac, which may result in a localized cellulitis. Chronic or recurrent dacryocystitis in adults may necessitate probing or dacryocystorhinostomy (DCR) because of resistant obstruction of the nasolacrimal duct related to

infection-associated scarring, dacryolith (calculus in the duct), trauma, or for intolerable epiphora resulting from tear duct laceration following medial orbital wall fracture. DCR is the establishment of a new tear passageway for drainage directly into the nasal cavity. The minimally invasive approach to DCR surgery includes the use of a transconjunctival incision, lasers, and endoscopic techniques. This approach to DCR is generally associated with less pain (Research Highlight) and low risk of infection.

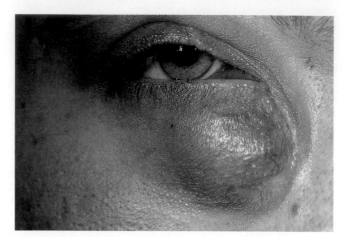

FIG. 18.30 Chronic infection of lacrimal sac (dacryocystitis) causes swelling of inner lower corner of eye socket.

RESEARCH HIGHLIGHT

Aromatherapy for Managing Pain, Anxiety, and Nausea

Pain management is a focus of TJC. Healthcare facilities are required to ask patients about their pain and provide appropriate care. Additional recommendations emphasize nonpharmacologic and multimodal strategies to help patients manage their pain. Such strategies are part of ERAS protocols. Nurses are often advocates for patients when it comes to assisting pain management and anxiety during visits to hospitals and ambulatory surgery centers.

Studies have been undertaken to research the effectiveness of alternative methods of managing pain, such as meditation and aromatherapy. Research has shown that certain essential oil scents improve pain, nausea, and anxiety. This study used inhalation administered aromatherapy in lavender, ginger, sweet marjoram, mandarin, or combination oils to patients admitted to the acute care setting.

During the study patients reported their pain, anxiety, and nausea levels on a 10-point scale before and after receiving aromatherapy. Pain, anxiety, and nausea levels were measured for each patient; the essential oils had varying effects on the three main measured symptoms. Pain had the largest decrease when sweet marjoram was used. To lower anxiety, lavender and sweet marjoram had equal effects. Ginger had the largest effect for combatting nausea.

Initial studies using essential oils have so far shown promising data for combining nontraditional pain management techniques to reduce the need for traditional medications. One method does not replace the other, but they can work in conjunction to have positive outcomes in acute care settings.

ERAS, Enhanced recovery after surgery; *TJC,* The Joint Commission.
Modified from Johnson JR et al: The effectiveness of nurse-delivered aromatherapy in an acute care setting, *Complement Ther Med* 25:164–169, 2016; Montgomery R, McNamara SA: Multimodal pain management for enhanced recovery: reinforcing the shift from traditional pathways through nurse-led interventions, *AORN J* 104(6S):S9–S22, 2016.

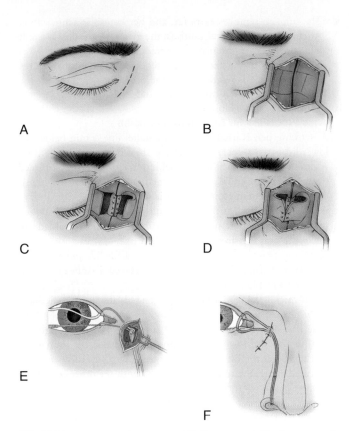

FIG. 18.31 Dacryocystorhinostomy. (A) Skin incision for dacryocystorhinostomy or dacryocystectomy. (B) Lacrimal sac and lacrimal bone exposed. Opening made in lacrimal bone and lacrimal crest. (C) Posterior flap of wall of sac sutured to posterior flap of nasal mucosa. (D) Anterior flap of wall of sac sutured to anterior flap of nasal mucosa (drawing is somewhat distorted for visualization of relative positions). (E) Canaliculi are intubated with Silastic tubes. (F) Tubes are secured to lateral nasal wall and allowed to slide back into nose.

Procedural Considerations

The nasal cavity is anesthetized topically with cocaine, 2% Polocaine, or Afrin nasal spray (oxymetazoline) soaked on cottonoids just before surgery. DCR may also require the use of Gelfoam soaked with 5000 units of thrombin to aid in hemostasis. Local or general anesthesia is used.

Operative Procedure

1. An external incision is made in the medial canthal area or inside the nose when an internal approach is used (Fig. 18.31).
2. Blunt dissection is carried through the orbicularis down to the nasal bone. The orbicularis is separated from the bone with a Freer elevator. The lacrimal fossa sac is exposed.
3. A hemostat is used to press an opening through the lacrimal bone. If this is unsuccessful, the anterior lacrimal crest is perforated with a power burr or mallet and chisel. The opening is enlarged to a 10-mm circle with a Kerrison rongeur, and hemostasis is obtained with bone wax if necessary.
4. The inferior punctum is dilated, and a probe is passed into the lacrimal sac.
5. The lacrimal sac and nasal mucosa are incised with H flaps. The posterior nasal mucous membrane flaps are sutured to the posterior lacrimal sac flap with 4-0 absorbable suture.

6. The first end of the wire stylet of a Silastic lacrimal duct intubation set is passed through the upper canaliculus, through the opening, and out through the nose (under the inferior meatus). The procedure is repeated for the lower canaliculus.
7. The anterior nasal mucous membrane flap is sutured to the anterior lacrimal sac flap with 4-0 absorbable suture to create a bridge over the Silastic tubing. The tubing remains in place until the sutures are absorbed, acting as a stent around which epithelial union between the lacrimal and nasal mucosa can occur.
8. The orbicularis is closed with 6-0 absorbable suture. Skin margins are approximated and closed with nonabsorbable 6-0 suture. Antibiotic ointment is applied to the incision.
9. The surgeon cuts the wire stylets off the Silastic tubing and ties the ends of the tubing together. The tubing is sutured to the lateral nasal wall with 6-0 nonabsorbable suture. The tubing is cut so that it retracts into the nostril. An absorbent sponge may be taped under the nostrils.

Surgery of the Eyelids

Oculoplastic procedures performed on the eyelids include treatment of chalazion, entropion, ectropion, dermatochalasis, and ptosis; biopsy and excision of eyelid tumors; and repair and reconstruction of eyelid trauma or postbiopsy damage.

Removal of Chalazion

Obstruction of the meibomian gland caused by secretions may lead to a chalazion, manifesting as a variably firm bump in the eyelid. Although chalazia can become infected, they are not primarily an infectious process. If persistent, incision and drainage of the chronic chalazion may be warranted.

Procedural Considerations

Incision of chalazion is often performed in an office setting, but pediatric and very anxious patients may require IV sedation. Local anesthesia, with 1:100,000 epinephrine in the local anesthetic, is usually used. The majority of chalazia are surgically approached from the conjunctival side of the tarsal plate, but cutaneous incisions or repair of friable cutaneous tissue may be required.

Operative Procedure (Transconjunctival Approach)

1. The surgeon everts the affected lid to expose the chalazion and applies a chalazion clamp (Fig. 18.32)
2. A vertical incision is made on the inner lid surface with a sharp blade; the lesion is curetted, or the chalazion wall is excised, in part or in toto.
3. Hemostasis is achieved through use of the bipolar ESU.
4. The wound is left open for drainage. Cutaneous sutures are placed when needed. Pressure eye patching may be performed.

Repair of Entropion

Entropion occurs when the eyelid margin inverts. It may cause significant corneal irritation, attributable to rubbing of inturned eyelashes against the ocular surface. The most common type is *involutional entropion,* in which laxity and degeneration of fascial attachments between the pretarsal muscle and the tarsus permit the pretarsal muscle to override the lid margin during contraction. *Cicatricial entropion* is attributable to contraction of either the upper or the lower tarsus and its conjunctiva, causing inturned lashes (trichiasis) to abrade the cornea. Commonly used surgical techniques for entropion repair include lateral tightening of a lax eyelid via either a tarsal strip procedure or a pentagonal wedge resection and suture eversion (via either a Wies or a Quickert suture technique).

Procedural Considerations

The causes of entropion vary, as do corrective procedures, depending on the pathologic process. Local topical and infiltrative anesthesia is typically used, and antiinfective ointment is applied postoperatively.

Operative Procedures

Blepharoplasty of Lower Lid for Involutional Entropion

1. Local anesthetic is injected into the lower lid through the conjunctiva using an angled needle.
2. The skin is marked, and an incision is made in the lateral canthus.
3. The orbicularis is dissected off the orbital septum.
4. The skin excision is extended across the lower lid.
5. The orbital septum is incised to expose fat pockets, which can be excised.

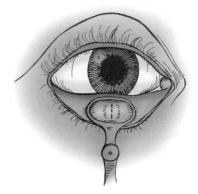

FIG. 18.32 Transconjunctival approach. Clamp everts eyelid during surgery for chalazion. Viscous contents of chalazion will be removed with curette.

6. The surgeon removes extra fat, and hemostasis is achieved.
7. After incising the lateral canthus, the lower lid is pulled laterally and shortened (tightened) to correct entropion.
8. The tarsus is reattached to the lateral canthal tendon, and the lower lid fascia is reattached to the orbicularis.
9. Excess skin is pulled up, marked, and excised.
10. Skin incisions are closed.

Wies Procedure for Cicatricial Entropion

1. A marking pen is used to draw a parallel line 4 mm below the lower lid margin; local anesthetic is then injected (Fig. 18.33).
2. A double-armed 4-0 nonabsorbable retraction suture is placed through the conjunctiva and lower lid 4 mm from the lateral canthus and 4 mm from the medial canthus.
3. A lid plate retractor is placed behind the lower lid as it is pulled up with the traction suture. The surgeon uses a #15 blade to make the skin incision on the marked line.
4. The lid plate retractor is placed in front of the lid, and the lower lid is everted using the traction suture. The conjunctiva is incised with the #15 blade.
5. A full-thickness blepharotomy is extended laterally and medially with scissors.
6. One end of a double-armed 4-0 suture is passed through the conjunctiva and lower lid tendons and between the orbicularis and tarsus on the medial aspect of the lower lid. This process is repeated approximately 4 mm laterally with the other end of the 4-0 suture.
7. Mattress sutures are placed and tied to evert the lower lid.
8. Excess skin is excised, and the skin incision is closed with 7-0 nonabsorbable suture.

Repair of Ectropion

Ectropion (sagging and eversion of the lower lid), usually bilateral, is common in older adults. Ectropion may be caused by the relaxation of the orbicular muscle and canthal tendons. Symptoms include tearing, conjunctival infection, irritation, and inadequate corneal

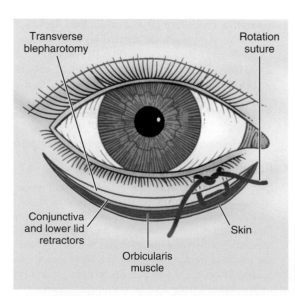

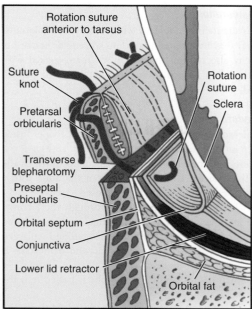

FIG. 18.33 Wies procedure for entropion. Placement of an everting mattress suture across a transverse blepharotomy.

protection leading to corneal injury. Surgery is indicated when facial paralysis is permanent or when scarring follows lacerations, lesions, or penetrating injuries and the cornea becomes exposed, resulting in ulceration and photophobia.

Procedural Considerations

The causes of ectropion vary, and corrective procedures also vary depending on the pathologic process. Local anesthesia is typically used, and antiinfective ointment and ice compresses are applied postoperatively. The Müller muscle conjunctival resection (MMCR) can be done with an internal approach by starting the incision from the inside lower eyelid.

Operative Procedure

Lateral Canthal Sling Procedure. This procedure repositions and tightens the lower lid in a horizontal direction (Fig. 18.34).

1. The lateral canthus is incised, and a strip of tarsus and lateral canthal tendon is isolated.
2. The tarsus/tendon is sutured to the periosteum along the inner surface of the lateral wall of the orbit, tightening the lid and correcting the ectropion.

Plastic Repair for Dermatochalasis

Dermatochalasis is a condition of drooping skin and herniated fat of the upper and lower lids that causes the skin of the upper eyelids to hang down over the palpebral fissure, sometimes obscuring vision. It may occur in older adults who have lost normal elasticity in the skin of their upper lids or in individuals who have persistent angioneurotic edema with stretching of the skin of the eyelids. If ptosis is present, it accentuates the condition. Dermatochalasis is corrected with blepharoplasty of the redundant skin of the upper or lower eyelids (refer to Chapter 22 for procedural considerations and the operative procedure for blepharoplasty).

Surgery for Unilateral or Bilateral Ptosis

Ptosis is true drooping of the upper lid. It may be congenital or acquired. In congenital ptosis there usually is developmental weakness of the levator muscle. The condition may be unilateral or bilateral. The child often compensates by raising the eyebrow or tilting the chin upward. Acquired ptosis can be neurogenic, myogenic, or involutional, which is manifested by a gradual stretching or dehiscence of the levator aponeurosis. The eyelid crease may be high or absent. Ptosis can affect both the visual field and the cosmetic appearance of the eye (Fig. 18.35).

Procedural Considerations

The objective of ptosis surgery is to achieve a good cosmetic result, expand the superior visual field, and restore function with elevation of the lid. Many surgical procedures have been devised, directed at the levator aponeurosis, frontalis muscle, or the levator-Müller muscle

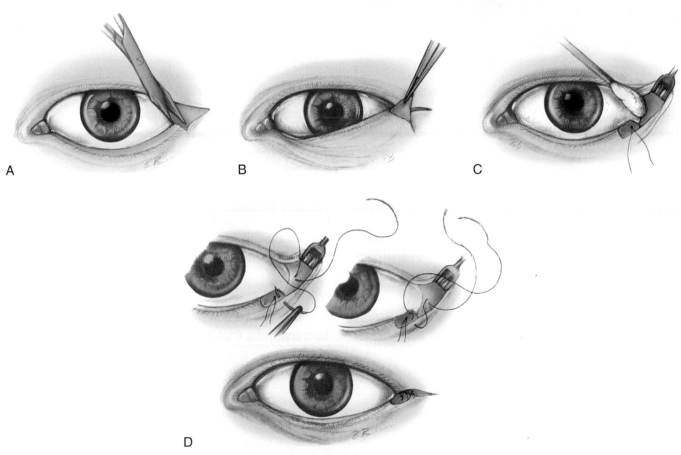

FIG. 18.34 Lateral canthal sling procedure for ectropion. (A) Cantholysis of the lower arm of the lateral canthal tendon is performed. (B) Horizontal laxity of the lid is relieved by stretching the lid temporally until it fits tightly against the globe. A tarsal lateral canthal tendon strip is isolated. (C) Using a cotton applicator, tissue is cleaned from the periosteum of the lateral rim of the orbit. (D) The tarsal tendon strip is sutured to the periosteum along the inner surface of the lateral wall of the orbit.

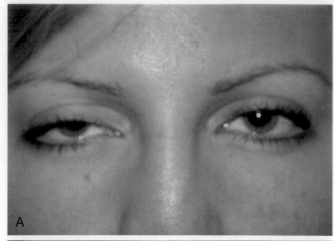

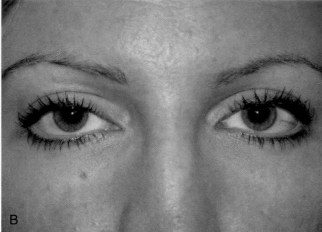

FIG. 18.35 Ptosis surgery before (A) and after (B).

complex. These muscles are the elevating forces of the upper lids. Local anesthesia may be preferred in cooperative individuals so that intraoperative adjustments can be made. Frontalis suspension uses fascia lata or synthetic materials to attach the tarsus to the frontalis, bypassing the ineffective levator muscle. Harvesting fascia lata requires an additional incision in the leg.

Operative Procedures
Levator Aponeurosis Repair
1. The existing or potential eyelid crease is marked. With the skin of the upper lid held taut, the skin incision is made (Fig. 18.36).
2. An incision is made through the orbicularis. The orbicularis is dissected off the orbital septum and the levator aponeurosis anterior to the tarsus.
3. The aponeurosis is incised across the tarsus and dissected off the orbicularis. The levator is reattached to the tarsus with interrupted 6-0 suture.
4. If the patient is awake, he or she is asked to look forward and sutures are adjusted as needed.
5. The pretarsal orbicularis is sutured to the aponeurosis to reconstruct the lid crease.
6. The skin is closed with a running 6-0 nonabsorbable suture.

Frontalis Suspension
1. The upper lid is marked, one incision is made in the lid crease, and two incisions are made above the eyebrow (Fig. 18.37).
2. A lid plate is placed behind the upper lid, the tarsus exposed, and the suspension material (fascia graft or a synthetic implant) secured to the tarsus with nonabsorbable sutures.
3. Using a Wright needle, the suspension material is passed away from the globe deeply into the orbital septum and out through one eyebrow incision.
4. The remaining end of the suspension material is passed in the same manner.
5. The pretarsal orbicularis is sutured to the tarsus to form the lid crease.
6. The lid incision is closed with a running 6-0 nonabsorbable suture.
7. The long end of the suspension material is passed under the skin between the brow incisions to complete the loop; the ends of the material are sutured together.
8. The brow incisions are closed with interrupted 6-0 nonabsorbable suture.

Excisional Biopsy

Excisional biopsy is removal of lesions for diagnostic examination. Basal cell carcinomas account for 95% of neoplastic lesions of the lid; the treatment of choice is excision with frozen-section analysis or Mohs technique.

Operative Procedure
Through-and-through excision of skin, muscle, tarsus, and conjunctiva is followed by careful structural closure of anatomic spaces. Depending on the type, extent, and location of the lesion, rotation flaps or free grafts may be necessary (see Chapter 22).

Plastic Repair for Traumatic Injuries

Lacerations of the lids, including damage to the inferior canaliculus, are repaired surgically. Paramount for success is careful approximation of the borders of the lid margin and the ends of a torn canaliculus.

Operative Procedure
Lacerations of the lid margin are closed with a 6-0 silk suture to align the gray line of the lid that lies between the lash follicles and the orifices of the meibomian glands. Once this anatomic line has been approximated, all other sutures are placed, maintaining the approximation. If the canaliculus has been lacerated, the lacrimal drainage system is intubated with a silicone tube and the canaliculus and lid are reconstructed around the tube.

Surgery of the Globe and Orbit

Surgery of the globe (eyeball) and orbit is usually performed because of trauma. Rupture of the eyeball may be direct at the site of injury or, more frequently, indirect from an increase in IOP that causes the wall of the eyeball to tear at weaker points, such as the limbus. When the intraocular contents have become so deranged that useful function is prohibited or the blind eye becomes painful, removal of the eye contents (evisceration procedure) or of the entire eyeball (enucleation) is indicated. If either procedure is required, an inert globe or a coralline hydroxyapatite (coral) implant may be inserted as a space filler and to aid in the movement of a prosthesis (artificial eye). Fractures of the orbit are discussed in Chapter 22.

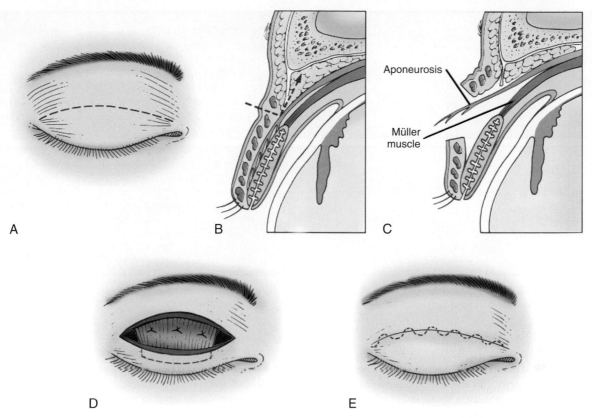

FIG. 18.36 Levator aponeurosis repair for ptosis. (A) Eyelid crease is marked. (B) Skin incision is made, and the orbicularis and orbital septum are divided while dissection proceeds toward the orbital rim. (C) The anterior surface of the tarsus is exposed, and the aponeurosis is separated from the Müller muscle. (D) The aponeurosis is reattached to the tarsus with partial-thickness permanent sutures. Lid contour and position are adjusted. (E) The eyelid crease is created by suturing the pretarsal orbicularis muscle to the aponeurosis, and the skin is closed.

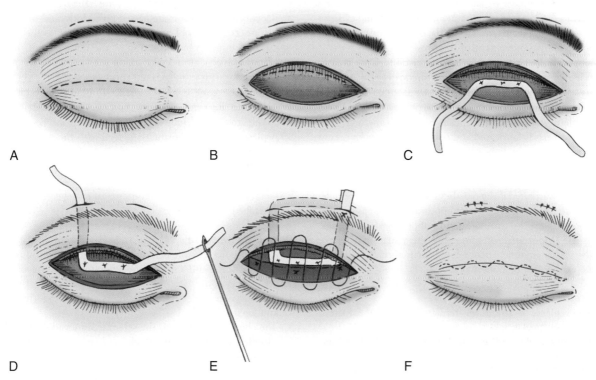

FIG. 18.37 Frontalis suspension for ptosis. One method used to suspend the eyelid from the brow.

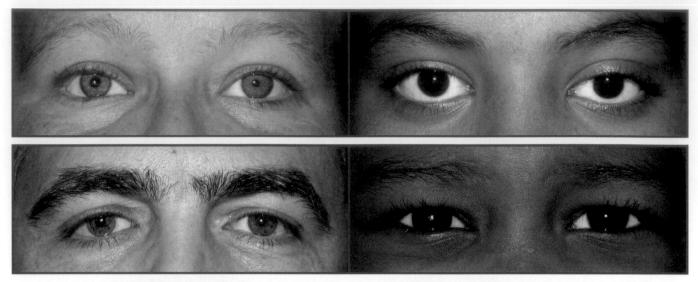

FIG. 18.38 Patients who have an enucleation can have excellent cosmetic results when fitted with an ocular prosthesis designed by a board certified ocularist.

Enucleation

Enucleation is removal of the entire eyeball, severing its muscular attachments and optic nerve. This life-altering procedure is indicated for a blind, painful eye; intraocular tumors; and as a last resort after trauma. Usually a round implant is inserted into the socket to replace the globe and provide support for a prosthetic eye. Sphere implants may be coralline (hydroxyapatite) or synthetic, although glass and silicone implants are still used. Hydroxyapatite, a lightweight coral-like material, may be used as the foundation for a prosthetic eye because its porous structure encourages fibrovascular ingrowth. The hydroxyapatite implant is wrapped in human donor sclera or Silastic sheeting before insertion into the orbital space. Synthetic porous polyethylene implants have the advantage of allowing the rectus muscles to be sutured directly to the implant, eliminating the wrapping and expense of donor sclera. Suturing rectus muscles to the orbital implant enables improved postoperative movement of the prosthesis.

The patient typically consults with an ocularist 4 to 6 weeks after enucleation or evisceration surgery for a prosthetic eye (Fig. 18.38). A temporary prosthesis may be inserted while a custom-made prosthesis is fabricated. The prosthesis fitting process takes about 7 hours to complete. A mold of the socket is made using a type of wax, and the prosthesis is fabricated and painted to match the seeing eye. The patient follows up 1 month later to ensure proper fitting, and then once per year to evaluate its size and to resurface (polish) the prosthesis to maintain the health of surrounding socket tissue. An appointment is warranted if the prosthesis becomes uncomfortable, feels rough to the touch, or changes in appearance, such as the lids appearing droopy or the eye turning in, out, up, or down. The nurse should stress the importance of protecting the visually viable eye with protective glasses anytime damage could occur, such as participating in sports, yard work, or housework.

Operative Procedure
1. The surgeon places a speculum retractor into the palpebral fissure.
2. The conjunctiva is divided around the cornea with sharp and blunt dissection.

3. The medial, lateral, inferior, and superior rectus muscles are divided, leaving a stump of medial rectus muscle. If a coralline hydroxyapatite implant with donor sclera is used, the four rectus muscles and two oblique muscles are identified and secured with 6-0 suture (to be used to reattach muscles to cut-out areas in donor sclera) before the muscles are disinserted. The two oblique muscles are similarly detached, but are often not subsequently secured to the orbital implant.
4. Using blunt-pointed curved scissors, retractors, hemostats, and forceps, the surgeon separates the globe from the Tenon capsule. The eye is rotated laterally by grasping the stump of the medial rectus muscle.
5. A large curved hemostat is passed behind the globe, and the optic nerve is clamped for 60 seconds. The hemostat is removed, the enucleation scissors are passed posteriorly, and the optic nerve is transected. The oblique muscles are severed as the eye is lifted out of the socket by the stump of the medial rectus muscle.
6. Hemostasis is achieved with either pressure via a sterile test tube or packing with saline-soaked sponges.
7. The muscle cone is filled with an implant; the rectus muscles may then be sutured to the surface. Tenon capsule and the conjunctiva are carefully closed over the implant in separate layers.
8. A plastic socket conformer is placed into the cul-de-sac.
9. A pressure dressing with eye pads is applied.

Evisceration

Evisceration is removal of the contents of the eye, leaving the sclera and attached muscles intact.

Operative Procedure
1. A sharp-pointed knife is inserted through the limbus anterior to the iris. The conjunctiva is not separated from the sclera as it is for enucleation.
2. The surgeon removes the contents of the eye (iris, vitreous, and lens).
3. The choroid adhering to the sclera is removed with curettes.
4. Bleeding is controlled with delicate hemostatic forceps, an ESU, and sutures.

5. A plastic or coral implant is placed within the empty shell.
6. Using nonabsorbable 4-0 or 5-0 suture, the surgeon approximates the conjunctival and scleral edges.
7. A pressure dressing is applied.

Exenteration

Exenteration is removal of the entire orbital contents, including the periosteum, for certain malignancies of the globe or orbit. The procedure may also include removal of the external structures of the eyelids.

Procedural Considerations

General anesthesia is usually administered.

Operative Procedure

1. Depending on circumstances, exenteration of the eye may include removal of the lids. An incision is made down to the orbital rim, through the periosteum, and around the entire orbit.
2. The surgeon frees the periosteum from the orbital walls and apex of the orbit with periosteal elevators.
3. The optic nerve is clamped, and the entire contents of the orbit are removed en bloc.
4. Hemostasis is obtained using the ESU and bone wax.
5. A skin graft or temporal muscle implant may be used to fill the orbital cavity or iodoform gauze is used to fill the cavity.
6. A pressure dressing is applied. The cavity is allowed to granulate.

Key Points

- Surgery on the eyes requires precision and detailed preoperative planning. A millimeter in eye surgery can mean the difference between a successful surgery and one with undesired results. The eyes work together binocularly, so surgery on one eye may yield decreased vision or issues in the second eye.
- Cataract surgery is the most performed ambulatory surgery in the United States and with advancements in technology can restore and even improve a patient's vision to reduce the need for eyeglasses.
- Glaucoma surgeries do not restore vision, but rather prevent further damage from the progressing disease. Patients with glaucoma may have limited peripheral vision that requires personnel, forms and papers, and medication bottles to be in their central field of vision to view.
- Retina issues are a serious threat to vision, and retina surgeries are often emergent in nature. A combination of injections and surgery may be needed to repair damage. Retina surgery may be needed after an initial unrelated eye surgery so detailed histories and review of medications and postoperative care are required.
- The cornea accounts for two-thirds of the refraction and is the first layer of the eye in the visual system. Damage from foreign objects or accidents is more likely to occur on the cornea.

Critical Thinking Question

You are assigned to the ophthalmology OR for the day and have seven cataract procedures scheduled for your room. The first three patients were on schedule but the fourth patient did not show up or call the surgery center to cancel, so the OR scheduling coordinator has moved the fifth and remaining two patients up in time to fill the gap. The fifth patient is checked in and ready for surgery and the surgeon is made aware of the changes. What factors must you consider and prepare for the remaining surgeries to avoid errors or delays?

℮volve *The answer to the Critical Thinking Question can be found at http://evolve.elsevier.com/Rothrock/Alexander.*

References

Alio J et al: Cataract surgery on the previous corneal refractive surgery patient, *Surv Ophthalmol* 61(6):769–777, 2016.

American Academy of Ophthalmology (AAO): *IOL implants: lens replacement and cataract surgery* (website), 2016. www.aao.org/eye-health/diseases/cataracts-iol-implants. (Accessed 28 January 2017).

American Academy of Ophthalmology (AAO): *Vision screening recommendations for adults 40 to 60* (website), 2014. www.aao.org/eye-health/tips-prevention/midlife-adults-screening. (Accessed 27 January 2017).

Association of periOperative Registered Nurses (AORN): *Guidelines for perioperative practice*, Denver, 2017, The Association.

Bausch + Lomb: *Barometer of global eye health study* (website), 2012. www.bausch.com/ecp/for-your-practice/fact-sheet. (Accessed 27 January 2017).

Betsy Lehman Center: *Advancing patient safety in cataract surgery: a Betsy Lehman Center Expert Panel Report* (website), 2017. www.betsylehmancenterma.gov/initiatives-and-research-medical-errors-massachusetts/cataract-surgery-report-massachusetts. (Accessed 30 January 2017).

Custer P et al: Building a culture of safety in ophthalmology, *Ophthalmology* 123(9):S40–S45, 2016.

Eye Bank Association of America (EBAA): *Frequently asked questions: corneal transplant* (website), 2015. http://restoresight.org/cornea-donation/faqs/. (Accessed 24 July 2017).

Food and Drug Administration (FDA): *Banned devices; powdered surgeon's gloves, powdered patient examination gloves, and absorbable powder for lubricating a surgeon's glove* (website), 2016. https://www.federalregister.gov/documents/2016/12/19/2016-30382/banned-devices-powdered-surgeons-gloves-powdered-patient-examination-gloves-and-absorbable-powder. (Accessed 27 July 2017).

Goodman T, Spry C: *Essentials of perioperative nursing*, ed 6, New York, 2017, Jones & Bartlett Learning.

Jabbarvand M et al: Endophthalmitis occurring after cataract surgery, *Ophthalmology* 123(2):95–301, 2016.

Mamalis N: Toxic anterior segment syndrome: role of enzymatic detergents used in the cleaning of intraocular surgical instruments, *J Cataract Refract Surg* 42(9):1249–1250, 2016.

Mayo Clinic Health Newsletter: *Glaucoma—A silent thief*, 33(8):1-3, 2015.

National Academies of Sciences, Engineering, and Medicine: *Making eye health a population health imperative: vision for tomorrow*, Washington, DC, 2016, The National Academies Press.

National Eye Institute (NEI): *Facts about cataracts* (website), 2016a. www.nei.nih.gov/health/cataract/. (Accessed 1 February 2017).

National Eye Institute (NEI): *Facts about floaters* (website). 2016b, nei.nih.gov/health/floaters/floaters. (Accessed 1 February 2017).

National Eye Institute (NEI): *Facts about retinal detachment* (website). 2016c, nei.nih.gov/health/retinaldetach/retinaldetach. (Accessed 1 February 2017).

National Eye Institute (NEI): *Macular pucker* (website). 2016d, nei.nih.gov/health/pucker/. (Accessed 1 February 2017).

Olson R: What exactly does femtosecond technology add to phacoemulsification based on objective studies to date?, *Am J Ophthalmol* 165:xii–xiv, 2016.

Shorstein NH et al: Decreased postoperative endophthalmitis rate after institution of intracameral antibiotics in a Northern California eye department, *J Cataract Refract Surg* 39(1):8–14, 2013.

The Joint Commission (TJC): *2017 national patient safety goals* (website), 2017. www.jointcommission.org/assets/1/6/2013_HAP_NPSG_final_10-23.pdf. (Accessed 27 January 2017).

Workman LM, LaCharity L: *Understanding pharmacology*, St Louis, 2016, Elsevier.

CHAPTER 19
Otorhinolaryngologic Surgery

ALLISON L. FLANAGAN

Otorhinolaryngology is the study and science of the human ear *(oto)*, nose *(rhino)*, and throat *(laryngo)*. It is a specialty that continues to evolve as a result of cutting-edge technology; high-powered surgical microscopes; narrower, flexible endoscopes; computer imaging; wound care improvements; and navigation systems that communicate with radiologic imaging. Such advances yield significant gains in improving the health and surgical outcomes of patients with physical ailments of the head and neck. This chapter comprehensively and respectively reviews perioperative care of patients undergoing surgical procedures to the ear, nose, head, and neck.

Surgical Anatomy
External, Middle, and Inner Ear

The ear is a sensory organ that identifies, localizes, and interprets sound as well as maintains equilibrium. Hearing is the sense by which sounds are appreciated. Referred to as the "watchdog of the senses," hearing is the last sense to disappear when one falls asleep and the first to return when one awakens. The physical nature of sound results from the compression and rarefaction of pressure waves and moving molecules, but the sensations humans actually experience are the product of complex mechanical, electrical, and psychologic interactions in the ear and central nervous system (CNS). Three anatomic segments—the external ear, middle ear, and inner ear—work together to provide hearing and balance (Fig. 19.1).

The *external ear* includes the auricle (or pinna) and external auditory canal and is composed of cartilage covered with skin. The auricles are fixed in position and lie close to the head; they concentrate incoming sound waves and conduct them into the external auditory canal. Both ears provide stereophonic hearing that allows very specific sound localization capabilities. Without binaural hearing, determining where sounds emanate can be difficult; this is a common problem for patients with unilateral or asymmetric hearing loss.

The external auditory canal, an S-shaped pathway leading to the middle ear, is approximately 2.5 cm in length in adults and shelters the tympanic membrane. Its skeleton of bone and cartilage is covered with very thin, sensitive skin. The canal lining is protected and lubricated with cerumen, which is a waxy substance secreted by sebaceous glands in the distal third of the canal. Cerumen helps trap foreign material and has a mildly acidic pH that reduces bacterial levels in the outer ear.

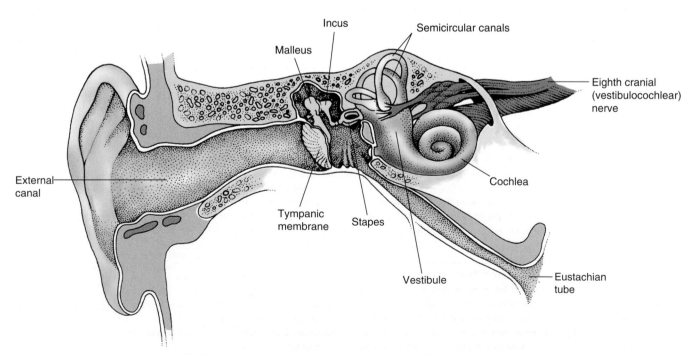

FIG. 19.1 Anatomic structures of the external ear, middle ear, and inner ear.

RIGHT TYMPANIC MEMBRANE

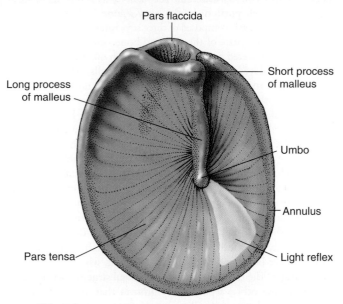

FIG. 19.2 Structural landmarks of the tympanic membrane.

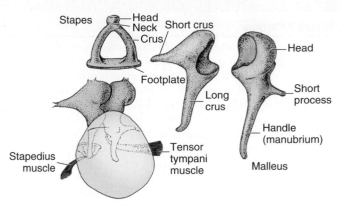

FIG. 19.3 Articulated ossicles of the right middle ear.

Located at the end of the external auditory canal is the *tympanic membrane* (eardrum) (Fig. 19.2). It is a thin structure with three distinct layers: an outer squamous epithelial layer in continuity with the skin of the external ear canal, a fibrous middle layer for strength and support, and a medial mucous membrane layer that is continuous with the lining of the middle ear.

The *middle ear* is filled with air, which flows from the nasopharynx through the eustachian tube. It is divided into three areas: the epitympanum (upper), mesotympanum (middle), and hypotympanum (lower). Posteriorly, the epitympanic portion of the middle ear communicates with the mastoid air cells of the temporal bone via the mastoid antrum. The mucous membrane of the middle ear is continuous with that of the pharynx and the mastoid cells, making it possible for infection to travel to the middle ear (otitis media) and mastoid cells (mastoiditis). The eustachian tube serves to aerate the air-filled spaces of the temporal bone and to equalize pressure in the middle ear with atmospheric pressure. It is normally closed at rest and actively opens during yawning, sneezing, or swallowing. A chain of three small articulated bones (ossicles) extends across the middle ear cavity and conducts vibrations (airborne sound waves) from the tympanic membrane across the middle ear into the oval window and the fluid-filled inner ear (Fig. 19.3).

The *malleus* (hammer) consists of a head, neck, handle, and short process. The handle and short process are attached to the undersurface of the eardrum, and the head articulates with the body of the incus in the upper segment of the middle ear called the epitympanum or "attic." The *incus* (anvil) consists of a body and long and short processes (see Fig. 19.2). The distal end of the long process of the incus is called the lenticular process, and it articulates with the capitulum (head) of the stapes, which is the third, innermost bone. The *stapes* (stirrup) consists of a head, neck, anterior and posterior crura, and a mobile footplate that is secured to the oval window by an annular ligament. The movable joints between these ossicles contribute to a lever system that amplifies the received sound and transmits and converts vibrations from ambient air to the fluid of the inner ear.

The inner ear is protected from loud noise by the *tensor tympani* muscle, which draws the drum inward to increase tension and restricts its ability to vibrate, and the *stapedius* muscle, which contracts and tightens the stapes in the oval window to reduce the intensity of vibrations passing through the ossicles into the inner ear. The middle ear and mastoid are supplied with blood from the branches of the internal and external carotid artery systems.

The *inner ear* is a membranous, curved cavity located in the petrous portion of the temporal bone; it contains hair cell receptors that provide us with both hearing and balance. The inner ear consists of a bony labyrinth filled with a watery fluid (perilymph) that surrounds and bathes a membranous labyrinth filled with another fluid with distinct electrolyte characteristics, called the endolymph. The bony labyrinth includes the cochlea and the vestibular labyrinth.

The *cochlea* resembles a snail shell. It is divided into three compartments: the scala vestibuli, which is associated with the oval window; the scala tympani, which is associated with the round window; and the cochlear duct. The scala vestibuli and scala tympani are filled with perilymph, whereas the cochlear duct contains endolymph. On the basilar membrane of the cochlea lies the organ of Corti, which is the neural end organ for hearing. Its neuroepithelium projects thousands of hair cells that are set into motion by vibrations passing through the ossicles and oval window to the perilymph. The hair cells convert the mechanical energy of wave movement from vibration in the perilymph into electrochemical impulses. The *vestibular labyrinth* is composed of the utricle, the saccule, and three semicircular canals, referred to as the *lateral, superior,* and *posterior canals.* They are positioned at right angles to one another and are responsible for detecting angular acceleration that can be elicited with any head or body movement. Each canal contains a sense organ (crista) that responds to fluid movement in the endolymph, which triggers impulses in the vestibular branch of the acoustic nerve. Cristae are stimulated by angular accelerations and movements, such as head turning. The maculae of the utricle and saccule of the vestibular labyrinth are gravity oriented. Linear accelerations are detected by the utricle and saccule; they both have a mat of sensory cells *(otoconia)* imbedded in a gelatinous material covered with calcium deposits. The weight of these otoconia constantly orients us to the direction of gravity. Their inertia gives information about linear accelerations. The combined signals from the cristae of the semicircular canals and the sensory cells of the utricle and saccule provide a sense of balance and orientation in space. The internal auditory branches of the basilar artery supply the inner ear.

Nasal Anatomy

The nose is covered with skin and is supported internally by bone and cartilage. The two external nares provide openings for the passage of air through the nasal cavity. These openings contain internal hairs for the filtration of coarse particles that are sometimes carried by air. The nose is divided into the prominent external portion and the internal portion known as the *nasal cavity* (Fig. 19.4). The chief purpose of the nose is to prepare air for use in the lungs.

The nasal bones and the frontal process of the maxilla form the upper portion of the external nose, and the lower portion is formed by a group of nasal cartilages and connective tissue covered with skin (Fig. 19.5). The nostrils and the tip of the nose are shaped by the major alar cartilages. The nares are separated by the *columella,* which is formed by the lower margin of the septal cartilage, the

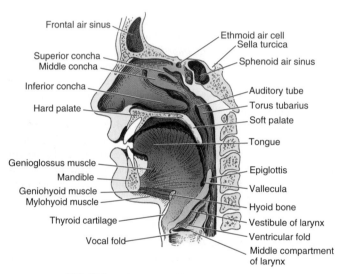

FIG. 19.4 Sagittal section of the face and neck.

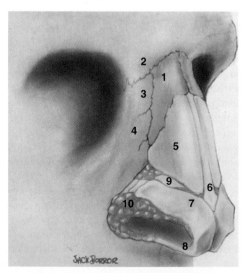

FIG. 19.5 Nasal bony framework. *1,* Nasal bone; *2,* frontal bone; *3,* lacrimal bone; *4,* maxillary bone; *5,* upper lateral cartilage; *6,* nasal septum; *7,* lower lateral cartilage, lateral crus; *8,* lower lateral cartilage, medial crus; *9,* sesamoid cartilage; *10,* fibrofatty tissue.

medial parts of the major alar cartilages, and the anterior nasal spine, all of which are covered with skin. The nasal cavity is divided medially into right and left portions by the *nasal septum.*

The *nasal septum* is composed of three structures: the nasal cartilage, the perpendicular plate of the ethmoid bone, and the vomer bone. The septum is covered by mucoperichondrium on either side, which contains blood vessels and mucus-secreting cells. The rich blood supply warms and moistens the air, and the sticky mucus traps dust, pollen, and other small particles.

The nasal cavity communicates with the outside by its external openings, called the *nares.* The nares open into the nasopharynx through the choanae. The nasal cavity is also associated with each ear, sharing the torus tubarius (opening of the eustachian tube in the nasopharynx) with the paranasal sinuses (frontal, maxillary, ethmoidal, and sphenoidal) through their respective orifices (meatus). The nasal cavity also communicates with the conjunctivae through the nasolacrimal duct. The nasal cavity is separated from the lingual cavity by the hard and soft palates (see Fig. 19.4) and from the cranial cavity by the ethmoids. It is held together by periosteal covering over bone and by the perichondrium, which extends over the cartilages. The turbinate bones of the nasal structure are arranged one above the other, separated by grooves that are composed of pseudostratified columnar ciliated respiratory epithelium. The turbinates act to increase the turbulence of airflow to humidify and regulate the temperature of air that is naturally inspired. This area is commonly referred to as the *sphenoethmoidal recess* and contains bony shelves known as the *superior, middle,* and *inferior meatus* or *turbinates* (Fig. 19.6).

The nasal sinuses serve as air spaces and communicate with the nasal cavity through the meatus. Anteriorly, on each side of the skull, the frontal sinus, the anterior ethmoidal sinus, and the maxillary sinus (antrum of Highmore) drain into the middle meatus; the posterior ethmoid and the sphenoid sinuses drain into the sphenoethmoidal recess (see Fig. 19.6).

Throat Anatomy

Oral Cavity

The *oral cavity* is composed of the mouth and salivary glands. The mouth is formed by the cheeks, the hard palate, the mandible, and the tongue. It extends from the lips to the junction of the hard and soft palates. The portion of the mouth outside the teeth is the buccal cavity, and that on the inner side of the teeth is the lingual cavity. The hard palate forms the upper boundary of the oral cavity. The hard palate is formed by the maxilla and palatine bones. The mandible and floor of the mouth form the lower boundary of the oral cavity (Fig. 19.7).

The *salivary glands* consist of three paired glands: the sublingual, submandibular, and parotid. They communicate with the mouth and produce saliva, which serves to moisten the mouth and initiate digestion of carbohydrates. The minor salivary glands exist in the submucosa of the cheeks, tongue, palates, and floor of the mouth, pharynx, lips, and paranasal sinuses.

The *sublingual gland* lies on the undersurface of the tongue beneath the mucous membrane on the floor of the mouth and the side of the tongue, on the inner surface of the mandible. The many tiny ducts of each gland separately enter the oral cavity on the sublingual fold.

The *submandibular gland* lies partly above and partly below the posterior half of the base of the mandible and on the mylohyoid and hyoglossus muscles. Its duct (Wharton duct) runs superficially

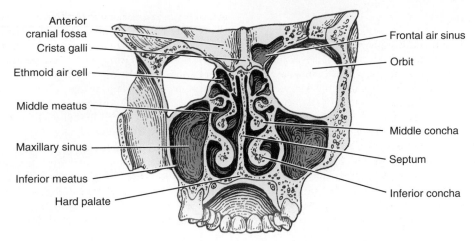

FIG. 19.6 Vertical section through the nose. Plane of the section passes slightly obliquely through the left first molar tooth and behind the second right premolar tooth. The posterior wall of right frontal sinus is removed.

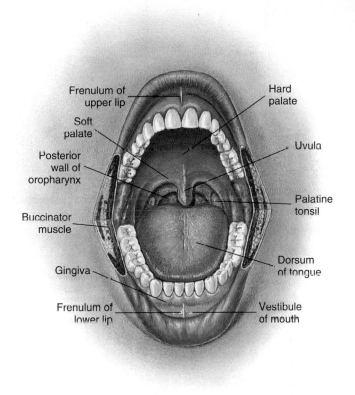

FIG. 19.7 Anatomic structures of the oral cavity.

beneath the mucosa of the floor of the mouth and enters the oral cavity behind the central incisors.

The *parotid gland,* the largest of the salivary glands, lies below the zygomatic arch in front of the mastoid process and behind the ramus of the mandible; it is divided into a superficial portion and a deep portion. The parotid duct (Stensen duct) pierces the buccal pad of fat and the buccinator muscle, finally opening into the oral cavity opposite the crown of the upper second molar tooth.

Pharynx

The pharynx extends from the posterior portion of the nose to the esophagus and larynx and serves as a channel for both the digestive and respiratory systems (Fig. 19.8). It is composed of muscular and fibrous layers with a mucous membrane lining. It is approximately 13 cm long and lies anterior to the cervical vertebrae and posterior to the nasal and oral cavities. The pharynx is associated above with the sphenoid sinus and the basilar part of the occipital bone, and it joins the esophagus below. Seven cavities communicate with the pharynx: the two nasal cavities, the two tympanic cavities, the mouth, the larynx, and the esophagus. The pharynx comprises three groups of constrictor muscles. Each muscle fits within the one below, and each inserts posteriorly in the median line with its mate from the opposite side. The constrictor muscles provide constriction of the pharynx for swallowing. Between the origins of the constrictor muscle groups are the so-called *intervals,* through which ligaments, nerves, and arteries pass. The pharynx is divided anatomically into three sections: the nasopharynx, the oropharynx, and the hypopharynx.

Nasopharynx

The nasopharynx lies posterior to the nasal cavity and extends over the soft palate. It communicates with the oropharynx through the pharyngeal isthmus, which is closed by muscular action during swallowing. Infection can spread from the nasopharynx to the middle ear through the eustachian tube.

Oropharynx

The oropharynx lies posterior to the oral cavity and extends from the palate to the level of the hyoid bone. The tonsils are situated on each side of the oropharynx and are lodged in a tonsillar fossa that is attached to folds of membrane-containing muscle. The palatine tonsils (a pair of oval structures) are the only lymphatic organs covered with stratified squamous epithelium. The lateral surface of each tonsil is usually covered with a fibrous capsule. The anterior and posterior tonsillar pillars join to form a triangular fossa, with the posterior lateral aspects of the tongue at its base. The lingual tonsils are lodged in each fossa. The adenoids, or pharyngeal tonsils, are suspended from the roof of the nasopharynx and consist of an accumulation of lymphoid tissue.

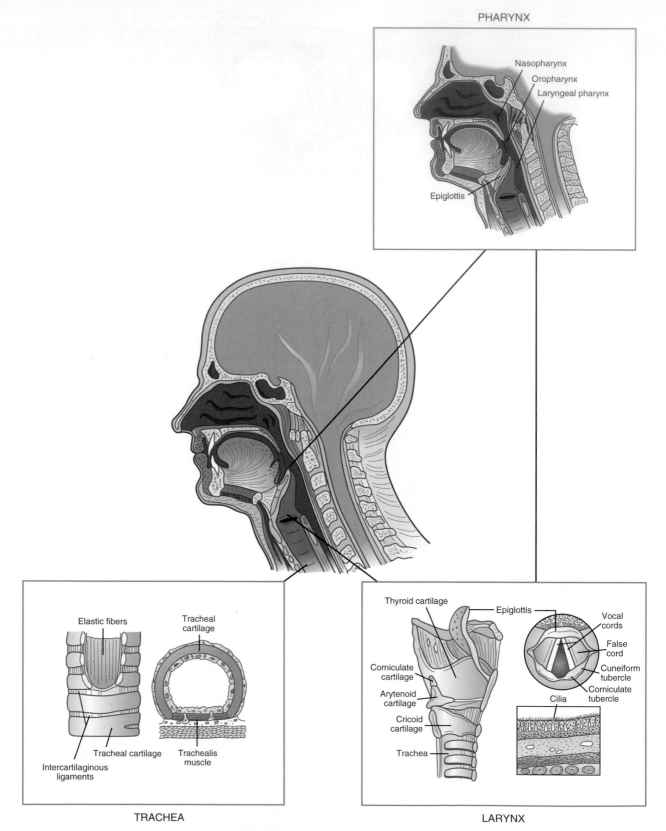

FIG. 19.8 Structures of the upper airway.

Hypopharynx

The hypopharynx extends from the hyoid bone and empties into the esophagus posteriorly and the larynx anteriorly. The piriform sinuses are bound medially by the arytenoepiglottic fold and laterally by the thyroid cartilage and hypothyroid membrane. The fossae are involved in speech.

Larynx and Associated Structures

Larynx

The larynx is a cartilaginous box that lays midline in front of the fourth, fifth, and sixth cervical vertebrae between the trachea and the root of the tongue, at the upper front part of the neck. The location of the larynx between the gastrointestinal (GI) and respiratory systems is strategic in protecting the airway during swallowing and breathing. The larynx has three main functions: as a passageway for respiration, as a valve to prevent aspiration, and as a vibratory source for vocalization.

The larynx can be divided into three portions: *supraglottis* (or upper portion above the true vocal cords), *glottis* (level of the true vocal cords), and *subglottis* (below the true vocal cords). The upper portion of the larynx is continuous with the pharynx above and includes the epiglottis, vallecula, and the laryngeal cartilages. Its lower portion joins the trachea. The skeletal structure provides for patency of the enclosed airway. The complex muscle action and arrangement of tissues within the larynx provide for closure of the lumen, to protect against trauma and entrance of foreign bodies, and for speech.

Laryngeal Cartilages

The skeletal framework of the larynx consists of cartilages and membranes. Of the nine separate cartilages, three are single and six are arranged in pairs. The main cartilages of the larynx include the thyroid, the cricoid, the epiglottis, two arytenoid, two corniculate, and two cuneiform. The thyroid cartilage, or Adam's apple, forms the anterior portion of the voice box. The cricoid cartilage is a complete cartilaginous ring that resembles a signet ring; it rests beneath the thyroid cartilage and supports the airway (see Fig. 19.8). The epiglottis is a slightly curled, leaf-shaped, elastic, fibrous membrane that is attached in the midline to the upper border of the thyroid cartilage. The epiglottis helps protect the larynx during swallowing. Contraction of the cricothyroid muscle pulls the thyroid cartilage and the cricoid cartilage to tighten the vocal cords and close the glottis. The arytenoid cartilages, which rest above the signet-ring portion of the cricoid cartilage, support the posterior portion of the true vocal cords.

Laryngeal Ligaments

The extrinsic ligaments of the larynx are those connecting (1) the thyroid cartilage and epiglottis with the hyoid bone, and (2) the cricoid cartilage with the trachea. The intrinsic ligaments of the larynx are those connecting several cartilages of the organ to each other. They are considered the elastic membrane of the larynx.

The mucous lining of the larynx blends with fibrous tissue to form two folds on each side of the larynx. The upper set is known as the *false vocal cords.* The lower set is called the *true vocal cords* because they are concerned primarily with the speaking voice and protection of the lower respiratory channels against the invasion of food and foreign bodies. The region of the larynx at the true vocal cord level is called the *glottis,* which is a triangular space between the vocal cords. During swallowing, the rising action of the muscular larynx, the closure of the glottis, and the doorlike action of the epiglottis all serve to guide food and fluid into the esophagus.

Laryngeal Muscles

The laryngeal muscles perform two distinct functions: the extrinsic muscles (Fig. 19.9) regulate the degree of tension on the vocal cords, and the intrinsic muscles open and close the glottis. The spoken voice also depends on the sphincter action of the soft palate, tongue,

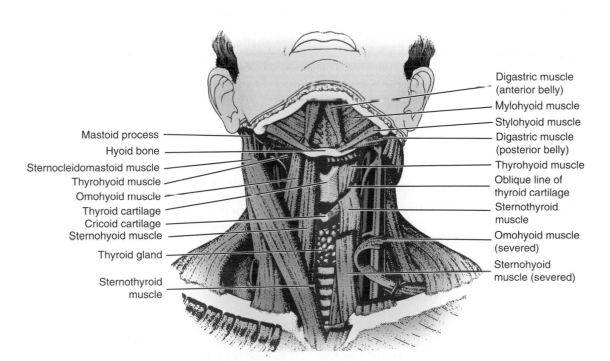

Mastoid process
Hyoid bone
Sternocleidomastoid muscle
Thyrohyoid muscle
Omohyoid muscle
Thyroid cartilage
Cricoid cartilage
Sternohyoid muscle
Thyroid gland
Sternothyroid muscle

Digastric muscle (anterior belly)
Mylohyoid muscle
Stylohyoid muscle
Digastric muscle (posterior belly)
Thyrohyoid muscle
Oblique line of thyroid cartilage
Sternothyroid muscle
Omohyoid muscle (severed)
Sternohyoid muscle (severed)

FIG. 19.9 Extrinsic muscles of the larynx.

and lips. The muscle action of the larynx permits the glottis to close either voluntarily or involuntarily by reflex action. The closure of the inlet by this mechanism protects the respiratory passages. The closure of the glottis and the action of the vocal cords are precisely coordinated to produce the voice.

Trachea

The trachea is a cartilaginous tube about 15 cm in length and 2 to 2.5 cm in diameter. It begins in the neck and extends from the lower part of the larynx, on a level with the sixth cervical vertebra, to the upper border of the fifth thoracic vertebra. It descends anteriorly to the esophagus, enters the superior mediastinum, and divides into right and left main bronchi. The trachea is composed of a series of C-shaped rings of hyaline cartilage. The posterior surface of the trachea is flattened rather than round because the cartilaginous rings are incomplete. The carina is a ridge on the inside of the bifurcation of the trachea. It is a landmark during bronchoscopy and separates the upper end of the right main branches from the upper end of the left main branches of the bronchi. Branches from the arch of the aorta—the brachiocephalic (innominate) and left common carotid arteries—are in close relation to the trachea. The cervical portion of the trachea is related anteriorly to the sternohyoid and sternothyroid muscles and to the isthmus of the thyroid gland.

Musculature of the Neck

A layer of deep cervical fascia surrounds the neck like a collar and is attached to the trapezius and sternocleidomastoid muscles. The sternocleidomastoid muscle extends from the upper part of the sternum and medial third of the clavicle to the mastoid process. The trapezius muscle extends from the scapula, the lateral third of the clavicle, and the vertebrae to the occipital prominence. The relationship of these muscles to each other and to the adjacent bone creates triangles used as anatomic landmarks.

The pretracheal fascia of the neck lies deep in the strap muscles (sternothyroid, sternohyoid, thyrohyoid, and omohyoid) and partially encloses the thyroid gland, trachea, and larynx. The pretracheal fascia is pierced by the thyroid vessels. It fuses with the front of the carotid sheath on the deep surface of the sternocleidomastoid muscle. The carotid sheath consists of a network of areolar tissue surrounding the carotid arteries and vagus nerve.

Laterally the carotid sheath is fused with the fascia on the deep surface of the sternocleidomastoid muscle; anteriorly it is fused with the middle cervical fascia along the lateral border of the sternothyroid muscle. Lying between the floor and roof of this triangular formation of muscles are the lymph glands and the accessory nerve. Arteries and nerves traverse and pierce this triangle.

Proximal Structures

Cranial Nerves

The trigeminal (fifth cranial) nerve supplies sensory innervation to the face, oral cavity, nose, nasal cavity, and maxillary sinuses. It provides motor innervation to the muscles of mastication.

The right and left facial (seventh cranial) nerves are responsible for all the movements of the facial muscles. Both nerves have a very complex and tortuous course from the brainstem to the motor endplates of the facial musculature. The facial nerve enters the internal auditory meatus along with the eighth (vestibulocochlear) cranial nerve and travels through the internal auditory canal, passing through the labyrinthine portion of the temporal bone to the geniculate ganglion, where it turns sharply and passes superior to the oval

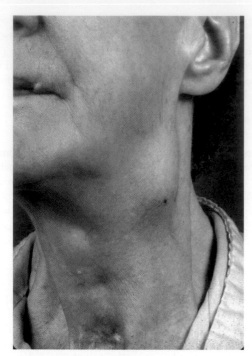

FIG. 19.10 Advanced cancer of the mouth with metastasis to the neck.

window. It then turns inferiorly through the mastoid and exits through the stylomastoid foramen. There are three primary branches of the facial nerve in the temporal bone: the greater superficial petrosal nerve controls lacrimation, the stapedial branch controls the stapedius muscle, and the chorda tympani nerve carries the taste sensation to the anterior two-thirds of the tongue.

The vestibulocochlear (eighth cranial) nerve connects the inner ear to the brain through its brainstem nuclei and ascending neural pathways. The recurrent laryngeal branch of the vagus (tenth cranial) nerve is the important motor nerve of the intrinsic muscles of the pharynx and larynx.

Lymphatic System

The lymphatic system serves both immunologic and circulatory functions. Interstitial fluid, which may contain bacteria, viruses, or tumor cells, is returned to the blood circulation through the lymphatic channels. As the lymph nodes trap the foreign matter, the nodes may become enlarged, infected, or the focus of metastatic cancer (Fig. 19.10).

The nasal cavity, the paranasal sinuses, and the pharynx drain into the retropharyngeal nodes. The mouth, lips, and external nose are drained by the submandibular nodes. The lymphatics of the tip and lateral aspects of the tongue drain to the submental nodes, and the posterior tongue lymphatics drain to the cervical nodes.

The lymphatic drainage of the neck can be divided into superficial and deep nodes (Fig. 19.11). Lymph nodes of the neck can be further classified into subzones. Level Ia nodes are submental nodes; level Ib nodes are submandibular nodes. Level IIa nodes are upper jugular nodes anterior to cranial nerve IX. Level IIb nodes are upper jugular nodes posterior to cranial nerve IX. Level III nodes are middle jugular nodes. Level IV nodes are lower jugular nodes. Level Va nodes are posterior triangle nodes of the spinal accessory group, and level Vb nodes are posterior triangle nodes of the transverse cervical artery and supraclavicular group. Level VI nodes are anterior tracheal nodes. Level VII nodes are superior mediastinum nodes.

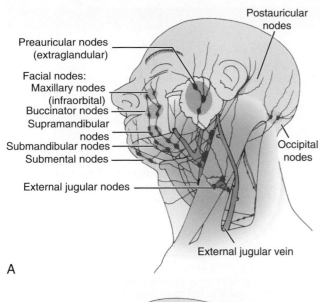

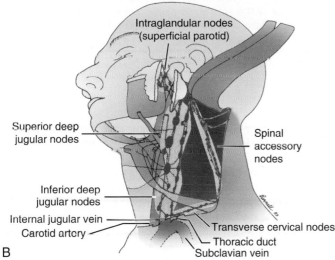

FIG. 19.11 Lymphatic drainage of neck. (A) Superficial cervical and facial nodal drainage patterns. (B) Deep cervical lymphatic drainage patterns. Note that the sternocleidomastoid muscle is reflected.

TABLE 19.1

Types of Hearing Loss

Classification	Definition	Causes
Conductive	Loss of hearing acuity resulting from failure to conduct sound from external ear to middle ear	Blockage of external canal with cerumen or foreign bodies Edema Trauma Infection Tympanic perforation Otosclerosis, ossicular chain fixation
Sensorineural	Loss of hearing acuity resulting from failure to conduct sound to inner ear (cochlea or acoustic nerve)	Ototoxic medications Exposure to loud noise Trauma Meniere disease Tumor Presbycusis Infectious disease (measles, mumps, meningitis)
Mixed	Loss of hearing acuity resulting from combination of conductive and sensorineural factors	Develops secondary to either conductive or sensorineural loss (e.g., patient with presbycusis and impacted cerumen)

Perioperative Nursing Considerations

Assessment

Assessment is a systematic and intentional process of collecting and interpreting data concerning a patient's health history and status with diagnoses related to the head and neck. Familiarity with otorhinolaryngologic conditions is essential for effective patient assessment. Information obtained helps develop nursing diagnoses, which direct nursing plans, interventions, and evaluation. A nursing preoperative assessment is usually obtained either in person during scheduled preoperative evaluation or by telephone before the day of surgery. The perioperative nurse should review this assessment as well as the physician's evaluation to prepare for patient care in the operating room (OR). The assessment should include a review of the following:

- *Communication status.* One in three people in the United States between the ages of 65 and 74 have hearing loss, and nearly half

of those who are over age 75 have difficulty hearing (NIDCD, 2016). Hearing loss may be classified as conductive, sensorineural, or mixed (Table 19.1). Nurses must determine the best way to communicate with the patient who is hard-of-hearing (Evidence for Practice). Patients who are unable to speak because of vocal cord dysfunction must be provided an alternate means of communication (e.g., pen and paper, erasable board). Nurses must assess for adaptive responses, such as lip reading, sign language, and written communication, and the effect of the patient's communication status on daily life (e.g., inability to hear traffic, alarms, or telephone; inability of voice to be heard because of hoarseness; voice volume issues; reluctance to communicate).

- *Respiratory status.* Observe and note the quality and character of respirations; observe and note the quality and character of the voice, such as hoarseness, "hot potato" voice (e.g., voice that lacks resonance, sounds muffled, and evidences a distortion of vowels, as if the speaker has a hot potato in his or her mouth), or hyponasal speech; note inspiratory stridor, expiratory stridor, hemoptysis, or dyspnea.

- *Physical status.* Observe problems in range of motion in all four extremities; note joint replacements, back or neck stiffness or pain, or trismus. Assess facial symmetry, landmarks, color, position, and presence of deformities, lesions, and nodules; note presence or absence of rhinorrhea or otorrhea. Note any cranial nerve involvement (e.g., inability to look downward, nystagmus, facial asymmetry, and facial paresis).

- *Presence of a mass.* Note the length of time the mass has been evident; note if the size of the mass decreased after antibiotic therapy; note a fixed mass versus a mobile mass.

- *Nutritional status.* Note any weight loss, including length of time weight loss occurred. Patients with diagnosed and undiagnosed

▮ EVIDENCE FOR PRACTICE

Aiding the Hearing Imparied Consume Music

With millions of people worldwide affected by some type of hearing loss, it has come to the attention of researchers that the impairment negatively affects aspects of the social life of deaf people. Music-centered situations such as concerts are not appealing to the hearing impaired. Music therapy is also not a viable for option for those looking for a holistic treatment plan or who simply need a stress reducer. The Auris System was created to provide a musical experience for people with hearing loss. The system can extract musical information from audio and create a representation of the music using different stimuli. The new media format can be interpreted by other senses, giving patients with hearing loss the ability to be reintegrated into activities that are centered around auditory stimuli.

Different solutions are being developed to aid patients with hearing loss consume music. The Model Human Cochlea uses musical representation in a vibrotactile display. The vibration is expressed through eight coils in the back of a chair with each row of coils representing a specific element of the music. Another approach includes the use of The Haptic Chair, which sends vibrations through contact speakers to the patient. The chair amplifies pure audio sound, allowing patients with partial deafness

to hear the audio through transducers vibrations. A visual display allows patients to follow different shapes and colors in coordination with the music. The visual display matches changes in pitch, timbre, and key changes. Visual stimuli can activate the auditory cortex in deaf patients. Video may be able to help deaf patients understand and consume music.

The Auris System uses a set of tools that converts audio into a new media consisting of synchronized tactile impulses. The system includes a chair, bracelet, the Auris Core, and Auris Controller. The chair is composed of four speakers and a subwoofer while the bracelet is made up of a series of vibration motors that will represent musical tones. The core receives the audio while the controller manages the functionality of the other components.

Researchers used both a questionnaire and EEG to test the effectiveness of the Auris System. The Auris System was utilized to expose participants to three different songs as soundtrack to a single video. As a result of the study, researchers concluded that with the use of the Auris System, deaf patients using tactile vibrations along with a video representation of the music can aid them in consuming music.

Modified from Alves Araujo F et al: Auris system: providing vibrotactile feedback for hearing impaired population, *Biomed Research International* 2017: article ID 2181380, 1-9, 2017.

---

neoplasms may be nutritionally depleted from dysphagia, tumor, chemotherapy, or radiation therapy.

- *Emotional status and anxiety level.* Observe for restlessness, poor eye contact, facial tension, or increased perspiration.
- *Pain.* Observe location and character of odynophagia (painful swallowing), sore throat, facial pain, or otalgia. Note preoperative medications and the time they were administered. Begin education for pain management before discharge.
- *Allergies.* Note allergic reactions to medications, foods, or latex.
- *Medication history.* Note medications taken by the patient for the presenting condition and any other diagnosed medical condition. Medications should include prescription medications; over-the-counter medications; vitamins; herbals; nutraceuticals; ototoxic drugs, including salicylates, aminoglycosides, furosemide, streptomycin, quinine, and ethacrynic acid; or any chemotherapy. Ensure key participants in the patient's care are aware of the medication history (Ambulatory Surgery Considerations).
- *Past responses to anesthesia.* Local anesthetics are often used either as the sole means of anesthesia for minor procedures or as an adjunct to procedures performed using monitored anesthesia care or general anesthesia. The patient's account of previous dental experiences with local anesthetics can provide a clue as to how the patient will respond to local anesthetic agents. Cardiac status should be noted because many surgeons use epinephrine as an additive to the local anesthetic to achieve vasoconstriction and minimize blood loss. The epinephrine effect may contribute to cardiac dysrhythmias and an increased potential for cardiac arrest.
- *Patient's knowledge and understanding of the surgical procedure.* Note questions and provide answers, or ask the surgeon to clarify information for the patient (Patient Engagement Exemplar). Review equipment and care (e.g., suctioning, packing, drains) that will be part of the postoperative regimen and possible

communication deficits related to the procedure (e.g., inability to speak after laryngeal procedures, decreased hearing after otologic procedures).

- *Patient's support system.* Note family members' names and their location during the surgical procedure, and explain that a nurse will communicate with them during the procedure regarding the patient (as applicable).

In addition to standard office diagnostic procedures performed by the surgeon, several other tests may be performed before the patient arrives in the OR. Study results of most significance to the perioperative team that should be available in the OR are listed under Laboratory Data in Appendix A. Radiology studies are described as follows.

Computed Tomography

Computed tomography (CT) scans are radiographic studies that visualize structures by producing serial sections, many times clinically referred to as "cuts," through planes of the head and neck. CT imaging provides visualization of bone, soft tissue, and adjacent intracranial and extracranial pathologic conditions. Intravenous (IV) injection of iodine contrast agents produces visual enhancement of some anatomic structures and pathologic tissues, including highly vascularized tumors. CT is the study of choice to assess intratemporal bone pathologic conditions and to evaluate the paranasal sinuses and adjacent structures. It is also used in the assessment of the oral cavity and neck.

Magnetic Resonance Imaging

Magnetic resonance imaging (MRI) is an imaging modality using powerful magnetic and radiofrequency waves to reproduce cross-sectional images of the human body without exposing the patient to ionizing radiation. On an MRI scan, fat and fluid produce high-intensity signals, which appear as bright areas, whereas bone

AMBULATORY SURGERY CONSIDERATIONS

Medication Reconciliation

Medication reconciliation is defined by The Joint Commission (TJC) as the comparison of medications a patient should be using (and is actually using) to the new medications that are ordered for the patient, and resolution of any discrepancies. Medication reconciliation is an important element of National Patient Safety Goal 3, Improve the Safety of Using Medication.

Reconciliation of medication information can prevent prescribing errors, such as duplicate prescriptions, incompatible medications, and overprescribing. The patient entering the perioperative setting may be at risk for medication errors because of decreased communication with the patient's primary care physician or other treating specialists. Otorhinolaryngologic patients may also have communication challenges (auditory or vocal) that increase the risk of error in obtaining an accurate medication history. In ambulatory surgery, perioperative nurses typically review the patient's medication history in the preoperative period and then review medications again in the postoperative or discharge phase. Nurses can positively affect patient safety and reduce the risk for prescribing errors by

following medication safety practices, using medication reconciliation processes, and implementing these risk-reduction strategies:

- Obtain a list of the medications the patient is currently taking when he or she is admitted to the hospital or is seen in an outpatient setting. This list may include medications taken at a scheduled time and as needed medications. Examples of medication information that may be collected include name, dose, route, frequency, and purpose.
- Compare the medication information provided by the patient to the medications ordered for the patient by the surgeon to identify and resolve discrepancies. Discrepancies include omissions, duplications, and contraindications.
- Provide the patient and/or family member with information on the medications he or she is taking when discharged from the hospital or at the end of the ambulatory encounter.
- Explain the importance of these medications to the patient and/or family member.

Modified from The Joint Commission (TJC): *Hospital national patient safety goals* (website), 2016. https://www.jointcommission.org/assets/1/6/2016_NPSG_HAP_ER.pdf. (Accessed 8 September 2016).

PATIENT ENGAGEMENT EXEMPLAR

Communication and Informed Consent

Patients have specific concerns when undergoing otorhinolaryngologic surgery. Ramos (2014) identified crucial concerns for patients and the need for education in these areas:

- Approximate length of incision
- Tubes in the nose
- Wound care
- Nutrition and ability to eat
- Breathing and mouth care
- Heparin injections
- Calcium deficiency
- Management of postoperative pain
- Voice changes
- Anticipated wait time for biopsy results

Keeping these concerns in mind it is important to remember that otorhinolaryngology patients may be at more risk for communication errors due to hearing or phonation. Paulson (2010) noted: "The idea of informed consent is often associated with the piece of paper signed before a procedure rather than the continuum of communication that happens during the course of the medical care of patients." Responsibility for explaining the surgical procedure, risks, benefits, and possible complications lies with the surgeon, but nurses can play an important role in ensuring the patient is fully cognizant of the implications of surgery and advocating for additional communication with the physician if necessary. Nurses can also discuss patient concerns and educate them before surgery. Some talking points and questions nurses can use to assess a patient's understanding of the informed consent process include the following:

- Tell me what health problem you are being treated for today.

- Can you describe in your own words what the physician will be doing to you?
- Tell me where on your body you will have surgery.
- Can you tell me in your own words what you expect to happen as a result of this surgery?
- Tell me what you think the risks are for this operation.
- What do you know about different ways to treat your problem?

TJC also suggests that healthcare workers can support the informed consent process through the following actions:

- Arrange for language services to help with treatment of patients whose preferred language is not English or who are deaf.
- Make sure that appropriate auxiliary aids and services are available during treatment of patients who have sensory impairments (e.g., hearing aids, speech-generating devices, alphabet boards, speaking valves, interpreters for the deaf, etc.).
- Provide AAC resources to help in treating patients with communication impairments (e.g., alphabet boards, picture boards, teletype for the deaf).
- Note the use of communication assistance in the medical record, and communicate needed aids and services to staff.
- Use informed consent materials that meet health literacy needs. Materials should be written at a fifth grade or lower reading level. Consider revising written materials to address the health literacy needs of all patients. Use readability tests; divide complex information into bullet points; and modify document font, layout, and design to improve readability.

AAC, Augmentative and alternative communication; *TJC,* The Joint Commission.
Modified from Ramos JE. *Preoperative education needs in ear, nose & throat clinic: a patient perspective* [dissertation]. Minneapolis, MN, Walden University (website), 2014. http://scholarworks.waldenu.edu/dissertations/105/; The Joint Commission (TJC): *Advancing effective communication, cultural competence, and patient- and family-centered care: a roadmap for hospitals* (website), 2010. www.jointcommission.org/assets/1/6/aroadmapforhospitalsfinalversion727.pdf. (Accessed 26 November 2016).

and air emit weak signals and appear as darkened areas. MRI is often used with CT imaging in a complementary fashion when evaluating lesions in and around bone for a variety of head and neck conditions, including tumors in the oral cavity, external auditory canal, middle ear, and mastoid.

Audiogram

Patients scheduled for otologic surgery may have undergone evaluation of their hearing through audiograms to determine whether they have normal hearing, conductive hearing loss, or sensorineural hearing loss (see Table 19.1). Two types of audiometric testing (pure tone and speech audiometry) are performed on patients with suspected hearing loss.

Nursing Diagnosis

Nursing diagnoses related to the care of patients undergoing otorhinolaryngologic surgery might include the following:
- Anxiety
- Acute Pain
- Ineffective Breathing Pattern
- Risk for Bleeding
- Disturbed Body Image
- Impaired Verbal Communication

Outcome Identification

Outcomes identified for the selected nursing diagnoses could be stated as follows:
- The patient will be able to identify factors that cause anxiety and verbalize an ability to cope.
- The patient will communicate adequate pain control and display absence of physiologic indicators of pain (e.g., tachypnea, tachycardia, pallor, hypertension).
- The patient will demonstrate effective breathing patterns.
- The patient will maintain a hematocrit level of 30 mg/dL or greater or a hemoglobin level of 12 to 14 mg/dL.

- The patient will experience a sense of self-worth and self-respect.
- The patient will establish an effective communication method with staff and family.

Planning

The development of a plan of care is based on the preoperative assessment, nursing diagnoses, expected outcomes, and the surgery being performed. Patients undergoing otolaryngologic procedures may have special communication needs that must be considered in planning effective care. The perioperative nurse should determine the best way to communicate with patients who have hearing deficits or impaired vocalization. Information given to the patient should be reinforced as needed throughout the perioperative experience. The OR environment must be quiet and free of any loud noise. Intraoperative noises, such as those from suction, electrosurgical units (ESUs), and other equipment, should be explained to the locally anesthetized patient before they are generated. This will help avoid startling the patient and adversely affecting the success of the surgery. Patients receiving local anesthetics need to remain still during the procedure, so providing for comfort measures becomes especially important. The room temperature should be regulated at a comfortable setting, and the patient should be adequately covered to maintain normal body temperature.

Preparation of the OR includes checking the availability and functional capacity of suction, the surgeon's headlight and light source, and the ESU. It is essential that the x-ray view box is in working order and appropriately located so that scans may be easily viewed by the surgeon during the procedure. In endoscopic cases the navigation tower and monitor should be rolled to the head of the table and tested to ensure proper functioning of the light source for the camera wands and suction. If the surgeon plans on videorecording the case, assurance that the video recorder is adequately working is needed before the start of the case.

A Sample Plan of Care for a patient undergoing otorhinolaryngologic surgery is shown.

SAMPLE PLAN OF CARE

Nursing Diagnosis
Anxiety

Outcome
The patient will be able to identify factors that cause anxiety and verbalize an ability to cope.

Interventions
- Assess the patient's level of anxiety (alertness, ability to comprehend, ability to perform ADLs).
- Maintain a calm and safe environment.
- Assist the patient in identifying possible sources of stress.
- Allow the patient to talk and ask questions. Assess the patient for desire for preoperative visit by people with altered communication methods.
- Inform the patient, family, and caregiver what to expect on the day of surgery and describe the environment of care (preoperative area, OR, postanesthesia care unit).

- Introduce members of the surgical staff. Explain activities performed by the nursing staff in simple language the patient can understand.
- Assure the patient that he or she will be informed before any procedure is done.
- Provide time for the patient, family, and caregiver to express fears and concerns. Provide factual, accurate information.
- Note expressions of distress and anxiety.
- Prevent unnecessary body exposure during transfer and positioning.
- Control external stimuli and noise levels.

Nursing Diagnosis
Acute Pain

Outcome
The patient will communicate adequate pain control and display absence of physiologic indicators of pain (e.g., tachypnea, tachycardia, pallor, and hypertension).

SAMPLE PLAN OF CARE—cont'd

Interventions

- Review with the patient normal coping mechanisms that are personally effective; support and encourage these during surgical intervention. As appropriate, consider nonpharmacologic measures such as guided imagery, music, and relaxation exercises.
- Describe the anticipated sequence of perioperative events.
- Explain that some initial discomfort (e.g., pinprick followed by slight burning and then numbness) may be felt during the administration of local anesthetic.
- Inform the patient before the injection of local anesthetic; provide support and reassurance; evaluate patient response.
- Observe for, document, and report any changes in the patient's vital signs (blood pressure, heart rate and rhythm, respiratory rate, oxygen saturation), skin condition, and mental status.
- Be aware of the maximum recommended dosage of local anesthetics and be alert for signs of allergic reactions or toxic responses.
- Ask the patient whether he or she is experiencing any pain; communicate the presence of pain sensation to the surgeon.
- Administer sedation or analgesics as ordered by the surgeon. Describe the purpose and expected response to the medication administered. Document medications administered.
- Verify with the patient that the desired response has been achieved.

Nursing Diagnosis
Ineffective Breathing Pattern

Outcome
The patient will demonstrate effective breathing patterns.

Interventions

- Assess respiratory status and breathing pattern. Monitor respiratory rate, rhythm, depth, and oxygen saturation (pulse oximetry). Maintain oxygen saturation at greater than 90%. Report any variances from normal.
- Note any restlessness, apprehension, agitation, lethargy, or repeated swallowing. Use a penlight to examine the throat for bleeding if nasal, oral cavity, or laryngologic procedures were performed. Notify the surgeon if bleeding is present.
- Have emergency medications and airway equipment available.
- Elevate the head of the bed (to decrease edema, which can interfere with breathing).
- Increase humidification with a bedside humidifier or a humidified facemask.
- Encourage the patient, family, and caregiver to increase frequency of oral hygiene.

Nursing Diagnosis
Risk for Bleeding

Outcome
The patient will maintain a hematocrit of 30 mg/dL or greater or a hemoglobin of 12 to 14 mg/dL.

Interventions

- Assist with the insertion of IV lines and fluid replacement therapy. Keep IV lines patent.

- Provide blood or blood products for fluid replacement; assist in replacement therapy and patient monitoring.
- Estimate blood loss on soft goods and drapes; communicate to anesthesia provider and surgeon.
- Record the amount of irrigation used.
- Document the contents of the suction canisters.
- Monitor and document hourly urine output (as applicable); communicate results of measurements.
- Observe for signs of shock (e.g., hypotension, abnormal ECG); report signs, and initiate corrective nursing actions.
- Observe for signs of excess blood loss (e.g., rapid, weak pulse; rapid respirations; cool, moist skin; early, slight rise in blood pressure); report signs and initiate corrective nursing actions.
- Collaborate with the collection and interpretation of intraoperative blood analyses.

Nursing Diagnosis
Disturbed Body Image

Outcome
The patient will experience a sense of self-worth and self-respect.

Interventions

- Acknowledge normalcy of emotional response to actual or perceived change in body structure or function. Experiencing stages of grief over loss of a body part or function is normal and typically involves a period of denial, the length of which is variable.
- Encourage the patient to verbalize feelings and self-perceived changes related to health status and surgical procedure.
- Involve the family or significant others in initial communication with patient.
- Encourage the patient to ask questions.
- Discuss referrals for support groups.

Nursing Diagnosis
Impaired Verbal Communication

Outcome
The patient will establish an effective communication method with staff and family.

Interventions

- Plan in advance to obtain necessary assistive devices or interpreters.
- Inform the entire healthcare team of the patient's communication challenges and any interpretive services to be used.
- Agree on a method of communication preoperatively to be used postoperatively. Suggestions include the following:
  - Writing with a pen or pencil and paper, or using an erasable board or picture board
  - Using hand signals or signs, body expressions
- Consult with the surgeon regarding requirements for voice rest.
- Place IV lines in the nondominant hand.
- Adapt written materials (e.g., consent forms, discharge instructions) as necessary; include visual information such as symbols, pictures, or diagrams to help understanding.

ADL, Activities of daily living; *ECG,* electrocardiogram; *IV,* intravenous.

Implementation

The nurse ensures the following interventions are instituted for the patient:

1. Using the institutional verification process immediately before surgery to identify the correct surgical site. This should include verifying the operative side and site with the patient or family and confirmation through review of the medical record, informed consent, diagnostic test reports, and other members of the surgical team during the time-out.

2. Verifying the patient has maintained nothing-by-mouth (NPO) status as directed and that requested laboratory studies are on the medical record.

3. Providing calm, careful, and comforting nursing measures to reduce the patient's anxiety. Allow the patient time to comply with requests, and explain the sequence of perioperative events.

4. Allowing patients who wear hearing aids to wear them to the OR. Carefully remove the hearing aids at the time of or after anesthesia induction, or leave them in place if local anesthesia is used. Prescription eyewear should be brought into the holding area because hearing-impaired patients may require them to assist in lip reading when instructions and procedures are explained. If the patient has impaired vocalization, the nurse should ensure that the patient's preferred method of communication (e.g., pen and paper, artificial larynx) is available. Disposition of any assistive devices brought into the OR must be documented on the record.

5. Protecting patients with impaired communication from injury. The perioperative nurse must control the environment because excess stimulation interferes with the patient's ability to hear, vocalize, and comply with instructions and explanations.

6. Reviewing instructions for patients receiving local anesthetics. The nurse reminds the patient of the need to remain immobile during the procedure and report any adverse symptoms related to the anesthetic. Symptoms of adverse drug reactions include skin changes, such as rash or itching; restlessness; unexplained anxiety or fearfulness; diaphoresis; and complaints of blurred vision, tinnitus, dizziness, nausea, palpitations or acute changes in heart rate, disturbed respiration, pallor or flushing, and syncope. Emergency drugs, suction apparatus, and resuscitation equipment, including a defibrillator should be readily available.

7. Remaining with the patient throughout the induction phase of anesthesia.

8. Performing any hair removal by clipping. Protect the patient's eyes during skin preparation.

9. Promoting normothermia through the use of thermal warming blankets, warming units, and warm IV and irrigating solutions.

10. Using graduated compression stockings and intermittent pneumatic compression devices to decrease the risk of deep vein thrombosis (DVT) and pulmonary embolism (PE) during long surgical procedures.

11. Documenting the serial number and lot numbers of any implanted materials according to institutional policy.

12. Initiating and documenting laser safety precautions if the laser is used (see Chapter 8).

Preoperative Room Preparation

Before the patient enters the OR, the nurse and scrub person (who may be a surgical technologist or a registered nurse) gather the equipment and supplies for the scheduled procedure. A well-organized surgical environment can significantly reduce anesthesia time and enable the perioperative nurse to spend more time attending to the patient's preoperative and intraoperative needs. Planning includes identifying equipment, instrumentation, furniture, and positioning accessories necessary to perform the surgery, such as the operating microscope, video system, monopolar and bipolar ESUs, suction, nerve integrity monitors, specialty instrument sets, prosthetic devices, drill and irrigation accessories, and the laser. A dedicated otorhinolaryngologic specialty storage cart centrally houses assorted prostheses, drill burrs and accessories, and dressing and packing materials, which contributes to efficient intraoperative care.

Positioning

The supine position with modifications is used during otorhinolaryngologic procedures. The perioperative nurse gathers the supplies necessary to ensure the patient's comfort in a supine position. Usually a foam headrest or a pillow for under the knees and warm blankets are included. The nurse pads the patient's extremities at pressure points and at major nerves. A pillow should be placed under the thighs, and the legs should be slightly angled to decrease pressure on the patient's back. Gel or foam heel pads are placed under the heels to prevent pressure ulcers. This positioning should be performed before the patient is anesthetized to ensure comfort. Although the incidence is low, the morbidity associated with ulnar neuropathy can be severe. Neuropathy, if permanent, results in the inability to abduct the fifth finger, diminished sensation in the fourth and fifth fingers, and eventual atrophy of the intrinsic muscle, creating a clawlike hand (Cassorla and Woo-Lee, 2015). Arms are placed on padded armboards or wrapped with gel pad wraps with the palms up and fingers extended. Armboards are maintained at less than a 90-degree angle to prevent brachial plexus stretch. If there are surgical reasons to tuck the arms at the side, the elbows are padded to protect the ulnar nerve, the palms face inward, and the wrist is maintained in a neutral position. A drape secures the arms. It should be tucked snugly under the patient, not under the mattress. This prevents the arm from shifting downward intraoperatively and resting against the OR bed rail. Placing IV lines in an arm that is to be tucked at the side should be avoided, but when this is not avoidable, patency of those lines must be ensured.

Otologic Surgical Positioning. Microscopes are used for most otologic procedures. Based on the design of the microscope and the OR bed used, the patient may be placed on the bed in the reverse position, with the head at the foot of the bed, to facilitate proper placement of the microscope mounted on a floor stand and to allow adequate space for the surgeon and assistant to be positioned on sitting stools near the surgical site.

The patient is placed supine with the operative side as close to the edge of the OR bed as possible, with the head turned and the operative ear upward. This positioning gives the surgeon access in viewing all areas of the middle ear and mastoid. One or more safety or restraining belts are used to secure the patient on the OR bed to ensure safety when turning or rotating the bed. During some procedures, such as mastoidectomy, the patient's head may be secured in position by placing tape across the head and attaching it to the frame of the OR bed. For other procedures, such as myringotomy, the patient's head may be immobilized and supported on a foam headrest. A donut-shaped foam head support helps immobilize the head and permits easy adjustment of the angle while the operating microscope is being used.

To protect the nonoperative ear, the perioperative nurse should ensure that it is in the center of the donut hole and that the headrest does not cause any pressure on the ear. The dependent arm on the nonoperative side must also be well padded and properly positioned to minimize pressure injury; the patient's body weight could cause injury when the OR bed is rotated laterally to optimize surgical access. Special consideration must be given when the patient's head is positioned for surgery, especially when general anesthetics are used. Extremes in neck extension and head torsion can cause injury to the brachial plexus or cervical spine. Other options to assist in patient positioning are determined by the otologic procedure to be performed and by the surgeon's preference. They may include ophthalmic headrests with a crescent-shaped pad, a padded horseshoe-shaped headrest, or a headrest with skull pins such as the Mayfield, which is used in certain neurologic procedures.

Positioning of the surgeon is equally important to the success of the surgery. The surgeon's chair should be positioned at a height and distance that allow comfortable access to the operative site. The use of hydraulic or electric chairs enables the surgeon to adjust the position to meet these needs.

Rhinologic Surgical Positioning. A standard headrest may be used to maintain the head in normal position but is not necessary. The entire bed is turned 180 degrees to allow the right-handed surgeon to work from the patient's right side, and the right arm is tucked in at the patient's side. The nurse pads the elbows to protect the ulnar nerve and places the palms facing inward and the wrist in a neutral position. Depending on the procedure, the patient's left arm may be maintained by the anesthesia provider and usually has the IV line placed in it for easier access. The anesthesia provider will be at the patient's head. Positioning the bed in the reverse Trendelenburg position greater than 45 degrees uses gravity to help minimize intraoperative bleeding. The scrub person may stand at the patient's head or near the patient's waist next to the surgeon's right arm (Fig. 19.12). The Mayo stand can be positioned at the head and to the side of the bed; however, it is most commonly positioned over the patient's chest, depending on where the scrub person is standing. If indicated for the procedure, the perioperative nurse assists with setting up the navigation towers and video monitor equipment at this time.

Oral Cavity/Pharyngeal/Laryngeal/Neck Surgical Positioning. The nurse assists with placing the patient in the supine position. A shoulder roll may be used for hyperextension of the neck. The

headrest should allow easy movement of the head from side to side yet maintain support. The patient's arms are often tucked at the sides as described earlier in this section to allow access of the surgical team to the operative site. If a microscope or video equipment is used, the OR bed may be turned to accommodate this equipment.

Anesthesia

Both the use of general anesthesia and the infiltration of a local anesthetic agent (local anesthesia) have advantages during otorhinolaryngologic surgery. General anesthesia provides airway control and allows the patient to remain still throughout the procedure, making surgery technically easier to perform, but requires particular attention to extremes in head positioning, possible air emboli, the control of bleeding, and, for otologic procedures, the effects of nitrous oxide in the middle ear. All anesthetics create an oxygen-rich atmosphere, and the perioperative team must consider the patient's safety in this environment (Patient Safety).

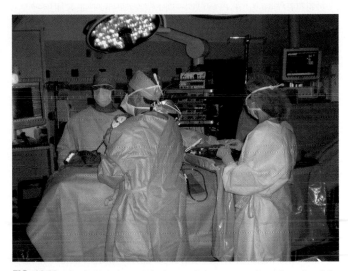

FIG. 19.12 Nasal procedure with the scrub person on the right side of the surgeon.

PATIENT SAFETY

Managing the Risk of Fire in Oxygen-Rich Environments

Surgical fires, although rare, can have devastating consequences for patients, staff, and the healthcare facility. Three elements must be present for a surgical fire to occur: heat source, fuel, and oxygen. All three of these elements are present in the OR. Prevention is key.

Surgical fires are especially devastating if they occur during surgery of the head, face, neck, and upper chest.

Estimates suggest there are approximately 700 fires each year with more than 500 cases that are unreported or near misses. Airway fires are more common in head/neck and ENT procedures including, but not limited to, tracheostomy and adenotonsillectomy.

Patients undergoing otorhinolaryngologic procedures are at greater risk for fire injury because of the proximity of the surgical field to high concentrations of oxygen. Devices used in this

specialty (e.g., lasers, fiberoptic light cables, ESU, high-speed surgical drills and burrs) further contribute to the risk by providing a heat source and fuel.

The tenets of fire safety are discussed in length in Chapter 2. Specific recommendations that the perioperative team should consider include the following:
- Awareness of risk factors. Oxygen vents into surgical field from facemasks, nasal cannulae, and uncuffed ETTs, which can then accumulate under surgical drapes. This creates an oxygen-enriched atmosphere within the proximity of the surgical site for otorhinolaryngologic procedures.
- Anticipating risk. The perioperative nurse and scrub person should collaborate before procedures to plan for risk and ensure that sterile saline is available on the surgical field, a holster is used for the active ESU electrode (and not placed on

Continued

PATIENT SAFETY

Managing the Risk of Fire in Oxygen-Rich Environments—cont'd

the drapes), and that the volume of extraneous noise is kept to a minimum so that the audio from the ESU or laser can be heard. The team should be well versed on how to extinguish a fire and locate evacuation routes if necessary.

- Implementation of specific safety protocols for the use of the laser or ESU in the airway include the following:
  - A laser-resistant ETT should be used in airway laser cases with the cuff of the laser tube filled with saline and colored with an indicator dye such as methylene blue. This will allow for the surgeon to know quickly if the integrity of the cuff has been compromised by the laser.
  - Cuffed ETTs should be used whenever possible for airway procedures. Before activating the ESU inside the airway, the surgeon should give the anesthesia provider adequate

notice that the ignition source is about to be activated. The anesthesia provider should reduce the oxygen concentration to the minimum required to prevent hypoxia, and the surgeon should wait a few minutes before using the ESU to allow the oxygen concentration to diminish. Suctioning the airway before cautery activation is also essential.

- Soft goods such as cottonoid or surgical patties should be moistened when used in oxygen-rich environments to reduce the ignition potential from sources such as the laser or ESU. Wet sponges (soft goods) should be packed in the back of the patient's throat and wet sponges or towels should be placed around the tube and/or surgical site, including the patient's face.

ENT, Ear, nose and throat; *ESU,* electrosurgical unit.
Modified from Akhtar N et al: Airway fires during surgery: management and prevention, *J Anaesthesiol Clin Pharmacol* 32(1):109–111, 2016; Spruce L: Back to basics: preventing surgical fires, *AORN J* 104(3):217–224, 2016.

Local anesthesia is used alone or as an adjunct to many procedures. Safe administration of medication is essential for achieving optimal outcomes. Lidocaine is frequently combined with epinephrine. A concentration of 1:200,000 provides maximum vasoconstriction, but some surgeons prefer a concentration of 1:100,000. Cocaine 4% topical solution is the second medication that is used commonly for rhinologic procedures. It is a good vasoconstrictor with the added benefit of anesthetic properties. Some surgeons use a nasal decongestant instead of cocaine for nasal vasoconstriction. These decongestants do not produce some of the cardiac effects seen with cocaine. Because nasal and sinus surgeries are performed in such a confined space, vasoconstriction becomes crucial for appropriate visualization of the surgical field. Hypertension can increase bleeding despite the use of vasoconstrictive agents and may need to be managed medically by the anesthesia provider intraoperatively if the field becomes compromised and surgery is impaired (Surgical Pharmacology).

For rhinologic procedures, before the patient arrives in the OR the nurse prepares a separate prep table, which includes a labeled container of the vasoconstrictor solution, x-ray–detectable cottonoid patties (usually ½ × 3 inches with attached strings), bayonet forceps, and a small nasal speculum. The surgeon soaks the cottonoid patties with the vasoconstrictor solution and usually packs the nose with the patties before prepping and draping to allow time for the vasoconstrictive properties to take effect. The patties are left in place. Some surgeons also inject local anesthetic at this time, but others may wait to inject at the time of surgery. Maximum vasoconstriction occurs in approximately 10 to 12 minutes after epinephrine is administered. If a local anesthetic is to be injected next, the prep table should also include a 10-mL Luer-Lok syringe, appropriate size needle (usually 25 gauge, 1½ inches), and labeled lidocaine (0.5%–2%, according to surgeon's preference). Additional syringes, needles, and labeled local anesthetic solution should be available on the sterile field for additional administration intraoperatively. Additional labeled cocaine solution and cottonoid patties should be available on the sterile field as well. The nurse and scrub person ensure that the cottonoid patties are counted before and at the end of the procedure. (If a pattie is placed extremely posterior along the nasal floor, it can slide past the palate and be swallowed or aspirated by the patient.)

Topical agents used in laryngeal surgery include epinephrine, phenylephrine hydrochloride, or cocaine. These agents may be applied on a cottonoid pattie or sprayed directly onto the vocal cords. Lidocaine 4% (Xylocaine) may be instilled into the trachea to decrease the cough reflex when it becomes an obstacle to a thorough physical assessment.

Local anesthesia combined with sedation or monitored anesthesia care (MAC) is often used for surgery in the premeatal region and for stapedectomy and uncomplicated middle ear procedures of less than 2 hours' duration, some rhinologic procedures, and some excisional neck procedures. Sedation should render the patient calm, comfortable, cooperative, and able to understand and communicate. Patients should not be overmedicated to the point of demonstrating obtunded reflexes or being out of touch with their surroundings. Documentation should follow institutional policy for recording intraoperative medications administered (AORN, 2016b).

Preparation of the Operative Site

If hair removal is absolutely necessary, clipping is preferred because shaving may injure the skin and increase the risk of infection. Postauricular and endaural incisions extending upward from the meatus require hair to be about 1 to 2 cm away from the proposed incision site so that hair will not be in the operative field. Long scalp hair is easily managed and kept out of the way with tape or lubricant. It is good practice to pull the top layer of hair out of the way and only clip under the hair, which helps maximize normal hair aesthetics postoperatively. Plastic adhesive drapes can be applied circumferentially around the proposed incision site, or a clear sterile drape can be laid over the entire surgical area. Parotid surgery may require hair removal from just below the temple to a line even with or slightly behind the pinna of the ear. Head and neck surgeries may require removal of hair on the chest to the nipple area on both sides. Thorough drying of the surgical area after the prep has been applied is critical for proper adhesion of the drapes to the skin so sterility is maintained throughout the operative procedure.

A povidone-iodine solution is generally used (unless the patient is allergic to iodine) to prep the surgical site for otologic and head and neck procedures. Povidone-iodine 10% solution is generally considered safe for the middle ear space and has not been found to

SURGICAL PHARMACOLOGY

Medications Commonly Used in Otorhinolaryngologic Surgery

Category	Dosage/Route	Purpose/Action	Adverse Reactions	Nursing Implications
Local Anesthetics				
Lidocaine, 0.5% or 1%	Local injection	Blocks pain and temperature fibers; used as medium to dilute epinephrine Local anesthetic	Cardiovascular, hypotension, confusion, dizziness, headache, somnolence, tremor, injection site pain, cardiac arrest, cardiac dysrhythmias, seizure	Contraindicated in hypersensitivity to amide locals Use with caution in CHF, bradycardia, hypovolemia, liver disease, renal impairment
Tetracaine (Pontocaine)	Topical: 0.25%–0.5% by nebulization or direct application	Blocks pain, suppresses gag reflex; local anesthetic	Pain, redness, irritation on initial contact	Solution must be refrigerated Frequently given by way of an atomizer. Remind patient not to eat, drink, or chew gum for at least 1 h after procedure or until cleared by physician; return of gag reflex should be determined before discharge from PACU
Benzocaine/ tetracaine/ butamben (Cetacaine)	Topical: Available in gel, liquid, and spray	Blocks pain, suppresses gag reflex; local anesthetic	Dry mouth, dizziness	Spray is given by way of metered applicator; 1- to 2-s spray is approximately 200 mg/s Should not be used over prolonged periods Remind patient not to eat, drink, or chew gum for at least 1 h after procedure or until cleared by physician; return of gag reflex should be determined before discharge from PACU
Benzocaine	Topical: Available in 20% gel and 20% spray	Blocks pain, suppresses gag reflex, local/topical anesthetic	Dry mouth, dizziness	Spray delivers 180–200 mg/s when container is full, 60–80 mg/s when inverted Remind patient not to eat, drink, or chew gum for at least 1 h after procedure or until cleared by physician; return of gag reflex should be determined before discharge from PACU
Lidocaine hydrochloride (topical)	Available as 4% solution, 2% viscous solution	Local anesthetic	High doses may cause cardiac dysrhythmias, minor burning and stinging of mouth and throat on initial contact	Provide patient with emesis basin to expectorate any secretions Patient may be instructed to gargle or swish with viscous solution to numb oral cavity in preparation for introducing Abraham cannula with 4% solution
Cocaine hydrochloride	4% topical swab; packing instilled into cavity or spray; may be applied directly to vocal cords or other laryngeal structures on pledgets to promote vasoconstriction	Local anesthetic (also used as vasoconstrictor)	CNS depression, CNS stimulation, anxiety, tachydysrhythmia, seizures; may interact with cannabis, promethazine (Phenergan), and St. John's wort	Contraindicated in hypersensitivity to cocaine products Use with caution in acutely ill patients or children, on severely traumatized mucosa, or when sepsis is present in area of intended application

Continued

Medications Commonly Used in Otorhinolaryngologic Surgery—cont'd

Category	Dosage/Route	Purpose/Action	Adverse Reactions	Nursing Implications
Vasoconstrictors				
Oxymetazoline hydrochloride (Afrin nasal spray, Neo-Synephrine 12 h, Nasacon)	Nasal spray: 4%	Nasal decongestant used for vasoconstriction	Headache, insomnia, nervousness, nasal congestion, rebound congestion, dry nasal mucosa, nasal stinging/ burning, sneezing, cardiac dysrhythmias, hypertension, tachydysrhythmia	Contraindicated in patients hypersensitive to oxymetazoline or other adrenergic agents, narrow-angle glaucoma Use with caution in patients with cardiovascular disease, concurrent MAOI or tricyclic depressant therapy, diabetes, hypertension, prostatic enlargement, thyroid disease
Epinephrine	1:100,000–1:200,000 1:1,000 (topical only)	Used for local anesthetic; vasopressor, topical antihemorrhagic	Palpitations, tachydysrhythmia, paleness and sweating, nausea and vomiting, asthenia, dizziness, headache, tremor, pain in eye, anxiety, apprehension, nervousness, dyspnea, cardiac dysrhythmias, hypertensive crisis, pulmonary edema	Should not be used in patients with hypersensitivity to epinephrine products, narrow-angle glaucoma (ophthalmic form) within 2 weeks of MAOI (inhalational form) Proceed with caution in presence of cerebrovascular insufficiency, diabetes, geriatrics, heart disease, coronary insufficiency, hypertension, thyroid disease, pregnancy
Topical Antibiotics				
Mupirocin (nasal Bactroban)	Topical: 2%	Antibacterial and lubricant for nasal packing, applied topically to skin incisions	Dermatologic, nasal stinging and burning, disorder of taste, headache	Do not use with patients hypersensitive to mupirocin products Prolonged use may result in overgrowth of nonsusceptible organisms including fungi; not intended for open wounds or mucous membranes Good for intranasal MRSA
Bacitracin	Topical ointment: 500 units/g	Antibacterial, topical antibiotic	Swelling, contact dermatitis, pruritus	Apply with sterile tip applicator or cotton swab
Ciprodex	Ciprofloxacin: 3 mg/mL Dexamethasone: 1 mg/mL (0.3%; dexamethasone 0.1%) 10 drops into the affected ear once a day for 7 days	Fluoroquinolone derivative; interferes with DNA gyrase with steroid combination		Has been shown in randomized clinical trials to be more effective at resolving acute OE than neomycin/polymyxin/ hydrocortisone
Ciprofloxin otic	Otic solution (Floxin Otic): 0.3% 10 drops into the affected ear once a day for 7 days	Fluoroquinolone derivative; interferes with DNA gyrase	Taste perversion, pruritus, site irritation; dizziness, earache, and vertigo in ~1% of patients studied	Commonly reported side effects include pruritus and bitter taste if used with a perforated tympanic membrane
Topical Antifungals				
Vosol	3 or 4 drops q6h until ears are dry and free of infection	A solution containing acetic acid (2%) in a propylene glycol vehicle containing propylene glycol diacetate (3%), benzethonium chloride (0.02%), and sodium acetate (0.015%)	Stinging on administration of an acutely inflamed ear from an external auditory infection	Contraindicated for the inner ear; ruptured TM

Medications Commonly Used in Otorhinolaryngologic Surgery—cont'd

Category	Dosage/Route	Purpose/Action	Adverse Reactions	Nursing Implications
Chloramphenicol powder 0.5%: reconstitute 25 mg/vial	2 or 3 drops 3 or 4 times per day for 7 days via powder insufflator	Dichloroacetic acid derivative	Prolonged use: headache, contact sensitivity, pruritus	Effective against yeast and bacteria, for chronic wet ears/mastoid cavity; commonly used in combination powder with tolnaftate and sodium sulfacetamide powder
Boric acid powder: reconstitute 7.5 g/15.375 g	1 or 2 drops 4–6 times per day for 7 days via powder insufflator	Weak acid; boron often used as an antiseptic	Repeated skin contact of damaged skin with boric acid can cause nausea, vomiting, diarrhea, loss of appetite, weakness, confusion, abnormalities in menstruation and hair loss	Avoid in children; toxicity and death reported with prolonged use. Avoid during pregnancy
Tolnaftate topical powder (1%)	A typical dosage is 3 or 4 drops into affected ear 4 times daily for 7 days via powder insufflator	A synthetic topical thiocarbamate antifungal agent	Skin irritation, allergic reaction	Effective in the treatment of fungal OE; commonly used in combination powder with chloramphenicol and sodium sulfacetamide powder
Sulfanilamide powder	A typical dosage is 3 or 4 drops into affected ear 4 times daily for 7 days via powder insufflator	Sulfonamides inhibit bacterial dihydropteroate synthase by competing with PABA. This action interferes with the conversion of PABA into folic acid, an essential component of bacterial development	Pruritus; limited data available	Effective in the treatment of fungal OE; commonly used in combination powder with chloramphenicol and tolnaftate powder
Steroids				
Triamcinolone acetonide (Aristocort, Kenalog)	Topical	Used topically to lubricate packs or expand packing	Hypertension, atrophic condition of skin	Use with caution in patients with hypertension, hypothyroidism, and pregnancy. Do not use with hypersensitivity to triamcinolone acetonide; local, viral, fungal, or bacterial infections
Cortisporin otic suspension (neomycin and polymyxin B sulfates/hydrocortisone)	Topical	Used after otologic surgery as an antiinflammatory/antibiotic agent	Itching, pain, stinging, burning, ototoxicity	When administering to patient, do the following: Tilt patient's head in opposite direction of affected ear. Instill prescribed number of drops toward ear canal, not directly onto eardrum (Tip: To promote correct placement of drops in children pull auricle down and posterior; in adults pull auricle up and posterior)

CHF, Congestive heart failure; *CNS*, central nervous system; *DNA*, deoxyribonucleic acid; *MAOI*, monoamine oxidase inhibitor; *MRSA*, methicillin-resistant *Staphylococcus aureus*; *OE*, otitis externa; *PABA*, para-aminobenzoic acid; *PACU*, postanesthesia care unit; *s*, second(s); *TM*, tympanic membrane.
Modified from Skidmore-Roth L: *Mosby's drug guide for nurses*, ed 11, St Louis, 2016, Mosby; Hodgson BB, Kizior RJ: *Saunders nursing drug handbook 2015*, St Louis, 2015, Saunders.

be ototoxic in animal studies; however, in the presence of a tympanic membrane perforation, swabbing of the ear canal skin is preferred to instillation or pooling in the ear canal to prevent large volumes of prep solution from entering the middle ear space. All other surgical prep solutions, such as chlorhexidine and alcohol, are considered ototoxic and should be strictly limited to the outer ear and surrounding skin. Head and neck procedures may involve extensive skin preparation and usually include the entire area from the chin to the nipples; it may also include a donor skin graft site if a defect or large flap coverage is anticipated. Some surgeons prefer the patient's face to be included in the prep, depending on the type of surgery anticipated and the site of the lesion. If a flap may be raised to reconstruct a defect, saline should be available to remove the discoloration from the skin to allow the surgeon to check for flap viability.

Prepping the nose and face may be done for rhinologic and laryngeal or oral cavity procedures, depending on the surgical procedure and institutional policy. These areas are considered "dirty" and not possible to prep as effectively as other surgical sites, such as an abdomen. The surgical field is maintained in sterile fashion, and these procedures usually have a "clean-contaminated" wound classification (see Chapter 4).

Facial Nerve Monitoring

Alteration of facial nerve function can be a direct consequence of parotid gland surgery. Despite improvements in surgical techniques, postoperative facial weakness is still a considerable complication from parotidectomy and has been reported to occur in up to 65% of patients (Mamelle et al., 2013). Facial nerve monitoring can be used to help the surgeon identify the nerve and decrease the risk of injury to the nerve. Audible facial nerve monitors are used intraoperatively during procedures in which the facial nerve is at risk. The system allows for assessment of the nerve's integrity after the gland has been removed.

The surgeon places electrodes into the facial muscles before the patient is draped. Consultation and communication with the anesthesia provider are essential because the use of muscle relaxants and long-term paralyzing agents must be avoided. In the setting of a tympanic membrane perforation, lidocaine should not be allowed to spill into the middle ear space when injecting the ear canal because temporary facial paralysis can ensue from topical anesthesia of a dehiscent facial nerve in the tympanic segment. Facial nerve monitoring is commonly used during acoustic neuroma and mastoid surgery (Fig. 19.13).

Draping

Barrier draping minimizes the risk of postoperative infection. Draping technique is based on the surgeon's preference and the procedure to be performed.

Otologic Procedure Draping. Draping may be minimal for procedures such as myringotomy. For major otologic procedures, plastic adhesive drapes are applied around the ear to keep the patient's hair out of the surgical field. A sterile, plastic aperture drape is placed over the surgical site with the ear exposed through the opening. The surgeon may elect to expose a portion of the face on the affected side to observe facial movement.

Three or four towels are draped over the aperture drape around the ear and may be secured with nonpenetrating towel clips. The scrubbed and gowned team unfolds a fenestrated drape over the patient, with the opening centered over the operative site. An alternative method is the use of a split sheet with the split end secured at the base of the ear and the open flaps wrapped around the patient's head. Disposable drapes with adhesive backing may be used to secure the sheet to the patient.

During mastoid surgery and for resections of acoustic tumors, fluid-collection pouches may be attached to the drape. These pouches will catch fluid runoff when drilling and irrigation are planned. The operating microscope is draped to extend the sterile field (Fig. 19.14).

Special consideration must be given to the selection of draping material used during ear surgery. Lint from drapes can be transferred to instruments and introduced into the ear. They act as a foreign body in the wound, causing the formation of granulomas in the middle and inner ear, and may contribute to irreversible hearing loss. Therefore lint-free drapes should be used.

Rhinologic Procedure Draping. Draping is done for most rhinologic cases. A small sheet with a towel on top of it is placed under the patient's head, and the towel is secured around the hairline with a nonpenetrating towel clip. A split sheet is then placed around the head. It is good practice to place a towel over the endotracheal tube (ETT) if one is in place; this helps prevent the adhesive portion of the split sheet from sticking to the ETT and inadvertently pulling on the tube after the procedure is completed and drapes are removed. Except during certain endoscopic procedures, the patient's eyes should be covered with moist gauze or towels if the patient is awake or taped closed if the patient has received a general anesthetic, protecting the eyes from nasal drainage or injury from instruments.

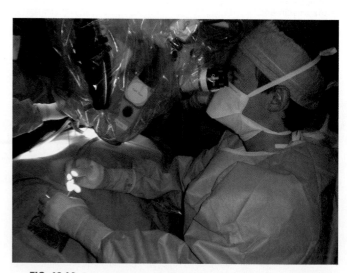

FIG. 19.14 Surgeon in correct seated position for otologic surgery.

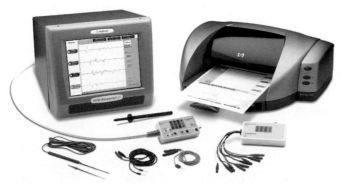

FIG. 19.13 Nerve integrity monitor system for intraoperative facial nerve monitoring.

Oral Cavity, Pharyngeal, Laryngologic, and Neck Procedure Draping. Draping of the patient for a laryngeal procedure for a benign lesion (intraoral approach) is minimal, with the primary focus being protection of the patient's eyes and face. This may be accomplished by (1) placing ointment in the patient's eyes; (2) taping the eyelids closed with a nonabrasive, nonirritating tape; (3) applying moist padding over the tape (if use of a laser is anticipated); and (4) placing self-adhering eye pads over the moistened pads. A head drape may be placed over the patient's face to expose only the lips and chin.

Draping for neck procedures often varies according to surgeon preference and is similar to the draping procedures described for rhinologic surgery. After the surgeon marks the incision site, the site is cleansed with antiseptic prep. Sterile towels are squared off around the field, then secured in place with either towel clips or staples. A "scrunched" towel may be set underneath the lobule of each ear onto the OR table to collect any drainage. A split sheet is then applied. Additional drapes may be needed if skin grafts or flaps are used for reconstructive procedures.

Surgical Microscope

A surgical microscope is often used to provide illumination and magnification for complex procedures to the ear, laryngeal surgery, or reconstructive free flap procedures after neck surgery. Several kinds of surgical microscopes with different attachments are available for otologic and laryngologic surgery. The microscope may be floor or ceiling mounted. Optimal light is provided by a xenon or halogen light source. Numerous types of monocular and binocular heads are available for the microscope. These heads may be fixed in a straight or angled plane, or they may be designed to be adjustable in an inclinable plane. For operations through an ear speculum, the microscope provides direct light and permits the surgeon to select a magnification of ×6, ×10, ×16, ×25, or ×40. A common eyepiece magnification for an otologic microscope is ×12.5, and the usual objective (lens) is 250- or 300-mm focal length (f). A 400-mm lens is used for laryngeal surgery. The total magnification is determined by multiplying the magnification of the eyepiece times that of the microscope body times that of the objective. The type of head and objective selected is based on the surgeon's preference. Microscopes equipped with a variable distance feature allow the surgeon to adjust the focal length from 200 to 400 mm without changing the lens objective. Video equipment may be attached to the microscope, which allows other team members to follow the procedure and to anticipate the necessary instrumentation. Before lenses are placed on the microscope they should be checked to ensure that they are free from lint, dust, fingerprints, and soil. The surgeon adjusts the microscope before it is draped for surgery and manipulates it during the procedure. The microscope is draped with a sterile cover for otologic surgery, but is often left undraped for laryngeal procedures. It is necessary to keep the drape material away from the light source fan of the microscope. Doing so allows cool air to continue to circulate and avoids overheating of the fan, which could prematurely burn out the lamp and cause a fire. When micromanipulators are secured to transmit laser energy to tissue through the operating microscope, special microscope laser drapes must be used. These drapes have an opening in the plastic at the base of the micromanipulator covering the objective, allowing laser energy to pass through the opening of the drape without burning the drape.

Care should be taken when removing the drapes from the microscope to avoid discarding the eyepieces with the drapes or dropping them on the floor. Eyepieces have been lost or damaged in this manner, necessitating costly repair or replacement.

When the microscope is not in use it should be kept in a locked, upright position and stored in an area that is away from traffic, free from dust, and properly ventilated. Ideally a set of eyepieces should be left in the scope to prevent the inside of the scope from becoming dusty. The microscope may also be covered with either a protective cover or a plastic bag.

Equipment and Instrumentation

Equipment that may be used in otorhinolaryngologic surgery includes an ESU (both monopolar and bipolar), a warming unit or other device to maintain normothermia, and headlights. Lasers assist in vaporization of scar tissue, granulomas, and cholesteatomas without damaging surrounding tissue and may be used for select otolaryngologic procedures. Lasers used in this specialty include the carbon dioxide (CO_2), potassium titanyl phosphate (KTP), erbium:yttrium-aluminum-garnet (Er:YAG), and neodymium:yttrium-aluminum-garnet (Nd:YAG) lasers. Lasers can be secured to the operating microscope and laser energy delivered to the tissue by means of a micromanipulator. Laser energy is delivered directly to tissue by fiberoptic probes, which can be navigated around obstructing structures.

For complex reconstructive procedures in the neck, a handheld Doppler unit (to determine the viability of blood vessels) or an electromyographic nerve monitor (to determine the location and quality of nerves) may be used.

Specimen cups, labels, and a marking pen should be available on the sterile field because often several specimens are obtained. Institutional procedure for correct patient and specimen identification should be followed (AORN, 2016e).

The basic principles of care, handling, and sterilization of instruments are discussed in Chapter 4. The instrumentation used in otorhinolaryngologic surgery is quite specific and is discussed with each surgical intervention. Head and neck instrumentation combines general surgical instruments and procedure-specific instruments. Many procedures use delicate microinstruments that should be handled individually and should not be allowed to physically contact each other. Fine tympanoplasty and stapedectomy instrumentation should be kept in special storage and sterilization trays. These trays help separate instruments, aid in quick identification, protect the instruments from damage, and facilitate handling during surgery. Instruments used in the path of the operating microscope may have an ebony glare-reducing finish. Handles of assorted knives and dissectors may be flat, hexagonal, or round for better gripping or handling during surgery. The shaft of these instruments may be straight, angled, or bayonet shaped.

Powered Equipment. A power sagittal saw is used for complex neck procedures. A power drill and assorted rotating burrs are essential for middle ear surgery and some sinus procedures. Many drills are commercially available that are pneumatically or electrically driven. Pneumatic drills must have high torque (power) and more than 20,000 revolutions per minute (rpm) (speed). Some surgeons believe electrically powered drills offer equal torque but better control of the drill tip.

A selection of burrs including assorted sizes of round cutting burrs and diamond polishing burrs should be available. A diamond burr cuts slowly and grinds the bone away rather than tearing into it; it is commonly used around vital structures. Cutting burrs assist in quickly removing bone from areas not close to vital structures. The grooves or teeth of burrs must be clean of bone dust. Bone-cutting burrs tend to clog more easily than coarse-toothed burrs. A sterile wire brush may be used to keep burrs clean intraoperatively. Bone dust must be prevented from settling in areas such as those in sta-pedectomy, tympanoplasty, endolymphatic sac, or fenestration surgery. A sterile field continuously flooded with irrigation solution helps lessen clogging of the burr and washes away bone dust.

Evaluation

Perioperative nursing care should be evaluated at the completion of the procedure before the patient is transported to the postanesthesia care unit (PACU) or ambulatory recovery area. If the patient has received a local anesthetic, the nurse will have had the opportunity to evaluate care on an ongoing basis, communicating with the patient throughout the procedure.

At the conclusion of the procedure, the nurse assesses the patient for any breathing difficulty. Patients who have undergone nasal surgery may have packing, which can inhibit breathing; however, the patient should be able to breathe normally through the mouth. Patients who have undergone oral cavity or laryngeal surgery are at risk for airway edema. The head of the PACU bed should be elevated before transport to the unit for all otorhinolaryngologic patients. Because of the proximity of the facial nerve to many structures within the anatomic field for otorhinolaryngologic procedures, the nurse must evaluate the patient's facial nerve function. This evaluation requires the patient's cooperation in smiling, closing the eye, and wrinkling the nose on the operative side. If facial palsy is observed and does not resolve within 2 hours of the procedure, it may be caused by surgical trauma. The nurse assesses skin integrity at positional pressure sites and the ESU dispersive electrode site and documents the findings. The amount of drainage present on any dressings is also noted.

During evaluation, the perioperative nurse determines whether the patient met the outcomes in the plan of care. Some outcomes can be reached during the preoperative and intraoperative phases of care; they are evaluated before the patient's discharge from the OR. Others require ongoing monitoring and measurement in the post-operative phase. A complete hand-off report allows the PACU or intensive care unit (ICU) nurse to detect significant changes in the patient's condition at an early stage. Special considerations should also be included, such as the necessity for flexion of the neck to avoid disruption of the suture line of the trachea in a patient who has undergone tracheal resection. Repeated swallowing should be noted because this may indicate posterior nasal or oral cavity bleeding. Part of the hand-off report to the PACU or nursing unit should include the following outcomes of care provided:

- The patient identified factors that caused anxiety and verbalized effective coping; frequent explanations were provided, which assisted in coping with an unknown environment.

- The patient communicated adequate pain management using a pain scale and demonstrated effective coping with the physical and psychologic effects of pain. Vital signs remained stable; there were no electrocardiogram (ECG) or CNS changes.
- The patient demonstrated effective breathing patterns. Respiratory rate and depth were within normal limits, and the respiratory pattern appeared effective with no cyanosis or other signs of hypoxia.
- Intraoperative bleeding was kept at a minimum during the case, keeping the patient safe from a dangerous amount of surgical blood loss.
- The patient verbalized understanding of anticipated postoperative alteration in the senses of hearing or smell and taste.
- The patient verbalized feelings regarding disturbances in body image, interacted positively with perioperative staff, main-tained eye contact, and identified personally effective coping strategies.
- The patient is able to communicate effectively (ongoing) and use an alternative method (specify) of communication.

Patient, Family, and Caregiver Education and Discharge Planning

Patient, family, and caregiver education is an important component of the age-appropriate and culturally sensitive care provided by perioperative nurses. Visual teaching aids, teaching brochures, and written discharge instructions provide the patient with knowledge of the surgery and what to expect during the postoperative period. Preoperative patient education includes preparing the patient for alterations in body image and function, if applicable to the planned procedure. Alternate methods of communication must be discussed before disruption of oral or laryngeal function, or hearing. The presence of edema, drains, or dressings; changes in mobility; side effects of surgery or anesthesia; possible complications of surgery; and the pertinent signs and symptoms of these complications must be discussed. The OR environment and presence of equipment should be described to the patient preoperatively to keep anxiety at a minimum. Specific instructions based on the type of surgery performed must be reviewed with the patient, focusing on important areas, such as management of pain and discomfort, restriction of activity levels, and observation for signs of infection. Printed information should be reviewed with the patient, and the patient should repeat back the key points that are essential to a successful recovery. By the time of discharge, patients and family members should have a thorough knowledge and understanding of what to expect during the postoperative recuperation period (Patient, Family, and Caregiver Education).

PATIENT, FAMILY, AND CAREGIVER EDUCATION

Patient Education for Otorhinolaryngologic Surgery

The following information is applicable to all otorhinolaryngologic procedures. Instructions unique to specific procedures are also included. Teaching is best accomplished using a variety of methods (e.g., conversation, printed materials, written instructions) and should include evaluation of the patient's understanding of the material, such as by having the patient or caregiver "teach-back" the concepts previously discussed.

Preprocedural Teaching: All Procedures
- Review the physician's explanation of the procedure and its purpose; encourage the patient to ask questions and to discuss any fears or anxieties. Discuss the need for informed consent for surgery and anesthesia.
- Tell the patient that NPO status must be maintained as directed by the anesthesia provider.

- Describe the OR environment and sequence of events that occur, explaining what the patient will see, feel, and hear during the perioperative experience.
- Provide information about what to expect if a local anesthetic is used (e.g., some discomfort may occur during the initial administration of a local anesthetic; if epinephrine is used with the local agent, the resulting weak, quivering feeling and increased heart rate are effects of the epinephrine and disappear after a few minutes).
- Remind the patient undergoing a local procedure that there will be pressure at some point but not pain. Encourage the patient to inform the perioperative nurse and surgeon if any discomfort is felt during the procedure. Discuss a mechanism to communicate when unable to speak. A gesture as simple as raising the hand nearest to the nurse monitoring the patient may be appropriate.
- Inform the patient that the skin will be cleansed with bactericidal soap or antiseptic solutions to remove bacteria.

Otologic/Laryngologic Procedures

- Review the use of an erasable board, paper and pencil, flash cards, or other communication board if applicable to the surgery performed.
- Encourage questions and verbalization of fears and anxieties regarding possible loss of voice or hearing.

Review of Postprocedural Care: All Procedures

- Explain that the patient will be in high Fowler position to lessen edema, improve coughing and deep breathing, and provide comfort. Advise patients to use pillows or a wedge to elevate the head by 30 degrees for the first 24 hours after discharge. Note that some patients use a recliner chair at home for comfort.
- Discuss the importance of frequent deep breathing and coughing.
- Explain the presence of any dressings and drainage tubes.
- Review pain management, encouraging the patient to use mild analgesics when possible.
- Remind the patient to limit the Valsalva maneuver (e.g., coughing, straining at stool) to prevent tissue damage or bleeding.
- Inform the patient that some bruising and swelling can be expected after many procedures, but will gradually subside.
- Note that some numbness may be noted postoperatively but gradually disappears.
- Discuss that heavy lifting or strenuous activity should be avoided until directed by the surgeon.

Rhinologic Procedures

- Inform the patient that if a nasal pack is inserted, there may be some difficulty in swallowing. When the patient attempts to swallow, a sucking action occurs in the throat because the packing does not allow air passage through the nose, creating a partial vacuum.
- Review the procedure for changing the mustache dressing (or drip pad) that is in place postoperatively to absorb any drainage. The dressing is usually a folded 2 × 2-inch gauze pad placed under the nose and secured by tape. Blood-tinged

secretions in the nasopharynx are normal in the first few hours after the procedure.
- Advise the patient that forceful nose blowing must be avoided for a time to prevent movement of the rearranged nasal structures. If necessary to clear nasal passages, the patient should sniff gently.
- Review the importance of humidification. As directed by the surgeon, patients may use a humidifier at home to reduce nasal dryness.
- Note that the sense of smell is diminished for a time after surgery but gradually returns.

Otologic Procedures

- Avoid rapidly moving the head, bouncing, or bending over for 3 weeks.
- Exercise caution when coughing or blowing the nose; open both the nose and mouth if sneezing is unavoidable.
- Avoid drinking through a straw.

Oral Cavity/Laryngologic Procedures

- Rinse the mouth as directed by the surgeon; avoid contact with agents that may inflame the mouth, such as mouthwashes that contain alcohol.
- Perform oral hygiene after each meal or as often as needed.
- Use a soft toothbrush, sponge brush, or gauze for oral care.
- Use and apply topical analgesics and anesthetics as ordered by the physician.
- Observe voice rest as directed by the surgeon.
- Use humidification to decrease dryness and increase comfort.

Home Care: All Procedures

Give both the patient and the caregiver *verbal* and *written* instructions. Provide them with the name and telephone number of a physician or nurse to call if questions arise. Use visual aids to assist in instruction.

- General information
  - Review any explanation about the procedure and any specific follow-up care.
  - Review the signs and symptoms that should be reported to the surgeon or nurse:
    - Infection of the incision: redness, drainage, pain, warm to touch
    - Fever
    - Dyspnea without exertion
    - Difficulty swallowing
    - Bleeding or discharge of clear fluid from the ear or nose
    - Vertigo that lasts more than 24 to 48 hours after surgery
- Discuss activity limits
  - Remind the patient to plan frequent rest periods.
  - Assist the patient to begin self-care as soon as possible.
  - Review any restricted activities such as driving, swimming or diving, and air travel.
- Emphasize follow-up care
  - Stress the importance of regular follow-up visits. Make sure the patient has the necessary names and telephone numbers to contact the surgeon.

NPO, Nothing-by-mouth.

Modified from Workman ML: Assessment and care of patients with ear and hearing problems. In Ignatavicius DD, Workman ML, editors: *Medical-surgical nursing: patient-centered collaborative care,* ed 8, Philadelphia, 2016, Saunders; Rebar CR et al: Care of patients with oral cavity problems. In Ignatavicius DD, Workman ML, editors: *Medical-surgical nursing: patient-centered collaborative care,* ed 8, St Louis, 2016, Saunders.

Surgical Interventions

Otologic Procedures

The majority of otologic procedures are performed either through the ear canal or from behind the ear. Incisions through the ear canal include endaural and transcanal approaches. The postauricular approach is made through an incision from behind the ear (Fig. 19.15).

Endaural Approach

The endaural incision is made in two steps, using a #15 blade on a knife handle. The first incision starts at the superior meatal wall about 1 cm in from the outer edge of the meatus and extends down the posterior meatal wall to the edge of the conchal cartilage. The second incision on the superior meatal wall extends upward to a point halfway between the meatus and upper edge of the auricle. This approach offers direct access to the external auditory meatus and tympanic membrane and may be used for meatoplasty, canalplasty, selected tympanic membrane perforations, and stapes surgery.

Transcanal Approach

The transcanal approach is used for those procedures that are limited to the mesotympanum, hypotympanum, and tympanic membrane. The incision entails a superiorly based tympanomeatal flap through the ear canal and involves making a semilunar canal skin incision anywhere from 2 to 10 mm lateral to the tympanic membrane. For exposure, the skin, fibrous annulus, and tympanic membrane are elevated as a unit. Posterior tympanomeatal flaps may be used in stapedectomy, labyrinthectomy, myringoplasty, tumor biopsy, ossiculoplasty, and removal of glomus tympanicum tumors. Congenital cholesteatomas are best approached superiorly, whereas perforations of the tympanic membrane are typically accessed through an inferior incision.

Transcanal endoscopic ear surgery can be used in patients with chronic ear disease for cholesteatoma removal and middle ear reconstruction, reducing the need for a postauricular incision and mastoidectomy. This is a very difficult approach, however, requiring one-handed dissection (Dedman et al., 2015).

Postauricular Approach

The surgeon makes the postauricular incision 2 to 5 mm behind the ear following the curve of the posterior auricular fold, providing wide-field exposure and a versatile and adaptable incision. It is commonly used for tympanoplasty procedures; it is also used to expose the mastoid process for a mastoidectomy, endolymphatic sac procedure, labyrinthectomy, or translabyrinthectomy resection of an acoustic neuroma.

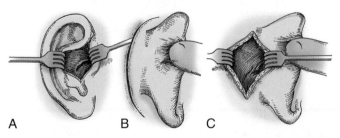

FIG. 19.15 Surgical incisions. (A) Endaural. (B) Postauricular. (C) Postauricular incision retracted.

Myringotomy

A standard myringotomy is an incision in the pars tensa of the tympanic membrane. Myringotomy is often accompanied by the aspiration of fluid under pressure in the tympanum, and the subsequent placement of small, hollow, pressure equalization tubes (PETs) (also known as *tympanostomy* or *myringotomy tubes*). It is indicated for acute otitis media (AOM) in the presence of an exudate that has not responded to antibiotic therapy. AOM occurs in 84% to 93% of all children. Otitis media with effusion (OME) occurs in 50% to 90% of children (Roditi et al., 2016). The majority of children with AOM have spontaneous resolution. OME is distinct from AOM, however, because it may still have a significant impact on speech, hearing, development, and quality of life. Hearing loss is a significant sequelae when fluid is present in the middle ear (OME).

If left untreated, hearing loss can affect language development. If the fluid persists more than 8 to 12 weeks and is accompanied by hearing loss, removal of the fluid and placement of ventilating tubes in the eardrum are necessary.

Otitis media, although more common in the pediatric population, is also seen in adults. Tympanic fibrosis is common in adults and is a result of repeated infections that occurred in childhood. AOM is a collection of infected pus in the middle ear. The patient may have severe pain and bulging of the tympanic membrane (Fig. 19.16). Failure to respond to oral antibiotics and analgesics or other complications, such as facial nerve paralysis, may require a myringotomy. By release of the pus or fluid, hearing is restored and the infection can be controlled. The procedure may be performed for chronic serous otitis media in which the presence of fluid in the middle ear produces a hearing loss. Frequently tubes are inserted into the tympanic membrane (Fig. 19.17) to allow ventilation of the middle ear. Myringotomy tubes may be used for the treatment of colds and fluid in the ear on a short-term basis (a few months), on an intermediate basis (6–18 months), and in long-term treatment (years) for chronic situations. Tubes may also be placed in patients undergoing hyperbaric therapy to prevent ear pain and tympanic rupture while in the hyperbaric chamber. Care must be taken to avoid getting water in the ears while the tubes are in place. Myringotomy is usually performed on an ambulatory surgery basis. A recent alternative to tube placement is CO_2 laser–assisted myringotomy, in which the laser energy is used to create a precise hole in the tympanic membrane. The hole remains open for 4 to 6 weeks. Laser-assisted myringotomy is done using a topical anesthetic and may be performed in the physician's office.

Procedural Considerations

Myringotomy with tube placement is considered a clean procedure. In adult patients the procedure may be performed using a topical anesthetic. Pediatric patients generally require general anesthesia. The surgeon may wear gown and gloves or gloves only, depending on the policy related to Standard Precautions at the institution in which the procedure is performed. Myringotomy procedures require a sharp knife for making incisions into the tympanic membrane. Sterile, disposable, single-use blades are supplied with integrated handles or as single blades that may be secured into reusable handles. Myringotomy blades are spear-, lancet-, and sickle-shaped and are a matter of the surgeon's preference. The instrument setup includes a myringotomy knife and disposable blade, assorted sizes of aural specula, ear curettes, suction tip and tubing, a delicate Hartmann forceps, metal aural applicators, a curved needle, a culture tube (if

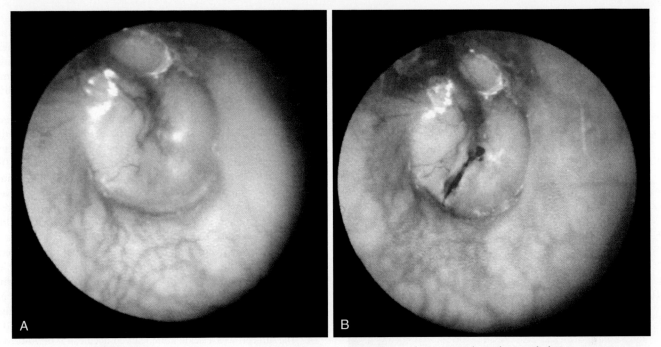

FIG. 19.16 (A) In purulent otitis media, pus under pressure pushes eardrum outward, resulting in bulging tympanic membrane. (B) Radial myringotomy incision.

cultures are to be taken), and myringotomy tubes (as applicable). Several types of disposable myringotomy tubes are available for implantation, depending on the length of time the surgeon wishes the tube to remain in place (see Fig. 19.17). After the tube falls out, the tympanic membrane incision usually heals.

Operative Procedure

1. With the patient's head and the surgical microscope in position, the surgeon inserts the aural speculum into the ear canal. The external canal is cleaned of excess cerumen using a wire loop curette. Using a sharp myringotomy knife, the surgeon makes a small, curved or radial incision in the anterior inferior quadrant of the pars tensa (see Fig. 19.2).
2. A culture may be taken to determine the type of organism present. Pus and fluid are suctioned from the middle ear.
3. The surgeon inserts the tube into the incision with alligator forceps or a tube inserter. Care should be taken to consult the manufacturer's directions for handling the tube.
4. Antibiotic drops (e.g., ofloxacin 0.3% otic) may be instilled after positioning the tube.
5. A cotton ball may be placed in the external canal at the end of the procedure.

Tympanoplasty

Tympanoplasty is the surgical repair of the tympanic membrane and the tympanum and the reconstruction of the ossicular chain. It is indicated for conductive hearing losses caused by perforation of the tympanic membrane as a result of trauma or infection, for ossicular discontinuity, for chronic or recurrent otitis media, for progressive hearing loss, and for the inability to safely bathe or participate in water activities as a result of perforation of the tympanic membrane with or without hearing loss.

Perforation of the tympanic membrane is the most common ear injury necessitating surgical intervention. Perforations may result from (1) direct injury (e.g., cotton applicators, pencil), (2) blow to the ear, and (3) injury from temporal bone fractures. Early diagnosis is the key to proper management.

Conductive hearing loss is caused by an obstruction in the external canal or middle ear, which impedes the passage of sound waves to the inner ear. It may be attributable to disease of the middle ear or tympanic membrane. Occasionally the tympanic membrane does not heal after myringotomy.

Ossicular discontinuity may result from chronic otitis media, trauma, or cholesteatoma, which is a skin cyst that erodes bone. Various methods and materials are used in constructing a closed, air-contained middle ear cavity and restoring a sound-pressure transforming action. Among these materials are high-density polyethylene, silicone, hydroxyapatite, and titanium prostheses.

Procedural Considerations

The ear is prepped and draped as previously described. An endaural or postauricular approach may be used. Both approaches provide similar functional results. The procedure most often is performed after the patient has been administered a general anesthetic.

Operative Procedure

1. The following three approaches may be used when performing a tympanoplasty:
   a. When an *endaural approach* is used, the surgeon introduces a Lempert speculum into the external meatus of the ear canal, and positions the microscope. The surgeon injects lidocaine with epinephrine postauricularly and into the external meatus and external auditory canal. The endaural incision is made as detailed previously and then the tympanomeatal incision is made using a sharp, round knife.
   b. When a *postauricular approach* is used, the surgeon injects lidocaine with epinephrine postauricularly. Next, the surgeon introduces an ear speculum and positions the microscope.

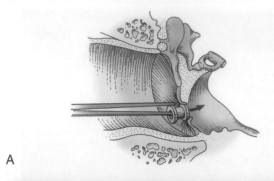

A

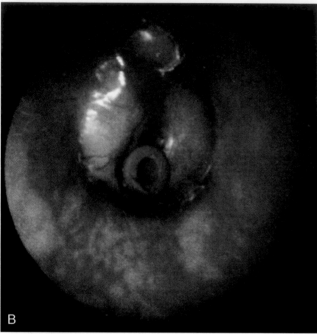

B

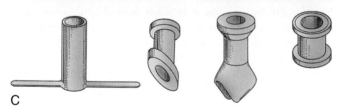

C

FIG. 19.17 (A) Tube (placed on end of alligator forceps) being inserted into tympanic membrane. (B) Tube in place. (C) Several types of plastic tubes that may be inserted into tympanic membrane. Purpose of the tubes is to aerate the middle ear and reduce middle ear infections.

Additional lidocaine is injected into the external auditory canal. The microscope head is moved from directly over the patient's ear. The surgeon incises the skin behind the fold of the ear with a #15 blade. Bleeding vessels are coagulated. An incision is then made into the periosteum down to the bone, and the periosteum is elevated from behind the incision with a Lempert elevator.

c. During the *transcanal approach,* the surgeon injects the four quadrants of the fibrocartilaginous canal with a 1% or 2% lidocaine solution with 1 : 100,000 epinephrine. An endaural speculum gently compresses the tissue edema resulting from the injection and assists in the placement of a speculum within the confines of the bony canal. A 30-gauge needle is used to inject the skin of the bony canal. Various canal incisions can be made, all of which accomplish the same goal of lifting the posterior ear canal skin and the tympanic membrane in continuity. Once the incisions have been made, the skin is elevated to the tympanic annulus, subcutaneous tissue at the tympanomastoid suture is dissected, and bleeding is controlled before the middle ear is reached.

2. At this point the surgeon or the assistant harvests a section of temporalis fascia for the graft material used in the repair of the tympanic membrane. Lidocaine with epinephrine may be injected under the fascia to separate it from the temporalis muscle. The surgeon uses a narrow Shambaugh elevator or duckbill elevator to separate the fascia and excises the amount needed using small, sharp scissors or a knife blade. The fascia is trimmed of excess tissue with small, sharp scissors and set aside to dry on a Teflon cutting block that is standard in most otologic instrument trays. Some surgeons prefer to thin the fascia by using a House Gelfoam press before placing the graft on the cutting block.

3. The canal skin may be elevated from the canal with a duckbill elevator, curved needle, gimmick, or similar microinstrument, or it may be removed (lateral/overlay tympanoplasty), depending on the size and location of the tympanic membrane perforation.

4. The surgeon uses a sickle knife, curved needle, 45- or 90-degree pick, or cup forceps to remove all the epithelium from the drum surrounding the perforation edges of the tympanic membrane in preparation for receiving the graft. This is referred to as "freshening the edges" and is a critical step in promoting reepithelialization of the graft.

5. If an edge of the perforation or tympanic membrane cannot be visualized because of the bony canal, the surgeon uses a microcurette or drill to remove the overhang of bone.

6. The middle ear is explored with a pick or similar instrument, and any epithelium is removed with an alligator, or cup, forceps. The surgeon inspects each ossicle to ensure that it is intact and mobile.

7. If the malleus or incus is diseased or eroded, it may be removed and replaced with a partial ossicular replacement prosthesis (PORP). Ossicles that are removed may be reshaped with the aid of a drill and small burr and replaced. If all ossicles are diseased or eroded, they may be removed and replaced with a total ossicular replacement prosthesis (TORP). This step is accomplished with microinstrumentation, such as Bellucci scissors, cup forceps, malleus nipper, incudostapedial joint knife, sickle knife, picks, and a curved needle.

8. The surgeon prepares the graft for insertion. The edges are trimmed with a #15 blade or sharp scissors to fit the shape of the ear canal and the size of the perforation. The surgical site is suctioned with a microsuction device. Hemostasis may be achieved by applying very small, epinephrine-soaked Gelfoam balls with an alligator forceps.

9. The surgeon selects the tissue for the repair. Different tissues, such as temporalis fascia or loose connective tissue, tragus perichondrium, and vein grafts, have been used for a tympanoplasty procedure. The most common tissue used is temporalis fascia. Most surgeons prefer to use autograft tissue, although homograft tympanic membranes have also been used. The risk of transmission of infectious disease has reduced homograft use. For easier manipulation, the graft may be dipped in water or saline before its insertion with alligator forceps. A gimmick, sickle knife, pick, curved needle, or similar microinstrument is used to position the graft into place. Small pieces of absorbable

gelatin sponge may be packed below the graft in the middle ear space to ensure support and position. The graft and tympanomeatal flap are then laid back into place and Gelfoam packing is used to secure the flap, remnant tympanic membrane, and graft in the proper position. This outer ear canal packing is left in place for 1 to 2 weeks postoperatively and removed in the surgeon's office.

10. The external ear canal is then packed with bioresorbable packing; moistened, absorbable, gelatin sponge pledgets; or antibiotic ointment.
11. The surgeon closes the incision.
12. A pressure dressing consisting of fluffed gauze placed around the ear and an elastic gauze wrapped around the affected ear and the head may be applied for the first 24 hours to reduce swelling. Commercially prepared postauricular incision dressings are available.

Mastoidectomy

Mastoidectomy is the removal of diseased bone of the mastoid process and mastoid space. Before the introduction of antibiotic therapy, mastoidectomy was commonly performed for infection. Although occasionally still performed to eradicate infection, it is more frequently used to treat cholesteatoma. Cholesteatoma is the result of accumulation of squamous epithelium and its products in the middle ear and mastoid. It occasionally forms a cystlike mass. As it expands it is destructive to the middle ear and mastoid. As a result, the diseased bone (ossicles and mastoid bone) must be removed to prevent recurrence of the cholesteatoma.

There are three types of mastoidectomy. A *simple mastoidectomy* is removal of the diseased bone of the mastoid with preservation of the ossicles, eardrum, and canal wall. This procedure is performed to eradicate chronic infections unresponsive to antibiotics or to remove cholesteatoma. A *modified radical mastoidectomy* is removal of the diseased bone of the mastoid along with some of the ossicles and the canal wall. The eardrum and some of the ossicles remain, leaving a mechanism for the patient to hear. A canal-wall-up mastoidectomy is similar to the modified mastoidectomy without removing the posterior ear canal wall. The benefit of a canal-wall-up mastoidectomy is that the patient's ear canal will appear and function normally. Canal-wall-down mastoid cavities require maintenance with removal of accumulated debris at least yearly.

A *radical mastoidectomy* is removal of the canal wall along with the ossicles and tympanic membrane. It is rarely performed except for unresectable disease. With either the modified radical or the radical mastoidectomy, a meatoplasty is performed to enlarge the ear canal opening. This facilitates cleaning the mastoid bowl that has been created.

Procedural Considerations

The surgical team preps and drapes the patient as for a tympanoplasty. An endaural or postauricular incision may be used, but most surgeons believe that the postauricular incision offers better exposure to all areas of the mastoid and middle ear. A drill is used to remove diseased bone and tissue. Facial nerve monitoring is used to alert the surgeon to the proximity of the nerve within the surgical field.

Operative Procedure

The operative procedure begins as described in steps 1 to 6 from the tympanoplasty procedure.

1. The surgeon uses a drill with a large cutting burr to drill the mastoid bone under direct vision. As the mastoid cavity is created, the scrub person should be able to anticipate changes needed in burr size. After the vital structures have been identified, diseased bone is removed by use of diamond burrs of the appropriate size. The surgeon may interrupt drilling to explore areas of the mastoid with a pick, curved needle or annulus elevator, or with other microinstruments to identify surrounding structures.
2. On completion of the mastoidectomy, the surgeon focuses on the middle ear. Diseased ossicles are removed, middle ear mucosa is inspected and removed if necessary, and all evidence of cholesteatoma is removed. Depending on the extent of the disease and the reliability that the patient will be available for follow-up care, the surgeon then reconstructs the ossicular chain or prepares the cavity created by a radical mastoidectomy. Some surgeons do not reconstruct at the time of mastoidectomy but reconstruct as a second-stage operation, which serves the added purpose of reexploring the middle ear and mastoid for residual or recurrent cholesteatoma.
3. The surgeon may pack the mastoid cavity and middle ear with an absorbable gelatin sponge or other bioresorbable material. The external auditory canal may be packed with bioresorbable material, an absorbable gelatin sponge, or antibiotic ointment.
4. The incision is closed and dressing applied in similar fashion to that used for postauricular tympanoplasty (as detailed previously).

Stapedotomy

Stapedotomy is removal of the stapes superstructure and creation of a fenestra (opening) in the fixed stapes footplate for treatment of otosclerosis and placement of a prosthesis to restore ossicular continuity and alleviate conductive hearing loss. Otosclerosis is the formation of abnormal bone around the stapes footplate, resulting in immobility of the footplate. Sound waves cannot be transmitted adequately through the oval window and round window to be changed into electrochemical impulses in the cochlea.

There are two types of procedures for replacing the immobile stapes. In *stapedotomy* the footplate of the stapes is not removed; only the superstructure is removed. A hole is made in the stapes footplate, and the prosthesis is secured laterally to the long process of the incus and positioned medially over the hole created in the footplate. A CO_2 laser may also be used for stapedotomy to create (drill) a hole in the footplate of the stapes for insertion of a prosthesis or to vaporize the stapedial tendon. Ideally, laser energy should be completely absorbed by the footplate and should not heat the perilymph or damage the inner ear (House and Cunningham, 2015). The laser stapedotomy offers improved postoperative hearing results while reducing postoperative dizziness and sensorineural hearing loss. An older procedure that is still used today, however, not as frequently as in years past, is the *stapedectomy*. In stapedectomy the entire stapes (superstructure and footplate) is removed, a graft is placed over the oval window, and a prosthesis is attached laterally to the long process of the incus and positioned medially on the graft over the oval window. Both of these procedures may be performed using MAC or local anesthesia for adults, enabling the surgeon to test hearing before the conclusion of the surgery. Certain patient populations, such as children and patients with anxiety, may find it difficult to remain immobile during the procedure, and general anesthesia is recommended in these populations to facilitate surgery and patient comfort.

Procedural Considerations

Various materials are used as the prosthesis for the stapes, and the most common are stainless steel, titanium, platinum, nitinol, and

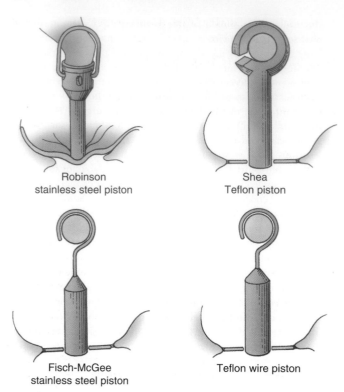

Robinson
stainless steel piston

Shea
Teflon piston

Fisch-McGee
stainless steel piston

Teflon wire piston

FIG. 19.18 Stapedectomy prostheses. *Top left,* Prostheses used after the footplate has been removed. *Top right and bottom,* Footplate had been "drilled" to accept a prefabricated piston precisely.

Teflon. The most common types are either bucket-handle or piston prostheses (Fig. 19.18). Both are secured to the incus and extend to the stapes footplate to reconstitute the ossicular chain. The use of stainless steel materials may present a risk for prosthesis displacement and subsequent sensorineural hearing loss if the patient undergoes MRI studies in the future.

The prosthesis of choice is determined by the surgeon's experience and preference. The scrub person must be aware of each step in the procedure and hand the instruments to the surgeon expediently. Because the oval window is left uncovered, some perilymph may leak from the inner ear into the middle ear. This leak subjects the patient to the possible complication of a sensorineural hearing loss postoperatively.

Microsuction tips (18–26 gauge) are used in this procedure because large suction tips may suction perilymph from the oval window, resulting in permanent hearing loss as well as promoting bleeding in the middle ear. After the incision and reflection of the flap, footplate hooks are used because the tips on picks are too large and long and may cause damage rather than assist in the procedure.

Operative Procedure: Stapedotomy

1. The surgeon or the assistant may harvest a temporalis fascia, fat, perichondrium, or vein graft at the start of the procedure to cover the oval window. Depending on the surgeon's graft preference, the ear, hand, or a portion of the abdomen may be prepped for the graft. Most surgeons use temporalis fascia or postauricular subcutaneous tissue because it is within the surgical field and easily accessible.

2. The ear speculum is introduced, and the microscope is appropriately positioned. The surgeon cleans any cerumen or debris from the ear canal and may gently wash the canal with physiologic irrigating solution.

3. The surgeon injects lidocaine with epinephrine into the ear canal.

4. An ear speculum is inserted, the tympanomeatal flap is created, and the tympanic membrane is reflected forward, exposing the middle ear.

5. If visualization of the ossicles is inadequate because of the overhang of bone, the surgeon may use microcurettes or a drill to remove enough bone to allow proper visualization. Attempts to save the chorda tympani nerve are made because it controls taste from the anterior two-thirds of the tongue. If this nerve obstructs the view of the stapes, it may on rare occasion be divided for exposure, and at the conclusion of the procedure the neural ends are reapproximated.

6. The surgeon may measure the distance from the incus to the stapes footplate at this time or after the removal of the stapes. It is accomplished with a depth gauge and done to ensure the proper fit of the prosthesis.

7. The incudostapedial joint is disarticulated to allow fracture and subsequent removal of the stapes, usually accomplished through the use of a joint knife or right-angled hook.

8. Both crura of the stapes are treated with a laser or fractured laterally, usually with a footplate pick or curved needle, and the superstructure is removed with alligator forceps. The surgeon may take this opportunity to ensure hemostasis, using tiny sponges soaked in epinephrine and applying suction with a microsuction tip. The laser helps coagulate middle ear vessels, improving hemostasis.

9. An opening is created in the footplate with a laser or a sharp footplate pick. If the footplate is extremely thick, a microdrill may be used. If a stapedectomy is to be performed, each half of the footplate is removed using a Hough hoe, footplate pick, or footplate hook.

10. The oval window is inspected to ensure that it is long enough, and then a measuring stick is used to approximate the correct size prosthesis required for reconstruction.

11. Holding the prosthesis with alligator forceps, the scrub person passes it to the surgeon. The prosthesis is introduced into the middle ear with the shaft resting against the oval window graft.

12. The wire is positioned over the long process of the incus using picks, Hough hoes, or footplate hooks. When the wire is in proper position, the surgeon crimps it onto the long process of the incus to ensure its attachment.

13. The surgeon may test the patient's hearing by softly whispering to the patient (if the procedure is performed with a local anesthetic) or by touching the malleus with a pick and observing for mobility of the malleus, incus, and stapes prosthesis (if performed with a general anesthetic).

14. Tiny pieces of the previously harvested graft tissue are then placed around the base of the prosthesis to ensure its stability. The surgeon uses alligator forceps, picks, a gimmick, and similar instruments to place the prosthesis.

15. The tympanomeatal flap is returned to its original location. The external ear canal may be packed with an antibiotic gel or ointment or a moistened, compressed gelatin sponge.

16. Cotton is placed in the concha of the ear, and an adhesive bandage or small dressing is usually applied to the graft site.

Ossicular Chain Reconstruction

Ossicular reconstruction may be required for long-standing recurrent ear infections. It is commonly performed for the replacement of the incus portion of the ossicular chain. There are many surgical techniques for ossicular reconstruction.

Natural and synthetic prosthetic materials are available for ossicular reconstruction or replacement. The autologous ossicle (incus or head of malleus) taken from the patient's ear is often used, particularly in children who do not have a cholesteatoma. A synthetic PORP or TORP is indicated for reconstitution of the ossicular chain.

Alloplastic materials for partial and total ossicular reconstruction prostheses are available. Hydroxyapatite is used in many prostheses because its mineral content is very similar to that of bone and it is well tolerated by the middle ear, decreasing extrusion rates. Because it is brittle, it is often combined with other materials to allow it to be more easily trimmed for a precise fit in the middle ear. Titanium is another material used frequently in middle ear prostheses. Titanium is ideal for ossicular reconstruction because of its properties of being rigid and lightweight. Regardless of the type of prosthesis used, the surgeon must sculpt or trim it to bridge the ossicular gap by simulating the ossicular configuration and preserving the lever mechanism of the middle ear.

Procedural Considerations

PORP refers to an ossiculoplasty with a strut from the head of the stapes to the tympanic membrane (or graft) or manubrium. TORP refers to a strut extending from the footplate to the tympanic membrane (or graft) or manubrium. The patient is prepped and draped as for stapedotomy or tympanoplasty.

Operative Procedure

The procedure steps are similar to those for stapedotomy, except that the stapes footplate is not removed or opened.

Labyrinthectomy

Labyrinthectomy is a procedure that eliminates the vestibular and auditory function of the labyrinth to relieve severe vertigo. The procedure is usually performed when the disease is unilateral, a shunt or decompression procedure has been ineffective, and the affected ear has severe or total loss of hearing. Because the inner ear is removed, the patient may be very dizzy for several days until the brainstem begins to compensate for the destroyed labyrinth. The operation also leaves the ear with no residual hearing.

Procedural Considerations

Labyrinthectomy is most commonly performed via the transmastoid approach. The patient is prepped and draped as described for the tympanoplasty or mastoidectomy procedure.

Operative Procedure

1. The surgeon creates a postauricular incision and performs a simple mastoidectomy.
2. The vertical segment of the facial nerve is identified, and the incus is disarticulated and removed.
3. Next, the surgeon drills and removes the horizontal, posterior, and superior semicircular canals. The neuroepithelium is completely removed from the ampullae of the three semicircular canals. The vestibule is exposed and the neuroepithelium from the utricle and saccule is removed.

4. The incision is closed in layers. An external pressure dressing of elastic gauze is applied.

Transmastoid, Translabyrinthine Approach

Procedural Considerations

The patient is prepped and draped as described for mastoidectomy. Preoperatively, ointments protect the eye and the eyelid is taped closed, or an adhesive bubble is placed over the eye to trap moisture. This protection is continued into the postoperative period unless a tarsorrhaphy (suturing the eyelid closed) is performed intraoperatively. Neurologic intensive care is required for the first 24 hours.

Operative Procedure

The operative procedure begins as described in steps 1 to 7 from the mastoidectomy procedure.

1. After completing the mastoidectomy, the surgeon continues the dissection using cutting and diamond burrs until the internal auditory canal and the posterior fossa bone are removed.
2. The bone immediately over the facial nerve is removed by the use of nerve excavators and picks.
3. Using a facial nerve knife, neurectomy knife, sickle knife, neurectomy scissors, or micropick, the surgeon incises the facial nerve sheath. The majority of surgeons do not incise the epineurium of the facial nerve, and decompression only is felt to be equally efficacious and less traumatic to the nerve itself.
4. The surgeon uses moistened, absorbable gelatin sponge; cottonoid patties; oxidized cellulose; bipolar ESU; or a combination of these to obtain hemostasis.
5. The incision is closed and a pressure dressing of elastic gauze applied.

Middle Cranial Fossa Approach

Procedural Considerations

The patient's hair is clipped almost to the midline on the affected side. Povidone-iodine solution generally is used for the prep, which includes the portion of the head that has been clipped, the affected side of the face, and the neck. The surgeon injects lidocaine with or without epinephrine subcutaneously above the ear to assist in hemostasis. The patient's eye on the affected side is protected as previously described.

Operative Procedure

1. The surgeon incises the temporalis muscle and elevates it with a Lempert, Shambaugh, or similar type of elevator.
2. Hemostasis is achieved by clamping and tying vessels or by electrocoagulation.
3. The surgeon drills a square of bone from the temporal bone to expose the middle cranial fossa dura. (The bone is saved for replacement at the end of the procedure.)
4. A self-retaining retractor with a blade for retraction of the middle fossa (e.g., Fisch middle fossa retractor, House-Urban retractor) is inserted.
5. After positioning the surgical microscope the surgeon elevates the dura from the floor of the middle fossa with a Freer elevator, a gimmick, or similar instruments.
6. When hemostasis is achieved and the blade is inserted over the dura to expose the middle fossa, drilling may proceed.
7. When the bone becomes quite thin, the surgeon may remove the remaining bone with excavators to avoid damaging the nerve sheath.

8. The facial nerve sheath can be incised with a facial nerve knife, neurectomy knife, neurectomy scissors, or microknife.
9. The retractor is removed when hemostasis is achieved, and the bone flap is replaced.
10. The temporalis muscle is approximated and sutured, the incision closed, and a pressure dressing applied.

Removal of Acoustic Neuroma (Vestibular Schwannoma)

Acoustic neuromas arise from the Schwann cells of the vestibular portion of the eighth cranial (acoustic) nerve and are therefore more appropriately termed *vestibular schwannomas*. These tumors are benign but may grow to a size that produces symptoms of cerebellar and brainstem origin. The majority of patients present with sporadic unilateral lesions and suffer from hearing loss and tinnitus, while approximately 5% develop bilateral vestibular schwannomas, which is the hallmark of neurofibromatosis type 2 (Sweeney et al., 2014).

Most patients experience unilateral tinnitus and hearing loss, which are the main symptoms of a possible acoustic neuroma. However, depending on the rate and direction of tumor growth, signs and symptoms may include hearing loss, tinnitus, vertigo, headaches, double vision, diplopia, decreased corneal reflex, decreased blink reflex, impaired taste, reduced lacrimation, facial paralysis, diminished gag reflex, vocal cord paralysis, atrophy or fasciculation of the tongue, weakness of the sternocleidomastoid and trapezius muscles, disturbance in balance and gait, hydrocephalus, lethargy, confusion, drowsiness, and coma.

Several surgery centers have developed great expertise in acoustic neuroma surgery, which requires the combined team of a neurologist and a neurosurgeon.

Procedural Considerations

The translabyrinthine approach for the removal of an acoustic tumor reduces mortality and morbidity and offers a good chance of saving the facial nerve if the tumor has not directly invaded it. The patient should be informed about the presence of a Foley catheter, arterial line, temperature probe, clipped hair, and graft-site incision. The patient's hair is clipped to the midline of the affected side. Some patients prefer to have the entire head clipped to facilitate wearing a wig. This option should be presented preoperatively to enable the patient to make a decision before surgery. The surgical team preps and drapes the patient as described for labyrinthectomy. The surgeon injects lidocaine (with or without epinephrine) subcutaneously behind the ear. A facial nerve monitor is routinely used in the excision of cerebellopontine angle tumors. An intermittent pneumatic compression device is used intraoperatively and for the first 24 to 48 hours postoperatively or until the patient is ambulatory to decrease the risk of DVT and PE.

Operative Procedure

1. The surgeon makes a postauricular incision slightly longer and more posterior than the incision for mastoidectomy and elevates the periosteum from the mastoid bone with a Lempert, Shambaugh, or similar type of elevator.
2. Self-retaining retractors are inserted, and the cortical mastoidectomy is begun with a large cutting burr.
3. The microscope is positioned, and the attic is opened to visualize the ossicles. The sigmoid sinus, middle fossa dura, and superior petrosal sinus are left in place with a thin covering of bone. The semicircular canals are exposed. The incus is removed with alligator forceps or cup forceps and suction.

4. The surgeon excises the semicircular canals with the drill. The utricle and saccule are removed, and the aqueduct of the vestibule is drilled out to expose the internal auditory canal 270 degrees circumferentially.
5. Using nerve excavators, Fisch dissectors, or picks, the surgeon removes the remainder of bone from the dura of the internal meatus, posterior fossa, middle fossa, and petrosal angle. The wedge of bone between the facial and superior vestibular nerves (Bill's bar) is removed.
6. The dura is opened with microscissors or a dura knife. The surgeon dissects the tumor with a gimmick, Freer microelevator, microinstrument, and bipolar forceps (with or without suction). Hemostasis is achieved with a moistened, absorbable gelatin sponge; cottonoid patties; oxidized cellulose; or the bipolar ESU.
7. The surgeon removes the tumor using pituitary cup forceps, long alligator forceps, and similar instruments.
8. Graft material (e.g., fat, fascia, or muscle) is obtained to pack the mastoid cavity created from the drilling. The packing is performed meticulously to avoid a cerebrospinal fluid (CSF) leak.
9. The surgeon closes the wound and applies a thick pressure dressing.

Assistive Hearing Devices

A variety of assistive devices are available to patients with hearing loss, including phone amplifiers, closed captioning broadcasts, Telecommunication Device for the Deaf (TDD), and electronic devices, such as hearing aids. Technology has evolved tremendously in the field of otology, enabling surgeons to use surgically implantable devices in the treatment of hearing loss. These devices have greatly benefited the recipients, allowing some to distinguish sounds for the first time. Research continues in this field to develop applications for conditions previously considered untreatable and to refine and improve existing technology.

Cochlear Implantation

Technologic advances have given the deaf patient new hope in the area of cochlear implantation. The device is implanted in the cochlea, with the receiver resting in the mastoid (Fig. 19.19). As the device receives sound through the receiver, it emits electrical impulses through the transmitter into the cochlea and along the acoustic nerve. These impulses are interpreted as sound in the auditory area of the brain, which is in the temporoparietal area of the cerebral cortex. The patient must be taught to interpret these sounds, which requires extensive training. A common speech-recognition test used to determine candidacy for a cochlear implant is the hearing in noise test (HINT), which tests speech recognition in the context of sentences. Pure-tone and speech audiometry tests are used to screen candidates. For individuals older than 2 years, the pure tone audiometry (PTA) for both ears should equal or exceed 70 decibels (dB). If the patient can detect speech with hearing aids in place, a speech-recognition test in a sound field of 55-dB HL sound pressure level (SPL) is performed. In children with prelingual deafness, cochlear implant candidacy is established when auditory skills fail to develop after amplification and aural rehab over a 3-month time period. Imaging with CT or MRI is performed before implantation to evaluate the inner ear, facial nerve, cochleovestibular nerve, brain, and brainstem. Results may alter the choice of side of implantation or raise other issues such as electrode selection (Lee, 2016).

Operative Procedure

1. A *modified postauricular incision is used*. The surgeon elevates the posterior flap, including the temporalis muscle, to expose the

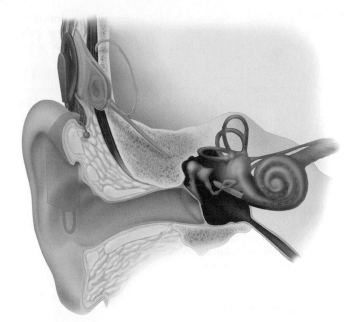

FIG. 19.19 Cochlear implant system. Sound is transformed into an electrical signal in a speech processor. The signal is transmitted from an external to internal induction coil, which is connected to an electrode implanted near the cochlear nerve.

underlying bone. The site of the internal receiver is identified, and the surgeon uses a special drill to create a circular depression in the squamous portion of the temporal bone to house the receiver.

2. A mastoidectomy is performed with preservation of the bony ear canal and opening of the facial recess.

3. The surgeon secures the internal receiver in the depressed area in the temporal bone, and introduces the intracochlear electrode through the facial recess via a cochleostomy into the cochlea. It is secured in place with a piece of temporalis fascia.

4. The wound is closed. The patient is observed for 2 to 4 weeks until the wound is completely healed. Then the external signal processor is fitted and programmed. This allows transmission of an electrical signal picked up at an ear-level microphone and processed in a microprocessor worn on the body.

Osseointegrated Bone-Anchored Hearing Implants

Conventional hearing aids transmit sound using air conduction and bone conduction. Traditional bone-conduction hearing aids are external and secured to the head with a spring device. Their design may make them uncomfortable and obtrusive, causing headaches and skin abrasions. The quality of sound is inferior, and they are associated with high battery consumption. Air-conduction devices use an earmold that fits into the ear canal. These devices may be contraindicated for patients with physical abnormalities that prevent the insertion of the earmold into the canal and for those who have chronic eczema, ear drainage, or inflammation in the ear canal. Osseointegrated bone-anchored hearing implants are designed for patients with moderate to severe conductive and sensorineural hearing loss (unilateral or bilateral). Ideally, implantable hearing devices should improve sound quality, provide comfort, improve appearance, and reduce the risk of chronic ear infections. Surgical implantation of hearing devices may be performed on an ambulatory basis using local or general anesthetics. The device is usually implanted in the ear with the best cochlear function.

Osseointegrated bone-anchored hearing implants (BAHA by Cochlear Limited, Sydney, Australia, and Ponto by Oticon Medical, Askim, Sweden) are considered a reliable and predictable adjunct for auditory rehabilitation in patients with chronic ear infections, microtia and congenital external auditory canal atresia, and single-sided deafness that cannot benefit from conventional hearing aids. The BAHA system consists of three components: a titanium implant, an external abutment, and an electronic sound processor. The device works by transmitting sound through bone to the inner ear bypassing both the external auditory canal and the middle ear. Surgical challenges faced by surgeons and patients include skin infection and/or overgrowth and proper surgical technique. Postoperative wound care plays an important role in the success of the procedure (Marfatia et al., 2016).

Rhinologic (Nasal) Procedures

Rhinologic surgery is performed to correct structural issues of the nose and to treat sinusitis and other conditions; it is also used as an adjunctive procedure to treat other disorders (e.g., pituitary neoplasms). Procedures that involve both internal and external nasal reconstruction can be done with local anesthetics, usually supplemented with IV sedation and analgesia. If the patient is particularly apprehensive or anxious, a general anesthetic may be more appropriate.

Treatment of Epistaxis

Patients with nasal bleeding usually control the problem themselves with direct pressure application. When their efforts fail, they seek help from their physician or an emergency department (ED). When more conservative measures (which involve vasoconstrictive agents and nasal packing) taken in the ED fail, surgical intervention becomes necessary.

When epistaxis occurs, the first step of treatment is to spray oxymetazoline nasal spray in both nares and apply direct pressure to the patient's nose. An initial hold of 15 minutes is recommended. Thereafter, inspection of the anterior nose and posterior oral pharynx should be performed to determine whether the site of bleeding is anteriorly based in the nose or posteriorly located deep in the nasal cavity. Evidence of a posterior bleed is usually demonstrated by a trickling flow of blood from the nasopharynx running down along the posterior pharyngeal wall during an oral inspection. Blood may also appear on the tongue and the patient may complain of swallowing blood. Anterior epistaxis characteristically trickles down the front of the face onto the upper lip. Anterior septum bleeds (in patients without coagulopathy), identified appropriately and timely, can often be easily controlled with silver nitrate sticks. If oxymetazoline spray and direct pressure fail to arrest the bleed, packing with nasal tampons or posterior packs should be considered. Various gelatin packing is available for selective patients. Brisk bleeding usually requires a nasal tampon or endoscopic surgical control, whereas slower oozing may be appropriately treated with oxymetazoline spray, direct pressure, and gelatin packing with close monitoring and follow-up.

The length of the pack should be based on the suspicion of where the bleed originates. Longer packing (8- or 10-cm packing) is considered when bleeds are more posterior in the nasopharynx. More anterior bleeds can be packed with 4.5-cm packing. Packing should be generously coated with antibiotic ointment and inserted in a horizontal angle following the floor of the nose. The packing is then sprayed with saline or oxymetazoline spray and expands. The patient should receive broad-spectrum antibiotics, such as oral third-generation

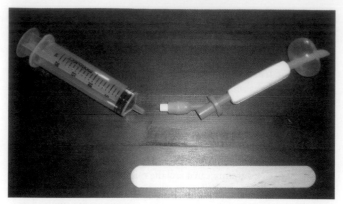

FIG. 19.20 Posterior nasal packing with syringe for balloon inflation.

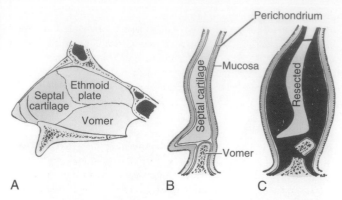

FIG. 19.21 (A) Primary components of septum. Incision line is for Killian-type submucous resection. (B) Septum with deviated cartilage and spur at junction of vomer and septal cartilage. (C) Resection of obstructive parts after careful elevation of the mucoperichondrium and mucoperiosteum.

cephalosporins, and is instructed to follow up in 2 to 3 days for removal of packing.

Balloon nasal packing has an exterior balloon along the tube length as well as an anchoring balloon on the end (Fig. 19.20). The anchoring balloon is first inflated, and then the pressure balloons are inflated to compress bleeding vessels. If commercial balloon sinus packing is not available, a Foley catheter may be used. A clamp can be placed on the Foley to prevent sliding back into the nasopharynx. Close attention to the ala must be observed to prevent alar necrosis. If this fails to stop the oozing and other hemostatic agents, such as gelatin-based packing, silver nitrate sticks, or oxidized cellulose, fail to halt the bleed, an endoscopic approach to control the epistaxis is warranted. The endoscopy is performed in the OR with the use of general anesthesia or conscious sedation. Occasionally ligation of the ethmoid, or internal maxillary artery, is necessary and should be considered for persistent bleeds. Embolization of the internal maxillary arteries may be considered as well. Endoscopic ligation of the sphenopalatine artery has been recently described and found to be useful in controlling persistent bleeds.

The setup for endoscopic control of epistaxis is the same as that for all nasal case prepping and draping. Using an endoscope, the surgeon focuses attention on the Kiesselbach plexus in the anterior nasal cavity and on the sphenopalatine artery because these are common sites of persistent bleeds. Suction ESU should be used to control any visual bleeding and to clear the nasal passages of clot or oozing. Other surgical options include transmaxillary artery ligation, internal maxillary artery ligation, anteroposterior ethmoid ligation, transnasal endoscopic sphenopalatine artery ligation, and submucosal supraperichondrial septoplasty and in extremely rare cases, ligation of the external carotid artery.

Nasoseptoplasty or Submucous Resection of the Septum

A nasoseptoplasty is straightening of either the cartilaginous or the osseous portions of the septum that lie between the flaps of the mucous membrane and the perichondrium. When the nasal septum is deformed, fractured, or injured, normal respiratory and nasal function may be impaired, interfering with airflow and sinus drainage. Deviations of the septum involving cartilage, bony parts (spurs), or both may block the meatus and compress the middle turbinate on that side, resulting in an obstruction of the sinus opening. Septal deviations tend to produce sinus disease and nasal polyps.

The objective of the procedure is to establish an adequate partition between the left and right nasal cavities, providing a clear airway through both the internal and external cavities of the nose.

Procedural Considerations

The procedure may be performed using local anesthesia, MAC, or general anesthesia. Regardless of the method chosen, the surgeon uses topical and injected anesthetics to aid in hemostasis. In most cases the surgeon wears a headlight to improve visualization of the intranasal structures.

Operative Procedure

1. The surgeon opens the nostril with a nasal speculum and incises through the mucoperichondrium of the septum with a #15 blade. Using a Freer elevator, the tissues are separated and elevated.
2. Deviated cartilage and bony, thickened structures are trimmed or removed with a septum punch and a nasal cutting forceps.
3. The surgeon trims the bony septal spurs with a punch forceps or chisel, gouge, and mallet. Suction is used to expose the field. Bleeding is controlled by insertion of additional cottonoid patties soaked with a topical hemostatic agent or by using an ESU.
4. The perpendicular plate of the ethmoid as well as the vomer may be removed by means of a suitable septum-cutting forceps (Fig. 19.21).
5. The incision is sutured with 4-0 absorbable atraumatic suture on a small, straight needle.
6. Plastic or Silastic nasal splints may be inserted to prevent adhesions and septal hematoma. Some surgeons use mattress sutures to provide a patent airway while maintaining support for the septum.
7. A mustache dressing (i.e., a piece of 2 × 2–inch gauze folded and placed below the nose and secured with tape across the face or bridge of the nose) is applied. A small ice bag (e.g., a surgical glove filled with ice) may be applied to the nose.

Closed Reduction of Nasal Fracture

The nose is the structure most susceptible to trauma because it is seated midface. The paired nasal bones are thin and project like a tent on the frontal process of the maxilla. If the trauma is caused by a direct frontal blow, usually both nasal bones are fractured, displaced outward, and depressed into the ethmoid sinus, and the septal cartilages become displaced. Noncontrast CT scans of the sinuses may be performed with protocols compatible with endoscopic navigation systems to provide an accurate sense of extension of deviation or possible injury to surrounding sinuses and structures.

Procedural Considerations

Simple nasal fractures often can be managed with topical and local anesthesia. However, as with most nasal procedures, if the patient is significantly anxious, general anesthesia may be necessary. Topical and local anesthetics are used with a general anesthetic to provide vasoconstriction and enhance visualization for the procedure. The surgical team preps and positions the patient for nasal surgery.

Operative Procedure

1. The surgeon packs the nose with cottonoid patties saturated with 4% cocaine. The local anesthetic is injected as previously described. When epinephrine is used, 10 minutes is the optimum time to wait for the effects of the hemostatic agent. This period of time will vary with other agents.
2. A Boies elevator is inserted into the nostril, and the nasal bones are elevated and molded into place by external manipulation (Fig. 19.22).
3. Nasal packing or a Denver splint may be used to stabilize the reduction because sometimes the bony fragments tend to return to a depressed status.

Sinus Surgery

Sinusitis can be either recurrent acute or chronic. It is caused by bacteria and fungi and may be associated with anatomic abnormalities of the nose, such as a deviated septum or poor drainage pathways from the sinuses. Medical management of acute bacterial sinusitis involves a course of appropriate antibiotic therapy for 10 days to 2 weeks. If a patient does not respond to medical treatment for acute bacterial sinusitis or if sinus complaints persist, surgical drainage of the sinuses is indicated. Traditionally open surgical treatments involved destructive procedures such as Caldwell-Luc, external ethmoidectomy and sphenoidectomy, and frontal sinus obliteration. Sinus procedures can be performed intranasally with or without the aid of endoscopes and video or through an open approach determined by which sinus cavity is involved. These procedures have been replaced by modern endoscopic sinus surgery. Noninvasive fungal sinusitis is treated by endoscopic removal. Invasive fungal sinusitis is frequently fatal and requires aggressive endoscopic debridement with a prolonged course of antifungals.

Functional Endoscopic Sinus Surgery

Functional endoscopic sinus surgery (FESS) provides a more purposeful approach to treat sinus disease. Procedures performed endoscopically decrease trauma to normal structures, reduce morbidity, and shorten the healing process for the patient. Endoscopic procedures offer an advantage over open procedures because of direct visualization of the tissue and anatomic structures. Dedicated endoscopic sinus and skull base suites present a popular option for FESS because of the ease of setup, use of multiple monitors, and rooms that free up floor space (Fig. 19.23).

FESS involves the endoscopic resection of inflammatory and anatomic defects of the sinuses while preserving natural function in a surgical procedure that is minimally invasive. Because of the anatomic relationship to the brain and orbit, this procedure has many risks, which should be incorporated into the informed consent process. FESS is considered to be a technically demanding surgery, and techniques vary significantly. Most surgeons prefer the endoscope to be attached to a video monitor, but some prefer to look directly through the eyepiece. The operative instruments are introduced into the nose alongside the endoscope.

If there is obstruction of outflow (e.g., allergy, septal deflection, spurs) between the mucosa and the sinus, mucociliary clearance is inhibited and secretions are retained in the sinus. This predisposes the patient to sinus infections and mucocele. The following sections are discussed with the understanding that they are more commonly performed endoscopically but may be done with an open approach as necessary. The purpose of FESS is to ensure adequate drainage of the sinuses by resecting tissue and creating increased aeration of the sinuses.

Procedural Considerations. FESS can be performed after induction of general anesthesia or MAC, depending on the surgeon's and the patient's preference. The setup for FESS is the same as the setup for any nasal surgery in terms of prepping, draping, and positioning. The instruments required are the basic nasal set, video equipment including monitor, and light source with the appropriate

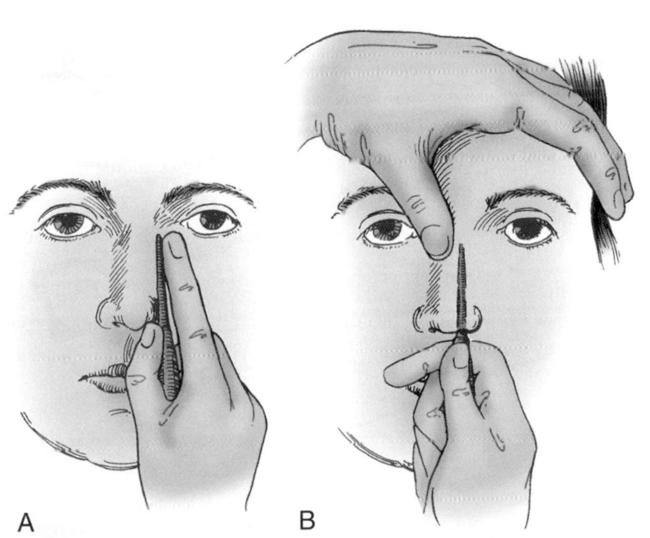

FIG. 19.22 Reduction of nasal fracture. (A) Boies elevator is placed along the lateral wall of the nose to a point below the nasofrontal angle. The distance to the ala is marked with the thumb. (B) The elevator is then placed under the depressed nasal bone, lifting it into position; the opposite thumb carefully exerts downward pressure on the elevated contralateral bone.

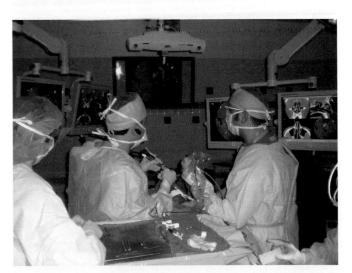

FIG. 19.23 Endoscopic suites demonstrating navigation systems and monitors.

light cord adapted to the type of endoscope used. The endoscopes used in sinus surgery are much like endoscopes used in other procedures. They are 4 to 5 mm in diameter and have different directions of view: 0, 30, 70, 90, or 120 degrees. Lenses are chosen based on the sinus to be operated on. Often if work is to be done in several sinus cavities, the surgeon may change lenses intraoperatively to obtain the optimal view in each cavity.

In addition to endoscopes, other instruments that may be used in FESS include endoscopic suction tips and suction elevators, biopsy forceps, forceps for retracting and cutting or excising tissue, and scissors. Patients undergo preoperative CT studies to determine the specific areas affected by the sinusitis. These CT scans should be available in the OR and will be referenced by the surgeon during the surgery (Fig. 19.24).

The video equipment is located at the head of the bed. The surgeon operates from the right side of the patient, the scrub person stands at the right of the surgeon, and the surgical assistant usually stands across from the surgeon on the opposite side of the table. More commonly the surgeon, the assistant, and the scrub person stand during the procedure. The rest of the surgical team can view the procedure on the video monitor.

Image-guided navigational systems are especially useful in revision sinus surgery, in which the familiar anatomy of the sinuses has been altered by previous surgery and the typical landmarks of the sinuses are now changed. From a safety standpoint and to reduce the risk of a revision surgery, many surgeons will not attempt a revision sinus procedure without having a navigational system available.

Several navigational systems are available, and many of these systems have applications for different types of surgeries, so the initial expense of the machine itself can be defrayed if it is shared with different surgical specialties, such as neurosurgery. Also technical components to facilitating this type of sinus surgery must be mastered by the perioperative nursing staff, who must develop competence in system setup, transfer of the CT scan data into the system, and perform maintenance procedures.

To avoid possible injury, the scrub person should pass instruments in the closed position and never over the patient's face. They should be passed smoothly and carefully so that the surgeon's eyes do not leave the endoscope or video monitor, limiting distractions. Some surgeons will request a suction-irrigation device that provides visualization of the sinus recesses by allowing simultaneous suction and irrigation of the operative field. Antifog solutions and endoscopic scrubbing devices are also used to improve visibility during the procedure.

Another consideration that is crucial to a successful outcome in FESS is to maintain the integrity of the patient's orbit. The patient's eyes must be visible to the surgeon at all times to avoid injury to the orbit or to immediately recognize injury if it occurs. The surgeon monitors for movement of the eyeball or appearance of an intraorbital hematoma.

Encroachment of the orbit can be recognized if yellow tissue is seen, because orbital fat is yellow. This finding should be communicated immediately to the surgeon. Another good technique is for the scrub person to place all tissue removed by the surgeon into a small labeled container of normal saline or lactated Ringer's solution on the surgical field. If any of the tissue floats, the surgeon should be notified immediately.

Balloon Sinuplasty

Balloon sinuplasty (Figs. 19.25 and 19.26) is an alternative surgical technique to FESS by which the paranasal sinus ostia are dilated open with a balloon catheter inserted over a guidewire or Lusk probe via direct visualization (video endoscopy) and then inflated into the ostia creating a patent ostium (Research Highlight). This procedure can only be performed on the frontal, maxillary, and sphenoid air cells. The ethmoid sinuses still need to be addressed by the endoscopic approach.

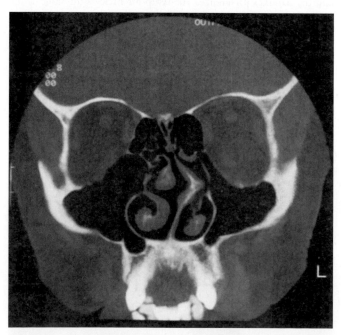

FIG. 19.24 Computed tomography scan of maxillary and ethmoid sinuses. Note septal deviation to the left, maxillary sinus ostia, turbinates, and ocular muscles.

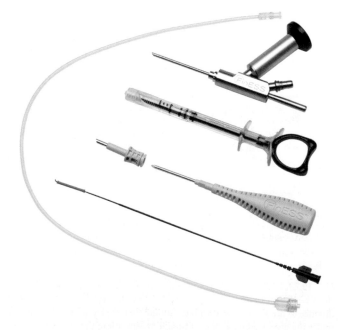

FIG. 19.25 Entellus procedure kit.

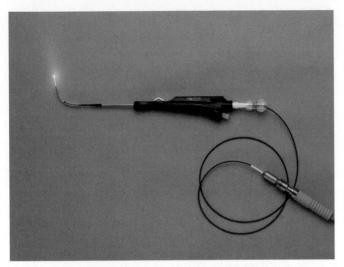

FIG. 19.26 Entellus express device with light fiber.

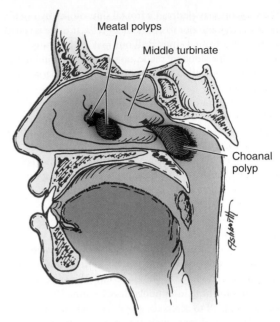

FIG. 19.27 Nasal polyps. A choanal polyp is usually single and originates in the maxillary sinus; however, most polyps are found in the middle meatus.

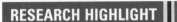

RESEARCH HIGHLIGHT

Balloon Sinuplasty and Chronic Sinusitis

The surgical management of sinusitis has been evolving over the last three decades. With the advent of the rigid nasal endoscope in the 1970s, surgeons worldwide favored functional endoscopic sinus surgery for the treatment of chronic sinusitis. This technique has become the standard of care. However, in 2004 balloon sinuplasty was introduced. This innovation was based on the principles of balloon angioplasty performed by cardiothoracic and vascular surgeons. The balloon sinus dilatational system required surgeons to pass a balloon catheter over a guidewire into a stenosed area in the sinuses and inflate a balloon, which in turns dilates the passage and restores natural sinus ventilation and drainage.

The principal aim of this study published in 2013 was to assess the efficacy and outcomes of balloon sinuplasty in a series of 20 patients with chronic sinusitis. These patients received follow-up over a period of 1 year. All patients in the study group had dramatic relief from their symptoms within the first postoperative week as reflected by the reduction in the Piccirillo's sino-nasal outcome test (SNOT) 20 scores. All patients were found to be symptom free during further follow-up as recorded by the low SNOT 20 scores. A larger study is required to establish the long-term outcomes of this technology.

Data from Raghunandhan S et al: Efficacy & outcomes of balloon sinuplasty in chronic rhinosinusitis: a prospective study, *Indian J Otolaryngol Head Neck Surg*, 65(S2):314–319, 2013.

Nasal Polypectomy

Nasal polyps are benign, grapelike clusters of mucous membrane and connective tissue lining the nose or sinuses. When the polyps become large, they obstruct the free passage of air, make breathing difficult, and cause a change in speech quality (Fig. 19.27). Endoscopic nasal polypectomies are often performed with other sinus procedures that also require removal of diseased tissue. Because of the aggressive nature of polyps, microdebriders are particularly helpful in these cases. They can greatly shorten surgical time by their mechanism of morcellating the polyp and removing it by immediate suctioning while controlling bleeding, as opposed to each polyp being manually extracted with an instrument in small pieces. Cases involving inverting papilloma (e.g., benign epithelial tumors that grow outward in finger-like projections in the nose) often recur and frequently require repeat polypectomies as symptoms recur.

Procedural Considerations. Nasal polypectomy setup is as for any intranasal procedure, with the addition of endoscopic equipment. Additional instruments may include a nasal polyp snare if a microdebrider is not used. Packing is typically not needed or used.

Operative Procedure

1. The surgeon applies topical anesthetic and administers the local anesthetic.
2. The lens of the endoscope is treated with antifog solution before the endoscope is introduced into the nose.
3. The surgeon enlarges the natural ostium of the maxillary sinus with a Lusk probe to provide physiologic drainage through the middle meatus. This creates a maxillary antrostomy and allows a larger drainage pathway into the ostiomeatal complex.
4. The diseased tissue is visualized through the endoscope, and the surgeon uses straight or angled true-cuts to remove it.
5. If an anterior ethmoidectomy is indicated, the surgeon inserts the endoscope into the ostiomeatal complex and performs the ethmoidectomy by taking small bites of the honeycombed bones with straight true-cuts and removing them manually or with suction. This reduces the many-celled ethmoid labyrinth into one large cavity to ensure adequate drainage and aeration.
6. A sphenoidotomy is created by biting an opening into one or both of the sphenoidal sinuses with a straight true-cut. It is usually performed only if sphenoid sinus disease is present on CT. Sphenoidotomies are often done with ethmoidectomies because once the ethmoid labyrinth is removed, the surgeon has excellent access through a lateralized middle turbinate exposing the sphenoidal sinuses.

7. The surgeon may perform a frontal sinusotomy by opening the frontal recess anterior to ethmoid air cells. If more severe disease is present, a frontal sinus drill-out may be indicated.

8. Because no incisions are made, no sutures are required. Epistaxis should be controlled endoscopically until it becomes a slow ooze.

9. Absorbable gelatin film or packing may be placed into the patient's middle meatus to maintain patency and reduce stenosis. If used, it is rolled into a cylindric splint and set in place with bayonet forceps. Some surgeons use nonabsorbable packing. An antibiotic ointment may be applied to the splint first, according to the surgeon's preference. The gelatin splints dissolve gradually, or they may be removed with irrigation.

10. A mustache dressing is applied.

Caldwell-Luc With Antrostomy

The purpose of an antrostomy is to establish a large opening into the wall of the inferior meatus, which ensures adequate gravity drainage and aeration. This large opening allows removal of the diseased tissues in the sinuses under direct vision. The Caldwell-Luc approach is also used to access the maxillary artery in cases of extreme epistaxis. The procedure requires an incision into the canine fossa of the upper jaw and exposure of the antrum for removal of bony diseased portions of the antral wall and contents of the sinus (Fig. 19.28).

Endoscopic Transnasal Repair of Cerebrospinal Fluid Leak

An abnormal communication between the subarachnoid space and nasal cavity results in CSF rhinorrhea. According to Janakiram and colleagues (2015), nearly 80% of CSF leaks occur as a result of accidental trauma. About 16% are iatrogenic and attributable to intracranial or sinonasal surgeries. Only 4% of leaks are spontaneous (nontraumatic) leaks.

Patients usually present with clear drainage from the nose. Laboratory analysis of the nasal discharge looking for CSF markers can confirm the diagnosis. Most traumatic cases resolve with bed rest; head elevation; and avoidance of coughing, sneezing, nose blowing, and so forth for 7 to 10 days. Persistent leaks and leaks identified during surgery require surgical management.

Oral Cavity/Laryngologic/Pharyngologic/Neck Procedures

Surgery of the Oral Cavity and Pharynx

The oral cavity is susceptible to both benign and malignant lesions, in part because of environmental risk factors. Oral malignancies can be linked to specific carcinogens, the most important being tobacco usage (without and in combination with heavy alcohol consumption). It is estimated by the American Cancer Society (ACS) that in 2016 about 48,380 people will be diagnosed with oral cavity or oropharyngeal cancer and 9,570 will die from these cancers. Incidence rates are more than twice as high in men as in women and are greatest in men who are older than 50 years. The recent rise in human papillomavirus (HPV)–linked cancer has risen dramatically over the past decades. HPV DNA is now found in about two out of three oropharyngeal cancers. The rising rate of HPV-related cancers is thought to be caused by changes in sexual practices, particularly an increase in oral sex (ACS, 2016).

Benign or malignant lesions of the tongue, floor of the mouth, alveolar ridge, buccal mucosa, or tonsillar area are excised depending on extensiveness of disease, involvement of surrounding vessels and nerves, and candidacy for surgery (Figs. 19.29 and 19.30). Benign or small malignant tumors of the oral cavity may be excised without a neck dissection, although in the presence of diagnosed or highly suspicious metastatic disease, a selective neck dissection may be performed in an effort to control a cancerous growth in the upper jugular lymphatic chain of the neck. Transoral robotic surgery (TORS) may offer an alternative approach in certain situations and may be associated with fewer complications than traditional procedures (Research Highlight) (Robotic-Assisted Surgery).

Before treatment of carcinoma of the floor of the mouth with involvement of the mandible, a CT scan or MRI of the face and neck should be obtained to evaluate extension of the disease. A portion of the tongue is resected and may require a combined operation with reconstructive surgeons. A tracheostomy, percutaneous endoscopic gastric tube, neck dissection, and composite resection

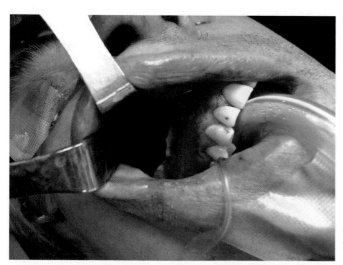

FIG. 19.28 Caldwell-Luc operation.

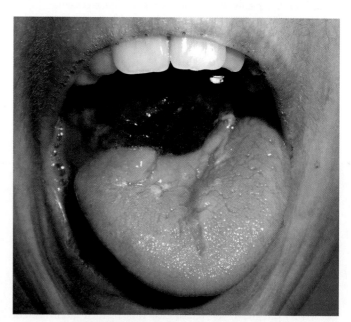

FIG. 19.29 Carcinoma of the dorsal tongue.

of both the mandible and the tongue with free flap reconstruction may be considered for extensive disease. When the primary intraoral lesion is confined to the tongue, a neck dissection and a hemiglossectomy are performed without resection of the mandible. In the presence of a lesion of the tonsil or an extensive lesion of the base of the tongue with pharyngeal wall involvement, resection of the mass may require removal of portions of the base of the tongue,

pharyngeal wall, and soft palate to secure an adequate margin of normal tissue around the lesion. In recent years nonsurgical management with chemoradiotherapy has advanced for select oropharyngeal tumors. A free flap may be considered to fill a soft tissue defect if one is created from surgical resection. Psychologic preparation of the patient is extremely important because these procedures may be done for a minor lesion in the oral cavity or may be the first stage of much more extensive surgery in the head and neck area. A supportive and accepting family is important to the patient because of the possibility of disfigurement after surgery.

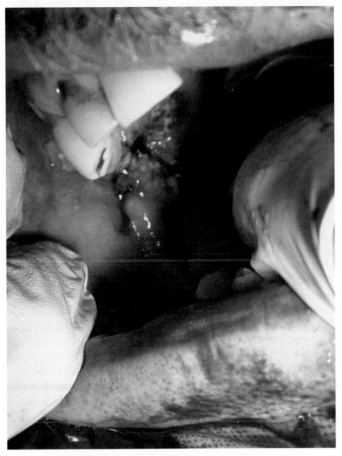

FIG. 19.30 Carcinoma of the right tonsil.

ROBOTIC-ASSISTED SURGERY

Transoral Robotic Surgery

Head and neck squamous cell carcinoma is the sixth most common malignancy in the world. Presenting symptoms include pain when swallowing, ear pain, bleeding, trismus (lockjaw), weight loss, night sweats, and weakness. The disease typically presents in the fifth decade of life or later; however, HPV-positive patients tend to present at a younger age. The main risk factors are tobacco use, alcohol, and HPV. TORS provides a mechanism to approach tumors of the upper aerodigestive tract through a natural body orifice, such as the mouth. The surgical robot is able to provide superior visualization and maneuverability compared with the traditional transoral approach. In otolaryngology this technique has been applied to malignant tumors of the oral cavity, thyroidectomies, tonsillectomy, and tongue cancer and tongue base surgeries. Positioning for robotic-assisted surgery is similar to positioning used for other otorhinolaryngologic procedures. After the patient is anesthetized, protective eye shields are placed over the patient's eyes. An instrument clamping arm is fastened to the side of the bed and attached to a Davis mouth gag that has been carefully placed into the patient's mouth. The robotic equipment is then positioned over the top of the patient's mouth or head. Additional information about robotic-assisted surgery is available in Chapter 8.

HPV, Human papillomavirus; *TORS,* transoral robotic surgery.
Modified from Helman SN et al: Transoral robotic surgery in oropharyngeal carcinoma, *Arch Pathol Lab Med* 139(11):1389–1397, 2015.

RESEARCH HIGHLIGHT

Complications After Transoral Robotic Surgery

TORS offers significant advantages over traditional open surgical approaches in oropharyngeal surgery. TORS is a minimally invasive approach with a magnified, three-dimensional view of the surgical field. TORS has been described for treatment of benign and malignant lesions of the oropharynx, hypopharynx, supraglottis, glottis, skull base, and parapharyngeal space. Researchers conducted a study to look at postoperative complications after TORS surgery. Complications found during their extensive study included patient death (from hemorrhage), hemorrhage, dehydration requiring readmission, aspiration pneumonia, airway obstruction, lingual nerve injury, hypoglossal nerve injury, tooth injury, fistula, and prolonged PEG tube dependency (>6 months). The most common complications were hemorrhage and tooth injury, followed by dehydration requiring

readmission and aspiration pneumonia. Arterial exposure is expected intraoperatively during TORS procedures and is typically controlled by clip application and electrocautery. Catastrophic postoperative hemorrhage is the most feared complication of TORS. It is important to protect the exposed carotid artery.

The most common indication for TORS in this particular study was oropharyngeal carcinoma, followed by obstructive sleep apnea as the second most common indication. The incidence of oropharyngeal carcinoma is rising because of HPV-associated squamous cell carcinoma. The overall complication rate after TORS in this study was 10.1%. Research completed by the authors of this study note that overall, reported complications of TORS are low, with sporadic reports of bleeding.

HPV, Human papilloma virus; *PEG,* percutaneous endoscopic gastrostomy; *TORS,* transoral robotic surgery.
Modified from Chia SH et al: Surgeon experience and complications with transoral robotic surgery (TORS), *Otolaryngol Head Neck Surg* 149(6):885–892, 2013.

Procedural Considerations

The patient is positioned supine with the shoulders elevated. Generally, endotracheal anesthesia is used, and a pharyngeal pack of moist gauze may be inserted in the mouth. Instruments and supplies vary, depending on the surgical intervention.

Operative Procedure

Although the procedure may be scheduled as a local excision, frequently lesions of the oral cavity require more extensive excision. The setup should be designed to include the instruments for a neck dissection, or they should be readily available. For some tumors of the oral cavity, a tracheostomy is performed to ensure a patent airway after surgery. A laser may be used to excise locally confined lesions of the oral cavity.

Salivary Gland Surgery

Disorders of the salivary glands typically fall into one of three categories: inflammatory, obstructive, and neoplastic. Benign and malignant tumors can occur in the salivary glands and usually present as a painless solitary neck mass. Diagnosis is made by imaging (e.g., ultrasonography, CT, MRI) and biopsy (initially with fine-needle aspiration). Overall, most salivary gland tumors are benign and can be treated with surgical excision. Bacterial inflammatory gland disorders typically affecting the parotid bacterial contamination from the oral cavity are thought to be the etiology. Predisposing factors include diabetes mellitus, hypothyroidism, and renal failure. Drainage of the abscess may be required. Mumps is the most common cause of viral disorders of the salivary gland. Vaccination, however, has reduced the incidence by 99% (Wilson et al., 2014). Neoplasms can be benign or malignant. Most are benign and slow-growing neck masses. These benign tumors, however, have a risk of malignant transformation and should be completely surgically excised. Malignant tumors are rare and are diagnosed after performing a biopsy. Perioperative nurses will facilitate surgical care for patients experiencing any of these conditions.

Excision of the Submandibular Gland

Excision of the submandibular gland is performed to remove mixed tumors and calculi associated with extensive chronic inflammation. An incision is made below and parallel to the mandible and extending to beneath the chin to remove the gland and tumor.

Procedural Considerations. The team positions the patient supine, with the affected side up. The instruments include a minor neck dissection setup. A set of lacrimal probes should also be added to the instrument setup if exploration of the submandibular (Wharton) duct is necessary during surgery. The perioperative nurse must ensure that no local anesthetic is delivered to the sterile field if identification of major nerves is anticipated. A nerve stimulator and bipolar ESU may be requested.

Operative Procedure

1. The surgeon makes a small skin incision below and parallel to the mandible, extending forward to beneath the chin (Fig. 19.31A). The platysma is incised with scissors; the skin flaps and undersurface of the platysma and cervical fascia covering the gland are undermined with fine hooks, tissue forceps, and Metzenbaum scissors (see Fig. 19.31B).
2. The mandibular branch of the facial nerve is retracted with a small loop retractor or nerve hook.
3. The surgeon elevates the submandibular gland from the mylohyoid muscle (see Fig. 19.31C). The edge of the muscle is retracted

anteriorly to expose the lingual veins and nerve and the hypoglossal nerve, which is identified and preserved.

4. The gland is freed by blunt dissection, and the submandibular duct is clamped, ligated, and divided with care to prevent injury to the lingual nerve.
5. The surgeon clamps, ligates, and divides the facial artery. The submandibular gland is removed (see Fig. 19.31D).
6. The wound is closed with interrupted absorbable sutures. The skin edges are approximated with nonabsorbable sutures. A drain is inserted into the submandibular bed and secured to the skin. Dressings are applied.

Parotidectomy

Parotidectomy may be performed to treat recurrent parotitis, but it is more commonly performed as part of the management of parotid gland tumors. In parotidectomy for tumor removal, the tumor and a portion of or the entire parotid gland is removed through a curved incision in the upper neck, in front of the earlobe, or through a Y-type incision on both sides of the ear and below the angle of the mandible. Even when a mass in the parotid gland is benign, the closeness of the facial nerve makes removing the entire mass surgically challenging (Fig. 19.32). The facial nerve exits the stylomastoid foramen, enters the substance of the salivary gland, and then bifurcates into the temporofacial and cervicofacial branches, variably communicating with the gland. These branches then further divide into the temporal, zygomatic, buccal, and marginal mandibular and cervical branches near the edge of the parotid. The gland is divided artificially into a *superficial* and a *deep* lobe according to its relationship to the facial nerve. The possibility of damaging the facial nerve (resulting in facial nerve weakness or paralysis) during the dissection of the gland should be considered carefully by all patients contemplating parotidectomy. Therefore the surgeon must understand that the most definitive way of avoiding damage to the facial nerve is to identify it early in the procedure. In addition, the patient should understand that a more radical procedure might be required if a malignant tumor is discovered to involve adjacent structures.

Procedural Considerations. The patient is positioned supine with the entire affected side of the face up. The entire side of the face, the mouth, the outer canthus of the eye, the ear, and the forehead are prepped and left exposed.

The instrument setup is a neck dissection set. The nurse ensures a nerve stimulator or nerve integrity monitor is available. A set of lacrimal probes should be included in the setup if exploration of the ductal system of the parotid is necessary during the course of surgery. Bipolar ESU may also be required.

Operative Procedure

1. The incision (Fig. 19.33) may extend from the posterior angle of the zygoma downward in front of the tragus of the ear and behind the lobule of the ear backward; the incision continues over the mastoid process and then downward and forward on the neck parallel to and below the body of the mandible (a chin incision also may be used). Bleeding vessels are controlled by hemostats and fine ligatures or with an ESU.
2. Using fine-toothed tissue forceps and scissors, the surgeon elevates the skin flaps as described for thyroidectomy (see Chapter 16) and retracts the flap with silk sutures fastened to clamps.
3. The surgeon exposes and retracts the upper portion of the sternocleidomastoid muscle. The auricular nerve is identified, and the lower part of the parotid gland is elevated with curved hemostats.

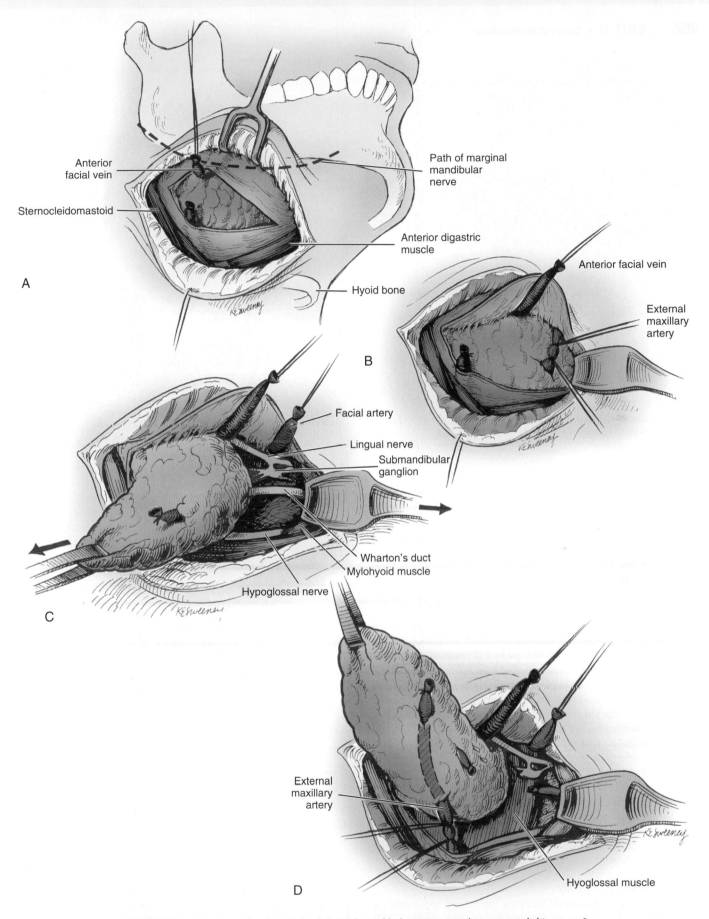

FIG. 19.31 Excision of submandibular gland. (A) Submandibular incision made in a natural skin crease 3 to 4 cm inferior to the mandible. The marginal mandibular nerve generally lies just superficial to the anterior facial vein. (B) The external maxillary artery is identified on the submandibular gland. (C) The mylohyoid muscle is retracted anteriorly and submandibular gland posteriorly. This exposes the lingual nerve, submandibular ganglion, and the Wharton duct. (D) The hypoglossal nerve, running between the hypoglossal and mylohyoid muscles. The external maxillary artery must be divided a second time.

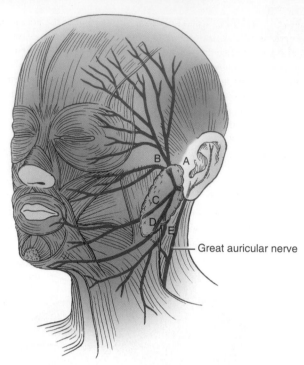

FIG. 19.32 Branches of facial nerve. *A,* Temporal; *B,* zygomatic; *C,* buccal; *D,* mandibular; *E,* cervical.

4. The superficial temporal artery and vein and external jugular vein are identified by means of blunt dissection. The surgeon dissects the parotid tissue from the cartilage of the ear and the tympanic plate of the temporal bone. The temporal, zygomatic, mandibular, and cervical branches of the facial nerve are identified and preserved.

5. The surgeon removes the diseased portion of the parotid gland, which can be superficial or deep.
   a. The *superficial portion* of the parotid gland containing the tumor is removed. In some cases the entire superficial portion is removed, followed by ligation and division of the parotid duct (Fig. 19.34).
   b. When the *deep portion* of the parotid gland must be removed, the facial nerve is gently retracted upward and outward and then the parotid tissue is removed from beneath the nerve. Kocher retractors are used to retract the mandible. The external carotid artery is identified. In many cases the internal maxillary and superficial temporal arteries are clamped, ligated, and divided.

6. The surgeon closes the wound in layers with absorbable suture. If a tissue defect is observed or anticipated overlying the resected portion of the parotid gland, abdominal fat may be harvested. A small drain is inserted, the skin is closed with fine nonabsorbable suture, and a pressure dressing may be applied depending on the surgeon's preference.

Uvulopalatopharyngoplasty

Uvulopalatopharyngoplasty (UPPP) is performed primarily to relieve obstructive sleep apnea (OSA) and snoring (Fig. 19.35). UPPP is not a substitution for the use of continuous positive airway pressure (CPAP), although the procedure may be considered when

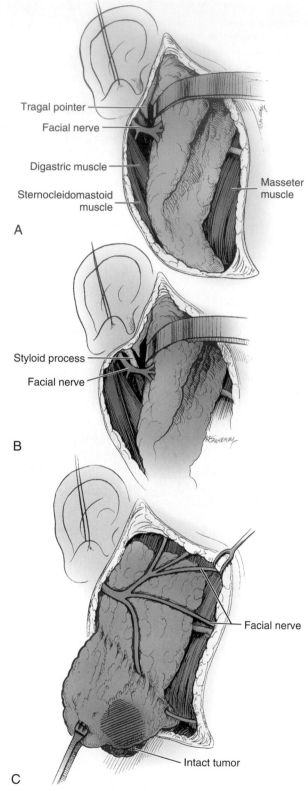

FIG. 19.33 Operative technique for parotidectomy. (A) Blunt dissection of parotid gland from the external auditory canal cartilage exposes the tragal pointer. The facial nerve lies approximately 1 cm deep and slightly antero-inferior to the pointer and 6 to 8 mm deep to the tympanomastoid suture line. (B) Facial nerve exits stylomastoid foramen to run anteriorly between the styloid process and attachment of digastric muscle to the digastric ridge. (C) Nearly completed process with tumor within intact superficial parotidectomy specimen.

conventional use of CPAP fails. Two or more of the following indications are reason to perform the operation:

- An O_2 saturation that drops below 80%
- Apnea index worse than 20
- Significant daytime sleepiness
- Heroic snoring (e.g., snoring that can be heard several rooms away), producing social or relationship problems
- Cardiac dysrhythmias, other than tachycardia or bradycardia, during sleep

Procedural Considerations. On occasion, tracheostomy may be performed with UPPP because of postoperative edema with subsequent risk of airway obstruction. The tracheostomy tube is removed and the incision is closed when the danger of postoperative edema and bleeding has passed. Because some of these patients are obese (causing the tissue of the pharynx to sag during sleep), preoperative planning should include obtaining an assortment of tracheostomy tubes, including extralong tubes, before the start of the procedure. Care must be taken in positioning the obese patient to ensure proper body alignment. Emergency tracheotomy or bronchoscopy should be anticipated in the event of airway obstruction after anesthesia induction. The surgeon may choose to administer a local anesthetic with the anesthesia provider monitoring the patient. The ease of intubation should have already been determined by this time, choosing the safest method of intubation (i.e., fiberoptic intubation, video laryngoscope). Once the method of intubation has been established and an airway is secured, a general anesthetic may be delivered. The team positions the patient supine with a shoulder roll to hyperextend the neck. If the tonsils are present, a tonsillectomy is performed

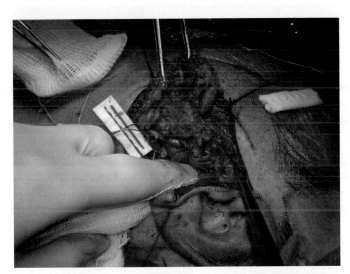

FIG. 19.34 Surgical removal of superficial parotid mass.

along with the UPPP. When inspecting the incision in the postoperative period, care should be taken not to disturb it with a tongue blade, if one is used to provide access for inspection. The patient must not use a straw for fluid intake because it might disturb the suture line. Gentle oral cavity rinsing is recommended several times daily to decrease the chance of postoperative infection and to increase patient comfort.

Operative Procedure

1. The surgeon inserts a McIvor mouth gag.
2. The surgeon may outline the tissue to be resected using an ESU blade. The incision may be completed with the ESU or with a #3 knife handle with a #15 blade or a #7 knife handle with a #12 blade. The incision is made in the soft palate and anteriorly to the tonsillar pillar (if the patient has not previously undergone a tonsillectomy) or posteriorly to the tonsillar pillars (if the patient has undergone a tonsillectomy) (Fig. 19.36).

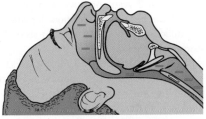

Patient predisposed to OSA

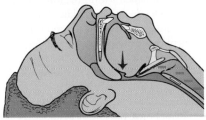

Apneic episode

FIG. 19.35 Sleep apnea syndrome is a condition in which airflow is temporarily obstructed during sleep. Airflow obstruction occurs when the tongue and the soft palate fall backward and partially or completely obstruct the pharynx. The obstruction may last from 10 seconds to as long as 2 minutes. During the apneic period the patient experiences severe hypoxemia (decreased PaO_2), hypercapnia (increased $PaCO_2$), and acidosis. These changes interrupt sleep and cause the patient to partially awaken. When the patient begins to awaken, the tone of the muscles of the upper airway increases. The tongue and soft palate move forward, and the airway opens. Apnea and arousals occur repeatedly during the night, separated by several normal breaths. The cause of sleep apnea is not definitely known. However, three factors appear to be involved: (1) shape of the upper airway, (2) neural control of the respiratory muscles, and (3) hormonal balance. *OSA,* Obstructive sleep apnea.

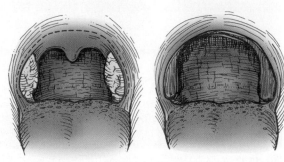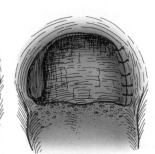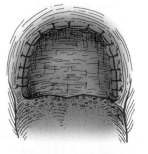

FIG. 19.36 Technique of palatopharyngoplasty as advocated by Simmons and associates.

3. Larger blood vessels may be clamped until the tissue is removed, or a suction coagulator or hand-controlled ESU handpiece may be used to obtain hemostasis as the tissue is excised.

4. After the tissue is removed and hemostasis is achieved, the surgeon uses absorbable sutures to approximate the edges of the mucosa. Depending on the surgeon's preference, 2-0 and 3-0 absorbable suture should be available. Needle holders should be long enough to allow the surgeon ease in delivering the atraumatic needle to the edges of the mucosa.

5. The surgeon irrigates the oral cavity and inspects the incision before the patient is transferred from the OR.

Tonsillectomy

Indications for tonsillectomy include sleep apnea and other obstructive breathing disorders, pharyngitis, chronic tonsillitis, and peritonsillar abscess. Tonsillectomy can relieve sleep apnea in 80% of patients (Gysin, 2013). When recurrent infections are documented in children (seven in 1 year, five in 2 years, or three in 3 years) some benefit from a tonsillectomy can be found. Indications for adult tonsillectomy include chronic infection, airway obstruction secondary to hypertrophy, and suspected neoplasms.

Pharyngeal obstruction is revealed by a history of sleep-disordered breathing. Mouth breathing, snoring, pauses in breathing, restless sleep, waking at night, and enuresis may be related to obstruction. Daytime somnolence and an inability to concentrate may also be indicators of poor sleep quality. Tonsil size is graded on a scale of 1 to 4, with 1 being contained within the tonsillar fossa, and 4 with the tonsils touching each other in the middle of the pharynx. Adenoids are not able to be visualized through the mouth, but symptoms of adenoid enlargement can include mouth breathing, nasal congestion, rhinorrhea, and hyponasal speech. Flexible nasolaryngoscopy and lateral neck radiography can aid in diagnosis of nasopharyngeal obstruction.

An additional reason for tonsillectomy would be a marked difference in size. Lymphoma on rare occasion may present in this fashion. Unusually enlarged tonsils in an immunosuppressed transplant recipient may also be indicative of posttransplant lymphoproliferative disorder.

Other indications include dysphagia from obstructing tonsils, halitosis from tonsilloliths, recurrent adenoiditis contributing to sinusitis, or otitis media.

Cold knife and snare technique with or without the ESU, and the harmonic ultrasound scalpel and bipolar radiofrequency ablation techniques may all be used for tonsillectomy. Both the harmonic ultrasonic scalpel and the bipolar radiofrequency wand cut and coagulate at the same time, resulting in very little blood loss. Hemostasis is achieved by the production of a protein plug in the end of the cut vessel from the ultrasonic or plasma energy of the devices.

Cold knife and snare is the oldest and most widely recognized method of tonsil removal. Bleeding must be controlled by other means such as electrocautery, vasoactive topical agents, packing, or placement of absorbable sutures.

The harmonic scalpel technique uses an ultrasonic generator that passes energy to a special titanium rod that vibrates at 55,000 times per second (Hz) for controlled vaporization of tissue. The ultrasonic energy forms protein plugs in the severed ends of blood vessels.

The bipolar radiofrequency technique can be used for both tonsillectomy and adenoidectomy. The technique vaporizes tissue and coagulates severed blood vessels. The wand in this unit contains both suction and bipolar ESU and is twice the diameter of the harmonic scalpel.

Procedural Considerations. The team positions the patient supine with the head hyperextended using a dropped headrest or a shoulder roll. The head must be secured on a donut-style headrest or on head pads. An oral ETT with a preformed bend, such as the Ring, Adair, Elwin (RAE), is used to facilitate visualization of the surgical field (Fig. 19.37). The neck is extended by placing a small roll under the shoulders. Typical draping includes a head drape and an impervious sheet over the patient; no prep is used. A tonsil instrumentation set is used. A harmonic scalpel setup and a radiofrequency ablation unit are required for their respective procedures.

Operative Procedure

Cold Knife and Snare Technique

1. The surgeon inserts a mouth gag retractor with a size-appropriate tongue blade, taking care to keep the tongue in the midline position with the ETT protected by the blade.

2. The posterior and lateral walls of the pharynx are carefully inspected and palpated to detect abnormally positioned vessels.

3. The tip of a 12F red rubber catheter is advanced through one of the nares, into the nasopharynx, and out through the mouth. The catheter is gently stretched, and the two ends are clamped snugly with a Kelly clamp near the upper lip to retract the soft palate forward.

4. Next, the surgeon places a throat pack in the posterior pharynx, ensuring it is easily retrievable at the end of the procedure.

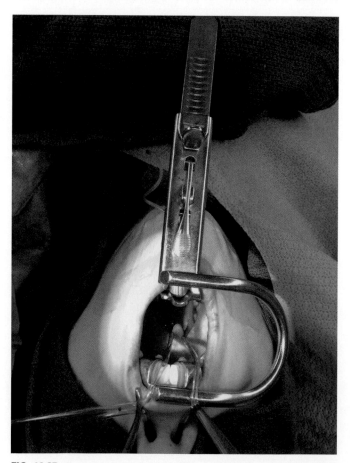

FIG. 19.37 Patient positioned for tonsillectomy with Davis mouth gag in place.

5. A tonsillar tenaculum is placed at the midpoint of the tonsil to apply medial traction on the tonsil, tenting the tonsil into the tonsillar fossae and oral cavity.

6. Using a curved tonsil knife, the surgeon makes an incision down to the palatoglossus muscle along the posterolateral aspect of the muscle in the plane of the muscle fibers and follows with blunt dissection starting from the superior portion of the tonsillar bed and working downward toward the lower one-third or inferior portion of the tonsillar bed.

7. A snare is applied over the tonsil, tightened, and then closed to bluntly dissect the tonsil from the tonsillar bed. The ESU is used along with sutures and packing to control bleeding.

8. At this point the mouth gag is released for a brief period, then reopened. The nasopharynx and oropharynx are reinspected to ensure that there is no further bleeding from vessels that may have been compressed by the opened mouth gag.

9. The oropharynx may be irrigated with 50 to 60 mL of normal saline solution to evaluate for additional signs of bleeding. The ETT cuff should be inflated, or the anesthesia provider should maintain positive pressure inflation during the irrigation to prevent inadvertent passage of the irrigation into the trachea.

10. The red rubber catheter is removed. The throat pack is removed. The mouth gag retractor is carefully removed from the oral cavity to prevent inadvertent extubation of the patient.

11. Dentition, temporomandibular joint mobility, and perioral skin are reinspected for inadvertent surgical complications.

Harmonic Scalpel Technique

1. Steps 1 to 5 from the cold knife and snare technique are performed.

2. The surgeon uses the blunt, curved back portion of the tip with extremely light downward pressure to dissect the tonsil from the bed, moving inferiorly or superiorly, depending on how easily the tonsil releases.

3. After the tonsil is completely released from the bed, the surgeon reapplies the tenaculum to facilitate removal of the tonsil from the palatopharyngeus muscle of the posterior pillar.

4. The surgeon controls any residual bleeding by placing the flat portion of the dissection tip against the bleeding site and gently tamponading the bleeding. Small amounts of capillary bleeding also can be controlled by lightly moving the activated tip over the bleeding site until the bleeding stops or a light char appears.

5. The tonsillar beds are painted with sucralfate liquid, and the self-retaining retractor is released to check for residual bleeding. The posterior throat pack is removed and the posterior pharynx is then thoroughly suctioned, if necessary.

Radiofrequency Tonsillectomy

1. Steps 1 to 5 from the cold knife and snare technique are performed.

2. The surgeon uses the tip of the wand to carefully dissect the anterior portion of the tonsil away from the surrounding muscle.

3. The surgeon controls any residual bleeding with the ESU portion of the device.

4. The tonsillar beds are painted with sucralfate liquid, and the self-retaining retractor is released to check for residual bleeding. The posterior throat pack is removed and the posterior pharynx is then thoroughly suctioned, if necessary.

Adenoidectomy

Children with polysomnogram-proven sleep disorder breathing and hypertrophic adenoids should have their adenoids assessed as a complete workup. Obstructive upper airways from hypertrophic adenoids can be easily evaluated using flexible nasopharyngoscopy by an otolaryngologist. Surgical removal of hypertrophic adenoids to relieve upper airway obstruction is often performed to create a patent nasal airway. Adenoidectomy by curette, ablation, radiofrequency, and powered microdebriders has been described in the pediatric otolaryngology literature. Hemostasis is achieved depending on the method chosen, by electrocautery, radiofrequency, or direct pressure (using angled mirrors or endoscopic visualization).

Laryngeal Surgery

Laryngeal surgery may be performed for diagnostic reasons or as a means of treatment for benign as well as malignant conditions (Fig. 19.38). This type of surgery involves both endoscopic and traditional "open" approaches and always has the potential to alter the patient's ability to communicate verbally in the postoperative period. As is the case with oral cavity malignancies, cancerous lesions within the laryngeal structures are often attributed to environmental factors, such as tobacco and alcohol use. Benign conditions, such as vocal cord polyps and nodules, are often treated with laryngeal surgery (Fig. 19.39).

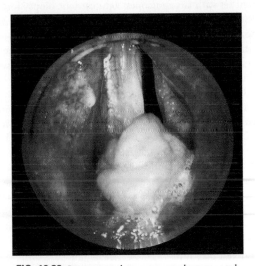

FIG. 19.38 Large granular tumor on the true cord.

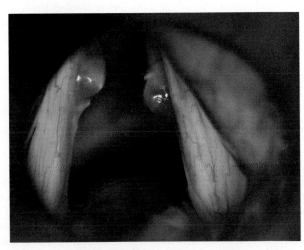

FIG. 19.39 Bilateral vocal cord polyps.

Endoscopic Procedures

Laryngoscopy. Laryngoscopy is direct visual examination of the interior of the larynx by means of a rigid, lighted speculum known as a *laryngoscope* to obtain a specimen of tissue or secretions for pathologic examination. Vocal cord visualization also may be accomplished in the office setting with a flexible fiberoptic nasopharyngolaryngoscope.

Procedural Considerations. Most rigid laryngoscopies are performed with the patient receiving a general anesthetic. If the patient is unable to tolerate general anesthesia, a local or topical anesthetic of lidocaine, tetracaine, cocaine, or benzocaine-tetracaine is administered. The patient should be sufficiently relaxed by reassurance and by pharmacologic preparation if the procedure is performed using local anesthesia. Sedatives may be administered before surgery. Immediate preoperative assessment should include the presence of any dental appliances and loose teeth and the condition of dental work. Any stiffness or immobility of the neck or shoulders should be evaluated. Respiratory problems such as asthma must receive careful attention. The patient should be cautioned about not eating or drinking after surgery until the gag reflex has returned and swallowing occurs without difficulty. The nurse or scrub person prepares a local anesthesia setup for the surgeon. An operative laryngoscope instrument set with laryngoscopes, light carriers, biopsy forceps, and telescopes is used.

If the surgeon wishes to perform a suspension laryngoscopy, a self-retaining laryngoscope holder is added to the instrument table, as well as microlaryngeal instruments, which include scissors, cup forceps, and alligator forceps. A special platform may be mounted onto the OR bed, or a Mayo stand may be placed above the patient's chest and over the OR bed to provide a place for the laryngoscope holder to rest. The surgeon normally uses the operating microscope with a 400-mm lens during suspension laryngoscopy. The team positions the patient supine to facilitate visualization of the vocal cords. A shoulder roll should be available if slight hyperextension of the neck is necessary to assist in visualization of the larynx. Laryngoscopy instrumentation should remain set up in the room until the patient is transferred because the equipment may be needed if the patient experiences laryngospasm postoperatively and requires intubation.

Operative Procedure

1. The anesthesia provider places moist gauze pads or tape over the patient's eyes to protect them from the instrumentation and to prevent injury and irritation from secretions during the procedure. The head may also be wrapped in a sterile towel. A sterile drape may be used to cover the patient. A tooth guard or moistened soft goods is placed to protect the patient's teeth.
2. The surgeon introduces the spatula end of the laryngoscope into the right side of the patient's mouth and directs it toward the midline; then the dorsum of the tongue is elevated so that the epiglottis is exposed.
3. The surgeon tips the patient's head backward, then lifts it upward as the laryngoscope is advanced into the larynx.
4. The larynx is examined, a biopsy is taken, secretions are aspirated, and bleeding is controlled.

Microlaryngoscopy. Microlaryngoscopy facilitates improved diagnosis and allows the surgeon to view with relative ease areas that previously were inaccessible or difficult to visualize. It may also be used for minor surgery of the larynx, especially for the removal of polyps or nodules on the vocal cords. (Intralaryngeal surgery using the laryngoscope is often referred to as *phonosurgery.*) Instrumentation may vary according to surgeon preference.

Procedural Considerations. If the procedure is done to remove polyps or nodules from the vocal cords, the patient must be cautioned to observe complete voice rest postoperatively. The patient should be provided with a pencil and paper or erasable board to aid in communication. The patient's restriction on speaking should be noted on the nursing plan of care and on the front of the chart.

The basic instrument setup for laryngoscopy is used. Microlaryngeal instruments and a self-retaining laryngoscope holder are added to the setup. The microlaryngeal instruments are 22 cm long to allow use with the microscope, and are long enough to keep the surgeon's hands out of the visual field. The patient's head is adjusted to allow visualization of the larynx. The surgeon usually adjusts the microscope. The microscope lens should have a 400-mm focal length. Focal length is the distance from the lens to the operative area and is the point at which the field can be clearly viewed through the microscope. Beyond this point the field becomes blurry. The 400-mm lens gives the surgeon a 40-cm focal length, or working distance.

Carbon Dioxide Laser Surgery of the Larynx. Surgeons often use the CO_2 laser to treat lesions of the larynx and vocal cords. This laser is efficient and has a high power output. The beam destroys tissue at a precise point with minimal destruction of the surrounding tissue. It is especially useful in surgeries such as removal of webs in the larynx, vocal cord papillomas, and carcinoma in situ of the larynx, as well as benign endobronchial lesions.

Procedural Considerations. The basic setup for laryngoscopy and microlaryngoscopy is used. All instrumentation used for laser laryngoscopy should be ebonized. A general anesthetic is usually administered. The operating microscope with a 400-mm lens is used, with the laser micromanipulator attached to the microscope head. The beam should also be tested for proper working order before use on the patient. Extreme care should be used when handling this delicate piece of equipment. A smoke evacuator should be used to remove the laser plume (a smokelike steam rising from the impact site); high-filtration laser masks should be worn by personnel. Where minimal plume is generated, central wall suction with an in-line filter may be used for plume evacuation (AORN, 2016a). All other laser precautions apply (see Chapter 8).

Adjunctive Procedures. Although the following procedures do not technically involve the larynx, they are often performed by otorhinolaryngologists in conjunction with laryngeal surgery and are of particular use in the diagnostic arena.

Bronchoscopy. The trachea, bronchi, and lungs are visualized directly with a rigid or flexible bronchoscope that has a fiberoptic lighting system. A rigid scope gives a larger viewing area, whereas a flexible scope is easily inserted into the patient and manipulated. (Bronchoscopy is fully described in Chapter 23.) The Nd:YAG laser may be used for lesions of the trachea or bronchi, depending on the type of lesion. Most diagnostic bronchoscopies are performed using topical anesthetics and moderate sedation, requiring careful patient monitoring by the perioperative nurse.

Esophagoscopy. Esophagoscopy is the direct visualization of the esophagus and the inner stomach organ. This procedure is used to observe the area for extension of tumor, to remove tissue and secretions for study, or to evaluate for second primary tumor sites.

Procedural Considerations. Esophagoscopy facilitates the diagnosis of esophageal carcinoma, diverticula, hiatal hernia, stricture, benign stenosis, and varices. Patients with suspected obstruction, symptoms of bleeding, or regurgitation may require endoscopy. The Nd:YAG laser may be used to treat some of these lesions. Esophagoscopy may also be used for therapeutic manipulations, such as removal of a foreign body or insertion of an esophageal bougie to treat esophageal stenosis. A set of rigid esophagoscopes, light carriers, biopsy forceps, and bougies is used.

Operative Procedure

1. The scrub person inserts the fiberoptic light carrier into the esophagoscope and attaches the fiberoptic light cord. A thin layer of lubricant is applied to the scope. The surgeon passes the scope into the mouth. The tongue, epiglottis, laryngeal inlet, and cricopharyngeal lumen are identified. If necessary, a person holding the patient's head may be required to tip the head backward while extending the neck anteriorly. Usually the esophagoscope is passed to the right side of the tongue, and the patient's head is turned slightly to the left.

2. When the scope has passed the inferior constrictor muscles, the patient's head is moved in various directions so that all areas of the esophageal wall may be examined.

3. Specimens of secretions from the esophageal lumen may be obtained with an aspirating tube and suctioning apparatus. In some cases saline may be injected through the esophagoscope's aspirating channel and the fluid withdrawn immediately for histologic study. A tissue biopsy may be taken. After biopsy the area is assessed for bleeding and the esophagoscope is then removed.

Triple Endoscopy (Panendoscopy). When laryngoscopy, bronchoscopy, and esophagoscopy are performed in a single session on a patient, the procedure is termed *triple endoscopy* or *panendoscopy*. The order in which the procedures are performed depends on the surgeon's preference. The purpose of triple endoscopy is usually diagnostic. While inspecting for a malignancy, the surgeon views the structures, takes specimens for biopsy, and possibly makes smears or washings of the suspect areas. For any of the previously mentioned endoscopic procedures, all equipment or instrumentation should be set up and be in working order (i.e., light carriers in place; light cables connected and working). Instrumentation to be used through the various scopes (i.e., suction tips, telescopes, and biopsy forceps) should be checked for appropriate length. Specimens taken during endoscopic procedures should be labeled and removed from the back table as soon as possible. In some instances it may be helpful to indicate on the label that the specimens are microscopic.

Open Neck and Laryngeal Procedures

Tracheostomy. Tracheostomy is the opening of the trachea and the insertion of a cannula through a midline incision in the neck, below the cricoid cartilage. A tracheostomy may be permanent or temporary. It is used as an emergency procedure to treat upper respiratory tract obstruction, which can be caused by bilateral vocal cord paralysis, swelling of the neck or airway caused by trauma, allergic reactions, or neoplasms. It is also used as a prophylactic measure in the presence of chronic lung disease, in extensive neck resections when massive upper airway edema is anticipated, or if radiation-induced edema is expected during the treatment of cancers involving the tongue and neck. Tracheostomy is also considered the gold standard for treating sleep apnea in which obstruction may occur. Tracheostomy may be performed to permit easy and frequent pulmonary toileting on patients having a difficult time managing and expectorating their own secretions. Additionally, tracheostomy should be performed on patients experiencing prolonged intubation to avoid overgrowth of granulation tissue and subsequent subglottic stenosis.

The nurse carefully evaluates the patient's psychologic status because of the altered body image, which may be temporary or permanent depending on the disease entity involved. Tracheostomy care should be explained carefully and thoroughly so that the patient will understand why self-care should be performed frequently. Reinforcement should be given regarding the ability to communicate with others by means of a pencil and paper or message board. As recovery progresses and secretions diminish, the patient can be shown how to occlude the opening of the tube for brief periods to be able to speak a few words. The patient also must be taught the mastery of tracheostomy self-care. If a tracheostomy tube with a disposable inner cannula is inserted, the nursing staff must ensure that the patient has replacement cannulae in the event occlusion or blockage occurs in the immediate postoperative period.

Procedural Considerations. Before tracheostomy tubes are inserted, the cuffs should be tested for air leaks by inflating and then deflating the balloon. Cuffed tracheostomy tubes are used on patients at risk for aspiration, patients receiving positive-pressure ventilation, or patients who have undergone skull base surgeries involving open communication of the sinuses into the intracranium, where it is desirable to avoid pneumocephalus. The patient is placed in a supine position, with the shoulders raised by a small rolled sheet to slightly hyperextend the neck and head. Using a skin marker, the surgeon marks a midline incision site halfway between the sternal notch and the cricoid cartilage, between the second and third tracheal rings. The neck is prepped and sterile drapes are applied. A soft suction catheter should be available on the sterile field for suctioning after the tube is inserted. An additional tracheostomy tube of the same size and the obturator should be kept with the patient at all times, in the event the tube becomes dislodged or plugged with secretions. This practice expedites changing the tracheostomy tube with minimal potential for complications to the patient.

Operative Procedure

1. The surgeon injects lidocaine with epinephrine into the subcutaneous tissue across the tracheotomy site previously marked with a surgical marker.

2. A horizontal incision is made with a #10, #15, or #11 blade. Soft tissues and muscle are divided, using blunt hemostats and sharp dissection through the platysma and the overlying strap muscles. The thyroid gland is identified; attention is directed to the isthmus with the intention of transecting this area of the gland. Occasionally the isthmus can be retracted from the surgical site without transection (Fig. 19.40).

3. The plane between the isthmus and the trachea is separated by the surgeon with a blunt hemostat, exposing the thyroid gland so the surgical assistant can carefully transect it with the ESU blade. This exposes the underlying tracheal rings (usually the second and third). In some cases two curved clamps may be inserted through this incision across the isthmus, and then the isthmus is transected.

4. The transected ends of the isthmus are oversewn or suture-ligated with absorbable sutures.

5. After identifying the trachea, the surgeon makes a horizontal incision with a #11 blade through the second and third tracheal rings. The incision is extended and the tracheostomy tube is inserted.

6. Two 2-0 silk sutures are then sewn into the trachea for future use during the first tracheostomy change. In two motions, one silk suture is inserted into the trachea, and then retrieved with the needle driver through the horizontal incision. This is then repeated with another silk suture through the bottom half of the horizontal incision.

7. Air knots (e.g., knots that are not snugged against the skin) are tied into each of the sutures and secured with tape onto the chest so they are ready for easy retrieval for retraction during the first

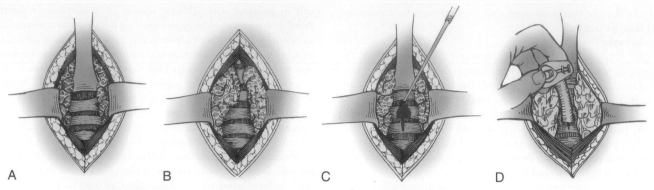

FIG. 19.40 Operative technique for elective tracheostomy. (A) Retractor exposing trachea by drawing the isthmus of the thyroid upward. (B) Alternative method to that shown in (A). Isthmus of thyroid is divided to expose the trachea. (C) Two tracheal rings are cut, and upper ring is partially resected. Tracheal hook pulls trachea from depth of wound nearer surface. (D) Insertion of tube.

tracheostomy change, about 5 to 7 days later. By tradition, one air knot is placed in the upper stay suture and two air knots are placed in the lower stay suture to allow for easy identification and proper retraction at the time of tracheostomy tube change or in the event of tracheostomy tube dislodgement. The air knots are cut and removed once the first tracheostomy change takes place.

Laryngofissure. Laryngofissure is an opening of the larynx for exploratory, excisional, or reconstructive procedures that cannot be accomplished endoscopically.

Procedural Considerations. A laryngofissure may be performed when access to the intrinsic larynx is necessary. The thyroid cartilages are split in the midline, and the true vocal cords and false vocal cords are incised at the midline anteriorly. A neck dissection instrument set is required, plus an oscillating power saw. A tracheotomy is performed as the first step of the procedure, and the tracheostomy tube is left in place postoperatively to ensure a patent airway.

Operative Procedure

1. The surgeon makes a transverse incision through the skin and first layer of the cervical fascia and platysma muscles, approximately 2 cm above the sternoclavicular junction or in the normal skin crease. The upper skin flap is undermined to the level of the cricoid cartilage, and the lower flap is undermined to the sternoclavicular joint.
2. Bleeding vessels are clamped with mosquito hemostats and ligated. The strap muscles are elevated and incised in the midline.
3. The surgeon cuts the thyroid cartilages with an oscillating saw, and visualizes the true vocal cords through an incision into the cricothyroid membrane. The true vocal cords are divided in the midline (anterior commissure), and the interior of the larynx is exposed.

Partial Laryngectomy. Partial laryngectomy is removal of a portion of the larynx. It is performed to remove superficial neoplasms that are confined to one vocal cord or to remove a tumor extending up into the ventricle or the anterior commissure or a short distance below the cord. A cancer confined to the intrinsic larynx is generally a low-grade malignancy and tends to remain localized for long periods. The patient should be prepared for an altered voice quality postoperatively as well as for the possibility of total laryngectomy if the tumor proves too extensive for partial resection. Types of partial laryngectomies include a vertical hemilaryngectomy, supraglottic laryngectomy, and supracricoid laryngectomy. With surgical excision

of the tumor along with postoperative administration of chemotherapy concurrently with external beam radiation therapy, it is possible to preserve some laryngeal function. The goal of partial laryngectomy is to avoid removing the entire larynx and to preserve the patient's natural swallowing ability. A successful partial laryngectomy should leave the patient with the ability to phonate, although usually with a more hoarse voice. The otolaryngologist must carefully stage the laryngeal cancer via a panendoscopy with biopsy and determine the overall candidacy of the patient who may receive a partial laryngectomy. If tumor extension does not warrant a partial laryngectomy, a total laryngectomy must be performed. Steps and procedural considerations for a total laryngectomy are described next.

Total Laryngectomy. Total laryngectomy is the complete removal of the cartilaginous larynx, the hyoid bone, and the strap muscles connected to the larynx and possible removal of the preepiglottic space with the lesion. A wide-field laryngectomy is done when there is a loss of mobility of the cords and to treat cancer of the extrinsic larynx and hypopharynx (Fig. 19.41). Malignant tumors of the extrinsic larynx are more anaplastic and tend to metastasize. When laryngeal carcinoma involves more than the true cords, a prophylactic (preventive) modified, or selective, neck dissection is done to remove the lymphatics. Depending on the extent and severity of disease in the neck, a radical neck dissection may be warranted, although it is rarely routinely performed.

Laryngectomy presents many psychologic problems. The loss of voice that follows total laryngectomy is traumatic for the patient, family, and caregiver. The patient may be taught to talk by using either an esophageal voice or an artificial larynx. The esophageal voice is produced by the air contained in the esophagus rather than by that in the trachea. Speech requires a sounding air column. With instruction and practice, the patient is able to control the swallowing of air into the esophagus and the reintroduction of this air into the mouth with phonation. The sounding air column is then transformed into speech by means of the lips, tongue, and teeth. A tracheoesophageal fistula facilitates insertion of a tracheoesophageal prosthesis or valve for the purpose of speech. This fistula may be created during the initial surgical procedure (primary tracheoesophageal puncture [TEP]) or at a later date when healing has occurred. Because the stump of the trachea is exteriorized to the skin of the neck to form a permanent stoma, all the patient's breathing is done directly into the trachea and no longer through the nose and mouth. The nose no longer moistens this air. Drying and crusting of the tracheal

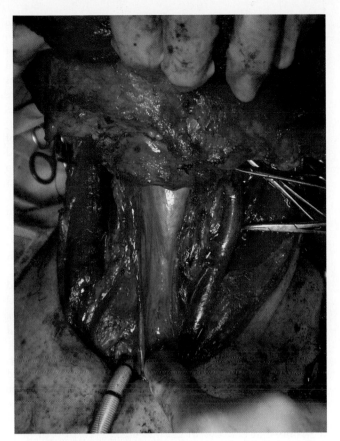

FIG. 19.41 Wide-field defect after removal of the larynx.

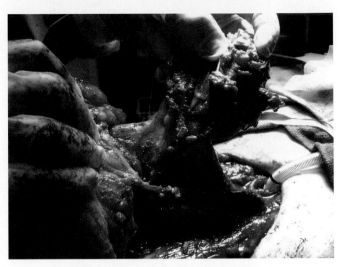

FIG. 19.42 Removal of the larynx en bloc.

secretions occur. Humidification may be provided with a humidified tracheostomy collar or a humidified moisture exchange system later during the healing process. The patient will be anxious to know about postoperative voice quality, which depends on the specific procedure performed.

Procedural Considerations. The team positions the patient supine with the neck extended and shoulders elevated by a shoulder roll or folded sheet. A general anesthetic is administered. Airway considerations are paramount when approaching a patient with laryngeal cancer. An awake tracheostomy may be performed initially to control the airway, and occasionally patients have previously placed tracheostomy tubes. If the tracheostomy is performed initially or is preexisting, the use of a cuffed, wire-reinforced, flexible ETT will ensure effective delivery of the anesthetic and give the surgical team flexibility as the larynx and trachea are manipulated during the surgical procedure. An effective suction apparatus is essential. The proposed operative site, including the anterior neck region, the lateral surfaces of the neck down to the outer aspects of the shoulders, and the upper anterior chest region, is prepped and draped in the usual manner. The instrument setup is a neck dissection set.

Operative Procedure

1. The surgeon makes a midline incision from the suprasternal notch to just above the hyoid bone. Skin flaps are undermined on each side. The sternothyroid, sternohyoid, and omohyoid muscles (strap muscles) on each side are divided by means of curved hemostats and a knife.
2. The suprahyoid muscles are severed from the portion of the hyoid to be divided. The hyoid bone is skeletonized with care

to preserve the hypoglossal nerves. Bleeding vessels are clamped and ligated.

3. The surgeon exposes and ligates the superior laryngeal nerve and vessels on each side with long, curved fine hemostats and fine ligatures.
4. Next, the isthmus of the thyroid gland is divided between hemostats. Each portion of the thyroid gland is dissected from the trachea with Metzenbaum scissors and fine tissue forceps. The superior pole of the thyroid is retracted. The superior thyroid vessels are freed from the larynx by sharp dissection. Sometimes one or both lobes of the thyroid gland are included in the resection for oncologic purposes.
5. The surgeon rotates the larynx. The inferior pharyngeal constrictor muscle is severed from its attachment to the thyroid cartilage on each side.
6. The ETT is removed. The trachea is transected with care to keep an adequate margin from the tumor. The upper resected portion of the trachea and the cricoid cartilage are held upward with Lahey forceps. A balloon-cuffed, wire-reinforced ETT is inserted into the distal portion of the trachea.
7. The surgeon frees the larynx from the cervical esophagus and attachments by sharp and blunt dissection. A moist pack is placed around the ETT to help prevent leakage of blood into the trachea.
8. The pharynx is entered. In most cancers of the intrinsic larynx, the pharynx is entered above the epiglottis. The surgeon extends the mucous membrane incision along either side of the epiglottis; the remaining portion of the pharynx and cervical esophagus is dissected well away from the tumor by means of fine-toothed tissue forceps, Metzenbaum scissors, knife, and fine hemostats. The specimen is removed en bloc (Fig. 19.42).
9. The surgeon inserts a nasal feeding tube through one naris into the esophagus; closure of the hypopharyngeal and esophageal defect is begun with continuous inverting fine 3-0 absorbable suture. The nasal tube is guided down past the pharyngeal suture line.
10. The pharyngeal suture line is reinforced with running horizontal or vertical mattress Vicryl sutures; the suprahyoid muscles are approximated to the cut edges of the inferior constrictor muscles.
11. The surgeon uses a knife and heavy scissors to increase the diameter of the tracheal stoma. The two portions of the thyroid

behind the tracheal opening are approximated with interrupted nonabsorbable sutures, obliterating dead space posterior to the upper portion of the trachea.

12. Using a blade, the surgeon makes a small puncture wound through the neck, lateral to the incision, using the tips of a hemostat inserted on the inner wound bed as a guide.

13. The hemostat is then stabbed into the puncture wound, grasping the distal drain tubing and pulling it through until the fluted portion of the drain is visible in the wound bed. The drain is trimmed and measured to fit into the wound.

14. The drain is secured to the skin just lateral to where the puncture wound was made, and an air knot is tied using square knots.

15. The surgeon closes the edges of the deep cervical fascia and the platysma separately.

16. Next, the surgeon inserts a laryngectomy tube into the tracheal stoma. A pressure dressing may be applied to the wound and neck, although some surgeons prefer leaving the wound without dressings to observe the skin flaps.

Radical Neck Dissection. In a radical neck dissection, the tumor, all soft tissue from the inferior aspect of the mandible to the midline of the neck to the clavicle end posterior to the trapezius muscle, and lymph nodes are removed en bloc from the affected side of the neck. This procedure is done to remove the tumor and metastatic cervical nodes present in malignant lesions as well as all nonvital structures of the neck. Metastasis occurs through the lymphatic channels by way of the bloodstream. Diseases of the oral cavity, lips, and thyroid gland may spread slowly to the neck. Radical neck surgery is done in the presence of cervical node metastasis from a cancer of the head and neck that has a reasonable chance of being controlled. Sentinel node biopsy may also be performed in conjunction with a neck dissection.

A prophylactic neck dissection implies an elective neck dissection when there is no clinical evidence of metastatic cancer in the cervical lymph nodes.

Procedural Considerations. The team positions the patient supine. General endotracheal anesthesia is induced before the patient is positioned for surgery. A shoulder roll may be placed to slightly hyperextend the neck, with the head slightly turned to the contralateral side. The head of the bed may be slightly elevated to reduce venous bleeding.

During the procedure the anesthesia provider works behind a sterile barrier at the patient's unaffected side. The preoperative skin prep is extensive, including the neck, lower face, and upper chest. The patient's neck is draped to leave a wide operative field. On occasion, local muscle flaps are harvested to cover and protect the carotid artery (as when a patient has received extensive previous radiation therapy). If this is the case, the thigh area is also prepped and draped with sterile towels in readiness for obtaining a dermal graft before closure of the neck wound. It is usually more convenient to use the thigh on the same side as the neck dissection. Patient, family, and caregiver education includes tracheostomy care (if applicable), pain management, care of the surgical incision, reportable signs and symptoms, healthful behaviors, and review of physical therapy exercises.

Operative Procedure

1. The surgeon may use one of several different incisions, including the Y-shaped, H-shaped, or trifurcate incision (Fig. 19.43), all of which aim for complete lymphadenectomy while preserving good, viable skin flaps.

2. The upper curved incision is made through the skin and platysma with a knife, tissue forceps, and fine hemostats; ligatures are

used for bleeding vessels. A monopolar ESU may be used to control skin edge bleeding.

3. The upper flap is retracted, then the vertical portion of the incision is made, and the skin flaps are retracted anteriorly and posteriorly with retractors. The anterior margin of the trapezius muscle is exposed by means of curved scissors. The flaps are retracted to expose the entire lateral aspect of the neck. Branches of the jugular veins are clamped, ligated, and divided.

4. The surgeon clamps the sternal and clavicular attachments of the sternocleidomastoid muscle with curved Péan forceps and then divides them with a knife. The superficial layer of deep fascia is incised. The omohyoid muscle is severed between clamps just above its scapular attachment.

5. Using sharp and blunt dissection, the surgeon opens the carotid sheath. The internal jugular vein is isolated by blunt dissection and then doubly clamped, doubly ligated with medium silk, and divided with Metzenbaum scissors. A transfixion suture is placed on the lower end of the vein.

6. Next, the common carotid artery and vagus nerve are identified and protected. The fatty areolar tissue and fascia are dissected and removed using Metzenbaum scissors and fine tissue forceps. Branches of the thyrocervical artery are clamped, divided, and ligated.

7. The surgeon dissects the tissues and fascia of the posterior triangle, beginning at the anterior margin of the trapezius muscle and continuing near the brachial plexus and the levator scapulae and scalene muscles. During the dissection branches of the cervical and suprascapular arteries are clamped, ligated, and divided.

8. The anterior portion of the block dissection is completed. The omohyoid muscle is severed at its attachment to the hyoid bone. Bleeding is controlled. All hemostats are removed, and the operative site may be covered with warm, moist laparotomy packs.

9. The surgeon severs and retracts the sternocleidomastoid muscle. The submental space is dissected free of fatty areolar tissue and lymph nodes, from above downward.

10. The deep fascia on the lower edge of the mandible is incised; the facial vessels are divided and ligated.

11. The submandibular triangle is entered. The submandibular duct is divided and ligated. The submandibular glands with surrounding fatty areolar tissue and lymph nodes are dissected toward the digastric muscle. The facial branch of the external carotid artery is divided. Portions of the digastric and stylohyoid muscles are severed from their attachments to the hyoid bone and on the mastoid. The upper end of the internal jugular vein is elevated and divided. The surgical specimen is removed.

12. The entire field is examined for bleeding, then irrigated with warm saline solution. If necessary, a skin graft may be placed to cover the bifurcation of the carotid artery, extending down approximately 4 inches, and sutured with 4-0 absorbable suture on a very small cutting needle.

13. Closed-wound suction drains are placed into the wound.

14. The surgeon approximates the flaps with interrupted fine nonabsorbable sutures or with skin staples. A bulky pressure dressing may be applied to the neck, depending on the surgeon's preference.

Modified Radical Neck Dissection. Modified radical neck dissection (Fig. 19.44) includes the en bloc removal of all node-bearing tissue in the anterior and posterior cervical triangles, the tail of the parotid gland, and cervical sensory nerves with sparing of the following

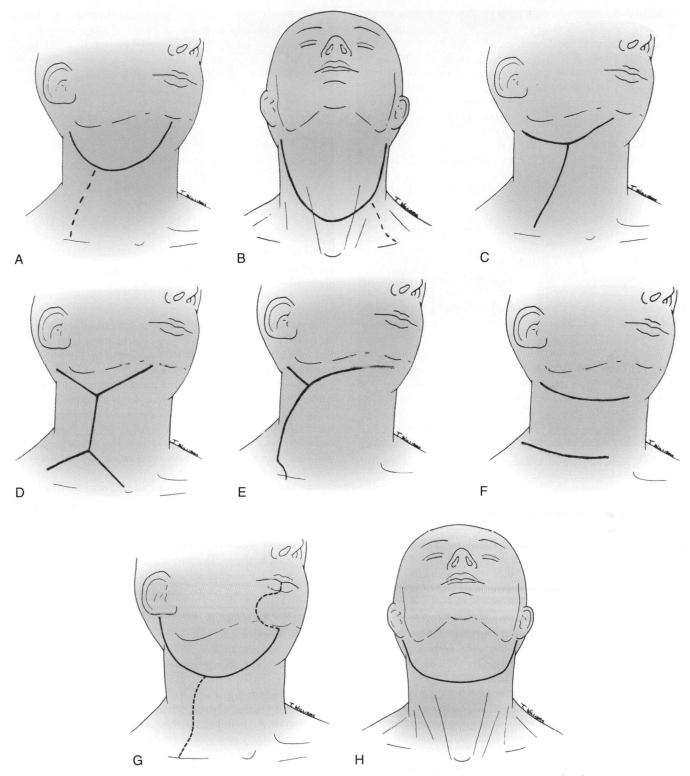

FIG. 19.43 Dissection incisions. (A) Latyshevsky and Freund. (B) Freund. (C) Crile. (D) Martin. (E) Babcock and Conley. (F) McFee. (G) Incision used for unilateral supraomohyoid neck dissection. (H) Incision used for bilateral supraomohyoid neck dissection.

structures: the sternocleidomastoid muscle, internal jugular vein, and eleventh cranial nerve. Depending on the extent of the cervical neck disease diagnosed by physical examination along with supportive imaging exams, a modified radical neck dissection is procedurally idealized first by the surgeon unless late-stage malignancy requires

a more extensive neck dissection, such as a radical. The goal of a modified neck dissection is to preserve as much of the normal anatomic structures of the neck as possible and remove only diseased neck content, tumor-invaded structures, and lymph nodes. Performing an appropriate neck dissection results in minimal morbidity to the

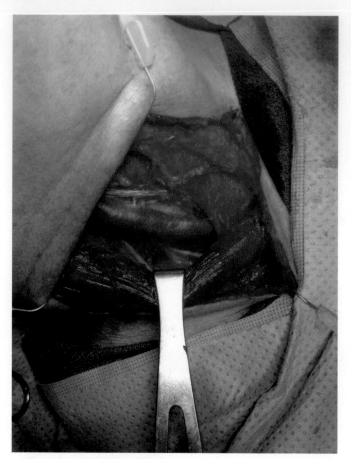

FIG. 19.44 Right modified neck dissection with retraction of the right sternocleidomastoid muscle exposing cranial nerves and jugular vein.

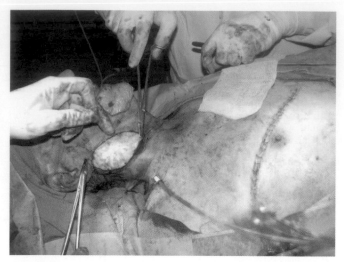

FIG. 19.45 Right pectoralis flap with two chest drains and one right neck drain.

patient, provides invaluable data to accurately stage the patient, and guides the need for further therapy.

Procedural Considerations. This modified type of neck dissection facilitates removal of a tumor and lymph nodes suspected of metastases and allows the patient a minimal defect and minimally impaired shoulder function. With radical and modified neck dissection, the surgeon and medical and radiation oncologists may decide on a course of postoperative radiation therapy or chemotherapy. The decision depends on the type and location of tumor, stage of disease, and patient's condition. Patients undergoing neck dissection are usually admitted overnight for observation of swelling, bleeding, or hematoma. A neck hemorrhage is an airway emergency and needs immediate attention.

Reconstructive Procedures. Depending on the surgical defect, head and neck surgical procedures to remove malignant tumors may also involve reconstructive procedures. The wound may be closed primarily, or local flaps and split-thickness skin grafts (as for facial and intraoral defects) or full-thickness skin grafts (as for nasal and facial defects) may be used. Split-thickness skin grafts and full-thickness skin grafts are ideal for small surgical defects.

Surgical flaps for the head and neck are chosen to fill surgical defects by their ability to survive in poorly vascularized areas. The surgeon chooses the surgical flap option (e.g., regional rotational, pedicled, or free microvascular) that provides the best aesthetic result for the patient based on location of the surgical defect, size of the defect, and vascular condition and whether bone, such as the fibula, needs to be harvested because of invasive disease.

Regional flaps, classified as either myocutaneous or fasciocutaneous, are typically rotated locally to fill large defects in the head and neck. Pectoralis major flaps raised on the long axis of the pectoral branch of the thoracoacromial artery are known for reliability, versatility, and strength (Fig. 19.45). A deltopectoral flap is usually used to fill cutaneous defects of the head and neck and is a pedicled flap based on the second and third perforating branches of the internal mammary artery. The latissimus dorsi flap is a pedicled flap or a free tissue transfer flap receiving its blood supply from the thoracodorsal artery, which arises from the subscapular axis, which can be used to fill large defects of the head and neck.

Free or microvascular flaps represent another reconstructive option for otorhinolaryngologic surgery. Perioperative nurses must incorporate the factors of increased surgical and anesthesia time (approximately 8–12 hours), positioning needs, and advanced equipment needs when planning care for the patient undergoing a free flap procedure. When the tissue is removed for the free flap, veins and arteries are microscopically connected, nerve grafts may be used, and bone must be connected with the use of plates and screws. The Doppler unit is also used intraoperatively and postoperatively to detect occlusions or spasms of the vessels.

The temporal arterial system provides a favorable donor site for head and neck reconstruction (Lam and Carlson, 2014). Temporoparietal fascial (TPF) flaps are popular among reconstructive surgeons in the oral and maxillofacial region. These flaps are versatile in the way that they encompass muscle, fascia, skin, and bone. According to Lam and Carlson (2014), advantages for using the TPF flap include minimal donor site morbidity, ease of harvesting, and versatility in flap defects. Complications include flap necrosis and alopecia long the incision line. Endoscopically assisted flap harvesting can minimize the risk of alopecia.

The radial forearm flap, based off the radial artery and accompanying paired venae comitantes, is the most commonly used free flap for oropharyngeal and osteocutaneous reconstruction, such as the reconstruction of defects of the floor of the mouth with or without partial or total tongue involvement (Fig. 19.46). If needed, radial bone may be harvested along with the skin paddle and fascia. It is important to note that all patients receive a preoperative Allen test.

The anterolateral thigh free flap (Fig. 19.47) is most often supplied by perforating vessels arising from the descending branch of the

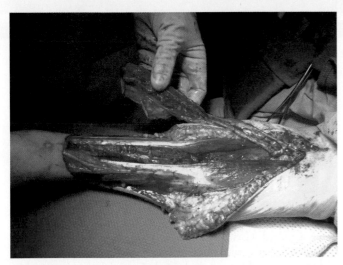

FIG. 19.46 Harvest of radial forearm osteocutaneous flap for repair of the mandible.

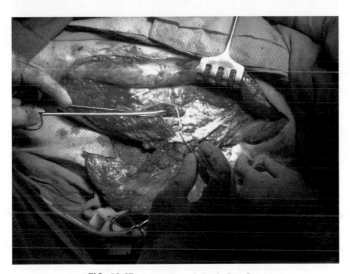

FIG. 19.47 Anterolateral thigh free flap.

lateral circumflex artery. Its potential bulkiness is deemed advantageous and can be harvested as a subcutaneous, fasciocutaneous, myocutaneous, or adipofascial flap, increasing its versatility. Fibula free flaps are commonly used in otolaryngology when tumor, osteonecrosis, or infection erodes or invades the mandible and reconstruction requires bone harvest.

Key Points

- The specialty of otorhinolaryngology focuses on disorders of the ear, nose, and throat.
- Patients undergoing otorhinolaryngologic surgery are considered a communication-vulnerable population because of possible deficits in hearing and phonation.
- Maintenance of the patient's airway is critical in many otorhinolaryngologic procedures.
- Perioperative nurses must be familiar with otorhinolaryngologic anatomy and a variety of surgical procedures and techniques to provide effective care to this patient population.
- Technology continues to evolve in this specialty, with new indications and experience with robotic-assisted surgery and other advancements in endoscopic techniques.

Critical Thinking Question

Mrs. B. is a 64-year-old smoker who arrived to the ED via a private vehicle with difficulty breathing. Mrs. B. had her fourth radiation treatment earlier in the day for an aggressive laryngeal tumor. The OR team responds to the page to assist the otolaryngologic surgeon on call. The patient is emergently brought up to the OR with signs of stridor, tachypnea, decreasing O_2 saturation, and increasing blood pressure and heart rate. What should the circulating nurse and scrub person anticipate needing to best assist the surgeon during this critical time?

⊖volve *The answer to the Critical Thinking Question can be found at http://evolve.elsevier.com/Rothrock/Alexander.*

References

American Cancer Society (ACS): *What are the key statistics about oral cavity and oropharyngeal cancers?* (website), 2016. www.cancer.org/cancer/oralcavityandoropharyngealcancer/detailedguide/oral-cavity-and-oropharyngeal-cancer-key-statistics. (Accessed 25 November 2016).

Association of periOperative Registered Nurses (AORN): Guideline for minimally invasive surgery. In *Guidelines for perioperative practice*, Denver, 2016a, The Association.

Association of periOperative Registered Nurses (AORN): Guideline for patient information management. In *Guidelines for perioperative practice*, Denver, 2016b, The Association.

Association of periOperative Registered Nurses (AORN): Guideline specimen management. In *Guidelines for perioperative practice*, Denver, 2016c, The Association.

Cassorla L, Woo-Lee J: Patient positioning and associated risks. In Miller RD et al, editors: *Miller's anesthesia*, ed 8, Philadelphia, 2015, Saunders.

Dedman MN et al: Development of a temporal bone model for transcanal endoscopic ear surgery, *Otolaryngol Head Neck Surg* 153(4):613–615, 2015.

Gysin C: Indications of pediatric tonsillectomy, *ORL J Otorhinolaryngol Relat Spec* 75(3):193–202, 2013.

House JW, Cunningham CD: Otosclerosis. In Flint PW et al, editors: *Cummings otolaryngology; head and neck surgery*, ed 6, Philadelphia, 2015, Mosby.

Janakiram TN et al: Endoscopic endonasal repair of sphenoid sinus cerebrospinal fluid leaks: our experience, *Indian J Otolaryngol Head Neck Surg* 67(4):412–416, 2015.

Lam D, Carlson ER: The temporalis muscle flap and temporoparietal fascial flap, *Oral Maxillofac Surg Clin North Am* 26(3):359–369, 2014.

Lee KH: *Indications for cochlear implants* (website), 2016. http://emedicine.medscape.com/article/857164-overview?pa=fc4IKJDv%2BoQJG5QJ1a9sUIuPl%62B Jt0qFup5HLthZtZ5QctlZkvm9N4vJA1hVl_e3Qsl1nrn59XpsOP7KBID2x-mJyTCgTLaddDjW30XNFYmyptyk%3D. (Accessed 27 September 2016).

Mamelle E et al: Supramaximal stimulation during intraoperative facial nerve monitoring as simple parameter to predict early functional outcome after parotidectomy, *Acta Otolaryngol* 133(7):779–784, 2013.

Marfatia H et al: Challenges during BAHA surgery: our experience, *Indian J Otolaryngol Head Neck Surg* 68(3):317–321, 2016.

National Institute on Deafness and other Communication Disorders (NIDCD): *Age-related hearing loss* (website), 2016. www.nidcd.nih.gov/health/age-related-hearing-loss. (Accessed 28 August 2016).

Paulson E: *A new look at informed consent: recent guidelines prompt patient-centered approach* (website), August 9, 2010. www.enttoday.org/details/article/806315/A_New_Look_at_Informed_Consent_Recent_guidelines_prompt_patient-centered_approach.html. (Accessed 22 August 2017).

Roditi RE et al: Oral antibiotic use for otitis media with effusion: ongoing opportunities for quality improvement, *Otolaryngol Head Neck Surg* 54(5):797–803, 2016.

Sweeney AD et al: Surgical approaches for vestibular schwannoma, *Curr Otorhinolaryngol Rep* 2(4):256–264, 2014.

Wilson KF et al: Salivary gland disorders, *Am Fam Physician* 89(11):882–888, 2014.

CHAPTER 20
Orthopedic Surgery

BARBARA A. BOWEN

The word *orthopédie* is derived from the Greek *orthos,* meaning "straight," and *paideia,* meaning "rearing of children." It was first used by Nicholas Andry in 1741 in the title for a book addressing the prevention and correction of skeletal deformities in children. Orthopedic surgery has been defined by the American Academy of Orthopaedic Surgeons' Board of Orthopaedic Surgery as "a broad based medical and surgical specialty dedicated to the prevention, diagnosis, and treatment of diseases and injuries of the musculoskeletal system" (ABOS, 2016).

Orthopedic surgery is an ever-changing field that is a challenge for the perioperative nurse. Technologic advances in the multitude of systems and hardware used have resulted in improved treatment of orthopedic disorders. In addition to understanding anatomic and physiologic responses, the perioperative nurse should have a general understanding of the concepts and purposes of these systems to provide the most safe and efficient care. Knowledge of the principles of bone fixation and healing and the relationship of bone and soft tissues provides a strong basis to ensure continued understanding of the care required for the orthopedic patient.

Surgical Anatomy

Anatomic Structures

The 206 bones of the body form the appendicular or axial framework that supports soft tissues, provides storage areas and reservoirs for minerals, and serves as a site for formation of blood cells (Fig. 20.1). The skeletal system is composed of varied elements, including bone, muscle, and associated structures.

Bone remains in a constant state of formation and resorption, preventing development of excessive thickness or thinness. These processes are related to individual metabolism and absorption of calcium, vitamin D, and phosphorus. Levels of minerals affect disease processes, causing bone changes. A layer of connective tissue called *periosteum* covers all bone. Bone formation at the cellular level is initiated by the osteoblasts. Osteocytes, which make up 90% of all cells in the adult skeleton, are responsible for maintaining bone. Osteoclasts resorb bone (Miller, 2016).

Muscles are masses of tissue that cover bones and provide movement to the skeletal system. Muscles interact with nerves, minerals, skin, and other connective tissue to contract and extend. Individual muscles are short or long and vary in diameter, depending on their position on a specific bone.

Ligaments, tendons, and cartilage also form the skeletal structures. Ligaments are bands of dense connective tissue that hold bone to bone. They provide stability to a joint by encircling or holding ends of bone in place. Tendons are tough, long strands of fibers that form the ends of muscles. They transmit forces to bone or cartilage without being damaged. Cartilage is a layer of elastic, resilient supporting tissue found at the ends of the bones. It forms a cap over the bone end to protect and support the bone during weight-bearing activities and provides a smooth gliding surface for joint movement. Cartilage is aneural (without nerves), alymphatic (without lymph tissue), avascular (without blood vessels), and high in water content. The lack of vascularity and loss of water from cartilage during a lifetime are causes of resulting degenerative disease, such as arthritis. Weight bearing and joint movements keep cartilage from becoming thin or damaged and help prevent degenerative conditions.

Joints are articulations where bones are joined to one another or where two surfaces of bones unite. Joints are classified by the type of material between them or according to movement. Material between joints is fibrous, cartilaginous, or synovial. The type of movement is synarthrotic (immovable), amphiarthrotic (slightly movable), or diarthrotic (freely movable). Synarthrotic joints are connected by fibrous tissue or ligaments (e.g., the suture type of joints holding the bones of the skull; connections between two bones, such as the radius and ulna). Amphiarthrotic joints are connected by cartilage. Joints of this type include the symphysis pubis, intervertebral joints, and manubriosternal joint. The majority of joints are diarthrotic; these are the only joints with one or more ranges of motion. These joints are lined with a synovial membrane and are called *synovial joints.* Examples include the knee, cervical vertebrae 1 and 2 (C1 and C2), the radius articulating on the wrist bones, the hip, and the shoulder.

The two types of bone tissue are *cortical* and *cancellous.* Cortical bone is the hard bone forming the outer shell (the main supporting tissue). Cancellous bone is soft and spongy and is located at the iliac crest, tibia, sternum, and the ends of long bones. It contains the red bone marrow for hematopoiesis.

Bones are divided according to their shape: long, short, flat, irregular, and round (Fig. 20.2). Long bones are present in the limbs and consist of a shaft and two ends; the ends generally flare out, are covered with articular cartilage, and provide a surface for articulation and musculotendinous attachment. Short bones, such as the carpals and tarsals (in the wrist and midfoot areas, respectively), are present where the structure is strong but limited movement is required. Flat bones are the scapula, the sternum, and the pelvic girdle. Irregular bones are found in the skull and vertebral column. Round bones, or sesamoid bones (resembling a sesame seed), are found within tendons. The patella is a large sesamoid bone; however, most are small, such as the two found on the head of the first metatarsal, which form the "ball" of the foot.

Long bones consist of a shaft (diaphysis) and two ends (epiphyses). The shaft is composed of compact bone. The epiphyses flare out

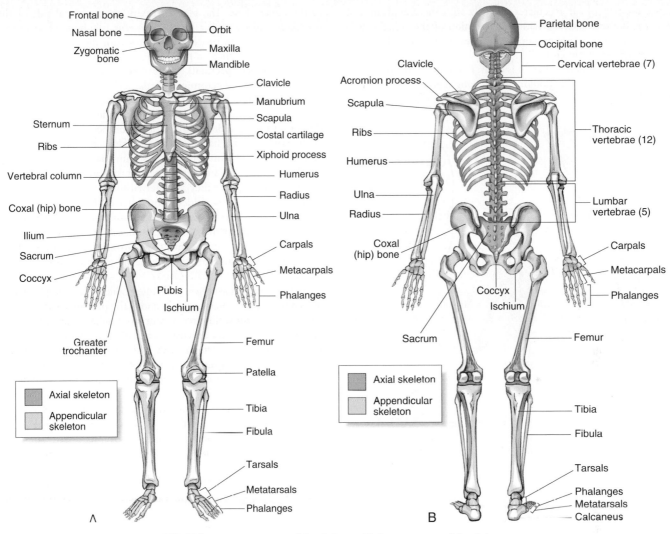

FIG. 20.1 (A) Anterior view of the skeleton. (B) Posterior view of the skeleton.

and consist of cancellous bone. They are covered by cartilage, which provides a cushion and offers protection during weight bearing and movement. Until skeletal maturity, a line of cartilage called the *epiphyseal plate* separates the epiphysis from the diaphysis. Fractures in this region by children can be devastating because they often lead to malformation and permanent limb shortening.

Trabeculae are located within cancellous bone and consist of an interconnecting network of bone oriented along the lines of stress. These structures are important for weight bearing, providing strength to withstand stress placed on the bone. The periosteum is a thin, outer covering of bone containing nutrient arteries for nourishment of bone cells. Disruption of these periosteal vessels after bone trauma can influence the ability of bone to heal. The haversian system consists of thousands of microscopic units found in the cortical bone. These units of matrix cells, canals, and conduits allow flow of nutrients and facilitate calcium absorption.

Vertebrae

Vertebrae form the longitudinal axis of the skeleton. The vertebral bodies are connected by several cartilaginous joints, which enable the vertebrae to flex, extend, or rotate while being held together. Intervertebral disks (IVDs) and ligaments connect the bodies of adjacent vertebrae. The ligamenta flava bind the laminae of adjacent vertebrae together. Other ligaments connect the spinous processes and vertebral bodies.

Seven cervical vertebrae form the skeletal framework of the neck, twelve thoracic vertebrae support the thoracic region, and five lumbar vertebrae support the small of the back. Below the lumbar vertebrae lie the sacrum and coccyx. Each of these bones is composed of fused vertebrae, five for the sacrum and four for the coccyx.

The vertebral column is curved. After birth there is a continuous posterior convexity. As development occurs, secondary posterior concavities develop in the cervical and lumbar regions, resulting in improved balance.

Each area of the vertebral column has specific bony structures. General features include a body (except the first two cervical vertebrae) on the anterior part. The posterior portion of the vertebrae consists of a neural arch formed by pedicles and laminae and the spinous and transverse processes.

Shoulder and Upper Extremity

The clavicle, which is a long, doubly curved bone, serves as a prop for the shoulder and holds it away from the chest wall. The clavicle rests almost horizontally at the upper and anterior part of the thorax, above the first rib. It articulates medially with the manubrium of the sternum and laterally with the acromion of the scapula; it is tethered to the underlying coracoid process of the scapula by the coracoclavicular ligaments.

The scapula (shoulder blade) is a flat, triangular bone that forms the posterior part of the shoulder girdle, lying superior and posterior

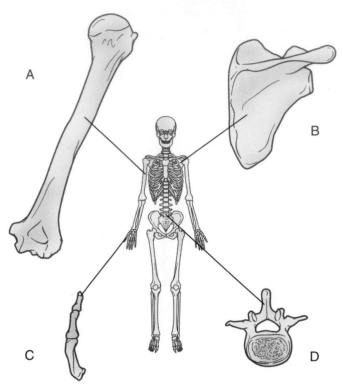

FIG. 20.2 Types of bones. (A) Long bones (humerus). (B) Flat bones (scapula). (C) Short bones (phalanx). (D) Irregular bones (vertebra).

to the upper chest. The glenoid cavity on the lateral side of the scapula provides a socket for the humerus (the bone of the upper arm). The acromion process articulates with the clavicle medially. The scapula is attached to the thorax by muscles.

The shoulder (pectoral) girdle consists of the glenohumeral, sternoclavicular, and acromioclavicular (AC) joints (Fig. 20.3). The glenohumeral joint has a multidirectional range of motion, whereas the latter two joints have limited motion. The AC joint, located at the top of the shoulder, is the articulation between the outer end of the clavicle and a flattened articular facet situated on the inner border of the acromion. The muscles immediately surrounding the shoulder joint are the supraspinatus, infraspinatus, teres minor, and subscapularis; together they are referred to as the *rotator cuff.* These muscles stabilize the shoulder joint, whereas the powerful deltoid, pectoralis major, teres major, and latissimus dorsi muscles move the entire arm. Shoulder girdle strength and stability are maintained by the soft tissue integrity and not the bony structures. A pathologic condition in this area can be the result of bone, soft tissue, or combined injury.

The humerus is the longest and largest bone of the upper extremity. It is composed of a shaft and two ends. The proximal end, or head, has two projections, the greater and lesser tuberosities (Fig. 20.4). The circumference of the articular surface of the humerus is constricted and is termed the *anatomic neck.* The anatomic neck marks the attachment to the capsule of the shoulder joint. The constriction below the tuberosities is called the *surgical neck* and is the site of most fractures.

The greater tuberosity is situated at the lateral aspect of the humeral head. Its upper surface has three impressions in which the supra-spinous, infraspinous, and teres minor tendons insert. The lesser tuberosity is situated in the anterior neck and has an impression for the insertion of the tendon of the subscapular muscle. The attachment sites for the rotator cuff, the tuberosities, are separated from each other by a deep groove (bicipital groove), in which lies the tendon of the long head of the biceps muscle of the arm. The tendon of

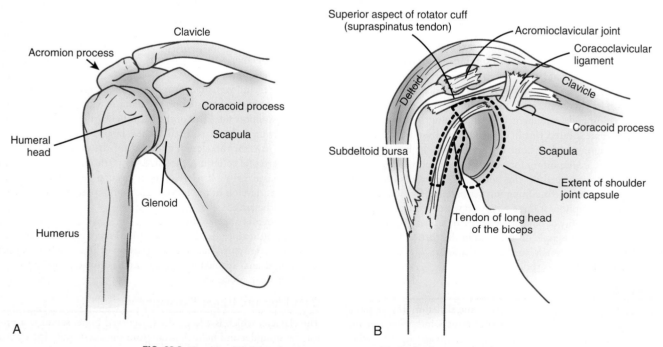

FIG. 20.3 Shoulder. (A) Joint showing anterior view. (B) Girdle showing articulations.

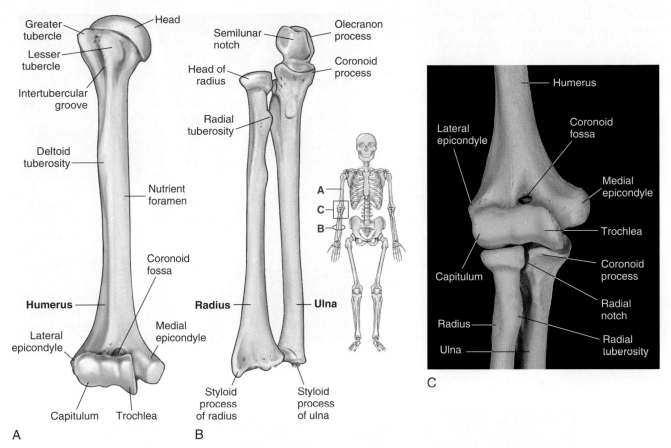

FIG. 20.4 Bones of the arm, anterior view, showing the humerus, radius, and ulna.

the pectoralis major inserts on the lateral margin of the bicipital groove, and the latissimus dorsi and teres major insert on the medial margin.

The distal humerus flattens and ends in a broad articular surface. The surface is divided into the medial and lateral condyles, which are separated by a slight ridge. On the lateral condyle, the rounded articular surface is called the *capitulum,* which articulates with the head of the radius. On the medial condyle, the articular surface is termed the *trochlea,* which articulates with the ulna.

The ulna is located medial to the radius. The proximal portion of the ulna, the olecranon, articulates with the trochlea of the humerus at the elbow. The radius rotates around the ulna. At the proximal end is the head, which articulates with the capitulum of the humerus and the radial notch of the ulna. The tendon of the biceps muscle is attached to the tuberosity just below the radial head. The distal end of the radius is divided into two articular surfaces. The distal surface articulates with the carpal bones of the wrist, and the surface on the medial side articulates with the distal end of the ulna.

Wrist and Hand

The skeletal bones of the wrist and hand consist of three distinct parts: (1) the carpals, or wrist bones; (2) the metacarpals, or bones of the palm; and (3) the phalanges, or bones of the digits (Fig. 20.5).

The eight carpal bones are arranged in two rows. The distal row, proceeding from the radial to the ulnar side, includes the trapezium, trapezoid, capitate, and hamate; the proximal row consists of the scaphoid (also called the *navicular*), lunate, triquetrum, and pisiform.

Functionally, the scaphoid links the rows as it stabilizes and coordinates the movement of the proximal and distal rows. Each carpal bone consists of several smooth articular surfaces for contact with the adjacent bones, as well as rough surfaces for the attachment of ligaments. The five metacarpal bones (long bones) are situated in the palm. Proximally they articulate with the distal row of carpal bones, and distally the head of each metacarpal articulates with its proper phalanx. The heads of the metacarpals form the knuckles. The phalanges, or fingers, consist of 14 bones in each hand, 2 in the thumb and 3 in each finger. Each phalanx consists of a shaft and two ends.

Pelvis, Hip, and Femur

The pelvis (Fig. 20.6) is a stable circular base that supports the trunk and forms an attachment for the lower extremities. It is a massive, irregular bone created by the fusion of three separate bones. The largest and uppermost of the three bones is the ilium, the strongest and lowermost is the ischium, and the anterior most is the pubis. Together these are termed the *os coxae,* or innominate bone.

The acetabular portion of the innominate bone and the proximal end of the femur (Fig. 20.7) form the hip, which is a ball-and-socket joint. The hip joint is surrounded by a capsule, ligaments, and muscles that provide stability. The iliofemoral ligament connects the ilium with the femur anteriorly and superiorly, and the ischiofemoral and pubofemoral ligaments attach the ischium and pubis to the femur, respectively. The acetabulum is a deep, round cavity that articulates with the head of the femur. The proximal end of the

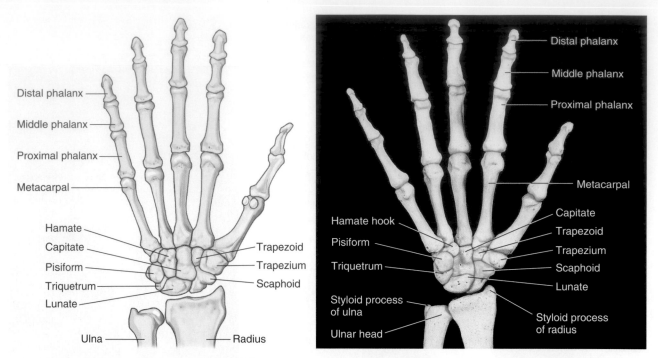

FIG. 20.5 Bones of the wrist and hand, palmar view.

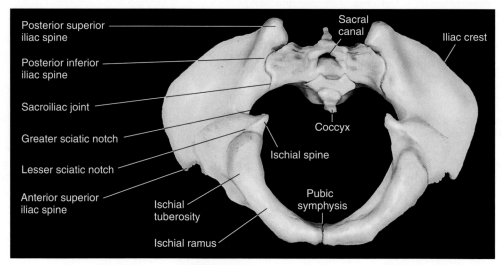

FIG. 20.6 Pelvis, superior view.

femur consists of the femoral head and neck, the upper portion of the shaft, and the greater and lesser trochanters (Fig. 20.8).

The greater trochanter is a broad process that protrudes from the outer, upper portion of the shaft and projects upward from the junction of the superior border of the neck with the outer surface of the shaft. It serves as a point of insertion for the abductor and short rotator muscles of the hip.

The lesser trochanter is a conical process projecting from the posterior and inferior portion of the base of the neck of the femur at its junction with the shaft. It serves as a point of insertion for the iliopsoas muscle. The lower end of the femur terminates in the two condyles. Anteriorly, the condyles are separated from one another by a smooth depression, called the *intercondylar,* or *patellar, groove,*

forming an articulating surface for the patella. Posteriorly, they project slightly, and the space between them forms the intercondylar fossa, which is a supporting structure for neurovascular structures.

The upper or condylar end of the tibia presents an articular surface corresponding with those of the femoral condyles. The articular surface of the two tibial condyles forms two facets that are deepened by the semilunar cartilage into fossae for the femoral condyles.

Knee, Tibia, and Fibula

The knee joint (Fig. 20.9) consists of two articulations. One articulation is between each condyle of the femur and the tibial plateau, and the other is between the patella and the femur. These areas are subject to degenerative changes, often requiring reconstructive surgery.

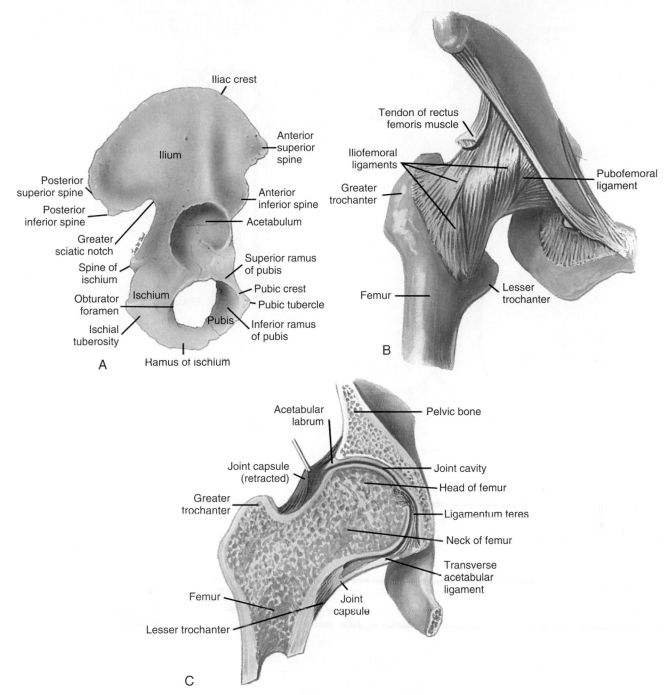

FIG. 20.7 Hip joint. (A) Coxal bone disarticulated from the skeleton. (B) Ligamentous structure. (C) Bone structure.

The bones of the knee joint are connected by extra-articular and intra-articular structures. The extra-articular attachments consist of the joint capsule, multiple muscular attachments, and two collateral ligaments. The intra-articular ligaments consist of the two cruciate ligaments and the attachments of the menisci.

The patella, or kneecap, is anterior to the knee joint in the intercondylar groove, or trochlea, of the distal femur. It is a sesamoid bone contained within the quadriceps tendon. The anterior surface of the patella is united with the patellar tendon as the tendon originates and inserts above and below the knee joint. The posterior surface of the patella articulates with the femur.

The capsule of the knee joint is attached proximally to the femoral condyles, and it is attached distally to the condyles of the tibia and to the upper end of the fibula. The capsule is reinforced anteriorly by the patellar and quadriceps tendon, on the sides by the medial collateral ligament (MCL) and lateral collateral ligament (LCL), and posteriorly by the popliteus and gastrocnemius muscles.

The cruciate ligaments (Fig. 20.10), consisting of two fibrous bands, extend from the intercondylar fossa of the femur to attachments anterior and posterior on the intercondylar surface of the tibia.

The menisci are interposed between the condyles of the femur and those of the tibia (see Fig. 20.10). Each meniscus is attached

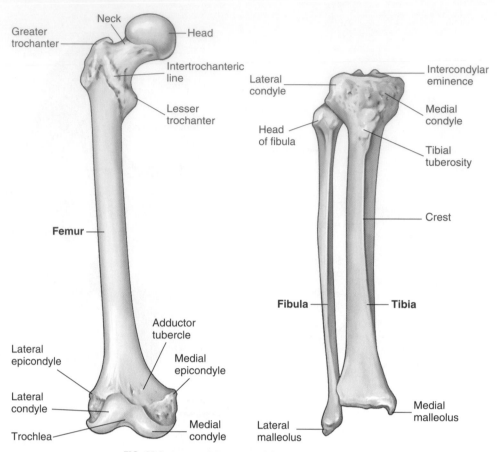

FIG. 20.8 Bones of the upper *(left)* and lower leg *(right)*.

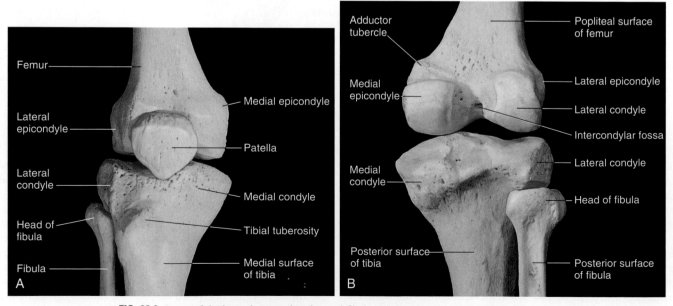

FIG. 20.9 Bones of the knee showing the tibia and fibula. (A) Anterior aspect. (B) Posterior aspect.

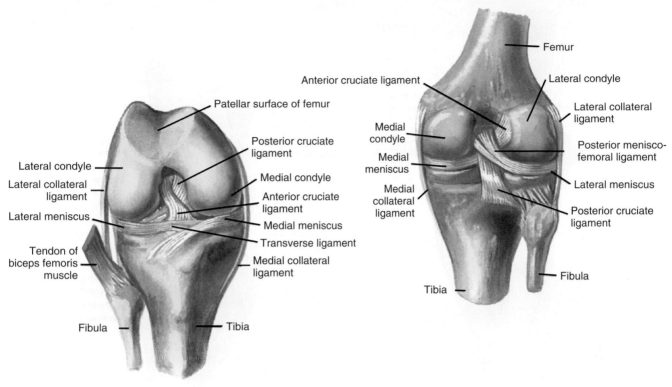

FIG. 20.10 Bony structures of the knee joint.

to the joint capsule. The ends of the cartilage are attached to the tibia in the middle of its upper articular surface. These structures are almost totally avascular, and degenerative changes are usually permanent.

Synovial membrane lines the capsule of the joint and covers the infrapatellar fat pad, parts of the cruciate ligaments, and portions of the bone. The portion of the knee joint cavity that extends upward in front of the femur is called the *suprapatellar pouch*, or *bursa* (Fig. 20.11).

The tibia is the larger and stronger of the lower leg bones. The fibula is smaller and located more laterally, articulating at the proximal end with the lateral condyle of the tibia. The proximal end of the tibia articulates with the femur to form the knee joint. Distally the tibia articulates with the fibula and with the talus, forming the ankle joint.

Ankle and Foot

The ankle is a hinge joint, formed by the distal end of the tibia and fibula and the proximal end of the talus. The tibia (medial and posterior malleoli) and fibula (lateral malleolus) form a mortise (notch) for the reception of the upper surface of the talus and its facets. The talus is an irregular bone consisting of a body, neck, and head. The bones are connected by ligaments that spread out from the malleoli to attach to the talus, calcaneus, and navicular bones (Fig. 20.12). A thin capsule surrounds the joint.

The bony framework of the foot (Fig. 20.13) comprises 7 tarsal bones, 5 metatarsal bones, and 14 phalanges. The calcaneus forms the heel and gives support to the talus. The cuboid bone articulates proximally and posteriorly with the calcaneus and distally with the fourth and fifth metatarsals and the third cuneiform bones.

The navicular bone articulates with the cuneiform bones, which lie side by side just anterior to it. The metatarsal bones articulate proximally with the tarsal bones and distally with the bases of the first phalanges of the corresponding toes. There are two phalanges for the great toe and three for each of the other toes.

Perioperative Nursing Considerations

Assessment

Assessment of the orthopedic patient is dynamic. Preoperatively, the nurse takes special care to document any functional losses that are caused by the disability. The social situation of the patient should also be documented both in the physician's office and again in the hospital chart, because this may affect discharge planning. Familiarity with orthopedic procedures and anticipated patient outcomes improves the ability to gather appropriate information and complete the nursing process. Obtaining patient-specific information from the physician also enhances the perioperative nursing assessment. The signed operative consent provides information to confirm the scheduled procedure or procedures and verify the operative site and side per The Joint Commission's (TJC) Universal Protocol for correct site surgery, which is now part of the National Patient Safety Goals (TJC, 2016). The consent is usually obtained before admission to the surgery suite and should be reviewed for accuracy and completeness.

Additional measures that should be undertaken to verify the correct operative side and site include marking the surgical site and having the patient verify the site with the surgeon during the marking process; using a verification checklist (which includes documents

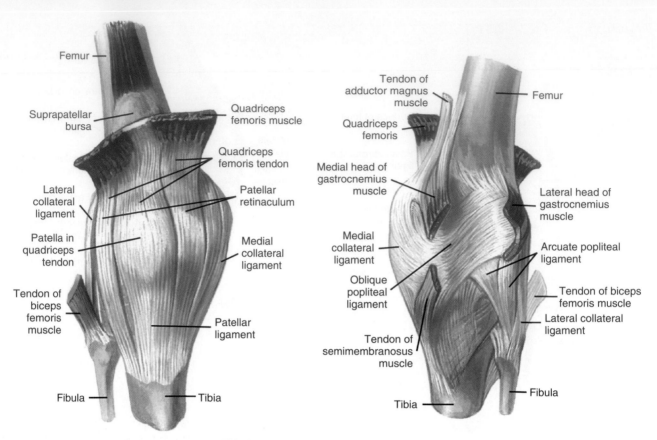

FIG. 20.11 Superficial aspect of the knee joint.

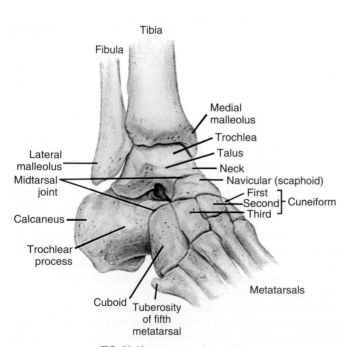

FIG. 20.12 Anatomy of the ankle.

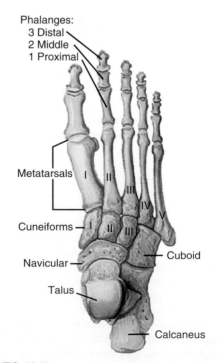

FIG. 20.13 Bones of the foot viewed from above.

EVIDENCE FOR PRACTICE

Universal Protocol for Preoperative Site Verification as Indicated for Orthopedic Surgery

The Joint Commission's Universal Protocol for correct patient, procedure, and surgical side and site as well as the AORN Position Statement on correct site surgery both emphasize verification and marking of the surgical site (or invasive procedure site), especially when it involves laterality, levels, or multiples. As part of this process, protocols are used to verify the correct patient; correct procedure; correct patient position; and availability of necessary equipment, implants, imaging studies/equipment, or other special requirements. These protocols are part of the preoperative verification process as well as the time-out before the start of the surgical procedure.

For surgery a recommended protocol may include:
- Preoperative skin marking of the procedure site.
- Preoperative films or images present in the OR or procedure room.
- A time-out, including patient identity (using two unique identifiers); procedure to be performed; correct patient position; correct procedure side, level, or site; and presence of necessary implants, imaging, equipment, or other special requirements.
- Provisions for delaying the procedure if there are any discrepancies by any members of the surgical team. If there are discrepancies, the procedure will not proceed until the institution's reconciliation procedure is initiated and the results of the reconciliation documented.
- Use of opaque instruments to mark the specific bony landmarks when intraoperative imaging is necessary. X-rays are taken and compared with the preoperative films or images by the surgeon performing the procedure.

AORN, Association of periOperative Registered Nurses.
Modified from The Joint Commission: *Universal protocol* (website). https://www.jointcommission.org/standards_information/up.aspx. (Accessed 17 September 2016).

such as the medical record, x-ray films, and imaging studies); using verbal verification by the patient of his or her identity, surgical site/side, and planned surgical procedure; confirming this information during the time-out by each member of the surgical team; and monitoring safe site protocol compliance with these procedures (Evidence for Practice).

The perioperative nurse reviews the patient record, noting relevant aspects of the history and physical examination; the nature of the problem and its onset; and results of radiographic studies, laboratory data, and other findings. He or she reviews the nursing history to determine physical, psychosocial, cultural, spiritual, and other needs. The nurse assesses the patient's range of motion, neurovascular status, and general condition. The patient's understanding of the surgical procedure and postoperative rehabilitation is determined, and patient education is begun.

Assessment information helps the nurse determine specific needs related to surgical positioning, skin preparation, equipment, instrumentation, and supplies. Environmental safety is also considered, including room temperature, traffic flow, lighting, and personnel attire.

The nurse communicates information with other members of the perioperative team. The information collected helps the perioperative nurse plan and coordinate activities, facilitate a smooth transition, and reduce operative time.

Nursing Diagnosis

Nursing diagnoses related to the care of patients undergoing orthopedic surgery might include the following:
- Anxiety
- Risk for Peripheral Neurovascular Dysfunction
- Risk for Perioperative Positioning Injury
- Impaired Gas Exchange
- Risk for Infection
- Risk for Hypothermia

Outcome Identification

Outcomes identified for the selected nursing diagnoses could be stated as follows:
- The patient will verbalize concerns and apprehension related to surgery and recovery.
- The patient will be free from peripheral neurovascular dysfunction.
- The patient will be free from perioperative positioning injury.
- The patient will maintain adequate ventilation and oxygen exchange.
- The patient will be free from postoperative surgical site infection.
- The patient will maintain appropriate body temperature intraoperatively.

Planning

The care of surgical patients undergoing any type of surgery requires planning for routine procedures that are always followed, as well as anticipating the unexpected. The perioperative nurse should be consistent and systematic in the planning process to expedite actual steps required to facilitate the surgical procedure. Care of the orthopedic patient presents unique challenges because of the psychosocial, physical, and technical aspects of patient care. Planning includes attention to environmental factors, positioning, transfusion supplies, equipment, and instrument needs, in addition to practices that will prevent complications.

The optimal environment is comfortable for the patient and surgical team. The patient should feel relaxed and secure enough to allow the surgical team to become his or her advocates during the procedure. Physical preparation of the environment changes with individual patients. At the time the procedure is posted in the operating room (OR), traffic flow is considered to determine room location. The temperature is selected for the procedure with consideration given to the age and general health of the patient, attire worn by the operative personnel (body exhaust suits), or use of polymethylmethacrylate (PMMA) (bone cement). The patient's temperature should be monitored for all but very brief surgical procedures, such as those lasting less than 30 minutes. To maintain normothermia, the perioperative nurse might consider using warming blankets preoperatively to prewarm the patient in the holding area, warming the ambient room temperature, warming intravenous (IV) fluids, warming the skin surface with a forced-air warming device intraoperatively, and using warm cotton blankets at the end of the surgical procedure.

Equipment and instrumentation needed for the procedure are planned before the patient's arrival in the OR; orthopedic procedures may vary significantly because of the patient's physical condition or age. It may be necessary to communicate with the manufacturer's representative to facilitate obtaining items needed for the procedure. It is common for healthcare industry representatives to bring requisite orthopedic instruments to the OR or to act as a product resource regarding new equipment. However, industry representatives must comply with all institutional policies and Association of periOperative Registered Nurses (AORN) standards and policy-defining requirements and procedures and restrictions that govern their presence in the OR (AORN, 2014).

The nurse reviews the procedural information to plan positioning and protective measures. Aseptic technique is essential in the perioperative environment and should be considered a priority when caring for the orthopedic patient. Osteomyelitis is an infection of the bone that can remain unrecognized for a long time and requires expensive, intensive treatment. Osteomyelitis can lead to severe bone loss and possible loss of a limb. Preventive measures, including administration of antibiotics within 60 minutes of the initial incision, have been demonstrated to be efficacious in preventing surgical site infection.

OR equipment such as defibrillators and resuscitative equipment must always be available, functional, and familiar to staff. This includes supplies needed for emergency treatment of a patient's condition, such as malignant hyperthermia or unanticipated blood loss. All medications and solutions along with their containers should be labeled both on and off the surgical field. Equipment alarms should be activated with appropriate settings and should be sufficiently audible. Orthopedic procedures may also require a change in the plan of care in the event of a fracture, damage to vascular integrity, or changes in the patient's condition, requiring an understanding of methods and equipment needed to manage these situations.

The nursing process requires continual reassessment and modifications. An effective plan entails communication, creating a culture that supports patient safety, creation of an optimal environment, and effective use of human and physical resources (AORN, 2016d). A Sample Plan of Care for a patient undergoing orthopedic surgery follows.

Implementation

Implementing care for the orthopedic surgical patient requires an understanding of anatomic, physiologic, psychologic, cultural, spiritual, and technical patient needs. Orthopedic surgical procedures demand special equipment, instruments, and psychomotor skills that differ from those required by other specialties. Implementation includes an understanding of the procedures, patient needs, periopera-

tive practices, and perioperative nursing interventions to protect the patient while delivering care.

The nurse should provide explanations to the patient about the intraoperative phase, including the anticipated sequence of events, personnel, environment, required positioning, and procedures such as administration of a regional anesthetic and application of a tourniquet. The patient may be alert during the procedure; therefore noise from power equipment and activities that will occur should be explained. Immobilization devices, such as splints, casts, braces, and drains, also should be explained.

Positioning and Positioning Aids

The orthopedic patient requires proper positioning on the OR bed or specialty bed to provide adequate exposure of the operative area, maintain body alignment, minimize strain or pressure on nerves and muscles, allow for optimal respiratory and circulatory function, and provide adequate stabilization of the body. Selection of position depends on several factors, including the type of procedure, the location of the injury or lesion, and the preference of the surgeon. Guidelines for placing the patient in the supine or recumbent position are followed (see Chapter 6), with modifications to facilitate the specific orthopedic procedure.

Procedures performed in lateral, prone, or modified positions require positioning aids and devices to support these positions. Patients undergoing surgical procedures risk neuromuscular and skin injury. The nurse's preoperative assessment should be thorough to plan the position, taking into consideration the prevention of neurovascular compromise, the potential for impaired chest excursion, and the danger of falls. The safety strap does not always provide adequate security, and other methods of securing the patient on the OR bed may need to be implemented. The surgeon is responsible for selecting the position and ensuring that adequate exposure can be obtained. The perioperative staff must understand the meaning of terms such as *flexion, extension, abduction,* and *adduction* when positioning the patient. The staff must also be thoroughly familiar with the function of the orthopedic surgical bed and its various attachments (e.g., the leg attachment for arthroscopy, the three-point positioner for lateral position, and positioning devices for shoulder procedures).

Many orthopedic operations require a device for holding the extremities. Various holders are available for both upper and lower extremities. Positioners used intraoperatively can be sterilized for

---

SAMPLE PLAN OF CARE

Nursing Diagnosis
Anxiety

Outcome
The patient will verbalize concerns and apprehension related to surgery and recovery.

Interventions
- Encourage verbalization of feelings, expression of fear, and questions about procedure, anticipated outcome, postoperative rehabilitation, pain management, and home care/self-care requirements.
- Explain anticipated routine activities (diagnostic studies, OR environment, preoperative holding area, PACU), and encourage questions.

- Encourage patient, family, and caregiver participation in decision-making activities related to discharge planning.
- Demonstrate respect, and attend to patient's individual needs and those of the family or significant others.
- Remain with patient; ensure other personnel are introduced.
- Provide comfort and care, for example, through the use of warm blankets, touch, and hand holding.
- Discuss any other concerns with the patient, family, and caregiver, and initiate appropriate referrals.

Nursing Diagnosis
Risk for Peripheral Neurovascular Dysfunction

Outcome
The patient will be free from peripheral neurovascular dysfunction.

SAMPLE PLAN OF CARE—cont'd

Interventions

- Complete and document a preoperative neurovascular assessment including skin color and temperature, pulses, motor strength and movement, and sensation; reassess and document at procedure conclusion.
- Position patient with proper body alignment, considering range of motion or any limitations in mobility.
- Protect vulnerable neurovascular structures and prevent pressure injury by properly padding bony prominences and pressure points.
- Pad the elbow, avoid excessive abduction, and secure arm gently on locked armboard to protect the brachial plexus.
- Pad the wrist and secure it gently on an armboard or at the patient's side to protect the radial nerve.
- Pad and tuck the arm carefully at the patient's side or on an armboard to protect the medial and ulnar nerves.
- Place a pillow at the knee (but not under it) and support the lower extremities to protect the peroneal nerve; ensure that restraining straps are not tight and do not compress the knee.
- Ensure equipment is kept off the lower extremities to protect the tibial nerve.
- Apply pneumatic tourniquet correctly, observing, verifying, and documenting procuro cottings and tourniquet inflation time.
- Provide padding (air mattress or gel pads) when long surgical times are expected or patients are predisposed to peripheral vascular compromise.
- Anticipate the needs of the patient and surgical team to minimize surgical time.

Nursing Diagnosis
Risk for Perioperative Positioning Injury

Outcome
The patient will be free from perioperative positioning injury.

Interventions

- Assess range of motion; identify joints at risk for injury caused by immobilization, pain, trauma, or arthritic or other disease processes.
- Position arthritic joints carefully to prevent strain.
- Observe and document condition of patient's skin before transfer to the OR bed and again at conclusion of procedure.
- Use proper lifting and transfer techniques when transferring the patient to and from the OR bed to prevent shearing forces on skin.
- Keep sheets on OR bed dry and wrinkle free.
- Ensure that personnel with knowledge of the patient's condition and equipment are available to supervise and assist with transfer of the patient.
- Use proper restraint devices to protect patients from falls or movement of the extremities.
- Avoid extending or flexing extremities beyond range of motion when there is resistance.
- Protect skin in dependent areas from pooling of solutions.
- Use positioning devices, such as pillows, to maintain position; use a small head pillow under the head if head and neck are normally bent slightly forward.
- Pad all dependent pressure sites; provide extra padding for patients with decreased circulation.
- Protect vulnerable neurovascular areas from compression.

Nursing Diagnosis
Impaired Gas Exchange

Outcome
The patient will maintain adequate ventilation and oxygen exchange.

Interventions

- Review preoperative evaluation of the patient's pulmonary status.
- Assist anesthesia provider in airway management.
- Ensure full chest excursion when positioning, particularly in the lateral and prone positions.
- Collaborate with anesthesia provider in monitoring vital signs, oxygen saturation, ventilation, cardiac rhythm, and blood loss.
- Complete a vascular assessment (pulse, sensation, movement, temperature, and color check) preoperatively, and compare with postoperative status.

Nursing Diagnosis
Risk for Infection

Outcome
The patient will be free from postoperative surgical site infection.

Interventions

- Confirm that the patient has complied with preoperative skin cleansing (as appropriate).
- Implement strict aseptic practices for preparing the patient's skin, draping the patient and equipment, opening supplies and equipment for the procedure, removing hair (only as necessary), and controlling traffic patterns in the OR.
- Prepare for pulsatile lavage or irrigation (as needed).
- Initiate antibiotic therapy preoperatively and/or intraoperatively per physician's orders; check for medication allergies before antibiotic administration.
- Implement procedure-specific activities, such as using body exhaust systems and pulsatile lavage.
- Anticipate equipment needs, and check equipment function; implement safety precautions when using equipment.
- Sterilize instruments according to policy and procedure and the manufacturer's guidelines.
- Handle implants according to manufacturer's recommendations.

Nursing Diagnosis
Risk for Hypothermia

Outcome
The patient will maintain normothermia intraoperatively.

Interventions

- Obtain and document baseline preoperative temperature.
- Initiate preoperative warming with either warmed blankets or forced hot air warming device.
- Maintain temperature in the OR between 68°F and 73°F (20°C to 23°C) if possible.
- Monitor patient temperature throughout the procedure.
- Use warming devices and warming blankets during the procedure.
- Warm fluids as necessary.
- Minimize patient exposure to room air.
- Place warm blankets on patient immediately after surgery.

PACU, Postanesthesia care unit.

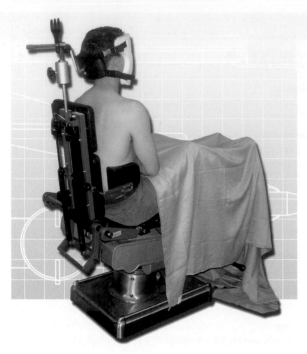

FIG. 20.14 Shoulder positioner allows distraction of the joint for visualization.

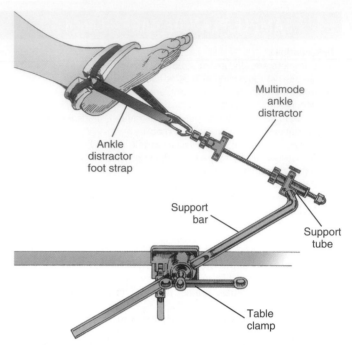

FIG. 20.16 Ankle distractor, noninvasive, for distraction of the joint and visualization.

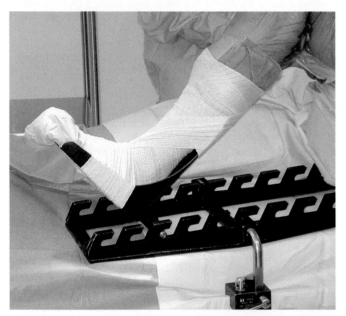

FIG. 20.15 Alvarado foot holder used during total joint procedures to position the extremity for exposure.

the procedure, resulting in the ability to reposition as needed throughout the procedure. These types of positioners include the shoulder positioner (Fig. 20.14), Alvarado foot holder (Fig. 20.15), and ankle distractor (Fig. 20.16). Many other orthopedic positioning devices are also available.

The lateral position is sometimes used for a total hip arthroplasty. Positioners such as the Wixson hip positioner and the Stulberg hip positioner will provide stability with lateral positioning of the patient

during surgery. Padded anterior and posterior supports may be positioned at the umbilicus and lumbar regions, respectively, to hold the patient in the lateral position. A vacuum beanbag positioning device can also achieve the lateral position. The nurse collaborates to ensure pressure points on the lateral area of the skull, ear, axilla, hip, knee, and ankle are adequately padded. The patient's feet are placed in the neutral position to prevent excessive plantar flexion or dorsiflexion. A conscientious effort should be made by the surgical team to avoid leaning on the patient during the procedure.

The patient is positioned prone for surgery on the posterior aspect of the body, including the spine; posterior portion of the shoulder, arms, and legs; and Achilles tendon; and for posterior iliac bone graft harvesting. This position presents a challenge for the anesthesia provider to monitor and manage the airway because of the potential for impaired chest excursion and gas exchange. The patient's extremities need to be moved through a normal range of motion when transferring and positioning into the prone position. Vascular integrity is always assessed before the patient is moved into position and reassessed after the patient is positioned; the nurse should note the quality of pulses, extremity warmth, and capillary refill.

The prone position is often attained with the use of adjunctive frames, such as the Wilson, Hastings, Canadian, Relton–Hall, Cloward saddle, or Andrews, or with the Andrews bed (Fig. 20.17). Each frame has qualities that meet the patient's or physician's needs. The Hastings and Andrews frames and the Andrews bed maintain the patient in a modified knee-chest position. The frames require assembly and are labor-intensive when positioning; some can be used only with certain beds. The Andrews bed is similar to the Andrews frame but has the attachments built in and is used exclusively for this position.

An OR fracture bed (Fig. 20.18) is generally used for femoral neck and shaft fixation. The team places the patient in supine or lateral position to allow exposure of the surgical site while maintaining

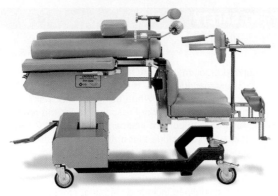

FIG. 20.17 Andrews bed used for prone positioning.

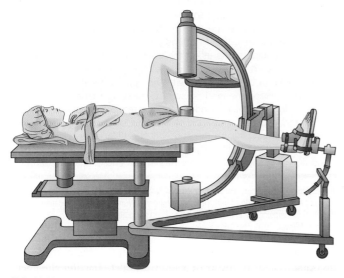

FIG. 20.18 Patient positioned on the orthopedic fracture bed for femoral neck, femoral shaft, or tibial fixation, with image intensifier in position.

alignment. The patient's legs are positioned on outriggers, allowing access by the image intensifier to obtain multiple radiographic views. Applying or releasing traction is performed to reduce the fracture or aid in intramedullary (IM) surgical techniques. Like all positioning devices, the fracture bed must be set up by experienced personnel and padded adequately. There are several moving parts that can cause injury if not operated properly.

If the patient is positioned supine, special attention must be paid to the arms. The patient's arms are placed on padded armboards with the palms up and fingers extended. Armboards are maintained at less than a 90-degree angle to prevent brachial plexus stretch. If there are surgical reasons to tuck the arms at the side, the elbows are padded to protect the ulnar nerve, the palms face inward, and the wrist is maintained in a neutral position (Spruce and Van Wicklin, 2014). A drape secures the arms and should be tucked snuggly under the patient, not under the mattress. This prevents the arm from shifting downward intraoperatively and resting against the OR bed rail.

Surgical Prep

A primary concern in orthopedic surgery is the prevention of infection. The orthopedic surgical prep must be meticulously performed using aseptic technique. Physicians often instruct patients to complete a scrub prep with an antimicrobial agent before arrival for surgery. The surgical prep for the orthopedic patient may include preoperative removal of hair from the surgical site. Surgical shave preps contribute to the possibility of infection caused by abrasion and cutting of the skin. If hair removal from the incisional site is ordered, it should occur immediately before surgery, using clippers or a depilatory (AORN, 2016b). Trauma patients require precautions during the skin prep to prevent further injury caused by solution contact with membranes or injury to the bone and soft tissue from movement.

Skin preparation is performed to remove microorganisms from the operative site. The site should be prepped with a broad-spectrum antimicrobial agent. The prep proceeds from the incision site to the periphery. Pooling of the prep solution beneath the patient or tourniquet must be avoided. Prep solutions should be allowed to dry before draping; this is a fire safety precaution and may be included in the time-out. The groin and anal areas should be isolated when the surgical site is on the upper third of the leg.

Devices such as leg stirrups may help support an extremity to complete a circumferential prep. When multiple extremities or other areas, such as a bone graft site, are prepped, cross-contamination of previously prepped areas must be prevented. Knowledge of aseptic technique and the ability to organize the activity are important in proper preparation of the surgical site.

Draping

Applying sterile drapes is the final step in preparing the patient for the operation. The surgeon and scrub person, who may be a registered nurse or surgical technologist, cover the patient's extremities with a cloth or water impervious stockinette, which is a cylindric drape that is rolled up the arm or leg. Impervious sheets are essential when large amounts of fluid are used, such as during arthroscopy and wound irrigation. Prefabricated disposable drapes with fenestrations for the upper and lower extremities are available.

Antimicrobial incise drapes can be used to isolate the surrounding area from the incisional site. Many of these drapes contain iodophor-impregnated adhesive, which slowly releases iodine during the procedure, inhibiting proliferation of organisms from the patient's skin. They are contraindicated for patients with an allergy to iodophors. An alcohol skin wipe may be done before placement of the antimicrobial incise drape.

Equipment and Supplies

Orthopedic ORs require a variety of special equipment and accessories in addition to routine OR equipment. Nitrogen-powered, battery-powered, and electrically powered equipment; video systems; pneumatic tourniquets; laminar airflow systems; x-ray equipment; lasers; and special orthopedic tables are included in the operative armamentarium. Manufacturers' pamphlets with illustrations and directions on equipment use and sterilization should be readily available for reference.

Radiographic Intervention. Radiographic intervention is widely used in orthopedic surgery. Many procedures require portable x-ray or fluoroscopy machines. Fluoroscopy, also known as *image intensification* or *C-arm,* allows the team to view the progression of the procedure, confirming fracture reduction or IM reaming of the humerus, femur, or tibia. An x-ray technician operates radiographic equipment. An understanding of equipment placement, function, and safety precautions is necessary. The perioperative nurse is responsible for communicating with the radiology personnel concerning the procedure, aseptic technique, and traffic flow in the OR. X-ray cassettes brought onto the sterile field are draped with a sterile plastic cover.

All personnel in proximity to the x-ray equipment should wear lead aprons and thyroid shields and should be monitored for exposure to radiation. The nurse takes measures to protect patients from direct and indirect radiation exposure, and documents them on the perioperative nursing record.

Pneumatic Tourniquets. Pneumatic tourniquets are frequently used for procedures involving the extremities. A tourniquet is a fabric-covered cylindric bladder inflated by compressed gas or ambient air. It applies circumferential pressure on arterial and venous circulation, which results in a relatively bloodless surgical field; this promotes visualization of structures during the procedure. Limb exsanguination is achieved by elevating the limb or by wrapping it, distally to proximally, with an elastic or Esmarch rubber bandage before tourniquet inflation. The majority of tourniquets used today are run by a microprocessor for regulation of pressure and time setting, providing both auditory and visual feedback for the user.

Tourniquet safety should be a priority; the surgical team should understand recommended parameters and precautions. Safety guidelines for the use of tourniquets include preventive measures and evaluation (AORN, 2016a). Preoperative assessment of the patient includes determining contraindications for use, including compartment syndrome, McArdle disease (e.g., glycogen storage disease), hypertension, or other vascular problems. If the tourniquet must be used for patients with these conditions, specific guidelines must be observed.

Before applying the tourniquet cuff, the nurse checks all components of the tourniquet equipment for proper functioning. Inflation pressures are established based on the systolic blood pressure, age of the patient, and circumference of the extremity. Duration of tourniquet inflation should be kept to a minimum. It is recommended in the average, healthy 50-year-old person to apply continuous tourniquet pressure less than 1 hour on the upper extremity and less than 2 hours on the thigh. Tourniquet pressure should not exceed the recommended maximum cuff pressure limits of 300 to 350 mm Hg for the thigh and 250 to 300 mm Hg for the arm and the lower leg. Netscher and colleagues (2017) noted the interval between inflation and deflation should be 5 minutes for every 30 minutes of tourniquet ischemia to minimize effects on muscle and nerves.

The tourniquet is placed on the extremity without compression on bony structures and superficial neurovascular structures. The person placing the cuff should ensure it is positioned as high as possible without pinching skinfolds. Soft padding or stockinette is wrapped around the extremity and kept free of wrinkles and gatherings beneath the cuff. Cuffs should overlap a minimum of 3 inches and a maximum of 6 inches; excess overlap can pinch skinfolds. A tourniquet cuff that is too short can loosen after inflation. Care must be taken to ensure that the line from the air supply to the cuff is not kinked.

Tourniquet equipment should be checked and calibrated periodically and serviced when problems arise. Injury from tourniquets may result from inadequate precautions, faulty preparation, or use of inaccurate equipment. The gauges and other related equipment should be checked with commercially available test equipment. Patient evaluation requires assessment of the extremity (skin color, temperature, pulses, movement, and sensation) after removal of the tourniquet. Abnormal findings need to be reported to the surgeon and documented (Patient Safety).

Traction. The surgeon uses traction preoperatively, intraoperatively, or postoperatively for prevention or reduction of muscle spasm, immobilization of a joint or body part, reduction of a fracture or

---

PATIENT SAFETY

Safe Tourniquet Use

Recommended practices from AORN help the perioperative nurse effectively manage cases that involve tourniquets. Patient safety is the primary concern when using tourniquets intraoperatively. All OR personnel responsible for the tourniquet should be familiar with current standards. The primary purpose of the tourniquet is to occlude blood flow to the extremity, providing a bloodless surgical site. Competency associated with the use of tourniquets should be demonstrated by the OR staff. All tourniquets should be maintained according to manufacturers' guidelines including cleaning, sterilizing, and testing. Disposable tourniquet cuffs are available for single use as are sterile, disposable exsanguinating tourniquets that do not require additional equipment for inflation. The surgeon applies the sterile exsanguinating tourniquet in the field and rolls it upward to the desired height. The rubber band within the fabric provides the tourniquet effect and produces the bloodless field. If inflating equipment is used, the integrity and function of the base unit should be tested before each use. Personnel are responsible for being familiar with the application of the tourniquet, recommended pressures, maximum times for inflation for extremities, and contraindications for tourniquet use. OR personnel must be aware of the risks of exceeding the time limits and should inform the surgeon at regular intervals of the tourniquet inflation time. The nurse is responsible for assessing and documenting patient outcomes at the end of the procedure.

AORN, Association of periOperative Registered Nurses.
Modified from Association of periOperative Registered Nurses (AORN): Guideline for care of patients undergoing pneumatic tourniquet-assisted procedures. *Guidelines for perioperative practice,* Denver, 2016, The Association.

---

dislocation, and treatment of a joint disorder. Traction alignment must be constant.

Various traction techniques can be used, including manual, skin, and skeletal (Fig. 20.19). In manual traction the hands provide the forces pulling on the bone being realigned. Skin traction uses strips of tape, digital straps, moleskin, or an elastic bandage applied directly to the skin. Common forms of skin traction are Buck extension and Russell traction. Skeletal traction applies forces directly to the bone, using pins. Manual and skin traction can be applied in the emergency department or patient room, whereas skeletal traction is applied preoperatively in the emergency department or in the OR.

Skeletal traction is often used in conjunction with the OR fracture bed, using the traction attachment to aid in reduction of a long bone fracture. Postoperatively the patient may be confined to bed with balanced skeletal traction using a Thomas splint (Fig. 20.20) and a Pearson attachment. Some cervical spine fractures or injuries may require Crutchfield or Gardner–Wells tongs or a cervical halo inserted directly into the skull to stabilize the vertebrae and reduce spinal cord damage or further injury. Application of skeletal traction requires the use of sterile supplies, including a traction bow, pins, and drill.

The perioperative nurse ensures the patient's postoperative bed is prepared with the correct traction frames. Nursing care of the patient in traction should include ensuring that the traction is continuous and skin tapes or skeletal pins are secured. The nurse checks the patient's neurovascular status routinely, including skin color, pulse, temperature, and sensation. Changes from baseline or normal value are reported to the surgeon.

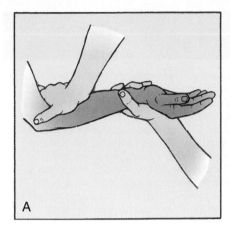
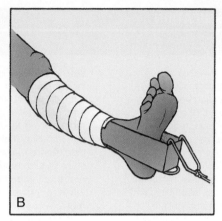
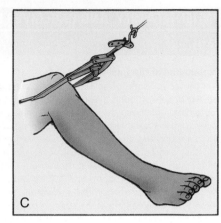

FIG. 20.19 Traction techniques. (A) Manual. (B) Skin. (C) Skeletal.

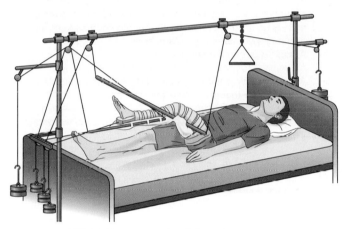

FIG. 20.20 Thomas splint balanced suspension.

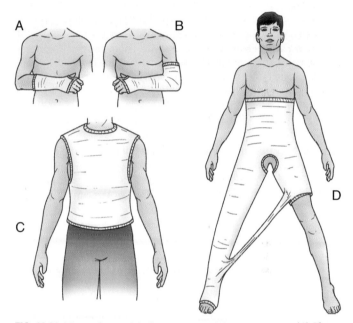

FIG. 20.21 Types of casts. (A) Short arm cast. (B) Long arm cast. (C) Plaster body jacket cast. (D) One and one-half hip spica cast.

Postoperative Immobilization. Postoperative immobilization may require use of a cast, splint, or other supplies designed for the specific anatomic part. A cast is a common method of immobilizing a fractured bone during healing (Patient, Family, and Caregiver Education). The forces of distraction, rotation, and malalignment can be overcome with the application of a cast. Closed reduction with a cast may be an option, minimizing the disadvantages and complications of open reduction, such as infection and tissue damage.

The surgeon uses plaster or synthetic materials such as fiberglass for casting. Plaster is less expensive, with a greater weight-to-strength ratio (it requires a greater weight of plaster to produce the same strength of fiberglass). Plaster casts may be burdensome if they are too heavy. They are routinely used as the primary cast after surgical procedures and are replaced later with a lighter fiberglass cast to promote patient mobility.

Casting material sets up and hardens rapidly when activated with water, and such a property necessitates that it be prepared with all necessary materials. Soft padding or stockinette is applied to the patient's extremity before the cast is applied to protect the skin from thermal injury while the plaster sets, as well as to protect the skin from undue abrasion and pressure. The plaster must be prepared, applied, and handled carefully and safely.

Fig. 20.21 shows types of casts. After wrist fractures the surgeon applies a short arm cast from below the elbow to the metacarpal heads. A long arm cast extends from the axilla to the metacarpal heads, immobilizing forearm or elbow fractures. The surgeon uses a short leg cast, applied from the tibial tuberosity to the metatarsal heads, to immobilize the ankle and foot. The long leg cast is used for fractures involving the femur, tibia, or fibula or for complicated ankle fractures. The femoral cast brace is used in the treatment of femoral shaft fractures.

A snug-fitting thigh cast and short leg cast are hinged at the knee joint. The cast brace is generally used after 4 to 6 weeks of skeletal traction after initiation of callus formation at the fracture site. A cylinder cast incorporates the leg from the groin to the ankle and is applied when complete knee immobilization is required. This is often required after surgery involving soft tissue reconstruction around the knee.

The hip spica cast is used when complete leg immobilization is desired. The patient's trunk, affected side, and unaffected side may all be incorporated into the cast. Spinal immobilization is accomplished with a body jacket.

PATIENT, FAMILY, AND CAREGIVER EDUCATION

Casts

Explanation of the Cast

The cast is only one of several devices used to promote the healing of broken bones. Surgeons also use traction and pins, or a combination of these three devices, to help heal broken bones. The cast has the advantage of being less expensive, requiring little care on the patient's part, and allowing the patient mobility. The cast also encloses and immobilizes the broken bone and injured soft tissues to prevent movement that could cause further injury and to keep the bone in place for proper healing. It may be made of plaster or of a synthetic material, such as fiberglass, and some fiberglass casts may be applied with a waterproof liner. Although the plaster cast is heavy, the surgeon can mold a plaster cast more easily for a close fit over severe injuries. The synthetic cast is lightweight and easier to move around.

Cast Care

- Keep a plaster cast dry; cover it or wrap it in a plastic bag when bathing or going out in the rain or snow.
- Check with the surgeon about immersing a fiberglass (or other synthetic) cast in water. The surgeon may permit immersion if there are no surgical wounds under the cast or if the cast has a waterproof lining.
- Maintain good skin care around the cast; however, do not:
  - Insert objects, such as a coat hanger, under the cast.
  - Put any creams, lotions, or powder inside the cast.

Things to Watch for and Report to Your Surgeon or Nurse

- Warm areas under the cast. The skin under the cast will feel warm at first because of the reaction that occurs during the setting process. However, warm areas on the cast later may indicate infection; notify the surgeon or nurse at once.
- Increased pain or soreness under the cast, particularly around a bony prominence such as the wrist or ankle not relieved by repositioning the body. Check the skin color and temperature periodically. When the tip of a finger or the big toe that extends from the cast is squeezed until it is white, the pink color should return within 4 to 6 seconds. If skin color does not return within 4 to 6 seconds or if the skin is red, blue, white, or otherwise discolored, notify the surgeon. If fingers or toes are cool, cover them. If they do not warm up in 20 minutes, call the surgeon. Call the surgeon immediately if any of these other symptoms occur:
  - Increase in swelling and pain. Some swelling is common at first. Your surgeon may have advised you to elevate the cast after it was applied. The cast should feel snug for the first 48 hours. If it continues to feel too snug and causes pain and swelling, call your surgeon.
  - A tingling or burning sensation.
  - An inability to move muscles around the cast.
  - A foul odor detected around the edges of the cast.
  - Any drainage that may show through the cast.
  - Any cracks or breaks in the cast.
  - Marked loosening of the cast, allowing the parts inside the cast to move fairly easily.

Modified from Clinical Key: *Cast care* (website). www.clinicalkey.com/#!/content/patient_handout/5-s2.0-pe_ExitCare_DI_Cast_Care_SportsMed_en. (Accessed 19 November 2016).

Splints may also be used for postoperative immobilization but are not circumferential and allow for swelling and closer observation of the surgical site.

Another immobilization device is the abduction pillow, used after total joint replacement. This prevents the patient's leg from adducting, or rotating internally, and the hip from flexing, which could cause dislocation of the hip. Further discussion of this and other devices is included with the descriptions of various surgical interventions.

Lasers. Laser application has been increasing in the field of orthopedics. Its use mandates safety precautions, certification, patient consent, and protective attire (see Chapter 8 for a full discussion of lasers and laser safety). Laser types include carbon dioxide, holmium:yttrium-aluminum-garnet (Ho:YAG), neodymium:YAG (Nd:YAG), potassium titanyl phosphate (KTP), erbium:YAG (Er:YAG), and excimer. Laser technique differs for use on bone, muscle, tendon, and cartilage. Lasers have been used successfully for osteotomy, revision arthroplasty (removal of PMMA), nerve and tendon repair, arthroscopy, and diskectomy.

Airflow Control. Airflow control in the orthopedic OR is critical to prevent introduction of microorganisms. Surgical site infections may result from airborne bacteria or transient bacteria from the patient or surgical team (AORN, 2016c). Laminar airflow is a system designed to provide highly filtered air and continuous air exchange for reducing airborne bacteria. Body exhaust suits are also used as a defense against airborne bacteria (Fig. 20.22). Aseptic practices, sterile technique, and conscientious behaviors in ORs using con-

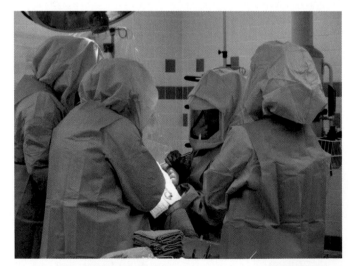

FIG. 20.22 Body exhaust system used in arthroplasty.

ventional airflow can be used to maintain low rates of surgical site infections.

Postoperative Management. The nurse begins planning the patient's postoperative management during the preoperative period. Special equipment may include continuous passive motion (CPM) machines, pain management devices and techniques, compression devices, and blood salvage. CPM machines stimulate the healing effect on articular tissues, including cartilage, tendon, and ligaments, without interfering with healing incisions over the moving joint. The benefits of CPM include inhibition of adhesion formation and joint stiffness, decreased pain and swelling, early functional range of motion, and decreased effects of immobilization. The device is applied early in the postoperative period.

Pain management may include insertion of an epidural catheter, use of a patient-controlled analgesia (PCA) pump, or local administration of pain medication through a pain pump. The advantages of using these techniques include rapid pain relief, increased patient satisfaction, and often less use of medication than with traditional intramuscular analgesics. These techniques can be used independently or in combination. In using the PCA pump, a predetermined IV dose of the prescribed pain medication is administered. It allows continuous infusion of analgesic as well as bolus administration when the patient feels it is necessary. Recent research demonstrates that the effectiveness of these pain management techniques combined with new multimodal approaches often result in better outcomes for the patient (Research Highlight).

Management of fluid and electrolyte balance may include use of intraoperative autologous transfusion or postoperative blood salvage. A potential problem with salvage of large amounts of blood is depletion of clotting factors; therefore coagulation problems should be identified preoperatively. Postoperative blood salvage is accomplished with a closed-drainage system. It requires a complete understanding of the system for safe use.

Instruments and Accessory Items

Orthopedic surgical procedures require an extensive inventory of instruments and implants and specific instruments to implant and apply hardware. Revision surgery requires that the perioperative staff be prepared with the appropriate tools and extractors needed to remove an old implant and have an understanding of equipment use. Preoperative planning is essential for orthopedic surgery.

Implant Inventories. Implant inventories include plates and screws, IM nails and rods, total joint implants, and a host of accessory items. Surgeon preference, patient population, and equipment cost are considered when selecting stock items. The surgical team must ensure these items are stocked in a timely fashion to prepare for consecutive implant use.

Inventory should be organized by manufacturer, type of implants (e.g., total hip, knee), and comparative sizes. Some may be provided on a loaner or consignment basis. Staff must be familiar with the varied types and refer to the manufacturer's information pertaining to each implant. Practices should ensure that the correct implant is opened on the operative field to prevent unnecessary expense or error in placement. Confirmation of the implant by the surgeon, scrub person, and perioperative nurse is essential before opening the implant onto the field.

Many different alloys are used in manufacturing implants. However, all devices implanted in a patient must be of the same metallic composition to prevent galvanic corrosion; internal fixation implants used during an orthopedic procedure should be of the same metal. Screws, for example, should be of the same composition as the metal plate affixed to the bone. Alloys used most frequently include stainless steel, cobalt-chromium, and titanium-vanadium-aluminum.

Internal fixation devices should never be reused. Resulting imperfections, such as abrasions or scratches, increase the potential for corrosion and weakening of the implant. Bending implants to conform to the contour of the bone should be avoided whenever

possible to prevent loss of strength. When bending is necessary, the proper bending press should be used. Once an implant is bent, it should not be reshaped or straightened; doing so may weaken the implant.

Orthopedic equipment and implants require special care, storage, and handling. When possible, implants should be individually wrapped and processed. Today's implants, excluding some plates and screws, are packaged separately by the manufacturer. During sterilization, implants should not be placed in a position in which knocking or bumping might occur. Appropriate sterilizing cases and trays should be used, and implants should be sterilized according to the manufacturer's instructions. An internal fixation device that

RESEARCH HIGHLIGHT

Pain Management After Total Joint Arthroplasty

Postoperative pain after TJAs can be significant for patients and challenging to manage. Traditionally, pain management was been geared toward unimodal methods (e.g., narcotic administration only), although complications are associated with this methodology. Bimodal methods combine two medications for analgesia, whereas true multimodal methods use three medications and may also involve nerve blocks. This study sought to determine whether the number of narcotic doses and length of hospital stay decreased when a multimodal approach was used. Additional outcomes considered were a reduction in complications related to narcotic use, immobility, and high pain levels.

The authors reviewed 10 pain management protocols from different facilities in developing their multimodal protocol as part of their study. They included 266 patients in the study; 95 patients represented the control group and the remainder underwent the study protocol.

The multimodal pain management protocol that was developed involved care providers administering pain medications before, during, and after surgery. Before surgery, the patient attended a total joint class, which included a review of the postoperative pain management protocol. On the day of surgery, patients received celecoxib and pregabalin orally. The anesthesia provider administrated a spinal anesthetic (with morphine unless contraindicated) after the patient arrived in the OR. The anesthesia provider also administered IV ondansetron and acetaminophen 30 minutes before the end of the procedure, and for patients undergoing total knee arthroplasty, the surgeon administered an intra-articular injection of ropivacaine and ketorolac. The nurses administered cold therapy in the immediate postanesthesia period and began a regimen of IV acetaminophen and ondansetron. Within 24 hours after surgery, oral medications were provided. Control group patients (determined by retrospective chart review) received spinal anesthesia and postoperative narcotics (e.g., morphine, hydromorphone, or fentanyl).

Analysis of the results showed the multimodal pain management protocol significantly reduced the total number of opioid doses and slightly reduced the number of days between surgery and discharge. Anecdotal information from patients treated with the multimodal approach showed better pain control, and quantifiable data showed these patients were able to participate in rehabilitation efforts earlier.

TJA, Total joint arthroplasty.
Modified from McDonald LT et al: Pain management after total joint arthroplasty, *AORN J* 103(6):605–616, 2016.

has become damaged as a result of improper storage or handling must be discarded.

The perioperative nurse assigned to orthopedic patients should have a working knowledge of the general types and sizes of implants that might be selected. Templates of radiographs are often made preoperatively, providing a general idea of the size of the implants needed.

The US Food and Drug Administration (FDA) requires strict guidelines in properly documenting and tracking implant devices. Documentation should include, but not be limited to, the patient's permanent record, the operative record, and an implant registry maintained by the OR. Many manufacturers now include mailers to return information to the company for data collection. Information to be recorded includes the lot and serial numbers and the manufacturer, size, type, and anatomic position of the implants used.

Orthopedic Instrumentation. Orthopedic instrumentation varies from very small to large instruments. Some procedures require multiple instrument containers (sets). Organization of instrument sets for multiple uses prevents the need for duplication and requires thoughtful consideration of anatomic and physiologic needs. When preparing for a procedure, the perioperative nurse should open the minimum number of instruments yet be prepared for unexpected or untoward events. Careful planning and preparation of instrumentation ensure efficient use of time and equipment.

Instruments that do not function properly (as a result of dullness, poor adjustment, lack of lubrication, damage, improper fit, or incomplete cleaning) are primary sources of complaints and problems in the OR. Instrument maintenance is vital to ensure availability for the procedure and ease in completion of the procedure. Instruments should be used for the intended purpose during the procedure. Movable parts should be lubricated after each cleaning and checked for cracks or damage after each use. The perioperative nurse is responsible for ensuring instruments are maintained and has knowledge of sterilization and packaging procedures.

The following basic bone instrument sets should be available in the orthopedic OR. Soft tissue instrument sets appropriate for the size of the anatomic site are used for procedures not requiring bone instruments or in addition to the sets. Additional instruments and special equipment are mentioned with the discussion of various surgical interventions:

- *Hip set:* Total hip arthroplasty or fractures of the neck and proximal femur
- *Total knee set:* Total knee arthroplasty or supracondylar and distal femoral fractures
- *Shoulder set:* Shoulder arthroplasty and other shoulder procedures
- *Large bone set:* Bone work on the large bones, including hip, knee, upper arm, and elbow
- *Extremity or small bone set:* Bone work on the hand or foot
- *Fusion or bone graft instruments:* Additional instruments necessary for an autograft

Powered Surgical Instruments. Powered surgical instruments used in the OR have eliminated the need for many hand-operated tools, reducing operative time and improving technical results. They are available as air-driven, battery-driven, or electrically driven equipment. Fingertip control provides the surgeon speed and power. Variable-speed saws, drills, and reamers offer wide flexibility. Power equipment has a safety control that prevents inadvertent activation; this should be engaged when passing the instrument to the surgeon or assistant. The perioperative nurse and scrub person should monitor the sterile field to make certain that powered instruments are not rested on the patient when they are not in use.

It is important to follow the manufacturer's recommended cleaning, sterilizing, and lubricating instructions. With proper care, powered surgical instruments have a long life span and many uses.

Suture Material. Suture material requires increased tensile strength and minimal degradability for the select type of tissue. Tendons and ligaments are fibrous, avascular tissues, resulting in a slower healing process than that occurring in tissues rich in blood supply. Absorbable suture may be used for sewing tendon or ligaments to bone. Nonabsorbable sutures, including polyester and surgical steel, are also used. For various ligament replacement grafts, a harvested tendon may be customized with multiple strands of suture material, increasing tensile strength and length of time until fibrous union occurs.

Polymethylmethacrylate. PMMA (bone cement) is an acrylic, cement-like substance composed of a liquid methyl methacrylate monomer and a powder methyl methacrylate-styrene copolymer. The powder component is 10% barium sulfate, US Pharmacopoeia (USP), which provides radiopacity to the finished product. The liquid monomer is highly flammable, and the OR should be properly ventilated. Caution should be exercised during mixing of the two components to prevent excessive exposure of OR personnel to the vapors of the monomer. This exposure can cause irritation of the respiratory tract and eyes. Personnel in a room in which methyl methacrylate is being mixed should not wear soft contact lenses. Many special hoods and mixing devices are available to minimize staff exposure to the fumes. Additionally, the use of antibiotic-impregnated PMMA bone cement has been shown to decrease the infection rates in total joint arthroplasty (Bosco et al., 2015).

Adverse patient reactions with PMMA include transitory hypotension, cardiac arrest, cerebrovascular accident, pulmonary and fat embolus, thrombophlebitis, and hypersensitivity reaction. Cardiac arrest and death, although uncommon, have resulted after insertion of bone cement. Adverse reactions have been attributed to a combination of factors, including a rise in IM canal pressure causing embolic phenomena, a possible chemical and blood reaction causing sudden hypotension, and certain preexisting patient conditions. More research is needed to discover the exact cause of adverse reactions. Patient care should include collaborating with the anesthesia provider before insertion of PMMA and then monitoring for side effects after insertion.

Medications

Antibiotics, hemostatics, and antibacterial agents are commonly used. Antibiotics are delivered intravenously, locally in irrigation solutions and injected directly into the surgical site postprocedure. Common antibiotics used in irrigation include polymyxin and bacitracin. Irrigation may also be delivered using pulsatile lavage, with antibiotics added to the solution. Hemostatic agents may include bone wax, gelatin foam, thrombin, microfibrillar collagen, and parecoxib sodium (Surgical Pharmacology). Parecoxib sodium is a liquid, sprayable hemostatic agent consisting of collagen, thrombin, the patient's own platelets, and fibrinogen. Antibacterial ointments are preimpregnated in gauze dressings from the manufacturer or are applied before the application of the dressing. Other medications used during orthopedic procedures include steroids, local anesthetics, antifibrinolytics, and normal saline. Local anesthetics are often injected near the end of the surgical procedure to minimize postoperative pain.

Protective Measures

Orthopedic procedures require caution as a result of the use of fluids for irrigation or bloody procedures. Personnel protective measures include handling items (blades, sharp instruments, bone) cautiously

SURGICAL PHARMACOLOGY

Medications Commonly Used in Orthopedic Surgery

Medication/Category	Dosage/Route	Purpose/Action	Adverse Reactions	Nursing Implications
Bupivacaine hydrochloride injection 0.5%	Injection via local infiltration, peripheral nerve block, and caudal and lumbar epidural blocks; 5-mL dose of 0.25% or 0.5% (12.5–25 mg); maximum dose 400 mg/day	Local anesthetic for pain management during surgery	Weak or shallow breathing; fast heart rate, gasping, feeling unusually hot; slow heart rate, weak pulse; feeling restless or anxious, ringing in the ears, metallic taste, speech problems, numbness or tingling around the mouth, tremors, feeling lightheaded	Monitor vital signs Patients should be informed in advance that they may experience temporary loss of sensation and motor activity
Bone wax	Topical application: 2.5 g	Sterile mixture of beeswax and isopropyl palmitate, a wax-softening agent, used to help control bleeding from bone surfaces	Delayed healing, increased infection and inflammation	Look for signs and symptoms of the adverse reactions postoperatively
Topical thrombin	5,000–20,000 IU applied topically on the bleeding area	Used to reduce bleeding and absorb blood	Incision site complications, increased bleeding times	Must be reconstituted before use

Modified from Hodgson BB, Kizior RJ: *Saunders nursing drug handbook 2015*, St Louis, 2015, Saunders; CP Medical. *Bone wax product insert* (website). http://cpmedical.com/wp-content/uploads/2012/07/BONE-WAX-INSERT.pdf. (Accessed 19 November 2016)

to prevent inadvertent punctures or cuts and wearing protective masks, eyewear, or a face shield as well as protective attire, including gowns and boots. Sharp bone edges are a hazard and can puncture gloves and skin. Double-gloving or protective gloves should be used to protect the patient and personnel.

Bone Banking

The American Association of Tissue Banks (AATB) accredits and periodically inspects bone-banking programs to ensure that specific standards are followed in the retrieval, processing, storage, and distribution of bone allografts (e.g., bone, ligament, cartilage, tendon, or section of skin that is transplanted from one person to another) (AATB, 2016). Allografts are frozen until use. Vacuum-sealed freezers are monitored with an alarm. When requested for a procedure, the bone allograft is delivered to the field, slightly thawed, cultured, and washed with an antibiotic solution. Banked bone is available in many shapes of cortical and cancellous tissue.

Records are maintained on both donors and recipients. Donor records provide the donor identification, medical history (with circumstances of death if applicable), laboratory results, and graft description. Recipient records include recipient identification, surgeon and organization implanting the graft, surgical procedure, culture results, and any adverse reactions. Like other implants, the recipient's operative record should include the name of the bone bank from which the allograft was received, type of allograft, tissue number, and expiration date if applicable.

Evaluation

Evaluation is an ongoing process throughout the procedure. The perioperative nurse evaluates the patient, considering the nursing diagnosis and achievement of identified outcomes. This part of the nursing process provides feedback regarding the effectiveness of the plan, its implementation, and alterations needed for improving patient care. Was the patient protected from peripheral neurovascular injury?

Was the patient free from perioperative positioning injury? Was adequate oxygenation maintained? Does the patient have more questions pertaining to recovery and rehabilitation? The answers will dictate whether there is a need to maintain or modify the plan. The evaluation information is shared with the nurse caring for the patient postoperatively to provide continuity of care.

The following sample outcome statements apply to evaluating care of the orthopedic patient when using the nursing diagnoses identified earlier in this chapter:

- The patient verbalized fears and feelings and indicated that anxiety and apprehension were lessened.
- The patient was free from peripheral neurovascular dysfunction on discharge to the PACU as evidenced by the presence of pulses, warmth of the extremity, good capillary refill, and intact movement and sensation.
- The patient was free from injury related to perioperative positioning as evidenced by maintenance of skin integrity and absence of reddened areas.
- The patient maintained adequate ventilation and perfusion as evidenced by blood gases, arterial saturation, oxygen saturation, and vital signs within normal limits.
- The patient was free from surgical site infection as evidenced by temperature within normal limits and a clean and dry incision site.

Patient, Family, and Caregiver Education and Discharge

Discharge planning and patient education should be initiated when the healthcare provider evaluates the patient for surgery. It should continue when the patient comes into contact with the healthcare system and should involve a multidisciplinary approach. A method of planning the overall care from preadmission to discharge is to place a patient on a clinical guideline or care path based on "best practice," which is a multidisciplinary case management tool. Best practices, such as enhanced recovery after surgery (ERAS) define

ENHANCED RECOVERY AFTER SURGERY

Enhanced Recovery After Surgery After Total Joint Arthroplasty

Total joint arthroplasty has used clinical pathways in the past with much success. These pathways have maximized patient outcomes and decreased length of stay. ERAS pathways allow changes in care leading to improved pain management secondary to multimodal therapy, accelerated physical therapy, and discharge to home once medically stable. By using ERAS for total joint surgery, length of stay has decreased from 76.6 hours to 56.1 hours with the trend toward outpatient total joint replacement. Patient selection is critical to good outcomes and decreased readmissions.

ERAS, Enhanced recovery after surgery.
Modified from Auyong DB et al: Reduced length of hospitalization in primary total knee arthroplasty patients using an updated enhanced recovery after orthopedic surgery (ERAS) pathway, *J Arthroplasty* 30(10):1705–1709, 2015.

the expected processes of care. Essentially they are strategies of care developed with the intent of encouraging physicians and other healthcare providers who care for the same surgical patient population to agree to a specific sequence of common interventions. Included with the clinical guideline on the patient's medical record is a set of orders that mirrors the guideline and allows the physician to make minor changes to the protocol. Receiving feedback from all disciplines involved in the patient's care and discharge planning is beneficial in reducing variance and improving efficiency, outcomes, and costs (Enhanced Recovery After Surgery).

For the patient undergoing orthopedic surgery, patient, family, and caregiver education and discharge planning in the following areas are essential: wound care and dressing changes, pain control, wound assessment, physical and occupational therapy, personal care, housekeeping, mobility, nutrition, prescriptions other than pain medication, extended anticoagulant therapy, application and removal of orthopedic appliances, and follow-up with a physician. Information concerning these content areas should be described, discussed, and reinforced with written instructions. Perioperative nurses should ensure that the patient, family, and caregiver understand the instructions, have the opportunity to demonstrate a requisite skill if that is part of home care and convalescence, and have time to ask questions and address concerns. A sample of written educational material that might be provided to the orthopedic surgical patient with a cast is presented in the Patient, Family, and Caregiver Education box on page 682.

Surgical Interventions

Allografts and Autografts

Bone grafting using allografts or autografts may be used (1) to fill cavities after removal of large amounts of bone that might result in instability, (2) to fill bony defects, and (3) to promote union of fractures at the time of open reduction. The type of graft used depends on the location of the fracture or defect, the condition of the bone, and the amount of bone loss as a result of injury. Bone grafts may be used for procedures involving revision of joints if there is significant bone loss caused by resorption or mechanical destruction after removal of bone cement.

The bone graft may be the patient's own bone (autogenous in origin and referred to as *autograft*) or bone obtained from a tissue bank (homogeneous in origin and referred to as *allograft*). Autografts are often harvested from the iliac crest, in which there is cortical and cancellous bone. Various harvesting techniques are used. Struts of cortical bone from the iliac crest can be fashioned to the desired shape and used in areas needing structural strength. The amount of cancellous bone is plentiful. It is used to promote bone growth in areas of defect. Local bone graft material may be taken from the site of injury. Allografts are used when bone is not available from the patient because of the lack of sufficient quantity or because a secondary procedure is undesirable for the patient.

Procedural Considerations

Cancellous grafts may be taken from the ilium, olecranon, or distal radius; cortical grafts may be taken from the tibia, fibula, iliac crest, or ribs. When the recipient site of an autogenous graft is diseased, instruments used for the recipient site must be separated from donor graft site instruments. The operating team must change their gowns and gloves to take the bone graft and again follow the procedure to prevent cross-contamination. The team positions the patient to allow exposure to the surgical site. A sandbag may be placed beneath the area for easier access.

The instrumentation for taking a bone graft includes soft tissue instruments and a bone graft set. Grafts may be harvested with hand instruments or power tools such as an oscillating saw. Power tools may be necessary if a uniformly shaped graft is needed to fill a defect. Because hemostasis is sometimes difficult to achieve as a result of the vascular nature of bone, wound drains may be desirable.

Operative Procedure

Harvest of Bone Graft

A cancellous bone graft consists of spongy bone usually taken from the anterior or posterior crest of the ilium. A cortical bone graft, consisting of hard, dense bone, is removed from the crest of the ilium or the tibia. The location of the crest of the ilium is subcutaneous, allowing exposure without difficulty.

1. The surgeon makes an incision along the border of the iliac crest, and strips, elevates, and retracts the muscles on the outer table of the ilium.
2. Strips of the iliac crest can be removed with an osteotome or oscillating saw.
3. A cortical window may also be made in the outer table, and the surgeon may use curettes or gouges to remove cancellous bone chips.
4. The surgeon may insert a drain before closing the wound in layers and applying a pressure dressing.

Electrical Stimulation

The healing process in bone involves several stages (Fig. 20.23). When a bone is damaged, such as during a surgical procedure or fracture, bleeding occurs. The amount of extravasated blood depends on the vascularity of the fracture site. The blood exudate infiltrates the surrounding area, where a clot is formed. Fibroblasts invade the hematoma and form a fibrin meshwork.

As osteoblasts invade the fibrin meshwork, blood vessels develop to build collagen. After several days, calcium deposits may form in the granulation tissue. These deposits eventually form new bone, known as *callus*. Within the callus, cartilage cells develop a temporary semirigid tissue that helps stabilize the bone fragments. The callus is immature bone that is remodeled by new connective tissue cells

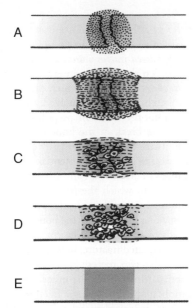

FIG. 20.23 Bone-healing process. (A) Hematoma formation. (B) Fibrin network formation. (C) Invasion of osteoblasts. (D) Callus formation. (E) Remodeling.

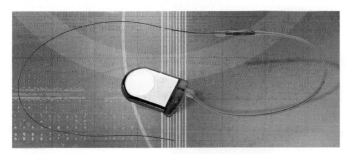

FIG. 20.24 Bone-growth stimulator used after procedures to induce bone formation.

(osteoblasts) of the periosteum and the inner membrane of the bone cavity. Through this process, mature bone is formed, excess callus is resorbed, and trabecular bone is placed.

After several months, depending on the age and physical condition of the individual, the bone becomes firmly united, although the ossification process is not yet completed. Complete union of the fractured bone or joint is determined by means of clinical and radiologic examination.

Healing of bone is classified by degree. *Delayed union* signifies that healing has not occurred within the average time. The average time depends on many factors, and delayed unions must not be considered nonunion until the healing process has ceased without bony union. *Malunion* signifies that the fracture has united with deformity sufficient to cause impairment of the function or a significant angulation of the extremity. *Nonunion* signifies that the process of healing has ended without producing bony union; in this case, electrical stimulation may be used.

Electrical stimulation is artificially applied electrical current that induces or influences the formation of new bone. Various types of stimulators (Fig. 20.24) are available for treatment of nonunion, including invasive (implantable), semi-invasive (percutaneous), and noninvasive (capacitance coupling). The bone stimulator of choice depends on the patient, pathologic condition, and the physician's comfort with the device.

The bone-growth stimulator is used in patients with high risk of nonunion. It can be used to provide electrical stimulation for treatment of nonunion, delayed union, congenital pseudarthrosis, and bone defects. It may be used with or without internal fixation devices, external fixation devices, or bone grafting. Patients who have undergone previous surgery, who have sustained significant tissue loss, or in whom bone grafting is contraindicated are candidates. Electrical stimulation requires long periods of immobilization of the site. This prolonged immobilization may impede rehabilitation.

Procedural Considerations

Instructions for implanting and components selected vary according to the type. The position of the patient depends on the implant site.

In addition to the implant of the surgeon's choice and the implant-specific instrumentation, a soft tissue set is used. Curettes, osteotomes, or bone rasps are used for bony debridement and to scarify the donor bed. Power drills with drill bits may be necessary to create access through the bone for the electrical leads.

Operative Procedure

1. The surgeon exposes the site and debrides it as necessary.
2. A bone slot is fashioned, spanning the nonunion site.
3. The surgeon makes a second incision about 8 to 10 cm from the first one and dissects the tissue. Before the generator is implanted, hemostasis must be achieved. The use of electrosurgical equipment may interfere with function of the bone-growth stimulator.
4. Using blunt or sharp dissection, the surgeon creates a subcutaneous channel for the cathode.
5. The surgeon guides the long cathode lead through the channel.
6. The generator is carefully implanted near the skin surface. The generator should be inserted into soft tissue, not against bone or metal fixation devices; it should not create a bulge beneath the skin.
7. The surgeon places the electrical coils in the prepared bone slot in equal lengths above and below the fracture site.
8. Cancellous bone grafts are placed between the coils if large bony defects are being treated.
9. Routine closure of the subcutaneous and skin tissue is performed.

After union has occurred (5–6 months), the surgeon removes the generator, usually under local anesthesia.

Fractures and Dislocations

A fracture is a break in the continuity of a bone. The care of fractured bones or dislocation of a joint is complicated when there is trauma to the soft tissues, including muscles, nerves, ligaments, and blood vessels. Bone diseases, which can increase the risk of a fracture, can be metabolic, infectious, or degenerative. Metabolic diseases are disorders of bone remodeling. The most common are osteoporosis, osteomalacia, and Paget disease, all of which may result in bone fractures. The most common infectious process is osteomyelitis. Degenerative musculoskeletal conditions are associated with aging. Osteoarthritis is the most common degenerative change.

Osteoporosis is one of the most common and serious of bone diseases and is responsible for more than 2 million fractures a year. Osteoporosis-related fractures most commonly occur in the hip, spine, and wrist, but any bone can be affected. About one in two women and one in four men older than age 50 will break a bone because of osteoporosis (NOF, 2016).

Osteoporosis is characterized by excessive loss of calcified matrix, bone mineral, and collagenous fibers, causing a reduction of total bone mass. Decreasing levels of estrogen and testosterone in the older adult result in reduced new bone growth and maintenance of existing bone. Inadequate intake of calcium or vitamin D; lack of weight-bearing activities, exercise, and physical activity; smoking; and caffeine intake are other contributing factors. Osteoporotic bone is porous, brittle, and fragile, fracturing easily under stress. This results in susceptibility to spontaneous fractures and pathologic curvature of the spine.

Osteomalacia is a metabolic bone disease characterized by inadequate mineralization of bone as a result of vitamin D deficiency, which leads to a reduced absorption of calcium and phosphorus. Risk factors for development of osteomalacia include malabsorption problems, vitamin D and calcium deficiencies, chronic renal failure, and inadequate exposure to sunlight. Medical treatment includes dietary supplements and exposure to sunlight.

Paget disease is a bone disorder affecting older adults. It is characterized by proliferation of osteoclasts and compensatory increased osteoblastic activity, resulting in rapid, disorganized bone remodeling. The bones are weak and poorly constructed.

Types of Fractures

Fractures are classified into two main groups: (1) closed and (2) open or compound. *Closed fractures* are those in which there is no communication between the bone fragments and the skin surface. *Incomplete closed fractures* are those in which the entire thickness of the bone is not broken but is bent or buckled, such as in greenstick fractures, which commonly occur in prepubertal children. *Open fractures* exist when the break in the bone communicates with a wound in the skin. These fractures are usually considered contaminated, requiring measures to control potential infection.

The many varieties of fracture architecture (Fig. 20.25) include (1) transverse fracture, in which the fracture line runs at a right angle to the longitudinal axis of the bone; (2) longitudinal and spiral fractures, which run along the length of the bone; (3) oblique fracture in which bone is twisted apart (similar except that oblique is shorter than spiral); (4) comminuted fracture, in which the bone fragments splinter into more than two pieces; (5) compression fracture, in which one fragment is driven into the other end and is relatively fixed in that position; and (6) pathologic fracture, in which a bone fractures easily because it is weakened by disease. A fracture in the

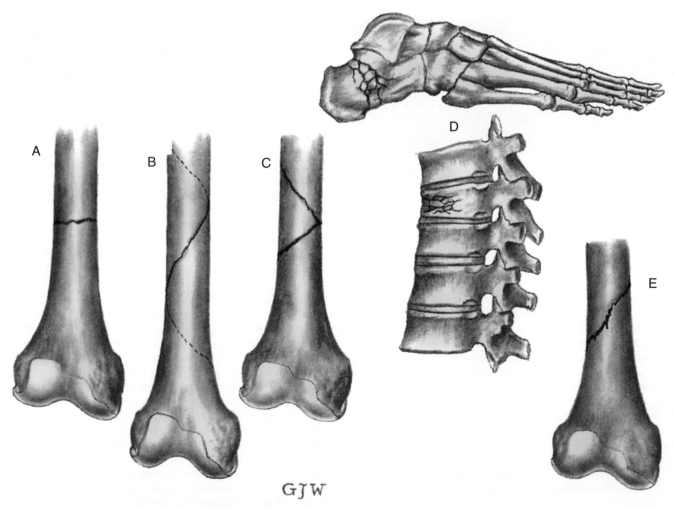

GJW

FIG. 20.25 Fracture types, which may be open or closed. (A) Transverse. (B) Longitudinal or spiral. (C) Comminuted. (D) Compression. (E) Oblique.

shaft of a long bone is described as being in the proximal, middle, or distal third or at the junction of one of these two divisions. A fracture of one of the bony prominences of the end of a long bone is described as a fracture of that prominence by name. Examples include a fracture of the olecranon, medial malleolus, or lateral condyle of the femur.

An epiphyseal separation occurs when a fracture passes through or lies within the growth plate of a bone. When this occurs in a child with immature bone, impediment to limb length and growth may occur. These injuries require immediate and expert treatment.

An avulsion fracture results in a ligamentous attachment remaining intact on a separated bone fragment. This may occur after joint dislocation or rotational injury, such as the femoral condyle separating from the tibial plateau. A dislocation (luxation) is a complete displacement of one articular surface from another. This injury can disrupt neurovascular structures, requiring immediate attention. A subluxation is a partial dislocation, often indicated by ligamentous instability.

Principles of Fracture Treatment

The purpose of fracture treatment is to reestablish the length, shape, and alignment of the fractured bones or joints and restore anatomic function. Acute fracture treatment is necessary to alleviate neurovascular compromise. The surgical team should consider the following principles when providing care for the patient: (1) the patient's extremity or fracture site must be handled gently, (2) initial general medical treatment must be provided, (3) equipment and personnel must be readily available to treat impending or existing shock and to control hemorrhage, (4) aseptic technique must be maintained, (5) positioning must allow adequate circulatory and respiratory function with adequate exposure, and (6) patient comfort must be considered.

The primary goal in treatment of an upper extremity fracture is to preserve mobility and restore range of motion, enabling the individual to perform skilled and delicate work. In fractures of a lower extremity, the objectives of surgery are to restore alignment and length and provide stability of the extremity for weight bearing.

In the presence of open fractures involving soft tissues, several associated conditions may arise, including (1) secondary hemorrhage, (2) infection, (3) severe damage to soft tissues, (4) damage to blood vessels and nerves, and (5) Volkmann contracture (ischemic paralysis).

Basic Treatment Techniques

Closed Reduction

The surgeon may treat fractures with closed reduction (manipulating the fragments into position without incising the skin). When possible this is the treatment of choice because it decreases the opportunity for infection, improves results (including bone union of the fracture), and minimizes the recovery period. Significant bone comminution, periosteal damage, or soft tissue entrapped within the fracture site may result in complications.

Procedural Considerations. The choice of anesthesia depends on the site of fracture and the patient's condition. A closed reduction can be performed with (1) infiltration of local anesthetic agent into the fracture site (hematoma block), (2) IV regional anesthesia (Bier block), (3) regional or spinal nerve block, or (4) general anesthesia. Closed reduction may take place before an open procedure to reduce the fracture site. Skeletal traction may also be applied to the fracture site, requiring a surgical skin prep and application of drapes. The perioperative nurse consults with the surgeon to determine the appropriate casting or brace materials and makes certain they are

readily available to prevent loss of fracture reduction. Instrumentation and supplies should be available in the event it is necessary to open the fracture site and apply fixation.

Operative Procedure
1. The surgeon uses manual traction to manipulate the fragments into alignment.
2. Reduction is confirmed using radiography (x-ray or fluoroscopy).
3. After reducing the fracture the surgeon immobilizes it with casting material or bracing techniques.

External Fixation

External fixation of fractures provides rigid fixation and reduction with the ability to manage severe soft tissue wounds. Because of the increased chance of infection in patients with an open fracture, external fixation is often the preferred treatment. Advantages of external fixation include the absence of casting material, fracture stabilization at a distance from the injury site, ability to perform subsequent procedures such as skin grafts or vascularized grafts, minimal joint interference, early mobilization, and the ability to use internal fixation or other skeleton-fixation devices at the same time or sequentially.

Indications for external fixation include the following: (1) severe open fractures, (2) highly comminuted closed fractures, (3) arthrodesis, (4) infected joints, (5) infected nonunion, (6) fracture stabilization to protect arterial or nerve anastomoses, (7) major alignment and length deficits, (8) congenital deformities, and (9) static contractures. External fixation provides a bridge between fracture reduction and insertion of an internal fixator such as an IM nail, allowing time for vascular recovery. Internal fixation can take place at a later date.

Many improvements have been made in the design and articulations of external fixation devices. The fixators can be applied to most anatomic sites. The available external fixators vary greatly in design; however, all contain three main components: (1) bone-anchoring devices (threaded pins, Kirschner wires), (2) longitudinal supporting devices (threaded or smooth rods), and (3) connecting elements (clamps and partial or full rings). Improvements have resulted in the use of lightweight and stronger materials, which are radiopaque, for use as connecting rods. The radiopaque feature prevents postoperative radiographic interference when viewing the fracture site for progress in healing.

The Ilizarov device uses principles of tension-stress and distraction to correct bone defects and limb-length discrepancies. It is not routinely used for acute fracture fixation; however, the principles and technique are similar. Limb length may be adjusted with gradual bone distraction of bone ends, stimulating new bone formation.

Procedural Considerations. External fixators are applied using sterile technique after the patient has been administered a general or regional anesthetic. Radiographic imaging ensures fracture reduction after closed manipulation; it also ensures proper pin placement. Because the incision site is small to allow introduction of pins, a soft tissue set appropriate to the site will be necessary. Many different external fixators are available for use. Some examples are shown in Figs. 20.26 and 20.27. Irrigation and debridement at the fracture site and surrounding soft tissue may be necessary if soft tissue is damaged, so pulsatile lavage with 3000 mL of normal saline solution should be available. The surgeon will use a power drill at the pin sites and a periosteal elevator if necessary for blunt or sharp dissection. An appropriate-size pin cutter should also be available to shorten the pins if the need arises. The dressing consists of an antibacterial ointment, antibiotic-impregnated gauze, or nonadherent gauze with gauze overwrap.

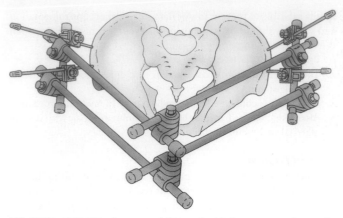

FIG. 20.26 AO/ASIF pelvic external fixator, double frame using tube-to-tube clamps.

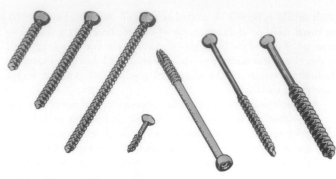

FIG. 20.28 Types of screws used for fixation with or without plating systems.

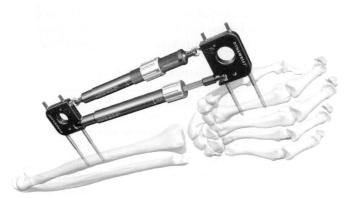

FIG. 20.27 Dynawrist dynamic wrist external fixator.

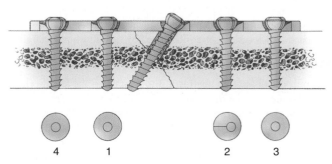

FIG. 20.29 Plating a closed forearm fracture using dynamic compression showing final position of the screw insertion.

Operative Procedure

1. The fracture is reduced manually.
2. The surgeon incises the skin.
3. Using a periosteal elevator, the surgeon dissects the periosteum from the bone if necessary.
4. The surgeon predrills the cortex, using a drill sheath to protect surrounding soft tissue.
5. Hand drilling or low-speed power drilling is used to insert the half-pins above and below the fracture.
6. Universal joints are slipped over the pins and joined with a connecting rod.
7. The surgeon tightens the frame using the appropriate wrenches.
8. Radiography or fluoroscopy is used to confirm reduction and alignment.
9. Dressings are applied to the pin sites.

Internal Fixation

Internal fixation is often the treatment of choice for correction of fractures of long bones or those in the hip region. Application of compression plates and screws and insertion of pins, IM rods, nails, or wiring are methods of internal fixation. Fractures of most anatomic parts in adults can be repaired using internal fixation.

Many principles and techniques apply when using internal fixation. Types of screws (Fig. 20.28) include cortical, cancellous, lag, pre-tapped, and self-tapping. Cortical bone screws have threads that are closer together and narrower than other types of threads. These threads run along the entire length of the screw and transfix bone, gaining purchase (grab) of bone cortex.

Cancellous bone screws feature threads that are broader and farther apart than those of cortical screws. Cancellous screws are used in cancellous bone, which is less dense than cortical bone; the bone accumulates within the threads to provide the purchase for fixation. Like cortical screws, cancellous screws can traverse fracture sites and hold plates onto bone. The screw threads do not completely traverse the bone through the opposite cortex. Cancellous screws are commonly used when fractures occur at the condylar ends of the shaft.

Plating of a fracture may occur with or without dynamic compression (Fig. 20.29). Dynamic compression uses screw and plate configurations to apply forces through the fracture site. Semitubular plates are less rigid and do not have the ability to produce dynamic compression. This type of plate is used in the forearm and fibula, where weight bearing, which could break the plate, is not a factor.

Closed Reduction With Percutaneous Pinning. The surgeon may reduce fractures using closed reduction methods of manipulation and traction combined with percutaneous insertion of pins, IM nails, or rods. Pins can be placed percutaneously (Fig. 20.30) to fix fractures involving the digits, wrist, elbow, and foot. A rod or nail is placed percutaneously (Fig. 20.31) in a large bone such as the humerus or femur. Closed reduction is, however, a misnomer because small openings in the soft tissue and bone are made to facilitate introduction of the devices. These incisions are considerably smaller than those created when repairing the fracture using open reduction. The advantages of closed reduction over open reduction and internal fixation (ORIF) are (1) a lower incidence of infection and (2) absence of additional soft tissue or vascular damage.

Open Reduction and Internal Fixation. ORIF provides exposure of the fracture site and uses pins, wire, screws, a plate and screw combination, rods, or nails to correct the fracture (Fig. 20.32). Surgeons use ORIF when they are unable to reduce a fracture by closed methods and skeletal traction is not indicated. The advantage

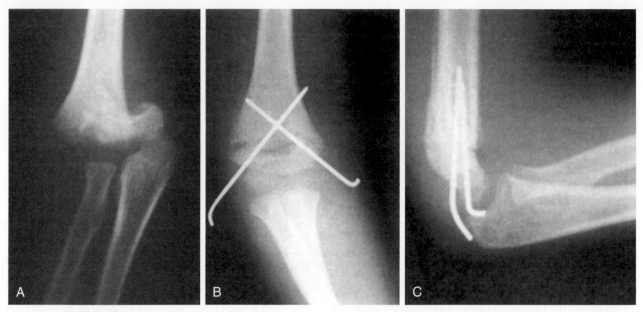

FIG. 20.30 Percutaneous pinning of a supracondylar fracture. (A) Severely displaced supracondylar fracture. (B and C) Treated by closed reduction and percutaneous pinning.

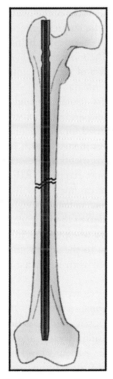

FIG. 20.31 Rod placement for femoral fracture.

is that anatomic alignment of the fracture can usually be obtained and verified through direct observation. Fractures that are comminuted or difficult to reduce can be more effectively treated using this technique. The incidence of infection and nonunion, however, is increased when the wound is opened.

The procedure varies for each anatomic site, using the principles for specific fixation devices. Several procedures described in the text

identify steps for completion of ORIF. Reference examples include the following:

- *Pin fixation:* Application of a unilateral frame
- *Wire fixation:* Reduction of patellar fracture, tension banding of the olecranon
- *Screw fixation:* Correction of scaphoid fractures
- *Plate and screw fixation:* Repair of a comminuted distal humeral fracture
- *Rod or nail fixation:* Correction of fractures of the shaft of the humerus, femoral shaft, or tibial shaft

Surgery of the Shoulder

Correction of Acromioclavicular Joint Separation

AC joint separation (Fig. 20.33), a common occupational and athletic injury, results from a force applied downward, most commonly from a fall, directly to the top of the shoulder. The ligamentous support of the distal clavicle in the form of the coracoclavicular, coracoacromial, and AC ligaments is disrupted. The result is either a posterior or a superior displacement of the lateral end of the clavicle.

The purpose of surgery in an acutely injured patient is to reestablish the proper relationship between the clavicle and the acromion, reducing long-term shoulder pain and increasing function. This is accomplished by replacing the coracoclavicular ligaments with heavy suture or Mersilene tape or by inserting a screw through the clavicle and into the coracoid process. It may also be necessary to stabilize the AC joint by placing a smooth Steinmann pin across the acromion and into the clavicle. Sometimes the distal end of the clavicle is also resected. If resection of the clavicle is the only treatment required, this may be completed arthroscopically. Shoulder arthroscopy is detailed in the Arthroscopy of the Shoulder section of Arthroscopy, page 745.

Procedural Considerations

The perioperative nurse assists in placing the patient in the supine or semi-sitting position with a sandbag or folded sheet under the

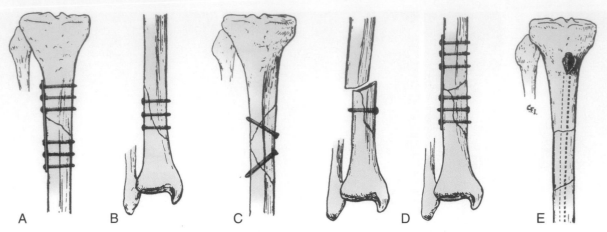

FIG. 20.32 Types of internal fixation for fracture repair. (A) Plate and screws for transverse or short oblique fracture. (B) Transfixion screws for long oblique or spiral fractures. (C) Transfixion screws for long butterfly fragment. (D) Fixation for short butterfly fragment. (E) Medullary fixation.

affected shoulder. The patient's shoulder is positioned slightly off the OR bed (Fig. 20.34) to allow full range of motion, or if mobility of the arm is unnecessary, a shoulder positioner is used. The head is turned to the opposite side, taking care not to overstretch the nerves of the brachial plexus. The scrub person assists with draping the patient's arm with a stockinette to the midhumeral level.

A soft tissue set and bone instrumentation specific for the shoulder are required. Depending on the technique used, bone screws and their instrumentation, free-cutting needles, bone-anchoring devices, and power instruments may be necessary.

Operative Procedure
Coracoclavicular Suture Fixation

1. A curved incision is made to expose the AC joint, the distal end of the clavicle, and the coracoid process.
2. The surgeon exposes the AC joint and removes any loose fragments or debris.
3. Mattress sutures are placed in the ruptured coracoclavicular ligaments but not tied.
4. The surgeon places drill holes in the clavicle above the coracoid in the anteroposterior (AP) plane.
5. A #5 nonabsorbable suture is placed beneath the base of the coracoid and superiorly through the two holes in the clavicle. With the joint reduced, the sutures are tied.
6. If instability is still a concern, the surgeon places small Kirschner wires across the AC joint, through the lateral border of the acromion. The ends of the wires are bent 90 degrees at the lateral border to prevent proximal migration.
7. The surgeon ties the sutures previously placed in the coracoclavicular ligaments.
8. The AC joint capsule and the origins of the deltoid and trapezius muscles are repaired.
9. A sling-and-swathe bandage is then applied to the extremity.

Correction of Sternoclavicular Dislocation

Traumatic dislocation of the sternoclavicular joint usually occurs from an indirect blow on the anterior shoulder while the arm is abducted. The clavicle most frequently is displaced anteriorly, but posterior or retrosternal dislocations can occur. Posterior dislocation can be more severe because injury to the trachea, esophagus, thoracic duct, and large vessels of the mediastinum is possible.

Except in severe cases, dislocation of the sternoclavicular joint is treated nonoperatively with manual traction and immobilization bandages.

Clavicular Fracture

Fractures of the clavicle are some of the most common bony injuries. These injuries rarely require surgical intervention. The majority of clavicular fractures are the result of an indirect or direct blow on the clavicle or shoulder. The most common site of clavicular fractures is the middle-third portion of the bone, mainly at the middle- and outer-third junction.

Clavicular fractures are usually treated by immobilization in a figure-of-eight splint. The chances of nonunion are greatly increased when open reduction is used for a clavicular fracture. The outcome may result in a bony prominence, which may be disturbing to the patient; the overriding fragments are resorbed with time.

Clavicular fractures may require ORIF after nonunion, neurovascular compromise that cannot be resolved with reduction, distal clavicular fracture with torn coracoclavicular ligaments in the adult, or persistent wide separation of the fragments with soft tissue entrapment. Surgery is necessary when the fracture is displaced enough to cause underlying damage to the vessels and brachial plexus. Open reduction is accomplished with a tubular plate and screws or IM pin fixation.

Procedural Considerations

The perioperative nurse assists with positioning the patient in the supine or semi-sitting position with a sandbag or folded sheet under the affected shoulder. The patient's head is turned to the opposite side, and care is taken to not stretch the nerves of the brachial plexus. The scrub person assists the surgeon with draping the entire extremity after it is prepped. Soft tissue instruments and bone instruments are used for dissection. Bone-reduction forceps and clamps are used to obtain reduction, and Kirschner wires may be used to temporarily hold the reduction. Permanent reduction is held with either Steinmann pins or plate and screws. A power drill is necessary to apply these. In the case of a nonunion, bone grafting is used.

Operative Procedure

1. The surgeon makes a 2.5-cm incision over the fracture site. The incision may need to be extended for comminuted fractures.

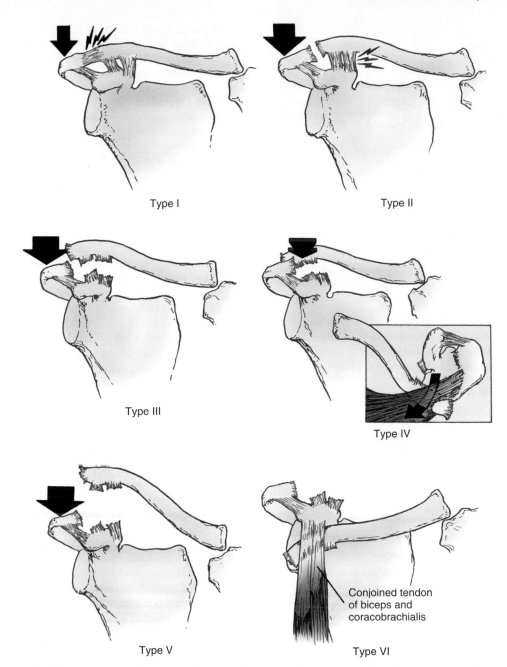

Type I   Type II

Type III   Type IV

Type V   Type VI

Conjoined tendon
of biceps and
coracobrachialis

FIG. 20.33 Classification of acromioclavicular injuries. *Type I,* Neither acromioclavicular nor coracoclavicular ligaments are disrupted. *Type II,* Acromioclavicular ligament is disrupted, and coracoclavicular ligament is intact. *Type III,* Both ligaments are disrupted. *Type IV,* Ligaments are disrupted, and distal end of clavicle is displaced posteriorly into or through trapezius muscle. *Type V,* Ligaments and muscle attachments are disrupted, and clavicle and acromion are widely separated. *Type VI,* Ligaments are disrupted, and distal clavicle is dislocated inferior to coracoid process and posterior to biceps and coracobrachialis tendons.

2. Dissection is carried down to the clavicle, taking care not to strip periosteum or disrupt vessels or nerves.
3. The surgeon exposes the fracture site and reduces the fracture with bone-holding forceps.
4. If pinning the clavicle is to be done, a Steinmann pin is passed into the medial fragment medullary canal and removed.
5. The pin is then passed in the same manner into the distal fragment.

6. The surgeon reduces the fracture again and uses a threaded Steinmann pin across the fracture site through both fragments to transfix it.
7. If plating the clavicle is to be done, a small semitubular plate is used with at least two screw holes on each side of the fracture site.
8. The surgeon strips a small portion of the periosteum from the clavicle so that a plate can be applied to the anterior surface.

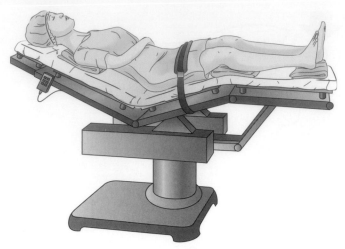

FIG. 20.34 Positioning for a surgical procedure on the shoulder with the patient in a semi-sitting position and support beneath the affected shoulder.

9. Extreme care must be taken when drilling screw holes to avoid damage to the subclavian vein and thoracic contents.
10. After closure, an immobilization sling is applied.

Correction of Rotator Cuff Tear

Most rotator cuff tears occur through the insertion of the tendinous fibers of the supraspinatus muscle that attaches onto the greater tuberosity of the proximal humerus. In severe tears the remaining tendons of the cuff, the subscapularis, infraspinatus, and teres minor, may also be involved. Supraspinatus syndrome, also known as *impingement syndrome,* can involve multiple pathologic conditions, such as calcium deposits, bicipital tendinitis, subacromial bursitis, tenosynovitis, and other nonarticular lesions along with a cuff tear. The approach to diagnosis and treatment is similar for both partial and complete rotator cuff tears.

Partial rotator cuff tears and impingement usually affect people in the middle decades of life or later and are often attributable to a long-term degenerative process. Complete tears of the rotator cuff may occur after accidental injury to younger patients, such as baseball pitchers and football quarterbacks. Patients with rotator cuff tears may not be able to initiate abduction of the shoulder because the stabilizing forces of the ruptured tendons on the humeral head are lost. Many rotator cuff tears can be treated conservatively with physical therapy and nonsteroidal antiinflammatory drugs (NSAIDs).

A variety of procedures may be performed for these conditions when conservative treatment is unsuccessful. Methods of repair depend on the size and shape of the tear. The common goal is to restore joint stability, alleviate pain, and allow the patient to return to normal activities. In some instances a significant reduction in preinjury activity may be permanent.

Procedural Considerations

The perioperative nurse assists the surgeon in positioning the patient in the supine or semi-sitting position with a sandbag or folded towel under the affected shoulder. The patient's head is gently turned to the opposite side, taking care to avoid undue stretch to the brachial plexus. A shoulder positioner can be used if intraoperative mobility of the arm is not a factor. In addition to a bone set and a soft tissue set, shoulder instruments are required. The remaining equipment needs depend on the severity of the tear. Minor tears may require

no more than heavy nonabsorbable suture. Major tears require a power drill and burr and possibly a microsagittal saw. Fixation may be gained with bone-anchoring devices. Free needles will be necessary if bone-anchoring devices are used.

Operative Procedure

1. The surgeon makes an anterosuperior deltoid incision and divides the coracoacromial ligament at the acromial attachment.
2. A subacromioplasty (resection of the undersurface of the acromion) is completed. This is also the primary treatment for impingement syndrome.
3. Small, simple tears can be repaired by suturing the torn edges with heavy nonabsorbable sutures.
4. Massive tears may require attaching the torn edges to the greater tuberosity using bone-anchoring devices.
5. If the defect cannot be bridged, the surgeon may transpose a flap from the subscapularis tendon and suture it to the supraspinatus and infraspinatus muscles.
6. If impingement is involved or solely the cause of a rotator pathologic condition, other measures involving the same approach are taken.
7. The surgeon excises any calcium deposits encased in the tendon to alleviate mechanical obstruction or performs an acromioplasty.
8. After closure, a sling is applied.

Patients with small tears may begin motion on the third to fourth postoperative day. Larger tears may require immobilization for 2 to 8 weeks.

Correction of Recurrent Anterior Dislocation of the Shoulder

The anterior fibers of the shoulder capsule become stretched and weakened as a result of frequent dislocations of the shoulder joint. The goals of surgical repair are to (1) prevent recurrence, (2) prevent surgical complications, (3) prevent creation of arthritic changes, (4) maintain joint motion, and (5) correct the problem. The surgeon selects the procedure appropriate for the patient's condition that will satisfy the conditions necessary to correct the problem.

Procedural Considerations

The surgeon and perioperative nurse place the patient in the supine or semi-sitting position with a sandbag or folded sheet under the shoulder. The patient's arm is draped free so that the extremity can be manipulated. The surgeon makes an anterior curved incision or a longitudinal incision in the anterior axillary fold over the shoulder joint, depending on the location of the tear and procedure planned. A soft tissue set and a bone set are required, as well as a set of instruments specific to shoulder surgery, power drill and burr, bone-anchoring devices, and free needles.

Operative Procedure

Bankart Procedure. For the Bankart procedure (Fig. 20.35), the scapula is not elevated with a sandbag or folded sheet. The surgeon reattaches the attenuated anterior capsule to the rim of the glenoid fossa with heavy sutures. The glenoid fossa rim is decorticated with a curette to provide a raw surface to which the capsule is attached. Special instruments designed for the Bankart procedure, such as a curved awl and humeral head retractor, facilitate the surgery, although the capsule may be attached with bone anchors, obviating the use of the awl. If the coracoid process is to be removed to obtain better operative exposure, a drill, bone screws, and washers should be available for reattachment. Postoperatively the extremity is immobilized

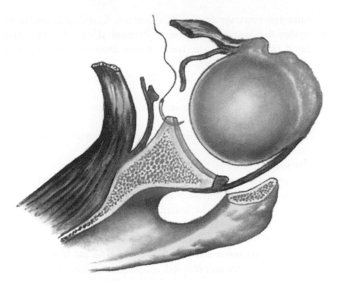

FIG. 20.35 Bankart procedure for restoration of shoulder stability. Holes are made in the rim of the glenoid, and the free lateral margin of the capsule is sutured to the rim of the glenoid. The medial margin of the capsule is sutured to the lateral surface.

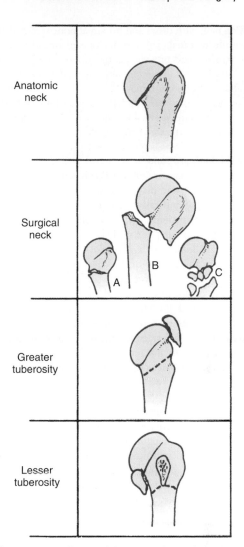

FIG. 20.36 Fractures and fracture-dislocations relate to the pattern of displacement. Fractures can occur in two, three, or four parts.

in a sling or shoulder immobilizer. Shoulder motion is begun 3 days postoperatively, and the patient may return to contact sports or heavy labor after approximately 6 months.

Putti–Platt Procedure. The steps of the Putti–Platt procedure are similar to those of the Bankart procedure in that the joint capsule is sutured to the glenoid rim. In addition, the Putti–Platt procedure requires the lateral advancement of the subscapularis. This produces a barrier against dislocation of the shoulder. This procedure is rarely useful when the anterior capsular mechanism is of poor quality.

The surgeon divides the subscapularis tendon 2.5 cm medially to its insertion. The glenoid and humeral head are inspected using palpation to assess osteochondral changes. The lateral portion of the subscapularis is sutured to the anterior glenoid rim. The medial portion of the subscapularis is sutured to the rotator cuff at the greater tuberosity. The layers of the shoulder joint are imbricated (overlapped); this technique is used often in soft tissue reconstruction. The incision is closed, and a shoulder immobilizer is applied. The immobilizer is worn for approximately 3 weeks. External rotation of the arm should be avoided immediately after the repair.

Bristow Procedure. In the Bristow procedure the coracoid process, along with the attached muscles, is detached and inserted onto the neck of the glenoid cavity, where it is attached with a screw through the subscapularis muscle. This stabilizes the anterior joint capsule and prevents recurrent dislocation. A Bristow procedure is considered an appropriate alternative when the anterior capsular mechanism is of poor quality. Disadvantages of this procedure are (1) internal rotation contracture, (2) inattention to labrum or capsule disorders, (3) potential for injury to the musculocutaneous nerve, (4) reduction of internal rotation power by shortening of the subscapularis muscle, (5) possible limitation of external rotation, (6) possible penetration of the screw into the articular surface of the glenoid, and (7) later development of early joint disease of the shoulder.

Correction of Humeral Head Fracture

Comminuted fractures of the humeral head (Fig. 20.36) with displacement may require ORIF with screws or pins or closed reduction

with a humeral nail or rod. However, if the fracture is badly comminuted, a prosthetic replacement is indicated. Traumatic or degenerative arthritic shoulder joints may be so painful or dysfunctional that a total shoulder joint replacement is necessary.

Extensive rehabilitation for the shoulder is required. Surgery should be performed as soon as possible because delay can allow time for increasing scar formation, contracture of the muscles, and increasing osteoporosis of the bone fragments. The shoulder is the most difficult joint in the body to rehabilitate because it has (1) the greatest range of motion, (2) a second space beneath the acromion that must be mobilized, and (3) many muscles that enter into complex movements.

Surgery of the Humerus, Radius, and Ulna

Fractures of the Humeral Shaft

Closed manipulation and immobilization usually reduce a fractured humerus as well as minimize the risk of nonunion and infection. When closed reduction is impossible or when nonunion of the fracture has occurred, surgery is indicated. The fracture is reduced and held with IM fixation, a compression plate, a lag screw, or a rigid locking nail, with distal and proximal bone screws that transfix the rod within the canal. This last device can control rotation of the fracture fragments and prevent distraction at the fracture site (Fig. 20.37). Multiple flexible nails may be used if more rigid nails are not available. A bone graft may be used, depending on both the extent of the fracture and the length of time since injury. Compression plating of shaft fractures is usually reserved for supracondylar involvement or when other treatment has failed.

Procedural Considerations

Fluoroscopy and permanent radiographs are required to ensure proper alignment, reduction, and placement of implants. The perioperative nurse arranges for intraoperative radiology support and a radiolucent OR bed before the patient's arrival in the OR suite. The surgeon and nurse position the patient supine with the body near the edge of the bed to facilitate moving the arm. The extremity is prepped and draped from the middle of the chest to below the elbow.

A soft tissue set and a large bone set are required. In addition, the IM fixation device of choice and the required instruments for its insertion are needed. PMMA may be used in the case of pathologic fractures. Instruments that are required for harvesting bone graft might be needed as well. A traction tray may be used to gain reduction. A power drill is necessary if screws are used to lock the device. Sterile x-ray cassette covers are needed for permanent intraoperative films.

Operative Procedure

Medullary Fixation: Antegrade Technique

1. Proper length and alignment of the fracture must be attained with traction. Nail length should ensure proximal burying to avoid subacromial impingement and be 1 to 2 cm proximal to the olecranon fossa. The surgeon makes a skin incision from the lateral point of the acromion over the tip of the greater tuberosity. The fascia is incised, and the greater tuberosity is palpated.

2. Using a small awl, the surgeon enters the greater tuberosity and confirms placement with fluoroscopy in both AP and lateral views.

3. The surgeon removes the awl and inserts a ball-nosed reamer guidewire, advancing it down the medullary canal (periodically verified with fluoroscopy). Confirmation is made with each step to ensure that the wires, reamers, or implant has not fractured through the cortex along the shaft.

4. The guidewire is advanced to within 1 to 2 cm of the olecranon fossa, avoiding distraction or shortening.

5. If Enders nails are used, each one is advanced in the same fashion as the guidewire.

6. Nail length can be determined by using a second guidewire of the same length held against what remains extended from the humerus. The difference between the length protruding and the length remaining on the second rod is the approximate length requirement of the humeral nail. Another method uses a nail-length gauge that is held directly against the upper arm, viewed with fluoroscopy, and read directly on the gauge.

7. Enders nails may be held directly against the arm and viewed with fluoroscopy to determine proper length. If Enders nails are used, the surgeon drives two or three nails down the shaft, across the fracture site, and into the distal fragment. Fluoroscopy is used to confirm proper placement and reduction.

8. If IM nailing is to be accomplished, the surgeon may use a cannulated reamer over the guidewire to ream the humerus. Reaming of the canal is completed in 0.5-mm increments. The

humerus becomes smaller in diameter. Reaming is gentle to ensure that protrusion through the bone does not occur. The bone is reamed 0.5 to 1 mm larger than the selected nail diameter.

9. The surgeon uses a medullary exchange tube to maintain fracture reduction.

10. The ball-tipped guidewire is replaced with a non–ball-tipped guidewire.

11. The medullary nail is assembled for impaction with the appropriate outrigger and drill guides.

12. The surgeon guides the nail into the proximal end of the humerus and uses the humeral nail driver to impact the nail within the canal. Care must be taken to avoid splitting the humerus or creating a supracondylar fracture by wedging the tip of the nail.

13. As the nail approaches and crosses the fracture site, the surgeon maintains manual reduction.

14. The scrub person attaches the proximal drill guide to the nail impactor with the nail coupled; the surgeon makes a stab wound in the skin and pushes the nail to reach the bone.

15. An 8-mm drill sleeve is inserted through the drill guide, followed by a 2.7-mm drill guide into the first guide.

16. The surgeon scores the cortex with the 2.7-mm trocar, and transfixing of the hole is completed with a 2.7-mm drill from the lateral to distal areas of the cortex.

17. The humeral screw-depth gauge is inserted and read directly to determine the appropriate screw size.

18. A 4-mm fully threaded humeral screw is inserted to the selected length. The surgeon confirms the screw position by inserting a guidewire down the end of the nail, where it is impeded by the transfixing screw.

19. Fluoroscopy is used to target the distal humeral locking screw.

20. The surgeon creates a second percutaneous access from the anterior to posterior cortex of the bone to the bone surface of the humerus.

21. With the freehand technique, the cortex of the bone is scored followed by insertion of the 8-mm handheld drill sleeve and the 2.7-mm drill bit.

22. The selected size of humeral screw is gauged and inserted. Placement is confirmed with fluoroscopy, and the impactor assembly is removed from the nail.

23. Full-view radiographs are obtained in both dimensions, and the wound is irrigated and closed.

NOTE: Many variations of approach and technique are used, depending on the complexity of the fracture and any associated injury. Often the fracture site may have to be opened if it is comminuted or will not reduce properly through closed techniques. The radial nerve or other neurovascular structures may become entrapped or traumatized, requiring exploration and repair.

Although this type of antegrade fixation, using locked rods, is preferred for this type of fracture, it is not the only method. Often a retrograde technique is used, with the patient in the prone or lateral decubitus position. The retrograde technique, used more commonly in the care of femoral shaft fractures, is described on page 708.

Distal Humeral Fractures (Supracondylar, Epicondylar, and Intercondylar)

Distal humeral fractures are classified into several types, depending on location and the presence or absence of articular involvement (Fig. 20.38). Supracondylar fractures of the humerus do not involve the articular surface and can generally be treated with closed reduction

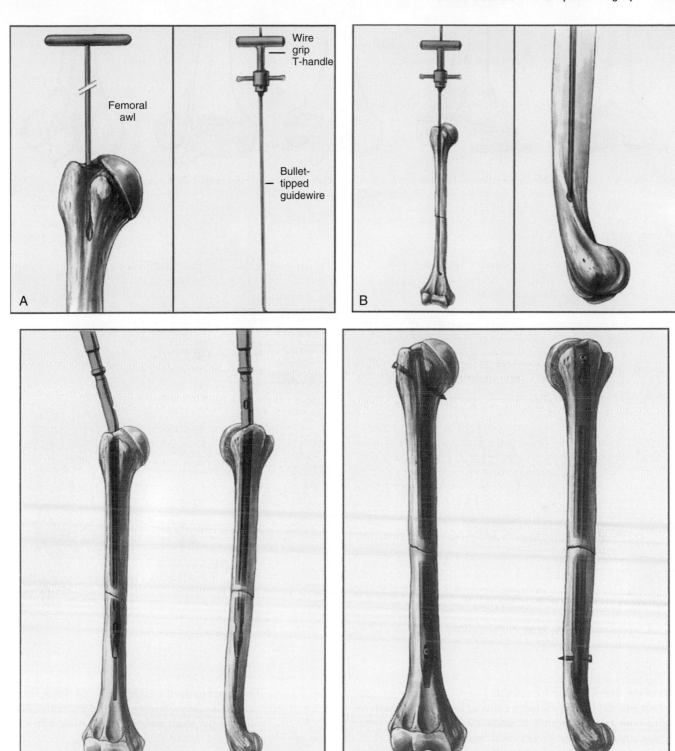

FIG. 20.37 Placement of the humeral rigid locking nail with distal and proximal screws. (A) After incision and exposure, a femoral awl is used to make an entry portal. (B) Guidewire is advanced into the center of the epicondylar region. (C) After reaming, the nail is advanced over the fracture site and seated. (D) Proximal and distal locking takes place after the correct screw placement is determined.

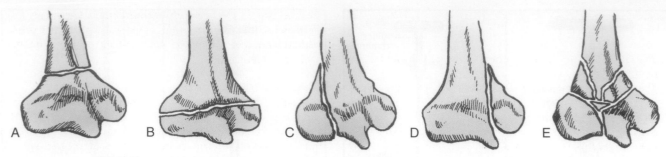

FIG. 20.38 Classification of distal humeral fractures. (A) Supracondylar. (B) Transcondylar. (C) Lateral condyle with trochlea. (D) Medial condyle. (E) Intercondylar with comminution.

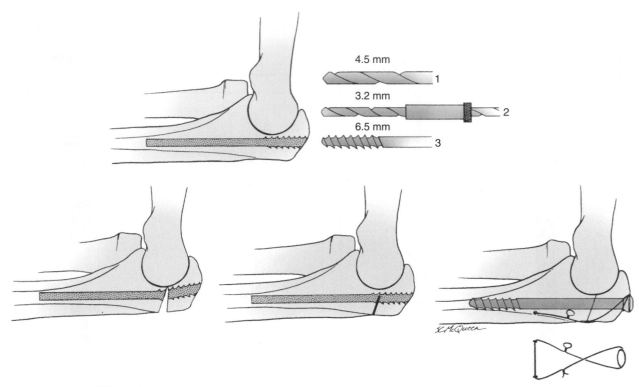

FIG. 20.39 Osteotomy of the olecranon with placement of a lag screw and tension band wire fixation.

and casting. Transcondylar fractures may or may not have articular involvement, and this will dictate treatment. Intercondylar fractures involve both condyles with a comminution of injury, are intra-articular, and present the greatest challenge for the surgical team. Fractures of the articular components (the capitulum and the trochlea) are usually the result of a fall on an outstretched arm. The force drives the radial head to shear off the capitulum, producing an intra-articular fragment. The lateral or medial condyles and epicondyles are also subject to fracture by various mechanisms.

Patients may present with a single isolated fracture or any combination, as previously mentioned. Neurovascular and other soft tissue trauma is considered in selecting the type of reduction and fixation. Screws, pins, a variety of different plates, and dynamic compression technique can be used for internal fixation. Certain fixation techniques of the distal portion of the humerus may require an osteotomy of the olecranon (proximal ulna) to properly align and affix hardware

(Fig. 20.39). The general goals of treating these injuries are to (1) maintain neurovascular integrity, (2) restore normal joint articulation, (3) preserve motion of the joint, and (4) correct other soft tissue injuries.

Procedural Considerations

Regional anesthesia can be used for procedures on the distal end of the humerus. Bone graft harvesting may require use of general anesthesia. The patient may be prone with the elbow flexed over a small table, supine with the arm over the chest, supine with the arm on a hand table, or in the lateral position. A tourniquet is placed before the surgical prep and inflated during surgery as needed.

A soft tissue set, a large bone set, and a bone graft set are needed, in addition to a compression set, bone-holding clamps, reconstruction plates, and smooth Kirschner wires. A power drill and Kirschner wire driver are needed to apply the hardware.

Operative Procedure
Open Reduction and Internal Fixation Comminuted Distal Humeral Fracture

1. The surgeon makes an incision over the distal humeral fracture site (Fig. 20.40).
2. The fracture is exposed and reduced using bone-reduction clamps and temporary small, smooth Kirschner wires, driving them across the fracture site with the power drill.
3. A cancellous bone screw is placed using drill and tap to transfix from one condyle to the other. The surgeon is careful not to violate the joint surface with the threads of the screw.
4. If the reduction is maintained, the surgeon removes the Kirschner wires.
5. A one-third tubular or reconstruction plate is contoured to the shape of the distal humeral fracture and applied to bridge the fracture fragments.
6. Throughout the entire procedure, the articular surface is periodically inspected to ensure integrity. The plates are held in place by hand while the patient's elbow is moved through its range of motion. The plates should not encroach on the olecranon or coronoid fossa (distal end of the ulna) because this limits flexion and extension of the arm.
7. The bone is drilled and tapped from one cortex to the other with the appropriate drill and tap. The screw is inserted and seated to the bone surface on the plate. This is done for all subsequent screws, observing the fracture site and articular surface.
8. Interfragmentary screws may be used in addition to the cortical screws spanning the condyles. If osteotomy of the olecranon was previously done for exposure, it is reattached using the tension band technique with a cancellous bone screw and heavy-gauge (18 or 20 gauge) wire (Fig. 20.41).
9. The surgeon irrigates the wound, places a drain (as needed), and closes the incision. A long arm posterior splint is applied.

Olecranon Fracture

If the olecranon fracture fragment is small, it may be excised and the triceps tendon reattached to the ulnar shaft. This does not result in loss of stability of the elbow joint. However, larger fragments must be reduced and held with internal fixation. Osteotomy of the olecranon is often done electively for surgical exposure (see previous section) and repaired in the same fashion as for a traumatic fracture.

Procedural Considerations

The patient is placed in the prone position with the arm on an armboard or hand table. A soft tissue set, a bone set, AO/ASIF (Swiss Association of Osteosynthesis/Association for the Study of Internal Fixation) instrumentation, heavy stainless steel wire (16 and 18 gauge in long lengths), a wire tightener, Kirschner wires, bone-reduction clamps, a power drill, and Kirschner wire driver are needed.

Operative Procedure
Tension Banding

1. The surgeon makes an incision over the olecranon and exposes the fracture (Fig. 20.42).
2. A drill hole is made in the distal fragment, traversing the bone.

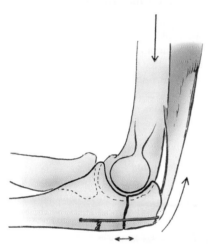

FIG. 20.41 Tension band technique used for repair of the olecranon.

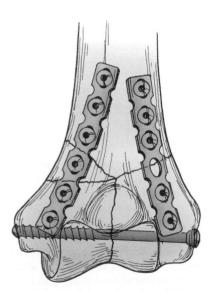

FIG. 20.40 Repair of the comminuted distal humeral fracture with 3.5-mm reconstruction plates.

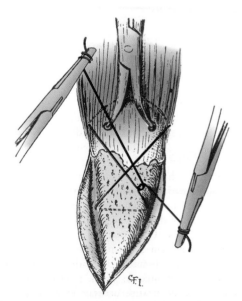

FIG. 20.42 Operative procedure: tension banding with stainless steel wire passed through drill holes; figure-of-eight adds stability to the fracture.

3. Stainless steel wire is passed through the drilled holes, crossed over, and pulled toward the tip of the olecranon.
4. After using the drill and tap, the surgeon uses a cancellous bone screw to attach the proximal fragment to the distal fragment, stopping short of totally seating the screw.
5. The surgeon pulls the wire and loops it around the exposed shaft of the screw while reduction is maintained manually or by using a reduction clamp. The wire can be tightened using the wire tightener. Two smooth Steinmann pins, bent over the exposed portion to hook the loop of wire, can substitute for the cancellous screws.
6. The remaining screw is threaded into the bone; the fracture site is observed for opposition.
7. The surgeon irrigates the wound and closes it. Drains are generally not necessary. A long arm posterior splint is placed.
   NOTE: Using this technique requires early active motion of the arm. Compression of the fracture site is achieved by moving the elbow through its range of motion and applying force by the hardware.

Transposition of the Ulnar Nerve

Transposition of the ulnar nerve involves freeing the nerve from a groove at the back of the medial epicondyle of the humerus and bringing it to the front of the condyle. The ulnar nerve is frequently divided or damaged after fracture or wounds to the elbow caused by trauma. Dislocation of the elbow may also cause ulnar nerve damage. Late traumatic neuritis may occur after an old injury, resulting in stretching of the ulnar nerve. The hand appears atrophied, and sensory loss is extensive. In severe cases, a claw hand deformity develops.

Procedural Considerations

The perioperative nurse assists with positioning the patient supine with the extremity slightly flexed on a hand table or over the chest. A tourniquet is applied to the upper arm, and the entire arm (fingers to tourniquet) is prepped and draped. A soft tissue set is required. Bone instruments may be required.

Operative Procedure

1. The surgeon makes an incision on the lateral aspect of the elbow near the epicondyle.
2. The fascia and the flexor carpi ulnaris muscle are divided.
3. The surgeon frees the ulnar nerve and dissects the medial intermuscular septum.
4. The nerve is then drawn anteriorly and placed deep into the brachialis flexor muscle origin.
5. The wound is irrigated and closed. A drain is not necessary. A short arm posterior splint is applied to the elbow postoperatively.

Excision of the Head of the Radius

Fractures of the radial head can be displaced or nondisplaced, segmental, or comminuted. Complications can arise when treatment is delayed, causing limitation of motion, pain, and posttraumatic arthritis. A congruous radial head is essential for proper rotation of the forearm at the elbow. Consequently in an adult it is necessary to excise the radial head if a severely comminuted fracture with angulation interferes with rotation. The radial head should never be excised in children. The outcome for the patient undergoing radial head excision may result in some permanent loss of pronation and supination of the forearm. Noncomminuted fractures that are easily reduced can be treated using closed reduction and casting.

Procedural Considerations

The patient is supine with the arm over the chest or on a hand table. A tourniquet is applied. A soft tissue set, a small bone set, and an oscillating microsaw with blades are needed.

Operative Procedure

1. The surgeon makes an incision on the shaft of the radius from 5 cm distal to the radial head, extending proximally over the lateral humeral condyle.
2. Dissection is continued between the extensor carpi ulnaris and extensor digitorum muscles onto the joint capsule.
3. With the head and neck of the radius exposed through the joint capsule, the surgeon irrigates the joint to clear bone debris and blood clots.
4. The surgeon excises the radial head just proximal to the radial tuberosity and removes all the periosteum to limit new bone formation. The remaining annular ligament is also excised. The fragments of the radial head should be saved and readily available so that they may be reassembled to ensure that all fragments have been retrieved.
5. The wound is closed, and a long arm posterior splint is applied with the elbow at 90 degrees.

Correction of Fractures of the Proximal Third of the Ulna With Radial Head Dislocation (Monteggia)

The Monteggia type of fracture presents with a proximal ulnar fracture and dislocation of the radial head. The fracture is rarely treated with open reduction in children. The open technique is often used to treat adults. A direct blow to the ulnar aspect or a fall while the arm is hyperextended produces this type of injury. If the open reduction approach is chosen, closed reduction of the radial dislocation is attempted and often is successful. At times the annular ligament may prevent reduction of the radial head dislocation, and open reduction becomes necessary. Deforming forces of the forearm vary, depending on the location of the fracture in relation to the insertion of muscles. These forces are often encountered when treating forearm injuries. The dynamic compression technique uses compression plates that are stockier and stronger than the semitubular plates mentioned earlier for distal humeral fractures. They are used to plate shaft fractures, where stress forces on the shaft are greater and stronger plates are required.

Procedural Considerations

The patient is placed in the supine position with or without a hand table. A tourniquet is applied and inflated as needed. A soft tissue set and a large bone set are required, as well as bone-reduction clamps and bone-grasping forceps, AO/ASIF instrumentation, plates and screws, and a power drill.

Operative Procedure

Fixation With Dynamic Compression Plate

1. The surgeon performs a closed reduction to reduce the radial head dislocation (Fig. 20.43).
2. An incision is made; the ulnar fracture site is dissected.
3. The surgeon strips the periosteum and reapproximates the fragments using bone-reduction and bone-grasping forceps.
4. The bone is assessed for placement of a small- or large-fragment dynamic compression plate (DCP), with at least three screw holes proximal and three distal to the fracture site.
5. A concentric (neutral) hole is drilled into the ulna (through one of the screw holes on the plate) to the opposite cortex.

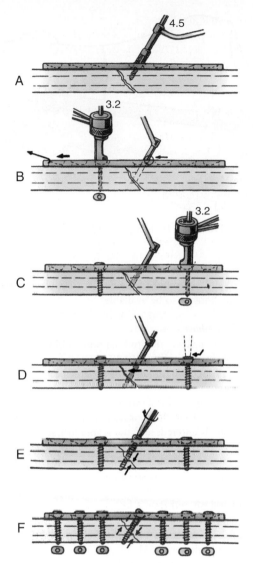

FIG. 20.43 Fixation with dynamic compression plate. (A) Gliding hole with drill bit. (B) Fracture is reduced, drill sleeve is inserted, the fracture is drawn together, a hole is drilled, and a screw is inserted in the neutral position to correct the fracture. (C and D) One screw is inserted in load position (eccentric) into the other fragment; as the screw is tightened, axial compression is generated. (E) Lag screw is inserted across the fracture site. (F) Remaining screws are inserted in the neutral position.

6. After the hole is gauged, the selected size of screw is inserted, with purchase of the opposite cortex ensured. The surgeon inserts a second screw on the opposite fragment in the neutral position.
7. On either side of the fracture site, an eccentric (loading) hole is drilled in the same fashion to the opposite cortex. The hole is gauged and tapped, and the screw is inserted.
8. The selected screw is entered eccentrically into the plate. As the screw seeks the center of the screw hole while riding the bevel of the screw hole, it compresses the fracture site. The surgeon tightens this screw completely and slightly loosens the other screws.
9. The fracture site is now visualized radiographically as the action of the screw in the plate compresses the fracture site.

10. The remaining bone screws are inserted following the same procedure.
11. The surgeon irrigates the wound and closes it; a drain may or may not be inserted.
12. A long arm posterior splint is placed with the arm in 110 to 120 degrees of flexion.

Correction of Colles Fracture With External Fixation

Colles fracture is a dorsally angulated fracture of the distal end of the radius. Most of these fractures can be managed successfully with closed reduction and immobilization, but external fixation is especially useful in the case of a comminuted intra-articular fracture. Internal fixation is indicated when the distal end of the radius is severely comminuted and displaced. In these cases, Kirschner wires are used for internal fixation.

Procedural Considerations
The team positions the patient supine with the arm extended on a hand table. Traction, via finger traps, may be required. A soft tissue set and a small bone set are required, along with a power drill, small elevator, and the external fixation device of choice. Fluoroscopy is necessary.

Operative Procedure
1. The surgeon makes small incisions as needed and places two pins through the second metacarpal, one at the base and the other distal-ward, a distance equal to the span between the openings in the fixator.
2. Two pins are placed in the radius 8 cm from the styloid.
3. The surgeon confirms pin placement radiographically in both the AP and lateral views.
4. A frame is constructed to incorporate all four pins.
5. Reduction of the fracture is obtained, and the surgeon secures the frame.
6. Postreduction films are obtained to check alignment and pin position.

Surgery of the Hand

Hand surgery has become highly specialized. The perioperative nurse encounters numerous procedures for treating bone, soft tissue, or both. Many of the techniques and principles used to treat large bone defects are used in the treatment of hand injuries. Hand procedures range from carpal tunnel release to complex digit reimplantation.

Tourniquets and regional anesthetics are often used for hand surgery. The OR team usually sits down at a hand table but may move to areas such as the iliac crest for bone grafting. The instruments for hand surgery are common to orthopedics but on a smaller scale. Many instruments and reconstruction systems have been developed primarily for hand surgery. Air- or battery-powered drills and saws are frequently used. The surgery often requires the use of eye loupes (glasses for magnification) or a microscope.

Carpal Tunnel Release

Carpal tunnel syndrome results from entrapment of the median nerve on the volar surface of the wrist; it is caused by thickened synovium, trauma, or aberrant muscles. Carpal tunnel syndrome is frequently seen in patients with rheumatoid synovitis or malaligned Colles fracture and is associated with obesity, Raynaud disease, pregnancy, and occupational injuries. The symptoms are pain, numbness, tingling of the fingers, and weakness of the intrinsic thumb muscles. These symptoms are usually reversible after the flexor retinaculum is incised so that the compressed median nerve is relieved. Carpal tunnel release may be completed endoscopically or by open incision.

Procedural Considerations

The team places the patient in the supine position with the arm extended on a hand table. A tourniquet is applied to the forearm or upper arm. A hand set is required. The endoscopic approach requires use of specialized equipment.

Operative Procedure: Open Approach

1. The surgeon makes a curvilinear, longitudinal volar incision from the proximal side of the palm, paralleling the thenar crease and extending to the crease of the wrist across the wrist joint.
2. The deep transverse carpal ligament is divided, taking care to avoid damage to the median nerve.
3. At this point the release is completed.
4. If indicated, the surgeon performs a tenosynovectomy.
5. The surgeon closes the wound and applies a compression dressing and volar splint.

Excision of Ganglions

A ganglion is a cystic lesion arising from a joint capsule or tendon sheath and containing glassy, clear fluid. Ganglions are most common on the dorsum of the wrist, palm of the hand, and dorsolateral aspect of the foot. Ganglions appear as firm masses that vary in size. They may resolve spontaneously but occasionally require excision because of discomfort or for cosmetic reasons.

Procedural Considerations

The perioperative nurse assists with positioning the patient supine with the arm extended on a hand table and applies the tourniquet as directed by the surgeon. A hand set is required.

Operative Procedure

1. The surgeon makes a transverse incision over the ganglion.
2. The ganglion is excised with a rim of normal joint capsule or tendon sheath at its base.
3. The surgeon irrigates the wound and closes it and applies a pressure dressing. A plaster splint may also be applied to immobilize the affected joint.

Correction of Carpal Fractures

Most fractures of the carpal bones are treated by closed reduction and immobilization. However, it is occasionally necessary to operate on a fracture because of acute instability, delayed union, or nonunion. The scaphoid is the most commonly fractured carpal bone. Internal fixation is accomplished with Kirschner wires, small compression screws, or mini fragment compression plates and screws. A bone graft from the distal end of the radius or olecranon may be taken.

For displaced or unstable scaphoid fractures, the Herbert bone screw (Fig. 20.44) has several advantages: (1) strong internal fixation, (2) compression at the fracture site with reversed threads at each end of the screw, and (3) reduced time required for external immobilization.

Procedural Considerations

The patient is supine with the arm extended on a hand table. A tourniquet is applied and fluoroscopy should be available. A soft tissue set and a small bone or hand set are required in addition to the Herbert screw set. If a mini fragment compression set is used,

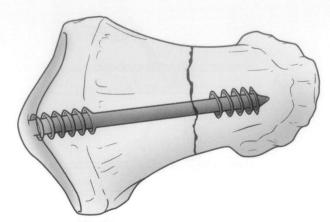

FIG. 20.44 Herbert bone screw placement.

a power drill and smooth Kirschner wires will also be needed. A bone graft set should also be available.

Operative Procedure

1. The surgeon makes a longitudinal skin incision over the palmar surface of the wrist (Fig. 20.45).
2. The superficial palmar branch of the radial artery is ligated and divided.
3. The surgeon incises the flexor carpi radialis tendon sheath and retracts it to expose the capsule of the wrist.
4. The capsule is entered, and the scaphoid fracture is identified and inspected to determine the need for bone grafting.
5. The surgeon manipulates the fracture to reduce it and inserts small Kirschner wires to temporarily hold the reduction.
6. The scaphoid fracture is reduced and held with the Herbert jig.
7. A short drill bit and then a long drill bit are inserted to create a channel for the screw.
8. The surgeon inserts the Herbert screw and turns it until it is seated within the scaphoid.
9. Bone graft is placed around the fracture site if needed. (The loss of significant bone can often be corrected by fashioning a strut of bone from graft.)
10. The wound is irrigated and closed.
11. A splint is applied with a thumb spica or long arm cast incorporating the thumb.

Surgery of the Hip and Lower Extremity

Fractures of the Acetabulum

Fractures of the acetabulum usually result from high-energy injuries such as motor vehicle accidents and falls with a landing on the extended extremities. The fracture is directly related to the force transmitted to the femoral head through the greater trochanter or lower leg. Management of these fractures can often present the surgical team with a complex and challenging task. Indications for internal fixation of acetabular fractures include (1) more than 2 mm of displacement, (2) presence of intra-articular loose bodies, (3) inability to reduce under closed methods, (4) unstable fractures of the posterior acetabular wall, and (5) open fractures. Internal fixation is usually delayed 3 to 10 days to allow time for the patient to be evaluated and clinically stabilized. Until internal fixation is undertaken, the fracture is reduced by means of closed methods and the patient is maintained in skeletal traction. General anesthesia may be required

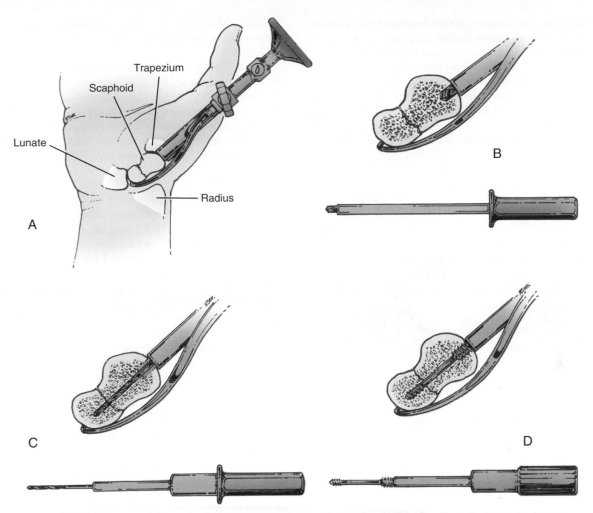

FIG. 20.45 Repair of the scaphoid. (A) Fracture site is exposed. (B) Alignment guide reduces the fracture and guides all subsequent instrumentation. (C) The screw hole is drilled by hand, and the tap is inserted. (D) The Herbert bone screw is inserted through the drill guide.

for closed reduction and placement of skeletal traction when the acetabular fracture is severely displaced or dislocated. The fractures are divided into five basic groups: (1) fractures of the posterior wall, (2) posterior column, or (3) anterior wall; (4) anterior column; and (5) transverse fractures (Fig. 20.46). Internal fixation is accomplished with reconstruction plates and screws, total hip replacement with bone grafting (see Total Hip Arthroplasty, page 721), or fusion if the fracture cannot be reduced.

Procedural Considerations

The surgical approach depends on the type and area of the fracture and the surgeon's preference. The perioperative nurse assists in placing the patient on a fracture or standard OR bed in the lateral or supine position. A general anesthetic is usually administered, but the procedure can be performed solely with a regional block or concurrent epidural infusion. Procedures of this magnitude can be lengthy and involve considerable blood loss. Appropriate measures should be taken to avoid complications from these factors. The room should remain warm, the patient protected from pressure injury, and red blood cell salvaging techniques used.

A soft tissue set, large bone and acetabular instruments, pelvic reduction clamps, reconstruction plates and screws (both 3.5 and 4.5 mm), plate-bending irons, and a femoral distractor are necessary. A total hip set should be available. Also needed are Kirschner wires and Steinmann pins, large-fragment bone screws, pulsatile lavage supplies, and power drill and reamer. Fluoroscopy may be used for this procedure.

Operative Procedure
Posterolateral Approach

1. The surgeon makes a lateral incision over the acetabular fracture site.
2. The joint is opened and the femur dislocated from the acetabulum.
3. The surgeon uses self-retaining or handheld hip retractors to maintain exposure of the acetabulum.
4. Femoral distraction or osteotomy of the trochanter may be used to improve visualization and access to the fracture.
5. The surgeon reduces the fracture using bone clamps, forceps, and a ball spike.
6. Reduction is accomplished in gradual steps using Kirschner wires to hold the fragments temporarily in place.
7. Reconstruction plates are fitted and contoured to the fracture site and secured with screws. The surgeon may also use long

cancellous lag screw fixation to provide interfragmentary compression, particularly in column fractures.

8. If necessary, a bone graft may be used for additional fixation. A femoral head allograft technique is sometimes used, in which the allograft is mushroomed to create a new acetabulum.

9. The surgeon uses pulsatile lavage to irrigate the wound with antibiotic solution to ensure the articular surfaces are free from loose bodies.

10. The wound is closed, drains are inserted, and pressure dressings are applied.

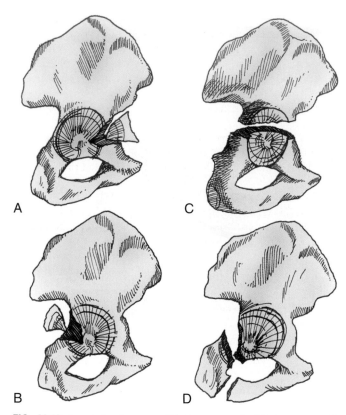

FIG. 20.46 Acetabular fractures. (A) Anterior wall. (B) Posterior wall. (C) Transverse. (D) Posterior column.

The leg is maintained in abduction and external rotation with traction. After the fracture is stabilized, traction is no longer necessary.

NOTE: If there is associated traumatic dislocation of the hip with the acetabular fracture, the dislocation should be treated promptly. The dislocation should be reduced as soon as possible and skeletal traction inserted if needed to maintain reduction. Acetabular fractures often accompany femoral shaft fractures, which also need to be treated concurrently with the surgeon's desired method (see Femoral Shaft Fractures: Internal Fixation, page 708).

Hip Fractures

Hip fractures are classified by anatomic location and can be categorized as femoral neck fractures, intertrochanteric fractures, and subtrochanteric fractures (Fig. 20.47), and these can each be subclassified. Fracture-dislocations also have a classification system and treatment protocol. Fractures of the greater or lesser trochanters alone are less common and can usually be treated nonoperatively.

Femoral neck fractures and intertrochanteric fractures commonly require ORIF. Femoral neck fractures are more common in women because of several factors, including osteoporosis. Most elderly patients require a comprehensive preoperative medical evaluation to define and treat anesthetic risks. However, efforts should be made to correct the fracture as soon as possible to avoid complications related to immobility, skin pressure, pulmonary congestion, and thrombophlebitis. Avascular necrosis and degenerative changes can occur as a result of diminished blood supply to the femoral head, resulting in irreversible changes. Buck traction may be placed preoperatively to reduce discomfort from muscle spasm caused by overriding of fracture fragments.

Manipulation, reduction, and internal fixation of these fractures are greatly facilitated by use of the OR fracture bed, which also permits adequate radiographic examination to determine placement of the internal fixation.

Intertrochanteric Fractures

Intertrochanteric fractures occur most frequently in older patients. The fractures usually unite without difficulty. However, because the lower extremity is externally rotated at the fracture site, internal fixation is necessary to prevent malunion. Internal fixation allows patients to be mobilized earlier, decreasing mortality and morbidity.

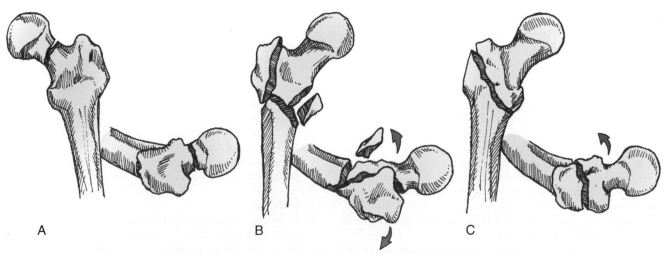

FIG. 20.47 Proximal femur fractures. (A) Midcervical. (B) Comminuted subtrochanteric. (C) Intertrochanteric.

Procedural Considerations. The patient is placed in the supine position on the OR fracture bed, and the surgeon reduces the fracture by manipulating the extremity and then confirming with fluoroscopy. Various internal fixation devices, including Ambi, Free-Lock, dynamic hip screw (DHS), and medullary fixation, may be used. Success of the procedure is determined by bone quality, fragment configuration, adequate reduction, implant design, and implant-insertion technique. Intraoperative blood loss is minimized because the hip joint is not opened.

A soft tissue set and a large bone set are required in addition to the compression hip screw instrumentation and implants, bone-reduction and plate-holding clamps, and a power drill and reamer.

Operative Procedure

Free-Lock Compression Plate and Lag Screw

1. The surgeon reduces the fracture as previously described (Fig. 20.48).
2. Reduction is checked in both the AP and lateral views with fluoroscopy.
3. The surgeon makes an incision from the greater trochanter distally to accommodate the length of the implant.
4. The dissection is completed through the fascia lata, and the vastus lateralis is exposed.
5. The reduction is visually confirmed and the surgeon inserts the guide pin after determining the angle plate to be used. A 135-degree angle plate is commonly used.
6. The surgeon ensures the pin is centralized in the femoral head approximately 1 cm short of the femoral articular surface, taking care not to enter the joint space because this might result in

arthritic changes. Further penetration of the pin through the acetabulum and into the pelvis can damage large vessels or bowel. If necessary, a second pin can be used to control rotation in high neck or unstable fractures.

7. Next the surgeon uses a conical cannulated drill bit over the guide pin to open the lateral cortex.
8. The depth gauge is placed over the guide pin. The size of the required lag screw is determined from the guide.
9. A double-barrel reamer is adjusted to correspond to the depth of the guide pin. The cortex is reamed over the guide pin to create a channel for the lag screw and barrel of the compression plate.
10. The lag screw channel is tapped to the full distance of reaming to allow proper seating of the lag screw, particularly in young patients with firm bone. Reaming depth of osteoporotic bone is reduced 5 mm, and the tap depth is reduced approximately 1 to 2 cm to allow sufficient screw purchase.
11. The surgeon may confirm the plate angle with a trial. Once confirmed, the nurse opens the implants (plate and lag screw) to the back table.
12. The scrub person assembles the plate, lag screw, and insertion wrench with the centering sleeve. A screw stabilizer is passed through the center of the insertion wrench and threaded into the lag screw.
13. The surgeon places the entire assembly over the guide pin and advances the lag screw to the desired depth with periodic verification with fluoroscopy. Penetration of the lag screw through the femoral articular surface must be avoided.

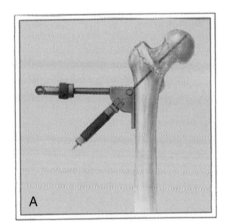
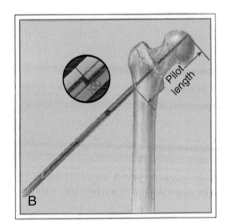
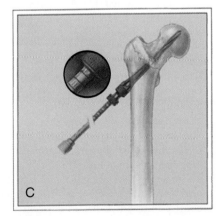
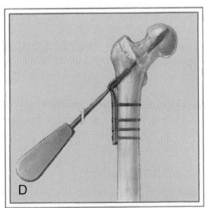

FIG. 20.48 Intertrochanteric fracture repair with compression plate. (A) Guide pin is inserted. (B) Depth of guide is measured. (C) Lag screw channel is reamed. (D) Tube/plate is applied, and lag screw is inserted.

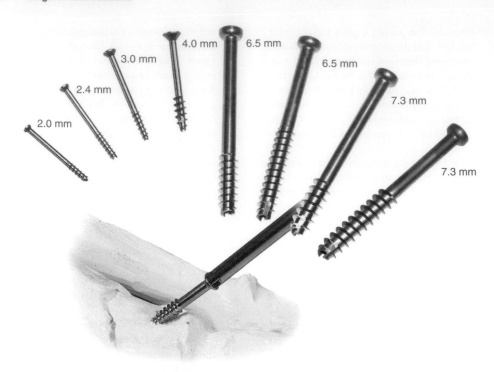

FIG. 20.49 Cannulated screw system.

14. The insertion wrench is disassembled, and the barrel of the compression plate is placed over the lag screw. The barrel of the plate should fully cover the lag screw. The plate is seated on the lateral femoral shaft.

15. The surgeon secures the plate to the shaft of the femur with plate-holding forceps. The guide pin is removed. At this point, traction can be released to allow compression of the fracture site.

16. Screw holes are made using the drill guide and a 3.5-mm drill bit. The length is determined, and cortical screws are inserted through the screw hole on the plate with sufficient purchase on the opposite cortex of the shaft. The top screw hole on the plate can accept a 6.5-mm cancellous screw, which can be angled for better purchase in comminuted fractures.

17. Traction is released if not done previously. The surgeon inserts a compression screw into the barrel of the screw and threads it into the back of the lag screw, compressing the fracture site. The compression screw exerts a powerful force. The amount of compression applied should correlate with the quality of the bone.

18. The wound is irrigated and closed. Two closed suction drains may be inserted during closure.

Weight bearing may begin as early as the first postoperative day, depending on reduction and quality of bone.

NOTE: Many of the same techniques and principles of long bone fracture fixation are used in treating various types of hip fractures. The different screw types, dynamic compression, and lag screw effect are described throughout the chapter.

Femoral Neck Fractures: Internal Fixation

Anatomic reduction is necessary before internal fixation of femoral neck fractures because of the high incidence of associated complications, such as nonunion and avascular necrosis of the femoral head. The degree of displacement, tamponade pressure from intracapsular bleeding, and delays in reduction and fixation can affect the blood supply to the femoral head. These factors contribute to the death of the femoral head and failed fixation. Growing children may sustain fractures through the epiphyseal growth plate (slipped capital femoral epiphysis). These injuries are treated by reduction and internal fixation of the femoral head, similar to the procedures used in the adult. The Garden and AO nomenclatures are the most popular classifications for grading the fractures. Pins of various designs, such as Knowles and Hagie, and universal cannulated screws (Fig. 20.49) are used for fixation (Fig. 20.50). In cases of severe comminution or avascular necrosis of the femoral head, the patient may require a prosthetic replacement (see Total Joint Arthroplasty, page 721).

Procedural Considerations

The perioperative nurse assists with positioning the patient on the OR fracture bed, and a general or regional anesthetic (spinal or epidural) is administered. Slight traction and external rotation are adjusted on the affected side. A soft tissue set and a large bone set are required, as well as the fixation device of choice with instrumentation, Kirschner wires, Cobra retractors, a power drill, and fluoroscopy.

Operative Procedure

Cannulated Screw Fixation for Nondisplaced Femoral Neck Fractures

1. The surgeon makes a 5-cm lateral incision over the greater trochanter and exposes the fracture.

2. The dissection is carried through the subcutaneous and fascial layers; the vastus lateralis is detached anteriorly and retracted, exposing the femoral neck.

3. The surgeon drives two guide pins into the middle of the femoral head, one anterior and one posterior, within 5 mm of subchondral bone; a third pin is placed adjacent to the medial cortex at a 135-degree angle. The surgeon is careful to not violate the articular surface.

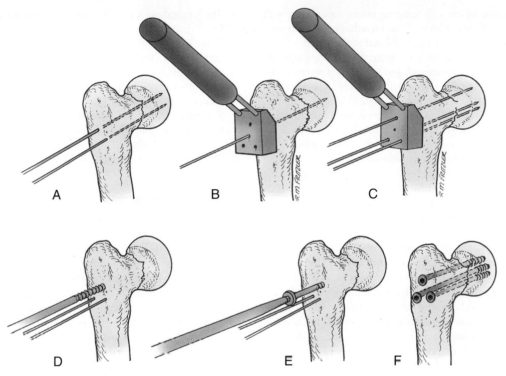

FIG. 20.50 Internal fixation with cannulated screws (AO technique). (A) Guidewire parallel to anteversion wire. (B) Guidewire placed over positioning wire through diamond-patterned positioning holes. (C) Guidewire placed through each outer triangle of holes. (D) Cannulated tap passed over guidewire to tap near cortex. (E) Large cannulated screw inserted over guidewire. (F) Remaining screws inserted in same manner.

4. The guide pins are measured for correct screw length, and the cannulated screws are inserted over the guide pin without applying compression until all are seated.
5. Compression of the anterior screws is completed first and the posterior screws last to avoid collapse of the posterior aspect of the neck.
6. The surgeon releases the traction and visualizes the fracture site with fluoroscopy while rotating the hip through a full range of motion.
7. Radiographs are taken to verify the position of the screws; the wound is irrigated and closed.
NOTE: Screw protrusion into the joint space can be disastrous to the articular surface. Radiopaque dye can be injected to rule out communication with the joint.

Femoral Head Prosthetic Replacement: Unipolar and Bipolar Implants

With the development of current cement fixation techniques and the evolution of the modular bipolar and monopolar design, the use of fixed endoprostheses such as the Austin–Moore and Thompson designs declined. During the early 1980s the bipolar system in conjunction with a cemented femoral stem became popular. Bipolar endoprostheses (Fig. 20.51) were introduced to reduce the shear stresses affecting the acetabular surface, decreasing the motion and friction between the prosthetic head and the acetabulum that is seen with conventional (unipolar) endoprostheses. A femoral head prosthesis is snapped into a rotating polyethylene-lined cup that, when inserted, moves as one unit. Friction occurs between the ball and plastic instead of between the head and the acetabulum. This was a revolutionary design in the mechanics of hip motion and

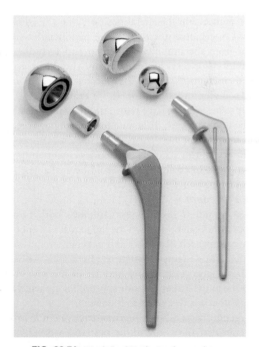

FIG. 20.51 Modular bipolar endoprostheses.

stresses. Some surgeons and engineers believe that bipolar motion subsides after fibrous growth has taken place, allowing for only unipolar motion. There have also been reports of bone resorption and subsequent prosthetic loosening in cases in which bipolar prostheses were used. Researchers are evaluating evidence of metallic head wear of the polyethylene cup, creating microscopic debris with a subsequent chemical lysis of bone. Thus there has been resurgence in the use of unipolar heads for femoral head replacement.

Trends in healthcare toward cost reduction precipitated the development of the *diagnosis-related group (DRG) prosthesis.* The modular design was retained, allowing for different combinations of head size, neck length, and stem size. Instead of being bipolar, the head is solid, or unipolar, and the stem is the result of a less costly manufacturing process. The most cost-effective prosthesis is still the original Austin–Moore design, which may be selected for those patients whose life expectancy is short and who have a minimal level of activity. If major deficiencies in the acetabular side of the joint are present, a total joint arthroplasty may be performed. In deciding between the hemiarthroplasty and total hip reconstruction, the patient's medical condition, age, and level of activity must be considered.

Current biomaterials, methods of fixation (cemented versus uncemented), prosthetic life, and modular components allow conversion of a hemiarthroplasty (reconstruction of one side of the joint) to a total hip arthroplasty, provided that the femoral component is adequately fixed. Depending on the patient's condition, the acetabulum may eventually require arthroplasty as a result of degenerative changes. Improved technology and surgical technique have increased the life span of implanted components. The portion of the implant that articulates within the acetabulum can be removed and replaced with a smaller femoral head. The acetabulum is then prepared for prosthetic implantation by various means of fixation. The ability to convert from hemiarthroplasty to total arthroplasty reduces the amount of surgery required.

Procedural Considerations

The patient is placed in the lateral position after the administration of a general or regional anesthetic. The perioperative nurse preps the patient from the umbilicus down to and including the foot. Instrumentation for total hip replacement should be available but not opened until inspection of the resected joint is completed to determine whether a total arthroplasty is required.

The soft tissue and the large bone sets are required, as well as the endoprosthesis instruments, trials, and implants. A power reciprocating or sagittal saw may be necessary. Templates or a caliper is used to measure the size of the femoral head. Bone cement and the supplies for preparing and inserting it also should be available.

Operative Procedure

Modular Austin–Moore Endoprosthesis. Both posterior and anterior approaches can be made to the hip to place an endoprosthesis. The posterior approach is quicker and generally involves less blood loss, but detractors suggest that there is a higher dislocation rate and a greater chance of infection because of the proximity of the incision to the anus. Although both approaches are widely used, the posterior approach is described as follows:

1. The surgeon makes a linear incision from 5 cm below the posteroinferior iliac spine toward the posterior aspect of the greater trochanter and distally along the posterior aspect of the proximal femur for 7 mm.
2. The capsule is entered, and the femoral head is removed and gauged with the template. Fragments that may be loose in the acetabulum or attached to the ligamentum teres are removed.
3. The surgeon inserts a trial cup into the acetabulum and applies axial compression while checking clearance of the extremity's lateral motion.

4. The femoral neck is fashioned to achieve an accurate prosthetic fit.
5. Using a punch, the surgeon opens the medullary canal from the femoral neck. The IM canal is reamed and rasped to accommodate the prosthesis.
6. After the canal is prepared, the surgeon inserts the prosthesis of choice with or without bone cement.
7. A unipolar or bipolar assembly is snapped onto the neck of the femoral stem. The height of the head determines the neck length and is selected after trial reduction.
8. The hip is reduced, and closure is accomplished in layers over suction drains.

Femoral Shaft Fractures: Internal Fixation

Fractures involving the femoral shaft are very common in today's orthopedic OR. Prolonged immobility, with its attendant complications, and disability can result if femoral shaft fractures are not managed appropriately. The femur is the largest principal load-bearing bone in the body. Fractures of the femoral shaft can be surgically treated with several available techniques. Considerations for treatment are type and location of fracture (location on shaft), the number of segments involved, the degree of comminution (Fig. 20.52), and the activity level of the patient. Femoral shaft fractures are often associated with ipsilateral (same-side) trochanteric or condylar fractures. Pathologic fractures often occur in this region.

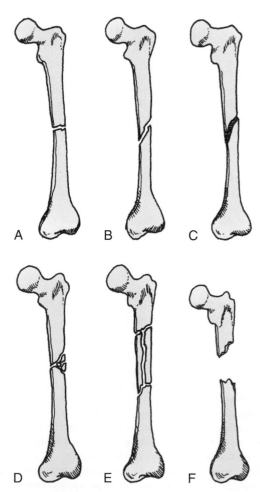

FIG. 20.52 Femoral shaft fractures. (A) Transverse. (B) Oblique. (C) Spiral. (D) Comminuted. (E) Longitudinal split. (F) Complete bone loss.

Possible treatment methods for femoral shaft fractures are closed reduction, skeletal traction, and femoral cast bracing. External fixation has limited use when fractures associated with surgical site infection or neurovascular compromise are treated, but it may serve temporarily until internal fixation can be performed. Although plates and screws are used for femoral shaft fractures, their use has been widely disputed because of complications such as bent or broken plates, refractures, and deep surgical site infections. IM fixation devices have become the preferred method of treatment. IM nails and rods increase the load sharing of the bone, making the implant less likely to fracture. Bone healing requires a load across the fracture site to promote osteosynthesis and prevent refracture. The open or closed method of IM nailing can be used with locked and nonlocked nails. Closed methods of IM fixation often minimize exposure of the surgical site and decrease surgical time, resulting in less opportunity for infection.

IM nail and rod designs vary and include the following: (1) flexible nails such as the Rusch or Enders type, (2) standard rods such as the Sampson and AO rods, and (3) interlocking nails (see Fractures of the Humeral Shaft, page 695) such as the Grosse–Kempf and Russell–Taylor varieties. Closed reduction and IM nailing with or without locking screws have become the method against which other methods are measured. Incidences of scarring, blood loss, and infection are all favorable. Fracture hematoma remains intact at the fracture site, which is important in bone healing, and the rate of bone union is increased.

Procedural Considerations

General or epidural anesthetics are used. The patient is placed on the OR fracture bed in the supine position, traction applied, and the fracture manually reduced and confirmed with fluoroscopy. If the fracture is profoundly unstable, the surgeon must take care during manipulation to prevent neurovascular complications. For open IM fixation, extra retractors and bone instruments may be required. For a percutaneous reduction, a soft tissue set and a large bone set are required in addition to the IM nail implants and associated instruments, a power reamer and drill, and long guidewires for reamers. This procedure requires the use of fluoroscopy. A skeletal traction tray with Steinmann pins may be necessary.

Operative Procedure

Russell–Taylor Rod With or Without Locking Screws

1. The surgeon makes an incision over the tip of the greater trochanter and continues it proximally and medially for 6 to 8 cm. The fascia of the gluteus is incised, and the piriformis fossa is palpated.
2. With a threaded guide pin followed by cannulated reamers or by use of an awl, the surgeon identifies the trochanteric fossa and penetrates the cortex. A 3.2-mm guide rod is inserted to the level of the fracture. A curved guide pin is available for more severely displaced fractures.
3. Under fluoroscopy, the surgeon advances the guidewire across the fracture site and into the distal fragment until the ball tip of the guidewire reaches the level of the epiphyseal scar. A second guidewire is held against the portion of the guidewire extending out of the proximal femur, and the length is measured. That measurement is subtracted from 90 mm (total guidewire length) to determine the length of the IM nail required.
4. The cannulated reamers are placed sequentially over the guidewire. The entire femur is reamed at 0.5-mm increments. The entire shaft, and especially the fracture site, should be visualized with fluoroscopy as the reamers pass.

5. The surgeon verifies the final reamer size with the reamer gauge. The femur is reamed 1 mm over the selected nail diameter. Inserting a nail in an inadequately reamed femur or inserting a nail that is too large can cause severe bone splitting and comminution.
6. The proximal screw guide/slap hammer is assembled onto the nail. The nail is oriented to match the curve of the femur.
7. Using the handle of the inserter, the surgeon controls the rotation of the nail and drives it into the femur. The nail is fully seated when the proximal screw guide is flush with the greater trochanter. The surgeon disengages the inserter from the slap hammer.
8. Using the power drill and correct drill sleeves, the surgeon drills a 4.8-mm hole through both cortices and measures the depth directly off the bit.
9. Through the appropriate drill sleeve, a 6.4-mm self-tapping locking screw is inserted and the drill sleeve is removed.
10. By fluoroscopy, the distal screw holes are confirmed as perfect circles on the screen. The distal targeting device is mounted on the nail, followed by the left or right adapter block. The adapter block is adjusted until the calibration reads the length of the nail. The crosshairs are aligned in the adapter to the holes in the distal nail, with confirmation by fluoroscopy.
11. The surgeon makes an incision through the adapter block over the distal femur to the lateral cortex. Following the same steps as those for placing the proximal screw, one or two distal locking screws are inserted. There are various freehand techniques for inserting distal locking screws.

Surgery of the Lower Leg (Distal Femur, Tibia, and Fibula)

Many procedures on the lower leg use the same principles of fracture fixation already mentioned. Meticulous detail is required to ensure proper alignment and optimal surgical results for the patient. As in the hip, fractures around the knee require secure fixation to allow bone healing, preserve motion, and provide joint mobility as early as possible. Fracture treatment for the various described injuries is based on location and the pattern of fracture. Methods of fixation for the distal end of the femur and proximal end of the tibia include pins, wire, compression plates, IM nails, supracondylar plates, and cannulated screws. Multiple-trauma patients with one or a combination of fractures may require more than one method of fixation. ORIF must ensure anatomic restoration of the joint surface and rigid fixation and allow early motion of the knee joint.

Most operations on the knee are performed with the patient in the supine position and the leg prepped and draped from the groin to the middle of the calf or including the entire foot. It is occasionally necessary for the surgeon to operate with the foot of the OR bed dropped and the patient's knee flexed to 90 degrees. Consequently it is important for the nurse to position the patient so that the knee is at a break in the bed; if it is necessary, the lower leg can then be flexed at the knee during the operation. A tourniquet is often used.

Femoral Condyle and Tibial Plateau Fractures

The joint surfaces are often involved with fractures of the distal end of the femur and proximal end of the tibia. Anatomic alignment of the articular surfaces is necessary to provide joint stability and decrease the chance of posttraumatic arthritis. Nonunion is the most common complication in supracondylar fractures, leading to failure of surgery. As with humeral head and hip fractures, it is important that the articular surfaces are reposed as close as possible to avoid future degenerative changes. Unfortunately these often cannot be avoided, and patients with this type of injury often face future joint arthroplasty and replacement (see Total Joint Arthroplasty, page 721).

Distal femoral fractures result in varying degrees of comminution. Condylar fractures can be unicondylar or bicondylar, with separation of both condyles (Fig. 20.53). Type A fractures are extra-articular. Type B are single condyle fractures in the sagittal or coronal planes, whereas type C fractures are T and Y configurations. Type C fractures have varying degrees of shaft and condylar comminution, presenting the greatest treatment challenge.

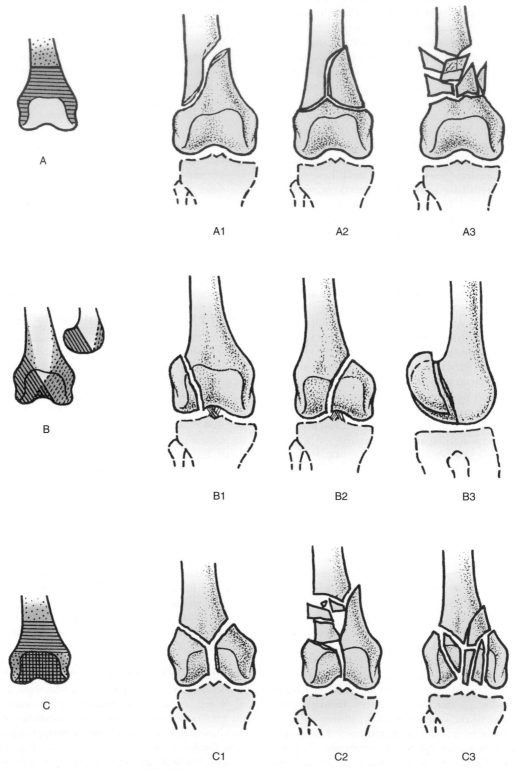

FIG. 20.53 Classification of fractures of distal femur.

Simple, nondisplaced distal femoral fractures can be treated with closed reduction and immobilization by casting if anatomic reduction is achieved. Nondisplaced extra-articular fractures can be treated with a hinged cast brace. Comminuted fractures in this region can also be treated in this manner if shortening and angulation are minimal. Traction can be used initially to augment this type of treatment. Distal femoral fractures are treated with open reduction if distal tibial traction and manipulation attempts fail. Flexible nails, locking IM nails, blade plates, condylar compression screws, and condylar buttress plates are accepted methods of treating condylar fractures. Attention must be given to the attachment of the cruciate ligaments, which originate in the condylar notch and may require fixation of a partial or full disruption as a result of the injury to the knee (see Arthroscopic Anterior Cruciate Ligament Repair, page 743).

Tibial plateau fractures historically have been attributed to bumper or fender injuries, but a variety of falls or other traumas frequently are the cause. Compression force of the distal end of the femur on the tibia produces the various types of plateau fractures. Commonly this occurs from abduction of the tibia while the foot is planted, driving the lateral femoral condyle into the lateral tibial plateau. There are several classification systems based on fracture and dislocation patterns. The general theme of these fracture classifications and examples of their treatment can be summarized by the following types (Fig. 20.54): (1) pure cleavage, unicondylar fracture; (2) cleavage fracture combined with local depression; (3) pure central depression; (4) medial condylar wedge with depression or comminution; (5) bicondylar but with continuity of diaphysis and metaphysis; and (6) comminution with dissociation of metaphysis from diaphysis. Fractures of the tibial plateau are often associated with dislocation, which may spontaneously reduce at the time of trauma.

Special attention must be given to the possibility of neurovascular insult, which must be addressed immediately. Elevation and fixation of the depressed fracture are the focus for treatment of plateau fractures. As with distal femoral fractures, the articular surfaces and cruciate insertion require reapproximation and fixation. Repair to the menisci and ligaments should occur simultaneously to prevent knee instability.

Blade plates, buttress plates, and cannulated screws are all methods by which fractures of the tibial plateau are fixed. Severe fractures are treated using multiple buttress plates and screws (Fig. 20.55). Bone graft from the iliac crest and fibular head autograft are often used when there is a significant amount of bone lost to comminution with proximal tibial fractures.

Supracondylar Fractures of the Femur

Fractures of the distal femur in the multitrauma patient are treated early to promote rapid ambulation, which decreases complications caused by immobility. In an effort to deliver quick fracture reduction and stabilization, many orthopedic trauma systems have been developed. Often these are the same systems used in daily orthopedic procedures with modifications to expedite implantation and fixation. Some of the IM devices do not require reaming.

Procedural Considerations

Initial stabilization of the patient may immediately precede the nailing procedure. Often other team members are attending to treatment of other systems. The perioperative nurse is challenged to control traffic, coordinate team efforts, and protect the patient from increased risk of infection by the inadvertent contamination of instruments and implants. The OR team places the patient in the supine position after induction of general or regional anesthesia. If possible, the patient is positioned on the OR fracture bed; if not, a radiolucent OR bed is used. A pneumatic tourniquet may be applied as high up on the femur as possible, taking care to protect the genitals during placement. The nail can be inserted using the closed or open technique.

The soft tissue set and large bone set are required, as well as the IM supracondylar nail implant (Fig. 20.56) and the instruments necessary for its insertion. A power drill, guidewires, IM rod set, and fluoroscopy also are needed. In addition, Steinmann pins, Kirschner wires, bone-reduction clamps, and a bone graft set should be available. Occasionally a primary total knee arthroplasty is performed, and the appropriate instruments should be available should that possibility exist.

Operative Procedure

Intercondylar Fracture of the Femur, T Type (AIM Supracondylar Intramedullary Nail)

1. The surgeon makes a standard midline skin incision with parapatellar arthrotomy. Depending on the degree of intra-articular extension, the incision may be as small as 2.5 cm or involve lateral eversion of the patella to gain visualization of the entire joint. Articular fractures are anatomically reduced and secured with 6.5-mm or 8-mm cannulated screws placed in the anterior and posterior aspects of the condyles to allow adequate space for the placement of the nail.

2. Using an awl, the surgeon makes an entry hole into the femoral canal just anterior to the femoral insertion of the posterior cruciate ligament (PCL). Care is taken to ensure anatomic alignment of the condyles to avoid varus or valgus femoral alignment.

3. The surgeon enlarges the hole with the nonadjustable step reamer to accept the largest diameter of the chosen nail. Further reaming of the canal is necessary only in the case of nonunion, when the canal is reamed 0.5 to 1 mm larger than the size of the selected nail.

4. The selected nail is attached to the screw-targeting jig, which is then locked into place by the jig adapter. Before the nail is inserted, the surgeon checks the alignment of the jig and nail holes by manually inserting the sheath and trocar through the selected holes.

5. The surgeon places the nail in the prepared canal and advances it retrograde either by hand or with gentle blows of a mallet on the jig adapter. The nail should be countersunk approximately 3 to 5 mm below the articular surface.

6. The screws may then be placed using the targeting jig and sheath and trocar assembly. The surgeon makes a small lateral incision and advances the sheath and trocar to the femoral cortex. A 5.3-mm drill bit is advanced through the medial cortex, and the length is measured from the calibrated drill bit or by use of a depth gauge. The appropriate 6.5-mm cortical screw is inserted, and the process is repeated for placement of the second screw.

7. The surgeon uses the same technique for proximal locking of the nail, taking care to use the appropriate holes in the targeting jig for the length of nail inserted. The 3.8-mm drill bit and 4.5-mm self-tapping screws are used to fill these holes after femoral rotation and alignment are confirmed with fluoroscopy.

8. The jig adapter and screw-targeting jig are removed, and an end cap is placed into the distal end of the nail. The surgeon irrigates the wounds and closes them in layers. A compression dressing is applied.

The patient begins range-of-motion and muscle-strengthening exercises on the first postoperative day. Care is taken to protect

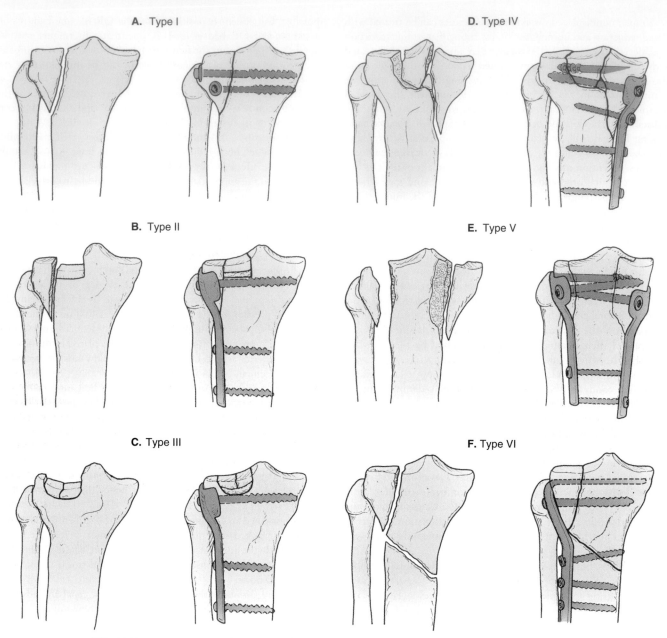

A. Type I

D. Type IV

B. Type II

E. Type V

C. Type III

F. Type VI

FIG. 20.54 Classification of fractures of the tibial plateau. (A) *Type I:* Pure cleavage fracture. (B) *Type II:* Cleavage combined with depression. Reduction requires elevation of fragments with bone grafting of resultant hole in metaphysis. Wedge is lagged on lateral aspect of cortex protected with buttress plate. (C) *Type III:* Pure central depression. There is no lateral wedge. Depression may also be anterior or posterior or involve whole plateau. After elevation of depression and bone grafting, lateral aspect of cortex is best protected with buttress plate. (D) *Type IV:* Medial condyle either is split off as a wedge or may be crumbled and depressed, which is characteristic of older patients with osteoporosis (not illustrated). (E) *Type V:* Note continuity of metaphysis and diaphysis. In internal fixation both sides must be protected with buttress plates. (F) *Type VI:* Essence of this fracture is a fracture line that dissociates metaphysis from diaphysis. Fracture pattern of the condyles is variable, and all types can occur. If both condyles are involved, the proximal tibia should be buttressed on both sides.

against varus and valgus stresses. The patient is discouraged from bearing weight on the extremity until there is radiographic evidence of healing.

Supracondylar Fracture (Compression Plate)

1. The lateral area of the distal end of the femur is exposed above and below the knee joint.
2. The surgeon reduces the fracture site and inserts multiple Kirschner wires for fixation.
3. Next, the surgeon places a calibrated Steinmann pin transversely across the condyles parallel to the joint line. The pin must stop 8 to 10 mm short of the medial cortex.
4. The length of the lag screw is gauged when it is read directly on the calibrated Steinmann pin, and adjustable double reamers are used to ream to this depth.
5. A lag screw is inserted across the condyles, followed by the compression screw.

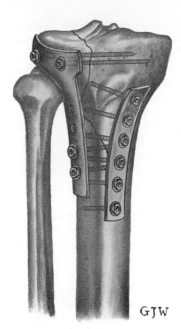

GJW

FIG. 20.55 Severe fractures are treated by use of multiple buttress plates and screws.

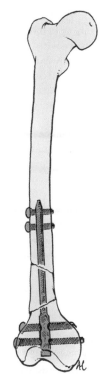

FIG. 20.56 Supracondylar nail.

6. The surgeon secures the plate to the femoral shaft with cortical bone screws and confirms the repair by fluoroscopy.
7. The surgeon irrigates the incision site and closes it. A knee immobilizer is placed.

Medial and Lateral Y-Type Tibial Plateau Fractures

1. The surgeon makes a long anterolateral incision, starting 2.5 cm above the superolateral aspect of the patella and tendon and proceeding distally around the patella to the anterior aspect of the tibia just below the tibial tuberosity. The distal end of the tibial shaft should be exposed.
2. The level of the prepatellar bursa is identified. The surgeon uses blunt dissection beneath the skin and retracts the proximal end of the tibia to expose it from midline medially to midline laterally.
3. The surgeon detaches the patellar tendon and exposes both the medial and lateral articular surfaces. The articular surface is reconstructed using temporary Kirschner wires. A contoured T-plate is attached to the medial aspect of the tibia using cancellous screws in the proximal portion and cortical screws in the distal portion. A smaller T-plate is inserted on the lateral side and secured in the same manner. The Kirschner wires are removed. Care should be taken to ensure that the screws do not interfere with each other as they traverse from opposite sides of the tibia.
4. The surgeon reattaches the patellar tendon using a 6.5-mm cancellous screw through the bone plug.
5. The surgeon closes the wound and immobilizes it at 30 degrees with a posterior splint.

Patellectomy and Reduction of Fractures of the Patella

Patellectomy was a frequently performed procedure until the early 1970s. It is possible to excise a portion of the patella (for comminuted fracture) or the entire patella (for painful degenerative arthritis) without significantly affecting ordinary activities. However, patellectomy has been shown to significantly reduce the power of extension as the joint extends, which is the most important function of the knee. Other complications associated with patellectomy are (1) slow return of quadriceps mechanism strength, (2) quadriceps muscle atrophy, and (3) loss of knee protection from the patella. Removal of the entire patella may result in relative lengthening of the knee extensor mechanism, which necessitates overlapping of the quadriceps tendon at the time of operation to prevent a lag in knee extension. Patellectomy should be performed only when comminution is extensive and reconstruction of the articular surface of the patella is not possible.

If the fracture consists of two large fragments that can be anatomically reduced, fixation is accomplished with a tension band, a circumferential loop technique, or bone screws. Tension band wiring produces compression forces across the fracture site and results in earlier union and immediate mobility of the knee.

Procedural Considerations

The patient is supine. The tourniquet is applied, and the leg is prepped and draped. A soft tissue set and a bone set are required, along with a power drill and bits, bone-reduction clamps, 18-gauge wire, heavy needle holders, and a wire tightener.

Operative Procedure

1. The surgeon makes a transverse curved incision over the patella.
2. Using sharp and blunt dissection the surgeon exposes the surface of the patella, the quadriceps, and the patellar tendons.
3. The joint is irrigated, and the fracture is reduced with bone-reduction clamps.
4. One length of wire is passed around the insertion of the patellar tendon and then around the quadriceps tendon. A second wire is passed more superficially through the bone fragments.
5. The fracture is overcorrected, and the wire is tightened with the wire tightener. In flexing the knee or contracting the quadriceps, the condyles press against the patellar fragments, producing compression at the fracture site.

Correction of Recurrent Dislocation of the Patella

Recurrent dislocation of the patella can be the result of violent initial dislocation or more commonly from underlying anatomic abnormalities. The underlying condition causes an abnormal excursion of the extensor mechanism over the femoral condyles. Dynamic forces, such as the vastus lateralis, and static forces, such as those arising from the shape of the patella, tend to displace the patella laterally. Dislocations occur when there are extreme displacing forces combined with internal rotation of the femur and flexion of the knee. If untreated, patellar dislocations will deteriorate the knee by causing abnormal patellofemoral articulation, chondromalacia, and meniscal tears.

Conservative treatment aimed at quadriceps strengthening may be indicated in some patients. Numerous procedures have been designed to realign the knee extensor mechanism. All the procedures include incising the lateral quadriceps tendon and shifting the insertion of the patellar tendon medially or distally to the original insertion of the tibia.

Procedural Considerations

The team places the patient in the supine position. The tourniquet is applied, and the leg is prepped and draped. A soft tissue set and a bone set are required, along with a large-fragment screw set, a power drill, a microsagittal saw, and osteotomes.

Operative Procedure

Patellar Realignment (Elmslie–Trillat)

1. The surgeon makes a lateral parapatellar incision beginning proximally to the patellar pole, laterally around the patella, and extending to 2 cm distally and just laterally to the tibial tuberosity.
2. A skin flap is developed and retracted medially to expose the capsule. A medial arthrotomy is completed, the joint is inspected, and any pathologic condition present is repaired.
3. The lateral retinaculum is released from the vastus lateralis proximally and the patellar tendon distally.
4. Using a ½-inch osteotome, the surgeon scores the tibial tuberosity medially and laterally, just below the fat pad and under the patella.
5. The surgeon continues the osteotomy using a microsagittal saw distally for 4 to 6 cm, and leaves the periosteum hinged at the distal-most part of the osteotomy.
6. The entire segment, with patellar tendon attached, is displaced medially and manually held in place while moving the knee through a range of motion. Tracking of the patella on the femoral groove is completed by systematically moving the knee medially in increments.
7. A cancellous bone bed is prepared at the point of reattachment of the tibial tuberosity.
8. The surgeon displaces the tuberosity medially and places a 6.5-mm cancellous bone screw.
9. The wound is irrigated and closed, and a long leg cylinder cast is applied. The cast is bivalved immediately.

Repair of Collateral or Cruciate Ligament Tears

The stability of the knee depends on the integrity of the cruciate and collateral ligaments. If any of these supporting structures are damaged, an unstable knee is likely unless properly repaired. Injuries to these supporting structures are usually not isolated. More frequently, several of the ligaments are injured at the same time. For example,

the injury commonly referred to as the "terrible triad" includes a torn anterior cruciate ligament (ACL), torn medial meniscus, and torn MCL.

The knee demonstrates grave disability with major ligamentous disruption. The *collateral ligaments* reinforce the knee capsule medially and laterally. They resist varus and valgus stresses on the knee. The *cruciate ligaments* control AP stability. Along with the ligaments, the muscle groups stabilize the joint and control movement. Because muscle strength is the first line of defense for the knee, damage is repaired to protect the ligaments. For optimum function of the joint, damaged structures should be reconstructed as close as possible to the original anatomic structures. If the knee is left untreated, osteoarthritis will develop.

Injury to a single cruciate ligament may not significantly compromise knee function. When the injury is combined with other injuries, surgery may be warranted. Surgeons may use various types of ligament grafts to replace or augment the cruciate ligaments. Autografts, allografts, and artificial substitutes are available. Ligament substitutes act as a scaffold, stent, or augmentation of the torn cruciate ligaments. Scaffolds support the soft tissue initially to allow ingrowth of the host tissue. Stents protect the joint from excessive stress while the permanent ligament substitute is healing. Augmentation, as by the patient's own iliotibial band, protects the graft initially after repair of a partial tear. Synthetic ligaments, which are less popular, include carbon-fiber grafts, polyglycolic acid material, Dacron, polyester, and polytetrafluoroethylene.

All synthetic grafts are subject to mechanical failure from weakening with fragmentation and synovitis. These are recommended for salvage procedures only when conventional reconstruction has failed and when other autogenous tissue is unavailable for substitution. Biologic materials from animals, such as bovine xenografts, are also available for ligament substitution, although they are subject to increased risk of infection, synovitis, and rejection. Homogeneous allografts are the substitute of choice for knee reconstruction when no autogenous graft is available from the patient. Disadvantages of homogeneous allografts include long-term weakening, possible rejection, and the possibility of infectious disease transfer.

Autogenous tissues are currently the substitute of choice, with the middle third of the patellar tendon and a block of patella being the most reliable. To minimize necrosis and maintain graft strength, the fat pad with its blood supply may be preserved along with the patellar tendon. Using this graft and other soft tissue autografts, the cruciate-deficient knee can be reconstructed arthroscopically. A combination of a torn ACL, medial meniscus, and MCL in the past often indicated the need for an open procedure (arthrotomy). With developing technology, many of these procedures can now be done arthroscopically. When reconstructing the cruciate ligament, the surgeon must have the graft biomechanically correct to maintain proper function. Many devices and systems are used to provide placement assistance and gauge appropriate graft tension. These devices are used either separately or in some combination. Although there are many variations, the principles are the same.

Procedural Considerations

The patient is positioned supine with a tourniquet applied to the upper area of the thigh. The perioperative nurse preps the patient from the upper area of the thigh down to and including the foot. Soft tissue instruments, arthroscopy instruments, ACL reconstruction instruments, Steinmann pins, reconstruction guides (Fig. 20.57), and a tension isometer are required. A power drill, microsagittal

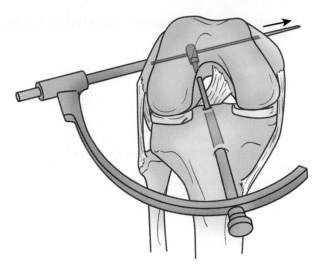

FIG. 20.57 Reconstruction guide used for ligament repair.

saw, and burrs are essential. The fixation device of choice also should be available. Meniscal repair instruments should be in the room.

Operative Procedure

Anterior Cruciate Repair. The surgeon performs an examination under anesthesia (EUA) immediately after induction of anesthesia, when the ligaments are completely lax, to evaluate the severity of the injury.

1. The surgeon makes a straight midline or slightly medial incision across the knee (Arthroscopic Anterior Cruciate Ligament Repair, see page 743).
2. Meniscus tears in the vascular zone (peripheral) are repaired with arthroscopic meniscal repair instruments or cutting needles with a heavy absorbable suture to repair the meniscofemoral and meniscotibial ligaments. If the meniscus is not repairable, the surgeon will perform a partial meniscectomy.
3. Using a power saw and osteotome, the surgeon harvests patellar and tibial bone plugs from the middle third of the patellar tendon.
4. A notchplasty is then performed, debriding and smoothing the lateral intercondylar wall with a burr and curette.
5. The surgeon uses the ligament guide to develop the femoral and tibial osseous tunnels and passes guidewires from the lateral area of the femoral condyle and tibial tubercle into the inter-condylar notch at isometric points near the anatomic attachment site of the ACL.
6. The pins are then overdrilled with cannulated drills as close to the size of the patellar tendon graft as possible. The tunnels are smoothed with a curette.
7. Sutures are placed through drill holes at both ends of the graft to pass the graft through the tunnels.
8. The surgeon passes the graft through the femoral and tibial osseous tunnels and fixes it at both ends with interference screws, staples, or polyethylene buttons.
9. The MCL and posterior oblique ligament are then individually repaired at their insertion sites with bone screws and spiked washers.
10. Additional extra-articular repair is done if necessary.
11. The surgeon closes the wound over intra-articular and subcutaneous drains, and a locking knee brace or knee immobilizer is applied.

Popliteal (Baker) Cyst Excision

Baker cysts occur in joints, frequently affecting the popliteal fossa. Baker cysts are often painful and can become very large, especially when associated with rheumatoid arthritis. Cysts in the popliteal fossa occur without a precipitating cause in children; in adults they often indicate an intra-articular disease process, such as rheumatoid arthritis, or a torn meniscus.

Procedural Considerations

In contrast to many other operative procedures on the knee, the patient is placed in the prone position. A soft tissue set and a bone set are required.

Operative Procedure

1. The surgeon makes an oblique incision in the popliteal area over the mass and divides the fascia to expose the mass.
2. Using blunt dissection, the surgeon frees the cyst and clamps it at the base of its attachment to the joint capsule.
3. The cyst is divided, and the pedicle is inverted and closed.
4. After the mass has been removed, the surgeon irrigates and closes the wound.

Postoperatively, the knee may be immobilized in extension with a posterior splint.

Correction of Fractures of the Tibial Shaft

The location of the tibia results in frequent exposure to injury. Open fractures are more common in the tibia than in other major bones because one-third of its surface is subcutaneous. Tibial shaft fractures are difficult to treat. The blood supply to the tibia is more precarious than that of other long bones because of its lack of enclosure by heavy muscle. The presence of hinge joints at the knee and ankle allows no adjustment for rotational deformity after fracture, so special care is required to correct for rotation during reduction and fixation. Rotational deformities are often seen. Delayed union, nonunion, and infection are fairly common complications. Closed reduction and casting provide excellent healing without significant complications, but this treatment can require casting for 6 months or more. Surgical reduction and internal fixation generally allow for earlier weight bearing and a shortened period of casting; however, the rate of complications is higher.

Generally torsional fractures seem to heal better and are more amenable to treatment than transverse fractures. It is theorized that twisting injuries cause less damage to endosteal vessels than that caused by transverse fractures, in which periosteum and endosteal vessels are torn circumferentially. The important prognostic indicators for tibial fractures are as follows: (1) the amount of initial displacement, (2) the degree of comminution, (3) the presence or absence of infection, and (4) the severity of soft tissue injury, excluding infection. As a rule, high-energy fractures, such as those caused by motor vehicle accidents or crushing injury, have a much worse prognosis than low-energy fractures, such as those caused by falls on ice or skiing accidents.

Because IM tibial nailings do not cause a significant increase in infections, external fixation of open tibial shaft fractures is less commonly performed. However, in the presence of gross contamination, severe soft tissue and vascular injury, bone infection, and delayed treatment, external fixation is the treatment of choice. The Ilizarov external fixation device is indicated when bone loss is significant and limb lengthening is required. Plate and screw fixation is another method in which tibial shaft fractures can be treated, although infection and nonunion of tibial shaft fractures are twice as likely with this method. Plate and screw fixation is indicated when intra-articular fragments of the knee and ankle are associated with the injury. Closed IM nailing is the treatment of choice in tibial shaft fractures because infection is less likely to occur and the periosteal blood supply is preserved. Static locking nails (locking both proximal and distal ends of the nail) are indicated for fractures with comminution, bone loss, and lengthening osteotomies. Dynamic locking nails (locking the end closest to the fracture site) are indicated for proximal or distal tibial fractures, nonunions, and malunions. Locking tibial nails include the Russell–Taylor and the Grosse–Kempf tibial nail.

The key to successful treatment of open tibial fractures, as in all open fractures, is meticulous and systematic debridement of all foreign matter and devitalized tissue. The surgeon is careful to minimize devascularization when reducing and fixing the fracture. Systemic antibiotics and those delivered by pulsatile lavage help reduce the chance of infection.

Procedural Considerations

The patient is usually administered a general or regional anesthetic while still on the hospital bed or the transport vehicle and then transferred to the OR fracture bed. The perioperative nurse assists with positioning the patient supine with the affected hip flexed approximately 45 degrees and the knee at 90 degrees. This positioning provides a horizontal orientation of the tibia. Using a calcaneal traction pin or table foot holder, traction is applied and rotational alignment obtained. After rotational alignment is obtained, a tourniquet is applied and the leg is prepped and draped. Some surgeons prefer to use a standard OR bed, breaking it at the knee. This obviates the need to insert the calcaneal traction pin and allows for easier maneuvering of the tibia during insertion of the locking screws.

A soft tissue set and a large bone set are required, in addition to the IM nail and insertion instruments of choice. A power drill and reamer driver are needed to use the necessary IM reamers. Fluoroscopy is needed as well. If open plating is being considered, the plates of choice and the large-fragment screws need to be available as well as bone-reduction clamps.

Operative Procedure

Closed or Open Tibial Intramedullary Nailing

1. If the open technique is required, the surgeon exposes the fracture site, reduces it, and irrigates it as necessary. Focus is then turned toward the nailing procedure (Fig. 20.58).
2. The surgeon makes a 5-cm incision medial to the patellar tendon to just below the tibial tuberosity.
3. Using a curved awl, the surgeon opens the medullary canal just proximal to the tibial tuberosity.
4. A guide rod (3.2 mm) is inserted into the shaft of the tibia down to the fracture site. The proximal fragment is reduced distally and the guide rod advanced into the distal fragment. Rod types include the straight guide rod for simple fractures, a curved guide rod for displaced fractures, and a cutting tip for an obstructed canal.
5. The length of the required nail is determined by the guide rod method (see Operative Procedure under Femoral Shaft Fractures: Internal Fixation, page 708) or by using the nail-length gauge and confirming with fluoroscopy.
6. With cannulated reamers over the guide rods, the surgeon reams the entire tibia 1 mm larger than the nail to be inserted. Inserting a nail too large for the canal can have a detrimental effect.

7. The driver, proximal drill, guide, and hexagonal bolt are assembled onto the tibial nail.
8. The surgeon inserts the nail over the guide rod and, with a mallet, drives it down the proximal fragment to enter the distal fragment, crossing the fracture site. The nail is not fully seated.
9. The guide rod is removed to prevent incarceration, and the surgeon completes the seating of the nail. The proximal tip of the nail should be flush with the tibial entry site.
10. Proximal locking is accomplished with the corresponding drill and tap through the proximal drill guide for 5-mm cortical bone screws.
11. Using the distal targeting device or a freehand technique, the surgeon inserts the distal screws. The 5-mm cortical bone screws are inserted, traversing the tibia through the tibial nail.
12. The surgeon irrigates the wounds. If bone graft is to be used, the surgeon places it around the fracture site and then closes the wound. Dressings are applied, and a cast or splint for immobilization may be applied.

Dynamization, or removal of either the proximal or the distal screws, may take place after 3 months for fractures that are stable but lack callus. Dynamization produces compressive forces at the fracture, promoting osteogenesis.

Tibial Dynamic Compression Plating

1. The surgeon makes a longitudinal incision large enough to accommodate the selected plate lateral to the tibial crest and exposes the fracture site.
2. The periosteum is stripped only enough for application of the plate. Circumferential stripping can diminish blood supply.
3. The surgeon reduces the fracture, places a plate across the fracture site, and secures the plate with bone-holding and plate-holding forceps. The plate may have to be contoured with a handheld or plate-bending press.
4. Using the neutral drill guide, the surgeon drills a 3.2-mm bicortical hole into the plate screw hole close to the fracture site, gauges it, and taps to 4.5 mm. The first bone screw is inserted, ensuring purchase of the screw on the opposite cortex.
5. Using the load drill guide (eccentric), the surgeon drills a second hole next to the fracture line in the opposite fragment. Drill and tap are accomplished as in the previous step. As the screw enters the bone, it will seek the center of the screw hole (the screw is eccentric, and the screw hole is beveled). The fracture site is brought under compression as the screw seats into the hole.
6. The wounds are irrigated. If bone graft is to be used, the surgeon places it around the fracture site and then closes the wound. Dressings are applied, and a cast or splint for immobilization may be applied.

Surgery of the Ankle and Foot

Correction of Ankle Fractures

Ankle fractures include fractures of the medial malleolus (tibia), lateral malleolus (fibula), and posterior malleolus (posterior aspect of the articular surface of the distal end of the tibia). They may or may not be associated with ligamentous injury. Ankle fractures can be classified in anatomic lines as unimalleolar, bimalleolar, and trimalleolar. Because medial malleolar and posterior malleolar fractures involve the distal weight-bearing articular surface of the tibia, open reduction and anatomic alignment are necessary. Fixation of the lateral malleolus is also important because it forms the ankle mortise (the socket formed by the distal tibia and fibula into which the body of the talus fits).

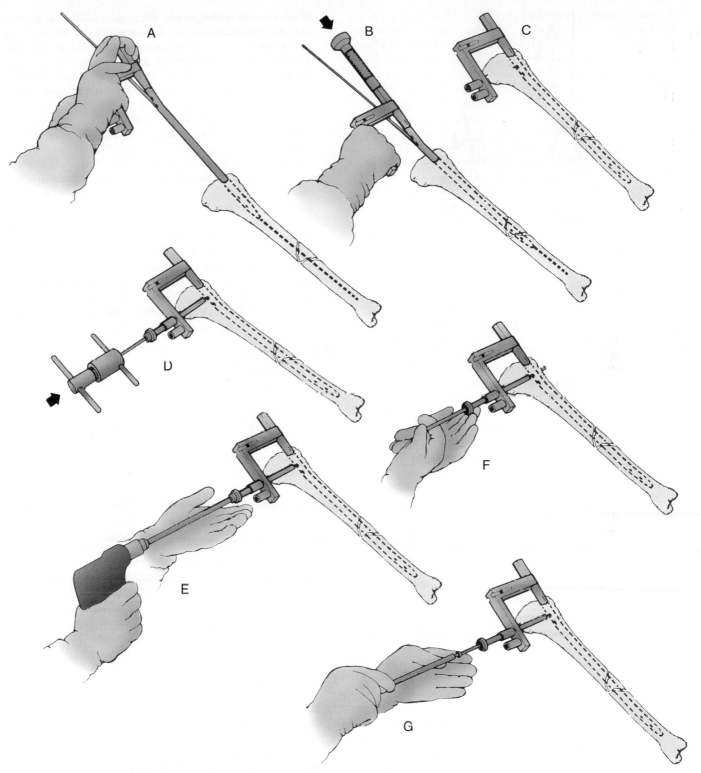

FIG. 20.58 Tibial intramedullary nailing. (A) Attachment of nail to proximal drill guide. (B) Driving nail over guide rod. (C) Final seating of nail with its tip flush with tibial entry portal. (D) For proximal interlocking, cortex is dimpled. (E) Depth measurements are made. (F) Locking screw length is confirmed. (G) Self-tapping screw is inserted through drill sleeve.

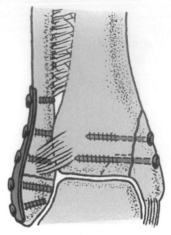

FIG. 20.59 Plate-screw placement for lateral malleolar fragment repair using one-third tubular plate.

Anatomic reduction prevents the occurrence of degenerative joint disease. Displaced fractures are treated with pins, malleolar or bone screws, or plates and screws (Fig. 20.59). Bimalleolar fractures can be treated with closed reduction and casting, but approximately 10% of these eventually develop a nonunion. The lateral malleolus (distal end of the fibula) is important for lateral and rotational stability of the joint. ORIF using Steinmann pins or screws placed obliquely into the tibia is a common technique. Lateral malleolar fractures can be fixed with the cancellous lag technique, which consists of overdrilling the first fragment and allowing compression of the fragments. Fracture of the lateral malleolus can also be treated with a Rush rod, inserted through the fragment and into the fibular canal. Compared with the other varieties of fractures, trimalleolar fractures require surgery more frequently. The posterior lip of the articulating surface of the tibia is usually involved and needs to be anatomically reduced to minimize degenerative changes. Cannulated screws can provide efficient reduction of a posterior fragment.

Procedural Considerations

The patient is in the supine position. The affected leg is prepped and draped after application of a pneumatic tourniquet. If the lateral ankle is involved, a padded sandbag is placed beneath the hip to internally rotate it. A soft tissue set; a small bone set; a small-fragment set with plates, screws, and pins; a power drill; and bone-reduction clamps are required.

Operative Procedure
Open Reduction Internal Fixation Trimalleolar Fracture
1. The surgeon makes medial and lateral incisions across the ankle.
2. The posterior malleolar fracture is exposed and reduced with bone-holding clamps and manipulation.
3. The surgeon inserts two Kirschner wires above the anterior tibial lip to temporarily reduce the fracture. The wires are directed anteriorly to posteriorly, to engage both fragments.
4. A drill hole is made anteriorly to posteriorly through both fragments. After measuring with a depth gauge, a malleolar, small cancellous, or other preferred screw is inserted through the fracture. The wires are removed.
5. The surgeon manipulates the lateral malleolar fracture into reduction.

6. If the fracture is oblique and not comminuted, the surgeon reduces it with one or two lag screws placed anteriorly to posteriorly. If the fracture is transverse, the surgeon inserts a long screw or medullary pin across the fracture line into the canal of the proximal fragment. A small semitubular or one-third tubular plate is applied if the fracture occurs above the syndesmosis.
7. Once the posterior and lateral malleolar fractures have been fixed, the medial malleolar fracture is finally reduced using bone clamps.
8. The reduction is held with two Kirschner wires while a hole is drilled through the medial malleolus into the metaphysis of the tibia.
9. Using a depth gauge, the surgeon determines the screw length. The malleolar screw is inserted across the fracture site and the Kirschner wires are removed.
10. If rotational stability is needed, the surgeon may add an additional smaller screw or compression wiring.
11. Intraoperative radiographs are taken in AP, lateral, and mortise views.
12. The wounds are irrigated and closed, and a short or long leg cast or splint is applied.

Triple Arthrodesis

The talocalcaneal (subtalar), talonavicular, and calcaneocuboid joints must be fused in patients with pronounced inversion or eversion deformities of the foot. Such deformities occur in clubfoot, poliomyelitis, and rheumatoid arthritis. Occasionally this operation is necessary for patients who have pain resulting from degenerative or traumatic arthritis, such as that occurring after intra-articular fractures of the calcaneus. Triple arthrodesis limits motion of the foot and ankle to plantar flexion and dorsiflexion.

Procedural Considerations

The perioperative nurse assists with positioning the patient in the supine position and preps the patient from the midcalf down to and including the foot. The perioperative nurse should consult with the surgeon before the procedure to determine whether bone grafting is anticipated so the patient's iliac crest area can be prepped.

A soft tissue set; a small bone set; a power saw, drill, or rasp; a bone graft set; and the AO compression plates and screws or bone staples to hold the fusion are required. Kirschner wires can be used to provide temporary fixation. A small lamina spreader is helpful in providing exposure.

Operative Procedure
1. An anterior or anterolateral approach is used.
2. The surgeon exposes the subtalar and calcaneocuboid joints and the lateral portion of the talonavicular joint.
3. The surgeon incises the capsules of the talonavicular, calcaneocuboid, and subtalar joints circumferentially to obtain as much mobility as possible. If this release allows the foot to be placed into a normal position, removal of large bony wedges is not required.
4. Using an osteotome, power saw, or power rasp, the surgeon removes the articular surfaces of the calcaneocuboid joint, the subtalar joint, and the talonavicular joint. The small lamina spreader is used to expose these surfaces. Care is taken to save all bone removed for later use in the fusion.
5. The removed bone is cut into small pieces to be used for bone grafting. If the quantity is insufficient, the surgeon will harvest

additional bone from the anterior ilium. Most of the bone is placed around the talonavicular joint and in the depth of the sinus tarsi.

6. Smooth Steinmann pins, staples, or screws are used for internal fixation.

7. The wound is closed over a suction drain. A short leg cast or splint is applied.

Bunionectomy

A bunion (hallux valgus) is a soft tissue or bony mass at the medial side of the first metatarsal head. It is associated with a valgus deformity of the great toe (Fig. 20.60). A bunion is caused by a basic structural defect of the foot, which predisposes to the development of this deformity. Ill-fitting shoes accentuate the situation and speed the development of bunions. Bunions are more common in women because of shoe styles, including high heels and pointed toes. Other factors that may contribute to this deformity are heredity, flat feet, foot pronation, longer first toe, muscle imbalance, and inflammatory disturbances of the feet.

Symptoms include pain on the dorsomedial aspect of the first metatarsal head or directly over the medial exostosis, swelling of the big toe, painful plantar callus, and plantar keratosis. Discomfort to the entire foot occurs as the forefoot becomes more fatigued and symptomatic, with pain radiating to the leg and knee.

Hallux valgus is treated with a variety of surgical procedures (Fig. 20.61), all of which remove the exostosis and attempt to realign the great toe by removal of bone, transfer of tendons, osteotomy of the first metatarsal shaft, or appropriate imbrication of soft tissue.

The goals of surgery are correction of the deformity (cosmesis), resection of the abnormal bony components (reconstruction), and restoration of normal or near-normal range of motion (function).

Procedural Considerations

The anesthesia provider administers a general or regional anesthetic, and a tourniquet is applied. The foot and leg are prepped and then draped using a sterile stockinette.

A soft tissue set, a small bone set, Kirschner wires, a power wire driver, and a microsagittal saw are required.

Operative Procedure
Keller Procedure

1. The surgeon makes a midline, straight, medial incision beginning at the neck of the proximal phalanx and extends it proximally.

2. Using blunt and sharp dissection, the surgeon exposes the joint capsule. A flap incision is made to expose the underlying hypertrophic bone found at the dorsomedial aspect of the first metatarsal head.

3. All soft tissue attachments are removed from the base of the proximal phalanx.

4. The surgeon uses a power-oscillating saw to resect the proximal third of the proximal phalanx.

5. Proper alignment of the toe is maintained as one or two 0.062-inch Kirschner wires are placed in the center of the medullary canal of the phalanx and then driven into the metatarsal head, neck, and shaft.

6. The surgeon irrigates and closes the wound. A bandage is applied to maintain the toe in the correct position.

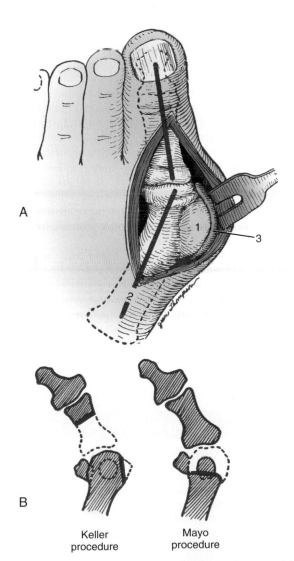

FIG. 20.60 Bunionectomy. (A) Bunion. *1,* Exostosis of metatarsal head; *2,* hallux valgus deformity; *3,* overlying bursa. (B) Operations for hallux valgus.

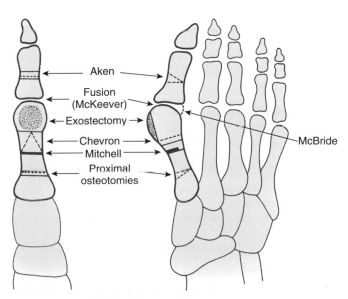

FIG. 20.61 Types of bunionectomies.

Correction of Hammer Toe Deformity

The term *hammer toe* is most often used to describe an abnormal flexion posture of the proximal interphalangeal joint of one of the four lesser toes. This deformity causes painful calluses to develop on the dorsal joints of the four lesser toes because the cocked-up digits rub against the shoes. Incising the long extensor tendon to the toes and fusing the proximal interphalangeal joint treat the deformities. A smooth Kirschner wire is frequently used to stabilize the fusion and position the toe properly during the postoperative period.

Procedural Considerations

The patient is positioned supine. An ankle tourniquet is applied. The foot is prepped and draped. A soft tissue set, a small bone set, Kirschner wires, and a power wire driver are required.

Operative Procedure

1. The surgeon makes an elliptic incision over the proximal inter-phalangeal joint measuring 5 to 6 mm wide with a 2-mm or 3-mm lateral extension on either side.
2. The capsular tissue of the distal third of the proximal phalanx and proximal interphalangeal joint is entered to expose the defect completely.
3. Using a small rongeur or microsaw, the surgeon resects the distal third portion of the proximal phalanx. After the capital fragment is excised, the surgeon debrides the remaining portion of the distal proximal phalanx with a rongeur or rasp.
4. Digital alignment can be maintained with small Kirschner wires.
5. The surgeon irrigates and closes the wounds. A sterile dressing and orthopedic shoe are applied for postoperative recovery.

Correction of Metatarsal Fractures

Metatarsal fractures occur in various sites. These fractures have a reduced healing potential because metatarsals consist mainly of cortical bone, which lacks vascularity. Treatment is determined by the extent of the fracture; the greater the displacement is, the greater the need for reduction. Generally transverse and short, oblique, midshaft fractures of the metatarsals are internally fixed because of their instability and displacement. Pins, wires, screws, and plates are used for internal fixation of metatarsal fractures. The simplest method is Kirschner wire fixation.

Procedural Considerations

The patient is placed in the supine position, a tourniquet is applied, and the foot is prepped and draped. A soft tissue set, a small bone set, Kirschner wires, and a power wire driver are required.

Operative Procedure

1. The surgeon makes a small incision over the fracture and identifies and retracts the distal fragment.
2. A smooth Kirschner wire is driven distally, exiting the skin.
3. The surgeon uses a wire driver to drive the wire proximally into the canal of the proximal fragment.
4. If the fracture is more complex or comminuted, the surgeon may cross two Kirschner wires through the fracture to transfix the fracture site.
5. The incision is closed, and a postoperative shoe is applied.

Metatarsal Head Resection

Patients with rheumatoid arthritis frequently have dorsally dislocated toes and prominent and painful metatarsal heads on the plantar surfaces of their feet. Excision of all the metatarsal heads commonly relieves the pain and corrects an associated bunion deformity.

Procedural Considerations

The patient is placed in the supine position, a tourniquet is applied, and the foot is prepped and draped. A soft tissue set, a small bone set, Kirschner wires, a power wire driver, and a power microsagittal saw are required.

Operative Procedure

Clayton Technique

1. A transverse plantar incision is made, and tissue is dissected to the metatarsal heads.
2. Using a microsagittal saw the surgeon removes the metatarsal heads and half the proximal phalanges.
3. The surgeon transects the extensor tendons; they are not repaired.
4. The skin is closed, and a dressing and postoperative shoe are applied.

Pelvic Fractures and Disruption

Patients with multiple trauma often present with multiple fractures that can be life-threatening. Complications of pelvic fractures include injury to not only major vessels and nerves but also major visceral organs, such as the intestines, bladder, and urethra. Factors influencing mortality include associated visceral injury, hemorrhage, and head injury.

Pelvic fracture classification is divided into three main groups (Table 20.1). *Type A fractures* are stable, without ring involvement (A1) or minimally displaced fractures of the ring (A2). *Type B fractures* are rotationally unstable and vertically stable and are also subclassified: B1 is an open book fracture, B2 has ipsilateral compression, and B3 has contralateral compression. *Type C fractures* are both rotationally and vertically unstable: C1 is unilateral, C2 is bilateral, and C3 is associated with the acetabulum. Radiographic films, computed tomography (CT) scan, and magnetic resonance imaging (MRI) all prove useful in determining the type and appropriate treatment for pelvic trauma.

Treatment is based on classification and may include closed manipulation and reduction or internal and external fixation. Internal and external fixation can be used concurrently in the treatment of some pelvic fractures.

Type A fractures are stable and can be treated nonoperatively. Type B1 fractures may be treated with external fixation or anterior plate fixation. Type C fractures usually require open procedures to

TABLE 20.1		
Classification of Pelvic Injuries		
Type A	Stable	
	A1: Fractures of pelvis not involving ring	
	A2: Stable, minimally displaced fractures of ring	
Type B	Rotationally unstable, vertically stable	
	B1: Open book	
	B2: Lateral compression: ipsilateral	
	B3: Lateral compression: contralateral (bucket handle)	
Type C	Rotationally and vertically unstable	
	C1: Unilateral	
	C2: Bilateral	
	C3: Associated with an acetabular fracture	

fix the fractures with plates and screws, and reduction of sacral disruptions with transiliac rods or screws. Type C fractures may be treated with external fixation when the patient is hemodynamically unstable and a quicker, simpler procedure is prudent.

External fixation is the most widely recommended treatment for type B fractures of the pelvis. A technique similar to that of external fixation of extremity fractures is done in the OR with anesthesia and sterile conditions. If external fixation is to be used, the earlier it is attempted the greater the chance of success.

Procedural Considerations

This procedure is often done during other emergent and trauma resuscitative efforts. The patient's entire pelvic area is prepped and draped. Pin placement is performed to complete the reduction. A soft tissue set is needed in addition to the external fixator of choice and the instruments for its insertion, including a power drill.

Operative Procedure

AO External Fixation

1. The surgeon reduces the pelvic disruption manually and confirms it radiographically. It may be impossible to completely reduce the disruption without skeletal traction using a distal femoral pin.
2. Kirschner wires are inserted percutaneously to determine the position of the pin placement, taking into consideration the inward and downward crest slope.
3. The surgeon places parallel rows of pins into the anterior iliac crest area by drilling the outer cortex and placing 5-mm half-pins medially and distally. The pins should enter cancellous bone between the outer and inner tables of ilium.
4. Three universal frames are placed over the pins as close to the skin as possible for maximum rigidity.
5. Optimal reduction of the fracture is visualized radiographically. The surgeon applies the crossbar, and compression and distraction maneuvers are used to maintain the reduction.
6. The surgeon removes the crossbar and applies the connecting rods with couplers.
7. After the couplers are in place, the surgeon reattaches the crossbar and tightens the joints of the frame.
8. The pin sites of tented skin are released. The wounds are dressed with iodine ointment and gauze.
9. The frames are left in place generally for 8 to 12 weeks.

Total Joint Arthroplasty

Arthroplasty of the joints is performed to restore motion of the joint and function to the muscles and ligaments. It is indicated in individuals with a painful, disabling arthritic joint that is no longer responsive to conservative therapy. In the past, the procedure was reserved for those with a less active lifestyle, and surgeons treated patients with reconstructive procedures such as arthrodesis or osteotomy because of the unknown life expectancy of the materials used in the manufacturing of the prostheses. Technologic advances in the prostheses used today allow the younger patient, or the very active older person, to undergo joint replacement. Many total hip and knee replacements are done each year. Improvements in implant design, materials, and fixation techniques are ongoing, as is research on enhancing soft and hard tissue healing.

The classic combination of metal on polyethylene is the mainstay of joint implants. Metals used in hip and knee implants include *cobalt-chromium* (weight-bearing femoral head) and *titanium* (stems of hips and tibial components). The acetabulum and tibial articulating surfaces continue to be substituted with *ultra-high-molecular-weight polyethylene* (UHMWPE), which provides superior wear characteristics. Other designs have emerged in total hip arthroplasty, including metal on metal and the use of ceramic femoral heads.

At one time it was thought that bone cement was the weak link in the longevity of a joint implant because of a relatively high rate of loosening of cement-fixed implants, especially in younger, more active patients. In response to this belief, alternative methods of fixation have been developed. One method involves the application of a precoat of PMMA to the femoral stem to enhance bonding of the prosthesis to the cement mantle. Another method involves the attachment of a porous metal surface to parts of the femoral stem and the entire outer surface of the acetabular component. Most of the porous surfaces are composed of multiple layers sintered in place, creating interconnecting, open pores among the various particles. This allows for the ingrowth of bone to occur, ultimately anchoring the prosthesis in place. "Porous coating" was an attempt to eradicate what was termed *cement disease*, which is a lysis of bone around the prosthesis causing early loosening. It is now believed that this condition is caused by "wear debris," or particulate matter being shed from metal-to-polyethylene interfaces, and not necessarily from the effects of PMMA.

Bone cement, or PMMA, has received considerable attention in the search for optimal bone-to-implant fixation. Cement seems to exhibit various degrees of porosity depending on mixing methods and cement pressurization within the canal. Bone cement must prevent motion at the implant interface. Porosity can lead to fatigue and fracture, which ultimately can lead to implant loosening. Local tissue effects of PMMA may include (1) tissue protein coagulation caused by polymerization, (2) bone necrosis caused by occlusion of nutrient metaphyseal arteries, and (3) cytotoxic and lipotoxic effects of nonpolymerized monomers.

Despite the high rate of success of total joint implantation over the years, there are numerous potential complications. They are generally divided into medical complications, mechanical complications, and infections. Medical complications include, but are not limited to, cardiac dysrhythmias, myocardial infarction, hemorrhage, and pulmonary emboli. Mechanical complications are implant breakage, loosening, and wear. Infection in the patient with a total joint implant is a catastrophic complication that usually requires additional surgery and prolonged hospitalization.

Most surgeons recommend the routine use of antibiotics in primary and revision joint arthroplasty. Antibiotic coverage is initiated preoperatively, continued during lengthy procedures, and administered for 24 to 48 hours postoperatively. The Surgical Care Improvement Project (SCIP) measures have been instituted by the TJC to prevent surgical site infections and are one of eight reportable Joint Commission eCQM measures (TJC, 2016). Pulsatile lavage systems with antibiotic irrigation are used to keep tissues moist, remove debris, and dilute bacteria that may be present.

Total Hip Arthroplasty

Total hip arthroplasty is a common orthopedic procedure performed on patients with hip pain caused by degenerative joint disease, rheumatoid arthritis, or avascular necrosis. A total hip replacement can be cemented, noncemented, or be a hybrid. Hybrids involve cementing one component, usually the femoral stem, and then inserting a metal-backed, porous-coated acetabular component in a press-fit state. Hybrid arthroplasty is a controversial procedure for two reasons. The first reason relates to research that demonstrates that wear debris is increased with the larger metal-to-polyethylene interface present in the metal-backed, porous-coated acetabular component. The second reason is cost. The metal-backed, porous-coated acetabular component is significantly more expensive than the all-polyethylene component. Consequently patient selection is very important in determining which type of component is best.

The primary function of the femoral component is the replacement of the femoral head and femoral neck after resection. The femoral head should ultimately sit where it reproduces the center of rotation of the hip. The neck length is variable and is built into several different heights of femoral heads that are eventually seated onto the Morse taper of the femoral stem. The version (implant rotation within the canal) is very important; too much anteversion or retroversion leaves the hip prone to dislocation. The normal position of the proximal femur is in 10 to 15 degrees of anteversion.

Femoral stems can be collarless or have collars that sit down on the resected femur. Collars produce forces on the bone and may be desired in cases of osteoporotic bone, in which bone genesis may be diminished because of the disease process.

Acetabular cups have also presented challenges in trying to maintain fixation within the socket. When cement techniques of the 1970s were used, femoral loosening plateaued about 5 years after surgery. Wear properties of the UHMWPE are also a concern. For this and other reasons associated with component failure, the idea of modularity was developed. Modular components, such as a polyethylene cup that snaps into a metal acetabular shell, greatly decrease the amount of surgery needed in the case of some revisions. In the case of excessive cup wear or a short femoral neck, surgery is minimized with the ability to exchange the modular components without removing the implants fixed to the bone.

Acetabular cups come with a textured back for cement fixation and may have standoff pegs to allow an appropriate cement mantle. Noncemented cups usually are porous coated and may have screw holes to aid in anchoring the less-than-stable cup. The presence of screw holes in an acetabular component is another controversial issue. Some believe that more wear debris is created with micromotion between the screw head and the cup as well as between the uneven surface of the screw and the polyethylene liner.

Prostheses are available for every patient's needs. Modular hip systems allow the orthopedic surgeon to choose from an array of interchangeable components that have been developed. Various femoral head sizes (22, 26, 28, and 32 mm) are available to maintain proper center of rotation. Acetabular cups may be snap fit, low profile, or deep profile, which adds additional thickness to the medial wall, in which bone loss may be significant.

With modular systems, unipolar or bipolar cups are also an option when the acetabular articular surface is relatively normal. The unipolar and bipolar cups with appropriate head sizes are designed to fit on various modular system stems.

Custom prostheses or revision and extra-long stems are available when bone loss is significant. These implants are used in cases of revision when fixation is needed farther down the femoral canal or in oncologic cases in which tumor and corresponding bone have been resected.

Younger, active individuals with strong, healthy bones are ideal candidates for noncemented total hip replacement arthroplasties. Elderly patients with osteoporosis and poor-quality bone are usually candidates for cemented components because their bones may lack the compressive strength to support weight-bearing forces.

Several different surgical techniques have been developed for total hip arthroplasty. Surgical techniques have improved over the years focusing on minimizing soft tissue insult. Regardless of the

technique, patient education is critical to optimize outcomes (Patient Engagement Exemplar).

Hip Reconstruction (Cemented)

Numerous implants are available for total hip implantation. Many of the implants can be used for the same surgical indications, and one implant may not function any better than another, provided that all other conditions and techniques are the same. The instruments required to implant any one device cannot be used for another. During the preoperative verification process and time-out, the perioperative nurse and scrub person collaborate to ensure that all the instrumentation is available.

PMMA adheres to the polyethylene and metal but not to the bone. It fills the cavity and interstices of the bone and forms a mechanical bond. PMMA is manufactured as a liquid monomer and a powder and is mixed under sterile conditions by the scrub person in the OR at the time of implantation. It usually takes 10 to 12 minutes to harden. Because of the potentially harmful effects of PMMA fumes to the nasal epithelium, an exhaust system should be used during the mixing process.

Procedural Considerations. The patient is positioned in the lateral decubitus position and secured in place with anterior and posterior bolsters. This position is essential to ensure correct anatomic placement of the acetabular cup. The perioperative nurse verifies that the patient's bony prominences are adequately padded. The skin prep is completed from the level of the umbilicus down to and including the foot; then the patient is draped. The radiographs are overlaid with the implant templates.

A soft tissue set and a large bone set are required. In addition, the total hip implants and corresponding instrumentation, acetabular reamers, hip retractor set, power reamer driver and saw, and pulse lavage with a 3-L bag of normal saline solution are needed. If PMMA is used, femoral canal suction wicks, a cement restrictor and its inserter, and PMMA including its mixing supplies will be needed. If a trochanteric osteotomy is performed, the equipment of choice for its reattachment will be required.

Revision of total hip arthroplasties requires the same instrumentation as for cemented total hip reconstruction in addition to cement removal instrumentation, fluoroscopy, and the revision implants and their corresponding instrumentation.

Operative Procedure

Cemented Modular Hip System, Posterior Approach

1. The surgeon makes an incision 2.5 cm distal and lateral to the anterosuperior iliac spine and curves the incision distally and posteriorly over the lateral aspect of the greater trochanter and lateral surface of the femoral shaft to 5 cm distal to the base of the trochanter.
2. The surgeon divides the tensor fasciae latae over the greater trochanter and carries this distally to the extent of the incision. Dissection is carried proximally between the interval of the gluteus medius and the tensor fasciae latae muscles.
3. The anterior fibers of the gluteus medius tendon are tagged and detached from the trochanter. The surgeon incises the capsule longitudinally along the anterosuperior surface of the femoral neck. In the distal part of the incision, the origin of the vastus lateralis may be either reflected distally or split longitudinally to expose the base of the trochanter and proximal part of the femoral shaft.
4. After completing the capsulotomy, the surgeon dislocates the hip. Adduction and external rotation present the femoral head anteriorly into the surgical site.
5. The surgeon places the femoral osteotomy guide over the lateral femur to identify the point on the femoral neck in which the osteotomy should be made. Some femoral osteotomy guides also gauge the neck length required. The surgeon marks the level and uses an oscillating or a reciprocating saw to complete the femoral osteotomy.
6. The femur is retracted to expose the acetabulum, allowing completion of the capsulotomy, and exposing the bony rim of the entire acetabulum.
7. The surgeon inspects the acetabulum, removes any osteophytes, and reams the articular cartilage with bone-conserving reamers in a circumferential manner. The smallest reamer is progressed in a graduated method 1 or 2 mm at a time until the cartilage is reamed down to expose osteochondral bone. A hemispheric shape and bleeding bone should result.
8. Remaining soft tissue is curetted from the floor of the acetabulum, and cystic areas are filled with cancellous bone from the femoral canal and packed with a bone tamp. Any other bone grafting of major bony defects is accomplished using the fixation method of choice (bone screws).
9. Several 6-mm holes are drilled into the floor of the acetabulum, aimed into the ilium, ischium, and pubis. Holes are undercut using curettes. These prepared holes act as anchoring areas for the bone cement.
10. Trial acetabular components are placed on the positioning device and positioned in the socket. The surgeon assesses the cup for size, position within the socket, and the relationship of the component compared with the bony margins of the acetabulum.
11. The prepared acetabular socket is lavaged, dried with wicks, and filled with cement that has been injected and pressurized with an injection gun. The surgeon positions the acetabular shell component and holds it motionless until the cement polymerizes. Extruded cement is trimmed from around the edge of the component. A polyethylene insert is later snapped into the shell.
12. A radiopaque sponge (soft good) is placed in the acetabulum to protect the component from bone debris and subsequent cement as attention is turned to the femur.
13. Dropping the patient's foot toward the floor and internally rotating and pushing the leg proximally exposes the proximal femur. The surgeon accesses the femoral canal using a box osteotome or trochanteric reamer followed by the T-handle canal reamer.
14. Beginning with the smallest broach, the surgeon alternately impacts and extracts the proximal femoral canal. Progressively larger broaches are used to crush and remove cancellous bone until cortical bone is reached. A broach that is not advancing should not be used because this could result in shattering the femur.
15. With the final broach seated to the desired depth in the canal, the surgeon prepares the femoral neck with a calcar reamer. The broach remains while the surgeon places the femoral trial component along with the various-sized head, neck, and offset trial components.
16. The trial component is removed, and the canal is lavaged and brushed to accommodate the PMMA.
17. The surgeon inserts a cement restrictor into the femoral canal. The femoral components are passed and assembled on the back table.
18. The cement is injected and pressurized within the femoral canal.
19. The femoral component, with the proximal and distal centralizers, is inserted into the canal with or without the femoral head.
20. The surgeon positions the appropriate size of femoral head onto the stem, and reduction is performed. The joint is taken through a range of motion to check for positioning, stability, and the limit to which dislocation occurs.
21. Depending on the surgeon and the surgical approach, the greater trochanter may or may not have been removed for exposure of the hip joint. If removed, it is reattached with 18-gauge wire or a cable grip system.
22. The surgeon closes the wound in layers over suction drains. The skin is closed with staples, and a sterile dressing is applied to provide compression to the wound.
23. An abduction pillow or splint is placed between the patient's legs postoperatively if stability of the joint is of concern.

Hip Reconstruction (Noncemented)

Fixation with a noncemented prosthesis is initially accomplished by a tight fit and intimate contact of the implants within bone of substantial strength. As with all prosthetic designs, it is essential to fill the medullary canal and wedge the prosthesis in as tightly as possible to provide temporary press-fit fixation. These prostheses closely follow normal anatomic shape. Only the instrumentation corresponding to the implant should be used. Precise machining of the femoral canal must be ensured. Acetabular components are usually press-fitted, but many systems provide holes for screw fixation if stability of the prosthesis is in doubt. Sufficient time is then allowed for the cancellous bone to heal by growing into the porous portions of the prosthesis.

The healing process requires the same amount of time as a long bone cortical fracture (approximately 3 months). The patient must be cautious after the procedure and protect the operative hip from excessive compression, rotation, and shear stresses.

Procedural Considerations. The position and incision are at the surgeon's discretion. The Anatomic Medullary Locking Hip System (AML) can be used with multiple surgical approaches including small incision surgery. The radiographs and implant templates are placed on the view box.

Operative Procedure

Noncemented Anatomic Medullary Locking Hip System

1. After the incision is made, the surgeon enters the capsule and dislocates the femoral head (Fig. 20.62).

2. The femoral head is removed at 45 degrees using an oscillating power saw. Double-angle, double-footed retractors are placed to expose and elevate the acetabulum (retractors are subject to surgeon's preference and patient position).

3. The surgeon uses a Kocher and knife to remove the remaining cartilage and soft tissue from the acetabulum. Next progressively sized acetabular hemispheric reamers are used to prepare the bone. The reamer heads themselves can be used as trials.

4. At this point, some surgeon's prefer to implant the acetabular cup and liner. Occasionally, screws will be used to hold the cup until ingrowth occurs.

5. Acetabular retractors are removed and replaced with femoral retractors such as double-angle, Cobra, or double-footed retractors.

6. A small straight curette is used to find the IM canal. The femoral reamer (with power) is then inserted down the IM canal.

7. The surgeon uses the femoral broaches sequentially to enlarge the canal.

8. Once the IM canal is broached, the femoral broaches are then used for trial insertion.

9. The surgeon may use a power calcar planer placed over the trunnion of the broach to contour the femoral neck.

10. A trial head and neck component is positioned onto the fitted broach, and a trial reduction is performed.

11. If trial reduction is satisfactory, the surgeon removes the trial components.

12. The femoral component is placed into the canal, and the modular head is seated on the trunnion.

13. Reduction of the hip is followed by standard closure with or without drains.

Minimally Invasive Total Hip Arthroplasty

Minimally invasive total hip arthroplasty (MITHA) has resulted in minimized scarring, reduced patient morbidity, a shortened hospitalization period, and an accelerated rehabilitation process (AAOS, 2016a). MITHA can be performed with a single or double incision. For a single incision, the patient is placed in a lateral position; the patient is supine for a double-incision procedure. With double-incision MITHA, the acetabular and femoral components are inserted through two small incisions, one anterolateral and one posterolateral, each approximately 5 cm long. The technique spares the muscles and tendons around the hip.

Procedural Considerations. As with any joint replacement, templates of the x-rays preoperatively are recommended. A regular OR bed with x-ray capability is used. The perioperative nurse should alert the radiology department that fluoroscopy will be used.

Equipment should be arranged carefully (Fig. 20.63). The patient is positioned supine with a small bolster placed under the pelvis on the operative side. The patient's entire leg, from above the waist to the ankle, is then prepped and draped in the usual fashion. The time-out includes confirmation of the correct patient, site, side, procedure, position, and implants.

Operative Procedure (VerSys Hip System)

1. The C-arm is used to define the femoral neck. The surgeon makes the anterior incision directly over the femoral neck from the base of the femoral head. The lateral femoral cutaneous nerve is identified and located, and then carefully retracted along with the sartorius using an Army Navy retractor. A second retractor is used for the tensor fasciae latae laterally. This exposes the lateral border of the rectus femoris.

2. The surgeon uses an electrosurgical unit (ESU) for hemostasis of the lateral femoral vessels. The Army Navy retractors are extended deeper as the rectus femoris is dissected with a #10 blade on a long handle. An extended blade ESU pencil may also be used.

3. The surgeon incises the femoral capsule and fat pad. A Cobb elevator is used to move the tissue medially underneath the rectus muscles and laterally off the femoral neck, allowing exposure of the capsule over the femoral neck.

4. Two curved lighted retractors are placed outside the capsule around the femoral neck, perpendicular to it. If additional leverage is needed, retractor handle extenders may be attached and used. The surgeon incises the femoral capsule in line with the femoral neck lateral to the midline to facilitate future placement of the head of the femoral prosthesis. Sutures can be used to retract the capsule so that the femoral head and neck are clearly visible.

5. Fluoroscopy may then be used to verify osteotomy position. Using the oscillating saw, the surgeon places a high femoral neck cut and uses a straight, 4-cm osteotome to complete it. A second cut is then made, and a threaded Steinmann pin is inserted to remove the small wafer of bone. This allows enough room for the surgeon to make the final femoral neck cut.

6. The surgeon uses fluoroscopy to check the angle and length of resection. It is important for the surgical team to help keep the leg in neutral position, especially during these cuts. The femoral head is then removed while the surgical assistant applies gentle traction on the leg.

7. Three lighted anterior retractors are placed: one superiorly in the line of the incision, over the acetabulum, and the second and third at 90-degree angles to the first. After the acetabulum is exposed, sharp and blunt dissection is used to remove remaining tissue and synovium.

8. Reaming starts with the acetabular reamer that is close to the template size. C-arm visualization is used during the reaming. After reaming is completed to the acceptable size, the trial components are placed to determine fit. C-arm images are used to confirm location and size. The positioning bolster is removed at this time. The appropriate-sized cup and liner are then chosen. The acetabular component is then seated using the offset shell inserter, retractors are removed, and the cup is impacted into place. Multiple images are taken to check the placement and position of the cup while impacting. The inserter is then removed. If screws are used, a drill, screws, drill guide, depth gauge, and flexible screwdriver will be required. After the cup and screws are in place, their position is again checked with fluoroscopy. The liner is inserted.

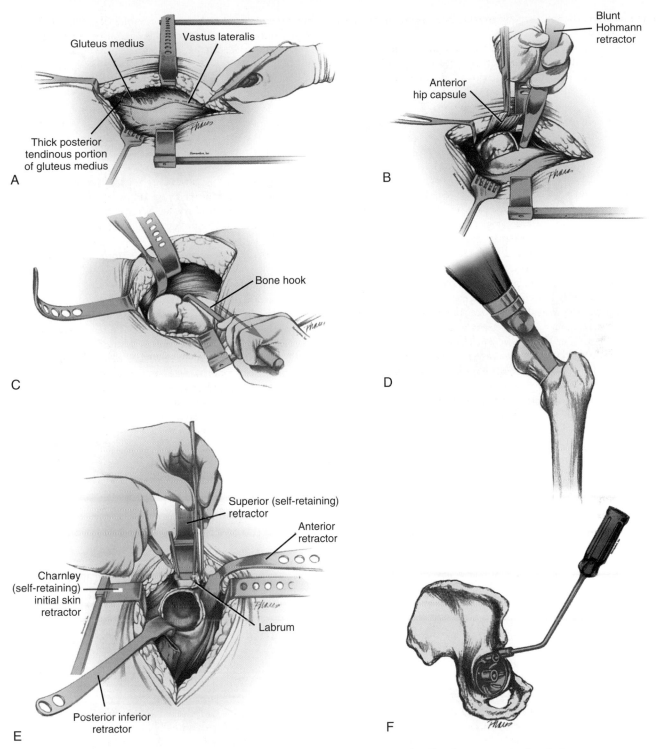

FIG. 20.62 Noncemented hip reconstruction. (A) After the incision, the Charnley retractor is placed, the tensor fasciae latae is incised, and the gluteus medius is detached. (B) An anterior capsulotomy is completed. (C) The hip is flexed, adducted, and externally rotated to dislocate from the acetabulum. (D) The femoral neck is cut by use of an oscillating saw blade. (E) The rim of the acetabulum is debrided of labrum, redundant capsule, and marginal osteophytes. (F) The acetabulum is reamed; after reaming, the appropriate drill guide is inserted into the acetabulum.   *Continued*

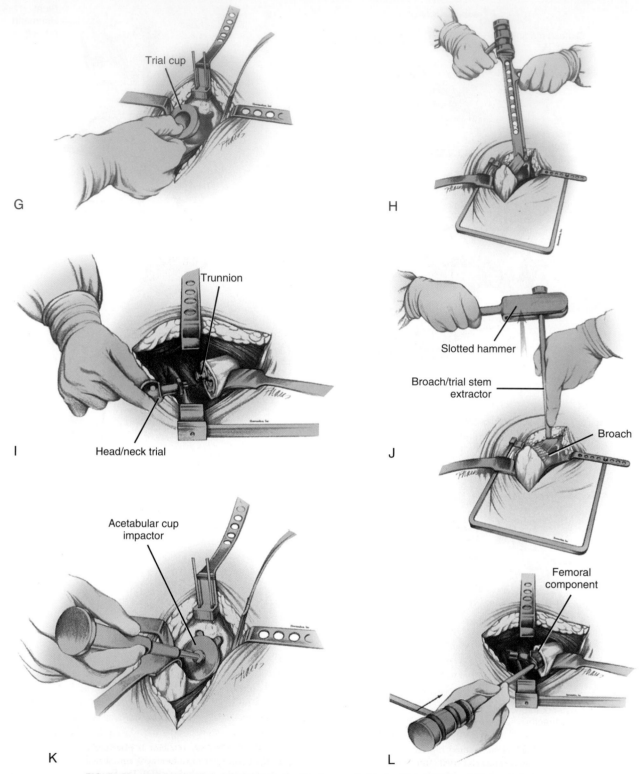

FIG. 20.62, cont'd (G) After drilling the holes for the acetabular fixation pegs, the trial acetabular cup is inserted. (H) The proximal wedge of cancellous bone is removed, and the appropriate size of femoral broach is introduced down the axis of the femoral canal. (I) The trial head is placed on the broach trunnion of trial reduction. (J) With the slotted hammer the femoral broach is extracted; the trial acetabular cup is removed. (K) Acetabular fixation pegs are seated, the acetabular cup is introduced, and the component is seated. (L) The femoral canal is irrigated with pulsatile lavage and dried with suction and soft goods. The femoral canal is plugged and filled with methylmethacrylate, and the femoral component is inserted.

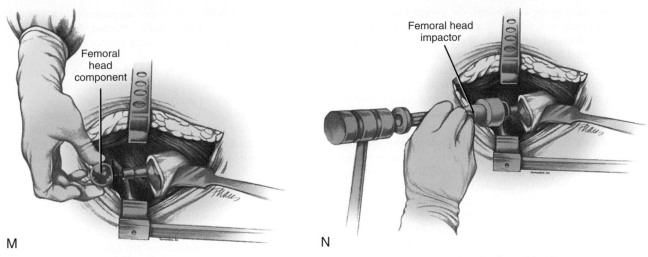

FIG. 20.62, cont'd (M) The femoral head component is placed on the trunnion. (N) The femoral head is impacted, the femur is reduced, and the wound is irrigated before closure.

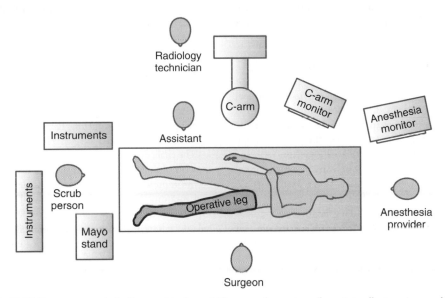

FIG. 20.63 Room setup, including positioning of C-arm and monitor, for minimally invasive total hip arthroplasty.

9. The second incision is found by direct palpation. The nonoperative leg is adducted. The operative leg is fully adducted, externally rotated, and flexed over the nonoperative leg. Location is verified by fluoroscopy. A stab wound is made in the posterior lateral buttock and extended to 1.5 to 3 cm as needed. Sharp dissection is used to spread the tissue along the coaxial pathway to the piriformis fossa.

10. Downward pressure is applied to the operative knee to elevate the trochanter. The surgeon inserts the tissue protector and reams the femoral canal beginning with the lateral reamers. All reamers should be inserted in the locked position. After the lateral reaming is complete, IM reamers are used. The surgeon uses fluoroscopy at regular intervals throughout the reaming process to ensure centralization in the canal. The tissue protector is then removed.

11. The surgeon rasps the canal, with the initial rasp two to three times smaller than the template size of the canal. The rasp is tapped into place until fully seated; its position is verified with fluoroscopy. The canal is rasped until proper sizing and positioning are obtained. The C-arm is used to check the final depth, fill, and positioning of the rasp with the apex of the calcar.

12. Trial reduction is done with the final rasp in place. The provisional head is placed on the rasp, and the hip is reduced by providing longitudinal traction and internal rotation. The surgeon moves the hip through a full range of motion. Fluoroscopy may be used to check the levels of the lesser trochanters for possible leg length discrepancies. Once trial reduction is complete, the rasp is removed by way of a posterior exit and the head through the anterior incision.

13. Two lighted anterior retractors are placed in the posterior incision to keep the tissue away from the stem as it is placed in the femoral canal. Once the implant is through the skin and properly rotated, the implant driver is attached. Gentle traction is placed on the leg in neutral abduction. Once the femoral component

is within the capsule of the hip, the patient's operative leg is repositioned; it is fully adducted, externally rotated, and flexed over the nonoperative leg. The stem is impacted until it is fully seated. Fluoroscopy is used to ensure proper seating and alignment.

14. The surgeon pulls the neck of the femur through the wound and places the trial head. Traction is placed on the hip, and the hip is then turned into internal rotation. Range-of-motion and leg length assessment is then done.

15. After the final trial reduction is performed, the surgeon dislocates the hip to put the final head in place. Hip dislocation is done using a dull bone hook and external rotation of the hip. Two sutures are placed in the capsule: one medially and the other laterally. This is done before the head is reduced to prevent the capsule from invaginating posteriorly. The prosthetic head can then be seated and impacted. Gentle traction and internal rotation are used to reduce the hip. A final range-of-motion and leg length assessment is performed.

16. The surgeon irrigates the incisions with antibiotic irrigation. A local anesthetic such as bupivacaine (Marcaine) may be infiltrated into the incision, the two previously placed sutures are tied, and additional sutures are placed to fully close the capsule. A drain may be placed.

Anterolateral Approach for Total Hip Arthroplasty

The anterolateral approach, between the hip abductor and the tensor fasciae latae, preserves the abductor muscles. It also provides additional inferior surgical field rather than a direct lateral approach and is better in preserving the soft tissue than a direct lateral approach.

Procedural Considerations. The team places the patient supine on the OR bed and places a hip bolster under the sacrum with the inferior edge of the bolster at the ischial tuberosity. A contralateral post is positioned at the opposite side of the torso. Both legs are draped with stockinettes within the sterile field. This surgical approach facilitates accurate component placement and leg length measurement intraoperatively. This approach also provides good visualization of the acetabulum with the aid of specific angled Hohmann retractors.

Operative Procedure

1. The surgeon makes an oblique incision between the anterosuperior iliac spine and the greater trochanter (or through a straight incision made at the anterior border of the trochanter). Visualization of the acetabulum is made with the angled Hohmann retractors. An osteotomy of the femoral neck is made, and a corkscrew facilitates the removal of the femoral head.

2. The Hohmann retractors are repositioned and the surgeon prepares the acetabulum for reaming by removing remaining cartilage with the Kocher clamp and knife. The acetabular reaming begins and progresses as the surgeon assesses for cup size and position within the socket. The prepared socket is then lavaged with antibiotic irrigation and the component is placed along the insert.

3. Hyperextension of the hip provides better access to the proximal femur and is accomplished by placing the operative leg under the nonoperative leg, held in place by the second assistant. Using an ESU and a bone hook, the surgeon releases the posterior capsule. Two double-footed retractors are placed over the greater trochanter between the bone and the abductor muscle. A small metal curette is used as a canal finder followed by a canal reamer.

4. The surgeon begins with zero femoral broach, impacting down the canal, followed by sequentially larger broaches until cortical bone is reached. With the final broach seated at the desired depth, the surgeon places the trial femoral and neck components. The

hip is reduced with traction and internal rotation, and the legs are straightened and leg lengths measured. Trial reduction with adjustment of the leg lengths is easily accomplished in the supine position.

5. After sizes are determined, the patient's leg is again positioned under the nonoperative leg and the Hohmann retractors replaced. The surgeon removes the trial components and lavages the femoral canal with antibiotic irrigation. The femoral component is inserted along with the trial femoral head; leg lengths are again measured. After the final size is determined, the femoral head is impacted. The surgeon reduces the hip and performs a final range of motion to check for stability in extension, adduction, and internal rotation.

6. The wound is lavaged and closed with a simple juxtaposition of the interval between the vastus lateralis, gluteus medius, and iliotibial muscle.

7. Superficial layers are then closed according to surgeon preference. Dressings are placed.

Total Knee Arthroplasty

Total knee arthroplasty is a surgical procedure designed to replace the worn surfaces of the knee joint. Patients complain of knee pain and instability. Degenerative osteoarthritis, rheumatoid arthritis, or traumatic arthritis can result in severe destruction of the entire knee joint, or only the medial or lateral compartments of the knee joint can deteriorate as a result of extreme varus or valgus deformity. Arthroplasty of the knee has been successful in relieving these symptoms. Success depends on patient selection, component design, surgical technique, and rehabilitation. Recent advances in knee arthroplasty include robotic-assisted surgery (Robotic-Assisted Surgery).

The challenge of finding the optimal knee implant is in reproducing the complicated range of motion of the knee. Motion of the knee occurs in three planes: flexion and extension, abduction and adduction, and rotation. Designs of total knees should allow preservation of the normal ligaments whenever possible while providing soft tissue balance when necessary to maintain stability.

Total knee implants may be classified into three different categories, according to the portions of the knee to be replaced. *Unicompartmental* implants are used to replace just one opposing articular surface (medial or lateral) of the femur and tibia. *Bicompartmental* designs, mentioned only to demonstrate the progression of total knee design, replace both the medial and lateral surfaces of the femur and tibia. Most of the total knee replacements completed today are *tricompartmental* implants, which replace not only the opposing femorotibial joint but also the patellofemoral joint.

The tricompartmental knees are further divided into three categories. *Unconstrained* prostheses have very little constraint built in between the femoral and tibial components and depend on the integrity of soft tissues to provide stability of the reconstructed joint. Where there is significant deformity and the need for soft tissue release, the surgeon may decide to use a *semiconstrained* prosthesis, which lends itself to more inherent stability necessitated by ligamentous deficiency. *Fully constrained* prostheses are linked together with pure hinges, rotating hinges, and nonhinged designs. They are used in the presence of considerable bone loss, instability, deformity, and revision surgery in which bone loss has been significant. Fully constrained prostheses do not provide a normal range of motion, and such a lack of motion leads to excessive wear, implant loosening, and breakage.

Methods of fixation of total knee implants include both cemented and noncemented techniques. The noncemented variety encompasses

ROBOTIC-ASSISTED SURGERY

Robotically Assisted Unicompartmental Knee Arthroplasty

Robotic-assisted surgery has led to improved accuracy of orthopedic implant positioning compared with conventional methods. It allows more accuracy with minimally invasive techniques and permits surgeons to tailor the surgical procedure to each individual patient's arthritic and kinematic needs. Surgical robots can be active, semiactive, or passive. Each level of robot autonomy versus surgeon control has potential benefits and limitations.

Lonner (2016) discussed the Navio PFS robotic system, which is a handheld, image-free, open-platform sculpting device. It is a semiautonomous system that augments the surgeon's movements, with safeguards in place to optimize both accuracy and safety.

Operative Procedure

1. The surgeon enters the capsule medially through a minimally invasive approach. The threaded pins are percutaneously inserted into the proximal tibia and distal femur and the attachment of optical tracking. Mechanical and rotational axes of the limb are determined by establishing the hip and knee centers and the center of the ankle.
2. The kinematic, AP, or transepicondylar axes of the knee are identified and selected to determine the rotational position of the femoral component. Osteophytes are excised, and the condylar anatomy is mapped out by painting the surfaces with the optical probes. A virtual model of the knee is created. In this way, intraoperative mapping supplants the predicate system that required a preoperative CT scan.
3. A dynamic soft tissue balancing algorithm is initiated. By adjusting the implant positions, including tibial slope, depth of resection, and anteriorization or distalization of the femoral component, virtual dynamic soft tissue balance can be achieved.
4. Either a 5-mm or 6-mm handheld sculpting burr is used to prepare the bone on the condylar surfaces. After bone preparation, the surfaces are assessed and trial components impacted into place for assessment of range of motion and stability. Limb alignment, range of motion, implant position, and gap balance can be quantified and compared with the preoperative plan. Once the knee is considered adequately aligned and balanced, the final components are cemented into place.

Modified from Lonner J: Robotically assisted unicompartmental knee arthroplasty with a handheld image-free sculpting tool, *Orthop Clin North Am* 47(1):29–40, 2016.

both porous bony ingrowth and press-fit designs. The choice of implant and method of fixation depend on the predisposition of the bone, the patient's age and activity level, and the surgeon's comfort with a particular technique. Previous designs did not retain the PCL, which led to increased joint instability. Newer designs allow the PCL to be retained. Some surgeons believe that the retention of the PCL dictates the need for absolute ligament balancing beyond what may be possible in the reconstructed knee.

In the interest of a more cost-effective use of medical resources, new designs have been developed for the less active patient with a shorter expected life span. The femoral component design is a symmetric design that can be used on either the left or the right knee. The tibial component is composed entirely of UHMWPE, lowering manufacturing costs. Both components are placed with the use of PMMA.

Procedural Considerations

The perioperative nurse assists with positioning the patient supine. A tourniquet is applied to the upper thigh. The surgical prep is completed. A soft tissue set and a large bone set; the total knee instruments, trials, and implants of choice; a power drill and saw; PMMA and cement supplies; and a pulse lavage are required.

Operative Procedure

NexGen Total Knee Arthroplasty

1. With the knee flexed, the surgeon makes a straight midline incision from 3 to 4 inches above the patella, ending at the patellar tubercle (Fig. 20.64).
2. The capsule is entered medially. After making a median parapatellar incision, the surgeon places Kocher clamps on both lateral and medial sides of the capsule, and reflects the patella laterally to expose the entire tibiofemoral joint.
3. Hypertrophic synovium and a portion of the infrapatellar fat pad are excised using a toothed forceps and knife or the ESU, and then the osteophytes are removed using a rongeur. This allows easy access to the medial, lateral, and intercondylar spaces and facilitates soft tissue releases, should the need arise.
4. The knee is flexed to 90 degrees, and Hohmann retractors are placed deep to the collateral ligaments and anterior to the posterior capsule as well as laterally to the patella to protect these structures during resection of the proximal tibia. A Richardson retractor is placed medially to protect the MCL.
5. The surgeon positions the distal cutting alignment guide extramedullary and parallel to the proximal tibial spine. Proper rotational alignment is established by positioning the appropriate malleoli wings parallel to the transmalleolar axis. The alignment rod is proximally placed just slightly lateral to the tibial tubercle.
6. The osteotomy saw is then used to resect the proximal portion of the tibia. The distal cutting guide is removed. Alignment is checked with a Gerber guide (spacer block with the alignment rod) by placing the guide on the tibia. This checks the tibial cut for valgus alignment. The tibia is then sized with templates.
7. Before proceeding further, the surgeon ensures that the extremity can be moved into normal mediolateral (ML) alignment in extension. If not, additional soft tissue balancing is performed until the normal mechanical axis is obtained.
8. The AP cutting guide is then used to size the femur. The guide yoke is attached to the AP block, and the yoke is slipped under the muscle anteriorly on the periosteum. The middle nail is hammered into place, while pressing down on the guide yoke. Then by pulling up on the yoke, the valgus alignment is achieved such that it is square with the tibial cut. The block is then nailed into place with two pins.
9. With the AP femoral guide in place, the surgeon positions right-angle retractors to protect the MCL and LCL. The anterior and posterior portions of the femur are resected. The tibial and femoral cuts are checked for balance and size at the same time with a tibial block.
10. After the flexion balance is determined, the distal femoral cutting block is set. The tensor, placed in flexion, is then slowly moved into extension. Tension is placed on the extension gap by dialing between 30 to 40 pounds of pressure on the tensor. The amount of pressure dialed on the tensor is based on the patient's size

and tightness of the ligaments. The distal cutting jig is then placed in the tensor. After the jig is secured, the surgeon drills two pin holes and removes the tensor. The distal cutting guide is then placed in the exact two pin holes made by the distal cutting jig. The knee is then flexed, and the distal portion of the femur is resected.

11. The surgeon uses the appropriate spacer block to ensure equal tension in flexion and extension.

12. The knee is placed in flexion; the femoral notch and chamfer guide are centered between the epicondyles and impacted until fully seated. Three anterior fixation pins secure the guide to the femur. The surgeon drills two ¼-inch holes into the distal end of the femur and cuts the anterior and posterior chamfers with the oscillating saw. The box osteotome is used to make the notch cut from the proximal end of the finishing guide. A power saw is used to resect the posterior femoral condyle remnants to ensure adequate flexion clearance. The femoral trial is then positioned.

13. The tibial size is reassessed using the tibial templates. The selected tibial template is then positioned rotationally and drilled, and

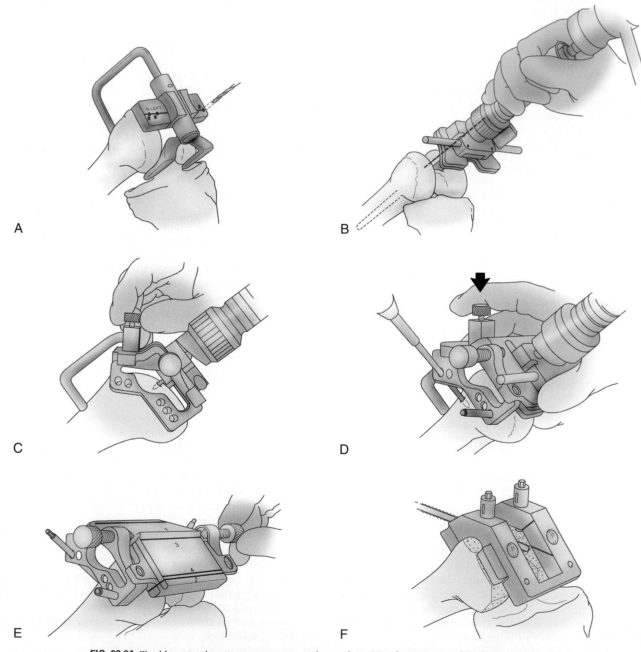

FIG. 20.64 Total knee implant, instrumentation, and procedure. (A) After exposure of the intercondylar notch, the femoral sizer is placed at the distal end of the femur. (B) After the femoral canal is reamed, the femoral intramedullary alignment guide is inserted and passed up the medullary canal. (C) Correct rotational alignment is maintained; the anterior femoral cutting guide is attached to the femoral intramedullary alignment guide. (D) The femoral cutting guide is mounted in place. (E) The femur is resected. (F) Femoral cuts are completed.

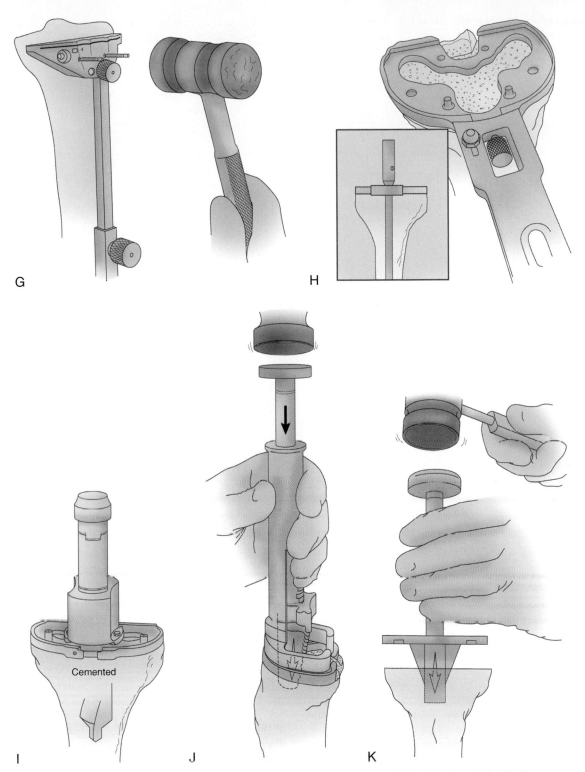

FIG. 20.64, cont'd (G) The tibial alignment guide is placed and secured, and the tibia is resected. (H) The tibia is sized. (I) The tibia is reamed. (J) The tibia is impacted. (K) The tibial trial is inserted.

Continued

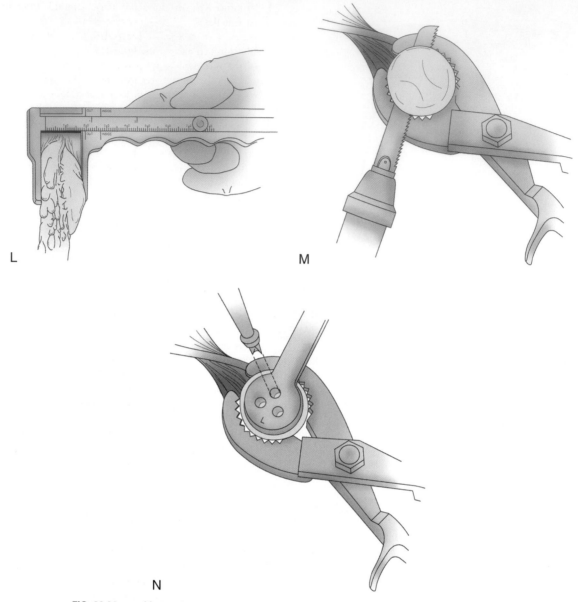

FIG. 20.64, cont'd (L) The patella is measured. (M) The patella is sized. (N) The patella is drilled.

the appropriate-sized centering punch is used to cut through the subchondral bone. The tibial trial is then placed.

14. The surgeon measures the patella and places two towel clips onto the distal and proximal portions of the patella tendon, and then performs the appropriate amount of resection. The patellar template is then placed over the resected surface, and the cruciate channels are created using the patellar drill through the slots in the template.

15. A trial reduction is performed. If this reduction proves satisfactory with regard to alignment and ligament laxity, the surgeon removes the trial components, irrigates with a pulsatile lavage, and places the permanent components. These can be inserted without bone cement, with bone cement, or with a combination of both.

16. Drains may or may not be placed in the joint depending on the surgeon's preference. The joint is closed, and a compression dressing is applied to the leg. The tourniquet can be released before closure or after the dressing has been applied.

Stryker Navigation Total Knee Arthroplasty
Procedural Considerations
During the surgical approach the company representative will initialize (set up) the Smart Tools instrumentation with the scrub person (Fig. 20.65). Healthcare industry representatives can provide valuable technical support to the perioperative team. Integration of surgical instrumentation and computers results in the ability to build a customized digital map of the patient's anatomy and navigate the surgical instruments according to this map. Successfully executed steps are marked with a blue checkmark and are graphically visualized. Proper setup is achieved when all Smart Tools are shown inside the camera's working space. Advantages to using a navigation system include the increased ability to verify the accuracy of cuts in less

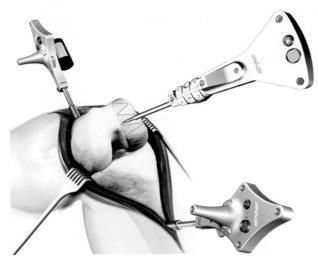

FIG. 20.65 Stryker navigation tracking equipment.

visible areas, decreased blood loss, and improved feedback to the surgeon about the patient's soft tissue balance.

A tourniquet, foot holder, and ESU are required. Antibiotics and heparin usually are ordered.

Operative Procedure

1. The capsule is entered medially. After making a median parapatellar incision, the surgeon places Kocher clamps on both lateral and medial sides of the capsule, and reflects the patella laterally to expose the entire tibiofemoral joint.
2. The surgeon begins to raise the medial flap using the ESU at the anterior tibia.
3. With a finger to retract medially, the surgeon places the tibial anchoring pin (self-tapping screws) at the distal aspect of the exposure. Drilling is then undertaken from the anterior to posterior tibial cortex using a 3.2-mm drill bit parallel to the joint line and rotated approximately 30 degrees medially.
4. Using a depth gauge, the surgeon rounds off to the size larger than measured (pins are available in 5-mm increments).
5. The scrub person places the pin on a T-handle for the surgeon to manually screw in the anchoring pin.
6. For the femoral anchoring pin, the surgeon next drills from the anterior to posterior femoral cortex, measures with a depth gauge, rounds up to the next larger size, and inserts the pin with a T-handle.
7. The blue tracker (B = bottom) is attached to the tibial pin and the green tracker to the femoral pin. Trackers should be placed so they are facing the camera attached to the navigation system.
8. The femoral head is registered. The hip is placed at 0 to 20 degrees of flexion and then at 45 degrees of flexion. As the leg is rotated, the light-emitting diode (LED) locations yield a set of data points relative to the size of the femoral head.
9. The distal femur is then registered. The medial and lateral condyles, the center of the knee, and the AP axis of the knee are digitalized to identify the articulating surfaces.
10. The proximal tibia is then registered. The center of the tibia, AP axis, and medial and lateral tibial plateaus are traced in a similar fashion to the femur, which identifies the slope of the tibia.

11. The knee is moved through its range of motion from full extension to full flexion. This kinematic datum is calculated and then recorded. Once data are recorded, the trackers are removed.
12. The surgeon excises any hypertrophic synovium and a portion of the infrapatellar fat pad using a toothed forceps and knife or ESU; the osteophytes are removed with a rongeur. This allows easy access to the medial, lateral, and intercondylar spaces and facilitates soft tissue releases, should the need arise.
13. The knee is flexed to 90 degrees, and Hohmann retractors are placed at the MCL and immediately anterior to the posterior capsule as well as laterally to the patella to protect these structures. A Richardson retractor is placed medially to protect the MCL. The surgeon uses a Kocher clamp and knife to resect the medial and lateral menisci as well as remnants of the ACL and PCL.
14. The surgeon places the navigated tibial cutting guide on the proximal tibia. A cutting guide is attached to the horseshoe device and then the blue tracker to the tibial anchoring pin and the green tracker to the femoral anchoring pin. With two pins, the guide is anchored. The position is confirmed with the navigation system, and the trackers and horseshoe device are then removed.
15. The surgeon uses a 5.5-mm round burr to open the tibial surface and then drive the keel punch slightly anteriorly. The guide and pins are then removed.
16. The horseshoe device is placed with the opening posterior on the distal femur with two pins. The distal femoral cutting guide is attached to the device, and the blue tracker is attached to the blue anchoring pins. Finally, the green tracker is attached to the femoral anchoring pins.
17. The surgeon manipulates the cutting guide to the distal femur. The first pin is driven into the guide and adjusted, and then the second and third pins are placed. The horseshoe and pins are removed. The saw is flushed with the cutting guide, the green top is attached, and the blue Gurba guide is set on the tibial surface to check the cuts.
18. The femoral 4-in-1 cutting guide is placed, and the pin is placed and cut with the saw. The LCL and MCL are protected with a finger or right-angled retractors and the pins are removed.
19. The surgeon places the Booth retractor over the tibia. After the notch guide and pin are placed, the surgeon cuts the tibia to an appropriate depth, using a saw as well as chamfer cuts. The pins and guide are then removed.
20. Next, the patella is measured; then two towel clips are placed onto the distal and proximal portions of the patellar tendon, and the appropriate resection is performed. The surgeon places the patellar template over the resected surface and creates the cruciate channels using the patellar drill through the slots in the template.
21. The surgeon places the trial components, attaches trackers, and moves the knee through a full range of motion. The trials and anchoring pins are then removed.
22. PMMA is prepared. Bone surfaces are irrigated with a pulsatile lavage, and the permanent components are placed. These can be inserted without bone cement, with bone cement, or a combination of both.
23. Drains are placed in the joint depending on the surgeon's preference. The joint is closed in the usual fashion, and a compression dressing is applied to the leg. The tourniquet can be released before closure or after the dressing has been applied.

Postoperative care consists of rapid mobilization and strengthening, with a target discharge of 2 to 3 days postoperatively.

Total Knee Revision Arthroplasty

Revision arthroplasty may be indicated if the patient's original knee replacement wears out or loosens, or fails as a result of repeated dislocation, infection, or trauma. Total joint revision can be a very demanding and complicated procedure. Attention to detail, anticipation, and preparation are essential. Important patient information includes the preoperative x-rays, bone scan, laboratory results (including aspiration results), and physical findings.

Procedural Considerations

The perioperative nurse assists with placing the patient in supine position with a footrest for the affected leg. An OR bed with x-ray capability is used. After the induction of anesthesia the surgeon performs an EUA. Although one of the most difficult aspects of revision surgery is that there is no clear-cut sequence of events, it is best, if possible, to approach revision surgery using the same logical sequence for each procedure. This allows all members of the surgical team to anticipate the steps in the procedure and the needs of the patient. In the case of revision arthroplasty for infection, antibiotics are held, usually at the surgeon's request, to allow for one final attempt to recover an organism. Tissue and fluid cultures are obtained when the initial incision is made through the capsule and into the joint space. Once the cultures are obtained, antibiotics are given.

Instrumentation includes a basic knee set, primary total knee instrumentation, and trials (in case only one portion of the prosthesis is revised); revision instrumentation to extract the components and cement; instrumentation and trials for the revision components; cementing system and extra cement (usually double the amount of cement used in a primary total knee arthroplasty); and power equipment including saw, reamer, and burrs.

Operative Procedure

The previous skin incision is usually used. This maintains adequate blood flow to the skin. A tourniquet cuff is applied after determining that there are no contraindications based on the patient's medical and surgical history.

1. Using a #10 blade, the surgeon incises through the scar from the original surgery.
2. With heavy-toothed forceps and blade, the surgeon undermines skin on each side of the incision; this allows the skin to be more easily closed at the end of the procedure.
3. After exposing the capsule, the surgeon uses a clean #10 blade to make a medial parapatellar incision into the joint. A Kocher is placed on the medial side of the capsule, and a towel clip is placed laterally, immediate to the patella, to aid with eversion.
4. Both tissue and fluid cultures are taken. Antibiotics are then administered by the anesthesia provider.
5. Using heavy-toothed forceps or a Kocher, the surgeon performs a synovectomy with a knife or the ESU. A clean dissection is needed to allow visualization of the bone-prosthesis interface and to remove any synovitis caused by polyethylene debris or metallosis, which is a nonsuppurative osteomyelitis that occurs around metal implants as a result of corrosion or hypersensitivity reaction.
6. The surgeon uses a periosteal elevator to peel away the medial ligament, which was stripped during the original surgery.
7. The knee is dislocated with posterior placement of a Hohmann retractor immediately behind the tibia. A second Hohmann retractor is placed laterally to the patella and LCL. Medially, a Richardson retractor provides protection of the MCL.
8. If possible, the surgeon removes the polyethylene tibia insert to allow better visualization and an increased work space.
9. Using an osteotomy saw with a small blade, the surgeon removes the tibial plate at the bone-prosthesis interface. If the saw is unable to complete the cuts, $\frac{1}{4}$-inch or $\frac{1}{2}$-inch curved osteotomes may be used to gain access to the posterior lateral corner. Cement is then removed from the canal using a Kocher clamp, $\frac{1}{4}$-inch straight osteotome, chisels, mallet, and curettes. If the cement is deep, a heavy-toothed alligator forceps may be required.
10. After the tibia and cement are removed, the surgeon recuts the tibia surface using an osteotomy saw and alignment guide. Sometimes the tibia is completely revised before the next step. If so, the tibial template, pins, mallet, and punch will be needed.
11. With the patella everted, the surgeon places a Booth retractor under the femur. Using a $\frac{1}{2}$-inch curved osteotome and mallet, the surgeon removes the femoral component. A $\frac{1}{4}$-inch curved osteotome may be required if there are metal pegs at the distal end on the femoral component or at the posterior edge of the prosthesis. A Gigli saw may also be used to remove the femur. After both sides of the prosthesis are loosened, it should fall off. If not, a femoral distractor will be used.
12. The surgeon removes any remaining cement using osteotomes, chisels, or the saw. Any cement in the canal will be removed with a Kocher clamp or alligator forceps.
13. Next, the posterior capsule is addressed. With the leg in extension, the surgeon places a lamina spreader between the femur and tibia. Using curettes and a rongeur, the surgeon removes the scar on the posterior capsule to improve postoperative range of motion.
14. After the capsule is released, attention is turned to rebuilding the femur. This is done by using a series of guides and trial components.
15. Augmentation of both tibia and femur components can be done using either metal augments or bone grafting. Balance between the femur and tibia is obtained first in flexion and then in extension.
16. The last component to be revised is the patella. Two towel clips are placed, distal and proximal on either side of the patella, and the button is removed, using a large-blade osteotomy saw. All poly buttons can be readily removed by this method. However, a metal-backed patella requires the additional use of a $\frac{1}{4}$-inch osteotome. Any remaining cement is removed from holes with a curette or 6-mm burr on a drill. The patella will be recut using a large-blade osteotomy saw.
17. The guide is placed on the patella, and the drill is used for new holes. The trial button is placed, the patella inverted, and the knee placed through a range of motion.
18. All components are removed, and the knee is irrigated with antibiotic solution using pulsatile lavage. The bone edges are dried with suction and clean sponges (e.g., soft goods) while the cement is being mixed.
19. Components can be cemented all at once or in stages, depending on the surgeon's preference.
20. The femur is usually cemented first. The surgeon places the Booth retractor under the femur and applies cement on the posterior phalanges of the femoral component and then on the distal edges of the bone. The component is placed on the end of the femur and impacted with an impactor and mallet. The cement is removed using glue knives anteriorly, laterally, and medially. Posterior glue is removed using curettes. The Booth retractor is then removed.

21. Hohmann retractors are placed posteriorly and laterally; a Richardson retractor can be placed medially if necessary. The surgeon applies cement to the tibia surface and the tip of the tibial stem. The tibial component is then placed and impacted. Remaining cement is removed using glue knives or bayonet forceps. The retractors are removed, and the knee is relocated.
22. Cement is applied to the patella in the predrilled holes as well as on the patella button itself. The button is placed on the patella and held with a patella clamp. Remaining cement is again removed using a glue knife or bayonets.
23. The surgeon inserts drains if indicated and closes the wound.

Total Shoulder Arthroplasty

Indications for total shoulder arthroplasty include degenerative joint disease, rheumatoid arthritis, posttraumatic arthritis, avascular necrosis, and fractures. In total shoulder replacement surgery the diseased bone and cartilage on the humeral head is removed, and a metal ball with a stem is placed in the proximal humerus and cartilage of the glenoid and replaced with a plastic socket (AAOS, 2016c).

Reverse total shoulder replacement can be performed when the patient has a large rotator cuff tear or the rotator cuff is not intact. A metal stem with plastic socket is placed in the proximal humerus, and the glenoid stabilizes the shoulder joint and allows the deltoid to raise the arm. The reverse total shoulder replacement allows other muscles, such as the deltoid, to do the work of the damaged rotator cuff tendons (AAOS, 2016b).

Procedural Considerations

The team places the patient in a 45-degree semi-Fowler position with the nonoperative arm on a padded armboard. The operative shoulder is positioned slightly off the OR bed to provide full access of the shoulder. A pillow is placed under the patient's knees at a 30-degree angle for back support, and heels are padded. The perioperative nurse verifies the patient's head and neck alignment and ensures it remains in neutral alignment throughout the procedure. The male patient's genitalia should be checked and freed of any pressure to avoid injury in the sitting position. The patient is secured to the OR bed with a safety strap and/or tape. The operative arm can be placed on a padded surface or in a hydraulic positioner during the procedure by the surgeon to ensure full extension and external rotation of the arm. Instrumentation includes a soft tissue tray, shoulder instrumentation tray, shoulder retractors, power drill and saw, cementing supplies, implants, trials, and pulse lavage (Taylor, 2016).

Operative Procedure

Total Shoulder Arthroplasty, Deltopectoral Approach

1. A 4- to 6-inch incision is made between the deltoid and pectoralis major muscles from the coracoid process of the scapula to the humerus (Fig. 20.66).
2. The surgeon dissects down to the deltoid and identifies and mobilizes the cephalic vein that runs down the deltopectoral groove. Branches of the vein may be cauterized.
3. The deltopectoral interval is separated exposing 1 inch of pectoralis tendon. The cephalic vein is retracted laterally with the deltoid.
4. The surgeon then dissects between the muscles and replaces the retractors under the deltoid laterally and the pectoralis major medially.
5. The superior pectoralis tendon is released 1 cm with ESU, and the surgeon visualizes the conjoined tendon.

6. The clavipectoral fascia is separated parallel to the conjoined ligament from the distal pectoralis major to the coracoacromial ligament proximally. Next, the surgeon abducts and internally rotates the arm to visualize the subacromial space.
7. The surgeon dissects under the coracoacromial ligament and places a retractor in the subacromial space. The subacromial and subdeltoid spaces are freed of any adhesions.
8. The surgeon takes care to identify the axillary and musculocutaneous nerves and places a retractor under the conjoined tendon to avoid these structures.
9. Next, the arm is externally rotated and the anterior humeral circumflex vessels are identified and coagulated along the inferior subscapularis.
10. The surgeon identifies the biceps tendon where it arises from beneath the pectoralis major tendon and exposes it.
11. The superior portion of the subscapularis is released by excising the rotator interval to the base of the coracoid.
12. The biceps is then sutured to the pectoralis major, and the proximal portion is removed and the subscapularis is tagged and reflected.
13. The surgeon releases the capsular insertion onto the humerus along the medial neck, avoiding the axillary nerve.
14. After the humerus is released, the surgeon dislocates the humeral head by placing an elevator between the glenoid and the proximal humerus and extending, externally rotating, and adducting the arm.
15. The surgeon removes any prominent osteophytes from the humeral neck and then removes the humeral head.
16. The surgeon prepares the humerus as indicated by the instrumentation system being used. A trial stem and humeral head are selected.
17. The glenoid is exposed with retractors in the posterior and inferior glenoid. The arm is placed in slight internal rotation, and the surgeon places a retractor gently between the inferior subscapularis and the axillary nerve.
18. The surgeon releases the inferior aspect of the subscapularis and places a retractor between the divide.
19. The anterior capsule is incised with a knife from the coracoid to the inferior scapularis, and retractors are placed to expose the glenoid.
20. The surgeon excises any labrum and remaining cartilage. Next, the surgeon prepares the glenoid by reaming, drilling, and sizing according to the instrumentation system being used.
21. The glenoid is then trialed for proper fit and compatibility with the humeral head trial. The trial is removed and the glenoid is irrigated while the cement is being prepared.
22. The surgeon pressurizes the cement into cancellous bone in the glenoid and then impacts the final component into place. Excess cement is removed.
23. After the cement cures, the surgeon reexposes the humerus and trials the humeral head with the stem to determine stability and neck length.
24. If necessary the humeral head and stem are assembled on the back table. Next, the surgeon uses an impactor and a mallet to implant the prosthesis. The humeral stem may be press-fit or cemented, depending on the patient's bone quality and stability.
25. After the shoulder is reduced and irrigated the surgeon repairs the subscapularis with heavy suture to prevent rupture. A layered wound closure is completed.
26. The arm is placed in an arm sling or shoulder immobilizer.

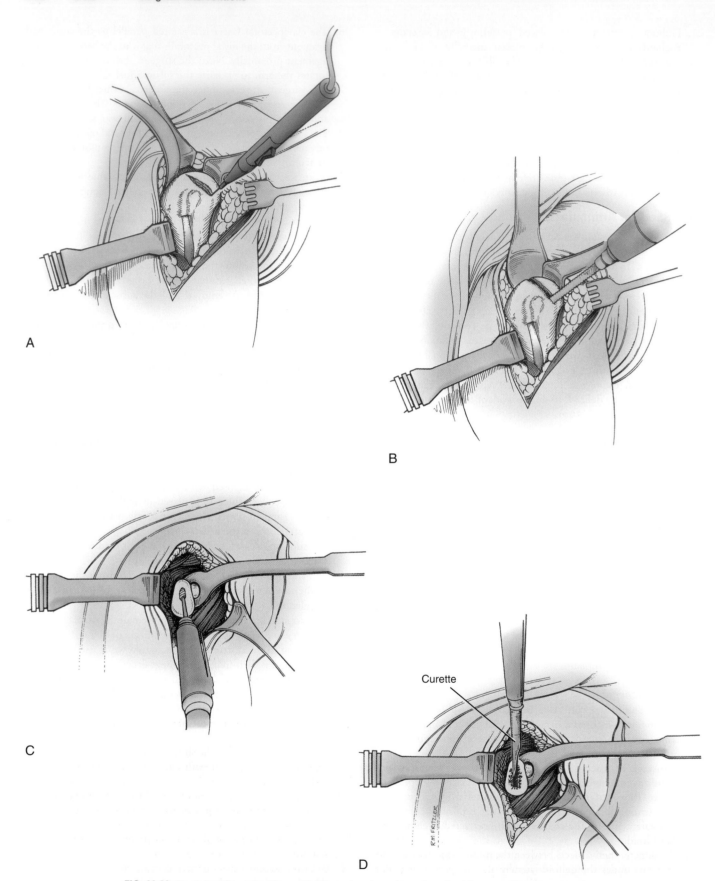

FIG. 20.66 Total shoulder arthroplasty. (A) The patient is positioned, and a deltopectoral incision is made to release the capsule. (B) The humeral head is removed with a reciprocating saw. (C) After exposure of the glenoid, a fenestration for the glenoid component is made. (D) The glenoid bow is curetted.

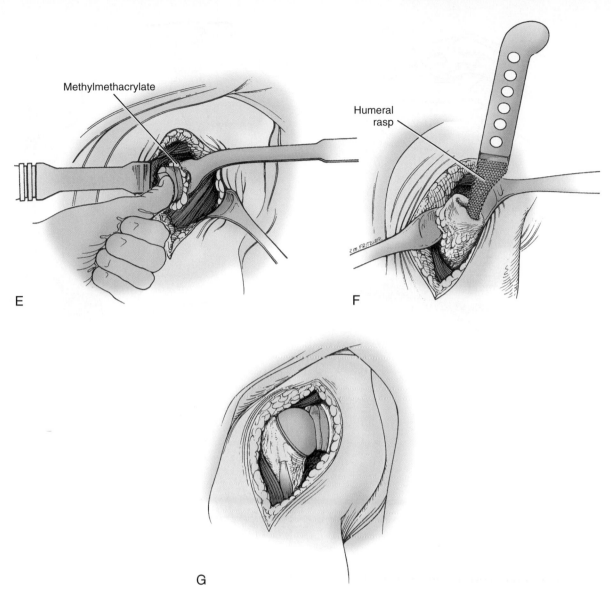

FIG. 20.66, cont'd (E) Cancellous bone is evacuated and cement impressed. (F) The humeral shaft is rasped. (G) The humeral component is inserted.

Operative Procedure

Reverse Total Shoulder Arthroplasty. Steps 1 through 27 of the total shoulder arthroplasty, deltopectoral approach are performed; however, the subscapularis takedown may not be needed.

1. The surgeon exposes more of the inferior glenoid for the positioning of the baseplate.
2. The surgeon prepares the glenoid according to the instrumentation system chosen, being sure to place the baseplate low on the glenoid. The glenosphere is then attached to the baseplate according to instrumentation guidelines.
3. The humerus is reexposed with retractors and the arm is externally rotated, extended, and abducted. Next, the surgeon inserts the final stem in the humerus with an impactor and mallet. The stem may be either press-fit or cemented.
4. The surgeon impacts the final polyethylene liner onto the humeral stem, and the shoulder is reduced. Range of motion and stability are assessed.
5. The wound is irrigated and the subscapularis may or may not be repaired before closing the wound in layers and applying a dressing.
6. The arm is placed in an arm sling or shoulder immobilizer.

Total Elbow Arthroplasty

Although not as prevalent as arthroplasty of the shoulder, knee, or hip, total elbow replacement (Fig. 20.67) is indicated for patients with traumatic lesions or excessive bone loss from rheumatoid or degenerative arthritis, resulting in elbow instability and pain or bilateral elbow ankylosis. The design of implants and methods of fixation for postoperative stability have presented challenges that have been overcome in arthroplasty of other joints but remain a challenge in elbow arthroplasty. Postoperative stability of the elbow implant depends largely on the soft tissues surrounding the joint. There are devices that provide more constraint for the patient with significant soft tissue laxity or loss of bone stock. The Coonrad–Morrey, Tri-Axial,

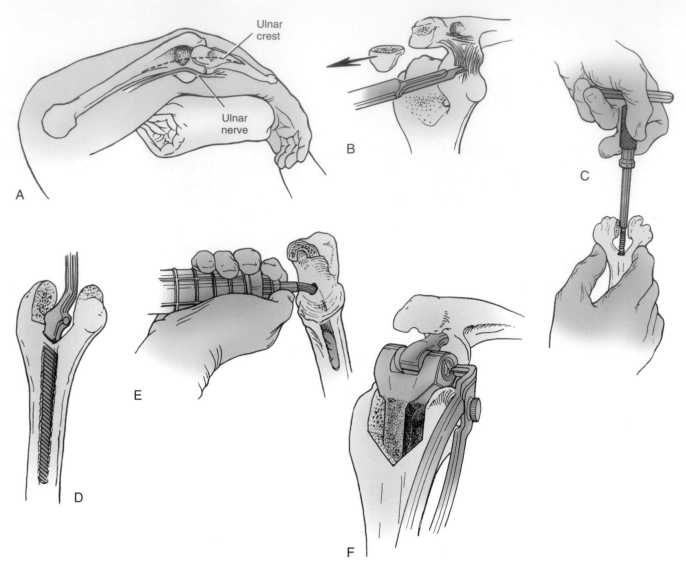

FIG. 20.67 Total elbow arthroplasty. (A) The arm is draped free, and the incision is made. (B) The tip of the olecranon is excised with an oscillating saw. (C) The canal is identified with a burr, and the canal is opened with a twist reamer. (D) The capitellum is measured and cut. (E) The medullary canal is cleaned and dried, and bone cement is inserted. (F) The ulnar prosthesis is inserted, followed by cementing and inserting of the humeral components.

and Pritchard–Walker are just a few of the total elbow prostheses available.

The prosthesis may be used with or without PMMA, depending on the quality of the diseased bone and the design of the implant. If PMMA is not used, bone grafting with local bone that has been resected may be used to help seat the ulnar component snugly and achieve adequate bony contact against the porous coating of the metal ulnar component. After elbow arthroplasty, patients with degenerative arthritis generally have better results than those with injury.

Procedural Considerations

The perioperative nurse assists with positioning the patient in the supine or semi-Fowler position with the arm over the chest. A tourniquet is applied and can be inflated if needed. The arm is prepped from shoulder to fingers and draped. A soft tissue set and

a small bone set; the total elbow implants and instruments; a power saw, drill, and burr; an awl; heavy-gauge wire; and a wire tightener are needed. PMMA and cement supplies as well as a pulsatile lavage system are required if the prosthesis is placed with the use of PMMA.

Operative Procedure

1. The limb is exsanguinated, and the tourniquet is inflated to the desired pressure.
2. The surgeon makes a midline posterior incision, protecting the ulnar nerve.
3. The triceps mechanism is elevated in continuity with the periosteum, and the elbow joint is explored.
4. The surgeon explores the distal end of the humerus, proximal end of the ulna, and radial head while preserving the collateral ligaments.

5. The midportion of the trochlea is removed to allow access to the distal end of the humerus; the medullary canal is opened with a high-speed burr, and the canal is entered with a twist hand reamer.
6. The distal end of the humerus is notched with the appropriate cutting guide.
7. A high-speed burr is used to drill through subchondral bone to allow access to the medullary canal of the ulna and serially ream the canal.
8. After the humerus and ulna have been prepared for insertion of the trial prosthesis, the surgeon evaluates the elbow for flexion and extension. Bony adjustments are made where necessary.
9. The surgeon irrigates with pulsatile antibiotic lavage to clean the canals of all bone fragments.
10. The canal is dried before implant insertion, and the preparation is checked before the cement is mixed to ensure that the correct size of component is available.
11. The surgeon inserts the cement into the canals followed by the prosthesis. Flexion and extension of the elbow are avoided until the cement has hardened.
12. Any bone graft that may be required is secured with wire or pins.
13. The tourniquet is deflated, and hemostasis is achieved.
14. The triceps mechanism is repaired. The incision site is irrigated and closed. A drain may be inserted.
15. A long arm posterior splint is applied with the elbow at 90 degrees.

Total Ankle Joint Arthroplasty

Indications for total ankle arthroplasty include: (1) failed arthrodesis, (2) bilateral ankle arthritis when arthrodesis has already been performed on one ankle, (3) after talectomy because of avascular necrosis, and (4) revision of a previous arthroplasty. Total ankle joint arthroplasty is reserved for older or more sedentary patients because long-term results tend be extremely poor. Ankle arthrodesis should be considered first in joint reconstruction. Total ankle replacement prostheses are made of high-density polyethylene and metal components.

Procedural Considerations

The team positions the patient supine and applies the tourniquet cuff. The leg is prepped and draped. A soft tissue set, a small bone set, the total ankle joint replacement instrumentation set and implants, a power drill and saw, a pulsatile lavage system, and PMMA cement and supplies are necessary.

Operative Procedure

1. The surgeon makes an anterior incision over the ankle joint (Fig. 20.68).
2. Using blunt and sharp dissection the surgeon exposes the tibiotalar joint and talus dome.
3. Once the center of the talus is identified and marked, a sizing template is used to mark the tibia.
4. A defect that is 1-inch wide by $\frac{3}{8}$-inch deep is made using the air drill. Anchoring holes can be made in the tibia. The template is positioned in the defect while the foot is distracted.
5. The talus is marked, and using a reciprocating saw the surgeon makes a groove that is $\frac{1}{2}$-inch deep by $\frac{3}{16}$-inch wide to accommodate the talar component.
6. A trial fit is performed to ensure that the talar unit is in the center of the talus and that the tibial unit is parallel to the plane of the floor, both centered over the dome of the talus.

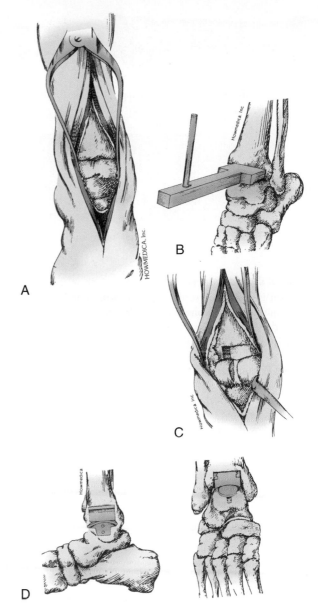

FIG. 20.68 Total ankle arthroplasty. (A) An anterior incision is made, and the tibiotalar joint and talus dome are exposed. (B) The sizing template is used to mark the tibia. (C) An air drill is used to create a defect, and anchoring holes are prepared. (D) Trial reduction is completed, and the talar and tibial components are cemented into place.

7. Once trial reduction is complete, the talar and tibial components are cemented into place.
8. The ankle joint is irrigated and closed, a drain inserted, and a posterior splint applied.

Metacarpal Arthroplasty

Metacarpal joint replacement is most often performed in patients who have pain or a disabling deformity associated with rheumatoid or degenerative arthritis of the metacarpophalangeal or interphalangeal joints. The results of rheumatoid reconstructive surgery are generally good, and pain can be eliminated and joint alignment and joint stability restored in the majority of patients. The greatest problems after surgery are weakness of grasp and pinch and progression of the disease in adjacent joints.

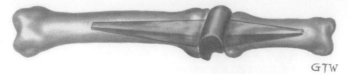

FIG. 20.69 Metacarpophalangeal implant.

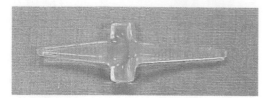

FIG. 20.70 Silastic implant for finger joint.

Procedural Considerations

The patient is positioned supine with the arm extended on a hand table. A tourniquet is applied, and the entire extremity is prepped and draped. A hand set, instrumentation for implants, and implants are required, as well as a high-speed burr.

Operative Procedure

1. Incisions are made on the dorsum of the appropriate fingers.
2. The surgeon excises the proximal and distal portions of the joints and reams the IM canals.
3. Sizers are used to facilitate a correct fit of the prosthesis.
4. Once the appropriately sized implant is determined, the surgeon positions it into the canal (Figs. 20.69 and 20.70) and makes tendon and ligament repairs as indicated to improve stability.
5. The joint is irrigated and closed, and a bulky dressing is applied.
6. A short arm posterior splint is applied for immobilization.

Metatarsal Arthroplasty

Silastic implantation is indicated in the treatment of deformities associated with rheumatoid arthritis, hallux valgus, hallux rigidus, and a painful or unstable joint.

Procedural Considerations

The patient is positioned supine. A tourniquet cuff is applied, and the entire extremity is prepped and draped. A small bone set is required, as well as the implant instruments and implants, a power wire driver, and the microsagittal saw.

Operative Procedure

1. The incisions are made over the appropriate joints.
2. The surgeon resects the proximal phalanx and removes exostosis from the metatarsal head.
3. The medullary canal is reamed, and trial implants are fitted.
4. The surgeon determines the appropriate sized metatarsal implant and seats it.
5. The wound is irrigated and closed.
6. A bulky compression dressing and orthopedic shoe are applied for early ambulation.

Arthroscopy

Progress and development of arthroscopy and arthroscopic procedures have changed the approach, diagnosis, and treatment of many joint ailments. Arthroscopic techniques require skill and accomplishment

in identifying three-dimensional relationships. The advantages of arthroscopic surgery surpass the disadvantages. Among the advantages are (1) decreased recovery and rehabilitation time; (2) smaller incisions; (3) less inflammatory response; (4) less postoperative pain, scarring, and extensor disruption; (5) reduced complications; (6) reduced hospital stay and cost; and (7) easier, more rapid surgical procedures (Ambulatory Surgery Considerations).

Disadvantages usually relate to the size and delicacy of the instruments. Maneuverability within a joint may be difficult and produce scuffing and scoring of the articular surfaces.

Improvements in scope and camera systems, sharper scope optics, and miniaturization have made operative arthroscopy a logical extension of diagnostic arthroscopy. Surgical arthroscopy has also been aided with the development of numerous second puncture instruments and devices to repair and excise defects. There are a multitude of motorized shaving and abrader systems. Irrigation systems provide regulated distention of the knee joint by infusing normal saline or lactated Ringer's solution. These systems may function by gravity flow or are mechanized with built-in microprocessors to monitor joint pressures and adjust accordingly. Lasers and ESUs can be used in tandem with arthroscopic equipment. Integrated video systems can record and store still and video images on film, tape, or digitally for education and documentation.

Arthroscopy is commonly performed on the knee, shoulder, and wrist. It is used less often in the elbow, hip, and ankle. Many corrective procedures that previously required an arthrotomy or other open procedure can be completed with the assistance of the arthroscope.

Arthroscopic equipment has certain requirements for care and handling (see Chapter 4 for equipment handling information). Fiberoptics, lenses, and cameras are heat sensitive, requiring consideration for sterilization. Temperatures and moisture generated by steam autoclaves can damage materials used in video equipment or deteriorate the sealant, making the moisture accessible to the lens. Alternatives to steam sterilization for this equipment are ethylene oxide, cold sterilization, and high-level disinfection (see Chapter 4 for a discussion of sterilization methods).

Two types of arthroscopy may be performed. *Diagnostic arthroscopy* is for patients whose diagnosis cannot be determined by history or physical examination or whose CT or MRI findings are insufficient to warrant surgical exploration. Diagnostic arthroscopy may be performed before an anticipated arthrotomy, and surgical treatment may be modified on the basis of the findings of the arthroscopic examination. *Operative arthroscopy* is for patients presenting with an intra-articular abnormality or ligamentous injury.

Arthroscopy of the Knee

The knee is the joint in which arthroscopy lends itself to the greatest number of diagnostic and surgical procedures. Arthroscopic surgery of the knee is indicated for diagnostic viewing, synovial biopsies, removal of loose bodies, resection of plicae, shaving of the patella, synovectomy, partial meniscectomy, meniscus repair, and ACL reconstruction. Anesthesia for knee arthroscopy may be general, spinal, or local. Tourniquet cuffs are often placed on the thigh but are inflated only if bleeding obscures the view. If there are no contraindications, an epinephrine solution may be injected at the portal sites or diluted into the distention fluid.

Procedural Considerations

The perioperative nurse assists with positioning the patient in the supine position on a standard OR bed. The surgeon may perform

AMBULATORY SURGERY CONSIDERATIONS

Arthroscopic Surgery

Ambulatory surgery has long been part of orthopedic surgery. Recent advances in minimally invasive surgery and postoperative pain management have led to even more orthopedic procedures being performed in an ambulatory setting.

The most important factor in ambulatory surgery is patient selection. Surgical, anesthesia, and nursing departments should work together to define the criteria to identify suitable candidates for ambulatory surgery.

Preoperative assessment can determine which patients are the best candidates for ambulatory surgery. Careful review of health history, social history, and potential limitations postoperatively is vital in the initial assessment. Special attention to mobility both preoperatively and postoperatively is key for the orthopedic ambulatory surgery patient. Patients who will experience significant limited mobility postoperatively, live alone with no help available postoperatively, and have multiple medical comorbidities are not ideal candidates for orthopedic ambulatory surgery. Patient education is initiated during the preoperative assessment. Gait training, pain management, postoperative instructions, and transportation should be addressed preoperatively as well as arrangements for any special equipment necessary for postoperative recovery. Attention to postoperative details before surgery will prevent delays with patient discharge postoperatively.

The anesthesia evaluation is done during preadmission testing during which the anesthesia provider will develop a plan of care best suited for the patient and the anticipated surgery. Patient comorbidities, length of procedure, and positioning during the procedure as well as the surgery itself are taken into consideration when establishing a plan of care.

Knee Arthroscopy

Knee arthroscopy is a common orthopedic ambulatory surgery procedure. New technology and approaches in surgery allow multiple procedures to be done through the arthroscope. As soon as the patient has been identified as a candidate for ambulatory surgery, preoperative planning for preadmission testing, anesthesia evaluation, and patient education begin. The popular choice of anesthesia is one of two types based on patient history. Choices include regional or general anesthesia. Many providers prefer regional anesthesia for knee arthroscopy because of the decreased complication rates postoperatively. On the day of surgery the history and physical are again reviewed with the patient. The surgical site is marked according to standards established by TJC and facility policy. The patient is taken to the OR, anesthetized, prepared, and positioned for surgery. With regional anesthesia, those patients who would like to remain alert during the procedure can do so, watch the surgery on the monitor, and even converse with the surgeon about the findings. When the procedure is complete the surgeon injects a local anesthetic into the joint to minimize pain. The length of the postoperative period depends on the regional anesthetic and the dose used. Patients will regain sensation and motion from trunk down to toes. Strength should be taken into consideration when gait training is initiated, and the nurse must ensure that the patient, family, and caregiver understand the use of assistive devices (e.g., crutches, canes, etc.) as well as application and removal of immobilizers (if prescribed). The nurse discharges the patient when discharge criteria have been met, physician orders have been reviewed with the patient, written discharge instructions and prescriptions have been given to the patient, and the responsible adult escort is present. Phone numbers for any emergency should be listed on both physician and hospital discharge sheets.

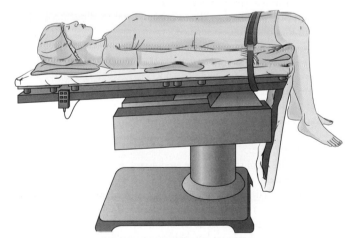

FIG. 20.71 Positioning for a knee arthroscopy to enhance visualization.

an EUA before the patient is placed in position for the arthroscopy. The foot end of the bed may be flexed 90 degrees (Fig. 20.71). A lateral post can be attached to the bed at the level of the midthigh. This post can provide a method of countertraction to open the medial side of the joint, providing better visualization of structures. After the leg is prepped the entire extremity is draped to allow complete range of motion and manipulation of the knee joint. The procedure requires specialized equipment for fluid collection and personnel protection.

Instruments and equipment needed for an arthroscopy depend on whether the procedure is diagnostic or operative. Diagnostic arthroscopy instruments include arthroscopy instrumentation; arthroscopes of 30 and 70 degrees; video with camera, light source, and peripheral equipment (Fig. 20.72); an arthroscopy pump and tubing (Fig. 20.73); inflow and egress cannulae (Fig. 20.74); 3-L bags of normal saline or lactated Ringer's solution; and a spinal needle. Operative arthroscopy instruments depend on the procedure planned. Arthroscopic powered shavers and abraders are almost universally used. Instruments specific for ACL reconstruction or meniscal repair will be needed if those procedures are planned.

Operative Procedure
Diagnostic Arthroscopy
1. The surgeon marks the anteromedial and anterolateral joint lines and portal positions with a skin marker.
2. The skin areas for portal placement are infiltrated with 1% lidocaine with 1:200,000 epinephrine. If the knee has an effusion, the surgeon aspirates it with a 16-gauge needle on a 60-mL syringe, followed by injection of a small amount of distending fluid.

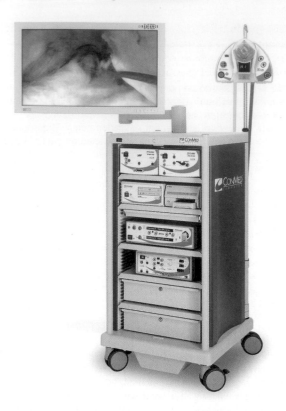

FIG. 20.72 Arthroscopy tower with video monitor, light source, camera, and shaver system.

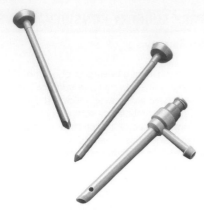

FIG. 20.74 Cannulae.

3. After creating a small stab incision with a #11 blade, the surgeon inserts the irrigation cannula and trocar into the lateral suprapatellar pouch near the superior pole of the patella. Lactated Ringer's or normal saline solution is connected to the cannula, and the joint is distended using gravity or a pressure-sensitive arthroscopy pump.

4. An additional stab incision is then made anterolaterally or anteromedially 2 to 3 mm above the tibial plateau or patellar tendon at the joint line. A sharp trocar and sheath are inserted through the stab wound and just through the capsule.

5. A blunt trocar is used to pass the sheath into the knee joint. The surgeon removes the trocar and inserts a 30-degree scope into the sheath. The light source and video camera are connected to the scope.

6. The inflow may remain in the suprapatellar area, and the egress tubing is connected to the arthroscope, or the position may be reversed.

7. A spinal needle can be introduced under direct vision to determine the best angle for an opposite portal for insertion of probes and operative instruments. The cruciate ligaments and menisci are probed to determine integrity and tears.

8. The scope is moved to the opposite portal to allow a complete examination to be performed.

9. The joint is irrigated periodically and at the end of the procedure to maintain good visualization and clear the joint of blood and tissue fragments.

10. The surgeon closes the portals with nylon or undyed polyglactin suture and ½-inch wound closure strips.

11. Bupivacaine (Marcaine) 0.25%, 30 mL, with epinephrine 1:200,000 may be injected intra-articularly to minimize bleeding and postoperative pain.

12. Gauze dressing, soft padding, and 4- and 6-inch elastic bandages are applied.

Operative Arthroscopy. Operative arthroscopy includes procedures for resection of synovial plica, patellar debridement, excision of meniscal tears, partial or total meniscectomy, lateral retinacular release, removal of loose bodies, abrasion or drilling of osteochondral defects, synovectomy, treatment of osteochondritis dissecans, meniscal repairs, and ACL reconstruction.

Arthroscopic Resection and Repair of Meniscal Tear. Menisci are important structures in the knee joint that distribute load across the joint and provide capsular stability. A tear in the meniscus is the most common knee injury requiring arthroscopic surgery. Although both menisci can sustain tears, the medial meniscus is injured much more frequently than the lateral one.

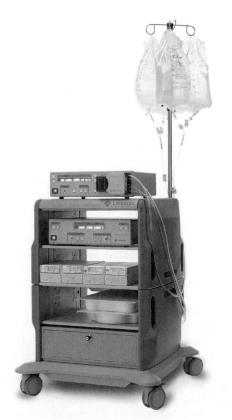

FIG. 20.73 Arthroscopy pump.

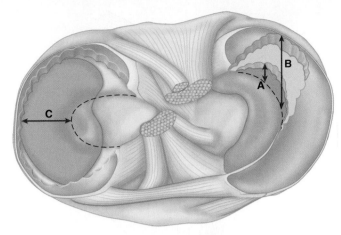

FIG. 20.75 Types of meniscal excision. *(A)* Partial meniscectomy. *(B)* Subtotal meniscectomy. *(C)* Total meniscectomy.

Treatment of meniscus tears is aimed at preserving the structures. Some minor tears heal with immobilization, but some persist and cause symptoms. In these more severe cases surgical intervention is necessary. A partial or complete meniscectomy may be necessary to alleviate troublesome symptoms such as locking, pain, and swelling (Fig. 20.75). Partial meniscectomy is preferred, leaving a peripheral rim to share load bearing and stabilize the knee. Complete meniscectomy removes all of this load-bearing protection and reduces knee stability. The goal is to leave an intact, balanced rim.

Arthroscopic meniscal repair is widely accepted as the standard of care. Arthroscopy provides better exposure than an arthrotomy and enables the surgeon to approach the meniscus from the inner margin, in which most tears begin. Suture repair is appropriate for meniscal tears occurring in the vascular zone (outer 10%–25%) that heal predictably with repair and immobilization.

Operative Procedure. The operative procedure begins as described in steps 1 through 9 of the diagnostic arthroscopy procedure.

1. Working and scope portals are determined. The lateral bucket handle tear is identified, displaced, and reduced with a probe.
2. The surgeon cuts the attachment of the anterior horn of the meniscus with a hook knife and clamps it with a grasper.
3. An accessory portal is determined with a spinal needle.
4. The surgeon maintains traction and twisting motions on the meniscal horn to present a better edge to divide the remainder of the tear. Various scissors or push knives can be used to complete resection.
5. The motorized shaver is used to trim any frayed edges of the meniscus.
6. Limited debridement of chronic tears is completed to clean the edges.
7. When the medial meniscus is to be sutured, the surgeon places a cannula next to the inner edge of the tear. Two long meniscal-stitching needles with synthetic absorbable suture are inserted into the cannula, through the meniscus, across the tear, and through the capsule.
8. The surgeon palpates the needle tips beneath the skin and makes a small incision to pull the suture out of the joint.
9. The sutures are tied over the capsule. Positioning the cannula enables either horizontal or vertical sutures to be placed.
10. After completing partial meniscectomy or suture repair, the surgeon irrigates the joint.

11. The incisions are closed, and the knee is lightly dressed and wrapped with soft rolled padding and elastic bandages.

Arthroscopic Anterior Cruciate Ligament Repair. The ACL is an important stabilizing structure of the knee and is the most frequently torn ligament. Injury is usually a result of simultaneous anterior and rotational stresses. Candidates for ACL reconstruction are active individuals with instability that is sufficient to interfere with their activities and that has failed to respond to bracing, rehabilitation, exercises, and other nonoperative treatment methods. The selected treatment method depends on the classification and severity of the tear, the experience and preference of the surgeon, and a history of a previous failed repair. According to Metzler and Johnson (2014) over 250,000 ACL reconstructions are performed each year in the United States.

ACL reconstruction may be intra-articular, extra-articular, or a combination of both. Arthroscopic repair causes less patellar pain and decreased disturbance of extensor mechanisms; therefore it is becoming the treatment of choice if there is no other significant capsular instability or gross disruption of the knee joint.

ACL repair most often involves replacement of the ligament with a substitute. Substitutes include autografts, allografts, and synthetic ligaments. Autografts are the method of choice, with a free central-third patellar tendon graft attached to patellar and tibial bone blocks used most often. The semitendinosus tendon and iliotibial band are sometimes used instead. Autografts may be used alone or augmented, although synthetic augmentation devices have fallen out of favor because of the development of chronic synovitis.

Procedural Considerations. Instrumentation for an ACL repair includes all instruments required for an operative arthroscopy. In addition, an ACL reconstruction guide system, fixation device of choice (bone screws, staples, spiked washers, or interference screws), bone tunnel plugs, a power drill, and microsagittal saw are needed. If the surgeon believes that isometric placement of the graft is important, a tension isometer will be needed, as well as a system for finding that intra-articular position.

Operative Procedure: Reconstruction of the Anterior Cruciate Ligament With Patellar Tendon Graft

1. The surgeon performs an EUA immediately after anesthesia induction to further evaluate the stability of the knee.
2. A diagnostic arthroscopy is then performed through the standard anteromedial and anterolateral portals.
3. Any meniscal tears or other intra-articular injuries are treated before attending to the ligament.
4. The surgeon debrides any remaining ACL tissue with a full-radius resector.
5. A notchplasty is then performed, widening the intercondylar notch with a 4.5-mm arthroplasty burr, rasp, osteotome, and curettes. Notchplasty aids in arthroscopic visualization and protects the graft from abrasion and amputation.
6. After preparation of the intercondylar area, the surgeon makes a small incision on the distal lateral aspect of the femur and extends the incision to the flare of the lateral femoral aspect of the condyle. A femoral aiming device is positioned, and a guide pin is inserted from the femoral site into the postero-superior region of the intercondylar notch at an isometric point (Fig. 20.76). Another small incision is made anteriorly, below the knee and medial to the tibial tubercle.
7. The tibial aiming device is positioned, and the surgeon inserts a guide pin from the anterior tibial incision into the intercondylar notch, anterior and medial to the center of the tibial anatomic attachment site of the ACL.

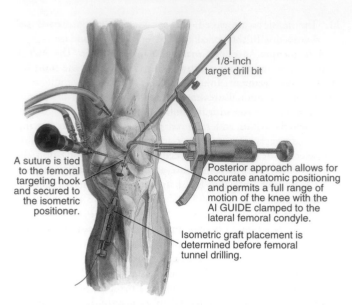

FIG. 20.76 Femoral aiming device positioned for anterior cruciate ligament reconstruction.

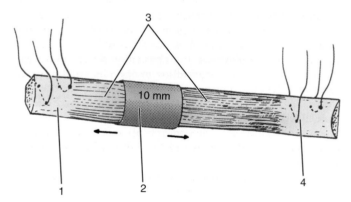

FIG. 20.77 Sizing tubes are used to determine the minimum diameter of tunnel necessary for passage of the graft.

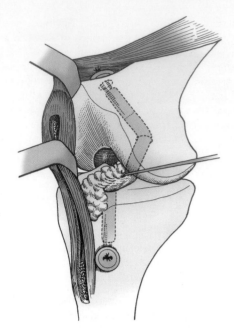

FIG. 20.78 Three drill holes are placed into each bone block of the patellar graft, and a heavy suture is placed into each drill hole.

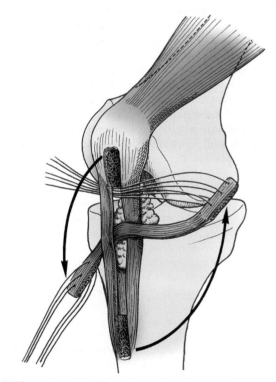

FIG. 20.79 A patellar tendon graft is affixed by tying of sutures over bone buttons at the tibial and femoral drill holes.

8. The surgeon replaces the pins with a heavy suture passing through the femoral and tibial pin sites.
9. Isometric placement of the guide pins is checked with a tensioning device that is attached to the heavy suture. The knee is moved through a range of motion to determine correct isometric measurement.
10. After isometric positioning is determined, the surgeon makes a longitudinal skin incision to the midline near the patellar tendon.
11. The central third portion of the patellar tendon with tibial and patellar bone plugs is harvested with a mini-saw and osteotome. The graft is sized to the appropriate width, usually 10 to 12 mm, using sizing tubes (Fig. 20.77).
12. Heavy nonabsorbable suture is placed through drill holes made at each end of the graft in the bone plugs (Fig. 20.78).
13. The guide pins are then reinserted and overdrilled with cannulae that are close in width to the prepared graft. Overdrilling establishes the tunnels so that they are in the center of the previous insertion sites of the ACL.

14. The surgeon smoothes the femoral and tibial osseous tunnels with curettes, a rasp, or an abrader. If the tunnels are made before the graft is harvested, they are temporarily occluded with bone tunnel plugs to minimize fluid extravasation.
15. Both ends of the graft are fixed with a barbed staple, bone screw with washer, interference screw, or ligament button (Fig. 20.79).

16. The incisions and joint are irrigated and closed.
17. A hinged knee brace may be applied over the dressing. The brace allows 10 to 90 degrees of motion.

Arthroscopic Posterior Cruciate Ligament Repair. Surgical procedures for tears of the PCL are considered if significant disabling instability has occurred. Patients usually return to adequate function without operative treatment. The arthroscopic procedure for repair of the PCL is similar to the technique used to repair the ACL, except that isometric placement is posterior within the joint and the femoral attachment is proximal to the medial epicondyle.

Arthroscopy of the Shoulder

Shoulder arthroscopy is a useful diagnostic and therapeutic tool in the management of shoulder disorders. It is particularly beneficial in evaluating and managing patients with chronic shoulder problems. Arthroscopy provides extensive visualization of the intra-articular aspect of the shoulder joint and is performed for removal of loose bodies; lysis of adhesions; synovial biopsy; synovectomy; bursectomy; stabilization of dislocations; correction of glenoid labrum, biceps tendon, and rotator cuff tears; and relief of impingement syndrome.

Procedural Considerations

The patient is either in the lateral position or in a sitting position using a "beach chair" positioner. The lateral position is maintained using a vacuum beanbag positioning device or lateral rolls with a kidney rest. Three-inch adhesive tape is secured across the patient's hips. Proper padding of the uninvolved axilla and lower extremity is important to prevent soft tissue or neurovascular problems. The affected extremity is placed in a shoulder suspension system, and Buck traction or a Velcro immobilizer is applied to the forearm to achieve adequate distraction to the glenohumeral joint. The extremity is abducted 40 to 60 degrees and forward-flexed 10 to 20 degrees, with 5- to 15-pound weights placed on the pulley system. Weight may be added to further distract the glenohumeral joint, taking care not to overstretch the axillary artery.

The shoulder is prepped and draped free, permitting full range of motion during the procedure.

The operative instruments and arthroscope commonly used for the knee may also be used in the shoulder, along with an 18-gauge needle, switching sticks, and a Wissinger rod. A variety of fixation devices (screws and tacks) can be used to repair bony defects and tears of the labrum.

Operative Procedure

1. An 18-gauge spinal needle is inserted through the posterior soft spot and directed anteriorly toward the coracoid process, in which the surgeon's index finger has been positioned (Fig. 20.80).
2. The glenohumeral joint is distended with normal saline or lactated Ringer's solution. This facilitates entry of the arthroscope.
3. The surgeon injects bupivacaine (Marcaine) 0.25%, 2 to 3 mL, with epinephrine 1:200,000 along the needle track to minimize bleeding.
4. With the needle removed, the surgeon makes a stab incision with a #11 blade over the needle site.
5. The surgeon introduces the arthroscope sleeve and sharp trocar through the posterior joint capsule.
6. After penetrating the capsule, the surgeon replaces the sharp trocar with a blunt obturator to enter the joint.
7. The surgeon inserts the arthroscope and attaches to inflow and outflow tubing, the video camera, and the light source.

8. Operative instruments are placed through an anterior portal that is established laterally to the coracoid process by using a Wissinger rod. A third portal can be established near the anterior portal or supraspinous fossa portal. Switching sticks are used to change portals.
9. The surgeon moves the arm and rotates it as needed to visualize various structures in and around the joint.
10. Glenoid tears can be repaired with the insertion of an absorbable fixation tack.
11. At the conclusion of the procedure, the joint is irrigated. The surgeon may inject a long-acting local anesthetic into the joint and subacromial space through the portal to minimize postoperative discomfort.
12. The puncture wounds are closed and dressed with a sterile 4 × 4 gauze pad. The patient's arm is placed in a sling for recovery.

Arthroscopy of the Elbow

The elbow joint is accessible to arthroscopic examination, although it requires more attention to detail than the knee because instruments must be placed through deeper muscle layers and close to important neurovascular structures.

Arthroscopy of the elbow, both diagnostic and operative, has become fairly routine. Indications for its use include extraction of loose bodies; evaluation or debridement of osteochondritis dissecans of the capitulum and radial head; partial synovectomy in rheumatoid disease; debridement and lysis of adhesions of posttraumatic or degenerative processes at or near the elbow; diagnosis of a chronically painful elbow when the diagnosis is obscure; and evaluation of fractures of the capitulum, radial head, or olecranon.

Procedural Considerations

General anesthesia is preferred to local anesthesia because it affords complete comfort to the patient and provides total muscle relaxation.

The perioperative nurse assists with placing the patient in either the supine or the prone position. In the supine position the forearm is flexed on an armboard or placed in a prefabricated wrist gauntlet connected to an overhead pulley device and tied off at the end of the OR bed. This provides excellent access to both the medial and lateral aspects of the elbow, allows the forearm to be freely pronated and supinated, and places the important neurovascular structures in the antecubital fossa at maximum relaxation.

A tourniquet is routinely used for hemostasis. The entire arm, including the hand, is prepped and draped.

The three portals most commonly used for diagnostic and operative arthroscopy of the elbow are the anterolateral, anteromedial, and posterolateral.

Operative arthroscopy instruments commonly used for the knee may also be used in the elbow. However, smaller diameter scopes and instruments may be desired instead.

Operative Procedure

1. The surgeon outlines the bony anatomic landmarks with a sterile marking pen before beginning the procedure. Lateral structures to be marked and identified are the radial head and the lateral epicondyle. The medial epicondyle is also marked.
2. An 18-gauge needle is inserted anteriorly to the radial head from the lateral side, and the joint is distended.
3. After distending the joint with approximately 15 to 30 mL of lactated Ringer's or normal saline solution, the surgeon makes a

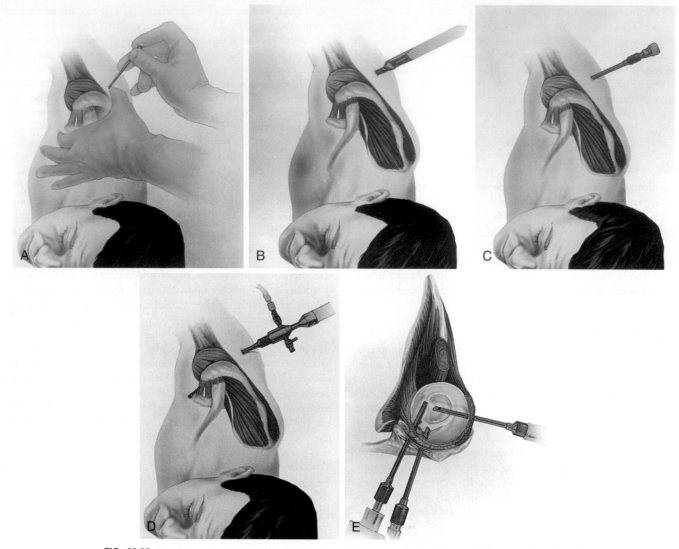

FIG. 20.80 Shoulder arthroscopy. (A) The spinal needle is inserted for dilation of the joint if indicated. (B) An incision is made over the glenohumeral joint. (C) The arthroscope sleeve and sharp trocar are inserted. (D) The arthroscope is inserted and attached to the inflow and outflow tubing, video camera, and light source. (E) Operative instruments are placed through the portal.

stab wound incision with a #11 blade and inserts the sharp trocar with cannula through the joint capsule.

4. The sharp trocar is replaced with the blunt obturator to provide safe entry of the cannula into the joint.

5. The surgeon replaces the blunt obturator with the scope and attaches it to the video and light source.

6. A second portal and third portal are established anteromedially and posterolaterally for triangulation. With the patient's elbow flexed to 90 degrees and adequate distention maintained at the time of insertion of the instruments, the surgeon displaces the neurovascular structures anteriorly. This provides a greater area above the medial and lateral humeral epicondyles in which to insert the various instruments.

7. Alternating the valve on the scope or using a separate 18-gauge needle with drainage tubing controls outflow and inflow.

8. After diagnostic and operative procedures have been completed, the joint is irrigated, the puncture sites are sutured, and a compression dressing is applied with soft rolled padding and elastic bandages.

Arthroscopy of the Ankle

The talocalcaneal articulations are complex and play an important role in the movements of inversion and eversion of the foot. The subtalar joints function as a single unit, but anatomically they are divided into anterior and posterior joints. The surgeon and perioperative nurse must be familiar with the extra-articular anatomy of the ankle to prevent neural or vascular damage.

Indications for ankle arthroscopy include osteochondral fragments or loose bodies, persistent ankle pain after trauma and despite adequate conservative treatment, biopsy, posttraumatic arthritis of the ankle joint, unstable ankle before lateral ligamentous reconstruction, and osteochondritis dissecans of the talus.

Procedural Considerations

General anesthesia is preferable because manipulation and distraction of the joint to obtain adequate arthroscopic viewing require muscle relaxation. The position of the patient is based on the surgeon's preference. The patient may be supine with the knee flexed approximately

70 degrees or supine with a sandbag under the buttock of the operative side. Ankle and thigh holders may be used; when better posterior visualization is necessary, a distractor may be used to increase the space between the tibia and talus. A tourniquet is placed around the upper thigh but is not used unless excessive bleeding, uncontrolled by irrigation, is encountered. Routine skin prepping and draping are done. Miniaturized instruments and needle scopes for the ankle are used.

Operative Procedure

1. Using a sterile marking pen, the surgeon outlines important extra-articular anatomic structures on the skin.
2. The surgeon examines the ankle joint, using the anterolateral portal. The anteromedial joint line is palpated, and an 18-gauge, 1½-inch needle is inserted into the joint.
3. Sterile plastic extension tubing is attached to the needle, and a 50-mL plastic syringe filled with normal saline is connected to the tubing to distend the joint. Approximately 15 to 20 mL is needed.
4. After intra-articular injection is confirmed by the ease with which the saline can be injected and by palpation of the joint as it is distended, the surgeon makes a small incision with a #11 blade over the site of the anterolateral portal.
5. A hemostat is then inserted and used to dissect to the capsule.
6. The surgeon places the sheath of the arthroscope and sharp trocar into the incision, angles them approximately 30 to 45 degrees laterally, and inserts them with a sharp plunge as joint distention is maintained. Entrance into the joint is felt as the sleeve and trocar "pop" through the capsule and is confirmed by the rush of saline on removal of the trocar from the sheath.
7. The arthroscope is inserted into the sheath, the needle is removed, and the plastic tubing and syringe are attached to the stopcock on the arthroscope sleeve. The video camera and light source are connected to the scope. Joint distention must be maintained.
8. Triangulation through other portals is easily done by first inserting the 18-gauge needle for localization while viewing with the arthroscope. Posterior viewing is done in the same fashion except that the patient is usually placed in the prone position and instruments are inserted through the posterior portals.
9. After the procedure is completed the surgeon irrigates the joint, closes the wounds with wound closure strips or a single suture, and covers the wound with a dressing and short leg compression elastic wrap.

Surgery of the Spine

Treatment of Back Pain

Back pain is a natural result of degenerative and arthritic change, punctuated by protrusion or rupture of a disk. It gradually progresses but may also disappear gradually. With aging, a degenerative disk-space narrowing or facet arthropathy begins to appear radiologically. The lower lumbar spine carries the burden of the body's weight; holds a person upright; and returns the body to the vertical position from sitting, lying, or a bent-over position. Degenerative changes, ruptured disk, and facet arthropathy develop at the lowest two limb segments, in which the greatest weight, torsion, and shearing stress occur. This degeneration sometimes extends into the upper and middle spine.

Cervical-spine degenerative disk narrowing also develops most often at the two lowest cervical spaces, which are also the levels of greatest stress resulting from movement of the head and neck.

Sometimes lumbar or cervical degenerative changes develop early from excessive repetitive movements or injury.

Epidural steroid injections, electrodes, stimulators, braces, or traction may be used to treat back pain. A natural recovery may result after 6 or 7 days of intense pain, subsiding between 6 weeks and 4 months. Motor and sensory deficits usually disappear with resolution of pain. The ability to recover without surgery depends on fragment size and compression on the nerve root. Neural compression remains the major indication for disk excision.

Spinal fusion is a consideration, usually for patients with demonstrable posttraumatic, postsurgical, rheumatoid, infectious, or neoplastic instability.

Lumbar Laminectomy

Procedural Considerations. After assessment the patient-specific plan of care is implemented. Radiographs are obtained. The perioperative nurse assesses the patient's bilateral pulses and range of motion in all of the extremities. Elastic wraps or intermittent pneumatic compression devices may be placed on the patients legs. The patient is positioned prone to eliminate lordosis, reduce venous congestion, and keep the abdomen free with chest rolls or special frames after inducing general anesthesia. Depending on the extent of the procedure, blood products may be required. The skin is prepped and the area draped. A spinal laminectomy set is used, in addition to a spinal retractor of choice and a bipolar ESU. Hemostatic adjuncts such as gelatin foam, oxidized cellulose strips, thrombin, and bone wax should be available. Antibiotic irrigation for the wound along with the use of topical vancomycin powder at the surgical site have shown to decrease surgical site infections in the spine while minimizing the systemic effects of the vancomycin (Research Highlight).

Operative Procedure

1. The surgeon makes a midline incision over the affected disk and carries it sharply down to the supraspinous ligament.

RESEARCH HIGHLIGHT

Effectiveness of Local Vancomycin Powder to Decrease Surgical Site Infections

SSIs remain a serious problem for patients undergoing surgical procedures. Infections after orthopedic surgery can be especially devastating. Preoperative administration of antibiotics is an accepted practice in orthopedics as is the topical application of antibiotics in irrigants and as additives to bone cement. This study provides a meta-analysis of the use of vancomycin powder to the wound bed in spinal surgery before closure.

Using observational studies, quasi-experimental studies and randomized clinical trials with control groups, researchers sought to determine the effectiveness of locally applied vancomycin powder in decreasing SSIs. After narrowing the search results, the analysis included 10 independent studies and 22 articles. Surgical procedures in the analysis included spinal surgery (8) and fusion, and cardiac (median sternotomy) procedures (2). No vancomycin-related complications were noted in the analysis.

The pooled results for all studies demonstrated the effectiveness of topical application of vancomycin to the wound bed in protecting against SSIs. The authors recommend additional studies to validate results as well as studies that investigate the use of vancomycin in procedures other than spinal operations.

SSI, Surgical site infection.
Modified from Chiang HY et al: Effectiveness of local vancomycin powder to decrease surgical site infections: a meta-analysis, *Spine J* 14(3):347–407, 2014.

2. The supraspinous ligament is incised, and the muscles are dissected subperiosteally from the spines and laminae of the vertebrae. These are retracted with a self-retaining retractor.
3. The surgeon denudes the laminae and ligamentum flavum with a curette.
4. A small part of the inferior margin of the lamina is removed with a rongeur.
5. The ligamentum flavum is grasped and incised where it fuses with the interspinous ligament, and this flap is then sharply removed to expose the dura.
6. The dura is then retracted medially, and the nerve root is identified.
7. Once identified, the nerve root is retracted medially so that the underlying posterior longitudinal ligament can be exposed.
8. The surgeon incises the posterior longitudinal ligament over the intervertebral space in a cruciate fashion and enters the disk space with a pituitary grasping forceps.
9. The disk material is systematically removed, taking care not to exceed the distance to the anterior annulus. A complete search for additional fragments of nucleus pulposus, both inside and outside the disk space, is then performed.
10. Residual bleeding is controlled with bipolar coagulation.
11. The surgeon closes the wound with absorbable sutures in the supraspinous ligament and subcutaneous tissue. Various non-absorbable sutures or staples are used for skin closure.

Minimally Invasive Spine Surgery

Advances in technology have made minimally invasive spinal surgery (MISS) available to certain patients. Candidates for MISS are carefully selected by the surgeon. Conditions that may be amenable to MISS include disk herniation, spinal stenosis, and kyphosis. The need to convert from MISS to the traditional incision must be discussed with the patient before the surgery, and the perioperative nurse and scrub person must prepare for that possibility. The microdiskectomy procedure, used to treat disk herniation, is described below.

Procedural Considerations

The perioperative nurse and scrub person ensure that all equipment is available and assembled before the patient's arrival into the OR. Equipment needed includes the C-arm, microscope, and radiolucent spinal table. After the administration of a general anesthetic, the patient is positioned prone on the radiolucent spinal table. Care is taken to ensure proper padding of bony prominences and proper positioning of extremities. The skin is prepped and draped. Instrumentation for MISS includes the tubular microdiskectomy set and the tubular retractor. A high-speed drill and hemostatic agents such as gelatin foam, thrombin, and bone wax should be available. The perioperative nurse places intermittent pneumatic compression devices on the patient's legs.

Operative Procedure

1. The surgeon inserts an 18-gauge spinal needle in the back at the level of the disk herniation and confirms the correct level with the C-arm.
2. The surgeon makes a 1- to 1.5-cm incision at the previously identified level.
3. A Cobb elevator and sequentially sized dilators are used to serially dilate the soft tissues, preserving the integrity of the muscles and ligaments.
4. The surgeon inserts a tubular retractor and connects the flex arm directly to the spinal table.

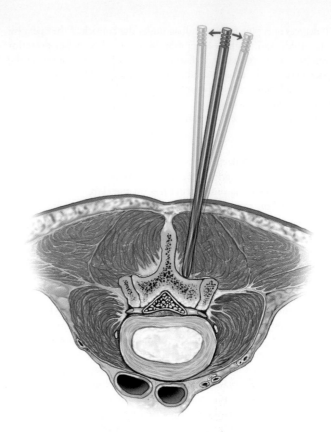

FIG. 20.81 Wanding maneuver is used to change the position of the tubular retractor and reach different areas of the spine.

5. The tubular retractor is used as a viewing portal to visualize and operate on the spine (Fig. 20.81).
6. The surgeon confirms the level again with x-ray and moves the draped microscope into position.
7. Using the long electrode on the ESU, the surgeon dissects the tissue.
8. A high-powered burr and/or assorted sizes of Kerrison punches are used to remove part of the caudal lamina.
9. After identifying the nerve roots, the surgeon enters the disk space and removes the extruded disk material with pituitary grasping forceps.
10. Gelatin foam and cotton pledgets are used to control bleeding along with the bipolar ESU.
11. The surgeon irrigates and closes the wound.

Pedicle Fixation of the Spine

Pedicle screw fixation (Fig. 20.82) is a method of surgical fixation of the spinal column. Screw fixation was initially used in an attempt to avoid postoperative external immobilization and prolonged bed rest. Pedicle screw fixation has been used most often in degenerative processes, particularly iatrogenic instability after decompression, degenerative and isthmic spondylolisthesis, and diskogenic disease. It is also indicated for tumor, trauma, degenerative spinal disorders, postoperative hypermobility, and infection.

Three basic approaches for fixation have been described as the procedure has evolved. Each has improved on the first, based on anatomic placement of the screw. Screw placement techniques include nontapping, line-to-line tapping, undertapping with incongruent

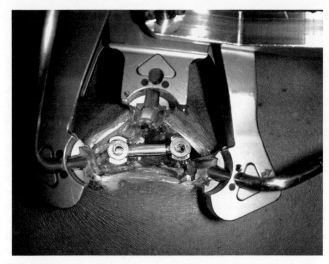

FIG. 20.82 Pedicle screw placement using the MaXcess retractor and SpheRx fixation system by NuVasive, Inc.

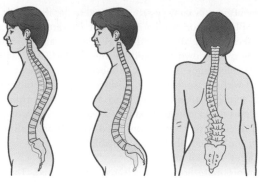

FIG. 20.83 Scoliotic deformity.

pitch, or undertapping with congruent pitch. Bohl and colleagues (2015) reported the results of these different techniques. Positioning and placement of the screw within the spine are established after direct visualization of the pedicle.

Procedural Considerations

After the administration of a general anesthetic, the patient is positioned prone. The skin is prepped, and drapes are applied. A spinal laminectomy set is used in addition to the instrumentation and implants of choice, a spinal retractor, power equipment such as a high-speed motorized hand tool, and hemostatic adjuncts such as gelatin foam, thrombin, bone wax and powdered fibrin sealant (Brooks, 2015). A bone graft set is needed to harvest a graft from the iliac crest.

Operative Procedure

1. The surgeon makes a standard midline incision. The surgeon follows the steps as described in the laminectomy procedure to expose the spine.
2. The areas of the pedicles to be fixated are located using external landmarks.
3. The surgeon removes the posterior cortical wall at the entrance site using a high-speed burr.
4. A Penfield dissector is used to identify the entrance hole through the pedicle.
5. The surgeon inserts a gearshift probe to identify the path into the vertebral body.
6. The hole is tapped (5.5-mm tap) and widened.
7. The surgeon places the screw(s). Guidelines for screw sizes are 7 mm for S1, L5, and L4; 6.25 mm for L3 and L2; and 5.5 mm for L1 and T12.
8. A posterolateral graft is performed, using graft strips from the iliac crest.
9. The surgeon contours the plate or rod to approximate the patient's physiologic lordosis. The longitudinal device is locked onto the screws in the appropriate position.
10. A screw-plate system may require oblique and transverse washers between the screw head and plate to provide a flush fit at the screw-plate interface.

11. The foramina are checked for patency before closure. The excess portion of the screw is cut close to the upper locking device.
12. A suction drain is placed; the wound is closed in layers.

Treatment of Scoliosis

Scoliosis is a three-dimensional deformity (Fig. 20.83) with lateral deviation of the spinal column from the midline; it may include rotation or deformity of the vertebrae. Types are congenital, juvenile, adolescent, and adult. School screening programs provide quick and simple detection. For effective treatment of scoliosis, early detection is critical.

Scoliosis can be idiopathic or congenital and may result from muscular or neurologic diseases or unequal leg lengths. Numerous posterior and anterior segmental spinal instrumentation systems are available for treating idiopathic scoliosis. Consequently fixation strategies are more complex than they were with Harrington instrumentation. The newer systems provide better sagittal control and more stable fixation, allowing quicker mobilization of the patient. On thin patients, however, the bulk of these implants may be a problem.

Posterior Spinal Fusion With Harrington Rods

Posterior spinal fusion is most frequently performed in adolescence, when the laterally deviated curve is still flexible. Harrington rods are internal splints that help maintain the spine as straight as possible until the vertebral body fusion has become solid. Distraction rods are placed on the concave side of the curve, and compression rods are placed on the convex side. On the convex side of the curve, three to eight hooks are inserted in the transverse processes of the vertebrae and pulled together with a threaded rod. In this way the scoliotic deformity can be corrected as much as the flexibility of the spine allows.

The posterior elements of the vertebrae are denuded of soft tissue, and the bone graft is added. Blood loss can be expected, and an accurate record of the loss must be maintained. After surgery the patient is placed in an immobilizing jacket.

Some disadvantages of the Harrington rod system over other systems are that there is only endpoint fixation, rod breakage is increased, fixation is less, sagittal plane curves are difficult to manage, distraction for correction is not always desired, and the patient is required to wear a postoperative cast or brace. Other systems have evolved from the Harrington rods that are used for correction of some scoliotic deformities. This technique, however, remains a feasible treatment of idiopathic scoliosis.

Procedural Considerations. The team positions the patient prone on a spinal table or a spinal frame to facilitate respiration. Before the procedure begins, an x-ray cassette is placed under the patient so that a radiograph for accurate identification of the vertebrae to be fused can be taken during the operation. A single straight longitudinal incision is made down the midline of the back. Because of the amount of bleeding, the skin and subcutaneous tissues are often infiltrated with a vasoconstricting solution, such as epinephrine.

Basic spinal instrumentation and bone graft instruments are required, plus the Harrington rod instrumentation. A large pin cutter, designed to cut large pins but provided with a small end so that it will fit in the wound, should be available.

Operative Procedure

1. The appropriate hooks are selected and inserted. The surgeon inserts a Harrington distraction rod of appropriate length through the two proximal self-adjusting hooks, which have been placed under the laminae.
2. A rod clamp is clamped onto the Harrington rod just below the hook, and a single regular spreader is used to obtain the first inch of distraction.
3. The Bobechko spreader is used to span over the first hook, closest to the smooth part of the rod, to apply distraction force on the most proximal hook.
4. The surgeon inserts two C-locking rings around the first ratchet immediately below the hook to prevent dislodgement of the hooks. The excessive length of protruding rod above the most proximal hook is removed with a rod cutter. The compression is tightened.

Luque Segmental Spinal Rod Procedure

The Luque segmental method uses smooth L-shaped stainless steel rods, usually $\frac{3}{16}$ or $\frac{1}{4}$ inch in diameter, with sublaminar wires placed at every level possible. It is more secure and longer than the Harrington rod system and was the first system to use multipoint fixation. Luque instrumentation applies corrective forces to the spinal segments at each level, spreading the corrective forces throughout the length of the deformity. Two Luque rods are wired to both sides of the spine. The rods are contoured to achieve no more than 10 degrees of increased correction beyond that exhibited on preoperative x-ray study.

Procedural Considerations. The patient is placed in the prone position as described for the Harrington rod procedure. Because of the amount of bleeding, the skin and subcutaneous tissues are often infiltrated with a vasoconstricting solution, such as epinephrine. Basic spinal instrumentation is required. In addition, Luque rods and instrumentation, a wire tightener and cutter, and bone graft instruments are needed.

Operative Procedure

1. The surgeon makes a straight, midline incision.
2. The ligamentum flavum is detached, exposing the neural canal.
3. The surgeon passes doubled stainless steel suture wire under the lamina.
4. Total bilateral facetectomies are made, forming posterolateral troughs for subsequent bone grafts.
5. Wedge osteotomies may be necessary in severe immobile curves to avoid stretching the spinal cord during correction.
6. The wire loop is cut, resulting in two separate wires at each level.
7. The surgeon secures the L bend to the base of the spinous process to prevent rod migration.
8. Initial placement of the convex rod is made, followed by initial placement of the concave rod.
9. Transverse wiring is done to add increased stability to the system.

10. Stabilization of the lumbosacral joint is corrected by bending the rods distally to form sacral bars.

Cotrel–Dubousset System Procedure

The Cotrel–Dubousset system provides three-dimensional correction of spinal deformities without sublaminar wiring and neurologic risks. This instrumentation permits distraction, compression, and derotation. The scoliotic curve is corrected by derotation and, at the same time, it restores the normal sagittal contours. In addition to correction of scoliosis, the Cotrel–Dubousset system can be applied to correct kyphosis or lordosis and to stabilize and rebuild the spine after tumor resection or after injury. No external support is necessary. The Cotrel–Dubousset system has no ratchets or notches. It consists of metallic rods with diamond crosscut patterns on which hooks and screws can be positioned in any position, level, or degree of rotation. The rod is held in the open hooks with blockers. The rods are then interlocked with devices for transverse traction. The Cotrel–Dubousset system was the forerunner to the systems used today, such as the Texas Scottish Rite Hospital (TSRH) system and the Isola system.

Procedural Considerations. The team places the patient in the prone position after induction of general anesthesia. Patient assessment and precautions for the prone position are initiated. Basic spinal instrumentation is required in addition to the Cotrel–Dubousset system and instrumentation as well as the instruments used for harvesting the bone graft.

Operative Procedure

1. Closed hooks are inserted at both ends of the surgical site, and open hooks are inserted at various levels between the closed hooks.
2. Decortication and facet excision are done at the remaining interposed vertebral levels for rod placement.
3. Bone graft is placed in the areas that will be under the rod.
4. The surgeon bends the appropriate concave rod to shape for sagittal-plane correction and manipulates it into the end hooks.
5. Stabilization along the length is achieved with blockers that anchor the rod into the open hooks.
6. Using the rod holders, the surgeon derotates the spine. The frontal-plane scoliosis curve becomes the sagittal-plane kyphosis.
7. Hooks are reseated for secure fixation.
8. To correct kyphosis, the surgeon bends the convex rod to shape and seats it.
9. Once the rods are placed, the surgeon applies the device for transverse traction (DTT), usually near the ends of the rods, to complete the stabilization.
10. Remaining bone graft is then applied to the fusion area.

Texas Scottish Rite Hospital Crosslink System

The TSRH crosslink system (Fig. 20.84) is a multicomponent stainless steel implant used to lock spinal rods together rigidly. Locking the rods increases construction stiffness and prevents rod migration. The system was originally designed for the Luque segmental system to prevent migration between the rods and wires before complete fusion occurred. By rigidly crosslinking the rods, loss of scoliotic correction was reduced. This system can also be used with the Harrington and Cotrel–Dubousset systems. Crosslinks are indicated when the rigidity of a spinal system alone is not sufficient to generate fusion in a reasonable amount of time.

Procedural Considerations. The patient is administered a general anesthetic and positioned prone. The skin is prepped, and drapes

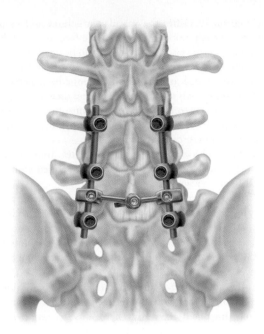

FIG. 20.84 Texas Scottish Rite Hospital crosslink system.

are applied. A spinal laminectomy set is used. Spinal instrumentation and implants, a spinal retractor, and power equipment such as a high-speed handheld tool are necessary. Hemostatic adjuncts such as gelatin foam, thrombin, oxidized cellulose, and bone wax should be available.

Operative Procedure
1. Eyebolts are placed on the spinal rods before the rods are implanted.
2. The surgeon secures the rods with hooks or wires, depending on the system used.
3. After the rods are positioned, cross plates of varying widths accommodating different rod-to-rod distances are bolted in place between the rods and nuts.

Anterior Spinal Fusion With Isola Instrumentation

The Isola anterior instrumentation is indicated in idiopathic scoliosis patients, approximately 10 to 30 years of age, with thoracolumbar or upper lumbar curves of 40 to 65 degrees. The procedure involves screw fixation into each vertebral body, complete disk excision and grafting, and segmental connection of the vertebral bodies. A semirigid rod connects the segments.

Procedural Considerations. The patient is positioned in a lateral decubitus position so that posteroanterior and lateral intraoperative radiographs can be taken. The anesthesia provider should ensure incomplete pharmacologic paralysis to allow for intraoperative neurophysiologic monitoring. In addition to a major soft tissue set and laminectomy set, the Isola instrumentation and implants, a vascular set, and power equipment are needed.

Operative Procedure
1. The surgeon approaches the spine through a transthoracic retroperitoneal (or retropleural retroperitoneal) approach, resecting the rib two vertebral levels above the upper instrumented vertebrae.
2. The sympathetic chain is mobilized laterally with the psoas.
3. The segmental vessels are temporarily occluded and, provided that there are no monitoring changes, ligated.

4. The disks are exposed to the far side to allow a full annulectomy. The bodies, however, are not exposed much beyond the midline.
5. A full 360-degree diskectomy and annulectomy are done, exposing the posterior longitudinal ligament.
6. The surgeon places the screws in the vertebral body, placing the end screws first. Care is taken to place the longitudinal axis of the screw parallel to the endplate and at the apex of the vertebral body.
7. Screw placement is started with an awl and continued with a 5.5-mm tap, continuing until the tip just exits the far side of the cortex. The first one-third of the hole is tapped with a 7-mm tap, and a 7-mm closed top screw with a washer is inserted. The screw must protrude through the opposite cortex by a thread or two. The same process is then repeated at the lower end vertebra.
8. The surgeon cuts the rod to the proper length and contours it to re-create the sagittal-plane angular position of the normal spine. It is then positioned in the end vertebra and used as a guide to locate the entry point for the intermediate screws.
9. Open-ended intermediate screws are inserted in a fashion similar to the end screws, taking care that their pathway is parallel to the end screws.
10. The rod is back entered through the upper screw and then the lower screw, and seated into the intermediate open screws. The open screws are capped, and the rod is rotated to place the sagittal-plane contour of the rod in the sagittal plane. An intermediate set screw is tightened to secure the new position of the rod.
11. As the remaining screws are tightened about the rod, it is essential that the disk spaces be opened completely. A Cobb elevator can be used to pry the disk space open.
12. Rib corticocancellous autograft is used to completely fill the disk spaces. The surgeon obtains the graft from the tenth rib (the usual site of entry), the twelfth rib (taken from inside the chest), and the eighth rib (taken from outside the chest).
13. The disk spaces are compressed to provide anterior column load sharing. Care should be taken to ensure that the set screws are visited at least twice for the end-closed connections and three times for the center-capped connections.
14. Closure is in the standard manner, using chest tubes if the chest has been entered or a retropleural closed wound drainage system if a retropleural retroperitoneal exposure has been done.
15. Postoperative care consists of an overnight intensive care stay with the patient sitting out of bed the next morning. A cast or brace is used at the physician's discretion. Activities are restricted for 6 to 12 months, until there is clear indication of graft incorporation.

Artificial Disk Replacement for Degenerative Disk Disease

Degenerative disk disease (DDD) occurs when the IVD is worn because of aging or trauma. Diskogenic back pain results from degeneration of the disk and is confirmed both by patient history and by radiographic studies. The IVD acts as the padding between the vertebrae. Once the IVD is worn out, pain, inflammation, and nerve impingement leading to numbness and muscle weakness can occur. Left untreated, nerve damage can be permanent. DDD occurs in 50% of people older than 40 years of age. Many patients are asymptomatic; however, those who are affected can be severely debilitated, changing their ability to cope with activities of daily living (ADLs) and affecting the quality of life. Artificial disk

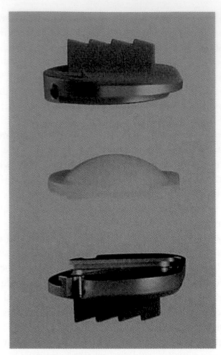

FIG. 20.85 Three components of the ProDisc.

replacement (Fig. 20.85) re-creates the natural disk function with preservation of spinal motion.

Procedural Considerations

The perioperative nurse and scrub person collaborate to ensure the availability of implants with the manufacturer's representative and reconfirm this during the preoperative verification process. Other considerations for this procedure include the use of a blood-salvaging system in both the intraoperative and postoperative periods. Templates of x-rays should be placed on the viewing box in the OR before the procedure. The patient is positioned supine on a Jackson bed with the right arm draped across the body. A C-arm is used to identify the disk or disks to be replaced in the marked areas. In many institutions, laminar airflow is used.

Operative Procedure

The two general anatomic routes for anterior exposure to the lumbar spine are retroperitoneal and transperitoneal.

The *retroperitoneal approach* can proceed from a variety of incisions, including vertical midline, paramedian, oblique, and transverse. This is determined by both the spinal level and the number of lumbar levels to be exposed. An infraumbilical transverse incision can accommodate most approaches to the L4-L5 and/or S1 disk levels, whereas a more obliquely oriented incision is favored for accessing disk levels above L4.

The *transperitoneal route* is not generally used except in extenuating circumstances (e.g., prior extensive retroperitoneal surgery or revisional spine surgery).

1. The surgeon creates a midline incision and places a fixed retractor system to move the small and large bowel out of the field and facilitate direct visualization of the abdominal cavity. Trendelenburg position can be used to assist with maintaining exposure.
2. For the L5-S1 level, the peritoneum superficial to the sacral prominence is incised.

3. The surgeon identifies the vascular structures and uses blunt dissection to tease open the area of the facet of the disk.
4. The middle sacral vessels generally need to be divided to complete the exposure. Excessive electrocoagulation should be avoided to decrease the risk of injury to the sympathetic nerves.
5. After the exposure is complete the surgeon uses a #3 long handle with a #15 blade to make an incision into the disk body.
6. The diskectomy is completed using a rongeur and curettes to remove remaining disk tissue.
7. Correct sizing is determined using templates. Trial instrumentation is inserted and correct placement is verified with AP and lateral C-arm views.
8. The trial is centered in the AP plane, and the marker appears as a plus sign aligned with the spinous process. On the lateral x-ray, a hole in the trial represents the center of rotation.
9. After verifying correct placement of the trial, the surgeon uses an ESU to mark the midline of the superior vertebral body and removes the trial.
10. Next, the pilot driver is aligned with the midline ESU mark.
11. The pilot driver that corresponds to the chosen footprint is then carefully impacted to verify the ability to accurately place endplates.
12. During this process lateral C-arm imaging is used to accurately monitor the depths of the pilot driver.
13. After the correct depth is achieved, the surgeon uses the slap hammer, removing the pilot driver from the disk space.
14. The endplate insertion tips are then attached to the corresponding superior and inferior endplates.
15. The endplates are then carefully inserted into the disk space with the assistance of the guided impactor.
16. The insertion is monitored with fluoroscopy to accurately control the posterior depth and verify the appropriate lordotic angle.
17. With the superior and inferior endplates in place, the surgeon uses the spreading and insertion forceps to open the disk space.
18. After appropriate distraction is achieved, the surgeon can use the size on the spacer to select the appropriate core trial.
19. The appropriate core insertion tip is loaded into the core insertion instrument, and the sliding core is inserted between the endplates.
20. The surgeon releases the distraction on the spreading forceps, which allows the endplates to close around and engage the sliding core.
21. The core insertion instrument is removed, and the final position verified using fluoroscopy (Fig. 20.86).
22. The wound is irrigated and closed.

Vertebroplasty and Kyphoplasty

Vertebroplasty and kyphoplasty are used for the treatment of vertebral compression fractures attributable to osteoporosis or pathologic conditions. Bone cement is injected into the vertebral body to decrease back pain and prevent further vertebral body height loss (Yimin et al., 2013).

Procedural Considerations

Patient selection is key in identifying appropriate candidates for this procedure. MRI is the most accurate radiologic diagnosis. Equipment includes C-arm, radiolucent procedure table, and x-ray vests for staff as well as vertebroplasty system and cement injection system. Bone biopsy needles should be available. The C-arm must provide a good quality image; all key bony landmarks should be clearly visible. Positioning of the patient requires careful vigilance to prevent skin

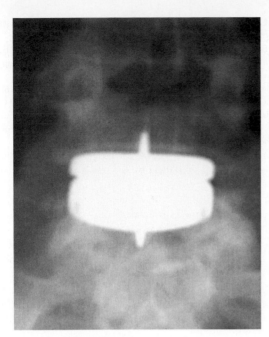

FIG. 20.86 Implanted ProDisc.

breakdown and nerve damage. After the administration of anesthetic, the patient is positioned prone with hyperextension of the vertebral compression fracture on the radiolucent procedure table. The patient is then prepped and draped and the C-arm is positioned.

Operative Procedure

1. Confirmation of the level of the vertebroplasty (or kyphoplasty) is determined by fluoroscopy.
2. The surgeon inserts the appropriate gauge bone needle (11- to 13-mm gauge for vertebroplasty; 8- to 10-mm gauge for kyphoplasty) at the desired level and confirms the correct level with fluoroscopy.
3. For kyphoplasty:
   a. The inflatable balloon tamp is placed. Available tamps are 10, 15, or 20 mm in length, and available styles are multidirectional, unidirectional, and bidirectional.
   b. After placing the tamp the surgeon gradually inflates the balloon to 50 pounds per square inch (psi) and then continues inflation in increments of 25 psi until the desired pressure is achieved and either there is height restoration of the vertebral body or the tamp is in proximity to the cortical margin. Pressure is monitored by a manometer.
   c. Once the tamp has reach maximum inflation, the surgeon deflates the balloon. A cavity is left within the vertebral body.
4. Cement is mixed and then injected through the bone needle using a 1-mL syringe under fluoroscopic control.
5. The needle is removed and a dressing is applied.

Key Points

- Preoperative preparation is key to prevent delays and cancellations on the day of surgery. This includes not only the patient and preoperative testing, paperwork, and education but also proper anticipation for the surgical procedure. Information regarding patient demographics, instrumentation and implants requested, and additional items such as bone grafts should be sent from the surgeon's office when the case is scheduled.

- All vendors should be notified of the scheduled cases to allow enough time to transport and properly sterilize instrumentation necessary for the surgery.
- Adherence to the SCIP guidelines for prevention of surgical site infection and venous thromboembolism is critical for this patient population.
- Care must be taken when transporting and moving patients to prevent any additional pain.
- Patient positioning and padding are crucial in preventing nerve injury and maintaining skin integrity.
- Trauma patients and their families need additional education and communication regarding the surgical process because of the critical nature of the surgery.

Critical Thinking Questions

Reviewing the surgical schedule the day before surgery, you notice your first patient has been on Coumadin but was told to discontinue the medication 5 days before surgery. Labwork was done while the patient was still on Coumadin, but no additional testing has been ordered. The patient is scheduled to arrive at 6:00 a.m. for a 7:30 a.m. incision time. What is the first thing you should do regarding this patient? What needs to be done before surgery to ensure a safe procedure for this patient? Who should you notify? Should the OR schedule be changed?

℮volve *The answers to the Critical Thinking Questions can be found at http://evolve.elsevier.com/Rothrock/Alexander.*

References

American Academy of Orthopaedic Surgeons (AAOS): *Minimally invasive total hip replacement* (website), 2016a. www.orthoinfo.org/topic.cfm?topic=A00404. (Accessed 1 October 2016).

American Academy of Orthopaedic Surgeons (AAOS): *Reverse total shoulder replacement* (website), 2016b. http://orthoinfo.aaos.org/topiccfm?topic=A00504. (Accessed 1 October 2016).

American Academy of Orthopaedic Surgeons (AAOS): *Shoulder joint replacement* (website), 2016c. http://orthoinfo.aaos.org/topiccfm?topic=A00094. (Accessed 25 September 2016).

American Association of Tissue Banks (AATB): *Standards for tissue banking,* McLean, VA, 2016, The Association.

American Board of Orthopaedic Surgeons (ABOS): *History of the American Board of Orthopaedic Surgery* (website), 2016. www.abos.org/about/history.aspx. (Accessed 19 September 2016).

Association of periOperative Registered Nurses (AORN): *AORN position statement on the role of the health care industry representative in the perioperative and invasive procedure setting* (website), 2014. www.aorn.org/Pos.Stat-Personnel -Health-Care-Reps-1pdf. (Accessed 25 September 2016).

Association of periOperative Registered Nurses (AORN): Guideline for care of patients undergoing pneumatic tourniquet-assisted devices. In *Guidelines for perioperative practice,* Denver, 2016a, The Association.

Association of periOperative Registered Nurses (AORN): Guideline for preoperative patient skin asepsis. In *Guidelines for perioperative practice,* Denver, 2016b, The Association.

Association of periOperative Registered Nurses (AORN): Guideline for a safe environment of care. In *Guidelines for perioperative practice,* Denver, 2016c, The Association.

Association of periOperative Registered Nurses (AORN): Guideline for transfer of patient care information. In *Guidelines for perioperative practice,* Denver, 2016d, The Association.

Bohl DD et al: Undertapping of lumbar pedicle screws can result in tapping with a pitch that differs from that of the screw, which decreases screw pullout force, *Spine* 40(12):E729–E734, 2015.

Bosco JA et al: Principles of antibiotic prophylaxis in total joint arthroplasty: current concepts, *J Am Acad Orthop Surg* 23(8):e27–e35, 2015.

Brooks M: *FDA approves Raplixa to help control bleeding during surgery* (website), 2015. www.medscape.com/viewarticle/844063. (Accessed 15 June 2016).

Lonner J: Robotically assisted unicompartmental knee arthroplasty with a handheld image-free sculpting tool, *Orthop Clin North Am* 47(1):29–40, 2016.

Metzler AV, Johnson DL: ACL Reconstruction: surgical approaches and anatomic considerations in 2014, *Curr Orthop Pract* 25(4):306–311, 2014.

Miller MD: *Review of orthopaedics*, ed 7, Philadelphia, 2016, Saunders.

National Osteoporosis Foundation (NOF): *Bone basics* (website), 2016. Washington, DC, National Osteoporosis Foundation. https://www.nof.org/preventing-fractures/general-facts/bone-basics/. (Accessed 9 October 2017).

Netscher D et al: Hand surgery. In Townsend CM, editor: *Sabiston textbook of surgery*, ed 20, Philadelphia, 2017, Saunders.

Spruce L, Van Wicklin SA: Back to basics positioning the patient, *AORN J* 100(3):298–303, 2014.

Taylor B: *Shoulder anterior (deltopectoral) approach* (website), 2016. www.orthobullets.com/approaches/12061/shoulder-anterior-deltopectoral-approach. (Accessed 1 October 2016).

The Joint Commission (TJC): *Universal protocol* (website), 2016. www.jointcommission.org/standards_information/up.aspx. (Accessed 10 October 2016).

Yimin Y et al: Current status of percutaneous vertebroplasty and percutaneous kyphoplasty–a review, *Med Sci Monit* 19:826–836, 2013.

CHAPTER 21

Neurosurgery

MAUREEN P. MURPHY AND DANA M. WHITMORE

Neurosurgery is a very diverse, complex, and challenging specialty. Brain surgery is performed for head injury, tumors, vascular disorders, hydrocephalus, epilepsy, and Parkinson disease. Neurosurgery also treats disorders of the spine from trauma and fractures, spinal cord injury, spinal stenosis, spinal tumors, and disk disease. Advancements in the highly technical field of neurosurgery are constant.

The perioperative team who cares for neurosurgical patients is challenged by the need to have a working knowledge of neuroanatomy, function, and clinical presentations of the many neurologic conditions that require surgical interventions. Understanding the surgical procedure to be performed allows the perioperative nurse and scrub person, who may be a registered nurse or surgical technologist, to anticipate and respond to the intraoperative needs of the patient and neurosurgical team, and to surgical complications if they arise. Given the range and complexity of today's neurosurgical interventions, an understanding of highly sophisticated equipment and instrumentation is necessary. Like all patients undergoing surgery, the neurosurgical patient is often vulnerable secondary to the presenting pathologic condition. For perioperative personnel to deliver sensitive, humanistic care in this highly technical environment, they must recognize and appreciate the individual's emotional and spiritual state, whether it is manifested by fear, pain, or grief. Reaching out and making the human connection allays the fear, moderates the pain, and facilitates the patient's grieving process. Information in this chapter will assist those working in neurosurgery to provide optimal patient care.

Surgical Anatomy

The nervous system is the most complex and least understood of body systems. It is divided structurally into the central nervous system (CNS) consisting of the brain and spinal cord and the peripheral nervous system (PNS), which encompasses every neurologic structure outside the CNS, including the cranial and spinal nerves. The brain and spinal cord are protected by the skull and vertebral columns, respectively. The cranial nerves originate within the brain and emerge through openings in the skull to run peripherally. The spinal nerves that emerge from the spinal cord through the vertebral foramina also run peripherally.

The nervous system is divided functionally into a voluntary system and an autonomic, or involuntary, system. It provides a means of communication for the rest of the body. The functions of all body systems depend in part on nervous system function. In turn, the nervous system depends directly on circulatory system function to obtain life-sustaining glucose and oxygen. Nervous system functions include motor and sensory functions, orientation, coordination, conceptual thought, emotion, memory, and reflex response.

Nervous system tissue is composed of vast amounts of neurons and far more neuroglial cells. Neurons are intercommunicating nerve cells that encode, conduct, and transmit information to other neurons, muscle, and glandular tissue (Fig. 21.1). They are composed of a body or soma with branches or extensions, called dendrites and axons, which communicate with other cells at synapses. Dendrites are short branches that conduct impulses toward the soma. Cell bodies and dendrites are mostly confined to areas of gray matter in the CNS. Axons are long branches, often encased in a white myelin sheath, that conduct impulses away from the soma. Axons pass into bundles of nerve fibers that tend to form tracts or pathways and are referred to as white matter. Tracts that cross midline to create a communication pathway from each side of the body to the opposite side of the brain are called commissures. Neuroglial cells support the neurons by creating and maintaining an appropriate environment in which neurons can operate efficiently. Glial cells include astrocytes, oligodendrocytes, ependymal cells, and microglia. The mutation of these cells can form a glioma, which is one of the more common brain tumors.

This chapter divides the nervous system into logical divisions within the framework of neurosurgical techniques. The brain and adjacent structures include the cranial nerves of the PNS, which are commonly encountered during brain surgery. Discussion of the spine and spinal cord includes the adjacent spinal nerves and the disks and ligaments that support the spine. Surgically significant pathology is incorporated with the normal anatomy of structures.

Brain and Adjacent Structures

Scalp

Scalp layers (Fig. 21.2) include skin, subcutaneous tissue, galea, and periosteum. Scalp skin is thick. The subcutaneous tissue, which is exceptionally dense, tough, and vascular, is firmly attached to the galea. Most of the blood vessels lie superficial to the galea. The subgaleal space contains loose areolar tissue that permits mobility of the scalp. It is in this bloodless plane that the standard craniotomy scalp flap is created. The pericranium, or outer periosteum of the skull, separates the galea from the cranium.

The arterial supply of the scalp comes from the external carotid artery through the superficial temporal, posterior auricular, occipital, frontal, and supraorbital branches. Most veins roughly follow the course of their corresponding arteries, except the emissary veins, which drain directly through the skull into the intracranial venous sinuses. The scalp, the extracranial arteries, and portions of the dura mater are the only pain-sensitive structures that cover the brain. The brain itself is insensate.

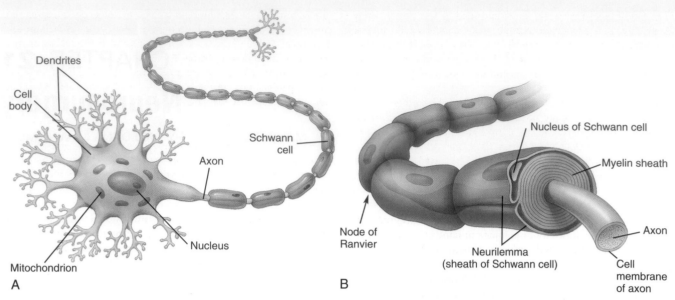

FIG. 21.1 (A) Many dendrites carry nerve impulses to the cell body, which then sends the nerve impulses along a single, long axon. Long axons are encased at intervals by a myelin sheath. (B) Segment of myelinated fiber in cross section, showing myelin sheath composed of several layers of myelin, which insulate the axon.

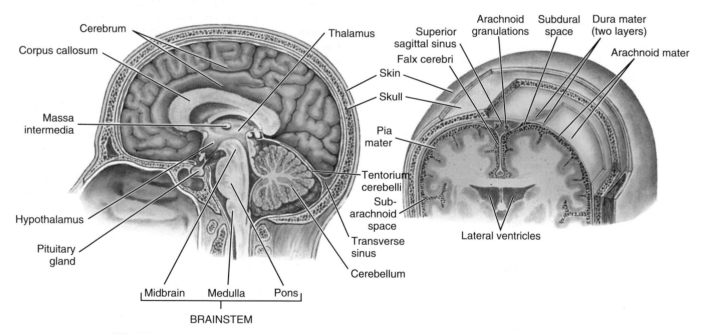

FIG. 21.2 Scalp is composed of the following layers: skin, subcutaneous tissue, galea, and periosteum. Skull bone has three tables: outer, diploë (or spongy layer), and inner. Dura mater lies beneath the skull and completely encapsulates the brain. Other structures are identified for reference and are described in text.

Skull

The skull provides protection for the brain. It is formed by 28 bones, most of which are paired although some in the median plane are single. Many of the bones are flat bones, consisting of two thin plates of compact bone encasing a spongy layer of cancellous bone containing bone marrow (see Fig. 21.2). Infants are born with two fontanelles. These are openings in the skull that are located both anterior and posterior to the parietal bones (Fig. 21.3). The posterior

fontanelle is generally closed by 2 months and the anterior by about 18 months after birth. The bones of the skull are joined by bony seams called *sutures*. Eight bones form the walls of the cranial cavity, which houses the brain. There are four single bones (frontal, occipital, ethmoid, and sphenoid) and four paired bones (temporal and parietal) (Fig. 21.4). The sagittal suture lies in the medial plane and joins the two parietal bones. The coronal suture joins the frontal and parietal bones. The squamous sutures border the squamous part of the temporal bones. The lambdoid suture joins the occipital and parietal bones. Skull bones vary in thickness and tend to be thinner where they are covered in muscles, for example, in the temporal and posterior fossae. The skull articulates with the first cervical vertebra to allow for flexion and extension of the skull. The skeletal surface landmarks of the head can be palpated and are commonly used to plan surgical approaches (Fig. 21.5).

The interior of the skull is anatomically divided into three cranial fossae: anterior, middle, and posterior. The anterior fossa is limited posteriorly by the sphenoid ridge, along which pituitary tumors and aneurysms of the circle of Willis are generally approached. The frontal lobes and olfactory bulbs and tracts lie in the anterior fossa. The temporal lobes lie in the middle fossa, which is shaped like a butterfly. The sella turcica, formed by the sphenoid bone, is the most central part of the middle fossa and houses the pituitary gland. The floor and lateral walls of the middle fossa are shaped from the greater wings of the sphenoid bone and parts of the temporal bone, which house the internal and middle ear structures. The posterior fossa,

the largest and deepest fossa, is formed by the occipital, sphenoid, and petrous portions of the temporal bones; the cerebellum and brainstem also lie here, as do many cranial nerves. The foramen magnum, the largest opening in the skull, provides passage for the spinal cord to join the brainstem in the posterior fossa. Numerous other openings exist in the base of the skull for passage of arteries, veins, and cranial nerves (Fig. 21.6).

Skull Fractures

The severity of skull fractures depends on the degree of resulting brain injury. Simple skull fractures can be serious if they cross major vascular channels in the skull. If vessels are torn, epidural or subdural hematomas may form. Depressed skull fractures require a surgical procedure to elevate the depressed bone. Open skull fractures should be irrigated copiously and closed to prevent infection. Basilar skull fractures may cause cerebrospinal fluid (CSF) rhinorrhea or otorrhea. A few patients with these CSF leaks require surgical repair if they do not resolve after 2 weeks.

Deformities of the Cranium

Craniosynostosis is the most common pediatric skull deformity seen and treated by the neurosurgeon. The phenomenon is a premature closure or lack of formation of cranial sutures, leading to cosmetic abnormalities, eventual life-threatening intracranial pressure (ICP) increases, and arrested brain development unless diagnostic and surgical interventions ensue. Cranial remodeling is most often undertaken during the first year of life, when brain capacity triples (see Chapter 26).

Meninges

The brain and spinal cord are completely enveloped by the meninges, which are three membranes that provide support and protection. The meningeal layers from superficial to deep are the dura mater, arachnoid mater, and pia mater (see Fig. 21.2). The space superficial to the dura is known as the epidural space. The cranial meninges are located between the skull and the brain.

The dura mater is a tough, shiny, fibrous membrane that is close to the inner surface of the skull and folds to separate the cranial

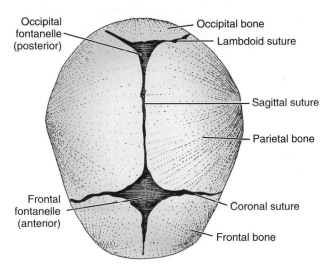

FIG. 21.3 Skull at birth viewed from above.

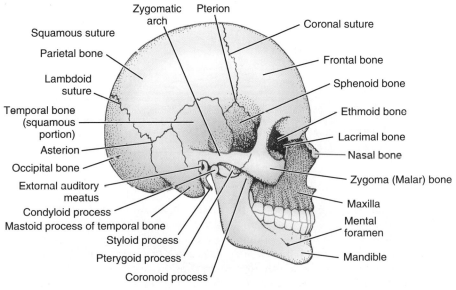

FIG. 21.4 Skull viewed from right side.

cavity into compartments. The largest fold is the falx cerebri, which is an arch-shaped, vertically placed, midline structure separating the right and left cerebral hemispheres (see Fig. 21.2). A smaller fold of dura mater, the falx cerebelli, separates the cerebellar hemispheres vertically. A transverse fold, the tentorium cerebelli, forms the roof of the posterior fossa. The tentorium supports the temporal lobe and occipital lobes of the cerebral hemispheres. Below the tentorium lie the cerebellum and brainstem. Structures above the tentorium are referred to as *supratentorial* and those below as *infratentorial* (Fig. 21.7). At margins of these dural folds lie large venous sinuses that drain blood from the intracranial structures into the jugular veins. Accidental breaching of a sinus during surgery can cause severe bleeding that is difficult to control and may put the patient at risk for a venous air embolism. Several arteries also lie within the layers of the dura. The largest is the middle meningeal, which is a source of serious epidural hemorrhage if torn by an overlying skull fracture. The rigid skull makes hemorrhage and swelling in the brain critical events. The volume of the intracranial cavity is fixed. Increasing the intracranial contents by a hemorrhage, tumor, or edema may lead to serious ICP problems. Pressure on brain tissue may cause irreparable damage.

Beneath the dura mater is a transparent membrane called the *arachnoid.* Although the outer layer of the arachnoid closely approximates the dura mater, the space between is considered the subdural space. The inner arachnoid layer forms innumerable weblike filaments that bridge to the surface of the brain (see Fig. 21.2). The arachnoid passes over the sulci and fissures of the brain, without dipping into them. The arachnoid is separated from the pia mater beneath it by the subarachnoid space, which is filled with CSF that bathes the brain. Around the base of the brain, particularly, this space becomes enlarged to form cisterns. The major intracranial nerves and blood vessels pass through these compartments. Intracranial approaches can be charted in terms of the basal cisterns.

The pia mater, the innermost membrane, closely follows the contours of the surface of the brain into the sulci and fissures. Only the microscopic subpial space separates the pia from the brain. The pia mater has a rich vascular network. Vascular fringes of pia mater project into the ventricles to form the choroid plexus of the ventricles, which produce CSF.

Brain

The anatomy of the brain, formally known as the encephalon, can be considered in multiple ways. Based on prenatal development, the

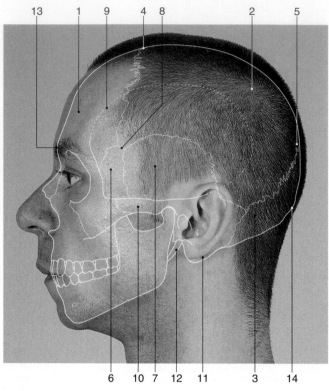

FIG. 21.5 Lateral aspect of the head: bones. *1,* Frontal. *2,* Parietal. *3,* Occipital. *4,* Bregma (anterior fontanelle). *5,* Lambda (posterior fontanelle). *6,* Greater wing of sphenoid. *7,* Squamous temporal. *8,* Pterion. *9,* Temporal lines. *10,* Zygomatic arch. *11,* Mastoid process. *12,* Styloid process. *13,* Glabella. *14,* External occipital protuberance.

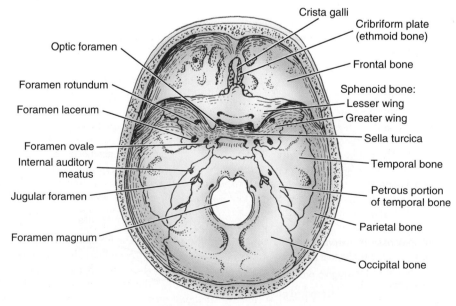

FIG. 21.6 Floor of cranial cavity.

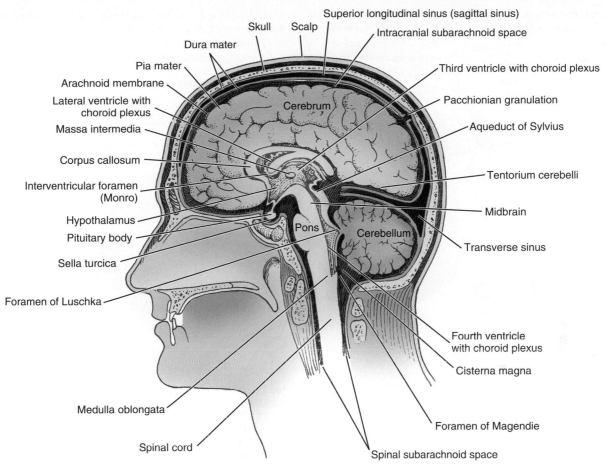

FIG. 21.7 Sagittal section of head showing cerebrospinal fluid spaces and their relationship to venous circulation and their principal subdivision of the brain and its coverings.

principal divisions from rostral (head) to caudal (tail), descending toward the spinal cord, are the forebrain or prosencephalon, the midbrain or mesencephalon, and the hindbrain or rhombencephalon. The rhombencephalon is subdivided into the cerebellum, the medulla oblongata, and the pons. The prosencephalon includes the diencephalon and the telencephalon, or cerebrum. The medulla oblongata, pons, and midbrain are collectively referred to as the brainstem (Fig. 21.8; see Fig. 21.7).

Cerebrum
The right and the left cerebral hemispheres are the largest parts of the brain and occupy the anterior and middle fossae. Each hemisphere is divided into frontal, parietal, occipital, and temporal lobes. The two hemispheres are separated by the longitudinal fissure and the falx cerebri but remain connected underneath the falx by a large transverse bundle of nerve fibers called the corpus callosum (see Fig. 21.8). Each of the cerebral hemispheres controls sensation and motor activity to and receives sensory stimuli from the opposite half of the body.

The convoluted surface of the cerebrum consists of gray matter, called the *cerebral cortex,* which contains the cell bodies of the many nerve pathways of the brain. The underlying white matter contains millions of myelinated nerve axons and is relatively avascular compared with the cortex. There are three types of nerve pathways, or fiber tracts: (1) commissural fibers, which pass from one cerebral hemisphere to the other; (2) association fibers, which connect regions of gyri and lobes longitudinally within a cerebral hemisphere; and (3) projection fibers, including the great motor and sensory systems, which run vertically to connect the cortical regions with other portions of the CNS.

The surfaces of the hemispheres form convolutions called *gyri* and intervening furrows called *sulci,* which serve as anatomic landmarks. Two sulci of particular anatomic importance during surgery are (1) the lateral sulcus, or sylvian fissure, which divides the temporal lobe from the frontal and parietal lobes, and (2) the central sulcus, or fissure of Rolando, which separates the frontal from the parietal lobe. The central sulcus also separates the motor cortex (precentral gyrus) from the sensory cortex (postcentral gyrus). The motor cortex lies anterior to the central sulcus, and the sensory cortex lies posterior to the central sulcus. Both the motor cortex and the sensory cortex can be represented by a topographically organized map called a homunculus, which proportionately represents each body part at the area of the gyri that controls it. The diagrams illustrate how the number of neurons corresponds to the degree of motor and sensory control required. For example, areas that need more fine motor control, such as the fingers and face, have a higher concentration of neurons than other areas. The left motor and sensory cortices control the right side of the body and vice versa (Fig. 21.9). Destruction of an area of motor cortex results in loss of voluntary motor function on the corresponding area of the opposite side of the body (Fig. 21.10).

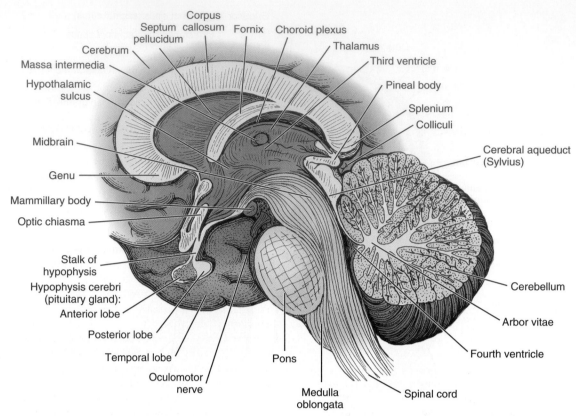

FIG. 21.8 Sagittal section through midline of the brain showing structures around the third ventricle, including corpus callosum, thalamus, and hypothalamus.

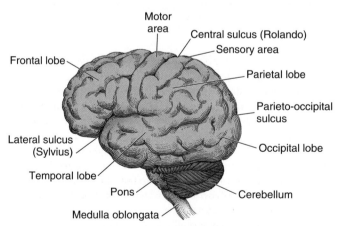

FIG. 21.9 Lateral view of cerebral hemisphere (showing lobes and principal fissures), cerebellum, pons, and medulla oblongata.

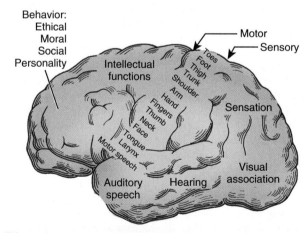

FIG. 21.10 Principal functional subdivisions of cerebral hemispheres.

The frontal lobe is anterior to the central sulcus and controls the higher functions of intellect and abstract reasoning, along with movement, language, and personality. Posterior to the central sulcus is the parietal lobe, extending back to the parieto-occipital fissure. This area contains the final receiving and integrating station for sensory impulses, such as pain and touch, from the contralateral side of the body. It is also involved with spatial relationships and object identification. The occipital lobe lies posterior to the parieto-occipital fissure. It receives and integrates visual impulses and registers them as meaningful images (see Figs. 21.9 and 21.10).

Inferior to the lateral sulcus, in the middle fossa, is the temporal lobe, which is involved with memory, speech, and smell. Lesions of the left temporal lobe in right-handed persons and in many left-handed persons may affect the comprehension and verbalization of words, resulting in aphasia. The insula (island of Reil) is an area of cortex that lies deep within the lateral sulcus and can be exposed when the upper and lower lips of the fissure are separated. The insula is believed to be involved with smell, taste, touch, and possibly language.

The limbic system consists of large parts of the cortex near the medial wall of the cerebral hemisphere (cingulate and parahippocampal

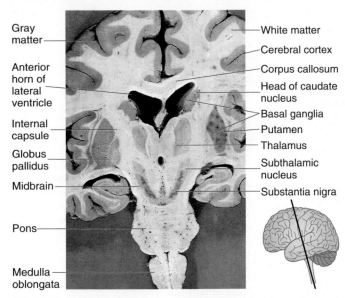

Gray matter — White matter
Cerebral cortex
Corpus callosum
Anterior horn of lateral ventricle — Head of caudate nucleus
Basal ganglia
Internal capsule — Putamen
Globus pallidus — Thalamus
Subthalamic nucleus
Midbrain — Substantia nigra
Pons
Medulla oblongata

FIG. 21.11 Oblique coronal section through the cerebral hemisphere and brainstem showing the disposition of gray and white matter, the basal ganglia, and the internal capsule.

gyri) along with the hippocampus, amygdala, and septum. It is closely and significantly connected with the hypothalamus. It has a diffuse distribution in the brain, and many components of the limbic system have overlapping functions. The hippocampus is critical for learning and memory. The amygdala regulates the perceptive and expressive aspects of emotional and social behavior. The limbic system affects endocrine and autonomic functions of the body, recent memory, emotions, behaviors, and motivational and mood states. Restlessness and hyperactivity may result from lesions of this area.

The basal ganglia are subcortical collections of nuclei (gray matter) that include the caudate nucleus, putamen, and globus pallidus (collectively referred to as the *corpus striatum*); the substantia nigra (which is located in the midbrain); and the subthalamic nucleus (part of the diencephalon). The basal ganglia influence movement and behavior through projections to the thalamus and brainstem and subsequently the cortex (Fig. 21.11). The basal ganglia function to promote and support patterns of behavior and movement that are appropriate in a given situation and to inhibit unwanted or inappropriate behavior and movements. Disorders of the basal ganglia are principally characterized by abnormalities of movement, muscle tone, and posture. Damage to these neural components may cause rigidity of the skeletal muscles and various types of spontaneous tremors.

Diencephalon

The diencephalon is composed of the thalamus, hypothalamus, epithalamus, and subthalamus and surrounds the third ventricle. The thalamus is the major relay station for incoming sensory stimuli. Except for some olfactory impulse transmission, all sensory information transmitted to the cerebral hemispheres is relayed through the thalamus. This is also true for motor pathways from the cerebellum and basal ganglia. Because of the central role of the thalamus in the perception of body sensations, surgical lesions can be made in this area in an attempt to alleviate pain.

Along the floor of the third ventricle is the hypothalamus (see Fig. 21.8), which is concerned principally with the autonomic

regulation of the body's internal environment and is intimately connected with the pituitary gland. It controls fluid and electrolyte balance, appetite, reproduction, thermoregulation, immune response, and many emotional responses. It influences levels of attention and consciousness. The pituitary gland is suspended from the base of the hypothalamus by the pituitary stalk. It secretes multiple hormones that are regulated by the hypothalamus. A pituitary tumor can result in a hormonal imbalance. It can also encroach on the optic chiasma, causing vision changes.

The subthalamus is a complex region of nuclear groups and fiber tracts, including the subthalamic nucleus, which is considered with the basal ganglia. The epithalamus consists of multiple nuclei and the pineal gland, an endocrine gland that regulates the circadian rhythm.

Brainstem

The brainstem consists of the midbrain, pons, and medulla oblongata. It is located in the posterior fossa and forms the floor of the fourth ventricle. It is the site of many ascending and descending fiber tracts that allow for communication among the structures of the brain and between the brain and spinal cord. All but 2 of the 12 cranial nerves attach to the brainstem. The short, stocky portion of the brain, between the cerebral hemispheres and pons, is the midbrain (see Fig. 21.7), also referred to as the *mesencephalon*. It is composed of the cerebral peduncles, the substantia nigra, numerous nerve tracts and nuclei, and association centers that control the majority of eye movements. Immediately below the midbrain is the pons, which contains control areas for horizontal eye movement and face movement. The medulla oblongata is continuous with the spinal cord at the foramen magnum. It contains the vital cardiovascular and respiratory regulatory centers (see Fig. 21.9). Damage to the brainstem is often devastating and life-threatening because it can affect movement, senses, consciousness, perception, and cognition.

Cerebellum

The cerebellum, which occupies most of the posterior fossa, forms the roof of the fourth ventricle (Fig. 21.12; see Fig. 21.8). It has two lateral lobes, or hemispheres, and a medial portion, the vermis. The fissures of the cerebellum are small and run transversely. The cerebellum is concerned principally with balance and coordination of movement. It has many complex connections with higher and lower centers and exerts its influence unilaterally, in contrast to the cerebral hemispheres, which act contralaterally. By splitting the vermis in the exact midline, a satisfactory exposure of tumors that lie in the fourth ventricle is obtained without sacrificing the important cerebellar functions.

Pathologic Lesions of the Brain

An estimated new 78,000 primary brain tumors were expected to occur in 2015, and an estimated 700,000 people in the United States were living with a primary brain and/or CNS tumor (ABTA, 2014). Brain metastases outnumber primary neoplasms by at least 10 to 1 and are the most common brain tumor in adults. Unfortunately, the exact incidence is unknown, but it has been estimated that 100,000 to 170,000 new cases are diagnosed in the United States each year (ABTA, 2014).

Multiple factors are suspected of playing a role in the pathogenesis of intracranial neoplasms. Early diagnosis simplifies surgical treatment because increased ICP and severe neurologic changes are not usually present. Brain tumors are either malignant or benign, depending on the cell type. Primary tumors generally do not resemble the

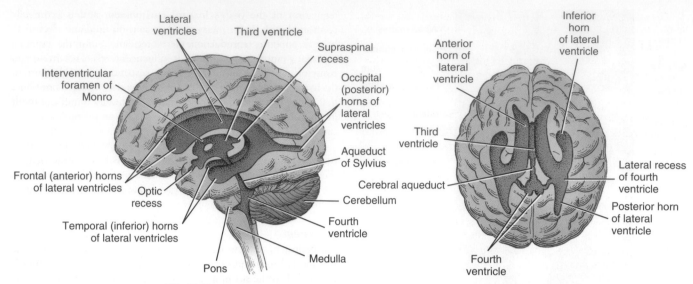

FIG. 21.12 Ventricular system showing its relationship to various parts of the brain.

carcinomas and sarcomas found elsewhere in the body and rarely metastasize outside the CNS. Both primary and metastatic tumors of the brain and its membranes are included in the term *intracranial tumors.*

Traditionally, tumors are classified by cell type; however, classification of brain tumors is an evolving process. The widely used World Health Organization (WHO) system lists more than 120 types of brain tumors (Louis et al., 2016). A brief description of a select list of brain tumors follows:

1. *Tumors of intraepithelial tissue* encompass gliomas, which are tumors believed to originate from neuroglial cells. Gliomas represent 27% of all brain tumors and 80% of all malignant tumors (ABTA, 2014).

   a. Astrocytomas represent 7% of all primary brain tumors and 75% of all gliomas (ABTA, 2014). They usually occur in the cerebellum of children and the cerebrum of adults. They are often cystic and discrete in children and infiltrating and ill-defined in adults. Astrocytomas are classified in the WHO system based on the principal cell type and on the degree of anaplasia as grade I to IV, with grade I being the more favorable type of tumor and grade IV being the most malignant. Glioblastoma multiforme (GBM), a grade IV astrocytoma, is an infiltrative, fast-growing, rapidly recurring cerebral tumor that occurs most frequently in the sixth and seventh decades of life. Glioblastomas represent 15% of all primary brain tumors, and account for about 55% of all gliomas (ABTA, 2014). It is one of the few tumors capable of invading both cerebral hemispheres by crossing the midline. Areas of necrosis are characteristic. Multiple studies have consistently demonstrated the benefits of radical surgical resection; however, because most of these tumors have finger-like tentacles, complete resection is difficult. Postoperative radiation therapy significantly improves survival. Even with aggressive multimodality therapy, median survival is approximately 14.6 months and 2-year survival is about 30% (ABTA, 2014).

   b. Oligodendroglioma, typically found in the cerebral hemispheres, is usually infiltrating but occasionally moderately well defined. It frequently presents in middle age with seizure. The incidence of oligodendrogliomas is approximately 2% of all primary

brain tumors, and represents 10% to 15% of all gliomas. Therapy usually consists of surgery followed by radiation therapy and chemotherapy (ABTA, 2014).

   c. Ependymoma occurs most frequently in children and is likely to arise in or near the ventricular walls. It commonly occurs in the fourth ventricle, where it abuts or involves vital medullary centers. It also frequently metastasizes into the subarachnoid spaces. This tumor accounts for 2% to 3% of gliomas in adults, and is the third most common brain tumor in children. Surgical resection followed by radiation therapy is the usual treatment. With treatment survival rates are approximately 67% to 80%; however, treatment in children may have significant side effects such as decreased intellect and learning problems (ABTA, 2014).

   d. Medulloblastoma is a fast-growing, rapidly recurring tumor of the vermis of the cerebellum and fourth ventricle that usually occurs in young children. It characteristically metastasizes into the subarachnoid spaces, usually spreading to the base of the brain by this route. It accounts for 2% of all primary brain tumors and 18% of childhood intracranial brain tumors. It is the most common malignant pediatric brain tumor (ABTA, 2014).

2. *Tumors of the meninges (meningiomas)* have become the most common primary brain tumor, representing 36.1% of all primary brain tumors (ABTA, 2014). They are usually benign, circumscribed, slow-growing tumors, arising from arachnoid cells with secondary attachment to the dura. Various factors have been implicated in the development of meningiomas. They typically involve the cortex and bone of the skull with growth. They can be very vascular and may adhere to the dural venous sinuses or major arteries, making their complete removal challenging. However, meningiomas often can be totally surgically removed.

3. *Tumors of the cranial nerves (vestibular schwannomas)* are benign; they usually arise from the neurilemma sheath cells of the vestibular portion of the eighth cranial nerve within the auditory meatus. The term *acoustic neuroma* is a misnomer. These tumors grow slowly to fill the cerebellopontine angle and may indent the brainstem. Presenting symptoms include hearing loss, tinnitus, facial numbness, and disequilibrium (NIDCD, 2016).

4. *Hematopoietic neoplasms and lymphomas* occur most often in the cerebral hemispheres, but may also involve CSF, the eyes, or the spinal cord (ABTA, 2014). CNS lymphoma represents 2.5% of all primary brain tumors, and the incidence has been rising over the past 20 years. The main role for surgery is for tumor biopsy. Stereotactic techniques are well suited for these often deep tumors. The standard treatment after biopsy is steroids to control brain swelling, chemotherapy, and radiation (ABTA, 2014).

5. *Germ cell tumors* occur in the midline (suprasellar and pineal region). Other than benign teratomas, all intracranial germ cell tumors are malignant and may metastasize by way of CSF and systemically. Tumors of the pineal region are very challenging to the neurosurgeon. Open microsurgery, endoscopy, and stereotactic biopsy are surgical options. Pineal region tumors often cause hydrocephalus. An endoscopic third ventriculostomy or a shunting procedure is routinely performed to alleviate the symptoms of hydrocephalus. The tumor itself is typically treated with radiation therapy and chemotherapy because of its location in the brain (ABTA, 2014).

   a. Germinoma is a neoplasm arising from germ cells. Survival with germinomas is much better than with nongerminomatous tumors (teratoma, embryonal cell carcinoma, choriocarcinoma).

   b. Teratoma is a congenital tumor containing embryonic elements.

   c. Embryonal cell carcinoma consists of a highly primitive group of neoplasms that arise in childhood. Predominantly large hemispheric masses involving deep supratentorial structures, these tumors are highly vascular and have poor prognoses. The primitive neuroectodermal tumor (PNET) is one such tumor.

   d. Choriocarcinoma is an extremely rare, very malignant neoplasm.

6. *Cysts and tumor-like lesions* include the following types:

   a. Epidermoid and dermoid cysts are developmental, benign tumors typically located in the suprasellar region.

   b. Colloid cysts are slow-growing benign tumors. They classically occur in the anterior third ventricle, blocking the foramen of Monro and causing obstructive hydrocephalus.

7. *Tumors of the sellar region* include the following types:

   a. Pituitary adenomas represent 9% to 12% of all primary brain tumors and can be classified as secreting or nonsecreting. *Nonsecreting* pituitary adenomas account for approximately 30% of pituitary tumors, usually occur in people in the fourth and fifth decades of life, and do not cause clinical hormone hypersecretion. They are typically large and cause hypopituitarism or blindness from regional compression. The usual treatment is endoscopic or microscopic transsphenoidal removal of the tumor. Radiation therapy or stereotactic radiosurgery may also be used. *Secreting* pituitary adenomas secrete excess quantities of pituitary hormones and account for 70% of pituitary tumors. The question of medical versus surgical treatment is ever present in the management of this group of patients. Adenomas may be further subdivided into microadenomas, which are less than 1 cm in diameter and may present with an increase in prolactin levels. Macroadenomas, which are larger than 1 cm, may present with an increase in growth hormone (ABTA, 2014).

      (1) Chromophobe tumors are relatively common in the anterior pituitary glands of adults. They cause compression of the pituitary, adjacent optic chiasma, and hypothalamus. Compression of the hypothalamus may lead to diabetes insipidus.

      (2) Eosinophilic adenomas are secretory, causing an excessive amount of growth hormone in the serum.

      (3) Basophilic adenomas are responsible for the excessive secretion of corticotropic, gonadotropic, and thyrotropic hormones. Acromegaly or, less commonly, Cushing syndrome may occur and cause the patient to seek help long before the tumor has expanded sufficiently to compromise the optic chiasma.

      (4) Prolactin cell adenoma exhibits considerable differences in clinical presentation, depending on the gender of the patient. In women of reproductive age, the onset of amenorrhea and galactorrhea with associated infertility is an obvious sign. The diagnosis of a prolactinoma is established early in the course. In men, the clinical endocrine symptoms, which include decreased libido and impotence, are not as conspicuous and initially may be disregarded by the patient. As a result, male patients frequently do not seek medical attention until the tumors are large and have spread beyond the confines of the sella turcica.

   b. Craniopharyngiomas account for 2% to 5% of adult intracranial tumors and 5% to 10% of childhood brain tumors (ABTA, 2014). They arise from the region of the pituitary stalk and typically contain both solid and cystic components. Calcification above the sella turcica is often seen radiographically. In addition to headache, vertigo, vomiting, and papilledema, diabetes insipidus and visual field changes are common. Although complete surgical removal is often impossible if it adheres to the carotid artery or hypothalamus, a subtotal resection with radiation offers favorable results.

8. *Metastatic tumors* are the most common brain tumor seen clinically, making up about half of brain tumors. They usually arise from carcinomas, more rarely from sarcomas, and occasionally from melanomas and retinal tumors. The most common sources are lung and breast cancer. The current principal options for treatment include whole-brain radiation therapy, surgery, stereotactic radiosurgery, and chemotherapy or immune-based therapy. The management of brain metastasis is complex and controversial with chemotherapy becoming increasingly used over the past few years; however, radiation therapy (whether or not surgery has taken place) still yields better results (ABTA, 2014). The most important prognostic variables are the extent of systemic disease and the patient's functional status and age. These factors, along with the size, number, and location of tumors, guide treatment decisions.

A brain lesion is diagnosed by history, neurologic examination, diagnostic studies (especially computed tomography [CT] scan and magnetic resonance imaging [MRI]), and biopsy. The manifestations of an intracranial tumor fall into two classes: those resulting from irritation or impairment of function in specific areas of the brain directly affected by the tumor and those resulting from diffuse increased ICP. The most common presentation of brain tumors is progressive neurologic deficit, usually motor weakness. Headache, seizures, vision loss, and hearing loss are also common presenting symptoms (ABTA, 2014).

Large left or bifrontal lobe tumors may cause striking personality changes and depressive symptoms. Lesions in the left frontotemporal region, where motor speech originates, lead to aphasia. Parietal lobe lesions may result in contralateral weakness and sensory changes, along with defects in the perception of objects. Occipital tumors produce hemianopic visual defects.

Cortical tumors frequently produce focal seizures of diagnostic value. The onset of epileptiform seizures in an adult is often associated with an intracranial neoplasm. Posterior fossa tumors often manifest their presence by blocking the CSF circulation, but they may also destroy cerebellar function, resulting in incoordination, ataxia, scanning speech, and deafness.

Treatment of brain tumors, although based on the characteristics of the tumor, can involve administration of steroids or antiepileptic medications, management of hydrocephalus, surgery, radiosurgery, radiation, and chemotherapy.

The presentation of multiple brain lesions in a patient is of grave concern, and an infective process should be considered along with the possibility of multiple tumors. Stereotactic biopsy of the lesion is most likely to provide a diagnosis. The operative team should use precautions to prevent the spread of an unknown infective process. Identification of the infective agent and process determines proper treatment.

Ventricular System and Cerebrospinal Fluid

Within the brain are four communicating cavities, or ventricles, filled with CSF. In the lower medial portion of each cerebral hemisphere lies a large lateral ventricle that resembles a wishbone and is separated anteriorly from its counterpart by a thin septum (see Fig. 21.12). Each lateral ventricle has a body and three horns: frontal, occipital, and temporal. Below the bodies of the lateral ventricles is a central cleft, or third ventricle. It communicates anteriorly with the lateral ventricles through the foramen of Monro and posteriorly with the fourth ventricle through the aqueduct of Sylvius, which is a long, narrow channel passing through the midbrain. The fourth ventricle is a cavity in the posterior fossa, between the cerebellum and the brainstem. In the roof of the fourth ventricle is the foramen of Magendie, an opening into the cisterna magna; at the lateral margins are the two foramina of Luschka, which open into the cisterna pontis. These cisterns are cavities that serve as reservoirs for CSF.

Much of the CSF originates in the choroid plexuses of the ventricles. These are tufted, vascular structures that allow certain fluid elements of the blood to pass through their ependymal linings. The choroid plexus is found along the floor in each lateral ventricle, on the roof of the third ventricle, and in the posterior portion of the fourth ventricle. Most of the fluid is formed in the lateral ventricles and flows through the interventricular foramen of Monro to the third ventricle and through the aqueduct of Sylvius to the fourth ventricle, where it escapes into the subarachnoid space of the basal cisterns through the foramina of Magendie and Luschka. From the basal cisterns the fluid flows around the spinal cord, over the cerebellar lobes, around the medulla and the base of the brain, and over the cerebral hemispheres in the subarachnoid space. The fluid is absorbed into the venous circulation through villi of the arachnoid (pacchionian granulations) into the great dural venous sinuses, particularly the superior sagittal sinus, and by diffusion through perivascular, perineural, and periradicular channels (see Fig. 21.7).

Spinal fluid bathes the brain and spinal cord, helps support the weight of the brain, and acts as a cushion for the brain and spinal cord by absorbing some of the force of external trauma. By variation in its volume, it aids in keeping ICP relatively constant. If the brain atrophies, the amount of CSF increases to fill the dead space; if the brain swells, the amount of CSF decreases to compensate for the increase in brain mass. The fluid can carry certain drugs to diseased parts of the brain. It does not, however, play a significant role in supplying nutrition to the structures that it bathes. The total amount of circulating CSF averages 150 mL in the adult. The ventricles contain about 25 mL, and the remaining CSF circulates in the cranial and spinal subarachnoid space. CSF is secreted at a rate of between 21 and 24 mL/hr, or approximately 450 mL/24 hr. This means that in an adult, CSF is recirculated about three times each day.

Pathologic Conditions Related to Cerebrospinal Fluid

CSF can be examined by the lab to provide diagnostic information. CSF is most commonly obtained by way of lumbar puncture (LP). Because the subarachnoid space surrounding the brain is freely connected to the subarachnoid space of the spinal cord, any abnormal increase in ICP will be directly reflected as an increase at the lumbar site. Tumors, infection, hydrocephalus, and intracranial bleeding can cause increased intracranial and spinal pressure. LP is contraindicated when ICP is increased from a suspected intracranial mass that is causing neurologic symptoms. In this situation the sudden reduction in pressure from the release of CSF could cause brain herniation. The ventricular fluid normally has a protein content of 5 to 15 mg/dL, whereas the protein content of spinal fluid is 25 to 45 mg/dL. These values may be considerably elevated in pathologic conditions of the CNS. The characteristics of normal spinal fluid are listed in Appendix A.

Elevations in CSF pressure can be caused by an expanding mass within the skull, such as a tumor, hemorrhage, or cerebral edema; an increase in formation or decrease in absorption of fluid, as in meningitis, encephalitis, and other febrile conditions; an increase in venous pressure within the skull from an obstruction to normal venous drainage; a blockage of absorption by inflammatory conditions of the arachnoid and perivascular spaces; any mechanical obstruction of the ventricular or subarachnoid fluid pathways; or decreased absorption of CSF. These pathologic conditions can cause a dangerous increase in ICP, which ultimately could result in brain herniation and death.

The rate of absorption and production of CSF is related to the osmotic and hydrostatic pressures of the blood. Intravenous (IV) injection of hypertonic mannitol, commonly used with a nonosmotic diuretic, can be used to pull fluid from tissue to the vascular space for excretion by the kidneys, resulting in systemic diuresis and a decrease in ICP.

Hydrocephalus is a condition marked by an excessive accumulation of CSF, resulting in dilation of the intracerebral ventricles in which CSF is synthesized and circulated. Enlargement of cerebral ventricles is the result of CSF blockage and interruption of CSF circulation or CSF reabsorption. The causes of hydrocephalus are many, including congenital conditions, aqueductal stenosis, tumors or cysts of the ventricular system, subarachnoid hemorrhage (SAH), posterior fossa tumors, or trauma with increased ICP. Noncommunicating (obstructive) hydrocephalus involves an obstruction of CSF pathways. In communicating hydrocephalus, the normal CSF pathways are open; however, there is an abnormality in CSF absorption with increased ICP. Normal-pressure hydrocephalus (NPH) is a chronic communicating adult-onset hydrocephalus that produces a normal pressure on random LP (NINDS, 2013). NPH most commonly develops in the elderly, probably because of abnormal CSF absorption; however, the cause may not be apparent. Symptoms of dementia, unsteady gait, and urinary incontinence are seen with normal-pressure and chronic hydrocephalus. Those with acute hydrocephalus present with headache, nausea, vomiting, drowsiness, and papilledema.

The appropriate surgical procedure depends on the precise type of hydrocephalus. Whenever possible, an obstructing lesion that causes hydrocephalus should be surgically removed. For some cases of obstructive hydrocephalus, endoscopic third ventriculostomy may be possible. With endoscopic third ventriculostomy, CSF can be diverted by surgically creating an opening at the floor of the third ventricle, eliminating the need for a shunt. Commonly, treatment of hydrocephalus in the adult and pediatric population is by placement of a ventriculoperitoneal (VP) shunt; however, it may be necessary to revise the shunt periodically as the child grows (Karajannis et al., 2016). With acute symptoms, temporary placement of an external ventriculostomy catheter used to measure the ICP and drain CSF may be preferred, postponing or eliminating the need for a permanent VP shunt.

Cerebral Blood Supply

The brain requires 20% more oxygen than any other organ to maintain its high level of metabolic activity. The arterial supply to the brain enters the cranium through the two internal carotid arteries anteriorly and the two vertebral arteries posteriorly. These communicate at the base of the brain through the circle of Willis (Fig. 21.13), which ensures continuity of the circulation if any one of the four main channels is interrupted. However, these connections are extremely variable and do not always have functional anastomoses. The main branches for distribution of blood to each hemisphere of the brain

from the internal carotid arteries are the anterior and middle cerebral arteries. Each artery nourishes a specific area of the brain (see Fig. 21.13). The anterior cerebral artery supplies the anterior two-thirds of the medial surface and adjacent region over the convexity of the hemisphere, including about half of the frontal and parietal lobes. The middle cerebral artery supplies most of the lateral surface of the hemisphere, including half of the frontal, parietal, and temporal lobes. The posterior cerebral artery, which originates at the basilar artery, supplies the occipital lobe and the remaining half of the temporal lobe, principally on the inferior and medial surfaces. The brainstem and cerebellum are supplied by branches of the basilar and vertebral arteries.

The cerebral veins do not parallel the arteries as the veins do in most other parts of the body. The external cortical veins anastomose freely in the pia mater, forming larger cerebral veins, and as such they pierce the arachnoid membrane, cross the subdural space, and empty into the great dural venous sinuses. A subdural hemorrhage after head trauma may arise from disruption of these bridging vessels; an epidural hemorrhage often results from lacerations of the middle meningeal artery, which is a branch of the external carotid artery that supplies the dura mater. The deep cerebral veins, which drain the interior of the hemispheres, empty principally into the great vein of Galen and the inferior sagittal sinus.

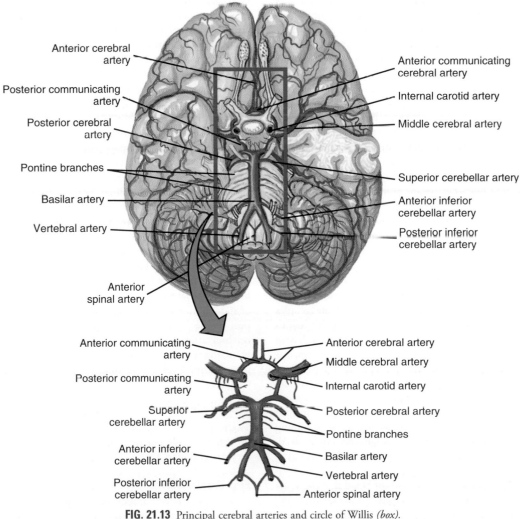

FIG. 21.13 Principal cerebral arteries and circle of Willis (*box*).

The blood transports oxygen, nutrients, and other substances necessary for the proper functioning of living tissue. The needs of the brain for oxygen and glucose are critical. The brain can store only small amounts of oxygen and energy-producing nutrients. Constant flow of blood to the brain must be maintained.

The brain uses oxygen in the metabolism of glucose, which is the chief source of energy. Protein and fat metabolism plays little part in energy production. In the face of an oxygen deficit, the survival time of CNS tissue is very short. In the presence of low levels of blood glucose, CNS function is compromised and unconsciousness results.

Generally, all factors affecting the systemic blood pressure indirectly affect the cerebral circulation. The brain normally receives 20% of the cardiac output. The cerebral blood flow is kept constant by an autoregulation phenomenon such that increases in blood pressure lead to vasoconstriction of cerebral arteries and decreases in blood pressure cause cerebral vasodilation to maintain a relatively constant cerebral blood flow. When the mean arterial pressure falls below 60 mm Hg, the autoregulation mechanism usually fails.

Vascular Pathologic Conditions of the Brain

Vascular lesions of the brain are most often diagnosed in people who present with acute, spontaneous intracranial hemorrhage.

Aneurysms. Aneurysms arise from a complex set of circumstances involving a congenital anatomic predisposition and local or systemic factors that weaken the arterial wall, leading to dilation. The majority of these lesions occur at the branching points of large subarachnoid conducting arteries. The greatest vulnerability to aneurysmal development occurs at points of vessel bifurcation. Acute SAH in this setting can lead to vessel vasospasm (with greatest risk at 4–10 days after the SAH), cerebral ischemia, hydrocephalus, increased ICP, diabetes insipidus, syndrome of inappropriate antidiuretic hormone (SIADH), respiratory failure, brain injury, and risk of rebleeding. The vessels of the circle of Willis are most often implicated, including the posterior communicating artery, anterior communicating artery, middle cerebral artery, carotid artery, posterior inferior cerebellar artery, vertebral artery, and basilar artery. Surgical intervention techniques are based on the characteristics of the aneurysm. Small neck aneurysms may be occluded using coils placed by means of interventional radiology techniques. Aneurysmal clipping by way of a craniotomy approach is most often used to treat broad neck aneurysms.

Vascular Malformations. Vascular malformations of the CNS are characterized by congenital lesions that have the potential to produce symptoms any time during the life of an individual with the malformation. Types of vascular malformations include arteriovenous malformations (AVMs), cavernous malformations, capillary telangiectasias, and venous malformations. AVMs are complex lesions in which direct shunting of arterial blood to the venous system occurs. The vascular channels are tightly packed and have a propensity to hemorrhage. Capillary telangiectasias are small vascular malformations commonly seen in the pons. They rarely bleed. Cavernous malformations are cystic vascular spaces, similar to capillary telangiectasias but larger and with a tendency to bleed. Venous malformations are the most common type, comprising anomalous veins, a single tortuous vein, or a number of smaller veins joining at a single point. These are considered benign and rarely bleed. Surgical excision of the cavernous malformation and the AVM is recommended.

Hematomas. Hematomas are collections of blood that coagulate to form space-occupying lesions. An intracerebral hemorrhage, the cause of stroke in many hypertensive patients, results in hematoma

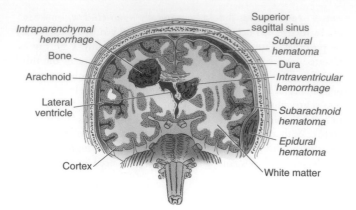

FIG. 21.14 Types of intracerebral hemorrhage (in italics).

formation most often in the basal ganglia, subcortical white matter, cerebellum, and brainstem. These hematomas compress vital structures, depress consciousness, and can be catastrophic. Intracerebral hematomas require emergent intervention or surgery to control the rising ICP. Patients who are deteriorating require emergent surgical intervention. Decompressive craniectomy is being more widely used by neurosurgeons for severe swelling, and ongoing studies are being performed to determine when the procedure should be performed (Heegaard and Biros, 2014).

Intracranial trauma (Research Highlight; see page 768) can cause a shearing of arterial and venous vessels, which results in hematoma collections in the epidural and subdural spaces. These space-occupying lesions raise ICP and often result in serious neurologic disruption (Fig. 21.14). Epidural hematomas are often the result of a blow to the head causing a tear in the middle meningeal artery, which lies on the dura under the skull. These arterial hemorrhages can be life-threatening in that they can cause rapid deterioration in the level of consciousness secondary to the size of the bleed and brain displacement by the hematoma (Fig. 21.15). In contrast to an epidural hematoma, a traumatic subdural hematoma usually results from venous bleeding and collects more slowly. Bridging veins in the subdural space are torn; blood escapes, dissecting a space between the dura and the arachnoid, and collects over one cerebral hemisphere (Fig. 21.16). Subdural hematomas may be acute, subacute, or chronic (Fig. 21.17). Chronic hematomas can often be evacuated through burr holes, but acute hematomas may require a craniotomy to remove the clot and control bleeding.

Cerebral Ischemia. Any area of the brain can become ischemic from an arterial occlusion or embolization. Symptoms may be gradual or sudden. Intracranial plaques most commonly form at the bifurcation of the internal carotid artery, into the middle and anterior cerebral arteries. In select cases, extracranial–intracranial arterial microanastomosis can be performed. Carotid endarterectomy can be performed for extracranial plaque of the carotid artery (see Chapter 24).

Cranial Nerves

Twelve pairs of cranial nerves arise within the cranial cavity (Fig. 21.18). Although they are part of the PNS, from a surgical standpoint they are considered with the head.

First Cranial Nerve

The olfactory nerve, a fiber tract of the brain, is located under the frontal lobe on the cribriform plate of the ethmoid bone. It transmits

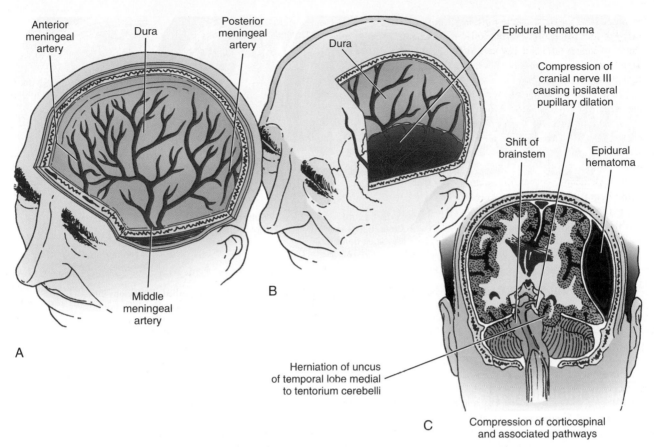

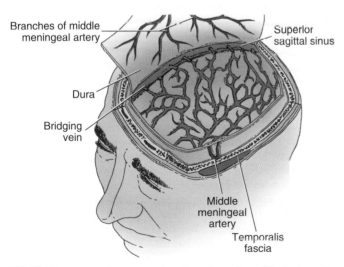

FIG. 21.15 Epidural hematoma is typically caused by trauma resulting in laceration of the middle meningeal artery (A). The typical traumatic epidural hematoma is caused by a laceration of this vessel. (B and C) Linear fracture of the squamous portion of the temporal bone has torn the middle meningeal artery, which has resulted in an epidural hematoma.

FIG. 21.16 Veins are shown extending from the surface of the brain to the superior sagittal sinus. Differential movement of the brain within the skull at the time of injury may tear one or more of these veins, leading to the formation of a subdural hematoma.

the sense of smell. Frontal lobe tumors, fractures of the anterior fossa of the skull, and lesions of the nasal cavity may affect the olfactory nerve.

Second Cranial Nerve

The optic nerve is a fiber tract of the brain. It originates in the ganglion cells of the retina and passes through the optic foramen in the apex of the orbit to reach the optic chiasma. A partial crossing of the fibers occurs there, so the fibers from the nasal half of each retina pass to the opposite side. Posterior to the chiasma, the visual pathway is called the *optic tract*. Still farther back it becomes the optic radiation. Lesions in various parts of this pathway produce characteristic defects in the visual fields. For example, a lesion near the chiasma usually destroys the temporal vision of each eye (bitemporal hemianopsia), whereas a lesion of the occipital lobe produces impairment of vision (homonymous hemianopsia), affecting the right or left halves of the visual fields of both eyes.

Lesions that affect the optic nerve and are treated by neurosurgery include primary gliomas of the nerve, pituitary tumors that press on the optic chiasma, and occasionally meningiomas of the optic nerve sheath or in the region of the sella turcica and olfactory groove. The optic nerves and chiasma are best exposed through a frontal craniotomy along the floor of the anterior fossa or through a frontotemporal approach along the sphenoid ridge. Cranial base

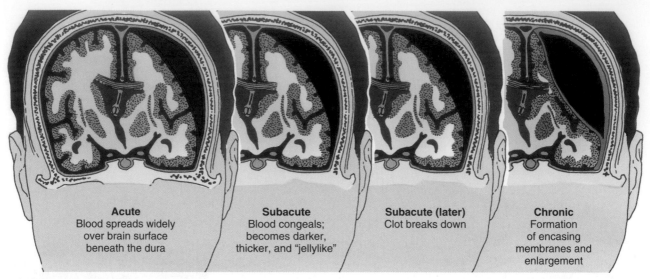

Acute	Subacute	Subacute (later)	Chronic
Blood spreads widely over brain surface beneath the dura	Blood congeals; becomes darker, thicker, and "jellylike"	Clot breaks down	Formation of encasing membranes and enlargement

FIG. 21.17 Subdural hematoma is liquid at first and subsequently clots. It is then reabsorbed or develops into a chronic subdural hematoma as a thick, vascular outer membrane. A thin, inner membrane develops around liquefying blood, starting about 2 weeks after injury. The chronic subdural hematoma enlarges as further bleeding occurs within it.

RESEARCH HIGHLIGHT

Impact of Head Trauma

Prevention and treatment of head injuries has been a topic of public health officials for decades. It is estimated that it costs (through direct and indirect costs) $76 billion annually to treat people in the United States with TBIs. The mechanisms of injury include but are not limited to motor vehicle accidents, assaults, sports injuries, and falls. Most injuries are seen in males younger than age 35, and men are twice as likely to sustain a head or spinal injury as women. Approximately 2.5 million people in the United States sustained a head injury in 2010. These head injuries can be classified as mild, moderate, or severe.

It is imperative that patients are evaluated as soon as possible for a neurologic injury when their cardiopulmonary status is stable. Head injury evaluations should also include a thorough assessment of the spine because 10% of individuals with severe head injuries also have a spinal cord injury. Assessments include using tools such as the Glasgow Coma Scale, the Abbreviated Injury Scale, the Trauma Score, laboratory studies, and imaging studies. Once all of the pertinent data are obtained, a treatment plan can be outlined that may include medical therapy, observation, or surgical intervention.

Preventative measures to prevent TBI include fall safety and motor vehicle safety education. Fall and motor vehicle crashes are the leading causes of head injury. Patients and hospitals benefit from adopting and implementing the Brain Trauma Foundation in-hospital guidelines for the treatment of adults with severe TBI. Research has showed that widespread use of these guidelines may aid in a 50% decrease in death rates.

TBI, Traumatic brain injury.
Modified from Centers for Disease Control and Prevention (CDC): *Traumatic brain injury and concussion* (website), 2016. www.cdc.gov/traumaticbraininjury/severe.html. (Accessed 26 November 2016).

approaches using an orbital osteotomy or orbital-zygomatic osteotomies improve access and exposure of the optic system.

Third, Fourth, and Sixth Cranial Nerves

The third, fourth, and sixth cranial nerves are three pairs of nerves, the oculomotor, the trochlear, and the abducens, respectively. They are conveniently considered together because they are the motor nerves to the muscles of the eyes. They are affected by many toxic, inflammatory, vascular, and neoplastic lesions. The third cranial nerve may be affected by aneurysms of the posterior communicating artery. Pressure against this nerve accounts for pupillary dilation when temporal lobe (uncal) herniation is present, resulting from increased ICP.

Fifth Cranial Nerve

The trigeminal nerve has two functions: (1) sensory supply to the forehead, eyes, meninges, face, jaw, teeth, hard palate, buccal mucosa, tongue, nose, nasal mucosa, and maxillary sinus and (2) motor innervation of the muscles of mastication. The sensory fibers that arise from cells in the trigeminal ganglion travel along the medial wall of the middle cranial fossa and then extend peripherally in three divisions: ophthalmic, maxillary, and mandibular. Behind the ganglion the fibers enter the brainstem by way of the sensory root. The motor root, which originates from cells in the brainstem, follows the course of the larger sensory component (Fig. 21.19).

Trigeminal neuralgia (tic douloureux) is characterized by excruciating, piercing paroxysms of pain, affecting one or more of the major peripheral divisions (see page 803 for additional information about trigeminal neuralgia and treatments).

Seventh Cranial Nerve

The facial nerve supplies the musculature of the face and the sensation of taste for the anterior two-thirds of the tongue. It originates in the brainstem, passes through the skull with the eighth nerve by way of the internal acoustic meatus, continues along the facial canal, and exits just posterior to the parotid gland. The nerve may be

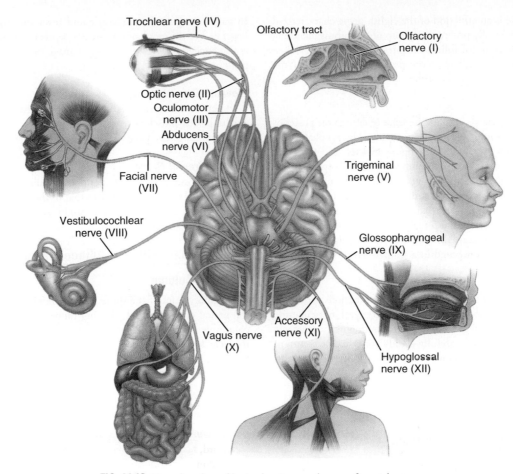

FIG. 21.18 Ventral surface of brain showing attachment of cranial nerves.

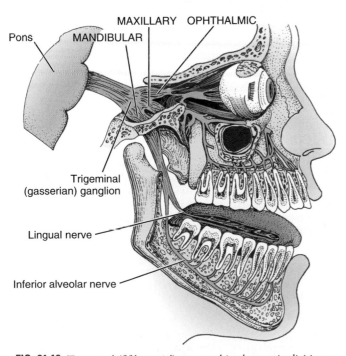

FIG. 21.19 Trigeminal (fifth cranial) nerve and its three main divisions.

damaged by vestibular schwannomas (e.g., acoustic neuromas), fractures at the base of the skull, mastoid infections, and surgical procedures in the vicinity of the parotid gland.

Bell's palsy, a facial lower motor neuron paralysis, can affect the seventh nerve. It may last for a few weeks to a few months, but recovery usually takes place. When permanent interruption of the nerve occurs, useful operations for restoration of function include spinal accessory-facial anastomosis and hypoglossal-facial anastomosis. These operations are performed high in the neck behind the parotid gland by use of the operating microscope.

Eighth Cranial Nerve

The acoustic nerve has two parts that are both sensory: the cochlear for hearing and the vestibular for balance. The former receives stimuli from the organ of Corti and the latter from the semicircular canals. The major surgical lesion of the eighth nerve is called a vestibular schwannoma (acoustic neuroma), which is a histologically benign tumor growing from the nerve sheath at its entrance into the internal auditory meatus. This tumor arises deep in the angle between the cerebellum and pons (cerebellopontine angle). Symptoms may include unilateral deafness, tinnitus, unilateral impairment of cerebellar function, numbness of the face from involvement of the fifth cranial nerve, and, late in the course, papilledema caused by increased ICP. The operative approach is usually through a retrosigmoid craniotomy, exposing the edges of the transverse and sigmoid sinuses.

Meniere disease is an affliction of the eighth nerve characterized by a recurrent and usually progressive group of symptoms including dizziness and a sensation of fullness or pressure in the ears. When medical measures fail to alleviate the problem, sectioning of the eighth nerve may be a surgical option.

Ninth Cranial Nerve

The glossopharyngeal nerve supplies the sense of taste to the posterior third of the tongue, supplies sensation to the tonsils and pharyngeal region, partially innervates the pharyngeal muscles, and primarily innervates the carotid sinus. Stimulation of the baroreceptors of the carotid sinus causes slowing of the heart, vasodilation, and decreased blood pressure. Its sensory component can be sectioned to treat a hypersensitive carotid sinus, or it can be sectioned in conjunction with the fifth nerve to treat painful malignancies of the face, mouth, and pharynx. The ninth cranial nerve lies near the eighth nerve in the posterior fossa and is exposed in a similar way.

Tenth Cranial Nerve

The vagus nerve has many motor and sensory functions, primarily including innervation of pharyngeal and laryngeal musculature, control of heart rate, and regulation of acid secretion of the stomach. In neck surgery the surgeon carefully avoids injury to the recurrent laryngeal branch because its injury results in vocal cord paralysis.

In gastric surgery the surgeon could sever the vagus nerve at the lower end of the esophagus to treat a peptic ulcer. The neurosurgeon is also concerned with preventing damage to the vagus nerve during posterior fossa surgery.

Eleventh Cranial Nerve

The spinal accessory nerve is a motor nerve to the sternocleidomastoid and trapezius muscles. To restore mobility to the face, it may be anastomosed to the peripheral end of a damaged facial nerve.

Twelfth Cranial Nerve

The hypoglossal nerve innervates the musculature of the tongue. Its neurosurgical interest is similar to that of the spinal accessory nerve.

Table 21.1 lists the function, origin, structures innervated, and assessment of the cranial nerves.

Spine, Spinal Cord, and Adjacent Structures

Vertebral Column

The primary roles of the spine are maintaining stability, protecting the neural elements, and allowing range of motion. The vertebral column has four distinct curves: cervical lordosis (a backward bend), thoracic kyphosis (a forward bend), lumbar lordosis, and sacral kyphosis. The spinal column consists of 33 vertebrae: 7 cervical, 12

TABLE 21.1

Understanding Cranial Nerves

Cranial Nerve	Function	Origin	Structures Innervated	Assessment
I: Olfactory	Sensory	Olfactory bulbs below frontal lobes	Olfactory mucous membranes	Ability to identify familiar odors
II: Optic	Sensory	Diencephalon	Retina of eye	Visual acuity Visual fields
III: Oculomotor	Motor	Midbrain	Medial, superior, and inferior rectus muscles of eye Inferior oblique eye muscles Sphincter of iris	Extraocular movements Pupillary reaction to light and accommodation
IV: Trochlear	Motor	Midbrain	Superior oblique muscle of eye	Extraocular movements
V: Trigeminal	Mixed	Pons	Sensory: Pain, touch, and temperature sensations in cheeks, jaw, and chin; corneal reflex Motor: Muscles of mastication	Sensation in forehead, cheeks, jaw, and chin Mastication
VI: Abducens	Motor	Pons	Lateral rectus muscle of eye	Extraocular movement
VII: Facial	Mixed	Pons	Sensory: Anterior two-thirds of tongue Motor: Muscles of face, forehead, and eye	Taste for anterior two-thirds of tongue Movement of facial muscles (smile) Facial symmetry
VIII: Acoustic (vestibulocochlear)	Sensory	Pons	Cochlear organ of Corti Vestibule and semicircular canals	Hearing acuity Balance
IX: Glossopharyngeal	Mixed	Medulla	Sensory: Posterior third of tongue Motor: Muscles of pharynx	Taste for posterior third of tongue Movement of pharynx Gag reflex Swallowing
X: Vagus	Mixed	Medulla	Sensory: Skin of external ear and mucous membranes Motor: Muscles of larynx, pharynx, and esophagus; thoracic and abdominal viscera	Movement of pharynx Gag reflex Cough
XI: Spinal accessory	Motor	Medulla	Sternocleidomastoid and trapezius muscles	Shoulder shrug Turn head
XII: Hypoglossal	Motor	Medulla	Tongue	Movement and strength of tongue

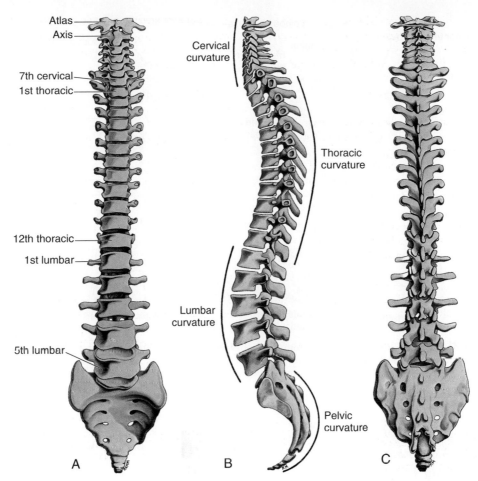

FIG. 21.20 Vertebral column. (A) Anterior aspect. (B) Lateral aspect. (C) Posterior aspect.

thoracic, 5 lumbar, 5 sacral (fused as one section), and 1 coccygeal, which may have 1 to 3 fused sections (Fig. 21.20).

The first cervical vertebra, or atlas, supports the skull. The second cervical vertebra, or axis, can be identified by its odontoid process, which is a vertical projection extending into the foramen of the atlas like a stick in a hoop. It rests against the anterior tubercle of the first cervical vertebra. Ligaments hold the two together but allow considerable rotational movement. The other cervical, thoracic, and lumbar vertebrae are more alike in structure. Each has a body, which is an oval block of bone situated anteriorly. An intervertebral disk, a fibrocartilaginous elastic cushion, separates one body from another (Figs. 21.21 and 21.22). The spinal cord lies in a canal formed by the vertebral bodies, pedicles, and laminae. Articular surfaces or facets project from the pedicles and form joints with the facets of the vertebrae above and below. Transverse processes extend laterally and serve as hitching posts for muscles and ligaments. Spinous processes extend posteriorly and can be palpated in most people. The vertebrae are held together by multiple ligaments and muscles (see Fig. 21.22). Motion of the spine occurs at the articular facets and through the elastic intervertebral disks. The intervertebral disks bond the adjacent surfaces of the vertebral bodies. Each disk consists of a fibrous outer annulus that contains the inner nucleus pulposus.

Spinal Cord

The spinal cord is protected by the bony framework of the spinal column. The dura mater is separated from its bony surroundings by a layer of epidural fat. Beneath the dura mater is the arachnoid, a continuation of the same structure in the head. The subarachnoid space contains CSF. A thin layer of pia mater adheres to the cord, and CSF also circulates from the fourth ventricle into the central canal of the cord.

The spinal cord is a downward prolongation of the brainstem, starting at the upper border of the atlas and ending at the upper border of the second lumbar vertebra (Fig. 21.23). The cord is oval in cross section and is slightly flattened in the anteroposterior diameter. A cross section looks like a gray H surrounded by a white mantle split in the midline, anteriorly and posteriorly, by sulci (Fig. 21.24).

The peripheral white matter carries long, myelinated motor and sensory tracts. The central gray matter consists of nerve cell bodies and short, unmyelinated fibers (see Figs. 21.23 and 21.24). The principal long pathways are the laterally placed pyramidal tracts, carrying impulses down from the cerebral cortex to the motor neurons of the cord; the dorsal ascending columns, mediating sensations of touch and proprioception; and the anterolaterally placed spinothalamic tracts, carrying pain and temperature sensations to the thalamus, which is the sensory receiving station of the brain (Fig. 21.25).

Spinal Nerves

At each vertebral level is a pair of spinal nerves, each consisting of an anterior and a posterior root (see Fig. 21.24). The anterior, or motor, root contains cell bodies that lie in the anterior horn of the spinal gray matter. The posterior, or sensory, root contains cell bodies

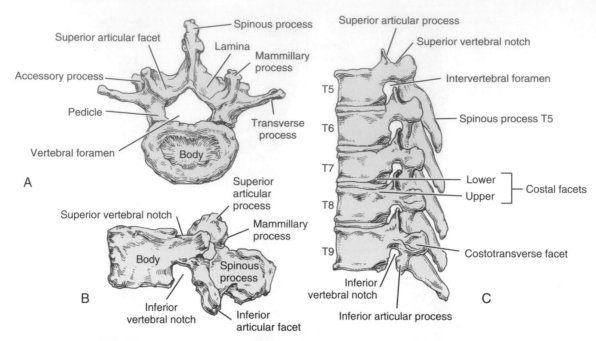

FIG. 21.21 (A) Fourth lumbar vertebra from above. (B) Fourth lumbar vertebra from side. (C) Fifth to ninth thoracic vertebrae, showing relationships of various parts.

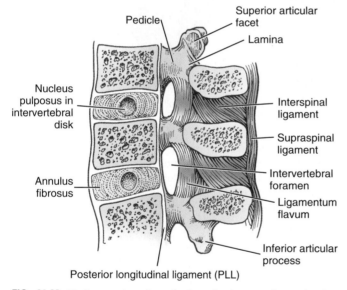

FIG. 21.22 Median section through three lumbar vertebrae, showing intervertebral disks (nuclei pulposi).

that lie in the spinal ganglia located in the intervertebral foramina, the opening through which the nerves exit from the spinal canal and emerge from the cord. The course of the cervical nerves is horizontal, but at each lower level they assume an increasingly oblique and downward direction. In the lumbar region, the course of the nerves is nearly vertical, forming the cauda equina (see Fig. 21.23). The normal segmental sensory distribution is valuable in the anatomic localization of sensory disorders (Fig. 21.26).

Dermatomes are bands of skin innervated by a sensory root of a single spinal nerve. Knowledge of these dermatomes aids the practitioner in locating neurologic lesions (Fig. 21.27).

Spinal Vasculature

The vasculature of the spinal cord and vertebral column is a rich, delicate network. The arterial blood supply to the spinal cord arises from the vertebral arteries as the anterior spinal artery and the posterior spinal arteries. These vessels branch and anastomose on both sides of the cord and within the substance of the cord. They also branch into anterior and posterior radicular arteries that form spinal rami as they accompany the spinal nerve roots through the intervertebral foramina.

A series of venous plexuses surround and innervate the spinal cord at each level in the vertebral canal. They anastomose with each other and form the intervertebral veins as they pass through the intervertebral foramina with the spinal nerves to join the intercostal, lumbar, and sacral veins. The lateral longitudinal veins near the foramen magnum empty into the inferior petrosal sinus and cerebellar veins. The venous network innervates the bony structures and musculature as well as the spinal cord and nerve roots. The perioperative nurse considers the possibility of venous bleeding during spinal surgery when planning care.

Pathologic Lesions of the Spinal Cord and Adjacent Structures

Surgery is performed to correct congenital malformations, traumatic injuries, tumors, abscesses, herniated and degenerative intervertebral disks, and intractable pain.

Meningocele

The most common congenital lesion encountered is a lumbar meningocele, or myelomeningocele, which is a failure of the union of the vertebral arches during fetal development. The fluid-filled, thin-walled sac often contains neural elements. This fetal anomaly is often diagnosed prenatally and is often seen with other CNS abnormalities, which include hydrocephalus, gyral abnormalities, and Chiari malformation of the hindbrain (see Chapter 26 for a discussion of the surgical treatment of meningocele).

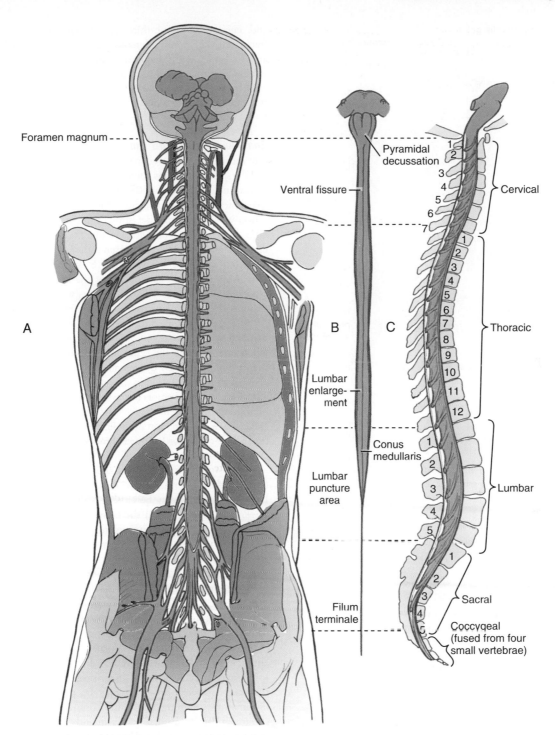

FIG. 21.23 Posterior view of brainstem and spinal cord. (A) Torso dissected from back is shown. Dura mater has been opened and cord exposed. Levels concerned can be easily determined by referring to ribs on left side of thorax. Cord proper terminates opposite the body of second lumbar vertebra (B) as conus medullaris. (B) Ventral surface of cord stripped of dura mater and arachnoid. It is symmetric in structure, two halves of which are separated by ventral fissure. This fissure stops at foramen magnum. Caudally, pia mater leaves conus medullaris as a glistening thread, or filum terminale. (C) Cord is exposed from the lateral side. Dura mater has been opened. Because the cord is shorter than the canal and spinal nerves exit through intervertebral foramina, one at a time, the lowest portion of the canal is occupied only by a bundle-like accumulation of nerve roots called the cauda equina. The caudal end of dural sac, enclosing spinal cord and cauda equina, lies somewhere between bodies of the first and third sacral vertebrae. Size and position of the three views of major vertebral levels is indicated by transverse lines for all three views.

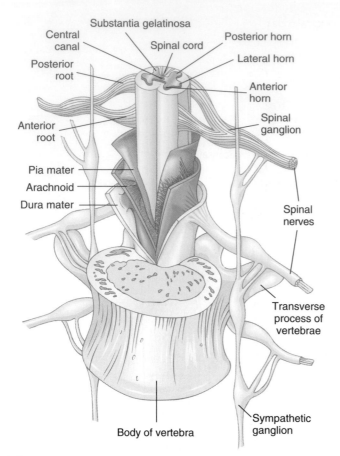

FIG. 21.24 Spinal cord, showing meninges, formation of spinal nerves, and relationships to vertebra and to sympathetic trunk and ganglia.

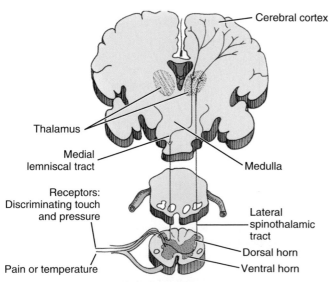

FIG. 21.25 Lateral spinothalamic and medial lemniscal neural tracts.

Trauma

Trauma to the spine is most commonly caused by motor vehicle crashes and falls. In blunt trauma patients, vertebral column fracture alone is more than 10 times more frequent than spinal cord injuries. The cervical spine is the most vulnerable to injury, and encompasses one-third of all traumatic vertebral column fractures (Martin and Meredith, 2017). Standardized trauma care and transport, early diagnosis, and closed reduction with surgical stabilization as necessary are part of spinal care focused on minimizing cord trauma and maximizing cord recovery. Spinal decompression, stabilization, and traction are all common interventions performed in trauma centers.

Spine and Spinal Cord Tumors

The most frequently occurring tumors of the spine are metastatic, and the spine is the most common site for skeletal metastasis. Although it is estimated that about 10% of cancer patients develop *symptomatic* spinal metastasis, approximately 5% to 30% of patients with systemic cancer will have spinal metastasis. Some studies have estimated that 30% to 70% of patients with a primary tumor have spinal metastatic disease at autopsy (Tse, 2016). Pain is the earliest and most prominent symptom, followed by weakness. Secondary spinal tumors most often originate from carcinomas of the lung, breast, prostate, and blood. Approximately 17% of patients with other primary tumors may experience cord compression as a result of spinal metastases. Metastases to the spine have a predilection toward the thoracic spine, followed by the lumbar and cervical areas. About 70% of symptomatic lesions are found in the thoracic region of the spine, particularly at the level of T4-T7. Of the remainder, 20% are found in the lumbar region and 10% are found in the cervical spine (Tse, 2016). Treatment goals for metastatic tumors of the spine are pain relief and preservation or restoration of neurologic function. Options include radiation, surgery, or a combination of these. Surgery involves both decompression of the spinal cord and nerve roots and stabilization of the spinal column.

Spinal tumors are classified according to location as *extradural* (outside the dura mater) or *intradural* (inside the dura mater). Intradural tumors may be either *extramedullary* (outside the cord) or *intramedullary* (within the cord). Although most spinal tumors are benign, metastatic tumors may be found in each category and are usually extradural. Other extradural lesions include lymphomas, lipomas, neurofibromas, chondromas, angiomas, abscesses, and granulomas.

Most intradural tumors are extramedullary and benign and, if diagnosed early before severe neurologic deficits occur, offer an excellent prognosis. They manifest their presence by pain of a radicular nature and various motor and sensory disabilities below their segmental locations. They are usually benign and originate from the dura mater and arachnoid surrounding the cord and from the root sheaths of spinal nerves. Schwannomas (neuromas) are especially common in the thoracocervical area and may be part of generalized neurofibromatosis. Meningiomas also commonly occur in intradural extramedullary locations. Less frequently, lipomas or other types of tumors are found. These tumors infiltrate the cord tissue and are much more difficult to remove than are extramedullary tumors. Of the intramedullary tumors, the most common are ependymomas and astrocytomas.

Cord tumors frequently produce spinal fluid blockage and can be pinpointed accurately with MRI. Intraspinal injection of contrast material (myelography) is another option for diagnosis. Often a standard laminectomy is used for exposure and removal.

Spinal Epidural Abscess

Spinal epidural abscess can develop from vertebral osteomyelitis; from infection originating at a distant source and transferred by the blood; or from direct inoculation caused by spinal surgery,

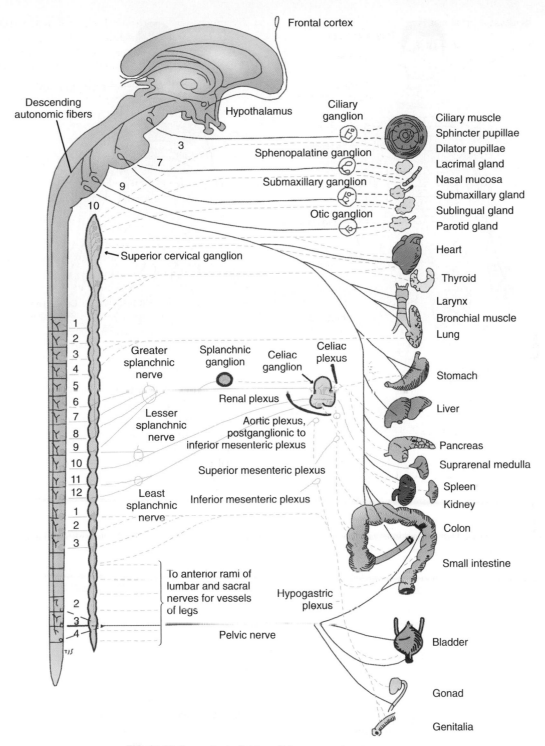

FIG. 21.26 Sympathetic division of the autonomic nervous system.

LP, or epidural administration of anesthetic. Patients who are immunosuppressed are especially at risk for epidural abscesses. Clinical presentation involves spinal and radicular pain and muscle weakness that can progress to paralysis. Epidural abscess is most easily diagnosed by MRI and typically treated with surgical decompression, culture, and irrigation, along with 4 to 8 weeks of IV antibiotic therapy.

Intervertebral Disk Disease

Intervertebral disk disease is the most frequently encountered neurosurgical problem. The axial skeleton bears both the body's weight and externally applied axial forces while maintaining mobility. Intervertebral disks serve as mechanical buffers that absorb axial loading, bending, and shear forces. Bipedal posture further stresses the intervertebral disks, leading to degenerative disk disorders. Disk

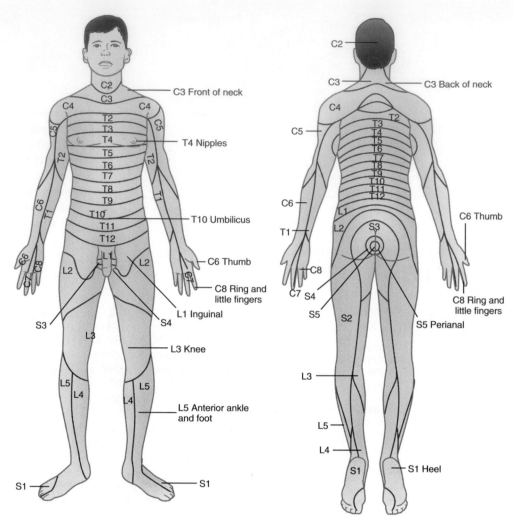

FIG. 21.27 Dermatomes innervated by posterior nerve roots and their correlation on the body; both anterior and posterior views are shown. *C,* Cervical; *T,* thoracic; *L,* lumbar; *S,* sacral.

rupture occurs with radial fissuring of the annulus. The nucleus pulposus then escapes, extending to the margin of the annulus and posterior longitudinal ligament. Once the nucleus pulposus protrudes beyond the perimeter of the disk space into the epidural space, it results in nerve root compression and radiculopathy (pain produced by pressure or traction on the nerve roots) (Figs. 21.28 and 21.29). Most disk protrusions occur at the L4-L5 and L5-S1 interspaces. Interventions include a medical trial of treatment with steroids and analgesics/narcotics; muscle relaxation; rest; epidural steroid injections; and, in failed cases, laminotomy or laminectomy with diskectomy. In far lateral disk herniations, percutaneous lumbar diskectomy is often an alternative to laminotomy.

Intractable Pain

Certain painful spinal lesions, usually of a malignant nature, can be controlled by use of epidural opiates, by use of fentanyl patches, or by temporary or permanent use of a medication pump. Another pain control procedure is to divide the pain fibers supplying the affected area. This may be accomplished by sectioning the sensory roots intraspinally (posterior rhizotomy) or by incising the spino-

thalamic tracts that carry pain and temperature impulses (anterolateral cordotomy). Alternatively, spinal cord stimulation of the affected area can be achieved with the placement of electrodes in the epidural space. A laminectomy for exposure is necessary to perform these surgical procedures.

Peripheral Nerves

The PNS consists of those structures containing nerve fibers or axons that connect the CNS with motor and sensory, somatic and visceral, end-organs. The PNS includes the cranial nerves (III to XII), the spinal nerves, the autonomic nerves, and the ganglia.

The 31 pairs of spinal nerves are each numbered for the level of the spinal column at which they emerge: cervical, C1 through C8; thoracic, T1 through T12; lumbar, L1 through L5; sacral, S1 through S5; and coccygeal, 1. The first pair of cervical spine nerves emerges between C1 and the occipital bone. The eight cervical nerves emerge from the intervertebral foramina between C7 and T1. The first thoracic nerves emerge between T1 and T2.

In the cervical and lumbosacral regions the spinal nerves regroup in a plexiform manner before they form the peripheral nerves of the

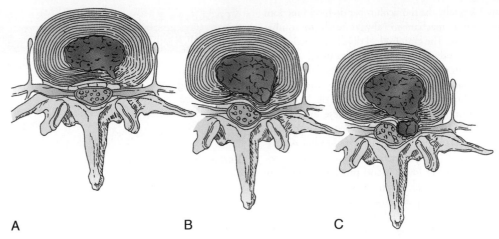

FIG. 21.28 Stages in the herniation of an intervertebral disk. (A) Tearing of the rings of the annulus fibrosus. (B) Protrusion of the disk against the nerve root. (C) Extrusion of part of the nucleus pulposus, with further nerve root compression.

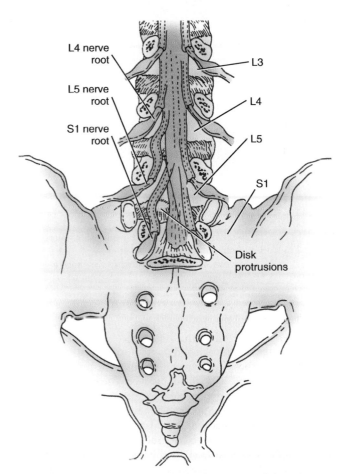

FIG. 21.29 Posterior view of the lower lumbar spine. A disk protrusion at L4-L5 on the left results in compression of the L5 nerve root where it leaves the dural sac but before it exits the spinal canal.

upper and lower extremities. Those in the thoracic region form cutaneous and intercostal nerves. The principal nerves of the upper plexus include the musculocutaneous, median, ulnar, and radial. Those of the lumbosacral plexus include the obturator, femoral, and sciatic.

Each spinal nerve divides into anterior, posterior, and white rami. Rami are primary divisions of a nerve. Anterior and posterior rami contain voluntary fibers; white rami contain autonomic fibers. Posterior rami further branch into nerves innervating the muscles, skin, and posterior surfaces of the head, neck, and trunk. Most anterior rami branch to the skeletal muscles and the skin of the extremities and anterior and lateral surfaces. In the process they form plexuses, such as the brachial and sacral plexuses. Spinal nerves contain sensory dendrites and motor axons; some have somatic axons, and some have axons of preganglionic autonomic motor neurons.

The autonomic (involuntary) nervous system consists of all the efferent nerves through which the cardiovascular apparatus, viscera, glands of internal secretion, and peripheral involuntary muscles are innervated (see Fig. 21.26). There is a major anatomic difference between the somatic and autonomic nervous systems. In the somatic nervous system an impulse from the brainstem or spinal cord reaches the end-organ through a single neuron. In the autonomic nervous system an impulse passes through two neurons: the first ending in an autonomic ganglion and the second running from the ganglion to the end-organ. Some of the ganglia lie adjacent to the vertebral column to form the sympathetic trunks or chains; others are closely associated with the end-organs.

The preganglionic neurons from the brainstem (which traverse along the cranial nerves) and those from the second, third, and fourth sacral segments to the pelvic viscera end in ganglia in proximity to their end-organs; thus their postganglionic fibers are very short. This is known as the *parasympathetic*, or *craniosacral*, division of the autonomic nervous system. The preganglionic fibers from the thoracic and lumbar spinal cord terminate in the paravertebral ganglia, making up the sympathetic chain, and their postganglionic fibers are relatively long. This is termed the *sympathetic*, or *thoracolumbar*, division of the autonomic nervous system.

The two divisions are distinct anatomically and physiologically. The chemical substance mediating transmission of impulses at most postganglionic sympathetic nerve endings is *norepinephrine*, and the neurotransmitter at all parasympathetic and preganglionic sympathetic neurons is *acetylcholine*.

The majority of organs have dual innervation, part from the craniosacral division and part from the thoracolumbar division. The functions of these two systems are antagonistic. Together they work to maintain homeostasis. Generally the thoracolumbar division functions as an emergency protection mechanism, always ready to combat physical or psychologic stress. The craniosacral division functions to conserve energy when the body is in a state of relaxation.

Stimuli arising from internal organs or from outside the body traverse visceral and somatic afferent nerve fibers to make reflex connections with preganglionic autonomic neurons in the brainstem and spinal cord. Such stimuli trigger activity of these involuntary systems automatically. When these automatic mechanisms break down or overact, surgery may be indicated. Thoracolumbar sympathectomy was once performed in hypertensive patients as an attempt to decrease blood vessel tone and lower blood pressure. Vagotomy can be performed to decrease acid secretion to the stomach in patients with peptic ulcers. Lumbar sympathectomy is used to relieve vasospastic disorders of the legs. T2 sympathectomy is done to relieve palmar hyperhidrosis (sweaty palms). See Chapter 23 for a discussion of thoracic sympathectomy.

Perioperative Nursing Considerations

Assessment

Neurologic Assessment Tools

A familiarity with basic neurologic assessment tools gives the nurse the ability to perform a standardized neurologic assessment that can be compared with the patient's previous assessments and easily communicated to other healthcare professionals. These tools can be used preoperatively to establish a baseline assessment. Postoperatively they can be used to establish a return to baseline and to assess postoperative neurologic stability. The postoperative condition of a neurosurgical patient can quickly deteriorate, so an adequate baseline assessment is essential. The Glasgow Coma Scale is commonly used to assess patients with brain injury (Table 21.2). Three indicators of cerebral function—eye opening, verbal communication, and motor response to verbal and noxious stimuli—are assessed, and the appropriate number of points for each is assigned and totaled. The best possible score is 15, and the worst possible score is 3. The Medical Research Council (MRC) Scale for Muscle Strength Grading can be used to assess muscle strength in the upper and lower extremities of spinal cord injury patients or patients who are having spine surgery (Table 21.3).

Preparation for Surgery

Communication among the perioperative team is essential for planning care for the neurosurgical patient in the operating room (OR). Information the perioperative nurse needs before the arrival of the patient in the OR includes the following:

- The patient's age, height, weight, level of consciousness, physical disabilities resulting from neuropathologic or other conditions, stability of spine, and communication barriers
- Diagnosis, allergies, medical clearance for surgery, and nothing-by-mouth (NPO) status
- Planned and possible surgical procedures
- Surgical and anesthesia consent signed by the patient or person with power of attorney for medical decisions (if the patient is unable to provide consent)
- Surgical site marked by the surgeon or a representative to designate correct side of head, level of spine, or other surgical site
- Diagnostic and lab studies done and reports needed at the time of operation

TABLE 21.2

Glasgow Coma Scale

	Points
Eye Opening	
Spontaneous	4
To speech	3
To pain	2
None	1
Verbal Communication	
Oriented	5
Confused conversation	4
Inappropriate words	3
Incomprehensible sounds	2
None	1
Motor Response	
Obeys commands	6
Localizes to pain	5
Withdraws to pain	4
Abnormal flexion	3
Abnormal extension	2
None	1

Modified from Gallagher RL: Assessment of the nervous system. In Ignatavicius DD, Workman ML, editors: *Medical-surgical nursing: patient-centered collaborative care*, ed 8, St Louis, 2016, Saunders.

TABLE 21.3

Medical Research Council Scale for Muscle Strength Grading

Grade	Strength
0	No muscle contraction
1	Trace of contraction
2	Active movement with gravity eliminated
3	Active movement against gravity
4	Active movement against gravity and resistance
5	Normal power

Modified from Daroff RB et al, editors: *Bradley's neurology in clinical practice*, ed 7, Philadelphia, 2016, Saunders.

- Specific surgical approach and position to be used
- Need for any special equipment, instruments, and supplies
- Amount of blood and blood products (fresh frozen plasma, platelets) ordered and available
- Need for radiologic support, neuromonitoring, intraoperative blood salvage unit, and image guidance
- Planned preliminary procedures such as LP, placement of lines (IV, central venous, arterial), and Foley catheter insertion
- Verification that all necessary personnel, equipment, and supplies are available
- A baseline, focused preoperative neurologic examination, which may include the following:
  - Mental status (level of consciousness, orientation, behavior, ability to follow commands)
  - Vision, pupil response, extraocular eye movements (EOMs), and hearing
  - Examination of sensation and motor strength of extremities
  - Area and intensity of pain

This information allows the perioperative nurse to properly plan and prepare for the surgery and to ensure the well-being of the patient. Preoperative assessment data are also used during the postoperative period as a means of measuring progress toward outcomes.

Diagnostic Procedures

Most patients will have undergone diagnostic procedures before arriving in the OR. Radiologic and other diagnostic studies are of great significance to the surgical team. The nurse should ensure that any pertinent radiographic images are available in the OR before the procedure begins. The surgeon can refer to these images to locate the pathologic condition, verify the correct surgical site, and plan the appropriate surgical approach and procedure. Diagnostic studies include the following:

1. *Plain x-rays.* X-rays of the spine can be used initially to identify injury to the spinal column. They are referred to intraoperatively to verify that surgery to the spine is being done at the correct level (Fig. 21.30).

2. *CT scan.* A CT scan uses x-ray studies, with or without instilled contrast medium, and computer technology to produce a sequential series of positive images of transverse sections of the brain and spinal cord in which differences in tissue density can be detected and deviations from normal identified. This study remains the criterion standard for evaluating acute head injury and is considered the first-line screening study.

3. *MRI.* Use of radiofrequency pulses in a powerful magnetic field yields high-resolution images of the human body and involves nonionizing radiation. Advances in MRI scanning provide enhancement of the scan with the use of gadolinium (contrast medium). A typical MRI study produces views of the brain featured as contiguous slices in three different planes. Axial cuts are from top to bottom. Coronal cuts are from front to back. Sagittal cuts are from side to side. The MRI is the gold standard for the diagnosis of tumors, abscesses, tissue/ligamentous injury, and disk herniation (Figs. 21.31 and 21.32).

4. *Stereotactic MRI or CT scan.* Placement of a stereotactic head frame (frame-based system) or fiducials (frameless system) before receiving a CT scan or MRI produces information that is registered into a computer. The goal of stereotactic surgery is to localize a point or volume in three-dimensional space. The surgeon uses the frame-based system by using an arc system mounted on the bed frame. This system allows the surgeon to access the target by different trajectories (Ortega-Barnett et al., 2017). The frameless system allows the neurosurgeon to see beyond the actual operative field by using an optical tracking device. This handheld device depicts in three planes on a computer screen where the surgeon is working in the brain relative to deeper structures beyond view.

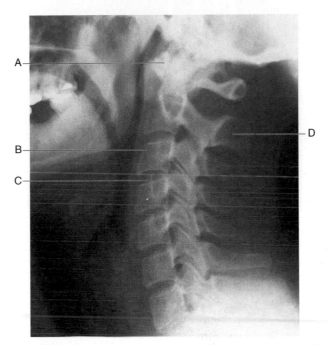

FIG. 21.30 Lateral x ray of the cervical spine *(A)* Anterior tubercle of the atlas (C1). *(B)* Cervical body. *(C)* Intervertebral disk. *(D)* Spinous process of the axis (C2).

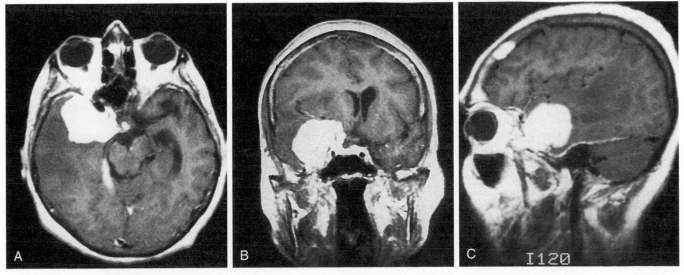

FIG. 21.31 Gadolinium-enhanced magnetic resonance image of a medial sphenoid wing meningioma in (A) axial, (B) coronal, and (C) sagittal planes.

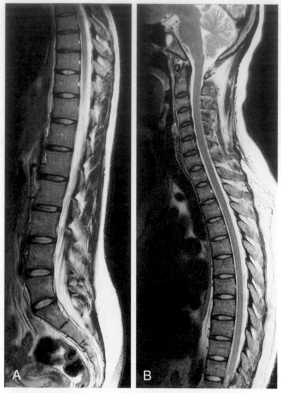

FIG. 21.32 Sagittal magnetic resonance image of (A) thoracolumbar spine and (B) cervicothoracic spine.

5. *Magnetic resonance angiography (MRA).* MRA is a noninvasive means of studying the cerebral vasculature. An MRA study is capable of detecting carotid stenosis, posttraumatic carotid artery dissection, AVMs, and aneurysms.

6. *Angiography (arteriography).* Injection of contrast medium into the brachial, carotid, vertebral, or femoral arteries is used to study the intracranial blood vessels for size, location, and configuration and to allow diagnosis of space-occupying lesions and vascular abnormalities.

7. *Digital subtraction angiography (DSA).* DSA is a computerized radiologic procedure. An IV rather than arterial injection is required; a contrast medium injection allows examination of selected arterial circulation. By using computer technology DSA provides an alternative to cerebral angiography for high-risk patients.

8. *Three-dimensional CT angiography.* Contrast-enhanced CT brain scan data are used to generate a three-dimensional image of the intracranial vasculature with minimal risk to the patient.

9. *Stereoscopic display of MRA.* Recent advances in MRI permit high-resolution imaging of blood flow. Projection angiograms can be produced to overcome the tomographic nature of conventional MRI scans. These angiograms are similar to plain x-ray films or digital subtraction angiograms in the demonstration of blood vessels, but the three-dimensional information inherent in them is partially lost in single projections. Stereoscopic image pairs allow the clinician to perceive the relative distance of vessels to one another. MRA permits perception of vascular anatomy in three dimensions.

10. *Myelography.* Contrast medium is injected into the spinal subarachnoid space and fluoroscopy is used to view the spinal cord, nerve roots, and spinal column and to demonstrate a defect involving these areas.

11. *Ultrasound.* Ultrasound is a noninvasive technique that uses high-frequency sound waves and a computer to create images of blood vessels, tissues, and organs. It is often used to assess the blood flow in the carotid artery. This procedure can be done in or out of the surgical suite. It can be used intraoperatively to localize intradural spinal cord tumors.

12. *Electroencephalogram (EEG).* An EEG is a procedure that records the brain's continuous electrical activity by means of electrodes placed on the scalp or intraoperatively on the brain.

13. *Evoked potentials (EPs).* EPs are procedures that record the brain's electrical response to visual, auditory, and sensory stimuli.

14. *Wada test (intracarotid amobarbital [Amytal] test).* The Wada test can be used before brain surgery to lateralize language, memory, and the dominant hemisphere. It can help lateralize seizure focus and assess the ability of the hemisphere with the lesion to maintain memory when isolated.

15. *LP.* A spinal needle is used to gain access to CSF in the subarachnoid space. Opening and closing pressures are measured to determine whether there is increased pressure surrounding the brain and spinal cord. This can help diagnose hydrocephalus or a spinal tumor. CSF is sent to the lab to evaluate for blood, infection, malignancy, and other neurologic diseases. LP is contraindicated when an intracranial mass is known or suspected because it can cause herniation of the brain in the presence of increased ICP.

Nursing Diagnosis

Nursing diagnoses are developed from interpreting and analyzing patient information to determine whether there are specific (actual) or potential (risk for) problems that the perioperative nurse needs to consider in the plan of care. Neurosurgery patients share common problems that the perioperative nurse should address. Nursing diagnoses related to the care of patients undergoing neurosurgery might include the following:

- Anxiety related to surgery or surgical outcome
- Deficient Knowledge related to diagnostic tests and surgical procedures
- Ineffective Breathing Pattern related to location of tumor, surgical position, or effects of general anesthesia
- Risk for Hypothermia
- Risk for Perioperative Positioning Injury

Outcome Identification

Outcomes identified for the selected nursing diagnoses could be stated as follows:

- The patient will verbalize that anxiety is reduced or controlled.
- The patient or family will verbalize an understanding of the diagnostic tests, surgical procedure, and postoperative plan of care.
- The patient will maintain effective breathing patterns.
- The patient will remain normothermic.
- The patient will be free from signs and symptoms of positioning injury.

Planning

Preparation can significantly reduce anesthesia time and intraoperative time for the patient, as well as physical and psychologic stress for the patient, surgeon, and perioperative nurse. Planning for the patient's care in the OR is based on the results of the nursing assessment and

PATIENT ENGAGEMENT EXEMPLAR

Healthcare Literacy

NAQC Guiding Principle Number 9 states:

Health care literacy and linguistically appropriate interactions are essential for patient, family, and clinicians to understand the components of patient engagement. Providers must maintain awareness of the language needs and health care literacy level of the patient and family and respond accordingly.

The US Department of Health and Human Services Health Resources and Services Administration defined health literacy as the degree to which individuals have the capacity to obtain, process, and understand basic health information and services needed to make appropriate health decisions. Neurosurgical patients are especially vulnerable if they are functioning at a decreased cognitive state secondary to their diagnosis. It is important that perioperative nurses do a thorough preoperative interview with the patient or the designated decision-maker to obtain his or her level of understanding of the diagnosis and treatment plan. Medical jargon should be avoided, and simple language explanations along with written materials should be used. For example, a consent may read "endoscopic transsphenoidal resection of pituitary adenoma." The perioperative nurse should assess the level of understanding of patients or designees by asking them to state the procedure in their own words. The patient may reply by saying, "The surgeon is going to use a scope to look up my nose and remove a tumor from my pituitary gland." A response such as this is considered health literate and appropriate. If the response is, "The surgeon is taking out a tumor from somewhere," then further discussion by all those involved in the care of the patient is essential.

NAQC, Nursing Alliance for Quality Care.

Modified from Health Resources and Services Administration (HRSA): *Health literacy* (website). www.hrsa.gov/healthliteracy. (Accessed 31 December 2016); Nursing Alliance for Quality Care (NAQC): *Fostering successful patient and family engagement: nursing's critical role* (website), 2013. www.naqc.org/WhitePaper-PatientEngagement. (Accessed 31 December 2016)

the identification of relevant nursing diagnoses. The plan of care then identifies desired outcomes derived from the nursing diagnoses; priorities are set and nursing interventions are designed to assist the patient to reach the desired outcomes. Nursing interventions identified for the patient's plan of care may include reassessment, teaching, counseling, referrals, and specific interventions to assist the patient in achieving patient care outcomes (Patient Engagement Exemplar). A Sample Plan of Care for a patient undergoing a neurosurgical procedure is provided.

Implementation

The perioperative nurse must determine that all personnel, equipment, instrumentation, and supplies necessary for a successful surgery are available. The nurse uses the information obtained through assessment of the patient and communication with the surgical team to provide individualized patient care. Neurosurgical patients vary in age from the very young to the very old. They often have special needs because of conditions such as mental status changes, spinal instability, spinal cord injuries, paralysis, other traumatic injuries, and pain. These conditions need to be considered at all times. Neurosurgery patients

who seem to be unconscious may actually be aware of their environment and unable to voice their concerns. The perioperative nurse should always talk to the patient and explain what is happening. Showing compassion and attempting to relieve the fears of the patient and his or her family are essential.

Equipment

Neurosurgical procedures require an extensive amount of equipment. The nurse must analyze the arrangement of the equipment in the OR to ensure that the sterile field is not compromised. Electrical equipment should be placed in proximity to electrical outlets, so that cords are out of high-traffic areas. Monitors should be in comfortable view of the surgeon. A microscope needs a clear path to the surgical field. The surgeon and surgical assistants may require specialized surgical chairs or sitting or standing stools to comfortably perform the surgery.

Operating Room Bed and Attachments. The nurse uses information about the proposed surgical procedure and desired surgical position to gather the proper OR bed, attachments, and positioning devices before the patient arrives in the OR suite. Perioperative nurses must anticipate needs that may arise during the surgery and prepare for them, considering questions such as the following: Is this the correct OR bed in the correct position with the correct attachments? If fluoroscopy will be used, is the base of the OR bed in a position that will accommodate the C-arm? A specialized OR table, such as a Jackson table or Andrews table or frame, may be required for posterior spine surgery. Skull clamps, skull pins, and tongs are commonly used for craniotomies and posterior cervical spine surgeries to stabilize the head and neck (Fig. 21.33). Occasionally a patient may come to the OR in a halo that was placed for preoperative stabilization of the cervical spine. At least part of the halo will need to be removed so the surgical site can be accessed. Compatible wrenches must be available to accomplish this.

Basic Equipment. Neurosurgical procedures typically require one special neurosurgical overhead instrument table, such as the Mayfield table (Fig. 21.34), or two large Mayo trays along with one long back table. Other basic equipment includes the following: an intermittent pneumatic compression device, a cooling-heating unit, one or two monopolar electrosurgical units (ESUs), a bipolar ESU, and a wall supply or tank of nitrogen with a special pressure gauge for operating air-powered instruments. Usually two suction units are required. Intraoperative blood salvage is used for most spine surgeries, unless infection or malignancy is suspected.

Neurosurgeons usually wear surgical loupes and a fiberoptic headlight, requiring a light source.

Operating Microscope. An operating microscope may be required for surgery during certain neurosurgical procedures. The operating microscope has revolutionized neurosurgery by providing intense light and magnification to areas that previously may have been inoperable or inaccessible. Microsurgery allows for greater surgical precision when operating in proximity to vital structures and has better surgical results. The perioperative nurse must be able to prepare the microscope for use in neurosurgery, and the surgeon must check it for focal length and focus before scrubbing. Disposable sterile drapes are available for the microscope, as are assistant and observer lenses. Cameras and closed-circuit television monitors are also available for use with the operating microscope.

Endoscopes. Surgeons use endoscopes to perform minimally invasive neurosurgery, such as endoscopic biopsy. The endoscope provides illumination and magnification of structures and an extended viewing angle. Perioperative nurses must be prepared to convert

SAMPLE PLAN OF CARE

Nursing Diagnosis
Anxiety related to surgery or surgical outcome

Outcome
The patient's anxiety will be reduced or controlled.

Interventions
- Broadly classify intensity of the patient's anxiety.
- Determine the patient's coping skills.
- Provide listening, reassurance, and information.
- Provide ongoing opportunity for questions or expression of concerns or fears.
- Involve other support systems (e.g., family, friends, social worker, chaplain).
- Assist the patient to use personally effective coping skills.
- Use touch (if welcomed by the patient) and eye contact during communication.

Nursing Diagnosis
Deficient Knowledge related to diagnostic tests and surgical procedures

Outcome
The patient, family, and caregiver will verbalize an understanding of the diagnostic tests, surgical procedure, and postoperative plan of care.

Interventions
- Determine knowledge level and desire for knowledge.
- Correct misinformation.
- Identify readiness and motivation to learn.
- Provide information regarding tests or surgery.
- Explain perioperative routine, postoperative recovery, and discharge plans.
- Base interventions on the patient's needs.

Nursing Diagnosis
Ineffective Breathing Pattern related to location of tumor, surgical position, or effects of general anesthesia

Outcome
The patient will maintain effective breathing patterns.

Interventions
- Provide appropriate positioning accessories, and assist in their placement.
- Collaborate with anesthesia provider and surgeon during positioning activities relevant to respiratory effectiveness.

- Determine the patient's comfort on the OR bed; provide comfort measures as appropriate.
- Maintain an open suction line.
- Observe respiratory rate, depth, and character.
- Encourage deep breaths and coughing.
- Communicate with the PACU regarding respiratory needs.
- Check airway patency frequently during transport to the PACU.

Nursing Diagnosis
Risk for Hypothermia

Outcome
The patient will remain normothermic.

Interventions
- Provide warm ambient OR temperature during surgical intervention.
- Provide warmed IV fluids and blood products.
- Provide body-warming system (e.g., warm air unit) during surgery.
- Keep the head covered or wrapped when possible.
- Monitor temperature with the anesthesia provider.
- Cover the patient with warm blankets at end of the surgical intervention for transport to the PACU.

Nursing Diagnosis
Risk for Perioperative Positioning Injury

Outcome
The patient will be free from signs and symptoms of positioning injury.

Interventions
- Assess the patient's physical limitations before positioning; make accommodations.
- Carefully pad and protect all prominences and sites that are vulnerable to neurovascular injury.
- Check all positioning devices for cleanliness, working order, and freedom from sharp edges.
- Collaborate with the OR team in placing positioning devices to maintain patient safety.
- Assess the patient at completion of surgery for areas of redness, blanching, or bruising.
- Communicate any findings to the PACU nursing staff.
- Document findings and follow-up with the patient, as applicable.

IV, Intravenous; *PACU*, postanesthesia care unit.

---

from a neuroendovascular procedure to an open procedure if it is determined that the surgery cannot be successfully completed endoscopically. An additional use for endoscopes is in open procedures to see areas that are otherwise visually inaccessible.

Radiologic Intervention. Radiology is commonly used intraoperatively for spine surgery. Typically a radiology technician operates the equipment. Lead aprons and thyroid shields must be worn or protective shields must be used by all staff in the OR as protection from radiation exposure. X-rays can be taken to check for proper positioning of the spine and to help the surgeon identify a specific level of the spine. This may be done before incision or after partial exposure of the spinous processes and laminae. In both cases an instrument or needle is used to mark a position on the spine, and an x-ray of the spine is taken. The x-ray enables the surgeon to

identify the level of the spine that is marked. The surgeon uses that information to identify the correct surgical level. A postoperative x-ray is also taken to verify that the surgery was done to the correct level of the spine.

With fluoroscopy, also called direct image intensification, a C-arm (covered with a sterile drape) is used to take a continuous x-ray that is portrayed on a monitor. This gives the surgeon the ability to view the spine and to directly view screws as they are being placed during an instrumented fusion. This ensures that spinal instrumentation for fusion is properly positioned in the correct levels. Fluoroscopy is also used for placement of nerve-stimulator electrodes in brain or spinal areas and stereotactic procedures.

Stereotactic and Image-Guided Equipment. Stereotactic and image-guided equipment is commonly used for neurosurgery. Either

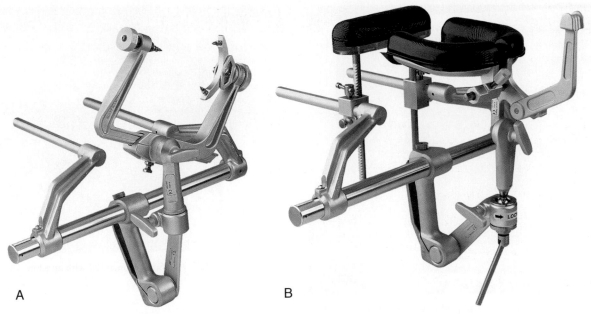

FIG. 21.33 (A) Three-pin fixation skull clamp (Mayfield) for stabilizing head during neurosurgical procedures. (B) Mayfield horseshoe headrest.

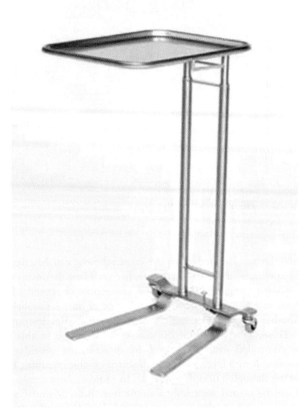

FIG. 21.34 Mayfield overhead instrument table.

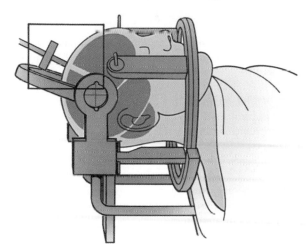

FIG. 21.35 Stereotactic procedure. Patient fitted with head frame before computed tomography or magnetic resonance imaging scanning.

accompanying attachments and instruments that must be available. The frameless image-guided system requires a monitor to display views of the brain or spine in three different planes: axial, coronal, and sagittal (Fig. 21.36).

Ultrasonic Aspirator. An ultrasonic aspirator (e.g., Cavitron ultrasonic surgical aspirator [CUSA]) may be used to emulsify and debulk a tumor with high-frequency sound waves. Various settings allow the surgeon to adjust the instrument to remove firm or calcified lesions, or soft masses. The ultrasonic aspirator provides hemostasis and spares adjacent nerves and vessels as it removes the tumor.

Equipment. The use of video cameras, recorders, and television monitors is invaluable to teach staff and enhance understanding of the surgical procedure by perioperative personnel who are otherwise unable to visualize the surgeon's actions directly. By viewing the operative field through the monitor, the experienced scrub person will be able to anticipate the neurosurgeon's next move and will therefore provide better assistance.

a frame-based (requiring a head frame skull attachment) (Fig. 21.35) or a frameless system can be used. Both systems use a computer to register points, based on information obtained from a stereotactic MRI or CT scan done preoperatively, to determine the least traumatic approach to the target (tumor, lesion, ventricle). Both systems have

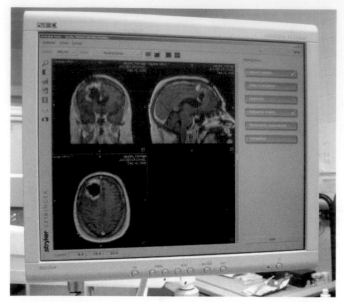

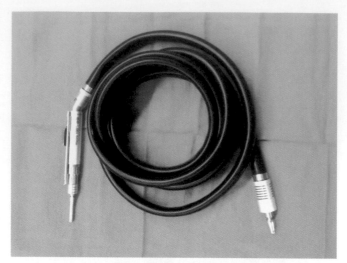

FIG. 21.37 Hall Surgairtome 200 with attachments.

FIG. 21.36 Frameless stereotactic image-guided navigation monitor showing the brain with tumor in three planes: coronal *(upper left),* sagittal *(upper right),* and axial *(lower left).*

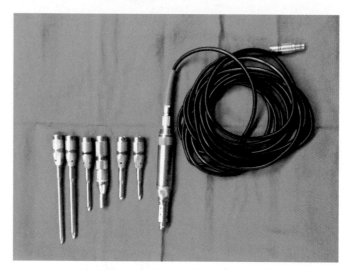

FIG. 21.38 Midas Rex drill with attachments.

Intraoperative Monitoring Equipment. Equipment for intraoperative monitoring, such as EEG, EPs, ICP, and Doppler, may also be required.

Instrumentation, Implants, and Supplies

Typically instrumentation used in neurosurgery is added to basic surgical instrumentation to make neurosurgical-specific trays, such as a basic craniotomy tray or a laminectomy tray. Specialized trays, instruments, or implants can be added based on the surgical procedure.

Powered surgical instruments are commonly used in neurosurgery. Multiple drills, drill bits, and accessories are available. These tools may be powered by air, battery, or electricity and are operated by a hand control or foot pedal. All drills have a safety control that should be engaged at all times the instrument is not in use. The perioperative nurse should monitor the sterile field to ensure that drills and other power equipment are not left lying on the patient. The use of drills makes bone work easier and reduces operating time. Irrigating the tip of the drill while it is in use prevents overheating of the tissue. By changing drill bits and attachments, different drills can be used to make burr holes, craniotomies, craniectomies, and holes for dural tack-up sutures. They can be used to thin bone for a decompression, to perform decortication for spinal fusion, to harvest hip graft, to shape bone grafts, and to make holes for plating and fixation systems.

The Hall Surgairtome 200 (Fig. 21.37) can be used for precision cutting, shaping, and repair of bone. Compressed nitrogen is the power source, as with other air-powered equipment. The Hall Surgairtome 200 can be used to widen the graft area in anterior fusions and to unroof the auditory canal in eighth cranial nerve surgery. For use in less accessible areas, such as the sphenoidal sinus, pituitary fossa, and vertebral bodies, attachments with 20- and 90-degree angles are available. A range of burrs and guards is available.

The craniotome offers a perforator drive for drilling burr holes. Both 12- and 7-mm perforators are available in disposable and reusable forms. The perforator driver attachment can be removed and a saw blade and dura guard attached to adapt the instrument for cutting a craniotomy bone flap. A cranioplasty burr and a skull contour burr as well as guards for each type of burr are available.

Another versatile pneumatic tool is the Midas Rex instrument (Fig. 21.38). The variety of disposable cutting tools of this foot pedal–controlled instrument and its attachments provides the neurosurgeon with a versatile bone dissector capable of cutting bone by sawing through it or drilling it away. In addition, large craniotomy flaps can be turned with only a single burr hole. Manufacturers' precautions and instructions must be followed for all powered instruments.

A variety of suction tips, retractors, and retractor systems are required for visualization. A transsphenoidal tray and instruments are required for that specialized approach. Microneurosurgical instruments may be needed for delicate brain or spinal cord surgery. Dural grafts and substitutes may be required to repair the dura. Aneurysm instruments, aneurysm clips, or hemostatic clips may be needed for neurovascular surgery. Titanium plates or wire is used to replace a bone plate after a craniotomy. Spinal instrumentation (plating and fixation systems) may be implanted, and bone grafts and substitutes may be used to promote spinal fusion.

Specific surgeries may require shunts or CSF reservoirs, implantable stimulators or pumps, endoscopes and endoscopic instruments, endovascular instruments, catheters, and coils. These supplies must be available if they are to be placed or implanted during surgery.

The perioperative team assembles instrumentation with consideration for each individual surgery and according to each individual surgeon's preferences. The instrument list for each procedure and neurosurgeon should be documented, referenced, and frequently updated in collaboration with the surgeon. Specific instruments are mentioned in the surgical procedure descriptions that follow.

Preliminary Procedures

A number of procedures or therapeutic measures are performed before the primary surgery begins. It is important that the perioperative nurse anticipate these procedures, understand why they are done, and be prepared to facilitate them.

Anesthesia Concerns. The anesthesia provider collaborates with the surgeon and nurses to provide appropriate care to the patient. The anesthesia provider must be aware of and plan for situations in which the neurosurgery patient may need to be awake during the surgery for intraoperative assessment. Anesthesia agents must be adjusted if intraoperative monitoring of EPs is to be done. If the cervical spine is unstable or unable to extend, endotracheal intubation may need to be done while the patient is awake. The position of the bed in the OR should be communicated to the anesthesia provider. For surgery of the head, the bed may be turned 90 degrees or 180 degrees away from the anesthesia machine to provide comfortable access to the surgical site. Anesthesia providers can prepare by having enough length on their tubing to make the turn while maintaining control of the patient's airway.

Anesthesia for neurosurgery requires sufficient IV access. The anesthesia provider may place a central line if peripheral IV lines are insufficient, or if the procedure requires the patient to be positioned in the sitting position. Increased risk of an air embolism during surgery exists when the patient is in a sitting position and when a venous sinus may be breeched. A precordial Doppler ultrasound or a pulmonary artery catheter may be placed to monitor for an air embolus. A catheter in the right atrium can be used to remove an air embolus in the heart. An arterial line may be placed for continuous monitoring of blood pressure and for drawing samples for arterial blood gas (ABG) analysis.

Antibiotic prophylaxis is administered within 60 minutes of incision time and continued at the appropriate dose schedule for at least 24 hours. The preoperative antibiotic dose is the most important dose in the prevention of postoperative infection. Generally a broad-spectrum cephalosporin is the antibiotic drug of choice, but this depends on the needs and allergies of the individual patient. In addition, antibiotics can be added to the irrigation fluid. Preoperative steroids may be given to minimize inflammation and edema when surgery involves the brain or spinal cord. Diuretics may be added for brain relaxation during surgery and to decrease ICP. To prevent seizures, antiepileptic drugs are typically given when the cerebral cortex is manipulated. Coagulopathies must be identified and corrected preoperatively.

For all but minor surgeries, a Foley catheter is inserted into the bladder to monitor urinary output during the procedure. It is essential when procedures are expected to be prolonged, when excessive bleeding is anticipated, or when diuretics are to be given intravenously,

so that the bladder does not become distended. A Foley catheter is needed by trauma patients for continual assessment of kidney function.

Stereotactic Image-Guided Navigation. To prepare for surgery on the brain, fiducials are placed on bony landmarks or points around the skull before a preoperative MRI or CT scan. Afterward the fiducials are left in place for entry into the OR. After the patient is anesthetized and positioned, a skull clamp is placed and an image-guided navigation arm is attached to the skull clamp. This provides a fixed point of reference. The arm should be out of the way of the surgical team to ensure that it will not be inadvertently bumped and moved from its fixed point during surgery, disrupting the navigation system and potentially making it useless. The location of the fiducials is registered into the computer, allowing the computer to align the preoperative images (of the CT scan or MRI) to the patient's head. The monitor then shows the location of the navigation probe (which is maneuvered by the surgeon) and its trajectory on all three planes (axial, coronal, and sagittal) of the CT or MRI (see Fig. 21.36). This enables the neurosurgeon to plan the approach to the target area and to navigate the surgical area using the navigation probe. After the registration process is complete, the fiducials can be removed so that the area can be prepped for surgery. A sterile sleeve is placed over the navigation arm when draping. The navigation system is used to find the target (tumor, lesion, ventricle) using the least traumatic trajectory. It also helps ensure that the desired amount of tissue is removed. The image-guided navigation system can also be used for spine surgery.

Neuromonitoring. An EEG can be used intraoperatively to view and record electrical activity by way of electrodes placed on the scalp or directly on the brain. It can be used to identify the location of seizure foci on the brain for possible resection. Nonconvulsive use of EEG monitors is used to monitor for burst suppression, which refers to a decrease in brain activity on the EEG monitor and may be related to hypoxemia-related hypoperfusion.

EPs record the brain's electrical response to visual, auditory, and sensory stimuli. They may be used intraoperatively to monitor hearing during resection of acoustic neuromas or to monitor somatosensory-evoked potentials (SSEPs) during some spine surgery. SSEPs may also be used to localize the primary sensory cortex in anesthetized patients. SSEPs involve placing needles in significant muscles of the patient and recording a baseline reading before the surgical incision. A significant change in EPs can indicate surgical invasion of the spinal cord, peripheral nerves, brainstem, or midbrain. To avoid permanent injury to the patient, the patient's position may need to be adjusted, or the surgeon may need to adjust retractors or instrumentation, alter a surgical approach, or decide that a subtotal tumor resection is necessary.

Lumbar and Ventricular Drains. The neurosurgeon may place a lumbar drain in the subarachnoid space of the lumbar spine to allow for CSF removal and intraoperative brain relaxation during aneurysm or tumor exposure. It may also be placed to prevent (or postoperatively, to treat) a CSF leak, which is most likely to occur after posterior fossa or transsphenoidal procedures. Alternatively, surgeons may place a ventricular catheter through a burr hole into a ventricle of the brain. In addition to providing the ability to drain CSF, a ventriculostomy provides the most accurate method of monitoring ICP. A transducer-tipped catheter system is a less accurate but less invasive method for monitoring. It does not allow for CSF drainage. With both the lumbar drain and the ventricular catheter, the nurse must ensure that stopcocks and clamps are properly positioned to avoid overdrainage of CSF, which could result in brain herniation. A separate surgical prep and setup are required for placement of these ICP devices.

Positioning

Many of the basic surgical positions described in Chapter 6 and their modifications are used in neurosurgery. The perioperative nurse must collaborate with the surgeon before the procedure to ensure the appropriate OR bed, attachments, and supportive positioning devices are available. Positioning devices that may be needed include a headrest, pillows, blankets, gel pads, a safety belt, tape, a shoulder roll (supine), an axillary roll (lateral), a beanbag (lateral), and chest rolls (prone).

Specialized neurosurgical headrests and skull clamps are commonly used for craniotomies and posterior cervical spine surgeries to support and stabilize the head and neck. They can be used with any body position. The basic unit of the neurosurgical headrest attaches to the frame of the OR bed after the standard OR bed headpiece has been removed. An articulated arm allows fine adjustments to the position of the head. A horseshoe-shaped headrest may be used. Alternatively, head clamps, skull pins, and tongs that are attached to the neurosurgical headrest bed attachment and provide maximum stability may be required (see Fig. 21.33). A variety of manufacturers provide an array of skull clamps for intraoperative cranial stabilization.

Standard skull clamps are molded of composite materials and stainless steel, and radiolucent skull clamps are made of a composite material that reduces artifact in procedures requiring x-ray (Integra, 2016).

Most skull clamps have three sterile pins that are placed in the skull clamp and covered with antibiotic or povidone-iodine ointment. Pins are available in adult and child sizes. Pins are not recommended for use in children less than 5 years of age, and it is at the discretion of the surgeon to determine which set of pins are appropriate for use on the patient (Integra, 2016). The surgeon or surgeon's assistant places the skull clamps on the patient's head after anesthetic is administered. The surgeon must place the skull clamp strategically in the skull to provide access to the surgical site and to avoid the frontal sinuses, the superficial temporal arteries, and the eyes. The pins on the clamp partially penetrate the outer table of the skull. If the prone position is used, the surgeon will place the skull clamp while the patient is supine. The surgeon supports the patient's head during the position change and adjusts the final head position after the patient is placed prone (Patient Safety).

After positional adjustments to the patient's body are complete, the skull clamp (and patient's head) is locked into the articulating arm of the headrest by someone other than the person who is supporting the head. The apparatus is tightened from proximal to distal and double-checked for security. After the patient's head is locked

---

PATIENT SAFETY

Preventing Injury When Using an Intraoperative Head Fixation System

Specialized bed attachments in conjunction with a skull clamp create a mechanical support system that is often used in head and neck surgery when rigid cranial stabilization is desired. Features of this device include the base unit (which attaches to the OR bed), cross bars, a swivel adaptor (reticulating arm), and the skull clamp. Only properly trained OR staff should be permitted to operate these devices. Mounting instructions for the bed attachment vary by OR bed manufacturer. The nurse must verify that the bed attachment is properly secured before the start of patient positioning.

Safe Application of the Skull Clamp

When the anesthesia provider has determined that the patient is ready for positioning, the designated member of the OR team will pin the patient's head with the skull clamp. The clamp consists of two skull pins in the rocker arm and one skull pin in the extension arm. When properly placed, the pins in the rocker arm are equidistant from the centerline of the patient's head and the single pin in the extension arm is exactly at the centerline. Improper positioning of the skull pins may cause serious injury to the patient. Special attention should be paid to avoid the areas of the frontal sinus, temporal fossa, blood vessels, and nerves. The person securing the skull clamp must ensure that the pins are at a 90-degree angle, the necessary pounds of clamping force are applied, and the rocker arm is in the "closed" position.

Safe Positioning

After the head is safely secured, the patient can be positioned for surgery. It is important that open communication exists among all members in the OR suite. Every member of the OR team plays a key role in the positioning process, and without good communication critical steps may be missed. Airway management

is vital, and the anesthesia provider must have control of the patient's airway at all times. All movements of the patient's head and body must first be cleared by the anesthesia provider. There must be at least three people responsible for positioning the head. One member of the anesthesia team monitors the airway, one member of the surgical team holds the patient's head within the skull clamp, and one member secures the reticulating arm of the bed attachment to the skull clamp. All the components of the bed attachment have a starburst locking mechanism, and it is critical that all teeth are engaged and locked securely. It is the responsibility of the team member holding the patient's head to do the final check to ensure all locking mechanisms are engaged properly. There should be no movement detected in any component of the system if secured properly. If even one component of the system is not properly engaged, the patient could be injured.

Postoperative Monitoring

When the procedure is complete and it is time to remove the patient from the fixation system, the same safety measures go into effect. The anesthesia provider maintains control of the patient's airway while one member of the surgical team holds the patient's head within the skull clamp, and a second member of the surgical team releases all the locking mechanisms of the reticulating arm. At this time either the standard headpiece of the OR bed can be reattached or the patient can be moved to the postoperative bed or stretcher. When the skull clamp is released, the surgeon confirms that all three pins are extracted from the patient's head and secured. If bleeding is observed from the pin site, the surgeon may apply pressure to control the oozing, or may use a monofilament suture to close the hole.

Modified from Integra: *Product information* (website). https://www.integralife.com/file/general/1453799329.pdf. (Accessed 25 September 2017); PMI: *DORO QR3 skull clamp–neurological head holder* (website). www.pmisurgical.com/cranial-stabilization/doror-skull-clamps/. (Accessed 13 September 2016).

into place, no positional adjustments can be made to the patient's body without first releasing the head. Not doing so could cause injury to the patient's cervical spine. If necessary, an image-guided navigation arm can be attached to certain skull clamps, and the positions of the fiducials are registered into the system before the patient is prepped.

The position of the patient's arms must also be considered. For cranial surgery, usually at least one arm is tucked so that the Mayo stand can be positioned over the patient. For cervical spine surgery, both arms are tucked so that the surgical site can be accessed from both sides of the bed. When the arms are tucked, the elbows are padded to protect the ulnar nerve, the palms face inward, and the wrist is maintained in a neutral position (AORN, 2016). A drape secures the arms. It should be tucked snuggly under the patient, not under the mattress. This prevents the arm from shifting downward intraoperatively and resting against the OR bed rail.

For thoracic and lumbar spine surgery, armboards can usually be placed out of the way of the surgeon and radiology equipment. Armboards are maintained at less than a 90-degree angle to prevent brachial plexus stretch.

As always, the nurse identifies any potential hazards and takes precautions to prevent them. Intermittent pneumatic compression devices are applied before induction of anesthesia to prevent deep vein thrombosis (DVT) unless they are contraindicated because of a known DVT. Pressure points must be identified and relieved. Joints must be maintained in functional alignment with no pressure or tension on superficial nerves and vessels. A warming or cooling blanket is applied for temperature control. An occlusive dressing applied over the eyes protects them from chemical burns and corneal abrasions that may occur from solutions used to prep the head. Keeping the head positioned above the heart minimizes bleeding when operating on the head.

Supine position or some modification of it can be used for approaches to the frontal, parietal, and temporal lobes; the anterior cervical spine; and the anterior lumbar spine. Lateral position can be used for an approach to the cerebellopontine angle in the posterior fossa, for anterior thoracic and lumbar spine surgery, and for posterior spine surgery. It can be used for lumbar sympathectomies and for placements of nerve stimulators and pumps.

Prone position and modifications of it can be used for access to the posterior spine and for suboccipital and posterior fossa craniotomies. A laminectomy frame or chest rolls are commonly used for prone position. The Jackson table permits access of the C-arm for intraoperative fluoroscopy of the spine. The Andrews table or frame can be used for a modified knee-chest position, which is useful for posterior lumbar spine surgery. The patient's hips and knees are flexed so that the lower body is supported primarily by the knees. The Hicks spinal surgery frame may be used to support this position and allow the abdomen to hang free. The chest is supported on a chest roll. Advantages of this position include decreased bleeding because of the collapse of epidural veins, better exposure resulting from hyperflexion of the spine, absence of pressure on the vena cava, and increased ease of ventilation. Operating time is usually reduced when this position is used. Disadvantages of the knee-chest position include the difficulty of maintaining physical stability on the OR bed, the increased possibility of patient hypotension, and the pooling of blood in the lower extremities.

The Fowler (sitting) position is used for some craniotomies involving a posterior or occipital approach. Advantages of this position include optimum visibility of the operative field and decreased blood loss because of the lowered arterial and venous pressures. Disadvantages

are the potential for orthostatic hypotension and air embolism. In the sitting position the venous pressure in the head and neck may be negative, predisposing the patient to air embolism. Other potential problems with this position include neck flexion with airway compromise and difficulty in achieving and maintaining functional alignment (see Chapter 6 for more information on the previously mentioned positions).

Skin Preparation

Prevention of infection is a primary concern in neurosurgery. An antiseptic skin prep is performed by the perioperative nurse, surgeon, resident, or surgical assistant. General principles and precautions cited in Chapter 4 apply to neurosurgical preps. Although studies have shown that shaving the surgical site can contribute to the possibility of infection, usually some hair removal is necessary when operating on the head and posterior cervical spine.

Hair removal from the head causes a disturbance in body image and can be upsetting to patients. A discussion and often a compromise regarding hair removal should take place between the surgeon and patient before the surgery, and an understanding should be reached as to how much hair will be removed. Hair that is removed is the property of the patient. It should be placed in a container, labeled with the patient's name, and kept with the patient after surgery.

Hair removal should be done as close to the time of skin incision as possible to decrease the possibility of surgical site infection. Whenever possible, minimal hair removal is recommended. It is possible to shave a 1- to 2-cm-wide area along the length of some craniotomy incisions after the hair is parted at the incision site. After the minimal shave, the hair can be combed away from the incision and held back with prepping solution or antimicrobial ointment. However, other craniotomies require more extensive hair removal. Electric hair clippers are preferred to razors because they are less irritating and less likely to nick the skin, which would predispose the area to infection. After hair removal the nurse should inspect the patient's skin carefully for any signs of inflammation or infection. If any such signs are noted, they should be reported to the surgeon immediately. The head and hair surrounding the planned incision can be prepped, even though the hair will be draped out of the operative field.

For surgery on the cervical spine it is possible to secure long hair on top of the head and remove neck hair with clippers to a level even with the top of the ears or to the occipital protuberance. Postoperatively, patients with long hair can comb it down over the shaved area until the hair regrows. Patients undergoing thoracic or lumbar spine surgery may not need to be shaved. If a bone graft from the hip will be taken for spinal fusion, that area must be prepped as well as the spinal incision area.

Many neurosurgeons mark the incision line with a marking pen or a marking solution and wooden stick. If a marking solution is used, indigo carmine, gentian violet, or brilliant green is recommended. Methylene blue should never be present in a neurosurgical OR because it produces an inflammatory reaction in CNS tissue.

Draping

In neurosurgical procedures, the right or left side of the head and the level of the spine must be specified. The surgical team should also check that the marking (initials) made to the surgical site in the holding area is in the operative field.

Draping for some neurosurgery procedures is complex and requires the cooperation of the surgeon, assistant, and scrub person. Four or more towels are placed around the operative site. They may be secured by disposable skin staples, small towel clips, or silk sutures on a cutting needle.

Draping for a craniotomy is challenging. If a minimal shave was done, an adhesive drape with staples placed around the shaved area near the incision can help to keep hair out of the incision. Towels can be contoured to the prepped area of the head and held in place with staples, leaving the operative site exposed. A craniotomy drape can then be placed over the towels. A sterile drainage bag below the incision will help to catch irrigation and blood and drain it into a suction canister. If a stereotactic head frame is used, the team confirms that the drapes do not interfere with the head frame attachments.

Prepping a hip graft incision site may need to be done with spinal fusion surgery. Two areas may need to be prepped and squared off with towels, which can be held in place with an adhesive drape. A partially unfolded three-quarters drape can be placed between the two planned incision sites before the universal or laparotomy drape is placed. A clamp can be placed over the prepped hip area to positively identify it. The drape can be cut over the prepped area, being sure not to cut an area of the drape that covers a nonsterile area. A second adhesive drape can hold the cut drape in place (see Chapter 4 for general draping procedures).

Hemostasis and Visualization

A few minutes before making the incision, the surgeon may inject the incision site with a local anesthetic agent, such as lidocaine or bupivacaine. Lidocaine has a more rapid onset and shorter duration of action than bupivacaine. Along with decreasing the effect of the stimulus of the skin incision, infiltration of the solution will apply pressure within the tissues and decrease bleeding at the time of incision. Using a local anesthetic that also contains epinephrine will constrict blood vessels to further minimize bleeding.

Meticulous hemostasis is particularly important in neurosurgery. Many methods are used to limit blood loss. A major consideration is control of hemorrhage from the highly vascular scalp. Skin edges along the wound are compressed with gauze sponges and fingers during the initial incision. Usually, this is followed by application of disposable scalp clips (Fig. 21.39). An automatic clip gun may be used to apply clips to include the galea and skin edge. The clips limit bleeding by applying pressure to the scalp edges. They remain

in place until closure. Placement of self-retaining retractors also helps control bleeding of the scalp.

Retraction is required for visualization. Self-retaining retractors such as cerebellar or Gelpi retractors can be used to retract skin, subcutaneous tissue, muscle, or the scalp. Suture can be used to retract the scalp or the dura of the brain or spinal cord. Blunt, malleable retractors are used on brain tissue. Table-mounted self-retaining retractor systems, such as the Greenberg, help the surgeon to see deep into the brain and may be used with a microscope.

Electrosurgery is routine for neurosurgical procedures. Perioperative nurses must understand the uses and hazards of the ESU and be familiar with the safety measures. Electrocoagulation current seals the blood vessels. To be effective the electrocoagulating current must contact the vessel in a dry field. For this reason, suctioning is necessary to remove blood as the contact is made between the instrument carrying the current and the bleeding point. A monopolar current is used to cut and coagulate tissue. It can be applied to forceps, a metal suction tip, or another instrument, which acts as a conducting tool. Monopolar electrosurgery is safe to use on the epidermis, dermis, galea, periosteum, muscle, and bone. It is used extensively for exposure of the posterior spine.

Bipolar ESUs provide a completely isolated output with negligible leakage of current between the tips of the forceps, permitting use of electrocoagulating current in proximity to structures where ordinary monopolar electrocoagulation would be hazardous (Fig. 21.40). It is safe to use the bipolar ESU to control bleeding on the dura of the brain and spinal cord and near vital nerves and vessels. The bipolar ESU can be used to maintain hemostasis and to dissect tissue in the brain. Ringer's or normal saline solution irrigation is often used during bipolar electrocoagulation to minimize tissue heating, shrinkage, drying, and adherence to the forceps. Some bipolar units have built-in irrigating systems. The use of the bipolar electrocoagulation technique allows hemostasis of almost any size vessel encountered.

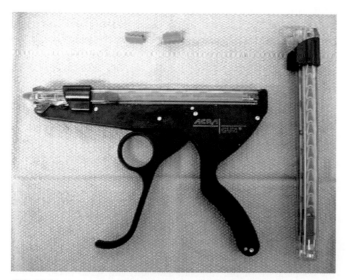

FIG. 21.39 Automatic clip gun, with disposable scalp clips and cartridge.

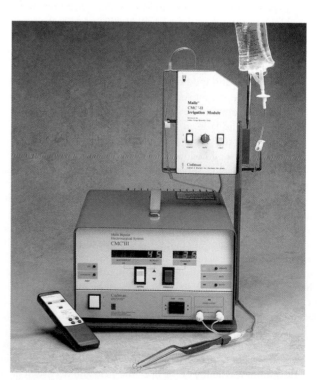

FIG. 21.40 Malis bipolar coagulator and bipolar cutter, with irrigation module.

Vessels as large as the superficial temporal artery, as well as those too small for suture or clip ligation, may be coagulated with bipolar units.

Suction is necessary to evacuate blood, CSF, and irrigation solution from the surgical site. Metal suction tips in multiple sizes, such as the Sachs, Frazier, and Adson, are used not only because they keep the wound dry but also because they can conduct electrocoagulation current from a monopolar unit to the bleeding point. Suction applied directly on normal neural tissue may be harmful and is avoided. Instead, a moistened cottonoid pattie may be placed between the suction tip and neural tissue for protection. Suction can be used to aspirate necrotic or traumatized brain tissue or soft brain tumors after a sample has been obtained for pathologic examination. It is also useful in evacuating abscess cavities, removing fluid from a ventricle or the subarachnoid space, holding a solid tumor during its removal, and applying compression to a bleeding vessel.

Bone wax is a hemostatic material that should be available for all cranial and spinal cord operations. Bone wax may be applied with the surgeon's fingertip or with the tip of an instrument such as a Freer or Penfield elevator. The surgeon firmly rubs or packs the wax into the bleeding surfaces of bone. Bone wax is commonly used in burr holes, along the edges of a craniotomy, and on the cut edges of the spine.

Soft goods (e.g., gauze sponges) are used to control bleeding before the skull or spinal canal is entered; however, they are coarse and can injure fragile tissues such as the brain and spinal cord. Instead, compressed, absorbent patties made of rayon or cotton (cottonoids) are used to control bleeding beneath the skull and around the spinal cord. Patties are also placed over delicate neural tissue for protection. It is far less traumatic to suction through a pattie than directly on the tissue. Patties are available in a variety of sizes, in both squares and strips, ranging from 4 to 6 inches long and from $\frac{1}{4}$- to 1-inch wide (Fig. 21.41). A supply of various sizes is typically moistened with irrigation solution or thrombin and offered to the surgeon on a waterproof surface. Patties have x-ray–detectable markers and strings attached and are included in the standard soft goods count.

Cotton balls moistened with irrigation solution or thrombin may be used as a temporary pack or tamponade in a bleeding tumor bed after a tumor has been removed. The gentle pressure of the cotton balls along with time and patience on the part of the surgeon may stop bleeding not controllable by other means. Cotton balls also have x-ray–detectable strings and are included in the soft goods count.

A variety of hemostatic clips are available and used by neurosurgeons to occlude both superficial and deep vessels. Unlike clips that were used in the past, hemoclips and Ligaclips are made of an alloy that is compatible with the MRI scanner. The scrub person removes the clips from a special cartridge with the appropriate applicator and passes them to the surgeon for application to a vessel. Such clips enable the surgeon to occlude vessels in areas difficult to reach by other means and to ligate superficial vessels of the brain before cutting them and without destroying any surrounding tissues. Clips are available in a variety of sizes. Numerous types of special clips are used for permanent or temporary occlusion of vessels or an aneurysm neck in the surgical treatment of an intracranial aneurysm (Fig. 21.42).

Neurosurgeons almost routinely use certain hemostatic agents in addition to mechanical hemostasis (Surgical Pharmacology). An absorbable gelatin sponge (Gelfoam) can be applied to an oozing surface, either dry or saturated with irrigation solution or topical thrombin. Larger pieces can be cut into a variety of sizes of strips and squares. Gelfoam is often followed by a pattie, which enables the surgeon to maneuver and compress it once it is in the surgical site. Gelfoam is absorbable and can be left in the body.

Oxidized regenerated cellulose is available in two forms: a rayon-like gauze (Surgicel) and a cotton-like form (Fibrillar). These are also absorbable hemostatic agents that are used to control bleeding from oozing surfaces, vessels, and sinuses in the brain. These hemostatic substances are presented in various sizes and shapes and are offered to the surgeon dry. The hemostatic material adheres to the bleeding area with gentle pressure.

Thrombin is a drug that can be topically applied to bleeding surfaces to achieve hemostasis. Typically, Gelfoam or patties are saturated with thrombin and placed on the oozing surface.

Irrigating the wound helps the surgeon identify active bleeding points and may facilitate hemostasis. A syringe with an angiocatheter tip may be used to deliver irrigation for microsurgery. Many neurosurgeons irrigate surgical wounds with an antibiotic solution before wound closure. The antibiotic is mixed with irrigation solution according to the surgeon's preference so that it is ready for use when needed.

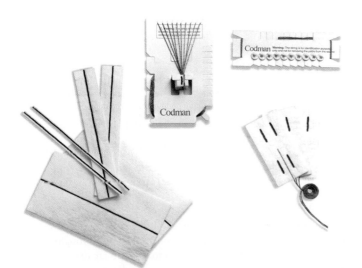

FIG. 21.41 Cottonoid patties.

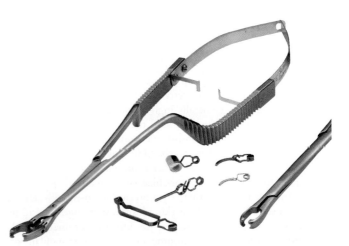

FIG. 21.42 Standard aneurysm clips and appliers.

Hemostatic Agents

Achieving hemostasis in delicate areas can be a challenge for the neurosurgeon. In addition to using meticulous technique to prevent bleeding, topical agents are routinely used as an adjunct to hemostasis. The perioperative nurse must be familiar with the agents used in this setting.

Medication/Category	Dosage/Route	Purpose/Action	Adverse Reactions	Nursing Implications
Topical thrombin/hemostatic agent	Bovine-derived thrombin: 1000- to 2000 units/mL applied directly to the source of bleeding or in conjunction with absorbable gelatin sponges	Catalyzes conversion of fibrinogen to fibrin	May cause fever or allergic-type reactions	Product is for external use only; not for intravenous use
Gelatin matrix (FloSeal)/hemostatic agent	Gelatin matrix granules and topical thrombin packaged as a kit with syringes and mixing bowl. Available in 5- and 10-mL kits. FloSeal is applied directly to the source of bleeding	Matrix particles form a composite clot that seals bleeding site; thrombin component converts fibrinogen in patient's blood to fibrin	Anemia, atrial fibrillation, infection	Product reaches maximum expansion at approximately 10 min. Excess product should be removed with gentle irrigation. Not for intravascular use
Absorbable gelatin sponge (Gelfoam)/hemostatic agent	Film, powder, and compressed sponge forms. Can be cut to the desired size and used directly at the site of bleeding	Absorbs and holds blood and fluid within its interstices; exerts physical hemostatic effect	Local infection and abscess formation	Should not be used in closure of skin incisions because it may interfere with healing of skin edges. Often moistened with saline or topical thrombin before use
Collagen hemostat (Avitene, Helistat, Instat)/hemostatic agent	Available in powder, sheets, or sponges. Powder is available in 0.5-, 1-, and 5-g containers. Applied directly to the site of bleeding	When in contact with a bleeding surface, attracts platelets that aggregate into thrombi, initiating formation of a physiologic platelet plug	Adhesion formation, allergic reaction, foreign-body reaction, inflammation, potentiation of infection	Apply dry. Excess material should be removed with irrigation and suction
Oxidized regenerated cellulose (Surgicel)/hemostatic agent	Fibrous, knitted, or sheer weave fabric. Can be cut to the desired size and used directly at the site of bleeding	Allows platelets and aggregates of thrombin and particulate blood elements to cling and form a coagulum that can act as a patch	Encapsulation of fluid, foreign-body reactions	Store at room temperature

Modified from LexiComp (website). www.crlonline.com/crlsql/servlet/crlonline. (Accessed 8 October 2016); Baxter: *FloSeal package insert product information* (website). http://floseal.com/us/pdf/FLOSEAL_Needle-Free_10mL_IFU.pdf. (Accessed 8 October 2016); Pfizer: *Gelfoam package insert product information* (website), 2012. www.pfizer.com/files/products/uspi_gelfoam_plus.pdf. (Accessed 8 October 2016). FDA: *Thrombin product information* (website). https://www.fda.gov/ucm/groups/fdagov-public/@fdagov-bio-gen/documents/document/ucm256531.pdf. (Accessed 26 September 2017); Bard: *Avitene product information* (website). https://www.scribd.com/document/316967453/avitene-microfibrillar-collagen-hemostat-product-brochure-pdf. (Accessed 26 September 2017).

Suture

Required suture will vary according to the surgery, the condition of the wound and patient, and the surgeon's preference. Suture can be used for retraction of the scalp for a craniotomy flap. Dura of the brain and spinal cord may be retracted, tacked up, and closed with braided nylon suture. Generally high tensile strength is needed for closure of the galea of the scalp and the fascia and subcutaneous tissue of the back. Braided, absorbable suture can be used in interrupted stitches to close these layers. Skin may be closed with subcuticular absorbable suture, with either a continuous or an interrupted suturing technique using a monofilament, nonabsorbable suture material such as nylon; alternatively, skin can be closed with staples. Whatever technique is used for skin closure, skin edges should be everted. A drain may be secured to the skin with a nonabsorbable suture such as nylon. In an environment of infection, monofilament, nonabsorbable suture is preferred.

Dressings

Applying dressings to wounds on the head is challenging, especially if a minimal shave was done. For larger incisions in particular, a head wrap can be the best alternative. A wrap helps keep the nonadherent dressing in place over the incision site and provides compression to prevent the formation of a postoperative hematoma. A smaller dressing can sometimes be held in place with a transparent dressing or tape. Applying a liquid adhesive to the skin before application of the dressing can help to hold it in place.

Evaluation

The identified outcomes from the established nursing diagnoses and interventions are evaluated on an ongoing basis throughout the perioperative period, and adjustments to the plan are made as necessary. Before leaving the OR, the nurse assesses the patient's postoperative skin integrity and performs a postoperative neurologic assessment for comparison with the preoperative assessment. In addition, the patient's outcomes from the identified nursing diagnoses are evaluated. If the outcomes were met, they may be communicated as follows:

- The patient expressed feeling less anxious, coped with perioperative routines adequately, and verbalized an understanding of the planned procedure or procedures.
- The patient or family verbalized knowledge of diagnostic and surgical procedures and had realistic expectations of tests, routines, and postoperative care.
- The patient maintained effective breathing patterns; ventilation was maintained, ABGs were within normal limits, and breath sounds were bilateral.
- The patient will continue to maintain a normal body temperature or undergo rewarming.
- The patient exhibited no signs and symptoms of pressure injury; sensation and motion were the same as preoperative functional levels; and respiratory status and blood pressure were maintained within expected parameters.

After the surgical procedure is completed, the team transports the patient to the intensive care unit (ICU) or postanesthesia care unit (PACU). The perioperative nurse provides the intraoperative documentation and a verbal report to the nurse receiving the patient.

Patient, Family, and Caregiver Education and Discharge Planning

Patient, family, and caregiver education is the key to helping the patient return to his or her optimal quality of life. As soon as the need for surgery is identified, a multidimensional education program should begin and include the patient's family. Teaching should address the psychosocial as well as the physiologic aspects of the patient's life. The plan should offer opportunities for the patient to develop new skills, coping mechanisms, and behaviors to adapt to aspects of temporary or permanent neurologic deficit.

Neurosurgery patients may experience a variety of deficits involving vision, hearing, swallowing, speech, motor, sensation, and mental status. Depending on the patient's pathologic condition and surgery, other physicians may observe the patient postoperatively along with the neurosurgeon. Neurologists, ophthalmologists, endocrinologists, cardiologists, radiologists, oncologists, and infectious disease physicians may be involved with managing the medical care of neurosurgery patients. Rehabilitation, physical, occupational, and speech therapists are instrumental in the recovery of neurosurgery patients. They also teach the patients and their families how to cope with temporary and lifelong deficits and how to improve their quality of life. Some patients may benefit from time spent in a rehabilitation facility before returning home. Patients with severe alterations in neurologic function may require long-term care.

The nurse plays an important role in teaching patients and family members how to look for and recognize potential postoperative complications, such as changes in mental status or behavior, progressive weakness, seizure activity, increasing pain, and signs and symptoms of infection. Routine discharge instructions should include information about newly prescribed medications and their potential side effects in addition to treatment options for postoperative and chronic pain (Patient, Family, and Caregiver Education). The nurse should also ensure the patient has instructions for the use of cervical collars, braces for spinal stability, and wound dressing changes when applicable.

The entire healthcare team is responsible for planning the transition from the acute care center to the patient's home or to a skilled nursing or rehabilitation facility. The patient, family, and caregiver need to be involved in every aspect of the neurosurgery patient's care and should be encouraged to ask questions and voice their concerns and opinions.

Surgical Interventions

Minimally Invasive and Specialized Neurosurgery Techniques

Microneurosurgery

Adaptation of the operating microscope for neurosurgery has resulted in improvement of many neurosurgical procedures and made new procedures possible. For years, neurosurgeons have worn magnifying loupes to see small structures. Loupes usually have a magnification of 2× or 3.5×. The microscope has a variety of magnifications ranging from 6× to 40×, providing flexibility and precision. The coaxial illumination overcomes the difficulties of lighting neurosurgical wounds.

Use of the microscope restricts the surgeon's field of vision and mobility; therefore the scrub person and surgical assistant must be actively engaged in the procedure and must be proficient. The operative field, unless video monitoring is available, cannot be seen. Surgical personnel must understand the surgical procedure and the corresponding anatomy, know the names and uses of all microinstruments, and be proficient at passing the instruments to the surgeon without delay. Each time the surgeon must look away and then back to the surgical field, open wound time and anesthesia time are increased while the surgeon becomes reoriented to the field. Therefore the assistance the scrub person gives the surgeon saves time and directly benefits the patient.

Microsurgical instruments have been modified and adapted to the requirements of neurosurgery. These instruments often possess the following characteristics: bayonet shape, so that the surgeon's hand remains outside the line of vision and the beam of the microscope light; finely sprung and fluted grip; long length for access to deep structures; and slender and delicate tips that occupy as little space as possible. Microneurosurgical instruments are expensive and fragile. Instructions for handling, cleaning, sterilizing, and storing these instruments should be followed. An instrument that is sprung, bent, dulled, hooked, or in any way damaged must never be handed to a surgeon for use but must be repaired or replaced. Instruments must be kept free from blood and tissue during use because the microscope also magnifies debris on the instruments, occluding the structure the surgeon is about to approach. Very fine microsutures are available.

Microsurgical techniques have been applied to cranial, spinal, and peripheral nerve operations. Some procedures in which microsurgery is of value are explorations of the posterior fossa, especially for tumors of the fourth ventricle or cerebellopontine angle, and removal of small acoustic neuromas, with resulting preservation of the facial nerve. Small-vessel endarterectomy, cerebral arterial bypass, cerebral aneurysm clipping, and excision of AVMs are performed using the microscope for visualization of the surgical site. Microsurgery also has advantages in the treatment of tumors and AVMs of the spinal cord.

Neuroendoscopy

Neuroendoscopy is a rapidly evolving field of minimally invasive surgery, where the goal is to minimize collateral damage without compromising the intended goal of surgery. The endoscope provides illumination and magnification of structures and an extended viewing

PATIENT, FAMILY, AND CAREGIVER EDUCATION

Discharge Planning for Spinal Surgery

When discharging patients, the nurse ensures that all postoperative instructions are clear and legible, including contact numbers for the surgeon and facility. The nurse should reinforce all written instructions, and ask the patient and caregivers to verbalize and demonstrate a clear understanding of the instructions.

Home Care
- Stress the importance of follow-up care. Advise patients when to schedule a follow-up appointment with the surgeon, and when to begin physical therapy.
- Review the signs or symptoms of infection that warrant immediate notification to the surgeon. They include a temperature of 101°F (38°C) or greater; increased swelling, redness, or tenderness around the incision site; and any drainage originating from the incision.
- Instruct the patient to seek immediate medical attention if he or she experiences the onset of a sudden and/or severe headache, weakness of the extremities, or changes in bowel or bladder function.

Wound Care
- Ensure that patients and caregivers are instructed on proper cleaning, inspecting, and dressing of the wound. Assure them that a small amount of swelling is normal and should continually decrease. Instruct patients to avoid soaking the wound, to shower only when cleared by the surgeon, and to discontinue the use of any lotions or oils on or near the incision site.
- Educate patients on the risk factors that contribute to delayed wound healing such as smoking, obesity, advanced age, diabetes, chronic steroid use, and malnutrition.

Activity
- Encourage walking and stair climbing as directed by the surgeon. Activity tolerance is generally patient specific and should be personalized as necessary.

- Review typical activity restrictions, such as prolonged travel or driving, sitting for longer than 30 minutes at a time, occupational limitations, strenuous exercise, lifting more than 10 pounds, and bending or twisting at the waist.

Pain Management
- Discuss how much pain, soreness, and stiffness are expected and the importance of contacting the surgeon if the pain is excessive. Over several months, back and leg pain should decrease, depending on the severity of pain preoperatively.
- Review all prescriptions and proper dosing. Discuss which over-the-counter medications, such as acetaminophen, are appropriate. Advise patients that the use of aspirin and NSAIDs, such as ibuprofen, may not be indicated for several weeks because they can cause bleeding.
- Offer pain-reducing activities, such as exercise, and relaxation techniques.

Diet
- Provide education for proper nutrition to promote wound healing.
- Encourage fluids, fruits, and fiber to help prevent constipation.

Special Instructions and Follow-Up Care
- Provide instructions for use of any braces or supports. Generally a brace should be worn at all times, except when showering and sleeping, until told otherwise by the surgeon.
- Advise patients to resume all preoperative medications unless otherwise noted.
- Provide prescriptions for new x-rays, CT scans, and MRIs according to the physician's orders.
- Discuss smoking cessation when appropriate. Stress the connection between smoking and delayed wound healing, and offer resources for smoking cessation.

CT, Computed tomography; *MRI,* magnetic resonance imaging; *NSAIDs,* nonsteroidal antiinflammatory drugs.
Modified from Albert T et al: *Discharge instructions for lumbar fusion surgery* (website). www.spineuniverse.com/treatments/surgery/lumbar/discharge-instructions-lumbar-fusion-surgery. (Accessed 9 October 2016).

angle. The surgical team must be prepared to convert from a neuroendovascular procedure to an open procedure if it is determined that the surgery cannot be successfully completed endoscopically.

Indications for neuroendoscopic surgery are many. Endoscopic tumor removal or CSF diversion through endoscopic fenestration, such as a third ventriculostomy, can be done for the treatment of hydrocephalus and can eliminate the need for a shunt. Interventricular tumors may be removed endoscopically. In addition, the endoscope can be used to assess adequacy of tumor removal and to identify tumor portions left behind or adherent to vital structures. Stereotactic and image-guided surgery (IGS) is often used with neuroendoscopy successfully. The endoscope is commonly used in the transsphenoidal approach for pituitary and sellar tumor resection (possibly in collaboration with an otolaryngology surgeon), for microvascular decompression, and for endoscopic biopsy of a lesion.

Endovascular Procedures

Several neurovascular disorders are amenable to endovascular intervention. The endoscopic approach is considered minimally invasive; therefore it is a reasonable option for patients who are not candidates for open surgical procedures because of age, health status, medical condition, or location of the lesion. Interventional neuroradiology uses fluoroscopy to gain access to the intracranial circulation by way of a percutaneous transfemoral catheter.

The endovascular approach to the treatment of both ruptured and unruptured cerebral aneurysms is endosaccular occlusion (Evidence for Practice). This is an excellent technique for aneurysms that are complex, have a neck that is too short for clipping, or are difficult to reach via traditional craniotomy.

Although surgical excision is still the standard treatment for intracranial AVM, surgical morbidity may be decreased by using endovascular embolization preoperatively in select cases. A specialized microcatheter is guided directly into the AVM via angiography. The abnormal blood vessels in the AVM are occluded from the inside by means of embolization. Several materials are used to cause embolization, including fibered titanium coils, polyvinyl alcohol particles, and fast-drying biologically inert glues. The AVM may effectively be devascularized and reduced in size through endovascular

Surgical/Endovascular Treatment of Ruptured Aneurysms

The Stroke Council of the AHA has formulated the following recommendations for the surgical/endovascular treatment of ruptured aneurysms:

- Endovascular coil occlusion of the aneurysm is appropriate if the aneurysm is deemed treatable by either endovascular coiling or surgical clipping.
- Reasonable consideration of the individual characteristics of the patient and aneurysm must be used in deciding the best means of repair.
- The patient should be managed in a surgery center offering both techniques.
- Either procedure should be performed to reduce the risk of rebleeding after the initial aneurysmal SAH.

Clipping

The surgeon performs a craniotomy (opening of a portion of the skull) and separates the aneurysm from the surrounding tissue. A small titanium clip, whose features are similar to those of a clothespin, is then placed across the base of the aneurysm. Once the clip is secured, blood can no longer enter or exit the aneurysm sac. The procedure is ideally performed within 72 hours of diagnosis. It is important to note that after rupture there is a 40% chance of death and 80% chance of disability. Early detection and treatment offer the best chances of survival.

Coiling

Also known as endovascular therapy, coiling is a less invasive treatment option. Especially for those patients who are in poor health, surgical intervention may pose a greater threat than the aneurysm itself. Coiling has proven to be a safe alternative to the traditional treatment of a craniotomy. This procedure does not involve opening of the skull, and is performed from inside the blood vessel. The radiologist inserts a catheter into the patient's groin, and guides it up toward the brain under fluoroscopy. A wire is then threaded into the catheter and directed into the aneurysm. Once inside the aneurysm the wire twists into small coils and continues filling the aneurysm sac until eventually the aneurysm is occluded (Ringer, 2016).

Previous studies, such as the ISAT in 2007, found that patients who were initial candidates for both types of procedures had better outcomes 1 year after endovascular coiling as opposed to surgical clipping. This study was, however, limited to only ruptured aneurysms (Ringer, 2016).

AHA, American Heart Association; *ISAT,* International Subarachnoid Aneurysm Trial; *SAH,* subarachnoid hemorrhage.
Modified from Mirza FA, Fraser AF: Subarachnoid hemorrhage. In Ferri FF, editors: *Ferri's clinical advisor 2017,* ed 1, Philadelphia, 2017, Elsevier; Ringer A: *Aneurysm embolization: coiling* (website), 2016. www.mayfieldclinic.com/PE-Coiling.htm. (Accessed 28 November 2016); Zuccarello M, Ringer A: *Aneurysm surgery: clipping* (website), 2016. www.mayfieldclinic.com/PE-clipping.htm. (Accessed 28 November 2016).

embolization, and when combined with microsurgery or stereotactic radiosurgery, the AVM may be completely eradicated.

Endovascular embolization is also advantageous when used as a preoperative treatment for select intracranial tumor resections. Highly vascular tumors, as well as tumors that are inopportunely positioned, can be devascularized using techniques similar to those used in the treatment of AVMs, decreasing blood loss and risk of hemorrhage during resection.

Intracranial stenosis has been deemed a high-risk disease in need of alternative therapies. Successful use of balloon angioplasty has been documented in mostly academic, high-volume centers, performed by highly skilled and experienced physicians. Although the results are encouraging, the technically demanding nature of the procedures carries substantial risk. The Wingspan stent has been approved by the US Food and Drug Administration (FDA) to treat symptomatic patients with intracranial stenosis greater than 50% that is refractory to medical therapies. The stent is implanted using the Wingspan technique. After balloon angioplasty, the radiologist inserts a self-expanding nitinol stent across the atherosclerotic lesion in the brain. Although the Wingspan system appears to be a viable treatment option, a high rate of restenosis has been reported, and its value is not yet firmly established. Continued studies show varying rates of restenosis and complications. The largest study to test its efficacy versus aggressive medical management was halted because of high rates of stroke and mortality in the stent cohort (Walker, 2012).

Intra-arterial thrombolysis for the treatment of acute ischemic stroke is a consideration for patients who have missed the 3-hour window for therapeutic IV thrombolysis. The endovascular route is used to deliver a high concentration of a thrombolytic agent directly to the site of the offending thrombus in combination with mechanical clot extraction. Intra-arterial thrombolysis is still being studied for its long-term value. It is recommended for selected patients with major ischemic stroke of less than 6 hours' duration caused by occlusion to the middle cerebral artery, and those who are being treated at hospitals with appropriate facilities (Biller et al., 2016).

Mechanical clot extraction is an endovascular technique that may be used alone or in conjunction with intra-arterial thrombolysis. Success rates are improved when both modalities are used. A typical retrieval device consists of a coil that is delivered to the thrombus site via endovascular microcatheter and screwed into the clot like a corkscrew to extract the clot. Mechanical clot extraction shows its best use for cerebral arteries demonstrating large or irregularly shaped clot burdens. Early generation devices have not been shown to improve clinical outcomes; however, newer generation devices have showed improved efficacy when used within 6 hours of onset. Further studies are currently under way (Kidwell and Jahan, 2015).

Stereotactic Radiosurgery

In stereotactic radiosurgery, stereotactic localization is coupled with delivery of ionizing radiation to destroy a lesion in the brain. Radiosurgery is technically noninvasive and has a low associated morbidity. The use of radiosurgery has increased, and success of treatment has improved with advancements in neuroimaging (CT and MRI) and computer technology. The goal of radiosurgery is to obliterate a relatively small intracranial target with a high irradiation dose while sparing adjacent and distant tissues. Radiosurgical instruments include the Gamma Knife, the Novalis, and the CyberKnife. With any of these techniques, using a stereotactic head frame along with the radiation delivery system allows for great precision (Baehring and Hochberg, 2016).

Radiosurgery can be used to treat AVMs, tumors, and trigeminal neuralgia. Best results are achieved for lesions smaller than 35 mm. Larger lesions or lesions involving or near cranial nerves can be successfully treated with a fractionated approach in which the radiation is precisely delivered in small daily fractions. This technique, called fractionated stereotactic radiotherapy (FSR), has been particularly useful for preserving vision and hearing. Patients with larger lesions often have symptoms of mass effect that are generally not improved with radiosurgery. Radiosurgery and FSR techniques have successfully sterilized a variety of intracranial lesions often with far less morbidity than a surgical approach (Robotic-Assisted Surgery).

ROBOTIC-ASSISTED SURGERY

Seizure Mapping and Deep Brain Stimulator

Although robotics have been around in surgery for some time, it is an emerging technology in neurosurgery. Minimally invasive techniques have been used for craniotomies and spinal surgery since the 1990s. Robotic technology (Renishaw Neuromate) is now being used for seizure-mapping surgery, deep brain stimulation, and brain biopsy procedures.

Before surgery, the patient undergoes a head CT with 2-D or 3-D imaging, MRI, and appropriate lab work. The day of surgery, members of the surgical team apply a stereotactic head frame under local anesthetic. The patient is then sent for a head CT with the stereotactic head frame in place. The radiology department and anesthesia providers should be made aware of the stereotactic head frame placement because this may alter their care plan. The neurosurgical team will map out placement of the EEG leads, deep brain stimulator lead, or biopsy entry location before the start of the procedure. Positioning is supine or lateral depending on the operative location. After the patient is positioned and the robot is locked in place, it is imperative that the patient or patient bed is not moved because the head frame is typically locked into place with the robot. Surgical tools needed may include a power drill, specialized trocars, guidewires, depth gauge, and anchor bolts. Electrocoagulation and suction may or may not be necessary because this is a minimally invasive procedure. After electrodes have been placed via the robot arm, electrode placement is confirmed via intraoperative 2-D or 3-D imaging. The deep brain stimulator battery is placed after placement is confirmed. Patients with EEG electrodes are sent to be monitored for seizure activity, typically while remaining in the hospital.

The role of robotics in neurosurgery is expanding throughout the world. Use of the robot for stereoelectroencephalography has been proven to be precise and safe for the placement of EEG leads for brain mapping.

EEG, Electroencephalography.
Modified from Cardinale F et al: Stereoelectroencephalography: surgical methodology, safety, and stereotactic application accuracy in 500 patients, *Neurosurgery* 72(3):353–366, 2013; Renishaw: *Neuromate stereotactic robot* (website), 2016. www.renishaw.com/en/neuromate-stereotactic-robot--10712. (Accessed 29 October 2016).

RESEARCH HIGHLIGHT

Deep Brain Stimulation for the Treatment of Parkinson Disease: Awake Versus Asleep

PD is defined as a progressive neurodegenerative disorder of unknown origin that is characterized by rigidity, tremors, postural instability, and bradykinesia. PD is an age-related disease, showing a gradual increase in prevalence beginning after age 50, with a steep increase in prevalence after age 60. Disease before 30 years of age is rare and often suggests a hereditary form of parkinsonism. Dopamine agonists appear to be the drug of choice to treat the disease in younger populations (between 40 and 70 years old). Over the age of 70, levodopa remains the gold standard. For those patients who remain responsive to levodopa, but experience a wearing off the drug's effects too quickly, or experience severe motor fluctuations, DBS may be a surgical option. DBS for PD has traditionally been performed in awake patients. Some patients are unable to tolerate awake surgery or extensive time off their medication to allow for neurophysiologic testing during traditional DBS implantation, which has previously limited surgical options for these patients. Recently, asleep image-guided lead placement using intraoperative MRI or CT for verification has been proposed as an alternative for patients unable or unwilling to undergo awake DBS surgery.

In 2015, the University of Wisconsin School of Medicine and Public Health conducted a retrospective chart review comparing PD patients who underwent asleep MRI-guided STN DBS lead placement (n = 14) and awake neurophysiologically guided STN DBS lead placement (n = 23). Both groups' LEDDs and complications at approximately 6 months of follow-up were compared, along with operative times. Both groups showed statistically similar reductions in LEDD at 6 months of therapy (38.27% for awake, 49.27% for asleep) and similar complications. Operative times were initially longer for MRI-guided DBS but improved with surgical experience. Asleep MRI-guided DBS placement is a new and viable option for PD patients unable or unwilling to undergo awake placement, with similar results in terms of LEDD reduction and complications.

DBS, Deep brain stimulation; LEDD, levodopa equivalent daily dose; PD, Parkinson disease; STN, subthalamic nucleus.
Modified from Saleh S et al: Awake neurophysiologically guided versus asleep MRI-guided STN DBS for Parkinson disease: a comparison of outcomes using levodopa equivalents, *Stereotact Funct Neurosurg* 93(6):419–426, 2015; Jankovic J: Parkinson disease and other movement disorders. In Daroff RB et al, editors: *Bradley's neurology in clinical practice*, ed 7, Philadelphia, 2016, Saunders.

Stereotactic Procedures

The goal of stereotactic surgery is to target a point or volume in three-dimensional space (Ortega-Barnett et al., 2017). This is accomplished with coordinate systems that provide a constant frame of reference. Radiographic modalities (CT, MRI) are used to navigate three dimensionally and locate and destroy target structures. Predetermined anatomic landmarks are used as guides.

Originally, special head-fixation devices were developed for stereotactic brain surgery (see Fig. 21.35). Since the early 2000s, frameless systems have surpassed frame-based techniques in popularity and versatility. These systems use fiducial markers that either affix temporarily to the skin or are implanted into the outer table of the skull, eliminating the need to mount a frame on the patient's head. These markers are visible on the imaging modality being used.

Both frame-based and frameless stereotactic systems use radiography, fluoroscopy, CT scans, or MRI to permit accurate placement of a probe directed at the target area. The preoperative images are aligned to the patient's head during surgery so that the surgeon has a better idea of the target area. Certain frame-based and frameless surgeries may performed with the assistance of a robot

(see Robotic-Assisted Surgery box). These include placement of depth electrodes for seizure mapping, deep brain stimulation, and biopsy.

The many common applications for cranial stereotactic surgery include craniotomies, transsphenoidal approaches, endoscopic surgery, needle biopsies, and therapeutic aspiration. It is also used for catheter placement and third ventriculostomy surgery. Spinal stereotactic surgery is used for screw placement and spinal cord lesions. Common target areas for the stereotactic approach include tumors, infectious lesions, vascular malformations, the basal ganglia, the thalamus, and anterolateral spinal tracts. Target areas can undergo biopsy, be destroyed by chemical or mechanical means, or be electrically stimulated (Research Highlight). Stereotactic procedures are also done to place electrodes in various regions of the brain to determine the site of origin of seizures.

For treatment of metastatic and primary tumors refractory to other treatments, or small tumors in difficult locations, a newly

FDA-approved device is being used intraoperatively. This procedure is called intraoperative MRI-guided laser interstitial thermocoagulation therapy (LITT). This procedure is done via a burr hole and laser probe. The laser probe is directly applied to tumor tissue in the brain, and high-intensity laser energy is administered to destroy tumor tissue (Baehring and Hochberg, 2016).

Procedural Considerations

As in most IGS, carts with a monitor and computer, along with accessory equipment and supplies, are required. A variety of stereotactic frame systems are available. The nurse must be familiar with the system in place at his or her institution. Frameless stereotactic surgery triggered a new era in surgical navigation and information delivery. This technology provides three-dimensional visualization of anatomic features with real-time localization information (see Fig. 21.36).

Operative Procedure

1. The surgeon places the patient's head into a halo head frame with a stereotactic cage before the surgery (framed stereotaxy). Alternatively, fiducials are placed on the patient's skull (frameless stereotaxy).
2. The patient is then transported for a CT or MRI scan of the brain. The target is identified, and computer coordinates are determined and recorded.
3. After the scan the nurse takes the patient to the OR with the frame or fiducials left in place. The stereotactic coordinates are registered or entered into the computer, and the surgeon performs the procedure through a burr hole. The stereotactic probe is guided by the computer, directing the surgical approach and trajectory (see Fig. 21.35).
4. The surgeon may introduce hollow cannulae, coagulating electrodes, cryosurgical probes, wire loops, and other lesion-producing or biopsy instruments through the burr hole for the destruction of areas in the brain. Temporary and permanent nerve-stimulator electrodes may also be introduced to augment the pain-control function of the CNS.

Surgical Approaches to the Brain

Burr Holes

A burr hole is the minimum exposure that can be made to gain access to the brain. Burr holes are necessary for many neurosurgical procedures. They are placed in the skull to remove a localized fluid collection secondary to head trauma that results in an epidural or subdural hematoma. A burr hole can be used to access the intracerebral ventricles for the following reasons: placement of a ventricular catheter to drain obstructed CSF; measurement of ICP; or establishment of a ventricular shunting system. Burr holes are often placed for many stereotactic procedures, such as stereotactic biopsy or placement of electrodes. Additionally, burr holes are also made before turning the bone flap in preparation for a craniotomy procedure.

Craniotomy

A craniotomy is the removal of a section of the cranium referred to as a bone flap. One or more burr holes are placed, and the dura is dissected away from the cranium. A craniotome with a dura guard attachment is used to excise a section of the cranium, exposing an area of the brain. The surgeon replaces the bone flap to its original location and secures it with wire or titanium plates and screws.

Multiple types of craniotomy incisions are used to expose different parts of the brain. Depending on the location of the pathologic condition, a craniotomy may be frontal, parietal, occipital, temporal, or a combination of two or more of these approaches. The pterional craniotomy is an extremely versatile approach to the anterior and middle fossae. It is useful to access lesions of the frontal or temporal lobes near the sylvian fissure or skull base. A craniotomy may be performed to evacuate intracranial hematomas not accessible through a burr hole, to control bleeding, to debulk or resect tumors, to excise or clip vascular lesions, to aspirate abscess formation, and to decompress cranial nerves.

When turning a scalp flap for a craniotomy, the surgeon may peel the scalp back off the pericranium. The surgeon elevates the bone flap with the overlying muscles still attached (osteoplastic) or strips the periosteum off the skull before the bone flap (free flap) is turned. The bone plate may be separated from the soft tissues, removed from the skull, and set aside for replacement at the end of the procedure. It is placed in an antibiotic solution and remains on the sterile field. The scrub person ensures that the bone flap stays separate from other items on the sterile field and alerts the perioperative circulating nurse and any relief scrub persons of its location to prevent it from being inadvertently discarded. If the bone is not separated from the soft tissues, it is reflected with the temporal muscle and soft tissues. If intracranial swelling is a major concern or the purpose for the craniotomy, the bone plate may not be replaced. If it is not replaced, it may be preserved by means of deep freezing, preservation in bactericidal solutions, sterilization, and preservation in a subgaleal pouch. A recent study found that the technique of storing the craniotomy graft in a subcutaneous location on the patient reduced graft devitalization and maintained the osteogenic viability (Singla et al., 2014).

Craniectomy

Craniectomy is the permanent removal of a section of the cranium using burrs and rongeurs to enlarge one or more burr holes. The surgeon performs a craniectomy to gain access to the underlying structures. This procedure may be required to remove tumors, hematomas, and infection of the bone. A suboccipital craniectomy, done with the patient in prone or lateral position, allows access to the posterior fossa. Titanium mesh may be used to repair the cranial defect. Craniectomy is also indicated as treatment for craniosynostosis in infants and young children. Severe head injuries with increased ICP can be treated with a craniectomy to give the brain room to swell.

Transsphenoidal Approach

The transsphenoidal route to the pituitary fossa is a less invasive means of removing tumors than the transcranial route. The approach can be performed via a small incision through the nose or through the gingiva under the upper lip. More recently, an endoscope has been used to assist with access through the sphenoid sinus into the pituitary fossa. Tumors of the parasellar region may also be accessed using this technique.

Surgery of the Brain and Cranium

Ventricular Catheter and Shunt Placement for Hydrocephalus

Hydrocephalus is a condition marked by an excessive accumulation of CSF resulting in dilation of the ventricular system (where CSF is manufactured and circulated) and increased ICP. Conditions that result in the development of hydrocephalus and CSF obstruction in both children and adults include congenital hydrocephalus, spina bifida, tumors, intracranial/intraventricular hemorrhage, aqueductal stenosis, and Chiari malformations. Hydrocephalus is treated by accessing the lateral ventricles for the insertion of a ventricle shunting system. The most commonly used methods to divert CSF from the ventricles are the externalized ventriculostomy catheter and the internalized VP shunt.

Placement of an externalized ventriculostomy catheter requires that a burr hole be made to access either the right or the left lateral ventricle. The ventricular catheter is passed into the ventricle. Flow of CSF is verified. The distal end of the catheter is tunneled beneath the scalp, posterior to the burr hole, externalized, and secured to the scalp with suture. The externalized end of the catheter is connected to an external drainage system, which allows for controlled CSF drainage and for ICP measurement. This system has allowed for temporary shunting in patients with elevated ICP and hydrocephalus from any cause. It is an invaluable adjunct in the clinical assessment and management of head trauma with increased ICP.

For more permanent control of hydrocephalus, an internalized ventricular shunt is placed. The type of shunt and the site of insertion are determined by the neurosurgeon. Three approaches for ventricular insertion are frontal, parietal, and occipital. Although the most common drainage site for an internalized shunting system is the peritoneum by way of open dissection or percutaneous trocar, there are other options. If drainage in the peritoneum is inappropriate because of infection or adhesions, other possible shunting techniques include ventriculovenous, ventriculoatrial, ventriculopleural, and lumboperitoneal (Badhiwala and Kulkami, 2017).

The VP shunt system components are a ventricular (proximal) catheter, a reservoir, a valve, and a peritoneal (distal) catheter. A unitized shunt has fewer separations and connections. The reservoir, if used, is inserted between the catheter and the valve. Access to the system through the reservoir enables the practitioner to assess the patency of the shunt, to obtain CSF for laboratory analysis, to introduce contrast medium for radiologic studies, and in some specific cases to inject medication into the shunt. The one-way valve system directs flow of CSF out of the ventricular system. Valves are available in a variety of different pressure and flow settings. Nonprogrammable valves and shunts are pressure controlled and open to release flow whenever the actual pressure exceeds the pressure that the valve is designed to open (the opening pressure). Some valves are flow controlled and attempt to maintain a constant flow despite pressure changes. Programmable valves and shunts allow adjustments to the opening pressure after the shunt is implanted, avoiding surgical procedures to change valves.

Procedural Considerations

The patient is placed in a modified supine position with a shoulder roll. The head is turned to the opposite side and supported on a donut. Hair is removed from the site in which the burr hole will be made to behind the ear and down to the neck. The burr hole site must be prepped, along with the neck, chest, and abdomen on the side of the shunt insertion.

The shunt unit should be handled with extreme care. As with all implantable devices, each manufacturer's specific instructions must be followed and care taken to keep the assembly free of lint or other foreign bodies that could cause a reaction in the patient's tissues. Lubricants are never used. Blood should be kept clear from the lumen of the catheter to prevent clotting and obstruction. The scrub person soaks the unit in normal saline and antibiotic solution and primes it at the surgeon's direction before implantation. Air trapping in the valve assembly should be avoided. The valve must be properly oriented to facilitate CSF flow from the ventricles to the peritoneum.

The surgeon may use an endoscope or stereotactic image-guided navigation system to locate small ventricles or to fenestrate the septum between ventricles, avoiding the need to place multiple ventricular catheters. Surgical technique for VP shunt placement is basically the same for adults and children (Fig. 21.43).

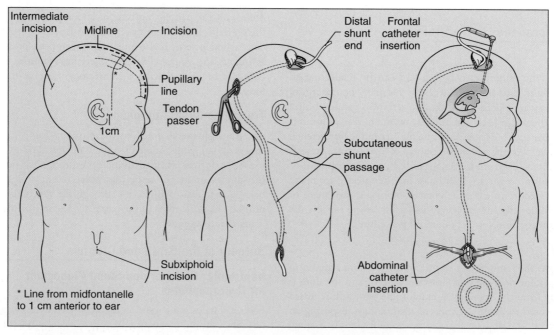

FIG. 21.43 Placement of a frontal ventriculoperitoneal shunt. The technique is similar for adult and pediatric patients. The patient is positioned, and coordinates are marked. The shunt is passed subcutaneously. The ventricular catheter and then the peritoneal catheter are inserted.

Operative Procedure

1. The surgeon makes a horseshoe-shaped incision to the right or left of midline, along the papillary line.
2. Scalp bleeding is controlled, and the skin flap is retracted.
3. The surgeon uses a periosteal elevator to clean the periosteum from the skull.
4. Next the surgeon uses a drill or cranial perforator to create a 1- to 2-cm burr hole. The dura is coagulated and incised. The surgeon uses the bipolar ESU to electrocoagulate the pia at the catheter insertion site.
5. The ventricular catheter with an introducer is inserted perpendicularly into the lateral ventricle approximately 4.5 cm in the infant and 6.5 cm in the adult. When the ventricle is penetrated, the surgeon removes the introducer, verifies the CSF flow, and attaches and secures the reservoir and valve with 2-0 silk ties.
6. A subcutaneous tunnel is created from the burr hole to a neck incision, where the peritoneal catheter is then connected.
7. The surgeon makes a subxiphoid or lateral abdominal incision and exposes the peritoneum.
8. Further tunneling is performed from the neck to the chest and abdomen, avoiding the nipples and umbilicus. The surgeon passes the catheter through the tunneling device to the abdominal incision. After spontaneous distal flow of CSF is verified, the distal end of the peritoneal catheter is passed into the peritoneal cavity, leaving enough length to allow for growth in the child and movement in the adult.
9. The catheter is secured to the peritoneum with a purse-string suture. All incisions are closed, with care taken not to puncture the shunt system with a suture needle.

Shunt failure can occur at any time, requiring any single portion of the shunt system or the entire system to be replaced. Obstruction, disconnection, malfunction, and infection are routine causes of shunt failure. Revising a shunt typically involves a troubleshooting process. Therefore it is best to prep and drape the patient to provide access to any and all portions of the shunt system. An infected shunt may be externalized until the infection is treated.

Evacuation of Epidural or Subdural Hematoma

After trauma, decompression of the brain, as well as removal and drainage of blood clots and collections of liquefied blood from above or beneath the dura mater, may be required. The need for hematoma evacuation is primarily determined by a declining neurologic status in the patient. Depending on the severity of the injury, evacuation can be accomplished through burr holes or a craniotomy. If elevated ICP is a major concern, the craniotomy plate may be temporarily removed from the skull to allow for swelling and prevention of brain herniation.

Operative Procedure: Burr Hole Placement for Evacuating a Hematoma

1. The surgeon makes at least two linear or small horseshoe incisions over the site of the lesion. Two or more burr holes are made.
2. The surgeon enlarges the burr hole with a Kerrison rongeur until adequate exposure is obtained.
3. If the hematoma is subdural, the surgeon incises the dura.
4. Clot and fluid are evacuated, and hemostasis is accomplished with the ESU or the use of hemostatic clips.
5. The surgeon irrigates through the burr holes using catheters or bulb syringes. Large amounts of irrigating solution are used until the return appears clear.

6. A drain or catheter may be inserted in the subdural or epidural space for postoperative drainage. Additional burr holes can be made as necessary during the course of the procedure to ensure complete evacuation.

Craniotomy

Procedural Considerations

Craniotomy is a technique for exposure of the brain to surgically treat intracranial disease. There are multiple types of craniotomy incisions. A key element of these operative approaches is patient positioning, which facilitates exposure, allowing complex procedures to be done through small bony windows with limited dural opening and minimum cortex exposure. A skull fixation device provides head stability and allows for rotation, flexion, and extension in the final head positioning. If frameless stereotactic image-guided navigation is used, registration of fiducials must be done. Careful planning of the incision is imperative for adequate exposure. As a rule, flaps that create a vascular pedicle should be avoided and linear or sigmoid (S-shaped) flaps should be used. This is particularly true for patients with malignant brain tumors who will be treated with radiation, steroids, and chemotherapy. A pedicle flap compromises the blood supply to the incision and, with these other treatments, increases the likelihood of wound infection.

Operative Procedure: Craniotomy for Tumor Resection

1. The surgeon infiltrates the incision site using a local anesthetic with epinephrine.
2. The surgeon and the assistant apply digital pressure along the skin edges as the surgeon incises the skin through the galea.
3. Raney scalp clips are applied to skin edges, and/or self-retaining retractors are placed. The ESU is used on the major scalp vessels for hemostasis.
4. The scalp flap is reflected in the subperiosteal plane with periosteal elevators or with a monopolar ESU device to divide muscle attachments. It is retracted up using devices that may include retractors, towel clips, suture, or rubber bands and supported with a scalp roll.
5. The surgeon places burr holes to expose the dura, which are then widened with curettes and Kerrison rongeurs. The dura is dissected from the cranium using a Woodson, Penfield, or Adson dissector.
6. The surgeon creates the craniotomy using a craniotome loaded with the footplate attachment as the assistant irrigates to cool the bone. The bone flap is carefully elevated from the dura and placed in irrigating solution on the back table.
7. Bone dust is irrigated away from the wound, and hemostasis is established. Bleeding edges of bone are waxed, and bleeding vessels in the dura are electrocoagulated with the bipolar ESU or occluded with thrombin-soaked Gelfoam and patties. The surgeon places hemostatic agents and patties around the craniotomy edges, and then places dural tacking sutures that will remain permanently to prevent postoperative epidural hematoma formation.
8. After hemostasis is achieved, the surgeon opens the dura with a #11 or #15 blade. A dural suture may be placed in the dura before incising it. This tents the dura, ensuring that the surface of the brain is not inadvertently nicked. A Woodson dissector and blade or Metzenbaum scissors are used to extend the dural incision. Bleeding from transected dural vessels can be prevented by coagulating them with the bipolar ESU before cutting them,

or to avoid shrinking of the dura, and hemoclips can be placed or vessels can be compressed with a hemostat.

9. The surgeon places a self-retaining retractor system. Cortical dissection is achieved using the bipolar ESU, microscissors, and suction, and the specific surgical procedure is completed. Samples of tumor are sent for pathologic study if applicable.

10. Hemostasis is established. Irrigation can be used to find bleeding sites in the brain. A resection cavity is lined with Surgicel and filled with irrigation. The anesthesia provider produces the Valsalva maneuver with the ventilator to verify hemostasis.

11. The surgeon closes the dura with a 4-0 suture (braided nylon or silk). Gaps in the dura can be repaired using muscle, pericranium, dural substitute, or pericardium. A central dural tacking suture may be placed, and Gelfoam may be placed over the dura.

12. The bone plate is fitted with titanium plates and screws and reconnected to the cranium, or it may be wired into place depending on the surgeon's preference.

13. Muscle/fascia is reapproximated and galea is closed with interrupted absorbable sutures. Skin is closed with suture or staples.

Operative Procedure: Pterional Craniotomy

1. The skin incision for the pterional craniotomy extends from the zygoma to the midline, curving gently just posterior to the hairline (Fig. 21.44).

2. The surgeon and the assistant apply digital pressure over folded sponges on both sides of the incision line. The skin and galea are incised in segments, with the length of each segment being equal to that over which the finger pressure is applied. The tissue edges are held with 6-inch toothed forceps as scalp clips are placed on the flap edges. Any remaining active arterial bleeding is controlled with the ESU. If the incision extends into the temporal area, bleeding in the temporal muscle is managed by electrocoagulation, hemostats, tamponade, or suture ligature. Mayo scissors can be used to incise temporal muscle and fascia.

3. The surgeon uses sharp or blunt dissection or electrodissection to remove the soft tissue off the periosteum. The scalp flap is reflected over folded sponges and retracted by use of small towel clips and rubber bands or by muscle hooks on rubber bands. In either case, the traction is maintained by securing the rubber band to the drapes with heavy forceps. The flap may be covered with a moist sponge and a sterile towel. Bleeding is controlled with the ESU (Fig. 21.45).

4. When a free bone flap is planned, the muscle and periosteum are incised. Muscle and periosteum are elevated with the skin-galea flap, reflected, and retracted as a unit, as described previously.

5. The surgeon incises the periosteum and muscle with a scalpel or the ESU except at the inferior margins, which are left intact to preserve the blood supply to the bone flap. The periosteum is stripped from the bone at the incision line with a periosteal elevator. Bone wax is used to control bleeding.

6. The scalp edges and muscle are retracted from the bone incision line by a Sachs or Cushing retractor. Two or more burr holes are placed (Fig. 21.46). A great deal of heat is generated by the friction of the perforator or burr against the bone. The assistant must irrigate the drilling site to counteract the heat and remove bone dust, which collects as the holes are made. A large-gauge suction tip is used to remove both irrigating solution and debris from the field. As the inner table is perforated and the dura exposed, tamponade of the burr hole may be achieved temporarily with bone wax or a cottonoid strip or pattie. Each hole is eventually debrided by a #0 or #00 bone curette or small periosteal elevator. The dura mater is freed at the margins with a #3 Adson elevator, #3 Penfield dissector, or right-angle Frazier elevator or similar instrument. The hole is irrigated and suction

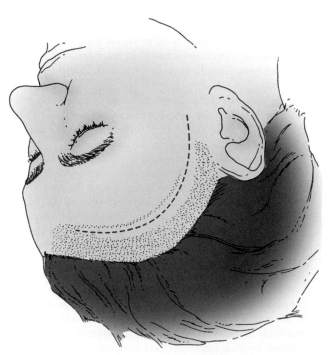

FIG. 21.44 Skin incision for a pterional craniotomy.

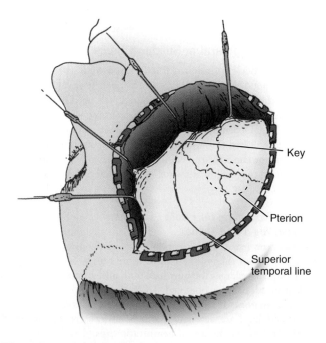

FIG. 21.45 Commonly used means of opening the scalp involves incision of the skin, galea, temporalis fascia, and muscle with reflection of the resultant flap in a single layer.

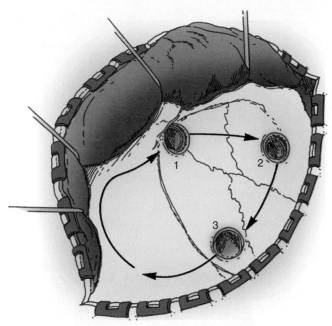

FIG. 21.46 Pterion craniotomy is performed with power instruments so that three burr holes are placed. The bone is cut as shown, exposing the frontal and temporal dura and the sphenoid ridge.

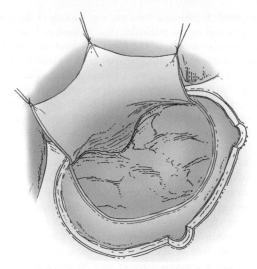

FIG. 21.47 Dura is opened and reflected back with stay sutures.

applied simultaneously. Active bleeding points in the bone are identified, and bone wax is applied.

7. When all burr holes have been made, the surgeon separates the dura mater from the bone with a dural separator, such as a #3 Penfield dissector. Dural separation is done to prevent tearing of the dura mater, especially over venous sinuses. An air craniotome or Midas Rex drill can be used for cutting the bone flap. Irrigation and suction are required as the bone flap is cut. Soft tissue edges are retracted with Sachs or Cushing retractors.

8. The surgeon lifts the bone flap (with muscle attached) off the dura mater with two periosteal elevators. Bleeding from the bone is controlled with bone wax. The bone flap is covered with a moist sponge, cottonoid material, and then a clean sterile towel and is retracted in the same manner as the scalp flap.

9. The dura mater is irrigated. Moist patties may be inserted between the dura mater and bone and folded back to cover the exposed bone edges. Epidural tack-up sutures are usually placed around the edge of the craniotomy defect to close the epidural dead space. Sterile towels may be placed around the operative site.

10. The surgeon opens the dura (Fig. 21.47). A dura hook or a dural stitch may be used to elevate the dura mater from the brain, and a small nick is made in the dura mater with a #15 blade. Alternatively, a small opening may be made in the dura mater without elevating it, after which the dural edges are grasped with two forceps with teeth and are elevated. A narrow, moist cottonoid strip is inserted with smooth forceps (bayonet or Cushing) into the opening to protect the brain as the dura mater is incised and elevated. The dural incision can be made with Metzenbaum scissors, special dura scissors, or a Rayport dura knife. Usually traction sutures are placed at the outer edge of the dura mater and are tagged with small bulldog clamps or mosquito hemostats. Sometimes the tag instruments are attached to the drapes to increase traction and keep tension on them.

As the dural veins are approached during dural opening, the surgeon ligates or coagulates them before cutting. Ligation is done with hemostatic clips such as Weck hemoclips, McKenzie clips, or Ligaclips. The brain surface is protected by moist cottonoid patties.

11. The surgeon appropriately places cottonoid patties and brain retractors, both self-retaining and manual, while working toward visualizing the particular pathologic entity.

12. Pituitary rongeurs as well as the CUSA or Sonopet (ultrasonic aspirator) may be needed for tumor removal. Also, a selection of dissectors, bayonet and Gerald forceps, and a bipolar ESU are used. Completely filled irrigating syringes and a full range of moist cottonoid patties and strips must be within easy reach of the surgeon and the assistant. After correction of the pathologic condition and control of bleeding, the brain may be irrigated with an antibiotic solution of the surgeon's choice.

13. The surgeon closes the dura mater using running or interrupted sutures of absorbable suture or black braided nylon. If necessary a dural graft may be used if a defect is present.

14. The bone flap is replaced and fixated with titanium plates and screws.

15. Periosteum and muscle are approximated with 2-0 or 3-0 absorbable suture. The galea is closed with the same sutures. Skin closure can be interrupted, or continuous suture, or skin staples.

Surgery for Intracranial Aneurysm

An aneurysm is a vascular dilation usually caused by a local defect in the arterial vascular wall, particularly at points of bifurcation. Vessels at risk within the brain involve those of the major circulation within and around the circle of Willis. Aneurysms are believed to arise from a complex set of circumstances involving a congenital anatomic predisposition enhanced by local and systemic factors. Aneurysmal rupture and hemorrhage into the subarachnoid space are frequently the first signs of an aneurysm, resulting in a sudden, severe headache described as "the worst headache ever" the person has ever had. Current neurosurgical techniques have made operations on intracranial aneurysms more feasible; however, the mortality rate is still as high as 40%. Furthermore, 66% of survivors have long-term cognitive impairment (TBAF, 2017). Hemorrhage and the cascade of ensuing cerebral trauma are the greatest hazards of the condition and of the operation. To minimize this, control of blood pressure as well as vascular supply to the region beyond the limits of the lesion may be required. Occasionally, control of the cerebral circulation at the level of the cervical carotid artery is desired. The artery may be exposed and controlled by means of preplaced ligatures or clamps that can be tightened to occlude the vessel if bleeding occurs at the aneurysm site during the operation. This is a separate preliminary surgical procedure.

Procedural Considerations

Aneurysm clips and appliers of the surgeon's choice must be included with the instrumentation. A variety of aneurysm clips are available; most are spring loaded (see Fig. 21.42, which illustrates a few of the clips and appliers). Clips may be classified as temporary or permanent, and both must be available with a minimum of two appliers for each type of clip. Temporary clips are commonly used to control giant aneurysms when it may be necessary to evacuate clot and debris before permanent occlusion can be accomplished (Fig. 21.48). Temporary clips may also be used to establish the best position for the permanent clip. Temporary clips should be discarded after use. Permanent clips are used to occlude the neck of the aneurysm. Aneurysm clips should not be compressed between the fingers. Clips should be compressed only by the surgeon when seated in their appliers. Once a clip has been compressed, it should be discarded. Clips that have been compressed may be sprung and may slip, causing complications such as bleeding or compression of another vessel or a nerve.

The full armamentarium of aneurysm-occlusion tools should be available for the surgeon. Along with clips, fast-setting aneuroplastic resinous material, a piece of temporal muscle, ligature carriers, or any other material requested by the surgeon should be in the room and ready to use. Fine silk ligatures and hemostatic clips, with or without bipolar electrocoagulation of the neck of the aneurysm, have also been used successfully.

A basic craniotomy setup is required in addition to the special items mentioned. Supplementary suction must be immediately available on the field to prevent hemorrhage from obscuring the surgeon's vision if the aneurysm dome ruptures during the operation. A blood salvage unit should be available for reprocessing blood for replacement when significant blood loss is expected.

Interventional radiology plays an important role in the management of intracranial aneurysms. Intravascular balloon occlusion and coiling of aneurysms by interventional radiologists are considerations in the treatment of aneurysms that meet the criteria for endoscopic therapy. The coils, composed of a soft platinum alloy, allow conformability to the dome of the aneurysm. A guide catheter is introduced into the femoral artery under fluoroscopy and advanced from the aorta into the vessel specific to the aneurysm. Coils are first introduced to outline the border of the aneurysm, and then smaller coils are added to fill the center of the aneurysm. Gradually, blood flow will be reduced, allowing the aneurysm to thrombose. Both the neurosurgeon and the radiologist work closely to diagnose and treat these life-threatening anomalies.

Operative Procedure

1. A frontal, pterional, or bifrontal craniotomy may be done to approach an aneurysm in the area of the circle of Willis. The bifrontal approach requires extra scalp clips and hemostatic forceps. All aneurysm instruments preferred by the surgeon must be included.

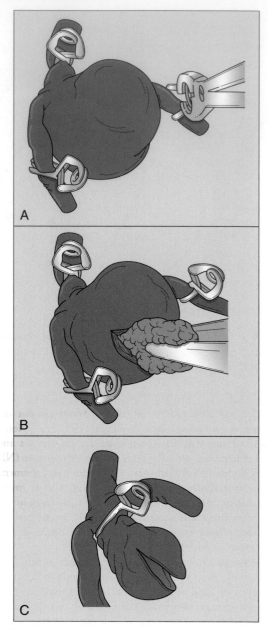

FIG. 21.48 Temporary arterial occlusion is often necessary in repairing complex large or giant aneurysms. (A) Temporary clips are placed on the feeder vessels. (B) The aneurysm sac is opened to allow evacuation of debris and thrombus. (C) Permanent clip in place.

2. After the dura mater has been opened, the surgeon places a self-retaining brain retractor and exposes the optic nerve and subarachnoid cisterns. The olfactory nerve may be electrocoagulated and divided with a long scissors for better exposure.
3. The scrub person and perioperative nurse position the operating microscope as directed by the surgeon. Microinstruments, including a micropolar bayonet, are used.
4. Bridging veins are coagulated with bipolar electrocoagulating forceps. Irrigation, which may be a part of the bipolar ESU, is necessary during bipolar electrocoagulation.
5. The surgeon uses microdissectors, hooks, elevators, scissors, knives, forceps, a diamond microknife, and an irrigating bipolar ESU to dissect the covering arachnoidal webs.

6. Careful dissection of the arachnoid and clear visualization of the neck of the aneurysm without rupture of the dome are the aims of the surgeon.

7. The surgeon identifies and frees the parent arteries so that they can be occluded with a temporary clip if necessary. Other structures, such as the optic chiasma and optic nerves, are identified.

8. As the surgeon works slowly toward the dome and neck of the aneurysm, the anesthesia provider may lower the patient's blood pressure for easier control of hemorrhage, should the aneurysm rupture. If the neck of the aneurysm can be isolated, the surgeon places a clip across it. Clips such as the Sundt-Kees and Heifetz have Teflon linings and can be used to approach the aneurysm from a 180-degree angle to avoid excessive manipulation and traction of the parent vessel, if the neck is on the underside of the vessel. These clips support the vessel and serve as a clip graft.

9. After clip placement, the surgeon may check the aneurysm sac by puncturing it with a needle to see if the clip pressure is adequate to stop blood flow to the aneurysm or to aspirate the aneurysmal contents.

10. As soon as the aneurysm has been occluded, the anesthesia provider returns the patient's blood pressure to normal and the surgeon checks the aneurysm site for bleeding. When the surgeon is satisfied that the operative field is dry, wound closure is begun.

Surgery for Arteriovenous Malformation

An AVM consists of thin-walled vascular channels that connect arteries and veins without the usual intervening capillaries. These vascular lesions may be microscopic or massive. AVMs are rare, affecting less than 1% of the population in the United States (NINDS, 2016). Malformations vary widely in size, area of involvement, and structure. Arteriovenous fistulas may be congenital or may result from trauma or disease. Vascular anomalies may also lead to subarachnoid or intracerebral hemorrhage or may have extensive irritative effects and cause focal or generalized seizures.

Procedural Considerations

AVMs are difficult to treat successfully. Feeding vessels can be clipped with or without partial removal of the lesion. Total removal, when possible, gives the best results. Microsurgical techniques have made total removal without devastating injury to surrounding brain tissue and vessels possible in many cases.

Other methods of treating these malformations include stereotactic radiosurgery with the Gamma Knife. Another method is preoperative embolization, which makes dissection much easier. Surgical glue, such as *N*-butyl cyanoacrylate and tantalum powder, is delivered by means of a catheter into the blood vessels before surgery. During the surgery, the glue is removed along with the AVM.

Operative Procedure

1. A supratentorial or infratentorial craniotomy is performed, depending on the location of the lesion.

2. The surgeon exposes the feeding arteries distant from the malformation, traces toward it, and then occludes the feeders by clipping, electrocoagulation, ligation, or laser beam coagulation.

3. The malformation is dissected out with suction and bayonet forceps. Additional vessels are clipped or coagulated along the way. Usually one or more draining veins are left to be ligated as the last step in the removal. Closure and dressing are as described for craniotomy.

Craniotomy for Suprasellar and Parasellar Tumors (Pituitary Tumor, Craniopharyngioma, Meningioma, and Optic Glioma)

Procedural Considerations

The preferred approach for pituitary tumors and some parasellar tumors is the less invasive transsphenoidal approach. However, for large and complex pituitary and parasellar tumors, a craniotomy may be indicated. A craniotomy setup is used with these additional pituitary instruments: Ray curettes (ring, sharp); angulated suction tips, right and left; large and small spinal needles, #22 or #24; small curettes, #0 through #4-0; and a 10-mL Luer-Lok syringe.

Extreme caution must be used in removing fluid from the capsule of a craniopharyngioma because the fluid is extremely irritating and may cause chemical leptomeningitis. Calcified pieces of tumor are dissected and removed in the same manner as the capsule of a pituitary adenoma. This is an extremely difficult procedure because of deposits on the carotid arteries, optic nerves, and optic chiasma. The tumor capsule is often left behind on the hypothalamus to avoid stripping off blood vessels supplying this structure. Many moist cottonoid patties are used to protect the surrounding areas from the cystic contents.

Suprasellar meningiomas usually arise from the tuberculum sellae just anterior to the optic nerves and chiasma. Tumor removal is similar to that of a pituitary adenoma except that the electrosurgical cutting loop may be used to excavate the interior of the tumor. After the tumor has been removed, the site of its attachment to the dura is thoroughly electrocoagulated to prevent recurrence. Other meningiomas arising at the base of the skull are treated by similar techniques.

Operative Procedure: Craniotomy for Pituitary Tumor Resection

1. The surgeon makes either a bifrontal or a unilateral incision into the frontal or frontotemporal region. Most unilateral approaches are performed from the right side.

2. Wet brain retractors over moist cottonoids are inserted for exposure of the optic chiasma and the pituitary gland. The frontal and often the temporal lobes are retracted. The olfactory nerve may be coagulated and divided with scissors.

3. A DeMartel, Yasargil, or Greenberg self-retaining retractor is placed to maintain exposure. Aneurysm clips and applicators should be available to control unexpected bleeding from major vessels. The microscope may be moved into place.

4. The surgeon uses the bipolar ESU for hemostasis around the tumor capsule and incises it with a #11 blade on a long knife handle; the tumor is removed with a pituitary rongeur or cup forceps.

5. Small stainless steel, copper, or Ray curettes, as well as suction, may be used during tumor removal.

6. A wide clip may be applied to the stalk of the pituitary, which may then be cut distally. A long angulated scissors is especially helpful for this.

7. If the tumor capsule is to be removed the surgeon uses bayonet forceps, cup forceps, nerve hooks, and suction to aid in the dissection.

8. Closure and dressing are as described for craniotomy.

Suboccipital Craniectomy for Posterior Fossa Exploration

The posterior occipital bone is perforated and removed using a drill and rongeurs, and the foramen magnum and arch of the atlas are exposed to remove a lesion in the posterior fossa (Fig. 21.49). Posterior

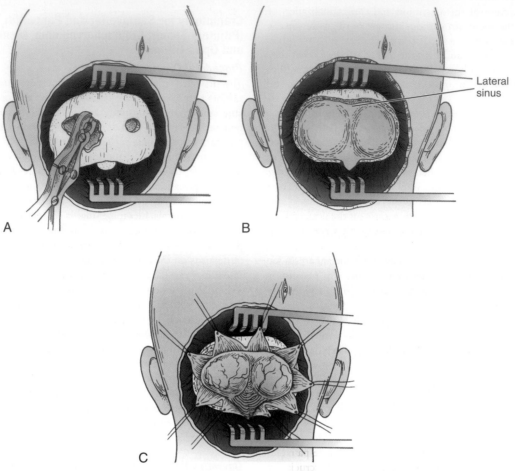

FIG. 21.49 Suboccipital craniectomy. (A) Craniectomy being performed. (B) Dura exposed. (C) Dura incised and cerebellum exposed.

fossa lesions include lesions in the cerebellum, the fourth ventricle, and the brainstem; posterior fossa meningiomas; and nerve sheath tumors.

Procedural Considerations

Depending on the type and size of the lesion, the exposure may be unilateral or bilateral. The operation may include the removal of the arch of the atlas. This approach gives the surgeon access to the fourth ventricle, the cerebellum, the brainstem, and the cranial nerves.

The prone position with the head of the OR bed elevated is the preferred position, but other positions may also be used. An extra-high instrument table or two Mayo stands and standing stool are necessary for the scrub person.

Operative Procedure

1. Before the initial surgical incision, the surgeon may make an occipital burr hole for placement of a ventricular catheter. This can be done as a separate procedure or concurrently with the procedure.
2. The incision may be made from mastoid tip to mastoid tip, in an arch curving upward 2 cm above the external occipital protuberance. Alternatively, a posterior midline incision can be used.
3. Scalp bleeding is controlled, and the skin flap is retracted with Weitlaner retractors.

4. The surgeon uses a periosteal elevator to free the muscles, and then divides them with an electrosurgical blade. The incision is deepened. A self-retaining retractor is used. The laminae of the first two or three cervical vertebrae may be exposed.
5. One or more holes are drilled in the occipital bone. A Midas Rex or Anspach drill is used to perform the craniectomy.
6. The surgeon frees the dura from under the bone. A double-action rongeur, Raney punch, Kerrison punch, or Leksell rongeur is used to enlarge the hole and smooth the edges.
7. Osseous and cerebellar venous bleeding is controlled at each step with bone wax, Gelfoam, and electrocoagulation to prevent air embolism.
8. Using a small brain spoon or cottonoid pattie to protect the brain, the surgeon extends the initial nick with scalpel or scissors. The dural incision is continued until the cerebellar hemispheres, the vermis, and the cerebellar tonsils can be visualized. Hemostatic clips are used on the dura mater as necessary. Dural traction sutures are placed.
9. The cisterna magna is opened, emptied of spinal fluid, and protected with a cottonoid strip.
10. The surgeon inspects the cerebellar hemispheres and controls bleeding with the bipolar ESU. A needle may be introduced through a small, coagulated incision into the cerebellar hemisphere in an attempt to palpate or tap a deep lesion.

11. Brain retractors over cottonoid patties are placed for exposure. The handle of the retractor must be kept dry to avoid slippage in the surgeon's hand. However, the inserted edge should be wet to prevent damage or tears in the brain surface. These retractors may be positioned in areas that control respiration or other vital functions, so every effort must be made to avoid jarring these instruments in the operative field. When the pathologic entity is identified, a self-retaining retractor may be placed.

12. Long bayonet forceps, bayonet cup forceps, pituitary forceps, suction, and the electrosurgical loop tips may be used to remove the lesion. Clips may be used to aid in hemostasis. A nerve stimulator may be used to identify cranial nerves; EPs for brainstem monitoring are not usual in routine practice.

13. After the lesion has been removed and bleeding controlled, the surgeon checks to ensure adequate hemostasis has been achieved. The anesthesia provider generates the Valsalva maneuver to increase venous pressure in the patient's head and facilitate identification of bleeding vessels.

14. The dura mater may be partially or completely closed. The cranial defect may be repaired with titanium mesh. The muscle, fascia, and skin are closed. A dressing is applied.

15. The patient must remain anesthetized until the supine position is achieved and the prongs of the headrest are removed. Particular attention must be given to the patient's head when these prongs are removed to prevent tearing the scalp or damaging the eyes.

Retromastoid Craniectomy for Microvascular Decompression of the Trigeminal Nerve

Trigeminal neuralgia (tic douloureux, fifth cranial nerve pain) is a condition characterized by brief, repeated attacks of excruciating, lancinating pain in the face. The etiology of this facial pain is believed to be the compression of the trigeminal nerve at its exit from the pons by an adjacent artery that has elongated over time to become wedged against the nerve, resulting in demyelination. Pain distribution follows one or all of the trigeminal nerve branches. It is characteristically severe, with a sudden onset, short duration, and paroxysmal nature. Triggers often precipitate the pain, such as touching the face, chewing, and talking. When pharmacologic measures fail, surgery to decompress the nerve is undertaken. Frequently more than one treatment is necessary during the course of the disease.

Procedural Considerations

The patient is in the supine, lateral, or sitting position, depending on the surgeon's preference. An endoscope can be used along with the microscope to improve visualization.

Operative Procedure

1. The surgeon makes a vertical retromastoid incision.
2. The soft tissue is freed from the bone with a periosteal elevator. The bone exposure is maintained with a self-retaining retractor.
3. A burr hole is created, and the dura mater is freed.
4. The surgeon uses a drill and rongeurs to enlarge the burr hole to a diameter of about 2½ inches.
5. Using a moist brain retractor, the surgeon retracts the dura mater overlying the pons and cerebellum.
6. A self-retaining brain retractor is placed deeper into the wound to retract the cerebellum. The microscope is used to provide light as well as magnification.
7. The surgeon identifies the pons, the superior cerebellar artery, and the trigeminal nerve.

8. Additional blunt dissection frees the vessel from the nerve. A synthetic microsponge is inserted between the vessel and nerve to maintain the separation.
9. The dura and cranial defect are repaired, the incision is closed, and dressings are applied.

Transsphenoidal Hypophysectomy

Endocrine pituitary disorders (such as Cushing syndrome, acromegaly, malignant exophthalmos, and hypopituitarism resulting from intrasellar tumors) as well as nonpituitary disorders (such as advanced metastatic carcinoma of the breast and prostate, diabetic retinopathy, and uncontrollable severe diabetes) have been successfully treated by transsphenoidal hypophysectomy (TSH). A transnasal or a sublabial incision can be used for rapid access to the sella turcica.

Endoscopy has been used to assist with access through the sphenoid sinus into the pituitary fossa. Otorhinolaryngologic surgeons can be consulted to assist the neurosurgeon with this approach. The endoscope and instrumentation access the sphenoid sinus by the transnasal route. Endoscopic transsphenoidal surgery eliminates the need for an incision and the need for a microscope. When the sphenoid sinus is reached, instruments and technique are similar to the microsurgical technique. Stereotactic image-guided navigation can also be used with the transsphenoidal technique.

All these approaches produce similar results. Complete extracapsular enucleation of the pituitary in cases of hypophysectomy and possible complete removal of small pituitary tumors, with the remaining normal portion of the gland left intact, can be achieved. Patients are relatively free from pain after surgery. No visible scar remains.

Procedural Considerations: Microsurgical Approach for Transsphenoidal Hypophysectomy

General endotracheal anesthetic, combined with a local anesthetic, is used. The surgical team places the patient in a semi-sitting position, with the head against the headrest. The surgeon may use a subnasal midline rhinoseptal approach or a transnasal route, both exposing the sphenoid bone, the sphenoid sinus behind the bone, and the sella containing the tumor. Frequently an otorhinolaryngologist assists the neurosurgeon in gaining access to the surgical site.

The face, mouth, and nasal cavity are prepped with an antiseptic solution. The surgeon infiltrates the patient's nasal mucosa and gingiva with a local anesthetic such as lidocaine with epinephrine with a concentration of 1:100,000 to initiate submucosal elevation and diminish oozing from the mucosa. A sterile adhesive plastic drape is applied to the entire face, with additional sterile drapes to ensure a relatively sterile operative field. Sterile soft goods (sponges) are placed in the patient's mouth so that only the upper gum margin is exposed.

Although sterile technique is used, this approach through the nose or mouth is technically not a sterile procedure. Therefore a separate sterile field and instruments must be maintained for adjunct procedures. The thigh or abdomen is prepped if a muscle or fat graft is to be taken. A lumbar drain may be placed preoperatively or postoperatively.

Specialized transsphenoidal instruments are required. The operating microscope is used for the cranial portion of the procedure. A fluoroscopy unit with C-arm may be used to verify the anatomic location of the sella.

Operative Procedure: Microsurgical Approach for a Transsphenoidal Hypophysectomy

1. Using the biopsy setup on a separate small Mayo table, the surgeon may take a small piece of muscle from the previously prepared

thigh or a fat graft from the abdomen to be used later in the procedure. This is kept in a moist sponge or soaked in antibiotic solution.

2. The surgeon creates an incision in the middle of the upper gum margin. The soft tissues of the upper lip and nose are elevated from the bone with an elevator, and the nasal septum is exposed. The nasal mucosa is elevated from either side of the nasal septum, which is flanked by the blades of a Cushing bivalved speculum. The transnasal approach avoids the sublabial incision, instead operating through a bivalve speculum inserted directly through the nares. The inferior third of the anterior cartilaginous septum and osseous vomer are resected, as is the floor of the sphenoidal sinus, exposing the sinus cavity. The floor of the sella turcica can then be identified.

3. The surgeon opens the floor with a sphenoidal punch, and incises the dura mater. The hypophyseal cavity should be opened only in patients undergoing surgery for pituitary adenoma. In these patients the gland is explored and the tumor is identified and removed.

4. The extracapsular cleavage plane is identified, and the superior surface of the pituitary is dissected until the stalk and the diaphragmatic orifice are found. Cotton pledgets are applied for exposure, hemostasis, and protection of structures.

5. Using a sickle knife, the surgeon sections the pituitary stalk and uses an enucleator to dissect the lateral posterior and inferior surfaces of the gland.

6. The gland is removed, and the sellar cavity may be packed to prevent CSF leakage. The packing is accomplished with muscle obtained previously from the thigh or with the fat graft previously obtained from the abdomen or thigh. The floor is reconstructed with cartilage from the nasal septum.

7. Antibiotic powder may be used and nasal packing introduced for 2 days. If a gingival incision is used, it is closed with suture of the surgeon's preference.

8. Some surgeons prefer to perform this operation by means of a lateral rhinotomy with a transantral-transsphenoidal approach.

Cranioplasty

Cranioplasty is performed for repair of a skull defect resulting from trauma, malformation, or a surgical procedure. The purpose of cranioplasty is to relieve headache and local tenderness or throbbing, to prevent secondary injury to the underlying brain, and for cosmetic effect.

Procedural Considerations

Repair of a skull defect may be performed acutely in clean cases. When a bone plate is removed for control of elevated ICP, it can be repaired after resolution of ICP issues. If the patient's bone plate was preserved, it could be replaced with microplates and screws.

The most common materials used for cranioplasty include titanium mesh and/or methyl methacrylate. Commercially prepared cranioplastic synthetics that supply the needed chemicals and mixing containers have simplified the procedures of shaping and molding the prosthesis. Sometimes heavy wire mesh is cut to the shape of the defect, and the methyl methacrylate is molded over the mesh.

Recent technologic advancements use CT scans to produce a computer-generated duplication of the defect. A properly sized prosthesis can be produced and sterilized before the surgery. After the defect is exposed, minor adjustments in the shape of the prosthesis can be made with a burr to achieve an optimal fit.

Operative Procedure: Cranioplasty Using Computer-Generated Prosthesis

1. Typically the old incision is reopened.
2. Keeping in mind that there is no bony protection between the scalp and the brain, the surgeon carefully elevates the scalp flap from the underlying scar, dura, and brain.
3. Bone edges are exposed with a curette, and the prosthesis is fitted to the defect using a burr. Debris is irrigated out of the wound.
4. The surgeon uses microplates and screws to secure the prosthesis in place.
5. The incision is closed as usual for craniotomy.

Operative Procedure: Cranioplasty Using Cranioplastic Material

1. A scalp flap is turned, and the bony defect is exposed.
2. The surgeon trims the edges of the defect, forming a ledge to seat the prosthesis.
3. After the bone defect has been prepared so that it is slightly saucerized, the methyl methacrylate is mixed by combining one volume of liquid monomer with one volume of the powdered polymer. When this has formed a doughy mass, it is dropped into a sterile polyethylene bag. The soft plastic is then rolled on a flat surface into the desired shape, leaving the thickness to the approximate depth of the skull edges. A sterile test tube, syringe barrel, or other round object can be used, although a stainless steel roller is preferred because of its weight and ease of use.
4. The soft cranioplastic material in the bag is placed over the skull defect and, through light pressing with the ends of the fingers, is fitted into the missing skull area. Assistants stretch the plastic bag as the surgeon molds the plate into the defect and forms an overlapping bevel edge. This overlapping fringe keeps the plate from falling inside the skull, in the same manner as the skull saucerization.
5. When the heat of the chemical reactions is evident, the surgeon lifts the plate out of the bony wound and removes it from the polyethylene bag. Cool saline should be used on the flap while the exothermic reaction takes place.
6. When the plate is cool enough to handle, the surgeon trims excess material and bone using rongeurs or a saw and places the plate in the cranial defect to check for fit.
7. The surgeon uses a craniotome to smooth the rough spots and bevel the edges so that the plate will blend gradually with the skull.
8. Mixing and fitting the plate take about 7 minutes, which is the same time needed for the cranioplastic material to harden. Sutures may be used to hold the plate in place, generally at three or more points.

Surgery of the Spine

Surgery of the spinal column is also discussed in Chapter 20.

Anterior Cervical Decompression and Fusion

Anterior cervical decompression and fusion (ACDF) is performed to treat cervical disk herniation or cervical spondylosis (degeneration in the spine) with myelopathy (disorder of the spinal cord) or radiculopathy (disorder of the nerve roots). Symptoms include pain in the neck, shoulders, arms, and hands; and weakness of the upper extremity. ACDF allows for direct decompression of the spinal cord as well as the reconstruction of the anterior column of the cervical spine (Amorosa et al., 2015). An ACDF entails a corpectomy (removal of a vertebral body), diskectomy, and fusion of the vertebral bodies.

Bone grafts for the fusion are obtained from the patient's iliac crest (autograft) or from a bone bank (allograft).

Procedural Considerations

Awake endoscopic intubation may be required if the patient's neck is unstable or does not readily extend. Neurologic monitoring is commonly used to prevent further injury during surgery. The patient is placed in the supine position, with a small shoulder roll placed horizontally for mild neck extension. The perioperative nurse ensures the patient's arms are tucked, and the hip is elevated for exposure if bone graft is to be taken from the iliac crest (Fig. 21.50). Intraoperative x-ray may be used to confirm the correct surgical site and verify placement of the graft and related hardware.

Operative Procedure

1. The surgeon may harvest the iliac crest bone graft before the neck procedure begins, or after exposure of the anterior cervical spine. An incision is made over the iliac crest, at least 3 cm posterior to the anterosuperior iliac spine. The skin and subcutaneous tissues are retracted with a Weitlaner retractor.
2. Soft tissue is dissected until the crest is reached and exposed.
3. The surgeon uses an osteotome or oscillating saw to remove the bone graft. The graft is soaked in antibiotic solution and set aside. The perioperative nurse initiates a sponge and sharps count for this portion of the procedure. After verification of a correct count, the surgeon irrigates and closes the wound and covers it with a sterile towel.
4. A transverse or horizontal skin incision is made on one side of the neck, directly over the involved cervical level.
5. A Weitlaner retractor is placed, and the surgeon uses sharp dissection to divide the platysma.
6. The medial edge of the sternocleidomastoid muscle is defined with the scissors by blunt and sharp dissection.
7. Using blunt finger dissection, the surgeon creates a vertical plane of dissection between the carotid artery laterally and the trachea and esophagus medially. This plane is held open with retractors.
8. The anterior surface of the spine is identified, and the long muscles of the neck are peeled off the anterior surface of the spine with periosteal elevators or peanut dissectors. The bipolar ESU is used for hemostasis.
9. A 20-gauge spinal needle is inserted a short distance into the disk space, and the location is confirmed radiographically.
10. Self-retaining retractors are inserted into the neck incision. Care is used to protect the carotid artery and the esophagus. A combination of sharp and dull blades is used to acquire the best retraction. If a toothed blade is used, the teeth are carefully hooked beneath the long muscle of the neck.
11. The surgeon uses a #15 or #11 blade on a #7 knife handle to incise the disk space; a pituitary rongeur is used to remove the disk material, which may be saved as a specimen. A vertebral spreader may be inserted into the vertebral space to widen the area. Residual disk material is removed with the rongeur (Kerrison or pituitary) or small curettes (angled or straight, #0 to #4-0) until the entire surface of both vertebrae is clean. A small burr may also be used until complete anterior decompression of the nerve root or dural sac is obtained. Nerve hooks may be used for demonstration of adequate decompression.
12. Next, the surgeon uses a depth gauge and caliper to measure the size of the interbody defect. The bone graft is cut and placed into the defect with a tamp and a mallet.
13. The anterior cervical plate and screws are secured to the vertebral bodies above and below the bone graft.
14. Lateral x-ray or fluoroscopy is performed to confirm location, degree of distraction, and alignment.
15. Hemostasis is obtained, and the wound is irrigated. A drain may be placed. The platysma is closed with absorbable suture. A subcuticular closure of the skin is done, and wound closure strips are applied.
16. A cervical collar is placed before the patient awakens.

Posterior Cervical Approach

Disorders of the cervical spine can cause radiculopathy, myelopathy, or both. Compression of the neural elements occurs most commonly as a result of disk herniation and/or osteophyte formation but can also be caused by congenital deformities, facet joint hypertrophy, infection, and neoplasm (Ament et al., 2013). The posterior cervical approach is used for laminectomy for decompression, intradural tumor removal, cordotomy, diskectomy, and fusion.

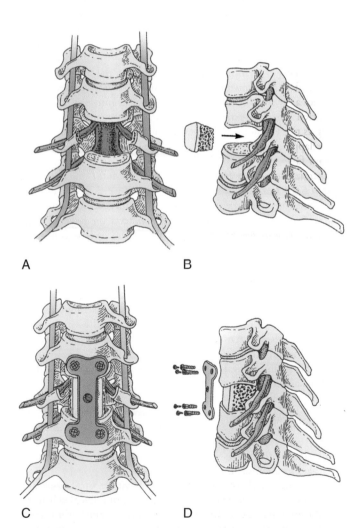

FIG. 21.50 Anterior cervical decompression and fusion. (A and B) Bone graft from the iliac crest or fashioned from bank bone is tailored to fit the site of corpectomy, resting on the vertebral endplates. (C and D) An anterior spinal plate and screws are secured to the vertebral bodies above and below the spanned segment to stabilize and promote a stable fusion.

Procedural Considerations

A patient with severe spondylosis may require fiberoptic intubation. Intraoperative neurologic monitoring should be used to detect a change in neurologic status. The patient is positioned prone with a three-pin skull clamp. The OR bed is positioned in slight reverse Trendelenburg position to encourage venous drainage. The patient's arms are tucked. If autograft bone graft is desired for fusion, the posterior iliac crest will be prepped. A cervical collar may be required postoperatively.

Operative Procedure

1. The surgeon palpates the cervical spinous processes as landmarks before creating a midline incision.
2. Soft tissue dissection is done, and a clamp is placed on the spinous process to verify the correct level with x-ray.
3. After placing self-retaining retractors to help gain exposure, the surgeon performs a subperiosteal dissection to the lateral margins of the involved facets using the ESU, suction, and a cervical Cobb elevator.
4. Hemostasis is maintained with the bipolar ESU, Gelfoam, and patties.
5. A laminectomy is performed using a drill, Leksell rongeurs, curettes, a nerve hook, and Kerrison punch rongeurs.
6. The surgeon removes the disk with pituitary rongeurs and curettes.
7. If a fusion is required, instrumentation and allograft or autograft may be needed.
8. The wound is irrigated. A drain may be placed and local anesthesia may be injected for postoperative pain control before the skin is closed.

Anterior Thoracic Approach

A transthoracic thalamotomy is done to access the spine for a thoracic diskectomy, burst fracture, osteomyelitis, and metastatic disease. Usually a thoracic or trauma surgeon assists the neurosurgeon in obtaining adequate exposure.

Procedural Considerations

The anesthesia provider may need to place a double-lumen endotracheal tube to allow for deflation of the lung for exposure of the higher thoracic levels. Lateral position with a beanbag is preferred. If intraoperative fluoroscopy is necessary, a Jackson table is needed. A beanbag interferes with fluoroscopy. The arch of the aorta is normally at the T4 vertebral level, and it becomes the descending aorta, traveling inferiorly along the left side of the vertebral bodies from T5 to T12 before passing through the diaphragm and becoming the abdominal aorta (Hiratzka and Brooke, 2013). For T1 to T4, a right-sided approach is preferred to avoid the aortic arch and heart. For T5 to T12, a left-sided approach is preferred because the aorta is safer to manipulate than the vena cava. If allograft is desired for fusion, prep the iliac crest.

At times, an anterior thoracic surgery is performed in combination with a posterior thoracic surgery. In this case the patient is repositioned prone after the completion of the anterior portion of the surgery. The posterior surgical site is prepped and draped, and the posterior portion of the surgery is completed.

Operative Procedure

1. The surgeon creates a thoracotomy incision and transects the latissimus dorsi and other muscles. A rib may be resected with a rib cutter to gain exposure.

2. The parietal pleura is opened, and a thoracotomy retractor is placed. If necessary, the anesthesia provider manually deflates the patient's lung.
3. A localization x-ray is done to verify the correct level. The parietal pleura is incised further onto the vertebral body and cleared with blunt dissection. Segmental vessels are ligated as necessary with hemoclips and transected to mobilize the aorta.
4. For diskectomy or decompression, a drill, rongeurs, and curettes may be needed. For spinal fusion, instrumentation and autograft or allograft may be used.
5. The wound is irrigated, and a chest tube is placed. The ribs are reapproximated with a rib approximator and sutured with heavy absorbable suture.
6. The fascia and subcuticular layers are closed.

Laminectomy

Laminectomy is removal of one or more of the vertebral laminae to expose the spinal canal. Laminectomy, hemilaminectomy, and the interlaminar approach are performed to reach the spinal canal and its adjacent structures to treat compression fracture, dislocation, herniated nucleus pulposus, and cord tumor, as well as for spinal cord stimulation. Section of the spinal nerves, including cordotomy and rhizotomy, requires similar surgical exposure.

Procedural Considerations

Laminectomy is performed with the patient in the prone or lateral position. It is performed on the cervical, thoracic, or lumbar spine. Laminectomy instruments include the basic neurosurgical set, the retractor of the surgeon's choice, and an assortment of specialty rongeurs. See Chapter 20 for a general discussion of the laminectomy procedure used to treat a variety of diagnoses.

Operative Procedure: Laminectomy for Intradural Spinal Cord Tumor

1. The surgeon creates a midline fascial incision, dissects both sides of the spinous processes, and reflects the bilateral paraspinous muscles, one side at a time. The level is confirmed with x-ray.
2. One or more Gelpi or Adson-Beckman self-retaining retractors are placed to maintain the bony exposure.
3. The surgeon performs a midline laminectomy and excises the spinous processes. Various rongeurs (e.g., Leksell) are used to remove the laminae after the edges are defined with a curette. A Midas Rex drill may also be used. The bone edges are waxed for bleeding.
4. The remaining flaval ligament is removed with scissors, scalpel, and a Kerrison rongeur. Epidural fat is removed so that the dura mater is fully exposed.
5. The surgeon places a wide, moist cottonoid pattie over the superficial soft tissues and muscle down to the bone bordering the exposed dura mater to provide additional hemostasis.
6. Intraoperative ultrasound may be used to verify the tumor's exact location beneath the dura.
7. The surgeon elevates the dura mater with a small hook and nicks it with a #15 blade. A grooved director is inserted beneath the dura mater, and the dural incision is extended over it using long forceps and fine scissors. Alternatively, the surgeon may lengthen the incision with Metzenbaum scissors. Traction sutures of 4-0 silk or braided nylon on dura needles are placed in the dural edges, and the cord is exposed (Fig. 21.51). The operating microscope may be used.

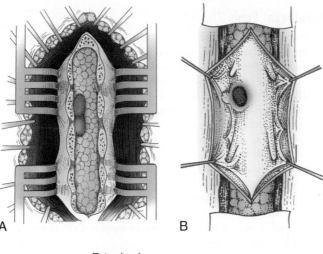

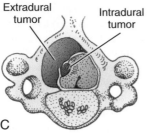

FIG. 21.51 (A) Laminectomy completed: dura mater and tumor exposed. (B) Dura mater incised and retracted, revealing pia arachnoid over spinal cord and part of tumor. (C) Diagram of cross section of tumor site and location of extradural and intradural pathologic areas.

8. The cord is explored for the pathologic area. Aspiration through a #22 needle on a plain-tipped syringe may be performed. Whenever possible, the tumor mass is dissected free and removed using suction, the dissecting scissors, the bipolar forceps, small (pituitary) scoops, curettes, pituitary rongeurs, or an ultrasonic aspirator. Bleeding is controlled with moist cottonoids, hemostatic clips, gelatin gauze, and topical hemostatics. Bipolar electrocoagulation is used around the nerves and spinal cord.

9. The surgeon irrigates the wound and obtains hemostasis, being careful to protect the spinal cord.

10. The dura mater is closed with a braided nylon or polytetrafluoroethylene (PTFE) suture.

11. The incision is checked for further bleeding, and the paraspinous muscles are approximated with absorbable suture. The remainder of the wound is closed.

Note: In the case of extradural tumors, invasion of the dura is avoided. Once the dura is opened from a tear or an incision, the surgeon may require that the patient remain flat for 24 hours or longer to allow healing of the dura.

Laminotomy

Laminotomy is the traditional approach to posterior microdiskectomy at the cervical, thoracic, and lumbar levels. Laminotomy is performed on the symptomatic side with resection of a small portion of the medial facet. The goal of this surgery is the resolution of leg pain with little to no residual back pain and a return to preinjury activity and lifestyle. The operating microscope has improved this surgical approach by offering magnification and illumination, which allows for smaller incisions and less tissue dissection. This surgical procedure

AMBULATORY SURGERY CONSIDERATIONS

Microdiskectomies

Microdiskectomies are one of several spinal surgeries performed to relieve pain caused by disk herniations. Patients selected for this specific procedure typically complain of leg pain longer than 6 weeks in duration, and receive minimal relief from prescribed pain medications or injections. A magnetic resonance image scan confirming the level of nerve root compression as well as a detailed history and physical will determine whether the patient is a candidate for surgery.

Ambulatory surgeries are designed for patients who have a nominal health history and pose minimal risk for operative complications. Microdiskectomies have the flexibility of being performed either in a same-day surgery center or in a hospital OR suite. The procedure is typically performed using a general or spinal anesthetic, depending on the needs of the patient. After the anesthesia provider has control of the airway, the patient is positioned prone for maximum operative accessibility. Positioning may take time, and it is essential that every precaution is taken to prevent patient injury. If the patient is awake, talking should be kept to a minimum, and OR traffic should be closely monitored by the perioperative nurse. Before making the incision the surgeon may inject a local anesthetic containing epinephrine into the lumbar spine to minimize bleeding intraoperatively.

The procedure is approximately 2 hours in duration, and many patients are able to return home the same day. Postoperative pain relief is maximized by the use of intraoperative topical steroids on the nerve root, local anesthetics, and prescribed oral pain medications.

Possible complications include bleeding, infection, and, on rare occasions, nerve damage. On discharge the patient is instructed to keep the surgical site clean, restrict activity, and notify the surgeon immediately if he or she experiences excessive pain, swelling, or discharge from the incision site. Follow-up appointments are generally scheduled 2 weeks after the procedure, and most patients can return to work after 4 to 6 weeks.

is associated with less postoperative discomfort and shorter hospital stays. The majority of patients who undergo this procedure can be discharged home on the same day (Ambulatory Surgery Considerations). See Chapter 20 for a full description of the surgical procedures for a discussion of diskectomy, disk replacement, and microdiskectomy.

Spinal Cord Stimulators

A spinal cord stimulator (SCS) is an implantable, nondestructive medical device used to treat chronic intractable pain of the trunk and limbs. The device generates an electrical impulse to the epidural space, which produces a tingling sensation that masks the perception of pain.

The goal of the stimulation is to lower the perception of pain, reduce medication use, increase function, and improve quality of life. Patients who are considered good candidates for an SCS placement undergo a trial to check for efficacy before permanent implantation. This trial may be standard open or percutaneous depending on the type of lead. Percutaneous trial lead placement may be performed under monitored anesthesia care (MAC) and local anesthetic with the patient participating by stating when and where he or she feels stimulation when testing the leads intraoperatively. The standard trial is generally performed in the OR using MAC or general anesthesia. During the trial a temporary percutaneous lead is placed and connected to an external pulse generator for approximately 3 to 7 days. The patient must experience at least 50% improvement in pain to be considered a candidate for permanent lead placement.

The permanent SCS lead is implanted into the epidural space, and the impulse generator (IPG), which is the device battery, is implanted in the abdomen or buttocks. The lead is positioned at a specific level of the spinal cord. The targeted level is determined by the individual patient's symptoms, and by information obtained from the trial. A thoracic SCS is placed for lower back and leg pain. A cervical SCS is placed for upper extremity pain. Peripheral nerve stimulators are an alternative or conjunctive neuromodulation technique that targets peripheral nerves.

Procedural Considerations

Lead placement must be assessed during the surgery. This can be done by waking the patient during the surgery and asking where the stimulation is felt. To secure the airway, lateral position is used with this method. Alternatively, electromyogram (EMG) monitoring may be used while the patient is under general anesthesia to verify motor responses in the targeted muscle groups. Fluoroscopy is also used to verify lead placement.

The surgeon determines the battery site and directs the patient's position accordingly. The prone position is used if the battery will be inserted into the subcutaneous tissue of the buttocks. The lateral position is used if the battery is placed in the subcutaneous tissue of the abdomen, or if the patient will be awakened during surgery. The perioperative nurse ensures that the SCS system, the product representative, and the fluoroscopy unit are available, and that the OR bed is compatible with fluoroscopy. The surgeon marks the operative site before the patient is prepped. The surgical prep includes the entire area from the lead placement site to the IPG site.

Operative Procedure

1. The surgeon makes a midline incision at the proper level over the spine and uses sharp and dull dissection through the subcutaneous tissues to reach the fascia.
2. Paravertebral muscles are then dissected off the spinous process and lamina. A self-retaining retractor is placed to provide a visual field.
3. Instruments such as punches and rongeurs are then used to perform a surgical laminectomy. The stimulator lead is placed in the epidural space. Proper placement is confirmed by testing with the stimulator programmer while waking and assessing the patient's perception of the stimulation, or while using EMG monitoring. Lead placement is also verified with fluoroscopy or x-ray. After testing is complete, the surgeon anchors the lead with a 2-0 nonabsorbable suture.
4. The surgeon creates a pocket in the subcutaneous tissue of the buttocks or the abdomen for IPG placement.
5. Using a tunneling device the surgeon tunnels the lead from the lead site to the battery location. The IPG is attached. Excess wire is protected by placing it beneath the IPG.
6. The IPG is anchored with 2-0 nonabsorbable suture to prevent migration.
7. Both incisions are irrigated and closed.
8. An abdominal binder is applied to compress the battery site.
9. A postoperative x-ray is obtained to confirm lead placement.

Intrathecal Pump Therapy

An intrathecal pump (ITP) is a specialized device that offers precise, targeted, and adjustable medication treatment for patients with spasticity and/or chronic pain. It delivers medication directly into the CSF via a small catheter attached to a pump.

The pump is controlled via a radiotelemetry link from an external programmer. This controls the rate and mode of infusion. The pump reservoirs are refilled with medication in the physician's office. Baclofen for spasticity or morphine sulfate for pain is most commonly used.

All patients are carefully screened for specific criteria, such as ineffective results or intolerable side effects with oral medication, limited functional abilities, no significant addiction history, and a diagnosed pathology. Contraindications for ITP therapy include active or frequent infections; medication allergy; failed screenings; and lack of patient reliability, resources, or support. ITP complications can include the following:

- Infection
- Mechanical failure
- CSF leak
- Overdose or adverse drug reactions

Each patient undergoes a trial injection that lasts 6 to 8 hours. Positive results must be noted before final implantation. Trials are performed in the physician's office; final implantation is performed in the OR using MAC or general anesthesia.

Procedural Considerations

The nurse ensures the availability of the ITP system and the prescribed intrathecal medication before the procedure. A representative from the manufacturer should be present to assist with pump programming. Intraoperative fluoroscopy is used to verify proper placement of the catheter, so a compatible OR bed is necessary. The surgeon will determine the patient's preference for pump placement (right or left abdomen) and mark the abdomen and back incisions. The back incision is typically marked at the area of L3-L4. The abdominal incision is marked strategically to avoid the belt line, umbilicus, and the iliac crest. The perioperative nurse assists with placing the patient in the lateral position, using pillows and side braces as positioning aids. The surgical prep extends from the posterior incision site to the abdominal pump site.

Operative Procedure

1. The surgeon makes an incision in the patient's back and extends it through the subcutaneous tissue to the fascia. Hemostasis is obtained with the ESU.
2. A Tuohy needle is inserted paraspinally and at a 30-degree angle through the fascia into the intrathecal space, usually at L3-L4. The surgeon confirms proper needle placement by removing the inner stylet of the Tuohy needle and visualizing a flow of CSF through the outer cannula.
3. The surgeon threads the catheter through the needle and feeds it to the proper level of the spine. This is determined by the patient's symptoms and the type of medication that will be administered. The catheter placement is verified under fluoroscopic visualization and is secured with anchors and a 4-0 nonabsorbable suture.
4. The abdominal incision is made to create a pocket approximately 2.5 cm deep subcutaneously for pump placement.
5. Using a tunneling device the surgeon tunnels the catheter from the back to the abdominal pocket. The flow of CSF is once again verified through the catheter before it is connected to the pump.

The pump is placed in the abdominal pocket and secured with 2-0 nonabsorbable suture to prevent migration.

6. Both the back and abdominal incisions are irrigated and closed.
7. Dressings are applied to both incisions, and an abdominal binder is secured. In the recovery area, the pump is set with the external programmer.

Additional spine techniques are covered in Chapter 20.

Key Points

- Perioperative nurses and scrub persons who care for neurosurgical patients are challenged by the need to have a working knowledge of neuroanatomy, function, and clinical presentations of the many neurologic conditions that require surgical interventions.
- The nervous system is divided functionally into a voluntary system and an autonomic, or involuntary, system.
- The nervous system is divided structurally into the CNS consisting of the brain and spinal cord and the PNS, which encompasses every neurologic structure outside the CNS, including the cranial and spinal nerves.
- The brain and adjacent structures include the cranial nerves of the PNS, which are commonly encountered during brain surgery. Discussion of the spine and spinal cord includes the adjacent spinal nerves and the disks and ligaments that support the spine.
- Surgical procedures to address disorders of the brain and spine are the cornerstone of the specialty. Brain surgery is performed to excise tumors, address trauma, and correct congenital and acquired conditions. Spinal surgery is performed to correct congenital malformations, traumatic injuries, tumors, abscesses, herniated and degenerative intervertebral disks, and intractable pain.
- Neurosurgical patients often have special needs because of conditions such as mental status changes, spinal instability, spinal cord injuries, paralysis, other traumatic injuries, and pain.

Critical Thinking Question

While interviewing Mr. J, who is scheduled for a right craniotomy and tumor resection, you discover that he is having a hard time answering your questions. He does not remember talking to the surgeon, or exactly what he was told about the treatment plan. You notice that Mr. J signed his surgical consent a month ago, and find the anesthesia provider is at the bedside assessing Mr. J and obtaining the anesthesia consent. You feel uneasy about Mr. J's level of understanding. What should you do?

evolve *The answer to the Critical Thinking Question can be found at http://evolve.elsevier.com/Rothrock/Alexander.*

References

Ament JD et al: Cervical microforaminotomy and decompressive laminectomy. In Cho D et al, editors: *Surgical anatomy and techniques to the spine*, ed 2, Philadelphia, 2013, Saunders.

American Brain Tumor Association (ABTA): *What now? First steps after receiving a brain tumor diagnosis* (website), 2014. www.abta.org/news/brain-tumor-fact-sheets. (Accessed 16 November 2016).

Amorosa LF, Vaccaro AR: Subaxial cervical spine trauma. In Browner BD et al, editors: *Skeletal trauma: basic science, management, and reconstruction*, ed 5, Philadelphia, 2015, Saunders.

Association of periOperative Registered Nurses (AORN): Guideline for positioning the patient. In Conner R, editor: *Guidelines for perioperative practice*, Denver, 2016, The Association.

Badhiwala J, Kulkami A: Ventricular shunting procedures. In Winn RH, editor: *Youmans neurological surgery*, ed 7, Philadelphia, 2017, Saunders.

Baehring JM, Hochberg FH: Primary nervous system tumors in adults. In Daroff RB et al, editors: *Bradley's neurology in clinical practice*, ed 7, Philadelphia, 2016, Saunders.

Biller J et al: Ischemic cerebrovascular disease. In Daroff RB et al, editors: *Bradley's neurology in clinical practice*, ed 7, Philadelphia, 2016, Saunders.

Heegaard WG, Biros MH: Head injury. In Marx JA et al, editors: *Rosen's emergency medicine*, ed 8, St Louis, 2014, Mosby.

Hiratzka JR, Brooke DS: Anterolateral transthoracic approaches to the thoracic spine. In Cho D et al, editors: *Surgical anatomy and techniques to the spine*, ed 2, Philadelphia, 2013, Saunders.

Integra: *Products for the neurosurgeon, 2010-2016* (website), 2016. https://www.integralife.com/file/general/1453799329.pdf. (Accessed 13 September 2016).

Karajannis MA et al: Primary nervous system tumors in infants and children. In Daroff RB et al, editors: *Bradley's neurology in clinical practice*, ed 7, Philadelphia, 2016, Saunders.

Kidwell CS, Jahan R: Endovascular treatment of acute ischemic stroke, *Neurol Clin* 33(2):401–420, 2015.

Louis DN et al: The 2016 World Health Organization classification of tumors, *Acta Neuropathol* 131(6):803–820, 2016.

Martin RS, Meredith JW: Management of acute trauma. In Townsend CM et al, editors: *Sabiston textbook of surgery*, ed 20, Philadelphia, 2017, Saunders.

National Institute on Deafness and Other Communication Disorders (NIDCD): *Vestibular schwannoma (acoustic neuroma) and neurofibromatosis* (website), 2016. www.nidcd.nih.gov/health/vestibular-schwannoma-acoustic-neuroma-and-neurofibromatosis. (Accessed 19 November 2016).

National Institute of Neurological Disorders and Stroke (NINDS): *Hydrocephalus fact sheet* (website), 2013. www.ninds.nih.gov/disorders/hydrocephalus/detail_hydrocephalus.htm. (Accessed 25 November 2016).

National Institute of Neurological Disorders and Stroke (NINDS): *Arteriovenous malformations and other vascular lesions of the central nervous system fact sheet* (website), 2016. https://www.ninds.nih.gov/Disorders/Patient-Caregiver-Education/Fact-Sheets/Arteriovenous-Malformation-Fact-Sheet. (Accessed 10 November 2016).

Ortega-Barnett J et al: Neurosurgery. In Townsend CM et al, editors: *Sabiston textbook of surgery*, ed 20, Philadelphia, 2017, Saunders.

Ringer A: *Aneurysm embolization: coiling* (website), 2016. www.mayfieldclinic.com/PE-Coiling.htm. (Accessed 28 November 2016).

Singla N et al: Histopathology of subcutaneously preserved autologous bone flap after decompressive craniectomy: a prospective study, *Acta Neurochir* 156(7):1369–1373, 2014.

The Brain Aneurysm Foundation (TBAF): *Brain aneurysm statistics and facts* (website), 2017. https://www.bafound.org/about-brain-aneurysms/brain-aneurysm-basics/brain-aneurysm-statistics-and-facts/. (Accessed 25 September 2017).

Tse V: *Spinal metastasis* (website), 2016. http://emedicine.medscape.com/article/1157987-overview. (Accessed 23 October 2016).

Walker EP: *Cardiology: FDA panel review may ground Wingspan Stent* (website), 2012. www.medpagetoday.com/cardiology/prevention/31805. (Accessed 25 November 2016).

CHAPTER 22

Reconstructive and Aesthetic Plastic Surgery

DONNA R. MCEWEN

Derived from the Greek word *plastikos,* which means to "mold or give form," plastic surgery is a medical specialty that restores or gives shape to the body. There are two different subspecialties of plastic surgery. *Cosmetic surgery* restores or reshapes normal structures of the body, to modify or improve appearance. *Reconstructive surgery* treats abnormal structures of the body caused by birth defects, developmental problems, disease, tumors, infection, or injury to restore function and correct disfigurement or scarring. As a surgical specialty plastic surgery owes much of its heritage to knowledge gained from the wars of the 20th century.

Approximately 15.9 million cosmetic surgical procedures were performed (by surgeons certified by the American Society of Plastic Surgeons [ASPS]) in 2015 (the latest year for which statistics are available), which is a 2% increase in both minimally invasive and surgical procedures. The top five surgical procedures were breast augmentation, liposuction, nose reshaping, eyelid surgery, and abdominoplasty. The top five minimally invasive procedures were botulinum toxin type A injections (e.g., Botox), soft tissue filler injection/insertion, chemical peels, laser hair removal, and micro-dermabrasion. Many cosmetic procedures are performed in outpatient settings (Ambulatory Surgery Considerations). Reconstructive plastic surgery, which improves function and appearance, was up 1%. The

top five reconstructive procedures were tumor removal, laceration repair, maxillofacial surgery, scar revision, and hand surgery. Breast reconstruction increased 4% over the previous year with more than 106,000 procedures performed (ASPS, 2015).

Surgical Anatomy

The specialty of plastic and reconstructive surgery requires the surgeon to have a thorough understanding of the anatomy and biology of tissue. Operative techniques are complex and are often completed in stages. The surgery also involves removing, reducing, enlarging, and recontouring tissue, as well as camouflaging scars into existing skin lines (Fig. 22.1). The tissues of the body can be transferred to use as various types of flaps. Free flaps are the transfer of tissue along with its vascular pedicle. When nerve is anastomosed with these flaps, they are called neurovascular free flaps. Flaps are used to cover defects or create new structures such as breasts, digits, or facial structures. Body parts can also be transplanted. The patient's self-esteem may improve as a result of the surgery, and the patient may feel more comfortable in public and social activities. The body changes as it ages. The patient's concern with aesthetics, the variety of acquired

---

AMBULATORY SURGERY CONSIDERATIONS

Patient Choices in Facility

There has been a dramatic shift toward encouraging patients to be more involved and informed in all of their healthcare decisions. Many organizations are focusing on active participation of patients in their own care. One aspect of this is choosing the outpatient facility for their plastic surgery. In keeping with this trend, the ASPS has developed a brochure, with an excerpt available online, to help patients choose a facility. The brochure includes the following information:
- *Types of facilities:* For ambulatory (discharge same day as surgery) procedures, the facility may be part of the surgeon's office, a surgical suite adjacent to the office, a free-standing facility, or part of a hospital.
- *Choice and benefits:* Some patients prefer not to stay overnight at a hospital. Cost savings and convenience along with added privacy and personalized care may be factors.
- *Accreditation:* As a result of the strict guidelines for equipment, staff, anesthesia services, and hospital access,

patients are encouraged to determine whether a facility is accredited because it could indicate the quality of the facility. (All ASPS member surgeons are required to operate in an accredited medical facility.)
- *Insurance:* Accreditation also affects financial aspects. Although facility fees are typically not covered by insurance providers for elective procedures, facility fees for reconstructive procedures may be covered. Reimbursement may be expedited for facilities that carry accreditation because the accreditation ensures that certain quality standards are met at that facility. Also similar services at a hospital generally cost more than in an ambulatory facility.
- *Individual considerations:* Each patient must discuss the options with his or her surgeon. Depending on medical history and condition requiring surgery, ambulatory surgery may not be appropriate for everyone.

ASPS, American Society of Plastic Surgeons.
Data from American Society of Plastic Surgeons (ASPS): *Patient safety do your homework: accredited facilities* (website), 2017. www.plasticsurgery.org/patient-safety?sub=Accredited +Facilities. (Accessed 22 January 2017).

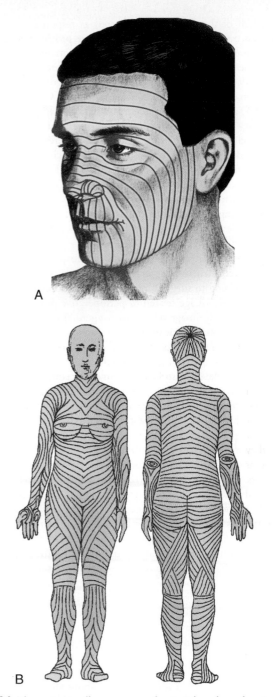

FIG. 22.1 The surgeon adheres to several principles when planning skin incisions, one of which is to reduce the amount of tension across the wound, thus minimizing scarring. Elective incisions should preferably parallel relaxed skin tension lines in the face (A) and the body (B). These lines are also referred to as Langer lines.

defects, the diversity of operative techniques, and the psychologic responses of patients offer unique learning experiences and challenges for perioperative nursing care.

Perioperative Nursing Considerations

The prospect of surgery, even elective, can produce anxiety and fear. Because it is so often associated with body image and self-esteem,

plastic and reconstructive surgery can trigger these emotions, especially when the proposed surgery is associated with potential disfigurement because of disease or trauma. Even a planned (desired) change in body image can be stressful. Many cosmetic surgery patients lack the traditional support system one comes to expect during illness and recuperation because of a desire for confidentiality or because cosmetic surgery is elective and may be viewed by friends or family as nonessential. In these situations the sensitivity of the perioperative nurse is critical.

Generally the nurse creates a therapeutic environment in the following ways: introducing himself or herself and other members of the surgical team; explaining all perioperative events and any sensations likely to be experienced; determining the patient's normal coping patterns; communicating with the patient in a calm, unhurried, and reassuring manner; encouraging the patient to verbalize feelings and concerns, and listening attentively; reducing distracting stimuli in the perioperative environment; providing reassurance and information about the progress of surgery (for awake patients); communicating progress reports to family; providing comfort measures (e.g., warm blankets, soft music of patient preference); and encouraging and assisting the patient to use personally effective coping strategies (e.g., meditation, guided imagery, relaxation) (Patient Engagement Exemplar).

Appropriate candidates for plastic surgery include those who have positive self-image but are bothered by a physical aspect that they would like to improve. After surgery these patients maintain their positive self-image. Another category of appropriate surgical candidates includes patients who have a physical defect or cosmetic flaw that has lowered their self-esteem over time. These patients require time to adjust (rebuild confidence) postoperatively and generally their self-esteem is strengthened, sometimes even dramatically. Patients who may not be suitable for plastic surgery include those in crisis or with unrealistic expectations; those who have an unwillingness to learn risks or unwillingness to change the behavior that led to the problem (e.g., a liposuction patient who continues to overeat); and those who are mentally ill/psychotic, delusional, or paranoid (ASPS, 2017).

The nursing process is dynamic, fluid, and complex. The nature of plastic and reconstructive surgery is rarely simple, routine, or predictable, and the nursing care must mirror that fact. Nursing care must include thorough and ongoing assessment, establishment of nursing diagnoses and outcomes, fastidious planning, superior implementation, and thoughtful evaluation. The perioperative nurse's goal is to produce positive, high-quality outcomes in an environment that is safe and nurturing and facilitate physical and emotional healing.

Assessment

As part of a holistic assessment, perioperative nurses consider physical and emotional factors of the planned procedure. A comprehensive review of the patient's chart is the first step. The presence of a signed and witnessed informed consent, a systems review and health history, pertinent laboratory and diagnostic data, interdisciplinary planning, anesthesia evaluation, and the surgical plan disclose vital information necessary to begin the assessment process. Visual assessment should include the patient's overall physical condition, the condition and integrity of the skin, nutritional status, and physical limitations. The next step is the patient interview, which includes checking patient identification, explaining the perioperative nursing role, and verifying the patient's understanding of the planned procedure. The perioperative nurse must be skilled in communication techniques

PATIENT ENGAGEMENT EXEMPLAR

Clinical Empathy

Creating a supportive patient-centered environment for care is especially important for the specialty of plastic surgery, in which patients may lack traditional support systems or are struggling with body image changes. An important consideration for patient-centered care is the relationship between healthcare providers and their patients. This relationship, as well as the patient's perceived healthcare provider's empathy, can greatly influence treatment outcomes and the patient's satisfaction with the care provided.

CE is a tool that can be used to foster patient-centered care. Sympathy, empathy, and compassion are similar but different; all capacities and compassionate acts result based on feeling. Sympathy refers to an individual's ability to share an emotion being experienced by another. Compassion enhances the empathy. In CE, more imaginative insight is required for the healthcare provider to understand what suffering from a particular pathology actually means from the patient's perspective. Although all three terms are often used interchangeably, it is important for the nurse to remember patients distinguish and experience them differently. Empathy can be expressed verbally or through respectful silence. Hashim (2017) recommends several techniques that may be useful in verbal expressions of empathy, including naming ("I can see that this makes you feel..."), understanding ("I can't imagine what that would feel like..."), respecting ("I respect your courage..."), supporting ("I am here to help you in any way I can..."), and exploring ("Tell me more...")

CE is beneficial for patients, but also for health providers. Literature suggests it helps with professional self-development and increased work satisfaction.

CE, Clinical empathy.

Modified from Hashim MJ: Patient-centered communication: basic skills, *Am Fam Physician* 95(1):29–34, 2017; Sinclair S et al: Sympathy, empathy, and compassion: a grounded theory study of palliative care patients' understandings, experiences, and preferences, *Palliat Med* 31(5):437–447, 2017; Wood D: *Nurses' compassionate care affects patient outcomes* (website), 2016. www.travelnursing.com/news/nurse-news/nurses-compassionate-care-affects-patient-outcomes/. (Accessed 28 January 2017).

to quickly establish a rapport with the patient. Greeting the patient by name in a calm, comforting manner, perhaps with a gentle, caring touch (if welcomed by the patient), and maintaining good eye contact will help establish the relationship needed to assess emotional status, body image disturbances, and anxiety level. Having a conversation with the patient may help reveal any barriers to communication or learning; religious, cultural, or other preferences; mental status; and insight into compliance. Other vital pieces of knowledge the nurse must obtain include the presence of realistic expectations and motivation for surgery, as well as support systems available to the patient.

An important component of the assessment phase of nursing care involves communication with the surgeon and anesthesia provider to determine the need for special equipment, supplies, sutures, or implants. The perioperative nurse should verify the procedure and position and, in the case of multiple procedures on the same patient, identify the planned order of surgeries.

Clear and effective hand-off communication is critical to patient safety. According to The Joint Commission (TJC), communication is the top contributing factor to medical error and sentinel events.

At least half of those incidents occurred as responsibility for the patient was transferred from one team of care providers to another. In the perioperative suites, handoffs occur as patients move to and from the operating room (OR), involving many different care providers for one patient (AORN, 2016c). TJC addresses communication in their National Patient Safety Goal 2 (Improve Staff Communication) (TJC, 2017) and through recommendations around effective handoffs. The primary objective of a handoff is to provide information about a patient's, client's, or resident's general care plan, treatment, services, current condition, and any recent or anticipated changes. Whatever form the hand-off communication takes at each facility, it must be standardized and provide a thorough discussion of patient history, issues, special needs, and precautions for safety, with opportunity for the receiving provider to ask questions.

Nursing Diagnosis

Nursing diagnoses related to the care of the patient undergoing plastic and reconstructive surgery might include the following:
- Anxiety related to surgical interventions or outcomes
- Deficient Knowledge related to perioperative process
- Disturbed Body Image related to congenital or acquired defect or developmental abnormality
- Risk for Ineffective Peripheral Tissue Perfusion related to surgical intervention
- Acute Pain related to surgical/invasive procedure
- Risk for Impaired Skin Integrity and injury related to positioning during surgical procedure
- Risk for Hypothermia related to procedure

Outcome Identification

Nursing diagnoses lead to the formulation of desired or expected patient outcomes. These are desirable and measurable patient states, including biologic or physiologic states; psychologic, cultural, and spiritual aspects; and the knowledge, behavior, or skills related to these states. As such, the patient outcome indicates progress toward or resolution of the nursing diagnosis. Outcomes should be mutually formulated with the patient, family, and other healthcare providers. Such formulations should be realistic, involve consideration of the patient's present and potential capabilities and resources, and provide direction for continuity of care, as well as determine satisfaction with that care. Outcomes identified for the selected nursing diagnoses could be stated as follows:
- The patient will verbalize management of anxiety.
- The patient participates in decision making affecting the perioperative plan of care.
- The patient will acknowledge feelings about altered structure or function.
- The patient has wound/tissue perfusion consistent with or improved from baseline level established preoperatively.
- The patient demonstrates knowledge of pain management.
- The patient will be free of injury and have intact skin integrity at the end of the procedure.
- The patient will maintain adequate body temperature.

Planning

The perioperative nurse designs a plan of care using critical thinking to integrate knowledge gained from the patient. The nurse should seek to create and maintain a culture and environment of safety for the patient, the OR, and all members of the surgical team during the planning process. A Sample Plan of Care for a patient undergoing plastic and reconstructive surgery follows.

SAMPLE PLAN OF CARE

Nursing Diagnosis
Anxiety related to surgical intervention or outcome

Outcome
The patient will verbalize management of anxiety.

Interventions
- Broadly classify the patient's anxiety (mild, moderate, or severe).
- Try to understand the patient's perception of the stressors or stressful situation or event.
- Identify contributing factors.
- Introduce self and other members of the surgical team.
- Explain all perioperative events and any sensations likely to be experienced.
- Determine the patient's normal coping patterns.
- Communicate with the patient in a calm, unhurried, reassuring manner.
- Encourage the patient to express feelings and concerns; listen attentively.
- Reduce distracting stimuli in the perioperative environment.
- Provide reassurance and information about the progress of the surgery (if the patient is awake), and implement a mechanism for family progress reports.
- Provide comfort measures (e.g., warm blankets, soft music that the patient prefers).
- Use touch as appropriate (e.g., softly stroking the hand).
- Encourage and assist the patient to use personally effective coping strategies (e.g., meditation, guided imagery, relaxation).

Nursing Diagnosis
Deficient Knowledge related to the perioperative process

Outcome
The patient demonstrates knowledge of the expected responses to the operative or other invasive procedure.

Interventions
- Determine knowledge level (assess knowledge and comprehension of new information and ability to apply in self-care activities); assess readiness to learn (evaluate factors that may affect abilities to learn or demonstrate knowledge).
- Provide instruction based on age and identified needs; identify barriers to communication and adapt instructions to these.
- Evaluate environment for home care; identify expectations of home care.
- Explain expected sequence of events related to perioperative care; include family members in preoperative teaching; identify family members' knowledge and provide education and support.
- Assess knowledge; provide and evaluate response to instructions (e.g., about wound care and phases of wound healing) (evaluate patient's/family members' understanding of instruction regarding perioperative experience and ongoing care, listening to explanations and observing return demonstrations, techniques of wound care, and signs and symptoms to report).
- Include patient, family members, and caregiver in discharge planning, including resources available to facilitate the rehabilitation process.
- Initiate institution's checklist policy for correct site surgery.
- Verify surgical consent with OR schedule and patient's statement of planned surgery.

- Solicit the patient's questions; answer or refer questions as appropriate.
- Explain the sequence of perioperative events and their purpose, as appropriate (e.g., holding area, OR attire, insertion of lines and attachment of monitoring devices, type of anesthesia, postanesthesia care unit [PACU], protocols).
- Provide printed material to reinforce patient education (e.g., preoperative routines, explanations of surgical intervention, postoperative management of pain, discharge instructions).

Nursing Diagnosis
Disturbed Body Image related to disease, congenital or acquired deformity, developmental abnormality

Outcome
The patient will acknowledge feelings about altered structure or function and identify effective, optimistic coping options.

Interventions
- Identify psychosocial status; elicit perceptions of surgery.
- Identify individual values and wishes concerning care.
- Assess coping mechanisms.
- Implement measures to provide psychologic support.
- Maintain patient's dignity and privacy (e.g., keep OR doors closed, only expose body as needed for care).
- Assist patient to identify and discuss feelings, stressors, and perception of physical deformity.
- Provide an environment (e.g., privacy, supportive listening) conducive to expression of feelings.
- Help patient identify significance of culture, religion, gender, and age on perceived changes in body structure or function or image.
- Determine patient's body image expectations and whether expectations are realistic; clarify unrealistic expectations or misconceptions.
- Convey sense of respect for abilities and strengths in coping with problems or concerns.
- Assist patient to separate physical appearance from feelings of personal worth, self-concept, and self-esteem (as appropriate).
- Refer the patient to other health professionals (e.g., clergy, social worker, psychiatric liaison) or support groups as appropriate.

Nursing Diagnosis
Risk for Ineffective Peripheral Tissue Perfusion related to surgical intervention

Outcome
The patient has wound/tissue perfusion consistent with or improved from baseline levels established preoperatively.

Interventions
- Assess factors related to risks for ineffective tissue perfusion (e.g., presence of diabetes, immunosuppression); assess history of previous radiation exposure.
- Evaluate postoperative tissue perfusion.
- Identify factors associated with an increased risk for hemorrhage or fluid and electrolyte loss (e.g., patients with recent traumatic injury, abnormal bleeding or clotting time, extensive surgical procedure, complicated renal/liver disease, and major organ transplant).
- Implement hemostasis techniques (provide supplies, instrumentation, and appropriate surgical techniques as needed to control hemorrhage).

Continued

SAMPLE PLAN OF CARE—cont'd

- Note any sensory or perceptual alterations in the affected body part, and document them.
- Maintain body temperature with the use of a warming device or reflective blankets, for example.
- Warm intravenous fluids, blood and blood products, and irrigating fluids.
- Increase the temperature in the OR as indicated.
- Collaborate with the anesthesia provider in monitoring the patient's core temperature.
- Apply compression stockings and antiembolic devices as indicated.
- Monitor tissue perfusion (e.g., by assessing blanching and capillary refill; using Doppler ultrasound), as prescribed; record results.
- Note any swelling, change in color or temperature, or drainage from graft sites before discharge from the OR.
- Provide warm blankets for the patient at the conclusion of the surgical procedure.
- Teach the patient or the family how to care for the incision, including signs and symptoms of infection and graft failure (as applicable).

Nursing Diagnosis
Acute Pain related to surgical procedure

Outcome
The patient demonstrates knowledge of pain management.

Interventions
- Assess pain control using validated pain scale.
- Identify cultural and value components related to pain (e.g., stoicism, alternative therapy, verbalization, meditation).
- Implement pain guidelines; provide pain management instruction (purpose; administration; and desired, side, and adverse effects of prescribed medications and nonpharmacologic techniques for managing pain).
- Evaluate response to pain management instruction and instruction about prescribed medications.

- Collaborate in initiating patient-controlled analgesia.
- Evaluate response to pain management interventions (physiologic parameters and subjective and objective findings) and response to medications.
- Implement alternative methods of pain control (diversified activities, therapeutic touch, meditation, breathing, and positioning to augment pain control methods).

Nursing Diagnosis
Risk for Impaired Skin Integrity and injury related to positioning during surgical procedure

Outcome
The patient will have intact skin and be free from injury.

Interventions
- Make sure all bony prominences are well padded with use of positioning devices.
- Monitor patient's extremities every 30 minutes during procedure.
- Maintain extremities in anatomic alignment during surgical procedure.

Nursing Diagnosis
Risk for Hypothermia related to procedure

Outcome
The patient will maintain adequate body temperature during surgical procedure.

Interventions
- Provide warm blankets before anesthesia induction.
- Monitor body temperature during surgical procedure with use of temperature probe.
- Use warming unit during procedure.
- Cover undraped parts of body during surgical procedure.
- Increase OR temperature before anesthesia induction and before extubation.

Implementation

The implementation phase typically begins with preparation of the OR and requires a thorough understanding of the procedure and the special needs of the patient, surgeon, and anesthesia provider. The perioperative nurse must continually monitor and reassess the patient as well as the needs of the perioperative team, implementing and documenting the delivery of care. Constant consideration is given to the safety of the patient and the perioperative environment during this phase.

Preparation of the OR Suite

Before transporting the patient to the OR, the perioperative nurse will assemble all necessary medical and surgical supplies, equipment, suture material, positioning aids, implantable devices, and medications. The nurse is responsible for ensuring that equipment is in working order, that emergency supplies are present, and that compressed gases are adequate. Depending on the procedure to be performed, the OR bed may need to be configured differently from the standard room setup. To minimize inefficiencies during the procedure the nurse should confirm with the surgeon and anesthesia provider the position of the bed and any proposed intraoperative changes to

the bed, room temperature, or room configuration. Plastic and reconstructive surgeons frequently use preoperative photographs of the patient when attempting to restore or modify appearance. These photographs help the surgeon maintain perspective because features may change as a result of surgical positioning. The nurse should collaborate with the surgeon to determine the best placement of these photographs for intraoperative viewing.

Equipment and Special Mechanical Devices

Essential equipment for any OR includes a fully functional bed that may be positioned for any number of special needs and also has accessory attachments, such as headrests and aids for extremity positioning. The room must also have well-positioned and numerous electrical outlets, good overhead lighting, suction equipment, mounted x-ray view boxes, and computer terminals for those facilities using electronic medical records. Stepstools, tables, chairs, hand tables, tourniquets, microscopes, and intravenous (IV) poles should be in appropriate supply and accessible.

Instrumentation. Basic instrument trays are available for the plastic surgery OR. A local procedure tray may include Bishop Harmon and Adson tissue forceps (with and without teeth); straight and curved iris, Stevens, and Metzenbaum scissors; fine mosquito

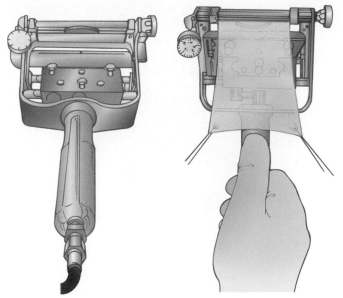

FIG. 22.2 Powered Brown dermatome.

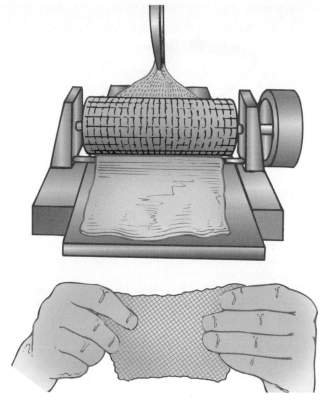

FIG. 22.3 Manual skin graft meshing device.

forceps; and skin hooks. Minor and major trays for plastic surgery may contain a range of tissue forceps, scissors, hemostats, and retractors. With the addition of instruments for specific surgeries and surgeons, these trays usually suffice for all plastic surgery operations. Adequate instrumentation should be available to avoid immediate-use sterilization.

Dermatomes. Dermatomes are used for removing split-thickness skin grafts (STSGs) from donor sites. There are three basic types: knife, drum, and electric and air driven (Fig. 22.2). Sterile mineral oil and a tongue blade should be available when STSGs are being obtained.

Skin Meshers. Several types of skin meshers are available, and each is designed to produce multiple uniform slits in a skin graft approximately 0.05 inch apart. These multiple apertures in the graft can then expand, permitting the skin graft to stretch and cover a larger area. Meshing also facilitates drainage through the graft, preventing fluid accumulation under a graft. The graft is placed on the carrier and passed through the mesher (Fig. 22.3). The manufacturer supplies sterile carriers for meshers. They are usually available in several sizes, which determine the expansion ratio of the skin graft.

Pneumatic-Powered Instruments. Pneumatic-powered instruments use an inert, nonflammable, and explosion-free compressed gas as their power source. The motor may be activated by a foot pedal or hand control. The various attachments should be sterilized as recommended by the manufacturer to prolong instrument life and ensure effective sterilization. The following attachments may be used in plastic surgery:

• Wire driver and bone drill
• Oscillating saw
• Reciprocating saw
• Dermabrader
• Sagittal saw

A pneumatic tourniquet with an inflatable cuff is used in most hand surgery procedures as well as in other upper and lower extremity surgical interventions. Safe use of the tourniquet is described in Chapter 20.

Hemostatic Devices and Equipment. Monopolar and bipolar electrosurgical units (ESUs) are commonly used in plastic surgery. The functionality of ESUs and the safety precautions to observe during their use are described in Chapter 8.

Harmonic ultrasonic devices are cutting instruments used during surgical procedures to simultaneously cut and coagulate tissue. They are similar to ESUs but superior in that they can cut thicker tissue, and they create less toxic smoke with less thermal damage.

Tissue fusion devices provide a combination of pressure and energy to create vessel fusion. They permanently fuse vessels up to and including 7 mm in diameter and tissue bundles without dissection or isolation an average seal cycle of 2 to 4 seconds. Seals withstand three times normal systolic blood pressure.

Fiberoptic Instruments. Examples of fiberoptic instrument attachments used in plastic surgery are a headlight for rhinoplasties, augmentation mammoplasties, and other procedures; a mammary retractor for augmentation mammoplasties; a rhytidectomy retractor; abdominoplasty retractors; and endoscopic face and forehead fiberoptic instrumentation.

Loupes. Loupes (Fig. 22.4) are magnifying lenses used by many plastic surgeons for microvascular surgery and nerve repairs and for numerous other instances in which cosmetic results are improved by the magnification effect. The nurse should inquire about the use of loupes before the surgeon dons a headlight because adjustments will need to be made to the headlight alignment if the loupes are required midprocedure. Adjusting or removing the headlight in midprocedure has the potential to contaminate the sterile field.

Microscope. The microscope is frequently used in nerve repairs and microsurgical anastomoses; the nerves or vessels to be repaired, such as in hand surgery, and the suture used to do so (sometimes 9-0, 10-0, or even 11-0 size) can be finer than human hair and thus

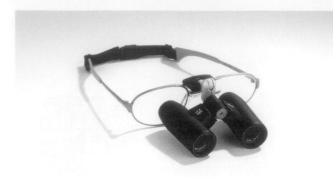

FIG. 22.4 Loupes from Carl Zeiss, used for magnification.

requires magnification. Although each microscope has different features, an important matter to avoid confusion is whether the surgeon control overrides the assistant view, or if each can separately adjust the field of view.

Wood Lamp. The Wood lamp is an ultraviolet lamp used in a darkened room to determine the viability of skin flaps. After IV injection of fluorescein, the blood vessels appear bright purple (the skin appears yellow). Sodium fluorescein is excreted in the urine, and patients should be informed of this.

Special Supplies. Surgeon-specific and procedure-specific special supplies are frequently added to instrument setups for plastic and reconstructive procedures. These commonly include the following: sterile marking pen or methylene blue; ruler; local anesthetic of choice for injection, with syringes and needles; and ESU, with active electrode (pencil) and tip of choice, with tip cleaner.

Sutures

Sutures range from permanent to absorbable and include monofilament and multifilament materials. The perioperative nurse should be a good steward of costly resources and verify the type and number of sutures needed before opening suture packages, as well as needle preference, to prevent waste. Many plastic surgical procedures have multiple techniques, each of which necessitates very specific suture choices. See Chapter 7 for further discussion and explanations.

Dressings

Dressings are an essential part of the operative procedure in plastic surgery and may contribute to the ultimate outcome of the surgical intervention. Dressings are usually applied while the patient is still anesthetized. Generally the dressing should accomplish the following five goals:

1. Immobilize the surgical part.
2. Apply even pressure over the wound.
3. Collect drainage.
4. Provide comfort for the patient.
5. Protect the wound.

Pressure dressings may be used to eliminate dead space, to prevent seroma and hematoma formation, and to prevent third spacing associated with liposuction and reconstructive procedures involving transfer of large muscle or tissue flaps. In some cases pressure can be achieved by the use of catheters or drains placed within the operative site and connected to closed-wound suction devices. In smaller wounds a Penrose drain or a butterfly cannula may be inserted into the operative site, with the needle end placed into a red-top tube, such as a blood collection tube, which has a vacuum (evacuated tube).

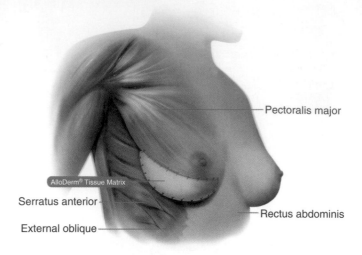

FIG. 22.5 AlloDerm.

The perioperative nurse should be familiar with common general dressings and supplies available in sterile form and various sizes.

In some instances, such as a free flap, transparent dressings are used so that the flap can be monitored and observed for vascular flow. Compression garments and support devices are also frequently used by plastic surgeons. Proper fit is essential to minimize vascular compromise. Compression garments are typically applied over a light dressing. A proper garment is selected based on its characteristics (e.g., fabric, stretch, softness, antimicrobial properties) and proper sizing according to measurement instructions. Educating patients of the needs and benefits of compression garment use as well as providing hints for their proper application (avoid ripping with long nails, instructions on how to don the garment) promotes comfort and compliance

Implant Materials

The range of materials available for implantation and augmentation in the specialty of plastic and reconstructive surgery has benefited from ongoing research and includes prosthetic and natural materials. Perioperative nurses are responsible for complying with tracking regulations for implantable materials and devices (Patient Safety).

Biologic materials (autogenous grafts) are preferred when available. Autologous human tissue successfully used includes fat, solid dermis, and collagen. A cellular collagen (AlloDerm regenerative tissue matrix) is a material that allows for a strong intact repair in breast reconstruction postmastectomy procedures by providing soft tissue reinforcement or replacement. Human cadavers are used as a source for AlloDerm (Fig. 22.5). This product is available in various sizes of sheeting and must be rehydrated in several steps. AlloDerm integrates with the body's tissue and helps prevent rejection over the long term, which allows for a safe and clinically optimal outcome (Acelity, 2017).

Implant failure may be directly linked to bacterial contamination; therefore meticulous aseptic technique with minimal handling is essential when using implants of any sort. Most alloplastic implants are presterilized from the manufacturer.

Anesthesia

A variety of anesthetic techniques are used with plastic surgery procedures. Local, regional, tumescent, conscious sedation, deep sedation, or general anesthesia may be used, depending on the type

PATIENT SAFETY

Tracking Medical Devices

A variety of implantable devices are used in aesthetic and reconstructive plastic surgery procedures. Tracking these devices is critical to patient safety because it facilitates mandatory recalls or notifications. Devices may be recalled for sterility issues, malfunction, or any event that is found to pose a serious health risk.

The FDA regulates the process of tracking medical devices and directs the tracking of devices whose failure would result in serious, adverse health consequences; devices that are intended to be implanted in the human body for more than 1 year; and devices that are life-sustaining and life-supporting and are used outside of a facility such as a hospital, nursing home, or ambulatory surgery center.

The perioperative nurse plays an important role in the accurate documentation of implantable devices for tracking purposes. Information that the nurse typically will gather for tracking purposes includes:

- Device identification (i.e., lot, batch, model number, serial number)
- Date of manufacture and shipping
- Name, address, telephone number, and social security number of the patient who received the device
- Location the device was implanted

- Name, address, and telephone number of the surgeon who is caring for the patient, if different from the prescribing physician

If an implantable device is sterilized within the sterile processing department of the facility, monitoring requirements include the use of a process challenge device containing a biologic indicator. The load should be quarantined until the result of the biologic indicator is determined. Documentation should include a record of the sterilizer load identification number on the patient's medical record, or the patient's name on the load record. Lot identification provides a method for tracing problems in the event of a recall. Immediate-use sterilization of implantable devices is not recommended.

Patients have the right to refuse tracking of their devices and may refuse to have their social security number used for tracking. The patient's consent for tracking should be obtained before the procedure. If the patient refuses to have the device tracked, the nurse will document the refusal along with the required product information and report this information to the manufacturer.

Under the Safe Medical Device Act, institutions must also report any incident of death or serious injury relating to the use of a medical device. Nurses should work within their institutional policies to report these incidents.

FDA, US Food and Drug Administration.
Modified from US Food and Drug Administration (FDA): *Medical device tracking–guidance for industry and Food and Drug Administration staff* (website), 2014. www.fda.gov/RegulatoryInformation/Guidances/ucm071756.htm. (Accessed 22 January 2017); US Food and Drug Administration (FDA): *Medical device reporting (MDR)* (website), 2016. www.fda.gov/MedicalDevices/Safety/ReportaProblem/ucm2005291.htm. (Accessed 22 January 2017); US Food and Drug Administration (FDA): *Mandatory reporting requirements: manufacturers, importers, and device user facilities* (website), 2016. www.fda.gov/MedicalDevices/DeviceRegulationandGuidance/PostmarketRequirements/ReportingAdverseEvents/ucm2005737.htm#3. (Accessed 22 January 2017).

of procedure, the patient's anesthetic history, the American Society of Anesthesiologists (ASA) physical status classification, and the surgeon's preference. Regardless of the type of anesthesia, patients should have baseline vital signs recorded and fully monitored, including blood pressure, heart rate, respirations, cardiac rate and rhythm, oxygen saturation, and end-tidal carbon dioxide ($ETCO_2$) pressure if indicated. When using oxygen on a head and neck procedure, oxygen must be temporarily shut off while the ESU is being used because of its flammability. If a local or regional anesthetic is used without an anesthesia provider, appropriate staffing should be determined based on patient assessment and nurse competency. The presence of a perioperative registered nurse whose sole responsibility is to monitor the patient may be warranted, depending on clinical assessment and patient behavior. This nurse must be sufficiently skilled in assessment and knowledgeable about the agents being used so that changes in the patient's status can be promptly reported and appropriate interventions to prevent complications can be initiated (AORN, 2015).

Injectable anesthetics are frequently used, not only for strictly local cases but also in conjunction with regional, sedation, and even general anesthesia. Local anesthetics (e.g., lidocaine, bupivacaine, prilocaine) act by reversibly blocking nerve impulses—they stop nerve conduction by blocking sodium channels in the axon membrane. When combined with a vasoconstrictor such as epinephrine, local blood flow is decreased and systemic absorption of the anesthetic delayed. This prolongs anesthesia time and reduces the risk of toxicity. Sodium bicarbonate also can be combined with local anesthetics to decrease pain during injection by changing the pH of the solution.

In addition, infiltration of a local anesthetic can help define tissue planes through hydrodissection. Use of epinephrine is contraindicated in areas with limited vascularity, such as digits, the penis, nasal tip, and ears. Additional information about the use of local anesthetics is found in Chapter 5.

Topical anesthetics used by the plastic surgeon include tetracaine (Pontocaine) 2% ophthalmic drops (for blepharoplasty or before application of eye shields), eutectic mixture of local anesthetics (EMLA) for penetration on intact skin (associated with laser surgery), and cocaine solution applied on neurosurgical patties for mucous membranes (for rhinoplasty).

Preoperative Skin Preparation

Most surgical interventions require that the operative site and adjacent areas be cleansed with an antibacterial soap before surgery. The surgeon may prescribe that the patient performs this treatment before surgery. Special attention is given to the fingernails for patients undergoing hand surgery; to hair for surgery of the head, face, or neck; and to oral hygiene for surgery in or near the mouth. The perioperative nurse should verify with the patient that the prescribed regimens have been performed. All body jewelry that pierces the skin should be removed before the skin prep. The operative site should be inspected for any rashes, bruises, open sores, cuts, or other skin conditions. Hair should only be removed if it interferes with the procedure. Shaving is avoided and clippers, not a razor, are used if needed, because shaving creates access for the entry of bacteria into the operative site (AORN, 2016b). The eyebrows and eyelashes, in particular, are left intact to preserve facial appearance and expression. The surgical site is marked before surgery by the surgeon to designate the correct site and to define landmark areas. Either a povidone-iodine solution, an iodine-alcohol mixture, chlorhexidine gluconate (CHG), or another broad-spectrum agent may be selected for the antimicrobial skin prep. The use of CHG should be avoided around the ears and eyes. It is important to place shields on the eyes and/or eye ointment if prepping the periorbital site or performing an extensive head and neck prep, and to place sterile cotton balls or kittners in the ear canals, and prevent pooling of the prep agent. If kittners or cotton balls are used, they must be included in the soft goods count. The perioperative nurse should query the patient regarding any allergies to antimicrobial agents. If indicated, the plan of care should be modified to avoid the use of these products. When prepping for a skin graft procedure, separate skin prep setups are needed for the graft and donor sites.

Positioning and Draping

The OR bed must be positioned so that the remaining space in the room can comfortably accommodate anesthetic equipment, members of the surgical team, instrument tables, and any adjunct equipment (hand table, drills, microscope, laser) to be used. The team positions the patient on the OR bed so that all operative sites may be appropriately exposed and the airway easily observed and accessed.

Before implementing any positioning changes, the perioperative nurse should verify the appropriate placement of the OR bed and the desired patient position. Adequate numbers of personnel and supportive positioning devices must be present. No changes should begin until the anesthesia provider gives permission. Although a majority of plastic surgical procedures are performed in the supine position, many also take place with the patient prone or lateral. Liposuction and postbariatric body contouring procedures may also require repositioning one or more times during surgery. Abdominal procedures may start supine and usually require repositioning to facilitate closure. With each new position, reassessment and documentation of the position and devices used to stabilize the patient should occur. Chapter 6 reviews patient positioning and appropriate safety measures for the supine, lateral, and prone positions, all of which may be used during plastic surgical patient care. The perioperative nurse pays particular attention to the patient's arms during positioning to ensure that they are placed on padded armboards with the palms up and fingers extended (for the supine position). Armboards are maintained at less than a 90-degree angle to prevent brachial plexus stretch. If there are reasons to tuck the arms at the side, the elbows are padded to protect the ulnar nerve, the palms face inward, and the wrist is maintained in a neutral position (AORN, 2016a). A drape secures the arms. It should be tucked snugly under the patient, not under the mattress. This prevents the arm from shifting downward intraoperatively and resting against the OR bed rail.

Correct draping procedures depend on the location of the operative site or sites. Disposable drapes (see Chapter 4) are often used because of their barrier qualities, ease of handling and storage, and versatility in adapting to a variety of plastic surgery procedures. Three frequently used draping techniques in plastic surgery are the head drape, chest drape, and hand drape. These draping configurations have the goal of providing maximum mobility of the operative part. The head drape includes a fluid-resistant drape that encircles the head and the addition of a drape to cover the remainder of the body. The following configurations represent methods of obtaining maximum accessibility and sterile coverage for facial surgery:

1. A barrier sheet, folded in half, and two towels are placed beneath the patient's head with the towels uppermost. The folded barrier sheet covers the headrest or head portion of the OR bed. One towel is brought around the patient's head on each side to cover all hair, leaving the entire face (and ears, as necessary) exposed; the towel is then secured with nonpenetrating towel clamps. For craniofacial procedures a towel folded lengthwise in quarters may be placed under the head to assist with moving the head from side to side. Two additional towels are then placed diagonally across the neck, just under the chin; they are secured to each other (with nonpenetrating towel clamps) in the middle over the neck and are secured on each side to the towel around the head. A full sheet is then added to cover the patient from neck to feet.

2. After the head portion of the drape is placed, a split, or U, drape is added to cover the patient from neck to feet.

Additional Considerations

Preparation is a key ingredient in success. Having backup supplies or equipment, sometimes as elementary as an extra bulb for the light source, can mean the difference in a positive outcome for the patient. Occasionally during the course of a procedure, a flap may become congested and fail, the anatomy may dictate a change in the surgical plan, or perhaps a preselected implant just may not be right. Flexibility, meticulous preparation, and a willingness to improvise and innovate will always serve the perioperative nurse well when working with plastic surgeons.

Evaluation

During the surgical intervention the perioperative nurse is constantly evaluating the patient's response to nursing interventions, anesthesia, and the surgery itself. Progress or lack of progress toward the identified patient outcomes is continually assessed. The results of this ongoing evaluation enable the perioperative nurse to reassess the patient, reorder priorities of patient care, establish new patient outcomes, and revise the perioperative plan of care.

At the conclusion of the surgical intervention the perioperative nurse reviews whether identified patient outcomes have been achieved. The patient's skin integrity is assessed; dressings are applied and their integrity is established before discharge from the OR. Any drains or tubes incorporated in the dressing should be noted. Infusion sites are inspected, and the type of infusing solution, flow rate, and amount infused are noted in the patient record. Local anesthetics, sedatives, or other medications received by the patient are similarly documented. The patient's response during the perioperative period is noted; any unusual or untoward responses are reported to the nurse in the PACU. Warm blankets may be provided, and the patient is gently moved to the transport vehicle. The patient who is recovering from general anesthesia is placed in a safe position on the vehicle; the awake patient should be assisted to a position of comfort.

The perioperative nurse, in collaboration with the anesthesia provider, should give the hand-off report to the nurse in the PACU. Areas requiring ongoing patient observation should be noted in this report; the patient's preoperative, intraoperative, and immediate postoperative statuses are also reported. Using the Sample Plan of Care introduced earlier in this chapter, the perioperative nurse may give part of the report based on patient outcomes. If they were achieved, they may be stated as listed under the Outcomes sections.

Patient, Family, and Caregiver Education and Discharge Planning

Education of the plastic surgery patient begins at the time of consultation. Anxiety inhibits the retention of information; therefore it is always helpful to have written information or other tools for the patient to use as a reference source, beginning with the preoperative instructions as well as postoperative information. The approach to teaching should lend itself to the patient's preferred learning style (e.g., auditory, visual). Specifics that should be addressed include pain management, self-care, diet, exercise, care of incisions and drains, return to the clinic for follow-up appointments, signs and symptoms of infections or complications, and how to reach the surgeon in case of an emergency.

Benefits of an effective education intervention are numerous; it serves to decrease anxiety, improves compliance, reduces the incidence of complications, empowers the patient to become an active participant in his or her own care, and maximizes independence, allowing the patient to more quickly return to an optimal state of health. The patient's readiness to learn, needs, and styles of learning must be assessed. A teaching plan should be individualized based on the desired outcomes of all parties. The teaching should be implemented in consideration of the patient's cultural, psychologic, physical, and cognitive factors.

Surgical Interventions

Reconstructive Plastic Surgery

Reconstructive plastic surgery seeks to restore or improve function after trauma, disease, infection, congenital anomalies, or acquired defects while trying to approximate an aesthetic appearance.

Removal of Skin Cancers

The three most common skin cancers are basal cell, squamous cell, and melanoma (McCance, 2017). Basal cell cancer accounts for the largest percentage of all skin cancers (Fig. 22.6A). If basal cell cancer is left untreated, it will grow locally, but rarely metastasizes (Box 22.1). Treated early, it may be cured by simple excision and closure (with pathologic diagnosis to ensure disease-free margins). The second most common form of cancer is squamous cell carcinoma. Squamous cell skin cancers are considered more aggressive (see Fig. 22.6B). Surgical treatment is the same as that for basal cell carcinomas. Melanoma accounts for the smallest percentage of skin cancers, but it is treated much more aggressively because of its invasive nature and high mortality rate (see Fig. 22.6C). Excision of melanoma may involve sentinel node mapping and excision. Early diagnosis of melanoma is imperative to successful treatment (Evidence for Practice).

Procedural Considerations

Consideration must be given to the type of skin cancer to be excised and the anticipated closure technique. Simple excision and closure with adjacent tissue is the simplest technique, requiring a local plastic tray accompanied by skin markers and an ESU, and usually involving use of a local anesthetic with epinephrine. A simple excision may be performed with the patient administered a local or general anesthetic or after induction of sedation. If additional procedures will be performed (e.g., reconstruction with skin graft, flap, or sentinel

---

BOX 22.1

Important Trends for Skin Cancer

Incidence

An estimated 3.3 million Americans were diagnosed with skin cancer in 2016. Of those cases, 8 or 10 are basal cell, with squamous cell carcinoma occurring less frequently. Malignant melanoma accounts for an estimated 76,380 cases per year.

Mortality

Total estimated deaths for 2016 were 10,130 from malignant melanoma and 3520 from other nonepithelial skin cancers.

Risk Factors

- Excessive exposure to ultraviolet radiation from the sun, including history of sunburns, tanning booths
- Fair complexion
- Occupational exposure to coal tar, pitch, creosote, arsenic compounds, and radium
- Exposure to human papillomavirus and human immunodeficiency virus
- Skin cancer negligible in African Americans because of heavy skin pigmentation

Warning Signals

Any unusual skin conditions, especially a change in the size or color of a mole or other darkly pigmented growth or spot or a sore that does not heal. Changes that occur over a month or so should be evaluated.

Prevention and Early Detection

Avoid sun when ultraviolet light is strongest (e.g., 10.00 a.m. to 3:00 p.m.); use sunscreen preparations, especially those containing ingredients such as PABA. Basal and squamous cell cancers often form a pale, waxlike, pearly nodule or a red, scaly, sharply outlined patch. Melanomas are usually dark brown or black pigmentation. They start as small molelike growths that increase in size, change color, become ulcerated, and bleed easily from a slight injury.

Treatment

The four methods of treatment are excisional surgery, electrodesiccation (tissue destruction by heat), radiation therapy, and cryosurgery (tissue destruction by freezing). For malignant melanomas, wide and often deep excisions and removal of nearby lymph nodes are required.

Survival

For basal cell and squamous cell cancers, cure is virtually ensured with early detection and treatment. Malignant melanoma, however, is more likely than other skin cancers to spread to other parts of the body. The 5- and 10-year survival rates for people with melanoma are 91% and 89%, respectively.

PABA, Para-aminobenzoic acid.
Modified from American Cancer Society (ACS): *Key statistics for basal and squamous cell skin cancers* (website), 2016. www.cancer.org/cancer/basal-and-squamous-cell-skin-cancer/about/key-statistics.html. (Accessed 21 January 2017); McCann SA et al: Structure, function, and disorders of the integument. In Huether SE et al, editors: *Understanding pathology,* ed 6, St Louis, 2017, Mosby.

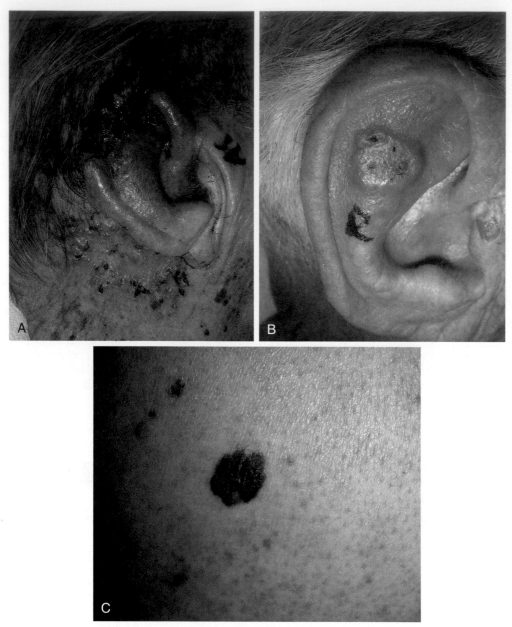

FIG. 22.6 (A) Basal cell carcinoma. (B) Squamous cell carcinoma. (C) Melanoma.

EVIDENCE FOR PRACTICE

Melanoma Awareness, Prevention, and Detection

Melanoma is a cancer that begins in the melanocytes (the cells responsible for skin pigment). Melanoma is more common in men than women and may develop anywhere on the skin or, less commonly the eyes, mouth, genitals, and anal area. Although the exact cause of developing a melanoma is not known, certain risk factors have been identified:

- UV radiation: Sunlight, tanning beds
- Moles: More than 50 = greater risk
- Fair skin: Fair skin, freckling, red or blond hair
- Family history: 10% have a relative with melanoma
- Immune system compromise: Taking antirejection medications after organ transplantation surgery
- Age: Increased risk in older adults

- Gender: Men more than women
- Previous melanoma: Increased risk for having another melanoma

Prevention

Limit UV radiation exposure:

1. Wear protective clothing (tight weave) and a hat with a broad brim.
2. Avoid too much sunlight; remember that it reflects off water, sand, concrete, and snow. Shade is good.
3. Use sunscreen with an SPF 15 or higher (daily use); apply 20 to 30 minutes before sun exposure; reapply every 2 hours; protect your lips.

▌ EVIDENCE FOR PRACTICE

Melanoma Awareness, Prevention, and Detection—cont'd

4. Do not forget your eyes. Look for sunglasses with 99% UV absorption.
5. Stay away from tanning beds and lamps. Try using self-tanning lotions.
6. Protect children with sunscreen. Their skin is fragile, and most damage to skin is acquired before the age of 18 years.
7. Take an inventory. Know your moles and what they normally look like so you can detect changes if and when they occur.

Know Your A-B-C-D-Es

- *Asymmetry:* one-half of the lesion looks different from the other side.
- *Border irregularity:* instead of a smooth edge, the border is ragged or irregular.
- *Color:* the color is usually irregular as well; may have a number of different hues and colors.
- *Diameter:* lesions larger than 6 mm have a greater chance of being a melanoma.
- *E:* enlargement and elevation.

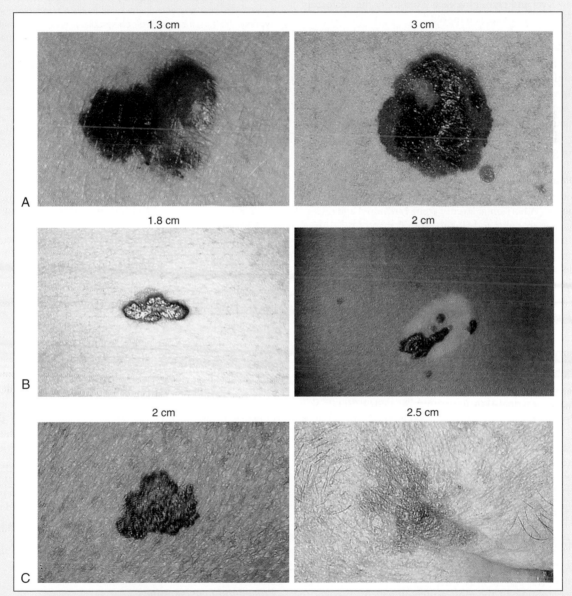

Malignant melanomas. Note presence of "ABCDE" characteristics (*a*symmetry, irregular *b*order, variation in *c*olor, *d*iameter >6 mm, *e*nlargement and *e*levation). (A) Superficial spreading melanoma. (B) Nodular melanoma. (C) Lentigo malignant melanoma.

UV, Ultraviolet.

Modified from American Cancer Society (ACS): *Melanoma skin cancer* (website), 2017. www.cancer.org/cancer/melanoma-skin-cancer.html. (Accessed 22 January 2017); Ignatavicius D et al: *Medical-surgical nursing: patient-centered collaborative care,* ed 8, St Louis, 2016, Elsevier; Niederhuber JE et al: *Abeloff's clinical oncology,* ed 5, Philadelphia, 2014, Elsevier.

node mapping), refer to those sections for additional procedural considerations.

Operative Procedure: Simple Excision

1. The site is marked, prepped, and draped.
2. The surgeon infiltrates the site with a local anesthetic.
3. The lesion is curetted or excised and may be sent for frozen section or pathologic diagnosis.
4. Hemostasis is obtained.
5. The surgeon closes the wound if necessary.

Mohs Surgery

Mohs surgery is a specialized technique used to treat basal and squamous cell skin cancers. The procedure involves excising the lesion layer by layer and examining each layer under the microscope until all the abnormal tissue is removed.

Procedural Considerations

Mohs surgery is usually completed on an ambulatory basis with the patient administered a local anesthetic. The procedure can be very time-consuming to accomplish, but it typically results in the preservation of the surrounding healthy tissue. Because the procedure is lengthy, patient preparation and comfort are essential to facilitate cooperation during the procedure. A minor plastic surgery set is required, along with fine (5-0 or 6-0) suture material.

Operative Procedure

Current procedures involve removal of all visible portions of the skin cancer lesion. A horizontal layer of tissue is removed and divided into sections that are color coded with dyes. A map of the surgical site is then drawn. Frozen sections are immediately prepared and examined microscopically for any remaining tumor. If tumor is found, the location or locations are noted on the map and another layer of tissue is resected. The procedure is repeated as many times as necessary to completely remove the tumor. The patient may be referred to a plastic surgeon for reconstruction of the defect after completion of the Mohs procedure.

Burn Surgery

A majority of burns result from exposure to high temperatures, which injures the skin. Flame, scalding, or direct contact with a hot object may cause thermal skin injury. Similar destruction of skin can result from contact with chemicals such as acid or alkali or contact with an electrical current. The latter, however, often involves extensive destruction of the underlying tissue and physiologic systems in addition to the skin. Approximately 486,000 burn injuries receive medical treatment yearly; 40,000 patients are hospitalized in the United States for burn injuries, with 30,000 of those admitted to the 128 hospitals with specialized burn centers (ABA, 2016).

Intact skin provides protection against the environment for all underlying tissues and organs. It aids in heat regulation, prevents water loss, and is the major barrier against bacterial invasion. The tissue injury resulting from a burn disrupts this normal protective function, resulting in local and systemic effects (Box 22.2). Therefore burn patients are some of the most acutely ill patients brought to the OR. The greater the degree of injury to the skin, expressed in percentage of total body surface area (BSA) and depth of burn, the more severe the injury. One method of measuring BSA in adults is by use of the "rule of nines" (Coffee, 2016) (Fig. 22.7).

Partial-thickness (first- and second-degree) burns heal by regeneration of skin from dermal elements that remain intact. First-degree

---

BOX 22.2

Pathophysiology of Burn Injuries

Thermal and chemical injuries disrupt the normal protective function of the skin, causing local and systemic effects. The extent of these effects depends on the type, duration, and intensity of exposure to the causative agent. With electrical burns, heat is generated as the electrical current passes through body tissues, causing thermal burns along the path taken by the current. Local damage is marked by histamine release and severe vasoconstriction, followed in a few hours by vasodilation and increased capillary permeability, which allows plasma to escape into the wound. Damaged cells swell and platelets and leukocytes aggregate, causing thrombotic ischemia and escalating tissue damage. Systemic effects, which are caused by vascular changes and tissue loss, include hypovolemia, hyperventilation, increased blood viscosity, and suppression of the immune system. The severity of the burn determines the extent of local and systemic effects. Severity is judged by the depth of the burn and the quantity of tissue involved. The depth of the burn is classified by degree. First-degree (superficial) burns affect the epidermis only; second-degree burns (split thickness) affect the epidermis and dermis; third-degree burns (full thickness) affect all skin layers and extend to subcutaneous tissue, muscle, and nerves; fourth-degree burns involve all skin layers, plus bone. The percentage of TBSA system of the American Burn Association classifies quantity as follows:

- *Minor burn:* Full-thickness burns over less than 2% of TBSA; partial-thickness burns over less than 15% of TBSA
- *Moderate burns:* Full-thickness burns over 2% to 10% of TBSA; partial-thickness burns over less than 15% to 25% of TBSA
- *Major burns:* Full-thickness burns over 10% or more of TBSA; partial-thickness burns over 25% or more of TBSA; any burn to face, head, hands, feet, or perineum; inhalation and electrical burns; burns complicated by trauma or other disease processes

TBSA, Total body surface area.
Modified from Jeschke MG, Herndon DN: Burns. In Townsend CM et al, editors: *Sabiston textbook of surgery: the biological basis of modern surgical practice,* ed 20, Philadelphia, 2017, Saunders.

---

burns involve the epidermis, which appears pink or red; sunburn is usually a first-degree burn. Second-degree burns, also called partial-thickness burns, involve the epidermis and some of the dermis. Full-thickness (third-degree) burns (Fig. 22.8) involve the epidermis, the entire dermis, and the subcutaneous tissues; they require skin grafting to heal because no dermal elements remain intact. Both partial-thickness and full-thickness burns may require debridement of necrotic tissue (eschar) before healing can occur by skin regeneration or grafting. An allograft may be used to cover the burned area during the initial healing process. However, the allograft must be carefully tested for immunodeficiency diseases. A xenograft (e.g., graft from a donor of a different species, such as pig skin) may also be used for covering the burned area.

Procedural Considerations

The essentials of skin grafting are discussed later in this chapter. This section deals only with the procedure for debridement of burn wounds.

A basic plastic instrument set is required, plus a knife dermatome, an ESU, topical thrombin solution, a pneumatic tourniquet for isolated extremity burns, and a topical antimicrobial agent of choice.

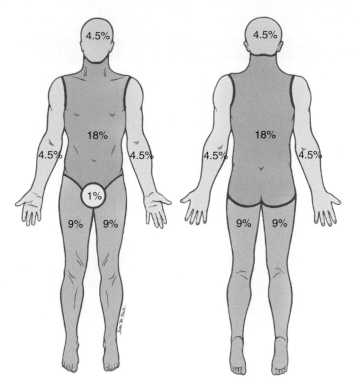

FIG. 22.7 The "rule of nines." The amount of skin surface burned in an adult can be estimated by dividing the body into 11 areas of 9% each.

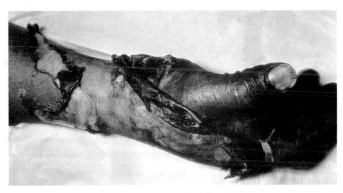

FIG. 22.8 Full-thickness thermal injury.

Because patients who have sustained burns are vulnerable to hypothermia from the loss of BSA, the perioperative nurse should ensure the temperature and humidity in the OR are increased and exposure is limited only to the areas related to the planned surgical event. Anesthesia is often induced while the patient is on the burn unit bed; transfer to the OR bed is done carefully and gently, with attention to maintaining the airway. Most burn patients arrive in the OR with dressings covering their wounds. The dressings are removed after the patient has been anesthetized to minimize pain and loss of body heat through the open burn wounds. Throughout the procedure, the temperature in the OR is constantly monitored to prevent hypothermia in the patient. The OR team caring for burn patients coordinates activities to prevent any delays in obtaining required equipment or supplies. The perioperative nurse will need to collaborate with the anesthesia provider in determining fluid replacement requirements. A variety of topical agents are used to dress burn wounds. Perioperative nurses must be familiar with these agents and their uses (Surgical Pharmacology).

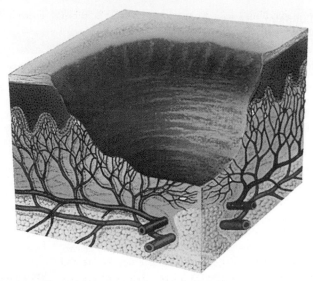

FIG. 22.9 Pressure ulcers often appear after blood flow to an area slows or is obstructed because of pressure on bony prominences. Infections often follow because lack of blood flow causes tissue damage or death.

Operative Procedure

1. The surgeon excises only affected damaged nonviable tissue down to underlying muscle fascia.
2. An alternative method is tangential excision of the burn wound, which is performed with a knife dermatome. This type of excision is usually carried down only to the bleeding subcutaneous fat, rather than to fascia.
3. Hemostasis is obtained with the ESU or use of topical thrombin solution.
4. Dressings saturated with the topical antimicrobial agent of choice are applied.

Although skin grafting may be done at the time of wound debridement, it is usually performed several days later, particularly in extensive burns.

Excisional Debridement

Excisional debridement is the act of removing dead or devitalized tissue to promote healing. Plastic surgeons use debridement in conjunction with treatment of injuries, trauma, and infection. Additional information on wound debridement may be found in Chapter 9.

Treatment of Pressure Injury

Pressure injury can result from prolonged compression of soft tissues overlying bony prominences (Fig. 22.9). However, whether excessive pressure is sufficient to create an ulcer depends on the intensity and duration of the pressure as well as on tissue tolerance. Prevention is the key, and avoiding pressure on bony prominences is most important in immobilized or paralyzed patients. Factors that contribute to pressure injury are immobility, sensory and motor deficits, reduced circulation, anemia, edema, infection, moisture, shearing force, friction, and nutritional debilitation (McGrath and Pomeranz, 2017). The most common sites of pressure injury are the sacrum, the ischium, the trochanter, the malleolus, and the heel. Pressure injury is different from chronic ulcers such as vascular, diabetic, and neurogenic ulcers. Surgical interventions for pressure injury are usually based on staging (see Chapter 6). Stage 3 injuries show full-thickness

SURGICAL PHARMACOLOGY

Topical Medications Used in Burn Therapy

Medication and Category	Dosage and Route	Purpose and Action	Adverse Reactions	Nursing Implications
Petroleum-based antimicrobials (bacitracin, polymyxin B, Neosporin)	Topical (500 units/g): Apply one to five times a day as directed	Partial-thickness burns Provides barrier protection to wound Has broad-spectrum antimicrobial action against gram-negative, gram-positive, and *Candida* organisms Minor skin abrasions, superficial infections, prophylactic postsurgical wounds	Rash, burning, inflammation, pruritus	Gently cleanse wound before application; evaluate for hypersensitivity reaction
Silver sulfadiazine (Silvadene)	Topical: Apply one or two times a day as directed	Deep partial to full-thickness burns Wound infection	Burning, stinging at treatment site; fungal superinfections may occur; toxic nephrosis possible with significant systemic absorption	Apply to cleansed, debrided burns using sterile gloves; keep burns covered with silver sulfadiazine at all times
Mafenide acetate (Sulfamylon)	Topical cream (1 g): Two or three times daily 11.1% cream: Penetrates thick eschar and cartilage 5% solution: Antimicrobial solution used to treat and prevent wound infections	Deep partial-thickness to full-thickness burns Wound infection Is bacteriostatic against gram-negative and gram-positive bacteria Diffuses through devascularized areas, is absorbed, and rapidly converts to a metabolite	Pain on application, metabolic acidosis, hypersensitivity rash, fungal growth	Discontinue when eschar no longer present; may need pain management during application
Silver nitrate (5% solution)	Topical: Apply two or three times per week for 3 weeks	Deep partial-thickness to full-thickness burns Wound infection Has poor penetration of eschar Is bacteriostatic against gram-negative and gram-positive organisms	Skin discoloration, pain on application, staining of clothes and linens, decreases in electrolytes	Apply with cotton-tipped applicator; treat only affected areas

Modified from Kizior RJ, Hodgson BB: *Saunders nursing drug handbook 2017*, St Louis, 2017, Saunders.

skin loss with injury to underlying tissue layers and may contain necrotic material. Thorough excisional debridement is performed, and IV antibiotic therapy is instituted. Although debrided stage injuries often heal on their own, surgical excision and closure may be done to prevent a lengthy spontaneous closure, which may result in a weak, unstable scar with resultant recurrence. Stage 4 injuries are the deepest, requiring more radical excisional debridement. Adequate soft tissue cover may be obtained by either split-thickness or full-thickness skin grafting or tissue flaps (Fig. 22.10). Tissue expansion may be used when there is not enough tissue adjacent to the ulcer site to provide flap coverage.

Although many techniques and flaps are surgical options, basic principles apply to all pressure injury procedures. The following procedure is for an adjacent flap.

Procedural Considerations

A basic plastic instrument set is required, as well as assorted sizes of osteotomes (straight and curved), a mallet, assorted curettes, a Key periosteal elevator, a duckbill rongeur, bone wax, the dermatome of choice, the ESU, a sterile marking pen, and a closed-wound drainage system. The patient is positioned and draped so that the pressure ulcer, adjacent flap donor site, and skin graft donor site are well exposed.

Operative Procedure

1. The area to be excised and the local flap are outlined.
2. The surgeon excises the ulcer along with the underlying bony prominence. Avascular bone is debrided using rongeurs, rasps, osteotomes, and curettes.
3. Large drains are placed into the defect left by excision of the ulcer and beneath the flap.
4. The flap is sutured in place.
5. A STSG generally is used to resurface the flap donor site.
6. A stent dressing is placed over the skin graft, and gauze dressings or a plastic spray dressing is applied over the suture lines of the flap.

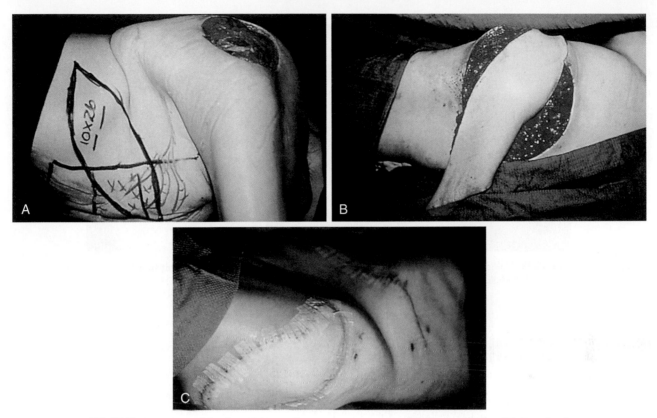

FIG. 22.10 (A) Rotational flap from abdomen for pressure sore coverage. (B) Placement of flap. (C) Completed coverage with flap placement.

Skin and Tissue Grafting

Skin grafting provides an effective way to cover a wound if vascularity is adequate, infection is absent, and hemostasis is achieved. Skin from the donor site is detached from its blood supply and placed on the recipient site, where it develops a new blood supply from the base of the wound. Color match, contour, and durability of the graft are all considerations in selection of an appropriate donor area. Other types of grafts that are available for surgical reconstruction include bone, cartilage, nerve, tendon, and autologous fat grafts.

Split-Thickness and Full-Thickness Skin Grafts

Skin grafts can be either STSGs or full-thickness skin grafts (FTSGs) (Fig. 22.11). Emerging research is also focused on perfecting techniques for epidermal skin grafts (Research Highlight). An STSG (or partial-thickness graft) contains epidermis and only a portion of the dermis of the donor site; its thickness varies. Although this type of graft becomes vascularized more rapidly and the donor site heals more rapidly than an FTSG, it may exhibit postgraft contraction, be minimally resistant to surface trauma, and be least like normal skin in texture, suppleness, pore pattern, hair growth, and other characteristics. An STSG may be meshed (Fig. 22.12); meshed grafts can expand to many times their original size. Meshing allows the graft to be placed on an irregular recipient area; however, its appearance may be aesthetically undesirable. An FTSG contains both epidermis and dermis. Any remaining subcutaneous tissue is trimmed before the FTSG is applied to the graft site. The advantages of this type of graft are that it causes minimal contracture, can be used in areas of flexion, has a greater ability to withstand trauma, can add tissue where a loss has occurred or where padding is required, and

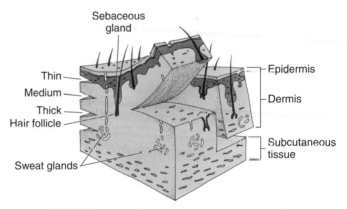

FIG. 22.11 Split-thickness and full-thickness skin grafts.

is aesthetically more acceptable than an STSG. The donor site can be closed primarily, leaving a minimal defect.

The donor site for an STSG heals by regeneration of epithelium from dermal elements that remain intact. Thus only a dressing is placed over this donor site. Because no dermal elements remain when an FTSG is taken, this donor site does not heal spontaneously. It heals either when the wound edges of the donor site are sutured together (primary closure) or when an STSG is applied over it. A scar remains at the donor site of a skin graft; therefore donor sites that are covered by clothing are generally chosen.

For a graft to survive, the vascularity of the recipient area must be adequate, contact between the graft and recipient bed must be maintained, and the graft-bed unit must be adequately immobilized.

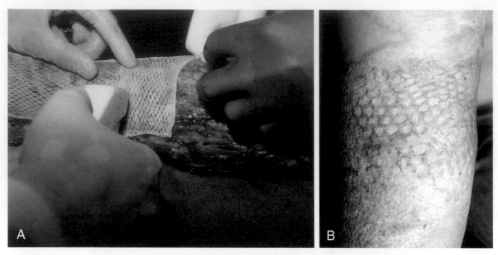

FIG. 22.12 (A) Split-thickness skin is meshed and used to cover a marginal wound. Minimal expansion is used, and the holes provide drainage. (B) Appearance of the graft after healing.

RESEARCH HIGHLIGHT

Epidermal Skin Grafts

Autologous skin grafts, such as full-thickness and split-thickness, have long been part of the reconstructive ladder as an option to close skin defects. Although they are effective in providing coverage, they require the need for a trained surgeon, use of anesthesia and OR, and creation of a wound at the donor site. These drawbacks can be overcome with the use of ESGs, which can be harvested without the use of anesthesia in an office setting and with minimal to no scarring at the donor site. A comprehensive search (Kanapathy, 2016) of studies on ESGs reviewed a total of 154 wounds in 134 patients. Of these, 73.1% of the wounds achieved complete healing with no reported donor-site morbidity, concluding that ESG offers a reasonable treatment option for wound healing.

ESGs consist of only the epidermal layer of skin and provide epidermal cells to the recipient area. They do not prevent wound contracture and therefore, like STSGs the major goal of epidermal grafting is to restore the functional integrity of the skin at the recipient site. However, distinct from other forms of skin grafting, ESGs do not require anesthesia to harvest, cause minimal scarring, and leave little to no donor-site morbidity. This eliminates the risk of anesthesia-related complications and makes epidermal grafting more practical and less expensive to obtain.

ESGs are an alternative when only epidermis is needed. Wound bed preparation, such as adequate granulation tissue formation, is necessary for reepithelialization to occur. Established treatment protocols for wounds are recommended to initially prepare the wound bed for ESGs. The patient and wound should also be assessed to ensure comorbidities are addressed and the

patient has the ability to heal such as adequate nutrition, vascular supply, and the absence of infection.

No pretreatment is required at the donor site. The donor site may be warmed and/or moistened before applying the harvesting device to speed up time to microdome formation. These warming/moistening techniques may be helpful in young patients and in individuals with darkly pigmented skin. The harvested microdomes can be transferred using a film dressing or a nonadherent silicone dressing, both of which can help manage wound exudate and prevent shifting of the grafts from the wound bed. Skin adhesives may also be used around the wound when using the film dressing.

Secondary dressings can, and should, be used over the wound after application of ESGs. These secondary dressings include compression and bolstering materials, compression wraps, and off-loading devices including total contact casting depending on the wound etiology and location. The purpose of the bolster is to keep the transfer dressing in contact with the wound, increase the surface area contact, and help prevent shearing. Negative pressure wound therapy can also be used to improve graft/wound bed contact.

For at least 1 week, ESGs should not be disturbed in any way and primary dressings should not be removed, although secondary dressings can be changed within 1 week, if needed. At the first few weekly dressing changes, debridement should not be performed, unless there is any negative change in the wound bed appearance, such as excessive maceration, infection, or necrosis. Given the thinness of the graft, the graft take may occur but may not be visible for up to 3 weeks after application.

ESG, Epidermal skin graft; *STSG,* split-thickness skin graft.

Modified from Edmondson O et al: To cellutome or not to cellutome? A patient reported outcome measure and cost evaluation study, *Int J Surg* 36(S1): S93, 2016; Hachach-Haram N et al: The use of epidermal grafting for the management of acute wounds in the outpatient setting, *J Plast Reconstr Aesthet Surg* 68(9):1317–1318, 2015; Kanapathy M et al: Systematic review and meta-analysis of the efficacy of epidermal grafting for wound healing, *Int Wound J* [Epub], 2017; Kirsner R et al: Clinical experience and best practices using epidermal skin grafts on wounds, *Wounds* 27(11):289–292, 2015.

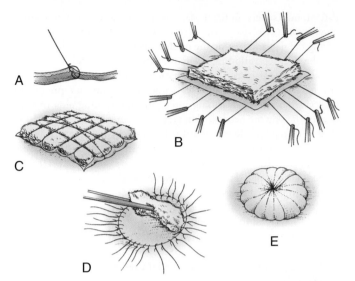

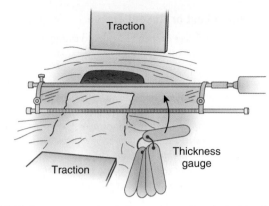

FIG. 22.14 Harvesting a split-thickness skin graft with the Humby knife.

FIG. 22.13 (A) Method of fixation of skin graft to edges of wound. (B) Nonadherent dressing is applied over skin graft, on top of which is placed a generous pad of acrylic fiber. (C) Long ends of suture are tied over fiber to produce area of pressure between graft and base. (D) Similar dressing is applied to circular graft. (E) Long suture ends are tied over circular graft (often called *stent dressing*).

Color, temperature, signs of infection, blanching of the skin, excessive pain and discomfort, edema, vasoconstriction, and venous congestion should be noted and any change documented and reported to the surgeon.

A stent or tie-over dressing is often placed over a skin graft (Fig. 22.13). This exerts even pressure, ensuring good contact between graft and recipient site. It also eliminates potential shearing forces at the graft and recipient site interface that might disrupt new blood vessels growing into the graft.

Procedural Considerations. A plastic local procedure instrument set is required, with the addition of a dermatome of choice, a skin mesher, sterile tongue blades, mineral oil, and a sterile marking pen. The team positions the patient so that both donor and recipient sites are well exposed. Both areas are prepped and draped to maintain adequate exposure and mobility, as required.

Operative Procedure

1. The recipient site is prepared as necessary. This step may involve excision of a benign or malignant skin tumor, debridement of an open wound, or release of a scar contracture.
2. Careful planning and marking before harvesting the graft from the recipient site are essential. Patterns matching intended recipient site and the donor site are outlined with a sterile marking pen.
3. STSGs are harvested with a knife dermatome or powered dermatome of the surgeon's choice (Fig. 22.14).
4. Counted soft goods (sponges) moistened in normal saline, an antibiotic solution, or a solution of 20 mg of phenylephrine HCl (Neo-Synephrine) per 1000 mL of normal saline may be applied to the donor sites to aid hemostasis. The scrub person, who may be a registered nurse or surgical technologist, ensures medication labels indicating strength are placed on all solutions to further identify all solutions on the sterile field. After hemostasis is obtained, the soft goods are removed, the count reconciled, and the donor site covered with the surgeon's preference, which could include Biobrane, xeroform, scarlet red, or OpSite.

5. If the graft is to be meshed, it is now applied to the skin mesh carrier.
6. The scrub person should make sure the graft is kept on the carrier and covered with moist gauze sponges to prevent drying and inadvertent loss of the graft. Meshed skin should not be removed from its carrier until it is applied directly to the recipient site. Whether applied as a sheet or meshed, the STSG may be sutured or stapled with a skin stapler. Nonadherent gauze is usually applied as the first layer of dressing over a graft. Moist dressings should be applied to all meshed grafts to prevent desiccation and loss of the graft.
7. Fat adherent to the graft is trimmed. The graft is applied to the recipient site and usually sutured at the edges, and these sutures are left long to tie over a stent dressing. Blood clots beneath the graft are removed by saline irrigation before the dressing is applied.

Composite Grafts

Composite grafts are composed of skin and underlying tissues that are completely separated from the blood supply of the donor site and transplanted to another area of the body. The survival of a composite graft depends on ingrowth of new blood vessels from the recipient site around the periphery of the graft. Therefore composite grafts are usually small so that no portion of the graft is more than 1 cm from its periphery. An example of compound tissues used as composite grafts is hair transplants, composed of skin, fat, and hair follicles, which are used to treat male pattern baldness. The term *composite* thus indicates a defect that requires a graft be transferred to the area to meet more than one type of tissue deficiency.

Procedural Considerations. A plastic local instrument set is required, plus a sterile marking pen. The patient is positioned, prepped, and draped such that adequate exposure of both donor and recipient sites is achieved.

Operative Procedure

1. When feasible, the surgeon makes a pattern of the recipient site and transfers it to the donor site.
2. The surgeon excises the composite graft and closes the donor site by approximating its skin edges or leaving it unsutured if appropriate.
3. Meanwhile, the composite graft is kept in a moist sponge until it is sutured to the edges of the recipient site.
4. Dressings of choice are applied to the composite graft and donor site.

Replacement of Lost or Absent Tissue

When coverage for a defect cannot be achieved through skin grafting, plastic surgeons rely on other techniques to replace tissue. Just as the flap has evolved, other techniques for tissue restoration through biologic tissue engineering have also evolved. Tissue engineering is defined by Leona and colleagues (2017) as:

> *The application of the principles and methods of engineering and the life sciences toward the development of biologic substitutes to restore, maintain, or improve function. The use of biologic dressings as well as scaffolds, stem cell therapy and gene therapy are a few examples of tissue engineering, in which new tissues are created rather than transferred.*

A discussion of flap techniques follows.

Flaps

The term *flap* refers to tissue that is detached from one area of the body and transferred to the recipient area with either part or all of its original blood supply intact. Because flaps carry their own blood supply, they generally are used to cover recipient sites that have poor vascularity and full-thickness tissue loss. Flaps are used for reconstruction or wound closure. They are useful for covering exposed bone, tendon, or nerve. They may be used if surgery through the wound may be necessary at a later date to repair underlying structures. Flaps containing skin and subcutaneous tissue retain more properties of normal skin and shrink less than skin grafts. Flaps, however, have some disadvantages, such as bulky appearance, failure to match tissue of the recipient site in texture or color, and the possibility of requiring multiple operations and prolonged hospitalization.

Flaps may be classified according to blood supply. *Random pattern flaps* consist of skin and subcutaneous tissue vascularized by random perforators with a limited length-to-width ratio. *Axial pattern flaps* have a well-defined arteriovenous supply along the long axis; they can be comparatively long in relation to width. Flaps may also be classified according to position or how they are rotated after elevation. *Advancement flaps* are cut and advanced to reconstruct a nearby defect. *Transposition flaps* are advanced along an axis that forms an angle to the flap's original position. *Rotation flaps* are similar to transposition flaps but are semicircular and rotate along a greater axis. *Island flaps* of isolated sections of skin and subcutaneous tissue are tunneled beneath the skin to new sites. *Pedicle flaps* were the forerunners of muscle and musculocutaneous flaps. These consist of skin and underlying muscle; they are very mobile and can be rotated into distant defects. *Free flaps* are actually a form of tissue transplantation. Using microvascular techniques, a defined amount of skin, muscle, or bone can be isolated, totally detached, and reattached at the recipient site by microvascular anastomoses between recipient site blood vessels and the major vessels that supply the flap. The vascular pedicle may contain functional nerves, yielding sensory flaps to provide protective sensation or motor flaps to restore function. Bone and joints may be transplanted as free flaps, as in the case of toe-to-thumb site transfers (see Fig. 22.22).

Procedural Considerations. The perioperative nurse should consult with the surgeon in advance of the procedure to determine the donor site, the patient's position(s), and the surgical sequence of the procedure. Generally the surgical site and flap area are marked preoperatively with the patient in a functional position because landmarks and aesthetics are influenced by surgical positioning. If marking is undertaken on the anesthetized and surgically positioned

patient, inaccuracies in tissue placement could occur. Flap procedures may involve two teams of surgeons working simultaneously: one raising the flap and closing the resulting defect, and the other preparing the site, repositioning the flap in its new site, and, in the case of a free flap, microscopically reanastomosing the blood vessels. For any lengthy procedure, a Foley catheter, intermittent pneumatic compression device, warming units, and positioning aids that are safe for the skin are needed. Skin grafts are sometimes used to achieve closure of the flap donor site; if this is anticipated, then the nurse and scrub person should add appropriate instrumentation for harvesting a skin graft. A plastic instrument set and surgeon's preference of dermatome and skin mesher should be available as well as any other equipment requests.

Operative Procedure: Advancement, Transpositional, Rotational, Island, and Pedicle Flaps

1. The recipient site is prepared in the same manner as for a skin graft.
2. Patterns matching the recipient and donor sites are drawn or marked.
3. The surgeon incises, elevates, and transfers the flap to the recipient site.
4. The edges of the flap are sutured to the periphery of the recipient site.
5. The surgeon repairs the flap donor site by approximating the skin edges directly or by covering the defect with a skin graft or another flap.
6. Drains are usually placed under flaps.
7. Dressings are applied with particular attention given to immobilization of the flap, which may require a stockinette, padding, or plaster of Paris.

Note: Before a pedicle flap is detached from the donor site, the surgeon evaluates the adequacy of circulation within the flap. One method to check circulation involves placing rubber-shod clamps across the base of the pedicle and injecting sodium fluorescein intravenously. After 10 minutes have elapsed, all lights in the OR are turned off and a Wood lamp is held over the flap to determine the presence or absence of fluorescence within the flap. Fluorescein may be injected locally for the same purpose.

Operative Procedure: Free Flaps. See Operative Procedure for free transverse rectus abdominis myocutaneous (TRAM) flap described under Reconstructive Breast Surgery.

Reconstructive Breast Surgery

According to the US Department of Labor (DOL), the Women's Health and Cancer Rights Act of 1998 (WHCRA) mandates financial coverage of all breast reconstruction–related procedures (DOL, 2014).

The loss of a breast because of cancer may have a devastating effect on a woman. Fortunately the option of breast reconstruction is available to virtually any woman who loses her breast to cancer. Reconstruction has the ability to offer hope and a return to wholeness and normalcy. Normal, of course, is subjective, and although breasts may be reconstructed, there is a wide range of outcomes, and it must be stressed that breast reconstruction is not a onetime surgery. Revisions are the rule, not the exception. Techniques and options continue to evolve and improve, and women have many options. Breast reconstruction may be offered at one of many times during this process: initially, at the time of mastectomy; before or after adjunct therapy; or even many years later. The important fact is that each woman and her oncologic status are individual, so the decision for reconstruction must be made according to the woman's wishes coupled with her most favorable circumstances. Reconstruction has no known effect on the recurrence of breast cancer. Breast reconstruction options include alloplastic (artificial materials such as breast implants), autogenous (flaps), or a combination of both. Flaps may be pedicle based or free flaps, requiring microsurgical techniques for their reconstruction.

Breast Reconstruction Using Tissue Expanders and Permanent Implants

Mastectomy may leave a shortage of skin that prevents creation of a breast mound. For these patients, extra tissue can be created locally with the use of tissue expanders (Fig. 22.15). Tissue expansion is a technique used to stretch normal tissue that is adjacent to a defect, mechanically creating redundancy of normal tissue to correct the defect. For breast reconstruction, the expander resembles the shape of a breast prosthesis. The expander has a metal-backed, self-sealing silicone valve at its dome. Another type of expander used less frequently has a small, dome-shaped reservoir with a fill tube that is positioned subcutaneously at a distance from the expander but connected to it. Following surgery, the tissue expander is gradually filled with percutaneous injections of normal saline during routine office visits. The expander may be filled as often as weekly, or it may remain unused until chemotherapy or radiation is completed. After the tissue expander is filled to the appropriate volume, it may be removed and replaced with a permanent reconstructive mammary prosthesis, either saline or silicone, as an ambulatory surgical procedure. Silicone can be used for breast augmentation for patients older than 22 years. If silicone is chosen, both the surgeon and the patient must participate in an adjunct clinical study at this time; the patient may opt out. Another option is the use of combination tissue expander and breast prosthesis, which remains in place after the desired amount of saline has been sequentially added. The benefit of this prosthesis is the ability to add or remove saline in case an adjustment proves necessary. The recent introduction of allografts helps achieve better shape and fast expansion and is less painful. A direct-to-implant or "one-step" approach can make it possible for some patients to undergo immediate reconstruction of the breast. A mastectomy that conserves a large amount of breast skin is best for this approach. The permanent saline or silicone implant is placed behind the pectoralis major muscle. AlloDerm (collagen sheeting)

is placed from below to provide coverage for the implant. Sometimes nipple sparing can also be accomplished depending on the location of the breast mass. Planning between the plastic and general surgeon preoperatively will determine the best procedure to be performed.

Procedural Considerations. A basic plastic set may be used with the addition of fiberoptic breast retractors. The team positions the patient supine with both arms extended on armboards. The surgeon marks both inframammary folds preoperatively. Both sides of the chest should be prepped and draped. The breast shape expander and sizers are supplied in a sterile package from the manufacturer and are available in a variety of sizes. If permanent saline or silicone implants are used, they will be ordered by the surgeon ahead of time. Meticulous sterile technique is required, and the expander/implant should be handled as little as possible. This procedure may be performed immediately after mastectomy or at a later date. Drains are usually placed to prevent hematoma and seroma formation, the latter of which could cause rotation or malposition of the tissue expander. If a surgical bra is used, care must be taken that it is not too tight and does not compromise circulation to the skin flaps. A breast band may also be used to hold the implant down and in place postoperatively.

Operative Procedure

1. Skin flaps are assessed for adequate blood supply, and then the pectoralis fascia is incised along its lateral border. The surgeon creates a submuscular pocket for the temporary expander or permanent implant by undermining the muscle over the sternal attachments and down over the lower ribs.
2. Allograft material may be used to bridge the gap created from the elevated pectoral and serratus muscles to the inframammary fold.
3. The tissue expander is tested before insertion for watertight integrity. The surgeon inspects the implant for defects.
4. After hemostasis is achieved, the surgeon checks the expander for integrity and then inserts it into the pocket. Muscle coverage is assessed, and if adequate the reservoir is positioned subcutaneously and connected, the wound is closed, and the expander is filled with sterile saline solution until slight blanching of the skin is achieved. The amount is recorded on the patient record.

Second-Stage Tissue Expander Breast Reconstruction

When the tissue expander has been expanded to the desired size, the patient is taken back to surgery for the next stage of her breast reconstruction. This is a relatively minor procedure in which the tissue expander is deflated and replaced with a permanent mammary prosthesis (Figs. 22.16 and 22.17A–B). At this time, if there is asymmetry of the opposite breast, surgery may be performed to create bilateral symmetry. The patient may require correction of breast ptosis through mastopexy, with or without the addition of a breast implant; alternatively, a reduction mammoplasty may be needed on the opposite breast. This procedure is usually performed on an outpatient basis in which the patient is administered a general anesthetic.

Breast Reconstruction Using Myocutaneous Flaps

Flaps are described by the types of tissue they contain, the blood supply of the tissues, and the method by which the flaps are moved from the donor site to the recipient site. *Myocutaneous* flaps are formed from skin, fat, and muscle. Options for breast reconstruction may include the latissimus dorsi and TRAM flap procedures, which are detailed in the following sections. An additional option is the superior gluteal artery perforator (SGAP) flap, which has become

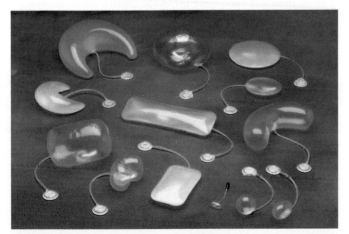

FIG. 22.15 Tissue expanders are inflatable plastic reservoirs of various shapes and volumes that are implanted under the skin. The skin over the expander is stretched during a period of several weeks as the expander is gradually filled by percutaneous injection of saline into an incorporated part of the remote-fill port. Expanders are useful for breast reconstruction.

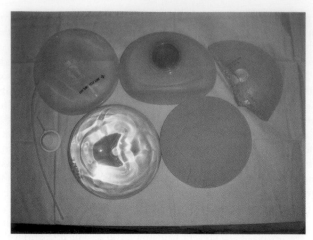

FIG. 22.16 While discussing options in the surgeon's office, samples of tissue expanders and textured and smooth saline and silicone implants are shown to patients for their selection.

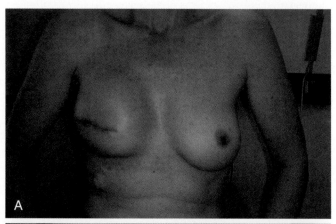

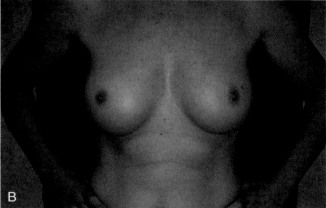

FIG. 22.17 (A) Tissue expander is used to create extra tissue after mastectomy so a breast mound can be created. (B) Postoperative result after tissue expander replaced with breast prosthesis.

more refined. Some women choose to use their own tissue for reconstruction because they prefer what they consider more realistic, which are supple breasts that would not need to be replaced or removed, which is possible with implants. The SGAP flap does require microsurgical skills and is not offered at all institutions. Factors for choosing reconstructive options include the patient's size

and availability of appropriate abdominal or gluteal tissue. Even very thin patients generally have enough skin and fat for the SGAP procedure, and the consistency of the buttock fat (thicker than abdominal) provides the more supple result. Positioning is especially challenging, and some operative efficiency may be achieved by using two OR beds.

Latissimus Dorsi Flap. The latissimus dorsi myocutaneous flap is used when significant tissue deficiency occurs after a mastectomy or when TRAM flap reconstruction is not an option. The latissimus dorsi muscle is a wide, flat muscle extending over the midthoracic portion of the back and inserting into the humerus. Its blood supply comes from the thoracodorsal artery and from perforators of the upper lumbar arteries and intercostal vessels. This rich vascularity allows the surgeon flexibility in orienting and positioning the flap to the pattern of the deficit on the anterior chest wall. Latissimus dorsi flaps are usually used in conjunction with a reconstructive breast prosthesis to create a more natural breast mound (Fig. 22.18).

Procedural Considerations. The surgeon marks the donor site of the latissimus dorsi with its skin island, along with the intended recipient site, before surgery with the patient in a sitting position. In the OR the patient is placed in a lateral position, donor side up, with the arm extended and safely supported. The perioperative nurse should assemble extra padding and positioning aids in preparation for the patient's arrival. After the donor muscle has been mobilized and exteriorized through the area of defect, the back incision is closed and the patient repositioned supine with the arm extended on an armboard. Instrumentation should include a basic plastic instrument set, fiberoptic breast retractors, vascular instruments, sterile marking pens, suction, and long tissue forceps and scissors. A Doppler unit and probe should be available.

Operative Procedure

1. Initially the island of skin is incised transversely across the back, being careful to ensure that a bra or bathing suit will cover the resulting scar.
2. The surgeon frees the muscle, subcutaneous fat, and fascia from the overlying skin by undermining so that part or all of the muscle may be mobilized.
3. The skin island and the muscle are then tunneled under the axilla to the chest wall. The insertion of the muscle on the humerus and accompanying blood vessels are left undisturbed. The latissimus dorsi muscle fills the space left by the missing pectoralis muscle.
4. The island of skin is oriented to the recipient site, and the surgeon sutures both into place.
5. A permanent mammary prosthesis is placed under the muscle before suturing to reconstruct the breast mound.
6. The wound is drained via a closed-wound drainage system.
7. The surgeon may reconstruct the nipple-areola complex by sharing the nipple on the unaffected side or by using groin, adjacent tissue, thigh, or auricular tissue. This can be done at the time of reconstruction or at a later date as a minor procedure with the patient administered a local anesthetic.
8. Dressings are applied. If a surgical bra is used, care must be taken not to compromise blood supply to the flap.

Transverse Rectus Abdominis Myocutaneous Flap. TRAM flaps are pedicle-based flaps used for breast reconstruction. The rectus muscle is the broad, wide abdominal muscle that reaches from under the ribs to the pubis, and either one or both sides of the muscle may be used for reconstruction. The blood supply (superior epigastric artery and vein) is carried within the muscle pedicle. The muscle along with its pedicle is severed at its most distal origins and pulled through a subcutaneous tunnel to the chest to form a breast. Although

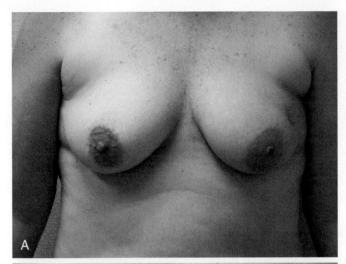

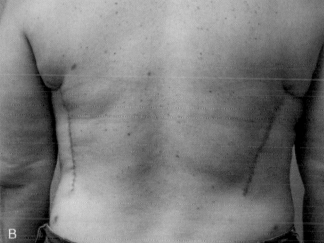

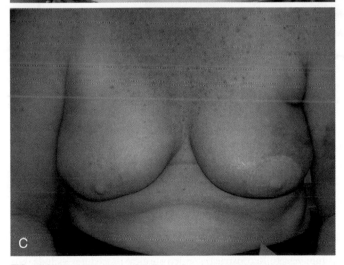

FIG. 22.18 Latissimus dorsi flap for breast reconstruction. (A) Preoperative view. (B) Healed bilateral back incisions. (C) Postoperative view with nipple reconstruction.

this procedure has the added benefit of an abdominoplasty, if there is inadequate abdominal tissue the patient may require a small mammary prosthesis.

The different types of TRAM techniques are based on blood supply, but the procedure still follows a basic format. As with other types of breast reconstruction, TRAM flaps may be performed immediately after mastectomy or planned for a later stage in the patient's recuperative phase.

Procedural Considerations. The surgeon marks the surgical landmarks preoperatively with the patient in a standing position. A basic plastic instrument set is used as for the latissimus dorsi flap. The patient is positioned supine with arms extended on armboards. Positioning the patient for this procedure is particularly difficult because of the need to promote closure of the abdominal wound, support circulation to the flap, and protect the patient from injury. The OR bed is often flexed, and additional padding of the lower extremities may be required. The skin prep should extend from the lower neck to midthigh.

Operative Procedure
1. The surgeon excises the skin from the mastectomy scar and makes the abdominal incision. The abdominal flap is dissected with care being taken not to shear the skin and subcutaneous tissue from its underlying muscle attachments (Fig. 22.19A).
2. The transverse rectus abdominis muscle is divided from its inferior-most attachment (see Fig. 22.19B).
3. The flap is rotated and passed through to its new location on the chest wall (see Fig. 22.19C–D) and sutured medially; the thinnest portion of the flap is superior and medial, and the thickest portion is inferior and lateral.
4. Because of the amount of tissue available, an implant is often unnecessary (see Fig. 22.19E).

Free Transverse Rectus Abdominis Myocutaneous Flap. The free TRAM flap is indicated when there is concern about the absence of one or both of the rectus muscles after the procedure or when there are concerns about vascularity, either with the pedicle used in the standard TRAM flap or with any other factors that may compromise vascularity of the flap. A newer technique of the free TRAM (deep inferior epigastric perforator procedure) has the advantage of not requiring the entire rectus muscle, because only a small portion of the rectus muscle that carries a segment of the deep inferior epigastric perforator vessels is needed to move with the fat and skin to its new location. It is also used when the buttock tissue (superior gluteal perforator flap) is planned to replace the absent breast or breasts.

Procedural Considerations. Care of the patient undergoing a free TRAM procedure is identical to that of patients undergoing pedicle TRAM flaps with the addition of the surgical microscope. Refer to the Procedural Considerations under TRAM. Two surgical teams may be used, one for harvesting and one for site preparation. Meticulous attention must be paid to positioning and protection from pressure injuries because of the length of the procedure. During the preoperative verification process, the perioperative nurse should determine whether the patient has made preoperative autologous blood donations and if the appropriate blood work has been performed.

Operative Procedure
1. The surgeon identifies, dissects, and isolates the recipient vessels.
2. Donor vessels are selected based on pedicle length, and the flap is prepared.
3. The anesthesia provider administers heparin to prevent clotting and vasospasm.
4. When the recipient vessels are ready, the surgeon severs the flap.
5. The microscope is positioned in place and draped with a sterile drape.
6. The free flap is transferred to the recipient site, and the surgeon anastomoses the blood vessels.

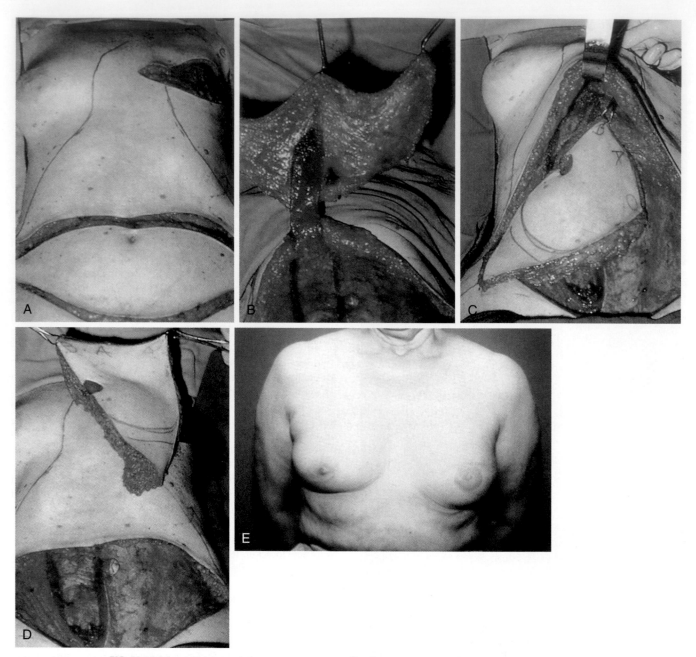

FIG. 22.19 Transverse rectus abdominis myocutaneous flap for postmastectomy breast reconstruction (see text for procedure).

7. The breast mound is shaped and sutured in place.
8. The donor site is closed, covering with a skin graft if necessary.

Nipple Reconstruction

Although nipple reconstruction can be performed at the time of breast reconstruction or replacement of the tissue expander with a mammary prosthesis, some surgeons prefer to wait and let the new breast tissues "settle" and mature to reconstruct the new nipple in the most accurate anatomic position. Generally this may take a minimum of 6 to 8 weeks. Tissue for the new nipple can be recruited locally by raising a flap or be grafted from the opposite nipple. The areola is reconstructed with skin grafting from the groin, buttock crease, or auricle (Fig. 22.20). The areolar skin may be tattooed to create a very pleasing nipple-areolar complex (Fig. 22.21A–B).

Microsurgery

The term *microsurgery* within the specialty of plastic and reconstructive surgery typically refers to procedures involving anastomosis of 1- to 2-mm vessels. Reconstructive microsurgical procedures include, but are not limited to, replantation of amputated body parts, repair of facial nerves, repair of lacerated nerves and blood vessels, treatment of extensive trauma to extremities and hands, reconstruction after removal of extensive cancers, and female-to-male transsexual reassignment. Today's surgeons skilled in microsurgery can successfully anastomose the ends of a vessel measuring less than 1 mm in diameter. The surgeon's use of an operating microscope or loupes for microsurgical procedures depends on the procedure to be performed, condition of the tissue, and personal preference. Endoscopic harvesting of

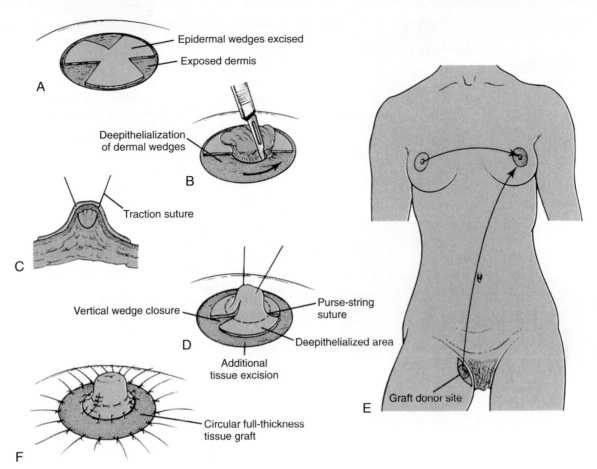

FIG. 22.20 (A) Circumferential demarcation of the nipple periphery with removal of dermal wedges. (B) Dermal wedges are deepithelialized from the rim toward the center. (C) A traction suture is used to elevate the central future nipple tip. (D) Traction is applied to the future nipple tip as the wedges are approximated to create a permanent projected surface. A purse-string suture is placed, and excess tissue is excised. (E) Possible full-thickness donor site areolar color match may be found in the labial folds. (F) The donor graft is measured, cut, and secured to the dermal ring of the neonipple-areolar complex.

tissues for microsurgical grafting is possible in some circumstances. Factors contributing to the success of microsurgery include (1) the individual and collective experiences of the surgical team and the members' ability to work together, relieving each other as necessary during long operations; (2) the surgeon's knowledge of the physiology of the microcirculation; (3) many hours of practice in the laboratory by the surgical team; and (4) the availability of proper microscopes, microvascular instruments, and microvascular suture.

Replantation of Amputated Body Part

Replantation is an attempt to reattach a completely amputated digit or other body part. Revascularization is the procedure performed on incomplete amputations, when the part remains partially attached to the body by skin, artery, vein, or nerve. Good candidates for replantation are those with the following amputations: (1) thumb, (2) multiple digits, (3) distal portion of hand at palm level, (4) wrist or forearm, (5) elbow and above the elbow, and (6) almost any body part of a child.

The success of digital replantation depends primarily on the microsurgical repair of one digital artery and two digital veins. Replantation of an amputated part is ideally performed within 4 to

6 hours after injury, but success has been reported up to 24 hours after injury if the amputated part has been cooled. Proper care of the amputated body part or parts before surgery is vital to successful replantation. The ultimate aim of replantation is the restoration of function beyond that provided by a prosthesis.

Procedural Considerations. A regional anesthetic is usually given to replantation patients if the anticipated length of surgery permits. Because of the length of these surgeries (12–16 hours), positioning is important. The perioperative nurse ensures that the OR bed and armboards are carefully padded with pressure-reducing materials to support the supine patient. The surgeon may request the room temperature be increased before the patient arrives because the warm room will reduce vasoconstriction in the extremities. A warming device is applied to maintain the patient's core body temperature. The surgeon usually brings the amputated part to the OR before the patient arrives to ensure ample time for preparation of it for replantation. The amputated body part should be maintained by wrapping it in saline-soaked gauze, placing it in an occlusive bag, and immersing it in a container of iced saline. The amputated part should not be in direct contact with the saline. If radiographs of the amputated body part and amputation site have not been taken

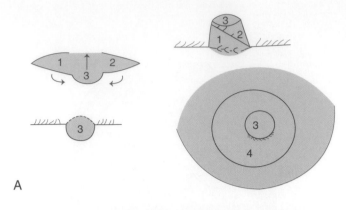

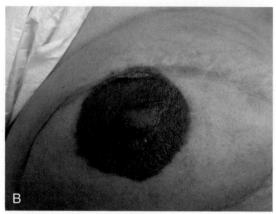

FIG. 22.21 (A) Breast nipple reconstruction. *1* and *2,* Wing flaps raised from side and wrapped around *3;* the central flap was raised superiorly; *4,* areolar skin created with skin grafted either from pigmented groin skin or from opposite areolar skin by tattooing. (B) Areolar tattoo.

before the patient's arrival in the OR, the perioperative nurse should arrange for these to be taken. Radiographic films are crucial to determine bone trauma and loss.

The hand drape (described later in this paragraph) can be applied to either upper or lower extremities, as required by the surgical procedure. Before a hand drape is placed, a pneumatic tourniquet cuff is often applied to the upper arm over padding. The patient is positioned supine on the OR bed, with the affected arm extended and supported on a hand table. While an assistant holds the patient's arm with both hands around the tourniquet cuff, the skin prep solution is applied from fingertips to tourniquet cuff. Care is taken to keep the cuff dry and free of solution. Then two folded barrier sheets are used to cover the hand table. The first sheet is placed with the folded edge nearest the patient (thus forming a cuff). A double-thickness, 4-inch stockinette is used to cover the extremity, and the edge is rolled over the tourniquet. The upper arm and upper half of the body are covered by a folded sheet, with the folded edge placed across the part of the stockinette that covers the tourniquet cuff. A small, nonperforating towel clamp that grasps the edge of the folded top sheet, the stockinette, and the edge of the cuff of the bottom sheet is placed on each side of the arm. This excludes the tourniquet cuff from the sterile field. The remainder of the body is covered with one or two additional sheets. A commercially prepared extremity drape that has an aperture incorporated into the drape also may be used.

Instrumentation includes a plastic hand instrument set, microvascular instruments, a Kirschner wire driver, Kirschner wires, an operating microscope, and a bipolar ESU.

Operative Procedure

1. The surgeon shortens the bone ends to eliminate tension on vascular anastomoses to be done later; the bone is stabilized by means of internal fixation with Kirschner wires.
2. Flexor and extensor tendon repairs are usually performed next.
3. The digital nerves are repaired with the aid of loupes or the operating microscope.
4. Using microsurgical instruments and techniques, the surgeon repairs the two digital veins followed by repair of one digital artery. If ischemic time has been prolonged, digital vessel repair may precede repair of tendons and nerves.
5. The skin is sutured.
6. A bulky supportive hand dressing is applied. A posterior splint may be placed.

Toe-to-Hand Transfer

The reconstructive procedure of toe-to-hand transfer involves surgical removal of a single toe or multiple toes and anastomosis of the vessels of the toes to those on the hand to restore finger and thumb functions. It is lengthy surgery (12–16 hours) and entails a two-team approach, one team is at the foot for toe removal, and one team is at the recipient site (the hand).

Procedural Considerations. The patient is placed in the supine position on the OR bed. The anesthesia provider administers an anticoagulation regimen during the anastomosis procedure. Two tourniquets are needed, one on the thigh of the operative foot and one on the operative arm. Both extremities are separately prepped and draped. Instrumentation includes a plastic hand set, microvascular instruments, power Kirschner wire driver, and Kirschner wires. Additional equipment includes the operating microscope, two tourniquet power sources, two bipolar ESUs, a sterile marking pen, and an Esmarch bandage.

Operative Procedure

1. The surgeon preparing the hand determines adequate blood flow and vessel location on the thumb site (Fig. 22.22A). This may prevent a needless amputation of the toe.
2. Appropriate skin flaps are incised to expose the veins on the dorsum of the hand and clamped with vessel microclips.
3. The radial artery or its branches are dissected out and prepared for anastomosis.
4. The surgeon locates and transfixes the flexor and extensor pollicis longus tendons.
5. The bone at the base of the thumb is prepared for the toe.
6. The nerves to the thumb are dissected out with adequate length for suturing without tension.
7. Using a racket-shaped incision the surgeon circumscribes the toe (see Fig. 22.22B). Next, the veins are isolated through the dorsal aspect and clamped with vessel microclips.
8. The extensor tendon is dissected proximally and transected over the base of the metatarsal.
9. The dorsalis pedis artery is dissected to the digital vessels with ligation of all branches of that vessel to prepare for the anastomosis.
10. On the plantar surface the digital nerves and flexor tendons are transected at levels of adequate length for anastomosis (see Fig. 22.22C).
11. The surgeon transects the toe at the level previously determined for adequate length of the thumb.

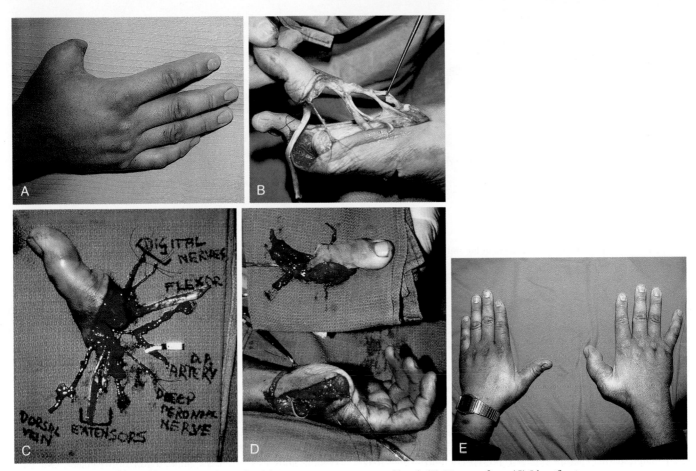

FIG. 22.22 Toe-to-hand transfer. (A) Preoperative appearance of hand. (B) Harvest of toe. (C) Identification of vessels and nerves. (D) Transfer of toe to thumb site. (E) Postoperative view of toe-to-thumb site transfer.

12. The toe vessels are anastomosed microsurgically to the thumb vessels. The toe is attached to the thumb area by Kirschner wires (see Fig. 22.22D).

An aesthetic and functionally effective hand can be achieved through this procedure (see Fig. 22.22E).

Reconstructive Maxillofacial Surgery

The need for maxillofacial surgery results from blunt or penetrating trauma, disease, or congenital anomaly. Regardless of the cause, the principles are the same: establishment of preinjury/predisease/normal anatomic dental occlusion, anatomic reduction, stabilization of the fracture, and healing for functional results. The technique and approach must be individualized to optimize the visual reduction (or reconstruction) of the procedure as well as minimize facial scarring and nerve injury, whether a mandibular free flap tissue and bone reconstruction or open reduction and internal fixation of any number and combination of facial fractures are performed. In addition to midface fractures, other common facial fractures include nasal, orbital (blow-out) floor, zygomatic, and mandibular fractures.

Procedural Considerations for Maxillofacial Surgery

The perioperative nurse should ask the surgeon about the precise injuries and the expected surgical treatment plan: open or closed reduction; intraoral or extraoral approach; the order of multiple procedures; need for intraoperative x-rays; and type, number, and sizes of screws and compression plates to be placed if rigid fixation

is to be used. Orbital fractures may require alloplastic implant material. Wire is used less frequently for immobilization because of the greater degree of stability afforded by plating systems. The patient's head should be immobilized and stabilized in a gel-type head ring; the position is almost always supine. Both eyes should be protected, and care must be taken not to displace endotracheal tubes. Instrumentation needs include a plastic surgery set, periosteal elevators, power drill for plating systems, bone hooks, Rowe disimpaction forceps (for maxillary fractures), an ESU, sterile marking pens, and suction. For application of arch bars, the nurse should assemble arch bars, wires, elastics, wire cutters, wire twisters, and dull retractors for good exposure of the teeth. A set of wire cutters should be sent to PACU with the patient and kept at the bedside in the event emergent access to the patient's airway becomes necessary.

Reduction of Nasal Fracture

Usually a closed reduction of the bony nasal fragments is performed by digital and instrumental manipulation. Occasionally an open reduction with interosseous wire fixation of nasal bone fragments is necessary. Procedural considerations and the surgical intervention are described in Chapter 19.

Reduction of Orbital Floor Fractures

The orbital floor is the eggshell-thin bone on which the eye and periorbital tissues rest. It separates the orbit from the maxillary antrum. Orbital floor fractures usually occur in combination with

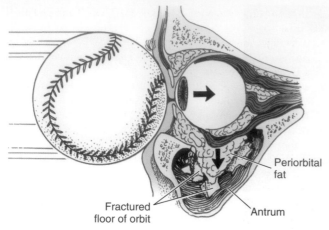

FIG. 22.23 A ball has struck the rim of the orbit and has pressed orbital contents backward, displacing fragments of bone into maxillary sinus. The inferior rectus muscle is incarcerated in the fracture. The inferior oblique muscle may also be involved.

fractures of the infraorbital rim (maxillary and zygomatic fractures). An isolated depressed orbital floor fracture with an intact infraorbital rim is called a *blow-out* fracture.

Fractures of the walls of the orbit may be caused by direct blows or by extension of a fracture line from adjacent bones. Isolated orbital floor, or blow-out, fractures usually occur after injury to the region of the eye by an object the size of an apple or an adult's fist (Fig. 22.23). Orbital contents herniated into the maxillary sinus, and the inferior rectus or inferior oblique muscle may become incarcerated at the fracture site. A Caldwell-Luc antrostomy may be done with reduction of the fracture from below, or the fracture site may be approached directly through the lower lid along the orbital floor; the prolapsed tissue is reduced, the orbital floor is reduced, and the orbital floor defect is bridged with bone grafts, molded metal implants, or plastic material.

Procedural Considerations. A graft set may be used for implantation of autogenous graft or synthetic graft materials of various sizes and thicknesses, along with a flexible narrow-width retractor. Interosseous wiring may be required for fractures of the frontozygomatic junction. Microplates and screws to stabilize fractures involving the fragile facial and orbital bones also may be used. A general anesthetic is usually administered.

Operative Procedure

1. The surgeon tests the maximum ocular rotation by exerting traction with a forceps on the tendon of the inferior rectus muscle to determine whether the inferior muscle sling is trapped in the fracture.
2. To distribute tension over the lower lid and stretch the orbicularis muscle, the surgeon inserts a traction suture through the lower lid margin.
3. With a #3 knife handle and a #15 blade, the surgeon incises the lower lid in the lid fold above the orbital rim.
4. The surgeon separates the skin from the orbicularis muscle and identifies the orbital septum by blunt dissection. Dissection is continued down to the periosteum of the orbital rim by means of scissors, loop retractors, elevators, and forceps.
5. The periosteum of the orbital rim is incised with a #15 blade. With periosteal elevators, the floor of the orbit is exposed and explored. When the fracture site is identified, bone spicules (needle-shaped bone fragments) are removed and the herniated

contents are freed from the maxillary antrum. The contents of the orbit are elevated by means of narrow-width, flexible retractors. A 4-0 traction suture is placed around the tendon of the inferior rectus muscle.

6. The surgeon obtains an autogenous graft taken from the patient's iliac crest or uses an alloplastic material of proper size to repair the bony defect. The material may or may not be anchored to the orbital rim by wire sutures.
7. The periosteum is carefully closed, the skin is closed, and a pressure dressing is applied.

Reduction of Zygomatic Fractures

Fractures of the zygoma (the cheek or malar bone) are corrected by either closed or open reduction. The two most common types of zygomatic fractures are depressed fractures of the arch and separation at or near the zygomaticofrontal, zygomaticomaxillary, and zygomaticotemporal suture lines, which constitutes a trimalar fracture. Although fractures of the zygoma can interfere with the ability to open and close the mouth properly, their chief consequence is a flattening of the cheek on the involved side, which results from a depressed trimalar or zygomatic arch fracture. Treatment is directed toward elevating the depressed fracture and maintaining the reduction. Closed reduction is the procedure used for treatment of zygomatic arch fractures, whereas most trimalar fractures are reduced by means of open reduction with internal fixation.

Procedural Considerations. A plastic instrument set, a Suraci zygoma hook elevator, and a jaw hook are required for a closed reduction. A basic plastic instrument set, along with the following instruments and supplies, is required for an open reduction: a Hall II air drill, stainless steel wires (#26, #28, and #30), the Suraci zygoma hook elevator, a jaw hook, a Kerrison rongeur, two Blair retractors, a bipolar ESU, a sterile marking pen, epinephrine 1:200,000 for injection, and a mini-plating rigid fixation set. The team positions the patient supine on the OR bed. A head drape is used.

Operative Procedure. The surgeon performs a closed reduction by elevating the depressed fracture with a percutaneous bone hook. Stabilization of a trimalar fracture may then be achieved by inserting a transantral Kirschner wire from the fractured side to the normal side.

The technique of open reduction of a trimalar fracture is as follows:

1. Incisions are marked along the lateral area of the eyebrow and lower eyelid over the zygomaticofrontal suture line and zygomaticomaxillary suture line (infraorbital rim) fractures, respectively.
2. After injection with epinephrine 1:200,000 for hemostasis, the surgeon incises along the premarked lines down to bone, and suture lines are identified and exposed.
3. The depressed zygoma is elevated with a Kelly hemostat or periosteal elevator placed behind the body of the zygoma through the lateral eyebrow incision. Bone hooks placed percutaneously or at the fracture sites may be used instead.
4. The surgeon drills holes into bone on each side of the fracture lines. Stainless steel wires are passed through the hole and twisted down tightly to maintain the reduction (reduction and stabilization of two of the three fractures are sufficient). Alternative methods of stabilization of the fractures are interosseous wiring of the zygomaticofrontal fracture and placement of a transmural Kirschner wire or stabilization with micro/mini plates and screws.
5. Using a subcuticular technique, the surgeon closes the incisions.
6. An eyepatch dressing may be applied.

Reduction of Maxillary Fractures

Midface fractures are usually classified according to a system developed in the early 1900s by Dr. Rene Le Fort: (1) Le Fort I, or transverse maxillary, fracture, which is a horizontal fracture that includes the nasal floor, septum, and teeth; (2) Le Fort II, or pyramidal maxillary, fracture (unilateral or bilateral), which is a type of fracture that often involves the nasal cavity, hard palate, and the orbital rim; and (3) Le Fort III, or craniofacial dysjunction, fracture, which is a type of fracture that includes both zygomas and the nose (Kelman, 2015) (Fig. 22.24). Like a mandibular fracture, a maxillary fracture also produces malocclusion. In addition, depending on the severity of the fracture, it may produce considerable deformity of the middle of the face, usually perceived as a flattening or smashed-in appearance.

Closed reduction with intermaxillary fixation suffices for treatment of Le Fort I and some Le Fort II fractures. The more severe Le Fort II and all Le Fort III fractures require open reduction in addition to intermaxillary fixation.

Procedural Considerations. The basic plastic instrument set is required as well as an air-powered drill; stainless steel wires (#25, #26, and #28); Rowe maxillary forceps, right and left; a Brown fascia needle; polyethylene buttons (for suspension wire pull-through for Le Fort III repair); a small foam-rubber pad; a sterile marking pen or methylene blue; an ESU; epinephrine 1:200,000 for injection; periosteal elevators; and a rigid fixation system. A separate Mayo setup for the application of arch bars is required, as described for reduction of mandibular fractures. The patient is placed in the supine position on the OR bed. A head drape is used.

Operative Procedure. The surgeon will apply arch bars either before or after the open reduction, or in some cases use them as the only mode of treatment in closed reduction. In addition to ligating the maxillary arch bar to the teeth, it must also be suspended from stable bones superior to the fractured maxilla (which is unstable). In Le Fort I fractures, suspension may be around both zygomatic arches by passage of percutaneous wires. In Le Fort II and Le Fort III fractures, the surgeon may place suspension wires through holes drilled bilaterally into the zygomatic process of the frontal bone. This requires incisions into both lateral eyebrow areas. The following description pertains to open reduction of Le Fort II and Le Fort III fractures:

1. After injection of epinephrine 1:200,000 for hemostasis, the surgeon makes bilateral incisions to expose the infraorbital rims and zygomaticofrontal suture lines.
2. The surgeon applies Rowe maxillary forceps intranasally and intraorally to disimpact and reduce the maxilla. Holes are drilled into bone on each side of fracture lines along the infraorbital rim (and zygomaticofrontal area for Le Fort III fractures, after reducing the zygomatic fractures).
3. Stainless steel wires are passed through these holes and twisted down tightly to maintain the reduction.
4. Suspension wires are passed from the eyebrow incisions, behind the zygomatic arches, and into the mouth with the Brown fascia needle. A pullout wire is looped through each suspension wire within the eyebrow incision, brought out through the skin near the hairline, and tied down over a polyethylene button and foam-rubber padding. Self-tapping screws, mini compression plates, and bone grafts may also be used, based on the surgeon's preference. Incisions are closed.
5. When indicated, reduction of a nasal fracture is then performed.

Reduction of Mandibular Fractures

The purpose of treatment for a mandibular fracture is to restore the patient's preinjury dental occlusion. With some types of fractures, a closed reduction with immobilization by means of intermaxillary fixation is sufficient for treatment. With a majority of mandibular fractures, however, an open reduction with wire fixation is necessary, plus supplemental intermaxillary fixation to achieve adequate immobilization for healing.

Intermaxillary fixation is most often accomplished when arch bars are applied to the maxillary and mandibular teeth. The surgeon places stainless steel wires (#24 or #25) around the necks of the teeth and ligates the wire around the arch bars to hold the latter in place. Latex bands are attached to the tongs on the maxillary and mandibular arch bars to fix the teeth in occlusion (Fig. 22.25). If the patient is edentulous, arch bars are attached to dentures or specially fabricated dental splints. The dentures or splints are held in place by means of wires placed around the mandible (for the mandibular arch bar) and through the nasal spine and around the

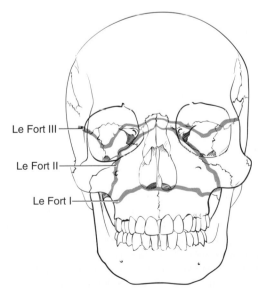

FIG. 22.24 Le Fort classification of fractures.

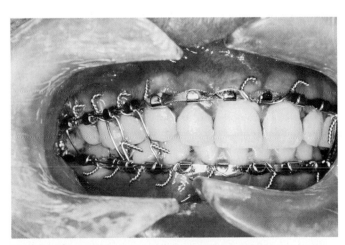

FIG. 22.25 Teeth in occlusion with arch bars in place. Tongs on arch bars will accept latex bands, which maintain occlusion for several weeks (wires around tongs are shown).

zygomatic arches (for the maxillary arch bar). Wire cutters must be sent with the patient to the PACU.

Procedural Considerations: Open Reduction. In addition to a basic plastic instrument set, the following instruments and supplies are needed for an open reduction of a fractured mandible: a Hall II air drill, two Dingman bone-holding forceps, a nerve stimulator, a sterile marking pen, stainless steel wires (#24, #26, and #28), an ESU, epinephrine 1:200,000 for injection, and a rigid fixation system.

For the application of arch bars or other types of interdental wiring techniques, a separate Mayo setup with the following instruments and supplies is required: a set of coil arch bars and latex bands; stainless steel wire (#25 or #26); wire suture scissors; a wire twister; Wieder tongue depressors, large and small; a Brown fascia needle (if dentures or splints are used); a Freer septal elevator; and a small drain.

If arch bars are applied before the open reduction is performed, this former setup must be kept completely separate from the instruments used for the open reduction. Because the mouth is a contaminated area, a complete change of gowns, gloves, and drapes is necessary after the intraoral procedure.

Operative Procedure

1. The surgeon may apply the arch bars before or after the open reduction.
2. A line inferior and parallel to the lower border of the mandible at the fracture site is marked, and the area is infiltrated with epinephrine 1:200,000 for hemostasis.
3. The surgeon places the incision to expose the inferior border of the mandible. The nerve stimulator may be used to aid in identification of the marginal mandibular branch of the facial nerve in fractures of the posterior body and angle of the mandible.
4. The fracture is reduced by manipulation. The surgeon drills holes into the mandible on each side of the fracture line with the Hall II air drill while an assistant holds the reduced fracture with the aid of Dingman bone-holding forceps.
5. The surgeon inserts stainless steel wire through the holes and twists them tightly to secure the fracture fragments in anatomic alignment.
6. In the event that rigid fixation is desired with the use of plates and screws, the appropriate drill bit, tap, and depth gauge are chosen. With these items the surgeon places the proper-size prosthesis, and the fracture is approximated, aligned, and placed in anatomic position.
7. The surgeon may place a small drain into the wound, and the wound is closed in layers (periosteum, platysma muscle, and skin).
8. The latex bands may be applied to the arch bars at this time but more frequently are applied later, after the patient is fully awake and reactive.
9. A moderate compression dressing is applied to cover the submandibular wound and drain.

Elective Orthognathic Surgery

A large number of patients have either acquired or congenital facial defects that affect the maxilla, the mandible, or both. The condition of many of these patients can be improved dramatically with orthodontic care; however, many also require surgical rearrangement of the maxilla or mandible.

Procedural Considerations. Psychosocial and functional deficits are related to abnormalities of the maxilla and mandible. Surgical correction of these defects can improve a patient's quality of life.

Surgery is usually delayed until an adequate number of permanent teeth are in place for postoperative immobilization. Coordinated preoperative and postoperative planning is of great importance to the success of these procedures. Meticulous oral hygiene is extremely important to prevent tooth decay and gum inflammation caused by food buildup between the wires and the teeth. Thorough tooth brushing with a child-sized soft-bristled toothbrush is recommended for cleaning. A home dental irrigator can also be useful in loosening food and debris trapped between the wires and elastic bands of the arch bars. A liquid diet that is high in protein and calories is recommended. The arch bars will be in place for 4 to 6 weeks. Commercial nutritional supplements are a convenient way to increase calories and protein because it is difficult to maintain weight on a liquid diet. An over-the-counter liquid multivitamin supplement is also recommended.

Operative Procedure

1. The surgeon applies arch bars for postoperative immobilization.
2. Intraoral incisions are made to provide exposure to the maxilla or mandible.
3. Using a saw, the surgeon cuts the maxilla or mandible as indicated by the patient's diagnosis.
4. Bone is advanced or set back to a predetermined position.
5. Bones are wired in place, with grafts placed in defects as needed.

Sex Reassignment Surgery

As our society changes, the needs of transsexual, transgender, and gender nonconforming individuals have become more prominent in the Western world. A *transsexual* individual is one who seeks to take on the social role of the other gender, either full or part time, often with the assistance of hormone therapy, surgery, or both. Transgender is defined as the condition in which an individual with chromosomes and internal and external organs associated with one gender identifies psychologically and socially with attributes of the opposite gender.

People may seek medical assistance in changing their physical sex to be congruent with their internal self-perception (Biggs and Chaganaboyana, 2016). Gender transition can involve social aspects such as changing appearance (including styles of dress and hair) and name, arranging new identity documents, or simply the use of a more suitable gendered pronoun. It can also involve a change in physical characteristics through hormones, plastic surgery, or sex reassignment surgery. Physical transition can facilitate social transition, enabling styles of dress, social activities, and (in many countries) changes in documentation that would not otherwise be possible (Winter et al., 2016).

Reassignment of gender by means of surgery is performed only after the patient has been treated with hormones of the opposite gender, has experienced a period of cross-gender living, and has had intensive psychiatric evaluation. Most institutions performing this type of surgery have gender-identity teams who evaluate and treat transsexuals. These teams usually include a variety of professionals: psychiatrist, psychologist, endocrinologist, plastic surgeon, urologist, gynecologist, and social worker.

The surgical techniques for assignment of male to female are technically easier. A breast augmentation may be performed if hormone therapy has not sufficiently changed breast size. Construction of the neovagina includes radical penectomy, bilateral orchiectomy, urethroplasty, perineal dissection, creation of a neovaginal vault, vaginoplasty, and vulvoplasty. Other procedures could include facial feminization, body contouring, and thyroid chondrolaryngoplasty ("tracheal shave").

The surgical technique for female to male is technically more difficult and requires multiple surgical procedures. Considerations that must be addressed are twofold: the neophallus must be constructed to (1) allow the patient to stand to void and (2) permit stimulation of a sexual partner during intercourse. This may require a radial artery forearm free flap with a later stage surgical insertion of a penile prosthesis for attaining an erection. Other plastic surgery procedures could include bilateral subcutaneous mastectomies, facial masculinization, body implants, and hair transplants.

Aesthetic Surgery

Aesthetic surgery may be performed after induction of general anesthesia, monitored anesthesia care, or local anesthesia with moderate sedation. The perioperative nurse must be qualified and prepared to monitor the patient during the procedure according to AORN *Guidelines for Perioperative Practice* (AORN, 2015). Baseline vital signs should be recorded in the OR record. A blood pressure cuff, pulse oximeter, and cardiac monitor electrodes should be placed (with staff capable of interpreting cardiac data). IV fluids should be administered. The OR should be kept quiet and patient privacy protected. Care should be taken to avoid conversation that could be misinterpreted by the patient.

Scar Revision

Scar revision involves the rearranging or reshaping of an existing scar so that the scar is less noticeable. The simplest form of scar revision is excision of an existing scar and simple resuturing of the wound. This may improve scars that are wide.

The Z-plasty is the most widely used method of scar revision (Fig. 22.26). It breaks up linear scars, rearranging them so that the central limb of the Z lies in the same direction as a natural skin line. Scars that are parallel to skin lines are less noticeable than scars that are perpendicular to skin lines. A contracted scar line can also be lengthened with a Z-plasty.

Procedural Considerations

A plastic local instrument set and a sterile marking pen are required. The procedure may be performed with the patient administered a local or general anesthetic. The patient is positioned, prepped, and draped so that the scar that is to be revised is well exposed.

Operative Procedure

1. The surgeon marks the pattern for the planned revision and injects local anesthesia.
2. The scar is excised.
3. The surrounding tissue is undermined, and the wound edges are approximated according to the surgeon's markings.
4. Dressings may or may not be applied.

Endoscopic Brow Lift

The aging process affects the area above the eyes and brows in several ways. Loss of skin elasticity can cause the appearance of a heavy brow and emphasize hooding of the upper eyelids. Repetitive muscle action results in horizontal forehead lines and furrows as well as creases between the brows. The goal of endoscopic brow/forehead surgery is to minimize the heaviness of the brow and improve the frown lines of aging, reduce upper eyelid hooding, reposition the eyebrows if necessary, and create a more youthful, refreshed appearance of the forehead and brow area, all through multiple, short incisions in the scalp.

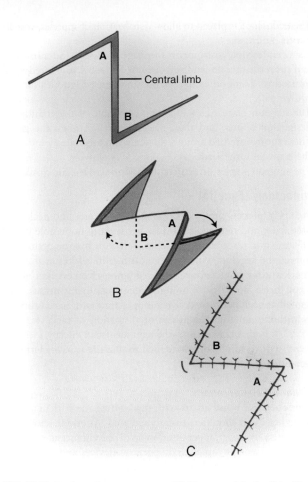

FIG. 22.26 Z-plasty for scar revision. (A) The central limb of the Z-plasty is over the scar that needs to be revised. (B) Two other limbs are incised, and each is equal in length to the central limb and diverging from it at an equal angle. The flaps are then transposed. (C) Flaps transposed, and original Z rotated 90 degrees and reversed.

Procedural Considerations

Positioning the patient with his or her head at the very top of the OR bed is necessary for good utilization and mobility of the endoscopic instruments. For patients with medium to long hair, the hair may be sectioned and tied with sterilized rubber bands to minimize interference with the planned incision. The surgeon marks the patient's incision lines and anatomic landmarks before the surgery. The entire head (scalp, face, ears, and neck) should be prepped and draped with impervious drape material. The patient's eyes may be protected with ointment and shields for the duration of the procedure; ear canals should also be protected from pooling of prep solution, irrigation, or blood. During preparation of the room, the perioperative nurse and scrub person perform a check of all endoscopic equipment to ensure it is functioning properly. Endoscopic instrumentation includes elevators, scissors, clamps, needle holders, camera, and light sources. Depending on the method of fixation, screws and accompanying instrumentation may be necessary.

Operative Procedure

1. The surgeon injects a local anesthetic and places three to five small incisions in the scalp (one midline and one or two paramedian).
2. Using blunt dissection, the surgeon elevates the forehead skin.

3. The endoscope is placed to allow visualization of muscles, vessels, nerves, and tissues.
4. Using endoscopic instruments the surgeon dissects the corrugator and procerus muscles and soft tissues. The soft tissue is redraped to produce a smoother appearance and desired repositioning of brows.
5. The surgeon places screws in the outer table of the cranium at designated points, and then places sutures through the galea. These sutures are tied around the screws to facilitate elevation of the brow and forehead.
6. The surgeon staples or sutures the scalp incisions for closure.

Rhytidectomy (Facelift)

As the aging process progresses, the skin of the face and neck may become loose and redundant. This is particularly noticeable in the "jowl" areas and just beneath the chin. A facelift may be performed to correct the sagging skin. The typical facelift addresses the face and neck and involves removal and redraping of excess skin of the face and neck after repositioning of the underlying muscle and platysma has been performed. The result is a smooth, rested appearance, without unnatural tightness or distortion of facial features (Fig. 22.27). Rather than excising the redundant skin directly, incisions adjacent to or within hairlines are used so that the scars are virtually indiscernible.

Procedural Considerations

The perioperative nurse assists with positioning the patient supine with the head and shoulders slightly elevated. Attention should be given to safety by using proper positioning to prevent pressure injuries, using intermittent pneumatic compression devices and a warming unit, and preventing eye injuries by using shields or eye ointment. The patient's ear canals are protected to keep blood and fluids from entering and causing irritation. Depending on the complexity of the procedure and planned surgical time, the nurse may insert an indwelling urinary catheter.

Specialized scissors of varying lengths should be available, along with smooth and toothed tissue forceps and various sizes of needle holders. A fiberoptic lighted retractor is standard for facelifts. To avoid immediate-use steam sterilization, contact with the surgeon or office staff should be initiated before the day of surgery to discuss special requests and ensure that instrumentation is prepared according to AORN standards and facility guidelines.

There are numerous techniques for rhytidectomy, and a well-prepared perioperative nurse will ask the surgeon about the specific technique to have the appropriate suture material and special needles available. The underlying superficial muscular aponeurotic system (SMAS) may be repositioned, the cheek may be elevated independently, the midface may be lifted, and there may or may not be accompanying liposuction. Facelift procedures are customized specific to the anatomic needs of the individual patient. The entire head, neck, ears, and scalp are prepped and draped.

Operative Procedure

1. The surgeon marks bilateral incision lines from the temporal scalp, around the earlobe, around the posterior margin of the auricula, and into the occipital scalp (Figs. 22.28 and 22.29).
2. The incision lines, both temples, cheeks, upper neck, and the submental area are injected with the local anesthetic agent.
3. The surgeon may inject wetting solution (e.g., tumescent) and perform liposuction on the neck, jowls, or cheeks before placing the incisions. The tumescent can assist in undermining the tissue (see Liposuction section, page 843).
4. After the incisions are made, the surgeon elevates the temporal and cheek skin. The SMAS is plicated cephalad and caudally, elevating and tightening the SMAS and platysma.
5. The surgeon elevates and repositions the malar pad; it is then anchored with suture.
6. The facial skin flap is then elevated in a superior and slightly posterior direction and tacked, and excess skin is trimmed at the flap edges.

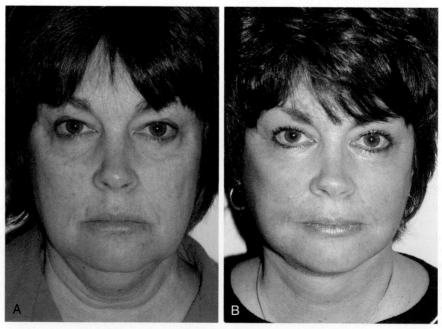

FIG. 22.27 (A) Preoperative and (B) postoperative rhytidectomy.

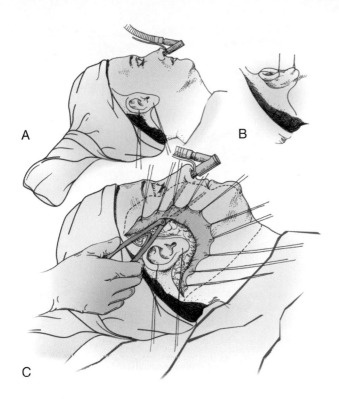

FIG. 22.28 Rhytidectomy: line of incision and undermining. (A) Traction sutures of 4-0 silk placed into auricle; temporal incision curved posteriorly for better support of upward pull. (B) Incision carried under earlobe and then curved posteriorly upward and then caudad toward midline. (C) Skin undermined almost to nasolabial fold, to area of mental foramen, and to midline of neck as far down as thyroid cartilage. Care is taken to avoid injury to submandibular branches of facial nerve and facial artery.

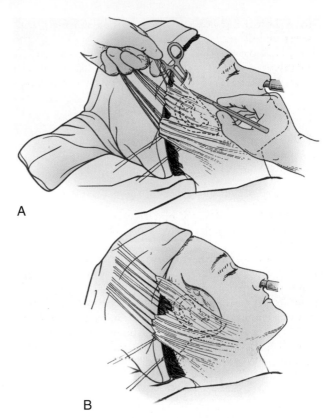

FIG. 22.29 Rhytidectomy: removal of superfluous skin. (A) Skin drawn upward to proper degree of tension, and incision made along posterior margin of clamp. (B) Incision continued upward around posterior margin of auricle and then backward to excise skin specimen.

7. Through a submental incision, the surgeon undermines the neck and identifies and plicates the platysmal bands. Excess tissue is trimmed and tacked postauricularly. Small drains are placed beneath the skin flaps and secured.
8. Incisions are closed in one or two layers. Fibrin sealant and/or a drain may be used before closure to aid in hemostasis.
9. The patient's hair is cleaned before the application of the dressing. A moderate pressure dressing is applied depending on surgeon preference.

Blepharoplasty

The aging process causes a sagging or relaxation of eyelid skin and the orbital septum. As the latter becomes weaker, it allows periorbital fat to bulge. These changes are perceived as baggy eyelids, which give the patient a chronically tired appearance. The goal of blepharoplasty is to improve the patient's appearance by removing excess eyelid skin, removing or repositioning bulging periorbital fat, and tightening and smoothing the muscles under the eye (Fig. 22.30). The upper eyelid skin can be so redundant that it encroaches on the patient's field of vision, and removal of excessive hooding of the upper eyelid skin may even improve peripheral vision. The upper eyelid crease may also be enhanced. Not all patients need removal of skin; for selected individuals, CO_2 skin resurfacing may be the procedure of choice to achieve a smoother appearance of the lower eyelid skin. Incisions in the subconjunctival mucosa of the lower lids are sometimes used for this group of patients if resection or repositioning of the periorbital fat is also indicated. Blepharoplasty is often performed with rhytidectomy. Blepharoplasty may be performed on both the upper and lower lids, upper lids only, or lower lids only.

Procedural Considerations

A plastic local instrument set is required. Delicate, short instruments are used, with special attention to scissors (curved Kaye blepharoplasty), fine Adson forceps with teeth, calipers, and fixation forceps. Webster needle holders are frequently desired. A bipolar ESU unit may be used. A needle tip for the active electrode may be requested if the monopolar ESU is used. (With the monopolar ESU, a lower setting is used. The perioperative nurse should verbally repeat back the settings requested by the surgeon.) Blepharoplasty is usually performed using a local anesthetic with monitored anesthesia care. The patient is in the supine position on the OR bed. The patient's face is prepped, and the head drape is used. Corneal shields may be used to protect the cornea.

Operative Procedure: Upper Lids

1. The surgeon marks the lines of incision and injects local anesthetic.
2. The incision is placed, and excess skin is removed. Hemostasis is obtained (Fig. 22.31A–C).
3. The surgeon trims the orbicularis oculi muscle and identifies and excises the septum orbitale. Excess periorbital fat is trimmed and coagulated.

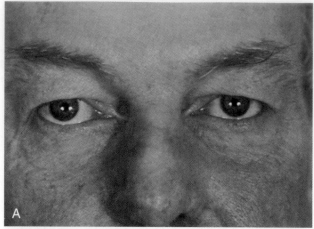

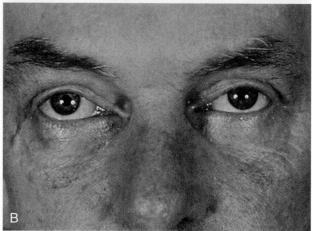

FIG. 22.30 (A) Preoperative and (B) postoperative blepharoplasty.

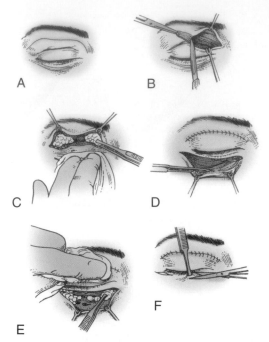

FIG. 22.31 Blepharoplasty for drooping eyelids. (A) Areas of proposed skin excision marked with methylene blue or a sterile marking pen. (B) Strip of skin excised from upper lid; fat pad shining through orbital fascia and orbicular muscle of eye. (C) Orbital fascia opened in two places (medially and laterally). Pressure on eyeball causes fat pads to bulge. They are eased out meticulously. (D) Upper lid incision sutured with continuous 6-0 suture material of choice. Orbital muscle fibers of lower lid are separated from skin. (E) Orbital fascia opened; fat pads bulge because of digital pressure and are teased out meticulously. (F) Skin tailored to fit and sutured.

4. Upper lid incisions are closed; and the surgeon repeats the procedure for the opposite upper lid.
5. Finely crushed ice on moist gauze 4 × 4 pads may be applied to the periorbital region; other means of reducing swelling, such as cold compresses or a hydrogel cold mask, may be similarly applied. Compresses are changed as often as they become warm.

Operative Procedure: Lower Lids

1. The surgeon marks the lines of incision and injects local anesthetic.
2. A subciliary incision (1 mm below eyelashes) is made and brought out in a natural line in the outer canthal skin.
3. The skin-muscle flap is raised, leaving a 3-mm strip of muscle attached to the tarsus (see Fig. 22.31D).
4. The skin-muscle flap is dissected down below the level of the orbital rim.
5. The surgeon incises the arcus marginalis, and redundant fat with the overlying septum orbitale is draped over the orbital rim (see Fig. 22.31E) and sutured.
6. Hemostasis is obtained. Skin is redraped in an upward and outward fashion with attention to prevention of ectropion.
7. Excess skin is trimmed (see Fig. 22.31F).
8. Lateral muscle is sutured to periosteum.
9. The surgeon closes the lower lid incision and repeats the procedure for the opposite lower lid.
10. Compresses are applied as described in the upper lid procedure.

Rhinoplasty

Deformities of the external nose and nasal septum may be congenital or secondary to previous trauma. The goal of rhinoplasty is to improve the appearance of the external nose. This is accomplished by reshaping the underlying framework of the nose, which allows the overlying skin and subcutaneous tissue to redrape over the new framework. Reshaping the nasal skeleton usually includes use of a rasp for dorsal hump reduction, partial excision of lateral and alar cartilages, shortening of the septum, and osteotomy of nasal bones. Rhinoplasty may be performed as an open procedure by making an external incision across the base of the columella, or it may be performed entirely through the nares by using internal incisions. Small external incisions at the alar bases are used to narrow the nares, and internal incisions placed alongside the base of the nasal bones are used to narrow the entire nose once the hump is removed or dorsum is incised. A full description of rhinologic procedures (including septoplasty and submucous resection, which are often performed with rhinoplasty) may be found in Chapter 19.

Laser Surgery

Common uses for lasers in plastic surgery include exfoliation, treatment of vascular malformations, removal of hair and tattoos, and tightening of collagen fibers in aging skin. A variety of lasers are available; selection of the appropriate laser depends on the patient's diagnosis because the effect of the laser on the skin tissue is dependent on its wavelength.

One of the most popular types of laser is the skin resurfacing, or CO_2, laser. Laser safety and procedures are described in great detail in Chapter 8.

Liposuction

Liposuction is a surgical technique designed to remove excess deposits of fat and improve the contour of the body (Fig. 22.32). It is not a treatment for obesity or simply a weight reduction procedure; rather, the ideal candidate is of normal weight and desires to remove localized fat that has proved resistant despite diet and exercise. By extension, liposuction patients must adhere to lifestyle changes (e.g., proper nutrition, adequate exercise) to maintain optimal results. Although most often associated with contour correction, liposuction may also be used for treatment of gynecomastia or to remove lipomas. Areas that may be suctioned include face, neck, back, breasts (not a replacement for reduction mammoplasty, only contour correction), waist, abdomen, midriff, flanks, upper arms, hips, medial and lateral thighs, knees, and ankles (Figs. 22.33 and 22.34).

Multiple techniques have been developed to enhance the final results as well as ease the removal of the fat. These techniques are not always used in isolation of each other; rather, some may be combined both to achieve the best possible outcome and to address the surgeon's preferences. Each procedure has specific equipment needed for that technique and often has highly specific cannulae and other instrumentation. Because multiple areas are usually treated, the perioperative nurse should determine the sequence of liposuction the surgeon prefers to be prepared for positioning.

Procedural Considerations

Immediate preoperative preparation includes asking the patient to stand while the area of deformity is outlined. The surgeon usually draws two lines on the skin surface, one delineating the major area of defect and the other placed a short distance outside the first area. These lines make it easier for the surgeon to make a smooth transition toward the normal tissue by adjusting the amount of fat removed from the center to the periphery of the deformity. The patient may remain standing and be prepped circumferentially with a spray bottle of antimicrobial skin solution. The perioperative nurse provides for the patient's privacy and uses appropriate measures to protect the patient from hypothermia.

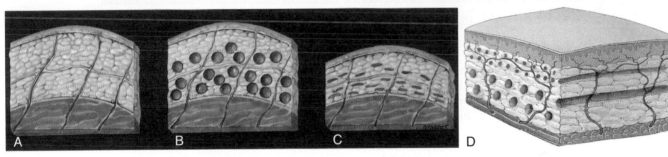

FIG. 22.32 (A) Normal appearance of excess fat. (B) Removal of deep fat by larger-diameter cannulae. (C) Corrected contour after removal of excess fat by liposuction. (D) Removal of superficial fat involves using narrower gauge cannulae.

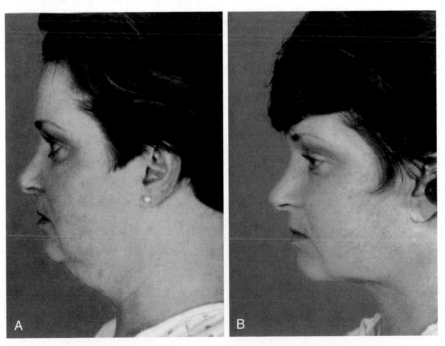

FIG. 22.33 Submental liposuction. (A) Preoperative. (B) Postoperative.

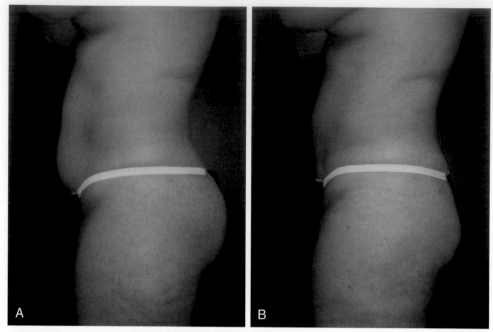

FIG. 22.34 Female 43-year-old patient. (A) Before and (B) 6 months after liposuction of the abdomen and buttocks.

Preoperative patient education should include a discussion of the compression garment, which is typically worn for 2 to 4 weeks postoperatively. Patients should also be informed about the likelihood of the puncture sites leaking tumescent solution during the first 24 hours of the postoperative period. Absorbent dressings are required to minimize soiling of clothing and bedding during this period as well as to maintain the cleanliness of the compression garment.

Depending on the areas targeted for liposuction, draping may require a good deal of innovation. Minimal instrumentation is necessary. A knife handle, towel clips, tissue forceps, scissors, clamps, and needle holder are used along with the suction cannulae specific to the proposed liposuction technique. A general anesthetic, moderate sedation, or epidural anesthetic may be used. However, the surgeon typically injects a medicated wetting solution into the fatty areas before removal because of concerns about large fluid volume shift and blood loss after lipectomy. The wetting solution contains IV fluid (e.g., lactated Ringer's), lidocaine, and epinephrine. Using more than 70 mL/kg of wetting solution for infiltration can lead to fluid overload; this may present as increased blood pressure, jugular vein distention, bounding pulses, cough, dyspnea, lung crackles, and pulmonary edema. For safety issues the nurse needs to communicate and verify with the surgeon the total lipoaspirate and volume of wetting solution used. Additionally, it is imperative that warmed wetting solution be used for suction-assisted lipectomy (SAL).

In the tumescent technique, large volumes of this solution are administered. The "super-wet" technique uses less solution. Usually the amount of fluid injected approximates the amount of fat to be removed; thus the name, which refers to the swollen and firm ("tumesced") state of the tissues when they are filled with solution. The perioperative nurse should inquire if the surgeon will be infiltrating tumescent solution and, if so, what ingredients are used for his or her technique. Also the nurse should ask whether the surgeon uses internal or external ultrasound (sound waves that liquefy fat) or power-assisted liposuction. One of the newer techniques is the use of vibration amplification of sound energy at resonance

(VASER)-assisted liposuction, which incorporates thermal energy to liquefy the fat, aiding greatly in its removal.

Operative Procedure

1. The surgeon places stablike incisions in concealed areas to access sites to be liposuctioned.
2. The tumescent solution is infused.
3. Depending on the technique, at this point either internal or external ultrasound or the VASER technique is performed at predetermined settings and length of time.
4. Liposuction is performed with the use of various sizes and lengths of cannulae. The cannula is attached to large-bore, firm suction tubing and connected to an aspirating unit. The high vacuum pressure caused by the unit causes the fat cells to emulsify so that they can be suctioned through the vacuum opening near the rounded tip of the cannula. Areas are usually cross-suctioned to achieve the best outcomes. Stab wounds may be closed with absorbable suture or left open to drain.
5. The patient's skin is cleaned, and bulky dressings and compression garments are applied.

Abdominoplasty

Abdominoplasty is particularly useful in improving the appearance (and to a certain extent, function) of persons who have lost a great deal of weight or who suffer from laxity of abdominal skin after pregnancy. Obesity produces distention and stretching of the skin of the abdomen. Weight loss reduces the volume of the underlying fat; however, it does not produce concomitant reduction in the excess surface area of the overlying skin, which results from destruction or insufficiency of elastic fibers in the skin. The rectus abdominis fascia is also stretched in obese patients, and weight loss does not restore its integrity.

There are several versions of the abdominoplasty procedure, and the choice of which technique to use depends on the degree of deformity of the abdominal skin and muscle. All techniques are designed to improve the appearance of the abdomen by tightening the abdominal area (abdominal wall/rectus muscles) and removing excess skin or fullness.

If there is minimal to no laxity of the skin and mostly fullness of the lower abdomen, then a "mini-abdominoplasty" may be indicated. With this technique it is not necessary to relocate or incise the umbilicus and a short incision, resembling a Pfannenstiel, may be effectively used. However, if there is laxity of the periumbilical and upper and lower abdominal skin accompanied by protrusion of the abdominal wall with diastasis (separation) of the rectus muscle, then full abdominoplasty is the procedure of choice. This version requires relocation of the umbilicus and an incision that stretches from hip to hip. Endoscopic abdominoplasty is another option if only muscle repair (correction of the diastasis deformity or shortening of the rectus muscles) is needed.

Procedural Considerations

A basic plastic instrument set is required, as well as extra retractors and clamping instruments, an ESU, and a sterile marking pen. Frequently tumescent anesthetic solution is added to minimize bleeding, reduce postoperative discomfort, and aid in dissection. The perioperative nurse should ask the surgeon about the use of tumescent as well as preference for ingredients. A lighted fiberoptic retractor should be available. Intermittent pneumatic compression devices or antiembolism hose are usually in place or applied in the OR. The patient is in the supine position with slight flexion at the hips. Draping is such that the entire abdomen, lower costal margins, upper thighs, and both anterior iliac spines are exposed.

Operative Procedure

1. The surgeon makes a low transverse abdominal incision across both inguinal areas laterally and the superior border of the mons pubis in the midline down to fascia.
2. A large flap of skin and subcutaneous tissue is elevated away from the fascia of the anterior abdominal wall.
3. The umbilicus is circumscribed and left in its normal position.
4. The surgeon elevates the abdominal flap until the xiphoid process of the sternum and the lower costal margins are reached.
5. If diastasis of the rectus abdominis fascia is present, the surgeon plicates it with suture from the xiphoid process to the mons pubis.
6. The flap of abdominal skin and subcutaneous tissue is pulled inferiorly, and excess tissue is excised.
7. A small incision is made in the midline of the flap to accommodate the umbilicus, which is then sutured peripherally to the flap.
8. Drains are inserted, followed by closure of the lower abdominal incision in layers.
9. Postoperatively the patient is placed in the hospital bed in high Fowler position.

Postbariatric Surgery Body Contouring

Successful bariatric surgery produces significant weight loss. The weight loss may result in a trunk that lacks waist and hip definition; ptosis of the mons pubis; and various degrees of skin, fat, and abdominal wall laxity. Upper and lower back rolls accompany the anterior truncal deformities; the buttocks are lower and lack fullness. Upper arms and thighs exhibit similar deformities.

Treatment is aimed at removing the excessive skin and creating a desirable body contour. Most patients are candidates for some form of circumferential recontouring (belt lipectomy) (Fig. 22.35) in combination with any number of other recontouring procedures:

brachioplasty (Fig. 22.36), thigh lifts (Fig. 22.37), and mastopexy. For the perioperative nurse, these surgeries offer a logistical challenge because of the combination of procedures and positioning required. The malabsorptive effects of the original bariatric surgery may compromise postoperative wound healing after body contouring procedures. Patients who undergo major recontouring procedures are at increased risk for postoperative complications. The perioperative nurse must be familiar with the complications relating to postbariatric surgery body contouring to provide comprehensive care for this unique group of patients (Research Highlight).

Procedural Considerations

Extensive measuring and marking are performed by the plastic surgeon in the preoperative area. The perioperative nurse should inquire about the ordering of the procedures and positioning. If more than one procedure is planned, intermittent pneumatic compression devices and a Foley catheter should be used once the patient arrives in the OR. During prepping and draping, attempts should be made to preserve the patient's body temperature. Repositioning is a standard part of these procedures. Pressure points should be well padded with appropriate positioning aids to maintain functional alignment and stable positioning. With each repositioning activity the patient must be reassessed for safety in terms of skin and nerve compression and competence of the grounding pad, Foley catheter, and all monitoring devices. A basic plastic surgery instrument set with additional towel clamps is used. Other supplies include a stapler for skin approximation, multiple drains, and an ESU. The surgeon may choose to use tissue adhesive products in combination with suture material to reduce the incidence of seroma. Compression garments may be applied, but care must be taken not to compromise the vascularity of the skin flaps.

Operative Procedure: Belt Lipectomy

Sites addressed are the abdomen, including mons pubis; upper and lower back; lateral trunk skin; buttocks; and lateral upper thighs.

1. The surgeon infuses dilute tumescent solution to aid in hemostasis and facilitate undermining of flaps.
2. Incisions are made and taken down to the level of the fascia, and flaps are elevated to previously marked margins. Liposuction cannulae without vacuum attachments may be used for undermining.
3. Liposuction is used if indicated for contouring only.
4. Muscle plication is performed when indicated.
5. The surgeon approximates and sutures the superficial fascia with permanent sutures.
6. Skin flaps are approximated, and excess skin is excised.
7. Closed-wound suction drains are inserted and secured with suture.
8. The patient is repositioned; depending on position at the start of the procedure, this could be lateral decubitus or supine.
9. Similar techniques are used for defects in areas presented by the new position and repeated until all areas are addressed, including relocation of the umbilicus.
10. The patient's skin is cleaned, incisions are dressed, and compression garments are applied per the surgeon's preference.
11. The patient is transferred to a stretcher or bed and placed in the flexed position.

Breast Surgeries

A variety of surgical procedures are available to enhance the aesthetic appearance of the breasts. Patients may choose to enlarge, reduce, and change the position of their breasts.

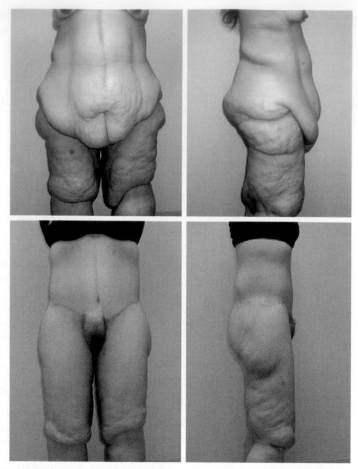

FIG. 22.35 Belt lipectomy and thigh liposuction. The patient was a 40-year-old woman 40 months after gastric bypass surgery with a weight loss of 269 pounds.

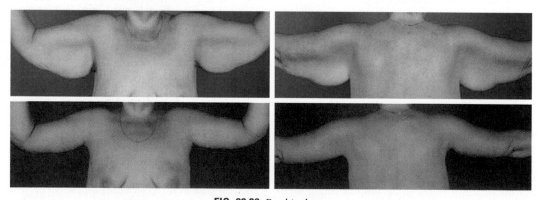

FIG. 22.36 Brachioplasty.

Augmentation Mammoplasty

Breast augmentation is performed for correction of hypomastia, to correct breast asymmetry, and to re-create the breast after mastectomy. A prosthesis is inserted to enlarge or form the breast mound.

Breast Implants. The two basic types of breast implants are saline filled and silicone gel filled. Both are approved by the US Food and Drug Administration (FDA) for elective breast augmentation; in November 2006 the FDA approved the use of silicone gel–filled breast implants for breast augmentation and breast reconstruction and revision surgeries (FDA, 2011).

Implants are configured into round or teardrop (also known as anatomic) shapes and may have a smooth or textured surface. The surfaces are designed to minimize capsular contracture and migration. The choice to use a round or an anatomic implant is based on the shape and form of the existing breast.

Procedural Considerations. The perioperative nurse verifies the style and size of implant and handles the implant according to the manufacturer's recommendations. Handling implants as little as possible assists in efforts to reduce the potential for implant contamination. A basic plastic instrument set is used, plus lighted fiberoptic

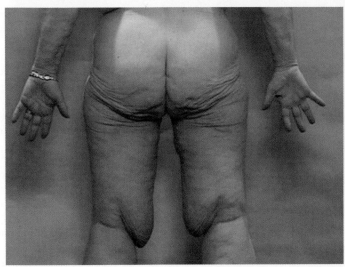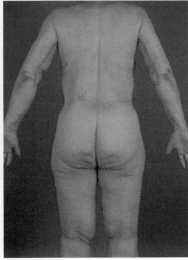

FIG. 22.37 Thigh lift.

RESEARCH HIGHLIGHT

Circular Abdominoplasty After Massive Weight Loss: Is It a Risky Procedure?

Body contouring after bariatric surgery is different from similar procedures in those who have not been obese. The deformity after bariatric surgery is more severe because the skin damage and associated loss of tone and elasticity do not recover, and the laxity is global. A number of procedures may be required. Various techniques are used for contouring:

- Panniculectomy is removal of excess skin and soft tissue from the abdominal wall without umbilical transposition. It is limited to removal of the overhanging pannus.
- Abdominoplasty includes panniculectomy with wide undermining of the upper abdominal flap and umbilical transposition. Unlike in a traditional abdominoplasty, a vertical ellipse or fleur-de-lis pattern of excision often is necessary to remove significant excess skin in the horizontal dimension superior to the umbilicus.
- Circumferential abdominoplasty, or belt lipectomy, may also be referred to as a lower body lift. It corrects the circumferential roll of excess tissue found in most patients by extending the abdominal resection around the sides of the abdomen to include the lower back. In the course of resecting this circumferential ring of tissue, the lateral thighs and buttocks are also lifted.

Among these procedures, many surgeons are wary of circumferential abdominoplasty because it is considered a major intervention with a high complication rate. This study (Modarressi et al., 2016) looked at 56 consecutive patients who underwent circumferential abdominoplasty after massive weight loss to assess for complication rate. Before weight loss, all were morbidly obese with a mean BMI of 45.8. For those who underwent bariatric surgery (95% of patients), the mean time between bariatric surgery and circular abdominoplasty was 3.3 years. Fifteen patients were active smokers. Seven patients had arterial hypertension, and five patients had type 2 diabetes. The mean age was 39.8 years and mean BMI was 25.7.

No general complications such as deep venous thrombosis, pulmonary embolism, or pneumonia occurred. The overall complication rate was 23.2% with nonsignificant difference between smokers and nonsmokers (26.7% versus 22%). Four infections (7.1%) were observed and treated conservatively with antibiotics. No skin flap necrosis was observed. Seven patients (12.5%) suffered from localized delayed wound healing, and only one (1.8%) needed early surgical revision under local anesthesia.

The authors concluded that circular abdominoplasty is a reliable procedure. Patient preselection is crucial for reducing the complication rate. Patients who have lost <45 kg, but achieved a low BMI (<30) at the time of body contouring, present a lesser operative risk and obtain a better aesthetic result.

Patient selection (e.g., BMI <30 kg/m²), precise preoperative planning and markings, and simple and careful surgical technique with minimal liposuction and undermining are crucial. Ensuring these key factors renders circular abdominoplasty a reliable and safe procedure, with low complication rates.

BMI, Body mass index.
Modified from McGrath M et al: Plastic surgery. In Townsend C et al, editors: *Sabiston textbook of surgery*, ed 20, Philadelphia, 2017, Elsevier; Modarressi A et al: Circular abdominoplasty after massive weight loss: is it a risky procedure? *J Plast Reconstr Aesthet Surg* 69(11):1497–1505, 2016.

retractors. The breast implants are packaged in sterile containers from the manufacturer and given to the scrub person when breast size is determined. Breast implants should only be filled with sterile injectable saline using a closed system designed for that purpose. The patient is supine. The arms may be extended on armboards to approximately 60 degrees. Prepping and draping are performed in the routine manner to expose the operative site.

Operative Procedure. The surgeon may perform augmentation mammoplasty through circumareolar, inframammary, axillary, or transumbilical incisions using an open or endoscopic approach. Depending on the anatomy of the patient and the surgeon's preference, breast implants may be placed subglandularly, subpectorally (Fig. 22.38), or biplanarly (partial muscle coverage).

Operative Procedure: Unfilled Saline Implants

1. The surgeon may inject local anesthetic to decrease bleeding and provide analgesia.
2. An incision is made, the pocket is dissected, and hemostasis is achieved.

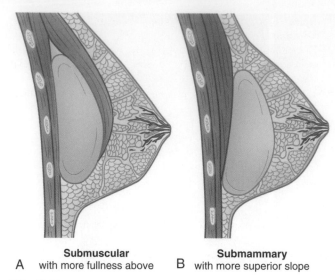

A **Submuscular** with more fullness above   **B** **Submammary** with more superior slope

FIG. 22.38 (A) Augmentation mammoplasty implant under muscle. (B) Implant under breast tissue.

3. The surgeon may use breast implant sizers (gel or saline) to evaluate the size of the pocket and determine the size of the final implant.

4. With the sizers in place, the anesthesia provider elevates the patient to the 90-degree position so the surgeon can evaluate the appearance from various angles and plan for any adjustments or revisions to the pocket.

5. The sizers are removed, and the surgeon finalizes the pocket.

6. The perioperative nurse verifies the implant type and size again with the surgeon and dispenses it to the sterile field.

7. The surgeon rolls the implant into a cylindric shape in preparation for insertion.

8. The pocket is irrigated with saline or antibiotic solution.

9. The surgeon inserts the implant and unrolls it, and after it is properly positioned, the surgeon inflates the implant with an appropriate amount of saline.

10. The procedure is repeated for the opposite breast.

11. The incision is closed in two layers.

12. The patient is cleaned, and bandages and a surgical bra are applied.

Capsulotomy

Capsule contracture occurs when the normal envelope of fibrous tissue around an implant gets thicker or tighter so that the implant no longer feels soft and pliant. If the degree of capsular contracture is great, there can be pain, distortion, and palpability or distortion of the implant. Capsular contracture occurs in approximately 15% of patients, and it is not possible to predict who will develop it or take preventive measures (McGrath and Pomeranz, 2017). Depending on the extent of the contracture, an open capsulotomy may be used to release the constrictive tissue, or a capsulectomy may be indicated to actually remove the tissue. Although patients receive education about capsule contracture as part of the informed consent process for breast augmentation, the actuality of the event may cause emotional distress for the patient. The patient may verbalize disappointment over the results and express fear related to additional postoperative changes in the appearance and functioning of the breast. In addition, the patient now faces the surgical and anesthetic

risks associated with a second surgical procedure and may also be struggling with a possible financial burden because these procedures may not be covered by the patient's health plan. An empathic and understanding approach is paramount to easing the patient's anxiety.

Procedural Considerations. The patient is prepared, positioned, and draped in the same manner as for breast augmentation.

Operative Procedure

1. The surgeon incises the skin and exposes the capsule.

2. The capsule is scored in multiple areas to achieve the desired release. Depending on the degree of contracture, circumferential incisions may be necessary to release the contracture.

3. If capsulotomy is not effective in releasing the capsule, a partial or full capsulectomy may be required to physically remove all or a portion of the capsule.

   a. The capsule is excised, and the breast implant is removed.

   b. The breast implant may be replaced in the same area, exchanged and replaced, or placed in a new pocket.

4. The site is irrigated with antibiotic solution. Drains are placed if a capsulectomy was performed.

5. The surgeon closes the incision in two layers.

6. The patient's skin is cleaned, and dressings are applied.

Reduction Mammoplasty

Reduction mammoplasty is indicated for the patient with macromastia with resulting back pain, intertrigo (chronic skin infection), or deep grooving in the shoulders from bra straps because of the weight of the breasts (Patient, Family, and Caregiver Education) (Fig. 22.39A). The procedure may also be performed to achieve symmetry after a mastectomy on the contralateral side. Excessive breast tissue and its overlying skin are excised, with reconstruction of the breast contour, size, shape, and symmetry (see Fig. 22.39B).

Procedural Considerations. A basic plastic instrument set is used with the addition of a "cookie cutter" areola marker or a "keyhole" pattern marker, a sterile marking pen, skin stapler, tape measure, baby Deaver retractors, and two closed-wound suction systems. An ESU and a scale for weighing specimens should also be available, and tissue from each side should be carefully weighed and marked appropriately. The perioperative nurse should ensure the scale is calibrated correctly before weighing any tissue. Numerous blades will be used if deepithelializing breast skin. If the nipple is removed and placed as a free nipple graft, extra suture will be necessary for tie-over bolsters. There are numerous choices in the reduction mammoplasty technique; therefore before opening suture or other supplies, the perioperative nurse should ask the surgeon which technique will be used. The surgeon will mark the skin to be excised and the new site for the nipple preoperatively with the patient in a sitting position.

The patient is supine with arms slightly extended on padded armboards. The hips should be positioned at the break in the OR bed so that the patient may be raised to a sitting position if necessary. Standard prepping and draping are done. Care should be taken not to remove the preoperative markings.

Operative Procedure. The standard reduction mammoplasty procedure is described below. If the surgeon is using the "short scar" technique, the breast tissue is incised and removed according to the technique chosen. The nipple pedicle technique, in which the nipple is mobilized and secured in a new position, may be chosen, or a free nipple graft may be used.

1. The surgeon incises and removes the skin between the new and the old nipple sites, with the nipple remaining attached to the underlying breast tissue. On patients with very large breasts, the

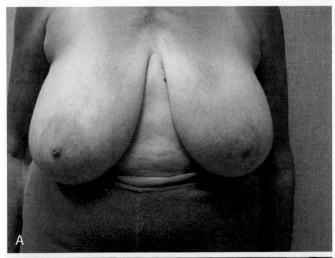

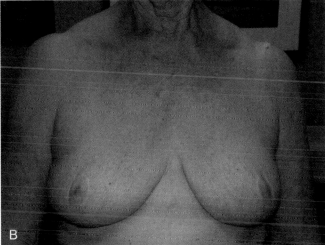

FIG. 22.39 (A) Preoperative view of reduction mammoplasty. (B) Postoperative view.

nipples are removed and then reapplied as free grafts when the reduction is complete.

2. The redundant segment of breast tissue inferior to the nipple is excised through an inverted-T incision. Tissue from each breast is weighed and kept separate.

3. The surgeon mobilizes the nipple and adjacent tissue and sutures them in place.

4. The medial and lateral skin edges are approximated in a vertical suture line inferior to the nipple.

5. The inframammary elliptic incision is trimmed and closed transversely. Closed-wound suction catheters may be placed. The wound is dressed.

Mastopexy

Breast ptosis (drooping) is corrected by moving the nipple to a more normal position and removing excess breast skin (Fig. 22.40). With mastopexy surgery there is usually minimal to no removal of breast tissue, although it may be necessary to add a breast implant to achieve the desired result.

Procedural Considerations. The surgeon marks the patient before surgery. Positioning is similar to that used for breast augmentation. Skin incision choices are periareolar only; periareolar combined with a vertical (known as a short scar or vertical mastopexy); the classic inverted T, which adds an inframammary incision to the previous incision; or the horizontal inframammary, which combines the periareolar and inframammary, leaving out the vertical component. Mastopexy may involve reduction of the skin envelope only or combine skin removal with glandular reshaping and placement in a more desirable position.

Operative Procedure

1. The surgeon places the initial incisions and then uses one or more of the following techniques to reduce the breasts:
   a. Excess skin is removed.
   b. The breast cone is reshaped by invagination of lower midbreast tissue.
   c. The lower submammary breast tissue pedicle is advanced below the breast tissue and tacked superiorly to the pectoral muscle.

PATIENT, FAMILY, AND CAREGIVER EDUCATION

Patient Education for Breast Reduction

General Information

Women with very large, pendulous breasts (a condition known as macromastia) can experience a number of physical and emotional problems. Macromastia is generally defined as excessive breast size, usually a bra cup size of D or larger. This condition is seen in young girls to middle-aged women. The condition probably is caused by hormonal factors but is also associated with obesity. Often there is a family pattern of large breasts.

Common Signs and Symptoms

- Breast size that is out of proportion to the torso and larger than the accepted norm
- Upper back and neck pain
- Shoulder pain
- Arm pain
- Breast pain
- Rashes and sometimes infections of the skin under the breasts
- Shoulder grooving from bra straps

- Hyperpigmentation (dark marks) in the bra strap lines
- Difficulty in finding bras or clothing that fits

Diagnosis

The surgeon will confirm the diagnosis of macromastia by examining the breasts carefully and relating the findings of the patient's history.

Treatment

- Women with large breasts have often tried custom bras and weight loss as a way of reducing breast size or adding support. Physical therapy and pain medications may also be used in an effort to relieve symptoms. After trying these methods without success, many women seek surgical help in the form of breast reduction surgery. Technically, breast reduction surgery is known as reduction mammoplasty.
- The best candidates for breast reduction usually have at least two of the symptoms listed in the previously mentioned Common Signs and Symptoms section.

Continued

PATIENT, FAMILY, AND CAREGIVER EDUCATION

Patient Education for Breast Reduction—cont'd

- Breast reduction surgery should be delayed if weight gain or loss is anticipated. The patient's weight should be stable at the time of the procedure.
- The aims of the operation are the following:
  - To remove enough breast tissue to be able to construct a normal-appearing breast mound.
- To reposition the nipple-areola complex in a suitable position in the "new" breast.
- There are many operations to reduce large breasts. A common technique is shown in the figures.

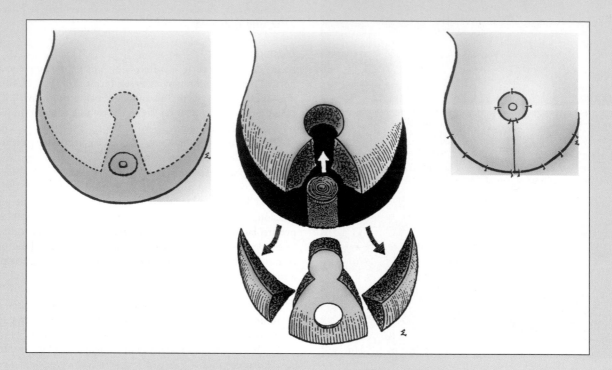

Preparing for the Operation

- The surgeon will examine and measure the breasts and will probably photograph the patient for reference during the surgery and afterward.
- A mammogram may be ordered if patient is 35 years or older or there is a family history of breast cancer.
- The patient should avoid smoking completely for at least 1 month before surgery. Smoking affects the blood vessels in the skin and can slow healing.
- A drug and alcohol consumption history should also be obtained before surgery (can be done during the history and physical).
- The surgeon may instruct the patient to avoid taking aspirin, nonsteroidal antiinflammatory drugs (ibuprofen [Motrin]), vitamin E, herbal supplements, fenfluramine, or phentermine at least 2 weeks before surgery. These substances may interfere with normal blood clotting or with the ability to heal after surgery.
- Before surgery the patient may want to do the following:
  - Wash hair (will not be able to shower or bathe immediately after surgery).
  - Arrange for temporary care for any house pets or children.
  - Move "daily use" items within arm's reach.
  - Fill any prescriptions from the surgeon.
- The following are common after this operation:
  - Decreased nipple sensation
  - Reduced ability to breastfeed

- Decreased ability for the radiologist to interpret mammograms performed after the surgery because of the scarring inside the breast
- Prominent scars

The Operation

- The area in which the incisions will be made on the breasts and the new position of the nipple-areola complex will be marked with dissolving ink while the patient is in a sitting position.
- Most women have general anesthesia for breast reduction. Some surgeons may perform the procedure with a local anesthetic and sedation.
- The operation generally takes 3 to 4 hours.

After Your Operation (Postoperative Instructions for the Patient)

- You will be taken to a recovery room and observed. When blood pressure, pulse, and breathing are stable, you will be taken to a regular hospital room.
- Your chest will be wrapped in elastic bandages or a surgical bra over gauze. Small plastic tubes called drains may be coming from the breast incisions and will be connected to small plastic bulbs. They drain any extra fluid that needs to come out.
- Many breast reduction surgeries are done as outpatient procedures, in which case you will go home after you wake up from the anesthesia and the pain is under control. In some cases you may stay in the hospital after surgery for a short period (1 or 2 days).

Patient Education for Breast Reduction—cont'd

- Recovery is different for every patient, but bed rest may only be needed for 1 or 2 days after the procedure. Even in the first 24 to 48 hours after surgery it is important for you to get out of bed and walk around every 2 hours during the day and early evening. Coughing, deep breathing, and incentive spirometry are also important to prevent atelectasis and pneumonia. Continuous bed rest after surgery may increase your risks for pneumonia or blood clots.
- As with any operation, complications are always possible. With this type of operation, they can include bleeding, infection, delayed wound healing, abnormal scarring, and shape irregularities.

Home Care

You will want to take it easy at first, but may walk about as you wish, even climb stairs, but should not overdo things. Avoid heavy exercise, heavy lifting, or stress on the upper body for 1 month. Items that can be helpful as you recover include the following:

- A body or sitting support pillow
- Cordless phone
- Variety of easy-to-cook or precooked meals
- Two or three loose-fitting robes or housedresses with snaps in the front and large pockets
- Slip-on shoes
- Soft sponge for bathing before showering is allowed
- Small containers for drinks (gallon containers are very heavy)
- A listing of physicians, pharmacy, and caregivers/helpers with telephone contact information. You should call the surgeon if any of the following occurs:
  - The incisions become red and inflamed, or have abnormal pain or excessive swelling.
  - You develop a temperature higher than 101.5°F (38°C).
  - You have any questions.

Modified from American Society of Plastic Surgeons (ASPS): *Breast reduction* (website), 2017. www.plasticsurgery.org/reconstructive-procedures/breast-reduction. (Accessed 25 January 2017). McGrath MH, Pomeranz J: Plastic surgery. In Townsend CM et al, editors: *Sabiston textbook of surgery: the biological basis of modern surgical practice*, ed 20, Philadelphia, 2017, Saunders.

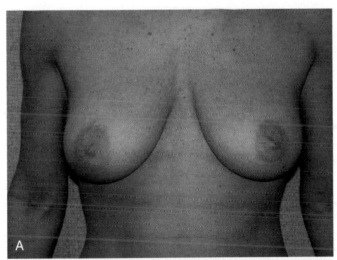
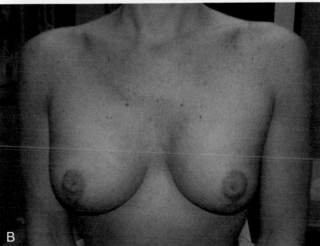

FIG. 22.40 Mastopexy. (A) Preoperative view. (B) Postoperative view; ptosis corrected.

d. Lower midbreast tissue is incised and overlapped.

e. A superiorly based (on the nipple-areolar complex pedicle) wedge tissue flap is created, turned under, and superiorly attached.

f. The upper pole of breast tissue is mobilized and advanced superiorly and tacked to the pectoral muscle fascia.

2. The breast may be sutured entirely at this time or approximated, and the same procedure is applied to the opposite breast, closing both at the end of the procedure.

3. The operative area is cleaned, dressings of choice are applied, and a surgical bra is applied.

Excision of Gynecomastia

Gynecomastia is a relatively common pathologic condition that consists of bilateral or unilateral enlargement of the male breast. It occurs primarily during puberty or after age 40 years. Although it may be produced by a variety of diseases or be the result of side effects related to certain medications, it is usually related to excessive hormone production or alterations in hormonal balance. It may also be seen in elderly men and in men after excessive use of marijuana. All subareolar fibroglandular tissue is removed, and the resultant defect is surgically closed (Fig. 22.41). The patient may be positioned in a supine position or semi-Fowler position, according to the surgeon's preference. Supplies and equipment needed are the same as those for a simple mastectomy, plus a basic plastic instrument set. Because SAL may be used for contouring, suction cannulae, associated supplies, and an aspirator should also be available. All breast tissue removed should be weighed and then sent for pathologic examination. Although infrequent, men are not immune to breast cancer.

Operative Procedure

1. The surgeon instills local anesthetic and makes a stab wound incision for introduction of the liposuction cannula.

2. Liposuction is performed. If satisfactory removal of breast tissue is accomplished, the incision is closed and a compression garment applied.

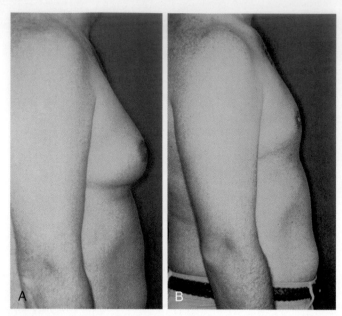

FIG. 22.41 (A) Preoperative view of gynecomastia. (B) Postoperative view after excision of gynecomastia.

3. If additional surgery is required, the surgeon makes a periareolar incision. Through this incision the fibrous and ductal attachments of the underlying glandular tissue to the nipple are divided.
4. A cuff of fatty tissue is left attached to the underlying nipple surface to protect the blood supply.
5. The surgeon dissects the breast tissue mass. Carrying the dissection to the pectoralis fascia is usually necessary to remove the entire mass.
6. Hemostasis is achieved.
7. Closure is performed, the area cleaned, and a compression garment applied.

Key Points

- There are two subspecialties in plastic surgery. Cosmetic surgery restores or reshapes normal structures of the body; reconstructive surgery treats abnormal structures of the body caused by birth defects, developmental problems, disease, tumors, infection, or injury.
- Plastic surgery is not limited to a single anatomic location or biologic system.
- Procedures involve removing, reducing, enlarging, and recontouring tissue and camouflaging of scars. Microsurgical techniques are often used.

Critical Thinking Questions

You are caring for a female patient who is undergoing tumescent liposuction of her abdomen, hips, and thighs under general anesthesia. About 30 minutes into the procedure the anesthesia provider notes that the patient is tachycardic with a widened PR interval and is hypertensive. As he informs the surgeon of these findings, the patient experiences a tonic-clonic seizure. What is the likely cause of the patient's clinical deterioration? How should the nurse intervene?

evolve *The answers to the Critical Thinking Questions can be found at http://evolve.elsevier.com/Rothrock/Alexander.*

References

Acelity Corporation: *AlloDerm select regenerative tissue matrix—the surgeons' choice, now with enhanced precision* (website), 2017. http://www.acelity.com/products/alloderm-select. (Accessed 22 January 2017).

American Burn Association (ABA): *Burn incidence and treatment in the U.S.* (website), 2016. www.ameriburn.org/resources_factsheet.php. (Accessed 22 January 2017).

American Society of Plastic Surgeons (ASPS): *Physician's guide to cosmetic surgery overview* (website), 2017. www.plasticsurgery.org/for-medical-professionals/resources-and-education/publications/physicians-guide-to-cosmetic-surgery/physicians-guide-to-cosmetic-surgery-overview?sub=Does+Your+Patient+Have+Realistic+Goals?#section-title. (Accessed 22 January 2017).

American Society of Plastic Surgeons (ASPS): *2015 plastic surgery statistics report* (website), 2015. https://d2wirczt3b6wjm.cloudfront.net/News/Statistics/2015/plastic-surgery-statistics-full-report-2015.pdf. (Accessed 22 January 2017).

Association of periOperative Registered Nurses (AORN): Guideline for care of the patient receiving local anesthesia. In *Guidelines for perioperative practice*, Denver, 2015, The Association.

Association of periOperative Registered Nurses (AORN): Guideline for positioning the patient. In *Guidelines for perioperative practice*, Denver, 2016a, The Association.

Association of periOperative Registered Nurses (AORN): Guideline for preoperative patient skin asepsis. In *Guidelines for perioperative practice*, Denver, 2016b, The Association.

Association of periOperative Registered Nurses (AORN): *Patient hand-off tool kit* (website), 2016c. www.aorn.org/guidelines/clinical-resources/tool-kits/patient-hand-off-tool-kit. (Accessed 22 January 2017).

Biggs WP, Chaganaboyana S: Human sexuality. In Rakel R, Rakel DP, editors: *Textbook of family medicine*, ed 9, Philadelphia, 2016, Saunders.

Coffee T: Care of patients with burns. In Ignatavicius DD, Workman ML, editors: *Medical-surgical nursing: patient-centered collaborative care*, ed 8, St Louis, 2016, Saunders.

Kelman RM: Maxillofacial trauma. In Flint PW et al, editors: *Cummings otolaryngology head and neck surgery*, ed 6, Philadelphia, 2015, Mosby.

Leona M et al: Wound healing. In Townsend CM et al, editors: *Sabiston textbook of surgery: the biological basis of modern surgical practice*, ed 12, Philadelphia, 2017, Saunders.

McCance KL: Cancer epidemiology. In Huether SE et al, editors: *Understanding pathophysiology*, ed 6, St Louis, 2017, Mosby.

McGrath MH, Pomeranz J: Plastic surgery. In Townsend CM et al, editors: *Sabiston textbook of surgery: the biological basis of modern surgical practice*, ed 20, Philadelphia, 2017, Saunders.

The Joint Commission (TJC): *Hospital national safety goals* (website), 2017. www.jointcommission.org/assets/1/6/2017_NPSG_HAP_ER.pdf. (Accessed 22 January 2017).

US Department of Labor (DOL): *Your rights after a mastectomy* (website), 2014. www.dol.gov/ebsa/publications/whcra.html. (Accessed 22 January 2017).

US Food and Drug Administration (FDA): *Silicone gel-filled breast implants* (website), 2011. www.fda.gov/MedicalDevices/ProductsandMedicalProcedures/ImplantsandProsthetics/BreastImplants/ucm063871.htm. (Accessed 22 January 2017).

Winter S et al: Transgender people: health at the margins of society, *Lancet* 388(10042):390–400, 2016.

Thoracic surgery, like other specialties, has evolved with the increased understanding of pathophysiology and development of improved surgical techniques and treatments. The thoracic specialty extends beyond the surgical arena into infectious disease, trauma, and oncology. Improved technology and the determination to treat diseases previously considered untreatable with operative and other invasive procedures continue to improve the recovery rate for patients experiencing thoracic diseases. As the ability to treat thoracic disease has improved, the responsibilities of the perioperative nurse have expanded as well.

Surgical Anatomy

The skeletal framework of the thorax is formed anteriorly by the sternum and costal cartilages, laterally by the 12 pairs of ribs, and posteriorly by the 12 thoracic vertebrae (Fig. 23.1). This airtight compartment is enclosed in the root of the neck by Sibson fascia and is separated from the abdomen by the diaphragm.

The sternum forms the anterior thoracic wall in the midline. It consists of three parts: (1) the upper part, or manubrium; (2) the body, or gladiolus; and (3) the lower cartilage, or xiphoid process. The manubrium articulates with the clavicles and the first two ribs on each side; the gladiolus articulates with the remaining true ribs by separate costal cartilages; and the xiphoid fuses with the gladiolus in early development and is attached to the diaphragm by the substernal ligament.

Normally the lateral walls of the thorax are formed by the 12 pairs of ribs. Posteriorly, each pair of ribs articulates with its corresponding thoracic vertebrae. Anteriorly, the first seven ribs articulate with the sternum. The eighth, ninth, and tenth ribs articulate with the costal cartilages of the rib above; however, the eleventh and twelfth ribs are not fixed to the costal arch (see Fig. 23.1).

The muscles of each hemithorax (Figs. 23.2 and 23.3) include the 11 external and 11 internal intercostal muscles, which fill the spaces between the ribs. An intercostal artery, vein, and nerve accompany each intercostal muscle. The arteries communicate with the internal thoracic artery anteriorly and arise from the aorta posteriorly. The intercostal veins follow the course of the arteries and communicate with the mammary veins anteriorly and with the azygos and hemiazygos veins posteriorly.

During surgery great care is taken to prevent injury to the intercostal nerves, which pass forward and alongside the posterior intercostal arteries and share the intercostal grooves on the inferior edges of the corresponding rib with the superior branch of the artery. When the nerve must be disturbed, an anesthetic agent may be injected to prevent postoperative pain.

The thoracic outlet is a junction bound anteriorly by the manubrium, anterolaterally by the first ribs, and posteriorly by the first thoracic vertebrae and posterior angles of the first ribs of the space. The great vessels of the head, neck, and arm pass through this space. Compression of these structures may cause thoracic outlet syndrome.

The mediastinum is divided into anterior, middle, and posterior compartments. The anterior mediastinum is bound anteriorly by the sternum and posteriorly by the pericardium and great vessels. It contains the thymus gland, lymph nodes, and pericardial fat. The middle mediastinum is bound anteriorly by the pericardium and great vessels and posteriorly by the anterior border of the vertebral bodies. The posterior mediastinum is bound anteriorly by the vertebral bodies and extends posteriorly to the chest wall.

The chest cavity is subdivided into the right and the left pleural cavities, which contain the lungs separated by the mediastinum, which lies medially between the two pleural membranes. The parietal pleura, the membrane that lines the inner surface of each hemithorax, is adjacent to the inner surfaces of the ribs posteriorly and the mediastinum medially and covers the surface of the diaphragm except at the central portion. Part of the parietal membrane is reflected back at the root of each lung to form a sac around it. This reflection is called the *visceral pleura.* The pleural space normally holds about 50 mL of pleural fluid, a serous secretion that provides lubrication between these two membranes to minimize friction during inspiration and expiration (Brashers, 2017).

The lungs are the essential organs of respiration. The base of each lung rests on the diaphragm, whereas its apex (upper end) projects into the base of the neck at a level above the first rib. The bronchus, the nerves, the lymphatics, and the pulmonary and bronchial vessels enter and leave the lung on the mediastinal surface in a structure

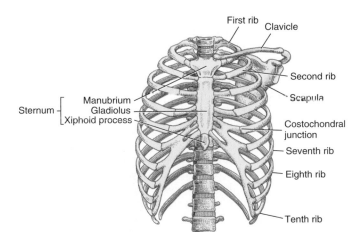

First rib
Clavicle
Second rib
Scapula
Costochondral junction
Seventh rib
Eighth rib
Tenth rib
Sternum {
Manubrium
Gladiolus
Xiphoid process

FIG. 23.1 Bony thorax.

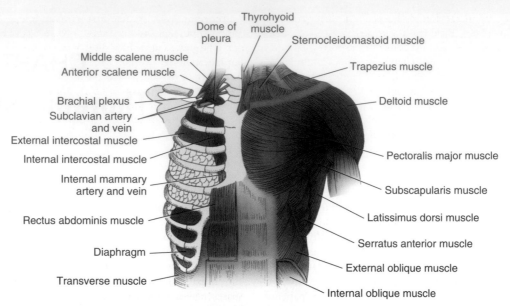

FIG. 23.2 Anterior view of thorax and contiguous portions of base of neck and anterior abdominal wall. *Right half,* Superficial layer of muscles and fascia; *left half,* relationships of deep muscles of neck and abdomen to rib cage, intercostal muscles, diaphragm, and internal mammary vessels; relationships of muscles, nerves, and vessels with first rib; and anterior relations of lung.

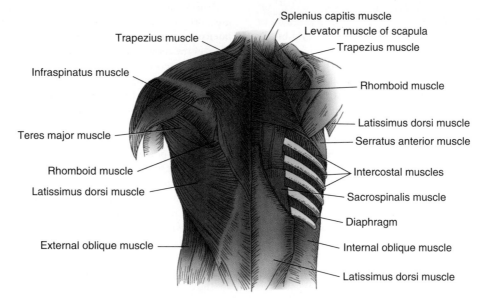

FIG. 23.3 Posterior view of thorax and contiguous portions of neck and abdominal wall. *Left half,* Superficial muscles; *right half,* deeper muscles.

known as the *hilum*, or *root*, of the lung. Deep fissures divide the spongy, porous lung into lobes. The primary bronchi divide and then subdivide into each lobe and eventually become bronchioles. The right lung has an upper, a middle, and a lower lobe; the left lung has only an upper and a lower lobe (Fig. 23.4). However, the lungs are similar in that each is composed of 10 major segments (Fig. 23.5). Each segment extends to the pleural surface, expanding in volume from its center to its peripheral edges. Each segment also has its own bronchus and branches of the pulmonary artery and vein.

The bronchial arteries, arising from the aorta, supply nourishment to the lungs. They vary in their number and course. The arrangement may include two branches to the left lung and one branch to the right lung, which later branches into two, or there may be one or two branches for each lung. The pulmonary arteries carry the blood to the pulmonary parenchyma, and the pulmonary veins transport the oxygenated blood to the left atrium.

The nerves of the lungs are a part of the autonomic nervous system (see Chapter 21). They regulate constriction and relaxation of the bronchi and of the blood vessels within the lungs.

Although the thoracic cavity is an airtight space, the lungs receive outside air through the nasal passages, trachea, and bronchi. The main function of the lungs is to exchange carbon dioxide for oxygen. Normally, as the thorax expands, the lungs also expand as air is drawn in; during expiration, the thorax relaxes and the lungs passively contract as air is forced out. Inspiration normally takes place when the intrathoracic pressure is slightly below atmospheric pressure (76 cm Hg, or 760 mm Hg) and when a partial vacuum exists between the parietal and visceral pleural (intrathoracic) surfaces. As the muscles of inspiration contract to enlarge the chest cage, the lungs passively follow the diaphragm and chest wall because of decreased intrathoracic pressure. The acts of inspiration and expiration are the result of air moving in and out of the lung, causing pressure to equalize with that of the atmosphere at the end of expiration.

The normal intrapleural pressure varies from −9 to −12 cm H_2O during inspiration and from about −3 to −6 cm H_2O during expiration. The greatest amount of air that can be expired after a maximum inspiration is termed the *vital capacity*, and the volume of gas remaining in the lungs after maximal expiration is *residual volume*. Size, age, gender, and pulmonary disease of the patient influence vital capacity. Any condition that interferes with the normally negative intrapleural pressure affects respiratory function.

Perioperative Nursing Considerations

Assessment

During assessment the perioperative nurse gathers information that is important to planning patient care. The nurse may begin data collection by identifying the patient and confirming the correct surgical site. A thorough review of the patient's medical record, including results of the history, physical examination, laboratory tests, other diagnostic workups, and the nursing history and assessment, is critical for subsequent care planning. The perioperative nurse assesses the patient's understanding of the disease process and of the anticipated procedure and confirms the patient has adequate support to assist him or her through the surgical experience and recovery. The nurse assesses emotional status because patients with a possible diagnosis of cancer may be very anxious. A focused assessment of the respiratory system should be included during the physical assessment with an emphasis on any increased frequency of cough, increase in sputum production, recurrent hemoptysis, malaise, shortness of breath, substernal chest discomfort, weight loss, poor appetite, status of nutrition, and hypoxia. As part of the assessment, the perioperative nurse may auscultate the chest and confirm the presence of crackles or wheezes on inspiration or expiration and documents findings in the medical record.

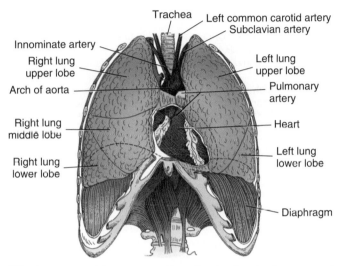

FIG. 23.4 Organs of thoracic cavity. Part of pericardium has been removed to expose the heart.

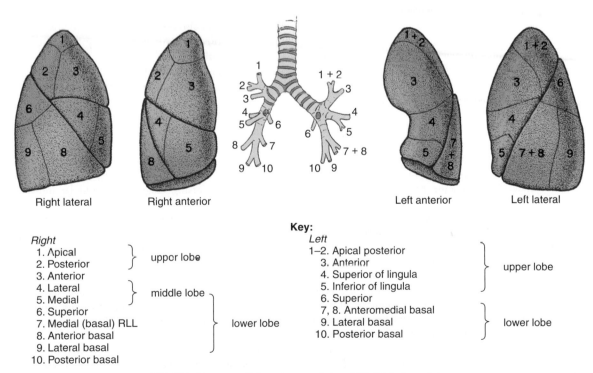

Key:

Right	Left
1. Apical ⎱ upper lobe	1–2. Apical posterior ⎱
2. Posterior ⎰	3. Anterior
3. Anterior	4. Superior of lingula ⎰ upper lobe
4. Lateral ⎱ middle lobe	5. Inferior of lingula
5. Medial ⎰	6. Superior
6. Superior	7, 8. Anteromedial basal ⎱
7. Medial (basal) RLL	9. Lateral basal ⎰ lower lobe
8. Anterior basal ⎱ lower lobe	10. Posterior basal
9. Lateral basal	
10. Posterior basal	

FIG. 23.5 Segments of the pulmonary lobes. *RLL,* Right lower lobe.

TABLE 23.1

Pulmonary Function Tests

Test	Purpose
FVC: Records maximum amount of air that can be exhaled as quickly as possible after maximum inspiration	Provides an indication of respiratory muscle strength and ventilatory reserve; often reduced in obstructive disease (because of air trapping) and in restrictive disease
FEV₁: Records maximum amount of air that can be exhaled in first second of respiration	Offers data about the degree of airway obstruction; effort dependent and declines with age; reduced in certain obstructive and restrictive disorders
FEV₁/FVC: Ratio of expiratory volume in 1 second to FVC	Provides a more sensitive indicator of obstruction to airflow; ratio is normal or increased in restrictive disease, but decreased in obstructive disease
FEF₂₅₋₇₅%: Records forced expiratory flow over 25%–75% volume (middle half) of FVC	This measure provides a more sensitive index of obstruction in smaller airways
FRC: Amount of air remaining in lungs after normal expiration	Increased FRC indicates hyperinflation or air trapping, which may result from obstructive disease.
TLC: Amount of air remaining in lungs at end of maximum inhalation	Increased TLC indicates air trapping associated with obstructive pulmonary disease; decreased TLC indicates restrictive disease
RV: Amount of air remaining in lungs at end of a full, forced exhalation	RV is increased in obstructive pulmonary disease, such as emphysema
DL_CO: Reflects surface area of alveolocapillary membrane	DL_CO is reduced when alveolocapillary membrane is diminished, such as in emphysema, pulmonary hypertension, and pulmonary fibrosis

DL_CO, Diffusion capacity of carbon monoxide; *FEF,* forced expiratory flow; *FEV₁,* forced expiratory volume in 1 second; *FRC,* functional residual capacity; *FVC,* forced vital capacity; *TLC,* total lung capacity; *RV,* residual volume.
From Pagana KD, Pagana TJ: *Mosby's diagnostic and laboratory test references,* ed 13, St Louis, 2016, Mosby; Rees HC: Assessment of the respiratory system. In Ignatavicius DD, Workman ML, editors: *Medical-surgical nursing: patient-centered collaborative care,* ed 8, St Louis, 2016, Saunders.

The review of diagnostic and laboratory tests may include the chest x-ray films, sputum analysis obtained during bronchoscopy, cytology reports, arterial blood gas (ABG) results (see Appendix A), and pulmonary function studies (Table 23.1). The chest x-ray film remains an indispensable diagnostic tool and is needed in the operating room (OR). This film outlines the lesion, if any is present, and defines its shape and space-occupying nature (e.g., tracheal shift). The presence of air in the hilar region, pleural effusion, or atelectasis may also be confirmed by radiologic evidence. Sputum analysis for culture and sensitivity may alert the perioperative nurse to an infectious process; cytologic examination may confirm a malignancy. The patient may have already undergone diagnostic bronchoscopy or mediastinoscopy; if so, the findings for acid-fast bacillus smear, culture, bronchial washing, and biopsy should be reviewed. Pulmonary function tests with a forced expiratory volume in 1 second (FEV₁) less than 1 L indicate the patient is at extremely high risk for pulmonary complications in the postoperative period. Computed tomography (CT) scans of the chest, as well as of the brain, liver, and abdomen, may reveal the presence or absence of metastasis, pleural calcification, thickening, or plaque. Radioisotope scans may have been done for similar reasons as the CT. Magnetic resonance imaging (MRI) detects vascular relationships to masses or vascular lesions. Positron emission tomography (PET) is a noninvasive study that is accurate in diagnosing malignant pulmonary nodules and lymphadenopathy. MRI and PET are sometimes performed to rule out metastasis of the lesion. Transbronchial needle aspiration is useful in diagnosing mediastinal lymphadenopathy and staging lung cancer. Ventilation and perfusion studies show the distribution of each function in the lung. These results assist the perioperative nurse in collaborating with the surgical team to maintain effective gas exchange during the surgical intervention. The results are also valuable in predicting postoperative respiratory function and metabolic responses. Patients hospitalized for surgery related to cancer may have received chemotherapy or radiation therapy before surgery. Assessment of the skin and the patient's general condition is important in preventing perioperative complications. The nurse should also assess the patient's pain tolerance to determine necessary teaching or tools that will assist in achieving positive postoperative outcomes.

The nurse assesses the patient's smoking history (including the use of cigars, pipes, tobacco, or controlled substances) and any exposure to secondhand smoke within the home and workplace. The nurse should also reinforce the need to abstain from tobacco after surgery (Rees, 2016). Patients may be sensitive if they have a history of tobacco use because of the assumed relationship between smoking and lung disease, so the nurse phrases questions in a nonjudgmental manner to respect any feelings the patient may have.

After a general and focused review of the patient's medical record and patient interview, the perioperative nurse formulates nursing diagnoses individualized for the patient's unique needs. These statements reflect problems that require perioperative nursing intervention, either independently or collaboratively, with other members of the surgical team. Nursing diagnoses should be individualized and prioritized for each patient.

Nursing Diagnosis

Nursing diagnoses related to the care of patients undergoing thoracic surgery might include the following:
- Impaired Gas Exchange related to surgical intervention
- Risk for Impaired Skin Integrity related to surgical positioning, length of surgical intervention, previous radiation, previous chemotherapy, or use of chemical antimicrobial agents on the skin
- Risk for Imbalanced Fluid Volume related to decreased surface area of the lung for perfusion and to administration of intravenous (IV) fluids during surgery

- Risk for Infection at surgical site related to inadequate secondary defenses (presence of existing disease process) and surgical disruption of tissues
- Acute pain related to surgical intervention

Outcome Identification

Outcomes identified for the selected nursing diagnoses could be stated as follows:

- The patient will experience adequate gas exchange during the surgical procedure.
- The patient's skin integrity will be maintained.

- The patient will maintain appropriate fluid balance.
- The patient will be free from postoperative surgical site infection.
- The patient's pain will be monitored and managed.

Planning

A Sample Plan of Care for a patient undergoing thoracic surgery is shown below.

Implementation

During implementation of the plan of care the perioperative nurse is concerned with both preparatory patient considerations (e.g.,

---

SAMPLE PLAN OF CARE

Nursing Diagnosis
Impaired Gas Exchange related to surgical intervention

Outcome
The patient will experience adequate gas exchange during the surgical procedure.

Interventions
- Determine the preoperative status of gas exchange by reviewing laboratory results and assessing the patient; report deviations from preoperative laboratory values and patient assessment findings.
- Obtain chest x-ray films for the intraoperative period.
- Verify that a double-lumen endotracheal tube with a soft, inflatable cuff is available for the anesthesia provider.
- Collaborate in obtaining equipment for and monitoring ABGs; document results.
- Obtain equipment for and assist with patient preparation for hemodynamic monitoring: ECG, CO_2 analyzer, pulse oximeter, arterial pressure line, and central venous pressure line; collaborate with the anesthesia provider in evaluating results provided by these monitoring devices during the procedure.
- Apply thermal unit (forced-air warming device or other device as available in institution); check equipment before procedure; monitor and note patient temperature during procedure.
- Collaborate in positioning the patient to provide access to the endotracheal tube, enable efficient ventilatory function, and prevent injury.
- Obtain and label specimens (e.g., ABG, blood count) to be sent to laboratory; document specimens sent, and evaluate results. Report abnormal values to the anesthesia provider and surgical team.

Nursing Diagnosis
Risk for Impaired Skin Integrity related to surgical positioning, length of surgical intervention, previous radiation, previous chemotherapy, or use of chemical antimicrobial agents on the skin

Outcome
The patient's skin integrity will be maintained.

Interventions
- Assess skin integrity and condition of the skin preoperatively. Document findings; report the presence of any lesions, rashes, cuts, nicks, or reddened areas.
- Determine the presence of preexisting conditions that could compromise skin integrity (e.g., age, obesity, diabetes, allergies, radiation therapy).
- Apply principles of positioning for efficient circulatory function for lateral or supine position during the procedure; pad and

protect vulnerable neurovascular bundles and dependent pressure areas.
- Assess the area in which the electrosurgical dispersive pad will be placed; clip any hair from the area if necessary. Document assessment and pad placement on the intraoperative record.
- Use clippers or a depilatory (check patient sensitivity) if hair must be removed from the operative site.
- Prevent pooling of skin prep solutions at the bedline, site of ECG electrodes, and electrosurgical dispersive pad.
- Observe and document skin integrity and condition postoperatively; compare with preoperative status.

Nursing Diagnosis
Risk for Imbalanced Fluid Volume related to decreased surface area of the lung for perfusion and to administration of IV fluids during surgery

Outcome
The patient will maintain appropriate fluid balance.

Interventions
- Insert indwelling urinary catheter; use aseptic technique.
- Monitor urinary output hourly during the procedure; report output less than 30 mL/hr.
- Provide access for administration of IV fluids; assist with fluid administration and insertion of lines. Keep lines protected and patent during positional changes.
- Monitor results of hemodynamic parameters; document and report appropriately.
- Monitor blood loss during the procedure; document and report appropriately.
- Provide blood or blood products for fluid replacement; assist in replacement therapy and patient monitoring.
- Observe for signs of shock (e.g., hypotension, abnormal ECG); report signs, and initiate corrective nursing actions.
- Observe for signs of excess blood loss (e.g., rapid, weak pulse; rapid respirations; cool, moist skin; early, slight rise in blood pressure); report signs, and initiate corrective nursing actions.
- Observe for signs of fluid excess (e.g., tachycardia, increased blood pressure); report signs, and initiate corrective nursing actions.

Nursing Diagnosis
Risk for Infection at surgical site related to inadequate secondary defenses (presence of existing disease process) and surgical disruption of tissues

Outcome
The patient will be free from surgical site infection.

Continued

SAMPLE PLAN OF CARE—cont'd

Interventions

- Administer preoperative antibiotics at least 1 hour before the procedure.
- Create and maintain a sterile field immediately before use; monitor the sterile field, and take corrective action if breaks in technique occur.
- Do not remove hair preoperatively unless the hair at or around the incision site will interfere with the surgical procedure. If hair must be removed, it should be done immediately before the surgical procedure, using clippers or a depilatory.
- Complete skin preparation at the incision site to decrease microbial contamination. Use an appropriate antiseptic agent, applied according the manufacturer's directions. The prepped area should be extensive enough to extend the incision or create new incisions or drain sites.
- Monitor traffic patterns; limit the number of people entering and leaving the OR.
- Administer prescribed antibiotics for irrigation and IV administration; check for patient allergies; record all medications administered by the perioperative nurse or scrub person (who may be a registered nurse or surgical technologist) at the sterile field.
- Assist anesthesia provider in maintaining the patient in a normothermic state.
- Using sterile gloves, apply sterile dressings to the surgical site before the drape is removed.

Nursing Diagnosis
Acute pain related to surgical intervention

Outcome
The patient's pain will be assessed, monitored, and managed.

Interventions

- Assess patient's current pain level and determine patient's perception of pain.
- Teach the pain assessment scale preoperatively.
- Provide education to the patient regarding the physiology of pain and the importance of treating pain before it becomes unmanageable.
- Discuss pain management techniques and options (i.e., oral, IM, IV medications, PCA, epidural use, intercostal blocks).
- Assist anesthesia provider in initiating pain control methods (i.e., epidural placement, nerve blocks).
- Assess pain before and after administration of pain medication or use of comfort measures (e.g., repositioning, applying support devices).
- Monitor the effects of pain management strategies, and document.
- Assess verbal and nonverbal cues during procedures requiring monitored anesthesia care and administration of local anesthesia.
- Teach pain control methods and medication uses and side effects before discharge.

ABG, Arterial blood gas; *ECG,* electrocardiogram; *IM,* intramuscular *IV,* intravenous; *PCA,* patient-controlled analgesia.

---

procedure explanation and teaching for the patient; verification of the patient, surgical procedure, and site; positioning; presurgical diagnostic interventions; draping) and the requirements of the surgical intervention (e.g., medication delivery; instrumentation equipment, and supply availability). These patient care needs are coordinated with the other nursing interventions identified in the specific patient's plan of care.

Positioning

The type of position used in thoracic surgery is determined by the operative procedure planned. Bronchoscopy is usually performed in the supine position, commonly with a shoulder roll. Thoracotomy can be performed with the patient in one of three common positions: (1) lateral for the posterolateral approach, (2) semilateral for the anterolateral approach (Fig. 23.6), and (3) supine for the median sternotomy approach. Arms are placed on padded armboards with the palms up and fingers extended. Armboards are maintained at less than a 90-degree angle to prevent brachial plexus stretch. If there are surgical reasons to tuck the arms at the side, the elbows are padded to protect the ulnar nerve, the palms face inward, and the wrist is maintained in a neutral position (AORN, 2016a). A drape secures the arms. It should be tucked snugly under the patient, not under the mattress. This prevents the arm from shifting downward intraoperatively and resting against the OR bed rail. A beanbag can be used to support the patient in the lateral decubitus position.

The prone position also can provide access in some procedures (see Chapter 6 for safe positioning interventions). Adequate padding and safe transfer should be implemented to prevent pressure injury.

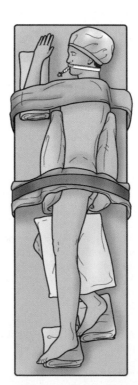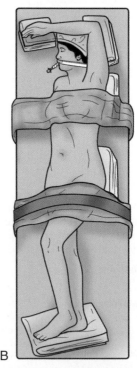

FIG. 23.6 Positions for thoracotomy incisions. (A) Lateral position for posterolateral incision. (B) Semilateral position for axillary or anterolateral position.

Draping

Draping may be minimal for bronchoscopic procedures. The principles of draping for other procedures (see Chapter 4) are followed in all other thoracic procedures. Drapes may consist of a fenestrated sheet or single sheets surrounding the incision site. To prevent instruments from falling from the field, the scrub person may place a magnetic pad on the drapes below the incision site when the patient is placed in lateral position. The perioperative nurse ensures a warming unit is in place before draping to maintain normothermia. Intermittent pneumatic compression devices are often applied to prevent the development of venous thromboembolism (VTE) (Research Highlight: Prevention of Postoperative Venous Thromboembolism in Thoracic Surgical Patients).

RESEARCH HIGHLIGHT

Prevention of Postoperative Venous Thromboembolism in Thoracic Surgical Patients

VTE can be a devastating postoperative complication, with about one-third of VTEs occurring postdischarge. The prevalence of VTE after lung resection is significant despite the current standard of care for in-hospital VTE prophylaxis. The majority of VTE events are asymptomatic and primarily occur in the postdischarge time frame. A recent study of patients undergoing lung resection for malignancy who received guideline-based VTE prophylaxis until discharge demonstrated a VTE prevalence of 12.1% (Agzarian, 2015).

The Caprini VTE RAM has previously demonstrated that "high-risk" patients were more likely to have a postoperative VTE in postoperative lung and esophageal cancer patients (Hachey, 2016). This follow-up study implemented the RAM protocol in thoracic surgical patients to evaluate adherence, safety, and VTE outcomes.

The Caprini RAM is comprised of about 40 VTE-related risk factors, such as history of VTE, current cancer diagnosis, recent surgery, and central venous access, each with an assigned weighted score. For patients at low risk (Caprini scores 0–4), no postdischarge prophylaxis is prescribed. For moderate risk patients (score 5–8), 10 days of total prophylaxis (including inpatient and outpatient days) is prescribed. For high-risk patients (scores ≥9), 30 total days of prophylaxis are recommended.

Despite significant variation in socioeconomic and cultural factors among patients, this study demonstrated high rates of adherence to prophylactic anticoagulation after discharge, supporting the general applicability of this VTE prevention protocol and suggesting that it is acceptable to patients. The overall VTE rate was 2.3%, with no postdischarge VTEs or adverse bleeding events.

This study on the prevention of postoperative VTE in thoracic surgical patients demonstrated that implementation of the Caprini RAM protocol is feasible and safe for both providers and postoperative surgical patients. Risk assessment across case types appears justified to identify those at high risk for VTE who may benefit from extended course prophylaxis.

RAM, Risk assessment model; *VTE*, venous thromboembolism.
Modified from Hachey K et al: Prevention of postoperative venous thromboembolism in thoracic surgical patients: implementation and evaluation of a Caprini Assessment Protocol, *J Am Coll Surg* 222(6):1019–1027, 2016; Agzarian J et al: Postdischarge venous thromboembolic complications following pulmonary oncologic resection: an underdetected problem, *J Thorac Cardiovasc Surg* 151(4):992–999, 2016; Hachey K et al: Caprini venous thromboembolism risk assessment permits selection for postdischarge prophylactic anticoagulation in patients with resectable lung cancer, *J Thorac Cardiovasc Surg* 151(1):37–44, 2016.

Instrumentation

Bronchoscopy instruments are designed to directly inspect and observe the larynx, trachea, and bronchi; to remove secretions; to obtain washings or tissue for bacterial and cytologic studies; or to remove tissue. They are also designed to remove foreign bodies. Both rigid and flexible bronchoscopes are available, with the rigid bronchoscope better suited for removing foreign bodies. Instrumentation for thoracic surgery includes the laparotomy instrument set (see Chapter 11) and specialty items. Instruments used for a thoracotomy or chest procedure include a combination of delicate and heavy instruments. Stapling equipment is commonly used. These devices require staplers and staple reload of appropriate sizes. The delicate instruments are used to cut tissue and vessels or to clamp tissue in an atraumatic manner. The heavier instruments are used for bone cutting, dissecting, or retracting. Instrumentation must also be available for hemostasis and suturing of all types of tissue. Newer technologies such as cryoablation, use of ultrasonic shears, and stereotactic ablative radiotherapy are emerging in the field of thoracic surgery (Research Highlight: Energy Devices in Thoracic Surgery, Present and Future).

The scrub person should determine the arrangement of items on the instrument table and Mayo stand; this arrangement should be an effective standard method that applies principles of work simplification and thorough knowledge of procedures. The possibility always exists that any incision may need to be extended to accommodate a more extensive procedure than was originally planned. Therefore the practice of performing an initial count is recommended for all procedures, including minimally invasive procedures such as laparoscopy or thoracoscopy (AORN, 2016b). Lengthy incisions are often required for thoracic procedures; therefore it is critical that an instrument count be performed before closure.

Equipment

In thoracic surgery a variety of equipment is used, including a forced-air warming unit, fiberoptic headlights, fiberoptic light sources, video equipment, intermittent pneumatic compression devices, and anesthesia supplies. To deflate the operative lung and ventilate the nonoperative lung, double-lumen endotracheal tubes are commonly used for thoracotomies.

The neodymium:yttrium-aluminum-garnet (Nd:YAG) or CO_2 laser can be used for treating tracheobronchial lesions with use of a bronchoscope. Obstruction of the mainstem bronchus and trachea caused by benign and malignant lesions can also be effectively treated with laser therapy. Use of laser equipment requires a thorough understanding of the equipment, the safety issues, the responsibilities (see Chapter 8), and the planned surgical procedure.

Monitoring

Monitored anesthesia care, local anesthesia, or topical anesthesia may be used during some bronchoscopic procedures. General anesthesia also may be used for bronchoscopic procedures as well as other thoracic procedures. Team members work in cooperation to constantly monitor laboratory results (e.g., ABGs), oxygenation, temperature, blood loss, and urine output. Monitoring intermittent pneumatic compression device settings and patient position also is important in providing safe patient care. Results are communicated with other team members and documented for continuity of care.

Blood Replacement

Blood replacement therapy during or after the procedure may be required because of extensive tissue dissection in a highly vascular area. The patient's blood type and amount of blood ordered should

Energy Devices in Thoracic Surgery, Present and Future

In the last decade, many energy devices such as ultrasonic shears, RFA, stereotactic ablative radiotherapy, argon plasma coagulation, and cryoablation have entered day-to-day practice in thoracic surgery. Some devices have proven and recognized applications, whereas others require further trials.

There is growing evidence that ultrasonic shears are effective and safe for pulmonary artery branch ligation of 7-mm diameter or less. Ultrasonic shears use both compression and friction to deliver mechanical energy to target tissue. This adaptive tissue technology reduces power output, potentially diminishing the risk of thermal injury while achieving adequate hemostasis. Additional studies are needed to confirm safety and further demonstrate decreased risk of iatrogenic pulmonary artery injury in VATS lobectomy.

Although surgery is the gold standard for stage I lung cancer, RFA is a treatment option for inoperable patients. RFA uses heat induced by an electrode placed in the lung tumor to induce cell death by a process called coagulation necrosis. It can be performed percutaneously, under conscious sedation and image guidance, and as an outpatient procedure or with a short hospital stay.

SBRT, which is also referred to as stereotactic ablative radiation therapy, has emerged as another important treatment option for inoperable stage I NSCLC over the last 10 years. This radiation technology allows accurate delivery of a very high dose to the tumor, while sparing normal adjacent tissue. A systematic review and pooled analysis was performed (Bi, 2016) to compare SBRT and RFA in inoperable stage I NSCLC. This systemic review and pooled analysis demonstrated that SBRT provided superior 1-, 2-, 3-, and 5-year local tumor control over RFA, even when corrected for patients' age and tumor size ≤3 cm. However,

caution should be taken because of the relatively limited number of RFA trials and short follow-up time. More studies with larger sample sizes for RFA treatment are needed.

APC has gained interest for the treatment of endobronchial lesions and for hemostasis. Most of its application is in the palliative context, but it is also one of the therapeutic options in the management of airway bleeding and the treatment of benign lesions. APC is useful in the chest or abdominal cavity for diffuse bleeding and is specifically useful in the treatment of diffuse bleeding from the chest wall after extrapleural resection or dissection. APC is a type of electrocautery device that requires specific equipment. The effect penetrates 2 to 3 mm deep in the tissue. This property of APC makes it an interesting energy source because its low penetration reduces risks of airway perforation.

Cryoablation freezes tissue using either nitrous oxide or liquid nitrogen. Repeated rapid cooling of tissue under 20°C results in cell death by causing intracellular ice crystal formation. Another mechanism of cell destruction results from ischemic necrosis as the microcirculation around the tissue significantly reduces blood flow from the freezing effects on microcirculation. Hence, cryoablation does not instantaneously destroy tissue; it takes days to weeks to reach full effect. The effect of cryoablation penetrates approximately 3 mm into the tissue. Cryoablation can achieve control of malignant airway lesions in non–life-threatening situations, and has been suggested as a possible curative treatment strategy for typical carcinoid tumors; however, this has not been validated in prospective controlled trials and is not considered standard of care for operable patients.

Novel applications of energy in thoracic surgery and refinement in technology will hopefully allow for safer and less invasive techniques for patients requiring thoracic surgical procedures.

APC, Argon plasma coagulation; *NSCLC,* non–small-cell lung cancer; *RFA,* radiofrequency ablation; *SBRT,* stereotactic body radiation therapy; *VATS,* video-assisted thoracoscopic surgery.
Modified from Goudie E et al: Present and future application of energy devices in thoracic surgery, *Thorac Surg Clin* 26(2): 229–236, 2016; Bi N et al: Comparison of the effectiveness of radiofrequency ablation with stereotactic body radiation therapy in inoperable Stage 1 non-small cell lung cancer: a systemic review and pooled analysis, *Int J Radiat Oncol Biol Phys* 95(5):1378–1390, 2016.

---

be noted before the procedure and its availability confirmed. During the procedure every effort should be made to control and monitor bleeding. If blood collection or reinfusion systems are used, the manufacturer's instructions and institutional protocols should be followed.

Chest Drainage Systems

Chest tube and chest drainage system management represents an important intervention for perioperative nurses. In the presence of restrictive and obstructive pulmonary disease, the lung may not fully expand or contract, causing a reduction in alveolar ventilation with resultant hypoxia. Other conditions that interfere with respiratory function are excessive accumulation of mucus, pleural effusions, a foreign body in a bronchus, closed pneumothorax (simple and tension types), open pneumothorax, hemothorax, and multiple rib injuries that produce paradoxical motion of the thoracic cage, or flail chest (Fig. 23.7).

The normal function of the lungs is supported by elasticity and negative intrapleural pressure. Collapse of the normal lung follows any condition that reduces or eliminates the negative intrapleural pressure if the lung is not adhering to the chest wall. When the pleural space is filled with air, the lung collapses because of the

loss of negative pressure. This action may cause complete collapse if the pressure within the intrathoracic (pleural) space becomes positive.

A diminished negative pressure or the occurrence of actual positive pressure in one pleural space may cause the mediastinum or trachea to shift toward the opposite side. When this occurs, not only does the affected lung collapse because of a positive pressure in the pleural space, but also the function of the lung on the opposite side may be impaired as a result of compression by the mediastinal shift. Tension pneumothorax can produce serious effects as air continues to escape from the lung into the intrapleural space. The air cannot return to the bronchi to be exhaled, increasing the intrapleural pressure. As the positive pressure continues to build, venous return to the heart is impaired and hemodynamic collapse may occur. When a large opening in the chest wall allows direct communication of the pleural space with atmospheric pressure, it may cause death if the mediastinum becomes mobile.

Paradoxical motion of the chest results from severe instability of the chest wall because of multiple and often bilateral rib fractures; with inspiration, partial collapse of the thoracic space occurs. The blunt injury that caused the multiple rib fractures also causes severe contusion of the lung itself. This contusion contributes to impairment

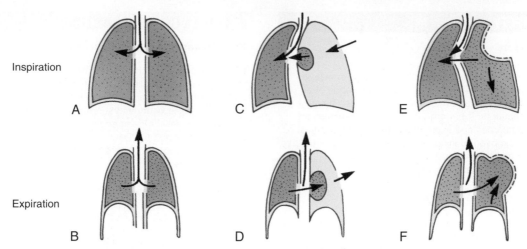

Inspiration

Expiration

FIG. 23.7 Pathophysiology of severe chest injuries. (A and B) Normal physiology of inspiration and expiration. (C and D) Open (sucking) wound of thorax. On inspiration, air at atmospheric pressure rushes in through a defect (C), collapsing the lung. Next, positive pressure causes mediastinum to shift, compressing the opposite lung. On expiration (D), air from lung on the uninjured side reenters collapsed lung and is rebreathed in next inspiration. Impaired cardiopulmonary function in the presence of a sucking wound of the chest is caused by (1) collapse of lung on injured side, (2) partial collapse of opposite lung, (3) increased functional dead space caused by rebreathing of unoxygenated air from collapsed lung, and (4) diminished venous return to right side of heart. (E and F) Primary effect of paradoxical motion resulting from flail or stove-in chest is diminution of pulmonary ventilation and extensive rebreathing from one lung to the other. Venous return to right side of heart is impaired. Appropriate treatment requires intubation of trachea and use of volume-limited ventilator.

of lung function by affecting gas exchange, which may result in severe, life-threatening hypoxia.

One or more chest catheters (tubes) may be inserted for postoperative closed-chest drainage. The chest tubes provide a conduit for drainage of air, blood, and other fluid from the intrapleural or mediastinal space and reestablishment of negative pressure in the intrapleural space (Patient Safety). Drainage systems use three mechanisms to drain fluid and air from the pleural cavity: positive expiratory pressure, gravity, and suction. The chest tubes are connected to a sterile water-seal or gravity drainage system. Water-seal suction may be necessary when a persistent air leak cannot be controlled by drainage alone. Several compact, disposable units are available. The disposable units have three or four compartments for drainage, water seal, and suction. The first chamber collects the drainage from the intrapleural space, the second chamber provides the water seal, and the third provides the suction control determined by the level of water (Fig. 23.8). If two chest tubes are inserted, they may be attached by a Y connector to a single drainage unit or may be attached individually to two separate units. Chest tubes may be removed when the air leak has been resolved and the volume of drainage remains at an acceptable level for 24 hours.

Documentation

The nurse's documentation of perioperative care includes a summary of preoperative assessment information that supports formulated nursing diagnoses, nursing interventions, and postoperative evaluation. Documentation for a patient undergoing a thoracotomy specifically addresses patient assessment information related to position of the patient, positioning aids used, medications administered, results of laboratory tests completed, special equipment used, urine output, blood replacement, insertion of chest tubes and drainage systems, and postoperative evaluation of patient care outcomes.

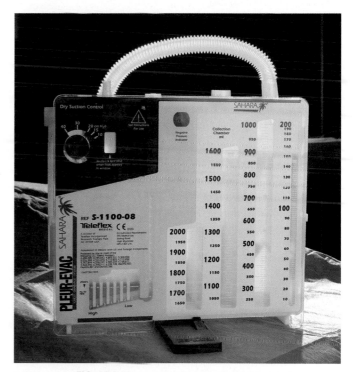

FIG. 23.8 Commercial chest drainage system.

Hand-Off Report

The patient is transferred from the OR to the postanesthesia care unit (PACU) after thoracotomy. The hand-off report to the PACU nurse is often a collaborative effort of the nurse and anesthesia provider. The perioperative nurse reports the procedure performed,

PATIENT SAFETY

Chest Tube Safety

Chest tube insertion is a life-saving procedure used to relieve tension pneumothorax or hemothorax, the accumulation of air or blood (fluid) under pressure in the pleural space, seen most often in trauma patients. If performed incorrectly, patients can suffer adverse outcomes and even fatal complications, and clinicians can be exposed to injury or infection.

Observations and recommendations:

- Trying to perform multiple procedures concurrently is a major source of error.
- Equipment trays should be positioned near the surgeon's dominant hand.
- A patient's discomfort can make it hard to do a sterile procedure. While adequate anesthesia is important, the patient may also need verbal and physical comforting. If a patient's movements cannot be controlled, the anesthesiology team should be called.
- Correct techniques can prevent damage to the lung and surrounding tissue, contamination of the wound, and leakage of fluid.
- Universal Precautions against bloodborne infections are crucial to protect clinicians and their patients. In US urban trauma centers, HIV rates among trauma patients are as high as 10%, and hepatitis C rates are as high as 15%, so Universal Precautions should be practiced for all chest tube insertions.

HIV, Human immunodeficiency virus.
Modified from Agency for Healthcare Research and Quality (AHRQ): *Problems and prevention: chest tube insertion* (website), 2014. www.ahrq.gov/research/findings/factsheets/errors-safety/chesttubes/index.html. (Accessed 3 February 2017).

particularly if it varies from the anticipated or scheduled procedure, and describes the patient's preoperative status, including anxiety level and understanding of the procedure, to assist the PACU nurse in meeting the emotional and educational needs of the patient. The nurse's description of the patient's position during the procedure provides criteria for assessment and evaluation of mobility. Results of immediate postoperative assessment, including skin integrity, location and type of dressing applied, location and type of drains, blood loss, fluid replacement, medications administered, and laboratory results obtained during the procedure, are reported by the nurse and anesthesia provider as a baseline control for assessment in the PACU. The perioperative care plan should be reviewed and patient outcomes reported.

Postprocedural Concerns

The patient's endotracheal tube may remain in place to maintain an adequate gas exchange. Gas exchange and effective ventilation are two immediate clinical needs after thoracotomy. Chest tubes are often connected to suction, except for postpneumonectomy procedures. The thoracotomy is considered a painful procedure and, when coupled with muscle injury, affects functional capacity. Anesthesia providers frequently use multiple techniques for pain management to improve the comfort level of the patient (Evidence for Practice).

Fluid volume overload can lead to acute life-threatening respiratory disease syndrome, which should be avoided. Monitoring urine output is important, but postthoracotomy patients should be maintained in a state of hydration that does not require a fluid bolus for low urine output.

EVIDENCE FOR PRACTICE

Pain Management After Thoracic Surgery

Pain management is the cornerstone of enhanced recovery after thoracic surgery care maps. This management consists of multimodal therapeutic strategies that aim toward enhanced postoperative recovery and shortened hospital stay.

Preoperatively, it is important to dedicate time during the preoperative period to discuss the perioperative pain management strategy, with specific attention to addressing patients' concerns.

Intraoperatively, TEA has historically provided effective postoperative analgesia but has unwanted side effects, including hypotension, urinary retention, nausea, and vomiting. Alternatives to TEA include PICB, paravertebral blockade, and wound infiltration using local anesthetics. Although early pain control is adequate, none of these approaches provides durable relief of pain after thoracic surgery because of the relatively short half-life of local anesthetics (approximately 5 hours). LipoB is a long-acting formulation of bupivacaine that is contained within slow-release liposomal vesicles. Originally approved by the US Food and Drug Administration in October 2011 for provision of local analgesia through wound infiltration, it has been shown to provide effective analgesia for thoracic surgery when used for PICB (Rice, 2015). LipoB may also be injected into the chest tube site or around a fracture should fracture occur.

General endotracheal anesthesia, with emphasis on IV anesthetics rather than inhalational agents, is also administered. The anesthesiologist administers acetaminophen 1000 mg IV, dexamethasone 4 mg IV, and ketorolac 30 mg IV before the completion of general anesthesia. Patients are extubated in the OR.

Postoperatively, patients may receive oral gabapentin, IV acetaminophen, IV ketorolac, oral famotidine, and oral tramadol. IV hydromorphone may be used if pain is not relieved with tramadol. The use of gabapentinoids and tramadol does not affect the anesthesia reversal process and the time to awakening. This pain control regimen reduces the reliance on narcotics, minimizing their side effects.

IV, Intravenous; *LipoB,* liposomal bupivacaine; *PICB,* posterior intercostal nerve blockade; *TEA,* thoracic epidural analgesia.
Modified from Mehran R et al: Pain management in an enhanced recovery pathway after thoracic surgical procedures, *Ann Thorac Surg* 102(6):595–596, 2016; Rice D et al: Posterior intercostal nerve block with liposomal bupivacaine: an alternative to thoracic epidural analgesia, *Ann Thorac Surg* 99(6):1953–1960, 2015.

Patients are often anxious about their limitations, the environment, and the results of the procedure. Patients and families will benefit from preoperative teaching about pain management techniques and use of the institution's pain assessment tool. Patients and families should also be encouraged to discuss their feelings and needs both before and after the surgical procedure. The perioperative nurse should facilitate notification of the patient's status to the family members during and as soon as possible after the procedure.

Evaluation

At the completion of the surgical procedure, perioperative nursing goals are evaluated. They may be restated as brief outcomes. For the goals identified for the patient undergoing thoracic surgery, outcomes could be stated as follows:

- The patient's gas exchange was satisfactory; ventilation/perfusion ratios were adequate as evidenced by laboratory results, and vital signs were within normal limits; skin, nailbeds, and mucosa were pink; lung fields were clear bilaterally; and chest excursion was normal.

- The patient's skin integrity was maintained; reddened or discolored skin and other signs of altered tissue perfusion were not present.
- Fluid balance was maintained; there were no fluid excesses or deficits; mental orientation was consistent with preoperative level; serum electrolytes and ABGs were within normal limits; urinary output was adequate.
- The patient will be free of signs and symptoms of surgical site infection.
- Pain will be managed and pain levels assessed.

Patient, Family, and Caregiver Education and Discharge Planning

Discharge status is determined by the type of procedure being performed and the patient's overall state of health. General patient concerns might include mobility and activity levels or restrictions, pain management, wound care, dietary recommendations, medication regimens, follow-up appointments, and any prescribed outpatient care or referrals. Both the patient and the family need specific instructions for discharge that relate to the specific procedure. Patients and their families are encouraged to partner with the healthcare team and to ask appropriate questions and establish lines of communication (Patient Engagement Exemplar). The nurse fosters patient autonomy and reviews all information verbally and provides it in written form, with verification of understanding and time for questions and concerns.

Patients are discharged within hours of a bronchoscopy. Their main concerns might be the results of biopsy and diagnosis. The

patient, family, and caregiver should be aware of the length of time until results will be available and the method used to obtain those results. Patients should also be reminded of the need to rest for 2 to 3 days after the procedure. Side effects might result from medications used for moderate sedation or untoward intraoperative outcomes (e.g., the patient may experience bloody sputum, difficulty breathing). In addition, patients should be reminded that their throats might feel numb 2 to 3 hours after the procedure and difficulty with swallowing will subside (Ambulatory Surgery Considerations).

AMBULATORY SURGERY CONSIDERATIONS

Ambulatory Thoracic Surgery

The concept of ambulatory surgical procedures is not new to the thoracic specialty; patients undergoing bronchoscopy or endoscopic sympathectomy have often completed their procedures on an outpatient basis. With the increased trend toward more minimally invasive procedures and improved technology to accomplish those procedures, the indications for ambulatory thoracic surgery are growing. Recent data support the notion that the majority of patients do not require hospital admission after a routine diagnostic thoracoscopy.

Operative thoracoscopy is surprisingly well tolerated by even chronically ill and frail patients who might otherwise be poor candidates for general anesthesia. Absolute contraindications to thoracoscopy include absence of a pleural space, chronic hypoxemia, or hypercapnia. Moderate-to-severe sleep apnea should also be considered a contraindication because patients are not typically intubated during operative thoracoscopy, increasing the risk of hypercapnic respiratory failure. Furthermore, the use of positive airway pressure would prevent adequate lung atelectasis and interfere with optimal inspection of the pleural space. Absence of anesthesia and surgical backup should also be considered absolute contraindications. A clear plan of action delineating the optimal sequence of interventions to effectively deal with such rare but potentially life-threatening complications in the outpatient setting is absolutely crucial to ensure patient safety and the long-term success of a medical thoracoscopy program.

Because a pneumothorax must be induced to perform a medical thoracoscopy, all patients need some form of air evacuation postprocedurally. Small- to medium-bore pigtail drains connected to suction at −20 cm H_2O for 1 hour have been found to be effective. A chest x-ray is done to confirm lung reexpansion. A very small residual pneumothorax may occasionally be seen; however, in the absence of an air leak, the drain may safely be removed. The patient's level of pain, amount of chest tube output, presence or absence of an air leak, and pneumothorax status must be closely monitored before the final determination for discharge that same day.

Essential teaching points to cover with the patient and caregiver include pain control, respiratory treatments (to include deep breathing and coughing as ordered by the surgeon), and activity. Because the chest wall has been entered, the nurse must emphasize the importance of seeking emergency care if the patient experiences difficulty breathing, sudden chest pain, palpitations, uncontrollable cough, or bloody sputum.

The patient is discharged once he or she has satisfied the requirements of the institution's postanesthesia care discharge scoring system.

PATIENT ENGAGEMENT EXEMPLAR

How Are You Doing?

Patients undergoing thoracic surgery are often faced with a life-threatening illness that must be dealt with quickly giving them little time to understand what is happening to them. With the fast pace of the surgical environment it is easy to get caught up in the operational aspects of surgery and forget to ask the patient simply "how are you doing?" and have a conversation about the impact of the surgery on family and on work, and identifying what the patient is concerned or worried about. The nurse should make an effort to find out what the patient is expecting and how he or she is coping with the possible outcomes of having thoracic surgery. Perioperative teams can be very efficient and fast and always follow safety precautions, but they can sometimes overlook important patient needs. If patients are away from home or their families are away from home, arranging a video call would be beneficial to patients and families who are anxious about the impending surgery. Patients can experience depression after surgery, and offering a counselor or psychiatrist to discuss emotions and well-being can be extremely beneficial. Surgical centers that are operationally excellent may still be missing the importance of patient engagement and identifying what is important to patients and how patient needs are being met. Patients should be considered part of the process and influence healthcare in a way that will improve outcomes for all.

Modified from Mulligan JP: Engaging Patients.org: *View from the other side of the stethoscope: the doctor as patient* (website), 2015. www.engagingpatients.org/paths-to-patient-centered-care/view-side-stethoscope-doctor-patient/. (Accessed 8 January 2017).

Modified from Kern J et al: Outpatient thoracoscopy: safety and practical considerations, *Curr Opin Pulm Med* 21(4):357–362, 2015.

After a surgical procedure such as thoracoscopy or thoracotomy, vigorous pulmonary toileting is encouraged, including use of a spirometer, deep breathing, and turning and coughing every 1 to 2 hours while awake. Patients will transfer to the chair or ambulate on the day of surgery; length of time until discharge might be a few days to 1 week or more. Patients who progress without difficulty after a thoracoscopy or thoracotomy will be monitored for drainage from the chest tubes and for pain management or complications. Postoperative air leaks or pulmonary infections will delay discharge from the healthcare setting.

The patient may be discharged with supplemental oxygen. This requires that the patient be weaned and demonstrate satisfactory ambulatory SaO_2 (i.e., percentage of saturation of arterial oxygen) rates of 88% to 90%, which will most likely be supervised by home-care nurses.

Enhanced recovery after surgery (ERAS) protocols, which emphasize a multimodal approach, seek to provide patients early recovery after surgery and are beginning to be used in thoracic surgery (Enhanced Recovery After Surgery).

Surgical Interventions

Endoscopy (Diagnostic or Therapeutic)

Endoscopy refers to examination of hollow body organs or cavities with instruments that permit visual inspection of their contents and walls. The endoscopic procedures pertinent to thoracic surgery are bronchoscopy, esophagoscopy, mediastinoscopy, and thoracoscopy. Each surgeon has preferences regarding the type of endoscope, positioning of the patient, type of anesthetic, and equipment. Invasive diagnostic or therapeutic measures enhance the decision to pursue surgical intervention by providing information related to the disease process, including histologic characteristics, location of the lesion, and lesion extent. Therapeutic endoscopy provides treatment by removal of a lesion or foreign body.

Standard Bronchoscopy Using a Rigid Bronchoscope

Standard bronchoscopy is the direct visualization of the mucosa of the trachea, the main bronchi and their openings, and most of the

---

ENHANCED RECOVERY AFTER SURGERY

An Emerging Trend in Thoracic Surgery

Enhanced recovery pathways seek to reduce patients' perioperative stress response and have been successfully and safely adopted globally in a variety of specialties including thoracic surgery.

Muehling and associates (2008) monitored patients who had undergone lung resection who were cared for using either a traditional treatment regimen or an ERAS treatment regimen. The researchers found the overall rates of pulmonary complications were 36% in the traditional group and 7% in the ERAS group, with lower rates of pneumonia, atelectasis, prolonged air leak, and pleural effusion.

As with all specialties, patient education is a critical component to the success of an ERAS program in thoracic surgery. Cessation of smoking and participation in an exercise regimen preoperatively are required in most programs. Early ambulation is critical, and patients are informed that they will walk a short distance within the first hour after extubation in the PACU. All interventions from the timing of extubation to pain management are designed to facilitate early ambulation, pulmonary hygiene, and maximum lung expansion.

Intraoperatively, the perioperative team works to prevent adverse outcomes related to hypothermia by minimizing skin exposure and using warming devices and warming irrigation solutions (AORN, 2016). Fluid administration is kept to a minimum to minimize the risk of pulmonary edema and ALI. This judicious use of fluids also minimizes the need for urinary catheters, decreasing the risk for catheter-associated urinary tract infection. Surgical insertion of a paravertebral catheter allowing a bolus dose of local anesthetic followed by a continuous infusion of local anesthetic, along with multimodal analgesia with NSAIDs and opiates, has been used effectively to manage postoperative pain after thoracic surgery (Gimenez-Mila, 2016).

Postoperatively, chest tube management is streamlined by placing the tube to water seal after a brief period of suction. Placing the tube to water seal eliminates the tubing associated with suction, providing increased freedom to ambulate. Respiratory therapists begin breathing exercises in the PACU, helping patients expand the lungs in a physiologic fashion rather than relying on suction. Oral intake also begins in the PACU if the patient has minimal postoperative nausea.

Discharge occurs when patients are hemodynamically stable, tolerating their usual diet, and their pain controlled by oral medication. The chest tube is removed if there is no air leak, and the quality and amount of discharge is within normal limits. The presence of an air leak does not necessarily preclude discharge, and patients may be discharged home with the chest tube in place with instructions on its care.

Schatz (2015) analyzed data from 750 patients cared for using the ERAS care approach. Patients undergoing a lobectomy had a postoperative stay of 1.9 days compared with the national average with 6.2 days. Patients undergoing a wedge resection stayed in the hospital 1 day compared with the reported average of 4.1 days. The rate of postoperative pneumonia postlobectomy was 2.6% compared with the national average of 4.3%. After wedge resection, patients had a 0% pneumonia rate (national average 1.3%). Atelectasis requiring bronchoscopy occurred 0% of the time compared with national averages of 4.5% and 0.7%, respectively.

Data suggest that ERAS techniques and interventions promote a more effective movement through the perioperative continuum while minimizing many of the postoperative complications associated with thoracic surgery.

ALI, Acute lung injury; *ERAS*, enhanced recovery after surgery; *NSAIDs*, nonsteroidal antiinflammatory drugs; *PACU*, postanesthesia care unit.
Modified from Association of periOperative Registered Nurses (AORN): Guideline for prevention of unplanned patient hypothermia. *Guidelines for perioperative practice*, Denver, 2016, The Association; Gimenez-Mila M et al: Design and implementation of an enhanced recovery program in thoracic surgery, *J Thorac Dis* 8(S1):S37–S45, 2016; Muehling BM et al: Reduction of postoperative pulmonary complications after lung surgery using a fast track clinical pathway, *Eur J Cardiothorac Surg* 34(1):174–180, 2008; Schatz C: Enhanced recovery in a minimally invasive thoracic surgery program, *AORN J* 102(5): 482–492, 2015.

segmental bronchi. It also includes removal of material for microscopic study if necessary.

Bronchoscopy is an integral part of the examination of patients with pulmonary symptoms such as persistent cough or wheezing, hemoptysis, obstruction, and abnormal radiologic changes. Common causes of bleeding (hemoptysis) are bronchiectasis, cancer, and tuberculosis. Congenital anomalies and suspected presence of a foreign body, especially in infants and children, are responsible for emergency examination of the respiratory tract.

The surgeon performs bronchoscopy to determine the presence of a lesion in the tracheobronchial passages, to identify and localize that lesion accurately, and to observe periodically the effects of therapy. It can be completed for dilating structures, debriding tumors, obtaining biopsies of masses, or evacuating clots. In suspected cancer, the aspirated secretions obtained by bronchoscopy may contain malignant cells.

Procedural Considerations

Flexible bronchoscopy on an adult patient may be completed after induction of local (topical) anesthesia or monitored anesthesia care; a child usually receives a general anesthetic. Patients undergoing rigid bronchoscopy should be administered general anesthesia. To reduce anxiety, the perioperative nurse should introduce members of the surgical team, explain intraoperative activities, and provide reassurance to the patient (Patient, Family, and Caregiver Education). The oral structures, including the teeth and lips, should be assessed for integrity. Loose teeth may require removal before or during the procedure.

The anesthesia provider or nurse providing moderate sedation may administer IV sedatives or analgesics during the procedure. See Chapter 5 for perioperative nursing considerations when the patient is receiving local or monitored anesthesia care. The topical (or local) anesthetic setup should include a headlight for visualization, laryngeal mirrors of various sizes, a lingual spatula, sprays with straight and curved cannulae, and anesthetic drugs, as ordered. Other items include the laryngeal syringe with straight and curved cannulae, Jackson cross-action forceps, and the Schindler pharyngeal anesthetizer, if desired. Luer-Lok 10-mL syringes and 20- and 22-gauge needles are needed for transtracheal injection. The scrub person ensures that all requested instrumentation is available to avoid delays and ensures the procedure is performed efficiently for the patient.

Anesthetic drugs frequently used for local or topical anesthesia are lidocaine (Xylocaine), procaine (Novocain), and tetracaine (Pontocaine, Cetacaine) with or without epinephrine. Pauses of 3 to 4 minutes are taken between applications of the anesthetic agent to the tongue, palate, and pharynx and then to the larynx and to the trachea. The surgeon or anesthesia provider applies the anesthetic agent by means of a spray or laryngeal syringe with a straight or curved cannula.

Some physicians prefer to have the patient sit upright and gargle with the topical anesthetic mixture, rinse it around in the mouth, and then expectorate it, producing a partial anesthesia of the buccal mucosa and pharynx.

For direct bronchoscopy, the surgeon or anesthesia provider uses a long metal cannula attached to a syringe to apply the anesthetic agent to the surface of the vocal cords; then the agent is injected through the anesthetized glottis into the trachea. This act causes the patient to produce a sharp, sudden cough. For intrabronchial anesthesia, a portion of the anesthetic agent is introduced through the bronchoscope.

The patient may be positioned either in the supine position—with the shoulders elevated on a small roll, gel pad, or a sandbag to gently extend the head and neck—or in the sitting position.

The setup includes the bronchoscope, telescopes of desired types, fiberoptic light cords, and the fiberoptic light source. Each standard scope requires a fiberoptic light carrier, cord, and light source. The scrub person ensures that duplicates of each, along with the appropriate replacement light bulbs for the light source, are available for immediate use. The light source should be tested before use. During a procedure, the perioperative nurse switches the light source to standby mode whenever it is not in active use to conserve the life of the bulb and promote cooling. The light source should be kept away from any flammable materials (e.g., radiopaque soft goods and drapes) to avoid creating a fire hazard.

Other supplies that will be needed are suction tubing, aspirating tubes, specimen collectors, soft goods carriers, and the desired type of forceps. The metal soft goods carrier consists of two parts: an inner rod, which has two jaws protruding from its distal end; and an outer band, which is screwed down on the inner rod so that a soft good can be held securely within the jaws. Small gauze soft goods are used to keep the field dry, remove secretions, and apply topical anesthetic agents. Cytologic specimen collectors, such as the Clerf or Lukens, are used to hold secretions as they are obtained. Aspirating tubes of different lengths and designs are used to remove secretions and collect material for microscopic examination and culture(s). The straight aspirating tube with one or two openings at the distal end is used to remove material from the pharynx, larynx, and esophagus. The curved aspirating tube with a flexible tip is used to remove secretions from the upper and dorsal orifices of the bronchi.

The surgeon uses various types of forceps to remove foreign bodies or tissues for histologic study. Biting-tip forceps may be used to secure tissue for pathologic study. Forceps with jaws that veer laterally at about a 45-degree angle from the instrument's axis permit visualization during the biopsy maneuver. Bronchoesophageal forceps consist of a stylet, a cannula with a handle, a screw, a locknut, and a setscrew. Forceps for laryngeal and bronchial regions are designed to remove tissue specimens. The nurse should prepare several specimen containers with the identifying patient information label, along with laboratory slips for specific requests. If brush specimens are collected, slides and alcohol are required.

The standard bronchoscope is a rigid speculum used for visualizing the tracheobronchial tree. The rigid bronchoscope might be selected for biopsy of a large central mass, for removal of a foreign object, or to control hemorrhage during biopsy of a vascular mass. The rigid bronchoscope remains the instrument of choice for removal of foreign bodies in infants and children. A fiberoptic light carrier is inserted into the bronchoscope to illuminate the distal opening. A side channel is incorporated into the bronchoscope to permit aeration of the lungs with oxygen or anesthetic gases. An additional device, the Sanders Venturi system, which is available to the anesthesia provider, provides adequate patient ventilation during bronchoscopies and laryngoscopies.

The surgeon risks exposure in the presence of communicable diseases. For this reason, the surgeon and assistants should wear facemasks and eye protection or a transparent shield attached to a headband (see Chapter 4 for specific transmission-based precautions). With increasing numbers of patients with tuberculosis, particulate respirators are recommended as protective devices. Aseptic technique is used to prevent cross-contamination.

Operative Procedure

1. The patient's head is positioned to optimize visualization of the bronchus—to the left when the right main bronchi are inspected and to the right when the left bronchi are inspected. The head is lowered for inspection of the middle lobe.
2. The surgeon places a tooth guard to protect the patient's teeth. The bronchoscope is inserted over the surface of the tongue, usually through the right corner of the mouth. The patient's lip is retracted from the upper teeth with a finger of the surgeon's left hand. The epiglottis is identified and elevated with the tip of the bronchoscope.
3. The surgeon passes the distal end of the scope through the true vocal cords of the larynx, and views the upper tracheal rings. A

small amount of anesthetic solution may be sprayed through the tube on the carina of the trachea and into the bronchus with the bronchial atomizer or spray. The patient's head is moved to the left to obtain a view of the right bronchi. The right-angle telescope is inserted with the light adjusted into the bronchoscope.

4. The segmental bronchial orifices of the upper right lobe bronchi are viewed, and the telescope is removed. The surgeon uses suction and aspirating tubes to clear the field of vision and remove accumulated secretions.
5. The surgeon inserts an oblique 45-degree-angle telescope or right-angle telescope and advances it to inspect the middle lobe branches. The patient's head is lowered to view the right middle lobe or turned to the right to view the left main bronchus.
6. Secretions are aspirated by the surgeon for study. Biopsy forceps are used if indicated; foreign bodies are removed with forceps.

The nurse encourages patients who have undergone bronchoscopy after administration of a local anesthetic to sit on the edge of the OR bed before transfer to the stretcher. An emesis basin and tissues should be provided for the patient's use. Assistance and support are provided to the patient to prevent a fall.

Postprocedural Concerns

Patient safety during and after endoscopy using topical anesthetics, local anesthetics, or monitored anesthesia care is a concern attributable to the medications administered. The gag reflex may not return for 2 to 3 hours. The patient may be positioned on his or her side or with the head of the bed elevated to promote secretion drainage. The patient should be restricted from any oral intake until the gag reflex has returned. During bronchoscopy, particularly with a rigid bronchoscope, teeth could be loosened or oral structures damaged. The lips, teeth, and oral mucosa should be examined to ensure undisturbed integrity. Patients are often anxious to know the results of the procedure, and they benefit from the perioperative nurse's openness and willingness to discuss when results might be available, as well as the patient's feelings and concerns.

Bronchoscopy Using a Flexible Bronchoscope

Flexible bronchoscopy is performed to view structures that cannot be observed with a rigid scope. Flexible bronchoscopy may be performed in addition to a standard rigid bronchoscopy or as an independent procedure. If performed independently, the patient may remain on the transporting stretcher during the procedure. Flexible bronchoscopy is completed for the same reasons as rigid bronchoscopy. Flexible fiberoptic telescopes permit visualization of the upper, middle, and lower lobe bronchi. They can be passed in patients with a jaw deformity or cervical bone rigidity with less difficulty than the rigid scope. A flexible bronchoscope can also be passed through the nares in an awake patient. Flexible fiberoptic bronchoscopes are more frequently used, as is video endoscopy.

Procedural Considerations

Patient considerations are as described for rigid bronchoscopy. Instruments and equipment used include the flexible bronchoscope, fiberoptic light source, flexible biopsy forceps, flexible brush (optional; if used, slides and alcohol are necessary to collect specimen), labeled specimen collectors, pathology requests, syringe for wash, and suction tubing with collection tube attached to collect the wash specimen.

Operative Procedure

1. The lubricated bronchoscope is passed through the adapter on the endotracheal tube, which is held secure by the anesthesia

provider. If local or monitored anesthesia care is used for the procedure, the lubricated bronchoscope may be passed nasally.

2. The suction tube is positioned with the specimen collector attached for collection of bronchial washings. When indicated, the suction tubing is connected to the bronchoscope; the container for collection is held securely in an upright position to prevent loss of the specimen through the suction tubing.

3. The surgeon or scrub person injects approximately 5 mL of saline solution into the channel. Suction is quickly reapplied. This procedure may be repeated as necessary.

After completion of the procedure, the perioperative nurse sends the specimens to the laboratory for analysis.

Electromagnetic Navigation Bronchoscopy

Electromagnetic navigation bronchoscopy (ENB) is newer technology that entails a minimally invasive approach to allow access to difficult to reach areas of the lung for biopsy. Standard flexible bronchoscopy is augmented with an image-guided localization device that assists in placing endobronchial accessories in the peripheral target areas of the lung. The electromagnetic system guides and steers the catheters beyond the reach of the bronchoscope to allow the surgeon to reach the lesion and obtain a biopsy of it (Marino et al., 2016). Potential complications are similar to those after traditional bronchoscopy. Clinical trials are in progress to evaluate adverse events, quality of life, and patient satisfaction with the procedure/technology. Trials will also collect data related to diagnostic yield and accuracy, repeat biopsy rate, tissue adequacy for genetic testing, and staging (Fulch et al., 2016).

Mediastinoscopy

Mediastinoscopy is the direct visualization and possible biopsy of lymph nodes or tumors at the tracheobronchial junction, under the carina of the trachea, or on the upper lobe bronchi or subdivisions. Mediastinoscopy may precede an exploratory thoracotomy in known cases of lung cancer or may be completed to assist in accurately staging the patient's lymph node status. Patients with positive findings may be treated with radiation or chemotherapy, as indicated. The mediastinoscope is a hollow tube with a fiberoptic light carrier. A fiberoptic light source with a light-intensity dial provides power and control of illumination.

Procedural Considerations

The setup for mediastinoscopy includes a set of instruments for incising, cutting, retracting, and suturing similar to those needed for a minor procedure. In addition, the desired type of mediastinoscope; fiberoptic light cords; fiberoptic light source; suction tubing; aspirating tubes; biopsy forceps; electrosurgical unit (ESU); and an 8-inch, 20-gauge endocardiac needle are required. Depending on institutional policy, a thoracotomy tray may be in the OR on standby in the event of uncontrolled bleeding after biopsy.

The anesthesia provider administers a general anesthetic agent and assists with positioning the patient as described for a tracheostomy (see Chapter 19).

Operative Procedure

1. The surgeon makes a short (approximately 2-cm) transverse incision above the suprasternal notch, and exposes and incises the pretracheal fascia.

2. Using blunt (digital) dissection, the surgeon tunnels anteriorly along the trachea into the mediastinum.

3. The surgeon introduces the mediastinoscope under direct vision deep to the fascial plane and advances it anterior to the trachea toward the mediastinum.

4. The scope is manipulated to visualize the tracheal bifurcation, bronchi, aortic arch, and associated lymph nodes.

5. Lymph node tissue is located for biopsy and aspirated with a small-gauge needle and syringe to verify that it is a nonvascular structure.

6. The surgeon inserts a biopsy forceps through the scope, and obtains a tissue specimen. Pressure can be applied to the excision site with a bronchus soft good on a holder. The mediastinum is reinspected for bleeding.

7. Subcutaneous tissue is sutured with absorbable sutures. The surgeon closes the skin with absorbable material on a small cutting needle.

8. A small dressing is applied.

Video-Assisted Thoracic Surgery

Video-assisted thoracoscopic surgery (VATS) is a minimally invasive operative technique. It uses an endoscopic approach to visualize the thoracic cavity for diagnosis of pleural disease or treatment of pleural conditions, such as cysts, blebs, and effusions; to biopsy mediastinal masses; to perform wedge resections, lobectomy, pericardectomy, lung volume reduction surgery (LVRS), and cervical sympathectomy; to obtain hemostasis; and to evacuate blood clots or divide adhesions. Pleurodesis with instillation of talc, tetracycline, or other sclerosing treatment can be accomplished through the thoracoscope (Surgical Pharmacology). VATS has many benefits, including the elimination of a thoracotomy incision, decreased pain, shortened hospital stay, and reduced morbidity. VATS also may be used in conjunction with robotically assisted thoracic procedures such as robotic lobectomy (Robotic-Assisted Surgery).

Procedural Considerations

Endoscopic instrumentation and equipment used for a thoracoscopy include 5- and 10-mm telescopes, light cord, camera, graspers, dissectors, scissors, ligators, and endoscopic soft tissue instruments (scissors, hemostats, suction tips, and retractors) and stapling devices. It is also advisable to have thoracic instrument trays set up in the event there is a need to convert to a thoracotomy. Accessory equipment for video (television monitors, recorder, printer, and light source for camera and scope) and insufflation is also used. The perioperative nurse will assist in positioning the patient supine, semilaterally, or laterally, depending on the anatomic structures involved.

Operative Procedure

1. The surgeon creates a 2- to 3-cm incision between the fifth and seventh intercostal spaces for insertion of the 10- or 12-mm trocar. The zero-degree telescope is inserted to view the site so that the approach can be determined.

2. If the procedure can be completed by thoracoscopy, the surgeon creates additional puncture sites for insertion of additional trocars to allow instrument manipulation. The size of trocars and types of instruments vary for the diagnosis.

3. After the selected procedure, the surgeon inserts a chest tube through one of the surgical puncture sites and secures it to the skin. Trocar sites are closed, and small dressings or adhesive skin tapes are applied.

Endoscopic Thoracic Sympathectomy

Hyperhidrosis is defined as excessive sweating, usually affecting the palms, axillae, and soles of the feet. It may also affect the face, groin,

Surgical Pharmacology

Agents for Chemical Pleurodesis

Pleurodesis is undertaken as a treatment for malignant pleural effusion and for unresolved T-type spontaneous pneumothorax. A variety of chemical agents can be administered intrathoracically to cause adherence of the pleural layers. Adherence of the pleural layers is thought to prevent the accumulation of pleural fluid in the case of pleural effusion and to prevent subsequent pneumothorax. Commonly used agents for chemical pleurodesis are listed. Other agents may be used according to the surgeon's preference, surgical region, and agent availability. Perioperative nurses should consult with the surgeon before the procedure to determine the agent used.

Sclerosing Agent	Indications	Clinical Efficacy	Adverse Reactions	Nursing Implications
Talc 2.5–10 g in 50–500 cc saline	Initial treatment for PSP and SSP	80%–95% efficacy; decreased pneumothorax recurrence to 0%–9%	Chest pain, fever, dyspnea, pneumonia, hemothorax, and ARDS	May be administered as a poudrage, aerosol, or slurry
Bleomycin 60 units mixed with 100–200 mg of lidocaine	Initial treatment for PSP and SSP	60%–85% efficacy	Pain, fever, neutropenia, potential toxicity from systemic absorption	Antineoplastics require special handling to reduce personal exposure Nurses should follow hospital policies and procedures for safe medication handling procedures
Cyclines Minocycline: 7 mg/kg Doxycycline: 500 mg in 100–200 cc of saline	Initial treatment for PSP and SSP Adjuvant treatment for PSP after VATS	70%–80% efficacy	Pain, fever, hemothorax, neutropenia	Requires several doses Determine whether patient is allergic to cycline medications before procedure
Silver Nitrate 	20 mL of 0.5% silver nitrate	75%–90% efficacy	Severe pain, transient alveolar inflammation in underlying lung, may induce systemic inflammation	Handle with care Solution stains skin and clothing
Iodopovidone 20 cc of 10% iodopovidone in 80 cc of saline	Initial treatment for PSP and SSP	65%–95% efficacy Decreased pneumothorax recurrence to 0%–6%	Severe pain, hypotension, empyema, possible thyroid uptake	Assess patient for allergies to iodine
Picibanil (OK-432)	Adjuvant treatment for PSP after VATS and initial treatment for SSP	95% efficacy Decreased pneumothorax recurrence to 5% after VATS	Chest pain and fever	Low virulence strain of *Streptococcus pyogenes* incubated with benzylpenicillin Assess for penicillin allergy

ARDS, Acute respiratory distress syndrome; *PSP,* primary spontaneous pneumothorax; *SSP,* secondary spontaneous pneumothorax; *VATS,* video-assisted thoracoscopic surgery.
Modified from Aronson JK: Minocycline and talc. In Aronson JK, editor: *Meyler's side effects of drugs,* ed 16, Amsterdam, 2016, Elsevier; Garrido V et al: Recommendations of diagnosis and treatment of pleural effusion, *Arch Bronconeumol,* 50(6):235–249, 2013; How C et al: Chemical pleurodesis for spontaneous pneumothorax, *J Formos Med Assoc* 112(12):749–755, 2013; Yendamuri S et al: Malignant pleural and pericardial effusion. In Sellke FW et al, editors: *Sabiston & Spencer surgery of the chest,* ed 9, Philadelphia, 2016, Elsevier.

or legs. Hyperhidrosis is widely unreported and undiagnosed; however, most individuals with the condition experience it in the axillary and palmar areas. Sweating is characterized as intolerable, and it typically interferes with daily activities. Familial history of hyperhidrosis is implicated in approximately 35% to 55% of cases (Moraites et al., 2014). Endoscopic thoracic sympathectomy (ETS) is a thoracoscopic intervention used to surgically treat hyperhidrosis. To treat palmar hyperhidrosis, the surgeon interrupts the sympathetic chain at the T2 level. Compensatory sweating, defined as increased sweating in other areas after the procedure, is the most common side effect of this procedure. The incidence of compensatory sweating varies after the procedure and may be classified as mild, which occurs in small amounts and is tolerable; moderate, which is defined as sweat that coalesces into flowing droplets; and severe, which is characterized by flowing sweat necessitating a change of clothing several times a day. Many patients who undergo ETS do so on an ambulatory basis or require only an overnight stay. The procedure can produce dramatic and immediate results and is associated with a positive outcome for

the patient. ETS may also be used to surgically treat pain syndromes (e.g., complex regional pain syndrome), facial blushing, and Raynaud syndrome.

Procedural Considerations

The team positions the patient supine, and the anesthesia provider inserts a double-lumen endotracheal tube. The patient may be repositioned into a lawn chair or upright position depending on the surgeon's preference. Video monitors are placed on each side of the patient to allow the surgeon an unobstructed view from either side, because the procedure is performed bilaterally.

Operative Procedure

1. The anesthesia provider deflates the patient's lung as directed by the surgeon.
2. The surgeon uses the blade to make a small (2 mm or less) incision between the patient's second and third ribs in the axillary plane.

ROBOTIC-ASSISTED SURGERY ▐▌

Moving Beyond Video-Assisted Thoracoscopic Surgery

Robotic-assisted thoracic procedures enhance the accuracy and safety of VATS. During traditional thoracotomy the surgeon's view is hampered by the size of the incision and rigidity of the chest wall. An advantage to the robotic-assisted approach is the superior three-dimensional view of the operative field and thoracic cavity, allowing the surgeon superior visualization, increased magnification, and better maneuverability. Smaller incisions are used for robotic surgery, so patients experience less postoperative pain and morbidity. A variety of robotic-assisted procedures are performed by specially trained surgeons, including mediastinal tumor resection, lobectomy, and sympathectomy. Continued advances in technology will allow for the development of additional applications and procedures within the thoracic specialty.

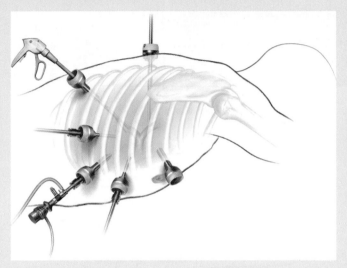

The arcs of rotation and management of the instrumentation for dissection within the chest, allowing surgical dissection to occur in small spaces. (From Kernstine KH et al: Robotic lobectomy, *Op Tech Thorac Cardiovasc Surg* 13(3):204.e1–204.e23, 2009.)

Refer to Chapter 8 for a general discussion of the equipment and instrumentation (e.g., robotic console, chassis) used for the procedure. In addition to preparing for the robotic procedure, the perioperative nurse and scrub person ensure that they have also gathered instrumentation and supplies to convert to an open procedure in the event an emergency arises or the surgeon is unable to complete the procedure through the minimally invasive approach. The nurse assists the anesthesia provider with inserting a double-lumen endotracheal tube and helps position the patient in the lateral position with the operative side up. After the patient is prepped and draped, the anesthesia provider places the patient in reverse Trendelenburg position. The nurse assists with positioning the robot, video monitors, and three-dimensional vision console equipment. The surgeon places the thoracoports based on the location of the lesion, inserts the scope, and then connects the dissecting instruments to the robot's instrument arms. A 3.5-mm endostapler is used to complete the bronchial transection.

VATS, Video-assisted thoracoscopic surgery.

---

3. Next, the surgeon inserts a disposable thoracic port through the incision, and then inserts a small (2-mm or 5-mm) telescope through the port.
4. The surgeon identifies the sympathetic chain at the T2 level (Fig. 23.9A–B) and uses endoscopic scissors to open the pleura.
5. The nerve is grasped with a bipolar forceps and divided with bipolar ESU (see Fig. 23.9C). Alternatively, clips may be applied to the nerve.
6. The port is removed, and a small thoracic catheter is inserted through the incision.
7. The surgeon closes the incision, and the lung is reexpanded. As the air is forced out of the pleural cavity, the catheter is removed and wound closure is completed.
8. The procedure is repeated for the opposite side.
9. Adhesive skin tapes are placed over the incision sites.
10. A postoperative chest x-ray film is obtained in the PACU to rule out any residual pneumothorax.

Lung Surgery

Thoracotomy

Thoracotomy involves an incision in the chest wall through a median sternotomy or a lateral or posterolateral incision for the purpose of operating on the lungs. Thoracotomy may be performed for a variety of benign and malignant conditions. Lung cancer (Fig. 23.10) is a common diagnosis for which a thoracotomy may be required. Patients with lung cancer may have specific treatment based on their tumor, node, and metastasis (TNM) characteristics. The TNM system defines tumor (T) as the size, location, and spread (pulmonary or extrapulmonary). The designation of nodes (N) refers to spread to a lymph node or group of lymph nodes. Metastasis (M) relates to metastatic tumor activity in distant organs (e.g., brain, liver) (Box 23.1). Staging is based on TNM findings (Fig. 23.11). Intraoperative patient care is similar for various thoracotomy procedures, with consideration of the patient's history and disease process, planned procedure, and

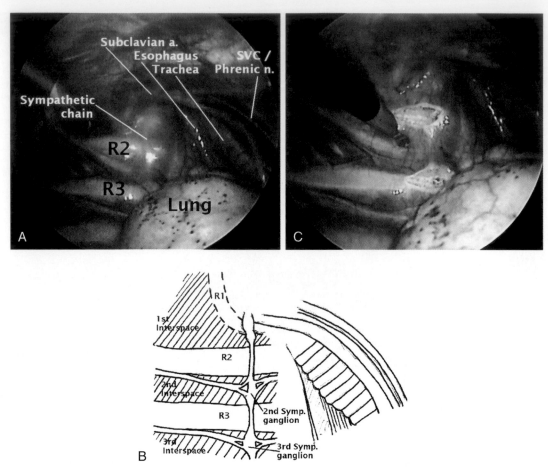

FIG. 23.9 (A) Thoracoscopic view of right superior posterior mediastinum. The sympathetic chain runs over the anterior surface of the posterior rib heads. The first rib is not visualized but can be palpated. (B) Schematic diagram. The first rib is outlined. The sympathetic ganglion and its rami are seen just below the respective rib level. (C) Sympathectomy over the right second and third ribs. The ganglia themselves are spared. *a,* Artery; *n,* nerve; *R1,* first rib; *R2,* second rib; *R3,* third rib; *SVC,* superior vena cava; *Symp,* sympathetic.

individualized patient needs. Basic thoracic instrumentation is used and may include a sternal saw and stapling devices. Preparation by the anesthesia provider with careful monitoring of the patient is a priority. Insertion of a double-lumen endotracheal tube, an arterial line for monitoring ABG samples, and a central venous line to ensure patent access for fluids are procedures performed by the anesthesia provider. An epidural catheter may be inserted for intraoperative and postoperative pain management. Patient preparation by the surgical team includes positioning and placement of devices for prevention of complications (e.g., intermittent pneumatic compression devices, warming devices, and insertion of a urinary catheter). The nurse is responsible for ongoing evaluation and communication of the patient's status to the family throughout the procedure.

Pneumonectomy

Pneumonectomy is the removal of an entire lung, usually to treat malignant neoplasms. Other reasons for this procedure include removal of an extensive unilateral bronchiectasis (e.g., irreversible dilation of the bronchi) involving the greater part of one lung, drainage of an extensive chronic pulmonary abscess involving portions of one or more lobes, removal of selected benign tumors, and treatment of any extensive unilateral lesion. Other resections are often combined with pneumonectomy, such as resection of mediastinal

lymph nodes, resections of portions of the chest wall or diaphragm, and removal of parietal pleura.

Operative Procedure

1. The surgeon incises the skin, subcutaneous tissue, and muscle with a blade and an ESU. Hemostasis is attained. If a rib is to be excised, bone instruments are required.
2. The ribs and tissue are protected with moist soft goods; the rib retractor is placed (Fig. 23.12) and opened slowly and gently.
3. The surgeon frees any peripheral adhesions to mobilize the lung and divides the pulmonary ligament. Dissection to the hilum of the involved lobe is performed.
4. The superior pulmonary vein is gently retracted, and the pulmonary artery is dissected.
5. The surgeon clamps the branches of the pulmonary artery and vein of the involved lobe, places double ligatures, and divides them with fine right-angled vascular clamps, scissors, and nonabsorbable suture. Alternatively, a stapling device may be used to ligate the vessels.
6. The inferior pulmonary vein is exposed by incising the hilar pleura and retracting the lung anteriorly. The inferior pulmonary vein is clamped, doubly ligated, and divided.

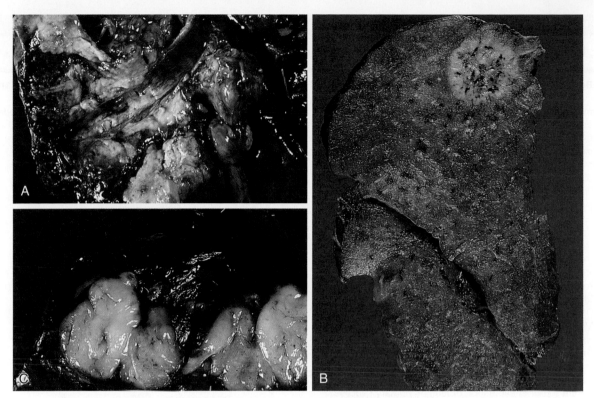

FIG. 23.10 Lung cancer. (A) Squamous cell carcinoma originating from the main bronchus. (B) Peripheral adenoma. (C) Small cell carcinoma.

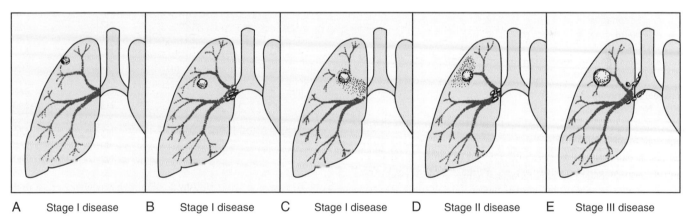

| A | Stage I disease | B | Stage I disease | C | Stage I disease | D | Stage II disease | E | Stage III disease |

FIG. 23.11 Staging of lung cancer by the tumor, node, and metastasis (TNM) system. (A and B) Stage I disease includes tumors classified as T1 with or without metastasis to the lymph node in the ipsilateral hilar region. (C) Also included in stage I are tumors classified as T2 but having no nodal or distant metastases. (D) Stage II disease includes those tumors classified as T2, with metastasis only to the ipsilateral hilar lymph nodes. (E) Stage III includes all tumors more extensive than T2 or any tumor with metastasis to the lymph nodes in the mediastinum with distant metastasis.

7. The surgeon applies a bronchus clamp and divides the bronchus near the tracheal bifurcation. The stump is closed with atraumatic nonabsorbable mattress sutures or bronchus staples. If staples are applied, the blade is used to complete division of the bronchus. The lung is removed from the chest.

8. The scrub person supplies normal saline to irrigate the pleural space and checks for hemostasis and air leaks during positive-pressure inspiration.

9. A pleural flap may be created and sutured over the bronchial stump. Other methods of securing the bronchus (such as placement of an intercostal flap) might be used.

10. Hemostasis is ensured in the pleural space.

11. The surgeon inserts chest tubes (28F to 30F) into the pleural space and exteriorizes them through a stab wound at the eighth or ninth interspace near the anterior axillary line (Fig. 23.13). An upper tube is inserted through a second stab wound if

BOX 23.1

Tumor, Node, and Metastasis (TNM) Definitions and Staging for Lung Cancer

T (Tumor) Descriptors

T0   No visible primary tumor

T1   Tumor <3 cm in diameter and completely surrounded by lung tissue; no evidence of tumor in main lung airways

T1a   Tumor <2 cm in diameter

T1b   Tumor >2 cm and <3 cm in diameter

T2   Tumor with one of the following characteristics:
>3 cm and <7 cm in diameter
Present in mainstem airway and >2 cm from where trachea divides to form the mainstem bronchi (main carina)
Invades the surface covering of the lung
Causes partial collapse or inflammation of the lung

T2a   Tumor >3 cm but <5 cm in diameter

T2b   Tumor >5 cm but <7 cm in diameter

T3   Tumor >7 cm
Tumor invades any of the following:
Chest wall
Diaphragm
Mediastinal surface
Heart surface
Tumor in the mainstem bronchi within 2 cm of but not involving the main carina
No whole lung collapse or lung inflammation
Separate tumor in same lobe of lung as primary cancer

T4   Tumor of any size that invades any of the following:
Mediastinum
Heart
Great vessels
Trachea
Esophagus
Spine
Carina
Separate tumor in different lobe of lung but on same side as primary cancer

N (Node) Descriptors

N0   No lymph node involvement

N1   Tumor involvement of hilar lymph nodes on the same side as the primary cancer

N2   Tumor involvement of subcarinal or paratracheal lymph nodes on the same side as the primary cancer

N3   Tumor involvement of paratracheal lymph nodes on the opposite side of the primary cancer

M (Metastasis) Descriptors

M0   No distant metastasis

M1   Distant metastasis

M1a   Separate tumor in opposite lung
Tumor in pleural fluid
Tumor in pericardial fluid
Tumor nodules on lung surface

M1b   Tumor in non-lung organs

Biopsy Methods for the Staging and Diagnosis of Lung Cancer

Biopsy Method	Accessible Lymph Node Stations
Endobronchial ultrasonography–guided fine needle aspiration	2, 3, 4, 7, 10, 11
Endoscopic ultrasonography–guided fine needle aspiration	4, 5, 7, 8, 9
Cervical mediastinoscopy	1, 2, 3, 4, anterior 7
Anterior mediastinoscopy	5
Extended cervical mediastinoscopy	6
Video-assisted thoracoscopic surgery	Ipsilateral mediastinal lymph nodes

Anatomic Stage/Prognostic Groups

Occult carcinoma	TX	N0	M0
Stage 0	Tis	N0	M0
Stage IA	T1a	N0	M0
	T1b	N0	M0
Stage IB	T2a	N0	M0
Stage IIA	T2b	N0	M0
	T1a	N1	M0
	T1b	N1	M0
	T2a	N1	M0
Stage IIB	T2b	N1	M0
	T3	N0	M0
Stage IIIA	T1a	N2	M0
	T1b	N2	M0
	T2a	N2	M0
	T2b	N2	M0
	T3	N1	M0
	T3	N2	M0
	T4	N0	M0
	T4	N1	M0
Stage IIIB	T1a	N3	M0
	T1b	N3	M0
	T2a	N3	M0
	T2b	N3	M0
	T3	N3	M0
	T4	N2	M0
	T4	N3	M0
Stage IV	Any T	Any N	M1a
	Any T	Any N	M1b

Modified from American Cancer Society (ACS): *Non-small cell lung cancer staging* (website), 2016. www.cancer.org/cancer/lungcancer-non-smallcell/detailedguide/non-small-cell-lung-cancer-staging. (Accessed 8 January 2017); Ankaru M, Keshavjee S: Lung cancer: surgical treatment. In Selke FW et al, editors: *Sabiston & Spencer surgery of the chest,* ed 9, Philadelphia, 2016, Saunders; Tan WW: *Non-small cell lung cancer* (website), 2016. http://emedicine.medscape.com/article/279960-overview. (Accessed 8 January 2017).

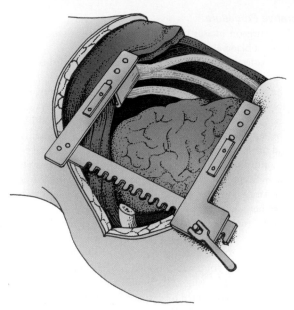

FIG. 23.12 Rib retractor placed for thoracotomy.

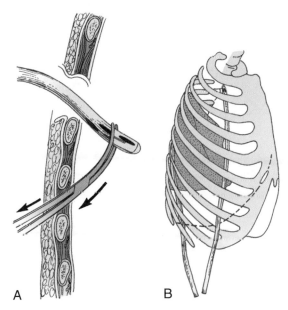

FIG. 23.13 (A) Introduction of chest drainage tube through a stab wound. (B) Placement of apical and basal drainage tubes after upper and middle lobectomy.

indicated to evaluate leaking air. The tubes are secured with heavy sutures and connected to water-seal drainage after closure of the pleural space.

12. The surgeon places the rib approximator (Fig. 23.14) and begins closure with interrupted sutures.
13. The muscle, subcutaneous tissue, and skin are closed. Drains are anchored to the chest wall with suture.
14. The dressing is applied.
15. Chest tube connections are secured with nylon bands or tape and labeled (anterior or posterior).

Lobectomy

Lobectomy is excision of one or more lobes of the lung. It is performed when the primary tumor is located in a particular lobe or to remove

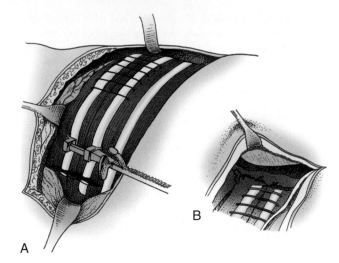

FIG. 23.14 (A) Rib approximator placed for closure of incision. (B) Heavy-gauge suture used for closure of ribs.

metastatic lesions when the tumor is peripherally located and hilar nodes are not involved. Other conditions affecting the lung and treated by lobectomy might be bronchiectasis; giant emphysematous blebs or bullae; large, centrally located benign tumors; fungal infections; and congenital anomalies.

Procedural Considerations

Basic thoracic instrumentation is used. The perioperative nurse assists with placing the patient in a lateral position for a posterolateral approach; the supine position may be used for upper and middle lobe resections. The procedure varies with the specific lobe to be removed depending on the anatomic structure.

Operative Procedure

1. The surgeon incises the skin, subcutaneous tissue, and muscle using a blade and an ESU. Hemostasis is attained. If a rib is to be excised, bone instruments are required.
2. The ribs and tissue are protected with soft goods. The rib retractor is placed and opened slowly and gently.
3. The surgeon enters the pleura and frees the peripheral adhesions with scissors, blunt dissection, or small folded soft good (sponge) on a forceps.
4. The hilar pleura is incised and separated.
5. The branches of the pulmonary arteries and veins are isolated; clamped; doubly ligated; and divided with fine, right-angled vascular clamps, scissors, and nonabsorbable suture. A stapling device may be used to divide the vessels as an alternative.
6. The surgeon identifies the main trunk of the pulmonary artery and the fissure between the lobes.
7. The bronchus clamp is applied. The remaining lung is inflated to identify the line of demarcation. The bronchus is divided with a blade or heavy scissors.
8. Bronchial secretions are suctioned.
9. The surgeon closes the bronchus with atraumatic nonabsorbable mattress sutures or bronchus staples. If staples are applied, a blade is used to complete division of the bronchus.
10. Incomplete fissures are divided between hemostats with fine Metzenbaum scissors. Edges may be sutured closed.
11. A pleural flap may be created and sutured over the bronchial stump (other methods of securing the bronchus may be used).

12. The pleural cavity is thoroughly irrigated with normal saline, and hemostasis is ensured. The remaining lobes are inflated to check for air leaks, and the degree of expansion of the remaining lobes is assessed.

13. The pleural space is irrigated, and the procedure is completed as described for a pneumonectomy.

Segmental Resection

Segmental resection is removal of one or more anatomic subdivisions of the pulmonary lobe. It conserves healthy, functioning pulmonary tissue by sparing remaining segments. Segmental resection is indicated for any benign lesion with segmental distribution or diseased tissue affecting only one segment of the lung with compromised cardiorespiratory reserve. The most common cause for removal is bronchiectasis. Other conditions requiring removal include chronic, localized inflammation and congenital cysts or blebs.

Procedural Considerations

Basic thoracotomy instrumentation is used. The perioperative nurse assists the surgical team in placing the patient in the lateral position.

Operative Procedure

1. The surgeon incises the skin, subcutaneous tissue, and muscle using a blade and an ESU.
2. The parietal pleura is incised with a blade and scissors. Adhesions are divided with sharp or blunt dissection.
3. The segmental artery is identified to provide accurate identification of the bronchus of the diseased segment.
4. The surgeon ligates the segmental pulmonary vein and branches.
5. The surgeon clamps the bronchus with the bronchus clamp, and the remaining lung is inflated. The intersegmental boundary is confirmed, and proper placement of the clamp is ensured.
6. The visceral pleura is incised around the diseased segment, beginning anterior to the hilum and progressing toward the periphery. Exposure is facilitated with a malleable or other type of retractor. The intersegmental vessels are clamped with thoracic hemostats and ligated.
7. The surgeon transects the segmental bronchus and closes the stump with atraumatic nonabsorbable mattress sutures or bronchus staples (Fig. 23.15).
8. Dissection is continued to separate segmental surfaces, and vessels are ligated as needed. The segment of the lung is removed.

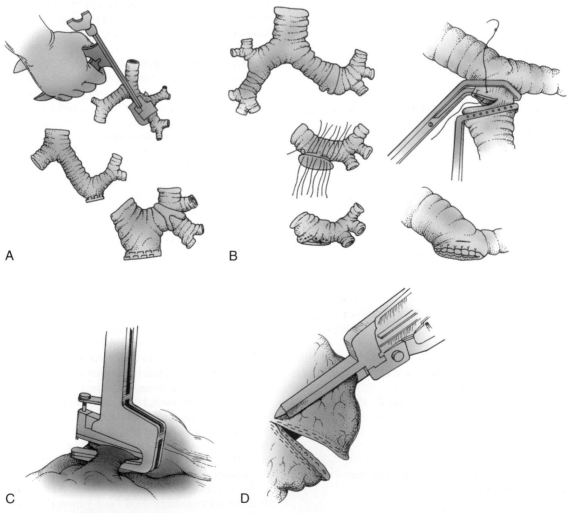

FIG. 23.15 (A) Staple suturing of bronchus. (B) Conventional suturing of bronchus; application of bronchus clamp and incision; closure of stump. (C) Staple suturing of pulmonary vessels. (D) Staple suturing of lung tissue (wedge resection or lung biopsy).

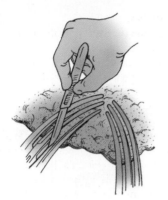
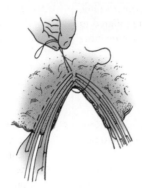
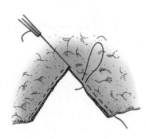

FIG. 23.16 Wedge resection. Clamps applied to edge of lung tissue to be excised with blade and sutured with a running suture and oversewn.

9. The anesthesia provider reinflates the lung and the surgeon irrigates with normal saline. Bleeding is controlled with ligatures or hemoclips.
10. The procedure is completed as described for pneumonectomy.

Wedge Resection

Wedge resection is removal of a wedge-shaped section of parenchyma that includes the identified lesion, without regard for intersegmental planes. The resection is also used for removal of small, peripherally located benign primary tumors and peripherally located inflammatory disease, as well as for biopsy in patients with chronic, diffuse lung disease.

Procedural Considerations

Thoracic instrumentation is used. The team positions the patient to allow access to the operative site with consideration of the area of lung to be resected.

Operative Procedure

1. The surgeon incises the skin, subcutaneous tissue, and muscle using a blade and an ESU.
2. The rib retractor is placed.
3. The wedge is outlined for excision, with a margin of normal tissue left, using one of the following techniques:
   a. Long hemostatic clamps are applied in three rows to outline the wedge. Excision is accomplished with a blade. The tissue is sutured with a running absorbable suture behind the clamps before removal. The edges of the tissue are oversewn with a continuous or interrupted suture (Fig. 23.16). The surgeon controls bleeding and secures the small bronchi with clamps and ligature. Large bronchi are ligated or sutured to prevent persistent air leak.
   b. The lobe is grasped with a lung clamp, and the thoracic stapling instrument is applied to the parenchymal portion of the lung. Staples are applied, and the wedge is excised with the blade. Staples are reapplied to the opposite side of the lesion adjoining the staple lines.
4. The specimen is removed. The surgeon checks for air leaks by irrigation and inspection. Bleeding is controlled with ligation or hemoclips. The procedure is completed as described for pneumonectomy.

Lung Volume Reduction Surgery

LVRS is an alternative surgical treatment for patients with chronic pulmonary emphysema (Fig. 23.17). The surgery is intended to increase expiratory airflow, maximal exercise capacity, and respiratory muscle strength, relieving dyspnea. The procedure may also be referred to as *lung volume reduction,* or *pneumoplasty.* Candidates for the procedure are those who have progressive, severe dyspnea secondary to pulmonary dysfunction; those whose medical management is ineffective; and those in whom disease distribution is limited to target areas of severity. The two most common operative approaches for LVRS are median sternotomy and VATS. Median sternotomy provides excellent bilateral exposure and flexibility, whereas the VATS approach has the advantage of a shorter hospitalization, fewer days of postoperative air leaks, and fewer days on the ventilator. Patients undergoing LVRS participate in vigorous pulmonary rehabilitation as a standard practice in preparation for surgery. Pulmonary rehabilitation programs not only improve airway clearance and diaphragmatic function but also ensure that optimal conditioning is achieved, which improves surgical outcomes, improves tolerance for surgery, and decreases postoperative complications.

Procedural Considerations

The basic thoracotomy setup and instrumentation are used, along with stapling devices, chest tubes, and a water-seal drainage system. A laser may be required, as may other materials for sealing the resected edges (e.g., bovine pericardium, collagen). Positioning is a particular concern for this patient population, who may be malnourished and are at increased risk for positioning injury. The perioperative nurse must collaborate with the surgeon and anesthesia provider to ensure that the best possible positioning practices are implemented.

Operative Procedure

1. The surgeon exposes the patient's lungs through a transverse anterior thoracotomy incision using the sternal saw to separate the sternum. Adhesiotomies are performed, and the inferior pulmonary ligaments are incised.
2. The anesthesia provider deflates the patient's lungs to allow for visualization of the portions of the lung in which air is trapped in emphysematous lung tissue.
3. A lung-grasping forceps is used to hold the portion of the lung to be excised. A surgical stapling device is lined with bovine pericardium and positioned on either side of the lung. The stapling of emphysematous lung tissue continues, and staple lines are overlapped to prevent air leaks. Alternative means of sealing the resection line include the use of a pleural flap or the application of collagen.
4. The anesthesia provider reinflates the lung to identify air leaks. If air leaks are found, the lung is deflated and the stapling procedure continues.

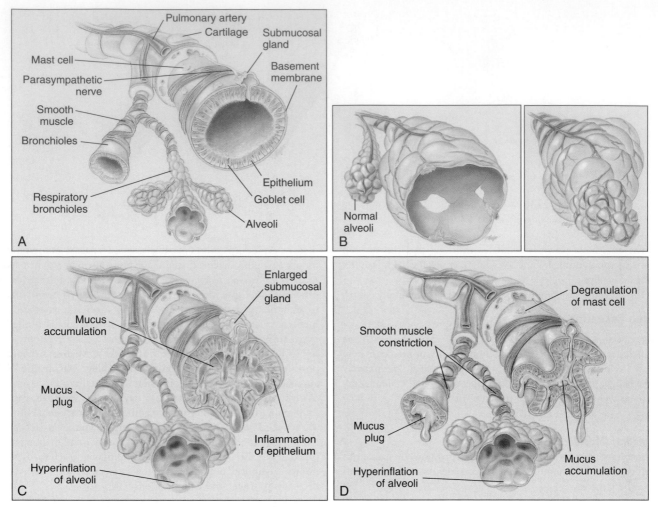

FIG. 23.17 Airway obstruction caused by emphysema, chronic bronchitis, and asthma. (A) The normal lung. (B) Emphysema enlargement and destruction of alveolar walls with loss of elasticity and trapping of air; *(left)* panlobular emphysema showing abnormal weakening and enlargement of all air spaces distal to the terminal bronchioles (normal alveoli shown for comparison only); *(right)* centrilobular emphysema showing abnormal weakening and enlargement of the respiratory bronchioles in the proximal portion of the acinus. (C) Chronic bronchitis: inflammation and thickening of mucous membrane with accumulation of mucus and pus leading to obstruction; characterized by cough. (D) Bronchial asthma: thick mucus, mucosal edema, and smooth muscle spasm causing obstruction of small airways; breathing becomes labored, and expiration is difficult.

5. One or two chest tubes are placed into each pleural space. The chest tubes are connected to water-seal drainage systems without suction.
6. The surgeon reapproximates the ribs and sternum using stainless steel surgical wire. The muscle layer, subcutaneous tissue, and skin are closed, and dressings are applied.

Biopsy

Lung biopsy is the resection of a small portion of the lung for diagnosis. The biopsy allows removal of relatively large specimens for microscopic examination of the lung tissue. Indications include (1) failure of closed methods (needle biopsy) for diagnosis and (2) the presence of small, localized lesions that can be removed by biopsy.

Procedural Considerations

In addition to the basic instrument setup, a rib retractor, a lung-grasping forceps, dissecting scissors, a chest tube and water-seal

system, and an endostapling device are required. More than one specimen container may be needed. The patient is positioned in a semilateral position for an anterolateral incision.

Operative Procedure

1. A short incision (approximately 5 cm) is made at the fifth intercostal space. The surgeon incises the pleura and retracts the ribs. Alternatively, a VATS approach may be used.
2. The lung is secured and exteriorized using a Duval lung clamp.
3. Using a Satinsky clamp or a stapling device, the surgeon segments the tissue to be biopsied. The tissue to be removed is excised with a blade. After application of the clamp, tissue edges are approximated with absorbable suture. If a larger piece of tissue is desired, a stapling device may be used as described under Wedge Resection.
4. Bleeding is controlled by the application of moist soft goods at the incision site. The area is irrigated and inspected for air leaks.

5. The chest tube (28F to 30F) is inserted and connected to suction.
6. The incision is closed, the chest tube is anchored to the chest wall, and a dressing is applied.

Decortication

Decortication of the lung is removal of any fibrinous deposit, cancer, or restrictive membrane on the visceral and parietal pleura that interferes with pulmonary ventilatory function. It may also be done in conjunction with a pleurectomy for patients with pleural-based tumors, such as mesothelioma. The procedure can result in significant blood loss and trauma to the lung. The objective is to allow full expansion of the lung to maximize its function.

Procedural Considerations

The basic thoracic instrumentation is used. The perioperative nurse assists with positioning the patient in a lateral position for a posterolateral incision.

Operative Procedure

1. The surgeon incises the skin, subcutaneous tissue, and muscle using a blade and an ESU.
2. A rib, usually the fifth or sixth, is stripped (Fig. 23.18) and resected.
3. The scrub person provides moist soft goods (e.g., sponges) to protect the ribs and tissue. The rib retractor is placed and slowly and gently opened.
4. Parietal adhesions are divided to the margins of the lung, mediastinal surface, and pericardium with thoracic scissors, forceps, and a moist small folded soft good (sponge) on forceps.
5. The fibrous membrane is incised and separated from the visceral pleura using blunt and sharp dissection, handling the tissues gently (Fig. 23.19). The procedure is completed as described for pneumonectomy.

Drainage of Empyema

The accumulation of pus in the pleural space (empyema) might be associated with acute or chronic infection. Acute empyema may result from a lung abscess, pneumonia, or infection after thoracotomy.

Parapneumonic effusions occur in 60,000 of patients annually with 50% resulting from pneumonia. The occurrence of empyema is more prevalent in older or debilitated patients (Perry and Linden, 2016). Empyema (other than a pure tuberculous type) must be drained to prevent fibrothorax, and patients with empyema may require further treatment with decortication. When the infection is not extensive or organized, it can be managed by placing a chest tube under a local anesthetic. Prolonged intrapleural infection results in chronic empyema, which can result in the formation of loculations and create additional complications such as mediastinal shift, swallowing difficulties, respiratory limitations, bronchus erosion, and chest deformity. Postoperative empyema or empyema occurring in immunosuppressed patients can be effectively treated with a rib resection and drainage.

Procedural Considerations

Basic thoracic instrumentation is used. The team positions the patient in a lateral position for an anterolateral incision. If a pleurodesis is to be performed for a simple pleural effusion, a catheter for instillation of the sclerosing agent is required. The chest cavity is irrigated profusely during and on completion of the procedure.

Operative Procedure

1. The surgeon incises the skin and tissues with a blade to expose the affected area of the lung. Suction is used to prevent spillage of drainage from the chest.
2. The adjacent rib may be resected, and the intercostal neurovascular bundle is divided.

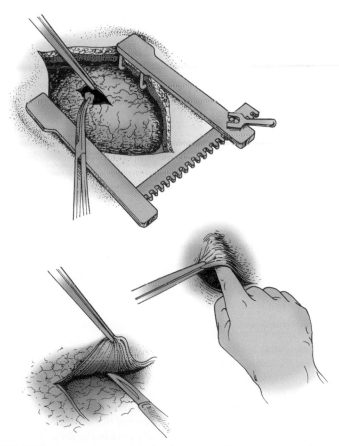

FIG. 23.19 Decortication. Methods of separating fibrous membrane from visceral pleura.

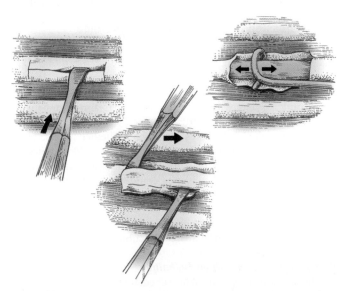

FIG. 23.18 Separation of muscles of rib with a periosteal elevator and rib stripper.

3. The underlying thickened pleura is incised and gross pus is evacuated. An inflammatory response might be created by stripping the parietal pleura from the visceral pleura by sharp or blunt dissection.
4. A large-bore catheter (46F) is inserted, and the sclerosing agent is instilled when indicated (see Surgical Pharmacology).
5. The surgeon closes the incision site as described for other thoracotomy procedures.
6. A dressing is applied.

Open Thoracostomy: Partial Rib Resection

Partial rib resection is removal of a portion of selected rib or ribs through an open thoracostomy incision to allow healing and reinflation of an infected lung. The procedure is performed for treatment of chronic empyemic lesions to establish a mechanism for continuous drainage.

Procedural Considerations

The basic thoracic instrument set and bone-cutting instruments are used. An ESU, chest tube, and water-seal drainage system are required, as are culture tubes for aerobic and anaerobic laboratory analysis. The patient is placed in a lateral position for a posterolateral incision. The surgical procedure can be completed with the patient administered a local anesthetic, but is most commonly performed under general anesthesia.

Operative Procedure

1. The surgeon incises the skin, subcutaneous tissue, and muscle using a blade and an ESU.
2. The rib is resected, and the pleura is incised. Suction is used to control anticipated drainage.
3. Aerobic and anaerobic swabs for culture and sensitivity are obtained. The chest cavity is irrigated.
4. A large chest tube may be inserted through the pleural opening. The incision is packed open.
5. The chest tube is secured with a suture of heavy-gauge material on a cutting needle.
6. The chest tube is connected to a water-seal drainage system, and connections are secured.
7. A dressing is applied. A number of layers of dressing may be necessary to absorb drainage.

Closed Thoracostomy: Intercostal Drainage

Closed thoracostomy is insertion of a chest catheter through an intercostal space for establishment of closed drainage. The procedure provides continuous aspiration of air, blood, or infectious fluid from the pleural cavity. It is indicated for treatment of spontaneous pneumothorax, traumatic hemothorax, pleural effusion, and acute empyema. Malignant pleural effusions (Fig. 23.20) may be managed by drainage and chemical pleurodesis by way of the thoracostomy tube.

Procedural Considerations

Thoracostomy as a singular procedure generally does not take place in an OR setting. The procedure is usually done with monitored anesthesia care and local anesthesia. A local anesthesia set, including syringes, needles, and an anesthetic agent of choice for local injection, is needed. The minor instrument set is used, in addition to disposable chest catheters, water-seal drainage system, two aspirating needles, and culture tubes. The patient is placed in a lateral or sitting position. Despite the administration of local anesthetic, thoracostomy can be uncomfortable for the patient. Administration of IV narcotic agents

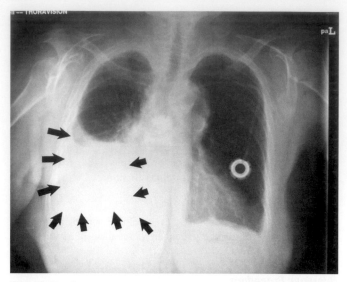

FIG. 23.20 Chest x-ray showing large right pleural effusion outlined by arrows.

at the time of the procedure may help prevent pain during performance of the procedure. The perioperative nurse should provide explanations and emotional support to the patient during the procedure.

Operative Procedure

1. The surgeon estimates the correct depth of insertion and marks the catheter. The operative site is anesthetized.
2. An aspirating needle attached to a syringe is introduced into the chest cavity to verify the presence of purulent drainage, air, or blood.
3. The surgeon incises the skin and introduces a clamp through the incision into the intercostal space and pleural cavity.
4. Next, the surgeon inserts a catheter through the incision site and clamps it to prevent egress of air as it is inserted into the cavity.
5. The incision site is sutured, and the catheter is secured.
6. The catheter is attached to water-seal drainage, and the tubing is secured. The clamp is removed, and a dressing is applied.

Decompression for Thoracic Outlet Syndrome

Thoracic outlet syndrome is a compression of the subclavian vessels and brachial plexus at the superior aperture of the thorax (Fig. 23.21). The first rib is the usual cause of the compression, because of either a congenital deformity or a traumatic injury that results in anatomic changes. Fibromuscular bands may also form between the cervical rib and other structures (i.e., scalenus tubercle) and cause compression. Symptoms depend on whether nerves, blood vessels, or both are compressed at the thoracic outlet. Decompression is accomplished through partial or entire removal of the rib using an open technique or video-assisted endoscopic techniques.

Procedural Considerations

Soft tissue and bone instrumentation is used. An ESU is required. The patient is positioned in a lateral decubitus position.

Operative Procedure: Open Technique

1. The surgeon incises the skin, subcutaneous tissue, and muscle using a blade and an ESU. Soft tissue dissection continues to identify the neurovascular bundle.

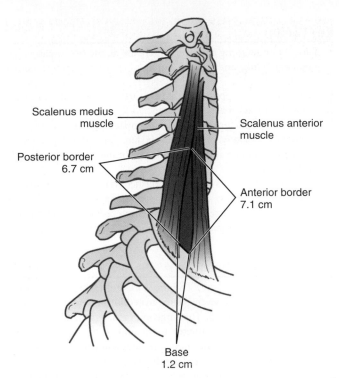

Scalenus medius
muscle

Scalenus anterior
muscle

Posterior border
6.7 cm

Anterior border
7.1 cm

Base
1.2 cm

FIG. 23.21 The scalene (anterior) triangle showing its measurements and the narrow space through which the neurovascular bundle passes.

2. The first rib is meticulously dissected subperiosteally using the periosteal elevator. A rib elevator, stripper, and rib raspatories may be required. Undue traction on the brachial plexus and damage to the subclavian artery or vein are avoided during the dissection.
3. A wedge is taken from the midportion, or the rib is removed in its entirety using rib shears.
4. A drain is placed, and the incision is closed. A dressing is applied.

Excision of Mediastinal Lesion

Excision of a mediastinal lesion involves removal of a lesion from the anterior, middle, and posterior sections of the mediastinum. Identifying the compartment is important for planning a surgical approach to the resection, for optimal exposure and access. Typically preoperative imaging will determine the location of the lesion. A mediastinoscopy may be a useful adjunct to help determine the diagnosis of an anterior mediastinal lesion. Indications for excision of a mediastinal lesion include miscellaneous cysts and tumors, thymoma, lymphoma, and neurogenic tumor.

Procedural Considerations

The thoracic instrumentation set is used. A procedure on the superior mediastinum might require use of thyroid instruments (see Chapter 16). An ESU and bone wax are needed. The perioperative nurse assists with placing the patient in a supine position for a median sternotomy incision (alternatively, lateral position may be used).

Operative Procedure: Thymectomy

1. The surgeon incises the skin, subcutaneous tissue, and muscle using a blade and an ESU.
2. The sternum is transected with a power saw or sternal knife. Bleeding is controlled at the bone edges with bone wax.

Alternatively, a transcervical approach may be used. Some surgeons have also used VATS or robotic-assisted approaches.
3. The thymus gland is dissected; vessels are clamped, ligated, and divided. The gland is removed.
4. The incision is closed. The sternum is reapproximated and closed with heavy wire. The skin is sutured closed. A dressing is applied.

Lung Transplantation

Since 1988 more than 30,000 lung transplants have been performed (UNOS, 2017). Indications for single-lung transplantation (SLT) include restrictive lung disease, emphysema, pulmonary hypertension, and other nonseptic end-stage pulmonary diseases. Double-lung transplantation (DLT) can be performed for many of these indications and is specifically indicated for patients with cystic fibrosis or patients with a chronic infection in end-stage pulmonary failure. The procedure involves the allografting of one or both lungs from a cadaver or donor who has met clinical criteria for brain death. Developments in SLT include donor contribution from living relatives for patients who have chronic disease and a high risk for death while waiting on the donor transplantation list. Contraindications for transplantation include multisystem disease other than the lung, history of carcinoma or sarcoma, current infection, significant renal or hepatic dysfunction, cigarette smoking within 3 or 4 months, drug or alcohol abuse, psychologic instability, or poor medication compliance. Although the surgical technique is increasingly successful, the application of lung transplantation techniques may be limited by donor supply. Questions regarding quality of life after transplantation and whether the single or double procedure is ultimately best for patients with chronic obstructive lung disease and primary pulmonary hypertension still remain. Issues also include the shortage of suitable donors, and improving methods for early detection of chronic rejection.

Procedural Considerations

Selection of the donor and recipients, preservation of the lung, and administration of anesthetic agents are considerations in this procedure. The nursing plan of care is modified considerably for each patient because nursing personnel are caring for two patients with different needs. Recipient patients will have been started preoperatively on immunosuppressive therapy and infection prophylaxis. The patient's positioning will vary for the techniques being used. The instrumentation is similar to that used for a thoracotomy. Cardiopulmonary bypass (CPB) may be required, as described in Chapter 25, along with the ESU, cold perfusion solution, and surgical stapling devices. The perioperative nurse will need to collaborate with the anesthesia provider because continuous hemodynamic monitoring, oximetry, and ventricular function assessment by transesophageal echocardiography (TEE) are all performed intraoperatively.

Operative Procedure: Single-Lung Transplantation
Donor Harvesting

1. The patient's skin is prepped from chin to knees and laterally to the midaxillary line. A median sternotomy incision is most commonly used. A thoracotomy may also be used.
2. The surgeon opens the pleura longitudinally posterior to the sternum, and divides the pericardium back to the hilum on both sides. The inferior pulmonary ligament is dissected, pleural adhesions are incised, and the proximal pulmonary arteries are dissected at their origin.
3. After heparinization and hypotensive anesthesia, the superior vena cava is ligated and divided and heavy silk ties are placed around each vessel.

4. The surgeon dissects the aortic arch free, and divides the ligamentum arteriosum. The anterior and inferior margins of the pulmonary artery are separated from the main artery and ascending aorta. Umbilical tapes are placed around the pulmonary artery and aorta. A purse-string suture is placed for infusion of the cardioplegia solution in the heart.

5. After cardioplegia and pulmoplegia are established, the heart is prepared for removal; veins and arteries are separated, and the heart is removed and placed in cold preservation solution.

6. Using blunt and sharp dissection, the surgeon dissects the pulmonary arteries free from the mediastinum to the hilum anteriorly and then posteriorly to the anterior aorta and hilum. The trachea is dissected free. The lungs are inflated before stapling and dissection. The lungs are removed and immersed in cold preservation solution.

7. The team provides postmortem care for the donor.

Recipient Preparation and Transplantation

1. The perioperative nurse assists with positioning the patient laterally for SLTs or in the supine position for bilateral lung transplants. The nurse also performs a wide skin prep for exposure of the chest and abdomen (nipple line to knees).

2. An incision is made. Usually a thoracotomy is created for SLTs. Bilateral lung transplants may be performed through bilateral thoracotomies, median sternotomy, or a clamshell incision. The conduct of the procedure depends on which lung is to be removed. If the right lung is being removed, the pulmonary vein is isolated extrapericardially; the pulmonary artery is isolated as close to the lung as possible. The surgeon may ligate and divide the azygos vein for additional exposure; the pulmonary artery is dissected.

3. If the left lung is being removed, the ligamentum arteriosum is divided.

4. The anesthesia provider collapses the lung to be removed, and the proximal pulmonary artery is occluded. If instability occurs after occlusion, CPB may be required. In some cases femoral bypass is initiated. If the patient remains stable, the pneumonectomy is performed.

5. Pulmonary veins are divided extrapericardially. The first branch of the pulmonary artery and descending branch are separated. The blood supply to the bronchus is preserved by not dissecting tissue around the bronchus.

6. The surgeon divides the bronchus and removes the lung. The pericardium is opened around the pulmonary veins to allow room for the atrial clamp.

7. Inferior and superior pulmonary veins are incised and joined.

8. Three anastomoses are completed for an SLT: bronchus to bronchus, pulmonary artery to pulmonary artery, and recipient pulmonary veins to donor atrial cuff. Techniques used to minimize bronchial anastomotic complications include shortening the donor bronchial stump, reinforcing the anastomosis with a vascularized tissue pedicle such as omentum or intercostal muscle pedicle flap, or using an intussuscepting bronchial anastomosis technique.

9. After anastomoses and restoration of circulation, the lung is fully inflated and observed. Chest tubes are placed and secured.

10. After closure of the chest the surgeon performs a bronchoscopy to remove secretions and to ensure that the anastomosis is intact.

Key Points

- Patients undergoing thoracic surgery are at risk for impaired gas exchange, imbalanced fluid volume, infection, and impaired comfort.
- Supine and lateral positioning are used most often to accommodate the different approaches for thoracic surgery.
- Correction of pneumothorax is an essential component of thoracic surgery. Perioperative nurses must be familiar with the physiology of pneumothorax and chest tube technology to provide safe patient care.
- Thoracic surgery may be accomplished via open or minimally invasive approaches; the use of robotic-assisted technology is evolving. Diagnostic endoscopy often precedes thoracic surgery.
- Malignant and nonmalignant conditions are treated with thoracic surgery.

Critical Thinking Question

You have just completed an ETS procedure on Ms. N., a 21-year-old who was diagnosed with severe palmar hyperhidrosis. No intraoperative complications were noted. The surgeon evacuated the air from Ms. N.'s chest cavity with a catheter at the end of the procedure and closed the incision. The anesthesia provider confirmed that Ms. N. had bilateral breath sounds and extubated her shortly after the team transferred her to the transport vehicle. While en route to the PACU, Ms. N. becomes agitated and complains she "can't breathe." On arrival at the PACU, the anesthesia provider notes that Ms. N. no longer has breath sounds on the right and orders a chest x-ray. What actions should you prepare for next?

ⓔvolve *The answer to the Critical Thinking Question can be found at http://evolve.elsevier.com/Rothrock/Alexander.*

References

Association of periOperative Registered Nurses (AORN): Guideline for positioning the patient. In Conner R, editor: *Guidelines for perioperative practice*, Denver, 2016a, The Association.

Association of periOperative Registered Nurses (AORN): Recommended practices for prevention of retained surgical items. In Conner R, editor: *Guidelines for perioperative practice*, Denver, 2016b, The Association.

Brashers VL: Structure and function of the pulmonary system. In Huether S, McCance K, editors: *Understanding pathophysiology*, ed 6, St Louis, 2017, Mosby.

Fulch EE et al: Design of a prospective, multicenter, global, cohort study of electromagnetic navigation bronchoscopy, *BMC Pulm Med* 16(1):60, 2016.

Marino KA et al: Electromagnetic navigation bronchoscopy for identifying lung nodules for thoracoscopic resection, *Ann Thoracic Surg* 102(2):454–457, 2016.

Moraites E et al: Incidence and prevalence of hyperhidrosis, *Dermatol Clin* 32(4):457–654, 2014.

Perry Y, Linden PA: Empyema. In Selke FW et al, editors: *Sabiston & Spencer surgery of the chest*, ed 9, Philadelphia, 2016, Saunders.

Rees HC: Assessment of the respiratory system. In Ignatavicius DD, Workman ML, editors: *Medical-surgical nursing: patient-centered collaborative care*, ed 8, St Louis, 2016, Saunders.

United Network for Organ Sharing (UNOS): *National data: transplants by donor type January 1,1988 - July 31, 2017* (website), 2017. https://www.unos.org/data/. (Accessed 19 August 2017).

CHAPTER 24

Vascular Surgery

PATRICIA WIECZOREK

Atherosclerosis continues to be one of the leading causes of death and disability in the Western world. It is estimated that peripheral atherosclerosis, including carotid, mesenteric, renal, and peripheral arterial disease (PAD) (also referred to as peripheral arterial occlusive disease [PAOD]), affects 8 to 12 million people in the United States. The prevalence of PAD increases with age affecting approximately 14.5% of adults over 69 years of age, with men being affected slightly more than women (Conte et al., 2015). This is particularly striking, given that by the year 2030 the percentage of the US population older than 65 years will range from 21% to 24% (Federal Interagency Forum on Aging-Related Statistics, 2016). Many of these people will require interventions for the syndromes of peripheral ischemia, aneurysm, and venous disease.

Interventional radiologic therapy for peripheral atherosclerosis has become common. Aortic procedures are now routinely performed with minimal mortality. Carotid endarterectomy (CEA) has also proven to be safe and effective. Peripheral angioplasty and bypass have a high initial success rate, but restenosis, graft failure, and progression of distal disease still lead to limb loss in certain patients after several years. Thus emphasis has been placed on decreasing morbidity and hospital stay associated with revascularization. Minimally invasive methods and strategies, including endovascular aortic aneurysm repair (Malas et al., 2014), carotid artery stenting (CAS) (Sgroi et al., 2014) (Research Highlight), stenting for lower limb ischemia, and percutaneous transluminal angioplasty (PTA) (Budge et al., 2016), have been developed, and their application and popularity increase. New technologies, such as miniature shavers and laser arthrectomy devices for arterial plaque, continue to be developed (Conte et al., 2015). Perioperative nurses must be prepared for the demands of patient care in vascular surgery. This chapter reviews surgical anatomy, perioperative nursing considerations, and surgical interventions for a variety of vascular procedures.

Surgical Anatomy

Basic knowledge of anatomy is essential when caring for perioperative patients with a vascular disorder. Fig. 24.1 depicts the principal arteries and veins of the body. Arteries and veins have three layers:
- Tunica intima (innermost layer)
- Tunica media (muscular middle layer)
- Tunica adventitia (fibrous outer layer)

Arteries differ from veins in function and slightly in structure (Fig. 24.2). Structurally, arteries have a thicker muscle layer and more elastic fibers than veins. The properties of elasticity and distensibility enable arteries to compensate for changes in blood pressure and volume. Because of the thicker muscle layer, severed arteries are

often capable of contracting and constricting enough to stop hemorrhage. In contrast, veins are more fragile than arteries, and whether its cause is traumatic or iatrogenic, venous bleeding may be difficult to control. Another difference is the presence of semilunar intimal folds, or valves, in veins that prevent backflow. Veins and arteries are nourished by a tiny network of vessels (the vasa vasorum), as well as from the intraluminal blood flow. Both are regulated by the autonomic nervous system, with veins having fewer nerve fibers than arteries. The two systems are connected (except for the pulmonary artery [PA] and pulmonary venous system): major arteries carry oxygenated blood, they branch into smaller arteries and arterioles, and then blood moves into capillaries to venules and to veins. The work of exchanging nutrients and metabolic waste is done at the capillary level.

Blood flow is a complex process that depends on many factors. Blood flows through arteries such that the blood in the center of the vessel moves faster than the blood at the periphery. Because the movement of the blood is in parallel lines, it is referred to as *laminar*. When flow is disrupted by an obstruction, stenosis, curve, or

RESEARCH HIGHLIGHT

Systematic Review and Meta-Analysis of Carotid Stenting Versus Endarterectomy for Carotid Stenosis: A Chronological and Worldwide Study

This meta-analysis comparing CAS versus CEA included 35 studies and encompassed 27,525 patients worldwide. Each study contained at least 10 patients and each was stratified into subgroups according to publication year, location of the study, and randomized and nonrandomized study designs. Factors such as lesion length, stent types, methods of endarterectomy (conventional or eversion, with or without patch), antiplatelet therapy, and clinical manifestation of patients (symptomatic or asymptomatic) were not considered in the present study.

The evidence suggests CEA is superior to CAS for freedom from stroke/death within 30 days of the procedure at 4- and 10-year follow-up examinations, for restenosis at 1 year, and for transient ischemic attack (TIA) within 30 days.

The authors presumed that the inferiority of CAS may be procedure related in which a guidewire is passed through atherosclerotic lesions with severe stenosis or total occlusion. Complications may also be associated with stent design, which incises the plaque and may cause small emboli.

CAS, Carotid artery stenting; *CEA,* carotid endarterectomy.
Modified from Zhang L et al: Systematic review and meta-analysis of carotid artery stenting versus endarterectomy for carotid stenosis: a chronological and worldwide study, *Medicine* 94(26):1–10, 2015.

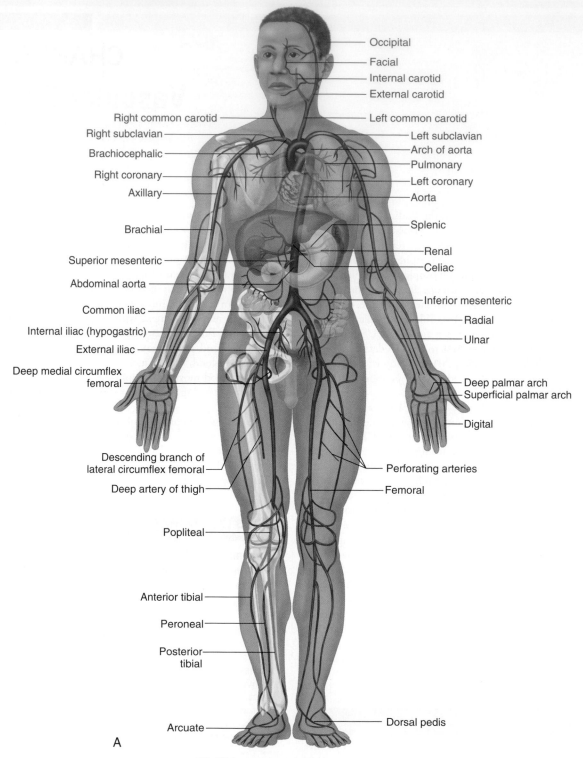

FIG. 24.1 (A) Principal arteries of the body.

bifurcation, the particle motion is referred to as *turbulent*. Turbulence may be evidenced by the presence of a bruit (e.g., turbulent noise), detected by auscultation, or detected by a characteristic Doppler signal. Flow depends on blood viscosity, vessel wall resistance, and the peripheral resistance of the arterioles. There must be a difference in pressures, or a pressure gradient, to allow blood to flow. The gradient is provided by the contraction of the left ventricle. The negative pressure created by the relaxed right ventricle assists in venous return by creating a suctioning effect, and the skeletal and visceral muscles help propel venous return toward the heart.

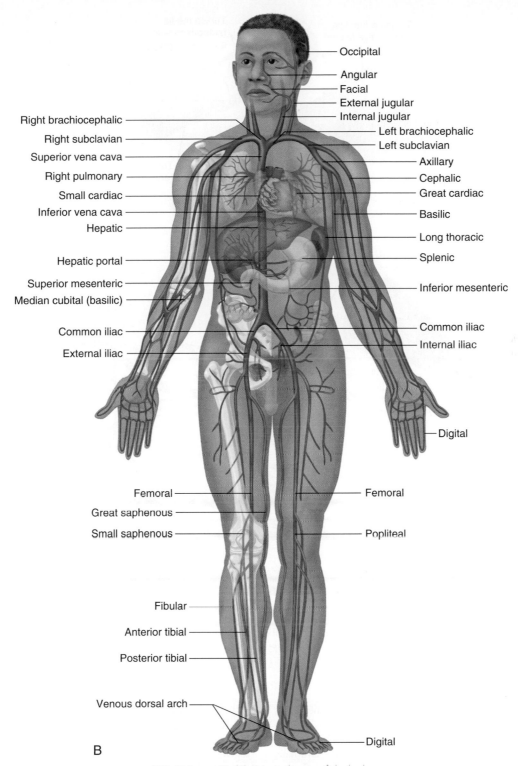

Occipital
Angular
Facial
External jugular
Internal jugular
Right brachiocephalic
Left brachiocephalic
Right subclavian
Left subclavian
Superior vena cava
Axillary
Right pulmonary
Cephalic
Small cardiac
Great cardiac
Inferior vena cava
Basilic
Hepatic
Long thoracic
Hepatic portal
Splenic
Superior mesenteric
Inferior mesenteric
Median cubital (basilic)
Common iliac
Common iliac
Internal iliac
External iliac
Digital
Femoral
Femoral
Great saphenous
Small saphenous
Popliteal
Fibular
Anterior tibial
Posterior tibial
Venous dorsal arch
B
Digital

FIG. 24.1, cont'd (B) Principal veins of the body.

Arterial Disease

Aneurysmal Disease

The most common cause of an arterial aneurysm is atherosclerotic degeneration of the arterial wall. The pathogenesis is a multifactorial process, involving atherosclerosis along with genetic predisposition, aging, inflammation, and localized activation of proteolytic enzymes (Conte et al., 2015). A true aneurysm is a dilation of all layers of the artery wall. A dissecting aneurysm results from a tear in the artery wall, allowing blood to dissect between the layers of the vessel wall. A false aneurysm, or pseudoaneurysm, is not an aneurysm but a disruption through all the layers of a vessel wall with the escaping

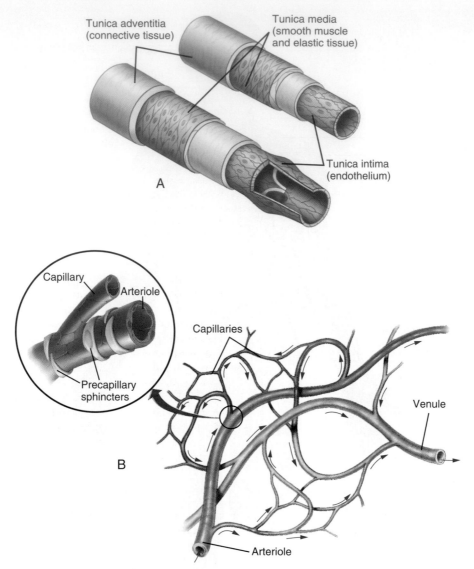

FIG. 24.2 (A) Layers of artery and vein. Drawings of a sectioned artery and vein show the three layers of large vessel walls. (B) Microcirculation. The smaller blood vessels, such as arterioles, capillaries, and venules, cannot be observed without magnification. Note that the control of blood flow through any particular region of a capillary network can be regulated by the relative contraction of precapillary sphincters in the walls of the arterioles *(inset)*. Note also that capillaries have a wall composed of only a single layer of flattened cells, whereas the walls of the larger vessels also have a smooth layer.

blood being contained by the perivascular tissues. False aneurysms may result from trauma, infection, or disruption of an arterial suture line after surgery. True aneurysms are most frequently found in the abdominal aorta but are also found in the thoracic aorta and iliac, femoral, and popliteal arteries. More men than women are affected, and aneurysmal disease tends to be a disease of older adults. As early as 1977, a familial tendency was observed that subsequent research verified; as many as 18% of patients with abdominal aortic aneurysms (AAAs) have a first-degree relative with a similar diagnosis (Conte et al., 2015).

AAAs, which account for most aneurysms, occur primarily between the renal arteries and the aortic bifurcation (Ignatavicius, 2015). An aneurysm involves intimal damage of the aorta and weakening of the tunica media (Conte et al., 2015) or elastic portion (collagen and elastin defects) of the arterial wall. Gradually the vessel wall in the damaged area expands and atheroma (i.e., plaque) develops within the aneurysm sac (Fig. 24.3). An AAA has minimal symptoms and is generally discovered on routine history and physical examination. In men, the diameter of the infrarenal aorta normally measures between 14 and 24 mm and in women it measures between 12 and 21 mm. An AAA is diagnosed if the diameter is 3 cm or larger for men or 2.6 cm or larger for females. Mortality is low with elective repair of the aneurysm (Research Highlight). Dissection and rupture of the aneurysm (aortic dissection) dramatically increases operative mortality because of the abrupt and massive hemorrhagic shock that accompanies the rupture. Aortic dissection is believed to arise from a sudden tear in the aortic intima, opening the way for blood to enter the aortic wall.

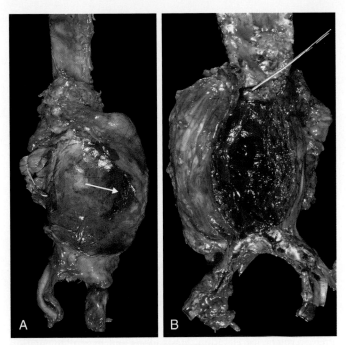

FIG. 24.3 Abdominal aortic aneurysm. (A) External view, gross photograph of a large aortic aneurysm that ruptured *(arrow)*. (B) Opened view. The wall of the aneurysm is thin and the lumen is filled with a large quantity of thrombus. The probe indicates the track of the rupture.

RESEARCH HIGHLIGHT

Comparison of Outcomes After Endovascular and Open Repair of Abdominal Aortic Aneurysms in Low-Risk Patients

The study's objective was to analyze perioperative and long-term outcomes of OAR and EVAR in patients identified as low risk using the Medicare scoring system for perioperative complications and death.

All elective infrarenal EVARs and OARs in the Vascular Study Group of New England database were reviewed from 2003 to 2014. There were 1070 EVAR patients and 476 OAR patients with a mean age of 67 and 65, respectively, included in the study. EVAR was associated with a lower perioperative complication rate (4.2% versus 26.5%). There were no statistical differences in the 30-day mortality (0.4% versus 0.6%) or 3-year survival rate (92.5% versus 92.1%) between the EVAR and OAR procedures. A Kaplan–Meier plot was constructed for evaluation of longer-term survival.

The findings of this study were consistent with other randomized trials involving both high- and low-risk patients.

EVAR, Endovascular aneurysm repair; *OAR,* open aneurysm repair.
Modified from Siracuse J et al: Comparison of outcomes after endovascular and open repair of abdominal aortic aneurysms in low risk patients, *Br J Surg* 103(8):989–994, 2016.

Acute Arterial Insufficiency

Arterial insufficiency may result from an acute occlusion, as in embolic disease, or from the rupture of an unstable atherosclerotic plaque, causing acute thrombosis of the vessel. Emboli usually arise from the heart as a result of atrial fibrillation but may occasionally result from a myocardial infarction (MI), during which a clot forms on the endocardium (the lining of the heart) in an area of

muscle damage. Atherosclerotic plaque can also break loose from other areas and result in an acute arterial blockage. Patients with acute arterial occlusion usually present with the onset of the six Ps: sudden severe *p*ain, *p*ulselessness, *p*aresthesia, *p*aralysis, *p*allor, and *p*oikilothermia (coolness) of an extremity (Ignatavicius, 2015). Heparin is the mainstay to prevent the enlargement of emboli while allowing time for collateral blood flow to develop. In the threatened limb, however, there are basically two options: surgical removal of the clot (embolectomy) or chemical removal of the clot with the use of a thrombolytic medication. If the limb reaches the point where the muscle is rigid, the limb is unsalvageable and amputation is a lifesaving procedure.

Chronic Arterial Insufficiency

Chronic arterial insufficiency occurs because of the deposition of calcium and cholesterol within the wall of the artery. Arteriosclerosis is a natural part of the aging process and occurs when the walls of the arterial vasculature undergo changes such as increased thickness and hardening, reducing the elasticity of the arteries. The decrease in elasticity should not be confused with atherosclerosis obliterans, which is a pathologic process that affects the intimal layer of the artery with the buildup of a fibrous plaque of lipids that can calcify and necrose. Atherosclerosis is the most common cause of PAD, with the probable mechanism being initial damage to the intima and subsequent activation and aggregation of the body's platelets. Inflammation follows, with the deposition of lipoproteins forming an atheroma. Calcification of this lesion leads to the development of an atherosclerotic plaque, resulting in inadequate muscle perfusion and ischemia (Budge et al., 2016). The process is a gradual one, and a localized lesion usually indicates systemic disease. The body develops a network of collateral vessels as an adaptive mechanism to supply the tissues with oxygenated blood. Many theories have been postulated to explain the process of atherogenesis. The inflammatory process of intimal injury, as just described, seems to be the current and most widely accepted hypothesis. Box 24.1 presents risk factors for atherosclerosis. A large number of vascular surgical procedures are used to treat the results of chronic arterial insufficiency.

Arterial Insufficiency: Cerebrovascular Disease and Stroke

Cerebrovascular accident (CVA or stroke) is a leading cause of death in the United States and most industrialized countries. In the United

States, approximately 795,000 people experience a new or recurrent stroke each year (CDC, 2015). Cerebrovascular disease may manifest itself as a TIA or as a major or minor stroke. A TIA is an episode of neurologic dysfunction that resolves in 24 hours. It may be caused by atheromatous debris or a thromboembolism from a carotid artery or the vertebral basilar system. Vascular lesions in the carotid artery occur primarily at the bifurcation of the common carotid artery into the internal and the external carotid arteries. The internal carotid artery supplies the brain with needed oxygenated blood. Obstruction in this arterial vessel leads to cerebrovascular insufficiency.

The right and the left carotid and vertebral arteries supply the brain (Fig. 24.4). The first major branch of the internal carotid artery is the ophthalmic artery. Thromboembolic events that affect this artery may result in visual disturbances, ocular TIAs, or "amaurosis fugax" (complete or partial loss of vision). Patients often describe amaurosis fugax as a curtain over a partial field of vision, usually at the top. Clinical conditions that generally indicate the need for a CEA are transient cerebral ischemia, asymptomatic severe stenosis, and stable strokes. Carotid disease may recur after a CEA. Redo surgery for restenosis poses the same complication risks as the original procedure.

Arterial Insufficiency: Peripheral Vascular Disease

The initial and most important symptom of vascular disease in the aortoiliac vessels and distal arteries is intermittent claudication. The term *claudication* is derived from the Latin word *claudicare,* which means "to limp." This is the most common symptom of lower extremity PAD and occurs distal to the arterial obstruction while the patient is exercising. Many patients are asymptomatic and do not experience pain. When this symptom does occur, it is typically located in the working muscle, occurs with the same amount of exercise each time, and is relieved with rest. This is referred to as functional ischemia; blood flow is adequate at rest but inadequate to sustain exercise. The increased muscle demand for oxygen with exercise cannot be met distal to the arterial obstruction. Anaerobic metabolism occurs, and muscle cramping develops. Walking difficulties are often seen in the elderly patient with PAD. Surgery is not usually performed for claudication unless it is unusually disabling.

The second symptom, rest pain, which is located in the foot, develops as the vascular disease progresses (Eun et al., 2015). At this stage the ischemia is termed *critical.* Rest pain occurs without exercise and is a constant discomfort, often aggravated at night. The body is now unable to meet the oxygen needs of distal tissues even at rest. Rest pain may be somewhat relieved by analgesics or by lowering the legs off the bed. Gravity assists in increasing the tissue perfusion and oxygen supply to decrease the pain. Unless the vascular disease is corrected, nonhealing ulcers and gangrene can develop. Gangrene occurs when the arterial vessels are unable to meet the oxygen needs of distal tissues even at complete rest.

Venous Disease

Acute Venous Insufficiency

Acute venous insufficiency is caused by a clot in the deep venous system, or deep vein thrombosis (DVT). Such venous insufficiency can be a diagnosis of DVT, phlebitis, thrombophlebitis, or phlebothrombosis, which merely indicates that there is a clot, usually in the lower extremity. Virchow, a pathologist, identified the three elements that trigger venous thrombosis. Referred to as Virchow's triad, these elements, or risk factors, are endothelial injury, venostasis, and hypercoagulability (Ignatavicius, 2015). The cause of hypercoagulability is sometimes unknown but is seen in patients with tissue trauma (e.g., surgery, burns, or stroke), malignancy, sepsis, pregnancy or estrogen use, and diabetes mellitus. The patient may be asymptomatic or present with limb swelling, pain, and a skin color change. The danger lies in the potential emboli migrating to the right ventricle and proceeding to the lungs. A pulmonary embolus (PE) can be fatal. The majority of pulmonary emboli cases are caused by DVT. The majority of these originate in the lower extremities. The use of heparin and bed rest is the usual medical treatment. In cases that preclude the use of systemic heparin or in which heparin is ineffective, surgical insertion of a vena cava filter (VCF) may be indicated.

Chronic Venous Insufficiency

Patients with chronic venous insufficiency (CVI) have not been treated surgically as often as patients with arterial disease for several reasons. CVI is generally not life- or limb-threatening. Improved imaging techniques (e.g., duplex ultrasonography) allow better diagnoses of the precise problem. The treatment of the majority of venous disorders is nonsurgical and aimed at increasing venous return and decreasing edema. CVI, which presents with stasis ulcers from postphlebitic syndrome, usually occurs in one leg. The leg is usually very swollen with a cyclic edema, which does not change visibly after overnight leg elevation. Stasis ulcers and hyperpigmentation usually are found in the "gaiter" area (e.g., midcalf to about 1 inch above the medial malleolus) on the leg. The condition is caused by incompetent perforator valves. The perforating veins connect the superficial and deep venous systems. The usual management is to apply 20 to 30 mm Hg of external pressure by means of special pressure stockings. Surgical interventions such as valvuloplasty (direct repair of the valve), valve transposition or transplantation (moving a valve from the arm to the leg), or perforator interruptions are occasionally performed but have had limited success. Patient selection is critical, and long-term results are mixed.

Diabetic and Vascular Foot Conditions

The severity of these conditions is conveyed by diagnoses and sequelae (e.g., necrotizing fasciitis, gas gangrene, ascending cellulitis, and infection with systemic toxicity or metabolic instability). Because patients with diabetes mellitus may have peripheral neuropathies, they may not feel and therefore not notice any tenderness or early signs of infection. These foot infections can lead to hospitalization and eventual lower extremity amputation for patients with preexisting ulcerations; surgical management is often required for the severe infections. The experienced surgeon determines when and how to intervene. Main principles for management include stabilization of the patient, adequate debridement along with antibiotic therapy, vascular evaluation and revascularization as necessary, delayed soft tissue reconstruction, and postoperative information and intervention for medical and surgical issues. In addressing all these aspects, the surgeon optimizes the possibility for limb salvage. This overview serves as a reminder to emphasize the importance of overall adherence in managing diabetes mellitus to prevent further complications (Hingorani et al., 2016).

These complex patients are best handled with multidisciplinary consultations to coordinate care and determine optimal timing for soft tissue reconstruction. Primary closure may not be an option, and secondary healing is not necessarily reliable. The proactive surgical approach aims to salvage the diabetic limb by improving overall health and to provide a stable, mechanically sound limb that will resist further breakdown once the patient is able to walk again. Patients need ongoing support and validation to prevent complications. Hospital

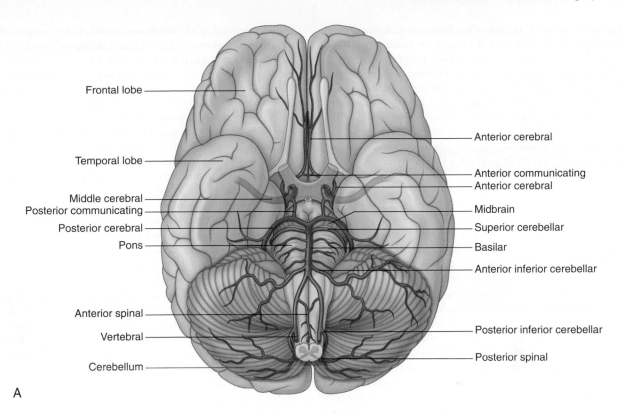

Frontal lobe

Temporal lobe

Middle cerebral
Posterior communicating
Posterior cerebral
Pons

Anterior spinal
Vertebral
Cerebellum

Anterior cerebral

Anterior communicating
Anterior cerebral
Midbrain
Superior cerebellar
Basilar
Anterior inferior cerebellar

Posterior inferior cerebellar

Posterior spinal

A

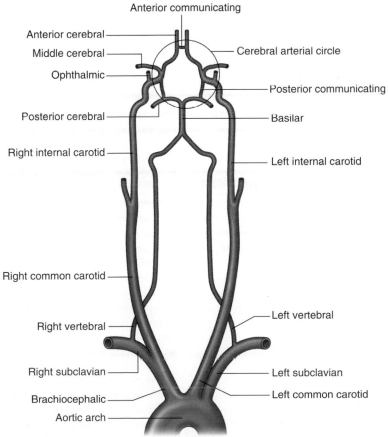

Anterior communicating

Anterior cerebral
Middle cerebral
Ophthalmic

Posterior cerebral

Right internal carotid

Right common carotid

Right vertebral

Right subclavian
Brachiocephalic
Aortic arch

Cerebral arterial circle

Posterior communicating

Basilar

Left internal carotid

Left vertebral

Left subclavian
Left common carotid

B

FIG. 24.4 Arteries at the base of the brain. (A) Diagram shows the cerebral arterial circle (of Willis) and related structures on the base of the brain. Note the arterial anastomoses. (B) Origins of blood vessels that form the cerebral arterial circle.

care focuses on dressing changes, wound care, physical therapy, limb position, and laboratory testing. Postoperative nursing care should provide instruction for follow-up and frequency of monitoring of the surgical results, ambulatory status, work and social restrictions, and bathing. Especially important for the perioperative nurse to review with the patient are identification of infection and ways of contacting the surgical team if problems arise (Hingorani et al., 2016).

Perioperative Nursing Considerations

Assessment

Nursing Responsibilities

A preoperative assessment is necessary for an adequate understanding of the patient's disease, the patient's response, and the proposed surgical procedure. Knowledge of vascular disease and its progression assists the perioperative nurse in performing a critical review of the comprehensive assessment and developing a plan of care for patients undergoing vascular surgical procedures.

The perioperative nurse should assess the patient, reviewing an already completed, current nursing assessment for the development and extent of vascular symptoms. The nurse must assess medical conditions, including cardiac, renal, and pulmonary disease; coagulation status; and allergies (Box 24.2), to ensure that the patient can tolerate a possible angiogram because the contrast medium is toxic and increased fluid volumes are needed if angioscopy or intraoperative angiography is planned. This is a shared responsibility of the nursing, surgical, and anesthesia providers. The patient's nutritional status, the patient's use of alcohol and tobacco, and the existence of any skin lesions should also be noted. Preoperative location, grading, and marking of distal peripheral pulses assist the perioperative nurse with intraoperative and postoperative assessment of tissue perfusion. In addition to the physical assessment, the nurse completes a cultural assessment because the patient's beliefs, values, and cultural practices could impact the plan of care (AORN, 2016). The cultural assessment

---

BOX 24.2

Review of Patient's Medical Record

The perioperative nurse should review the patient's medical record, confirming or obtaining information for the following items:

- Correct and current medical record/chart
- Surgical consent
- History and physical examination
- Baseline vital signs (including height and weight)
- Mental status
- Medications
- Allergies or adverse reactions to medications, topical agents, or other substances (e.g., latex)
- Skin tone and integrity
- Physical limitations
- Laboratory data (e.g., prescribed bloodwork, electrocardiogram report, urinalysis, ultrasound or x-ray studies, and other pertinent tests)
- Religious, cultural, ethnic preferences
- Nursing plan of care or other notations from transferring nurse
- Presence or disposition of prosthetic devices (e.g., hearing aids, dentures, glasses)

---

includes language used for communication, family support, diet and food habits, religious beliefs, and health beliefs and practices (AORN, 2016). An area of specific concern related to cultural/religious beliefs for vascular surgery patients is the willingness to receive blood products if needed. The nurse shares pertinent information gathered during the assessment phase with the rest of the surgical team, including the scrub person, as appropriate.

The nurse greets the patient by name and verifies identification using two unique identifiers. When possible, the patient should confirm such identification. Identification must also be confirmed by the name band, medical record, surgical consent, operating room (OR) schedule, and marked surgical site. Safety is always the first priority. The surgical procedure must be confirmed and the patient's understanding of the procedure and associated risks assessed; inaccuracies or misconceptions must be clarified before proceeding with surgery. Written consent is designed to protect the patient by providing written clarification of the proposed procedure. The National Quality Forum (NQF) identified Safe Practice 10 for informed consent, recommending that each patient (or legal surrogate) be asked to "repeat-back" what he or she has been told during the informed consent discussion (Prochazka et al., 2014). Consents that are valid and obtained freely from a competent person remain in effect for as long as the person still agrees to the surgery or procedure. This may vary by institutional modification.

The nurse assesses patient comfort before continuing the interview and assessment. This reflects caring and will promote nurse–patient rapport and facilitate obtaining accurate and complete information. The acuity of the patient's condition will also affect the order of priority of the assessments and interactions. After reviewing the results of the patient's physical examination, the perioperative nurse should verify signs and symptoms of vascular disease that need to be considered during intraoperative care. Muscle and skin atrophy, the presence of tissue ulceration or necrosis, pain, neurovascular status, skin color and temperature, and other integumentary changes should be noted. Elderly, cachectic, or obese patients are at increased risk for pressure injuries.

The perioperative nurse should assess the patient's mental status and determine the level of understanding and emotional response to the surgery. Patients with vascular disorders usually have systemic disease, and the fear of a stroke (if the patient is having a carotid procedure), amputation (if the patient has an ischemic limb), or other complications may be a realistic concern. A skin assessment should include notation of color, integrity, pain, and pulses. Any musculoskeletal problems that preclude patients moving themselves to the OR bed and any weaknesses that may have resulted from a stroke or that would modify the positioning for surgery should be noted. Correction of misunderstandings is possible only if the perioperative nurse identifies the patient's current level of knowledge and understands his or her cultural needs (AORN, 2016). Identification of the patient's fears and concerns helps with planning supportive nursing interventions.

Vascular surgery can be lengthy. The nurse must consider the effects of hypothermia during long procedures. The patient's extremities should be assessed for color, temperature, and strength of pedal pulses before the surgical procedure so that baseline data will be available for comparison with perioperative assessment data. This assessment evaluates tissue perfusion distal to the arterial obstruction.

Preoperative Tests

A variety of tests may be required to plan for surgical interventions. Segmental pressure measurements give partial anatomic information

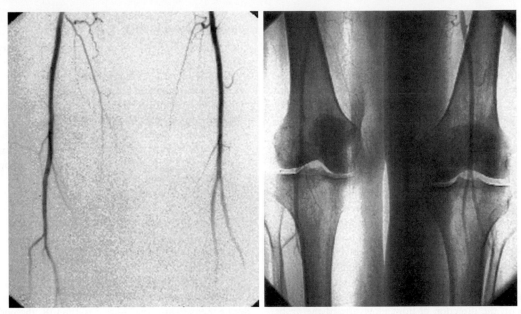

FIG. 24.5 Digital subtraction angiography.

in that they assist in locating lesions. Hemodynamic tests provide information on the flow of blood, such as that to the brain or an extremity, and the effects on flow caused by a vascular lesion.

Angiography. Invasive diagnostic tests may be performed preoperatively to identify the extent and location of the patient's peripheral vascular disease (Eun et al., 2015). The introduction of a contrast medium through a catheter into the arterial or venous system of the patient facilitates this visualization. Angiography also involves injecting a contrast medium into the patient's arterial system and taking serial radiographs of the movement of the dye through the arteries. Digital subtraction angiography (DSA) is one such technique that uses a computer along with contrast medium injection to make the image (Fig. 24.5). Usually one side of the film shows the bone for orientation, and the other side subtracts the density of the bone and soft tissue to allow a clearer view of the vessels. Arteriography provides information on arterial anatomy and the location of stenotic or occluded vessels and assists the surgeon in planning bypass procedures. A venogram (contrast venography) is performed to show venous abnormalities in extremities, the vena cava, and the hepatic and renal systems. Ascending venography can differentiate between acute and chronic thrombosis and can define anatomy. Descending venography assesses valve competence of the lower extremities

Doppler Scanning. The Doppler effect is the change in the frequency of echo signals that occurs whenever there is a change in the distance between the sources of a sound and the receiving object. The probe, or transducer, is aimed toward the blood vessel at an angle of 45 to 60 degrees. This directs an ultrasound beam that is reflected back to the probe by moving red blood cells (RBCs). The velocity of the flow of cells is converted into an audible signal heard through a speaker. The signal is described as a swishing sound. The sound is called a signal, not a pulse. The tip of the probe is made of an element called a ceramic piezoelectric crystal, which can send, receive, and convert signals when an electric current is applied. The element becomes thicker and thinner, resulting in a pressure wave converted to an audible signal. The simplest form is the continuous

wave (CW) Doppler probe. It has two elements: one sends a high-frequency wave, and the other receives it. In a pulsed Doppler probe, the same element sends and receives signals. The pulsed Doppler probe has the advantage of being able to differentiate among vessels of different depths. A normal arterial Doppler signal is either biphasic or triphasic. The first sound corresponds to systolic flow and is forward moving and of high velocity. The second sound is related to early diastole and has a lesser reversal of flow. The third sound is later diastole and is smaller, forward flowing, and of a lower velocity. The pitch is described as rising quickly in systole and dropping quickly in early diastole. An abnormal signal, indicating stenosis or occlusion, is heard as low pitched and monophasic. These abnormal arterial signals may sound like venous signals.

The Doppler probe can provide information in three forms: the audible signal, a visible graph printout similar to an electrocardiogram (ECG) tracing, and a spectral analysis that appears on a screen and may be recorded on paper as well. The Doppler transducer is the most widely used instrument for vascular study. It has the advantages of being readily available, inexpensive, and easy to use. A small, portable battery unit is durable and can be transported and stored easily. When the probe is used on intact skin, a water-soluble gel is needed to conduct a signal. Probes can be used directly on a vessel intraoperatively. The probes are heat sensitive and must either be sterilized according to manufacturer's instructions or be inserted into a sterile sleeve or probe cover. If they are handled gently, the probes have a reasonable life span. Care must be taken to protect the sensitive tip from being dropped or crushed. The biggest drawback of the Doppler probe is a negative finding in the presence of a stenotic lesion pronounced enough to produce a flow disturbance resulting in an altered signal.

A bruit is a sound disturbance that is sometimes described as a low-pitched, blowing sound. It can be heard through a stethoscope over an area of blood flow turbulence that occurs at points of vessel stenoses. Bruits do not provide information on the extent of a lesion—only that an abnormal flow may exist. They occur at points of significant stenosis and are not heard when severe flow restriction or total flow occlusion occurs. The Doppler probe is noninvasive and painless for patients.

Ultrasonography. Ultrasonography is done to obtain information about structures through the emission of high-frequency sound waves. These sound waves are reflected, or bounced back, to the probe or transducer that emits them and are electronically transformed into an image.

B-Mode Ultrasonography. B-mode is brightness modulation, a technique in ultrasound imaging that projects a two-dimensional image on an oscilloscope screen. The image appears as dots from the echoes of the signal. The strength of the echo is shown by the intensity and brightness of the dots on the screen.

Duplex Ultrasonography. A duplex ultrasound machine is a combination of the pulsed Doppler image and the so-called real-time B-mode image ultrasonogram. "Real time" simply refers to the image projecting current, undelayed information. B-mode image is best when the probe is perpendicular to the vessel, but the Doppler probe does not pick up signals at a perpendicular angle. Some manipulation of the probe angle is required to obtain the best results. Color duplex imaging converts the detected signals caused by blood flow into a color, depending on the direction of flow. Flow toward the probe may be displayed as red, away from the probe as blue, and turbulence as multiple colors. This imaging provides both hemodynamic and anatomic information. The technology is also used in transesophageal echocardiography (TEE) and is the diagnostic method of choice for venous insufficiency.

Pulse Volume Recording or Sequential Volume Plethysmography. A plethysmograph measures and records the changes in the sizes and volumes in extremities by measuring the blood volumes at blood pressure cuffs placed at intervals along the extremity. The methods include electrical impedance, mercury in Silastic strain gauges, and air or fluid displacement. This test, which is used to determine the location of an arterial lesion and estimate the severity of the disease, requires careful limb positioning and a cooperative patient. A negative study is a good predictor of low risk for PE.

This test is inexpensive, has good predictive value, and is accurate in detecting thrombosis. It has the disadvantage of a high rate of false-positive results in the presence of old DVT, heart failure (HF), and external compression.

Magnetic Resonance Imaging. Magnetic resonance imaging (MRI) measures the behavior of atoms in a strong magnetic field. This test provides detailed and three-dimensional images of anatomy for evaluation of carotid, aortic, and lower extremity disease (Eun et al., 2015). An MRI provides more detail than ultrasonography or computed tomography (CT) scan and avoids the complications of contrast medium injection and exposure to x-rays. MRI is contraindicated for patients with preexisting implantable devices.

Nursing Diagnosis

Nursing diagnoses related to the care of patients undergoing vascular surgery might include the following:
* Anxiety related to the surgical intervention and its outcomes
* Risk for Perioperative Hypothermia related to surgical exposure and anesthesia
* Risk for Deficient Fluid Volume related to loss of body fluids
* Risk for Impaired Skin Integrity and Ineffective Peripheral Tissue Perfusion related to surgical positioning, presence of vascular disease, and vascular clamping

Based on the perioperative nurse's assessment, identification and prioritization of nursing diagnoses aid in the development of an individualized plan of care.

Outcome Identification

Outcomes identified for the selected nursing diagnoses could be stated as follows:
* The patient will have all questions answered, will verbalize decreased anxiety and understanding of surgical procedure and perioperative routines, and will exhibit increased relaxation as shown by facial expression or other body language.
* The patient's body temperature will remain within normal limits as evidenced by postoperative temperature equivalent to preoperative level and absence of postoperative shivering.
* Fluid balance will be maintained as evidenced by postoperative pulses equivalent to preoperative level, hourly urine output of at least 30 mL, and good skin turgor.
* Skin integrity will be maintained. Skin temperature and color will be within normal limits. No skin injury lesions will be evident, and the electrosurgical unit (ESU) dispersive pad site will be intact.

Planning

Before the patient is transported to the OR, the perioperative nurse should confirm blood availability for the patient, identify if an autologous blood salvage machine is needed for blood conservation, and procure the necessary supplies and equipment for the intended surgical intervention. Because the need for intraoperative arteriography or fluoroscopy for endovascular procedures is a possibility, the patient with a vascular disorder should be positioned on an appropriate OR bed with x-ray capabilities. The perioperative nurse needs to coordinate the availability of x-ray department personnel. Appropriate contrast media, catheters, and impermeable sterile x-ray covers must be available. Radiation-protection devices, such as lead aprons and shields, should be used for the patient when possible and for surgical team members. A typical plan of care for a patient undergoing vascular surgery, using the suggested nursing diagnoses, is seen in the Sample Plan of Care on page 891.

Implementation

Site Verification: Time-Out

Patient safety is of utmost importance. It is the entire surgical team's responsibility to verify that the correct patient is receiving the correct procedure on the correct site immediately before the start of any surgical procedure. The surgical site needs to be marked and visible after draping if laterality is involved. The time-out is a requirement of The Joint Commission. During the time-out, the patient's name, procedure, site verification, and laterality are reviewed. Other items that may be discussed include the consent, anesthesia plan/concerns, the patient's allergies, antibiotics ordered, the patient's position, required instruments and special equipment, availability of blood, and anticipated length of the procedure. Such briefings improve team communication and intraoperative patient care (Hicks et al., 2014).

Intraoperative Monitoring

Intraoperative monitoring for patients with vascular disorders includes the use of the basic ECG, pulse oximeter, and blood pressure cuff. For patients undergoing saphenous vein stripping or amputation, these are usually adequate. For lengthy procedures, such as arterial bypass or reconstruction, the anesthesia provider usually places an arterial line into the radial artery. This line is kept open by a pressurized heparin drip line attached to a transducer, and a waveform monitor reads the systolic and diastolic pressures. The monitor calculates the

SAMPLE PLAN OF CARE

Nursing Diagnosis
Anxiety related to the surgical intervention and its outcomes

Outcome
The patient will have all questions answered. The patient will verbalize decreased anxiety and understanding of surgical procedure and perioperative routines. The patient will exhibit increased relaxation as shown by facial expression or other body language.

Interventions
- Include the family, significant others, or both in explanations of perioperative routines.
- Allow time for patient's questions; provide explanations, or make appropriate referral.
- Observe verbal and nonverbal indications of anxiety; assist the patient with anxiety-reducing/coping techniques that have proven effective in the past, such as meditation, prayer, rhythmic breathing, music, self-guided imagery, massage, and relaxation.
- Encourage expression of concerns and fears; clarify any misperceptions, and reinforce information provided by other members of the healthcare team.
- Provide emotional support and comforting nursing measures (e.g., touch, a warm blanket).
- Demonstrate warmth, calmness, and acceptance of the patient's anxiety.
- Maintain a quiet environment; minimize distractions.
- Document patient's reactions.
- Maintain awareness of specific cultural beliefs or needs.

Nursing Diagnosis
Hypothermia related to surgical exposure and anesthesia

Outcome
The patient's body temperature will remain within normal limits as evidenced by postoperative temperature equivalent to preoperative level and absence of postoperative shivering.

Interventions
- Limit the patient's physical exposure; expose only those body surfaces required for skin preparation.
- Cover the patient's head with a blanket or cap.
- Use a warming device (e.g., a forced-air warming unit).
- Provide the anesthesia provider with a fluid warmer.
- Consult with the anesthesia provider regarding the patient's temperature.
- Use warm saline for irrigation.
- Provide warm blankets at the end of the surgical procedure.

Nursing Diagnosis
Risk for Deficient Fluid Volume related to loss of body fluids

Outcome
The patient's fluid balance will be maintained as evidenced by postoperative pulses equivalent to preoperative level, hourly urine output of at least 30 mL, and good skin turgor.

Interventions
- Determine the availability of replacement blood or blood products.
- Assist with the insertion of IV lines and fluid replacement therapy. Keep IV lines patent.
- Estimate blood loss on soft goods (i.e., sponges and drapes); communicate to the anesthesia provider and surgeon.
- Initiate autotransfusion or use of an autologous blood salvage unit as required.
- Record the amount of irrigation used.
- Document the contents of the suction canisters.
- Monitor and document hourly urine output (as applicable); communicate results of measurements.
- Collaborate with the collection and interpretation of intraoperative blood analyses.

Nursing Diagnosis
Risk for Impaired Skin Integrity and **Ineffective Peripheral Tissue Perfusion** related to surgical positioning, presence of vascular disease, and vascular clamping

Outcome
The patient's skin integrity will be maintained. Skin temperature and color will be within normal limits. No skin injury lesions will be evident, and the ESU dispersive pad site will be intact.

Interventions
- Assess and document the patient's preoperative skin condition and tissue perfusion.
- Position the patient on a pressure-reducing mattress on the OR bed.
- Collaborate with the anesthesia provider in modifications of surgical position required for access to airway and monitoring devices.
- Keep OR bed sheets dry and wrinkle free.
- Pad all bony prominences.
- Maintain body alignment.
- Place restraining straps snugly but not tightly.
- Protect vulnerable neurovascular bundles from compression.
- Monitor and record tissue perfusion (e.g., color, temperature, pulses) as required.
- Elevate drapes off the patient's toes; use appropriate positioning accessories.
- Implement safety precautions for proper use of ESU.
- Reassess and document the patient's postoperative skin condition and tissue perfusion.

Arterial procedures, especially those that involve the aorta, may place the patient at risk for significant blood loss. The perioperative nurse should confirm the availability of ordered blood-replacement products. The use of rapid infusion systems or blood salvage equipment should be determined and planned.

ESU, Electrosurgical unit; *IV,* intravenous.

---

mean arterial pressure (MAP), which aids in the evaluation of the perfusion of systemic and cardiac circulation. This arterial line also allows easy access for collecting specimens for arterial blood gas (ABG) analysis. Continuous assessment of the patient's arterial pressure is a critical part of the surgical procedure. Pulmonary capillary wedge pressure, as an index of left atrial pressure (LAP), may be monitored depending on the patient's physiologic status. A general anesthetic may be administered and the patient intubated; local or regional anesthesia may also be used, depending on the surgical intervention. Epidural catheters may be placed to provide intraoperative anesthesia that can be augmented to accommodate increased surgical time, as opposed to a spinal anesthetic, which provides a finite period of anesthesia. Epidural catheters may be left in place postoperatively for pain management as well. Because many patients undergoing vascular surgery have generalized atherosclerotic disease, the perioperative nurse should be constantly alert for cardiac dysrhythmias and blood pressure changes. Acid-base balance and pulmonary gas exchange are assessed from the ABG analysis.

The anesthesia provider may also place a central venous pressure (CVP) catheter or PA catheter, usually by way of the right internal jugular vein. The CVP line allows assessment of blood volume and vascular tone. The PA catheter monitors cardiac output, fluid balance, and the cardiac response to medications. PA catheters are commonly used for patients undergoing aortic surgery or for patients with cardiac disease.

A TEE may be used to monitor the heart noninvasively during aortic surgery. The device looks similar to a bronchoscope and can be passed down the esophagus to provide an ultrasonic image. The cardiac structures, blood flow, wall motion, and great vessels can be observed. Use of TEE requires highly skilled personnel and may be unavailable in all surgical settings.

Electroencephalographic (EEG) monitoring is used for patients undergoing a CEA and allows for immediate observation of the slowing of brain waves caused by cerebral ischemia or reduced perfusion. The surgeon may elect to place a temporary shunt in the artery if this occurs during clamping, potentially reducing the chances of perioperative stroke.

The perioperative nurse inserts a urinary catheter for many procedures, including the following: if the proposed procedure involves the renal arteries or clamping of the aorta above the renal arteries; if considerable blood loss is anticipated; if the planned procedure time is lengthy; or whenever spinal or epidural anesthesia is used, because they delay the patient's ability to void voluntarily. Urinary catheterization facilitates accurate hourly measurements of urine during and after the surgical procedure and assists in the assessment of renal perfusion and fluid status.

Positioning

Positioning of the patient undergoing vascular surgery is of particular importance because of restricted circulation distal to the area of arterial obstruction and a generalized state of poor circulation. Particular care must be exercised in positioning elderly patients (see Chapter 27). Awareness of joint range-of-motion limitations attributable to immobility or joint surgery is critical even for a procedure as routine as urinary catheter insertion. Again, preoperative assessment can prevent injury and decrease OR time. Whenever possible, the perioperative nurse should have the patient demonstrate the ability to assume the position for the proposed procedure and provide feedback. A footboard may be applied to the OR bed to prevent the weight of drapes resting on the patient's lower extremities. A head support may be used to position the head. A roll may be placed between the scapulae. For surgical procedures involving a lower extremity, the patient's thigh may be externally rotated and abducted with the knee flexed. A small bolster may be used under the knee to support the patient's leg. Proper skeletal alignment during surgery prevents injury to the neuromuscular system. The nurse pays close attention to the skin overlying bony prominences, especially the heels, sacrum, and elbows, and uses the proper supports and pads to prevent pressure and potential positioning injury to the patient. If the procedure will be lengthy, a pressure-reducing mattress or pad can be placed on the OR bed to help prevent patient injury. Arms

are placed on padded armboards with the palms up and fingers extended. Armboards are maintained at less than a 90-degree angle to prevent brachial plexus stretch. If there are surgical reasons to tuck the arms at the side, the elbows are padded to protect the ulnar nerve, the palms face inward, and the wrist is maintained in a neutral position (Sorensen et al., 2016). A drape secures the arms. It should be tucked snuggly under the patient, not under the mattress. This prevents the arm from shifting downward intraoperatively and resting against the OR bed rail. During the procedure the perioperative nurse and scrub person continually monitor the sterile field to ensure heavy instruments and drapes do not rest on the patient's body and cause pressure injuries.

Skin Preparation and Draping

Skin preparation for vascular surgery may be extensive. The patient's hair should be removed preoperatively only if it interferes with the procedure; if hair removal is necessary, it should be done immediately before the surgical procedure using clippers (Evidence for Practice), not a razor. For carotid surgery, a nurse or surgeon preps the patient from the ear and chin on the affected side to below the clavicle (Fig. 24.6A). For abdominal aortic surgery, the patient's skin is prepped from the nipple line to the midthigh area (see Fig. 24.6B). For peripheral vascular surgery on the lower extremities, the nurse or surgeon preps the patient from the umbilicus to the feet. The patient's legs are prepped circumferentially. It is important that alcohol-based prep solutions are allowed to dry completely before applying the surgical drapes and starting the surgical procedure.

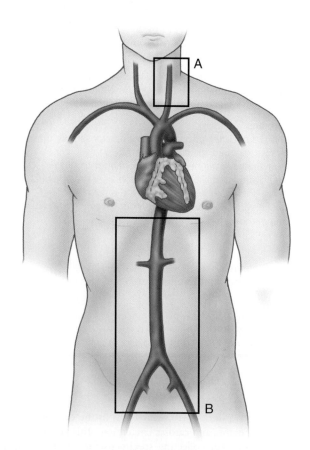

FIG. 24.6 Surgical skin prep (A) for carotid endarterectomy and (B) for abdominal aortic aneurysm procedures.

Draping should permit the surgeon free access to involved areas. For example, abdominal surgery may also require exposure of the groin region for possible exploration of the femoral arteries. A femoral-popliteal bypass on one leg may require access to the other leg for saphenous vein harvesting. Impervious drapes should be used to prevent contamination of the surgical field from blood and irrigation fluids.

Medications and Solutions

In vascular surgery, several medications may be present on the sterile field at any given time (Surgical Pharmacology). These may include heparin, heparinized saline, protamine sulfate, and papaverine

---

EVIDENCE FOR PRACTICE

Reducing the Risks of Surgical Site Infections: Preoperative Hair Removal

SSIs can be devastating to patients. An infection may mean a prolonged hospital stay, additional surgical procedures, or even death in an extreme case. A systematic literature review showed that clinical studies done in the early 1990s indicated that shaving with a razor increased the frequency of SSIs and that using clippers is the preferred method for hair removal when hair removal is deemed necessary. The increased SSI risk associated with shaving versus clipping is attributed to microscopic cuts in the skin that later serve as foci for bacterial multiplication. The CDC developed guidelines to reduce the risks of surgical site infections using this evidence of best practice from the literature. Following the CDC's recommended guidelines for hair removal to reduce the risks of SSIs equates to providing optimal patient care.

CDC, Centers for Disease Control and Prevention; SSI, surgical site infection.
Modified from Lefebvre A et al: Preoperative hair removal and surgical site infections: network meta-analysis of randomized controlled trials, J Hosp Infect 91(2):100–108, 2015; Mangram A et al: Guideline for prevention of surgical site infection, 1999. Hospital Infection Control Practices Advisory Committee, Infect Control Hosp Epidemiol 20(4):250–278, 1999.

---

hydrochloride, as well as local anesthetic medications and contrast dye. All medications and solutions on and off the sterile field must be labeled (Brown, 2014). Heparin is the most common medication used in vascular surgery and may be given as an intravenous (IV) bolus by the anesthesia provider for systemic anticoagulation. When administered parenterally, heparin has a rapid onset of action, peaks in minutes, and has a 2- to 6-hour duration. Because it is metabolized in the liver and excreted by the kidneys, the effects of heparin may be prolonged in patients with liver and renal disease. The anticoagulant effects may be monitored by measurement of the activated partial thromboplastin time (APTT) or partial thromboplastin time (PTT). Patients are given anticoagulants just before the placement of a vascular clamp to prevent a thromboembolic event. The effects of systemic heparin may or may not need to be reversed at the end of the surgical procedure. Monitoring the activated clotting time (ACT) intraoperatively provides useful data for judging the need for reversal or additional medication. The effects of heparin can be reversed by the administration of protamine sulfate.

Because protamine sulfate is derived from fish sperm and testes, caution is advised when administering it to patients who are allergic to fish or who have received protamine-containing insulin. One milligram of protamine neutralizes 100 mg of heparin. The dose should be calculated to offset half of the last dose of heparin. Protamine must be given slowly, at a maximum rate of 50 mg in 10 minutes, or dyspnea, flushing, bradycardia, and severe hypotension may occur. Another reason for monitoring heparin dose is that protamine, given in the absence of circulating heparin, acts as an anticoagulant and could delay hemostasis intraoperatively.

Heparinized saline solution is often used during vascular surgery for irrigation. It may be used to irrigate a blood vessel lumen during surgery, usually after the patient has been systemically heparinized. It is also commonly used to flush the lumen of tubes used to shunt blood. The strength of the heparin solution will vary according to the manufacturer's recommendations for certain implant devices or by the surgeon's preference. A reasonable range is 250 to 1000 units in 250 mL of normal saline.

SURGICAL PHARMACOLOGY

Medications Used in Vascular Surgery

Medication/Category	Dosage/Route	Purpose/Action	Adverse Reactions	Nursing Implications
Heparin/anticoagulant	5000 units IV for systemic anticoagulation during a surgical procedure (IV bolus), followed by maintenance infusion based on ACTs	Prevention of blood clot formation by inactivating thrombin and preventing the conversion of fibrinogen to fibrin	Hemorrhage, thrombocytopenia, abnormal liver function tests, hypersensitivity, allergic reaction	Increased bleeding
Protamine sulfate/antiheparin agent	IV: 1 mg of protamine neutralizes not less than 100 USP heparin units given over a 10-min period	Neutralization of heparin	IV administration may cause sudden decrease in blood pressure, bradycardia, and anaphylactic reactions. This medication must be infused slowly	Patients with a fish allergy may develop hypersensitivity to protamine. Overdose may cause increased bleeding
Papaverine hydrochloride/alkaloid	IV or intramuscular IV: 1–4 mL (30 mg/mL)	Smooth muscle relaxant, reduces vasospasm	Slight rise in blood pressure, increase in heart rate, excessive sedation, skin rash, abdominal discomfort, nausea, vomiting, weakness	Should be used with caution in patients with glaucoma

ACT, Activated clotting time; IV, intravenous injection; USP, United States Pharmacopeia.
Modified from Prescriber's Digital Reference (PDR): Physicians' desk reference (website). www.pdr.net/. (Accessed 23 September 2016).

Surgeon preferences differ regarding solutions with which to distend, irrigate, or store vein grafts. Some surgeons prefer a cold solution to decrease the metabolic demands of the vessel, whereas others believe this may lead to spasm. Spasm may be of particular concern when working with the small vessels of the distal leg or foot. Papaverine hydrochloride (HCl) may be added to a heparinized saline solution for its direct antispasmodic effect on the smooth muscle of the vessel wall and for its vasodilating properties. A reasonable dose is 120 mg in 250 mL of saline. The pressure of a handheld syringe to distend vein grafts has been viewed as a potential cause of graft failure or graft stenosis because this causes endothelial damage. Papaverine HCl, as a smooth muscle relaxant, allows distention at a lower pressure and may decrease the risk of injury. Concentrations for infiltration range from 0.05 to 0.6 mg/mL, or 12.5 to 150 mg per 250 mL of solution.

Topical hemostatic agents may be needed. Absorbable hemostatics are effective by creating an environment that promotes the adhesion of platelets. For example, an absorbable gelatin sponge may be applied to a bleeding surface to provide a matrix into which clots form. It may be applied dry, moistened with saline, or soaked in a topical thrombin-saline solution; 100 to 2000 National Institutes of Health (NIH) units of thrombin per 1 mL of saline or blood may be applied to control bleeding.

Infections of prosthetic vascular grafts are rare but extremely serious. Infection may be life-threatening for patients with aortic grafts or may be limb-threatening in lower extremity procedures. Protecting the prosthetic graft from contact with the skin is essential to prevent bacterial contamination. Prophylactic IV antibiotics that provide coverage for any likely organisms to be encountered in the procedure should be administered within 1 hour before the surgical incision (Tillman et al., 2013). In some institutions medical staff–approved protocols are available for selection of the appropriate antibiotic.

Vascular Prostheses

Vascular grafting materials and techniques are of major importance to the field of vascular surgery for bypass procedures and reconstruction. The understanding, study, and comparison of new prosthetic grafts; utilization and preparation of autogenous grafts; and knowledge of long-term patency rates are critical to improving patient outcomes. Grafts are made in various sizes and configurations; they may be straight, tapered, or Y-shaped (i.e., bifurcated); or they may be pieces of material cut for use as a patch. The arteriotomy from a CEA may be closed primarily or with a patch of either vein or synthetic fabric. In aortic surgery a straight tube or a bifurcated synthetic graft is used. Dacron (polyester) grafts are the usual choice and have been used successfully for many years. Large vessels, such as the aorta, have high flow rates and thus have a low incidence of thrombus formation and excellent graft-patency rate. Desirable characteristics for vascular grafts are that they are reasonably priced, readily available in a variety of sizes, suitable for use anywhere in the body, biocompatible and hypoallergenic, and able to survive repeated sterilizations. Grafts should be easy to handle and last a lifetime while permitting blood passage without clotting or infection.

Prosthetic grafts are nonantigenic; tissue incorporates well, which helps prevent infection, and such grafts generally resist thrombosis. For years, knitted polyester grafts were preferred over woven polyester because they were easier to handle, although they had to be preclotted because of their high porosity. Woven grafts are somewhat stronger and bleed less through the fabric interstices but can be less flexible. Newer grafts have been developed to incorporate the best of both

by using velour polyester. They are often impregnated with albumin, collagen, or gelatin to provide ease in handling without the need to preclot. The scrub person ensures the graft is preclotted by submerging it into a basin containing a small quantity of the patient's own blood collected before systemic heparinization. This makes the graft impervious by allowing fibrin to fill in the fabric spaces.

The other popular prosthetic material is polytetrafluoroethylene (PTFE), which is available in straight, tapered, and bifurcated styles of varying lengths and may have external support rings to prevent compression. These grafts do not stretch, and needle-hole bleeding may be troublesome.

Cryopreserved saphenous vein grafts are commercially available for patients who have no veins available because of previous bypass procedures, saphenous vein stripping, or poor quality or size of available veins. The nurse and scrub person must follow the manufacturers' instructions for rinsing these grafts to remove all traces of preservative.

Volumes have been written about vascular grafts, and the reader should consider this chapter an introduction only. The American National Standards Institute (ANSI), the US Food and Drug Administration (FDA), and the Association for the Advancement of Medical Instrumentation (AAMI) are a few of the organizations active in setting standards and regulating usage and development of grafts.

Autogenous vein grafting for infrainguinal bypass is considered the criterion standard. Undamaged endothelial cells inhibit the clotting mechanism by the natural release of fibrinolytic substances and plasminogen factors. Two methods of grafting veins have been extensively studied, and the results are not totally conclusive that one method is better than the other. These are the in situ graft and the reversed vein graft. The in situ method leaves the vein in its place, side branches are ligated to prevent arteriovenous fistulas, and the valves that would impede arterial flow are disrupted with instruments specifically designed to cut valves, called *valvulotomes* (Fig. 24.7). Reoperation is more frequent with the in situ method because of missed valves and residual arteriovenous fistulas. Reversal of a vein graft is performed per the surgeon's preference or when it must be harvested from the contralateral limb. Vein grafts are used in below-knee (BK) bypass procedures. Above-knee (AK) bypasses may

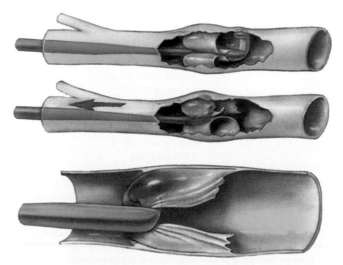

FIG. 24.7 Valve incision with valvulotome.

use PTFE or other synthetic grafts for vein sparing, or they may be used in high-risk patients who may not tolerate the longer vein harvesting or have a life expectancy of less than 3 years. *Atraumatic* clamps with rubber, plastic, or hydrostatic jaw clamps are used to protect vein grafts from injury. Distal bypasses, particularly those in patients with diabetes, are more successful today as a result of improved tissue handling. The surgeon may also use the pneumatic tourniquet as an alternative to clamping the vessels.

Sutures

Most vascular sutures are made of synthetic nonabsorbable materials, such as Dacron, polyester, PTFE, and polypropylene. Vascular sutures have swaged-on needles of various sizes and are available in sizes 0 to 10-0. The suture may be single armed or double armed (i.e., a needle on one or both ends). The size and curve of the needle depend on the vessel and its location. Teflon felt or leftover pieces of graft material (synthetic or vein) may be used as pledgets or buttresses under a suture. They are used when tissue is friable to keep the suture from tearing through or when an anastomosis leaks and needs a better seal. The pledget may be loaded onto the vascular suture or added by the surgeon to a suture already in use. The pledget remains on the suture line (Fig. 24.8).

Vascular Monitoring Equipment

Assessing blood flow through diseased vessels by palpation is often difficult. Physical assessment of the patient's hemodynamic status

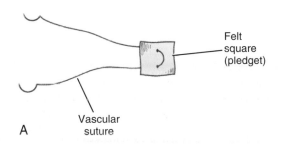

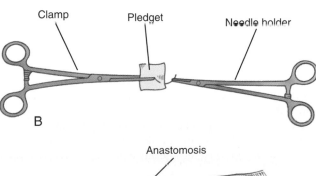

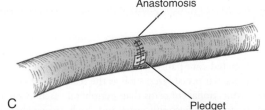

FIG. 24.8 Pledgeted suture. (A) Double-armed vascular suture prepared with pledget. (B) Technique for surgeon to add pledget to suture already in use. (C) Appearance of suture line with pledget in place.

during surgery can be further complicated by spasm of the vessel walls, the cool environment of the OR, and alterations in blood pressure caused by hemorrhage. Therefore the surgeon often uses vascular monitoring equipment to evaluate tissue perfusion and flow. The Doppler device is critical when pulses cannot be palpated. With a coupling gel, the unsterile Doppler probe can be placed on the patient's skin distal to the surgical site. Some probes can be sterilized and used within the sterile field to assess the flow in an arterial graft or determine whether the blood supply to the intestines or other structures is intact after aortic surgery. Along with providing an audible signal, the Doppler probe can provide a permanent record of the sound if a recorder is attached.

An EEG accurately determines reduced cerebral perfusion during a CEA. This enables the surgeon to decide whether to use a temporary shunt in the carotid artery or if the patient can tolerate clamping. Sterile IV tubing connected to an arterial transducer can also be used to check pressure gradients intraoperatively. The stump pressure of unclamped carotid arteries before thromboendarterectomy can also determine the need for intraoperative shunting. Trained personnel are necessary to operate this equipment.

Instrumentation

Most vascular procedures begin with a basic laparotomy set (for scissors, clamps, and retractors) and a vascular set. Items specific to each surgical procedure are then added. For abdominal surgery, a large self-retaining retractor should be added. Additional individually wrapped, sterile aortic clamps; some long clamps (cystic duct and right angle); and long forceps for larger patients should be available in the OR. Smaller vascular clamps and vascular bulldog clamps should also be kept sterile in the OR. For peripheral procedures, a variety of Weitlaner self-retaining retractors should be available. Carotid surgery requires carotid shunt clamps, shunts, microforceps, and dissectors for peeling plaque from the artery. The surgeon may use the saphenous vein as a graft conduit by removing and reversing it or by using it in situ. A variety of instruments are available for disrupting the valves to permit arterial flow in the in situ procedure. Amputations do not require vascular instrumentation. A minor basic set and appropriately sized bone instruments are needed.

Documentation

During the implementation of perioperative nursing care, documentation of patient problems and nursing actions addressing these identified problems is important. Every patient is identified and assessed for allergies, the surgical procedure is verified, and any other interventions performed by the nurse for patient safety and mandated by institution policy are documented. A brief mental status and neurologic assessment are especially important for vascular patients who are at risk for stroke. For a patient undergoing vascular surgery, documentation may include the preoperative and postoperative assessment of the integrity of the patient's skin, the presence or absence of peripheral pulses, the surgical position and positioning devices used, fluid intake and output measurements, and the achievement of patient goals. During surgery various local anesthetic medications and irrigating solutions, such as thrombin, antibiotic, and heparin solutions, may be used. The scrub person ensures that each medication or solution container on the sterile field is labeled with the medication name, strength, and amount. Labels should be verified by two qualified individuals if the person preparing the medication is not the person administering it (Brown, 2014). The perioperative nurse maintains an accurate record of the solutions used and the amounts administered. The recording of ischemic times is captured when vascular clamps are applied and removed from arteries. The type, size, and serial and lot numbers of vascular implants should be documented according to institutional policy and procedure.

Evaluation

Evaluation is an ongoing process during which the perioperative nurse determines the extent to which the patient goals are met. Patient evaluation is continuous as the perioperative nurse assesses, observes, and appraises the results of nursing interventions. The conclusion of the intraoperative phase is the transfer of the care of the vascular surgical patient to colleagues in the postanesthesia care unit (PACU) or the intensive care unit (ICU). A nursing hand-off report should be given, which includes identification of the patient, the surgical procedure performed, any allergies or special needs, location of surgical wounds and drains, and the achievement of patient outcomes.

Some of the desired patient outcomes are achieved at the end of the intraoperative phase of surgical patient care. Others require ongoing evaluation during the postoperative phase. Because perioperative nursing practice is collaborative, the perioperative nurse develops a plan of care that extends from the admission to the surgical suite through safe recovery from surgery. Some goals can be measured immediately on discharge from the OR; others require the collaboration of the PACU or unit nurse for final evaluation. The perioperative nurse thus develops and contributes to a comprehensive, holistic plan of patient care. Such planning and measurement of outcomes provide evidence of quality patient care and provide a mechanism of communication and continuity of care with other healthcare professionals.

Outcomes identified for the stated nursing diagnoses could be stated as follows:

- The patient verbalized an understanding of the surgical procedure and routines. All questions were answered to the patient's satisfaction. The patient appeared calmer as evidenced by facial expression and other body language.
- The patient's temperature remained within normal limits.
- The patient's fluid balance was maintained. Intake and output measurements were documented.
- The patient's skin remained intact, with no lesions or reddened areas; skin color, temperature, and turgor were adequate.

Patient, Family, and Caregiver Education and Discharge Planning

All surgical patients need basic instruction on care of their wounds, identification of the signs and symptoms of infection, review of medications (Patient Safety), schedule of follow-up appointments, and procedure for contacting healthcare providers. Proper handwashing should be reviewed and emphasized to prevent wound infection. Patients who have undergone a lower extremity arterial bypass are most interested in information that will assist them in recognizing, preventing, and managing complications. They need instruction on incision care and bathing to optimize incision healing. Many have had experience with slow healing of wounds because of their arterial disease. Pain, sleep disturbances, and fatigue have been identified as important topics for instruction. Patients are often capable of identifying their discharge learning needs in the preoperative period. Patients should be taught to manage the discomfort of incisions and leg swelling to prevent sleep disturbances. The need to balance activity and rest should be emphasized. Patients in the immediate postoperative period are often receptive to counseling on risk-factor

Teaching the Patient Discharged Home With Prescribed Anticoagulant Therapy

Anticoagulant therapy is prescribed to prevent the formation of blood clots. The length of time a patient is prescribed anticoagulant therapy depends on the underlying condition for which it is prescribed. It can be of short duration or lifelong. The patient and family or other caregiver should be provided with both verbal and written instructions. These should include the condition requiring anticoagulation therapy; reasons and benefits of therapy; name of the anticoagulant prescribed along with dosage, time of administration, and side effects; importance of follow-up monitoring; compliance issues; potential for any medication interactions; and safety precautions. After the patient and family member or other caregiver is instructed, they should "teach-back" information in their own words. In this way the nurse can verify their understanding. Additional helpful information to provide includes the following:

- Use only an electric razor or hair removal cream for shaving; do not use a straight razor.
- Take precautions to avoid injury. For example, do not use tools such as saws or hammers, which could lead to an accident. Avoid contact sports and other hazardous activities that can increase the risk of tissue injury.
- Report any signs and symptoms of bleeding, such as excessive bleeding from cuts; blood in urine, stool, or vomit; nosebleeds; bleeding from the gums; excessive menstrual bleeding; unusual bruising for unknown reasons; a change in mental status; dizziness; severe headache; or blurred vision.
- Take the prescribed dose of medication at the precise time it is prescribed to be taken.
- Do not stop taking the medication abruptly; the surgeon usually tapers this medication gradually.
- Carry or wear a Medic Alert bracelet or tag, and carry information in your wallet naming the specific medication.
- Avoid eating foods high in vitamin K, such as tomatoes, dark leafy vegetables, bananas, and fish.
- In the event of a missed dose, do not make up for any missed dose or double-up on doses. Call your physician if you are unsure about what to do in the event of a missed dose.

Modified from Ignatavicius DD: Care of patients with vascular problems. In Ignatavicius DD et al, editor: *Medical-surgical nursing: patient-centered collaborative care*, ed 8, St Louis, 2015, Saunders.

modification such as cessation of smoking and control of hypertension, diabetes, and stress (Eun et al., 2015). Assisting the patient in setting realistic goals without overwhelming demands is usually most productive. Patients must believe that their efforts will make a difference in improving their quality of life for lifestyle changes to be sustained.

Patient, family, and caregiver education related to postoperative activities and discharge planning for vascular procedures varies. Following an integrated care pathway improves efficiency and length of stay. Major vascular procedures, such as the resection of an AAA, have different educational concerns than peripheral vascular surgery. Patient, family, and caregiver education and discharge teaching for various procedures are presented in the Patient, Family, and Caregiver Education box and should be tailored to the patient's cultural needs (AORN, 2016).

PATIENT, FAMILY, AND CAREGIVER EDUCATION

Education for Various Vascular Procedures

Abdominal Aortic Aneurysm Resection

Postoperative care procedures include the following:

- Maintain intubation and ventilation for 12 hours (varies with setting and surgeon preference).
- Monitor cardiac, respiratory, and renal function.
- Maintain NPO status and nasogastric tube placement until bowel signs and flatus return; diet is advanced as tolerated.
- Perform hourly assessment of lower extremity perfusion.
- Assess pain: Provide pain relief via epidural and/or PCA; provide periods of rest.
- Promote bed rest, with the patient out of bed on postoperative day 1 and ambulating on postoperative day 2.

Discharge planning education includes the following instructions to the patient:

- Feelings of fatigue are normal and take weeks to resolve.
- Incision care: Showering is permitted; use soap and water only, and pat dry. Protect incision from oils, lotions, and powder. If wound closure strips are in place, showering is permitted. The strips will peel away in about 5 to 7 days.
- Activity is allowed with specific restrictions per surgeon:
  - Avoid lifting more than 5 to 10 pounds for 6 weeks to allow abdominal healing.
  - Walk to increase strength and improve circulation; progress gradually.
  - Climb stairs and walk outside as desired.
  - Avoid sitting for more than 1 or 2 hours.
  - Avoid crossing legs.
  - Obtain permission from surgeon before driving. Driving is usually permitted after the first office visit and when pain medication is discontinued.
- Stop smoking because it has a profound effect on vascular disease and wound healing.
- Follow the surgeon's instructions regarding dietary recommendations and medication use.
- Check with the surgeon about antibiotics, which may be prescribed before any endoscopic procedures, surgery, or dental procedures.
- Notify the surgeon of the following: changes in wound (e.g., redness, swelling, increased tenderness, bleeding, drainage), fever, and change in bowel habits.

Endovascular Abdominal Aortic Aneurysm Repair

Postoperative care procedures include the following:

- Transfer the patient from the OR to the PACU.
- Monitor cardiac, respiratory, and renal function.
- Assess peripheral pulses every 15 minutes for 1 hour, every hour ×4, every 2 hours ×4, and then every 4 hours (in general).
- Assess the presence of abdominal or back pain, sensation, and movement in the lower extremities.
- Provide pain management as ordered (encourage the patient to request pain medication).
- Transfer to a general nursing unit within 2 hours.
- Advance the patient from clear liquid to regular diet the first evening after surgery. The patient is NPO after midnight for ultrasound examination on day 2, with regular diet resumed after the examination.
- Perform gradual ambulation three times on day 1 (within 4–6 hours after surgery) and ambulation at will on day 2.
- Discharge to home generally on day 2.

Discharge planning education includes the following instructions to the patient:

- Showers are permitted; tub soaks are not.
- Intercourse is permitted as comfortable, with no restrictions.
- No driving is permitted until cleared by surgeon.
- No lifting more than 5 pounds is allowed for 6 weeks.
- Soap and water on sterile wound closure strips is permitted; strips will gradually fall off.
- Stair climbing is permitted.

Arterial Reconstructive Procedures of the Lower Extremity

Patient, family, and caregiver education and discharge planning include the following instructions to the patient:

- Diabetes and hypertension control is very important.
- Smoking should be stopped because it has a profound effect on vascular disease and wound healing.
- Signs and symptoms of graft failure may include the absence of a pulse in the extremity.

  Implement a foot care program as noted below:
  - Inspect daily (use mirror-assistive methods, or have a family member help).
  - Observe for cracks, ulcers, blisters, rashes, or discoloration.
  - Trim nails properly for prevention of ingrown toenails.
  - Wear properly fitting shoes (avoid walking barefoot).
  - Avoid tight socks or hose.
  - Perform incision care to avoid infection and promote wound healing.
- Apply ACE wraps for leg swelling (normal after surgery) per surgeon's instructions.
- Realize that sleep disruption and fatigue are normal after surgery. Ongoing pain management is important; pain levels should decrease gradually.
- Drive only with the surgeon's approval after follow-up office visit (approximately 2 weeks postoperatively).
- Avoid heavy lifting, vigorous exercise, or prolonged upright sitting; walking, stair climbing, and going outside are permissible as able.
- Do gentle range-of-motion exercise of the leg to prevent flexion contractures.
- Shower as permitted by the surgeon.
- Resume previous diet; follow special diets (e.g., diabetic, low salt, low fat) per the surgeon's instructions.
- Call the surgeon for any of the following: return of preoperative symptoms; wound changes (e.g., redness, swelling, drainage, pain); fever; change in color, temperature, sensation, or use of leg, foot, or toes.
- Check with the surgeon about antibiotics, which may be recommended before any dental or endoscopic procedures if a synthetic graft was implanted.

Carotid Endarterectomy

- Teach the patient about the possibility of reperfusion headaches (patients may fear that they are having recurrent symptoms unless they know about this possibility).
- Explain that if there are no postoperative complications, discharge to home will occur within 24 to 48 hours after surgery.
- Explain that activity may return to normal as tolerated and driving may be resumed when neck discomfort no longer restricts range of motion and the surgeon has examined patient 2 weeks postoperatively.

Continued

PATIENT, FAMILY, AND CAREGIVER EDUCATION

Education for Various Vascular Procedures—cont'd

- Explain that fatigue for 4 to 6 weeks after surgery is normal.
- Explain incision care: Keep the incision clean and dry; may shower with transparent dressing in place. Remove transparent dressing in 3 or 4 days. Wash the incision with soap and water; pat gently to dry. Avoid the use of powder and lotion. Do not shave over the incision until it is well healed.
- Explain that numbness around the incision and extending to the ear is normal, as well as mild swelling.
- Teach the patient about any cranial nerve deficits that may be the result of manipulation of nerves during surgery. Assist the patient in understanding the difference between an intraoperative stroke and cranial nerve deficits; that is, nerve injury or trauma from surgical manipulation occurs on the same side as surgery except for eye symptoms. Use diagrams and pictures to review pertinent anatomy.
- Encourage relevant lifestyle changes as indicated (e.g., low-cholesterol diet, review of diabetic diet, smoking cessation).
- Teach the patient, family, and caregiver to observe for and report any new symptoms, TIAs, mental status changes, personality changes, or speech difficulties.
- Explain that if a synthetic patch is in place the patient will need antibiotics before dental procedures or endoscopic procedures. Instruct the patient to notify dentists and other healthcare providers of this need.
- Explain that if a vein was used for a patch, occasional swelling in the leg may occur. If this occurs, elevate leg above the level

of the heart. Swelling may take 4 to 6 weeks to completely resolve.

Vena Cava Filter Insertion (Inferior Vena Caval Interruption)

Postoperative patient teaching for VCF insertion includes the following:

- Do not bend leg for about 8 hours if femoral vein insertion site is used.
- Avoid strenuous activity or lifting more than 5 pounds.
- Expect that bruising of the insertion site may occur because this is common in patients who are or have been receiving anticoagulant therapy.
- Inspect the incision site for bleeding; apply pressure using appropriate method if bleeding at insertion site occurs.
- Report signs of local infection or significant bleeding.
- Elevate the affected leg and wear elastic stockings to relieve lower extremity swelling, which may be a temporary side effect of the underlying DVT.
- Understand the purpose of and proper way to wear support stockings.
- Report sudden or severe leg swelling.
- Follow instructions for DVT prophylaxis.

Varicose Vein Surgery

- Provide instruction on the proper way to wrap an ACE bandage, the timing of rest and leg elevation, and how to apply manual pressure if bleeding occurs.
- Remind the patient that walking is permitted, but sitting should be limited as should standing in one place. Legs should be elevated when sitting.

DVT, Deep vein thrombosis; *NPO,* nothing by mouth; *PACU,* postanesthesia care unit; *PCA,* patient-controlled anesthesia; *TIA,* transient ischemic attack.

Surgical Interventions

Arterial Surgical Interventions

Abdominal Aortic Aneurysm Resection

Abdominal aortic aneurysmectomy is surgical obliteration of an aortic aneurysm, which may or may not include the iliac arteries, with insertion of a synthetic prosthesis to reestablish functional continuity. The majority of AAAs begin below the renal arteries (infrarenal), and many extend to involve the bifurcation and common iliac arteries. Severe back pain, along with symptoms of hypotension, shock, and distal vascular insufficiency, usually indicates rupture and represents a true emergency condition. The prime surgical consideration when a rupture occurs is the control of hemorrhage by occlusion of the aorta proximal to the point of rupture. AAAs are usually asymptomatic and are found on routine physical examination. They occur more frequently in men than in women. Aneurysmal disease is caused by a disruption of the tunica media, which structurally weakens the aortic wall. Aneurysmal aortas are found to have a significantly decreased amount of collagen and elastin in the vessel wall. Rupture carries less than a 50% death rate for patients in stable condition with a contained rupture. Risks from AAA surgery include massive hemorrhage and hypotension, injury to the ureters, renal failure, spinal cord ischemia, and death. Because peripheral vascular disease is a manifestation of a systemic disorder, it is not surprising that

patients with aneurysms often have concomitant coronary artery disease. Patients are at risk of myocardial ischemia, MI, hypotension, and hypertension. MI is the leading cause of death after AAA repair; therefore it is imperative that a patient with cardiac symptoms or ECG abnormalities have a thorough preoperative cardiac assessment.

The perioperative nurse must be alert to the fact that at the time the aortic clamp is released to permit distal flow, "de-clamping shock" or severe hypotension may occur. This may be attributable to the presence of inadequate volume replacement, the sudden reestablishment of flow to dilated distal vessels, or the release of acidic metabolites. De-clamping shock and hemorrhage have been proposed as causes of renal failure from acute tubular necrosis.

Patients undergoing a major vascular procedure, such as an open AAA repair, may benefit from the implementation of enhanced recovery after surgery (ERAS) protocols, which include decreased postoperative medical morbidity and decreased postoperative hospital length of stay (Enhanced Recovery After Surgery).

Procedural Considerations

The patient is positioned supine. General endotracheal anesthesia is used. The anesthesia provider inserts a central venous catheter and arterial line. After inserting the urinary catheter, the perioperative nurse preps the fields for a midline abdominal incision, and the scrub person assists with draping to permit access to the groin region for possible exploration of femoral arteries. The nurse ensures the patient's pedal pulses are marked before the beginning of the procedure

ENHANCED RECOVERY AFTER SURGERY

Open Abdominal Aortic Aneurysm Repairs

ERAS programs have been introduced to accelerate the postoperative recovery of surgical patients by decreasing the surgical stress response. In vascular surgery, minimally invasive endovascular repairs for AAAs is an important component, but patients undergoing an open AAA can benefit as well.

According to Feo and colleagues (2016), ERAS programs that include opioid-sparing anesthesia analgesia, early oral feeding, and early mobilization after an open AAA repair reduced postoperative medical morbidity, intensive care unit readmissions, hospital lengths of stay, and improved functional recovery.

AAA, Abdominal aortic aneurysm; *ERAS*, enhanced recovery after surgery.
Modified from Feo C et al: The effect of an Enhanced Recovery after Surgery program in elective retroperitoneal abdominal aortic aneurysm repair, *J Vasc Surg* 63(4):888–894, 2016.

so that they may be located easily when the surgeon requests a check of the pulses. This assessment of pulses can be done manually or with a Doppler probe.

Operative Procedure: Transperitoneal Approach

1. The surgeon makes a long midline abdominal incision (Fig. 24.9A) from the xiphoid process to the symphysis pubis and achieves hemostasis.
2. An abdominal self-retaining retractor is inserted into the wound. The surgeon and assistant retract the patient's small bowel, including the duodenum, to the right; they may place it outside the abdomen and cover it with moist laparotomy packs for better exposure.
3. The retroperitoneum overlying the aneurysm is incised and extended superiorly to expose the aneurysm and also inferiorly over the bifurcation and beyond the iliac arteries. Metzenbaum scissors, smooth forceps, and hemostats are used.
4. Careful blunt and sharp dissection is used to expose the aorta above the aneurysm to permit placement of an aortic clamp while avoiding the renal artery and ureters. The surgeon inspects the iliac vessels and bifurcation for evidence of small aneurysms, thrombosis, and calcification.
5. The anesthesia provider administers a dose of heparin intravenously, and the surgeon applies and closes an aortic clamp such as a DeBakey, Fogarty, or Satinsky around the aorta. Opening of the aneurysm is undertaken with a blade or electrosurgical blade and heavy scissors (see Fig. 24.9B).
6. The aneurysm is completely opened, and all atheromatous and thrombotic material is removed. The aneurysm walls may be excised but usually are left in place for eventual coverage of the prosthesis. In either case, the posterior aspect of the aorta is left intact (see Fig. 24.9C). The surgeon controls bleeding, especially from the lumbar vessels, which enter posteriorly, by oversewing their orifices with vascular suture.
7. At the direction of the surgeon, the scrub person prepares the prosthetic graft of appropriate size for insertion. If the aneurysm does not involve the aortic bifurcation, a straight tubular graft is used; otherwise, a bifurcated or Y-shaped graft is necessary. Preclotting of a knitted graft may be accomplished by immersing

the graft into a small quantity of the patient's own blood before systemic heparinization, or a manufactured graft impregnated with collagen, albumin, or gelatin may be used.

8. The aortic cuff is prepared for anastomosis by irrigating it with heparinized saline solution and by removing all fibrotic plaques. One or two vascular sutures (double armed) are used to accomplish the anastomosis by a through-and-through continuous suture (see Fig. 24.9D). Additional interrupted sutures may be needed if the anastomosis leaks on completion. A strip of Teflon felt may be used along the suture line for reinforcement.
9. The surgeon opens and inspects the distal vessels for back-bleeding, and may inject heparinized saline solution to prevent clotting.
10. Each limb of the graft is anastomosed to the iliac artery, using a smaller vascular suture and similar technique (see Fig. 24.9E). After the first side of the anastomosis has been completed, blood is permitted to circulate and the remaining limb of the graft is clamped to prevent leaking during the last part of the anastomosis.
11. The aneurysm may be closed over the graft.
12. The surgeon closes the peritoneum to exclude contact of the intestine with the graft, and then closes the abdominal wound.

Endovascular Abdominal Aortic Aneurysm Repair

More common than the traditional open repair is the endovascular aneurysm repair (EVAR) in which the surgeon introduces the prosthetic endograft or stent graft into the aneurysm through a surgically exposed femoral artery and fixes it in place to the nonaneurysmal infrarenal neck and iliac arteries with self-expanding or balloon-expandable stents rather than sutures (Fig. 24.10). A major abdominal incision is thus avoided, and patient morbidity related to the procedure is much reduced. The benefits of this procedure are a hospital stay of 1 to 2 days, a rapid return to normal physical activity, and a reduction in the mortality and complication rates compared with those of the conventional surgical procedure (Malas et al., 2014). The procedure may also be applicable to high-risk patients.

A number of commercially manufactured stent grafts have been developed since the first EVAR was performed in 1991, using a Dacron graft sutured onto balloon-expandable Palmaz stents. Early tubular grafts have largely been replaced by modular bifurcated grafts that have expanded the applicability of this therapy. Different graft configurations, depending on the anatomic problem, are available. For patients with an AAA that is limited to the aorta and in whom there is both a neck between the renal arteries and the aneurysm and a neck between the lower portion of the aneurysm and the iliac bifurcation, a graft of tubular configuration is available. For those patients in whom the abdominal aneurysm extends to the iliac bifurcation, a bifurcated or Y-shaped graft is available. For those patients who have both an AAA and an aneurysm of one or both iliac arteries, a tapered tube graft that excludes both the aortic aneurysm and one iliac aneurysm is usually selected. The technical details of endovascular repair vary with each specific device, but the general principles are similar. Candidates for this procedure include patients with a proximal infrarenal neck at least 1 to 2 cm in length and common iliac arteries for proximal and distal fixation of an endograft, without excessive tortuosity and with appropriate iliofemoral access. Long-term follow-up data are ongoing, and patients undergoing this procedure should understand that prolonged follow-up with periodic imaging will be required and that reintervention may become necessary (Malas et al., 2014).

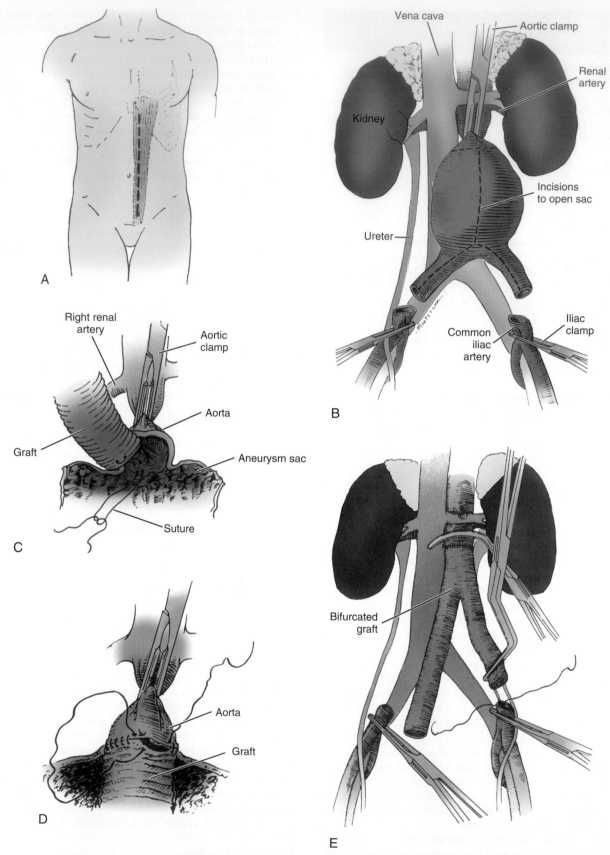

FIG. 24.9 Resection of abdominal aortic aneurysm. (A) Midline abdominal incision. (B) Aneurysm sac is opened. (C) Prosthetic graft is sewn to back wall of aorta, creating a cuff. (D) Completion of aortic graft anastomosis. (E) Iliac artery anastomosis.

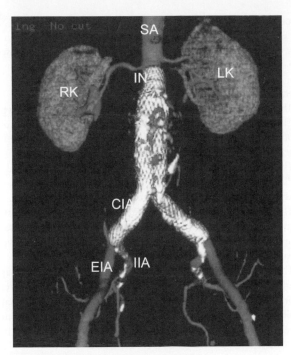

FIG. 24.10 Endovascular abdominal aortic aneurysm repair involves aneurysm exclusion with an endoluminal aortic stent graft introduced remotely, usually through the femoral artery. An endovascular graft extends from the infrarenal aorta to both common iliac arteries, preserving the flow to the internal iliac arteries. *CIA,* Common iliac artery; *EIA,* external iliac artery; *IIA,* internal iliac artery; *IN,* infrarenal aortic neck; *LK,* left kidney; *RK,* right kidney; *SA,* suprarenal aorta.

Procedural Considerations

The team positions the patient supine on a radiolucent OR bed with a special marker board. The board has remotely controlled radiopaque cursors that are used to fluoroscopically detect proximal and distal positions for graft deployment. An ample supply of lead gowns needs to be available. The anesthesia provider may administer a general anesthetic or an epidural anesthetic. If an epidural anesthetic is used, mechanical ventilation is available in case conversion to the traditional surgical procedure is required. The anesthesia provider inserts a central venous catheter and an arterial catheter for hemodynamic monitoring. The perioperative nurse inserts a urinary catheter and ensures that the patient's abdomen and groin areas are prepped and draped to allow conversion to the traditional surgical technique if necessary.

Operative Procedure

1. The surgeon performs bilateral groin cutdowns and dissects both common femoral arteries.
2. After the anesthesia provider administers IV heparin, the surgeon clamps the right common femoral artery, performs an arteriotomy, and introduces an 8F sheath into the right external iliac artery.
3. The left femoral artery is punctured, and the surgeon places a 12F sheath into the left external iliac artery. An angiocath is inserted, and an arteriogram is obtained to clearly mark the renal arteries and aortic bifurcation. The final length of the device to cover the aorta from the renal arteries to a suitable section of the common iliac arteries is chosen.
4. A snare is introduced into the aorta through the left femoral artery, and a pull wire is introduced into the aorta by way of the right femoral artery. The pull wire is snared above the aortic bifurcation and retracted into the left iliac artery. This step is done to help position the limbs of the graft into the iliac arteries.
5. The surgeon inserts the grafting device into the right femoral artery, advances it into the proximal part of the aorta, and positions it above the aortic bifurcation. Fluoroscopy is used to determine proper position of the stent.
6. The device is exposed by retracting a covering jacket, and the graft limbs are positioned in the iliac arteries. The hooks of the graft become attached to the walls of the aorta and the iliac arteries as the attachment systems are deployed.
7. The balloon on the device is inflated to secure the proximal attachment system to the aorta and the contralateral and ipsilateral systems to the iliac arteries.
8. An arteriogram is obtained to confirm proper positioning and complete exclusion of the AAA. Ideally, the graft is positioned to occlude the inferior mesenteric artery to prevent persistent blood flow within the aneurysmal sac.
9. After all the sheaths are removed, the surgeon closes the wounds with subcuticular sutures.

Percutaneous Transluminal Angioplasty

PTA is performed with a local anesthetic and minimal sedation as a same-day surgery admission. Although initially performed only in the common iliac artery for stenosis, PTA is routinely used to treat short-segment occlusions as well as external iliac lesions. Iliac artery PTA may be particularly useful to help improve inflow before a more distal surgical reconstruction.

The use of iliac artery stents has begun to play an increasing role in the management of patients with aortoiliac occlusive disease. Iliac artery stents are most useful after initial suboptimal results from PTA, but they are used primarily in the treatment of complex lesions. When PTA is not an option, a number of surgical alternatives are available. Depending on the condition of the patient and the patient's pathologic anatomy, the options include aortobifemoral bypass, aortoiliac thromboendarterectomy, axillofemoral bypass, iliofemoral bypass, and femorofemoral bypass.

Femoropopliteal and Femorotibial Bypass

Femoropopliteal bypass is the restoration of blood flow to the leg with a graft bypassing the occluded section of the femoral artery. The bypass may be a saphenous vein or straight synthetic graft. The patient must have a patent outflow artery for a successful bypass procedure. If popliteal patency is doubtful, artery exploration is necessary as the first procedure. Involvement of the popliteal artery may necessitate the exposure and use of the tibial vessels for the lower anastomosis. If this occurs, the procedure could require the use of microvascular instruments and technique.

Procedural Considerations

The team positions the patient supine. The hip is externally rotated and abducted with the knee flexed. Prepping and draping include the entire groin and leg. The instrument setup includes the basic minor and vascular sets, plus the following: Gelpi retractors, Garrett or Weitlaner retractors, a device to tunnel, and supplies and equipment for operative arteriograms.

Operative Procedures
Exploration of Common Femoral Artery

1. A vertical incision, extending downward about 3 to 5 inches along the medial aspect of the thigh, is made by the surgeon

over the femoral artery below the inguinal area, and the field is exposed with a self-retaining retractor.

2. The surgeon locates the common femoral artery and dissects it in both directions for complete exposure.

3. The scrub person supplies moist umbilical tapes or vessel loops, which the surgeon passes around the common femoral, the superficial femoral, and the deep femoral arteries.

Exploration of Above-Knee Popliteal Artery

1. The surgeon makes a vertical incision along the medial aspect of the lower area of the thigh. If the popliteal artery is diseased, an additional incision below the knee is made to expose the distal popliteal artery.

2. A Weitlaner retractor is used to retract the muscles and expose the artery.

3. The surgeon flexes the patient's knee, dissects the popliteal artery, and passes a moist umbilical tape around the popliteal artery. Arteriograms may be performed at this time if doubt exists about the patency of the popliteal artery or distal arterial tree.

4. The saphenous vein is exposed via joined femoral and popliteal incisions the length of the thigh or through multiple short incisions along the medial area of the thigh. If the vein is suitable, the surgeon resects the necessary length or prepares it for in situ grafting. If a prosthesis will be used, the surgeon determines the length and size and the scrub person preclots the graft as previously described.

5. The surgeon ligates the side branches of the saphenous vein with fine silk. Finally, because of venous valves, the vein is reversed so that the end originally in the groin is anastomosed to the popliteal artery.

6. If a synthetic graft is used, the surgeon passes a tunneling device beneath the sartorius muscle from the popliteal fossa to the groin.

7. The graft is carefully pulled through the tunnel and positioned to prevent kinks or twists.

8. The anesthesia provider administers IV heparin to the patient before the surgeon applies a vascular clamp to the femoral artery. An incision is made into the femoral artery with a #11 blade and extended with a Potts angulated scissors.

9. The graft is anastomosed to the artery with fine vascular sutures.

10. The patient's knee is flexed, and the surgeon places vascular clamps on the popliteal artery at the site of the distal anastomosis.

11. An incision is made into the popliteal artery as explained for femoral arteriotomy.

12. The graft is sutured to the popliteal (or tibial) artery, and before completion, the femoral occluding clamp is momentarily opened to eliminate air and debris.

13. All occluding clamps are removed, and the surgeon assesses the graft for anastomotic leaks.

14. The incision is closed as described previously.

Femoropopliteal Bypass In Situ

In situ femoropopliteal bypass is the restoration of blood flow to the leg, bypassing an occluded portion of the femoral artery with the patient's saphenous vein, which remains in place. The procedure includes incising the venous valves and interrupting the venous tributaries. The adequacy of the patient's saphenous vein may be validated before the surgical procedure by an ultrasound duplex scan. Varicose veins or a previous saphenous vein ligation and stripping are contraindications to the procedure. The advantages of a vein-bypass procedure include increased graft availability and improved patency. A disadvantage is the time-consuming aspect of this technique.

Procedural Considerations

The surgeon uses microvascular scissors, a valvulotome, or an in situ valve cutter kit to incise the valves within the vein. An angioscope may be used to monitor the lysis of valve leaflets.

Operative Procedure

1. The procedure is similar to that for a femoropopliteal bypass. The surgeon extends the groin incision downward over the course of the saphenous vein. A skin bridge may be left between the groin and the popliteal incisions.

2. The saphenous vein is exposed and divided at its proximal and distal ends. Venous tributaries are occluded with vessel clips, such as hemoclips, or fine nonabsorbable sutures.

3. The surgeon passes a valvulotome from below to the top, usually through side branches. The valvulotome is used to incise the internal valve (see Fig. 24.7). In angioscopically assisted bypass, valve lysis is done under direct vision.

4. The saphenous vein is distended with heparinized saline, papaverine, or heparinized blood to identify any valvular obstruction or open venous tributary. Another pass of the valve cutter alleviates the obstruction. Open branches of the saphenous vein can also be ligated with vessel clips or fine nonabsorbable sutures.

5. The incompetent saphenous vein is used to bypass the occluded segment of the femoral artery (see steps 8 through 14 of the femoropopliteal bypass procedure described under Exploration of Above-Knee Popliteal Artery).

Femorofemoral Bypass

Femorofemoral bypass is an extraanatomic (a route that is outside the normal path) bypass that is performed to restore blood flow to one leg when an inflow procedure is necessary but a major aortic procedure is undesirable. This type of bypass procedure is also used when the surgical risks for the patient are high because of a complicated medical condition or there are technical problems with the procedure (Fig. 24.11). Studies continue to examine the long-term patency rate and outcomes for this patient population. Severe cardiac or pulmonary disease may prevent the patient from undergoing a more extensive procedure. Subcutaneous vascular grafting is an option in these conditions because the procedure bypasses normal vascular anatomy and can be performed using a local anesthetic with adjunct moderate sedation and analgesia. The patient must have one good iliac artery for inflow for a femorofemoral bypass to be considered. Another extraanatomic procedure that can be done in these instances is an axillofemoral bypass involving the subcutaneous placement of a prosthesis from the axillary artery to the femoral artery on the same side (Fig. 24.12).

Procedural Considerations

The perioperative nurse assists with positioning the patient supine on the OR bed with a small pad placed under each knee. The area prepped for surgery extends from the umbilicus to midthigh area. The patient's genitalia are covered with a sterile towel.

Operative Procedure

1. A longitudinal incision is made by the surgeon over each femoral artery from the inguinal ligament to just below the femoral bifurcation.

2. Each common femoral artery, superficial femoral artery, and deep femoral artery is dissected free, mobilized, and secured with umbilical tapes or vessel loops.

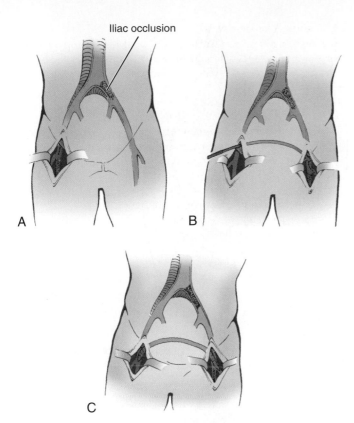

FIG. 24.11 Femorofemoral bypass to restore blood flow to left leg. (A) Left iliac artery occlusion and right femoral artery exposure. (B) Exposure of the right and left femoral arteries: tunneling device creating a path for the graft in the subcutaneous tissue. (C) Femorofemoral bypass graft in place.

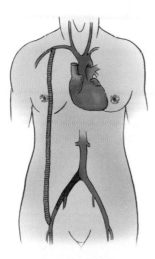

FIG. 24.12 Axillofemoral bypass graft for right iliac artery occlusion.

3. The surgeon creates a graft tunnel between the two femoral arteries across the symphysis pubis in the subcutaneous tissue with digital dissection, scissors dissection, or the passage of a clamp or tunneling device across the preperitoneal space.
4. A Dacron or PTFE vascular graft is passed through the subcutaneous tunnel with care to prevent kinking of the graft.
5. The anesthesia provider administers IV heparin, and the surgeon places vascular clamps on the common femoral, superficial femoral,

and deep femoral arteries. A longitudinal arteriotomy is made in the common femoral artery.
6. The surgeon performs an end-to-side anastomosis using nonabsorbable vascular sutures to join the graft with the common femoral artery. A similar anastomosis is done on the other side.
7. After the clamps are released and flow is restored, the patient's pulses are checked with a sterile Doppler; the perioperative nurse may be asked to assess the patient's feet for warmth and color.
8. The surgeon closes the femoral incisions.

Arterial Embolectomy

Arterial embolectomy uses an incision made in the affected artery to remove thromboembolic material and restore blood flow. Emboli may be clot particles, a foreign body, air, fat, or a tumor that circulates through the bloodstream and becomes lodged as the vessel decreases in size. More often the direct source is a cardiac mural thrombus, associated with cardiac or vascular disease. Pain or numbness distal to the obstruction is the initial symptom, accompanied by other signs of vascular occlusion, such as pallor and absence of pulses.

Procedural Considerations

The patient is placed in the supine position, the skin area is prepped, and draping is completed to permit access to the affected area. The instrument setup includes the basic instrument and vascular sets, including embolectomy catheters and irrigation catheters. Heparinized saline is required.

Operative Procedure: Femoral Embolectomy

1. After making a groin incision the surgeon exposes the femoral artery to permit the application of vascular clamps (Fig. 24.13A–B).
2. An incision is made into the artery with a #11 blade and a Potts scissors. The surgeon carefully inserts an embolectomy catheter through the incision beyond the point of clot proximally and distally. The balloon is inflated, and the surgeon withdraws the catheter along with the detached clot (see Fig. 24.13C–D).
3. As backflow is obtained, the surgeon applies a vascular clamp below the arteriotomy.
4. The artery may be flushed by injection of heparinized saline solution through a small irrigating catheter. Angioscopy or an arteriogram may be requested at this time (see Fig. 24.13E).
5. The arterial closure is completed with vascular sutures (see Fig. 24.13F). The wound is closed, and dressings are applied.

Amputation

Amputations involving the lower extremity are performed to eliminate ischemic, gangrenous, necrotic, or infected tissue; relieve pain; and promote maximum independence (Patient Engagement Exemplar). Amputations may be necessary because of trauma or malignancy or when the lower limb cannot be salvaged by arterial reconstruction. In the immediate postoperative period, patients may experience phantom limb pain in the area where the limb has been amputated. This pain is described as shooting, burning, throbbing, stabbing, or squeezing. Phantom limb pain may recur, but less frequently, in the months after surgery (Virani et al., 2015).

Procedural Considerations

It is critical to verify the correct limb for this procedure. Because amputations are often performed with the patient administered a regional anesthetic, the perioperative nurse must be sure that the patient does not witness the wrapping or transport of the amputated limb. Toes or partial foot amputations may be done in certain

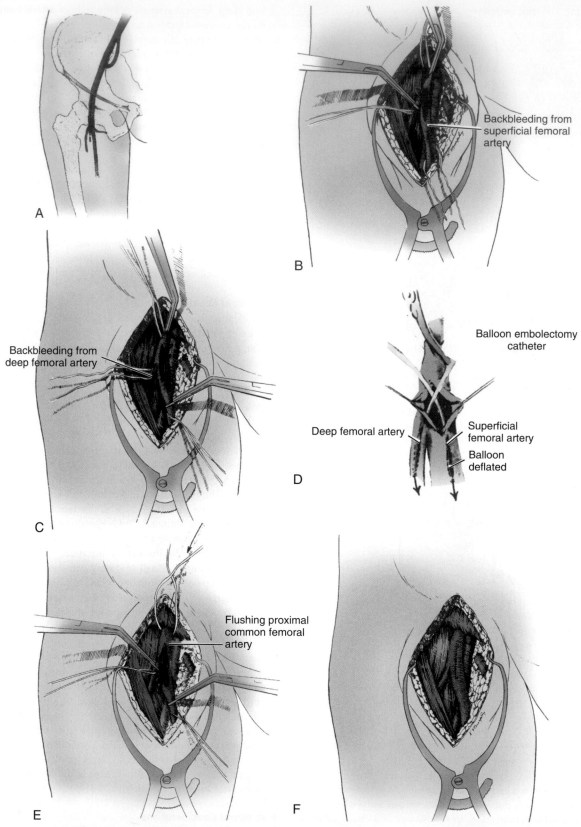

FIG. 24.13 Femoral embolectomy. (A) Femoral arteriotomy. (B) Clamp on common femoral and deep femoral (profunda femoris) arteries. Backflow of blood from superficial femoral artery (SFA) is checked. (C) Clamp on common femoral artery and SFA. Backflow of blood from deep femoral artery is checked. (D) Balloon embolectomy catheters are passed into SFA and profunda. (E) Proximal (common femoral) artery is unclamped and flushed. (F) Arteriotomy is closed.

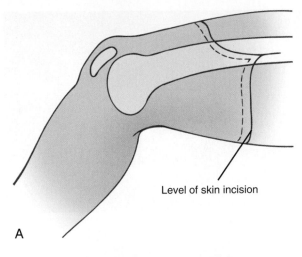

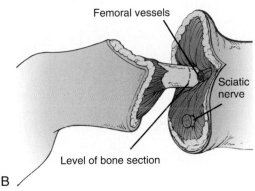

FIG. 24.14 Leg amputation, above knee, through the middle third of the thigh. (A) Level of skin incision. (B) Level of bone resection.

instances, but often a BK or AK amputation is indicated. A Syme amputation, through the ankle, is seldom performed because of improved prosthetics and rehabilitation that favor midcalf amputation. The level is based on the health of the patient, level of vascularity, and potential for healing and rehabilitation. Severe infection or bacteremia may require amputation as a lifesaving procedure. Operative risks for amputation are higher than those for reconstruction, possibly because of more extensive vascular disease. BK amputations are best done at the junction of the upper and middle thirds of the lower leg. This allows for an immediate postoperative prosthesis, aids in better healing, and may reduce phantom limb pain. AK amputations may be at the middle or lower third of the thigh. Flaps are tailored to provide fascial and skin coverage to cushion the smoothed end of the bone. Meticulous hemostasis and drainage are needed to decrease hematoma formation because healing is both problematic and critical in these patients. Individuals with diabetes are at highest risk for amputation because of their neuropathy, altered response to infection, and vascular insufficiency.

Operative Procedure

1. The surgeon determines the level of amputation and marks the incision line to create a long posterior flap for a BK amputation.

For an AK amputation, the anterior and posterior flaps are fairly equal in size (Fig. 24.14).

2. Blood loss may be reduced by using a sterile tourniquet after the leg is raised to drain venous blood. The tourniquet is inflated, and the surgeon makes the incision and divides the muscle and soft tissue. The periosteum is raised with an elevator.

3. The surgeon cuts the bones, the tibia with a Gigli or oscillating saw and the fibula with a bone cutter, and bevels their anterior aspect and smoothes them with a rongeur and rasp. The specimen is handed off the field.

4. The stump is gently irrigated, and hemostasis is achieved.

5. A closed-wound drainage system may be inserted.

6. Fascia is closed with interrupted sutures.

7. Skin is approximated and closed with interrupted suture or staples.

8. An immediate postoperative stump dressing may be applied to prevent flexion contracture.

Carotid Endarterectomy

CEA is the removal of an atheroma (plaque) at the carotid artery bifurcation to increase cerebral perfusion and decrease the risk of embolization and consequent stroke (Sgroi et al., 2014). In most settings the patient is discharged on the first postoperative day. Lessening the likelihood of any transient or permanent neurologic deficit is a major concern during a CEA. The use of a temporary carotid artery shunt (Fig. 24.15), such as an Argyle or Javid shunt, allows for continuous blood flow through the carotid artery and to

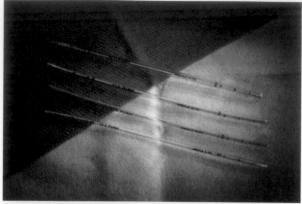

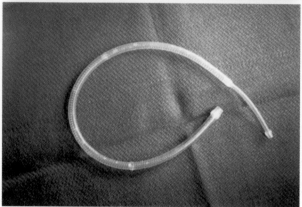

FIG. 24.15 Examples of temporary carotid artery shunts that are used to permit blood flow during carotid endarterectomy procedures.

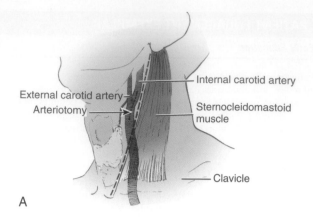

A

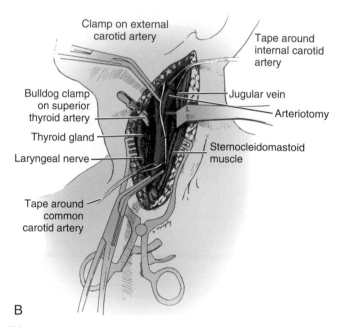

B

FIG. 24.16 Left carotid endarterectomy. (A) Incision and anatomy. (B) Exposure of carotid bifurcation.

the brain. Some disadvantages in using this temporary device are that additional dissection is necessary for its placement and that there is a possibility of dislodging debris when the shunt is inserted. Also it is difficult to view the endarterectomy endpoint and suturing a patch is more difficult.

Two techniques that facilitate continual assessment of cerebral perfusion are the use of a cervical plexus block for anesthesia and the use of EEG. A conscious patient with a cervical plexus block can be observed for neurologic deficits encountered during the procedure. The patient who is administered a general anesthetic can be monitored with an EEG. If either method demonstrates reduced cerebral perfusion, the surgeon may decide to use a temporary carotid artery shunt. The shunting device should always be available and sterile at the beginning of the procedure.

Procedural Considerations

The perioperative nurse assists with positioning the patient supine on the OR bed with the head supported on a head support. The patient's head is turned away from the operative side, and the neck may be slightly hyperextended. A roll may be placed between the scapulae.

Operative Procedure

1. The surgeon makes a longitudinal incision over the area of the carotid bifurcation (Fig. 24.16A) and places a Weitlaner self-retaining retractor for exposure.
2. With Metzenbaum scissors, the surgeon dissects the soft tissue to expose the carotid artery and its bifurcation (see Fig. 24.16B).

3. A moistened umbilical tape or vessel loop is passed around the vessel for ease of handling. Systemic heparin is given to the patient by the anesthesia provider.
4. The surgeon clamps the external, common, and internal carotid arteries.
5. The surgeon uses a #11 blade to create an arteriotomy over the stenotic area and lengthens the incision with a Potts angulated scissors to expose the full extent of the occluding plaque.
6. Using a blunt dissector, the surgeon dissects the plaque or plaques free from the arterial wall. Heparin solution is used as an irrigant to clean the intima.
7. The surgeon closes the arteriotomy with fine vascular sutures. A synthetic (polyester or PTFE) or autogenous (vein) patch graft may be used to restore the arterial lumen if it is small (Fig. 24.17). Before complete closure, blood flow is temporarily restored through the arteries to wash away any free plaques, air, or thrombi. For this to be done, the occluding clamps are opened and closed individually, with flushing of any debris away from

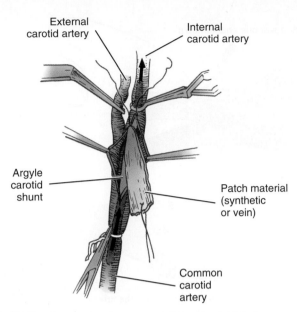

FIG. 24.17 Left carotid endarterectomy illustrating initial placement and suturing of a patch (a shunt is in place).

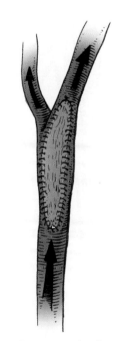

FIG. 24.18 Left carotid endarterectomy (patch angioplasty) with patch sewn in place. Arrows show the direction of blood flow.

the internal carotid artery. The closure of the arteriotomy is completed (Fig. 24.18).

8. The occluding clamps are removed from the external and common carotid arteries; the internal carotid artery clamp is removed last. This sequence ensures that any minor debris missed will be flushed harmlessly into the external rather than the internal carotid artery.

9. Additional interrupted sutures may be needed to control leakage.

10. A closed drainage system is inserted by way of a separate stab incision.

11. The wound is closed, and dressings are applied.

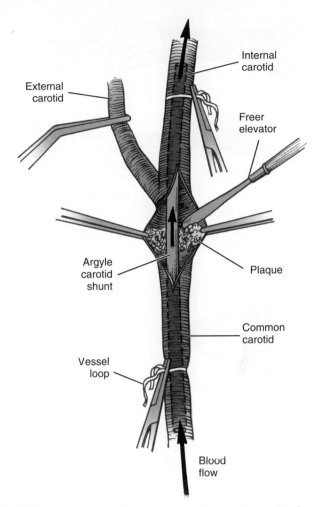

FIG. 24.19 Left carotid endarterectomy. Argyle carotid shunt in place to allow blood flow to the brain. Stenotic plaque being removed with Freer elevator.

Carotid Endarterectomy With Shunt

Operative Procedure

The operative procedure begins as described in steps 1 through 5 of the CEA procedure.

1. To maintain cerebral blood flow the surgeon inserts either a piece of tubing (polyethylene or Silastic) with a suture tied around its center or a commercially prepared shunt device into the common carotid artery and the internal carotid artery. The surgeon then stabilizes the tube or shunt with vessel loops or shunt clamps (Fig. 24.19).

2. The surgeon removes the plaque as described for CEA and the arteriotomy is closed with or without a patch.

3. Before the arteriotomy closure is completed, the surgeon releases the shunt clamp or vessel loop on the internal carotid artery and removes the shunt. The external carotid occluding clamp is removed, followed by the common carotid artery clamp, and, last, the internal carotid artery occluding clamp.

4. The wound is closed, and dressings are applied.

Arteriovenous Fistula

Arteriovenous fistulas (direct connections between an artery and a vein) are the standard means of vascular access for long-term renal

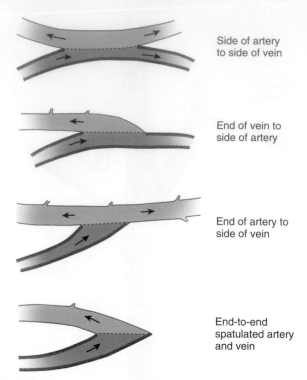

FIG. 24.20 Four types of anastomoses between radial artery and cephalic vein.

Side of artery to side of vein

End of vein to side of artery

End of artery to side of vein

End-to-end spatulated artery and vein

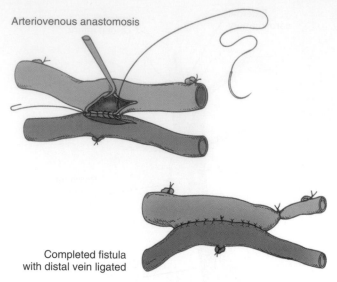

Arteriovenous anastomosis

Completed fistula with distal vein ligated

FIG. 24.21 Arteriovenous anastomosis. The artery is anastomosed to the vein.

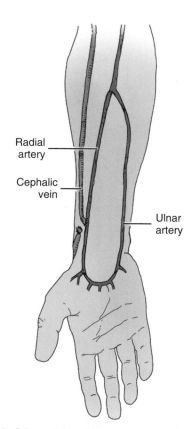

Radial artery

Cephalic vein

Ulnar artery

FIG. 24.22 End of the cephalic vein anastomosed to the side of the radial artery at a site superior to the usual location of the radiocephalic fistula. This technique can be useful if the distal radial artery is small or the cephalic vein at the wrist is thrombosed.

dialysis (McGrogan et al., 2015). The dilated vein can then be used for direct cannulation with large-bore needles for hemodialysis. This method is preferable to an external shunt, which carries a high risk of thrombosis and infection. The best access is achieved using the patient's own vessels and creating a subcutaneous connection between the artery and vein, referred to as an arteriovenous shunt, or bridge fistula. Other choices include using a bovine carotid artery, a human umbilical vein graft, or a synthetic vascular graft, usually PTFE. Four anastomoses that can be created between the artery and vein are side of artery to side of vein, end of artery to side of vein, end of vein to side of artery, and end of vein to end of artery (McGrogan et al., 2015) (Fig. 24.20). The Brescia-Cimino fistula is a connection between the radial artery and cephalic vein at the wrist (Fig. 24.21). A basic principle of creating a fistula is to start in the distal arm and move proximally with subsequent fistulas. These include ulnar artery to basilic vein and brachial artery to brachial or cephalic vein (Fig. 24.22).

Arteriovenous shunts are indicated for long-term renal dialysis access. Patients with end-stage renal disease have their creatinine clearance levels observed. When the creatinine clearance level falls to 10 mL/min, a Cimino fistula may be created in anticipation of the need for dialysis. A Cimino (or Brescia-Cimino) type of fistula has proved to have the longest patency and lowest infection rate. It is created to connect the patient's artery to a vein that will dilate and become thick walled (its muscle layer hypertrophies). This occurs from the high rate of blood flow delivered by the connection to the artery. The arterialization, or maturation process, necessary to allow the fistula to withstand the repeated needle punctures of dialysis takes about 3 weeks.

Bridge fistulas do not need to mature and, therefore, are available for immediate dialysis use. For connections between an artery and a vein that are in proximity, a U-shaped graft is placed. Grafts that are far apart require a straight or slightly curved graft. Although the saphenous vein, an umbilical vein graft, and the bovine carotid artery are often used, PTFE grafts work the best and are most commonly used for bridge fistulas. Some surgeons prefer to use a specially designed PTFE step graft, or tapered graft. These have a

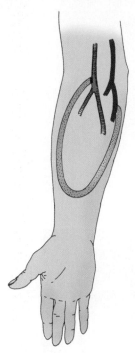

FIG. 24.23 An example of a loop fistula. A synthetic graft has been used to create a loop brachiocephalic fistula.

short segment of 4 mm in diameter at one end and the majority of the graft with a 7-mm diameter. This graft may avoid an output or flow rate that is so high it causes cardiac overload. Primary sites for bridge fistulas include the upper arm between the brachial artery and axillary vein and the forearm between the brachial artery and antecubital vein or between the brachial artery and basilic vein (Fig. 24.23). The axillofemoral graft for dialysis is reserved for those patients who have exhausted other fistula sites. A regular-walled (versus a thin-walled) graft is placed from the axillary artery to the common femoral vein. PTFE grafts can be used immediately, but it is recommended to wait 2 weeks for anastomotic healing to occur.

The side-to-side fistula was the original subcutaneous method introduced by Brescia in 1966. The side-to-side fistula is technically the easiest to perform and creates the highest flow rate. The arterial end-to-vein side fistula has a lower flow rate. The arterial side-to-vein end fistula is technically more difficult to create but has a lower incidence of venous hypertension. The end-to-end construction has the lowest rate of venous hypertension but also has the lowest flow rate. There is a trend toward performing fewer side-to-side fistulas and more artery side-to-vein end fistulas.

Because the patency of fistulas is limited, dialysis patients return for revision or embolectomy in attempts to salvage their function. Unfortunately the success rate for salvage is low and access may be better managed by the creation of another site or a bridge fistula. Risk factors for complications include female gender, African American race, increased age (older than 65 years), and presence of diabetes. Treatment for the most common complication, stenosis, is surgery. Stenosis usually results in thrombosis. Stenosis most often involves the venous anastomosis, and a patch angioplasty is usually performed to revise a thrombosed fistula. Other complications include aneurysm and pseudoaneurysm formation, infection, subclavian steal syndrome, and high-output HF.

Venous Surgical Interventions

Vena Cava Filter Insertion

VCF insertion entails the partial occlusion of the inferior vena cava with an intravascular filter, such as a Greenfield filter, inserted under fluoroscopy using a local anesthetic or moderate sedation and analgesia (monitored anesthesia care). VCFs are generally placed in the OR or angiography suite with fluoroscopic guidance. The Greenfield device offers the option of jugular or femoral vein insertion, and the correct kit must be selected. Box 24.3 gives indications for a caval filter (DeYoung and Minocha, 2016). Several types of filters have been used, as illustrated in Fig. 24.24. The Greenfield filter is the most successful and widely used device, and the mortality and morbidity have been extremely low. The device has progressed from an early design that required an incision and venotomy to the current percutaneous titanium VCF. The filter maintains a patent vena cava but prevents PE by trapping the emboli at the apex of the device.

Procedural Considerations

The perioperative nurse assists the patient to the supine position on a radiopaque OR bed to permit fluoroscopic visualization at the level of the renal veins. This procedure may be performed in the OR, radiology suite, or ICU for critical patients. The patient's head is turned to the left for jugular vein insertion, or the groin is exposed for femoral vein insertion. The right femoral vein is preferred over the left because the anatomy of the left vein often makes threading the filter more difficult. The nurse ensures that local anesthetic, heparinized saline to flush the device, and contrast media are available.

Operative Procedure

1. The right groin area is prepped and draped and infiltrated with local anesthetic.
2. An 18-gauge entry needle is used for right femoral venotomy.
3. The surgeon inserts the guidewire and advances it to a level above the renal veins under fluoroscopic guidance.
4. The sheath or dilator is inserted over the guidewire after all device lumens have been flushed with heparin solution.
5. The surgeon removes the sheath and inserts and advances the introducer catheter to the implantation site.
6. The introducer catheter carries the preloaded, radiopaque carrier capsule. The sheath is retracted, the filter is discharged, and the sheath is removed.
7. Pressure is applied to the puncture site for approximately 5 minutes or until hemostasis is achieved.

Vein Excision and Stripping

Varicose veins are enlarged and distended veins that are visible and palpable beneath the skin. Varicose veins are described as primary

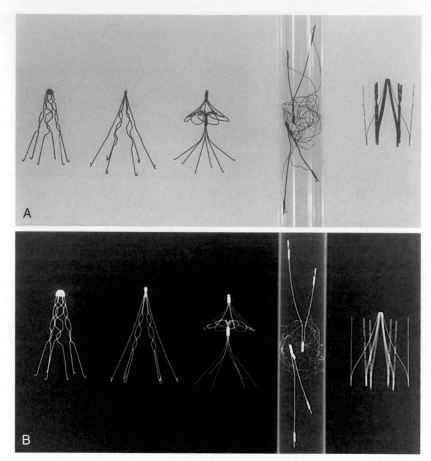

FIG. 24.24 Vena cava filters. (A) Actual filters. (B) Radiographic images. *Left to right,* Kimray-Greenfield, titanium Greenfield, Simon nitinol, Gianturco bird's nest, and Vena Tech.

or secondary. Primary varicose veins are more prevalent and are not associated with a pathologic condition of the deeper venous system, that is, postthrombotic syndrome or a history of DVT. Secondary varicose veins are believed to be a result of insufficiency of the deep venous system. Disease may prevent the normal functioning of these valves, resulting in distention; as the vein wall weakens and dilates, venous pressure increases and the valves become incompetent. The veins gradually become dilated. Veins in the lower extremities are most frequently affected, particularly the long saphenous vein. Risk factors include female gender, increased age, pregnancy, geographic location, and race (more prevalent in Caucasians).

Dilation of the saphenous vein produces venous stasis, which may be followed by secondary complications, such as stasis ulcers. Venous obstruction causes an increase in venous pressure, which leads to an increase in capillary pressure. This causes fluid to leak from the capillaries and produce edema. The objective of surgical intervention is to remove the diseased veins, thus preventing ulceration, secondary edema, pain, and fatigue in the extremity.

Procedural Considerations
Before sedation or entrance into the OR, the patient should stand and the varicose veins should be marked with an indelible marker. This ensures adequate visualization for complete removal of the varicosities because the patient is often placed in the Trendelenburg position intraoperatively to decrease venous congestion, which could

interfere with visualization of the varicosities. The perioperative nurse assists with positioning the patient on the OR bed in a supine position with the legs slightly abducted. Ligation or stripping of the lesser saphenous veins and branches may require placing the patient in the prone position. In the stab avulsion technique, multiple small (2- to 3-mm) incisions are made over the identified varicosities, and the affected vein segments are removed (Fig. 24.25). Stripping indicates removal of a long segment of vein by means of a special device (Fig. 24.26). Drapes are placed to enable flexing and lifting at the knee. Instruments include a basic minor instrument setup, plus the following: Weitlaner self-retaining retractors, #11 blades, skin hooks, mosquito hemostats, vein strippers with various tips available, and elastic bandages. Endovenous laser ablation (EVLA) is an innovative nonsurgical procedure for varicose veins and offers patients an alternative treatment to surgical vein stripping (Ambulatory Surgery Considerations).

Operative Procedure
1. The surgeon makes an incision in the upper area of the thigh, parallel to the crease in the groin, and clamps and ligates any bleeding vessels.
2. The saphenous vein is identified and isolated. Margins of the wound are separated with a Weitlaner self-retaining retractor.
3. The surgeon double-ligates the saphenous vein branches with black silk ties, or they are transfixed, clamped, and divided. The

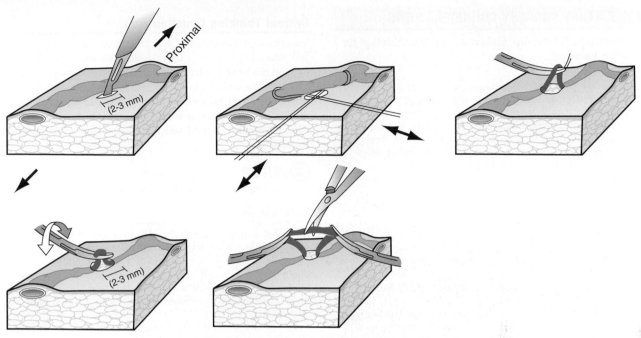

FIG. 24.25 Technique of stab avulsions of varicosities.

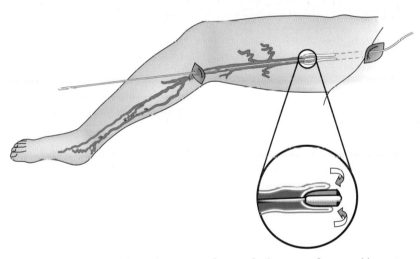

FIG. 24.26 Inversion stripping of the saphenous vein for superficial venous reflux caused by an incompetent saphenofemoral junction.

proximal stump is dissected upward to the point at which it enters the femoral vein, where it is carefully ligated.

4. If the saphenous vein is to be excised, the surgeon makes an incision at its distal portion at the ankle, and the vein is identified, ligated, and divided.

5. A vein stripper is inserted and advanced to the proximal end of the vein in the groin, where it is secured with a heavy suture, and the tip is attached.

6. As the surgeon pulls the stripper up the leg, external compression is applied by the assistant or scrub person.

7. Tributaries may be excised through numerous small incisions along the course of the vein.

8. The surgeon closes the groin wound in layers, and other small incisions are closed with skin sutures or staples. Dressings and circular compression bandages are applied.

AMBULATORY SURGERY CONSIDERATIONS

Postdischarge Follow-Up: Endovenous Laser Ablation for Varicose Veins

EVLA is an innovative nonsurgical procedure for varicose veins that offers an alternative treatment to the often painful surgical ligation (or stripping) of veins, which is performed with the patient administered a general anesthetic and often has a long recovery time. During EVLA, by delivering laser energy through a fiberoptic catheter, a particular vein is sealed to prevent blood flow. The catheter is inserted into the vein with ultrasound guidance. The entire procedure can be done in 1 hour as an ambulatory surgery procedure with the patient administered a local anesthetic. After the procedure is completed, the skin puncture site is approximated with an adhesive strip. A graduated compression stocking or wrap is applied to the affected extremity from the base of the toes to the groin; it is constantly kept in place for 2 weeks and thereafter for 6 weeks when ambulatory to help maintain occlusion of the vein. Immediate and frequent ambulation is encouraged to decrease the incidence of DVT formation.

An important consideration for vascular procedure patients in the ambulatory setting is postoperative and discharge education. Patients need detailed instructions regarding recovery and convalescence because this phase is not complete on discharge. These instructions should include possible complications, activity level, wound care, pain management, and the plan for follow-up. Postoperative phone calls, 24 to 48 hours after discharge, have proven beneficial to identify any adverse events and answer patient questions. In a study by Brenn and colleagues (2016), postoperative phones calls after surgery provided greater patient satisfaction and better outcomes. Although all patients received detailed education, new questions arose. The postdischarge phone call can stress the importance of wearing the compression stocking or wrap to prevent complications.

DVT, Deep vein thrombosis; *EVLA,* endovenous laser ablation.
Modified from Kabnick L, Sadek M: Varicose veins. In Cronenwett J et al, editors: *Rutherford's vascular surgery,* ed 8, Philadelphia, 2014, Saunders; Brenn BR et al: Outpatient outcomes and satisfaction in pediatric population: data from the postoperative phone call, *Paediatr Anaesth* 26(2):158–163, 2016.

Key Points

- Atherosclerosis continues to be one of the leading causes of death and disability in the Western world. It is estimated that PAD affects about 8 to 12 million persons in the United States.
- The prevalence of PAD is approximately 14.5% of the adult population over 69 years of age. This is particularly striking, given that by the year 2030 the percentage of the US population older than 69 years will increase to 21% (Federal Interagency Forum on Aging-Related Statistics, 2016).
- Many of these people will require surgical interventions for the syndromes of peripheral ischemia, aneurysm, and venous disease.
- Perioperative nursing assessments should take into consideration risk factors of PAD including hypertension, diabetes, obesity, and physical inactivity and use this information to plan the intraoperative and postoperative plan of care.
- Also of importance is to maintain skin integrity during the surgical skin prep to reduce the risks for surgical site infections.

Critical Thinking Question

Your first case is an elective CEA. During the preoperative assessment you note the patient is a 68-year-old male who states he has been in good health and is very active. His medical history includes mild hypertension and smoking. The patient expresses he has tried to stop smoking on his own without success. He has normal range of motion of all extremities as well as his neck. Based on your assessment, what information would you incorporate into your postoperative teaching plan?

evolve *The answer to the Critical Thinking Question can be found at http://evolve.elsevier.com/Rothrock/Alexander.*

References

Association of periOperative Registered Nurses (AORN): *Cultural awareness tool kit* (website), 2016. http://aorn.org/guidelines/clinical-resources/tool-kits/cultural-awareness-tool-kit. (Accessed 23 September 2016).

Brown L: Medication administration in the operating room: new standards and recommendations, *AANA J* 82(6):465–469, 2014.

Budge J et al: Acute and chronic limb ischaemia, *Surgery* 34(4):183–187, 2016.

Centers for Disease Control and Prevention (CDC): *Stroke facts 2015* (website), 2015. www.cdc.gov/stroke/facts.htm. (Accessed 22 September 2016).

Conte M et al: Society for vascular surgery practice guidelines for atherosclerotic occlusive disease of the lower extremities: management of asymptomatic disease and claudication, *J Vasc Surg* 61(3):2S–41S, 2015.

DeYoung E, Minocha J: Inferior vena cava filters: guidelines, best practices, and expanding indications, *Semin Intervent Radiol* 33(2):65–70, 2016.

Eun J et al: Measures to reduce unplanned readmissions after vascular surgery, *Semin Vasc Surg* 28(2):103–111, 2015.

Federal Interagency Forum on Aging-Related Statistics: *Older Americans 2016: key indicators of well-being* (website), 2016. www.agingstats.gov/docs/LatestReport/OA2016.pdf. (Accessed 21 September 2016).

Hicks C et al: Improving safety and quality of care with enhanced teamwork through operating room briefings, *JAMA Surg* 149(8):863–868, 2014.

Hingorani A et al: The management of diabetic foot: a clinical practice guideline by the Society for Vascular Surgery in collaboration with the American Podiatric Medical Association and the Society for Vascular Medicine, *J Vasc Surg* 63(2):3S–21S, 2016.

Ignatavicius DD: Care of patients with vascular problems. In Ignatavicius DD, Workman ML, editors: *Medical-surgical nursing: patient-centered collaborative care,* ed 8, St Louis, 2015, Saunders.

Malas M et al: Perioperative mortality following repair of abdominal aortic aneurysms: application of a randomized clinical trial to real-world practice using a validated nationwide data set, *JAMA Surg* 149(12):1260–1265, 2014.

McGrogan D et al: Arteriovenous fistula outcomes in the elderly, *J Vasc Surg* 62(6):1652–1657, 2015.

Prochazka A et al: Patient perceptions of surgical informed consent: is repeat back helpful or harmful?, *J Patient Saf* 10(3):140–145, 2014.

Sgroi M et al: Experience matters more than specialty for carotid stenting outcomes, *J Vasc Surg* 60(2):542–543, 2014.

Sorensen E et al: Operating room nurses' positioning of anesthetized surgical patients, *J Clin Nurs* 25(5–6):690–698, 2016.

Tillman M et al: Surgical care improvement project and surgical site infections: can integration in the surgical safety checklist improve quality performance and clinical outcomes?, *J Surg Res* 184(1):150–156, 2013.

Virani A et al: Caring for patients with limb amputation, *Nurs Stand* 30(6):51–60, 2015.

CHAPTER 25

Cardiac Surgery

PATRICIA C. SEIFERT AND CATERIA DAVIS-BRUNO

Cardiac surgery has consistently reflected innovation and advanced technology since the mid-20th century. These changes have encouraged clinicians to refine anastomotic techniques, investigate new routes to achieve cardiopulmonary bypass (CPB) and vascular repair, design more tissue-friendly instrumentation, and create operative arenas that embrace aspects of both the classic operating room (OR) and the newer interventional suites, as well as hybrid ORs that combine both traditional and interventional components. Common procedures performed in hybrid ORs include electrophysiology (EP) procedures, percutaneous management of valvular lesions, placement of occlusion or umbrella devices to close atrial or ventricular septal defects (VSDs; or to capture potentially embolic thrombi), insertion of percutaneous ventricular assist devices (VADs), and stenting of thoracic or abdominal aortic aneurysms and dissections (Nussmeier et al., 2015; Szelkowski et al., 2015). Growing use of hybrid ORs has stimulated cardiac clinicians to expand their skill sets and develop closer working relationships with colleagues in the cardiac catheterization, EP, and interventional radiology laboratories (Nussmeier et al., 2015).

The traditional focus during surgery, that of the technical expertise and experience of the surgeon, has expanded to include the entire perioperative care team. The primary role of this team is to provide evidence-based care to patients and to prevent harm (Elmadhun et al., 2016).

Other advances in surgery have included the growth of precise, three-dimensional diagnostic images; improved monitoring of neurologic and renal function; effective blood conservation strategies; refined anesthetic and cardiac drugs; and an overall greater understanding of the causes and treatment of glucose abnormalities, antibiotic-resistant infections, and other complications that affect patient outcomes (Nussmeier et al., 2015).

Cardiac surgery outcomes continue to improve. As performance improvement initiatives have increased, quality of care has risen. Other trends that have affected cardiac surgery significantly, in addition to quality outcomes, include heightened emphases on safety, education, staff competence, and cost-effectiveness. These advances promote robust inclusion of patients and families in care processes that focus on desired outcomes. The importance of the patient is emphasized in national measures of quality, evidenced by the Hospital Consumer Assessment of Healthcare Providers and Systems (HCAHPS) (Nussmeier et al., 2015).

This chapter describes both traditional and more innovative treatment options for coronary artery disease (CAD), valvular dysfunction, thoracic aneurysms and dissections, conduction disturbances, heart failure, and end-stage cardiac disease. Therapeutic interventions may use laser, radiofrequency (RF), or cryothermal energies. Investigative alternatives, such as stem cell therapy and viability testing, are just a few options used to induce cardiac revascularization at the cellular level. Still evolving, these areas of investigation demonstrate great promise (Acker and Jessup, 2015).

Surgical Anatomy

The heart (Fig. 25.1) is a four-chamber muscular pump that propels blood into the systemic and pulmonary circulatory systems. It sits within a pericardial sac within the mediastinum, which lies between the lungs, posterior to the sternum, and anterior to the vertebrae, esophagus, and descending portion of the aorta. The diaphragm is located below the heart (Fig. 25.2). The heart has attachments at the aorta, pulmonary artery (PA), superior and inferior venae cavae, and the pulmonary veins. Its ventricles are relatively mobile, enabling the surgeon to rotate the walls of the ventricles and the apex of the left ventricle (LV) to assess (and graft) coronary arteries to the lateral and posterior aspects of the myocardium.

The cardiac wall consists of three layers: the epicardium or outer lining; the myocardium or muscular layer, which is an important functional layer; and the endocardium or inner lining (Fig. 25.3). The left ventricular muscle layer has the most depth (i.e., thickness) of the four chambers and can generate the greatest pressure, which is required to pump blood into the circulatory system.

Two-thirds of the heart is positioned to the left of the midline, and the remaining third is to the right of the midline. Although functionally divided into right and left halves, the heart sits rotated to the left, with the right side anterior and the left side relatively posterior. Injury to the anterior chest (e.g., from blunt force or stab wounds) is likely to damage the right ventricle (RV). This may prove significant for myocardial repair because the RV has lower pressures than the left, thus allowing additional time for repair before exsanguination.

Each half of the heart contains an upper and a lower communicating chamber called the atrium and ventricle, respectively. The right atrium (RA) receives desaturated blood from the inferior and superior venae cavae and from coronary circulation via the coronary sinus. The left atrium (LA) receives oxygenated blood from the lungs by way of the pulmonary veins. From both atria, blood then flows through the atrioventricular (AV) valves into the ventricles.

The LV pumps oxygenated blood into the major vessels of the *systemic circulatory system* by way of the aorta and its main branches to the head, upper extremities, abdominal organs, and lower extremities. The right and left internal mammary arteries (IMAs), used as grafts during coronary artery bypass graft surgery (CABG), branch off the subclavian arteries and course behind and parallel to the edges of the sternum. The arteries of the circulatory system subdivide into arterioles and eventually into capillaries and the individual cells,

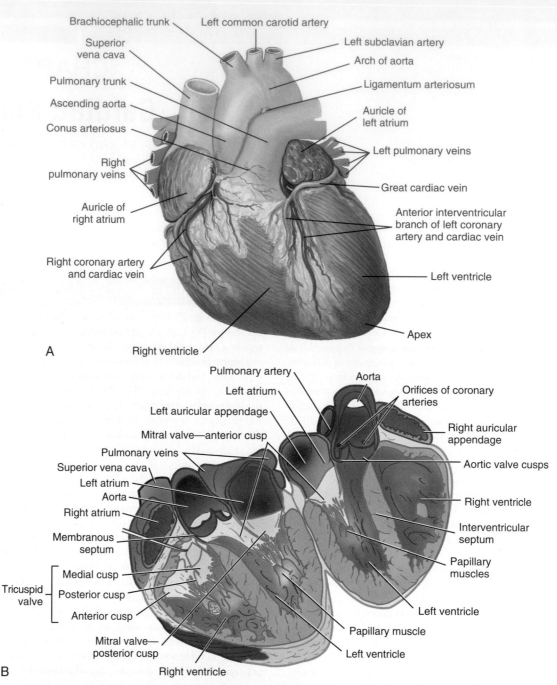

FIG. 25.1 (A) Anterior view of heart illustrates major vessels and chambers. (B) Drawing of a heart split perpendicular to the interventricular septum illustrates the anatomic relationships of the leaflets of the atrioventricular and aortic valve and the receiving chambers (atria) and the pumping chambers (ventricles). Systemic venous blood returns to the heart by way of the inferior and superior venae cavae. It enters the right atrium, flows through the tricuspid valve into the right ventricle, and ejects through the pulmonic valve (not shown) into the pulmonary circulation. The blood oxygenates in the lungs and returns to the left atrium through the pulmonary veins. From the left atrium it flows through the mitral valve into the left ventricle, where it ejects through the aortic valve into the aorta and systemic circulation.

in which internal respiration and metabolic exchange occur. From the cells and capillary beds, desaturated blood flows into the venules and veins and finally returns to the RA.

In the *pulmonary circulatory system,* blood pumps from the RV through the pulmonary valve into the main PA. The PA divides into the right and left pulmonary arteries, which further subdivide into

the arterioles and capillaries of the lungs. External respiration occurs in the capillary beds and the alveoli, in which carbon dioxide exchanges for oxygen. Freshly oxygenated blood from the lungs then flows through the pulmonary veins into the LA.

Coronary circulation (Fig. 25.4) supplies oxygen and nutrients to, and removes metabolic waste from, the myocardium; internal

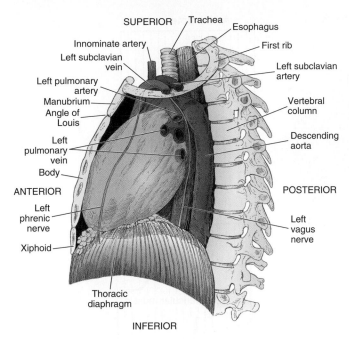

FIG. 25.2 Regions of the mediastinum.

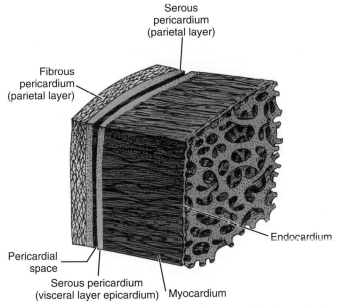

FIG. 25.3 Cross section of cardiac muscle showing its three layers (endocardium, myocardium, epicardium) and pericardium.

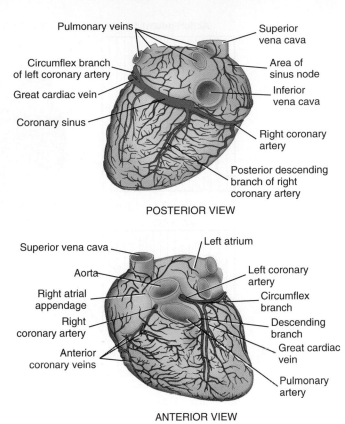

FIG. 25.4 Anterior and posterior surfaces of the heart, illustrating the location and distribution of the principal coronary arteries and veins.

respiration occurs in the *myocytes*. The heart receives its blood supply from the left and right coronary arteries, which originate in the corresponding left and right sinuses of Valsalva, behind the cusps of the aortic valve in the ascending aorta. The left main coronary artery divides into the left anterior descending (LAD) coronary artery and the circumflex coronary artery; with the right coronary artery (RCA), these arteries are the three main vessels of the coronary arterial system.

In coronary arteries affected by CAD, focal or diffuse atherosclerotic plaques develop and progressively enlarge, diminishing myocardial blood flow and oxygenation, which produces ischemic pain in many,

but not all, cases. Occlusion of a coronary artery by expanding atherosclerotic lesions causes myocardial infarction (MI) and irreversible damage to the region of the myocardium perfused by the obstructed artery. CABG procedures increase blood flow to the affected ischemic areas by attaching a bypass graft conduit to the artery distal to the narrowed portion of the artery. A totally occluded (infarcted) artery does not benefit from bypass surgery because the myocardial injury is irreversible if not treated (e.g., via revascularization) within 6 hours (Windecker and Piccolo, 2016). The main coronary arteries sit in the epicardium, which facilitates accessibility during bypass procedures. From these arteries arise the septal perforators and other branches that penetrate the entire myocardium. The cardiac veins empty into the RA via the coronary sinus; the thebesian veins, prominent in the walls of the RA and the RV, open directly into these chambers.

From the medulla oblongata, nerve impulses to the heart travel along the middle cervical nerve, which is composed of sympathetic fibers, and the vagus nerve, which is composed of parasympathetic fibers. Sympathetic fibers increase the force and rate of contraction, whereas parasympathetic fibers control heart rate. Running vertically along the right and left sides of the pericardium are major branches of the phrenic nerve, which innervate the diaphragm and stimulate it to contract. To protect the diaphragm, identifying the phrenic nerve is important in procedures that involve incision or excision of the lateral pericardium. Within the myocardium itself, certain areas of tissue undergo natural modification to form a *conduction system* (Fig. 25.5). The process of excitation and contraction originates in the sinoatrial (SA) node, located in the area in which the superior vena cava (SVC) meets the RA. The impulse spreads to the atria

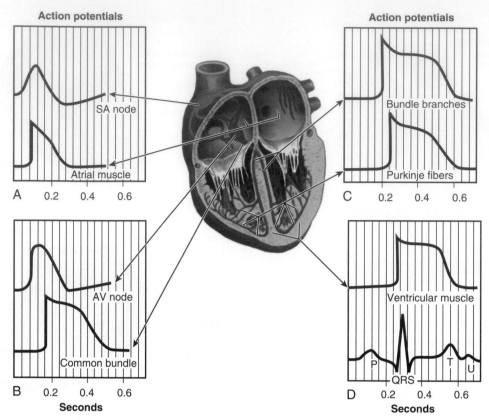

FIG. 25.5 (A) Heart with normal conduction pathways and transmembrane action potential of sinoatrial *(SA)* node. (B) Atrioventricular *(AV)* node (AV junction). (C) Bundle branches. (D) Ventricular muscle.

through internodal pathways and travels to the AV junction (which contains the AV node) located medial to the entrance of the coronary sinus in the RA, close to the tricuspid valve. From the AV junction, the impulse spreads to the bundle of His, which extends down the right side of the interventricular septum. The bundle of His divides into the right and left bundle branches, which terminate in a network of fibers called the *Purkinje system.* Purkinje fibers are spread throughout the inner surface of both ventricles and the papillary muscles, which when stimulated produce contraction of the heart muscle. Thus the location of conduction tissue is clinically significant during surgical repair of atrial or VSDs.

During myocardial contraction and relaxation, spiral fibers of the heart contract and relax (Fig. 25.6A). To prevent regurgitation of blood, the four cardiac valves (see Fig. 25.6B–C and Fig. 25.7) open and close to maintain unidirectional blood flow. The AV valves are between the atria and the ventricles. The right AV valve is called the *tricuspid valve* and contains three leaflets (or cusps). The left AV valve, called the *mitral valve,* consists of two leaflets (see Fig. 25.6). Each AV valve is a complex system consisting of a fibrous annulus surrounding the valve orifice, the valve leaflets, the chordae tendineae, the atrium, and the papillary muscles, which anchor the valve to the inner ventricular wall (see Fig. 25.1). The mitral valve annulus is a dynamic structure with a three-dimensional "saddle" shape, which has stimulated the design of newer prosthetic annuloplasty rings (Jarrett et al., 2016a). When the ventricle contracts, these muscles and the chordae tendineae, which are connected to the valve leaflets, prevent the leaflets from everting into the atrium. All parts of the system must function for the valve to work properly. If the shape of the ventricle has been changed by dilation or hypertrophy,

for example, the altered ventricle impairs ventricular function. Conditions such as hypertension, myocardial injury, and aortic stenosis (AS) promote a pathologic *remodeling* of the heart that can lead not only to valvular dysfunction but also heart failure and malignant dysrhythmias (Otto and Bonow, 2015).

The semilunar valves are at the outlets of the LV and RV. These valves are known as the *aortic* and *pulmonic* valves, respectively. They open and close passively with cyclic fluctuations in blood pressure (BP) and volume that occur during systole and diastole.

Abnormalities such as stenosis, insufficiency, or a combination of both, impair mechanical function of the valves. Stenosed valves have leaflets that are fibrous and stiff, with uneven and adherent margins. Regurgitant, insufficient, or incompetent valves, such as those with leaflet degeneration or perforations, dilated annuli, or ruptured chordae tendineae, produce regurgitation of blood into the originating chamber. These conditions, or a combination of stenosis and insufficiency, strain the myocardium by increasing intracardiac pressure, volume, and workload. The sound of blood flowing through a narrowed or incompetent valve produces an abnormal sound called a *murmur.*

Any of the four valves may be deformed congenitally. Acquired valvular heart disease most commonly affects the mitral and aortic valves and appears to worsen with increased stress associated with the higher pressures within the left chambers of the heart. Although rare, primary tumors of the heart may impair valve function by partially occluding a valve orifice, causing incomplete closure of the leaflets. Portions of the tumor may break off and embolize. Most tumors are benign; the most common is cardiac myxoma. Patients with myxomas can have a variety of symptoms. Classic findings,

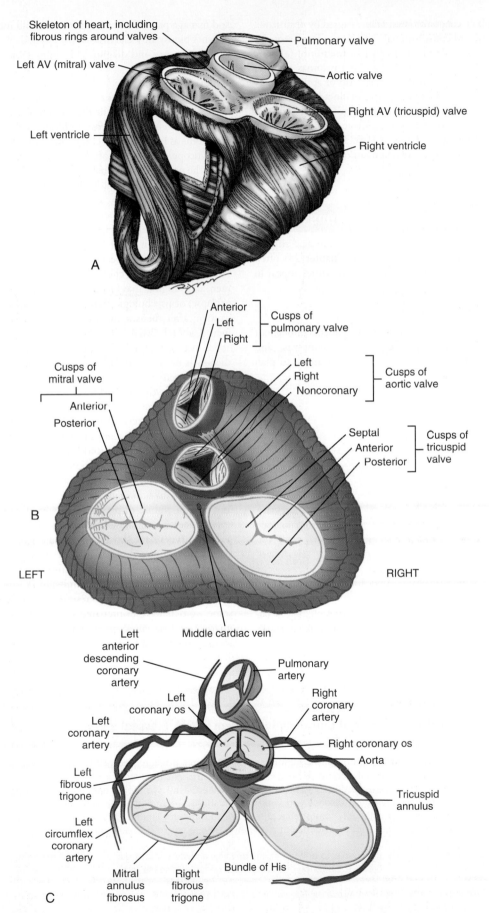

FIG. 25.6 (A) Location of the heart valves in relation to the spiral fibers of the myocardium. (B) Superior view of cardiac valves: pulmonary *(top)*, aortic *(middle)*, mitral *(bottom left)*, and tricuspid *(bottom right)*. (C) Superior view of valves in relation to coronary arteries and conduction tissue. *AV,* Atrioventricular.

however, include emboli, congestive heart failure caused by obstruction of cardiac blood flow, and constitutional symptoms. These sequelae are related to the location, size, and mobility of the tumor (Shapira and Reardon, 2016). The incidence of cardiac myxomas peaks at 40 to 60 years of age, with a female-to-male ratio of approximately 3:1. They account for 50% of all benign tumors in adults (Lenihan and Yusuf, 2015). Diagnostic imaging can identify many of these lesions, but the lesion may not cause symptoms to motivate a person to seek medical treatment (McManus, 2015). Lenihan and Yusuf (2015) advised that the only definitive treatment of a cardiac myxoma is surgical removal.

Perioperative Nursing Considerations

Specialized nursing considerations that apply to thoracic surgery (see Chapter 23) and to vascular surgery (see Chapter 24) often also apply to cardiac surgery. Pediatric cardiac procedures appear in Chapter 26.

Assessment

As the severity of pathologic changes varies among patients throughout life, knowledge of physical status, psychosocial concerns, and functional health patterns enables the perioperative nurse to plan

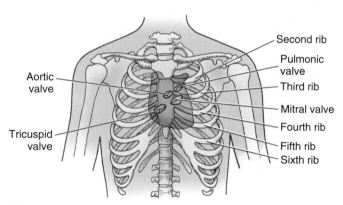

FIG. 25.7 Anatomic position of cardiac valves. Note relationship of left ventricular apex to fourth and fifth ribs, which is a frequent site for minimally invasive incisions.

and manage patient care. Assessment should include a review of the patient's biopsychosocial history, the physical examination, and results from laboratory and diagnostic imaging tests.

History

The history includes information about the patient's health status as well as the response to the disease and the recommended intervention or interventions. Patients with cardiac disease may display such symptoms as ischemic chest pain (angina pectoris), fatigue, dyspnea, and syncope. Depending on their severity, these *subjective* symptoms affect the patient's functional status and ability to engage in activities of daily living; the original New York Heart Association's Functional Classification System (Box 25.1) (New York Heart Association, 1994) is often used to assess functional ability. Updates to the classification system by the American Heart Association (AHA, 2014) also include information about heart failure as well as *objective* measurements such as x-rays and echocardiograms.

Atypical ischemic chest pain is more likely in women than in men, and angina may arise from vasospastic angina, mitral valve prolapse, or psychologic factors. CAD is unusual in premenopausal women; after menses ends, however, the risk is similar to that of men (Caboral, 2013; Gulati and Mertz, 2015). Controversy exists about menopausal hormone therapy. Estrogen hormone replacement therapy is not recommended in postmenopausal women, according to the Women's Health Initiative (WHI), a set of clinical trials whose results were first published in 2002 (Bope and Kellerman, 2017b) (Evidence for Practice). Greater emphasis is being placed on the effectiveness of interventions and on evidence supporting those interventions. Effective control of BP, diabetes management, and maintenance of optimal lipid levels are significant risk reduction interventions for women (Caboral, 2013).

Women undergoing CABG also face unique challenges and experiences. According to Caboral (2013), women may minimize any pain or public display of illness in an attempt to preserve an appearance of normalcy. In addition, American Heart Association (AHA) surveys have shown that a majority believe they can reduce their risk of heart disease through therapies with no established benefit; they even may not tell significant others about impending surgery until the day before admission. Postoperatively, they may wish to return home early to resume regular activities. Once home, some women were unprepared for the limitations they face, both physical and social; Bope and Kellerman (2017b) recommended focused advice, support, and education.

BOX 25.1

New York Heart Association's Functional Classification System (NYHA Classes) and Associated Objective Evidence

Class I   Patients with cardiac disease do not display symptoms of syncope, undue fatigue, dyspnea, or anginal pain with ordinary physical activity; no objective evidence of cardiovascular disease (e.g., normal electrocardiogram)

Class II   Patients with cardiac disease are comfortable at rest but display the Class I symptoms during ordinary physical activity; objective evidence of minimal cardiovascular disease (e.g., minimal mitral valve regurgitation on echocardiography)

Class III   Patients with cardiac disease, although comfortable at rest, are considerably limited functionally and display symptoms with less-than-ordinary exercise; objective evidence of moderately severe cardiovascular disease (e.g., ischemic electrocardiographic changes)

Class IV   Patients with cardiac disease are unable to engage in any physical activity without discomfort and may have symptoms of cardiac insufficiency even at rest; objective evidence of severe cardiovascular disease (e.g., enlarged heart shadow on x-ray)

Modified from The Criteria Committee of the New York Heart Association: *Nomenclature and criteria for diagnosis of diseases of the heart and great vessels*, ed 9, Boston, 1994, Little, Brown.

EVIDENCE FOR PRACTICE

Women and Cardiovascular Disease

Guidelines and interventions that may be useful to prevent CVD in women include the following:

Lifestyle Interventions
- Avoid smoking and environmental tobacco smoke.
- Engage in at least 150 minutes of exercise per week.
- Consume a diet rich in fruits and vegetables, high-fiber foods, and fish; avoid or limit high saturated fats or trans fatty acids, cholesterol, alcohol, sodium, and sugar.
- Maintain BMI of <25 kg/m^2.

Major Risk Factor Interventions
- Maintain close to optimal blood pressure of 120/80 mm Hg.
- Use appropriate pharmacotherapy to control hypertension, diabetes mellitus, renal disease, and high level of lipids and lipoproteins.

Guidelines and interventions that may *not* be useful or that may be harmful in preventing CVD in women include the following:

Menopausal Therapy, Supplements, and Aspirin
- Hormone therapy should *not* be used for the primary or secondary prevention of CVD.
- Antioxidant supplements.
  - Vitamin supplements (e.g., vitamins E, C, and beta-carotene) should not be used to prevent CVD.
- Folic acid supplementation should be used in the childbearing years to prevent neural tube defects but *not* be used for primary or secondary prevention of CVD.
- ASA for MI in women younger than 65 years of age: routine use of ASA in healthy women older than 65 years of age may be useful to prevent ischemic stroke and MI if use outweighs

risk of GI bleeding. ASA may also be useful in women with certain forms of AF and who have a contraindication to warfarin.

Guidelines and interventions that may be useful in women undergoing CABG include the following:

Use of Internal Mammary Artery
- IMA is associated with significant reduction in mortality (compared with CABG using venous conduits alone); less use of IMA in women.
- At least one IMA used to bypass stenotic coronary artery; bilateral IMA associated with reduced morbidity and mortality.

Use of Off-Pump Coronary Artery Bypass Graft Surgery
- Less use of off-pump CABG in women.
- Comorbid conditions in women affecting surgical intervention:
  - Greater incidence of diabetes mellitus, hypertension, hyperlipidemia, chronic renal insufficiency, COPD.
  - Increased risk of bleeding.
  - Women tend to be older at time of surgery.
  - Hyperglycemia increases risk in women.
  - Greater incidence of concomitant valvular disease.
- Surgical outcomes: equivocal.
  - Perioperative mortality may differ depending on studies (when data adjusted for age and comorbidities).
  - Evidence that women use more resources than men: intra-aortic balloon counterpulsation, vasopressors, mechanical ventilation, dialysis, blood products.
  - Women less likely to be completely revascularized.
  - Women tend to have smaller body surface area and hearts, and smaller coronary arteries.

AF, Atrial fibrillation; *ASA*, aspirin; *BMI*, body mass index; *CABG*, coronary artery bypass graft surgery; *COPD*, chronic obstructive pulmonary disease; *CVD*, cardiovascular disease; *GI*, gastrointestinal; *IMA*, internal mammary artery; *MI*, myocardial infarction.

Modified from Bope ET, Kellerman RD: Women's health. In Bope FT, editor: *Conn's current therapy*, Philadelphia, 2017, Elsevier; Gulati M, Mertz CNB. Cardiovascular disease in women. In Bonow RO et al, editors: *Braunwald's heart disease: a textbook of cardiovascular medicine*, ed 10, Philadelphia, 2015, Saunders; Caboral MF: Update on cardiovascular disease prevention in women, *Am J Nurs* 113(3):26–33, 2013; Mozzafarian D et al, on behalf of the American Heart Association Statistics Committee and Stroke Statistics Subcommittee: Heart disease and stroke statistics—2016 update: a report from the American Heart Association, *Circulation* 133(4):e38–e360, 2016.

A CVD risk factor profile (Box 25.2) is helpful to plan care for hospitalization and discharge by focusing on areas that require further patient education. For example, diabetes is a risk factor because it affects the vascular system, may retard healing, and may predispose the patient to infection. Of special concern are the epidemic growth of type 2 diabetes in particular and the role of hyperglycemia in general. Although type 2 diabetes formerly was considered an adult-onset disease, children are increasingly vulnerable because of a greater incidence of increased body weight, sedentary lifestyle, and accelerated insulin resistance (Bansal et al., 2017; Omer et al., 2017; Rhee et al., 2014). Altered glucose metabolism (absent diagnosed diabetes mellitus) has shown a significant correlation to atherosclerosis; control of hyperglycemia during CABG is an important strategy to reduce the risk of adverse clinical outcomes (Nussmeier et al., 2015; Omer et al., 2017; Rhee et al., 2014).

In addition to elevated lipid or cholesterol levels, inflammation increasingly has been implicated in the development of CAD. In particular, elevated homocysteine levels (which increase platelet aggregation) and high C-reactive protein (CRP) levels have been implicated (CRP is a biologic marker for inflammation and is

associated with increased risk for CAD) (Omer et al., 2017; Rhee et al., 2014). Additional risk factors include metabolic syndrome (central obesity, hypertension, insulin resistance, and dyslipidemia) and obesity (Omer et al., 2017; Rhee et al., 2014). Hypertension and obesity increase the workload of the heart; obesity may also increase the risk for postoperative infection because adipose tissue vascularizes poorly. Further, a growing percentage of the population is aging. Age, in and of itself, rarely contraindicates intervention, but comorbidities often associated with older individuals constitute additional risk factors and areas (e.g., cognitive impairment, depression, decision-making capacity), which may require investigation (Omer et al., 2017; Rhee et al., 2014).

Among the newer biomarkers for CVD are the *natriuretic peptides*, which are cardiac hormones synthesized and secreted by the atrium (atrial natriuretic peptide [ANP]) and the ventricle (B-type natriuretic peptide [BNP]). Natriuretic peptides have a regulatory effect that causes myocardial relaxation in response to acute increases in ventricular volume. Measurement of circulating peptides is increasingly used to identify heart failure and sudden cardiac death. Another biomarker under intensive study as a risk factor is lipoprotein(a)

Risk Factors for Coronary Artery Disease

Nonmodifiable

- Age
- Male (but postmenopausal women have risk similar to that of men)
- Heredity, genetic makeup, family history
- Race
- Menstrual status (estrogen levels may be modifiable; postmenopausal women have risk similar to that of men)

Modifiable

- Elevated levels of serum cholesterol and other lipids
- Hypertension
- Cigarette smoking
- Obesity, metabolic syndrome
- Diabetes mellitus
- Psychologic stress
- Personality type
- Physical inactivity

Newer, Novel Contributing Factors

- Elevated homocysteine levels (increase platelet aggregation)
- Inflammation (the atherosclerotic process is associated with inflammation)
- High CRP level (CRP is a marker for inflammation associated with atherogenesis)
- Periodontal disease (a marker for inflammation and possible infection)
- Atrial and ventricular natriuretic peptides (hormones secreted by the atria and ventricles in response to volume expansion and fluid retention; predictive of a variety of cardiac problems)

CRP, C-reactive protein.
Modified from Bachmann JM et al: Association between family history and coronary heart disease death across long-term follow-up in men: The Cooper Center Longitudinal Study, *Circulation* 125:3092–3098, 2012; Bonow RO et al, editors: *Braunwald's heart disease: a textbook of cardiovascular medicine*, ed 10, Philadelphia, 2015, Saunders; The Emerging Risk Factor Collaboration: C-reactive protein, fibrinogen, and cardiovascular disease prediction, *N Engl J Med* 367(14):1310–1320, 2012; Yang Q et al: Trends in cardiovascular health metrics and associations with all-cause and CVD mortality among US adults, *JAMA* 307(12):1273–1283, 2012.

(Lp[a]), which is identified from genetic studies as a causal link to MI; niacin has been shown to reduce the level of Lp(a) in some individuals (Tester and Ackerman, 2014).

Genetic risk factors for CAD and other cardiac disorders have been identified and are undergoing extensive study (Thanassoulis et al., 2013; Tester and Ackerman, 2014). Genetic studies have created a burgeoning body of knowledge about genetic mutations associated with risk factors, such as CRP, and possible pathways linking inflammatory processes with CAD (Thanassoulis et al., 2013; Tester and Ackerman, 2014). Genetic risk variants mediate their risk in multiple ways. Indeed, researchers have discovered that there are more unknown mechanisms than known mechanisms such as those associated with hypertension or lipids (Thanassoulis et al., 2013; Tester and Ackerman, 2014). Soon, an integral component of the preoperative assessment likely will include a genetic profile.

The risk for complications and major adverse cardiac events (MACEs) after cardiac surgery also appears to vary somewhat depending on gender (Gulati and Mertz, 2015). Investigations of risk factors in men and women for sternal wound infection have identified three significant risk factors that occur at significantly different rates in men and women: smoking, use of a single IMA, and age more than 70 years. Smoking and the use of a single IMA for bypass grafting are more common risk factors in men compared with women, but women tend to be older than men at the time of surgery (Gulati and Mertz, 2015). Fewer MACEs arose in women undergoing CABG surgery without the use of CPB (off-pump procedures) compared with surgery with CPB; however, malignant ventricular dysrhythmias (e.g., ventricular tachycardia), a calcified aorta, and preoperative renal failure are poor prognostic signs in women (Gulati and Mertz, 2015).

In addition to health status and risk factors, the perioperative nurse reviews patient medication history with particular attention to vasoactive drugs, anticoagulants, and other medications that can affect surgery. Nurses should note that patients taking ASA and other antiplatelet drugs (such as 2b/IIIa inhibitors) may require intraoperative replacement of platelets. Lipid-lowering drugs (statins) have shown cardiovascular benefits, but in high doses (i.e., 80 mg, compared with moderate doses of 40 mg), they have been associated with new-onset diabetes mellitus (Backes et al., 2016). Patients taking herbal medicines may be at risk for increased bleeding, hypoglycemia, or other complications, depending on the specific side effects of some herbal drugs (see Chapter 30).

Patient knowledge of CVD and related risk factors and their effect on functional, physiologic, and psychologic status should be part of the perioperative nursing assessment. The patient's personal strengths, external resources, and coping strategies are important subjects to discuss along with relevant cultural, ethnic, spiritual, or religious beliefs. A thorough risk assessment can help to reduce postoperative complications (Thanavaro, 2015).

Physical Examination

Physical assessment provides the perioperative nurse with baseline information about potential problems that might require intervention. Normal, age-specific changes in very young (see Chapter 26) and elderly (see Chapter 27) populations must be differentiated from pathologic conditions.

In addition to age-specific changes, a growing number of adults with acquired heart disease underwent surgery in childhood to repair congenital cardiac lesions (Webb et al., 2015). For example, patients with a previous Blalock-Taussig shunt for tetralogy of Fallot (see Chapter 26) may have altered pulmonary and subclavian artery anatomy. Likewise, patients with a mechanical closure device inserted for an atrial septal defect (ASD) may be at risk for endocardial injury if the heart is retracted or otherwise manipulated too forcefully. The nurse must be aware that anatomic anomalies associated with the original congenital defect, or its subsequent repair, may mandate changes to the original surgical plan. Consultation with the surgeon alerts the cardiac team to anticipate different anatomy (and surgical landmarks), special supplies and prosthetic materials, and potential complications.

Before a review of systems, it is helpful to assess the patient's functional capacity. How are activities of daily living accomplished? What barriers make independent living difficult? How are activities performed when there are disabilities? What support systems and educational resources are available? Answers to these and other questions alert the nurse to the need for referrals and other resources to help the patient achieve optimal outcomes.

A systems review often starts with the skin. The appearance of the skin offers clues to cardiovascular status. Dryness, coolness, diaphoresis, paleness, edema, poor capillary refill, bruising, and petechiae may reflect impaired cardiovascular function. Visual problems and headaches may relate to inadequate cardiac output, atherosclerotic disease, peripheral vascular disease, aortic valve stenosis, or medications such as digitalis. Chronic or local infection must be identified; if untreated, these are potential sources of postoperative infection. Nutritional status assessment (including metabolic syndrome) helps determine increased risk for infection, skin breakdown, impaired wound healing, and other complications.

The patient's level of consciousness, memory, comprehension, and emotional status also require assessment. Confusion, restlessness, slurred speech, numbness, and paralysis may signal impaired perfusion. The perioperative nurse should note their presence preoperatively and communicate this to nurses receiving the patient postoperatively.

During respiratory assessment, note the use of accessory muscles or nostril flaring and auscultate breath sounds. Adventitious sounds such as crackles and wheezes may point to pulmonary edema. Orthopnea, shortness of breath, or dyspnea may require elevation of the head of the stretcher and assistance during transfer onto the OR bed. If the patient is receiving oxygen, the flow rate and method of administration should be noted.

Alleviating pain is a prime consideration in the care of the cardiovascular patient because pain is a myocardial stressor. A patient with angina may arrive in the OR after nitroglycerin tablets have been administered or transdermal patches applied. Cold also increases the workload of the heart because shivering that accompanies chilling elevates the metabolic rate; the patient should be kept warm.

Heart sounds, murmurs, and friction rubs provide clues to congenital, ischemic, valvular heart disease, or pericarditis. The patient may experience palpitations. Apical, radial, and femoral pulses also reflect cardiac function, and their rate, rhythm, and quality should be noted. The presence of cyanosis or peripheral edema should also be noted.

BP is an important assessment element. The hypertensive patient may have left ventricular hypertrophy, and the hypotensive patient may display changes in neurologic, gastrointestinal (GI), and renal function. BP should be checked bilaterally. Unequal pressures in the arms may be a contraindication for the use of the IMA as a bypass graft on the side of the lower BP, in which perfusion may not be optimal. Radial and ulnar artery pulses should be checked bilaterally when the radial artery is to be used as a bypass graft. Patients with dissections or aneurysms may have unequal carotid, femoral, brachial, or radial artery BPs when the lesion occludes one or more of these vascular branches.

Cardiac function affects all the body's organ systems. Therefore assessment of the patient should be comprehensive whenever possible. A thorough assessment also alerts the physician and perioperative nurse to the need for special diagnostic tests and laboratory procedures.

Diagnostic Studies

Most patients referred for surgery have had clinical evaluations, including invasive and noninvasive studies (Box 25.3). After the history and physical assessment, a resting electrocardiogram (ECG) follows. An exercise ECG (stress test) is often undertaken because ST segment changes indicating myocardial ischemia may be apparent only during or after exercise. In patients with intractable dysrhythmias, EP studies may help locate irritable atrial or ventricular foci that can be surgically ablated, excised, or controlled with pharmacologic therapy. EP studies also may determine the need for internal defibrillators or antitachycardia devices. Bradycardia may indicate the need for pacemaker insertion.

BOX 25.3

Diagnostic Tests Commonly Performed for Cardiovascular Disorders

Noninvasive

- Resting ECG
- Exercise ECG (stress test)
- Chest radiography
- Echocardiogram (TTE, TEE)
- Epiaortic ultrasound (sternum already opened)
- Carotid Doppler echocardiogram
- Resting MUGA
- Exercise thallium
- Exercise MUGA
- CT scan
- PET scan with stress
- CMRI, MRA

Invasive

- Aortography
- Arteriography
- Digital subtraction angiography
- Electrophysiology
- Cardiac catheterization
- Ventriculography
- Endomyocardial biopsy

CT, Computed tomography; *CMRI,* cardiovascular magnetic resonance imaging; *ECG,* electrocardiogram; *MRA,* magnetic resonance angiogram; *MUGA,* multiple uptake gated acquisition; *PET,* positron emission tomography; *TEE,* transesophageal echocardiogram; *TTE,* transthoracic echocardiogram.

Modified from Bonow RO et al, editors: *Braunwald's heart disease: a textbook of cardiovascular medicine,* ed 10, Philadelphia, 2015, Saunders; Pagana KD, Pagana TJ: *Mosby's manual of diagnostic and laboratory tests,* ed 5, St Louis, 2014, Elsevier.

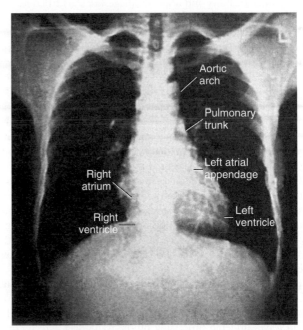

FIG. 25.8 Anteroposterior chest radiograph (normal).

Chest radiography provides information about the size of the cardiac chambers, thoracic aorta, and pulmonary vasculature as well as the presence of calcium in valves, pericardium, coronary arteries, and aorta (Fig. 25.8). Lateral chest radiographs of patients with prior sternal surgery show the chest wires and extent of pericardial

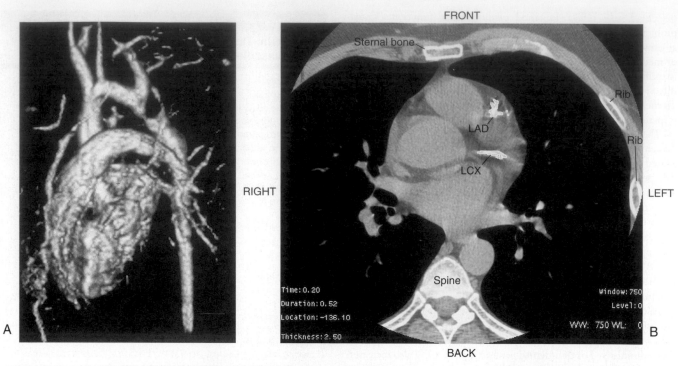

FIG. 25.9 (A) Three-dimensional reconstruction of a contrast medium–enhanced magnetic resonance angiogram of the thoracic aorta, illustrating a severe coarctation (narrowing) of the aorta. (B) High-resolution cross-sectional computed tomography scan of the heart, illustrating calcification within the left anterior descending *(LAD)* coronary artery and left circumflex *(LCX)* coronary artery.

adhesions. Magnetic resonance imaging (MRI) enables assessment of myocardial viability and also can image vascular structures with MRI angiograms that provide great clarity (Fig. 25.9A). In patients with suspected aortic or other vascular abnormalities, a computed tomography (CT) scan of the chest with intravenous (IV) injection of a contrast medium creates x-ray serial "slices" of the body area under study (see Fig. 25.9B). CT angiography is especially useful to image the aorta and the great vessels. CT images of the coronary arteries are used increasingly to identify areas of coronary calcification (shown in Fig. 25.9B), a recognized cardiovascular risk factor. Durhan and colleagues (2015) demonstrated the value of coronary artery calcium scoring to identify patients who may be asymptomatic for CAD, but are at risk for increased mortality.

CT scans may be contraindicated in very unstable patients because their position in the tubelike scanner makes patient access difficult. Less frequently performed is arteriography with radiographic contrast dye to determine the size and location of the lesion and the site of the intimal tear in aortic dissections (Fig. 25.10); digital subtraction angiography (DSA) provides clear images and requires less contrast material.

Echocardiography is a noninvasive test that evaluates heart structure and function by transmitting sound waves to the heart and measuring those sound waves reflected back to the transducer (Fig. 25.11). Sound waves undergo processing by the transducer, which creates visual images of the structure's movements. This test enables assessment of ventricular and valvular function before, during, and after surgery, and determination of the degree of valvular stenosis or regurgitation. It can also demonstrate tumor, thrombus, or air in the ventricular or atrial cavities. Two-dimensional and color-flow Doppler techniques have greatly enhanced functional assessment of valvular performance and carotid artery stenosis. Echocardiography is the gold standard

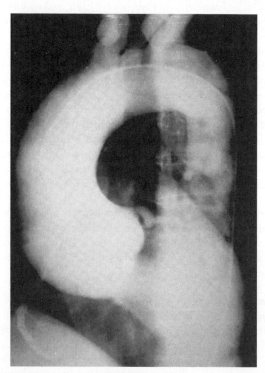

FIG. 25.10 Aortogram of ascending aortic dissection, with aortic valve insufficiency. Note regurgitation of dye into left ventricle.

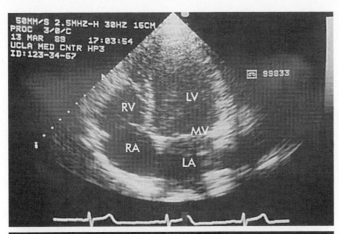

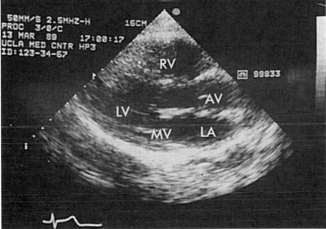

FIG. 25.11 Two-dimensional echocardiography showing two views of the cardiac chambers. *LA,* Left atrium; *LV,* left ventricle; *MV,* mitral valve; *RA,* right atrium; *RV,* right ventricle.

TABLE 25.1

Transesophageal Echocardiography Findings

Monitoring hemodynamic function	Assess ventricular, valve function, thoracic aorta; diastolic dysfunction; identify retained intracardiac air (to guide removal); guide insertion of IABP, VAD
Intraoperative evaluation	Valve function, cardiac structures, thoracic aorta; identify calcium and/or atheromas in area of aortic arterial cannulation site; guide cannulation entry into aorta; evaluate postrepair/postreplacement valve function, valve regurgitation
Measurement	Blood flow velocity

IABP, Intra-aortic balloon pump; *VAD,* ventricular assist device.
Modified from Bonow RO et al, editors. *Braunwald's heart disease: a textbook of cardiovascular medicine,* ed 10, Philadelphia, 2015, Saunders; Nussmeier NA et al: Anesthesia for cardiac surgical procedures. In Miller RD et al, editors: *Miller's anesthesia,* ed 8, Philadelphia, 2015, Churchill Livingstone.

to diagnose mitral stenosis, and its use to assess other valvular disorders and congenital heart disease (CHD) is widespread. Transesophageal echocardiography (TEE) also allows evaluation of the effectiveness of valve repairs and other surgical procedures (Table 25.1). Radionuclide imaging illustrates wall motion and blood flow through the

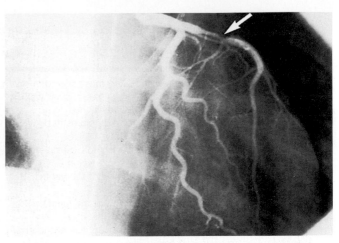

FIG. 25.12 Right anterior oblique view of left coronary artery injection demonstrating high-grade stenosis of the left anterior descending coronary artery *(arrow)* at the lead of the first septal perforator.

heart and quantifies cardiac function. Patients generally tolerate these noninvasive techniques well, especially when they may be too unstable to withstand a cardiac catheterization. These techniques may also serve to complement catheterization.

Cardiac catheterization provides definitive information about the extent and location of ischemic heart disease, acting as an adjunct to echocardiography, to diagnose valvular heart disease (Kern, 2016). A radiopaque plastic catheter is inserted retrograde through the aortic valve into the left side of the heart by a percutaneous puncture or a cutdown to the vessels of the brachial artery (Sones technique) or the femoral artery (Judkins technique). The right side of the heart is approached percutaneously via the superior or inferior vena cava. To perform coronary angiography that demonstrates intracoronary anatomy, a contrast medium is injected into the coronary ostia. Obstructions (Fig. 25.12), flow, and distal perfusion are assessable. Ventriculography illustrates contractile weaknesses of the ventricles as well as shunting and regurgitation of blood. These studies enable assessment of the degree of myocardial dysfunction and planning for interventions such as CABG, valve repair or replacement, repair of congenital anomalies, and cardiac transplantation. The cardiologist can compute the orifice of a stenosed valve or determine the degree of regurgitation of an incompetent valve.

Ventricular, atrial, and pulmonary pressures are recorded, and cardiac output and ejection fraction estimated (Box 25.4 and Table 25.2). Oxygen saturation of cardiac chambers and the ratio of pulmonary to systemic blood flow (Q_p/Q_s) are calculated for patients with shunts and congenital or acquired defects. Cinearteriograms record the movement of the heart, and cut films or digitized versions of the cines may be displayed during surgery.

The cardiac catheterization laboratory also performs percutaneous coronary interventional (PCI) therapies for evolving and acute MIs (Morrow and Boden, 2015). Coronary thrombolysis with fibrinolytic drugs can dissolve fresh blood clots and reopen (i.e., recanalize) the artery; antiplatelet agents such as ASA, dipyridamole, and clopidogrel often can block platelet aggregation that otherwise can lead to restenosis. Percutaneous transluminal coronary angioplasty (PTCA) followed by insertion of intracoronary (bare metal or drug-eluting) stents is often performed to dilate and maintain the patency of the recanalized artery. In many instances these interventions may obviate the need for surgical bypass grafting, although the progressive

BOX 25.4

Hemodynamic Concepts

Afterload: Impedance, or resistance, the heart must overcome to pump blood into the systemic circulation; left ventricular wall tension during systole; systemic vascular resistance.

Cardiac index: Cardiac output corrected for differences in body size.

Cardiac output: Amount of blood (in liters) ejected by left ventricle per minute; product of heart rate times stroke volume.

Contractility: Inotropic state of the heart; ability of the ventricle to pump.

Ejection fraction: Percentage of end-diastolic volume ejected into systemic circulation; indicator of ventricular function.

Preload: Volume and pressure of blood in the ventricle at the end of diastole. Central venous pressure measures right-sided heart preload; pulmonary artery wedge pressure indirectly measures left-sided heart preload.

nature of CAD may eventually lead to patients requiring surgical revascularization.

EP studies enable diagnosis of conduction disturbances and allow therapeutic interventions, such as RF or cryologic ablation of foci producing atrial fibrillation (AF) or accessory pathways seen in Wolff-Parkinson-White syndrome. Insertion of a pacemaker for bradydysrhythmias or an internal cardioverter defibrillator (ICD) for ventricular tachydysrhythmias commonly occurs in EP laboratories. Insertion of these devices, however, may require an OR when percutaneous access is unfeasible or when concomitant cardiac surgery is to be performed.

Laboratory Tests

Preoperative laboratory (lab) tests enable assessment of physiologic function (see Appendix A). Hematologic tests include a detailed coagulation profile to uncover hemorrhagic disorders. In patients who have been taking ASA or dipyridamole, platelet activity is decreased; this alerts the perioperative nurse to anticipate prolonged bleeding requiring replacement. After determination of blood type, an appropriate order to the blood bank follows. The blood undergoes testing for viral contamination and for cold antibodies that could produce agglutination of the patient's blood during surgery and after patient cooling to hypothermic temperatures. A monitored blood refrigerator stores blood brought to the OR before surgery. Although autotransfusion techniques have reduced the use of blood bank products, the occasional, emergent need for blood requires immediate availability of blood bank packed red blood cells (RBCs).

Liver and kidney function test results may be abnormal in patients with chronic heart failure, possibly because congestion related to right heart failure in the former and reduced blood flows in the latter occur with some frequency (Pagana and Pagana, 2014). Progressive improvement in hepatic and renal function often follows successful operative intervention. Statins and other cholesterol-reducing drugs can adversely impair hepatic function; review liver function results (He et al., 2014). Blood glucose levels require testing, monitoring, and control, especially in patients with impaired glucose metabolism and both type 1 and type 2 diabetes.

Additional perioperative laboratory work may include arterial blood gases and enzyme biomarkers of myocardial damage (e.g.,

troponin I and troponin T; creatine kinase MB isoenzyme, known as *MB bands*), particularly with persistent angina (Canty, 2015). Troponin levels are the focus of a revised definition of MI. This new definition incorporates specific troponin levels and at least one of the following criteria: symptoms of ischemia, new ST/T wave changes or left bundle branch block on the ECG, pathologic Q waves on ECG, evidence of loss of viable myocardium or regional wall motion on diagnostic images, and documentation of an intracoronary thrombus (O'Gara et al., 2013). This new definition differentiates between infarction and injury. The distinction is important not only to plan treatment but it also may affect the ability to obtain insurance and participate in secondary prevention (He et al., 2014).

Pulmonary function tests may help determine baseline data and plan postoperative care. The use of extracorporeal circulation and associated inflammatory responses, as well as stasis of lung secretions that accompany prolonged surgery, may impair postoperative respiratory function.

Nursing Diagnosis

After a comprehensive review of individual patient data, the perioperative nurse identifies relevant nursing diagnoses. Nursing diagnoses related to the care of patients undergoing cardiac surgery might include the following (AORN, 2017; Seifert, 2017):

- Decreased Cardiac Output related to emotional (fear), sensory (pain), or physiologic (electrical, mechanical, or structural) factors
- Risk for Infection related to surgical incision(s), catheters and intravascular lines, and altered cardiac function
- Risk for Perioperative Positioning Injury related to, for example, preexisting musculoskeletal disorder, lengthy surgical procedure, and preexisting conditions
- Risk for Contamination related to break in aseptic technique, preexisting infection, self-contamination (e.g., contamination by patient's own groin material)
- Risk for Bleeding related to surgical incision(s), tissue dissection, altered coagulation function, and inadvertent hypothermia
- Deficient Knowledge related to physiologic effects of the cardiac disorder, proposed surgical procedures, and immediate perioperative events
- Risk for Impaired Tissue Integrity (myocardial, peripheral, renal, and cerebral) related to surgery, hypothermia, CPB, or surgical particulate or air emboli

Outcome Identification

Outcomes identified for the selected nursing diagnoses could be stated as follows:

- The patient's cardiac function will be consistent with or improved from preoperative baseline levels as evidenced by hemodynamic indicators (BP, oxygenation, and ECG) within expected range; warm, dry skin; and urine output more than 30 mL/h.
- The patient will be free from signs and symptoms of infection at the surgical or other incisional sites as evidenced by absence of redness, edema, purulent incisional drainage, or untoward postoperative temperature elevation.
- The patient will be free from signs and symptoms of injury related to surgical position as evidenced by the absence of acquired neuromuscular impairment and tissue damage.
- The patient will be free from signs and symptoms of contamination as evidenced by maintenance of aseptic technique, timely treatment for preexisting infection, separation of "clean" and "dirty" areas of the field, and confirmation of integrity of implants (e.g., prosthetic heart valves, vascular grafts).

TABLE 25.2

Cardiac Catheterization Data

Hemodynamic Data	Normal Values		
Flow			
Cardiac output	3–6 L/min		
Cardiac index	2.8–4.2 L/min/m^2		
Ejection fraction	60%–70%		
Left ventricular end-diastolic volume	90–180 mL		
Stroke volume	60–130 mL/beat		
Stroke volume index	35–70 mL/beat/m^2		
	Systolic	**Diastolic**	**Mean**
Resistances (Wood Units)			
Systemic vascular resistance	<20	—	—
Total pulmonary resistance	<3.5	—	—
Pulmonary vascular resistance	<2.0	—	—
Shunts (Q$_p$/Q$_s$)			
Pulmonary flow/systemic flow	—	1:1	—
% Oxygen Saturation			
Venae cavae	—	70	—
Right atrium	—	70	—
Right ventricle	—	70	—
Pulmonary artery	—	70	—
Pulmonary veins	—	97	—
Left atrium	—	97	—
Left ventricle	—	97	—
Aorta	—	97	—
Valve Orifices (Adult) (cm^2)			
Aortic	2–4	—	—
Mitral	4–6	—	—
Tricuspid	10	—	—
Pressures (mm Hg)			
Venae cavae	—	—	0–5
Right atrium	—	—	2–6
Right ventricle	20–30	0–5	
Pulmonary artery	15–28	5–16	10–15
Pulmonary artery wedge pressure	—	—	4–12
Left atrium	—	—	4–12
Left ventricle	90–140	0–5	
Left ventricular end-diastolic pressure	—	—	4–12
Aorta	120–140	60–80	70–90
Brachial artery	90–140	60–90	—
Femoral artery	125	75	—
	Findings		
Angiographic Data			
Coronary arteries	Anatomy/function of coronary vascular bed; distal coronary flow; AV fistula; atherosclerosis; anomalous origin of coronary arteries		
Ventriculography	Anatomy/function of ventricles and associated structures; LV aneurysm; congenital abnormalities; valvular stenosis/regurgitation; shunts		
Valvular angiography	Intact mitral/tricuspid complex; valvular incompetence/stenosis/regurgitation		
Pulmonary angiography	Pulmonary embolism; congenital abnormalities		
Aortography	Patency of aortic branches; normal mobility, competence, and anatomy of aortic valve; aneurysms: saccular, fusiform; origin of aortic dissection; shunts or anomalous connections; congenital defect or obstructions		

AV, Arteriovenous; *LV*, left ventricle.
Modified from Pagana KD, Pagana TJ: *Mosby's manual of diagnostic and laboratory tests*, ed 5, St Louis, 2014, Elsevier; Bonow RO et al, editors: *Braunwald's heart disease: a textbook of cardiovascular medicine*, ed 10, Philadelphia, 2015, Saunders; Kern MJ: *Cardiac catheterization handbook*, ed 5, Philadelphia, 2011, Saunders; Nussmeier NA et al: Anesthesia for cardiac surgical procedures. In Miller RD et al, editors: *Miller's anesthesia*, ed 8, Philadelphia, 2015, Churchill Livingstone.

- The patient will be free from excessive bleeding as evidenced by chest tube drainage less than 100 mL/h, dressings dry and intact, normal coagulation function studies (or undergoing replacement treatment for deficient clotting factors), and normal body temperature.
- The patient will demonstrate knowledge of the physiologic responses to the cardiac disorder (at his or her level of understanding), the proposed surgical treatment, and the immediate perioperative events as evidenced by verbalization of disease state, purpose of surgery, sequence of events, anticipated outcomes, and recovery process.
- The patient's myocardial, peripheral, renal, and cerebral tissue integrity will be adequate or improved as evidenced by the absence of new electrocardiograph manifestations of infarction, the presence of palpable peripheral pulses, adequate urine output, and a clear or improving sensorium postoperatively.

Additional nursing diagnoses based on individual patient assessment should have a corresponding outcome statement. Each criterion evidences achievement of the outcome. Outcome evaluations should be documented in the perioperative record. Some outcome achievements will occur after the surgical procedure; others will require ongoing evaluation in the postoperative period for adequate measurement. The evaluation section affirmatively mandates ongoing goal measurement by the use of the word "will" rather than stating the outcome as "having been" achieved.

The nursing interventions in the Sample Plan of Care incorporate data elements from AORN's PNDS (Petersen, 2011). With increasing emphasis on correlating patient outcomes with clinical interventions, the PNDS is a valuable resource by which to demonstrate the nurse's ability to influence positive patient outcomes.

Planning

After establishing the diagnoses and outcomes, the perioperative nurse devises a plan of care to achieve the goals set. Patient, family, and caregiver needs, elicited from interviews when possible, are integrated into the planning. The perioperative nurse should then identify criteria specific to the patient for each of the stated outcomes. A Sample Plan of Care follows.

SAMPLE PLAN OF CARE

Nursing Diagnosis
Decreased Cardiac Output related to emotional (fear), sensory (pain), or physiologic (electrical, mechanical, or structural) factors

Outcome
The patient's cardiac function will be consistent with or improved from preoperative baseline levels as evidenced by hemodynamic indicators (BP, oxygenation, and ECG) within expected range; warm, dry skin; and urine output more than 30 mL/h.

Interventions
- Identify baseline cardiac status.
- Use monitoring equipment to assess cardiac status.
- Identify and report the presence of internal cardiac devices.
- Institute anxiety-reduction measures, address fear-producing concerns, clarify misconceptions, and answer questions.
- Measure pain level with pain scale; provide comfort measures and pharmacologic interventions as ordered; confirm and document degree of pain relief, measures used, and any medications administered.
- Check results of clotting function, coagulation profile, and electrolyte values; report abnormalities.
- Monitor BP (arterial, CVP, PAWP) and ECG.
- Maintain an adequate supply of and assist with administration of replacement blood or blood products.
- Have inotropic and antidysrhythmic medications available; assist with administration; document same according to institutional protocol.
- Monitor, report, and record urine output and chest tube drainage; keep tubes and catheters patent.
- Have available defibrillator (with appropriate internal and external paddles and settings), external defibrillator patches, fibrillator, external pacemaker, temporary epicardial pacemaker leads, and appropriate ECG cables for cardioversion, and intra-aortic balloon pump.
- Evaluate postoperative cardiac status.

Nursing Diagnosis
Risk for Infection related to surgical incision(s), catheters and intravascular lines, and altered cardiac function

Outcome
The patient will be free from signs and symptoms of infection at the surgical or other incisional sites as evidenced by absence of redness, edema, purulent incisional drainage, or untoward postoperative temperature elevation.

Interventions
- Verify that the prescribed preoperative prophylactic antibiotic has been administered within 1 hour of the surgical incision; document same according to institutional protocol.
- Assess individual patient risk factors for infection.
- Encourage and reinforce previous teaching regarding deep breathing and coughing exercises.
- Classify surgical wound and document according to institutional protocol.
- Implement and maintain aseptic technique.
- Initiate and maintain traffic control.
- Minimize the length of an invasive procedure by prioritizing, organizing, and planning care.
- Completely drape central line insertion sites.
- Perform skin preparation, using care to prevent pooling of solution; implement fire safety precautions during prepping. Prepare anatomic area to knees (or lower if leg vein needed) with antimicrobial antiseptic agent; document same according to institutional protocol.
- Use depilatories or electric clippers to remove hair at the surgical site; avoid shaving with razors.
- Monitor aseptic technique; correct breaks; accurately reclassify surgical wound on perioperative nursing record if a break in technique occurs.
- Have available prescribed topical antibiotics; document their administration according to institutional protocol.
- Manage culture specimen collection as indicated; use safe specimen management practices. Document specimens collected according to institutional protocol.
- Protect from cross-contamination.
- If the OR bed is raised, lowered, or turned from side to side, take measures to maintain sterility of field.
- Protect sterility of closed urinary drainage system.
- Maintain continuous surveillance.

SAMPLE PLAN OF CARE—cont'd

- Provide or apply surgical dressings to the wound and invasive line and device sites.
- Maintain sterility of instrument setup until patient is discharged from the OR.
- During patient rewarming, avoid excessive heat loss: cover exposed areas, irrigate with warm solutions, and increase room temperature.
- Use forced-air warming systems before and after period of induced hypothermia.
- Monitor for signs and symptoms of infection.

Nursing Diagnosis

Risk for Perioperative Positioning Injury related to, for example, preexisting musculoskeletal disorder, lengthy surgical procedure, and preexisting conditions

Outcome

The patient will be free from signs and symptoms of injury related to surgical position as evidenced by the absence of acquired neuromuscular impairment and tissue damage.

Interventions

- Obtain and prepare appropriate positioning and pressure redistribution accessories; verify that these are clean and in working order.
- Identify any physical alterations that require additional precautions for procedure-specific positioning.
- Verify the presence of prosthetics or corrective devices; document same according to institutional protocol.
- Position the patient, maintaining proper body alignment.
- Pad and protect vulnerable neurovascular bundles and dependent pressure areas. Consider a heel suspension device and slight flexion of the patient's knees to prevent heel pressure in lengthy procedures (supine position).
- Prevent pooling of skin preparation agents at bedlines and skin folds (obese patient).
- Pad thermal blanket to prevent direct contact with patient skin.
- Keep all OR bed surfaces dry and free of wrinkles.
- Ensure patency and security of peripheral and central lines, catheters, and ESU dispersive pad on positional changes.
- Have adequate personnel to assist with patient transfer to and from the OR bed and positional changes; lift (do not pull) patient during all positioning maneuvers.
- Safely secure patient to OR bed; ensure that safety straps are not too tightly placed yet maintain patient stability.
- Confirm correct position during time-out.
- Evaluate for signs and symptoms of injury related to positioning.

Nursing Diagnosis

Risk for Contamination related to break in aseptic technique, preexisting infection, self-contamination (e.g., contamination by patient's own groin material), and cross-contamination (e.g., moving from leg area to chest without changing gown and gloves; heater-cooler water contamination)

Outcome

The patient will be free from signs and symptoms of contamination as evidenced by maintenance of aseptic technique, timely treatment for preexisting infection, separation of "clean" and "dirty" areas of the field, confirmation of integrity of implants (e.g., prosthetic heart valves, vascular grafts).

Interventions

- Monitor asepsis; correct as indicated (e.g., change contaminated glove).
- Identify patient infection (e.g., MRSA).
- Confirm that antibiotics have been infused before incision.
- Confine and contain instruments used in the groin or leg.
- Change gown and gloves when moving from lower extremities to chest or after moving from one side of OR bed to other side (e.g., after holding the heart).
- Confirm that temperature-sensing package inserts have not changed (indicating ambient temperatures too high or too low for proper prosthesis storage).
- Document implants according to institutional protocol.
- Direct the heater-cooler's vent exhaust away from the surgical field.
- Establish, confirm, and maintain regular cleaning, disinfection, and maintenance schedules for heater-cooler devices according to the manufacturers' IFU.

Nursing Diagnosis

Risk for Bleeding related to surgical incision(s), tissue dissection, altered coagulation function, and inadvertent hypothermia

Outcome

The patient will be free from excessive bleeding as evidenced by chest tube drainage less than 100 mL/h, dressings dry and intact, normal coagulation function studies (or undergoing replacement treatment for deficient clotting factors), and normal body temperature.

Interventions

- Review results of clotting function and coagulation profile; report abnormalities.
- Check patient history for use of anticoagulant medication and other drugs affecting bleeding time and clotting function.
- Measure and report blood loss (e.g., suction, sponges).
- Use autotransfusion system per protocol.
- Have topical hemostatic agents available.
- Monitor, report, and record chest tube drainage; keep tubes patent.
- Before postoperative transfer, alert surgeon to chest tube drainage in excess of 100 mL/h.
- Maintain adequate supply and assist with administration of replacement blood, blood products, and clotting factors.
- Follow institutional protocol for allergic blood reaction (as applicable).
- Adjust room temperature as needed; room temperature should be warm (68°F–75°F [20°–24°C]) before and after completion of CPB.
- Monitor for development of inadvertent perioperative hypothermia.
- Evaluate for signs and symptoms of excessive bleeding.

Nursing Diagnosis

Deficient Knowledge related to the physiologic effects of the cardiac disorder, proposed surgical procedures, and immediate perioperative events

Outcome

The patient will demonstrate knowledge of the physiologic responses to the cardiac disorder (at his or her level of understanding), proposed surgical treatment, and immediate perioperative events as evidenced by verbalization of disease state, name of and purpose of surgery, sequence of events, anticipated outcomes, and recovery process.

Continued

SAMPLE PLAN OF CARE—cont'd

Interventions

Explain or describe the following events; solicit feedback from patient:

- Purpose and expectations of surgery
- Disease state producing need for surgery
- Sequence of events during perioperative period
- Recovery and rehabilitation process
- NPO status
- Administration and effects of preoperative medication
- Transport to OR
- Preoperative unit
- Insertion of peripheral, arterial, and venous lines
- OR environment (temperature, room furniture and equipment, sounds of monitors and other machines, staff functions, induction of anesthesia)
- Skin preparation
- Anticipated length of surgery
- Minimally invasive versus standard cardiac procedures
- Surgical ICU and patient status (e.g., unable to talk while intubated and plans for alternative methods of communication)
- Assess knowledge regarding wound care and phases of wound healing.
- Provide information about wound care and anticipated phases of wound healing.
- Determine patient's desire for additional knowledge (respect denial).
- Answer questions; clarify misperceptions.
- Know where family or significant others will be waiting during surgery; provide communication per institutional protocol.

Nursing Diagnosis

Risk for Impaired Tissue Integrity (myocardial, peripheral, renal, and cerebral) related to surgery, hypothermia, CPB, surgical particulate, or air emboli

Outcome

The patient's myocardial, peripheral, renal, and cerebral tissue integrity will be adequate or improved as evidenced by absence of new ECG manifestations of infarction, presence of palpable peripheral pulses, adequate urine output, and a clear or improving sensorium.

Interventions

- Identify baseline tissue perfusion.
- Assess factors related to risks for ineffective tissue perfusion.
- Place padded thermia blanket on OR bed.
- Preoperatively, provide warm blankets or active-warming device.
- Expose only those body areas required for surgical intervention.
- Use forced-air warming systems during period requiring normothermia (keep patient warm before and after arrest; warm throughout for "warm heart" surgery).
- Monitor patient's temperature (esophageal, pulmonary, rectal, bladder, or ventricular septal).
- Adjust room temperature as needed.
- Inspect CPB lines for patency and presence of particulate matter; alert the surgeon as indicated.
- Use solutions of appropriate temperature when irrigating the heart (cold during hypothermia arrest; warm before and after arrest); warm throughout for warm heart surgery.
- Avoid large ice particles on the heart.
- Evaluate postoperative tissue perfusion.

BP, Blood pressure; *CPB,* cardiopulmonary bypass; *CVP,* central venous pressure; *ECG,* electrocardiogram; *ESU,* electrosurgical unit; *ICU,* intensive care unit; *IFU,* instructions for use; *MRSA,* methicillin-resistant *Staphylococcus aureus; NPO,* nothing by mouth; *PAWP,* pulmonary artery wedge pressure.

Implementation

Additional considerations may prove useful to implement the perioperative plan of care for patients undergoing cardiac surgery.

Safety Considerations

The safety of the perioperative patient is a primary responsibility of the nurse. Among important National Patient Safety Goals (NPSGs) is compliance with "briefing," "debriefing," and other components of The Joint Commission's (TJC) Universal Protocol (TJC, 2017). The protocol consists of a checklist that addresses critical components (i.e., patient identification, confirmation of surgical procedure, availability of anticipated devices such as heart valves) that form the basis of a safe operation. Of special importance is promotion of a work culture that encourages asking questions and sharing information.

Equipment must function properly and undergo routine testing by the biomedical engineering department. Supplies should be used according to manufacturers' instructions for use (IFU), and instruments should be regularly scrutinized to ensure that there are no burrs that could injure tissue, that the jaws of vascular and other clamps align properly, and that all pieces are accounted for at the end of surgery. Toxic material, such as the glutaraldehyde storage solution for bioprosthetic valves, should be thoroughly rinsed before implantation. Monitoring aseptic practices of team members as well as visitors is important to safety.

Staff safety is also important (see Chapter 3). Personal protective equipment (PPE) should be worn consistently and properly. Gloves should be used by personnel whenever contact may occur with blood or other body fluids. Injury from inadvertent effects of electrical, chemical, and other potentially hazardous materials within the OR can be minimized by reinforcing safe practices.

Special Facilities

The OR must be large enough to accommodate bulky, highly specialized equipment while maintaining aseptic technique. Multiple electrical outlets, auxiliary lighting, and additional suction outlets should be available. Ceiling-mounted, mobile booms for housing electrosurgical units (ESUs), headlight sources, suction, medical gases, electrical outlets, and other items can reduce floor clutter and enhance the safety of the environment for patients and staff.

A growing number of hybrid suites have been designed that combine the traditional surgical environment and the fluoroscopic imaging capabilities of interventional cardiology laboratories (Fig. 25.13). A typical hybrid procedure may consist of a surgical coronary anastomosis under direct vision or with robotic assistance, combined with percutaneously inserted coronary artery stents under fluoroscopy. Endovascular aneurysm repair (of the thoracic and abdominal aorta) and percutaneous aortic valve insertion via fluoroscopic imaging are among other procedures performed in hybrid ORs (Chikwe et al., 2017).

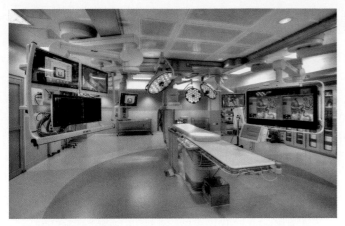

FIG. 25.13 Cardiovascular hybrid operating room.

Instrumentation and Equipment

The basic setup described for thoracic procedures (see Chapter 23) is used, along with specialized cardiovascular instruments and equipment.

Vascular clamps, designed to occlude blood flow partially ("partial occlusion clamp") or completely ("cross-clamp"), must be maintained in good condition if they are to prevent fracture of the delicate tunica intima of blood vessels and still retain their specific holding qualities. There are many variations in construction of vascular instruments. Jaws may consist of single or double rows of fine, sharp or blunt, teeth or special crosshatching or longitudinal serrations. The working angles of the clamps also vary. All clamps are designed to hold vessels securely, without causing trauma.

Minimally invasive surgery (MIS) requires special instruments to access the heart through smaller incisions in the anterior and lateral aspects of the chest wall. Retractors, dissecting instruments, suturing devices, coronary artery stabilizers, and vascular clamps are available (Fig. 25.14).

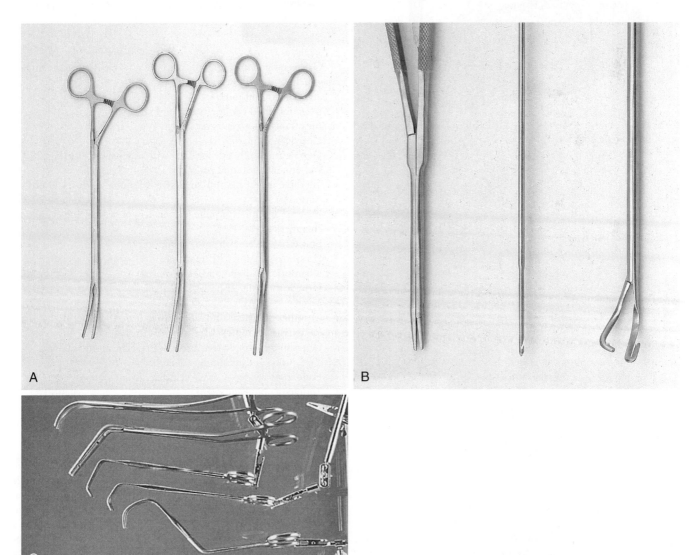

FIG. 25.14 (A) Transthoracic DeBakey vascular clamps, designed to pass through the chest wall by way of smaller incisions for minimally invasive procedures. (B) Close-up views of minimally invasive needle holder, trocar/suture puller, and knot slider. (C) Cardiovascular clamps (*top to bottom*) Semb suture passer, Fogarty cross-clamp (angled), Beck partial occlusion clamps (medium and small), Lambert-Kay partial occlusion clamp.

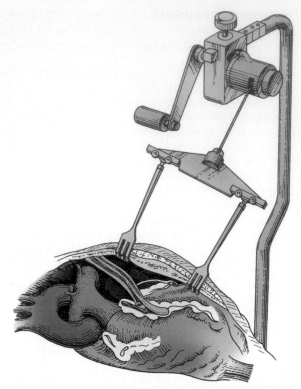

FIG. 25.15 Retractor used to elevate sternal border for exposure of the internal mammary artery.

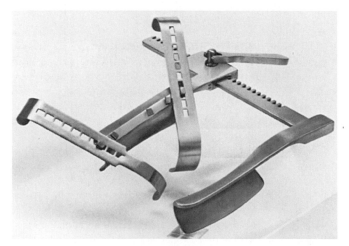

FIG. 25.16 Sternal self-retaining retractor with attachments for left atrial retraction during mitral valve replacement.

Sternal and rib retractors are selected to meet specific needs. IMA retractors expose the retrosternal artery bed by elevating the sternal border (Fig. 25.15). Some sternal retractors have attachments to provide improved exposure of the LA during mitral valve replacement (MVR) (Fig. 25.16). Handheld retractors can also expose the LA or RA or the aortic root. Special rib spreaders provide exposure for mini-thoracotomy procedures. Coronary artery stabilizer systems with left ventricular apical suction retractors are widely used for beating heart coronary bypass surgery (described later).

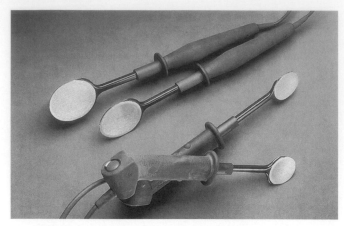

FIG. 25.17 Internal defibrillator paddles are available in an array of sizes and designs: the paddles may be activated through the handles or by pressing the button on the defibrillator. Smaller internal paddles are used for infants and children.

Other equipment commonly used (or available) for cardiac surgery may include the following:

- Sternal saw and motor
- Irrigation fluid cooling/warming machine
- Autotransfusion/cell saver system
- Electrical fibrillator
- Direct current (DC) defibrillator with internal paddles (Fig. 25.17) and adhesive external pads
- Thermia unit (mattress or active warming such as forced-air warming)
- External and internal pulse pacemaker generator (single and dual chamber)
- Epicardial pacemaker leads (temporary)
- Pump oxygenator/CPB machine
- Fiberoptic headlight and light source
- Intra-aortic balloon pump (IABP)
- Mechanical VADs
- Cryothermal energy ablation source (for AF surgery)
- RF energy ablation source (for AF surgery)
- Ultrasonic cutting/coagulation device (Harmonic scalpel)
- TEE probe and monitor
- Endoscopic, video-assisted vein harvesting system
- Thoracoscopic equipment
- Video equipment

Lasers (for transmyocardial laser revascularization) and robots (for valve repair) may also be found in a cardiac OR.

Suture Materials

A variety of nonabsorbable cardiovascular sutures with atraumatic needles are available. Synthetic sutures of Teflon, Dacron, polyester, or polypropylene are usually selected for insertion of prostheses and for vascular anastomoses. Most sutures are double-armed with a needle on each end. Given the numerous stitches required for prosthetic valve repair and replacement, alternately colored suture and slotted, numbered suture holders may help avoid confusion. Polytetrafluoroethylene (PTFE) sutures can be used for replacement of mitral valve chordae. Vessel loops and umbilical tapes are commonly used to identify and to retract blood vessels and other structures. Wire (monofilament or twisted cable) commonly is used to

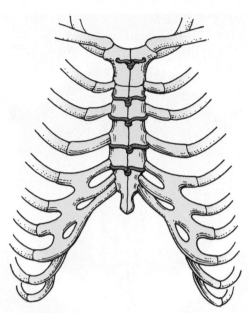

FIG. 25.18 Technique for wire closure of the sternum. A variety of closing mechanisms are available. These may consist of monofilament wire (shown), twisted wire cables, or (in some instances) plates and screws. In selected patients in whom disruption may be anticipated, such as elderly, obese, or malnourished patients, two or more heavy bands of nylon may be passed around the sternum and secured by a twisted stainless steel wire in addition to the wire sutures. Figure-of-eight technique may be used to reinforce weak sternum.

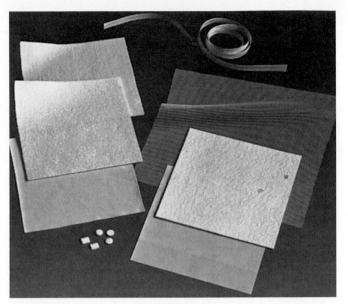

FIG. 25.19 Assorted prosthetic materials to repair intracardiac and extracardiac defects: tapes, Teflon and Dacron patches, and pledgets.

approximate the sternum (Fig. 25.18), with plastic, metal, or nylon bands occasionally added to reinforce fragile bone. Skin staplers may be used to close skin incisions; a staple remover must accompany the patient to the postanesthesia area if staples have been used for skin closure.

Supplies

The following supplies are used in most cardiac procedures. Depending on the surgeon's preferences, other items may be added or substituted.

- Rubber shods (placed on the tips of hemostats to protect suture clamped by the hemostat)
- Pill sponges (small gauze dissector sponges; also called peanuts, pushers, and kitners)
- Various sized Silastic or polyvinyl chloride tubing
- Tourniquet catheters
- Disposable drapes
- Foot-controlled and hand-controlled ESU pencils, ultrasonic scalpel
- Adapters, connectors, stopcocks
- Extra syringes and needles for injections, infusions, and blood samples
- Sterile marking pen to identify anastomotic sites and mark grafts
- Cotton gloves (worn by assistant to retract heart and expose target coronary artery); some surgeons prefer a sling to pull up the heart to expose the coronary arteries
- Suture organizer (to keep valve sutures in correct order)
- Irrigation cannulae
- Disposable vascular (bulldog) clamps
- Coronary occluders and stabilizers
- Autotransfusion supplies
- Chest tubes, chest drainage system

- Topical hemostatic agents
- Femoral arterial BP supplies (hypodermic needle, guidewire, stopcocks, pressure tubing)
- IABP insertion supplies (hypodermic needle, guidewire, vascular dilators, stopcocks, pressure tubing, and IABP catheter)
- CPB and myocardial protection cannulae, tubing, connectors, stopcocks

Prosthetic Material

In addition to these general supplies, special supplies are needed to repair or replace cardiovascular structures. Intracardiac patches, heart valves, and synthetic grafts should be handled with care to prevent damage or the introduction of foreign materials. Teflon, a fluorocarbon fiber, and Dacron, a polyester fiber, come in a variety of meshes, fabrics, felts, tapes, and sutures, and it is possible to combine them with other materials in prosthetic heart valves (Fig. 25.19).

Teflon patches are made in a variety of forms for intracardiac and outflow tract use. Varying degrees of firmness, thickness, and porosity are available for specific uses. Low reactivity, strength retention, and tissue acceptance are important considerations when selecting such patches.

Use of Dacron arterial tube grafts is common in cardiac surgery, although reinforced expanded PTFE grafts are also available. There are two types of Dacron grafts: knitted and woven. Woven prosthetic grafts are usually used when the patient has been fully heparinized because the interstices of woven grafts are tighter than those in knitted grafts and bleeding is usually less. Compared with woven grafts, the advantages of knitted grafts are that they do not fray as readily, they are easier to handle, and they reendothelialize more quickly. Grafts come in a variety of sizes and may be straight or bifurcated (Fig. 25.20). Knitted and woven grafts impregnated with collagen to reduce interstitial bleeding are useful in the thoracic aorta and do not have to be preclotted, even when the patient is fully heparinized for cardiopulmonary bypass (CPB). Graft sizers are available to determine correct size.

Specially designed tube grafts for the aortic arch incorporate prosthetic branches for the head vessels (brachiocephalic, left common

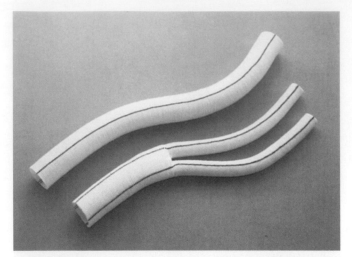

FIG. 25.20 Straight and bifurcated arterial tube grafts.

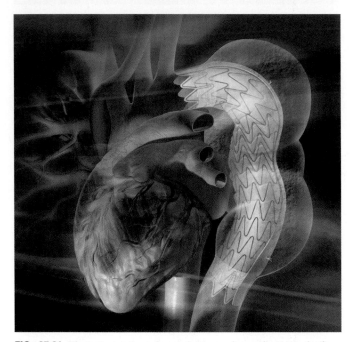

FIG. 25.21 Thoracic aortic endovascular stented prosthesis made from expanded polytetrafluoroethylene. Insertion of the compressed device is percutaneous through the femoral artery by a delivery catheter, guided to the desired position in the thoracic aorta under fluoroscopy. After confirmation that its position is correct, the device expands automatically on deployment from the delivery catheter. The delivery catheter is then withdrawn, and hemostasis of the femoral incision site follows.

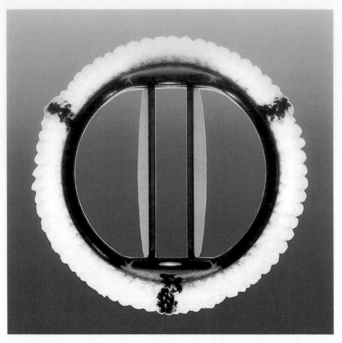

FIG. 25.22 St. Jude Medical bileaflet tilting disk valve prosthesis.

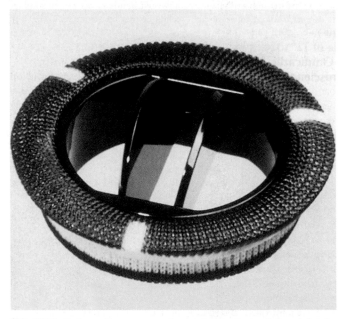

FIG. 25.23 Carbomedics supraannular aortic prosthesis, designed for the small aortic root.

carotid, and subclavian arteries). Tube grafts for replacement of the aortic root and ascending aorta are available with preformed sinuses of Valsalva incorporated into the prosthesis (David, 2016).

Endovascular, expandable stented tube grafts are available for both the abdominal aorta and the descending portion of the thoracic aorta (Fig. 25.21). The endovascular graft is inserted percutaneously into the femoral artery and advanced to the desired position in the abdominal or descending thoracic aorta, where the prosthesis is opened, implanted, and secured (Ehrlich et al., 2013; O'Gara, 2014; Szeto and Bavaria, 2016).

Valve Prostheses

Valve prosthesis selection depends on multiple factors: hemodynamics, thromboresistance, durability, ease of insertion, anatomic suitability, and patient acceptability; cost, patient outcome, and value are also important (O'Gara, 2014). Most mechanical prostheses use a tilting disk design. Prosthetic valves allow complete closure with slight regurgitation to prevent stasis of blood (Figs. 25.22–25.24). Prosthetic valves are manufactured with an attached annular sewing ring (often made of Dacron). The surgeon places sutures into the native valve annulus and then into the prosthesis sewing ring. The sewing ring

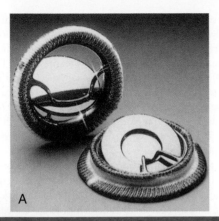

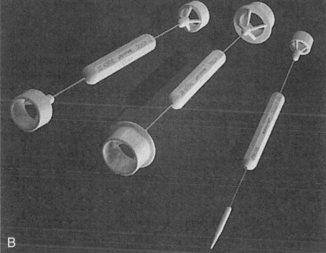

FIG. 25.24 (A) Medtronic-Hall tilting disk valve prosthesis. (B) Double-ended sizing obturators for the Medtronic-Hall prosthesis *(left and center)* and probe *(right)* to test leaflet movement. All valve prostheses have sizing obturators specific to the prosthesis itself.

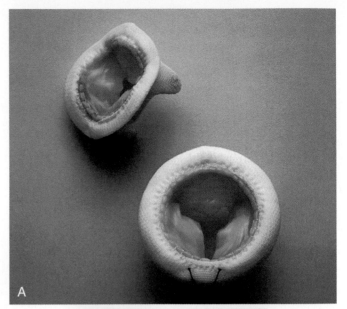

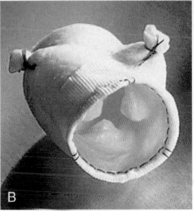

FIG. 25.25 (A) Medtronic Mosaic porcine aortic *(top)* and mitral *(bottom)* bioprostheses. (B) Stentless porcine aortic valve. The absence of a stent and sewing ring provides a greater orifice area through which blood can flow.

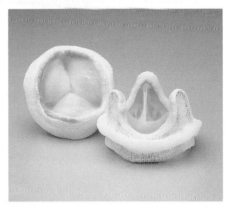

FIG. 25.26 Carpentier-Edwards bovine pericardial aortic bioprosthesis.

occupies space within the valvular orifice and may affect the amount of flow through the valve orifice. This is especially significant in the small aortic root (the location of the valve annulus). Aortic prostheses, especially in smaller sizes (e.g., 21 mm), tend to have minimal sewing ring material to avoid taking up space to minimize cardiac reduction of cardiac output that can flow through the prosthetic orifice.

When blood flow through the prosthetic valve fails to meet metabolic demands, a *prosthesis-patient mismatch* is said to exist (O'Gara, 2014). The deleterious effect of such a mismatch eventually produces deterioration of cardiac function. Thus surgeons select the prosthesis with the best hemodynamics for the patient. If a suitable prosthesis is unavailable, the surgeon may opt to perform a procedure to enlarge the aortic root to insert a larger, more hemodynamically suitable valve.

Bioprostheses derive from porcine, bovine, or equine tissue (Figs. 25.25–25.27). Porcine valves consist of an aortic valve from a pig that can be sutured to a Dacron-covered stent (see Fig. 25.25A); alternatively, the porcine aortic valve may be "stentless" (without a sewing ring) to enhance the hemodynamics, especially in patients with a small aortic root (see Fig. 25.25B). The bovine (calf) (see Fig. 25.26) pericardial bioprosthesis is created by cutting leaflet-shaped pieces from the pericardium and sewing them onto a Dacron ring. Alternatively, a bovine pericardial prosthesis (Kocher et al., 2013)

can be rapidly deployed by sliding the valve into position in the aortic annulus and inflating the frame to sit firmly in place (three commissural stitches also help to anchor the prosthesis). The equine (horse) (see Fig. 25.27A) pericardial prosthesis is created by cutting pieces of the pericardium, shaping the pieces into a tube, and attaching

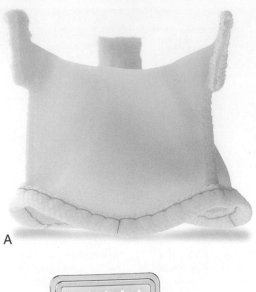

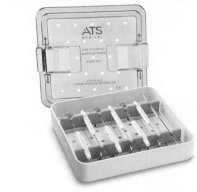

FIG. 25.27 (A) ATS Medical equine pericardial aortic prosthesis. (B) Obturators for ATS Medical 3f prosthesis.

the prosthesis to a ring of Dacron material. The advantage of these biologic valves is that administration of long-term anticoagulants is not necessary in most patients. Obturators to size prosthetic valves as well as valve holders are specific to the prostheses (see Figs. 25.24B and 25.27B). Tables 25.3 and 25.4 compare mechanical and biologic prosthetic heart valves, respectively. Tissue-engineered heart valves may offer a future potential cure for valvular heart disease (O'Gara, 2014).

Transcatheter, percutaneously inserted aortic valves come from bovine pericardium (Fig. 25.28). These may be inserted in a hybrid OR with fluoroscopy.

Aortic valve allografts (homografts) pose little or no risk of thromboembolism, offer optimal hemodynamic function, require no anticoagulation drugs, and raise virtually no risk of sudden catastrophic failure. Moreover, they demonstrate a lower incidence of infective endocarditis than that found in mechanical or biologic valves, and their long-term durability is comparable with that of bioprostheses. Allograft root replacement is also a valuable technique in the context of prosthetic valve endocarditis. The entire ascending aorta and valve (Fig. 25.29) or the valve alone (Fig. 25.30) may be inserted. Allografts are cryopreserved and must be thawed in saline according to the vendor's protocol before implantation. Because stentless aortic valves (see Fig. 25.25B) are more available than allografts, they are increasingly preferred for aortic root replacement.

Conduits consisting of mechanical or biologic aortic valves attached to a tube graft (Fig. 25.31) are used in procedures such as repair of aortic dissections requiring replacement of the aortic valve and ascending aorta. If vein grafts must be inserted into the conduit or if a direct coronary ostial anastomosis is required, the surgeon uses an electrocoagulator to make the opening into the graft and at the same time heat seal the cut edges of the prosthesis. Conduits with biologic valves interposed between tube graft materials may be used when patients are at increased risk for bleeding complications associated with the need for chronic anticoagulation therapy. Allograft conduits may be used for these procedures as well.

TABLE 25.3
Mechanical Valve Prostheses[a]

	Tilting Disk	
	Medtronic-Hall, Omniscience	**St. Jude Medical, Carbomedics**
Model/description • Advantages	• Spherical (single) tilting disk • Long-term durability • Good hemodynamics in all sizes • Low profile	• Bileaflet tilting disk • Long-term durability • Good hemodynamics in all sizes • Low profile • Low TE rate for mechanical valve
• Disadvantages	• Anticoagulation required • Potential for sudden thrombosis • Noisy • Higher risk of TE in mitral position • If warfarin (Coumadin) must be discontinued, there is increased risk of catastrophic thrombosis	• Anticoagulation strongly recommended • Potential for sudden thrombosis • Some noise • Higher risk of TE in mitral position • If warfarin (Coumadin) must be discontinued, there is increased risk of catastrophic thrombosis
• Special considerations	• Sizers and handles specific to prosthesis; must be sterilized	• Sizers and handles specific to prosthesis; must be sterilized • Frequently used in children needing mechanical prosthetic valve

[a]All prostheses should be stored in a cool, dry, contamination-free area. Resterilization is no longer recommended. The Starr-Edwards ball-and-cage valve is no longer available; clinicians occasionally still may encounter a patient with a ball-and-cage valve.
TE, Thromboembolism.
Modified from Otto CM, Bonow RO: Valvular heart disease. In Bonow RO et al, editors: *Braunwald's heart disease—a textbook of cardiovascular medicine*, ed 10, Philadelphia, 2015, Saunders.

TABLE 25.4

Biologic Valve Prostheses

| | Heterograft (Xenograft) | | |
	Heterograft/Xenograft	Allograft	Transcatheter Heterograft Valve
	Stentless Porcine Bioprostheses	**Stented Porcine Heterograft; Bovine and Equine Pericardial Valve Prostheses**	**Allograft (Homograft; Human Cadaver Valve)**	**Transcatheter Aortic Valve Replacement (Bovine, Porcine, or Equine)**
Model/ description	For use in aortic position Stentless (aortic): No sewing ring; includes porcine aortic root valve with coronary ostial branches	Pericardial valve used in aortic position; porcine heterograft used in aortic, mitral, and tricuspid positions Porcine heterograft (from excised pig aortic valves; leaflets attached to sewing ring) Aortic bovine and equine pericardium (cut and shaped into trileaflet valve)	Aortic valve allograft (cadaver, organ donor, excised cardiomyopathic heart from transplant recipient; mitral valve allograft also available)	For use in aortic position; trileaflet bovine pericardial valve mounted within a frame and placed into a delivery catheter; inserted via the femoral artery (occasionally through the subclavian artery) and guided fluoroscopically with TEE into the aortic position Two types: Self-expanding device placed into a nitinol frame (see Figs. 25.28 and 25.66); balloon-expandable device placed into a chromium frame (see Fig. 25.67)
Advantages	Incidence of TE very low; anticoagulation rare after AVR Stentless has excellent flow, especially in small aortic annulus (≤21 mm) No hemolysis Excellent hemodynamics; use may avoid need for aortic root enlargement Central flow Gradual failure allows elective reoperation Little residual gradient; durability good after age 60 years Stentless graft has many advantages of allograft valves	Incidence of TE very low; anticoagulation rare after AVR No hemolysis Good hemodynamics in all sizes Central flow Gradual failure allows elective reoperation Residual gradient minimal Slower rate of calcification in patients 60 years or older	Incidence of TE very low; anticoagulation rare; used for AVR and MVR No hemolysis Excellent hemodynamics (especially with stentless technique) Central flow Gradual failure allows elective reoperation No residual gradient —	Suitable for elderly patients (e.g., >80 years old) with severe aortic stenosis deemed unsuitable for surgical therapy No hemolysis Good hemodynamics Central flow Gradual failure Little residual gradient —
Disadvantages	Durability may be less than 15 years Accelerated fibrocalcific degeneration in children, patients with hypertension, or patients needing chronic renal dialysis Cross-clamp time and CPB longer than insertion of stented valve because of greater complexity of subcoronary insertion	Durability not yet established In small aortic root of large body, may produce prosthesis-patient mismatch Accelerated calcification may be a problem in children, renal patients, or those with hypertension	Limited availability Insertion technique more complex than stented valve Possible immunologic reaction (current decellularization process strips cells from graft and reduces immune response) —	Long-term durability not yet established; outcomes beyond 2 or more years not known; insertion technique more complex; potential injury to access vessels; higher stroke rate; paravalvular leak is a problem with newer sewing cuffs Requires fluoroscopy; requires radiation protection (lead aprons, etc.); long-term durability not yet established; significant initial learning curve

Continued

TABLE 25.4

Biologic Valve Prostheses—cont'd

	Heterograft (Xenograft)			
	Heterograft/Xenograft		**Allograft**	**Transcatheter Heterograft Valve**
	Stentless Porcine Bioprostheses	**Stented Porcine Heterograft; Bovine and Equine Pericardial Valve Prostheses**	**Allograft (Homograft; Human Cadaver Valve)**	**Transcatheter Aortic Valve Replacement (Bovine, Porcine, or Equine)**
Special considerations	Sizers and handles specific to prosthesis; must be sterilized before insertion; must be rinsed in saline to remove storage solution before insertion; follow manufacturer's IFU for rinsing; frequent irrigation recommended to prevent drying Diets low in calcium recommended for children, renal patients	Sizers and handles specific to prosthesis; must be sterilized before insertion; must be rinsed in saline to remove storage solution before insertion; follow manufacturer's IFU for rinsing; frequent irrigation recommended to prevent drying Diets low in calcium recommended for children, renal patients	No specific sizers; may use sizers for heterografts; cryopreserved allograft must be thawed per protocol; used for aortic or MVR; stent can be attached if indicated for use in other positions	No specific sizers; sizing via fluoroscopic imaging; potential radiation risks to patient and staff; need fluoroscopy, trained staff to run fluoroscopic machine, contrast media, and radiation protection

AVR, Aortic valve replacement; *CPB,* cardiopulmonary bypass; *IFU,* instructions for use; *MVR,* mitral valve replacement; *TE,* thromboembolism; *TEE,* transesophageal echocardiography.
Modified from Otto CM, Bonow RO: Valvular heart disease. In Bonow RO et al, editors: *Braunwald's heart disease: a textbook of cardiovascular medicine,* ed 10, Philadelphia, 2015, Saunders; O'Gara PT: Prosthetic heart valve. In Otto C editors: *Valvular heart disease—a companion to Braunwald's heart disease,* Philadelphia, 2014, Saunders.

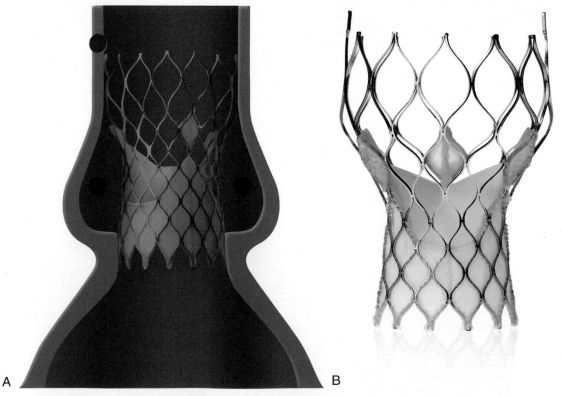

A   B

FIG. 25.28 Percutaneous aortic valve. (A) Diagram of bioprosthesis situated in the aortic valve annulus. (B) Valve frame with implanted bioprosthesis.

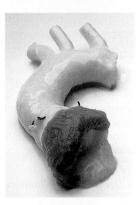

FIG. 25.29 Aortic allograft with aortic valve and arch vessels attached.

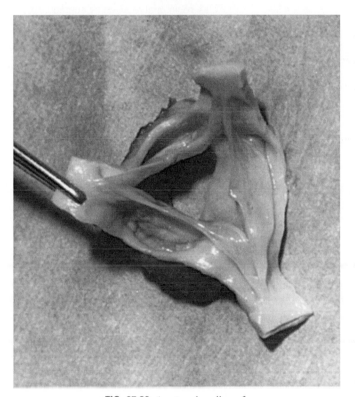

FIG. 25.30 Aortic valve allograft.

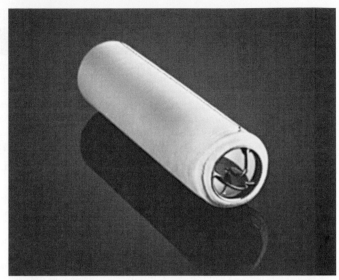

FIG. 25.31 Valved conduit with Medtronic-Hall tilting disk valve prosthesis.

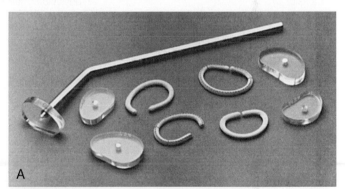

A

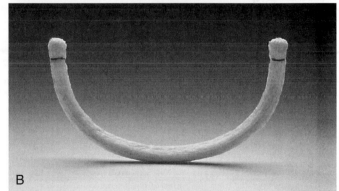

B

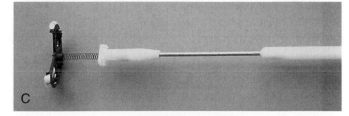

C

FIG. 25.32 (A) Carpentier-Edwards "classic" tricuspid and mitral annuloplasty rings, sizers, and sizer handle. The tricuspid rings bear notches in the area corresponding to conduction tissue in the tricuspid annulus to avoid suture injury. (B) Cosgrove annuloplasty ring. (C) Ring attached to ring holder and handle.

Although allografts and stentless bioprostheses may minimize prosthesis–patient mismatch and avoid the complications associated with prosthetic mechanical valve replacement, valve repair rather than replacement is preferred, particularly for mitral and tricuspid valve lesions. Numerous mitral valve rings and bands are available for both surgical and interventional percutaneous repair procedures. Consult with the surgeon about the intended prosthesis as well as alternative devices should another prosthesis be required (Otto and Bonow, 2015). When repairing the native valve with an annuloplasty ring, specific obturators are used to size the annulus (Fig. 25.32A–C). Ensure that the sizers appropriate for the prosthesis are available.

Additional safety considerations include storing prosthetic materials in a clean, protected environment and using them according to manufacturers' instructions. Before implantation, biologic valves (including the biologic valves within transcatheter aortic valve replacement [TAVR] systems) must be rinsed in three saline baths

TABLE 25.5

Valve-Rinsing Procedures for Biologic Heart Valves

Glutaraldehyde storage solution is used for many (but not all) bioprostheses, and rinsing procedures for its removal vary among bioprosthetic heart valve manufacturers. The amount of rinsing solution in each rinse basin, the number of basins, and the time for each rinse (and the total time of the rinsing baths) should be followed according to each manufacturer's instructions. Some manufacturers recommend a *fourth* basin for storing the bioprosthesis until implantation. The following sampling of rinsing processes reflects the differences among manufacturers' recommended rinsing procedures. The person rinsing the valve should collaborate with the circulating nurse when following the instructions for that particular valve. Given the wide variation in the following procedures, it is critical to check the manufacturers' instructions every time a bioprosthetic valve requires preparation for implantation.

Description	Number of Rinse Basins	Amount of Fluid in Each Basin	Rinse Time per Basin	Comments/Additional Information
Pericardial (equine) aortic valve (ATS Medical)	4	Minimum 500 mL physiologic saline	30 s in first three basins (total: 90 s/1.5 min)	Allow bioprosthesis to remain in fourth basin until required by surgeon
Pericardial (bovine) valve (Sorin Mitroflow)	3	Minimum 300 mL physiologic saline	2 min in the three basins (total: 6 min)	Allow bioprosthesis to remain in third basin until required by surgeon
Pericardial (bovine) valve (St. Jude Medical Epic)	3	Minimum 500 mL physiologic saline	10 s in each of the first two basins (total: 20 s)	Allow bioprosthesis to remain in third basin until required by surgeon
Pericardial (bovine) valve (Edwards Lifesciences Perimount Magna)	2	Minimum 500 mL physiologic saline	1 min in each of two basins (total: 2 min)	Allow bioprosthesis to remain in second basin until required by surgeon
Porcine valve (Medtronic Mosaic)	2	Minimum 500 mL physiologic saline	15 s in each of two basins (total: 30 s)	Allow bioprosthesis to remain in second basin until required by surgeon
Porcine valve (Medtronic Hancock)	2	Minimum 500 mL physiologic saline	15 s in each of two basins (total: 30 s)	Allow bioprosthesis to remain in second basin until required by surgeon
Porcine stentless valve (Medtronic Stentless Freestyle)	3	Minimum 500 mL physiologic saline	2 min in each basin (total: 6 min)	Allow bioprosthesis to remain in third basin until required by surgeon
Pericardial (bovine) valve (Sorin Freedom Solo)	None; rinsing not required because prosthesis not stored in glutaraldehyde	Not applicable	Not applicable	Although bioprosthesis does *not* require rinsing, it should be kept moist with physiologic saline to prevent drying
Pericardial (bovine) transcatheter heart valve (Edwards Lifesciences Sapien)	2	Minimum 500 mL physiologic saline	1 min in each basin (total: 2 min)	This is a bioprosthetic valve used for TAVR in patients at high risk for open-chest surgery Keep bioprosthesis moist with physiologic saline to prevent drying
Pericardial (porcine) transcatheter heart valve (Medtronic CoreValve)	3	Minimum 500 mL physiologic saline	2 min in each basin (total: 6 min)	This is a bioprosthetic valve used for TAVR in patients at high risk for open-chest surgery Keep bioprosthesis moist with physiologic saline to prevent drying

s, Seconds; *TAVR,* transcatheter aortic valve replacement.

to remove the glutaraldehyde (or other) storage solution. The prescribed number of baths, the amount of physiologic fluid in each rinsing bath, and the recommended rinsing time for each bath vary among bioprosthetic manufacturers (Table 25.5). Adhere to the specific manufacturer's IFU for each prosthesis. Some bioprostheses do not require rinsing because their storage is in a physiologically neutral solution (i.e., not glutaraldehyde). However, before and during insertion, all bioprostheses should be kept moist with saline. Mechanical valves should be protected from scratching and other injury.

Preinduction Care

After transfer to the OR, a focused preoperative assessment commences. The perioperative nurse reviews the medical record for a duly signed and witnessed informed consent form, advance directives, laboratory results, diagnostic data, and other pertinent information and confirms patient identity and the intended operation, including identification and confirmation of site and side, and required position. Verification of which leg (i.e., right or left) will serve for vein harvest in bypass patients may not be necessary if this decision depends on the surgeon's preference, rather than on a specific clinical indication. Some institutions, however, may require site marking of bypass harvesting sites, and the nurse should comply with institutional policy.

Preoperatively, cardiac surgical patients may exhibit more stress and anxiety than other surgical patients. Perioperative nurses should anticipate and prepare for this because stress and anxiety increase myocardial oxygen consumption. Efforts to reduce the family's stress and anxiety level are also important. Family members may ask questions about the surgery and the immediate postoperative appearance of the patient. It is helpful to prepare the family for some of the physical changes (e.g., edema, multiple tubes and lines) they can expect to see postoperatively and to encourage talking and

PATIENT ENGAGEMENT EXEMPLAR

Interacting With Families

The patient, a 50-year-old male, is accompanied by his wife and two teenage children. They are in the cardiac surgery preoperative area. Teenage children are very focused and protective about their family. You should initially recognize and answer any questions of the spouse, but also be alert to the children's concerns and fears. They will ask very direct and pointed questions that must be answered as truthfully and candidly as possible. When there is no answer (e.g., "Is my dad going to die?"), avoid making claims that you cannot substantiate. Allow the questioner to talk about specific fears, and address them; if there is a specific medical question, contact the physician (surgeon and/or anesthesia provider) to respond to the questioner. You can also discuss some of the precautions taken to protect the family member (e.g., sterile technique, having the necessary supplies, safe positioning, time-out). The OR remains foreign territory for many people.

The following is a possible scenario when the nurse provided patient-centered care:

RN: "Hello Mr. Jones, my name is Trish Seifert and I am a registered nurse. I will be in your room during surgery. Is this your family?" (nods toward older woman and a teenage male and female)
PATIENT: "Yes, my wife, Susan, my daughter Beth and son Jack."

RN: "Hello Mrs. Jones...Beth...Jack." [addressing children primarily] "Your dad will be in the OR for a few hours [confirms surgeon's time estimation]; we will call you if that time changes. Sometimes there are delays and we don't want you to worry if you don't hear from us when you expect to hear. I also want to tell you a bit about what your dad will look like when you see him after surgery. As we discussed before, we cool the body during surgery and use medication that keeps your dad comfortable and somewhat unconscious. When you see him right after surgery, he is going to look pale and feel cool and clammy. And he'll be *wired for sound*; there will be lots of tubes and catheters in your dad. These are important because they give us important information about what is going on inside his body. Most of these tubes will be gone in about 48 hours. Don't let his appearance and all the tubes stop you from touching your dad—patting his arm or hand. Also don't hesitate to talk to your dad; he will be medicated but his hearing is the first sense to come back. So he may not respond to your words, but I am sure that it will be a positive experience for him, and for you both. And don't hesitate to ask any questions. The nurses in the intensive care unit are terrific and can answer most of your questions. And if they can't, they'll find someone who can. I have worked with these nurses for many years. We'll all take good care of your dad."

---

touching the patient, even if the patient seems unable to respond (Patient Engagement Exemplar). The AHA and the Society of Thoracic Surgeons (STS) provide patient information about cardiac procedures and surgeries, and after reviewing their sites, patients (and family members) may have additional questions or concerns (AHA, 2016; STS, 2009).

In addition to communication with the patient, members of the team prepare the patient by ensuring vascular access for pressure monitoring and medication infusion. They insert a peripheral arterial pressure line and venous infusion lines. They may use a local anesthetic at insertion sites and may inject an IV sedative. Occasionally, a patient's response to sedation results in impaired respiration, as evidenced by shallow respirations, decreased oxygen saturation, and a reduced respiratory rate (e.g., 8 breaths/min or less) (Nussmeier et al., 2015; Reich et al., 2017). The nurse noticing these respiratory changes can call a rapid response team (RRT) to assess the patient and initiate treatment before the patient develops more serious reactions, such as cardiopulmonary arrest; the RRT may consist of anesthesia providers and staff in the immediate preoperative area rather than a specific hospital-wide RRT. Initiating a "rapid response" is an important aspect of enhancing a culture of patient safety.

Admission to the Operating Room

Depending on the patient's response to sedative medications received preoperatively, the patient may require assistance onto the OR bed. Warm blankets should be provided for comfort and to reduce shivering; ensure that blanket temperature does not produce thermal injury.

After application of ECG leads and the pulse oximeter finger cot, padding of the hands, elbows, and feet follows. The perioperative nurse confirms that the peripheral arterial pressure line functions properly, repositions the arm if necessary in collaboration with the anesthesia provider, and confirms that pulse oximetry functions properly. Additional monitoring devices appear in Table 25.6. A time-out commences.

Anesthesia Induction

The choice of anesthetic agent or agents depends on the cardiovascular effects of the anesthetic, the patient's hemodynamic status and general health, and the anticipated length of stay (LOS) in the surgical intensive care unit (SICU). Newer, fast-acting anesthetic agents are used to "fast-track" patients postoperatively, during which the patient may undergo extubation in the OR or very shortly after admission to the SICU, to speed recuperation (Kaplan et al., 2017; Nussmeier et al., 2015).

Anesthesia induction, a most critical element of the procedure, requires close monitoring of the patient, especially for patients with ventricular ischemia from congenital or acquired disease. Anesthetic management focuses on maintaining an adequate cardiac output by keeping myocardial oxygen demand low and oxygen supply high (Kaplan et al., 2017; Nussmeier et al., 2015) (see Chapter 5 for additional considerations related to anesthesia care monitoring).

Medication Safety

In addition to anesthetic medications, anesthesia providers use many other drugs to produce vasodilation or vasoconstriction, enhance heart rate and contractility, promote anticoagulation, effect diuresis, and provide antibiotic prophylaxis. Antibiotic prophylaxis to prevent infection in the cardiac patient is an important consideration, and the nurse should confirm that antibiotic infusion has occurred before surgical incision. Antibiotic selection should align with evidence-based recommendations. Reasons for exceptions to standard antibiotic

TABLE 25.6

Perioperative Patient Monitoring

Monitoring Device	Location	Measures
ECG	• Lateral, posterior electrode placement	• Electrical activity of heart
Arterial line	• Peripheral radial artery	• Arterial blood pressure (direct)
	• Central femoral artery	
	• Aorta (with needle attached to pressure tubing, or with sensor in bypass circuit or IABP)	
BP cuff	• Upper arm	• Arterial BP (indirect)
CVP	• RA	• RA pressure (e.g., CVP)
PA catheter (Swan-Ganz)	• RA (proximal port)	• RA pressure (e.g., CVP)
	• RV (midline port)	• RV pressure
	• Distal PA (distal port)	• PA and PAWP
		• Indirect measure of left atrial and LV pressure
		• CO
LA line	• Left atrium	• LA, LV pressure
Pulse oximeter	• Finger, earlobe	• Oxygen saturation of arterial hemoglobin
Urinary drainage catheter	• Urinary bladder	• Urine output, renal perfusion/function, temperature
Temperature probes	• Esophagus	• Temperature (core and peripheral)
	• Nasopharyngeal	
	• Urinary bladder	
	• Rectum	
	• Ventricular septum	
	• Bypass circuit	
	• Tympanic	
	• Face/forehead (adhesive patch)	
Neurologic monitoring	• Head	
EEG		• Electrical activity of brain; awareness
Transcranial Doppler		• Detects cerebral arterial emboli
BIS		• Detects anesthesia awareness
Cerebral oximetry		
TEE	• Esophagus	• Measures cerebral tissue oxygen saturation with sensors placed bilaterally on patient's forehead
		• Cardiac function, presence of air, integrity of valve repair
Epiaortic ultrasound	• Ascending aorta	• Amount of calcium within aorta (assists with location of calcium-free area for placement of aortic cross-clamp)

BIS, Bispectral index; *BP*, blood pressure; *CO*, cardiac output; *CVP*, central venous pressure; *ECG*, electrocardiogram; *EEG*, electroencephalogram; *IABP*, intra-aortic balloon pump; *LA*, left atrium; *LV*, left ventricle; *PA*, pulmonary artery; *PAWP*, pulmonary artery wedge pressure; *RA*, right atrium; *RV*, right ventricle; *TEE*, transesophageal echocardiogram.
Modified from Kaplan JA et al: *Kaplan's cardiac anesthesia: the echo era*, ed 7, Philadelphia, 2017, Saunders; Nussmeier NA et al: Anesthesia for cardiac surgical procedures. In Miller RD et al, editors: *Miller's anesthesia*, ed 8, Philadelphia, 2015, Churchill Livingstone.

protocol need to be documented and communicated (Elmadhun et al., 2016). Communication failure is a common contributor to adverse events (Research Highlight: Effective Communication).

An additional safety precaution is ensuring proper labeling of all medications on and off the field (including irrigating fluids and H_2O). Of particular importance are heparinized solutions, papaverine (to reduce spasm in IMA and radial artery conduits), saphenous vein infusions, and topical hemostatics (Levy et al., 2016). Containers and syringes are labeled, and the circulating nurse and scrub person visually and verbally should confirm drug name, dose, route, strength, and end date of every medication passed onto the sterile field (Hodgson and Kizior, 2013) (Surgical Pharmacology).

Monitoring

Extensive monitoring of hemodynamic and other variables is the norm during cardiac surgery (see Table 25.6). After intubation (or before, depending on the anesthesia provider's preference), insertion of additional pressure lines to measure central venous pressure (CVP)

and pulmonary artery pressures (PAPs) may follow. Central line–associated arterial bloodstream infections (CLABSIs) have lessened with adherence to practices that minimize infection (e.g., maximal barrier draping during insertion) (Gallegos et al., 2016) (Patient Safety).

Peripheral, central arterial, and venous pressures usually are monitored directly via transducer and oscilloscope. Perioperative nurses may need to collaborate in central line(s) preparation and placement. Then they should observe ECG monitors for signs of ventricular irritability, such as ectopy or tachycardia, and be prepared to assist with defibrillation of the patient if necessary. If the patient cannot be resuscitated, the chest must be opened rapidly and internal cardiac massage performed to decompress the heart and to perfuse the circulatory system.

An indwelling urinary catheter is inserted to measure urine output and to monitor renal function, especially during and after CPB. The urinary catheter may contain a thermistor temperature probe. Urinary catheters, however, place the cardiovascular surgical patient at risk

RESEARCH HIGHLIGHT

Effective Communication

The Joint Commission has reported that failure in communication and human factors are the two leading root causes of sentinel events that result in operative and postoperative complications. One proposal to improve communication and to reduce the possibility of error is to use standardized time-outs, checklists, and preoperative briefings. The World Health Organization (WHO) implemented a tool called the Surgical Safety Checklist, which is aimed at providing a standardized approach to practice and sharing of information. The WHO Surgical Safety Checklist has been associated with reduced rates of death from 1.5% to 0.8% and complications from 11% to 7% among patients undergoing noncardiac operations. The components of the WHO checklist include a standardized approach for three time-outs: before induction of anesthesia, before skin incision, and before the patient leaves the OR. Many team performance and communication tools have been developed, but there is no consensus about which approach is optimal.

Teamwork failures in cardiac surgery are commonly attributed to communication issues, leading to a lack of role clarity among team members, resource waste, tension, procedural violations, and errors. Preoperative briefings are intended to establish a dialog and provide an opportunity for all OR personnel to confirm and exchange information, identify concerns, and anticipate problems that may arise. For example, communication from surgeon to anesthesia provider about antibiotic selection is most effective when it occurs in a standardized fashion. Pharmacy staff also needs to be in the communication loop to ensure that drug preparations are available for timely infusion and completion before surgery. A short, structured briefing decreases the frequency of flow disruptions, enhances team knowledge about the procedure, and limits miscommunications among staff.

Modified from Elmadhun NY et al: Clinical quality and safety in adult cardiac surgery. In Sellke FW et al, editors: *Sabiston and Spencer's surgery of the chest*, ed 9, Philadelphia, 2016, Saunders; Fann JI et al: Human factors and human nature in cardiothoracic surgery, *Ann Thorac Surg* 101(6):2059–2066, 2016; Haynes AB et al: What do we know about the safe surgery checklist now?, *Ann Surg* 261(5):829–830, 2015; The Joint Commission Online: *Patient safety* (website), 2014. www.jointcommission.org/assets/1/23/jconline_April_29_15.pdf. (Accessed 4 February 2017).

SURGICAL PHARMACOLOGY

Medications Commonly Used During Cardiac Surgery

Medication/Category	Dosage/Route	Purpose/Action	Adverse Reactions	Nursing Implications
Heparin	For initiation of CPB: 300–400 units/kg (bolus) injected via central line or injected directly into RA	Systemic anticoagulation; prevents thrombosis of blood in CPB circuit; blocks activation of thrombin (and intrinsic clotting cascade)	Excess heparin can increase bleeding; possible allergic reaction	Ensure that heparin is infused before initiating CPB; if resuming CPB after reversal of heparin with protamine sulfate, confirm that patient has been reinfused with heparin; maintain ACT greater than 500 s
	For irrigation: 5000 units (per mg) in 500 mL of 0.9% NS	Topical irrigation		
Protamine sulfate	Can vary from 1–1.3 mg to 4 mg for every 100 units of heparin; infused through IV line	Reverse heparin; heparin antagonist	Potential for allergic reaction	If the patient's hemodynamic status requires reinstituting CPB, confirm that heparin has been reinfused; in some patients who are sensitive to protamine sulfate, heparin reversal proceeds without protamine; should have been administered slowly (over 5 min or more); heparin can rebound and may require additional protamine and/or laboratory tests to check platelet and fibrinogen levels
Papaverine	For IMA: 30 mg/mL in injectable NS; injected directly into IMA by surgeon	Antispasmodic (used to minimize spasm in IMA)	Potential for allergic reaction	Use a blunt-tipped needle to prevent injury to the artery
	For radial artery: 60 mg in 45 mL autologous blood; injected by person harvesting artery			

Continued

SURGICAL PHARMACOLOGY

Medications Commonly Used During Cardiac Surgery—cont'd

Medication/Category	Dosage/Route	Purpose/Action	Adverse Reactions	Nursing Implications
Bacitracin (or other topical antibiotic)	50,000 units in 1 L of NS Topical: Poured or applied with bulb syringe	Antibiotic (antibacterial) used for prophylaxis	Potential for allergic reaction	May be poured or applied with bulb syringe onto surgical site
Hemostatic agents: Mechanical	Gelatin, collagen, cellulose, polysaccharide: applied topically	Compresses tissue and absorbs blood; provides scaffold for clots to form; promotes hemostasis; halts bleeding in presence of active flowing blood; used for diffuse bleeding	Potential for allergic reaction	Examples: Gelfoam, Surgicel, Oxycel; has little hemostatic effect on heparinized patients
Hemostatic agents: Active	Bovine or human pooled thrombin; applied topically	Promotes platelet activation and initiation of clotting cascade	Potential for allergic reaction	Example: FloSeal
Hemostatic agents: Flowable	Bovine gelatin and human plasma; porcine gelatin; applied topically	Initiates clotting cascade through activation on contact with blood	Potential for allergic reaction	Examples: Gelfoam, thrombin; gelatin has little hemostatic effect on heparinized patients
Hemostatic agents: Fibrin sealant	2-mL or 5-mL packages; human pooled plasma; applied topically	Mixes fibrinogen, thrombin, and clotting factors to generate a clot; emulates final stages of clotting cascade	Potential for allergic reaction	Examples: Tisseel, Hemaseel; effective in patients with coagulopathies or who are on anticoagulants
Sealants: PEG	Becomes a gel and seals bleeding site; applied topically	Creates barriers to prevent leakage from tissues; used for vascular reconstruction	Potential for allergic reaction	Examples: Coseal, FocalSeal
Adhesives: Cyanoacrylate	Cyanoacrylate; applied topically	Adjunct to sutures or staples; used to attach tissues to each other	Potential for allergic reaction (especially in patients with bovine or glutaraldehyde allergies)	Example: Dermabond
Adhesive: Albumin and glutaraldehyde	Bovine serum albumin and 10% glutaraldehyde; applied topically	Glutaraldehyde and albumin form a strong adhesive	Potential for allergic reaction	Example: BioGlue
Vein solution	1000 mL Plasma-Lyte, 4000 units heparin, 120 mg papaverine; injected into vein graft	Provides physiologic solution for distending vein graft	Potential for allergic reaction	Ensure that solution is clear of particulate matter when transferring to field

ACT, Activated clotting time; *CPB*, cardiopulmonary bypass; *IMA*, internal mammary artery; *IV*, intravenous; *NS*, normal saline; *PEG*, polyethylene glycol; *RA*, right atrium.
Modified from Hodgson BB, Kizior RJ: *Saunders nursing drug handbook 2013*, Philadelphia, 2013, Saunders; Kaplan JA et al: *Kaplan's cardiac anesthesia*, ed 7, Philadelphia, 2017, Saunders; Miraflor E, Harken AH: Cardiovascular pharmacology. In Cameron JL, Cameron, AM, editors: *Current surgical therapy*, ed 12, Philadelphia, 2017, Elsevier; Nussmeier NA et al: Anesthesia for cardiac surgical procedures. In Miller RD et al, editors: *Miller's anesthesia*, ed 8, Philadelphia, 2015, Elsevier.

for a urinary tract infection (UTI) (Research Highlight: CAUTI After Cardiovascular Surgery). The most important risk factors for developing a catheter-associated UTI (CAUTI) is substandard hand hygiene, maintenance care, and prolonged use (CDC, 2015; Edivete et al., 2016). Therefore catheters should only be used for appropriate indications and should be removed as soon as they are no longer needed.

Placement of temperature probes, usually in the esophagus, nasopharynx, rectum, or on the forehead, is common. Temperatures also can be secured from the PA catheters and the arterial infusion line of the bypass circuit. Ventricular septal temperatures can be recorded by insertion of a needle probe while the patient's heart is arrested. Monitoring cerebral oxygenation and the level of anesthesia awareness frequently occurs.

The skin requires careful inspection before placement of ECG and ESU dispersive pads. Bony prominences, such as the coccyx and the back of the head, need padding to prevent pressure necrosis from hypoperfusion and hypothermia during bypass. Elderly patients are especially vulnerable to skin breakdown and require additional precautions to avoid pressure injuries (Kaplan et al., 2017). Monitoring aseptic practice is an important infection control strategy.

Positioning

The supine position provides optimal exposure for CPB and surgery to repair the heart and great vessels. In addition, respiratory impairment and discomfort lessen with this approach (Kern, 2016; Lytle, 2016). When using the supine position, hands and arms are tucked

Preventing Central Line–Associated Bloodstream Infections

Cardiac surgery patients routinely undergo insertion of central venous lines to monitor cardiac function and to infuse medications. Unfortunately, central venous lines have been associated with significant bacterial colonization, local infection at the site of insertion, and bloodstream infection. According to the CDC, CLABSIs result in thousands of deaths each year and billions of dollars in added costs to the US healthcare system. Research identified a number of effective strategies to reduce the risk of catheter contamination during insertion and throughout the time that the catheter remains in place. This research has led to a small number of evidenced-based practices, known as "central-line bundles." When these strategies are used together, 65% to 70% of potential CLABSIs are prevented.

- Follow recommended central line insertion practices to prevent infection when the central line is placed, including:
  - Perform hand hygiene.
  - Apply appropriate skin antiseptic.
  - Ensure that the skin prep agent has completely dried before inserting the central line.
  - Use all five maximal sterile barrier precautions: sterile gloves, sterile gown, head covering, mask, large sterile drape.
- Once the central line is in place:
  - Follow recommended central line maintenance practices.
  - Wash hands with soap and water or an alcohol-based hand rub before and after touching the line.
  - Remove central line as soon as it is no longer needed. The sooner it is removed, the less likely the chance of infection.

CDC, Centers for Disease Control and Prevention; *CLABSI,* central line–associated bloodstream infection.
Modified from Centers for Disease Control and Prevention (CDC): *Central line-associated bloodstream infections: resources for patients and healthcare providers* (website), 2011. www.cdc.gov/hai/bsi/clabsi-resources.html. (Accessed 4 February 2017); Yokoe DS et al: A compendium of strategies to prevent healthcare-associated infections in acute care hospitals: 2014 updates, *Infect Control Hosp Epidemiol* 35:967–977, 2014.

CAUTI After Cardiovascular Surgery

A UTI is the most common type of healthcare-associated infection reported to the National Healthcare Safety Network. It involves any part of the urinary system, including urethra, bladder, ureters, and kidney. About 75% of UTIs acquired in the hospital are associated with a urinary catheter. Edivete and colleagues (2016) assessed the impact of a multifaceted intervention on the incidence of CAUTI on cardiovascular surgical patients. The team conducted an interventional study during 18 months, divided into three consecutive 6 month periods. During these periods (phases 1–3), researchers observed insertion in the OR, verifying the use of hand hygiene before and after the procedure, sterile gloves, a sterile field, sterile lubricant, and antiseptic solution to clean the genital area. The staff was provided training on CAUTI prevention measures. The staff received adherence feedback, and researchers determined the incidence of CAUTI. Initial observations confirmed that hand hygiene was the procedure most often omitted, followed by failure to connect the collection bag to the catheter before insertion. Observations continued, more than 94% of the nurses were trained, and researchers found that during postintervention (phase 3), adherence to hand hygiene and to maintenance care improved significantly. CAUTI incidence declined, and urinary catheter utilization ratios remained constant.

CAUTI, Catheter-associated urinary tract infection; *UTI,* urinary tract infection.
Modified from Centers for Disease Control and Prevention (CDC): *Catheter-associated urinary tract infection (CAUTI)* (website), 2015. www.cdc.gov/hai/ca_uti/uti.html. (Accessed 4 February 2017); Edivete RA et al: Catheter-associated urinary tract infection after cardiovascular surgery: Impact of a multifaceted intervention, *Am J Infect Control* 44(3):289–293, 2016.

ous, fluoroscopically guided endovascular repairs of descending thoracic lesions, patient positioning in supine position is the norm (and not in the lateral position traditionally used for open procedures). Thoracotomy positioning aids should be available to position arms and legs per the surgeon's selected protocol (see Chapter 6 for a thorough discussion of surgical positioning).

Prepping and Draping

For procedures requiring excision of the saphenous vein, prepping (prep) extends from the jaw to the toes and includes the anterior (or lateral) area of the chest, abdomen, groin, and legs. Legs and feet are prepped circumferentially and the chest and abdomen from bedline to bedline.

In procedures without saphenous vein excision, prep extends to a level below the knees to provide access to the femoral artery or saphenous vein in the thigh area. Some surgeons prefer to have both legs prepped circumferentially for all cardiac procedures. Femoral artery access may be required for arterial pressure monitoring or insertion of an IABP. Saphenous vein exposure facilitates access if need for a bypass conduit appears. In lateral position, the patient is prepped bedline to bedline, anteriorly and posteriorly at least to the knees.

After prep, patient draping follows so that anterior areas of the chest, abdomen, and inguinal area are accessible. The perineum is covered, and a towel folded lengthwise creates a "belt," which is placed across the umbilicus to connect the side drapes. When excising the saphenous vein, both legs remain exposed; only the feet are covered. When draping, consider placement of bypass lines so that they remain securely attached and do not become contaminated. A

along either side of the body. The legs may be "frog-legged" slightly to provide access to the femoral arteries for insertion of pressure lines and IABP lines or to excise the saphenous vein. Measures to avoid pressure injury (especially in the elderly, debilitated, or obese patient) include padding the coccyx and applying heel protectors. Measures to protect the occipital area from pressure injuries include placing pillows under the head and repositioning the head during surgery. Significant factors associated with the development of pressure injuries include preexisting diabetes mellitus; lower preoperative hemoglobin, hematocrit (Hct), and serum albumin levels (Kaplan et al., 2017); and the presence of IABPs.

Semilateral position may prove optimal for thoracoabdominal aneurysms to expose both the descending thoracic and abdominal aorta. Thoracotomy position is common for some MIS procedures including surgery on the descending thoracic aorta; elevation of the right or left side of the chest with a roll or other positioning device provides adequate exposure for one or more small thoracotomy incisions. The presence of severe mediastinal adhesions may also require this approach in some repeat valve operations. For percutane-

small drape or towel may cover the groin when access to it is not immediately necessary. If the femoral artery needs to be accessed, the drape or towel can be discarded. Similarly, placement of towels over the legs after saphenous vein excision reduces inadvertent cooling.

Incisions

Surgeons use a variety of incisions. The standard median sternotomy is most common, but mini-sternotomy, mini-thoracotomy, or full thoracotomy incisions are frequent alternatives, depending on surgeon preference and the specific procedure (Fig. 25.33).

Median Sternotomy. The skin incision for full median sternotomy extends from the sternal notch to the linea alba below the xiphoid process (Fig. 25.34). Occasionally a shorter sternal incision is made for aortic valve replacement (see Fig. 25.33A, upper portion).

For mini-sternotomy, the surgeon partially divides the sternum with a saw, starting from either the sternal notch or the xiphoid process (depending on the cardiac structures to be exposed), and a sternal retractor is then inserted (see Fig. 25.33A). If the IMA or the saphenous vein will be used, it is made available at this time. The pericardium is incised and the pericardial edges retracted with six to eight sutures sewn to the subcutaneous tissue; this technique enhances exposure by elevating the heart and creates a well to contain irrigation solutions.

In repeat sternotomy, adhesions from a previous cardiac operation require dissection. The surgeon divides the sternum with an oscillating saw and dissects retrosternal tissue free. Increased risk of fibrillation from manipulation of the heart and bleeding and laceration of the RV provides the rationale for exposing the axillary artery (AA) or groin vessels (i.e., femoral vein and artery) before sternotomy. Further, authorities suggest that the perfusion team be in the OR during opening in the event that rapid initiation of CPB becomes necessary (Lytle, 2016). In addition, disposable defibrillation patches, applied preoperatively to the left lateral chest and the right upper posterior

chest, can be activated for defibrillation if the heart has not been exposed. Sterile external paddles also may be available.

Three-dimensional CT scans of the chest in real time illustrate various chest structures, extent of retrosternal adhesions, previous bypass grafts, and number of chest wires to be removed. Anteroposterior and lateral chest radiographs also may be available.

These images assist the surgeon and other members of the surgical team to anticipate and prepare for rescue interventions (Lytle, 2016). The preoperative briefing is important to confirm not only the "usual" plan, but also to consider specific interventions unique to the patient's history of surgeries.

On occasion a patient presents for repeat mitral valve surgery. If the original repair was through a thoracotomy incision, sternal adhesions may prove minimal or nonexistent, and the special precautions associated with repeat sternotomy may be unnecessary. Conversely, if the original chest incision was a sternotomy, a right or left lateral thoracic incision may provide better exposure because fewer adhesions are likely.

Mini-Thoracotomy. For minimally invasive cardiac procedures, a variety of smaller incisions (up to approximately 4–8 cm) and ports can be used. These include anterolateral chest incisions small enough for the insertion of specially designed instruments (see Fig. 25.33B), video cameras, and robotic arms. These smaller incisions in the right or left anterior thorax can be used to access, for example, the aortic or mitral valve, the LAD coronary artery, and the left atrial appendage. Performance of MIS cardiac procedures using smaller incisions under direct visualization or, increasingly, by means of video assistance, is common.

Cardiopulmonary Bypass. The temporary substitution of a pump oxygenator for the heart and lungs permits the surgeon to stop the heart to perform cardiac procedures under direct vision in a relatively dry, motionless field. It also allows the surgeon to manipulate the heart with no attendant risk for producing ventricular fibrillation

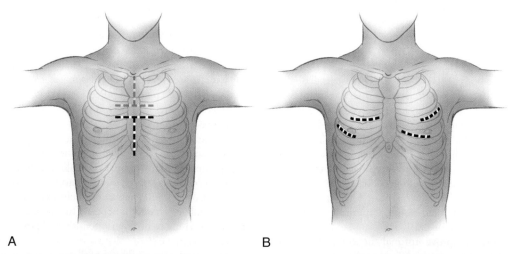

A   B

FIG. 25.33 Minimally invasive approaches in cardiac surgery. (A) Partial sternotomy, upper and lower. Both vertical and transverse incisions may be used (with care to avoid injury to the internal mammary artery). (B) Small, precise thoracotomy incisions may be used for specific surgeries. Right third interspace: aortic valve; right fourth interspace: tricuspid valve, mitral valve, atrial fibrillation, septal defects; left third interspace: left atrial appendage access during atrial fibrillation surgery; left fourth interspace: beating heart surgery for myocardial revascularization of the left anterior descending coronary artery and minimally invasive direct coronary artery bypass.

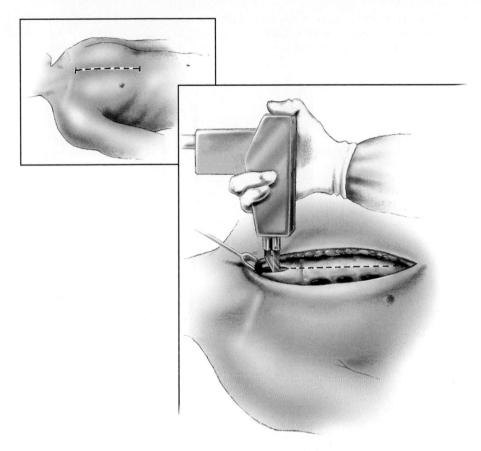

FIG. 25.34 Median sternotomy with sternal saw. *Upper left:* midsternal incision line; *lower right:* sternal division with saw.

or reduced cardiac output that otherwise could jeopardize perfusion to the myocardial, peripheral, and cerebral tissues (Toeg and Rubens, 2016).

Under some circumstances, it is possible to access the anteroapical portion of the heart without excess manipulation of the heart. Special retraction and stabilization devices (described later) allow the surgeon to create CABGs to the anterolateral coronary arteries without the use of CPB and induced cardiac arrest. This enables surgery to be performed on a beating heart (discussed later).

In traditional CPB circuits, systemic venous return to the heart flows by gravity drainage through cannula placed in the SVC and inferior vena cava (IVC) or through a single two-stage cannula in the RA into tubing connected to the bypass machine. Blood is oxygenated, filtered, warmed or cooled, and pumped back into the systemic circulation through a cannula placed in the ascending aorta. An array of arterial and venous cannulae are shown in Fig. 25.35A–E.

Arterial Cannulation. Often, the arterial inflow vessel to the body (commonly the ascending aorta) is cannulated first to have direct and prompt access for blood transfusion should it be necessary (Fig. 25.36A–F). Occasionally the AA (Grocott et al., 2017) (Fig. 25.37) or the femoral artery (Fig. 25.38) is used.

Venous Cannulation. Venous return to the RA can be captured with two cannulae: one placed into the SVC and the other into the IVC (Fig. 25.39A–B). Bicaval cannulation enables almost complete emptying of the heart, which is desirable during surgery in the right side of the heart and when temperature gradients created by relatively warmer returning blood need be minimized. A two-stage cannula

(see Fig. 25.39A, right side of figure) can also be used when complete emptying of the atrium is not required (such as during many aortic valve replacements). Completed cannulation with a two-stage venous cannula is shown in Fig. 25.40.

Bypass Circuits. With the CPB circuit (Fig. 25.41), the pump (Fig. 25.42) oxygenates the blood; consequently, the lungs need not function and may be deflated to provide better exposure of the mediastinal structures. Bypass circuits using percutaneous institution of femoral vein–femoral artery CPB allow MIS or conventional open procedures (Fig. 25.43) as well as emergency procedures in environments not conducive to traditional CPB (e.g., the cardiac catheterization laboratory, the intensive care unit [ICU], or emergency department). Thin-walled, wire-reinforced percutaneous catheters inserted into the femoral vein can increase resistance and impede gravity drainage; therefore assisted drainage using suction is often added to the circuit to achieve adequate venous return.

Other advances include the use of heparin-bonded bypass circuits and tubing. This reduces, but does not obviate, heparin required to achieve systemic anticoagulation, and it can reduce bleeding and the associated need for blood products. Efforts to reduce platelet destruction and the inflammatory response by coating components of the CPB circuits with phosphorylcholine and other materials have shown encouraging results (Grocott et al., 2017).

By diverting blood from the heart, CPB also decompresses the ventricles, reducing myocardial wall tension, which is a significant determinant of myocardial oxygen demand. This effect is evident with CPB or other means of ventricular support that aim to "rest"

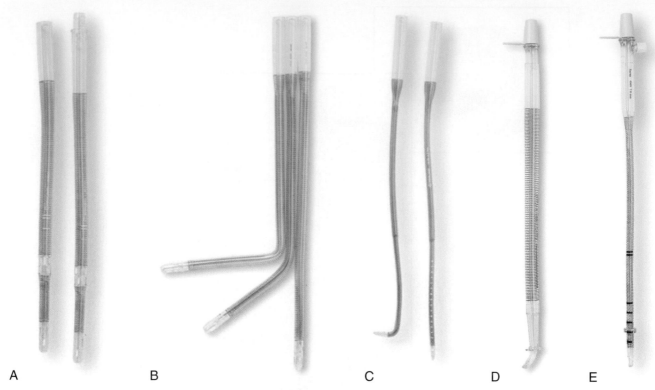

A   B   C   D   E

FIG. 25.35 Arterial and venous perfusion cannulae. (A) Venous return cannula, dual-stage. (B) Malleable venous return cannula. (C) Pediatric venous cannula. (D) Sarns Soft-Flow aortic cannula with suture flange. (E) Aortic cannula Soft-Flow, extended. Venous cannulae have a larger bore compared with aortic cannulae to facilitate gravity drainage into the bypass machine. Venous cannulae often have wire-reinforced walls to prevent crimping of the cannula (which would cause an immediate drop in venous return and subsequent reduction in cardiac output).

the heart. Further decompression results by venting the LV to remove air and accumulated thebesian and bronchial venous return as well as systemic return flowing around the venous cannulae (Fig. 25.44). Insertion of the venting catheter is into the LV via the right superior pulmonary vein or, less common, through the left ventricular apex. The venting line connects to the suction lines of the bypass machine. Insertion of a small venting catheter into the ascending aorta to remove air is also possible. Occasionally, a vent is inserted into the PA. The aim of venting is to reduce the incidence of gaseous microemboli. Ambient air removal is also achievable in cases when the heart is opened (e.g., in valve surgery) with the insertion of a CO_2 gas diffuser; the gas insufflates into the pericardial well. The CO_2 gas dissolves in blood about 25 times faster than room air; CO_2 retained within the cardiac chambers is better tolerated than ambient air and potentially less harmful to tissue. Specifically, CO_2 insufflation use aims to decrease gaseous microemboli in the circulation. A study by Chaudhuri and associates (2012) showed no difference in neurocognitive outcomes, but did show fewer gaseous emboli and a shortened period of de-airing (at least 3 minutes shorter).

Improved bypass technology also reduces the incidence of bypass-related microemboli and cellular injury with the use of finer filters for air and particulate emboli and moderation of siphoning pressure strength (Groom et al., 2009). Membrane oxygenators incorporated into the bypass circuit (see Fig. 25.41) perform gas exchange (CO_2 removal and oxygen addition to the blood) more efficiently and less traumatically. Gases diffuse through a semipermeable membrane

that separates the oxygenating gas and the venous blood. Although membrane oxygenators preserve platelet and RBC function better than older "bubble" oxygenators, there remains considerable morbidity associated with the use of CPB. Extracorporeal circulation may cause fluid retention and intercompartmental fluid shifts, multiple organ dysfunction, showers of microemboli, inflammatory responses, and unique bleeding complications (Groom et al., 2009). The mechanisms of injury likely relate to exposure of the blood to abnormal surfaces of the bypass circuit, hypothermia, shear forces, and altered blood flow. These can initiate a systemic inflammatory response (complement activation), which releases vasoactive substances.

Attempts to minimize inflammatory reactions have focused on modifying activation of platelets and blood factors that play a major role in initiating the response (Kaplan et al., 2017). To avoid complications associated with CPB, clinicians have stimulated greater use of "beating heart" (off-pump) techniques for myocardial revascularization. It should be noted, however, that off-pump techniques are not used for procedures requiring the heart to be opened (e.g., mitral valve surgery, left ventricular aneurysm repair) because air within the opened chamber would embolize to the brain. CPB enables the heart to be isolated from systemic circulation so that after repair completion (and before cross-clamp removal), various venting techniques can remove residual air effectively.

Two pumps are available, roller pumps and centrifugal pumps. Roller pumps have roller heads that propel blood forward by

Text continued on p. 951

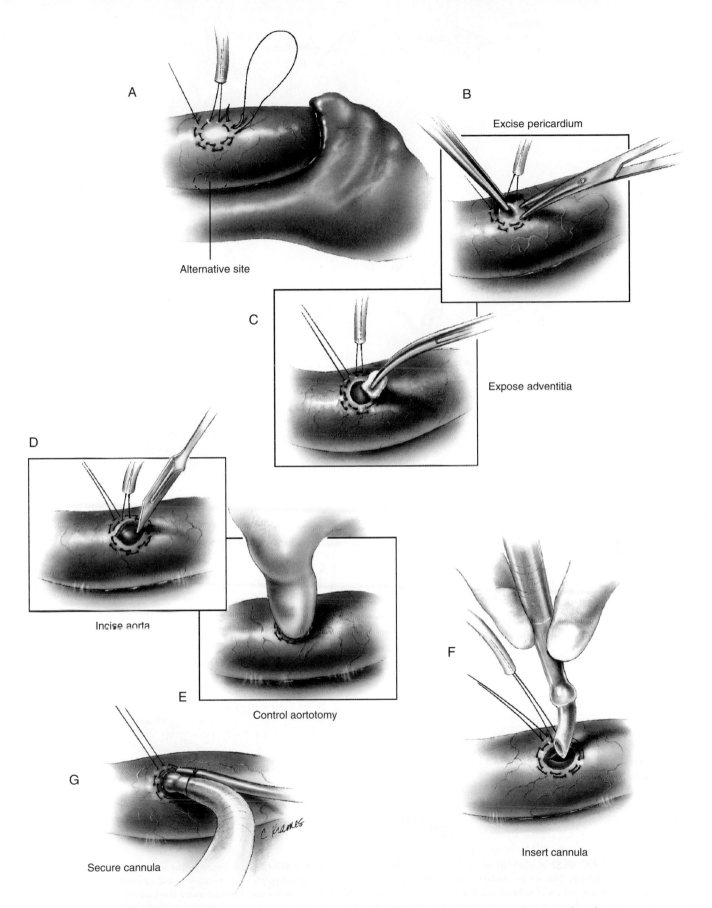

FIG. 25.36 Aortic cannulation. (A) Concentric purse-string sutures in the anterior ascending aorta; lateral alternative site shown. (B) Pericardium excised. (C) Exposure of adventitia. (D) Aorta incised. (E) Finger placed over aortotomy to minimize bleeding. (F) Insertion of cannula. (G) Cannula and tourniquet secured.

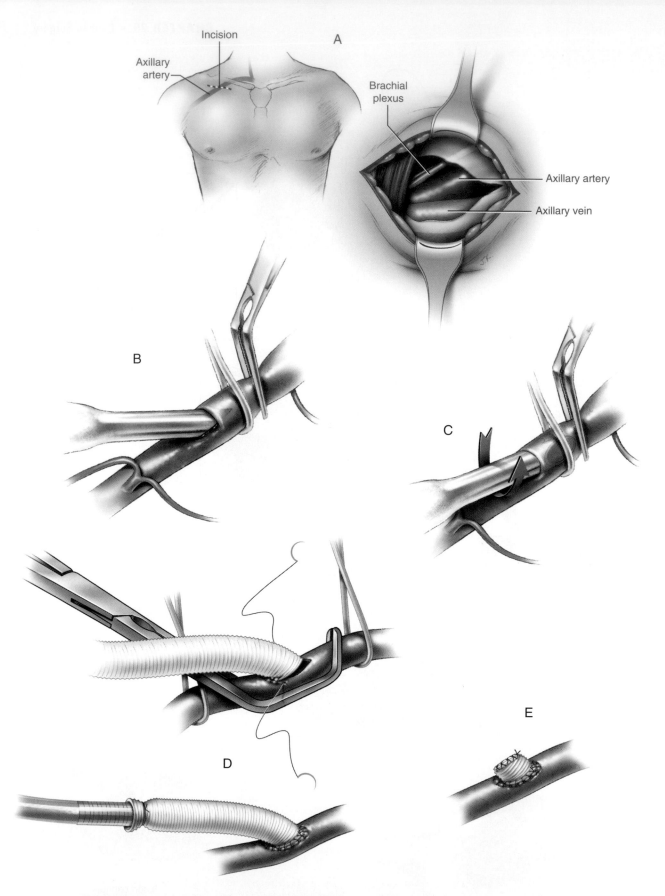

FIG. 25.37 Axillary artery cannulation. (A) Incision line; location of right axillary artery and vein, brachial plexus. (B) Artery clamped and umbilical tape applied to encircle artery, then artery incised and cannula inserted directly into artery while vascular clamp opened. (C) The cannula is rotated and advanced into position; the umbilical tape can be tightened around the cannula to achieve hemostasis; (D) Alternative method uses a prosthetic vascular graft anastomosed to the artery; cannula inserted through graft. (E) After cannula is removed, excess graft material is cut and the remaining graft is oversewn.

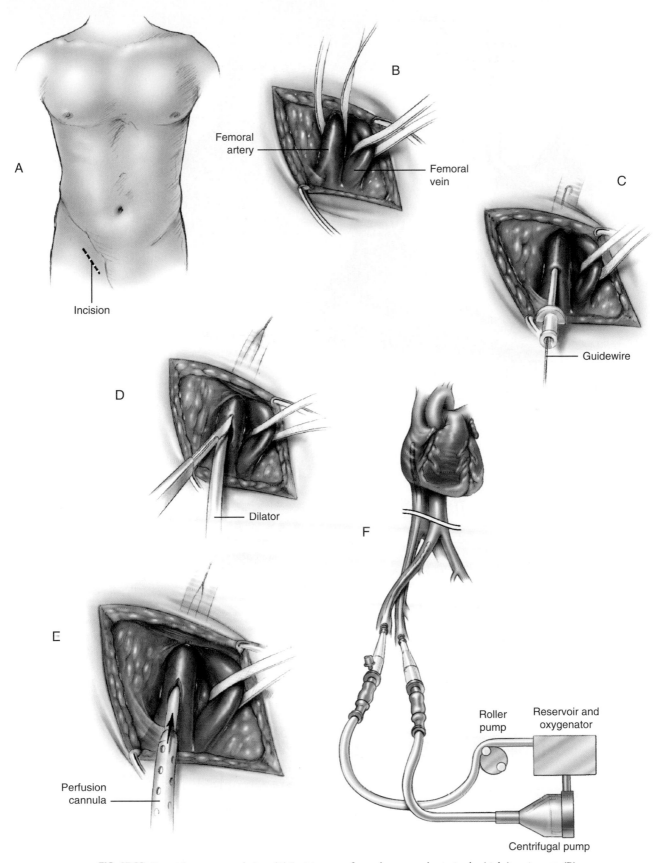

FIG. 25.38 Femoral artery cannulation. (A) Incision over femoral artery and vein in the (right) groin area. (B) Umbilical tapes placed around femoral artery (left) and vein (right). (C) Using Seldinger technique, a needle is inserted into the artery and a guidewire threaded through the needle into the artery. (D) One or more dilators is threaded over the guidewire (to enlarge the arterial lumen) and guided into position in the artery (a short incision in the arteriotomy can enhance passage of the cannula and prevent tearing of the vessel wall). (E) The cannula is inserted over the dilator and advanced into position, the guidewire is removed, and cannulation of the femoral vein is performed in a similar manner (but dilators are usually not needed). (F) The arterial and venous cannulae are connected to their respective bypass tubing lines to initiate bypass.

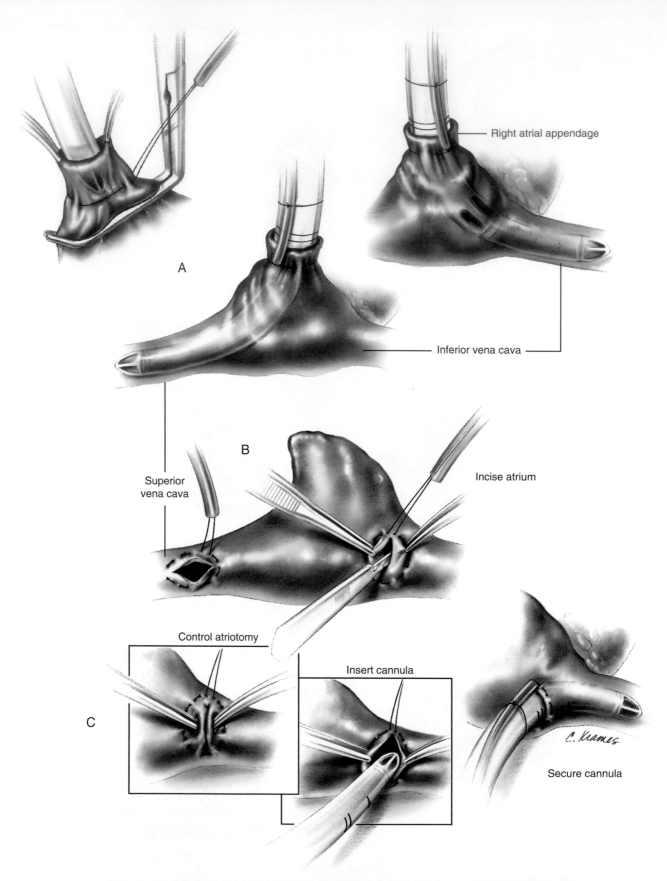

FIG. 25.39 Bicaval and single venous cannulation. (A) A purse-string suture is sewn into the right atrial appendage, tourniquet placed, partial occlusion clamp applied, appendage tip is amputated with scissors, and the superior vena cava (SVC) cannula inserted *(middle drawing)*. The tourniquet is tightened and heavy silk tied around cannula and tourniquet. A single, two-stage cannula *(right drawing)* can be inserted through the appendage and the tip of the cannula threaded into the inferior vena cava (IVC). The two-stage cannula has drainage holes in the portion of the cannula sitting in the body of the atrium (this drains blood returning from the upper body); the distal tip has holes that drain blood returning from the lower body. (B) Occasionally the opening for the SVC cannula is made over the SVC area, and an SVC cannula with a right angle is used for tricuspid valve surgery. Purse-string, tourniquet, and stab wound incision over inferior area of lateral wall allows cannula insertion into the IVC. (C) To minimize bleeding from atriotomy, atrial openings are closed with clamps or forceps until cannula can be inserted.

Labels in figure: Right atrial appendage; Inferior vena cava; Superior vena cava; Incise atrium; Control atriotomy; Insert cannula; Secure cannula; A; B; C

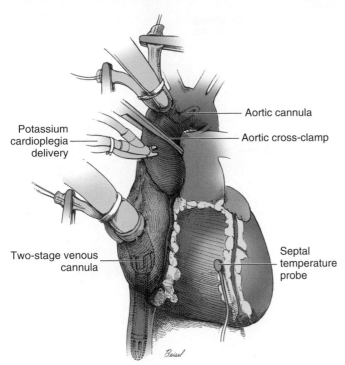

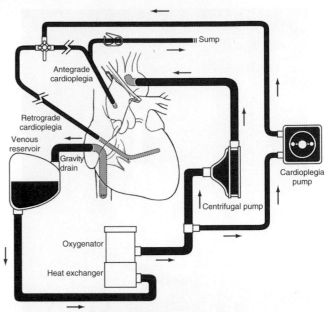

FIG. 25.40 Diagram showing aortic and venous cannulae during aortic cross-clamping. Also shown is antegrade cardioplegic solution delivery catheter in the aorta proximal to the cross-clamp and a temperature probe. The single (two-stage) venous cannula has openings in the distal end of the cannula to drain the inferior vena cava; the openings in the midportion (right atrial area) of the cannula drain the superior vena cava and the coronary sinus venous return.

FIG. 25.41 Cardiopulmonary bypass circuit. Venous blood is drained by gravity from the right atrium or venae cavae into an oxygenator that incorporates a blood reservoir and a heat exchanger, which warms or cools the blood as needed. Ventilating gas flows into the oxygenator, removes carbon dioxide, and adds oxygen to the blood. Saturated blood leaves the oxygenator and is pumped from the reservoir into the arterial system by the use of a centrifugal pump. Filters and monitors are incorporated into the circuit. Additional roller pumps are used to suction shed blood from the pericardial well and the intracardiac chambers (cardiotomy suckers); the blood is returned to the cardiotomy (venous) reservoir. A roller pump is used to deliver cardioplegia.

compressing blood-filled tubing against a smooth metal housing. Centrifugal pumps use cones or blades that rotate at high speed to produce forward flow. Both pumps produce some hemolysis from turbulence and shear forces, but careful calibration and minimal use of connectors can provide relatively atraumatic flow for short periods (e.g., less than 6 hours). Arterial blood flow on bypass is largely nonpulsatile, although modifications to the pump can simulate phasic (systolic/nonsystolic) flow (Grocott et al., 2017); arterial BP usually appears as a mean arterial waveform on the oscilloscope during CPB.

Suction lines, ordinarily used during CPB, return shed blood to the venous reservoir and the oxygenator. These lines may combine conventional handheld suction and ventricular decompression lines or sumps (see Fig. 25.44). Before initiation of CPB, the entire extracorporeal circuit must be primed and rendered free of air to prevent air emboli.

Priming solution is usually a combination of colloid and crystalloid fluids with a balanced electrolyte component. Priming volumes (i.e., within the CPB circuit) are generally between 1400 and 2000 mL. When the patient's blood volume mixes with the prime, there is some hemodilution and a subsequent reduction of Hct levels. Advantages of hemodilution include reducing the number of homologous serum reactions and providing better perfusion of capillary beds, which is a result of reduced blood viscosity. Hct levels as low as 25% may suffice during CPB, but once CPB ends, transfusion of RBCs may be needed to enhance the blood's oxygen-carrying capacity.

Low-weight, low-Hct patients may not tolerate hemodilution well. One method to decrease hemodilution is to use the *rapid autologous prime* (RAP) technique. First, the perfusionist shortens the length of bypass tubing to reduce the volume of prime solution in the CPB circuit. The surgeon then inserts an arterial cannula into the aorta and connects it to the arterial tubing leading to the bypass machine. Before initiation of bypass, the perfusionist allows a predetermined amount of the patient's arterial blood to drain from the line to fill part of the bypass circuit and then clamps the circuit; unclamping follows at bypass initiation (Grocott et al., 2017).

The amount and kinds of drugs used in priming solution vary, but the addition of heparin to block clot formation in the bypass circuit is routine. Anticoagulation monitoring is usual during bypass, as is adding more heparin as needed to maintain an activated clotting time (ACT) that exceeds 600 seconds. Addition of other ingredients to maintain normal pH and electrolytes is also common.

A current concern has arisen with *Mycobacterium chimaera* infections associated with heater-cooler systems used during cardiac surgery (Research Highlight). Water in the systems is used to cool or warm the patient. Although the water does not contact the patient directly, aerosolization or entry of contaminated water into other parts of the system may increase risk of infection (Sommerstein et al., 2016). Perioperative nurses are encouraged to communicate with their perfusion colleagues and infection prevention professional to review heater-cooler systems and minimize the risk of infection.

Finally, team members must estimate arterial blood flow rates according to the patient's height, weight, and body surface area. Arterial and venous pressure values and the results of blood gas determinations dictate flow adjustments.

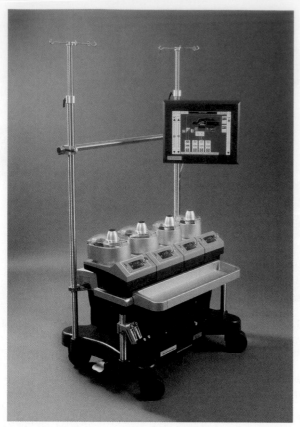

FIG. 25.42 Cardiopulmonary bypass pump. (From Terumo Cardiovascular Systems Corporation.)

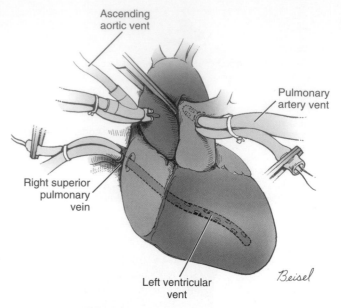

FIG. 25.44 Types of venting catheters.

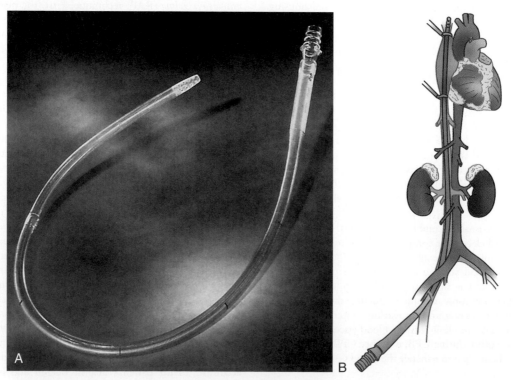

FIG. 25.43 (A) Venous endovascular cannula. (B) The catheter tip is inserted into the femoral vein and threaded to the right atrium; the distal tip is positioned in the superior vena cava to drain the upper body.

RESEARCH HIGHLIGHT ||

Mycobacterium chimaera Infections Associated With Heater-Cooler Systems

Heater-coolers are commonly used during cardiothoracic surgeries, as well as during other medical and surgical procedures, to warm or cool a patient to optimize medical care and improve patient outcomes. The devices include water tanks that provide temperature-controlled water to external heat exchangers or warming/cooling blankets through closed circuits. Although the water in the circuits does not come into direct contact with the patient, there is potential for contaminated water to enter other parts of the device or to aerosolize, transmitting bacteria through the air and through the device's exhaust vent into the environment and to the patient.

A European study describes a link between *M. chimaera* clinical samples, from several infected cardiothoracic patients, with samples from the heater-cooler devices used during these patient's procedures, and with environmental samples from the device manufacturer's production and servicing facility in Germany. The study suggests a direct link between the *M. chimaera* to which the European patients were exposed and became infected with during open-chest cardiac surgery and the heater-cooler model (the Sorin Stockert 3T).

M. chimaera, a type of NTM, is classified as a slow grower yet may cause serious illness or death. The caveat is that it is difficult to detect because infected patients may not develop symptoms or signs for months or even years.

Recommendations for Healthcare Facilities and Staff

The FDA recommends that facilities and staff using heater-cooler units continue to implement the following measures to help reduce risk to patients:

- Strictly adhere to cleaning and disinfection instructions provided in the manufacturer's device labeling. Ensure you have the most current version of the IFU readily available.
- Do not use tap water to rinse, fill, refill, or top off water tanks because this may introduce NTM organisms. Use only sterile water or water that has been passed through a filter of less than or equal to 0.22 microns for the device or when making ice needed for patient cooling during surgical procedures. Deionized water and sterile water created through reverse osmosis is not recommended because it may promote corrosion of the metal components of the system.
- Direct the heater-cooler's vent exhaust away from the surgical field to mitigate the risk of aerosolizing heater-cooler tank water into the sterile field and exposing the patient.

- Establish regular cleaning, disinfection, and maintenance schedules for heater-cooler devices according to manufacturers' instructions to minimize the risk of bacterial growth and subsequent patient infection.
- Develop and follow a comprehensive quality control program for maintenance, cleaning, and disinfection of heater-cooler devices. Your program may include written procedures for monitoring adherence to the program and documenting setup, cleaning, and disinfection processes before and after use.
- Immediately remove from service heater-cooler devices that show discoloration or cloudiness in the fluid lines/circuits, which may indicate bacterial growth. Consult your hospital infection control officials to perform the appropriate follow-up measures and report events of device contamination to the manufacturer and to the FDA via MedWatch.

Recommendations for Patients

- Be aware of the following:
  - In the United States most CPB procedures involve the use of a heater-cooler device.
  - Heater-cooler devices are important in patient care and, in appropriately selected patients, the benefits of temperature control necessary during open-chest cardiothoracic procedures generally outweigh the risk of infection transmission associated with using these devices.
  - The FDA has received reports of patient infections associated with exposure to *M. chimaera* when contaminated 3T heater-cooler devices were used during surgery.
  - *M. chimaera* infections are difficult to detect because symptoms or signs of infection may not appear for months to years after initial exposure.
  - There may be an increased risk of infection if you received a heart valve, graft, LVAD, or any other prosthetic product/material or had a heart transplant.
- If you have undergone CPB, be aware of the possible signs and symptoms of NTM infection. These may include fatigue, fever, pain, redness, heat, or pus at the surgical site; muscle pain; joint pain; night sweats; weight loss; abdominal pain; nausea; and vomiting.

The FDA continues to investigate infections associated with heater-coolers. Although infections associated with *M. chimaera* in heater-coolers are rare, healthcare facilities should take steps to mitigate the risk of infection.

CPB, Cardiopulmonary bypass; *FDA*, Food and Drug Administration; *IFU*, instructions for use; *LVAD*, left ventricular assist device; *NTM*, nontuberculous mycobacterium.
Modified from Centers for Disease Control and Prevention (CDC): *Contaminated devices putting open heart patients at risk* (website), 2016. www.cdc.gov/media/releases/2016/p1013-contaminated-devices-.html. (Accessed 7 March 2017); Centers for Disease Control and Prevention (CDC): *Contaminated heater-cooler devices* (website), 2017. www.cdc.gov/HAI/outbreaks/heater-cooler.html. (Accessed 7 March 2017); Haller S et al: Contamination during production of heater-cooler units by *Mycobacterium chimaera* potential cause for invasive cardiovascular infections: results of an outbreak investigation in Germany, April 2015 to February 2016, *Euro Surveill* 21(17), 2016; Sommerstein R et al: Transmission of *Mycobacterium chimaera* from heater-cooler units during cardiac surgery despite an ultraclean air ventilation system, *Emerg Infect Dis* 22(6):1008–1013, 2016; US Food and Drug Administration. *Heater-cooler devices* (website), 2016. www.fda.gov/MedicalDevices/ProductsandMedicalProcedures/CardiovascularDevices/Heater-CoolerDevices/ucm20082725.htm#_blank. (Accessed 7 March 2017).

Myocardial Protection

Improved cardiac surgery results are attributable largely to progress made in protecting the myocardium. Coronary circulatory interruptions, ischemia, and hypoperfusion accompanying induced cardiac arrest are often necessary to permit the surgeon sufficient time to repair cardiac lesions under direct vision. Without measures to protect the myocardium during these periods, irreversible damage can result. The main protective strategies are cooling the heart (and the rest of the body) to reduce metabolic demand, rapidly arresting the heart

to preserve myocardial energy resources, and restoring intracellular homeostasis (e.g., by correcting pH, oxygen, and electrolyte imbalances) to avoid postischemic reperfusion injury (Kaplan et al., 2017).

Hypothermia. Hypothermia in cardiac surgery is the deliberate reduction of body temperature for therapeutic purposes. A moderate degree of hypothermia to 82.4°F (28°C) permits reduction of oxygen consumption by 50%. At 68°F (20°C), there is a further reduction of about 25%. The heat exchanger of the heart-lung machine achieves systemic circulatory cooling. When very cold temperatures (less than

68°F [20°C]) are desired for myocardial protection in prolonged, complex procedures, additional surface cooling of the heart with topical application of cold saline/slush or continuous irrigation of the pericardial wall comes into play. Avoiding large ice chips in pericardial irrigating fluids prevents injury to the phrenic nerve within the right and left lateral pericardium and other cardiac tissue. Insulation pads placed behind the heart can reduce heat conduction from relatively warmer organs. Transmural cooling of the heart is achieved with cardioplegia (discussed in the following section).

Ventricular fibrillation can occur during the cooling process, although it is less likely at temperatures greater than 89.6°F (32°C). Other complications relate to the adverse effects that hypothermia has on coagulation and wound healing; these effects may delay hemostasis after heparin reversal and affect recuperation (Kaplan et al., 2017).

Cardioplegic Arrest. Rapidly arresting the heart during diastole is beneficial because an arrested heart uses less energy than a fibrillating or beating heart. Cardioplegia with hypothermia can reduce energy requirements even further. Providing a warm terminal bolus of cardioplegia helps avoid reperfusion injury (caused by oxygen free radicals and lactic acid buildup) by providing oxygen and other nutrients to the heart.

Cardioplegia Delivery. Cardioplegic arrest occurs by infusing the coronary arteries with a 39.2°F to 50°F (4°C–10°C) solution containing potassium (2–50 mEq/L) and buffering agents to counteract ischemic acidosis. Potassium acts to depolarize the myocardial cell membrane and arrests the heart in diastole.

Delivery of the solution may be by antegrade or retrograde routes (Figs. 25.45A–D and 25.46). *Antegrade* delivery requires insertion of a needle into the aortic root proximal to the aortic cross-clamp; the cardioplegic solution infuses under pressure to close the aortic valve leaflets. The only remaining route for the solution is into the right and left coronary arteries and the coronary circulation (see Fig. 25.40). If the aortic valve does not close properly, the cardioplegic solution will flow into the left ventricular chamber, causing distention. In such cases, direct cannulation of the coronary ostia is performed. Direct infusion into vein grafts protects the myocardium distal to coronary lesions and enhances transmural cooling. *Retrograde* infusion requires placement of a catheter transatrially into the coronary sinus; perfusate enters the coronary venous system and flows through the myocardial circulation, leaving through the coronary ostia. Retrograde infusion is especially useful when coronary artery obstructions and left ventricular hypertrophy are present.

When the heart arrests sufficiently, the ECG reflects a straight line; when electrical activity appears on the monitor (as fine fibrillation), the cardioplegic solution is reinfused to continue cooling as desired (about every 15–20 minutes).

MIS techniques for myocardial protection also have been developed. Percutaneously inserted catheters can infuse antegrade cardioplegic solution through a catheter threaded into the aortic root; likewise, a catheter inserted into the internal jugular vein and then passed into the SVC, the RA, and the coronary sinus can infuse retrograde cardioplegic solution.

Circulatory Arrest. In highly complex procedures, such as those involving the aortic arch, it may be impossible to place an occluding clamp across the aorta. In these cases circulatory arrest may be used to maintain a dry operative site. As all blood flow will be interrupted, protection of myocardial, cerebral, and other tissues from ischemia requires additional measures.

The patient undergoes cooling with the heat exchanger to about 65°F (18°C), at which point the bypass pump is turned off. Incision

and repair follow. A suction catheter can remove the small amount of collateral drainage entering the field. With repair complete, air removal follows.

Cerebral Perfusion. Circulatory arrest also poses risks to the brain. Cerebral protection, cerebroplegia, is by infusion of oxygenated blood to the brain. *Antegrade* cerebral perfusion occurs via insertion of cannulae directly into the innominate artery, the right common carotid artery, or another branch of the aortic arch. *Retrograde* cerebral perfusion is by use of a cannula that has been Y-ed to the SVC drainage cannula that connects to the arterial infusion line. Once blood flow stops during circulatory arrest, the venous line is clamped, the connection to the arterial line is opened, and the retrograde cerebral perfusion line infuses cerebroplegia into the head vessels. Blood returning from the head (through the carotid or vertebral arteries) is suctioned from the field.

Termination of Cardiopulmonary Bypass

Near the end of the repair, the heart is allowed to rewarm while the perfusionist rewarms the patient systemically with the oxygenator's heat exchanger. Air is evacuated from the LV and the proximal portion of the aorta. Removal of the cross-clamp follows. The heart often converts spontaneously to sinus rhythm, but internal (or external) defibrillation may be necessary. Temporary epicardial pacing wires may be sutured to the right atrial appendage or the RV; these remain postoperatively if the patient has transient bradycardia, supraventricular tachycardia, or other dysrhythmias. AF is a common postoperative complication associated with a greater risk of embolic events and increased LOS (Bainbridge and Cheng, 2017).

When the heart is contracting and the lungs are being ventilated, the patient undergoes gradual weaning from CPB. Reduction of venous flow is gradual, accomplished by reduced clamping of the venous line or lines, and the perfusionist effects a commensurate reduction in arterial flow. When heart action is sufficient and systemic and pulmonary BP is stabilized, the bypass terminates and the cannulae is removed.

Active measures to promote body heat retention and to enhance clotting mechanisms, immune function, and oxygenation follow. It is suggested that maintenance of normothermia after termination of CPB reduces the risk of postoperative infection (Grocott et al., 2017).

Closing

After achieving hemostasis, a team member inserts catheters into the pericardium to drain mediastinal shed blood. Entry into either or both pleurae requires the insertion of chest tubes to drain shed blood entering from the pericardium and to create negative intrapleural pressure to facilitate lung expansion. The tubes connect to a water-seal drainage system or an autotransfusion drainage system by using straight or Y-connectors. Chest tube drainage of greater than 100 mL/h requires investigation of possible causes (Bainbridge and Cheng, 2017). The clinician anticipates such excess drainage by ordering possible blood studies in advance to determine whether clotting factors require replacement, hemostasis of anastomoses is present, or bypass conduits require exploration. Reopening the chest may be necessary to control bleeding.

Chest closure in median sternotomy requires wire sutures (see Fig. 25.18). The wire sutures are twisted, excess wire is cut, and the wire ends are buried into the sternal periosteum. Some surgeons use small metal crimpers to approximate and hold the wires (rather than twisting and burying the wire ends). In a frail sternum, a long sternal closing wire may be threaded longitudinally along the right and left lateral margins of the sternum; the crossed sternal wires insert through

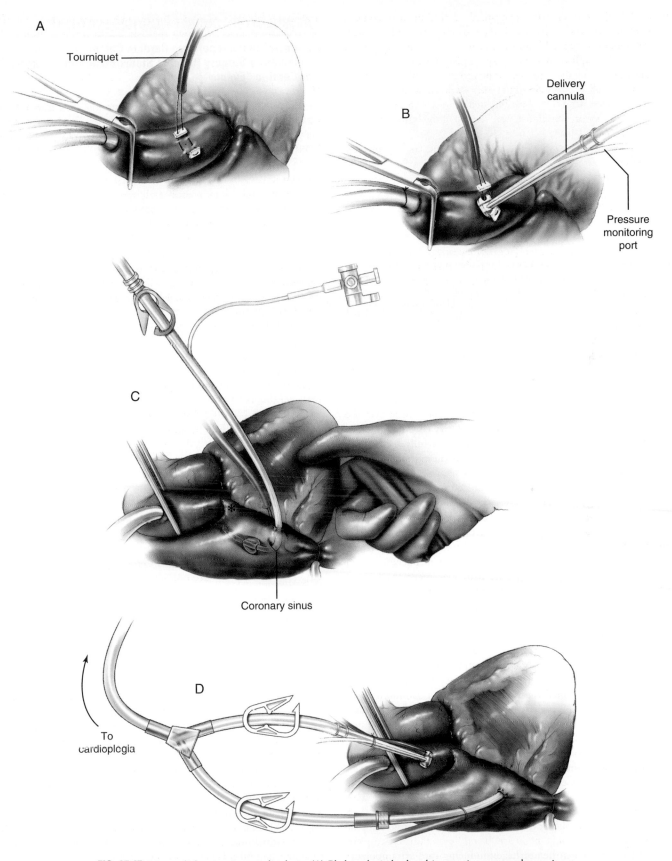

FIG. 25.45 Myocardial protection: cardioplegia. (A) Pledgeted stitch placed in anterior aorta and tourniquet applied. Cross-clamp placed (note arterial infusion cannula distal to clamp). (B) Stab wound made inside stitch and antegrade cardioplegia catheter inserted proximally to the cross-clamp. (C) Retrograde cardioplegia catheter is inserted transatrially through a stab wound in the purse-string and maneuvered into the coronary sinus. The coronary sinus pressure is monitored; its pressure should remain less than 50 mm Hg. (D) Antegrade and retrograde cardioplegia catheters are Y-ed so that the surgeon can selectively deliver cardioplegia through either route.

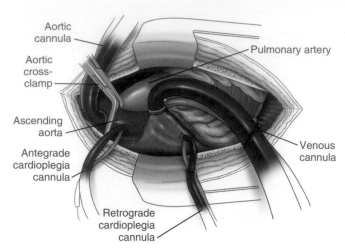

FIG. 25.46 View of cannulated heart from the surgeon's perspective. The cross-clamp isolates the aortic root and coronary blood vessels from the systemic circulation. This creates a closed circuit and allows the administration of cardioplegia without allowing the systemic blood from washing the cardioplegia out of the coronary circulation during induced arrest. This enables the surgeon to create a bloodless field.

the longitudinal wires and then are approximated to close the sternum. This reinforces the sternal closure and reduces the possibility of sternal dehiscence.

In some thin patients with little subcutaneous tissue over the sternum, one (or more) of the sternal wires may continue to cause irritation and discomfort after the sternum has fully healed. For these patients the surgeon may remove the wire during an ambulatory surgical procedure. The surgeon makes a small incision over the wire, dissects down to the wire, cuts it on the anterior surface, pulls it out of the sternum, and closes the incision. An ambulatory procedure to remove a keloid (an overgrown, elevated, and rounded scar) is also possible (Berman et al., 2015; Bope and Kellerman, 2017a). Patients may choose plastic repair if scarring poses personal or professional concerns (Ambulatory Surgery Considerations).

Closure of the linea alba is with suture. Placement of a layer of sutures approximates the fascia over the sternum, and closure of subcutaneous tissue and skin follows. If metal staples are used on the skin, a staple remover should accompany the patient to the recovery area. The clinician closes thoracotomy incisions in standard fashion.

Before transferring the patient, the perioperative nurse transfers information to the receiving unit, usually the cardiovascular SICU, with a telephoned report. Fig. 25.47 lists commonly supplied information. The patient's special concerns and fears, as well as significant physiologic alterations, should be communicated (Seifert, 2017).

Perioperative documentation follows standard protocols and includes a description of the procedure performed, identification of medications administered by the nursing team, and all implanted material (with lot and serial numbers) to ensure compliance with the Safe Medical Devices Act.

Postoperative complications associated with cardiac surgery appear in Table 25.7.

Excessive or sudden hemorrhage producing cardiac tamponade usually requires an organized, competent, rapid response to control hemorrhage and to achieve hemostasis (Bainbridge and Cheng, 2017; Kaplan et al., 2017).

AMBULATORY SURGERY CONSIDERATIONS

Decreasing Postoperative Cardiac Complications in Ambulatory Surgery Patients Status/Postcardiac Surgery or Cardiac "Events"

Perioperative nurses are increasingly aware that their cardiac patients may require future noncardiac surgery. The following steps are recommended to promote a safe ambulatory surgery experience for patients who previously underwent cardiac surgery.

Step 1
Patients scheduled for ambulatory surgery procedures should be at least 1 year post-MI, have anesthesia approval for age limits or body mass index greater than the facility's inclusion/exclusion criteria as a special exception, and conform to facility guidelines.

Step 2
Patients with a cardiac history are required to have the following:
• Preoperative screening and clearance from a cardiologist
• Thorough review of current medications, their use, continuance, and discontinuance.

Step 3
Patients should have an anesthesia screening *before* surgery, not only to reduce same-day cancelations, but also to determine whether the patient should undergo surgery. Screening should include the following:
• History and physical examination
• Information about medications, activity level, compliance with prescribed regimens, and other pertinent items

Step 4
The patient's plan of care should be based on the health history, presence of cardiac and noncardiac symptoms, need (or lack of need) for ECG monitoring or laboratory tests, and use of beta-blockers or DVT preventive measures. Other interventions include monitoring the patient's oxygenation and BP, and placing a magnet over an existing pacemaker (to deactivate and prevent injury to the device) if ESU energy is to be used.

BP, Blood pressure; *DVT,* deep vein thrombosis; *ECG,* electrocardiogram; *ESU,* electrosurgical unit.
Modified from Cunningham B: Ambulatory takeaway. In Thanavaro L: Cardiac risk assessment: decreasing postoperative complications, *AORN J* 101(2):201–212, 2015.

Evaluation

Evaluation of perioperative care includes determination of whether the patient met the outcomes identified in the plan of care. Such evaluation assists perioperative nurses to determine the success of nursing interventions designed for a specific patient. Evaluations become the basis for future plans for similar patients. Documentation of the evaluation should appear in the perioperative record. For the plan of care presented in this chapter, outcome statements might be the following:

• The patient's cardiac function is consistent with or improved from baseline levels established preoperatively, as evidenced by BP within expected range; warm, dry skin; and urine output more than 30 mL/h.
• The patient is free from signs and symptoms of infection at the surgical site(s) as evidenced by absence of redness, edema, purulent drainage, or untoward postoperative temperature elevation.

Patient Transfer Report

PROCEDURE (include source of autogenous grafts) _____   on-pump _____   off-pump _____

Endoscopic vein harvest   yes ___ no ___ N/A ___

MONITORING DEVICES (LOCATION)

CVP _____   Arterial Line_____   SWAN _____   Peripheral _____

LA _____   Other_____

HEMODYNAMICS

BP _____   PAP _____   PAD _____   PAWP _____   CO _____   CI _____   CVP _____   Svo$_2$ _____

INTRAOPERATIVE OCCURRENCES

BLOOD LOSS _____   URINE _____   DYSRHYTHMIAS _____   BYPASS

PROBLEMS _____   DEFIB X's _____   LO TEMP _____   HI TEMP_____

CROSS-CLAMP TIME _____   PUMP TIME _____

BLOOD: GIVEN _____   AVAILABLE _____   AUTOTRANSFUSION TOTALS: _____ mL _____ Units

COMPONENTS: FFP _____   PLATELETS _____   CRYO _____

ADDITIONAL ORDERED (TYPE) _____

MEDICATIONS

NEO _____   DOPAMINE _____   DOBUTAMINE _____   LIDOCAINE _____   NITRO _____

LEVOPHED _____   EPINEPHRINE _____   NITROPRUSSIDE _____   INOCOR _____

DDAVP _____   OTHER _____

TUBES/DRAINS: MEDIASTINAL _____   PLEURAL (Rt/Lt) _____

EPICARDIAL LEADS: ATRIAL _____   VENTRICULAR _____

PACING: YES/NO   RATE_____

LABS:

K+ _____   Na+ _____   Glu _____   Hgb _____   Hct _____

PATIENT CONCERNS _____

ADDITIONAL INFORMATION _____

ICU BED # _____   ETA _____

REPORTED BY _____

To _____   TIME _____

BP, Blood pressure; *CI,* cardiac index; *CO,* cardiac output; *CRYO,* cryoprecipitate; *CVP,* central venous pressure; *DDAVP,* 1-deamino-8-D-arginine vasopressin (e.g., desmopressin); *ETA,* estimated time of arrival; *FFP,* fresh frozen plasma; *Glu,* glucose; *Hct,* hematocrit; *Hgb,* hemoglobin; *K+,* potassium; *LA,* left atrium; *Na+,* sodium; *NEO,* Neo-Synephrine; *NITRO,* nitroglycerin; *PAD,* pulmonary artery diastolic pressure; *PAP,* pulmonary artery pressure; *PAWP,* pulmonary artery wedge pressure; *Svo$_2$,* percent saturation of mixed venous blood; *SWAN,* Swan-Ganz (pulmonary artery) catheter.

FIG. 25.47 Patient transfer report.

- The patient is free from signs and symptoms of injury related to the surgical position as evidenced by the absence of acquired neuromuscular impairment and tissue damage.
- The patient is free of contamination from external and internal sources; there were no documented lapses in sterile technique, no preexisting infections, or no other episodes of contamination.
- The patient is free from excessive bleeding as evidenced by chest tube drainage less than 100 mL/h, dressings dry and intact, normal coagulation function studies (or undergoing replacement treatment for deficient clotting factors), and normal body temperature.
- The patient demonstrated knowledge of the physiologic responses to the cardiac disorder (at his or her level of understanding), the proposed surgical treatment, and the immediate perioperative events as evidenced by verbalization of disease state, purpose of

surgery, sequence of events, anticipated outcomes, and recovery process.
- The patient's myocardial, peripheral, and cerebral tissue integrity are adequate: there are no new ECG manifestations of infarction, peripheral pulses are palpable, and sensorium is improving after extubation in the OR.

Patient, Family, and Caregiver Education and Discharge Planning

The cardiac service admits many patients on the day of surgery; therefore teaching sessions are scheduled before admission, along with preoperative laboratory testing. Perioperative nurses should include details about the surgical procedure, sights and sounds that the patient may face, and anesthesia care. With hospital LOS shortened

TABLE 25.7

Complications of Cardiac Surgery

Body System	Complication	Treatment Measures
Cardiovascular	Bleeding	Transfusion
		Replacement of clotting factors
		Control of hypertension
		Maintenance of normothermia
		Possible return to OR for exploration and hemostasis
	Cardiac tamponade	Release of constricting blood via chest tube insertion or operative exploration
	Myocardial ischemia/infarction	Monitor ECG for ischemic changes
		Measure serum enzymes
		Minimize oxygen demand
		Administer medications to reduce cardiac workload and dysrhythmias
		Insertion of an IABP
	Dysrhythmias	Administer antidysrhythmic drugs
		Correct electrolyte imbalances
		Correct acid-base imbalances; hypovolemia
		Use pacemaker therapy
		Cardiovert or defibrillate as necessary
		Maintain adequate CO
Pulmonary	Hemothorax/pneumothorax	Maintain chest tube patency
		Check chest tubes for air leaks
		Insert additional chest tube (pleural or mediastinal)
	Atelectasis/pneumonia	Check ventilator settings and endotracheal tube
		Suction endotracheal tube
		Monitor breath sounds
		Monitor pulse oximetry
		Obtain chest x-ray film
		Elevate head of bed
		Ensure proper function of NG tube
		After extubation, encourage mobilization and use of incentive spirometry
		Frequent staff handwashing
	Pulmonary embolus	Frequent patient mouth care
		Implement institution's DVT protocol; use mechanical compressions devices such as graduated compression stockings or IPCDs
		Assess for acute chest pain and SOB
		Perform radiologic examination
		Possible surgical embolectomy
	Failure to wean from ventilator	Maintain aggressive pulmonary toilet
		Elevate head of bed 30 degrees
		Monitor pulse oximetry
		Frequent mobilization (even while on ventilator)
		Pain and anxiety management
		Incentive spirometry once extubated
		Possible tracheostomy
Kidneys	Renal insufficiency/failure	Promote adequate CO, renal perfusion
		Monitor urine output
		Diuretics for oliguria
		Administer volume (vs. drugs) to increase renal perfusion
		Possible dialysis
GI	Ileus	Assess bowel sounds and distention
		Maintain NG tube function
		Progress diet slowly
	GI bleeding	Maintain NG tube function to differentiate upper and lower GI bleeding
		Stress ulcer prophylaxis
		Monitor complaints of nausea
		Use extra caution with anticoagulants
Neurologic	Stroke	Avoid hypotension
		Assess neurologic function
		Restart preoperative antidepressant drugs
	Neurocognitive dysfunction/ postcardiotomy delirium	Avoid hypoperfusion
		Correct metabolic derangements
		Avoid hypoxemia
		Orient frequently to time and place
		Discontinue medications that may promote delirium
		Ensure a safe environment

TABLE 25.7

Complications of Cardiac Surgery—cont'd

Body System	Complication	Treatment Measures
Immune	HAI	Frequent staff handwashing
		Strict aseptic technique
		Dressing care, urinary catheter care
		Early removal of central lines, urinary catheters, chest tubes
		Administer antibiotics
	Mediastinitis	Strict aseptic technique
		Administration of antibiotics
Metabolic	Hyperglycemia/hypoglycemia	Limited blood transfusion
		Glucose (hyperglycemic) control
		Possible return to OR for debridement and muscle flap repair
		Avoid hyperglycemia (maintain glucose at less than 200 mg/dL)
		Avoid hypoglycemia
		Monitor for potential rebound from insulin administered during surgery

CO, Cardiac output; *DVT*, deep venous thrombosis; *ECG*, electrocardiogram; *GI*, gastrointestinal; *HAI*, healthcare-associated infection; *IABP*, intra-aortic balloon pump; *IPCD*, intermittent pneumatic compression device; *NG*, nasogastric; *SOB*, shortness of breath.
Modified from Szelkowski LA et al: Current trends in preoperative, intraoperative, and postoperative care of the adult cardiac surgery patient, *Curr Probl Surg* 52(1):531–569, 2015; Seifert PC: Care of the cardiac surgical patient. In Odom-Forren J, editor: *Drain's perianesthesia nursing: a critical care approach*, ed 7, St Louis, 2017, Saunders.

to 3 to 5 days, patient education and preparation for home care maintenance has become even more critical to enhance positive patient outcomes. The perioperative nurse acts to reinforce, review, clarify, and add to important information and instructions the patient, family, and caregiver or significant others need to plan for surgery, recovery, and discharge. Although patients undergoing repeat operations have some experience with cardiac surgery, they often continue to have unmet educational and emotional needs. Changes in the patient's disease, alterations in surgical techniques, and the introduction of newer devices may require changes in expectations. Articles about endovascular thoracic repairs, endoscopic vein harvesting, and percutaneous aortic valve replacement, in less technical language, are available widely online; technology-savvy consumers can download information about many aspects of cardiac surgery, and nurses should be prepared to answer questions and clarify common misconceptions. An area of currently intense patient interest is MIS and comparisons of on-pump and off-pump techniques (Patient, Family, and Caregiver Education).

In addition to specific information about the perioperative period, the cardiac patient's preoperative state of mind is worthy of consideration. Having the patient complete a preoperative mental health status questionnaire, or being aware of the results of a previously completed questionnaire, can provide insight into the patient's frame of mind and serve as an opportunity to change pessimistic attitudes to a more positive state of mind. Patient attitudes can be affected negatively by the anticipation of pain, as well as by hesitation to complain of pain or to request pain medication. Perioperative nurses need to anticipate these normal fears and encourage patients to ask for pain medications to facilitate early postoperative ambulation, deep breathing and coughing, and other activities that promote recovery. Sharing such information with staff in the receiving unit during the hand-off report is entirely proper and good practice (see Fig. 25.47).

The hand-off report should include specific information to optimize recuperation. For example, patients undergoing prosthetic (e.g., mechanical) valve replacement need to know they will require long-term anticoagulation therapy. Important information includes drug dosage, reportable signs and symptoms of complications and side effects (e.g., bleeding, poor healing), and a follow-up protocol to monitor bleeding times.

Assessment of the patient's ability to cough and to breathe deeply is important; further, the patient needs instruction to use a cough pillow or splinting techniques. The patient also needs to know about required lifestyle changes and to express feelings about these modifications. The perioperative nurse should verify that the patient knows reportable signs and symptoms associated with the specific procedure and understands prescribed medications, including medication name and dosages, potential side effects, and signs and symptoms of complications (see Table 25.7). Any misconceptions should be corrected or referred to an appropriate source. The family or significant other's ability and willingness to assist the patient in home care maintenance should be queried; referrals to an agency for assistance at home may be appropriate.

Quality of life is an important concern for patients. Although objective measures are often used by clinicians to determine the patient's level of satisfaction with the quality of care received, measuring the patient's quality of life after surgery has been largely limited to evaluating angina relief and return to work. Other important variables, however, may affect quality of life positively or negatively, and nurses can assist patients with recovery and recuperation by incorporating these variables into the discharge plan. For example, quality of life for family caregivers also is an important consideration because shortened lengths of stay may force patients to depend more heavily on others to assist them with recuperation. Thus support for caregivers is an important adjunct to patient recovery.

Nurses can help patients to set realistic postoperative goals and develop strategies for appropriate lifestyle changes. The subjective perceptions of patients usually accurately reflect the patient's quality of life. At times when quality of life is perceived as less than optimal (e.g., during a difficult recuperation), the nurse can reassure the patient, family, and caregiver that physical, emotional, and psychologic improvement is a progressive process. A patient's perception and the clinical indications for treatment may not be the same, but clinicians should recognize that the patient's definition of quality of life is valid in its own right and it should be addressed whenever feasible.

PATIENT, FAMILY, AND CAREGIVER EDUCATION

Patient Teaching Considerations for Minimally Invasive Surgery (On-Pump/Off-Pump)

	Beating Heart/Off-Pump	Arrested Heart/On-Pump
Definition	CABG without CPB or induced cardiac arrest; HR and contractile force may be pharmacologically reduced; stabilizer used at anastomotic site; apical retractor used to expose lateral and posterior coronary arteries	CABG with CPB and endovascular technique for CPB and induced cardiac arrest
Indications	Multiple-vessel disease, angioplasty contraindicated, medical problems, poor anatomy, accessible target arteries, previous CABG with blocked grafts	Multiple-vessel disease; angioplasty contraindicated; need to stop heart to enhance technical precision, accessible target arteries, valve, or other cardiac disease requiring entry into a heart chamber
Contraindications	Intramyocardial lesions, hemodynamic instability	Highly complex lesions, posterior targets
Incisions	Sternotomy or mini-sternotomy (cephalad or caudad); one to three small right or left rib or submammary incisions	One to four small rib incisions, one or two groin incisions, one or two neck incisions
CPB	No, available on standby	Yes
Cardioplegia	No	Yes
Procedure time	2 h or more	2 h or more
Hospital LOS	2–5 days (vs. 4–6 days for sternotomy)	3–5 days (vs. 4–6 days for sternotomy)
Advantages	Avoids CPB, ischemic arrest, and hypothermia; may enable more complete revascularization with postoperative insertion of intracoronary stents into posterolateral coronary arteries in cardiac catheterization laboratory ("hybrid" procedure); may reduce MACE in patients with LMCAD	Allows repair of more complex lesions without technical challenge of a moving heart; better able to produce more complete revascularization; significantly reduces air embolism as a result of opening cardiac chambers
Potential complications and disadvantages	Learning curve technically more challenging; may cause VF; may have to revert to standard sternotomy with CPB and induced arrest; may be more technically challenging in females	Learning curve technically more challenging; may have to revert to standard sternotomy; potential for endovascular injury to cannulated blood vessels
Discharge planning	Anticipated faster recovery of 1–2 wk (vs. 4–12 wk for sternotomy), earlier ambulation, need to identify reportable signs and symptoms (angina, difficulty breathing, and infection)	Anticipated faster recovery of 1–2 wk (vs. 4–12 wk for sternotomy), earlier ambulation, need to identify reportable signs and symptoms (angina, difficulty breathing, and infection)

CABG, Coronary artery bypass graft; *CPB*, cardiopulmonary bypass; *HR*, heart rate; *LMCAD*, left main coronary artery disease; *LOS*, length of stay; *MACE*, major adverse cardiac event; *VF*, ventricular fibrillation.

Modified from Grocott HP et al: Cardiopulmonary bypass management and organ protection. In Kaplan JA et al, editors: *Kaplan's cardiac anesthesia: the echo era*, ed 7, Philadelphia, 2017, Saunders; Morrow DA, Boden WE: Stable ischemic heart disease. In Bonow RO et al, editors: *Braunwald's heart disease: a textbook of cardiovascular medicine*, ed 10, Philadelphia, 2015, Saunders.

Surgical Interventions

The following section describes surgery for acquired forms of heart disease. It describes both traditional "open" procedures and MIS techniques. Performance of open procedures is through a median sternotomy incision using aortocaval CPB (see Figs. 25.40 and 25.41) and antegrade-retrograde cardioplegia (see Figs. 25.45 and 25.46) with routine chest drainage and closure. MIS procedures include descriptions of CPB, saphenous vein harvesting, CABG, AF, and MVR. Performance of these procedures may be through a median sternotomy or an anterior left or right thoracotomy; some approaches, however, may be via cephalad or caudal mini-sternotomy.

Extracorporeal Circulation Procedures

Operative Procedures

Aortocaval Cannulation by Sternotomy

1. The surgeon makes a longitudinal pericardial incision, and retraction of the pericardial edges is by suture to the chest wall.

2. If the aorta is to undergo cannulation for arterial blood return to the patient, the surgeon partially dissects it from the PA.

3. The surgeon next places two concentric purse-string sutures in the aorta and one purse-string suture in the RA (or in each venae cava) for eventual placement of perfusion cannulae. Tourniquets are placed over the suture ends and held with a hemostat.

4. For ascending aortic cannulation, the aorta is incised inside the purse-string sutures with a knife (the surgeon places a finger over the aortotomy); the cannula is inserted, and the purse-string sutures are firmly secured with the tourniquet. It is important to have the distal end of the cannula clamped before it is inserted into the aorta to prevent back-bleeding from the aorta. To prevent air emboli, the arterial connection is made under a saline drip or by having the perfusionist slowly pump priming solution out of the arterial line. Arterial cannulation generally occurs before caval cannulation so that direct access for blood replacement is available if needed.

5. Venous cannulation occurs in one of the following ways:
   - *Single, two-stage cannulation for venous return to the pump-oxygenator:* An incision is made into the right atrial appendage,

and the two-stage cannula (see Fig. 25.40) is inserted into the atrium. Placement of the distal end is into the IVC. A tourniquet secures the purse-string suture, and the catheter is permitted to fill partially with blood before being connected to the venous line.

- *Double cannulation:* Double cannulation requires a second incision into the atrial wall within the purse-string suture; the cannulae are placed in the IVC and SVC (see Fig. 25.35). To force all venous return into the cannulae, umbilical tapes with tourniquets may be placed around each cava and then tightened. This forces systemic venous return to enter the cannulae, producing total CPB.

6. In procedures requiring greater exposure of the RA (e.g., tricuspid valve surgery or closure of ASDs in adults), a right angle cannula may be inserted into the SVC to provide better RA exposure for the surgeon.

Femoral Vein–Femoral Artery Cannulation

1. A vertical or oblique incision is made into the femoral triangle, exposing the femoral vein and artery. Umbilical compression tapes are passed around the vessels, above and below the proposed venotomy and arteriotomy. Vascular clamps may be applied above and below the incision into each vessel, or, a Seldinger technique may be used to introduce the arterial cannula (see Fig. 25.38).

2. The surgeon may place a purse-string suture into the femoral artery. A needle is then inserted into the artery, followed by a guidewire. The needle is removed and dilators threaded over the guidewire to enlarge the artery. After removal of the dilators, a perfusion catheter (occluded distally with a tubing clamp) is inserted retrograde into the arteriotomy as the proximal clamp or tourniquet is released. The proximal tourniquet is tightened and the cannula is connected to the arterial line.

3. The surgeon incises the femoral vein, and a venous catheter is inserted into the vein as the proximal clamp or tourniquet is released. After the cannula is in place, the proximal tourniquet is tightened to prevent bleeding from the venotomy. Occlusion of the cannula at the distal end with a tubing clamp occurs to prevent bleeding from the cannula. Connection of the cannula is made to the venous line and the tubing clamp removed.

Minimally Invasive Cannulation. Femoral cannulation techniques apply here. Femoral arterial cannulation is as just described. Venous drainage is with an extended catheter inserted into the exposed femoral vein, and the distal tip is advanced to the SVC to the inferior portion of the RA (Fig. 25.48). Side ports along the distal portion of the cannula allow drainage of blood from the SVC, the RA, and the IVC. Given higher resistance to drainage flow compared with right atrial cannulation, a centrifugal pump or vacuum-assisted drainage incorporated in the CPB circuit augments venous drainage. These MIS techniques also apply to newer percutaneous procedures (e.g., catheter-based aortic valve replacement).

Pump Oxygenator Preparation. After completion of arterial and venous connections and securing of lines, bypass slowly begins and the desired flow rate is gradually achieved. Arterial infusion calibration matches venous outflow to maintain consistent cardiac output and blood volume. Perfusion flow adjustments follow as required throughout the operation (Grocott et al., 2017).

Axillary Artery Cannulation

Although infrequently used for arterial perfusion, the right AA is a useful cannulation site when the ascending aorta cannot undergo cannulation because of aneurysm or dissection or when circulatory

arrest is necessary for surgery on the aorta (see Fig. 25.37). Another use occurs in the presence of acute or chronic aortic dissection, when retrograde flow through the femoral artery may produce femoral artery dissection and malperfusion of the central organs (e.g., brain, kidneys). The AA is usually free of atherosclerosis and has excellent collateral flow from the thyrocervical trunk to the suprascapular and transverse cervical arteries, which helps avoid upper extremity ischemia during cross-clamping (Grocott et al., 2017). Use of the AA for cannulation also facilitates antegrade cerebral perfusion during hypothermic arrest. The artery can undergo direct cannulation, but the risk of dissection favors indirect cannulation via an 8- to 10-mm Dacron tube graft anastomosed to the artery.

The patient is supine with a roll under the shoulders to enhance access to the artery; tilting the OR bed to the left provides better exposure of the artery during cannulation. Positioning of the right arm is next to the body with the elbow flexed slightly; extension of the arm on an armboard is proper in some procedures, depending on surgeon preference. Avoidance of severe traction and manipulation is the norm to prevent injury to the brachial plexus.

Cannulation Procedure

1. Exposure of the right axillary (or subclavian) artery is by a small incision below and parallel to the midportion of the right clavicle. The tissue is dissected toward the insertion of the pectoralis minor muscle and the deltopectoral groove; the pectoralis major muscle is dissected and divided, and the axillary vein and underlying artery exposed and gently mobilized for about 2 cm.

2. The brachial plexus is located cephalad to the vessels (see Fig. 25.37A); manipulation is avoided to protect the plexus during cannulation and the operative procedure.

3. The surgeon may cross-clamp the artery, incise the vessel, and insert the cannula (see Fig. 25.37B–C).

4. An alternative is to apply a partial occlusion clamp to the artery and anastomose an 8- to 10-mm Dacron tube graft end-to-side to the artery with 4-0 or 5-0 polypropylene suture (see Fig. 25.37D). A straight arterial cannula is inserted through the graft, and a heavy silk tie or umbilical tape is tied around the graft over the cannula to prevent bleeding.

5. A slow initiation of arterial flow follows. Comparison of BPs via both the right and left radial arteries must confirm the absence of a pressure gradient; after confirmation, arterial flow is increased to the initial desired rate of 2.2 to 2.8 L/min/m².

6. Completion of bypass and removal of the AA cannula: After CPB ends, the arterial cannula is gradually withdrawn and the AA graft is clamped (or ligated with two large metal clips); the graft is cut a few millimeters above the artery and oversewn with polypropylene suture (see Fig. 25.37E). The surgeon carefully avoids narrowing the AA or leaving a large graft "stump" (which could become a source of emboli) during closure.

Cardioplegic Delivery

Antegrade Cardioplegia. Placement of a pledgeted suture and tourniquet is into the anterior ascending aorta proximal to the aortic cross-clamp, followed by insertion of a needle-tipped catheter (see Fig. 25.45A–B). Flushing of both the catheter and the cardioplegic tubing removes residual air. The catheter tubing is often Y-ed into a vent line so that alternatively the needle can infuse the cardioplegic solution into the aortic root or vent air and blood from the aorta and LV. Individual lines incorporated into the antegrade infusion system can infuse the coronary bypass graft or grafts selectively. Handheld cardioplegic cannulae can infuse cardioplegic solution directly into the coronary ostia, but the risk of injuring ostial tissue

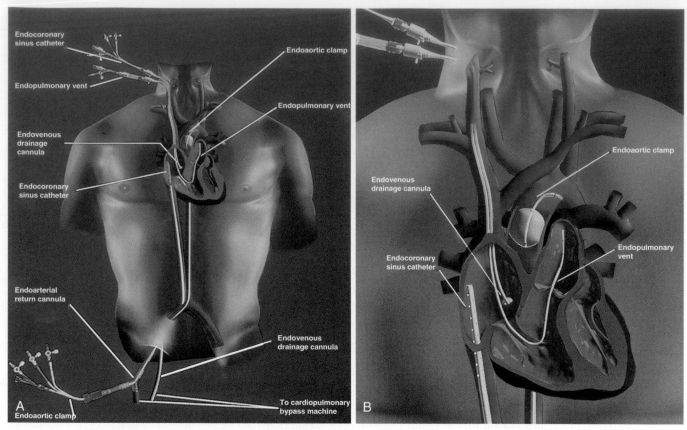

FIG. 25.48 (A) Endovascular cardiopulmonary bypass and myocardial protection system (see text). (B) Intracardiac placement of catheters.

usually favors this technique when retrograde delivery cannot be achieved.

Retrograde Cardioplegia. A purse-string suture is placed into the lateral wall of the RA and a tourniquet applied to the suture. The surgeon makes a stab wound into the atrium, and insertion and palpation of the retrograde catheter into the coronary sinus follow (see Fig. 25.45C). Blood is aspirated from the catheter, and the catheter is connected to the flushed retrograde infusion line and to a pressure line. Infusion pressure should be between 20 and 45 mm Hg (Grocott et al., 2017). Because a full RA facilitates insertion of the catheter, insertion occurs before initiation of CPB when possible. If the patient is already on CPB, the surgeon can fill the atrium by clamping the venous drainage line momentarily, diverting blood into the heart (see Fig. 25.45D) for the completed antegrade-retrograde cardioplegia circuit.

Minimally Invasive Endovascular Antegrade-Retrograde Cardioplegia. A system of endovascular multilumen catheters designed to infuse solutions, vent air and blood, measure intravascular pressures, and occlude the aorta may be used (see Fig. 25.48). Fluoroscopy or TEE confirms proper catheter placement.

The intravascular aortic catheter has three lumens. The first lumen has an inflatable balloon at the tip that, when inflated inside the vessel, occludes the aorta and serves as an internal "cross-clamp." The second lumen either infuses antegrade cardioplegic solution or vents the ventricle. The third lumen measures aortic root pressure. The catheter is introduced into the femoral artery and advanced into the ascending aorta. Either the femoral artery used for arterial inflow or the contralateral femoral artery is used.

A triple-lumen coronary sinus retrograde cardioplegic catheter inserts percutaneously through the jugular vein into the SVC. Fluoroscopy guides the catheter into the coronary sinus. One lumen allows manual catheter balloon inflation, another lumen infuses retroplegic solution, and the third lumen measures coronary sinus pressure.

A third catheter serves as a venting and decompression device. It inserts into the jugular vein (through a separate sheath from the retrograde catheter) and advances into the main PA.

These catheter systems allow surgeons to use MIS techniques to treat lesions, such as mitral valve stenosis, which cannot be performed safely with a beating heart.

Termination of Cardiopulmonary Bypass

1. After the intracardiac procedure ends, evacuation of all air from the LV follows. A warm dose of cardioplegic solution may be given, after which the cross-clamp is removed. The warm solution dilates the coronary vascular bed and enhances coronary perfusion after removal of the cross-clamp.
2. Defibrillation is often spontaneous with removal of the aortic cross-clamp and the entry of warm blood into the coronary circulation. If fibrillation persists, internal defibrillation is necessary. Endovascular MIS procedures require external defibrillation with sterile external paddles or patches. Temporary epicardial pacing wires attached to the atrium and to the ventricle adjust the heart rate and optimize cardiac output.
3. Venous flow to the pump is reduced. Arterial flow is also reduced to equal the reduced venous return. When heart action is sufficient

and systemic arterial BP stabilizes, venous return further reduces and the patient is taken off bypass by clamping all lines and stopping the pump.

4. On removal of the cannulation catheters, the purse-string sutures are tightened and tied. Hemostasis may require additional sutures.

5. Chest tubes are inserted into the pericardium (and the pleural cavity if the pleura has been opened).

6. Administration of protamine sulfate (a heparin antagonist) follows.

7. The pericardium is usually left open so that accumulating drainage does not produce cardiac tamponade.

Closure of Femoral Incisions

1. The femoral catheters are removed, and the arteriotomies are closed with nonabsorbable cardiovascular suture. Removal of any compression tapes and bulldog clamps, if used, follows.

2. Closure of the incision is with absorbable sutures and of the skin, with interrupted or continuous sutures. Closure is performed in multiple layers (e.g., fascia, subcutaneous tissue) to avoid seroma formation.

3. Dressings are applied to all incisions.

Pericardiectomy

Pericardiectomy is partial excision of an adhered, thickened fibrotic pericardium to relieve constriction of compressed heart and large blood vessels. Adhered portions of a scarred, thickened pericardium restrict diastolic filling and myocardial contractility. As the pericardial space is obliterated and calcification of the pericardium occurs, the heart is further compressed. Ascites, elevated venous pressure, decreased arterial pressure, edema, and hepatic enlargement result. In most patients etiology is unknown, although there are documented cases caused by chronic pericarditis, which may be of tubercular, rheumatic, viral, or neoplastic origin. Either supine or left lateral position may be used for a left anterolateral thoracotomy.

Procedural Considerations

The use of CPB is rare for pericardiectomy, but the surgeon may request it on a standby basis. Dissection of extensive adhesions contributes to increased bleeding, and packed RBCs should be readily available. Supplies and instruments for bypass should be available.

Operative Procedure

1. The team hypoinflates the lungs to enhance exposure of the heart. Identification and protection of the right and left phrenic nerves follow. The surgeon incises the pericardium.

2. Removal of the outer, thickened pericardium is as indicated. Cartilage scissors are available. The surgeon carefully dissects fibrous portions adhering to the atria and ventricles with dry dissectors and scissors. Caution is taken to prevent perforation of the atria and RV; thus the result may be small islands of retained, adherent pericardium.

3. Dissection continues, exposing and freeing the large blood vessels as indicated.

4. Placement of drainage catheters is near the heart or through the pleural spaces; connections to the water-seal drainage system follow.

Surgery for Coronary Artery Disease

The growth of MIS techniques (including off-pump CABGs) and PCIs is most evident in the treatment of CAD. When compared with PCI with stent insertion, CABG remains the standard of care for patients with left main or three-vessel CAD (Bakaeen et al., 2014; Teramoto et al., 2017). Revascularization procedures for ischemic myocardium also include an expanding array of options, such as port-access, robotic, endoscopic, and video-assisted procedures using smaller thoracic or sternal incisions (Table 25.8) (Al-Atassi et al., 2016). A combination of both traditional CABG surgical techniques and fluoroscopically guided PCI is appropriate in hybrid ORs. Hybrid ORs are also appropriate for transcatheter aortic valve implantation, arrhythmia surgery (e.g., for AF), and congenital surgery (Chikwe et al., 2017).

Off-pump CABG is gaining popularity as are procedures using CPB with MIS systems (Morrow and Boden, 2015). Revascularization procedures can be performed using a variety of on-pump or off-pump techniques and approaches (see Table 25.8). Advantages of MIS techniques, with or without CPB, include more cosmetic incisions, less perioperative bleeding, fewer surgical wound infections, and earlier postoperative ambulation.

A number of studies related to off-pump CABG show apparently conflicting results. The Randomized On/Off Bypass (ROOBY) trial showed increased repeat revascularization and fewer grafts compared with the on-pump group (Omer et al., 2017). A newer study, the CABG Off or On Pump Revascularization Study (CORONARY) trial showed more positive results (Teramoto et al., 2017; Omer et al., 2017). Some reasons offered for the differences include fewer experienced surgeons (residents were frequently the primary surgeon), more MIs and coronary reintervention, and fewer bypass grafts in the ROOBY trial (Omer et al., 2017). Some early advantages in the off-pump group demonstrated in the CORONARY trial were that surgeons were experienced with off-pump techniques, and more high-risk patients were included (e.g., older females, patients with aortic calcification or renal disease); available long-term data should make the relative advantages and disadvantages more evident (Bakaeen et al., 2014).

In patients with ST elevation myocardial infarction (STEMI), CABG surgery within 6 hours of symptom onset may be appropriate if they are not in cardiogenic shock and are not candidates for fibrinolysis or PCI. On-pump or off-pump techniques and temporary mechanical assistance demonstrate improved survival rates. In the acute phase of STEMI, the efficacy of CABG may prove limited (O'Gara et al., 2013; Wessler et al., 2015).

Standard surgical treatment of CAD includes myocardial revascularization with CABG by use of the left or right thoracic IMA, greater saphenous vein, radial artery, and other autogenous arterial and venous conduits. CABG can alleviate angina pectoris and prolong life in patients with CAD of the left main and LAD coronary arteries (Alexander and Smith, 2016; O'Gara et al., 2013). Selection of the IMA demonstrates excellent long-term patency (Alexander and Smith, 2016; Smith et al., 2014). This result has promoted the use of arterial conduits such as bilateral IMAs (Dorman et al., 2012), and the radial artery, especially in diabetic patients. Use of both IMAs is best when used by experienced surgeons in younger, nondiabetic, nonobese patients (Omer et al., 2017), but early work by Dorman and colleagues (2012) demonstrated no increased morbidity and mortality in diabetic patients receiving bilateral mammary grafts.

The saphenous vein remains an effective conduit when the need for multiple grafts appears. Endoscopic saphenous vein harvest occurs frequently; emergency surgery may preclude the endoscopic technique in favor of the faster, traditional open excision of the vein, but more recently trained clinicians may have learned only the endovascular technique; hence, they are able to perform rapid vein endoscopic harvesting (Aranki and Shopnick, 2011; Dacey, 2012).

TABLE 25.8

Thoracic Incisions

Incision	Position	Possible Indications	Special Patient Needs
Median sternotomy: Incision along center of sternum (sternal notch to xiphoid process)	Supine	Most adult cardiac procedures except those on branch pulmonary arteries, distal transverse aortic arch, and descending thoracic aorta; OPCAB	Padding for hands, elbows, feet/heels, back of head, dependent bony prominences
Mini-sternotomy: Partial upper or lower sternal incision starting either from sternal notch or from xiphoid process and extending to midportion of sternum; LESS	Supine	MAS, or OPCAB procedures	Same as median sternotomy
Parasternotomy: Resection of right or left costal cartilages (from second to fifth cartilage, depending on surgical target)	Supine; small roll may be placed under affected side	Left: MAS CABG Right: MAS CABG, valve procedures	Same as median sternotomy; risk of postoperative chest wall instability
Anterolateral thoracotomy: Curvilinear incision along subpectoral groove to axillary line	Supine with pad or pillow under operative site; arm supported in sling or overarm board; arm on unaffected side may be tucked at side if surgically necessary	MAS, MIDCAB, trauma to anterior pericardium and left ventricle; repeat sternotomy	Padding for extremities; pillow or other device to elevate affected side; armboard or sling for arm on affected side; padding for arm if tucked
Left anterior mini-thoracotomy; right anterior mini-thoracotomy: One or more small incisions (or ports) on left or right side	Supine with small roll under affected side	Left: MAS, MIDCAB, port access for robotic surgery Right: MAS valve procedures, surgery for atrial fibrillation ("mini-maze"); port-access for robotic surgery	Same as anterolateral thoracotomy
Lateral thoracotomy: Curvilinear incision along costochondral junction anteriorly to posterior border of scapula	Placed on side with arms extended and axilla and head supported; knees and legs protected	Lung biopsies; first-rib resection; lobectomy	Armboard, overarm board, axillary roll, padding for pressure sites on dependent side and extremities, pillow between legs; sandbags, straps, wide tape, or other devices to support torso
Posterolateral thoracotomy: Curvilinear incision from subpectoral crease below nipple, extended laterally and posteriorly along ribs almost to posterior midline below scapula (location of intercostal incision depends on surgical site); used less frequently with availability of VATS techniques	Lateral with arms extended and axilla and head supported; knees and legs protected	First-rib resection; lobectomy	Similar to needs for lateral thoracotomy
Transsternal bilateral anterior thoracotomy ("clamshell"): Submammary incision extending from one anterior axillary line to the other across sternum at fourth interspace	Supine	Bilateral lung transplant; emergency access to heart when sternal saw not available	Same as median sternotomy; requires transection of left and right IMA
Subxiphoid incision: Vertical midline incision from over xiphoid process to about 10 cm inferiorly (may divide lower portion of sternum to enhance exposure)	Supine	Pericardial drainage, pericardial biopsy, attachment of pacemaker electrodes, MAS	Same as median sternotomy
Thoracoabdominal incision: Low curvilinear incision on left side extended to anterior midline, continued vertically down abdomen	Anterior thoracotomy with chest at 45-degree angle to OR bed; abdomen supine	Thoracoabdominal aneurysm	Same as anterolateral thoracotomy

CABG, Coronary artery bypass graft; *IMA,* internal mammary artery; *LESS,* lower-end sternal splitting; *MAS,* minimal access surgery; *MIDCAB,* minimal access direct coronary artery bypass; *OPCAB,* off-pump coronary artery bypass; *VATS,* video-assisted thoracoscopic surgery.
Modified from Association of periOperative Registered Nurses (AORN): *Guidelines for perioperative practice,* Denver, 2017, The Association; Bojar RM: *Manual of perioperative care in adult cardiac surgery,* ed 5, Oxford, 2011, Wiley-Blackwell; Doty DB, Doty JR: *Cardiac surgery: operative technique,* ed 2, Philadelphia, 2012, Elsevier; Roselli EE: Reoperative cardiac surgery, *Texas Heart Inst J* 38(6):669–671, 2011.

BOX 25.5

Alternative Conduits for Use as Coronary Bypass Grafts

- Splenic artery
- Lesser saphenous vein
- Cephalic vein
- Basilic vein
- Greater saphenous vein allografts (homografts)
- Synthetic grafts (e.g., Dacron, PTFE)

PTFE, Polytetrafluoroethylene.
Modified from Kaplan JA et al: *Kaplan's cardiac anesthesia: the echo era,* ed 7, Philadelphia, 2017, Saunders.

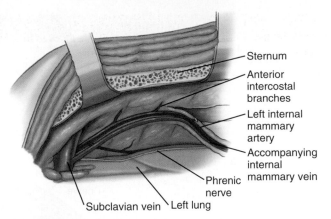

FIG. 25.49 View of internal mammary artery (IMA) and accompanying veins during dissection. Bleeding from side branches is controlled by vascular clips on the IMA side and electrocoagulation on the sternal side. A no-touch technique is important to achieve an atraumatic harvest of the vessel. Dilute solution of papaverine is sprayed onto or into the lumen of the IMA to dilate the artery and reduce muscular spasm. The IMA pedicle is placed in the pleural cavity until needed for anastomosis.

Performance of radial artery excision via endoscopic techniques is more frequent. Use of the radial artery as a second graft in conjunction with the IMA has shown benefits in older (e.g., greater than 70 years old) patients (Habib et al., 2012) and in both men and women, although long-term survival advantage was relatively lower in women (Bope and Kellerman, 2017b). The increasing number of reoperations for CAD has also stimulated use of alternative conduits (Box 25.5).

Distal and proximal anastomotic devices offer the potential for easier bypass procedures. These devices may use grasping hooks that attach the vein to the aorta, magnets, or coupling systems. Clampless devices or "no-touch" techniques may reduce the risk of disrupting aortic atherosclerotic plaque, which can dislodge and embolize after application of a vascular occlusion clamp (Morrow and Boden, 2015).

Dysrhythmias and AF in particular are common after CABG, and these can lead to hemodynamic compromise, systemic embolism, the need for extended anticoagulation therapy (with attendant risk of bleeding), cardiac pacing, patient discomfort and anxiety, and increased cost and LOS. Preoperative administration of beta-blockers is effective to reduce the incidence of postoperative AF; beta-blockers should be reinstituted (absent contraindications) after CABG as soon as possible to reduce the effects of AF. Giving amiodarone may reduce the incidence of AF in patients with contraindications for beta-blockers or in those at high risk for postoperative AF (Hillis et al., 2011).

Increasing recognition of gender differences in the planning, treatment, and outcomes in men and women is apparent in a growing number of practice guidelines for CABG (Hillis et al., 2011; Gulati and Mertz, 2015) (see Evidence for Practice). In particular, guidelines for women focus on use of the IMA, glycemic control, avoidance of anemia and hypothyroid states, avoidance of hormone replacement therapy, and use of off-pump CABG techniques.

Other ischemia-related disorders (including heart failure) that can benefit from surgery include postinfarction VSD, mitral regurgitation (MR), and certain ventricular (e.g., tachycardia) and supraventricular (e.g., AF) dysrhythmias (O'Gara et al., 2013).

Coronary Artery Bypass Grafts With Arterial and Venous Conduits

Operative Procedure

Coronary artery instruments supplement the basic setup for cardiac surgery.

1. Performance of a median sternotomy is as described previously.
2. Conduit preparation:
    a. *IMA.* A special retractor, such as the one shown in Fig. 25.15, elevates the sternum to expose the IMA. The surgeon dissects the IMA from its retrosternal bed to obtain the necessary length (Fig. 25.49). Heparin is administered, after which the surgeon clamps the exposed artery, cuts the IMA caudal to the clamp, and confirms that blood flow through the IMA is adequate. The surgeon may inject papaverine (or another antispasmodic drug) into the IMA lumen with a blunt-tipped needle and then occlude the tip of the IMA with a small bulldog clamp. The surgeon may wrap the pedicle with a papaverine-soaked sponge and store the vessel in the left (or right) pleural space until needed. Ligation of the remaining clamped portion of the distal IMA is done with a tie to prevent back-bleeding. Increasingly, both right and left IMAs are used, even in patients with diabetes, because of improved glucose control in this population. Heparin is given before clamping and cutting arterial grafts to prevent intraluminal thrombosis.
    b. *Endoscopic IMA dissection.* This can occur through thoracic ports (see Table 25.8) inserted into the left anterior thorax at the level of the fourth intercostal space. Ligation of arterial branches and venous tributaries is done with hemostatic clips and electrocoagulation.
    c. *Radial artery.* Generally the surgeon takes the artery from the patient's nondominant arm; adequate blood flow through the ulnar artery is confirmed commonly by Doppler. The surgeon may remove the artery endoscopically or through a longitudinal incision beginning 3 cm distal to the elbow crease lateral to the biceps tendon and ending 1 cm before the wrist crease (Fig. 25.50). The surgeon then exposes and mobilizes the artery with a vessel loop and harvests it as a free graft with adjacent veins and fatty tissue. Ligation of the artery occurs proximally and distally after systemic heparinization. Injection of papaverine into the lumen reduces spasm. The surgeon closes the arm incision; team members may dress it, reposition the arm along the patient's side, and apply more drapes to maintain sterility of the field.
    d. *Gastroepiploic artery.* Rarely used, but when need for an additional arterial conduit appears the surgeon may choose

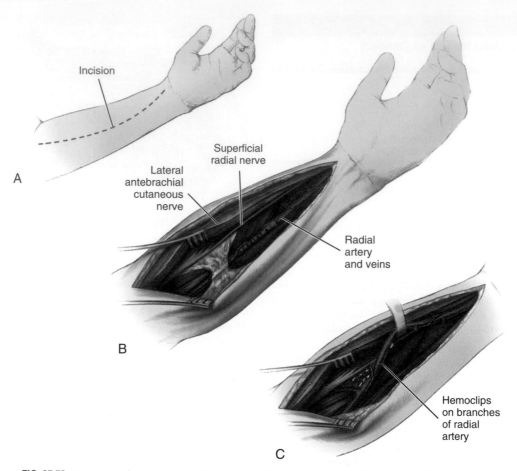

FIG. 25.50 Dissection of radial artery. Before removal of the radial artery, the Allen test is performed to ensure that the ulnar artery will provide sufficient blood flow to the hand if the radial artery is excised: the radial and ulnar arteries are compressed to produce blanching of the hand. The ulnar artery is released while compression is maintained on the radial artery. The skin on the palm of the hand should immediately become red as blood flow is restored through the ulnar artery to the hand. (A) Incision line. (B) Deep forearm dissection exposes the radial artery and vein pedicle. (C) Radial artery pedicle is mobilized, and the multiple side branches are clipped. The artery is removed and may be irrigated with a vasodilator. A continuous intravenous infusion of diltiazem helps prevent vasoconstriction of the artery.

to use the gastroepiploic artery, although required entry into the peritoneum to dissect the artery increases the risk of postoperative complications (Fig. 25.51).

e. *Saphenous vein.* Harvesting of the necessary length of saphenous vein is from one or both legs, either with video-assisted endoscopic techniques or, less commonly, by traditional open incision (Fig. 25.52). Tributaries on the leg side undergo ligation, electrocoagulation, or clipping. After dissection frees the saphenous vein, the surgeon removes it and ligates tributaries on the vein side. The distal end of the vein is identified to place the vein in a reversed position so that the semilunar valves do not interfere with blood flow. The vein undergoes flushing with heparinized blood or saline and must remain moist until needed.

3. With the endoscopic technique, saphenous vein harvesting is achieved through one to three incisions over the vein at the knee and at the ankle and groin if necessary. The surgeon locates the vein under direct vision; excision of the remaining length of vein is with a 5-mm angled endoscope and endoscopic scissors. An endoscopic clip applier and bipolar ESU seal tributaries on the leg side. Once vein removal is complete, the surgeon ligates

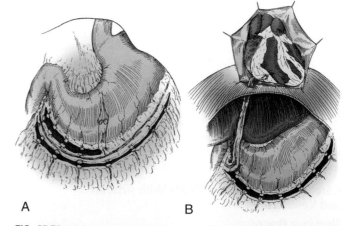

FIG. 25.51 Right gastroepiploic artery mobilization. (A) Branches to the stomach are divided with clamps and ties; omental branches may be divided with a staple gun. The gastroepiploic pedicle is isolated proximally to its origin from the gastroduodenal artery. (B) The pedicle is brought up into the pericardium and anastomosed to the right coronary artery (shown here). The artery can also be grafted to the distal right and left anterior descending coronary arteries.

the vein tributaries with silk ties. The leg is then wrapped with a pressure bandage to reduce postoperative tunnel dead space and to minimize fluid accumulation.

4. CPB with mild hypothermia begins. Antegrade-retrograde cardioplegic solution is infused after the aorta is cross-clamped.

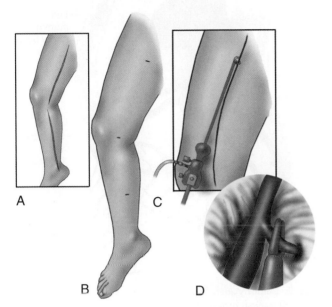

FIG. 25.52 Excision of greater saphenous vein. (A) Traditional open incision. (B) Incision sites (ankle, knee, and groin) for video-assisted, endoscopic vein harvesting. (C) Endoscope inserted into medial knee incision and used to dissect the vein. (D) Venous tributaries may be divided and electrocoagulated or clipped on the leg side; silk ties are commonly used on the vein side.

(Note: If CABG is performed without CPB, there is no patient cooling; CPB standby is usually available.)

5. Coronary anastomoses using the saphenous vein, free arterial grafts, and in situ arterial grafts (e.g., IMA and gastroepiploic artery) follow as described:

   a. The surgeon identifies the affected coronary artery, makes a small incision into the artery, and bevels the graft conduit to approximate the incision (side-to-side jump grafts may be appropriate as well).

   b. Completion of anastomoses is with fine cardiovascular sutures (Fig. 25.53). Before completing each anastomosis, the surgeon may probe the distal coronary artery to ensure patency.

6. Additional anastomoses are performed in a similar manner.

7. The distal anastomosis of the IMA to the coronary artery is as described for the anastomosis of the saphenous vein graft to the coronary artery. No aortic (proximal) anastomosis is necessary because the IMA remains attached proximally to the subclavian artery. Because the IMA has demonstrated superior long-term patency, and the LAD coronary artery is a critical source of blood to the LV, the surgeon commonly attaches the IMA to the LAD coronary artery.

8. Aortic anastomoses:

   a. Proximal aortic anastomoses may be performed with a partial occlusion clamp, but more often performance of anastomoses occurs during a single aortic cross-clamping to avoid excessive manipulation of the aorta that could lead to intimal injury or dislodgement of atherosclerotic material. Increasingly, assessment of the aorta is with epiaortic ultrasound before beginning the anastomoses to identify proximal anastomotic sites relatively free of atherosclerotic plaque. After completion of the proximal anastomoses, the surgeon removes the aortic cross-clamp and defibrillates the heart. Assessment of the

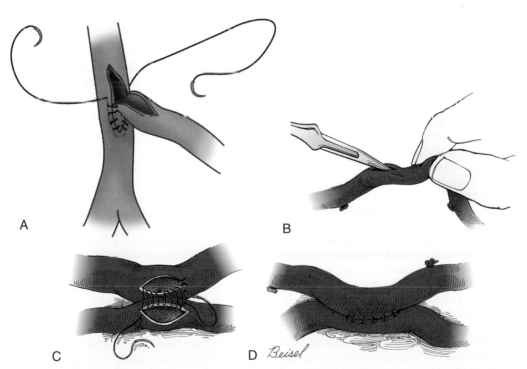

FIG. 25.53 (A) End-to-side coronary anastomosis with bypass graft conduit. (B) Arteriotomy made with #11 blade is shown. (C) Vein-to-coronary side-to-side coronary anastomosis. Double-ended suture used to create anastomosis. (D) Completed anastomosis. Side-to-side anastomoses are used to make more than one attachment of a conduit to an artery, especially when there may be insufficient available conduit material.

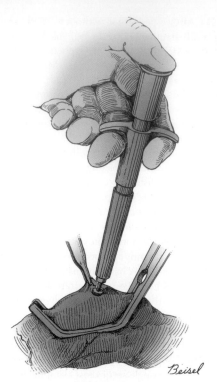

Beisel

FIG. 25.54 Proximal anastomosis of bypass graft. A partial occlusion clamp isolates the portion of the ascending aorta in which the aortotomy is to be made with the punch.

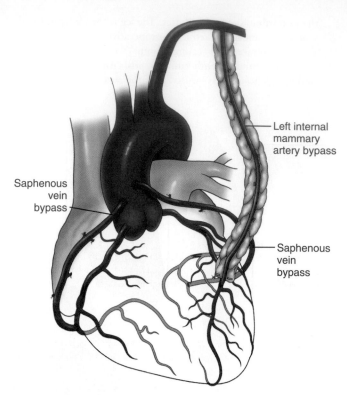

Left internal mammary artery bypass

Saphenous vein bypass

Saphenous vein bypass

FIG. 25.55 Coronary artery bypass grafts with reversed saphenous vein grafts and the left internal mammary artery.

aorta is especially helpful during *beating heart surgery* (usually through a median sternotomy), which requires proximal aortic anastomoses (with saphenous vein or other free graft) to be completed while the heart is contracting. After identification of a suitable site (i.e., relatively free of plaque), the proximal anastomoses may follow with a partial occlusion clamp. An angled vascular clamp partially occludes the aorta, and the surgeon resects a small segment (approximately the diameter of the vein graft). The surgeon performs the aortotomy with a knife blade and enlarges the opening with a punch (Fig. 25.54).

b. Anastomosis of the conduit is end-to-side to the aorta with fine vascular sutures (Fig. 25.55). Removal of the partial occlusion clamp (if used) follows, so that the proximal portion of the vein graft can fill with blood. Needle aspiration of the vein graft prevents air from entering the coronary circulation.

c. When performing proximal anastomoses during a single period of cross-clamping, aspiration from the grafts removes air before removal of the cross-clamp.

9. Marking the aortic anastomoses of the vein grafts with radiopaque clips or rings may follow to aid future identification.

10. CPB ends and closure of the sternum follows.

11. MIS procedures:

a. Performance of MIS direct coronary artery bypass (MIDCAB) occurs, albeit less frequently, in patients with lesions (e.g., narrowings in the LAD and diagonal coronary arteries), which are easily accessible through an anterior thoracotomy. Beating heart procedures performed through a median sternotomy allow surgeons to access lateral and posterior arteries. When using endovascular CPB and cardioplegic solution, it is possible to graft more lateral and posterior arteries (e.g., obtuse marginal and right coronary arteries) because ventricular fibrillation secondary to stimulation of the heart obviates with induced cardioplegic arrest. The surgeon may call for insertion of a double-lumen endotracheal tube to hypoventilate the left lung to enhance visualization of the LAD (and the IMA) while ventilating the right lung sufficiently to oxygenate pulmonary blood flow.

b. With off-pump CABG, cardiac contraction may pose technical difficulty for the surgeon to create a precise anastomosis. Coronary stabilizers reduce the motion of the heart in the vicinity of the anastomosis (Fig. 25.56). These stabilizing attachments fit onto the retractor, freeing the surgeon's hands to suture the anastomosis. Left ventricular apical suction cups allow retraction of the apex, exposing lateral and posterior coronary arteries (see Fig. 25.56). Although early off-pump procedures used beta-blockers and adenosine to achieve pharmacologic cardiac motion reduction, newer stabilizers have reduced the need for these drugs. Bleeding from the arteriotomy, resulting from the heart's continued beating, can obscure the field. To counteract this, the surgeon may use a fine mist of humidified CO_2 gas sprayed over the anastomotic site, elastic coronary artery tourniquets, or Silastic shunts to control bleeding.

c. Thoracic port-access procedures can be performed with a robot and endovascular catheters. Anastomoses can be created with video-assisted thoracoscopic techniques. If the surgeon desires or requires better visualization, conversion to a median sternotomy is an option.

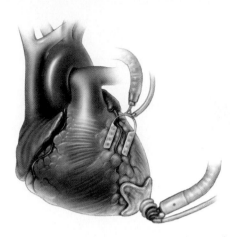

FIG. 25.56 Coronary anastomotic site stabilizer used during beating heart bypass surgery. The vacuum-assisted horseshoe-shaped stabilizer foot reduces the movement of the beating heart and isolates the target coronary artery site for anastomosis. The apical suction cup enables apical retraction.

Ventricular Aneurysmectomy

Left ventricular aneurysmectomy (LVA) is excision of the aneurysmal portion of the LV and its reinforcement with synthetic patch material. LVA is a form of left ventricular reconstruction to optimize cardiac function. An aneurysm of the LV occasionally develops after a severe MI; the aneurysm consists of thin scar tissue that replaces part of the myocardium and may rupture spontaneously. The LV undergoes remodeling when the scar stretches as a result of left ventricular pressure and forms an aneurysm (AHA, 2016). The aneurysm usually adheres to the pericardium; it may not be possible to dissect it free until CPB commences.

Procedural Considerations

Patient positioning is supine. Setup is the same as that described for open-heart surgery, with the addition of synthetic patch material; Teflon felt pledgets; and 0, 3-0, and 4-0 cardiovascular sutures. Occasionally, additional Teflon felt strips bolster the suture lines. Patch closure of the ventriculotomy (endoaneurysmorrhaphy) is more common than traditional excision, plication, and oversewing of the ventricular tissue because patch closure better preserves the geometry of the LV. Mortality remains very high, at approximately 30% (AHA, 2016).

Operative Procedure

The surgeon performs a median sternotomy, and CPB begins as previously described.

Endoaneurysmorrhaphy Technique (Doty and Doty, 2012)

1. The surgeon incises the aneurysmal wall, inspects the anatomy, and carefully removes any clot (Fig. 25.57A).
2. After identifying viable LV tissue, the surgeon places a purse-string suture around the circumference of the viable tissue (see Fig. 25.57B).
3. The surgeon creates a patch (Teflon, pericardium, or a combination of the two materials) and sews it to the area circumscribed by the purse-string suture (see Fig. 25.57C).
4. The surgeon closes the aneurysm scar over the repair (see Fig. 25.57D).

Traditional Technique (Doty and Doty, 2012)

1. The surgeon incises the aneurysmal wall, inspects the anatomy, and carefully removes any clot.

2. Aneurysmal tissue is excised to an area of viable LV wall tissue.
3. The resulting ventriculotomy is closed by plicating the residual tissue between strips of Teflon felt, using interrupted mattress sutures.
4. A second layer of closure stitches, reinforced with Teflon, may be performed to ensure hemostasis.

De-airing

1. A catheter inserted into the right superior pulmonary vein may vent the LV; after de-airing the ventricle, removal of the catheter and closure of the incision follow to end the procedure.

Postinfarction Ventricular Septal Defect

Ventricular septal or free wall rupture is a catastrophic complication of MI, creating an acute left-to-right shunt and cardiac failure requiring early surgical repair. Use of a prosthetic patch or pericardial tissue (Fig. 25.58) to close the defect follows. Felt strips and plicating sutures can reinforce the suture line. Insertion of percutaneous occlusion devices is via the transcatheter route in the cardiac catheterization laboratory (Webb et al., 2015).

Surgery for Heart Failure

Patients with heart failure associated with ischemic coronary disease may benefit from CABG (compared with medical treatment) (Stone et al., 2017). Additional interventions include mitral valve repair (see following section) for ischemic MR, mechanical and biologic support, and cardiac transplantation (described later) (Acker and Jessup, 2015).

Surgery for the Mitral Valve

Mitral *stenosis* (MS) is a narrowing of the valve orifice that impedes forward blood flow. It is often caused by rheumatic fever, especially in poor and developing countries (Castillo and Adams, 2014; Schoen and Gotlieb, 2016). The normal orifice area of the valve is about 5 cm². As the disease progresses, the mitral valve becomes a narrow slit in a fibrotic plaque, severely limiting blood flow into the LV. MS causes a rise in pressure and dilation of the LA. This pressure transmits throughout the pulmonary vascular bed, with subsequent pulmonary hypertension, right ventricular hypertrophy, and possible tricuspid valve regurgitation (Otto and Bonow, 2015). The major symptoms of MS are dyspnea, fatigue, and orthopnea. Late findings are severe pulmonary congestion and right ventricular failure. A diastolic murmur is characteristic, and AF is not unusual. Thromboembolism may result from stasis of blood in the left atrial appendage.

Mitral *regurgitation* occurs when the valve leaflets do not close properly or when the leaflets perforate and blood escapes back into the LA during ventricular systole. Isolated MR is most commonly associated with posterior leaflet prolapse (Castillo and Adams, 2014). Common causes of MR are myxomatous degeneration and as a secondary result of aortic valve stenosis. Other causes of MR are degenerative, ischemic, and dilated cardiomyopathy. During ventricular diastole, blood regurgitated into the LA augments blood volume entering the LV. Additionally, MR may accompany MS or be attributable to leaflet tears, annular dilation, or elongated or ruptured chordae. Ischemic heart disease may produce papillary muscle dysfunction, which prevents sufficient anchoring of the leaflets in the closed position. Symptoms are primarily dyspnea on exertion and easy fatigability related to pulmonary congestion.

The surgeon's selection of the procedure (repair or replacement) depends on mitral valve anatomy, stage of disease, presence or absence

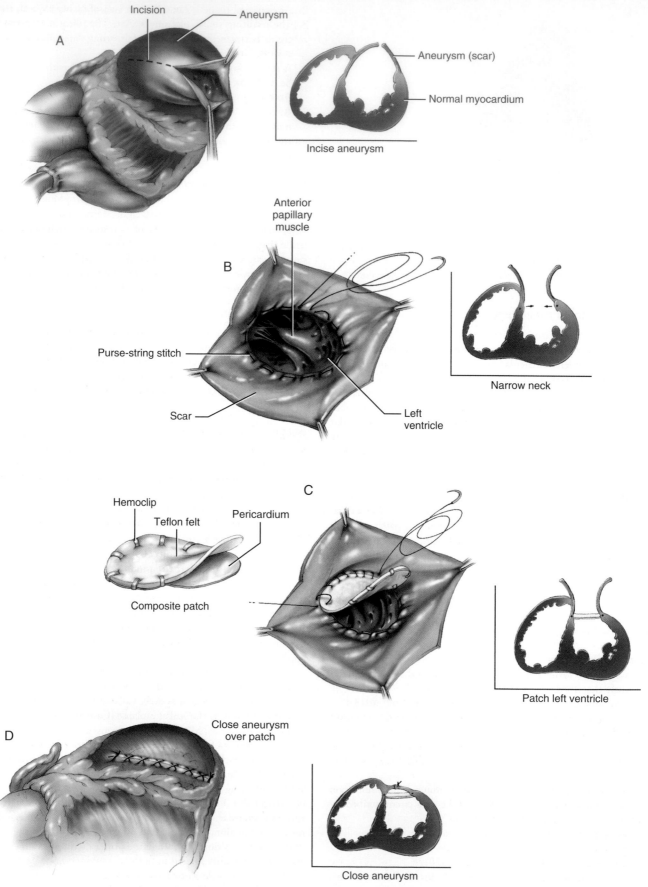

A

Incision — Aneurysm

Aneurysm (scar)

Normal myocardium

Incise aneurysm

B

Anterior papillary muscle

Purse-string stitch

Scar

Left ventricle

Narrow neck

C

Hemoclip

Teflon felt

Pericardium

Composite patch

Patch left ventricle

D

Close aneurysm over patch

Close aneurysm

FIG. 25.57 Repair of left ventricular aneurysm (see text).

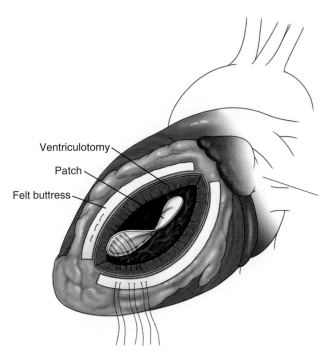

FIG. 25.58 Patch repair of acute ventricular septal defect after myocardial infarction.

of calcification, history of thromboembolism and dysrhythmia, the patient's ability to tolerate long-term anticoagulation therapy (required after insertion of a mechanical valve prosthesis), and the patient's willingness to undergo reoperation if a bioprosthesis deteriorates. Improvements in imaging capabilities with two-dimensional, three-dimensional, and color flow Doppler echocardiography have enabled surgeons to diagnose more precisely and subsequently identify the most appropriate repair procedure. Improved imaging has also fostered development of a consistent nomenclature to describe specific segments of the mitral valve leaflet anatomy. Building on the classic 1983 study of Carpentier, surgeons commonly divide each mitral leaflet into an alphanumeric system: (1) The *anterior* leaflet is divided into three sections that are designated from the lateral to the medial position (left to right): *A1* (lateral), *A2* (middle), and *A3* (medial), and (2) the *posterior* leaflet is divided into three sections that are designated (left to right): *P1* (lateral), *P2* (middle), and *P3* (medial) (see mitral valve in Fig. 25.6B). The goal of this system is to provide consistent descriptions for planning, performing, and documenting care for this highly variable, complex, and dynamic structure.

Consistency in description also promotes reproducibility of the reparative procedures performed to preserve the native valve. Mitral valve repair is widespread because complications associated with prosthetic replacement and anticoagulation therapy do not arise. The technique selected is tailored to the unique pathophysiologic findings; therefore the surgeon carefully evaluates the leaflets and related structures at the time of surgery before deciding which procedure to perform. Given the possibility that the valve may have to be replaced, instruments (and prostheses) for replacement as well as repairs are available. Also included are atrial handheld or self-retaining retractors, obturators to size prosthetic rings and valves, sizer or prosthesis handles, and special sutures if requested. Surgeons often use bicaval cannulation to enhance exposure of the operative field and decompress the heart. The use of TEE establishes a cardiac functional baseline and confirms efficacy of the repair both after the

cross-clamp is removed and the heart resumes beating, and after bypass is discontinued. Intraoperatively, TEE is used to assess left ventricular function and detect the presence of air (seen as white specks) within the cardiac chambers.

Mitral Valve Repairs

Open Commissurotomy of the Mitral Valve for Mitral Stenosis

Open commissurotomy is separation of fused, adhered leaflets of the mitral valve. It may be performed in younger patients to delay more intrusive surgery (such as extensive, prosthetic repair or replacement).

Procedural Considerations. The patient is positioned supine for a median sternotomy. Setup is the same as that described for open-heart procedures, with addition of mitral valve instruments.

Operative Procedure

1. The surgeon performs a median sternotomy, and bicaval cannulation follows for CPB.
2. The surgeon incises the LA and inspects the valve; in some cases the surgeon may use a transseptal approach (RA to LA).
3. Using vascular forceps and scissors or a knife, the surgeon separates fused leaflets and can use a dilator to enlarge the mitral valve orifice.
4. Reinspection of the valve for any resultant insufficiency occurs next.
5. The surgeon may choose to insert an annuloplasty ring to reinforce the repair (described in the next section).
6. Closure of the LA is with a continuous cardiovascular suture.

Mitral Annuloplasty for Mitral Regurgitation

Mitral annuloplasty is reduction of a dilated annulus by inserting a prosthetic ring. Although clinicians commonly assumed that only the posterior leaflet was subject to annular dilation, it now has been demonstrated that the anterior portion also can be affected. Prostheses are available to repair the entire circumference of the annulus (see Fig. 25.32A) or only the posterior leaflet (see Fig. 25.32B). The techniques (and associated prostheses) introduced in the 1980s by Carpentier (1983) and others continue to expand.

Operative Procedure

1. The surgeon incises the LA, after which sump suctions inserted into the atrial cavity remove blood and decompress the heart.
2. Inspection of the annulus, leaflets, chordae, and the rest of the mitral complex follows (Fig. 25.59A).
3. If generalized annular dilation appears, the surgeon inserts an annuloplasty ring; a C-shaped ring may address dilation affecting the posterior leaflet (see Fig. 25.32B). An obturator determines the appropriate size ring. The surgeon places interrupted sutures in the valve annulus and then into the corresponding position in the ring (see Fig. 25.59B). As the stitches are tied, excess annular tissue of the posterior leaflet draws up evenly against the prosthesis (see Fig. 25.59C).
4. The surgeon may select a "classic" mitral annuloplasty ring (that encircles the entire annulus) and attaches it in a manner similar to that as described previously (see Fig. 25.59D–E).
5. The surgeon inspects the valve for competency; use of a bulb syringe filled with saline to distend the ventricle confirms competence of the valve leaflets. Closure of the LA follows.

Mitral Valvuloplasty Repairs for Mitral Regurgitation

Mitral valvuloplasty is repair of the valve leaflets or related structures. Selection of the appropriate repair for perforated or redundant valve leaflets or for shortened or elongated chordae tendineae requires careful

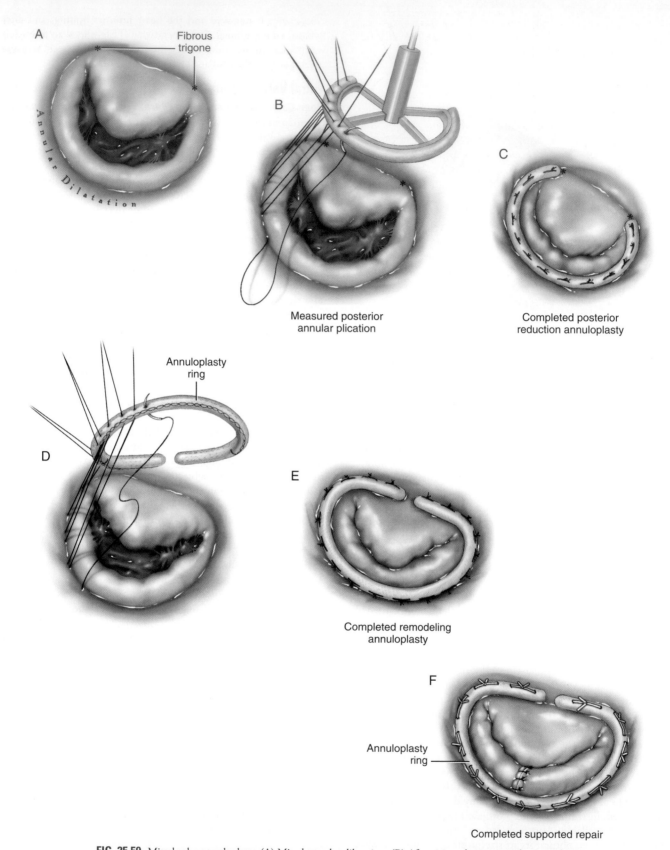

FIG. 25.59 Mitral valve annuloplasty. (A) Mitral annular dilatation. (B) After sizing, the surgeon places stitches into the annulus and the partial ring prosthesis (attached to a holder). (C) The stitches are tied and excess suture material cut. (D) Another type of ring can be used to "remodel" the mitral annulus. (E) stitches are placed, tied, and cut as in (C). (F) Quadrangular portion of excess posterior leaflet resected and remaining leaflet sudges plicated. A supporting annuloplasty ring is inserted.

assessment and evaluation of the abnormalities present. Historically, most mitral valve repairs have focused on the posterior leaflet, but a number of anterior leaflet repairs have been developed.

Operative Procedure

1. The surgeon can patch perforated leaflets with pericardium.
2. Redundant, prolapsed *posterior* leaflet tissue is resectable. The surgeon sews cut edges of the posterior leaflet together and plicates the corresponding annular segment to close the posterior leaflet defect. An annuloplasty ring, inserted to reinforce the leaflet repair, also reduces annular dilation (see Fig. 25.59F).
3. Shortened, fused chordae tendineae can be lengthened and mobilized by dividing them into secondary chordae or by incising the tip of the papillary muscles.
4. The surgeon can also implant redundant tissue of elongated chordae into the papillary muscle head or, rarely, fold it over itself, secured with a suture.
5. *Anterior* leaflet prolapse is a greater challenge and traditionally has indicated valve replacement. A small triangular resection of the anterior leaflet (reinforced with annuloplasty ring insertion) can be performed as well.
6. PTFE suture can replace elongated or ruptured chordae (Fig. 25.60).
7. Surgical use of a chordal flip procedure (Fig. 25.61) can reestablish chordal attachment to the *anterior* leaflet. The surgeon cuts a section of the posterior leaflet with attached chordae, swings it over to the anterior leaflet, and sews it onto the anterior leaflet. Closure of the remaining posterior leaflet defect with suture follows, as described previously.
8. The edge-to-edge technique (Alfieri technique) is used to repair mitral valves with bileaflet prolapse (i.e., both the *anterior* and *posterior* leaflets are incompetent, producing severe MR). The surgeon approximates the free edges of the mitral leaflets, then places a figure-of-eight suture (or percutaneously delivered clip) in the central (or lateral) portion of the apposed leaflets. This creates a double-orifice mitral valve that often significantly reduces MR and preserves the native valve. Frequently an annuloplasty ring supplements the Alfieri technique (Otto and Bonow, 2015).

Investigators have experimented with percutaneous mitral valve repair using various devices and delivery methods. In a transcatheter procedure that echoes the Alfieri technique, the interventionist implants a clip that approximates the edges of the mitral leaflet (Gross and Weiss, 2015). Although a number of innovative percutaneous techniques have developed—and succeeded in, for example, aortic valve replacement (see next)—the complex nature of the mitral valve apparatus, consisting of the annulus, leaflets, chordae tendineae, papillary muscles, and LV, poses particular challenges to successful percutaneous mitral valve repair and, conversely, to avoiding injury to the valve components and other cardiac structures (Otto and Bonow, 2015).

Mitral Valve Replacement

MVR is excision of the mitral valve leaflets and replacement with a mechanical or biologic prosthesis. Bioprostheses are increasingly the choice for valve replacement because of three improvements: improved bioprosthetic durability, fewer valve-related complications, and decreased mortality associated with reoperative valve replacement (Schoen and Gotlieb, 2016).

During MVR, the surgeon often retains the mural (posterior) leaflet, and associated chordae and papillary muscles, to maintain left ventricular geometric configuration, enhancing postoperative ventricular function. If possible, the surgeon also may retain the anterior leaflet if it does not interfere with prosthetic function and is not too heavily calcified.

Surgeons choose to perform median sternotomy in most cases, but right thoracotomy incisions are useful in selected cases (e.g., reoperation, especially in patients with CABG IMA and vein grafts

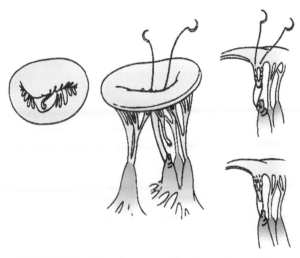

FIG. 25.60 Chordal replacement with polytetrafluoroethylene.

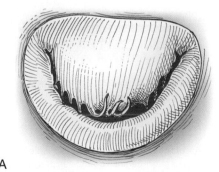
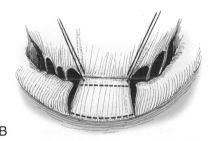

A   B

FIG. 25.61 Chordal flip procedure. Although portions of the posterior leaflet can be resected with success, the same is not true of the anterior leaflet because the shape of the valve and the coaptation margin are altered. (A) When there are ruptured chordae of the anterior leaflet of the mitral valve, the flip procedure can be used to reestablish chordal support for the anterior leaflet. (B) A portion of normal posterior leaflet tissue with attached chordae is cut, swung over, and sewn onto the flail segment of the anterior leaflet.

to the left ventricular coronary circulation). Minimally invasive approaches to heart surgery are becoming more common. The totally endoscopic mitral valve technique (Robotic-Assisted Surgery) is a current option for patients needing MVR or repair. Benefits include improved visualization and less distortion of the valve (Yarboro and Kron, 2016).

Interventional MVR (transcatheter mitral valve replacement [TMVR]) using balloon-expandable mitral prostheses may widen the options for treating mitral valve disease (Guerrero et al., 2016). Although early results show significant adverse events (39.7%

30-day all-cause mortality; 9.3% LV tract obstruction), TMVR is an option for high-risk patients with limited treatment options (Guerrero et al., 2016).

These advances have improved the view of the surgical field and provided better exposure for the repair or replacement of the mitral valve. Robotic mitral valve repair is complex surgery, requiring focus and coordination between the entire surgical team (McCarthy and Guy, 2016). Encouraging results confirm the feasibility and safety of these techniques and pave the way for the development of less invasive operations (Jarrett et al., 2016a, 2016b).

ROBOTIC-ASSISTED SURGERY

Preparing for Totally Endoscopic Robotic Mitral Valve Surgery

To assess valve and heart function and determine the type of mitral valve repair required, the cardiac surgeon orders and reviews the following:

- Transthoracic echocardiogram or TEE
- Right and left heart catheterization reports
- Thorough and complete H&P examination
- Functional assessment of the valve leaflets and subvalvular components
- Evaluation of the severity of the mitral regurgitation
- Preoperative ultrasound study of carotid arteries
- CT evaluation (with contrast) of vessels from neck to femorals (determines ability to undertake remote cannulation)
- A complete metabolic panel
- PFTs
- Chest x-rays
- Coronary angiogram

Preparation for Cardiopulmonary Bypass

After preliminary preparation (such as a nursing assessment, patient prewarming with a thermal device or warm blankets, reassurance and other comforting measures, and insertion of lines by the anesthesia provider), room set up commences. The patient is brought into the OR and a time-out takes place. Monitoring equipment is connected and secured, and general anesthesia begun. After the patient's airway is secured, the team places the patient in Trendelenburg position to produce venous distention of the neck veins. Using sterile technique and ultrasound guidance, the anesthesia provider enters the right internal jugular vein with a small-bore access needle then introduces a guidewire through the access needle. The needle is removed. A specialized guidewire is then inserted and threaded to the desired position in the SVC. This is necessary for SVC cannulation, which is undertaken preoperatively in this robotically assisted surgery.

Preparation for final patient positioning requires that the surgical team move the patient to the right side of the OR bed then roll the patient to the left. The right chest and hips are elevated, and a roll is placed under the right thorax. The patient's right arm is placed on a thoracic arm support, attached at the patient's head, in a position level with the OR bed. This provides posterior extension of the shoulder. Last, the hips are rotated slightly to approximate supine position. The anesthesia provider protects the patient's head and neck and IV lines during all positioning maneuvers. This positioning technique exposes the

anterior and midaxillary lines at the level of thoracic interspace 4 to provide access for the left robotic arm.

Surgical Port Placement

To provide adequate exposure for operating instrumentation and an endoscopic view of the surgical field, endoscopic ports and angiocatheters are required. The surgeon uses the following:

a. One 12-mm port for the endoscope
b. Two 8-mm ports for the right and left robotic arms
c. One 8-mm port for the atrial retractor
d. One 15-mm metal working port
e. Three angiocatheters for suture retraction

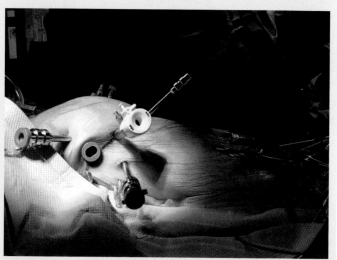

From McCarthy J, Guy TS: Totally endoscopic robotic mitral valve surgery, *AORN J* 104(4):293–306, 2016.

Surgical Procedure Overview

1. Cannulation
2. Institute CPB
3. Achieve cardiac arrest
4. Surgeon returns to robot console
5. Surgeon begins robotic-assisted procedure

CPB, Cardiopulmonary bypass; *CT*, computed tomography; *H&P*, history and physical; *IV*, intravenous; *PFT*, pulmonary function test; *SVC*, superior vena cava; *TEE*, transesophageal echocardiography.
Modified from McCarthy J, Guy TS: Totally endoscopic robotic mitral valve surgery, *AORN J* 104(4):293–306, 2016; Jarrett CM et al: Robotic and minimally invasive mitral valve surgery. In Sellke FW et al, editors: *Sabiston and Spencer's surgery of the chest*, ed 9, Philadelphia, 2016, Saunders; Yarboro LT, Kron IL: How I teach mitral valve surgery, *Ann Thorac Surg* 101(5):1641–1643, 2016.

Procedural Considerations

Although the surgeon may intend to implant a specific type of prosthesis, patient-related factors (Box 25.6) or prosthetic valve complications (Box 25.7) may compel modification of the plan. Additionally there is a greater focus on patient ideas about the ideal prosthetic heart valve (Box 25.8) (O'Gara, 2014). Nurses can incorporate all these ideas into their patient teaching.

A complete range of the surgeon's preferred valves should be available, as well as saline to rinse the glutaraldehyde storage solution from biologic prostheses, if used. Pledgeted sutures of alternating colors are used, and suture holders should be available as well, to keep the stitches in the correct order. Venting catheters and aspirating needles remove air from the heart and ascending aorta. The surgeon may choose to use a small dental mirror after implanting a bioprosthesis to ensure that sutures are not caught in the struts of the valve.

Operative Procedure (Double Venous Cannulation Is Used)

1. With the aorta first cross-clamped, infusion of cardioplegic solution through the aortic root or retrograde through the coronary sinus follows.
2. The surgeon incises the LA along the interatrial groove to expose the mitral valve (Fig. 25.62A).
3. The surgeon carefully assesses the valve and excises the anterior leaflet. Retention of the posterior leaflet and occasionally the anterior leaflet enhances ventricular configuration and postoperative function. Rongeurs are available to debride heavy calcification; loose debris is removed. The surgeon retains a margin of the valve annulus to insert fixation sutures to the prosthesis (see Fig. 25.62B).
4. A valve sizer determines the correct size of the prosthesis, which then is delivered to the field.
5. The surgeon places nonabsorbable cardiovascular sutures (15–20 or more) in the annulus of the valve and then into the sewing ring of the prosthesis.
6. The sutures are held taut (and moistened with saline) as the surgeon guides the prosthesis into position and secures it; the sutures are tied and cut (see Fig. 25.62C).
7. Partial closure of the atriotomy is with continuous nonabsorbable sutures. The patient is placed in Trendelenburg position and the lungs inflated to remove air from the pulmonary veins and atrium. Air aspiration from the LV is through a hypodermic needle inserted into the left ventricular apex or through the vent catheter, and completion of the atrial closure follows.

Endoscopic, video-assisted, robotic mitral valve surgery, described previously, has progressed from technical curiosity to acceptable methods, albeit with a significant learning curve, for intracardiac, telemanipulated valve repair. Surgeons have performed both mitral valve repair and replacement with these techniques (Fig. 25.63), as well as procedures to correct other intracardiac structural lesions (Jarrett et al., 2016a, 2016b; McCarthy and Guy, 2016; Peltz, 2013).

BOX 25.6

Patient-Related Factors and Risks for Valve Surgery

- Age
- Gender
- Residence
- History of atrial fibrillation
- Endocarditis (preoperative)
- Connective tissue disorders (e.g., myxomatous changes)
- Congenital anomalies (e.g., bicuspid aortic valve)
- Enlarged left atrium
- Left atrial thrombus
- Coronary artery disease
- Left ventricular function (e.g., functional class, myocardial infarction, heart failure)
- Syncope
- Mismatch between native valve orifice and patient body size (insufficient cardiac output for metabolic demands)
- Anticoagulation therapy compliance
- Comorbid conditions, preexisting medical problems (e.g., diabetes mellitus, hypertension, hepatic or renal disease)
- Valve lesion, anatomic anomalies
- Previous cardiac surgery

Modified from Otto CM, Bonow RO: Valvular heart disease. In Bonow RO et al, editors: *Braunwald's heart disease: a textbook of cardiovascular medicine*, ed 10, Philadelphia, 2015, Saunders; O'Gara PT: Prosthetic heart valve. In Otto C, editor: *Valvular heart disease—a companion to Braunwald's heart disease*, Philadelphia, 2014, Saunders.

BOX 25.7

Valve-Related Risks and Complications

- Thromboembolism, stroke
- Anticoagulation-related hemorrhage
- Prosthetic valve endocarditis
- Mismatch between prosthetic valve orifice and patient body size (inadequate cardiac output)
- Periprosthetic leak
- Perivalvular regurgitation
- Prosthetic failure
- Injury to heart or vascular access vessel (for percutaneous, transcatheter valve devices)

Modified from Otto CM, Bonow RO: Valvular heart disease. In Bonow RO et al, editors: *Braunwald's heart disease: a textbook of cardiovascular medicine*, 2015, Saunders; O'Gara PT: prosthetic heart valve. In Otto C, editor: *Valvular heart disease—a companion to Braunwald's heart disease*, Philadelphia, 2014, Saunders; Peltz M: Surgery for valvular heart disease. In Antman EM, Sabatine MS, editors: *Cardiovascular therapeutics—a companion to Braunwald's heart disease*, Philadelphia, 2013, Saunders.

BOX 25.8

Patients' Ideas of the Ideal Heart Valve

The prosthesis should:
- Cure the valve disease
- Function like a normal valve
- Improve the patient's lifestyle
- Last as long as the patient

The valve replacement operation should be:
- Performed with low morbidity and mortality
- Nondamaging to other components of the cardiovascular system
- Associated with a short hospital stay
- Affordable
- Possible via the percutaneous route

Follow-up requirements should:
- Require minimal laboratory testing and procedures
- Require minimal therapy

Modified from O'Gara PT: Prosthetic heart valve. In Otto C, editor: *Valvular heart disease—a companion to Braunwald's heart disease*, Philadelphia, 2014, Saunders.

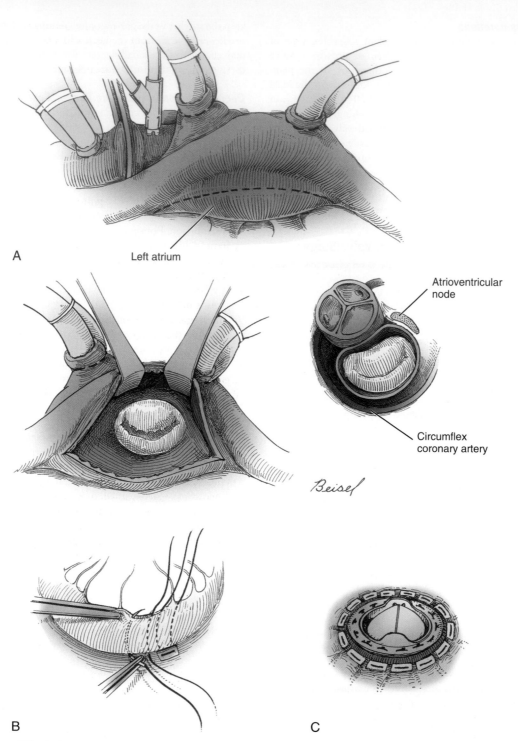

A   Left atrium

Atrioventricular
node

Circumflex
coronary artery

Beisel

B   C

FIG. 25.62 Mitral valve replacement. (A) Line of incision and cannulation for bypass, anatomic relationship between mitral and aortic valves with location of conduction node, and exposure of valve. (B) Placement of pledgeted double-armed sutures in native valve annulus. (C) Completed valve replacement.

Surgery for the Tricuspid Valve

Functional results of significant aortic or mitral valve disease necessitates most tricuspid valve surgery (Mestres et al., 2016; Rosengart and Anand, 2017). When right-sided pressures have increased significantly because of chronic tricuspid regurgitation, the surgeon will look for a patent foramen ovale and the potential for a right-to-left shunt, which could allow an air embolus to travel to the LV (Mestres et al., 2016).

Among treatment options for tricuspid valve disease are suture annuloplasty, ring annuloplasty, and valve replacement with either a biologic or mechanical prosthesis. Percutaneous approaches continue to be investigated (Mestres et al., 2016; Schoen and Gotlieb, 2016; Peltz, 2013).

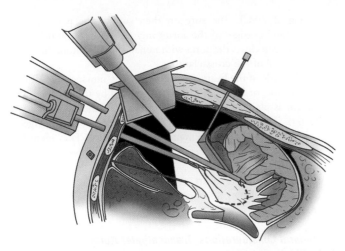

FIG. 25.63 The 1-cm robotic instrument arms are placed through the chest wall. A transthoracic retractor arm elevates the interatrial septum toward the sternum. The three-dimensional camera is placed through a 4-cm incision, which also serves as a working port for the assistant.

Like the mitral valve, the tricuspid annulus is saddle shaped, and techniques to repair the valve also must consider anatomic configuration for optimal repair. Annuloplasty ring insertion is preferable to suture annuloplasty (which does not offer the support provided by the annuloplasty ring) (Mestres et al., 2016).

Tricuspid Valve Annuloplasty

Tricuspid valve annuloplasty reduces a dilated annulus with a prosthetic ring. Tricuspid valve regurgitation may arise from bacterial or viral endocarditis, the presence of a pacemaker or defibrillator lead through the valve annulus, or the functional result of mitral or aortic valve disease. After mitral valve correction, tricuspid valve function may return to normal, although this result is subject to question (Mestres et al., 2016). Preoperatively, if tricuspid annular dilation is diagnosed as severe, ring repair (similar to mitral annuloplasty) or valve replacement may be appropriate. The surgeon takes care to avoid injury to the conduction tissue in the area of the AV node. A PA pressure line may not be inserted before surgery to avoid interference with the surgical site (and potentially be caught in the right atrial suture line); insertion of the PA pressure line may follow completion of surgery.

Patients with significant tricuspid stenosis or regurgitation, failed tricuspid annuloplasty, or significant leaflet damage may require insertion of a prosthetic biologic or mechanical valve (Castillo and Adams, 2014; Mestres et al., 2016). There are no specific tricuspid prosthetic valves; rather, the surgeon uses a *mitral* prosthesis to replace the patient's native tricuspid valve.

Operative Procedure

1. Double venous cannulae are inserted so that they do not cross one another in the RA, and occluding tapes are tightened around the cavae and cannulae to prevent venous return from entering the RA and obscuring the surgical site. A right-angled venous cannula may be placed into the SVC to enhance exposure.
2. The surgeon opens the RA longitudinally to expose the tricuspid valve. Inserted sump suctions remove coronary sinus drainage.
3. For ring annuloplasty, insertion of a prosthetic ring in a manner similar to that used for mitral valve annuloplasty follows (see Fig. 25.59).
4. For valve replacement, the surgeon selects the desired prosthesis and inserts it in a manner similar to that for MVR (see Fig. 25.62).
5. Saline injected into the ventricle tests competence of the repair; TEE is also used.
6. Closure of the RA is with nonabsorbable suture.

Surgery for the Pulmonary Valve

Adult pulmonary valve surgery is unusual, although patients with genetic deformities or those who have undergone repair of congenital pulmonary valve or right ventricular outflow tract obstruction may present with significant pulmonary valve disease (Otto and Bonow, 2015). Generally mild or moderate pulmonary stenosis (PS) produces few symptoms. For patients with severe PS, treatment options include valvulotomy or valve replacement via percutaneous or standard surgical techniques. Generally, surgeons insert an aortic bioprosthesis or an allograft for valve replacement.

Surgery for the Aortic Valve

Aortic *stenosis* produces obstruction to left ventricular outflow. Whether caused by rheumatic fever, a congenital bicuspid valve, or calcification, the fused valve leaflets present increasing resistance to left ventricular outflow, increasing pressure inside the LV. Histopathologic and clinical data suggest that calcified AS is not a "degenerative" passive process; rather it is an active and possibly inflammatory disease process (Otto and Bonow, 2015) with genetic association (Thanassoulis et al., 2013).

To compensate for the increased pressure load, the ventricle hypertrophies so that it can generate sufficient pressure to eject blood through the narrowed opening. When disease is severe, large pressure gradients are often measured during cardiac catheterization, with differences in systolic pressures between the ventricle and the aorta reaching 50 mm Hg or more. In early stages of the disease, a systolic ejection murmur may be heard, but patients are rarely symptomatic. Eventually, fatigue, exertional dyspnea, angina pectoris, syncope, and congestive heart failure may develop, presenting a grave prognosis. Although infrequent, sudden death may be the first sign of AS in asymptomatic patients who are not well monitored (Osnabrugge et al., 2013; Otto and Bonow, 2015; Schoen and Gotlieb, 2016).

In developing countries, aortic *insufficiency* (AI), a form of regurgitation, often arises from rheumatic fever or aortic root disease (e.g., aortic dilation preventing leaflet coaptation); other causes include calcific AS in older patients (the fixed lesion prevents complete closure of the stiffened leaflets), infective endocarditis (causing perforation of one or more leaflets), and trauma. Although *repair* of the aortic valve is challenging because of the precise closing mechanism of the valve leaflets, aortic valve reparative techniques have proved successful in selected patients (Otto and Bonow, 2015). Total valve excision and replacement with a prosthesis or an allograft are common. Transcatheter aortic valve implantation occurs increasingly in a hybrid OR as do mini-sternotomy incisions performed for isolated aortic valve replacement (Chikwe et al., 2017; Schoen and Gotlieb, 2016).

Prosthetic selection depends on achieving appropriate hemodynamic function in relation to body size. The small aortic root (e.g., less than 21 mm) presents challenges to provide an adequate cardiac output. In patients with a small aortic annulus and large body mass (patient/prosthesis mismatch), the surgeon selects a prosthesis that will provide flow adequate to meet the body's needs. The stentless aortic valve (see Fig. 25.25B) is advantageous because there is little sewing ring to reduce output, offering excellent hemodynamic function. Patch enlargement of the small aortic root is another option (described in the following operative procedure) when the patient's own pulmonary valve is used as an autograft to replace the aortic valve; replacement of the pulmonary valve can also be with an allograft (David, 2016; Otto and Bonow, 2015).

Aortic Valve Replacement

The surgeon excises the aortic valve and replaces it with a mechanical or biologic prosthesis or an aortic valve allograft or autograft. Insertion of a percutaneous valve may be with fluoroscopic guidance.

Procedural Considerations: Traditional Aortic Valve Replacement

To the basic setup, the following may be added: aortic valve instruments, aortic valves, sizers, and holders; coronary sinus retrograde-infusion cannula and venting catheters; saline and three basins to rinse the glutaraldehyde storage solution from bioprostheses; and a saline bath to thaw frozen allografts.

Operative Procedure

1. After institution of CPB (a two-stage venous cannula is often used), insertion of a left ventricular vent is placed through a stab wound into the right superior pulmonary vein, with the tip then advanced into the LV. Insertion of a retrograde cardioplegia catheter into the coronary sinus follows (Fig. 25.64A).

2. The aorta is cross-clamped. If AI is present, the initial bolus and subsequent cardioplegic solution infuses retrogradely. Occasionally, direct coronary perfusion (see Fig. 25.64B) is done if insertion of a retrograde catheter is not possible; the surgeon refrains from direct perfusion when possible, to avoid the risk of injuring the coronary endothelium. If AS is present, infusion of the initial bolus of cardioplegic solution may be performed by needle through the aorta into the aortic root. After arrest of the heart, the surgeon opens the aorta.

3. The surgeon first inspects the native valve and then carefully excises it to avoid injury to the annulus and underlying structures (see Fig. 25.64C). Calcium is debrided from the annulus with scissors or rongeurs, or both. Narrow packing used in the LV can confine any small, loose, calcified fragments that could subsequently embolize. Team members frequently wipe instruments clean with a moist sponge.

4. After sizing the annulus, selection of the proper prosthesis follows, as does attachment of a prosthesis holder.

5. If the surgeon has selected a biologic valve, it is delivered to the field and rinsed typically in three saline baths in accordance with the manufacturer's instructions. Biologic valves should be kept moist with frequent saline rinsing, but they should *not* be immersed in antibiotic solution.
   a. If using an allograft, once delivered to the field, it thaws in saline baths according to protocol.
   b. If using a mechanical valve, the team protects it from scratches or other damage.

6. Implantation of the new valve follows, using a technique similar to that earlier described for MVR (see Fig. 25.64D–E).
   a. If the aortic annulus is too small to accept a prosthesis of adequate size, enlargement of the annulus and proximal portion of the ascending aorta is possible. The surgeon places a patch of bovine pericardium or Dacron graft longitudinally in the proximal anterior ascending aorta where the aortic annulus has been incised (Fig. 25.65A–B). The valve prosthesis is sutured to the natural annulus and then to the patch (see

Fig. 25.65C). The surgeon then sutures the patch to the remaining edges of the aortotomy (see Fig. 25.65D).

7. The surgeon closes the aorta with nonabsorbable sutures followed by removal of the cross-clamp.

8. The left side of the heart de-airs by vent, by moving the OR bed side to side, or by other maneuvers chosen by the surgeon. The patient is placed in Trendelenburg position and lung inflation follows. The heart is not allowed to eject blood until the surgeon is satisfied that no air remains within the LV. TEE identifies residual air. The heart is defibrillated if it does not resume beating spontaneously.

9. Rewarming of the heart continues, removal of the venting catheter or catheters follows, and the chest is closed in the routine manner.

Procedural Considerations: Transcatheter Aortic Valve Replacement

Patients with severe, symptomatic AS, who have comorbid conditions that pose a high risk for open-chest surgery, are candidates for this procedure (Chikwe et al., 2017; Osnabrugge et al., 2013), although lower risk patients are increasingly referred by physicians for transcatheter replacement (Rosato et al., 2016). Performance of TAVR is via femoral access obtained in a hybrid OR or cardiac catheterization laboratory with fluoroscopy and intravascular ultrasound (IVUS) available. CT images also should be available for immediate review. If there is severe iliac or femoral tortuosity, atherosclerosis, or calcification, an axillary or LV transapical approach may prove appropriate (Abdel-Wahab et al., 2015; Chikwe et al., 2017; Osnabrugge et al., 2013).

Basic TAVR setup includes the following:
- Endovascular aortic valve instruments
- Femoral access instruments
- Percutaneous aortic valve (e.g., bovine [see Fig. 25.28], equine, or porcine pericardial prosthesis compressed either into a self-expanding system [see Figs. 25.28 and 25.66]) or a balloon-expanding system [Fig. 25.67]); the perioperative nurse confirms the valve size required by the surgeon.
- Valve deployment accessories
- Lubricants for catheters (follow manufacturer's IFU for lubricants)
- Guidewires and other catheters
- Contrast media
- X-ray protection (e.g., lead aprons)

Operative Procedure

1. The surgeon inserts a cannula over a guidewire into the femoral artery and threads the catheter up the aorta to the aortic valve.

2. The surgeon checks and confirms landmarks fluoroscopically.

3. The aortic valve is inserted through the catheter and threaded to the area of the aortic valve.

4. The surgeon positions the valve in the aortic annulus; depending on the type of device, the valve is released and self-expands (see Figs. 25.28 and 25.66), or the balloon expands the device (see Fig. 25.67). The surgeon then looks for perivalvular leaks. If leaks appear, the surgeon can adjust the self-inflating valve device (see Figs. 25.28 and 25.66); if the balloon-expanding device is used (see Fig. 25.67), another device of the same type is placed within the previously inserted device (currently this device cannot be repositioned).

5. Closure of incisions follows.

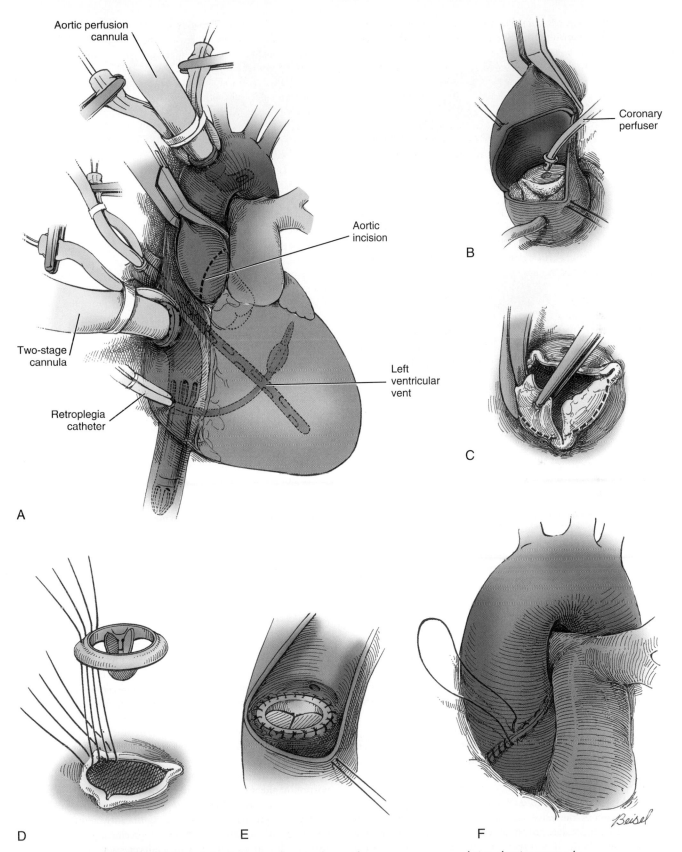

FIG. 25.64 (A) Cannulation for aortic valve procedures with two-stage venous cannulation, showing retrograde cardioplegia and vent sites. Note incision line. (B) If retrograde cardioplegia is not used, handheld coronary ostial catheters can deliver antegrade cardioplegic solution. (C) Diseased valve is completely excised. (D) Sutures are placed in the valve annulus and the prosthetic sewing ring. (E) Stitches are tied and cut. (F) Closure of the aortic suture line.

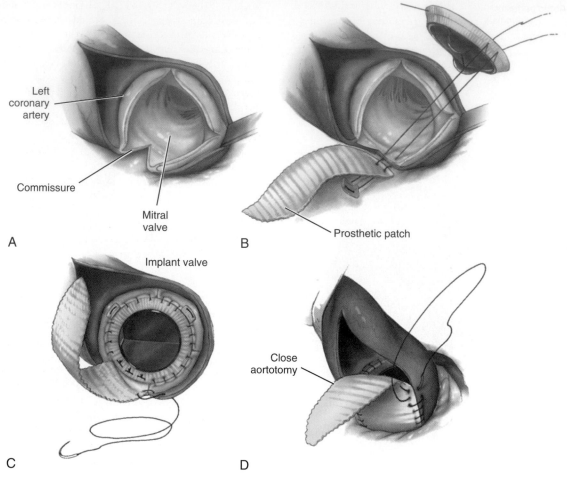

FIG. 25.65 Technique for aortic enlargement (Nicks-Nuñez operation). (A) The aortotomy is extended through the commissure separating the left and noncoronary cusps. (B) A prosthetic patch is sewn into the cut portion of the aorta and into the prosthetic valve. (C) The prosthetic valve is seated, and the stitches are tied and cut. (D) The patch is incorporated into the aortotomy closure.

Combined Surgery

When combining CABG with aortic valve replacement, the procedure usually occurs in the following order:

1. The diseased valve is excised, the annulus is sized, and the prosthesis is selected.
2. The surgeon performs distal coronary anastomoses.
3. Insertion of the prosthetic valve follows.
4. The surgeon closes the aorta (or LA in MVR).
5. Insertion of the proximal coronary anastomoses into the aorta follows, after which the aortic cross-clamp is removed.

Double Valve Replacement

When *both the aortic and mitral valves are to be replaced,* the surgeon first excises the valves and sizes the annuli. The surgeon implants the mitral valve prosthesis first and then implants the aortic valve prosthesis. If the aortic prosthesis was inserted first, the firm prosthetic aortic annular ring might cause cardiac injury and make insertion of a mitral prosthesis more difficult. Closure of the aorta follows, and after sufficient de-airing of the LV, the LA is closed.

Surgery for the Thoracic Aorta

Aneurysms may result from atherosclerosis, trauma, infection, or cystic medial degeneration (David, 2016; Szeto and Bavaria, 2016; Tracci and Cherry, 2017). *Atherosclerosis* affects large and medium arteries with tunica intima deposits of plaques containing cholesterol, lipoid material, and lipophages. Atherosclerosis generally affects the smaller arteries, rather than the aorta. *Arteriosclerosis* is a condition characterized by loss of elasticity and by thickening and hardening of the arteries. Both conditions may lead to aneurysm formation within an artery.

Thoracic aortic aneurysmectomy is excision of an aneurysmal portion of the ascending aorta, aortic arch, or descending thoracic aorta and replacement with a prosthetic graft or valve-graft conduit. Collagen-impregnated grafts have significantly reduced interstitial bleeding and obviated the need for preclotting techniques. It is also possible to use an allograft (cadaver segment of aorta) or an autograft (patient's own PA) to replace the affected aorta (a graft replaces the PA).

Aortic *dissection* is a unique condition related to a tear in the tunica intima of the aorta that exposes underlying degenerative changes in the tunica media layer of the artery. Intraluminal blood flow penetrates and flows through the tear, resulting in subsequent dissection of the tunica media (David, 2016). As blood passes between the layers of the wall, it forms a false channel; as the channel extends and enlarges, it can obstruct blood flow through the aorta and its branches, or the aorta can rupture, causing severe hemorrhage (Fig. 25.68A–B). Surgical intervention becomes necessary when presenting symptoms indicate a compromised circulation or danger of rupture. Generally, medical management with hypotensive agents to reduce stress on the vessel is the preferred initial treatment until surgical repair can be performed. Aneurysms and dissections of the descending thoracic aorta often undergo repair with endovascular prostheses (Ehrlich et al., 2013; Luozzo et al., 2013).

Aneurysms are characterized morphologically as follows: (1) saccular, a sac type of formation with a narrowed neck projecting from the side of the artery, or (2) fusiform, a spindle-shaped formation with complete circumferential involvement of the artery. *Dissections* can be characterized in at least two systems according to type, origin, and extent of the lesion (Table 25.9).

Procedural Considerations

Several methods of surgical treatment appear in the classic study by Crawford (1990). When an ascending aortic aneurysm or aortic dissection produces annular dilation with consequent aortic valve insufficiency, a modified Bentall-DeBono procedure may be used with a composite graft-valve conduit; reimplantation of the coronary ostia may be performed to replace the aortic valve and the aneurysmal aorta (David, 2016) (Fig. 25.69). Retrograde cardioplegia is usually used to arrest the heart; if necessary, selective coronary infusion is an option. The Bentall-DeBono procedure requires reimplanting the right and left coronary ostia into the prosthetic graft; in patients with documented CAD, the surgeon may anastomose vein grafts to the affected coronary artery and attach them proximally to the prosthetic graft.

Positioning, instrumentation, and the type of CPB depend on the location of the aneurysm or dissection. Often patients with dissections present emergently, requiring immediate intervention. The perioperative nurse minimizes delays by asking some basic questions to presage appropriate preparation and intervention to promote an effective outcome.

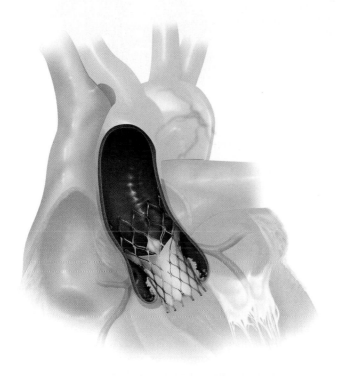

FIG. 25.66 Transcatheter self-expanding aortic valve in the aortic root.

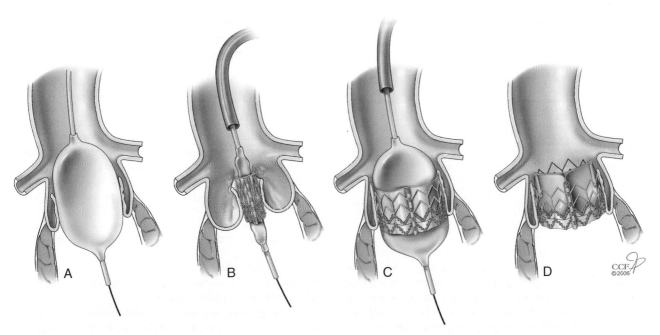

FIG. 25.67 Percutaneous insertion of transcatheter aortic valve. (A) Percutaneously inserted balloon catheter; balloon is inflated to enlarge aortic annulus. (B) Compressed valve positioned in aortic annulus. (C) Balloon inflation opens the valve in the aortic position. (D) After valve is deployed, the balloon is deflated and removed.

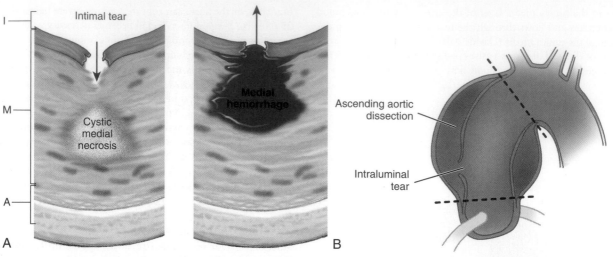

FIG. 25.68 Aortic dissection. (A) Proposed mechanism of the initiation of an aortic dissection (*A*, adventitia; *M*, media; *I*, intima). (B) Intimal tear in the ascending aorta causing a dissection.

TABLE 25.9

Commonly Used Classification Systems to Describe Aortic Dissection

Type	Site of Origin and Extent of Aortic Involvement
DeBakey	
Type I	Originates in ascending aorta and extends at least to aortic arch and often beyond it distally
Type II	Originates in and is confined to ascending aorta
Type III	Originates in descending aorta and extends distally down aorta or, rarely, retrograde into aortic arch and ascending aorta
Stanford	
Type A	All dissections involving ascending aorta, regardless of site of origin
Type B	All dissections not involving ascending aorta
Descriptive	
Proximal	Includes DeBakey types I and II or Stanford type A
Distal	Includes DeBakey type III or Stanford type B

Modified from David TE: Surgery of the aortic root and the ascending aorta. In Sellke FW et al, editors: *Sabiston and Spencer's surgery of the chest*, ed 9, Philadelphia, 2016, Saunders; Szeto WY, Bavaria JE: Endovascular therapy for thoracic aortic aneurysms and dissections. In Sellke FW et al, editors: *Sabiston and Spencer's surgery of the chest*, ed 9, Philadelphia, 2016, Saunders; Harris KM et al: Correlates of delayed recognition and treatment of acute type A aortic dissection: the International Registry of Acute Aortic Dissection (IRAD), *Circulation* 124(18):1911–1918, 2011; Svensson, LG et al: Aortic valve and ascending aorta guidelines for management and quality measures: executive summary, *Ann Thorac Surg* 95(4):1491–1505, 2013.

To initiate CPB, the atrium undergoes cannulation for venous return, and use of the femoral or AA affords arterial inflow because the weakened ascending aorta cannot be cannulated safely. Deep hypothermia with circulatory arrest and cerebroplegia offer protection of the heart and brain during procedures to address particularly complex lesions of the aortic arch, in which placement of a cross-clamp is difficult. Cerebral oximetry monitors oxygenation of the brain.

Traditionally, during open repair of descending thoracic aortic aneurysms, the heart is not arrested; it continues beating to perfuse the upper body. It is possible to institute a femoral bypass to perfuse the kidneys and lower extremities with maintenance of normothermia. Hypothermic CPB is available to repair complex descending and thoracoabdominal aneurysms to provide protection against paralysis and renal, cardiac, and visceral organ system failure. Increasingly, an endovascular stent is used (see Fig. 25.21) for aneurysms and dissections (Ehrlich et al., 2013; Luozzo et al., 2013; Szeto and Bavaria, 2016); insertion of the prosthesis is through the femoral artery, guided via fluoroscopy, to the area of the descending aortic aneurysm or dissection.

In complex lesions involving the ascending aorta, arch, and descending aorta, the ascending aorta and arch may be repaired using an open technique. Repair of the descending aorta may be achieved with an endovascular graft (Luozzo et al., 2013; David, 2016; Szeto and Bavaria, 2016).

Repair of Ascending Thoracic Aortic Aneurysm or Dissection

Procedural Considerations

To the basic setup are added aneurysm instruments. Valve instruments; coronary instruments; and an array of tube grafts, valves, or valved conduits should be available. Preference is for bicaval cannulation, but if the cavae cannot be accessed safely because of increased risk of injury to the enlarged aneurysm, the femoral vein affords initial venous drainage. Once control of the aneurysm is at hand, the femoral venous line can be Y-ed to a vena caval cannula. If there is normal aortic tissue in the distal potion of the ascending aorta, distal to the aneurysmal or dissected tissue, the surgeon can insert the arterial cannula into that area (Fig. 25.70A). Femoral arterial cannulation may be required if the aorta cannot be used for cannulation.

Operative Procedure

1. The patient's position is for median sternotomy.
2. Cannulation for CPB follows.
3. The surgeon opens the sternum and inspects the aneurysm.
4. The surgeon assesses the condition of the aortic annulus.
   a. If the aortic annulus is not involved, the surgeon may incise the aneurysm longitudinally and anastomose a woven graft proximally and distally to the healthy aorta (see Fig. 25.70B–C).

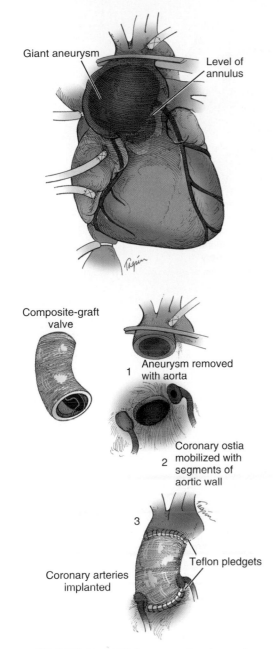

Giant aneurysm

Level of annulus

Composite-graft valve

1 Aneurysm removed with aorta

2 Coronary ostia mobilized with segments of aortic wall

3

Teflon pledgets

Coronary arteries implanted

FIG. 25.69 Bentall-DeBono procedure (see text).

BioGlue may be applied for hemostasis (see Fig. 25.70D). Additionally, felt strips may be incorporated into the anastomosis to bolster friable tissue.

b. If the aortic annulus is involved, the surgeon incises the ascending aorta to the annulus and then excises the aneurysm. Excision of the valve leaflets follows, and the annulus is measured. The proximal end of a valved conduit is inserted. The surgeon uses an electrocoagulator to create openings in the graft at the location of the right and left coronary ostia, which are then mobilized and anastomosed to the graft. If there is concomitant CAD, saphenous vein grafts are inserted. The surgeon sutures the distal end of the conduit to healthy aorta (see Fig. 25.69).

5. Bypass ends, and closure of all incisions follows.

Repair of Aortic Arch Aneurysm
Procedural Considerations

Aneurysm instruments and woven grafts are available. If the surgeon chooses deep hypothermia, the patient's head may be covered with bags of ice at the beginning of the procedure to reduce cerebral oxygen demand. Precautionary measures (e.g., padding) to prevent frostbite are in place. The location of the aneurysm determines positioning. Access to aneurysms of the proximal arch is through a median sternotomy; distal arch aneurysms may require a modified thoracotomy position to optimize exposure. Selective cerebral perfusion may be used during circulatory arrest to perfuse the brain. *Antegrade* cerebral perfusion can be achieved by infusing arterialized blood through one or more catheters into aortic arch vessels (i.e., aortic arch [Fig. 25.71A], brachiocephalic artery, or left common carotid artery). *Retrograde* cerebral perfusion can be achieved via the superior vena caval venous line Y-ed off the arterial line; arterial blood slowly infuses through the SVC line into the cerebral circulation while the surgeon anastomoses the distal aorta.

Operative Procedure

1. The RA and the right AA (see Fig. 25.71A–B) or femoral artery are cannulated. The patient is cooled to achieve hypothermic arrest, and the surgeon places a cross-clamp on the distal ascending aorta (see Fig. 25.71A).
2. After the patient is cooled to the desired temperature, the surgeon may cross-clamp the arch vessels individually or institute circulatory arrest (obviating the need for cross-clamping).
3. The surgeon selects the appropriately sized tube graft. Depending on the anatomy and the condition of the aortic tissue, the surgeon can choose to use a straight tube graft or one with side branches, if planning to individually anastomose the "head vessels" (Kouchoukos et al., 2013).
4. After hypothermic arrest is initiated, an "island" of superior aortic tissue is created that contains all three arch vessels (the common origin of the brachiocephalic, left carotid, and left subclavian vessels) (see Fig. 25.71B).
5. An appropriately sized graft is selected and anastomosed to the descending thoracic aorta (see Fig. 25.71C).
6. An oval-shaped piece of the graft matching the aortic arch island is excised and the surgeon anastomoses the graft to the island (see Fig. 25.71D).
7. De-airing is performed and bypass is reinstituted with arterial flow perfusing head vessels and the descending thoracic aorta and branches (see Fig. 25.71E).
8. The proximal aortic anastomoses are completed (see Fig. 25.71E).
9. The surgeon completes the replacement and may apply BioGlue for hemostasis (see Fig. 25.71F) (Doty and Doty, 2012; Luozzo et al., 2013; Svensson et al., 2013).
10. The patient rewarms, and after de-airing the graft, the patient undergoes weaning from bypass.
11. Closure of all incisions follows.

Repair of Descending Thoracic Aortic Aneurysm
Procedural Considerations

Both *endovascular* and *open* procedures are described below. *Endovascular* repair (see Fig. 25.21) of descending thoracic aortic aneurysms and dissections largely has supplanted the traditional open technique, although anatomic considerations may increase the difficulty of placing the straight endovascular tube graft into the angled portion of the proximal descending aorta (just distal to the

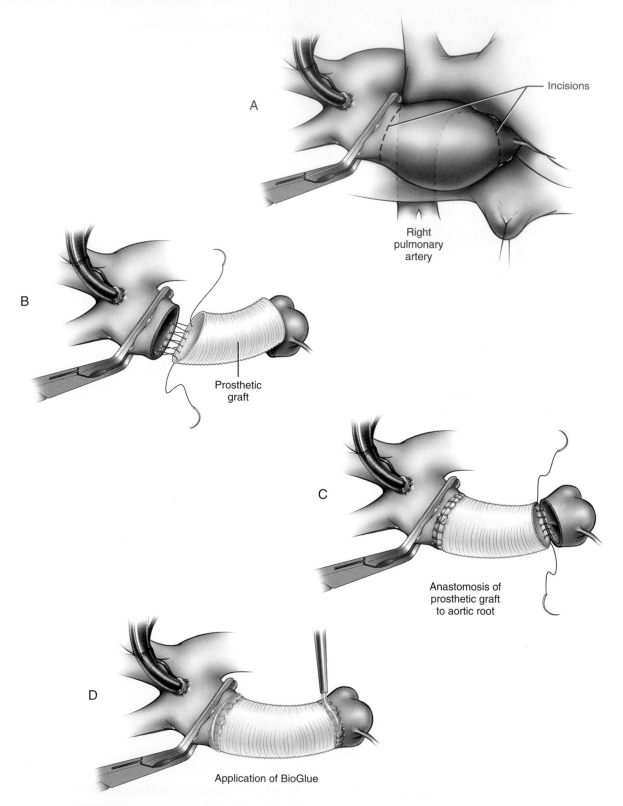

A

Incisions

Right
pulmonary
artery

B

Prosthetic
graft

C

Anastomosis of
prosthetic graft
to aortic root

D

Application of BioGlue

FIG. 25.70 Replacement and graft repair of ascending aorta. (A) Proximal and distal incisions. (B) The correct diameter-sized graft is selected and cut to the appropriate length for the anatomy. The distal anastomosis is performed first. (C) The graft is anastomosed proximally (with excess graft material removed). (D) The anastomotic sites are tested for hemostasis and reinforced with BioGlue.

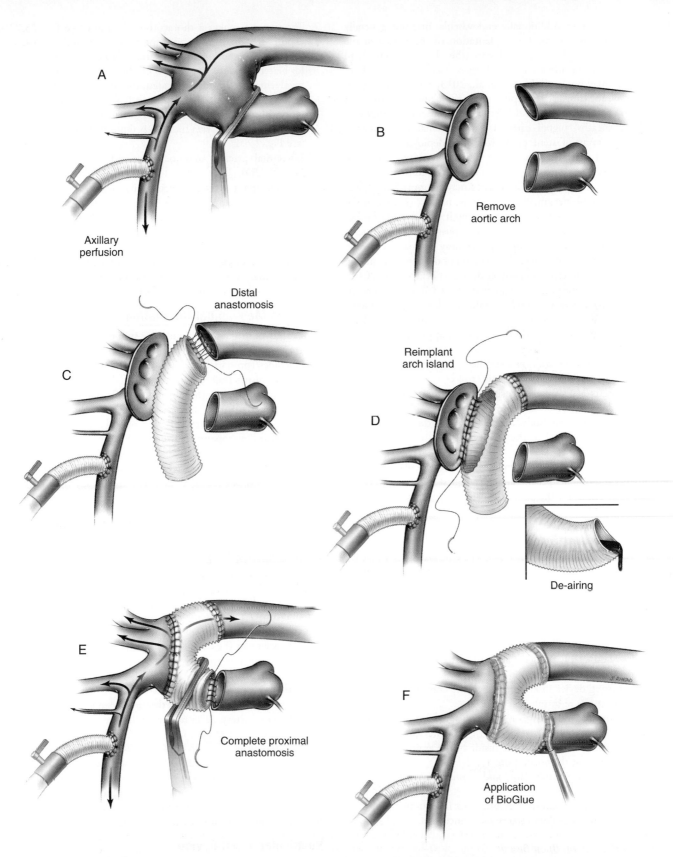

FIG. 25.71 Repair of aortic arch aneurysm. (A) Axillary artery cannulated for arterial inflow; ascending aorta is cross-clamped. (B) The arch vessels are removed as an "island." (C) A prosthetic graft is initially anastomosed distally to the descending aorta. (D) The arch vessel island is anastomosed to the opening created in the prosthetic graft. (E) The proximal anastomosis is completed. (F) BioGlue is applied to anastomotic sites.

left subclavian artery). Additionally, endovascular insertion generally requires nondiseased tissue for implantation of the device in the areas proximal and distal to the lesion (the "landing zones"); in patients with diffuse atherosclerotic disease or extensive dissection, viable tissue may not exist (Ehrlich et al., 2013; Szeto and Bavaria, 2016). It is not unusual to deploy more than one graft to cover the lesion. Setup includes endovascular instruments, guidewires, introducer sheaths, pigtail catheters, intravascular dye, dilators, catheters, an array of stent graft sizes, and deployment devices. Performance of the procedure occurs with fluoroscopy, usually on an OR bed that allows imaging without extensive bed manipulation. Radiation precautions apply. Guidewires may be more than 6 feet in length; the scrub person, therefore, must protect sterility of the distal portion of the guidewire by anchoring it with towels or other sterile objects when not being used. The postoperative period is considerably shorter than that for a thoracotomy approach. Potential complications include bleeding and migration of the device (requiring adjustment and/or insertion of another device) (Ehrlich et al., 2013). Although there is some evidence (Luozzo et al., 2013) that open repair (described next) may be preferable to endovascular repair in patients younger than 60 years, clinical and technical improvements have expanded the indications for the endovascular approach (Szeto and Bavaria, 2016).

For *open* repair, thoracotomy instruments and supplies are added to the basic setup; additional long aortic cross-clamps may be needed. Prosthetic grafts are available. Positioning of the patient is for a left posterolateral thoracotomy. Use of femoral vein–femoral artery bypass perfuses the lower body. In this situation, the heart perfuses the upper body proximal to the aneurysm, and normothermia is maintained.

If the surgeon uses hypothermic CPB with circulatory arrest, instruments and supplies per the surgeon's request should be available. Protective coverings for the patient's head, face, and extremities are used to avoid frostbite.

Operative Procedure: Endovascular Repair

1. The surgeon secures access to one or both femoral arteries via percutaneous (Seldinger) or cutdown technique. The surgeon inserts a hypodermic needle into the femoral artery and passes a guidewire through the needle into the aorta. Fluoroscopy images the aortic lumen and measures targeted segments of the aorta. The hypodermic needle is removed and a sheath inserted, through which the device will be inserted.
2. A delivery catheter housing the graft is inserted into the descending aorta.
3. A monitoring device inserted through the contralateral femoral artery can measure intraluminal pressures.
4. Using fluoroscopy, the surgeon guides the graft into position and deploys it into the aorta (see Fig. 25.21). The device self-expands; a balloon can inflate against the inside of the graft to secure the prosthesis against the aortic lumen.
5. Fluoroscopy images the aorta and confirms exclusion of the aneurysm/dissection.
6. Removal of deployment devices and other intraluminal catheters and wires follows as does closure of all incisions.

Operative Procedure: Open Repair

1. Cannulation for femoral vein–femoral artery bypass commences; a left groin incision is made for cannulation of the femoral artery for arterial infusion and femoral vein for venous drainage (Fig. 25.72A).

2. The surgeon makes a thoracotomy incision (see Fig. 25.72B), exposes the aneurysm, and inspects the surrounding structures. Occasionally, the surgeon may make *two* thoracotomy incisions for better access to, and control of, the aorta. Assessment of renal involvement follows; if indicated, the surgeon directs institution of measures to protect the kidneys (e.g., local cooling).
3. Normothermic femoral bypass is initiated.
4. Longitudinal aneurysm incision is done and aorta sizing follows (see Fig. 25.72C).
5. Intercostal arteries may be preserved or some ligated (see Fig. 25.72D).
6. The surgeon inserts a woven graft, creates a proximal aortic anastomosis, and reattaches selected intercostal arteries (see Fig. 25.72E).
7. Traditional distal suture anastomosis is undertaken (see Fig. 25.72F).
8. Distal anastomosis is completed with reinforcing collar and residual aneurysmal tissue closed around the graft to separate it from the lung (to avoid possible fistula formation [see Fig. 25.72G]).

Assisted Mechanical Circulation

Availability of mechanical circulatory support (MCS) has expanded the treatment for heart failure into a rapidly growing specialty that also includes coronary artery revascularization, left and right ventricular reconstruction, circulatory assist device implantation, and cardiac transplantation (Stone et al., 2017; Aaronson and Pagani, 2015). Formerly, VADs were reserved only for those patients who could not be weaned from CPB after open-heart operations or had end-stage cardiomyopathy. Current indications and choices include a variety of active and passive devices to support circulation for short, intermediate, and long-term use (Aaronson and Pagani, 2015). Use of VADs is not only for "destination" therapy (i.e., implanted permanently) and as a "bridge to transplantation," but also for recovery (Stone et al., 2017). The evolution of MCS and the success of MCS devices for destination therapy (especially continuous flow devices) have enabled mechanical devices to compete with cardiac transplantation (Aaronson and Pagani, 2015; Stone et al., 2017).

Intra-Aortic Balloon Pump

The most widely used short-term device is the IABP, which is a percutaneously inserted device. The IABP (Fig. 25.73) uses the principle of counterpulsation to increase coronary blood flow and decrease afterload (i.e., the resistance the ventricle must overcome to open the aortic valve).

Operative Procedure

1. A flexible guidewire is passed through a percutaneous needle into the femoral artery. After removing the needle, graduated dilators are inserted over the guidewire to dilate the overlying tissue and the artery wall.
2. The IABP catheter (with furled balloon) inserts into the artery and advances to a position just distal to the left subclavian artery. The surgeon marks the catheter at the proximal end with a silk tie to measure the distance the catheter should be inserted.
3. The balloon is unfurled and activated.

Ventricular Assist Device

An expanding array of VADs are available. Their position may be internal or external, they may be electrically or pneumatically powered, they may be pulsatile or nonpulsatile, and they may require warfarin anticoagulation. Most devices allow ambulation and some enable the patient to be discharged from the hospital (Stone et al., 2017). As designed, VADs augment cardiac output from the left (LVAD), right (RVAD), or both (biventricular [BiVAD]) ventricles and decrease workload of the heart by diverting blood from the ventricle or ventricles to an artificial pump that maintains systemic perfusion.

Patients with an LVAD (Fig. 25.74A–K) benefit from the resulting enhanced anabolism, ambulation, and improved organ function. Complications (e.g., bleeding, thromboembolism, infection, device failure) persist, but they have lessened with newer VADs (Stone et al., 2017).

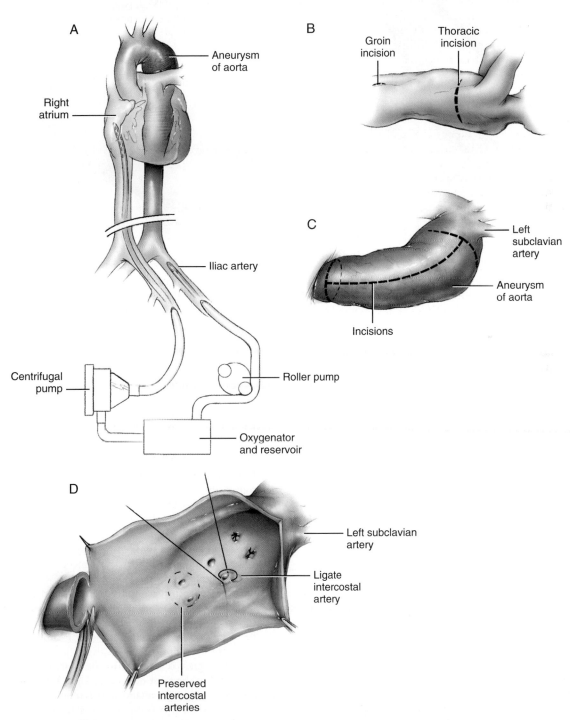

FIG. 25.72 Repair of descending thoracic aortic aneurysm. (A) Femoral vein–femoral/iliac artery bypass established. (B) Patient placed in a semilateral position, exposing left thorax and left groin area (to expose femoral vein/iliac artery). (C) Aneurysmal portion of descending aorta (lines illustrate areas of incision). (D) Opened aorta showing intercostal arteries; some arteries may be ligated and some may be preserved.

Continued

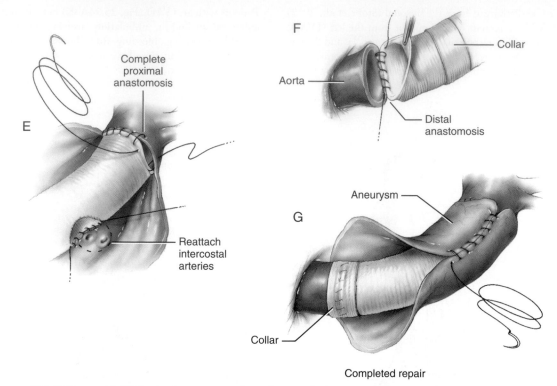

FIG. 25.72, cont'd (E) Proximal anastomosis of prosthetic graft; the intercostal arteries to be preserved and reattached are connected to an opening created in the graft. (F) The distal anastomosis is completed; a hemostatic collar may be attached. (G) The completed repair with an attached distal collar. The aneurysmal aortic wall is closed over the graft.

Among the designs are the axial flow pump, which inserts into the LV to propel blood flow (see Fig. 25.74L). The distal end anastomoses to the descending aorta. Miniaturized centrifugal pumps, totally implantable pulsatile devices incorporating a transcutaneous energy transmission (and power regeneration) system, and artificial hearts are additional devices used to treat heart failure (Ewald et al., 2016).

Procedural Considerations

Insertion of an assist device may be indicated for patients who cannot be weaned from CPB, or device insertion may be a scheduled procedure. Depending on the device, its components must be collected and prepared according to the manufacturer's IFU. Components may include external centrifugal pumps; internally powered assist devices (see Fig. 25.74); or wholly implantable systems with transcutaneous, rechargeable power sources. Perioperative nurses need to be aware of changes in device technology, possible troubleshooting scenarios, and potential complications (Nowotny et al., 2016).

The LVAD described in the following section is approved for support of the LV when right ventricular function is normal. Prosthetic valves incorporated into the circuit maintain unidirectional blood flow. All VADs differ, and preparation should be specific to the particular device. In preparation for VAD insertion, perioperative nurses should discuss VAD type, insertion considerations, graft preclotting, need for topical hemostatic agents (see Surgical Pharmacology), possible complications, and troubleshooting scenarios with the surgeon before the start of the procedure.

Operative Procedure
Thoratec Heartmate Left Ventricular Assist Device

1. The surgeon makes a median sternotomy incision, extended to the umbilicus, and creates a preperitoneal pouch for placement of the assist device (see Fig. 25.74A).
2. CPB commences. The surgeon clamps the aorta and anastomoses the graft to the ascending aorta (see Fig. 25.74B). The surgeon inspects the atrial septum for defects (or a patent foramen ovale), which are closed if found.
3. The left ventricular apex is mobilized and an opening created in the apex (see Fig. 25.74C).
4. The surgeon inserts a connector into the apex and sews the flange to the surrounding left ventricular myocardium with pledgeted sutures (see Fig. 25.74D–F).
5. The surgeon then makes an opening into the diaphragm near the location of the apical connector and inflow conduit. Passed through the diaphragm, the conduit undergoes attachment to the assist device. The inflow conduit is attached to the apical connector (see Fig. 25.74G–I).
6. The aortic graft is attached to the outflow conduit, which is connected to the assist device (see Fig. 25.74G–I).
7. Tunneling of the percutaneous driveline runs to the left lower quadrant, where it exits through the skin. The driveline connects to a drive console (see Fig. 25.74J) or to an electric lead (see Fig. 25.74K). Blood flows from the left ventricular apex, to the device, and back into the body through the aortic conduit.
8. If an *axial flow pump* is inserted into the LV to propel blood flow (see Fig. 25.74L), the distal (graft) end is anastomosed to

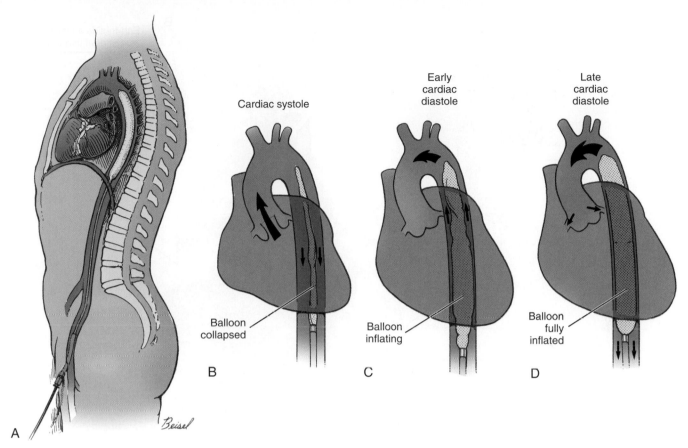

FIG. 25.73 Phases of balloon pumping. (A) Balloon inflation occurs from closure of aortic valve to the end of diastole. Inflation causes retrograde flow of blood in the aorta, increasing coronary perfusion pressure without increasing myocardial work or oxygen demand. Inflation also causes antegrade flow, increasing mean arterial pressure, renal flow, and cerebral flow. (B) Balloon deflation occurs from just before opening of aortic valve to closure of aortic valve. Deflation encourages antegrade flow, decreasing afterload or resistance to left ventricular ejection. Deflation also decreases oxygen required by left ventricle, shortens systolic ejection, and increases stroke volume. (C and D) When the balloon reinflates, the cycle is repeated.

the ascending aorta; the outflow component is inserted into the LV apex in a manner similar to that for the LVAD.

9. CPB ends, and closure of incisions follows.

To remove or replace the pump, the patient returns to the OR, the surgeon reopens the sternotomy and removes the cannulae, and then removes or replaces the device.

Total Artificial Heart

Although *destination therapy* for patients with VADs has improved, it has not replaced the need (nor the demand) for a total artificial heart (TAH), which continues to undergo refinement and implantation in patients with end-stage biventricular failure. Complications associated with thromboembolism and infection have lessened, but not ended, with technical and material refinements of VAD systems. Use of long-term RVADs or LVADs has increased as a bridge to cardiac transplantation by supporting circulation until a suitable donor heart appears (Stone et al., 2017).

Two examples of the TAH are the AbioCor TAH and the Syn-Cardia CardioWest (Ewald et al., 2016; Stone et al., 2017). The AbioCor TAH uses a centrifugal pump powered by an internal battery (rechargeable via transcutaneous energy source). The CardioWest

TAH uses two pneumatically driven pumps containing mechanical tilting disk valves. This TAH requires a chest anteroposterior diameter of at least 10 cm and a large body surface area, so the device is appropriate only for larger patients (Stone et al., 2017).

Heart and Heart-Lung Transplantation

Heart Transplantation

Orthotopic transplantation (replacing one heart with another) is most commonly performed; less common are heterotopic (piggyback) and combined heart-lung procedures (Fig. 25.75). Recipient and donor selection, immune response, and infection control are important considerations. Older recipients and donors (older than 65–70 years) have demonstrated acceptable morbidity and survival (Acker and Jessup, 2015). There also is a growing need for transplantation in patients who reach adulthood with CHD; perioperative nurses should review the medical and surgical history and discuss the proposed surgery with the surgeon to anticipate anatomic anomalies related to CHD and its surgical correction.

Modification of the traditional transplantation technique (i.e., atrial–atrial anastomoses or *biatrial technique*) was developed to

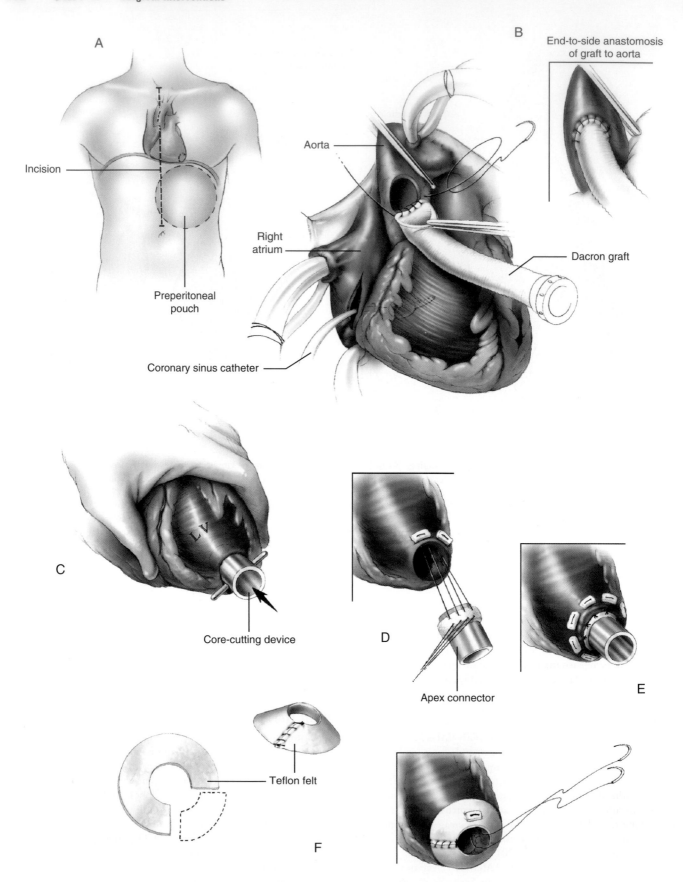

A

Incision

Preperitoneal
pouch

B

End-to-side anastomosis
of graft to aorta

Aorta

Right
atrium

Dacron graft

Coronary sinus catheter

C

LV

Core-cutting device

D

Apex connector

E

F

Teflon felt

FIG. 25.74 Left ventricular assist device (see text).

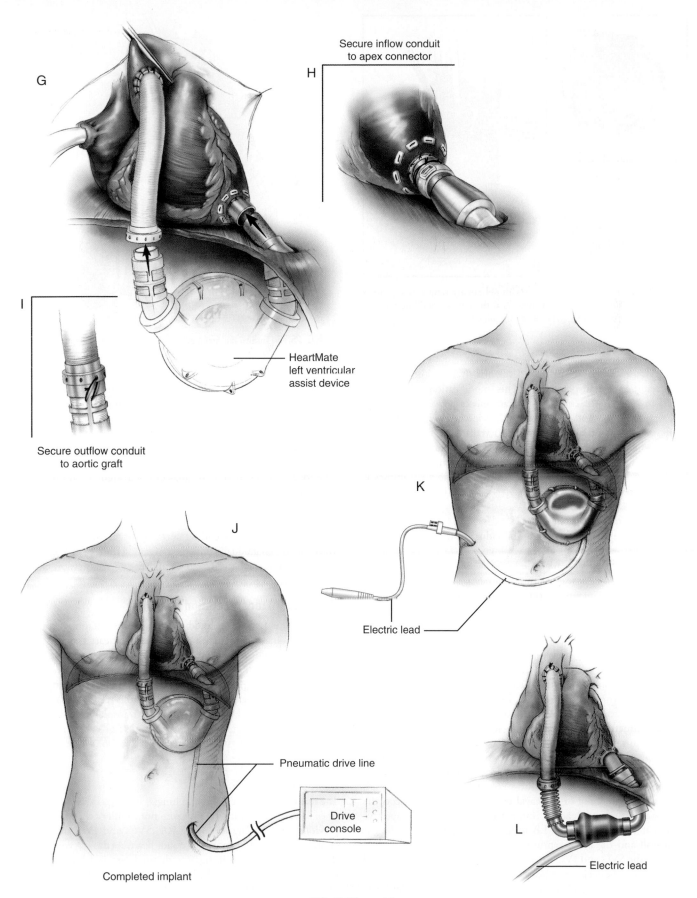

G

H

Secure inflow conduit
to apex connector

HeartMate
left ventricular
assist device

I

Secure outflow conduit
to aortic graft

J

Completed implant

Pneumatic drive line

Drive
console

K

Electric lead

L

Electric lead

FIG. 25.74, cont'd

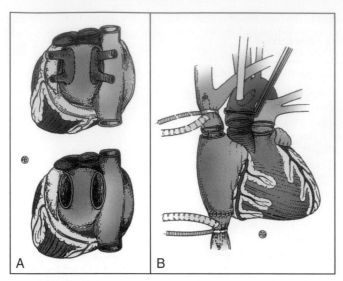

FIG. 25.75 (A) Heart transplantation with pulmonary venous anastomoses on right or left side, and caval anastomoses at the superior and inferior vena cavae. (B) Aorta and pulmonary artery are joined last.

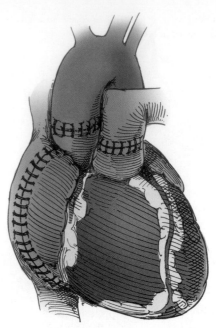

FIG. 25.76 Traditional atrial anastomosis for heart transplantation.

reduce dysrhythmias and tricuspid valvular dysfunction associated with traditional transplantation. This modification (the *bicaval technique*) consists of end-to-end anastomoses between the donor and recipient SVC and the donor and recipient IVC, producing a more physiologic atrial contribution to ventricular filling and less distortion of the mitral and tricuspid annuli (Murray et al., 2017). If there is tricuspid insufficiency, ring annuloplasty may be performed on the donor heart. Performance of PA and aortic anastomoses is in the traditional manner.

Procedural Considerations

Donor and recipient each require individual instrument setups.

Operative Procedure

Donor Heart. Exposure of the donor heart is through median sternotomy. The surgeon dissects the aorta, PA, and venae cavae. After occlusion of the venae cavae, the surgeon opens the LA to decompress the ventricle, after which rapid cooling and arrest of the heart follow.

Heart excision is by incision of the SVC and the IVC, the LA, the aorta, and the PA. The team immediately places the donor heart into cold saline and transports it to the site in which the recipient will receive it. If other organs (e.g., lungs, liver, kidneys, pancreas) are to be procured simultaneously, heart procurement team members must coordinate removal of other organs with their respective colleagues (Murray et al., 2017).

Recipient Heart. The recipient undergoes bypass with cannulation of the IVC and the SVC; caval tapes are placed around the cavae. Cooling of the patient is to about 89.6°F to 93.2°F (32°C–34°C), followed by tightening of the caval tapes. The surgeon dissects the pulmonary trunk and aorta immediately above their respective semilunar valves; incises the LA to leave intact portions of the left atrial wall and the atrial septum of the recipient; incises the RA, retaining the SVC and IVC for anastomosis to the donor heart; and then removes the recipient's heart.

The team places the donor heart in the pericardial well. The surgeon next performs pulmonary anastomoses (see Fig. 25.75A).

The SVC and IVC are anastomosed with running cardiovascular sutures (see Fig. 25.75B). Similar joinders of the donor and recipient aortas and pulmonary arteries are next. Removal of air from the left side of the heart follows. Before suturing the PA, the surgeon carefully inspects all caval and atrial suture lines for significant bleeding areas, after which the cross-clamp is removed. Fig. 25.76 illustrates the traditional (but less frequently anastomosed) right atrial suture line; aortic and pulmonary anastomoses are similar to the technique just described.

A single DC shock usually is effective to defibrillate the ventricles. A needle vent in the ascending aorta allows residual air to escape. The patient then gradually undergoes weaning from bypass. Cannulae are removed from the venae cavae and the aorta. Incision closures are as described previously.

Heart-Lung Transplantation

Newer techniques for lung and heart-lung transplantation incorporate the bicaval anastomoses used for orthotopic heart transplantation and also use bibronchial anastomosis to reduce bleeding and to enhance airway integrity. To maximize allocation of scarce donor organs, transplant procedures for the lungs may use a single lung or bilateral lungs; heart-lung transplantation is relatively rare, largely because of increased frequency of lung transplantation (Quinlan et al., 2017). Preservation of the *donor's* sinus node and the *recipient's* recurrent laryngeal, vagus, and phrenic nerves is an important surgical consideration.

Operative Procedure

The recipient's diseased heart and lung(s) undergo excision separately or *en bloc*, during which care is taken not to injure the major nerves previously listed. The recipient's RA, SVC, and IVC are saved to create bicaval attachments to the donor heart. As the surgeon transects the bronchi, the team brings the donor heart and lungs onto the field. Placement of the right lung is in the right pleural space and of the left lung in the left pleural space. The surgeon performs bronchial and the bicaval anastomoses, and rewarming begins. Aortic anastomosis follows; the aorta is de-aired and the cross-clamp is removed (Murray et al., 2017).

Surgery for Conduction Disturbances

Disturbances of the conduction system affect the rate, rhythm, and effectiveness of the contracting heart. Clinicians and researchers have developed surgical techniques to treat a variety of supraventricular dysrhythmias (e.g., AF and Wolff-Parkinson-White reentry tachycardia) and both ischemic and nonischemic ventricular tachydysrhythmias (e.g., ventricular tachycardia or fibrillation). Preprocedural electrophysiologic mapping of the patient's conduction pathways identifies and locates aberrant pathways, tachydysrhythmias, and the existence of additional pathways, as well as the effects of medications on a particular dysrhythmia. Indications for pacemaker implantation (including resynchronization therapy) and antitachycardia-antifibrillation devices have been expanded. Many (but not all) pacemaker and ICD insertions now occur in the EP laboratory or the cardiac catheterization suite (Cheng et al., 2017).

Ablation procedures for AF normally occur in the EP lab. Depending on the anticipated locus of the problem, the electrophysiologist inserts a catheter percutaneously into the femoral vein or artery and threads the catheter retrograde to the RA or LA and ventricle. The electrophysiologist tests various areas of the heart in an attempt to reproduce the dysrhythmia and then ablates the area of the heart in which the rhythm disturbance originates. Postoperative considerations are similar to those for AF surgery. Surgical correction normally occurs in the OR.

AF is the most common sustained cardiac dysrhythmia, with a prevalence in the United States ranging from approximately 2.7 to 6.1 million; AF is expected to rise in prevalence to between 5.6 and 12 million by 2050 with the gain of the US population (AHA, 2016). AF was considered a "benign" condition in the past, but serious consequences associated with the dysrhythmia have made it the subject of intense study. AF interferes with the atrial kick (which contributes a significant amount of "preload"), and the dysrhythmia can lead to insufficient cardiac output. Moreover, stasis of blood within the atria promotes the formation of thrombus (clotting), which leads to cerebrovascular accident (CVA) or pulmonary embolism (PE).

Although *intermittent* AF commonly follows CABG, it is potentially preventable by treatment with amiodarone, beta-blockers, angiotensin-converting enzyme (ACE) inhibitors, and nonsteroidal antiinflammatory drugs. Treatment includes restoration of sinus rhythm (when possible), control of ventricular rate, and administration of anticoagulants (Cheng et al., 2017).

Techniques to treat *continuous* AF have arisen based on research demonstrating that the pulmonary veins are an important source of ectopic beats that can initiate paroxysms of AF. Surgical interventions for AF have expanded beyond Cox's original maze procedures (Cox et al., 1991), in which the surgeon sutured extensive atrial incisions to create a maze through which electrical impulses were directed from the SA node to the AV node. Early research by Cox demonstrated that electrical impulses are unable to cross incised and sutured tissue and consequently cannot regenerate reentry circuits producing the dysrhythmia. Cox revised the cut-and-sew technique of the initial maze procedures with a cryosurgical technique to ensure creation of transmural lesions in the vicinity of the pulmonary veins and in other areas of the heart that generate impulses producing AF. This "mini-maze" can be performed through a sternotomy or via an MIS thoracic route; the mini-maze requires placement of fewer lesions in the left and right atria. Current focus is on selective ablation (with cryotherapy, ultrasonic or RF energy sources) of tissues surrounding, for example, the pulmonary veins to reestablish normal conduction pathways (Cheng et al., 2017).

Surgery for Atrial Fibrillation (The Maze Procedure)

Surgery for AF occurs through open sternotomy or right minithoracotomy incisions (Cheng et al., 2017). The perioperative nurse ensures appropriate supplies (including energy sources) are available. By creating small areas of scar tissue in the cardiac muscle, electrical impulses, unable to cross scar tissue, must follow an alternative conduction path, or maze.

Operative Procedure: Sternotomy

1. The surgeon performs a midline sternotomy.
2. Cannulation of the superior and inferior venae cavae follows for total CPB.
3. The surgeon occludes the ascending aorta, and cardioplegic solution infuses through the aortic root and into the coronary arteries.
4. After performance of a right atriotomy, ablation of the first set of lesions in the RA occurs (Fig. 25.77A).

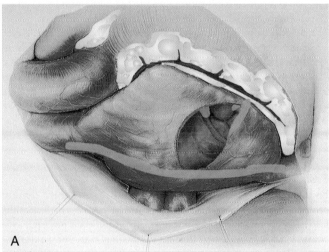

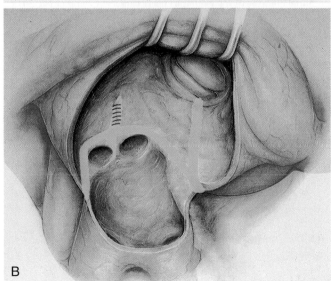

FIG. 25.77 (A) First lesion set for maze procedure. (B) Second lesion set for maze procedure.

5. A left atriotomy follows, as does ablation of the left atrial lesions (see Fig. 25.77B).
6. After closure of the atriotomies, the aorta is unclamped.
7. CPB discontinues, followed by removal of the cannulae.
8. Chest tubes and pacing wires are inserted, and the wound is closed.

Operative Procedure: Mini-Thoracotomy

1. The patient's position is supine, but tilted slightly to the left with a roll under the right rib cage; placement of the right arm is on an armboard at a right angle less than 90 degrees (Fig. 25.78).
2. The surgeon makes a 5- to 7-cm incision in the right submammary area in the fourth intercostal space and another incision for exposure.
3. Exposure of the right femoral vein and artery for CPB is by groin incision.
4. The anesthesia provider deflates the right lung and the surgeon opens the pericardium and tacks the pericardial edges to the chest wall.
5. The surgeon accesses the IVC and SVC.
6. The surgeon cannulates the femoral vein and artery and then places a purse-string suture into the SVC, followed by a venous cannula through the purse-string into the SVC.
7. Before instituting CPB, the surgeon creates the right atrial lesions.
8. After the surgeon completes the right atrial lesions, the perfusionist initiates CPB; the surgeon then cross-clamps the aorta and arrests the heart (with a retrograde cardioplegia catheter inserted through the right atrial wall into the coronary sinus).
9. The surgeon makes the left atrial lesions.
10. CPB discontinues and the cannulae are removed.
11. Chest tubes and pacing wires are inserted and the incisions closed.

Postoperative Considerations

Postoperatively, patients undergo monitoring for heart rhythm problems. In patients treated for AF, it may take up to 3 months for the heart to resume beating normally. Additional postoperative considerations include monitoring for bleeding, infection, and other potential complications related to heart surgery (Cheng et al., 2017).

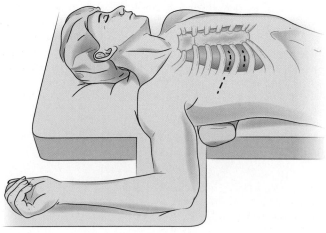

FIG. 25.78 Mini-thoracotomy position and incisions for minimally invasive maze procedure.

Insertion of Permanent Pacemaker

A permanent pacemaker (pulse generator and electrodes) initiates atrial or ventricular contraction, or both. Complete heart block and bradydysrhythmias (i.e., slow heart rates) are the most common indications for pacemaker implantation. A temporary pacemaker is also possible to remedy acute forms of heart block and dysrhythmias that occasionally occur during and after cardiac surgery (Cheng et al., 2017).

Insertion of Transvenous (Endocardial) Pacing Electrodes

Positioning of the patient is supine and the anesthesia provider monitors the ECG. Because lethal dysrhythmias can occur, a defibrillator must be available. Because the procedure requires fluoroscopy, a portable image intensifier is used or the procedure occurs in the special studies section of the radiology or cardiac catheterization department. Setup requires a minor set of instruments with vascular dissecting and tunneling instruments, as well as an introducer set, testing instruments, and supplies (e.g., alligator cables). Often the pacemaker representative will bring a pacing system analyzer (PSA).

Using local anesthesia, the surgeon puts the patient in Trendelenburg position to engorge the vein for easier access and to avoid air emboli and makes a skin pocket close to the subclavian vein. A venotomy is performed and a guidewire threaded to the desired cardiac chamber, after which the needle is removed. The pacing electrode inserts through a dilator and advances under direct fluoroscopic vision into the RA, through the tricuspid valve, and into the RV. The surgeon places the electrode in the trabeculae carneae cordis of the right ventricular apex and tests the electrode with alligator test cables and the PSA to confirm proper placement and function. If inserting a dual-chamber pacemaker, the surgeon entraps the second lead in the RA appendage. The electrode(s) are attached to the pulse generator, which is placed into the pocket. A tunneling device can thread the electrode to the pocket. Closure of the incision is in layers with absorbable sutures.

The development of a leadless, intracardiac transcatheter pacing system avoids transvenous leads as well as the need for a pacemaker pocket. The device combines the electrodes and the lithium-powered generator into a small device that is percutaneously delivered to, and implanted into, the RV. These newer devices can reduce the incidence of lead fracture and infection of the generator pocket (Reynolds et al., 2016).

Insertion of Myocardial (Epicardial) Pacing Electrodes

A subxiphoid left anterior thoracotomy approach or sternotomy approach is used. The subxiphoid process and left upper quadrant area are infiltrated with an anesthetic agent. The surgeon makes a small transverse incision below the xiphoid process and extends it down to the linea alba. Creation of a tunnel is under the xiphoid process to the pericardium, which is incised to expose the heart. The pacing electrode, mounted on its carrier, screws into the ventricular myocardium, followed by removal of the carrier. The remainder of the procedure is the same as that described for insertion of the endocardial electrode.

For the sternotomy approach, the surgeon opens the mediastinum for the concomitant cardiac procedure and chooses an area of myocardium for the pacing electrodes. The electrode tips either screw into or are sutured to the myocardium and attached by an appropriate cable to an external pulse generator or PSA for testing.

Creation of the pocket and subcutaneous tunnel is as described for insertion of the endocardial electrode.

Cardiac Resynchronization Therapy

Dual-site pacing of both the RV and LV is another treatment for patients with dilated cardiomyopathy and heart failure (Acker and Jessup, 2015). Cardiac resynchronization therapy (CRT) uses leads placed on the RA and the RV. An electrode introduced transvenously into the coronary sinus and extended into the great cardiac vein (or a tributary) to a position in the left side of the heart achieves left ventricular pacing; this electrode functions as the second ventricular lead. The three electrodes connect to the pacemaker generator. Resynchronization improves the mechanical pumping action between the RV and LV and optimizes AV synchrony; as a result, hemodynamic function improves in heart failure patients.

The *transvenous* or the *epicardial* approach may be used to place the electrodes. The transvenous route is most common because it does not require a major thoracotomy or general anesthesia and is, therefore, safer for high-risk patients. Permanent epicardial electrodes may be placed during cardiac operations when the chest is opened and the heart is exposed; if a permanent pacemaker is required, however, it is likely to be inserted transvenously during the postoperative period (temporary electrodes placed during surgery achieve pacing). To avoid opening the sternum, a subxiphoid approach to place epicardial leads is possible.

Insertion of Internal Cardioverter Defibrillator

Surgery or pharmacologic intervention may not prevent malignant ventricular dysrhythmias (ventricular fibrillation and ventricular tachycardia) in people who survive sudden cardiac death. The ICD is an electronic device designed to monitor cardiac electrical activity and deliver prompt defibrillator shocks. The ICD differs from a pacemaker because the ICD senses ventricular tachycardia or fibrillation, whereas the pacemaker senses asystole. ICD models are capable of tiered therapy, in which increasingly stronger impulses are delivered depending on the underlying dysrhythmias; some devices can also terminate AF. These devices are capable of pacing as well as defibrillating (pacing cardioverter defibrillators [PCDs]). Although the purposes of pacemakers and ICDs differ, their respective surgical procedures are similar (e.g., transvenous access, testing).

The ICD device consists of a generator and sensing and defibrillator electrodes. Many ICD electrodes consist of transvenous electrodes inserted into the generator similar to a transvenous pacemaker system. The addition of myocardial or thoracic subcutaneous patches is possible if transvenous catheters alone cannot defibrillate the heart adequately. Patients with previously applied defibrillator patches may present for patch removal; perioperative nurses should prepare for emergency intervention if excessive bleeding or lethal dysrhythmia appears. EP studies performed before and after insertion enable diagnosis of the dysrhythmia and evaluation of device function, respectively.

The transvenous route with fluoroscopy is common, and insertion is similar to that described for transvenous pacemaker insertion. Tunneling of the free ends of the lead system is to the generator, implanted in a subcutaneous pocket in the chest wall. After testing the device, closure of the incisions concludes the procedure.

Key Points

- Cardiac surgery is increasingly moving toward interventional procedures that use minimally invasive approaches and percutaneous access routes.

- Therapeutic interventions may use laser, RF, and cryothermal energies.
- The heart is a four-chamber muscular pump that propels blood into the systemic and pulmonary circulatory systems. It sits within a pericardial sac within the mediastinum, between the lungs, posterior to the sternum, and anterior to the vertebrae, esophagus, and descending portion of the aorta.
- Each half of the heart contains an upper and a lower communicating chamber called the atrium and ventricle, respectively.
- The pulmonary circulatory system pumps blood from the RV through the pulmonary valve into the main PA.
- The coronary circulation supplies oxygen and nutrients to, and removes metabolic waste from, the myocardium.
- To prevent regurgitation of blood, the four cardiac valves open and close to maintain unidirectional blood flow. Any of the four valves may be deformed congenitally or subject to acquired valvular heart disease.
- Because the severity of pathologic changes varies among patients throughout the life span, knowledge of physical status, psychosocial concerns, and functional health patterns enables the perioperative nurse to plan and manage patient care.
- In addition to health status and risk factors, the perioperative nurse reviews patient medication history with particular attention to vasoactive drugs, anticoagulants, and other medications that can affect surgery.
- After a comprehensive review of individual patient data, the perioperative nurse identifies relevant nursing diagnoses, from which the perioperative plan of patient care derives.
- Safety of the cardiac surgery patient is a primary responsibility of the perioperative nurse.

Critical Thinking Questions

In the middle of the night, the on-call cardiac surgery nurse receives a page to "come in for an aneurysm." Some of the immediate questions that come to the nurse's mind concern the type of aneurysm (or dissection) and comorbid conditions the patient may present with. One of the first considerations is aneurysm location, because that affects positioning, instrumentation, tissue perfusion, and other interventions. The differences among types of aneurysms and dissections are crucial for the nurse to know. The location can be in the ascending aorta, the aortic arch, the descending aorta, or a combination of sites. It is important to prepare for the patient and set up the OR appropriately, promptly, and efficiently. (1) Describe the instrumentation, equipment, prosthesis, and accessory items or supplies you would anticipate for an ascending aortic aneurysm, an aortic arch aneurysm, and a descending thoracic aortic aneurysm. (2) What comorbid conditions would you consider important to your plan of care? (3) What infection prevention strategies and special safety considerations would you implement for each type of patient? (4) What are essential items to include in your hand-off report?

⊝volve *The answers to the Critical Thinking Questions can be found at http://evolve.elsevier.com/Rothrock/Alexander.*

References

Aaronson KD, Pagani FD: Mechanical circulatory support. In Bonow RO et al, editors: *Braunwald's heart disease: a textbook of cardiovascular medicine*, ed 10, Philadelphia, 2015, Saunders.

Abdel-Wahab M, Jose JR: Transfemoral TAVI devices: design overview and clinical outcomes, *EuroIntervention* 11:W114–W118, 2015.

Acker MA, Jessup M: Surgical management of heart failure. In Bonow RO et al, editors: *Braunwald's heart disease: a textbook of cardiovascular medicine*, ed 10, Philadelphia, 2015, Saunders.

Al-Atassi T et al: Coronary artery bypass grafting. In Sellke FW et al, editors: *Sabiston and Spencer's surgery of the chest*, ed 9, Philadelphia, 2016, Saunders.

Alexander JH, Smith PK: Coronary-artery bypass grafting, *N Engl J Med* 374(20):1954–1964, 2016.

American Heart Association (AHA): *Cardiac procedures and surgeries* (website), 2016. www.heart.org/HEARTORG/Conditions/HeartAttack/Treatmentofa HeartAttack/Cardiac-Procedures-and-Surgeries_UCM_303939_Article.jsp# .WGYE8VMrL3g. (Accessed 15 February 2017).

American Heart Association (AHA): *Classes of heart failure* (website), 2014. www.heart.org/HEARTORG/Conditions/HeartFailure/AboutHeartFailure/ Classes-of-Heart-Failure_UCM_306328_Article.jsp. (Accessed 15 February 2017).

Aranki SF, Shopnick B: Demise of open vein harvesting (editorial), *Circulation* 123(2):127–128, 2011.

Association of periOperative Registered Nurses (AORN): *Guidelines for perioperative practice*, Denver, 2017, The Association.

Backes JM et al: Statin-associated diabetes mellitus: review and clinical guide, *South Med J* 109(3):167–173, 2016.

Bainbridge D, Cheng DCH: Postoperative cardiac recovery and outcomes. In Kaplan JA et al, editors: *Kaplan's cardiac anesthesia*, ed 7, Philadelphia, 2017, Saunders.

Bakaeen FG et al: Trends in use of off-pump coronary artery bypass grafting: results from the Society of Thoracic Surgeons Adult Cardiac Surgery Database, *J Thorac Cardiovasc Surg* 148(3):856–864, 2014.

Bansal M et al: Assessment of cardiac risk and the cardiology consultation. In Kaplan JA et al, editors: *Kaplan's cardiac anesthesia*, ed 7, Philadelphia, 2017, Saunders.

Berman B et al: Keloid management. In Robinson JK et al, editors: *Surgery of the skin*, ed 3, Philadelphia, 2015, Elsevier.

Bope ET, Kellerman RD: Diseases of the skin. In Bope ET, editor: *Conn's current therapy*, Philadelphia, 2017a, Saunders Elsevier.

Bope ET, Kellerman RD: Women's health. In Bope ET, editor: *Conn's current therapy*, Philadelphia, 2017b, Saunders Elsevier.

Caboral MF: Update on cardiovascular disease prevention in women, *Am J Nurs* 113(5):26–33, 2013.

Canty JM: Coronary blood flow and myocardial ischemia. In Bonow RO et al, editors: *Braunwald's heart disease: a textbook of cardiovascular medicine*, ed 10, Philadelphia, 2015, Saunders.

Carpentier A: Cardiac valve surgery: the "French Correction," *J Thorac Cardiovasc Surg* 86(3):323–337, 1983.

Castillo J, Adams DH: Mitral valve repair and replacement, including associated atrial fibrillation and tricuspid regurgitation. In Otto CM, Bonow RO, editors: *Valvular heart disease—a companion to Braunwald's heart disease*, ed 4, Philadelphia, 2014, Saunders.

Centers for Disease Control and Prevention (CDC): *Healthcare associated infections: catheter-associated urinary tract infections (CAUTI)* (website), 2015. www.cdc.gov/hai/ca_uti/uti.html. (Accessed 9 February 2017).

Chaudhuri K et al: Carbon dioxide insufflation in open-chamber cardiac surgery: a double-blind, randomized clinical trial of neurocognitive effects, *J Thorac Cardiovasc Surg* 144:646–653, 2012.

Cheng A et al: Cardiac electrophysiology: diagnosis and treatment. In Kaplan JA et al, editors: *Kaplan's cardiac anesthesia*, ed 7, Philadelphia, 2017, Saunders.

Chikwe JO et al: Procedures in the hybrid operating room. In Kaplan JA et al, editors: *Kaplan's cardiac anesthesia*, ed 7, Philadelphia, 2017, Saunders.

Cox JL et al: The surgical treatment of atrial fibrillation. III. Development of a definitive surgical procedure, *J Thorac Cardiovasc Surg* 101(4):569–583, 1991.

Crawford ES: The diagnosis and management of aortic dissection, *JAMA* 264(9):2537–2541, 1990.

Dacey LJ: Endoscopic vein-graft harvest is safe for CABG surgery, *JAMA* 308(5):512–513, 2012.

David TE: Surgery of the aortic root and the ascending aorta. In Sellke FW et al, editors: *Sabiston and Spencer's surgery of the chest*, ed 9, Philadelphia, 2016, Saunders.

Dorman MJ et al: Bilateral internal mammary artery grafting enhances survival in diabetic patients: a 30-year follow-up of propensity score-matched cohorts, *Circulation* 126(25):2935–2942, 2012.

Doty DB, Doty JR: *Cardiac surgery: operative technique*, ed 2, Philadelphia, 2012, Elsevier Saunders.

Durhan G et al: Does coronary calcium scoring with a SCORE better predict significant coronary artery stenosis than without? Correlation with computed tomography coronary angiography, *Eur Radiol* 25(3):776–784, 2015.

Edivete RA et al: Catheter-associated urinary tract infection after cardiovascular surgery: impact of a multifaceted intervention, *Am J Infect Control* 44(3):289–293, 2016.

Ehrlich MP et al: Midterm results after endovascular treatment of acute, complicated type B aortic dissection: the Talent Thoracic Registry, *J Thorac Cardiovasc Surg* 145(1):159–165, 2013.

Elmadhun NY et al: Clinical quality and safety in adult cardiac surgery. In Sellke FW et al, editors: *Sabiston and Spencer's surgery of the chest*, ed 9, Philadelphia, 2016, Saunders.

Ewald GA et al: Circulatory assist devices in heart failure. In Mann DL, editor: *Heart failure—a companion to Braunwald's heart disease*, ed 3, Philadelphia, 2016, Saunders.

Gallegos MM et al: Anesthesia and intraoperative care of the adult cardiac patient. In Sellke FW et al, editors: *Sabiston and Spencer's surgery of the chest*, ed 9, Philadelphia, 2016, Saunders.

Grocott HP et al: Cardiopulmonary bypass management and organ protection. In Kaplan JA et al, editors: *Kaplan's cardiac anesthesia*, ed 7, Philadelphia, 2017, Saunders.

Groom RC et al: Detection and elimination of microemboli related to cardiopulmonary bypass, *Circ Cardiovasc Qual Outcomes* 2(3):191–198, 2009.

Gross WL, Weiss MS: Non–operating room anesthesia. In Miller RD et al, editors: *Miller's anesthesia*, ed 8, Philadelphia, 2015, Churchill Livingstone.

Guerrero M et al: Transcatheter mitral valve replacement in native mitral valve disease with severe mitral annular calcification, *JACC Cardiovasc Interv* 9(13):1361–1371, 2016.

Gulati M, Mertz CNB: Cardiovascular disease in women. In Bonow RO et al, editors: *Braunwald's heart disease: a textbook of cardiovascular medicine*, ed 10, Philadelphia, 2015, Saunders.

Habib RH et al: Late effects of radial artery versus saphenous vein grafting in patients aged 70 years or older, *Ann Thorac Surg* 94(5):1478–1484, 2012.

He LY et al: Correlation between serum free fatty acids levels and Gensini score in elderly patients with coronary heart disease, *J Geriatric Cardiol* 11(1):57–62, 2014.

Hillis LD et al: ACCF/AHA guideline for coronary artery bypass graft surgery: a report of the American College of Cardiology Foundation/American Heart Association Task Force on Practice Guidelines developed in collaboration with the American Association for Thoracic Surgery, Society of Cardiovascular Anesthesiologists, and Society of Thoracic Surgeons, *J Am Coll Cardiol* 58(24):E123–E210, 2011.

Hodgson BB, Kizior RJ: *Saunders 2013 nursing drug handbook*, Philadelphia, 2013, Saunders.

Jarrett CM et al: Future systems and novel visualization techniques. In Sellke FW et al, editors: *Sabiston and Spencer's surgery of the chest*, ed 9, Philadelphia, 2016a, Saunders.

Jarrett CM et al: Robotic and minimally invasive mitral valve surgery. In Sellke FW et al, editors: *Sabiston and Spencer's surgery of the chest*, ed 9, Philadelphia, 2016b, Saunders.

Kaplan JA et al, editors: *Kaplan's cardiac anesthesia*, ed 7, Philadelphia, 2017, Elsevier Saunders.

Kern MJ: *Cardiac catheterization handbook*, ed 6, Philadelphia, 2016, Saunders.

Kocher AA et al: One year outcomes of the surgical treatment of aortic stenosis with a next generation surgical aortic valve (TRITON) trial: a prospective multicenter study of rapid deployment aortic valve replacement with the Edwards Intuity Valve System, *J Thorac Cardiovasc Surg* 145(1):110–116, 2013.

Kouchoukos NT et al: *Cardiac surgery*, ed 4, Philadelphia, 2013, Elsevier Saunders.

Lenihan DJ, Yusuf SW: Tumors affecting the cardiovascular system. In Bonow RO et al, editors: *Braunwald's heart disease: a textbook of cardiovascular medicine*, ed 10, Philadelphia, 2015, Saunders.

Levy JH et al: Blood coagulation, transfusion, and conservation. In Sellke FW et al, editors: *Sabiston and Spencer's surgery of the chest*, ed 9, Philadelphia, 2016, Saunders.

Luozzo GD et al: Open repair of descending and thoracoabdominal aortic aneurysms and dissections in patients aged younger than 60 years: superior to endovascular repair?, *Ann Thorac Surg* 95(1):12–19, 2013.

Lytle BW: Re-Do Coronary artery bypass surgery. In Sellke FW et al, editors: *Sabiston and Spencer's surgery of the chest*, ed 9, Philadelphia, 2016, Saunders.

McCarthy JR, Guy TS: Totally endoscopic robotic mitral valve surgery, *AORN J* 104(4):293–306, 2016.

McManus B: Primary tumors of the heart. In Bonow RO et al, editors: *Braunwald's heart disease: a textbook of cardiovascular medicine*, ed 10, Philadelphia, 2015, Saunders.

Mestres CA et al: Surgical treatment of the tricuspid valve. In Sellke FW et al, editors: *Sabiston and Spencer's surgery of the chest*, ed 9, Philadelphia, 2016, Saunders.

Morrow DA, Boden WE: Stable ischemic heart disease. In Bonow RO et al, editors: *Braunwald's heart disease: a textbook of cardiovascular medicine*, ed 10, Philadelphia, 2015, Saunders.

Murray AW et al: Anesthesia for heart, lung, and heart-lung transplantation. In Kaplan JA et al, editors: *Kaplan's cardiac anesthesia*, ed 7, Philadelphia, 2017, Saunders.

New York Heart Association. The Criteria Committee of the New York Heart Association: *Nomenclature and criteria for diagnosis of diseases of the heart and great vessels*, ed 9, Boston, 1994, Little, Brown.

Nowotny BH et al: Ventricular assist device implantation: perioperative nursing considerations, *AORN J* 103(4):389–403, 2016.

Nussmeier NA et al: Anesthesia for cardiac surgical procedures. In Miller RD et al, editors: *Miller's anesthesia*, ed 8, Philadelphia, 2015, Churchill Livingstone.

O'Gara PT: Prosthetic heart valve. In Otto C et al, editors: *Valvular heart disease—a companion to Braunwald's heart disease*, Philadelphia, 2014, Saunders.

O'Gara PT et al: 2013 ACCF/AHA guideline for the management of ST elevation myocardial infarction: a report of the American College of Cardiology Foundation/American Heart Association Task Force on Practice Guidelines, *Circulation* 127(4):529–555, 2013.

Omer S et al: Acquired heart disease: coronary insufficiency. In Townsend CM et al, editors: *Sabiston textbook of surgery*, ed 20, Philadelphia, 2017, Saunders.

Osnabrugge RL et al: Aortic stenosis in the elderly: disease prevalence and number of candidates for transcatheter aortic valve replacement: a meta-analysis and modeling study, *J Am Coll Cardiol* 62(11):1002–1012, 2013.

Otto CM, Bonow RO: Valvular heart disease. In Libby P et al, editors: *Braunwald's heart disease*, ed 10, Philadelphia, 2015, Saunders.

Pagana KD, Pagana TJ: *Mosby's manual of diagnostic and laboratory tests*, ed 5, St Louis, 2014, Elsevier Mosby.

Peltz M: Surgery for valvular heart disease. In Antman EM, Sabatine MS, editors: *Cardiovascular therapeutics—a companion to Braunwald's heart disease*, Philadelphia, 2013, Saunders.

Petersen C, editor: *Perioperative nursing data set*, ed 3, Denver, 2011, The Association.

Quinlan JJ et al: Anesthesia for heart, lung, and heart-lung transplantation. In Kaplan JA et al, editors: *Kaplan's cardiac anesthesia*, ed 7, Philadelphia, 2017, Saunders.

Reich DL et al: Monitoring of the heart and vascular system. In Kaplan JA et al, editors: *Kaplan's cardiac anesthesia*, ed 7, Philadelphia, 2017, Elsevier Saunders.

Reynolds D et al: A leadless intracardiac transcatheter pacing system, *N Engl J Med* 374(26):533–541, 2016.

Rhee J et al: Coronary artery disease. In Reed AP, Yudkowitz FS, editors: *Clinical cases in anesthesia*, ed 4, Philadelphia, 2014, Elsevier Saunders.

Rosato S et al: Transcatheter aortic valve implantation compared with surgical aortic valve replacement in low-risk patients, *Circ Cardiovasc Interv* 9(5):e003326, 2016.

Rosengart TK, Anand J: Acquired heart disease: valvular. In Townsend CM et al, editors: *Sabiston textbook of surgery*, ed 20, Philadelphia, 2017, Saunders.

Schoen FJ, Gotlieb AI: Heart valve health, disease, replacement, and repair: a 25-year cardiovascular pathology perspective, *Cardiovasc Pathol* 25(4):341–352, 2016.

Seifert PC: Care of the cardiac surgical patient. In Odom-Forren J, editor: *Drain's perianesthesia nursing: a critical care approach*, ed 7, St Louis, 2017, Saunders.

Shapira OM, Reardon MJ: Tumors of the heart. In Sellke FW et al, editors: *Sabiston and Spencer's surgery of the chest*, ed 9, Philadelphia, 2016, Saunders.

Smith T et al: Does the use of bilateral mammary artery grafts compared with the use of a single mammary artery graft offer a long-term survival benefit in patients undergoing coronary artery bypass surgery?, *Interact Cardiovasc Thorac Surg* 18(1):96–101, 2014.

Society of Thoracic Surgeons (STS): *What to expect after heart surgery* (website), 2009. www.sts.org/sites/default/files/documents/pdf/whattoexpect.pdf. (Accessed 9 February 2017).

Sommerstein R et al: Transmission of *Mycobacterium chimaera* from heater-cooler units during cardiac surgery despite an ultraclean air ventilation system, *Emerg Infect Dis* 22(6):1008–1013, 2016.

Stone ME et al: Mechanical assist devices for heart failure. In Kaplan JA et al, editors: *Kaplan's cardiac anesthesia*, ed 7, Philadelphia, 2017, Saunders.

Svensson LG et al: Aortic valve and ascending aorta guidelines for management and quality measures: executive summary, *Ann Thorac Surg* 95(4):1491–1505, 2013.

Szelkowski LA et al: Current trends in preoperative, intraoperative, and postoperative care of the adult cardiac surgery patient, *Curr Probl Surg* 52(1):531–569, 2015.

Szeto WY, Bavaria JE: Endovascular therapy for thoracic aortic aneurysms and dissections. In Sellke FW et al, editors: *Sabiston and Spencer's surgery of the chest*, ed 9, Philadelphia, 2016, Saunders.

Teramoto T et al: Successful revascularization improves long-term clinical outcome in patients with chronic coronary total occlusion, *Int J Cardiol Heart Vasc* 14:28–32, 2017.

Tester DJ, Ackerman MJ: Genetics of long QT syndrome, *Methodist DeBakey Cardiovasc J* 10(1):29–33, 2014.

Thanassoulis G et al: Genetic associations with valvular calcification and aortic stenosis, *N Engl J Med* 368(6):503–512, 2013.

Thanavaro L: Cardiac risk assessment: decreasing postoperative complications, *AORN J* 101(2):201–212, 2015.

The Joint Commission (TJC): *2017 National patient safety goals* (website), 2017. www.jointcommission.org/standards_information/npsgs.aspx. (Accessed 9 February 2017).

Toeg HD, Rubens FD: Cardiopulmonary bypass: technique and pathophysiology. In Sellke FW et al, editors: *Sabiston and Spencer's surgery of the chest*, ed 9, Philadelphia, 2016, Saunders.

Tracci MC, Cherry KJ: The aorta. In Townsend CM et al, editors: *Sabiston textbook of surgery*, ed 20, Philadelphia, 2017, Saunders.

Webb GD et al: Congenital heart disease. In Bonow RO et al, editors: *Braunwald's heart disease: a textbook of cardiovascular medicine*, ed 10, Philadelphia, 2015, Saunders.

Wessler JD et al: Updates to the ACCF/AHA and ESC STEMI and NSTEMI guidelines: putting guidelines into clinical practice, *Am J Cardiol* 15(5 Suppl):23A–28A, 2015.

Windecker S, Piccolo R: Myocardial revascularization for left main coronary artery disease, *J Am Coll Cardiol* 68(10):1010–1013, 2016.

Yarboro LT, Kron IL: How I teach mitral valve surgery, *Ann Thorac Surg* 101(5):1641–1643, 2016.

CHAPTER **26**

Pediatric Surgery

MICHELE CLEMENS SMITH AND SUSAN M. SCULLY

Pediatric surgery is a highly specialized and unique area of perioperative nursing in which the patients provide a unique challenge. Pediatrics includes the neonate; infant; child adolescent; and with recent advances, the fetus.

The pediatric patient often needs surgery for congenital anomalies that threaten life or the ability to function. Syndromes and the postpremature infant often need continuing surgical interventions. Trauma also affects a child's health far more often than adults. It is important to recognize that the difference between pediatric care and adult care is not just a size issue; from birth onward, the body and organs exist in a continual state of development, and multiple physiologic changes occur with age. Major areas of distinction are the airway and pulmonary status, cardiovascular status, temperature regulation, metabolism, fluid management, and psychologic and cognitive development. Family-centered care is also crucial to the care of pediatric patients because they are separated from their families, and management of anxiety of the patient, family, and caregiver is paramount to a successful outcome.

The advancement of improved diagnostic, imaging, and interventional technology; the development of new anesthetics and pharmacologic agents for pain management; and the creation of even smaller and more delicate instrumentation have revolutionized perioperative care of the pediatric population. Numerous pediatric surgeries that were once approached as open procedures are now being done with minimally invasive techniques, resulting in shorter hospital stays and faster recovery times. Off-site surgery in neonatal units and pediatric intensive care units (PICUs) is also becoming a way of caring for critically ill patients. Improvements in the transport of critically ill children and the intensive care management of neonatal and pediatric patients as well as the development of new surgical procedures are also saving more lives. Yet they are presenting medical professionals with a new and unique set of problems as complex, medically fragile children are now surviving into adulthood.

Pediatric Surgical Anatomy

Airway and Pulmonary Status

Respiratory mechanics alter dramatically from infancy to adulthood, resulting from increases in airway size, transformations in the rigidity of airway and chest structures, and major changes in neuromuscular status. A proportionally large head, a short neck, and a large tongue in relation to jaw size create more of a challenge for airway management. The glottis is very anterior, moving from the level of the second cervical vertebra to the level of the third or fourth vertebra in the adult. The epiglottis is floppy and more curved, and the vocal cords are slanted anteriorly. The airway forms an inverse cone with the narrowest portion at the cricoid cartilage until 8 years of age; endotracheal tube size is therefore very important because a tube that passes easily through the glottis may be too tight at the subglottic area, compromising the child's airway in the immediate postoperative period because of swelling. The infant is an obligate nasal breather, and the chest wall of an infant is very compliant, leading to increased work of breathing with any type of airway compromise. Infants also have type 2 respiratory muscle fibers until age 2 years, which fatigue more easily than type 1 muscle fibers. Premature infants are at risk for postanesthetic apnea until 60 weeks after conception age. There is a depression in the CO_2 response curve in infants; compared with an adult, the respiratory rate does not increase as readily in response to a rising CO_2 level, although all ages undergo a CO_2 response depression related to inhalational agents and narcotics. One of the most important considerations is that children have a much smaller pulmonary functional residual capacity; a child becomes hypoxic more quickly if the airway is lost. Alveolar maturation is not complete until 8 years of age. Smaller airways have higher resistance; airway resistance decreases approximately 15 times from infancy to adulthood, again with a major change occurring around 8 years of age. It is important to note that smaller airways can become compromised with even a minor amount of swelling. An additional consideration in the pediatric setting is loose teeth. Loose teeth are common in children ages 5 to 14 years; a dislodged tooth is a potential airway foreign body risk.

Cardiovascular Status

The most dramatic changes in the cardiovascular system occur at birth with the transition from fetal circulation. Even in full-term infants, persistent transitional circulation may occur. Heart rate is the predominant determinant of cardiac output in infants and children; bradycardia drastically decreases cardiac output and requires swift intervention. There is a decreased cardiac compliance because of a lower proportion of muscle to connective tissue until age 1 to 2 years, making infants preload insensitive. Young children are predisposed to parasympathetic hypertonia (increased vagal tone), which can be induced by painful stimuli such as laryngoscopy, intubation, eye surgery, or abdominal retraction. Attention to blood loss in young patients is very important because the patient's total blood volume is very small. Blood volume in neonates is 80 to 90 mL/kg, at 1 to 6 years it is 70 to 75 mL/kg, and at age 6 years to adult it is 65 to 70 mL/kg. At birth, 70% to 90% of the hemoglobin is fetal hemoglobin with a high affinity for oxygen. It is normal for hemoglobin levels to fall at about 2 to 3 months of age (physiologic anemia) to a hematocrit level of 29% and a hemoglobin level of 10 mg/dL as the infant's body begins to produce its own blood cells. A cardiology evaluation is essential if a murmur is auscultated. A murmur can be from a patent foramen ovale, which normally closes at 3 to 12 months; a patent ductus arteriosus (PDA), which can be present for up to 2 months; a previously undetected cardiac anomaly; or an innocent flow murmur. The evaluation is critical because anesthetic agents cause vasodilation and potentiate cardiac dysrhythmias.

Temperature Regulation

Infants and young children are most at risk of hypothermia because of their increased body surface area-to-weight ratio and thin fat layer (Evidence for Practice). Cold stress leads to increased oxygen consump-

---

EVIDENCE FOR PRACTICE

Preventing Unplanned Perioperative Hypothermia in Children

Unintentional perioperative hypothermia resulting in a core body temperature lower than 37°C (98.6°F) has been shown to cause serious patient complications such as surgical site infections, decreased incision-site healing, increased blood transfusions, and death. Reports of pediatric adverse outcomes resulting from perioperative hypothermia are limited but include cardiac arrhythmias, hypoglycemia, increased oxygen demand, metabolic acidosis, tissue hypoxia, and ischemia (Kim et al., 2013). Infants and children have a greater risk of developing unplanned hypothermia caused by limited stores of subcutaneous fat and a less effective regulatory capacity. Current published estimates of pediatric perioperative hypothermia range from 4.2% to 60% (Kim et al., 2013).

A recent study (Beedle et al., 2017) looked at the effectiveness of an evidence-based CPG to maintain normothermia for the pediatric population. Before full implementation of the CPG, the authors established a baseline occurrence of unplanned hypothermia at 16.3%.

Perioperative staff attended a lecture and completed self-directed learning modules before implementation of the CPG. A temporal artery thermometer was assigned to each child and traveled with the child through all phases of perioperative care. Nurses measured temperatures at the beginning and end of each phase of perioperative care for a total of eight documentation points. Children found to have a body temperature of ≤36°F (96.8°F) received nurse-initiated warming interventions as outlined by the CPG (warm blankets, forced-air warming, warm mattress). Temperature trends helped establish the importance of assessing the temperature at the designated documentation time points outlined in the CPG. Two of the lowest temperature assessment points included the end of the intraoperative period and the start of the PACU period. This finding establishes the continued importance of assessing temperatures as the child transitions to the PACU. Implementation of the CPG resulted in an unplanned hypothermia rate of 1.84%.

The clinical implications of this research study include the importance of consistent CPG implementation and the application of evidence-based guidelines to improve outcomes in pediatric surgical care.

CPG, Clinical practice guideline; *PACU,* postanesthesia care unit.
Modified from Association of periOperative Registered Nurses (AORN): Guideline for prevention of unplanned patient hypothermia. In: *Guidelines for perioperative practice,* ed 16, Denver, 2017, The Association; Beedle S et al: Preventing unplanned perioperative hypothermia in children, *AORN J* 105(2):170–183, 2017; Kim P et al: Perioperative hypothermia in the pediatric population: a quality improvement project, *Am J Med Qual* 28(5):400–406, 2013.

---

tion, resulting in hypoxia, respiratory depression, acidosis, hypoglycemia, and pulmonary vasoconstriction. Hypothermia alters drug metabolism, prolongs the action of neuromuscular blockers, and delays emergence from anesthesia. The child's temperature must be monitored continuously throughout the intraoperative experience. An axillary temperature probe is acceptable for short procedures in healthy children; an esophageal or rectal temperature probe provides more accurate monitoring of the child's temperature for longer cases. Hyperthermia should also be avoided because it leads to increased oxygen consumption and increased fluid losses.

It is vital to maintain normothermia in children, and the easiest way to do this is by exposing only the area on which surgery is being performed. Additional thermoregulatory interventions include altering the room temperature before the child enters the room and using a warming blanket. An overhead heater can be used during the anesthetic induction and patient preparation period immediately before prepping and draping. Coving the patient's head with a hat, blanket, or plastic also aids in temperature regulation. The anesthesia ventilation circuit can be heated and humidified, as can insufflated carbon dioxide during minimally invasive surgical procedures. For surgical procedures with large areas of exposure, warmed solutions should be available for use instead of room temperature solutions. Intravenous (IV) solutions can also be warmed before administration (AORN, 2017). The use of an impermeable plastic adherent incisional drape also keeps the patient temperature regulated because less area is exposed, and it also keeps fluids from collecting around the surgical site.

Metabolism

Infants have a higher basal metabolic rate than adults, and it is greatest at 18 months. Most importantly, children younger than age 2 years have immature liver function; pharmacologic response is altered, and there is slower hepatic clearance, decreased hepatic enzyme function, and decreased protein binding. Medication distribution is different in neonates and infants compared with older children and adults because of an increased percentage of total body weight and extracellular body fluid. Infants have an immature blood-brain barrier and decreased protein binding, which results in an increased sensitivity to sedatives, opioids, and hypnotics.

Fluid Management

Renal function at birth is immature, and the ability of the kidneys to concentrate urine is limited, so the infant is much more prone to dehydration. Complete maturation of renal function occurs at about 2 years. Compared with an adult, a child has a higher body water weight, a higher body surface area, and an increased metabolic rate, resulting in increased fluid requirements per kilogram of body weight. Despite these significant points, it is also important to remember that the body weight of the child, the length of time without fluids, and surgical losses are the primary factors in the calculations of the child's hydration needs.

Psychologic Development

A child's comprehension of and responses to the environment are based on developmental age. A key factor is that a child's developmental age does not necessarily match his or her chronologic age. Nursing care should be tailored to the developmental age of the child to optimize the child's ability to understand the situation, to minimize the stress and anxiety of the child and family, and to facilitate the development of a trusting and supportive medical relationship. The types of fears are also related to the child's level

TABLE 26.1

Developmental Stages

Approximate Ages	Piaget Stage	Erikson Stage	Developmentally Based Fears	Appropriate Nursing Interventions
Infancy to 1 year (Erikson) Infancy to 2 years (Piaget)	Sensorimotor Uses senses and motor skills to understand world Develops memory; begins to imitate others	Trust versus mistrust, develops belief that world can be counted on to meet basic needs Who to trust? Identifies strangers at 7–8 months	Separation	Use soothing voice; sing, hold child, give child objects to hold to provide distractions Meet child, family without touching child at first Allow personal item into OR for comfort/security
Toddlerhood	Preoperational Use of symbols, creative play (can pretend) Is very egocentric	Autonomy versus shame, doubt Develops free will; increasing control of their bodies Feels regret, sorrow for inappropriate behavior	Separation Forced dependence	Give only simple choices; involve child in actions when possible, use distractions, sing songs child may recognize Allow personal item into OR for comfort/security
Early childhood, preschool	Preoperational	Initiative versus guilt Begins to explore, imagine Feels remorse for actions Thinking dominated by perceptions; distorted reasoning	Separation Body mutilation	Magical thinkers, use stories during induction Likes colorful Band-Aids Allow child to handle unfamiliar objects to decrease stress (e.g., mask, pulse oximeter probe) Allow personal item into OR for comfort/security
Middle childhood, elementary school age (Erikson) Ages 7–11 years (Piaget)	Concrete operations Uses symbols, logic, principles to solve problems Classifies, sorts everything	Industry versus inferiority Beginning to understand time and unseen body functions Is cooperative; desires recognition for achievements	The unknown Body mutilation Inadequate performance	Provide simple information to decrease stress Be honest at all times Do not expect child to act like an adult yet Allow personal item into OR for comfort/security
Adolescence, puberty	Formal operations Uses logical and abstract thinking Understands hypothetical concepts	Identity versus role diffusion Peer group has increased importance Body image, clothing, activities help define identity	Altered body image Death	Query patient about concerns; offer information to decrease fears Provide as much privacy as possible if disrobing is necessary Use mental imagery to decrease stress Offer to hold hand to provide comfort; personal item still permitted

From Derieg S: An overview of perioperative care for pediatric patients, *AORN J* 104(1):4–10, 2016; Wilson D, Hockenberry M: *Wong's clinical manual of pediatric nursing*, ed 8, New York, 2017, Elsevier.

of psychologic development. Predictable stages mean predictable behaviors. The stages of growth have been described from a variety of different aspects. Dr. Jean Piaget described the stages by changes in cognition and the ability to think, and Dr. Erik Erikson based the stages on psychosocial and emotional needs. Their work provides an excellent guideline for assessing the pediatric patient's developmental level to use appropriate interventions (Table 26.1).

Perioperative Nursing Considerations

Assessment

The initial patient assessment provides information necessary to develop a plan of care specific to the needs of each pediatric patient related to age, developmental level, and diagnosis. The unique aspects of care of the pediatric surgical patient revolve around the fact that the child is constantly growing and changing. The perioperative nurse must have a good understanding of the normal physical and

psychologic parameters for pediatric patients and be able to recognize and act on deviations from these parameters. Table 26.2 presents normal vital sign ranges for infants and children.

In addition, the perioperative nurse must be familiar with normal growth and developmental factors for each age group. On any given day, the perioperative nurse may care for a variety of pediatric patients ranging from neonates through adolescents. In some instances, children undergoing an ambulatory surgical procedure may visit the operating room (OR) complex and ambulatory surgery area with their families 1 to 2 weeks before surgery, depending on the child's developmental level and the availability of a preoperative pediatric education program. If the child has a complex medical history or an extensive surgical procedure is planned, the child and family members will meet with a member of the anesthesia team during this advance visit. Various materials and videos are available on the Internet that are informative and provide a child-friendly perspective. There are many developmentally age-appropriate tools about surgery for children that can promote a better acceptance and understanding

TABLE 26.2
Pediatric Vital Signs

Age	Heart Rate (Beats/min)	Respirations (Breaths/min)	Systolic Blood Pressure (mm Hg)
Newborn	100–150	30–55	50–70
Infants to 2 years	80–120	25–40	70–88
2–6 years	70–110	20–30	88–94
6–10 years	60–95	16–22	94–102
10–16 years	60–85	12–20	80–111

Modified from Wilson D, Hockenberry ML: *Wong's clinical manual of pediatric nursing*, ed 8, New York, 2017, Elsevier.

PATIENT, FAMILY, AND CAREGIVER EDUCATION

The Role of the Nurse Educator and Child Life Specialist in Supporting Education

In the pediatric setting, patient, family, and caregiver education is accomplished through many avenues. Patient, family, and caregiver education manuals, electronic interactive materials, and hospital-based Internet sites contain teaching and information that include but are not limited to explanations of conditions, procedures, diagnostic studies, and home management techniques. These materials also contain lesson plans that a provider can access before providing teaching to a patient or family at the bedside or in a family learning center.

Many institutions have family learning centers on site that adopt teaching and learning techniques to suit both inpatient and outpatient clients and their families. A patient may be referred to the family learning center in preparation for discharge so that medical care can be effectively managed at home. Family learning centers promote learning in a safe, quiet environment with one-to-one instruction by a nurse educator. Care is simulated using mannequins, models, and other realistic tools and validated by return demonstration from the patient or caregiver. In addition, patients and caregivers are provided with feedback and additional materials to support the management of medical care in the home environment.

Institutions may also assign child life specialists to pediatric units and floors. Child life specialists are experts in child development who promote effective coping through play, preparation, education, and self-expression activities. They provide emotional support for families and encourage optimum development of children facing a broad range of challenging experiences, particularly those related to healthcare and hospitalization. Understanding that a child's well-being depends on the support of the family, child life specialists provide information, support, and guidance to parents, siblings, and other family members. They also play a vital role in educating caregivers, administrators, and the general public about the needs of children under stress.

AMBULATORY SURGERY CONSIDERATIONS

Guidelines for Pediatric Ambulatory Surgery

Candidates for ambulatory surgery in a pediatric institution should:

- Be categorized as either class I or class II in accordance with the American Society of Anesthesiologists (ASA) guidelines; in some cases, patients who are categorized as class III may be eligible for ambulatory surgery with the approval of the medical director or attending surgeon
- Be older than 6 months of age; patients older than the age of 18 who are followed by a physician on staff may have surgery at the ambulatory surgery center with the approval of the medical director and surgeon-in-chief

Procedures that are eligible for scheduling in ambulatory surgical settings should:

- Be no more than 4 hours in duration and have a total of 4 hours of direct supervised recovery unless exceeded by patient condition demands that cannot be anticipated before surgery
- Be able to be performed using local or regional anesthetics, MAC, or general anesthetic with a duration of less than 4 hours
- Be able to be performed without the risk of extensive blood loss, major prolonged invasion of body cavities, or direct involvement of major blood vessels

MAC, Monitored anesthesia care.
Modified from Children's Hospital of Philadelphia: *Ambulatory surgery policy and procedure manual*, 5.2.1 approved surgical procedures for ambulatory surgical centers; *Ambulatory surgery policy and procedure manual*, 2.1.1 patient selection criteria for the ambulatory surgery center, Philadelphia, 2014.

of the perioperative process. Facility tours are not always a feasible option, but most pediatric institutions have a thorough program that follows the preoperative and postoperative plan on their hospital websites. These are often developed by child life specialists (Patient, Family, and Caregiver Education) in conjunction with medical staff and are updated frequently. Many pediatric centers also have smartphone and tablet applications with comprehensive materials for parents and caregivers.

Occasionally the child's history and physical, surgical consent, and any necessary tests or labwork are done in advance in the surgeon's office setting, and the child and family have no introduction to the surgical experience until the day of surgery. Depending on local practice, information related to the child's scheduled procedure may be sent home with the family from the surgeon's office or mailed to the family the week before the surgery is scheduled. The surgical facility generally contacts the family the day before surgery to inform them when the child should arrive at the facility and to review preoperative eating and drinking instructions. In these instances, the initial interview performed by the perioperative nurse is especially crucial to provide a thorough, documented assessment of the child's growth (height and weight), current physical status (vital signs, heart and breath sounds, skin integrity), current medication history, allergies, nothing-by-mouth (NPO) status, recent illnesses, current medical concerns, and behavioral responses to the interview process. The perioperative nurse confirms the intended surgical procedure as well as correct site confirmation with the child and family as it is written on the surgical consent as well as their understanding of the operation. This information is critical to the nursing plan of care during the surgical procedure.

Children may undergo surgery at ambulatory surgery facilities or in a hospital setting. Certain criteria must be met for children to qualify for surgery at an ambulatory facility (Ambulatory Surgery Considerations). The nurse reviews the patient's chart, giving particular attention to the patient's age, developmental level, diagnosis, and intended surgical procedure. Current nursing diagnoses and the ongoing plan of care are examined. If the child is an inpatient, a discussion with the primary nurse can facilitate data collection, assist in providing continuity of care, and provide the perioperative nurse with information regarding preoperative education previously provided. The perioperative nurse can meet the child and any family members present at the time of the visit. The interview can be used to gather information helpful to develop the intraoperative plan of care and to decrease the anxiety related to the child's impending surgery by providing a familiar face on the day of the procedure. The focus of this visit is to discuss the perioperative process, and not always to provide preoperative education regarding the surgery. In pediatric centers in the inpatient setting, the primary nurse, child life therapist, or clinical nurse specialist may provide preoperative education. During the preoperative visit the perioperative nurse can explain, at a developmentally appropriate level, what the child will experience in the preoperative, intraoperative, and postoperative phases of care. The perioperative nurse may briefly describe the roles of various staff members who will be a part of the team responsible for the child's care in the OR. Common concerns that families express are the length of time that they will be separated from their child and their child's pain management. Explanations to children should be provided within a developmental framework, taking into account each child's cognitive and psychosocial abilities. Medical play items, audiovisual aids, puppets, and photographs are all helpful in the education process (Panella, 2016).

The perioperative nurse who will be participating in the intraoperative care of the child will review the patient's information and meet with the patient and the family before the child is transferred to the OR. In addition to reviewing the documentation, the nurse validates the patient's identification using two patient identifiers; confirms that the surgeon has marked the child's surgical site per institutional protocol; and seeks verbal verification from the patient, parent, or legal guardian about the scheduled procedure, making sure that it matches what is written on the surgical consent (Fig. 26.1). If implants are to be used, availability must be confirmed before the patient's transport to the surgical suite. Frequently children will be given premedication 20 to 45 minutes before their transportation to the OR. Premedication such as midazolam can greatly decrease

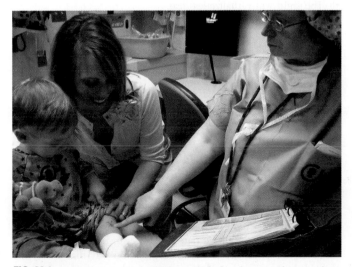

FIG. 26.1 Perioperative nurse and parent verify that the surgical site marking on a pediatric patient matches consent.

a child's anxiety, minimizing the stress of separation for both child and family. The surgeon and anesthesia provider will each meet with the child and family, usually while the OR is being prepared for the patient. The perioperative nurse will assess the child's psychologic state, review the intended surgical procedure with the child and family, and ensure that they have no additional questions or concerns. A final communication among the anesthesia provider, surgeon, and nursing staff for the room confirms the team's state of readiness for the delivery of care before the nurse transports the child to the OR.

Informed Consent

Informed consent must be obtained before administrating anesthesia or performing surgery. For children younger than age 18, consent must be obtained from one of the following individuals: a legal parent (biologic parent whose parental rights have not been terminated) or an adoptive parent who has completed the adoptive process. Foster parents of children in the custody of a child and youth agency (CYA) are not permitted to give consent; rather, consent should be obtained from the CYA social worker or appropriate legal representative. Legal guardians should be encouraged to bring any supporting documentation of legal guardianship or ability to consent for the child's medical care on the day of surgery. Perioperative nurses should review the chart for documentation of legal guardianship and ensure that the appropriate individual signs each document. For patients over the age of 18 who are still receiving treatment at a pediatric facility, an Advanced Directive should be provided and documented accordingly. For patients over the age of 18 who are considered unable to sign consents, an appropriate letter designating a person able to consent and make decisions is needed and should be reviewed by the hospital legal advisors.

When emergency situations arise and the need for treatment is immediately necessary to prevent serious or permanent impairment of the patient's health or to preserve the life of a patient, surgery may be performed without consent of the legal guardian. In the event that a legal parent is unable to be located or unable or unwilling to provide informed consent, a court order may be obtained to permit treatment. A pediatric patient who is an emancipated minor (e.g., legally under the age of consent but recognized as having the legal capacity to consent) can give valid consent. It is important for children to develop a trusting relationship with medical professionals and that these older children are in agreement (within their developmental capabilities) with their family's decision regarding surgery. Risk management and legal departments can assist in clarifying questions or conflicts specific to informed consent.

Child Abuse and Neglect

Perioperative nurses are obligated to screen all pediatric patients for abuse or neglect. Child abuse and neglect results from any of the following: physical injury, sexual abuse or exploitation, or negligence or maltreatment (Manga et al., 2015; Child Welfare Information Gateway, 2013). Child abuse is found in all segments of society, crossing cultural, ethnic, religious, socioeconomic, and professional groups. The perioperative nurse is in a unique situation to assess for the presence of abuse because the patient will be disrobed in the OR. Box 26.1 lists the clinical manifestations of child abuse. Every state has a child abuse law that dictates legal responsibility for reporting abuse and suspicion of abuse, and nurses are mandated reporters. Penalties, in the form of either fines or jail time or both, can be imposed on mandatory reporters who fail to report cases of suspected child abuse and neglect as required by the reporting laws. State laws also may impose penalties on any person who knowingly

BOX 26.1

Clinical Manifestations of Child Abuse and Neglect

Skin Injuries

Skin injuries are the most common and easily recognized signs of maltreatment of children. Human bite marks appear as an ovoid area with tooth imprints, suck marks, or tongue thrust marks. Multiple bruises in inaccessible places are indications that the child may have been abused. Bruises in different stages of healing may indicate repeated trauma. Bruises that take the shape of a recognized object are generally not accidental. Bruises do not typically occur in nonmobile children.

Traumatic Hair Loss

Traumatic hair loss occurs when the child's hair is pulled or used to drag or jerk the child. The result of the pulling on the scalp can cause the blood vessels under the skin to break. An accumulation of blood can help differentiate between abusive and nonabusive loss of hair.

Falls

If a child is reported to have experienced a routine fall but appears to have severe injuries, the inconsistency of the history with the trauma sustained indicates suspected child abuse.

External Head, Facial, and Oral Injuries

Cuts, bleeding, redness, or swelling of the external ear canal; facial fractures; tears or scarring of the lip; oral, perioral, and/or pharyngeal lesions; loosened, discolored, or fractured teeth; dental caries; tongue lacerations; unexplained erythema or petechiae of the palate; and bilateral black eyes without trauma to the nose may all indicate abuse.

Deliberate or Unexplained Thermal Injuries

Immersion burns, with a clear line of demarcation; multiple small circular burns, in varying stages of healing; iron burns (showing iron pattern); diaper area burns; and rope burns suggest intentional harm.

Shaken Baby Syndrome

A shaken baby may suffer only mild ocular or cerebral trauma. The infant may have a history of poor feeding, vomiting, lethargy, and/or irritability that occurs periodically for days or weeks before the initial healthcare consult. In 75% to 90% of cases, unilateral or bilateral retinal hemorrhages are present but may be missed unless the child is examined by a pediatric ophthalmologist. Shaking produces an acceleration-deceleration (shearing) injury to the brain, causing stretching and breaking of blood vessels, which results in subdural hemorrhage. Subdural hemorrhage may be most prominent in the interhemispheric fissure. However, cerebral edema may be the only finding. Serious insult to the central nervous system may result, without evidence of external injury.

Unexplained Fractures and Dislocation

Posterior rib fractures in different stages of healing, spiral fractures, or dislocation from twisting of an extremity may provide evidence of intentional injury in children.

Sexual Abuse

Abrasions or bruising of the inner thighs and genitalia; scars, tearing, or distortion of the labia/hymen; anal lacerations or dilation; lacerations or irritation of external genitalia; repeated urinary tract infections; sexually transmitted disease; nonspecific vaginitis; pregnancy in young adolescent; penile discharge; and sexual promiscuity may provide evidence of sexual abuse.

Neglect

The symptoms of neglect reflect a lack of both physical and medical care. Manifestations include failure to thrive without a medical explanation, multiple cat or dog bites and scratches, feces and dirt in the skinfolds, severe diaper rash with the presence of ammonia burns, feeding disorders, and developmental delays.

Modified from McCarthy K: Health problems of toddlers and preschoolers. In Hockenberry M, Wilson D, editors: *Wong's essentials of pediatric nursing*, ed 10, St Louis, 2017, Elsevier.

---

makes a false report of abuse or neglect (Child Welfare Information Gateway, 2013).

Nursing Diagnosis

Nursing diagnoses related to the care of pediatric patients undergoing surgery might include the following:
- Anxiety related to separation from family and friends
- Fear related to developmental level (fear of the unknown, fear of painful procedures and surgery)
- Risk for Infection related to surgical intervention and other invasive procedures
- Risk for Hypothermia related to loss of body surface heat to environment and immature temperature-control mechanisms

Outcome Identification

Perioperative nursing care is predicated on relevant nursing diagnoses and their corresponding desired outcome. Outcomes should be measurable with criteria by which to judge their attainment. Thus for the desired outcome, "The patient will demonstrate some ability to manage anxiety," and measurable criteria (e.g., the child will have posture, facial expressions, gestures, and activity levels that reflect decreased anxiety and will demonstrate increased focus) might be identified.

Outcomes identified for the selected nursing diagnoses for the pediatric patient could be stated as follows:
- The child will demonstrate some ability to manage anxiety.
- The child will verbalize less fear.
- The child will remain free from signs and symptoms of surgical site and invasive procedure site infection.
- The child will be maintained in a state of normothermia.

Planning

Assessment data, combined with information about the planned surgical procedure, enable perioperative nurses to anticipate requirements for surgical positioning, instrumentation, equipment and supplies, medications, and activities necessary for the provision of safe, competent care for the pediatric patient. Knowledge of the child's developmental level allows the nurse to plan her or his approach and interactions with the child and family (Fig. 26.2). The perioperative nurse identifies criteria appropriate to the child and surgical setting for each of the desired outcomes (Sample Plan of Care).

The perioperative nurse must also develop a trusting relationship with the child and his or her parents, family, or legal guardians. The nurse must explain the events of surgery in a way that allows the child and accompanying adults to better understand what to expect on transfer to the OR. Honest answers are used to minimize anxiety

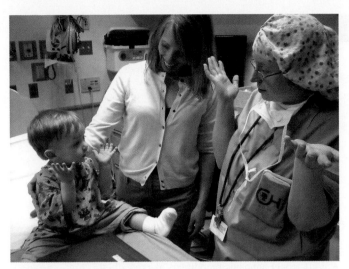

FIG. 26.2 Perioperative nurse engages in play with a toddler during preoperative assessment.

of the patient and the family. Taking the time to establish confidence and trust with the patient, family, and caregiver contributes to increased outcomes and satisfaction.

Infants, reliant on family to meet their basic needs, are difficult to pacify when NPO for surgery. The facility should provide rocking chairs, pacifiers, warm blankets, and simple distractions such as music or toys. Preoperative teaching should include telling the family to provide fluids for the infant until the deadline for NPO status. Unnecessary delays should be avoided at all costs. Parents may need reassurance and support during the period immediately before surgery.

The toddler or preschooler fears parental separation and abandonment. Toddlers fear, among other things, strangers, the dark, and machines. They attribute lifelike qualities to inanimate objects, believing that the objects, like them, have feelings. Thus a blood pressure cuff that squeezes the child's arm may be perceived to be doing so because it is angry with the toddler. Toddlers may also believe that their skin holds their body together; anything that violates the skin integrity is feared. For this reason, bandages are very important. Toddlers and preschoolers interact with the environment using their senses. To integrate this into the patient's care, the perioperative nurse should give the toddler the opportunity to touch and play with objects that he or she will encounter. An example is to give the child a small anesthesia mask to put on his or her teddy bear. Sensory information should be provided in a soft, gentle voice (i.e., what the toddler will see, feel, touch, and hear). A security object is extremely comforting. The OR should be quiet, and background noise should be controlled. Instruments that are frightening should be kept from view. To allow quick induction of anesthesia the toddler should be transferred into the surgical suite when the room and staff are completely prepared (Patient Engagement Exemplar).

The school-age child may still perceive hospitalization or surgery as a punishment but can evaluate painful intrusive actions in terms of logical function (e.g., getting an IV line hurts, but then I can get medicine in it to make me feel better). Feelings of inadequacy may be associated with something the child thinks he or she should be expected to do or know. Fear of body injury or mutilation, loss of control, and fear of the unknown characterize this developmental stage. These children benefit from simple, concrete explanations in familiar terms; a book or other teaching aid can be helpful. The concepts of time and unseen body functions can now be incorporated

in the explanations. The child should be allowed to make choices when possible (e.g., letting the child decide in which hand to place the IV line or which flavor to add to the anesthetic mask).

Adolescents may fear altered body image, peer rejection, disability, and loss of control or status. The fear of death is more prevalent in this age group than any other, and adolescents may find explanations of monitoring and safety measures reassuring. They need as much privacy as possible, and their attempts to be independent should be respected (e.g., walking into the OR instead of being wheeled in on a stretcher if the patient has not been sedated). The adolescent may not wish to show any fear; questions might not be answered while the parents are present. Information and explanations should be provided as reasonably and truthfully as possible. If appropriate, some choices should be allowed, such as wearing underwear to the OR. Patient care procedures that violate privacy, such as hair removal, skin preparation, or insertion of an indwelling urinary catheter, should be conducted after the patient is anesthetized. Modesty should be respected, and only the exposed surgical site should be uncovered.

Key points in providing perioperative care to pediatric patients include remaining alongside the child until the child is anesthetized, keeping the room quiet during induction, accepting a child's need to express fear and fearful behaviors (e.g., crying), and using simple words without double meanings to explain care. Security objects should remain with the child until induction has been completed. A child's behavior during induction is likely to be the same during emergence; thus all attempts should be made to provide calm, reassuring care. Parents should be alerted to delays in the surgery schedule, and in some instances, the child may be allowed to have clear fluids if the surgery is delayed by several hours.

Implementation

Implementing the nursing plan of care includes continual reassessment of the patient's needs as well as the efficient execution of activities

SAMPLE PLAN OF CARE

Nursing Diagnosis
Anxiety related to separation from family and friends

Outcome
The child will demonstrate some ability to manage anxiety; a toy or other comfort/security object will remain with the child, and he or she will cooperate with requests.

Interventions
- Provide an atmosphere of warmth and acceptance for both child and family members.
- Maintain a calm and relaxed manner. Talking with the child and being calm and smiling can provide comfort. Engage the child in conversations about his or her likes and family.
- Explain to the child when he or she will be reunited with the parents.
- Speak softly and slowly. When speaking, try to get down to the child's eye level so he or she can see your face. Do not assume you were understood. Repetition may be necessary.
- Allow the child to keep familiar comfort and security objects (e.g., toy, blanket).
- Administer preoperative sedation as prescribed; note effects.
- Encourage parents to stay with the child as long as permitted and according to their wishes.
- Encourage parents to hold child until child falls asleep, if desired (may vary according to institution policy).
- Offer reassurance through touch if welcomed and culturally appropriate.

Nursing Diagnosis
Fear related to developmental level (fear of the unknown, fear of painful procedures and surgery)

Outcome
The child will verbalize less fear; he or she will respond in an age-appropriate manner to comfort measures and recognize that the perioperative nurse is present to help.

Interventions
- Assess the child's growth and development, noting any variations from expected normal age-appropriate maturational levels.
- Provide preoperative education for the child and family, using audiovisual aids such as photographs, drawings, items for medical play, or a tour of the surgical suite.
- Provide explanations according to the child's level and the parent's level of understanding; use age-appropriate terminology that is familiar to the child, such as for body function.
- Place unfamiliar equipment out of the child's view to decrease fear.
- Encourage the child to handle items that may seem strange or threatening.
- Reassure the child that certain body parts can be removed without producing harm (e.g., blood, tonsils, appendix).
- Provide ongoing age-appropriate explanations for procedures/events during the perioperative period. Do not try to explain everything at once; instead, explain procedure by procedure.
- Allow choices whenever possible, such as wearing pajamas or clothing to the OR.
- Respect need for modesty; expose only those body parts necessary.

- Provide diversion activities to decrease fear.
- Be honest about the possibility of pain or discomfort; do not lie to the child.
- Reassure the child that you are there to help and care for him or her.

Nursing Diagnosis
Risk for Infection related to surgical intervention and other invasive procedures

Outcome
The child will remain free from signs and symptoms of infection at the surgical site and invasive procedure sites; the surgical site will heal by first intention, and white blood cell count and differential will remain within normal limits.

Interventions
- Administer antibiotic prophylaxis as prescribed.
- Follow Standard Precautions.
- Maintain aseptic technique, and monitor members of the surgical team for breaks in technique.
- Teach family members signs and symptoms of surgical site infection:
  - Redness
  - Swelling
  - Warmth
  - Tenderness
  - Pain
- Teach family members the importance of and proper handwashing techniques.
- Apply dressing to the surgical site before sterile drapes are removed to prevent contamination of incision.

Nursing Diagnosis
Risk for Hypothermia related to loss of body surface heat to environment and immature temperature-control mechanism

Outcome
The child will maintain normothermia as evidenced by body temperature within normal limits/expected range.

Interventions
- Adjust room temperature approximately 1 hour before arrival of the child: 78.8°F to 80.6°F (26°C to 27°C) for infants and newborns; 73.4°F to 75.2°F (23°C to 24°C) for older children.
- Keep the child covered as much as possible.
- Consider wrapping lower extremities in soft gauze or stockinette and encasing in a plastic bag for newborns and infants.
- Place knit hats, blankets, or plastic over the patient's head.
- Provide a radiant heat lamp for use during placement of monitoring lines, induction of anesthesia, positioning, skin prep, and draping.
- Use warmers during administration of intravenous fluids and blood products and surgical irrigation; temperature settings should not exceed 100.4°F (38°C).
- Monitor body temperature by rectal, esophageal, tympanic membrane, or other automatic temperature-monitoring device.
- Document temperature at prescribed intervals; take appropriate action for temperature extremes.
- Begin to warm the room as the procedure is ending and before undraping the patient.

that facilitate the surgical intervention. Remaining with the child during induction, positioning, and prepping the surgical site; creating and maintaining a sterile field; collecting and documenting specimens; and administering medications are all part of helping to provide a safe environment for the pediatric surgical patient. Making sure that the pediatric patient's family receives regular updates of the child's status is also a part of the perioperative nurse's responsibilities and will decrease their anxiety and help foster a sense of trust in the healthcare professionals caring for their child.

Instrumentation

The same types of instruments used in adult surgery are used in pediatric surgery. However, pediatric instruments are usually shorter, have more delicate or less pronounced curves, and are smaller. A complete range of instrument sizes is necessary to make the appropriate size available to each child because pediatric patients can range in size from less than 1 to more than 100 kg. Fewer instruments are normally required because incisions in children are shorter and shallower than those in adults. Use of basic instrument sets, grouped according to types of surgery performed (e.g., minor, major), facilitates instrument counts. Instrument sets may also be grouped according to categories of patient size (e.g., infant, pediatric, adolescent, and adult). These sets are easily adapted to the patient's needs as well as the surgeon's preferences and eliminate unnecessary instruments from the sterile field.

Sutures

A variety of sutures are used with the pediatric population because of the wide range of patient size; needles from size 1 to 7-0 are routinely stocked. Both absorbable and nonabsorbable sutures on cutting and tapered needles are used. The most frequently used sizes are 3-0 to 5-0 with ½- and 3/8-circle needles. A growing trend is the use of antibiotic-coated suture (Research Highlight). Skin staples are rarely used. Many skin incisions are closed with subcuticular techniques, over which adhesive strips or cyanoacrylate glue is then applied. The use of tape to apply dressings is done conservatively because of the delicate nature of children's skin; frequently, either a small transparent or an elastic net dressing is used to hold gauze dressings in place.

Anesthetic Considerations

Anesthesia is approached differently in pediatric patients than it is in adults. The equipment and supplies are scaled down to match the size of the patient, and different anesthesia circuits and delivery systems may be used. Adult facilities that provide anesthesia to pediatric patients should consider developing a mobile pediatric intubation cart that houses the appropriate-sized equipment and devices necessary to care for the anesthetized child.

The most common technique used in the pediatric population is a general inhalational anesthetic administered by facemask, laryngeal airway, or endotracheal tube. Selection of the endotracheal tube involves several considerations: the tube must be large enough to permit ventilation but small enough to minimize damage to the trachea while maintaining a seal to prevent aspiration.

Microdrip IV tubing and burettes are commonly used to avoid the administration of excess fluids in pediatric patients younger than 8 years, and only 500-mL bags of IV solution are used. The patient's IV line is usually started in the OR after induction with mask anesthesia, depending on the patient's diagnosis and medical history. Patients who require emergency surgery who have not been NPO, have increased intracranial pressure, an unusually difficult airway,

---

| **RESEARCH HIGHLIGHT** |

Triclosan-Containing Sutures for Reducing Surgical Site Infections in Children

Antimicrobial suture technology involves the coating or impregnation of synthetic, absorbable, sutures with the antiseptic, triclosan. A recent meta-analysis of 13 randomized clinical trials (Guo, 2016) involving more than 5000 patients demonstrated that triclosan-coated sutures are associated with lower risk of SSIs than conventional uncoated sutures when used in adult surgery. An additional meta-analysis (Leaper, 2016) suggested use of these sutures may also result in significant savings across various surgical wound types.

Because interventions in adult populations can have different effects compared with those in children, trial results cannot be directly extrapolated between adult and pediatric populations. Children have different physiologic characteristics and different risk factors for surgical site infections.

A double-blind, randomized, controlled trial looked at 1633 children who were undergoing various surgical procedures to assess the efficacy of suture material coated or impregnated with the antiseptic agent triclosan compared with standard suture material (Renko, 2017).

The outcome reviewed was the occurrence of a superficial or deep SSI. Superficial SSI was defined as occurring within 30 days of the operation and involving only skin or subcutaneous tissue. Deep SSI was defined as present if it occurred within 30 days of the surgical procedure (or longer if implant is in place and the infection appears to be related to the operation), was related to the procedure, and involved deep soft tissues, such as the fascia and muscles. SSI occurred in 20 (3%) of 778 patients allocated to receive triclosan-containing sutures and in 42 (5%) of 779 patients allocated to receive control sutures. The patients in the triclosan group had less need for revision of the wound, fewer visits to the physician or readmissions to the hospital, and fewer antimicrobial courses to treat SSIs than did the patients in the control group.

Use of triclosan-containing sutures effectively reduced the occurrence of all SSIs compared with normal sutures. The results align with the results of meta-analyses of previous studies in adults.

SSI, Surgical site infection.
Modified from Dennis C et al: Suture materials—current and emerging trends, *J Biomed Mater Res A* 104(6):1544–1559, 2016; Guo J et al: Efficacy of triclosan-coated sutures for reducing risk of sutures for reducing risk of surgical site infection in adults: a meta-analysis of randomized clinical trials, *J Surg Res* 201(1):105–117, 2016; Leaper DJ et al: Meta-analysis of the potential economic impact following introduction of absorbable antimicrobial sutures, *Br J Surg* 104(2):134–144, 2017; Renko M et al: Triclosan-containing sutures versus ordinary sutures for reducing surgical site infections in children: a double-blind randomised controlled trial, *Lancet Infect Dis* 17(1):50–57, 2017.

---

neuromuscular disease, or have been identified as a malignant hyperthermia (MH) risk require an IV placement before anesthesia induction. If the IV line is started before induction, measures should be taken to lessen the discomfort, such as an intradermal injection of 1% buffered lidocaine or saline at the site or the application of topical anesthetic creams. If possible, the surgical team should allow the child the option of sitting up or lying down during IV placement; if developmentally appropriate, hold the child's hand and tell the child about each step in the placement of an IV line.

Preoperative sedation is generally accomplished by the oral administration of midazolam. Midazolam can be given orally, nasally, rectally, intramuscularly, or intravenously. Oral midazolam should be administered in a flavored base to mask the bitter taste. The accepted dose is 0.5 mg/kg with a maximum dose of 10 mg. Relaxation is noted 15 to 45 minutes after administration. The child should be kept in a safe, observable environment after being medicated (Patient Safety). Depending on institutional policy, a parent may be present during induction to comfort the child and decrease the child's anxiety. The perioperative nurse should provide the parent an explanation of how the OR will appear and who will be present in the OR, how the child's anesthesia induction will be performed, and how the parent services provider or child life therapist should be present to escort the parent to and from the OR so that the perioperative nurse can focus on providing care for the patient after the child has been anesthetized.

Distraction methods during the induction of anesthesia can help minimize a child's stress and anxiety. Singing softly, telling a story, and, for the older child, providing a relaxing mental image are effective diversion techniques.

MH, although very rare, may be more prevalent in the pediatric population as a result of the administration of inhalational anesthetics and succinylcholine. In addition, physiologic conditions present in some pediatric patients are associated with a higher risk of MH. These conditions include congenital myopathies such as central core disease, some congenital neuromuscular diseases, and King-Denborough syndrome (Litman, 2016). Careful assessment of family history is essential to identify patients at risk for developing MH. The management of an MH crisis is described in Chapter 5.

PATIENT SAFETY

Fall Risk

The Joint Commission has identified Falls Prevention as one of its National Patient Safety Goals and several patient fall prevention algorithms and care plans are available. Administration of midazolam greatly increases the fall risk of children of all ages. The desired outcome of preoperative sedation is a relaxed state with reduced anxiety. Although having an altered level of consciousness, pediatric patients are able to maintain their airway, follow simple commands, and respond to tactile stimulation. It is this alteration in mental status that puts the patient at risk for falls in the perioperative setting.

Measures to reduce falls should include but are not limited to:
- Educating the patient, family, and caregiver about the effects of preoperative sedation; dizziness, drowsiness, slurred speech, blurred vision, and hiccups
- Encouraging older children to void before medication administration
- Placing the patient's bed or stretcher at the lowest point and placing the side rails upright; explain to children that they must stay in bed after they have been medicated so they do not fall and hurt themselves
- Allowing toddlers and small children to sit in a parent's lap with the parent securely holding them with both arms around the child; when the child feels too heavy, placement in the bed or stretcher is necessary

Modified from The Joint Commission (TJC): *Sentinel event alert* (website), 2015. http://www.jointcommission.org. (Accessed 31 January 2017); Murray E et al: Implementing a pediatric fall prevention policy and program, *Pediatr Nurs* 42(5):256–259, 2016.

Pain Management

In the past, many common fallacies existed about pain in the pediatric population. Some of these mistruths were that infants do not feel pain, children have better pain tolerance than adults, children cannot tell the healthcare provider where they hurt, children always tell the truth about pain, children become accustomed to pain or painful procedures, and narcotics are more dangerous for children than they are for adults. Research into this important area has revealed that infants do demonstrate behavioral and physiologic indicators of pain. Compared with adults, children have less pain tolerance, and their pain tolerance increases as they mature. Children are able to indicate pain, and children as young as 3 years can use pain-rating scales. Often children may not admit to having pain because they may believe that others know how much they hurt, or they fear receiving an injection. Children may also feel that pain and suffering are punishment for some misdeed, or they may not know what the word *pain* means. Children do not become accustomed to pain or painful procedures. They actually may demonstrate increased behavioral signs of pain with repeated procedures. Developmental level, culture, coping ability, temperament, and activity levels influence the behavioral manifestations of pain exhibited by the patient. Narcotics are no more dangerous for children than they are for adults and are not excluded as a treatment modality. The evaluation of a pediatric patient's level of pain is performed using a variety of assessment tools (pain scales) that are based on the age and developmental level of the child. Often these scales are tested for reliability and validity. In infants and nonverbal children, evaluation is based on physiologic changes and observation of behaviors. Children with verbal skills are able to articulate pain.

Questioning the child provides the most reliable indicator of pain. Children who may not be familiar with the word *pain* may be more comfortable with words like "ouch" and "hurt." It may also be helpful to ask the child to point to where it hurts. The Face, Legs Activity, Cry, Consolability (FLACC) Scale is a measurement used to assess pain for children between the ages of 2 months and 7 years or individuals who are unable to communicate their pain. FLACC in combination with a numeric pain scale can also be used to develop a customized pain behavioral scale for children with intellectual disability. Parents can be asked to recall one of the child's prior painful episodes and think about unique pain clues in association with the FLACC categories. The parent can then rate the behavior for each of the categories on a scale of 1 to 10 (Jacob, 2013). The FACES pain scale uses cartoon faces with a variety of expressions ranging from happy to crying. The child selects the face that best describes his or her pain (see Chapter 10). The Oucher scale has a numeric component and a component similar to the FACES scale but uses actual photographs of children. The adolescent pediatric pain tool (APPT) is a line drawing of a body; the child marks the drawing where he or she has pain (Jacob et al., 2014). Other tools include Likert-type scales rating pain on a score of 0 (no pain) to 10 (worst pain) or incorporate several components of pain assessment (subjective and objective data).

Physiologic indicators of pain, such as increased blood pressure, respirations, and heart rate and restlessness, are the same for children as for adults but may not be as reliable, except in neonates and nonverbal children. These indicators may also reflect anxiety or fear and should not be the sole indicator used to determine pain. Children may also tug or hold painful areas or show preference to a painful extremity.

Parental involvement in pain management is important. Parents know their child's normal behavior and can provide input into the behaviors being exhibited in the perioperative setting. Parents should be queried about the child's previous experiences with pain and be taught the nonverbal behaviors that may indicate pain.

Nurses should investigate all complaints of pain or discomfort and be sensitive to behavioral and nonverbal cues to determine treatment. Postoperative pain should be assessed after all surgical procedures, regardless of their nature. It is also critical to assess and document the child's response to the interventions provided for relief of pain.

Effective pain management requires a willingness to use a variety of methods and modalities to achieve optimal results. Pharmacologic methods include the administration of analgesics, both narcotic and nonnarcotic. Patient-controlled analgesia (PCA) is an option for children. It is safe, effective, and highly satisfactory from the viewpoint of patients and their families (Litman, 2016). Nonpharmacologic methods include distraction, relaxation, guided imagery, behavioral contracting, and cutaneous stimulation. Nonpharmacologic methods should never be used as substitutes for appropriate medication administration; instead, they should be used to enhance pain management.

Evaluation

The perioperative nurse evaluates care provided throughout the perioperative period. At the conclusion of the surgical intervention, the skin is inspected, especially at dependent pressure points, contact with medical devices, and at the site of the electrosurgical dispersive pad. Inspection is performed to detect any reddened, irritated areas or evidence of compression injury. If povidone-iodine or chlorhexidine gluconate preparations were used for skin prep, the area needs to be checked for any signs of chemical irritation. The patient's temperature is reassessed. The cardiopulmonary status is closely monitored as the child emerges from anesthesia. The perioperative nurse should assist the anesthesia team during emergence, remaining at the patient's bedside. Warm blankets are provided, hydration status is evaluated as replacement fluids continue to be administered, and fluid output is noted. The child is transferred to and positioned on the stretcher, crib, neonatal intensive care unit (NICU) warmer, or ICU bed; the airway and respiratory effort are reassessed before departing the OR. Tubes, IV lines, drains, and drainage devices must be carefully protected during the move from the operating bed. Supplemental oxygen is often given during transport from the OR to the PACU for pediatric patients.

The perioperative nurse provides a hand-off report to the PACU nurse, focusing on the condition of the child, the response to surgery and anesthesia, the presence of catheters and drains, the quality and amount of wound drainage, a description of the dressings applied, and any special needs. Part of this report should focus on the outcomes established in the perioperative plan of care. For the plan of care presented in this chapter, the outcomes might be as follows:

- The patient demonstrated decreased anxiety.
- The patient responded in an age-appropriate manner to comfort measures and exhibited decreased fear.
- The patient was protected from infection related to operative intervention; principles of asepsis and infection control were maintained.
- The patient's temperature was maintained in the desired range during the perioperative period.

The perioperative nurse may receive further feedback on the child's progress after the child is discharged from the PACU; information may be relayed by the surgeon, unit nurse, or anesthesia provider. This type of informal feedback helps the perioperative nurse collect additional data regarding effectiveness of the plan of care, providing information about the achievement of identified outcomes.

Patient, Family, and Caregiver Education and Discharge Planning

Patient, family, and caregiver teaching varies significantly based on the type of surgery performed. As noted, some hospitals provide special preoperative teaching and hospital tours for pediatric patients and their parents. Some information may be discussed with the child and family at the time of the office visit, when the surgery is scheduled. For same-day procedures, the day-surgery nursing staff might teach postoperative care immediately before patient discharge. Basics of postoperative care are reviewed with the parents at this time. In some cases, written material may be provided (Box 26.2). Parents should be advised to be alert for certain signs and symptoms during the postoperative recovery period that could indicate an infectious process, such as fever, pain, nausea, redness around the incision area, drainage from the wound, or difficulty breathing. These signs and symptoms may develop days or even weeks after surgery. It is important that parents understand the necessity of not ignoring any of these signs and symptoms and of reporting them to the surgeon promptly so that an early diagnosis can be made and treatment prescribed. Although discharge information depends on the type of surgery performed, it typically includes recommendations about activity restrictions, return to school or daycare, wound care, bathing or showering, diet, and follow-up appointments. The printed discharge instructions are reviewed with the parents, and their understanding is verified. This time should provide the family with an opportunity to ask questions or seek clarification of the instructions.

BOX 26.2

Sample Discharge Instructions

- Leave the wound open to the air.
- Do not apply any creams or ointments to the wound for 14 days.
- Clean the incision three times a day using a paper towel, mild soap, and water. Do this three times a day for 2 weeks, then just daily. Do not rub the incision. Gently clean the area in a circular motion with mild pressure. Remove the soap with a wet paper towel and pat dry. Do not use terry cloth washcloths. The fabric loops may snag and pull on stitches.
- Do not allow the incision to be under water for the first 2 weeks after surgery.
- Allow your child to shower the day after surgery.
- Monitor the stitches. If they are clear, they will dissolve and do not need to be removed. If they are blue or black, they need to be removed about 10 to 14 days after the surgery. Your surgeon will tell you how long they need to be in.
- Call the surgeon's office soon after going home if you need an appointment for stitch removal.
- Schedule a follow-up appointment in 4 to 6 weeks for a postprocedure visit.
- Check the wound daily. It is normal to have some redness around the stitch holes or on the incision line. Call the surgeon's office if you notice that the area around the outside of the incision is red, hot, or tender or has pus draining from it. Also call if your child has a fever greater than 101.5°F (38°C).

Modified from Children's Hospital of Philadelphia: *Hernia discharge family teaching sheet,* 2014.

Phone numbers for the surgeon and the main hospital are provided in case the family has concerns or questions during the child's recovery period at home. An appointment for the child's follow-up visit may be made before discharge, or the parents are instructed to call the physician's office to schedule an appointment.

Surgical Interventions

As mentioned, children require surgery for congenital malformations, an acquired disease, or trauma. The field of pediatric surgery is further subdivided into all the specialties. Several surgical procedures that may be designated pediatric are presented in previous chapters of this text under particular specialty headings. The surgical interventions presented here represent procedures that are most commonly performed on children.

Vascular Access

Vascular access in pediatric patients may be established intraoperatively for short-term (weeks) or long-term (months, years) use. Examples of short-term use include peripherally inserted central catheters (PICC lines) for antibiotic therapy. Central venous lines or implanted ports are placed for long-term access to provide parenteral nutrition, chemotherapy, bone marrow transplantation, or multiple IV access lines for the critically ill patient. Neonates and children born at low birth weights are at highest risk for catheter-associated infections as a result of their compromised immune status (Segal et al., 2014). National and consumer organizations are exerting pressure on hospitals to implement practices aimed at reducing and eliminating catheter-associated infections in all patients (Anderson et al., 2014).

Central Venous Catheter Placement

The preferred site of placement for central venous access is the external jugular vein. The internal jugular vein may be chosen if the external jugular vein has been used or is too small. From the cannulation site the catheter is tunneled under the skin about 5 to 10 cm. This is done to inhibit contamination of the bloodstream from frequent dressing changes. Subcutaneous ports are placed in a similar fashion. In cases in which the internal or external vein sites are unavailable, the catheter may be placed into the external iliac vein by way of a cutdown in the greater saphenous vein. In these cases, the catheter is tunneled into the abdominal wall.

Procedural Considerations

The manufacturer's instructions for handling and preparing the catheter must be followed. The catheter must not contact lint or other foreign matter. Before insertion the catheter is flushed and filled with heparinized saline (1 unit of heparin to 1 mL of saline) to prevent air bubbles from entering the circulatory system and to eliminate blood clots in the catheter lumen. Fluoroscopy is used to confirm proper placement of the catheter; lead shielding must be provided for patient and staff.

The child is appropriately positioned as dictated by the site chosen for cannulation and the area is prepped and draped.

Operative Procedure: External Jugular Vein Site

1. The surgeon uses a needle and syringe to puncture the external jugular and aspirates to confirm blood flow.
2. The syringe is removed from the needle, and a guidewire is fed through the needle into the vein. An intraoperative x-ray is taken to confirm correct position.
3. Once the position is confirmed, the surgeon makes an incision over the insertion site. A silver probe or tendon passer is used to create a tunnel beneath the skin to the desired exit site of the catheter. A second incision is made over the tip of the probe or passer.
4. The implantable end of the catheter is attached to the end of the passer or probe and pulled through the subcutaneous tunnel. The catheter is cut to a desired length.
5. The needle is removed from the vein, leaving the guidewire in place. An obturator is placed over the guidewire, and the wire is removed. The catheter is placed through the obturator into the vein, and an intraoperative x-ray is taken to confirm position.
6. The catheter is secured at the exit site on the chest wall with nonabsorbable sutures, flushed with heparinized saline (10 units of heparin to 1 mL of saline), and clamped.
7. An occlusive transparent dressing is placed over the catheter site. The catheter is coiled under this dressing to avoid tension on the line and accidental displacement.

Minimally Invasive Surgery

Improvements in instrumentation and the development of equipment in smaller sizes have resulted in the evolution of minimally invasive surgery (MIS) from that of a rapidly growing field to one of routine practice in the pediatric surgical arena. Much like the adult population, many traditional "open" pediatric surgical procedures are being replaced by MIS procedures. Advantages of MIS include diminished postoperative pain, improved cosmetic results, decreased prevalence of adhesion formation, accelerated recovery periods, and shorter hospital stays as in the adult population.

Despite the technical congruence with adult MIS procedures, the pediatric populations undergoing these procedures have specific needs that must be satisfied to promote positive outcomes. Anesthesia providers must take the size and age of the patient into consideration because of the risk of physiologic compromise related to insufflation. Likewise, steps are taken intraoperatively to decrease the likelihood of intra-abdominal injury, such as insertion of an appropriate size Foley catheter to decompress the bladder or application of graduated compression stockings or intermittent pneumatic compression devices to prevent deep vein thrombosis for adolescents.

Common pediatric MIS procedures for general surgery include diagnostic laparoscopy, pyloromyotomy, splenectomy, gastric fundoplication, and cholecystectomy. Thoracoscopic approaches may be used for the correction of pectus excavatum, effusions, lung biopsy, sympathectomy, and closure of a PDA. Procedures that are currently increasing in prevalence include choledochal cyst excision, lobectomy for congenital cystic adenomatoid malformation (CCAM), and repair of congenital diaphragmatic hernia (CDH) and tracheoesophageal fistula (TEF). Minimally invasive procedures in other disciplines include (but are not limited to) ventriculoscopy, which can be used to view the ventricles of the brain; functional endoscopic sinus surgery (FESS); and ureteral reimplantation and pyeloplasty, both of which may involve the use of a surgical robotic system (Robotic-Assisted Surgery). Although MIS is now considered common in the pediatric setting, the ability to convert to an open procedure should always be maintained with correct instrumentation available and an instrument count performed before incision. Insufflation flow rate should be set to the lowest acceptable level for achieving pneumoperitoneum and increased slowly to prevent adverse physiologic effects (decreased end-tidal CO_2, decreased SpO_2, tachycardia, cyanosis, arrhythmias) associated with CO_2 embolism.

ROBOTIC-ASSISTED SURGERY ▮▮

An Alternative to Open Surgery for Pediatric Patients

The use of robotic-assisted surgery in pediatrics is increasing in line with the advancements in robotic technology. Pediatric urologic surgeons were early adopters of minimally invasive surgery; however, these techniques were associated with a steep learning curve and considerable physical strain on the surgeon. Difficulties were exacerbated in smaller children and the pure laparoscopic approach was not broadly accepted.

The robotic-assisted laparoscopic (RAL) surgery concept, using a master–slave platform that is under the control of the surgeon, carries well-known advantages, as fully described fully in Chapter 8.

The most commonly performed urologic robotic-assisted pediatric surgeries are:

- Pyeloplasty (see page 1013)
- Ureteroneocystostomy
- Nephroureterectomy
- Partial nephrectomy

Although robotic-assisted urologic surgery has higher hospitalization costs, it offers a minimally invasive alternative for several of these procedures, as laparoscopic approaches to these procedures have not been widely adopted. The decrease in postoperative length of stay after robotic urologic procedures supports the potential benefit of the robotic approach. Other potential benefits of robotic-assisted surgery, such as decreased risk of small bowel obstruction, improved cosmesis, and higher patient satisfaction, may offset the higher costs associated with robotic-assisted urologic surgery in children.

Modified from Weiss DA, Shukla AR: The robotic-assisted ureteral reimplantation, *Urol Clin North Am* 42(1).99–109, 2015; Mahida JB et al: Utilization and costs associated with robotic surgery in children, *J Surg Res* 199(1):169–176, 2015.

Laparoscopic Pyloromyotomy for Pyloric Stenosis

Pyloric stenosis (Fig. 26.3) is the most common cause of gastric outlet obstructions in children and is the most common condition requiring surgery in the newborn. Signs and symptoms of high gastrointestinal (GI) obstruction appear at 2 to 6 weeks of age. The first sign is bile-free projectile vomiting after feeding. The infant usually fails to gain weight adequately, and there may be a severe loss of body fluids and electrolyte imbalance, evidenced as hypochloremic, hypokalemic metabolic alkalosis. After the diagnosis of hypertrophic pyloric stenosis is made, either through physical examination or by imaging techniques, surgical intervention is planned. Electrolyte imbalances must be corrected before surgery. The Fredet–Ramstedt pyloromyotomy for pyloric stenosis is an open procedure that involves the incision of the muscles of the pylorus to treat congenital hypertrophy of the pyloric sphincter that is obstructing the stomach. However, laparoscopic pyloromyotomy has replaced the open procedure as the standard for repair.

Procedural Considerations

The stomach is emptied just before induction of anesthesia, and the nasogastric tube is removed to guard against reflux of gastric contents around the tube during induction. The patient is positioned transverse on the OR bed so that the operating surgeon stands at the patient's feet. A video monitor is positioned above the patient's head. The abdomen is prepped and draped and trocar sites are injected with a local anesthetic. Appropriate-sized instrumentation and sterile supplies must be available, along with imaging equipment.

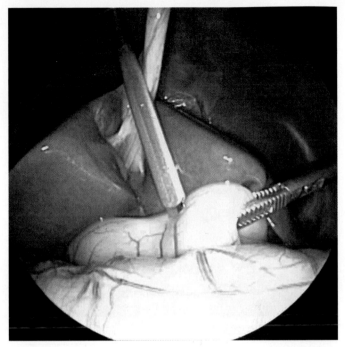

FIG. 26.3 Pyloric stenosis.

Operative Procedure

1. The surgeon makes a small incision in the umbilicus and places a 3-mm or 5-mm trocar through it to accommodate the telescope. Insufflation tubing is attached to this trocar and the abdomen is insufflated (maximum pressure of 10 mm Hg).
2. Using a #11 blade, the surgeon makes a small stab incision laterally, slightly above the umbilicus on each side.
3. The 3-mm laparoscopic instruments are passed directly through the stab incisions.
4. The surgeon makes an incision in the serosa on the anterior wall of the pyloric mass from the duodenal junction proximally to a point proximal to the area of hypertrophied muscle using an arthroscopic knife and laparoscopic grasper. The circular muscle is spread with the 3-mm laparoscopic pyloric spreader on the submucosal base so that all muscle fibers are completely divided (Fig. 26.4).
5. The anesthesia provider injects 60 to 120 mL of air into the stomach through an orogastric (OG) tube to ensure that there are no air bubbles at the pyloric incision.
6. The umbilical incision is closed using absorbable suture and cyanoacrylate glue applied to each incision.

Laparoscopic Fundoplication

Fundoplication is indicated for infants and children who experience severe gastroesophageal reflux (GER). The cause of GER in these patients is believed to be an inadequate antireflux barrier. The antireflux barrier normally consists of a combination of anatomic and physiologic factors, including sufficient amount and strength of muscle fibers located in the lower esophageal sphincter, adequate length of the abdominal esophagus, and a high-pressure zone in the lower esophagus. An incompetent antireflux barrier can result in life-threatening complications, including obstructive apnea, aspiration pneumonia, esophagitis, and failure to thrive. GER can be medically or surgically managed. Medical management relies on proton pump inhibitors (PPIs) to reduce the production of stomach acid. With

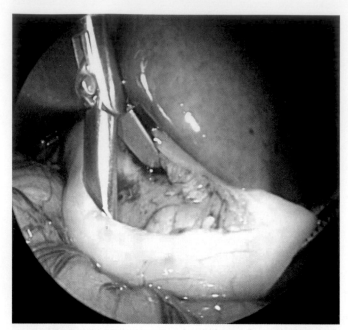

FIG. 26.4 Laparoscopic pyloromyotomy.

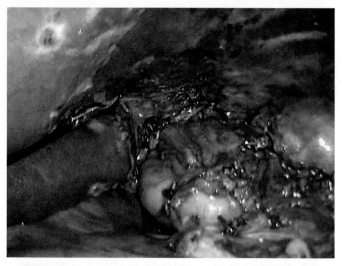

FIG. 26.5 Laparoscopic fundoplication, 270-degree (Toupet) wrap.

successful medical management of GER, surgery to correct the antireflux barrier may be avoided.

In certain cases, however, surgical intervention outweighs the benefit of medical management. Children who are more likely to benefit from surgical management of GER include those suffering from erosive esophagitis or volume regurgitation and patients who have had an adverse reaction to PPIs. Nissen fundoplication (NF) has historically been the most common surgical treatment of GER and has become one of the most common operations performed by pediatric surgeons. Surgical management of GER is accomplished by open or laparoscopic fundoplication technique. The Nissen is a complete 360-degree wrap with an antireflux valve created at the fundus of the stomach. With a complete fundoplication, the created valve inhibits the regurgitation of gastric contents into the esophagus, decreasing or diminishing GER (Fig. 26.5). The Toupet fundoplication

is a partial 270-degree dorsal wrap creating an adaptable reflux valve that grows and adapts with the patient, allowing restoration of function. This valve maintains normal physiologic actions such as burping and vomiting when necessary, minimizing the postoperative complications of gas, bloat, and retching that are common with NF.

Procedural Considerations

The patient is positioned supine for induction of general anesthesia. The anesthesia provider inserts an OG tube, which serves as a stent for the wrap during the procedure. After the endotracheal tube location is confirmed and secured, the patient is moved to the foot of the OR bed and positioned in low lithotomy position using stirrups and protective padding. The operating surgeon stands in the area between the patient's legs. A video monitor is positioned above the patient's head. The abdomen is prepped and draped and trocar sites are injected with local anesthetic. Appropriate-sized instrumentation and sterile supplies must be available, along with the appropriate imaging equipment.

Operative Procedure

1. The surgeon creates an umbilical incision and places a port. The abdomen is insufflated with CO_2 gas. A telescope is placed and the abdomen is inspected for gross abnormality. Additional incisions and ports are placed to accommodate the instrumentation.
2. Retraction is used to elevate the liver away from the stomach, and gastrohepatic connections are cut from the right crus. The crus is carefully dissected away from the esophagus, taking care to preserve the integrity of the peritoneum.
3. The surgeon uses a blunt dissector to create a retroesophageal tunnel for the esophageal length. The hiatus is reapproximated and tightened using endoscopic suturing devices.
4. A 270-degree (Toupet) wrap is completed. Two sutures incorporate the esophagus, stomach, and crus at the 10 and 2 o'clock positions on the diaphragmatic hiatus. Four sutures create intra-abdominal esophageal length with stitches anchored at the gastroesophageal (GE) junction, giving the fundoplasty the appearance of a "hot dog in a bun."
5. The OG tube is removed, and a final barrel suture is placed at the posterior portion of the wrap to anchor it to the right crus and keep it from unwrapping.
6. The stomach is inspected again to rule out gross abnormality or injury, then desufflated. Incisions are closed in layers using absorbable suture and sealed with cyanoacrylate glue.

Endoscopic Correction of Pectus Excavatum: Nuss Procedure

Pectus excavatum (funnel chest) is a visually obvious defect of the sternum, seen as a deep depression on the chest as a result of posterior displacement of the sternum (Fig. 26.6). It is usually associated with kyphosis. The defect may be asymmetric, most often deeper on the right side, with sternal angulation. In a majority of cases surgical treatment is cosmetic; impaired cardiorespiratory function is the underlying reason for surgical intervention in fewer cases. The procedure is most commonly performed in patients between 10 and 16 years of age, about the time when children become embarrassed to undress in front of peers. Rigid fixation has become a choice for correction of the defect, in which a metal bar and retaining stabilizer are inserted to gain chest wall stability and prevent recurrence. The bar and stabilizers are maintained for approximately 3 years. Other treatments may cosmetically correct the situation over the short term but usually result in progressive retraction of the sternum.

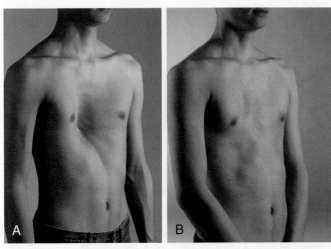

FIG. 26.6 Repair of pectus excavatum. (A) Preoperative. (B) Postoperative.

Procedural Considerations

Adolescent endoscopic instrumentation is used along with a camera, telescopes, corresponding thoracic instrumentation, and a fixation rod. The patient is positioned supine with the arms positioned along the sides and the elbows flexed 90 degrees and propped so that they are anterior to the chest. The hands are propped so that they are anterior to the elbows. The upper chest is elevated on a soft roll or sheets. A Foley catheter may be placed, and the patient is prepped and draped.

Operative Procedure

1. The surgeon measures the patient's chest to determine the size of the stabilization bar to be used, and bends an aluminum template to the desired shape of the chest. A stainless steel bar is bent to match the aluminum template using plate benders.
2. Two lateral chest incisions are made in line with the deepest part of the pectus, and subcutaneous pockets are created.
3. A port is placed into the left chest through which gentle insufflation takes place.
4. The surgeon makes an incision via the subcutaneous pocket to pass the Lorenz introducer. The introducer is positioned through one side of the chest, across the mediastinum, and out the other side using thoracoscopic visualization techniques.
5. A doubled tracheostomy tape is placed at the end hole of the introducer and brought through the anterior mediastinal tunnel. The tracheostomy tape is then tied to the stainless steel bar, which is brought through the chest using the same tunnel and flipped using a flipping device. Chest configuration is checked for correction, contour, and symmetry.
6. A side bar (strut) is placed on each side of the bar and a stainless steel wire is wrapped around the main bar both medially and laterally. Nonabsorbable sutures are placed between the chest wall and the end holes of the side and main bars. The suture knots are buried within the holes, and the thoracic cavity may be irrigated with antibiotic irrigation.
7. The wounds are closed in layers using absorbable suture, and a chest x-ray is obtained postoperatively to rule out pneumothorax.

Thoracoscopic Surgery for Patent Ductus Arteriosus

PDA is a condition in which the ductus arteriosus fails to close within 24 to 48 hours after birth. Symptomatic PDA can be treated medically or surgically. When pharmacologic treatment is ineffective or contraindicated, the only solution for PDA closure is an invasive treatment, especially when heart failure (HF) is present. This requires thoracoscopic equipment and supplies, including 0- and 30-degree, 4- and 2.7-mm telescopes, depending on the surgeon's preference and the patient's age and size. The endoscopic instruments, made smaller for the pediatric patient, include an electrocoagulation hook; Castroviejo-type scissors; graspers and right-angle clamps; fan lung retractors of varying sizes, either medium or medium-large; large endoscopic clip appliers; trocars with ports; and suction tip, preferably one that has a porthole to occlude when suction is required. Instrumentation for closure of PDA by thoracotomy is also set up in case the thoracoscopy fails or a complication arises and the chest needs to be opened emergently.

Procedural Considerations

Before the procedure the video monitors are set up on either side of the OR bed. The patient is placed in a right lateral position.

Operative Procedure

1. Usually four small incisions are made along the line of the posterolateral thoracotomy incision and ports are introduced.
2. The surgeon inserts the telescope. The first assistant holds the lung retractor while the second assistant holds the camera.
3. A grasper is used to elevate the pleura overlying the aorta near the insertion of the PDA and pulmonary artery, and careful dissection is begun with electrocoagulation. Suction is required to keep the area of dissection clear to enhance the surgeon's vision.
4. When the ductus has been clearly identified, a right-angle clamp may first be introduced and a tie applied to the duct. The clip applier is then inserted, and clips are applied.
5. Transesophageal or transthoracic echocardiography is performed by a cardiologist before closure of the porthole incisions to ensure closure of the ductus. The surgeon inserts a chest tube into the pleural space, the lungs are inflated, and the chest tube is removed; alternately, a chest tube may be left in place before porthole incision closures.

Robotic-Assisted Laparoscopic Pyeloplasty

Robotic-assisted laparoscopic pyeloplasty is commonly performed for children with ureteropelvic junction (UPJ) obstruction. The robotic-assisted technique is contraindicated in patients weighing less than 6 kg, an untreated urinary tract infection (UTI), and anatomical limitations (Tasain et al., 2015).

Procedural Considerations

The team positions the child in a modified flank position at a 45- to 60-degree angle with the affected kidney side up and the body supported with gel rolls or a beanbag. The nurse confirms that all pressure points are protected, and pillows are placed between the legs. Patients are secured to the table with tape applied below the knee, at or just below the hip, and just below the nipple line. The setup of the robotic system is completed before the patient being brought to the OR, and video monitors are placed accordingly. The nurse ensures that appropriate robotic instrumentation as well as laparoscopic and minor sets are available.

Operative Procedure

1. The surgeon places an 8.5-mm umbilical trocar to accommodate the telescope. The superior trocar is placed in the midline between

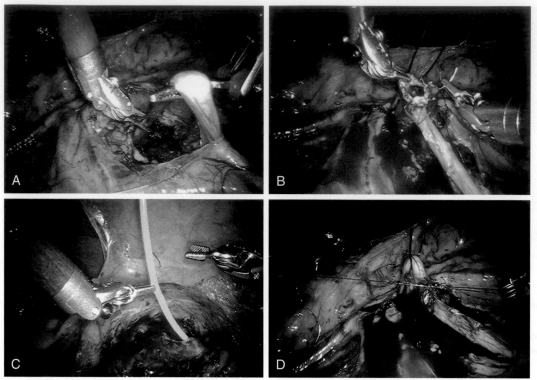

FIG. 26.7 Robotic-assisted pyeloplasty. (A) Ureter is dissected. (B) Anastomosis started at the apex of the ureter. (C) Stent is placed. (D) Completed anastomosis.

the umbilicus and the xiphoid and the inferior trocar is placed lateral to the rectus in the midclavicular line. The team brings the robot over the patient's chest and shoulder and places the camera and instruments in the corresponding arms.

2. After the surgeon reflects the bowel, attention is turned to the kidney. A transmesenteric incision is usually possible for left pyeloplasty, and the colon often has to be reflected on the right. In transmesenteric approaches, a small incision is made in the mesentery of the colon near the UPJ taking care to avoid mesenteric vessels (Fig. 26.7A).

3. The surgeon uses blunt dissection to expose the renal pelvis and ureter and spatulates the ureter laterally for about 1 to 2 cm leaving the UPJ attached to the ureter.

4. A hitch stitch may be passed through the abdominal wall to the renal pelvis just below the costal margin to expose and stabilize the UPJ.

5. The surgeon completes the anastomosis with 6-0 or 5-0 poliglecaprone 25 sutures. The anastomosis is started at the apex of the ureteral spatulation, which is secured to the most dependent portion of the renal pelvis (see Fig. 26.7B). The posterior anastomosis is completed first using a running suture.

6. A ureteral stent (see Fig. 26.7C) may be placed at this time. The surgeon places a 14-gauge angiocatheter through the abdominal wall to direct a stent down the ureter.

7. The surgeon completes the anterior anastomosis (see Fig. 26.7D) and closes the incisions.

Fetal Surgery

The expansion of prenatal diagnosis centers for mothers with problem pregnancies has resulted in earlier detection of fetal malformations,

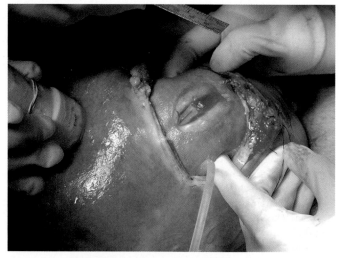

FIG. 26.8 Exposed fetal myelomeningocele.

such as CDH, myelomeningocele (MMC), and twin-to-twin transfusion syndrome (TTTS) (Figs. 26.8 and 26.9). One of the most significant advances in pediatric surgery is in the field of fetal surgery, which includes closed (percutaneous), minimally invasive (fetoscopic), open, and ex utero intrapartum therapy (EXIT) procedures (a specialized delivery technique originally developed to deliver babies who have undergone tracheal occlusion for CDH). One of the most recent fetal surgeries adopted in the United Sates includes fetoscopic endotracheal occlusion (FETO) (Research Highlight). Research has

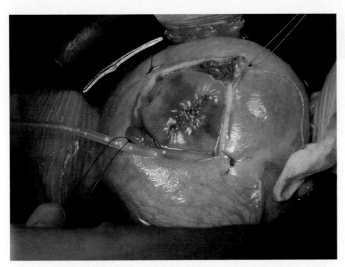

FIG. 26.9 Completed fetal myelomeningocele repair.

been a cornerstone of the fetal surgery discipline because performing fetal interventions without supporting research puts both the mother and fetus at higher risk for morbidity or mortality.

The type of anomaly and its immediate danger to the fetus determines the options for the pregnancy available to the family: allow nature to take its course and deliver at term, fetal surgery when the anomaly is life-threatening or when significant morbidity exists such as in MMC, or interruption of the pregnancy before 24 weeks' gestation. Criteria for consideration of fetal intervention include (Partridge and Flake, 2012) the following:

1. Ability to accurately establish a prenatal diagnosis
2. Evidence of a well-defined natural history of the disorder
3. Presence of a correctable lesion that, if left untreated, could result in fetal demise, irreversible organ dysfunction before birth, or severe postnatal morbidity
4. Absence of severe associated anomalies
5. Acceptable risk-to-benefit ratio to both the mother and the fetus

Descriptions of some defects that can be repaired prenatally are described in Table 26.3.

Procedural Considerations

The most important factor to consider when preparing for fetal surgery is that two patients are undergoing surgery: the mother and the fetus. The perioperative nurse must understand the maternal and fetal anatomy and pathophysiology as well as the entire operative procedure and potential risks to both patients to respond to emergencies such as fetal bradycardia, placental abruption, or other maternal–fetal complications. Perioperative nurses must also possess knowledge of fetal resuscitation medications as they prepare the field for any emergency.

Preparation of the fetal surgery OR is extensive, and usually involves multiple setups and specialized instrumentation and equipment. The concept of teamwork is of the utmost importance because the multidisciplinary approach to care extends into the OR. Multiple attending surgeons participate in the very small surgical field, and the procedures are performed within a short window of operating time. EXIT procedures necessitate an additional scrub and circulator team who assume responsibility for supporting the fetal airway during bronchoscopy, intubation, and tracheostomy.

RESEARCH HIGHLIGHT

Congenital Diaphragmatic Hernia

Advances in intrauterine fetal surgery unlock the possibility to increase the quality of life for many children. CDH occurs in 1 in 2500 to 4000 live births. A majority of CDH are on the left side and 40% are associated with other structural anomalies. Ultrasound increased the number of babies diagnosed prenatally, which in turn increased the chance of survival with diligent planning for the time of birth.

European doctors have been performing FETO procedures since 2000. In the FETO procedure, a small balloon is fetoscopically placed into the fetal trachea which decreases pulmonary hypoplasia by increasing the pressure in the fetus's chest, preventing organs from migrating into the thorax and allowing pulmonary development.

Survival rates of infants with CDH who received the FETO procedure are higher at both 30 days and 6 months of age than the survival rates of infants with CDH who did not undergo the FETO procedure. There are, however, increased complications in the pregnancies of the patients receiving intrauterine surgery. These complications include premature rupture of membranes, preterm birth at <37 weeks' gestation, and lower gestational age at birth (approximately 2 weeks) when compared with the pregnancies of patients not receiving intrauterine surgery. Furthermore, the infants who were not treated with fetal surgery suffered increased pulmonary arterial hypertension and pulmonary hypoplasia after birth.

This procedure, although offering remote hope to some parents of fetuses with CDH, is in the infancy stages itself. There is a high learning curve for the surgeons who perform this procedure. In addition, there is a lack of standardization between facilities as to when and how the balloon is removed. This lack of standardization would need to be studied to determine whether one removal technique is better for the patient's outcome. Currently the balloon can be removed fetoscopically during pregnancy before the onset of labor or can be removed during delivery of the fetus via the EXIT procedure.

FETO procedures have begun to be performed at hospitals in the United States. Diligent research is required to confirm the real benefits of FETO versus postnatal treatment. With the success of fetal surgery for the repair of a myelomeningocele it is possible to envision increasing the quality and quantity of life for fetuses with CDH.

CDH, Congenital diaphragmatic hernia; *EXIT,* ex utero intrapartum therapy; *FETO,* fetoscopic endotracheal occlusion.
Modified from Araujo J et al: Procedure-related complications and survival following fetoscopic endotracheal occlusion (FETO) for severe congenital diaphragmatic hernia: systematic review and meta-analysis in the FETO era, *Eur J Pediatr Surg* 27(4):e1, 2016.

Similar to any surgical procedure, perioperative team members who care for patients undergoing fetal surgery must be able to demonstrate critical judgment, organization, and prioritization skills. Circulating nurses and scrub persons who choose to participate in fetal surgery cases receive additional, specialized, simulation-based training that is both case and equipment specific. Precepted experiences in the circulating and scrub role are beneficial in promoting skill acquisition and competency achievement for fetal surgeries, which are considered a low-volume, high-risk surgery.

Minimally Invasive Fetal Surgery

TTTS can be treated by amnioreduction and placental laser ablation. Bipolar cord coagulation (BCC) and radiofrequency ablation (RFA)

TABLE 26.3

Defects That May Be Repaired Prenatally

Diagnosis	Definition	Treatment Modality
CCAM	Microcystic: Solid appearing Macrocystic: Grossly cystic; less predictable growth pattern can grow rapidly Fetal hydrops and placentomegaly may jeopardize maternal health ("maternal mirror" syndrome, in which the mother's condition mirrors that of the sick fetus)	Microcystic CCAM with hydrops may be effectively managed with steroids If steroids do not correct hydrops, open resection is offered Macrocystic CCAM may respond to thoracocentesis, thoracoamniotic shunting, or open lung resection
Giant neck mass	A large tumor in the neck that can compress the fetus's airway (e.g., cervical teratoma) Lymphangioma May compress esophagus, leading to polyhydramnios and preterm labor	EXIT procedure For babies at or near term, cesarean section to resection, postnatal sclerotherapy
HLHS	A range of congenital cardiac malformations that have in common underdevelopment of the left-sided heart structures Malformations include aortic valve atresia and stenosis with associated hypoplasia or absence of the left ventricle	Laparotomy without hysterotomy for percutaneous fetal aortic valvuloplasty continues to be studied
SCT	Fetal SCT may be cystic, solid, or mixed in its sonographic appearance (caused by mixed areas of tumor necrosis, cystic degeneration, hemorrhage, or calcification) Prenatally diagnosed SCT associated with fetal hydrops (excess fluid retention from high-output cardiac failure) can be rapidly fatal in utero; high-output cardiac failure is related to "vascular steal" from the high blood flow through the tumor Fetal hydrops and placentomegaly may jeopardize maternal health (maternal mirror syndrome, in which the mother's condition mirrors that of the sick fetus)	Steroid therapy can help manage the effects of preterm delivery. Sulindac (Clinoril) can help manage hydrops Cyst decompression Fetal surgery or EXIT procedure in cases in which increasing CCO and placentomegaly (caused by vascular steal and resulting high output failure) are present For babies at or near term, cesarean section to resection, postnatal sclerotherapy
MMC	Failure of the neural tube to close, resulting in protrusion of spinal cord and surrounding nerves from the open vertebrae The developing spinal cord and nerves are continuously exposed to amniotic fluid and friction over the course of gestation, which results in progressive neurologic injury	Fetal surgery or postnatal surgery options dependent on selection criteria
TRAP sequence	A rare complication of identical twinning in which one twin lacks a functioning cardiac system and is dependent on the twin with the fully functioning cardiac system (the "pump" twin) "Reversed perfusion" occurs when blood enters the acardiac/acephalic twin through its umbilical artery and exits through the umbilical vein (opposite of normal blood supply) The pump twin sustains increased cardiac demands that result in increased cardiac output, overproduction of urine, and ultimately, polyhydramnios	Fetoscopy to gain access to the fetus BCC or RFA to nonviable twin
TTTS	A rare and serious complication in identical twins who share a placenta that has abnormal connections between the two twins' blood vessels The smaller (donor) twin pumps blood to the larger (recipient) twin The recipient twin produces excess urine and is at risk for polyhydramnios and hydrops The donor twin produces less urine and is at risk for oligohydramnios and a small or absent bladder	Amnioreduction Fetoscopic placental laser surgery Selective reduction by BCC or RFA as a last option when the at-risk twin faces imminent demise; protects the co-twin from neurologic impairment or demise

BCC, Bipolar cord coagulation; *CCAM,* congenital cystic adenomatoid malformation; *CCO,* continuous cardiac output; *EXIT,* ex utero intrapartum therapy; *HLHS,* hypoplastic left heart syndrome; *MMC,* myelomeningocele; *RFA,* radiofrequency ablation; *SCT,* sacrococcygeal teratoma; *TRAP,* twin reversed arterial perfusion; *TTTS,* twin-to-twin transfusion syndrome.
From Children's Hospital of Philadelphia (CHOP): *Center for fetal diagnosis and treatment: conditions we treat* (website). www.chop.edu/service/fetal-diagnosis-and-treatment/fetal-diagnoses. (Accessed 18 February 2017).

are used to treat TTTS when the at-risk twin faces imminent demise. Regardless of the type of fetoscopic procedure, mothers who have fetuses with TTTS receive monitored anesthesia care (MAC), antibiotics, and an infiltration of a local anesthetic at the surgery site. Surgery is performed using continuous ultrasound guidance.

When TTTS is treated using selective placental laser coagulation, the recipient twin undergoes amnioreduction by needle aspiration before inserting a fetoscopic sheath. The fetoscopic sheath is attached

to a rapid fluid infusion warmer or pump and has a side port that accommodates a diode laser fiber. The surgeon inserts the fetoscope into the amniotic cavity of the recipient twin and is directed to the placental cord insertion site using ultrasound guidance. The branching vessels are followed in the direction of the donor twin until the collapsed intertwin membrane is identified. Blood vessels crossing from the donor side across the collapsed intertwin membrane are mapped. Vascular anastomoses with the recipient twin side are laser photocoagulated on continuous power with 0.5- to 1-second power bursts. After completion of the first pass, the region is remapped and reevaluated to identify additional anastomoses, and the process is repeated until no additional anastomoses are identified. The laser is removed and amnioreduction is completed on the recipient twin. Antibiotics are infused into the amniotic space, and the insertion site on the uterine wall is assessed for bleeding and membrane separation. The maternal stab wound is approximated and closed with cyanoacrylate glue and covered with a transparent dressing. Postoperatively, fetal heartbeats are confirmed and assessed in both twins using ultrasound and Doppler velocimetry.

Fetal intervention continues to be studied in fetuses with cardiac conditions such as aortic stenosis (AS) with evolving hypoplastic left heart syndrome (HLHS) (Sala et al., 2014). The complexity of the procedure determines whether IV sedation with local infiltration at the surgery site or general anesthesia is used. A mini-laparotomy without hysterotomy provides imaging or access to perform an aortic valvuloplasty to alter the in utero history of AS with evolving HLHS (Sala et al., 2014). The end result of percutaneous intervention alters left heart physiology and growth and allows postnatal survival with biventricular circulation (Sala et al., 2014). Postnatal repair of HLHS is described in a later section of this chapter detailing surgery for congenital heart disease.

The type of surgery and degree of intervention dictate how long a mother remains hospitalized after surgery. For example, typically a 4-day length of stay is incurred after open fetal surgery, whereas for a fetoscopic procedure, mothers stay overnight, then stay at a nearby facility, such as a Ronald McDonald house, and return in a week. If all is well, the mother is discharged to home. After discharge the mother is instructed to remain on bed rest for 2 weeks, and activity is restricted for an additional 3 to 4 weeks. Activity may be gradually increased if there are no concerns noted during follow-up appointments. Mothers are provided with discharge instructions including information regarding medications, preterm labor, and recovery.

Open Fetal Surgery

Mothers undergoing open fetal surgery or an EXIT procedure require deep general anesthesia to provide uterine relaxation to prevent placental abruption. These mothers also receive antibiotics and an epidural before incision. Examples of diagnoses in which open fetal surgical procedures may be indicated include CCAM in the presence of hydrops, sacrococcygeal teratoma (SCT) with high-output cardiac failure, and MMC (see Figs. 26.8 and 26.9). CCAMs grow primarily between 20 and 28 weeks' gestation and may jeopardize maternal health ("maternal mirror" syndrome), in which the mother's condition mirrors that of the sick fetus. In cases of maternal mirror syndrome, the only cure is delivery. Frequent ultrasound follow-up provides critical information about growth of the mass and is able to detect early development of hydrops. The CCAM volume ratio (CVR) can determine the likelihood of hydrops developing (Box 26.3). If the mass remains large, but no hydrops develops, then an EXIT procedure or cesarean section to mass resection may be warranted. Postnatal repair of SCT and MMC is described later in this chapter.

Open fetal surgery is performed using a low, transverse maternal laparotomy to expose the uterus. An ultrasound probe with a sterile drape is then used to map the placental edges to identify the uterine hysterotomy site. The uterine hysterotomy is performed using a uterine stapling device that has absorbable staples and allows the thickened midgestation uterus to be opened bloodlessly (Fig. 26.10). This type of incision requires a cesarean section delivery for this and

BOX 26.3

Congenital Cystic Adenomatoid Malformation Volume Ratio

Congenital pulmonary airway malformation (CPAM) volume to head circumference (HC) ratio (CVR); CVR is also used to measure CPAM volumes (which includes congenital cystic adenomatoid malformation [CCAM]):

$$CVR = (length \times width \times height \times 0.52)/HC \text{ [all measurements in centimeters]}$$

Current studies have conflicting CVR cutoffs. Depending on the study, a fetus has an 80% chance of developing hydrops with a CVR <1.6 or >2.0.

Modified from Euser AG et al: Comparison of congenital pulmonary airway malformation volume ratios calculated by ultrasound and magnetic resonance imaging, *J Matern Fetal Neonatal Med* 29(19):3172–3177, 2016.

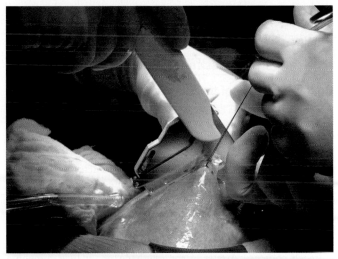

FIG. 26.10 Specially designed stapler used to quickly open the uterus during fetal surgery.

all subsequent pregnancies. Fetal oxygen saturation is monitored using pulse oximetry on the exposed limb. The fetus receives an IV line and an intramuscular shot of muscle relaxant and narcotic. Throughout the surgery the uterine cavity is continually filled with lactated Ringer's solution warmed to 37°C. A rapid infusion warmer and pump is used to maintain adequate uterine volume and to prevent umbilical cord compression and potential placental abruption. Postoperatively, preterm labor is of great concern, and uterine contractions, fetal heart rate, and fetal electrocardiogram (ECG) are continually monitored. Tocolytic medications are titrated to control uterine contractions. The nurse ensures the mother receives education in self-monitoring of uterine contractions. Tocolytic therapy is continued on an outpatient basis. Frequent fetal ultrasounds are performed postoperatively to monitor fetal well-being, amniotic fluid volume, and the adequacy of surgical repair.

Ex Utero Intrapartum Treatment

In cases in which the prenatal diagnosis confirms difficulty in obtaining a fetal airway (such as in giant neck masses) or difficulty ventilating a baby (such as in large CCAMs), the EXIT procedure may be warranted. After placing the epidural, the anesthesia provider administers antibiotics and deep general anesthesia. The surgeon then performs a maternal laparotomy and hysterotomy. Every attempt is made to use a stapling device to create an extended low-transverse incision. Patients should not get pregnant for 2 years after this delivery. It is feasible for patients to deliver vaginally after this uterine incision, however, it is strongly recommended that the patient delivers via scheduled cesarean section for all subsequent pregnancies because of the increased risk of uterine rupture.

With the use of halothane to promote uterine relaxation, utero-placental blood flow and gas exchange are maintained allowing appropriate time for execution of these life-saving procedures (Moldenhauer, 2013). The potential catastrophic event is in turn converted to a controlled, planned procedure. The appropriate surgery is then performed on the fetus while still on placental support (e.g., bronchoscopy, laryngoscopy, tracheostomy, resection of mass). The placenta is removed and residual blood clots are cleared, the hysterotomy and the maternal laparotomy are closed, and a sterile dressing is applied. After the baby is removed from placental support, he or she is taken to a stabilization room for resuscitation or to the adjacent OR for immediate surgical mass resection specific to diagnosis and related condition.

General Surgery: Gastrointestinal Procedures

Repair of Atresia of the Esophagus

Esophageal atresia is a congenital anomaly that may develop between the third and sixth weeks of fetal life. Several types are recognized, with the most common being an upper segment of esophagus ending in a blind pouch and a lower segment of esophagus communicating by a fistula with the trachea (TEF). Ideally this defect is recognized prenatally by ultrasound, but more often the diagnosis is made in the first 36 to 48 hours of life. Symptoms of esophageal atresia include excessive salivation, choking during feeds, and respiratory distress. Prompt surgical intervention allows the child to breathe and eat without the danger of aspirating mucus, saliva, feedings, or stomach contents. Atresia of the esophagus is repaired through a right retropleural thoracotomy, with closure of the TEF and anastomosis of the segments of the esophagus.

Procedural Considerations

A bronchoscopy is performed to promote accurate placement of the endotracheal tube before surgical repair. Intraoperative imaging studies with radiopaque feeding tubes may also be performed to determine the extent of the atresia. The team then positions the patient for a right thoracotomy and preps and drapes. A major instrument and a thoracotomy set are required with the appropriate-sized chest tube and a drainage system.

Operative Procedure

1. The surgeon enters the chest through the fourth intercostal space. Removal of the rib is not necessary (Fig. 26.11A).
2. The pleura is gently dissected off the chest wall (see Fig. 26.11B).
3. As the dissection proceeds posteriorly, the azygos vein is identified, which is reflected inferiorly after its highest intercostal branches are divided to expose the fistula beneath (see Fig. 26. 11C).
4. The surgeon passes an umbilical tape or vessel loop under the fistula to apply traction gently (see Fig. 26.11D). Dissection of the mediastinum begins with the TEF and distal end of the esophagus. The vagus nerve is an important landmark for the distal end of the esophagus.

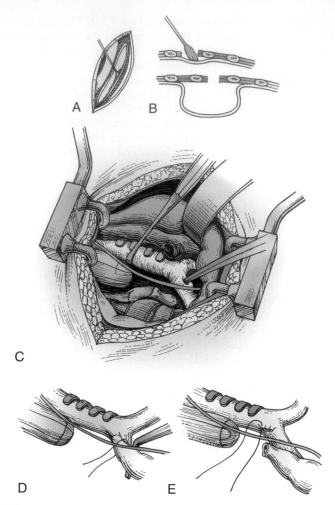

FIG. 26.11 Repair of atresia of the esophagus. (A) Incision at fourth intercostal space. (B) Dissection of pleura off chest wall. (C) Identification and division of azygos vein to expose fistula beneath. (D) Traction applied to fistula. (E) Transection of fistula leaving 3-mm cuff on trachea.

5. The fistula is clamped and transected, leaving a thin cuff of esophageal tissue on the tracheal side to allow closure of the trachea without narrowing it and compromising the lumen of the airway (see Fig. 26.11E).
6. To close the fistula, interrupted nonabsorbable sutures are used.
7. The surgeon dissects the upper esophageal pouch, and passage of a nasogastric tube by the anesthesia provider aids in its identification. The proximal pouch is identified and dissected as needed to allow it to reach the distal esophageal segment with minimal tension for anastomosis (Fig. 26.12A). At this point the surgeon decides whether to attempt primary anastomosis.
8. After transecting the blind proximal pouch (see Fig. 26.12B and C) primary anastomosis is performed with nonabsorbable suture, taking full-thickness bites along anterior and posterior borders (see Fig. 26.12D). Some surgeons prefer the Haight, or two-layer, anastomosis (Fig. 26.13). The inner layer is composed of the upper pouch mucosa sutured to the full thickness of the distal esophagus. The muscular sleeve of the upper esophagus is then pulled down over the inner anastomosis and sutured to the muscular layer of the inferior esophagus. The incision is irrigated with saline.

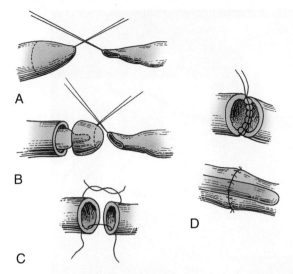

FIG. 26.12 Primary repair of atresia of the esophagus: single-layer repair. (A) Traction applied to proximal and distal portions of esophagus. (B) Blind proximal pouch transected. (C) Full-thickness bites of anterior and posterior borders. (D) Repair completed with Replogle tube in place to allow adequate lumen of esophagus.

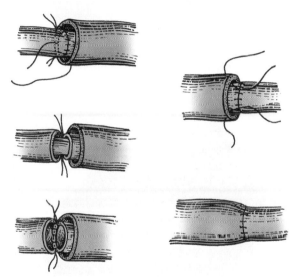

FIG. 26.13 Haight anastomosis. Mucosal layer of proximal pouch sutured to full thickness of distal esophagus. Muscular sleeve of upper pouch pulled down over inner anastomosis and sutured to muscle of distal esophagus.

9. The surgeon places a chest tube near the anastomosis through a posterior stab wound and secures it with sutures to prevent it from putting direct pressure on the anastomosis.
10. The surgeon closes the muscle layers and fascia and skin
11. The skin is closed with a continuous absorbable suture. The incision is approximated with cyanoacrylate glue or topical skin adhesive and wound closure strips.

Gastrostomy

Gastrostomy is the establishment of a temporary or permanent channel from the gastric lumen to the skin to permit gastric emptying, liquid feeding, or retrograde dilation of an esophageal stricture. The procedure may be completed as a separate procedure or be performed with other surgical procedures to facilitate care of the patient after

surgery. A growing number of surgeons are inserting low-profile (e.g., button) devices on initial creation of the gastrostomy because these are preferred for children receiving long-term feedings through the device. Low-profile devices, which protrude slightly from the abdomen, are more cosmetically acceptable and allow more mobility for the child. A gastrostomy tube can be placed in the OR as an open or laparoscopic procedure (Fig. 26.14). The laparoscopic technique allows direct visualization of the stomach, minimizing or eliminating the risk of accidental colon interposition and perforation. It also removes the need for secondary exchange to a skin-level or balloon-based device 3 to 6 months later (McSweeney et al., 2016). The laparoscopic surgical procedure is described in the following section.

Procedural Considerations

A minor instrument set, size-appropriate laparoscopic equipment, and a gastrostomy feeding catheter (G-tube) are required. The nurse ensures the patient is positioned carefully and the skin is protected from injury because children needing gastrostomy tubes often have accompanying comorbidities requiring surgery.

Operative Procedure

1. The surgeon marks the anticipated exit site for the G-tube before insufflation. This is usually near the greater curve of the stomach because it does not interfere with the pylorus or the duodenum.
2. After making an umbilical incision and inserting the camera port the surgeon visualizes the stomach.
3. Next, the surgeon makes an incision over the exit site and mobilizes the stomach with a nontraumatic grasper.
4. Hitch stitches are placed through the abdominal wall and on either side of the projected G-tube placement and secured (see Fig. 26.14A).
5. The surgeon then accesses the stomach via an introducer needle followed by a guidewire. The stoma tract is serially dilated, and a gastrostomy tube is then placed over the guidewire (see Fig. 26.14B and C).
6. The external suspending sutures are then tied over the sides of the gastrostomy tube to secure the tube in place. The tube may be used in 24 hours and the external sutures are later removed in 3 to 10 days following the procedure after the stoma tract has had time to mature (see Fig. 26.14D).

Repair of Pediatric Intestinal Disorders

There are many intestinal disorders in infants and children that require surgical intervention. Because most of these disorders present with fever, generalized malaise, decreased appetite, nausea, vomiting (sometimes bilious), diarrhea, abdominal distension, electrolyte imbalances, and altered vital signs (Fig. 26.15), they are often difficult to diagnose as infants and young children are often unable to communicate or are limited with descriptions. Often by the time of surgical intervention, the patient is quite compromised and surgery is performed emergently. Laparoscopic repair is occasionally attempted, but usually as an assistive technique before laparotomy. Contraindications to laparoscopy include peritonitis, hemodynamic instability, and severe bowel distension (Dominguez et al., 2014). Depending on the surgical findings, either an anastomosis or ostomy is performed. Ostomies are reversed when the child's condition improves.

Necrotizing Enterocolitis

Necrotizing enterocolitis (NEC) is a condition that manifests with the death of the intestinal lining and sloughing of corresponding

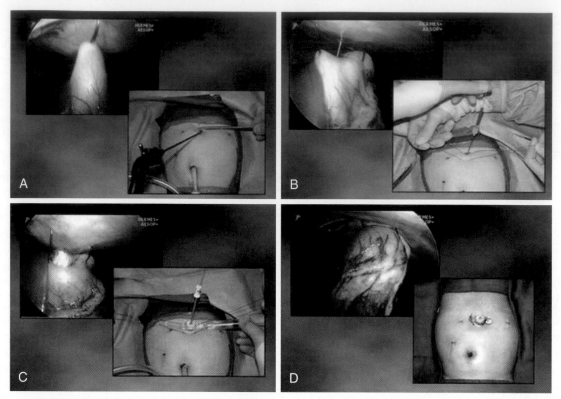

FIG. 26.14 Laparoscopic gastrostomy tube placement. (A) Hitch stitches are placed to bring stomach to abdominal wall. (B) Guidewire is placed in preparation for the dilator. (C) G-tube placed with dilator. (D) Secure gastrostomy tube.

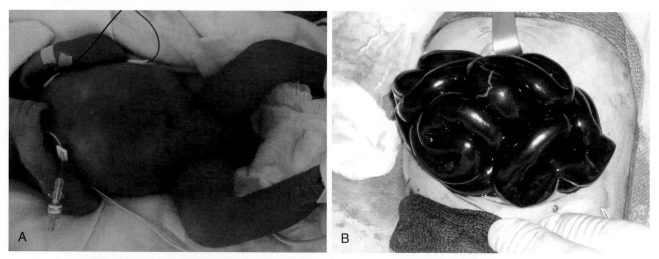

FIG. 26.15 Infants with intestinal disorders (e.g., necrotizing enterocolitis) often have abdominal distension. (A) Infant with abdominal distension. (B) Necrotic bowel.

tissues. Its exact cause is unknown, but it is suspected that NEC may result from two mechanisms: decreased blood flow to the bowel, which prevents the bowel from secreting the protective mucus that protects the GI tract; or bacteria within the intestine. It primarily affects premature newborns. The mainstay of treatment is intestinal rest with prohibition of enteral feeding during NEC, antibiotics, and intestinal decompression, as well as other supportive therapy as needed. Some patients with NEC may require surgery (see Fig. 26.15B).

Intussusception

Intussusception is the telescopic invagination of a portion of intestine into an adjacent part, with mechanical and vascular impairment (Fig. 26.16). The most common site for intussusception is the ileocecal junction. Intussusception in most children is idiopathic; in others, causes may include Meckel diverticulum (Fig. 26.17), polyps, or hematoma of the bowel. Intussusception is the most common cause of small bowel obstruction in children (Maki et al., 2014). It is relieved by reduction of invaginated bowel by the hydrostatic pressure of a barium enema or by laparotomy and manual manipulation. Early diagnosis and reduction are essential to bowel viability.

Malrotation

Intestinal malrotation is a congenital anomaly of rotation of the midgut. The incidence is 1:6000 live births (Bales et al., 2016). In malrotation, the small bowel is found predominately on the right side of the abdomen, the cecum is displaced to the epigastrium, and the ligament of Treitz is displaced inferiorly and rightward. Fibrous Ladd bands course over the horizontal part of the duodenum causing obstruction (Fig. 26.18A). The small intestine has an unusually narrow base; therefore the midgut is prone to volvulus (see Fig. 26.18B). An incidental appendectomy is performed because children have a 1 in 12 incidence of developing appendicitis (Bales et al., 2016).

Atresias

Atresias or narrowing of the intestinal tract occur mainly in infancy. With improved prenatal diagnostics, atresias, especially duodenal atresia, can be diagnosed before birth and intervention can occur earlier with better outcomes for the infant. Duodenal atresia complicates 1 per 10,000 live births and accounts for 25% to 40% of all intestinal atresias (Bales et al., 2016). Jejunoileal atresia and colonic atresias happen with much less frequency (Fig. 26.19).

Procedural Considerations

A major instrument set and pediatric bowel clamps are required along with intestinal staplers and suture for anastomosis. The patient is positioned supine, and routine prepping and draping of the abdomen are done. Surgical impermeable plastic adherent incisional drapes should be used to minimize irrigation and fluids collecting around the patient.

Bowel Resection

Operative Procedure

1. The surgeon makes an abdominal incision.
2. The intestines are explored to determine the location of the obstruction. The surgeon must examine the entire bowel to rule out multiple areas of involvement in patients with atresia or stenosis. If suspicious findings are found, specimens are sent fresh immediately to the pathology laboratory to further studies.
3. Resection is performed as indicated, and either the bowel is anastomosed by suture for neonates and infants or an intestinal stapler for older children.

Ostomy Creation

Operative Procedure

1. A transverse incision usually is preferred, and the surgeon enters the abdomen in the right upper quadrant for a transverse colostomy and ileostomy or the left lower quadrant for a sigmoid colostomy.

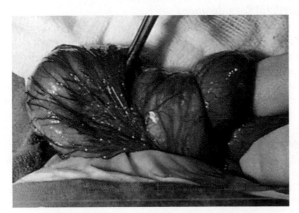

FIG. 26.16 Operative view of intussusception.

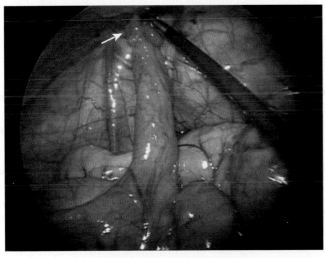

FIG. 26.17 Meckel diverticulum *(arrow)*.

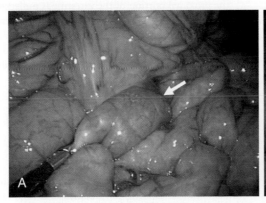
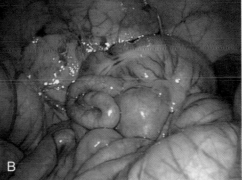

FIG. 26.18 Malrotation. (A) Ligament of Treitz *(arrow)* is seen to the left of the patient's midline. (B) Location of the cecum in the right lower quadrant.

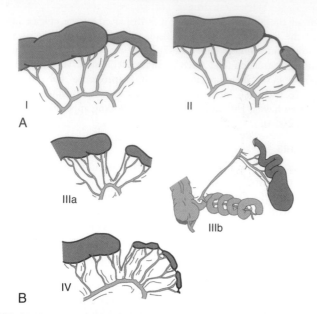

FIG. 26.19 Intestinal atresia. Classification of intestinal atresia. *I*, Mucosal obstruction caused by an intraluminal membrane with intact bowel wall and mesentery; *II*, blind ends are separated by a fibrous cord; *IIIa*, blind ends are separated by a V-shaped mesenteric defect; *IIIb*, "apple-peel" appearance; *IV*, multiple atresias.

2. The loop of intestine is freed of peritoneal attachments until it can be brought easily through the abdominal wall without tension.
3. The surgeon sutures the edges of the mesentery to the parietal peritoneum, and the serosa of the colonic loop is sutured with fine absorbable suture materials to the peritoneum and fascia as well as to the skin.
4. The ostomy may be sutured immediately. Some surgeons prefer to close the skin under an ostomy loop; others prefer to suture mucosa directly to skin edges. This decision may depend on the location of the ostomy. An important point is that each layer must be securely attached to the serosa of the colon to prevent evisceration and prolapse.

Resection and Pull-Through for Hirschsprung Disease

Hirschsprung disease is characterized by the absence of ganglion cells in a distal portion of the bowel. The distal colon is more frequently involved, but the disease may encompass the entire colon, with a less favorable prognosis. The absence of ganglion cells results in a lack of peristalsis. The normal proximal colon becomes dilated with stool because intestinal contents do not pass through the involved segment normally. The child presents with an abnormally distended abdomen. Barium enema reveals proximal distention of the colon and then a transition zone in which the bowel appears funnel shaped, followed by the distal aganglionic segment, which is narrowed. The child is taken to the OR for a leveling colostomy (a colostomy placed at the level at which ganglion cells begin and where there are no hypertrophic nerves). Multiple frozen-section biopsy specimens from the muscularis of the proximal portion of the colon are taken to determine the presence of ganglion cells. The colostomy is performed at the most distal portion of the colon that contains ganglion cells. Some surgeons prefer a routine right transverse colostomy at this time and delay frozen-section biopsy specimens until the time of the definitive procedure. Resection and pull-through for Hirschsprung

disease, the definitive surgical procedure, consists of the removal of the aganglionic portion of the bowel and anastomosis of the normal colon to the anus. The child is returned to the OR for the definitive repair at 1 year of age if clinical and nutritional status permits.

The procedure may be done laparoscopically or by an open approach. The Soave procedure of endorectal pull-through uses internal bypass of the involved segment. The internal sphincter muscle of the anus is kept intact for continence.

Procedural Considerations

The patient is prepped and draped from the nipples down to and including the buttocks, genitalia, perineal area, and upper thighs to permit positioning for the perineal stage without redraping. (Before prepping, the rectum may be irrigated with warm saline solution.) An indwelling catheter is inserted to keep the bladder empty during the operation. A major instrument set and pediatric intestinal clamps are needed.

Operative Procedure

1. A left paramedian incision that includes the sigmoid colonic stoma, if present, is made.
2. The surgeon frees the stoma from the abdominal wall and mobilizes the left portion of the colon. (If there is no sigmoid colonic stoma, the extent of aganglionic intestine is established by biopsy and frozen section, and all involved colon is excised. If a stoma is present and the area has already been established as normal, the colon above it constitutes the proximal end of the resection.)
3. The mesocolon and the vessels of the intestine to be resected are divided close to the intestine, with care taken to preserve the blood supply to the rectum (Fig. 26.20A).
4. The mucosal tube is freed from the outer muscular layers by sharp and blunt dissection (see Fig. 26.20B).
5. A muscular sleeve is transected, and 4-0 nonabsorbable traction sutures are placed on the distal edge (see Fig. 26.20C). The mucosa is stripped down to the anus. The depth of the dissection may be checked by inserting a lubricated finger into the anus (see Fig. 26.20D).
6. When the mucosa is adequately freed, the perineal phase is started. The surgeon dilates the anus and retracts it with Allis forceps. A circumferential incision is made, and the mucosal stripping is completed (see Fig. 26.20E).
7. The proximal portion of the intestine is pulled through the rectal muscular sleeve and out the anus (see Fig. 26.20F). If the portion of colon to be resected is large, it is excised abdominally before the proximal portion of the intestine is pulled through the anus.
8. Absorbable sutures are used to secure the seromuscular layers of the intussuscepted colon to the rectal muscular cuff. The surgeon divides the colon into axial or longitudinal quadrants, and an anastomosis is performed with 3-0 absorbable sutures (see Fig. 26.20G).
9. The abdominal phase of the operation is completed by approximating the proximal edge of the muscular cuff to the seromuscular layer of the colon (see Fig. 26.20H). The abdomen is closed in the routine manner.

Repair of Imperforate Anus

Congenital imperforate anus (Fig. 26.21) presents in a variety of forms, classified as low, intermediate, and high lesions, depending on how far the pelvis descends into the rectum. Baby girls commonly have low lesions, and baby boys primarily exhibit intermediate or

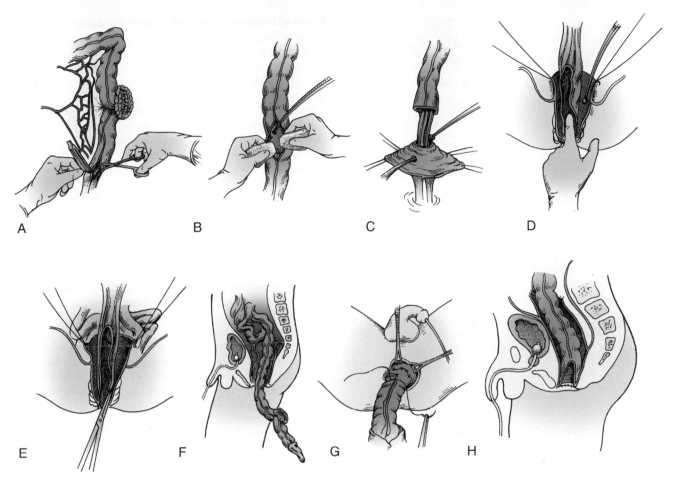

FIG. 26.20 Pull-through for Hirschsprung disease. (A) Dissection of mucosal tube begun through longitudinal incision. (B) Blunt dissection with sponges used to dissect entire circumference of tube. (C) Muscular sleeve transected. (D) Depth of dissection determined by insertion of finger into anus. (E) Circumferential incision made. (F) Mucosal tube and proximal portion of colon and stoma pulled through rectal muscular cuff. (G) Anastomosis performed among all layers of colon and anal mucosa. (H) Anastomosis completed.

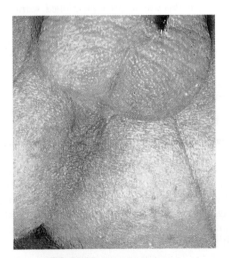

FIG. 26.21 Imperforate anus.

high lesions. A covered anus and anovulvar fistula is an example of a low lesion. Intermediate and high lesions consist of a blind rectal pouch, a "flat bottom," and a posterior urethral fistula or a fistula to the bladder. This type is the most prevalent and the most difficult to repair. An imperforate anus is repaired by establishing colorectoanal continuity through the external anal sphincter and closure of fistulas, if present.

Repair of Low Imperforate Anus in a Girl: Anal Transposition

Procedural Considerations. The patient is placed in the lithotomy position. A Foley catheter is inserted, and the perineum is prepped and draped. A major instrument set is required, with the addition of both a nerve and a muscle stimulator. The anesthesia provider must avoid the use of neuromuscular blocking agents for the nerve and muscle stimulator to work during the surgical procedure.

Operative Procedure

1. An electrical stimulator is applied to elicit muscle contractions and serve as a guide to the midline of the anus. The goal is to leave equal innervated tissue on both sides of the anus so that the child will be continent of stool.

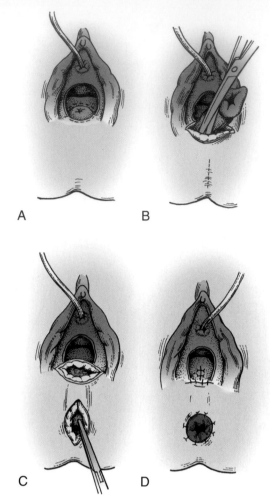

FIG. 26.22 Anal transposition. (A) Fistula excised by means of oval incision. (B) Dissection of bowel from surrounding structures. (C) Vertical midline incision at site of true anus, identification of external sphincter fibers, and mobilized rectum pulled down through subcutaneous tissue to new location. (D) External sphincter sutured to rectal mucosa. A new anus is constructed with interrupted sutures through all layers.

2. Stay sutures are placed in the fistula, and it is excised using an oval incision (Fig. 26.22A).
3. The surgeon dissects the bowel free from surrounding structures, taking care not to damage the vagina (see Fig. 26.22B).
4. When the dissection is complete, the surgeon makes a vertical midline incision at the opening of the true anus and identifies the fibers of the external sphincter (see Fig. 26.22C).
5. The mobilized rectum is pulled down through the subcutaneous tissue to its new location.
6. The surgeon amputates the end of the fistula. Using 4-0 nonabsorbable interrupted sutures, the surgeon sutures the external sphincter to the rectal serosa.
7. Using 4-0 absorbable suture, the surgeon constructs a new anus with interrupted sutures through all layers (see Fig. 26.22D).
8. A drain may or may not be placed in the anterior incision before it is closed in layers with interrupted 4-0 absorbable sutures.
9. Using a Hegar dilator, the surgeon calibrates the size of the new anus after closure.

Repair of Intermediate or High Imperforate Anus: Posterior Sagittal Anorectoplasty

When an intermediate or high imperforate anal anomaly presents, surgical intervention is indicated within 24 to 48 hours of birth. A transverse or sigmoid colostomy is performed to irrigate the hiatal lumen and to remove meconium plugs while allowing proximal colon function. The posterior sagittal anorectoplasty (PSARP) is the definitive surgical procedure and is performed when the condition and size of the child permit, which is usually around 1 year of age.

The PSARP is a highly technical procedure that uses electrostimulation throughout and may require position changes.

Procedural Considerations. The team positions the child prone with the hips flexed. Adequate padding must be placed under the hips to avoid compression injury to the femoral nerves. A major instrument set and a nerve stimulator are required.

Operative Procedure

1. The surgeon uses the electrostimulator to locate the true anus (Fig. 26.23) and makes a midsagittal incision through the skin from the midsacrum to the anterior border of the anal site. The incision is continued through subcutaneous tissue until the external sphincter muscle layers are identified.
2. Using electrostimulation, the surgeon identifies and dissects the fibers midsagittally, exactly in the midline.
3. A midsagittal split of the coccyx is performed, and the striated muscle complex found beneath the coccyx is incised sagittally, along with the visceral endopelvic fascia. Electrostimulation is used to aid in identifying muscle complexes.
4. Next the surgeon identifies the rectal pouch and urethra and incises the bowel vertically to expose the fistulas.
5. The fistula is closed in layers: first the mucosa with interrupted absorbable sutures and then the muscle layer with 5-0 nonabsorbable sutures.
6. The rectum is mobilized and tapered to allow its placement within the muscle complexes. Tapering consists of excising a wedge of bowel from either the ventral or the dorsal surface. The edges are approximated, and the mucosal and the muscularis layers are closed.
7. Again using electrostimulation, the tapered rectum is placed deep within the muscle complex, and the muscles are reconstructed. The seromuscular layer of the bowel is incorporated into these sutures to keep it securely positioned within the muscle complex.
8. The external sphincter muscles and coccyx are reapproximated.
9. Excess bowel is trimmed before it is secured to the skin edges of the anus and closed.

General Surgery: Hernias

Umbilical Hernia Repair

Umbilical hernias are frequently seen in pediatric populations. These hernias are also common in premature infants and are corrected by repair of the defect in which the intestine protrudes at the umbilicus. An umbilical hernia is always covered by skin. Small umbilical hernias may be left untreated. They usually close within a few months to 1 year. If surgical repair is required in a large fascial defect, it may be delayed until the child is at least 2 years of age; some surgeons delay repair until 5 years of age.

Procedural Considerations

Surgical correction of an umbilical hernia may be an ambulatory surgical procedure. A general anesthetic is used. A minor instrument

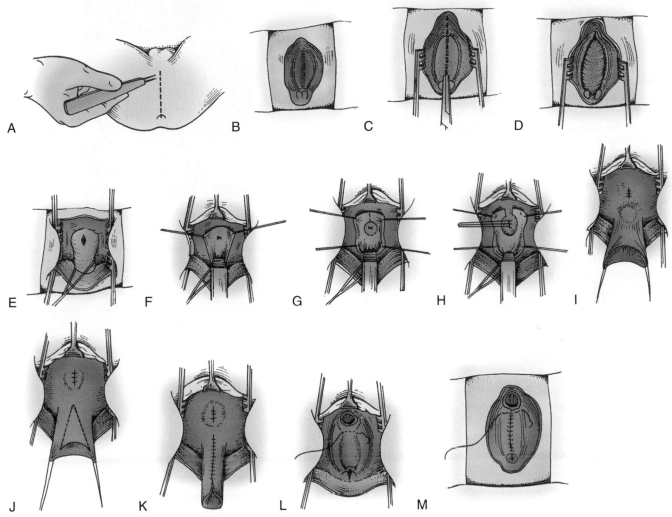

FIG. 26.23 Posterior sagittal anorectoplasty. (A) Line of incision and electrical stimulation to determine appropriate anal site. (B) Midsagittal incision through coccyx and external sphincter fibers of anus, showing striated muscle complex deep to anal site. Subcutaneous external sphincter extending about halfway to coccyx, superficial external sphincter inserting on coccyx, and levator deeper in midline. (C) Right-angled forceps beneath levator ani. (D) All layers of striated muscle partially retracted laterally to expose visceral endopelvic fascia. (E) Sagittal incision in terminal bowel after proximal dissection around rectum and placement of tape around rectum proximally. (F) Retracted rectotomy showing fistula site. (G) Semicircumferential incision through mucosa-submucosa for placement of first sutures to close fistula. (H) Completed closure of fistula orifice. (I) Stippled area where muscular bowel wall is left in place and clear area above where peritoneum may be encountered. (J) Extent of anterior wedge resection for tapered repair of rectum *(dotted line)*. (K) Approximation of tapered edges of rectum. (L) First and deepest suture for approximation of levators to establish beginning of canal. (M) After reapproximation of levator ani to coccyx, interrupted sutures are placed in edges of superficial external sphincter muscle.

set is required. Several variations in technique have been used; an infraumbilical approach is most common, and its description follows.

Operative Procedure

1. The surgeon makes an incision below the umbilicus through the skin and subcutaneous tissue.
2. Next, the surgeon mobilizes flaps of skin and subcutaneous tissue to expose the rectus fascia and hernia protrusion.
3. The hernia sac, which is between the rectus muscle sheaths in the midline, is completely freed from all surrounding structures.
4. The hernia sac may be invaginated, dissected free and ligated, or excised.

5. The surgeon closes the peritoneum with interrupted suture. Each suture is tagged and then closed all at once.
6. The two edges of the rectus fascia are approximated using interrupted sutures.
7. The surgeon performs a subcuticular closure of the skin and applies a pressure dressing over cyanoacrylate.

Inguinal Hernia Repair With Laparoscopic Exploration of Opposite Side

An inguinal hernia is a protrusion into the inguinal canal of a sac that contains the intestine. The testis develops high on the posterior wall of the abdomen. It gradually descends into the scrotum. Before the testis enters the inguinal canal, the processus vaginalis projects downward but retains communication with the peritoneal cavity. The upper part of the processus does not project downward; the remaining sac constitutes an indirect inguinal hernia. In a female child, a similar hernia sac is contiguous with the round ligament.

Procedural Considerations

A minor instrument set is used. A laparoscope may be used to visualize the contralateral (i.e., opposite) side because it is not uncommon for inguinal hernias to occur bilaterally. The patient is positioned supine, and routine prepping and draping procedures are followed.

Operative Procedure

1. The surgeon makes an incision over the inguinal area in the direction of the skin crease.
2. The subcutaneous tissue is opened, and hemostats are placed on bleeding vessels, which are then ligated or coagulated.
3. The surgeon identifies the external ring, and uses small scissors to free and clean the external oblique fascia.
4. Using a #15 blade, the surgeon opens the external oblique fascia and frees the upper flap. The lower flap is freed to expose the inguinal ligament.
5. Cord structures are opened at the upper end of the cord. Two forceps are used to grasp tissues at the same level and to separate them.
6. The hernia sac is grasped with a hemostat, and structures of the cord are peeled downward and away from the sac with forceps until the sac is freed. Care is taken to protect the spermatic cord and major vessels as the sac is freed.
7. After the sac is opened, the surgeon's pulls the sac upward. The upward traction is maintained with two or three hemostats.
8. If laparoscopic exploration of the contralateral side is indicated, a 20-gauge IV catheter is inserted over the opposite inguinal area. The insufflation tubing is connected and CO$_2$ instilled. The surgeon explores the contralateral side using a 2.7-mm telescope.
9. The sac is ligated with 3-0 nonabsorbable sutures, and excess sac is removed. Repair of the inguinal canal may be done with nonabsorbable sutures.
10. The subcutaneous tissue is closed with interrupted fine sutures; closure of the skin is done with fine nonabsorbable subcuticular sutures. Cyanoacrylate glue is applied.
11. If a bilateral hernia is diagnosed, steps 1 through 10 are repeated on the contralateral side.

General Surgery: Abdominal Procedures

Gastroschisis Repair and Omphalocele

An omphalocele is the protrusion of abdominal viscera outside the abdomen through a defect in the umbilical ring into a sac of amniotic membrane and peritoneum at the base of the umbilical cord. There is no skin covering (Fig. 26.24). Gastroschisis is the protrusion of the viscera through a defect in the abdominal wall to the right of the umbilical cord. No amniotic membrane or peritoneum covers the defect.

Omphalocele occurs during the eleventh week of fetal life when the viscera fail to withdraw normally from the exocoelomic position to occupy the peritoneal cavity. The resulting abdominal wall defect can vary in size from 2 to 15 cm. The sac may contain only a few loops of bowel, or nearly all the intestines and the liver and spleen.

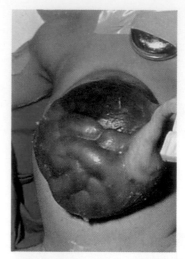

FIG. 26.24 Newborn with giant omphalocele containing liver and intestine.

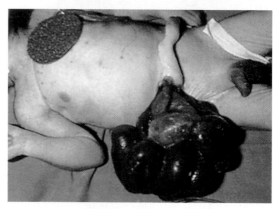

FIG. 26.25 Gastroschisis. A large amount of small intestine has eviscerated through a defect to the right of a normal-appearing umbilical cord. No sac is visible, and the intestine is thickened, edematous, and ischemic in areas.

Associated anomalies can include disorders of the cardiac, musculo-skeletal, genitourinary, and nervous systems, along with malrotation and abnormal fixation of the bowel (Fig. 26.25).

Direct closure is the treatment of choice for both gastroschisis and omphalocele. Treatment consists of inserting a nasogastric tube to prevent distention and aspiration and beginning IV access with fluid resuscitation and antibiotic therapy. Surgical intervention is necessary to prevent rupture of the sac, infection, or both. If intrauterine rupture of the sac has occurred, the newborn is kept warm, and the bowel is inspected for perforation and torsion but care must be taken to keep it moist by various means.

Omphaloceles and gastroschisis are repaired by placement of the viscera in the abdominal cavity, with reconstruction of the abdominal wall. Surgical procedures for omphaloceles may be primary or staged (Schuster procedure). Synthetic mesh may be used as a barrier to create tension that helps push the internal organs into the abdominal cavity. In some cases of gastroschisis, a silo is applied to the defect. The silo is made of a flexible ring that sits inside the abdomen and its size is gradually decreased to facilitate movement of the organs back to the abdominal cavity. Silo material may be prepackaged and kept at the patient's bedside if the patient is unable to tolerate an immediate trip to the OR.

Procedural Considerations

Particular attention to maintaining body temperature is essential because of the massive exposed surface area from which body heat can be lost. The use of nitrous oxide as an anesthetic agent is avoided during this procedure because it causes increased gas in the intestine, which in turn makes the reduction of abdominal contents into the peritoneal cavity very difficult. Repeated rectal irrigation with warm saline to evacuate meconium from the bowel may be performed before the abdominal prep to aid in bowel decompression.

Gastroschisis Repair With Silo Placement

Procedural Considerations

A major instrument set is required. The patient is positioned supine for the procedure. The abdomen, umbilical cord, and sac are gently prepped with povidone-iodine. This procedure may be performed at the bedside if the neonate is too unstable to transport.

Operative Procedure

1. The surgeon examines the bowel and measures the size of the defect to determine the silo size. The silo is applied so that the flexible ring is positioned inside the abdomen (Fig. 26.26).
2. The patient returns to the OR every 48 hours for a reduction of the silo, which is accomplished by decreasing the size of the ring to help guide the contents back into the abdominal cavity.
3. The height of bowel in the silo and length of reduction are measured with each procedure. When the amount of bowel remaining in the silo is 1 cm or less, the defect is closed. The silo is trimmed, and the spring-loaded ring is removed. The wound site and bowel are inspected and cleaned with surgical prep material.
4. The surgeon closes the defect using synthetic purse-string sutures or, if the defect is too large, running sutures that begin at each end of the wound and meet in the middle to preserve the umbilical cord stump.

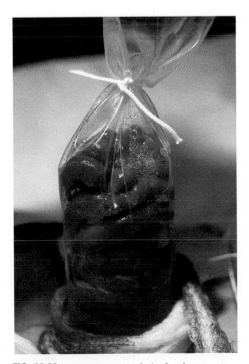

FIG. 26.26 Operative view of silo for the intestines.

5. The inferior aspect of skin is wrapped around the stump and secured with absorbable suture. Any redundant skin is trimmed and the stump is ligated using nonabsorbable suture.

Omphalocele Repair

Procedural Considerations

The patient is positioned supine for the procedure and the abdomen is prepped as described for silo placement.

Operative Procedure

1. The surgeon dissects the amnion of the omphalocele circumferentially from the dermis.
2. The umbilical vein is identified and ligated with absorbable suture. Umbilical cord structures and arteries are dissected and ligated with absorbable suture, and then oversewn with nonabsorbable suture.
3. Organs connected to the omphalocele are dissected, reduced (if necessary), and mobilized, and the internal mucosal layer is closed with running nonabsorbable suture.
4. The outer muscular layer is closed with interrupted nonabsorbable suture, organs are returned to the peritoneal cavity, and fascia is closed with interrupted nonabsorbable suture.
5. If necessary, an umbilicoplasty may be performed using interrupted absorbable suture.

In certain cases in which the defect is of medium to large size, a primary closure may not be accomplished. In these situations a staged procedure (Schuster procedure) is done using prosthetic reduction. In the first stage the patient is taken to the OR and positioned and prepped as previously described. Then the following steps are performed:

1. The sac is excised, and the umbilical vein and arteries are ligated.
2. A gastrostomy may be performed at this time.
3. A barrier is then created with Silastic mesh. The mesh is secured through all layers of the edge of the defect using a continuous locking nonabsorbable suture. The open end of the barrier is closed in the same manner.
4. The surgeon closes the open end of the cylinder with umbilical tape or, alternatively, attaches to a specifically designed roller clamp.
5. The mesh barrier suture line and edge of the defect are wrapped with roller gauze dipped in an iodophor solution. The patient is transferred to an open isolette, and the silo is suspended from the top of the isolette. Plastic wrap is applied to the barrier to prevent heat loss. The patient is then transported to the NICU, in which daily reduction of abdominal contents is performed by adding a lower tie of umbilical tape or by adjusting the roller clamp. The abdominal viscera are gradually reduced over several days, taking care to avoid respiratory compromise from abdominal distention. When reduction has successfully approached skin level, the patient is returned to the OR for the final stage of repair.
6. The mesh barrier is removed, and the remaining abdominal contents are brought into the peritoneal cavity. The peritoneal fascia is closed with interrupted nonabsorbable sutures. The skin is closed with interrupted nonabsorbable suture. In an attempt to create the appearance of an umbilicus, a purse-string suture is used to close the inferior 2 cm of incision.

Correction of Biliary Atresia: Hepatic Portoenterostomy (Kasai Procedure)

Biliary atresia is a congenital defect that results from nonpatent extrahepatic bile ducts. Bile is unable to drain from the liver to the small intestine, leading to eventual cirrhosis and death. The Kasai procedure is the construction of a bile drainage system by use of an intestinal conduit. This procedure is indicated in patients with extrahepatic biliary atresia who are younger than 3 months. All atretic segments of the existing bile ducts are removed. An intraoperative cholangiogram and frozen-section biopsy of the hepatic duct remnant are included in the surgical procedure.

Procedural Considerations

The team positions the patient supine. A major instrument set is required as well as radiopaque dye and catheter for the cholangiography.

Operative Procedure

1. The surgeon makes a right upper quadrant incision and exposes the gallbladder.
2. A small catheter is placed into the gallbladder and secured with a purse-string suture. Radiopaque dye is instilled into the gallbladder, and fluoroscopy is done. The surgeon observes for free flow of the dye through the ducts and into the duodenum, which occasionally is seen. These patients are then categorized as having correctable biliary atresia. In such situations, a liver biopsy is performed and the incision is closed. More commonly, however, there is a very small amount of flow or none at all, for which the Kasai or extended portoenterostomy procedure is performed. This involves an extended lateral dissection around the porta hepatis with a very wide anastomosis.
3. The surgeon mobilizes the gallbladder and atretic bile ducts and dissection/exposure of the porta hepatitis (Fig. 26.27A).
4. After the common bile duct remnants are severed from the duodenal side, the dissection proceeds cephalad and the portal bile duct remnants are freed from the underlying structures.
5. The portal vein and hepatic artery are encircled with vessel loops. Several small vessel branches between the portal vein to the fibrous remnant are identified and divided between ligatures (see Fig. 26.27B).
6. The portal bile duct remnants are dissected proximal to the anterior branch of the right hepatic artery on the right side and as far left as the entrance of the obliterated umbilical vein into the left portal vein.
7. The fibrous cone is sharply transected at the level of the posterior surface with scissors or a scalpel and is removed. The fibrous cone should have an extensive transected surface, which allows a wide anastomosis (see Fig. 26.27C).
8. The end of the Roux-en-Y limb is anastomosed around the transected end of the fibrous remnant. Sutures should not be placed into the transected surface of the bile duct remnant because minute bile ducts may be present. As much of the transected hilar surface as possible, including all potentially usable remnants of the intrahepatic ducts in the area between and beneath the branches of the right and left portal veins, is incorporated in the anastomosis. It is important to retract the right and left portal veins and hepatic arteries to allow extensive reception of the biliary remnant and a wide portoenterostomy.
9. The proximal portion of the jejunum is generally used as the intestinal conduit. A meticulous anastomosis is performed at the porta hepatis as previously identified by using a single running layer of absorbable sutures. The conduit is exteriorized with a double-barreled Roux-en-Y approach.
10. A drain is placed, and the incision is closed in layers.

If this procedure is not successful, the patient may be a candidate for liver transplantation.

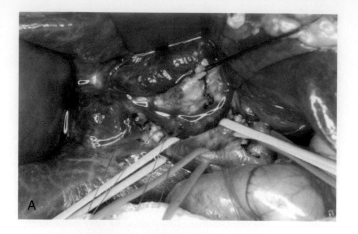

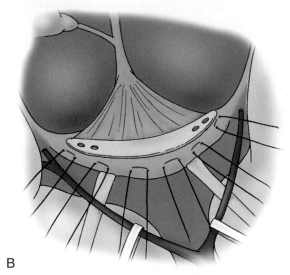

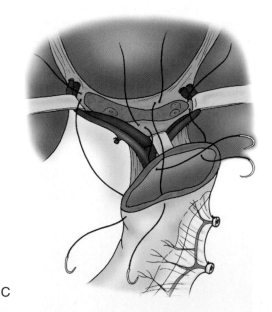

FIG. 26.27 Kasai procedure. (A) Initial mobilization of the gallbladder and atretic bile ducts and dissection/exposure of the porta hepatis. (B) Portal bile duct remnants dissected 5 mm or 6 mm proximal to the anterior branch of the right hepatic artery and as far left as the entrance of the obliterated umbilical vein into the left portal vein. (C) End of the Roux-en-Y limb anastomosed around the transected end of the fibrous remnant.

Repair of Congenital Diaphragmatic Hernia

A CDH is repaired by replacement of the displaced viscera into the abdominal cavity with surgical correction of the diaphragm defect (Fig. 26.28). The conventional surgical repair is through the abdomen, although small defects can be repaired thorascopically. The concurrence of intra-abdominal abnormalities is somewhat high in infants with diaphragmatic hernia; therefore treatment is facilitated with an abdominal approach. It is technically easier to extract the viscera from below than to push them out of the thorax. The abnormal intrathoracic intrusion of the abdominal viscera usually causes severe compromise of intrathoracic pulmonary and vascular activities. Therefore urgent restoration of more normal intrathoracic and intra-abdominal relationships is the rule in these newborns. The lung may be hypoplastic because of prolonged compression in utero by the displaced abdominal viscera. A residual intrapleural space usually remains for a few days after surgery.

Procedural Considerations

In severe cases the patient may be given extracorporeal membrane oxygenation (ECMO) (see page 1063) for several days before repair of the defect. This procedure may be performed at the bedside, especially if the patient's pulmonary status requires nitric oxide ventilation or the patient is still on ECMO. Direct suturing of the margins of the defect is possible, but insertion of prosthetic synthetic or biosynthetic sheeting is occasionally required and should be available. This procedure may be performed at the bedside, especially if the patient's pulmonary status requires nitric oxide ventilation or ECMO.

Operative Procedure

1. The surgeon makes a subcostal incision on the side of the defect, going through all muscle layers.
2. The abdominal viscera are withdrawn from the chest and held downward through the abdominal wound. Because abnormalities of abdominal viscera, such as malrotation, are associated with diaphragmatic hernia, the organs are carefully inspected at this time. If a malrotation is found, the surgeon may repair it if the patient's clinical condition permits.
3. The defect is then carefully inspected, including a search for a hernia sac, which is present in less than 5% of cases. If a sac is identified, it is excised.
4. The surgeon identifies the posterior and anterior rims of the diaphragm, and primary closure is performed with mattress sutures of nonabsorbable material. If the rim of tissue is too small for mattress sutures, ample nonabsorbable sutures are used. Occasionally, reinforced synthetic sheeting may be needed if sufficient diaphragm is not available for primary closure (Fig. 26.29).
5. The abdominal wall is then closed, followed by subcutaneous tissue and skin closure. In severe cases the patient may be given ECMO for several days before repair of the defect. The patient is returned to the OR within 7 days for repair of the ventral hernia.

Pancreatectomy

Pancreatectomies are performed in the pediatric population for congenital hyperinsulinism (CHI). This is the most common form of hypoglycemia in the neonate. Untreated it can have severe neurologic effects and even result in death. A number of causes exist. Some forms of CHI will resolve and are considered transient, whereas others arise from genetic defects and become lifelong chronic conditions. Genetic identification of mutations of the pancreatic beta cells, which regulate insulin, has helped to better identify the genetic differences in CHI and which types are responsive to medical management. The KATP genetic defect has been found to be nonresponsive to medical management of hypoglycemia; thus a pancreatectomy, either near total or partial for focal lesions, is indicated (Ferrara et al., 2016). The procedure for a total pancreatectomy for CHI is described in the following section.

Procedural Considerations

Multiple specimens are sent to the pathology laboratory for frozen-section analysis throughout the procedure to confirm the extent of the disease. The patient is positioned supine with the hips slightly elevated.

Operative Procedure

1. The surgeon makes a transverse supraumbilical incision and places an intra-abdominal retractor.
2. The body and tail of the pancreas are exposed for biopsy for analysis by frozen section.
3. The hepatic flexure of the colon and the duodenum are exposed for additional biopsy and frozen section.
4. If results indicate the need for total pancreatectomy (large nuclei in islet cells), the dissection is begun at the pancreatic tail and then extended to the body and head.

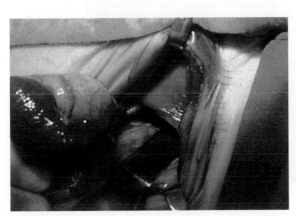

FIG. 26.28 Defect in the posterolateral aspect of the left diaphragm (diaphragmatic hernia).

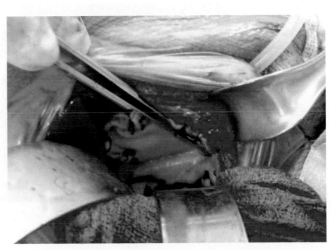

FIG. 26.29 Repaired congenital diaphragmatic hernia.

5. A vessel loop is used to isolate the common bile duct, and care is taken to preserve duodenal blood supply to the pancreatic head during dissection. Once the uncinate process is mobilized from behind the superior mesenteric vessels and the common bile duct is dissected away from its entry point into the duodenum, the pancreatic head is freed.

6. A pancreatectomy is performed and blood supply to the duodenum is evaluated. In the event that a pancreatic remnant remains, it is ligated using nonabsorbable interrupted horizontal mattress sutures. Omentum is tacked down to the dissected area, and the gallbladder is milked to evaluate patency and test for bile leak.

7. Occasionally, a gastrostomy tube may be placed for nutritional support

8. The abdominal incision is closed in layers using nonabsorbable suture for fascia and absorbable sutures for subcutaneous and subcuticular tissue. The incision is dressed with cyanoacrylate glue or topical skin adhesive and wound closure strips.

General Surgery: Resection of Tumors

Nearly two-thirds of childhood cancers occur as solid tumor malignancies. As is always the case, the therapy administered depends on the type of tumor. Examination and judicious investigation of all unusual masses are imperative. Thorough diagnostic workup and prompt definitive treatment may result in cure, even if the tumor is malignant. Chemotherapy and radiation therapy are adjuncts to surgical excision of tumors.

Resection of Wilms Tumor

Wilms tumor, also known as nephroblastoma, is the most common intra-abdominal childhood tumor. It presents as a painless mass whose enlargement may laterally distend the abdomen (Fig. 26.30). The child may be asymptomatic or may have weight loss, malaise, or abdominal pain. Nephroblastomas may cause obstruction of the vena cava, hepatic veins, or renal veins.

Procedural Considerations

The child is positioned supine with a roll under the affected side. Both chest and abdomen are prepped. Careful attention should be given when handling tumor and lymph nodes to avoid tumor spillage.

Operative Procedure

If the tumor is operable, the following aspects are important:

1. The transabdominal approach, which may be extended to a combined transabdominal-transthoracic approach, is used to inspect abdominal contents and clamp the vessels of the renal pedicle before tumor dissection.

2. All suspicious lymph nodes are removed and sent to pathology.

3. The surgeon explores the opposite kidney before dissecting the tumor.

4. Because of its proximity to the kidney, the adrenal gland is usually removed.

5. The abdominal cavity and viscera are thoroughly inspected for evidence of tumor extension or metastases. Extensive surgery may include partial colectomy or partial resection of the diaphragm.

6. The abdominal incision is closed in layers using nonabsorbable suture for fascia and absorbable sutures for subcutaneous and subcuticular tissue. The incision is dressed with cyanoacrylate glue or liquid adhesive and wound closure strips.

Resection of Neuroblastoma

Neuroblastoma is the third most common childhood cancer after leukemia and brain and nervous system cancers. It arises from neural crest tissue and can develop anywhere sympathetic nerve tissue is found; the most common sites are the retroperitoneum and adrenal medulla. The mass is usually firm, irregular, and nontender. It is a silent tumor in its early stages and metastasizes rapidly, often to the lymphatics, liver, skin, bone marrow, lung, brain, or orbits. Treatment includes an operation to ligate the tumor's blood supply and remove as much of the tumor as possible, as well as chemotherapy and radiation.

Resection of Sacrococcygeal Teratoma

An SCT is a tumor that originates early in embryonic cell division. The tumor consists of cell types from more than one embryonic germ layer. Teratomas range from benign, well-differentiated cystic lesions to solid, malignant lesions. The sacrococcygeal area is the most common extragonadal site of teratoma, usually presenting as a large protuberance rising from that site (Fig. 26.31). It may be irregular or symmetric, may vary in size, and may be pedunculated.

An SCT is usually resectable but may undergo malignant changes if not removed early in life. SCTs can be resected prenatally using

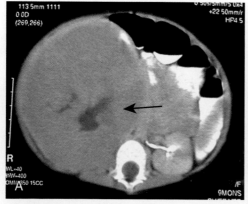
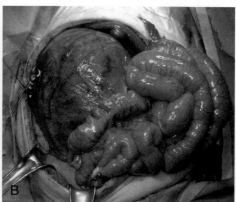

FIG. 26.30 (A) Computed tomography scan of the abdomen shows a large right-sided Wilms tumor *(arrow)* in an infant who subsequently underwent biopsy. (B) The tumor was not primarily resected secondary to size and adherence to surrounding structures.

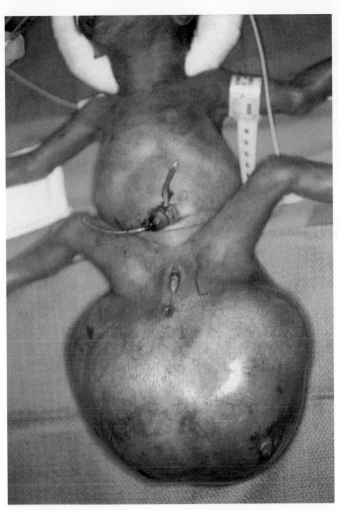

FIG. 26.31 Infant with large sacrococcygeal teratoma.

fetal surgery techniques or postnatally. Tumors resected in the newborn period show microscopic evidence of malignant cells, but surgical cures have been achieved. Early surgical resection is important because these tumors are not sensitive to irradiation and are only temporarily responsive to chemotherapy.

The tumor is in the area of the sacrum and coccyx but may extend into the pelvis or abdomen. Resection is usually feasible by placing the patient in the jackknife position and excising the tumor mass and coccyx en bloc. In cases in which the tumor extends high into the pelvis, an abdominal incision also may be required.

Genitourinary Surgery

Pediatric Cystoscopy

Pediatric cystoscopy is endoscopic examination of the lower urinary tract of pediatric patients. The major difference between adult and pediatric cystoscopy is the size of the instruments used and consideration of the small, delicate orifices of the pediatric patient. Indications for pediatric cystoscopy include UTIs, enuresis, urethral valves, vesicoureteral reflux (VUR), diverticula, bladder neck contractures, bladder tumors, stone treatment, and urinary tract obstructions.

Procedural Considerations

The cystoscopy setup has the same type of components as those for the adult cystoscopy patient (see Chapter 15), except that the size of the cystourethroscope system is specific to the pediatric patient's needs.

Each pediatric cystourethroscope is designed to fit specific component parts and is very delicate. Therefore the perioperative nurse must be familiar with the proper use of the system and handle the components carefully. The resectoscope loop is commonly used to resect urethral valves and occasionally bladder tumors. The cold knife (cutting blade without electrosurgery) may be used with the resectoscope to cut urethral strictures and occasionally resect a urethral valve.

After induction of anesthesia, the child is placed in a lithotomy or frog-leg position and prepped and draped according to established procedure.

Operative Procedure

The surgeon lubricates and inserts the pediatric cystourethroscope through the urethra into the bladder. The video monitor is placed over the patient. The light cord, camera, and irrigation tubing are attached to the telescope and cystoscope, and the procedure is performed.

Circumcision

Circumcision is the excision of the foreskin (prepuce) of the glans penis. Circumcision may be done for therapeutic reasons or for perceived prophylactic benefits; it may also be done for religious reasons, as is required in specific faiths. Provision should be made to observe the religious needs and preferences of the parents.

Therapeutic indications include correction of phimosis or paraphimosis or treatment of balanoposthitis. Phimosis is a condition in which the orifice of the prepuce is stenosed or too narrow to permit easy retraction behind the glans. Balanoposthitis is characterized by an inflamed glans and mucous membrane with purulent discharge and may require circumcision. Paraphimosis is a recurrent condition in which the prepuce cannot be reduced easily from a retracted position.

Procedural Considerations

Newborns are generally positioned on a specially constructed board that facilitates restraint by immobilizing the limbs and exposing the genitalia. Although it was once thought that circumcision caused infants little pain, the neonatal foreskin contains mature nerve endings that allow for the transmission of pain. Measures to ameliorate the pain of the procedure include local dorsal penile nerve block, a ring block with buffered lidocaine and bupivacaine, or the topical application of a local anesthesia cream. Older children require general anesthesia.

For infants, the setup includes small, fine instruments, a Gomco clamp of the appropriate size, and a Mogen clamp or a Plastibell. The Plastibell technique uses a plastic ring and suture tied around the foreskin like a tourniquet. The excess tissue is trimmed, and in about 5 to 8 days the ring falls off. For older patients a circumcision clamp is not needed, and only a specialized urology instrument set is used. Dressings are surgeon specific and range from a gauze wrap, petroleum gauze, or an antibacterial ointment.

Operative Procedure

1. If the prepuce is adherent, the surgeon may use a probe or hemostat to break up adhesions (Fig. 26.32). The prepuce is clamped in

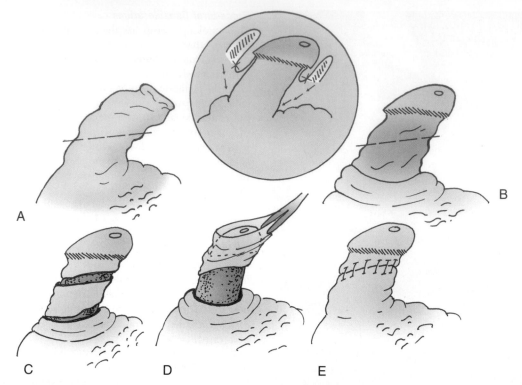

FIG. 26.32 Circumcision. (A) Initial incision made in the shaft. (B) Second incision made in subcoronal sulcus. (C) Amount of tissue to be removed. (D) Removal of tissue. (E) Shaft skin sutured to subcoronal skin.

the dorsal midline and incised toward the coronal mucosa margin, leaving about 5 cm of coronal mucosa intact. A similar procedure is performed ventrally. The two incisions are then joined circumferentially. Alternatively, a superficial circumferential incision is made in the skin with a scalpel at the level of the coronal sulcus and mucosa at the base of the glans. The redundant skin is undermined between the circumferential incisions and removed as a complete cuff.

2. Bleeding vessels are coagulated by low-setting monopolar or bipolar coagulation, or clamped with mosquito hemostats and tied with fine absorbable ligatures. Before closure the area may be cleansed with an appropriate antiseptic solution.

3. The surgeon approximates the raw edges of the skin incision to a coronal cuff of mucosal prepuce, generally with interrupted absorbable sutures. The wound is usually dressed with petrolatum gauze or an antibiotic ointment. A penile block with bupivacaine is often done for immediate postoperative pain, providing a more comfortable postoperative course.

Hypospadias Repair

Hypospadias is a developmental anomaly characterized by a urethral meatus that opens onto the ventral surface of the penis proximal to the end of the glans (Fig. 26.33). There are varying degrees of hypospadias (Box 26.4). The meatus may be on the ventral surface of the glans, on the corona, anywhere along the shaft, in the scrotum, or even in the perineum. The more proximal the opening is, the greater the degree of chordee (downward curvature of the penis). Chordee is caused by fibrous bands that extend from the hypospadiac urethral meatus to the tip of the glans and represent the abnormally developed urethra. In some cases of clinical curvature, however, these fibrous bands may not be present. Although these curvatures are still termed *chordee,* they are not true fibrous chordee.

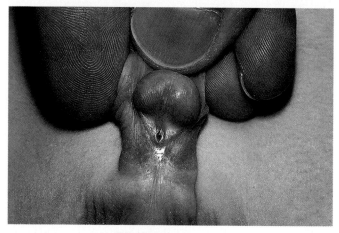

FIG. 26.33 Hypospadias.

The principal methods of hypospadias repair are meatoplasty and glanuloplasty, orthoplasty (release of chordee to straighten the penis), urethroplasty (reconstruction of the urethra), skin cover, and scrotoplasty. Because of variations of the defects, the technique of surgical repair is often made after the artificial erection is performed. Pediatric urologists must be well versed in multiple techniques to address all variants of the defect (Murphy, 2014) (Fig. 26.34). The meatoplasty and glanuloplasty incorporated (MAGPI) is described.

Procedural Considerations

The majority of patients are infants and toddlers, so preoperative interventions to protect them are implemented. The team places the patient supine with his legs apart. Urine may be diverted with a urethral catheter intraoperatively. The instrument setup varies

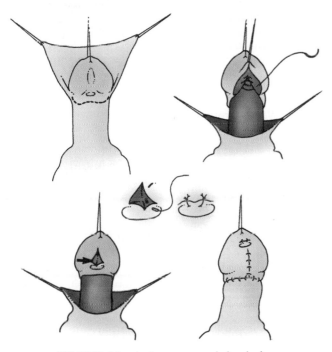

FIG. 26.34 Meatal advancement and glanuloplasty.

according to the surgeon's preference. A specialized hypospadias tray with fine plastic surgery instruments and occasionally ophthalmic instrumentation is used; 4F to 8F catheters and fine diameter suture are also required. The surgeon often wears optical loupes and occasionally uses a microscope. A small-diameter catheter (6F) is left in place for several days. After surgery, the repaired penis is dressed with a nonadherent dressing with an adhesive dressing over it.

Meatoplasty and Glanuloplasty Incorporated Procedure
Operative Procedure

1. The surgeon makes a subcoronal circumferential incision about 8 mm proximal to the meatus and corona. The skin is stripped back from the phallus by subcutaneous dissection.
2. A bridge of tissue between the meatus and glanular groove is made, with a transverse closure of the dorsal (upper) meatal edge to the distal glanular groove.

3. Three traction sutures are placed where the foreskin stops, at the apex of the ventral meatus (on the lower side) and lateral areas of the glans.
4. The surgeon sutures the edges of the glans together ventrally in a V configuration, and the redundant edges are excised. Vertical mattress sutures are used to approximate the glans beneath the meatus.
5. If foreskin is excessive the surgeon may trim it, followed by a sleeve style of reapproximation of the penile skin. If a ventral skin defect is present, a rotational skin flap closure is used.
6. An indwelling catheter is placed, and the wound is dressed.

Epispadias Repair

An epispadias is a congenital anomaly characterized by a urethral opening on the dorsum of the penis. The surgical procedures used in the correction of epispadias depend on the extent of the deformity. In mild, incomplete defects the repair is the same as a simple hypospadias repair. Complete deformity is always associated with urinary incontinence because of little or no development of the bladder neck; thus the operation is much more involved. The least severe forms of the exstrophy-epispadias complex are (1) balanic epispadias, in which the urethra opens on the dorsum of the glans, and (2) penile epispadias, in which the urethra opens on the shaft of the penis. The more severe variety, which occurs when the urethra opens on the proximal end of the shaft or in the penopubic position, is generally associated with severe dorsal chordee and urinary incontinence.

Procedural Considerations

The setup for an epispadias repair is the same as that described for hypospadias repair.

Bladder Exstrophy Repair

Bladder exstrophy repair corrects a more severe form of epispadias, in which the anterior bladder wall as well as the roof of the urethra are absent. Bladder exstrophy is always accompanied by wide separation of the rectus muscles of the lower abdominal wall and by diastasis of the pubic bone with anterior displacement of the anus. Repair of bladder exstrophy requires an adequate-sized bladder for ultimate continence to be achieved. It is preferable to perform this procedure in the neonatal period.

Procedural Considerations

The patient is placed in a supine position, and the abdomen and thighs are prepped and draped. Instruments are the same as those required for hypospadias repair.

Operative Procedure

1. The surgeon makes an incision around the exposed bladder medial to the paravesical neck mucosa. The incision is carried distally across the epispadial urethra distal to the verumontanum. The paravesical mucosa is preserved for urethral lengthening. The bladder is then freed from the rectus fascia and the peritoneum. The dorsal chordee is released, and the mobilized paravesical mucosa is apposed in the midline and sutured to the proximal end of the urethra just distal to the verumontanum.
2. The bladder wall is closed vertically in two layers with absorbable sutures, and a suprapubic tube is inserted for drainage.
3. The bladder neck is loosely reconstructed by approximating the interpubic ligament, which extends between the proximal end of the phallus and the pubic bone.

Hydrocelectomy

A hydrocele is an abnormal accumulation of fluid contained within the tunica vaginalis of the scrotum. Excessive secretion or accumulation of hydrocele fluid may be the result of infection or trauma. A hydrocelectomy is the excision of the tunica vaginalis of the testis to remove the enlarged fluid-filled sac. In older patients the procedure is performed through a scrotal incision.

Procedural Considerations

The patient is positioned supine. A minor instrument set is required.

Operative Procedure

1. The surgeon makes an anterolateral incision in the skin of the scrotum over the hydrocele mass. Bleeding is controlled with an electrosurgical unit (ESU).
2. Small retractors may be placed, after which the fascial layers are incised to expose the tunica vaginalis. The surgeon uses fine scissors, forceps, and blunt dissection to dissect the hydrocele and deliver it through the incision. The sac is opened, and the fluid contents are aspirated.
3. The surgeon inverts the sac so that it surrounds the testis, epididymis, and distal cord. Excess tunica vaginalis is excised, and the edges of the tunica are sutured with a continuous absorbable suture behind the testicle. The testicle is "bottled" by the inverted tunica vaginalis, and this may then be returned to the sac.
4. The scrotal incision is closed in layers with absorbable sutures and cyanoacrylate glue is applied. A fluff compression dressing contained in a scrotal support helps reduce postoperative scrotal edema in adolescents.

Orchiopexy

An orchiopexy is the surgical placement and fixation of the testicle in a normal anatomic position in the scrotal sac. If the testis fails to descend into the scrotum during gestation, it is considered undescended. An undescended testis becomes arrested somewhere along its normal path of descent. If it is palpable in a position other than its normal path of descent, its position is considered to be ectopic.

A retractile testis is one that has fully descended into the scrotum but retracts out of it as a result of contraction of the cremaster muscle. Gentle manipulation allows replacement of the testis in the most dependent portion of the scrotum. Retractile testes require no surgical or hormonal treatment.

All testes that are undescended after 1 year, including those that are unresponsive to hormone injections, require surgical placement in the scrotum for optimum maturation (Fig. 26.35). Laparoscopic exploration may also be used to determine position, existence, or size of a "hidden" testis.

Procedural Considerations

The setup is the same as that described for hydrocelectomy. Prepping and draping include the lower abdomen, genitalia, and upper thighs.

Operative Procedure

1. An inguinal incision is generally used for exploration of undescended testes. Most undescended testes are located in the superficial inguinal pouch or inguinal canal.
2. The external oblique aponeurosis is opened through the external inguinal ring to expose the inguinal canal; the gubernacular attachments of the undescended testis are dissected free as high as the internal inguinal ring or into the abdominal cavity.
3. The surgeon frees all adhesions and the associated inguinal hernia sac to lengthen the cord so that the testis is allowed to reach the scrotal cavity. The hernia sac is transected, twisted, and ligated with sutures.
4. To draw vessels into the inguinal canal, more proximal to the scrotum, the floor of the inguinal canal may have to be divided at the internal ring. The lateral portion of the internal ring is closed to prevent herniation. A scrotal pocket is created, and the testis is anchored in a normal anatomic position within the scrotum with absorbable sutures.

Orchiopexy may be accomplished using a variety of surgical approaches. The dependent portion of the undescended testis may be sutured to the base of the scrotum with absorbable sutures exteriorized through the scrotal wall. The most popular method is to anchor the testis into a dissected subdartos pouch. In this procedure a small midtransverse scrotal incision is made, and the skin and dartos muscle are dissected to create a pouch. The testis is then moved through a small hole in the dartos into the subdartos pouch and anchored in position by the traction suture. The overlying skin of the subdartos pouch is closed with fine absorbable suture material. The inguinal incision is repaired in layers with absorbable suture. The skin is closed with a subcuticular suture, and cyanoacrylate glue is used for dressing.

Repair of Vesicoureteral Reflux

VUR is defined as the retrograde flow of urine from the bladder to the ureter and even to the kidney pelvis. Children are usually initially diagnosed with the occurrence of a febrile UTI. The workup for reflux includes a renal bladder ultrasound with prevoid and postvoid views as well as a voiding cystourethrogram (VCUG). The VCUG is used to grade the reflux, with grade I being the least and grade V being the most extensive reflux. Children with VUR are given prophylactic antibiotics and checked yearly. Children with unresolved reflux or breakthrough infections will probably require repair of the reflux. There are two types of repair. Grade V may require a ureteral reimplant deeper into the bladder wall. This is either done with an open laparotomy or laparoscopic with robot assistance, if available. For lower grade reflux the most common approach is the minimally invasive approach of cystoscopy with injection of dextranomer/hyaluronic acid copolymer (Deflux) at the ureteral orifice into the bladder wall. Deflux is a sterile biodegradable gel that is injected around the opening of the ureter to create a valve. The valve facilitates urine drainage into the bladder while preventing backward flow into the ureter. Deflux is gradually replaced by body tissues, so the integrity of the valve is maintained over time. If the reflux is more severe, the child may require reimplantation of the ureter into the bladder wall. This is often performed as an ambulatory surgical procedure.

Procedural Considerations: Deflux

The setup for Deflux injection includes the same basic instrument setup as described for cystoscopy including a 10F offset cystoscope, light cord with a light source, cystoscopy fluid delivery tubing, Deflux needle, syringe of Deflux, and camera and monitor for the surgeon to view the procedure. The offset scope is the key to a good injection because the lens is offset at approximately a 45-degree angle, and the port to insert the needle through the scope comes straight off the end of the scope. The patient is placed in the dorsal lithotomy position for the procedure.

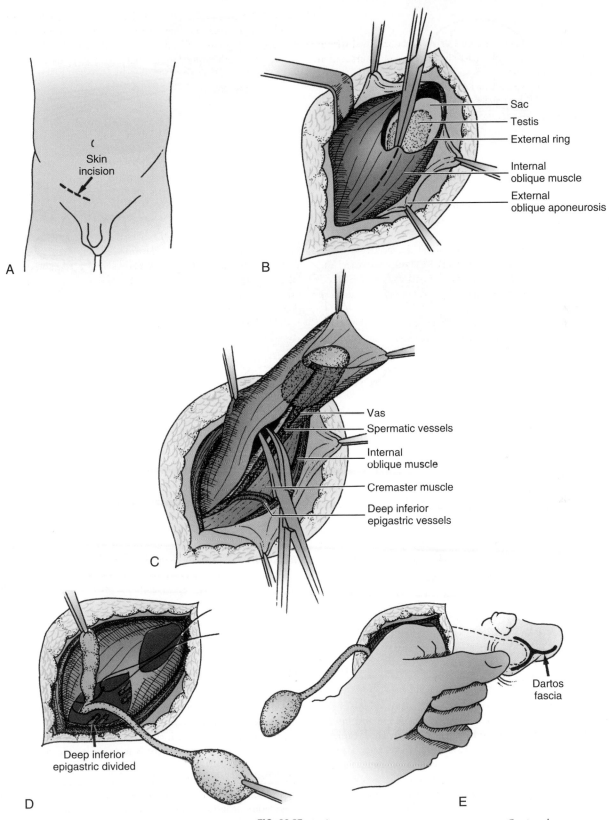

FIG. 26.35 Orchiopexy.   *Continued*

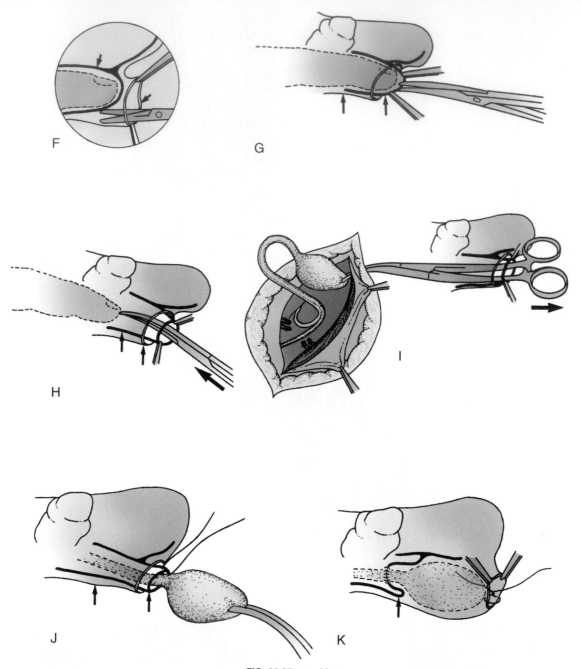

FIG. 26.35, cont'd

Operative Procedure

1. The surgeon lubricates the offset cystourethroscope and inserts it through the urethra into the bladder. The light cord, camera, and irrigation tubing are attached to the cystoscope, a urine specimen for culture is obtained, and an examination is performed.
2. The bladder is partially filled to allow for visualization.
3. The irrigation fluid is jetted into the ureteral orifice, opening it wide (hydrodistention), then the needle is introduced under the mucosa of the midureteral tunnel at the 6 o'clock position. The surgeon positions the needle tip just under the urothelium and advances it 4 to 5 mm in the submucosal plane of the ureter. Deflux is then injected until a prominent bulge appears, and the orifice has assumed a volcano-like shape.

4. The needle is kept in position for 15 to 30 seconds after the injection to prevent extravasation of Deflux.
5. The needle is removed, the bladder is decompressed, the scope is removed, and the patient is returned to the supine position.

Otorhinolaryngologic Procedures

Three common otorhinolaryngologic procedures in the pediatric population include myringotomy with insertion of pressure equalizing tubes, tonsillectomy, and adenoidectomy. These procedures are explained in greater detail in Chapter 19.

Foreign-Body Removal

In the normal course of exploration and play, children often ingest foreign objects or place objects in their noses or ears. Most foreign

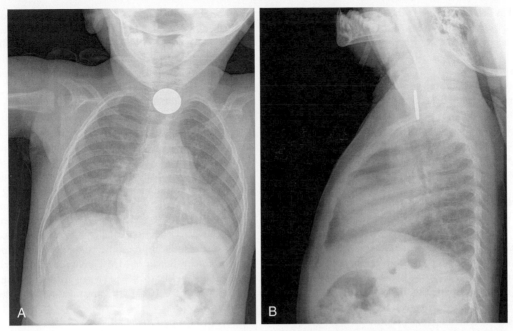

FIG. 26.36 (A) Anteroposterior view of coin trapped in esophagus. (B) Lateral view.

bodies that are ingested pass safely through the digestive tract without incident and do not need to be removed. If the foreign body is sharp, is caustic (i.e., batteries), or becomes lodged (Fig. 26.36), it may need to be removed by esophagoscopy (see Chapter 19) or through an open procedure.

The external ear canal and nose are other areas of interest to curious children. Common objects placed in the nares and external ear canal are dried beans, buttons, plastic objects, metals, food, erasers, nuts, seeds, and button batteries. Items placed in the ear can cause bleeding and difficulty with hearing. An insect found in a child's ear may indicate neglect and possible unsafe living conditions. Social services should be involved to determine whether a child abuse investigation is warranted.

A high index of suspicion should be raised in the child with unilateral rhinorrhea, nasal crusting, and air outflow obstruction as a nasal foreign body often causes these symptoms. Foreign bodies in the nose and ear may require removal in the OR setting with conscious sedation or a general anesthetic.

The most significant risk of foreign-body ingestion is aspiration. Children are more prone to aspiration than adults because their laryngeal sphincters are immature; they do not have molars to chew all foods adequately; and they often run, shout, and play with objects in their mouths. Commonly aspirated food items include candy/gum, peanuts and other nuts, seeds, popcorn, hot dogs, vegetable matter, meat matter, and fish bones. Commonly aspirated nonfood items include coins, toy parts, crayons, pen tops, tacks, nails, needles, pins, beads, and screws. Aspiration may produce a complete or partial airway obstruction (Fig. 26.37). Foreign objects in the respiratory tree are removed by means of rigid or flexible bronchoscopy (see Chapter 23).

Excision of Branchial Cleft Cyst/Remnant/Sinus Tract

Congenital branchial cleft anomalies are remnants of the branchial arch apparatus that failed to disappear during early embryologic development. At approximately 5 weeks' gestation, the branchial arches are associated with an external cleft of ectodermal origin and

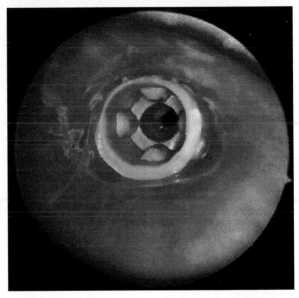

FIG. 26.37 Foreign body causing partial airway obstruction.

an internal pouch of endodermal origin. Anomalies that remain from incomplete resolution can be in the form of a branchial cleft cyst, a sinus, or a fistula. The location of branchial cleft anomalies ranges from the preauricular area (type 1) to the lateral neck along the sternocleidomastoid muscle (types 2–4). A cyst may not become apparent until later in childhood, typically during times of acute infection or possible abscess formation, and can occur anywhere along the course of a branchial sinus tract or fistulous tract. A sinus tract usually has an external opening to the neck, generally along the anterior border of the sternocleidomastoid muscle. A fistula has both an external opening and an internal opening; the internal opening is usually in the area of the pyriform sinus near the tonsil on that side. Excision of the branchial cleft anomaly is indicated if it is cystic or if it has become infected. The infection must be treated before surgical excision; if an abscess is present an incision and drainage may be needed.

Procedural Considerations

Imaging studies such as computed tomography (CT) or magnetic resonance imaging (MRI) are helpful to determine the presence of an associated tract. The patient is positioned supine with a roll under the shoulders to slightly extend the neck. A surgical drain, such as a rubber band, is frequently placed. Antibiotics are usually given intraoperatively before surgical incision. Description of a branchial cyst (type 2) excision follows.

Operative Procedure

1. A transverse skin crease overlying the lesion and 1.5 cm below the margin of the mandible is selected. The surgeon injects the proposed incision line with a local anesthetic.
2. The surgeon makes the skin incision through the skin and subcutaneous tissues.
3. The platysma muscle is divided with electrocautery.
4. The tissues overlying the cyst are gently dissected with fine forceps and small scissors or a small gauze peanut.
5. The cyst is gently grasped with a Babcock clamp. Surrounding tissue is dissected free from the cyst using small scissors to spread between the cyst capsule and surrounding tissue and then to cut through fibrous attachments.
6. If a pedicle or fibrous tract is identified, it is followed as far cephalic as possible before it is clamped, cut, and tied with absorbable sutures.
7. A small rubber band drain is usually placed to prevent accumulation of fluid or blood in the dissected cavity. A suture is attached to the distal end of the drain; the drain is removed within 24 hours.
8. The surgeon closes the wound in layers, finishing with subcuticular sutures, and adhesive strips.

Neurosurgical Procedures

Neuropathologic conditions requiring surgical intervention can be found in any age group. The most common problems requiring neurosurgical procedures in infants and children include meningocele, MMC, encephalocele, craniosynostosis, hydrocephalus, brain tumors, and trauma. The surgical approach, instruments, and equipment required for brain tumors and trauma are relatively similar to those required for adults; consequently, the majority of these procedures are as described in Chapter 21.

Myelomeningocele and Meningocele Repair

MMC (Fig. 26.38) is a form of spina bifida that is always associated with Chiari type II malformations. It occurs because of a congenital flaw in the neural tube closure at approximately 8 to 12 days after conception. The failure of the neural tube to close correctly causes a defect in the posterior elements of the lumbar vertebrae, fascia, and dura, allowing the meninges, spinal cord, and nerve roots to protrude out in a sac or cyst through the skin. The developing spinal cord and nerves are continuously exposed to amniotic fluid over the course of gestation, which results in progressive neurologic injury. There is always some degree of paralysis and loss of sensation below the defect. The amount of disability depends on the vertebral level of the spina bifida and frequently includes loss of bladder and bowel function and hydrocephalus, requiring ventriculoperitoneal shunts. Meningoceles are similar to MMCs but not as neurologically devastating: meninges

and cerebrospinal fluid (CSF) protrude into the defect but not the spinal cord. Although fetal repair of MMC is now an accepted treatment, it is not always feasible for patients. Lack of prenatal care, late prenatal care, and regional access to a hospital with a fetal surgery program are some obstacles in treating MMC prenatally.

Procedural Considerations

Infants born with either of these defects need to be given broad-spectrum antibiotics immediately after birth and taken to the OR within 24 hours for closure of the defect. Nursing care includes ensuring the area of the defect is covered with sterile gauze kept moistened with normal saline solution; positioning the infant so that the defect is not compressed; and maintaining the infant's body temperature, which is a more difficult task because of the need to keep the exposed defect moist. A very high percentage of children with this defect develop an allergy to latex; surgical closure and all subsequent surgical procedures should be performed in a latex-free environment. Repair of MMC may occur prenatally or postnatally. Conditions specific to prenatal repair are discussed in the Fetal Surgery section (see page 1017). The postnatal repair is described next.

Operative Procedure

1. The surgeon makes an elliptical incision around the defect.
2. The pearly epithelial tissue around the neural placode is dissected. Retention of the epithelial tissue can lead to formation of a postoperative epidermoid.
3. The surgeon performs blunt dissection following the nerve tissue on the ventral side of the placode down to the spinal canal.
4. The dura is then separated from the fascia.
5. Using small-diameter nonabsorbable sutures, the surgeon closes the dura over the neural placode.
6. The fascia is dissected from the muscle layer.
7. Nonabsorbable suture is used to close the fascial layer over the dura.
8. The muscle layer is then closed, followed by skin closure.

Craniectomy for Craniosynostosis

Craniosynostosis is the premature fusion of one or more cranial sutures. The condition can occur as part of a syndrome or as an isolated process. Craniosynostosis is characterized as "simple" when only one suture line is involved and "compound" when two or more suture lines are involved. The defect occurs in utero, and the exact etiology remains unknown. The purpose of the cranial sutures is to allow the calvaria to bend during the birth process and to allow the skull to expand to accommodate normal brain growth during infancy. The normal brain is finished growing by 2 years of age; at this time fusion of the cranial sutures normally begins. The fusion process is complete by 8 years of age.

The sagittal suture runs in the midline of the skull, connecting the anterior fontanelle to the posterior fontanelle. Premature closure of this fontanelle produces an elongation of the skull in the antero-posterior plane. Surgical intervention involves a linear strip crani-ectomy to excise the sagittal suture line from the anterior fontanelle to the lambdoidal suture line. Surgery is generally performed on the infant between 6 weeks and 6 months of age, with the best cosmetic results coming from the earlier repair. A craniectomy for sagittal synostosis is described.

Procedural Considerations

The patient is positioned supine using a cerebellar headrest. Additional measures are needed to maintain the patient's normal body

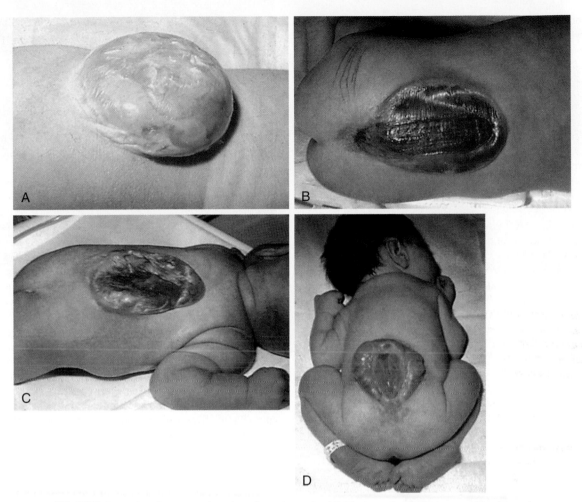

FIG. 26.38 Examples of meningocele and myelomeningoceles. (A) Meningocele. Lesion is covered by skin and meninges. (B) Myelomeningocele. Neural component evident at central strip of lesion. (C) Thoracolumbar myelomeningocele. (D) Severe myelomeningocele. Neural tissue in center represents the open spinal canal.

temperature; room temperature should be elevated, and a forced-air warming blanket should be used. An overbed warmer should be used during anesthesia induction and IV placement.

Operative Procedure

1. A sinusoidal incision is made midway between the anterior and posterior fontanelles from ear to ear, just posterior to the pinna.
2. The surgeon elevates the scalp off the skull anteriorly and posteriorly to expose the anterior fontanelle, posterior fontanelle, and asterion. The pericranium remains attached to the skull to minimize bleeding.
3. A burr hole is made on each side of the sagittal suture on the lambdoidal suture.
4. A craniotome drill attachment is used to cut anteriorly to the anterior fontanelle on each side of the sagittal suture. The surgeon uses a rongeur to cut across the sagittal suture and connect the burr holes.
5. The surgeon uses a Cobb periosteal elevator to carefully dissect the sagittal suture off the underlying dura.
6. A burr hole is placed at the asterion on each side. The craniotome is used to make a curvilinear cut just posterior to the coronal suture.

7. The parietal bone is then "greensticked" (fractured but leaving the periosteum intact) laterally.
8. The skin is closed with absorbable sutures.

Ventriculoatrial and Ventriculoperitoneal Shunt Insertion

Hydrocephalus is characterized by excess production of CSF or is associated with a blockage in the ventricular drainage system. Early intervention is indicated in infants to prevent cranial distortion caused by the increasing size of the ventricles (Fig. 26.39).

The two most widely used pediatric surgical procedures to divert excessive CSF from the ventricles to other body cavities from which it can be absorbed are ventriculoatrial (Fig. 26.40) and ventriculoperitoneal shunts. See Chapter 21 for complete information related to these two procedures.

Orthopedic Procedures

Pediatric orthopedic surgery may encompass the following areas: spine disorders, sports medicine, cerebral palsy, musculoskeletal tumors and injuries, foot and ankle disorders, limb length discrepancy, hip disorders, hand surgery, limb deficiency, thoracic insufficiency, and trauma. The majority of instrumentation, equipment, and procedural considerations are similar to those described in Chapter 20. Nonetheless, there are treatment modalities and procedures that

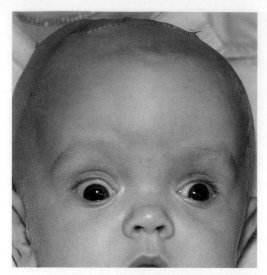

FIG. 26.39 Infant with hydrocephalus.

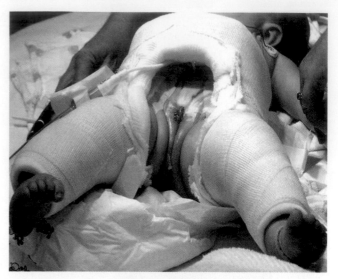

FIG. 26.41 Spica cast.

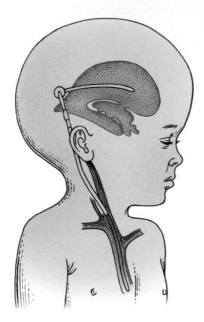

FIG. 26.40 Placement of ventriculoatrial shunt.

are more commonly performed in the pediatric population than in the adult population. Procedures for developmental dysplasia of the hip (DDH) abductor and adductor tenotomy and thoracic insufficiency syndrome (TIS) are described in this section.

Repair of Developmental Dysplasia of the Hip

Until recently, dislocation of the hip seen in newborns was referred to as congenital dislocation of the hip. DDH is a progressive condition in which the hip structures fail to develop adequately. Because the pathologic process leading to hip dysplasia may not be present or identifiable at birth, periodic exams of every infant's hips are essential at each routine baby examination until the child is 1 year old. About 1% of infants have dislocated, dislocatable, or subluxatable hips: 60% of DDH cases occur in females, and 60% of all cases involve only the left hip (Schmitz et al., 2016). DDH encompasses the entire spectrum of abnormalities involving the growing hip, ranging from simple dysplasia to dysplasia with subluxation or

dislocation of the hip joint. The goal of DDH management is to achieve and maintain a concentric reduction of the femoral head within the acetabulum to provide the optimal environment for the normal development of both structures. When proper alignment is disrupted, soft tissue and bony changes cause contractures of the hip muscles, a shallow acetabulum, and possibly a deformed femoral head. Treatment of congenital dislocation of the hip varies depending on the age of the patient and the stability of the hip. A Pavlik harness is the most commonly used nonoperative device in infants. If the Pavlik harness fails, the patient is taken to the OR and anesthetized for a closed reduction of the hip (proper positioning of the femur head within the acetabulum) confirmed by intraoperative arthrogram and fluoroscopy, with application of a spica cast (Fig. 26.41). Failure of closed reduction and immobilization necessitates an open reduction with an adductor tenotomy to allow adequate abduction to reduce the femoral head; after surgery, children younger than 2 years are then placed in a postreduction spica cast. For children older than 3 years the surgeon may need to perform a shortening varus femoral osteotomy (derotational osteotomy) to facilitate reduction of the femoral head into the acetabulum. In addition, if the acetabulum coverage is inadequate, a pelvic realignment (pelvic osteotomy) procedure may be necessary. Many of the pediatric orthopedic plating systems offer congenital dysplastic hip implants, which can be used in the reconstruction. The choice of femoral versus pelvic osteotomy is sometimes a matter of the surgeon's preference (Fig. 26.42).

The patient most often is in the lateral position for these procedures. An anterior incision is usually made for open reduction, whereas a lateral incision is made for the subtrochanteric femoral osteotomy. A soft tissue set and bone set (appropriate for age) are required as well as an oscillating saw, a wire driver, Steinmann pins, blade plate implants, and instrumentation.

Operative Procedures

Derotational Osteotomy for Developmental Dysplasia of the Hip. A derotational osteotomy is performed when the femoral head is improperly seated in the acetabulum.

1. The surgeon places the femur in internal rotation.
2. The distal fragment is rotated externally to place the knee and foot straight ahead.

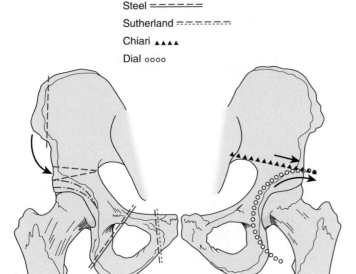

Salter – – – – –
Pemberton – · – · – ·
Steel ══════
Sutherland ═·═·═·═·═
Chiari ▲▲▲▲
Dial ○○○○

FIG. 26.42 Osteotomies for developmental dysplasia of the hip.

3. If the patient is a young child, the osteotomy is frequently performed in the supracondylar region, and the patient is immobilized in a plaster spica cast.
4. For an older child, the osteotomy is frequently done in the subtrochanteric region and the osteotomized fragments are held with an osteotomy blade plate or an intermediate compression screw. Immobilization may not be necessary.

Pelvic Osteotomy for Developmental Dysplasia of the Hip
1. The surgeon performs an osteotomy from the sciatic notch to the anterior margin of the ilium, superior to the acetabulum resulting in complete division of the wing of the ilium.
2. The ilium is then wedged down to increase the depth of the acetabulum when the osteotomy site is opened and a bone graft is inserted.
3. The surgeon uses heavy suture to close the capsule and applies a spica cast for postoperative immobilization.

Tenotomy and Lengthening Surgery

Tenotomies and lengthening procedures are commonly recommended for children with cerebral palsy to treat contractures or because the spasticity of these muscles makes mobility and abduction and adduction of the extremities difficult (Schmitz et al., 2016). These procedures also may be recommended as treatment for groin injuries when traditional medical treatment has failed. After the tendons are cut, the affected extremity may be immobilized in a cast, brace, or splint to allow for healing and promote normal growth patterns. In other cases, a dressing may be applied without immobilization. The procedure may be performed open (as described here) or using percutaneous techniques.

Procedural Considerations

The patient is positioned supine for the procedure with the affected extremity or extremities draped free for prepping and draping.

Operative Procedure
1. The surgeon makes a medial groin incision and lengthens the adductor longus, gracilis, and adductor brevis to improve hip abduction.
2. The pectineus adductor brevis interval is exposed to locate the iliopsoas tendon. The iliopsoas tendon is divided to correct hip flexion contractures.
3. Wounds are irrigated and closed using absorbable suture, and cyanoacrylate glue is applied to each incision line.

Thoracic Insufficiency Syndrome

TIS is a congenital condition characterized by severe deformities of the chest. Fused ribs, a hypoplastic thorax, and congenital scoliosis prevent normal breathing, lung growth, and lung development (Fig. 26.43). Until the vertical expandable prosthetic titanium rib (VEPTR) was developed there was no method for treating this condition that could account for a child's growth, and mortality was common. These children often have decreased respiratory function, with some requiring mechanical ventilation, and have poor growth and nutritional status (Mayer et al., 2016). The goal of surgical intervention is to increase thoracic volume, correct the scoliosis, improve thoracic function, and maintain these through the growth of the child (Fig. 26.44). Devices are attached perpendicularly to the patient's natural ribs (superior attachment point) and to more caudal ribs, a lumbar vertebra, or to the ilium (inferior attachment point). This is done through a standard thoracotomy incision by performing an opening wedge thoracotomy. This procedure is considered controversial because complications from VEPTR surgery are more common than most surgeries (Campbell, 2011).

VEPTR complications are frequent and are most likely to occur in patients with more significant spinal curves and in those with normokyphotic or hyperkyphotic curves. Infection is a common complication of VEPTR treatment, ranging from 10% to 32% based on prior reports. The variability in infection rate indicates a need for guided efforts to standardize best practices for infection control in VEPTR surgery (Garg et al., 2016). Many complications require additional surgery but most can be managed without loss of the VEPTR or treatment goals. A multidisciplinary approach with good attention to nutrition, tissue coverage, and surgical technique may be the best means of minimizing complications (Waldhausen, 2016).

Procedural Considerations

The VEPTR procedure involves an extensive setup. Often, these patients have a tracheostomy and are supported by mechanical ventilation. Neuromonitoring is necessary. Because of the high complication rate, room traffic is restricted and the setup happens after the patient is in the OR. Because TIS is associated with multiple physical deformities, the team positions the patient prone while taking care to prevent musculoskeletal and integumentary injury. Fluoroscopy is used during the case to confirm instrumentation placement. The VEPTR procedures are the primary procedure, expansion procedure, and replacement procedure. The primary procedure is discussed here.

Operative Procedure: Primary
1. The surgeon makes a J-shaped thoracotomy incision without disrupting the periosteum overlying the ribs.
2. The paraspinal muscles are elevated medially to the tips of the transverse process, and the scapula is elevated to expose the middle and posterior scalene muscle.

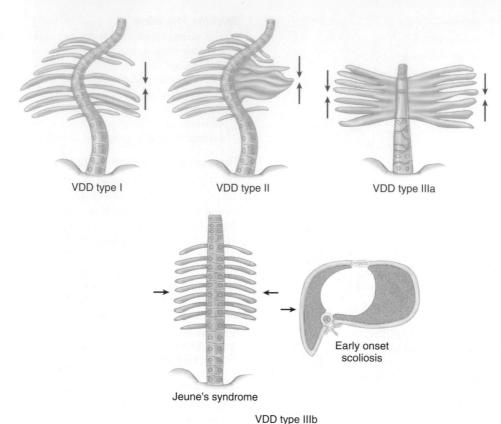

VDD type I   VDD type II   VDD type IIIa

Jeune's syndrome

Early onset
scoliosis

VDD type IIIb

FIG. 26.43 Types of thoracic insufficiency syndrome. *VDD,* Volume depletion deformity.

3. The surgeon identifies the cranial rib to be used as the cranial point of attachment and confirms it with fluoroscopy. Because of the risk of brachial plexus impingement, the first rib is not used as the cranial point of attachment.

4. A 1-cm incision is made into the intercostal muscles above and below the rib where the cranial rib support will attach and the periosteum is dissected.

5. The surgeon places the underside of the cranial rib support into the space between the periosteum and the rib. The rib support is rotated into the correct position, and the closing half ring around the ribs is attached and secured.

6. After the superior and inferior points of attachment have been chosen, an opening wedge thoracotomy is performed through the fused ribs at the apex of the thoracic deformity from the tip of the transverse process to the costochondral junction.

7. The surgeon cuts a transverse osteotomy from the transverse process to the sternum and separates the fusion mass into multiple longitudinal sections of the approximate width of normal ribs in the patient.

8. Next, the surgeon gently distracts the chest wall at the site of an opening wedge thoracotomy. Additional resection of medial fused ribs may be required if distraction is difficult.

9. The surgeon measures the distance between the cranial rib and either the thoracolumbar junction or the chosen caudal rib to determine the appropriate extension bar size.

10. The extension bar is attached to the endpoint at the iliac spine, lumbar spine, or rib.

11. Before closure, the surgeon brings the scapula to the approximate anatomic position, and the pulse oximeter reading on the recumbent arm and the neuromonitor is checked for signs of acute thoracic outlet syndrome.

12. The surgeon places a bone block of autograft, usually from rib resection from the superior lamina to the top of the hook, anchoring it with a single-level fusion.

13. To hold the hook in place until the bone block fuses, the surgeon wraps a #1 polypropylene suture around the shank of the hook and underneath the posterior spinous process at that level.

14. The surgeon closes the iliac crest incision, pulling the released abductor muscles over the S-hook to provide coverage and sutures them in place. Two subcutaneous closed suction drains are used in the thoracostomy incision.

Plastic and Reconstructive Surgery

Cleft Lip Repair

The normal upper lip is composed of skin, underlying orbicularis oris muscle, and mucosa. Two skin ridges are situated near the midline of the central philtrum of the lip. The vermilion (red portion of the lip) peaks at the philtral ridge on each side and gently curves downward as it reaches the midline to form Cupid's bow. A deficiency in tissue (skin, muscle, and mucosa) along one or both sides of the upper lip or in the midline results in a cleft at the site of this deficiency. The deficiency of tissue present with a cleft lip results in

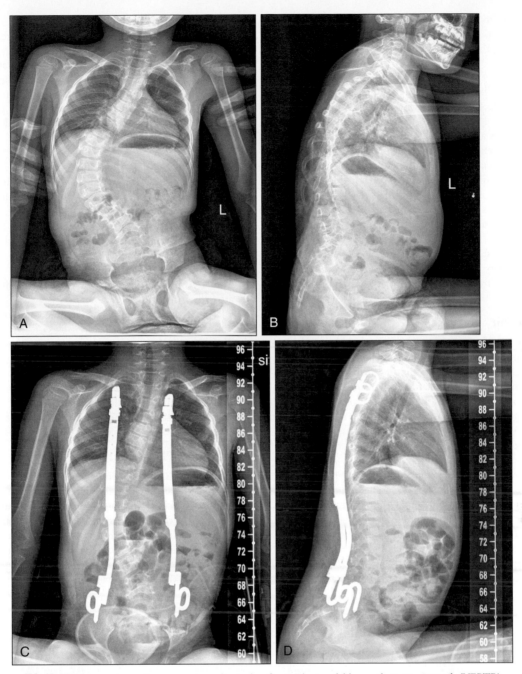

FIG. 26.44 Preoperative and postoperative radiographs of vertical expandable prosthetic titanium rib (VEPTR) instrumentation for thoracic insufficiency syndrome. (A) Anterior and (B) lateral views of a patient with thoracic insufficiency syndrome. (C) Anterior and (D) lateral views after VEPTR insertion.

distortion of Cupid's bow, absence of one or both philtral ridges, and distortion of the lower portion of the nose. Cleft lip is usually associated with a notch or cleft of the underlying alveolus and a cleft of the palate.

Cleft lip repair is most often performed when the infant is about 3 months of age. Timing of the repair follows the "rule of 10": the infant is 10 weeks of age, weighs 10 pounds, and has a hemoglobin level of 10 g/dL. Early surgical correction aids in feeding and

infant–parent bonding. Lip repair is directed toward rearrangement of existing tissues to approximate the normal lip as closely as possible. Some considerations also may be given to correcting the nasal deformity at the time of the cleft lip repair.

Procedural Considerations

A plastic surgery instrument set is required along with small scalpel blades. The OR bed is usually reversed to create more knee room if the surgeon prefers to sit during the surgery. The patient is placed in the supine position, with the head at the edge of the OR bed. The face is prepped with povidone-iodine and a head drape is used.

Operative Procedure

Many techniques for cleft lip repair are in common use. One type is illustrated in Fig. 26.45. The following steps are applicable to all lip repairs:

1. Normal landmarks are identified and marked. Precise measurements, taken with calipers and a ruler, are made so that corresponding points can be marked along the cleft.
2. The surgeon may infiltrate the lip with a local anesthetic. Incisions are made along the markings for the repair.
3. The surgeon dissects the abnormal musculature.
4. Additional dissection along the maxilla and nose may be performed.
5. Closure is accomplished in three layers: muscle, skin, and mucosa. Adhesive strips may be used and elbow restraints are placed to prevent the infant from putting his or her hands and fingers in his or her mouth.

Cleft Palate Repair

The palate is composed of the bony or hard palate anteriorly and the soft palate posteriorly. The alveolus borders the hard palate. A separation or cleft of the palate occurs in the midline and may involve only the soft palate or both hard and soft palates. The alveolus may be cleft on one or both sides.

The major function of the soft palate is to aid in the production of normal speech sounds. An intact hard palate is necessary to prevent escape of air through the nose during speech and to prevent the egress of liquid and food from the nose.

Cleft palate repair is usually performed when the child is 6 months old and should be completed before the beginning of speech. Variable factors, including the child's weight and the possibility of other disease processes, can affect surgery timing. The various operations used to achieve surgical closure of the palate all use tissue adjacent to the cleft (in the form of flaps), which is shifted centrally to close the defect (see Fig. 26.45).

Procedural Considerations

A basic plastic surgery instrument set is required, plus the following special instruments: Dingman mouth gag with assorted blades; Blair palate hook; palate knives; Blair palate elevators; and Fomon lower lateral scissors, short and long. The team positions the patient supine with the head at the edge of the OR bed, which is turned 180 degrees. The face is prepped with povidone-iodine, and a head drape is used. The head of the OR bed may be dropped one notch.

Operative Procedure

One of the most frequently used cleft palate repairs is illustrated in Fig. 26.46. The following steps are common to all palate repairs:

1. The surgeon inserts the Dingman mouth gag. Maintenance of the position of the endotracheal tube is crucial at this point. The surgeon may also insert a throat pack to absorb blood that may drain into the throat.
2. The outlines of the palatal flaps are marked.
3. The surgeon injects the palate with local anesthetic and the flaps are incised and elevated.
4. Closure is in three layers: nasal mucosa, muscle, and palatal mucosa.
5. The surgeon places a large horizontal mattress traction suture through the body of the tongue. If the patient experiences upper airway obstruction after extubation, traction is placed on this suture to pull the tongue forward, rather than insert an airway that might harm the palate repair. The throat pack is removed. The tongue stitch is removed in the PACU when the patient is awake.

Creation of a Pharyngeal Flap

When abnormal speech (velopharyngeal insufficiency) results despite a cleft palate repair, a secondary surgical procedure may be necessary to improve speech. Primarily an excess of air escaping through the nose during speech characterizes typical "cleft palate speech." This hypernasality often results from insufficient bulk or movement of the muscles of the soft palate. To decrease or eliminate this problem, tissue from the pharynx, in the form of a pharyngeal flap, is added

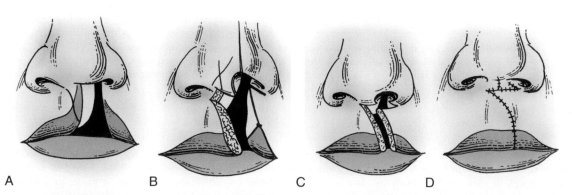

A   B   C   D

FIG. 26.45 Rotation-advancement method to correct complete unilateral cleft of lip. (A) Rotation incision marked so that the Cupid's bow-philtral dimple component will rotate down into normal position; flap advances into columella to form the nostril sill. (B) Dimple component has dropped down, and the second flap has advanced into columella. (C) Flap is being advanced into rotation gap, while skin-roll flap is interdigitated at mucocutaneous junction line. (D) Scar is maneuvered into strategic position where it is hidden at nasal base and floor and at philtrum column, and then it is interdigitated at mucocutaneous junction.

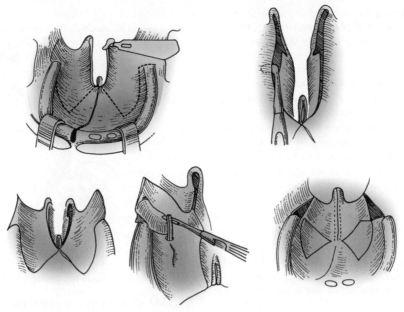

FIG. 26.46 Closure of cleft of soft palate by V-Y (Wardill–Kilner) palatoplasty. A V-shaped incision is made on oral side of the palate. Mucoperiosteal flaps are elevated on oral and nasal sides, with preservation of blood vessels. A Y-shaped closure (in three layers) closes cleft and lengthens palate.

to the soft palate. This flap also reduces the size of the opening between the oropharynx and nasopharynx, decreasing or eliminating the nasal escape of air during speech.

A pharyngeal flap repair may be done at any age, but most are done before the patient is 14 years old. A pharyngeal flap also may be part of primary cleft palate repair.

Procedural Considerations

Positioning, draping, and instruments are the same as those described for cleft palate repair, with the addition of two 12F red rubber catheters.

Operative Procedure

1. The Dingman mouth gag is inserted. A throat pack may be inserted.
2. The surgeon injects the palate and posterior wall of the pharynx with local anesthetic.
3. The palate is incised, and the pharyngeal flap is incised and elevated.
4. The pharyngeal wall donor site may be sutured or left open.
5. The pharyngeal flap is sutured to the palate, and the palate is closed.
6. A traction suture is placed through the body of the tongue. The throat pack is removed. The tongue stitch is removed in the PACU when the patient is awake.

Total Ear Reconstruction

An absent external ear presents the surgical team with the objective of developing or restoring a part of the appearance that will help with self-esteem and confidence in daily interactions as well as enhance hearing because the external ear funnels sound waves from the environment into the inner ear. Emotional support is a key aspect of the plan of care for these patients.

The external ear consists of skin, subcutaneous tissue, and cartilage. The surgical procedure to create an external ear involves the retrieval

of rib cartilage, carving the cartilage, placing the newly fashioned ear on the side of the patient's head, and skin grafting and dressing of the operative sites, with continual assessment and reassessment of the preoperative sketches made of the patient's ear in relation to facial structure. This can be accomplished as a one-stage procedure or as a sequence of surgeries. For congenital defects, the ideal time for initiating the procedure is between 6 and 10 years of age. In the case of traumatic loss of the external ear the time is individually determined. The use of tissue expanders may be considered in some cases to stretch the skin surface required to cover the ear.

Procedural Considerations

A basic plastic surgery instrument set is required, with the addition of rib graft instrumentation for autologous rib cartilage retrieval in total ear reconstruction. A sterile Doppler probe with sterile conduction gel should be available for intraoperative use. The surgeon creates preoperative sketches of the ear using unexposed x-ray film placed over the ear. Symmetric and anatomic landmarks are vital considerations in the patterns developed for the reconstruction. When the sketches are complete, the films are sterilized, with care not to remove the markings made by the surgeon. The patient is positioned supine with the arms tucked securely at the sides. Appropriate padding and protection of vulnerable neurovascular bundles and pressure sites are critical. Use of a pneumatic intermittent compression device and a forced air warming unit over the lower half of the patient's body should be considered because of the anticipated length of the procedure. Before the skin prep the surgeon assesses the vascular integrity of the temporoparietal flap with an unsterile Doppler probe and conduction gel and marks the incision sites. Infiltration of the operative sites is done with local anesthetic. Epinephrine is not recommended for use in the area of the flap because of the possible obliteration of the vascular complexes present. The patient's face and torso are prepped with povidone-iodine. A standard head drape and a split drape (or U drape) for the patient's torso allow the team access to the auricular area and chest, respectively.

Operative Procedure

1. The surgeon lifts a temporoparietal fascia flap and uses a sterile Doppler probe to assess the vascular integrity of the flap.
2. The chest wall is incised, and the rib cartilage segments are removed, taking care to preserve the perichondrium. This encourages bone growth and helps prevent a chest wall defect.
3. The surgeon determines the pleura is intact before closing the chest. Saline is instilled into the wound; if bubbles appear, the pleura is not intact; a chest tube is then inserted and attached to a chest drainage system. If the integrity of the pleura is in question, an intraoperative chest x-ray film may be taken to assess for a pneumothorax. If the pleura is intact, the surgeon closes the wound and injects local anesthetic into the intercostal incision area.
4. While one team closes the chest, another team begins the process of carving the rib cartilage for the ear reconstruction. The previously marked radiographs are crucial aids for the artistic abilities of the surgeon, providing a blueprint for the sculpting phase of the procedure.
5. If a skin graft is taken, then the donor site is covered with a dressing of choice.
6. Hemostasis is maintained with an ESU, topical thrombin, and infiltration of local anesthetic.
7. The flap covers the sculpted ear, and the skin graft is used to cover any exposed areas.
8. Next, the surgeon places drains and attaches them to closed-wound suction, or gauze stents wrapped with nonadherent gauze are sutured in place behind the ear. Soft, bulky dressings are applied to the ear and secured with a head wrap of rolled gauze. Standard dressings are applied to the chest wall.

Otoplasty

This congenital deformity in which the ear protrudes abnormally from the side of the head is generally the result of an absent or insufficiently pronounced antihelical fold of the external ear. The various methods of otoplasty are an attempt at correction by creating an antihelical fold that positions the ear more normally (Fig. 26.47). Protruding ears may be unilateral or bilateral. An otoplasty is generally performed for children who are uncomfortable or self-conscious about the deformity, which usually occurs in the elementary school years.

Procedural Considerations

A plastic surgery instrument set is needed. The patient is placed supine on the OR bed, and a head drape is used, leaving both ears well exposed. The patient's head is turned with the affected ear up and with the lower ear well-padded to avoid pressure injury.

Operative Procedure

1. The antihelical fold is created when the external ear is bent backward. The surgeon marks the position of the antihelical fold by placing 25-gauge or straight needles through the ear from anterior to posterior, applying methylene blue to the tips of the needles, and withdrawing them to mark the cartilage within.
2. The surgeon excises an ellipse of skin from the posterior surface of the ear after it has been infiltrated local anesthetic.
3. The ear cartilage is usually incised near the antihelical fold, and the anterior surface of the cartilage is scored to allow it to bend backward.
4. The surgeon places sutures to hold the cartilage in its new position.
5. The skin incision is closed.

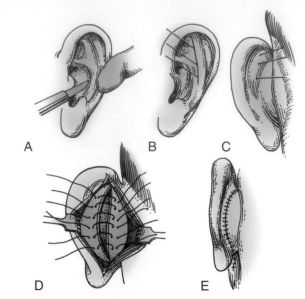

FIG. 26.47 Otoplasty for correction of protruding ears. (A) Antihelix defined by application of pressure to ear. (B) Position of antihelical fold marked by the passage of straight needles through ear. (C) Needle points visible along posterior surface of ear with ellipse of skin to be excised marked. (D) Section of ear cartilage incised and scored or excised with sutures placed to hold cartilage back. (E) Posterior ear incision sutured.

6. A drain may be placed to aid in the skin's adherence to the cartilage framework beneath.
7. A nonadherent dressing, such as petroleum gauze or cotton coated with antibiotic ointment, is usually placed in front of and behind the ear, followed by fluffed gauze and a bulky dressing made of rolled gauze to exert moderate compression on the ear.

Repair of Syndactyly

Syndactyly refers to a congenital webbing of the digits of the hands or feet. It is occasionally seen in association with other abnormalities, such as extra fingers or toes (polydactyly), or with bony abnormalities. In syndactyly with normal digits a web of skin joins adjacent fingers but each finger has its own tendons, vessels, nerves, and bony phalanges. Although the skin web may appear loose, a deficiency in skin is always present when surgical separation is performed. Plans for taking a skin graft (usually full thickness) should always be made. Surgical separation of syndactyly is performed at any time, usually after approximately 12 months of age (Fig. 26.48).

Toe syndactyly is less often treated surgically than finger syndactyly because proper function of the foot does not require fine movements of individual toes. Although the setup and description that follow are for the repair of finger syndactyly, they can also be applied to the repair of toe syndactyly.

Procedural Considerations

A hand surgery instrument set is required, plus a sterile marking pen, a pediatric pneumatic tourniquet, and an Esmarch bandage. The patient is placed supine on the OR bed with the affected arm extended on a hand table. A hand drape is used, and the affected hand and wrist are prepped and draped as well as both inguinal areas (donor sites for full-thickness skin grafts). Some surgeons prefer to use the wrist or forearm as donor sites.

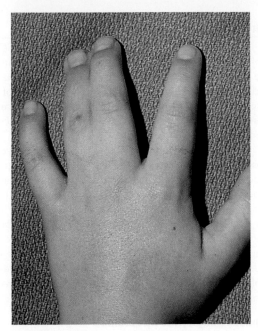

FIG. 26.48 Syndactyly involving third and fourth fingers.

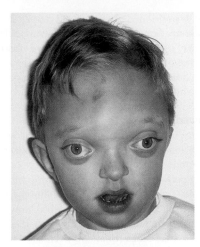

FIG. 26.49 Crouzon disease.

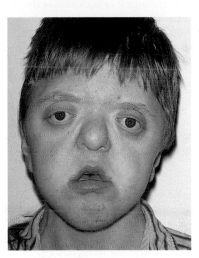

FIG. 26.50 Apert syndrome.

Operative Procedure

1. The surgeon incises the skin and elevates small flaps at the sides of fingers and in the web.
2. After the flaps have been sutured into position, patterns of areas of absent skin on the sides of fingers are made and transferred to the skin-graft donor site.
3. The skin graft is taken; if a full-thickness skin graft is used, it must be defatted before the graft is sutured in place.
4. Skin grafts are sutured to fingers.
5. Stent dressings are placed over the skin grafts. The entire hand is immobilized in a bulky dressing or in a long arm cast.

Orbital-Craniofacial Surgery

Some congenital anomalies involve the orbital-craniofacial skeleton. These include hypertelorism, in which the distance between the orbits is increased as seen in Crouzon disease and Apert syndrome. Crouzon disease is characterized by premature closure of the cranial sutures, resulting in an abnormally shaped skull, exophthalmos and hypertelorism, parrot's beak nose, and maxillary hypoplasia. Apert syndrome includes the same craniofacial deformities as Crouzon disease as well as syndactyly or other hand anomalies. Advances in plastic surgery make surgical correction of some of these deformities possible.

Binocular vision is normal in humans. It involves the coordinated use of both eyes to obtain a single mental impression of objects. Binocular vision is usually absent in craniofacial anomalies because of the increased distance between the orbits. The purposes of orbital-craniofacial surgery are to provide the patient with binocular vision by moving the orbits closer together and to provide the patient with a more acceptable appearance by moving the bones of the orbital-craniofacial skeleton into a more normal position. Correction of the deformity seen in Crouzon disease (Fig. 26.49) and Apert syndrome (Fig. 26.50) involves a surgically created Le Fort III maxillary fracture.

Although an extracranial approach may be used, an intracranial approach is used in most cases; therefore a neurosurgeon and a plastic surgeon perform these operations through a bifrontal (coronal) craniotomy. A tracheostomy may be done before the start of the procedure. Bone grafts from hips or ribs may be necessary to augment areas of bone deficit, which result from movement of the craniofacial skeleton.

Procedural Considerations

These operations are usually performed on children. They are very extensive procedures, often lasting several hours. Blood loss may be considerable. Postoperative complications, such as cerebral edema or meningitis, can be formidable. The perioperative nurse must pay particular attention to the following important details: (1) insertion of a Foley catheter into the patient's bladder before the operation is started, (2) positioning of the patient on the OR bed so that all bony prominences are well padded, and (3) availability of accurate means for measuring blood loss. Use of sequential compression devices and warming devices should also be anticipated.

A basic plastic surgery instrument set, craniectomy instruments and supplies (see Chapter 21), plastic hand instrumentation, and tracheostomy instruments and supplies are required. A high-speed drill, saws, and general orthopedic instrumentation are also needed. A separate setup is necessary for obtaining the bone graft.

The patient is positioned, prepped, and draped as described for bifrontal craniotomy (see Chapter 21). The entire face is left exposed, however, and may temporarily be covered with a plastic drape until the portion of the operation requiring access to the face is reached. The bone-graft donor site is also prepped and draped so that both iliac crests and the lower ribs are exposed.

Operative Procedure

1. Tracheostomy, if required, is performed first, followed by application of arch bars (when indicated as in Crouzon disease and Apert syndrome).
2. The surgeon performs a bifrontal craniotomy with craniectomy.
3. Bilateral orbital osteotomies (Fig. 26.51A) into the anterior cranial fossa are performed. Bilateral conjunctival (lower eyelid) and labiogingival sulcus incisions (for Crouzon disease and Apert syndrome) are made for orbital and maxillary osteotomies.
4. The surgeon moves the bones of the orbital-craniofacial region (see Fig. 26.51B), based on measurement of the intercanthal distance (in hypertelorism) or occlusion of the teeth (in Crouzon disease and Apert syndrome).
5. Bone grafts may be taken from the calvaria, ribs, or hips to augment areas of bone deficit, which result from movement of the craniofacial skeleton.
6. Bone grafts are fixed in place with interosseous wires and by means of intermaxillary fixation applied to arch bars (for Crouzon disease and Apert syndrome) (see Fig. 26.51C). Rigid plate-and-screw fixation is another option.

The craniotomy, conjunctival, intraoral, and bone-graft donor site incisions are closed and dressings are applied.

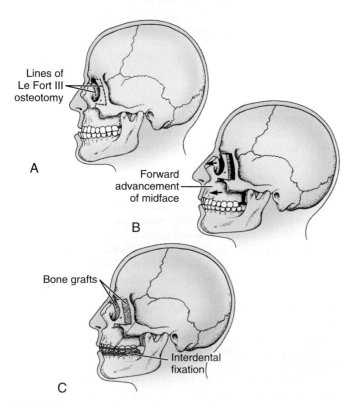

FIG. 26.51 (A–C) Steps in surgical correction of Crouzon disease deformities.

(labels on figure: Lines of Le Fort III osteotomy; A; Forward advancement of midface; B; Bone grafts; Interdental fixation; C)

Pediatric Ophthalmic Surgery

Although the anatomy of the eye remains the same (see Chapter 18), children experience different eye conditions than adults that are specifically related to vision development in the brain. Vision develops in the brain until approximately 9 years of age. It is affected by eyes that are not straight or do not focus correctly. Therefore it is imperative that any vision problems are detected and corrected early.

Pediatric ophthalmologists participate in specific programs of study that focus on examination and care of childhood vision problems and structural disorders of the eye as well as surgical management of disorders such as congenital nasolacrimal duct obstruction, pediatric cataracts, ptosis, strabismus, pediatric glaucoma, and eye injuries. It is not uncommon for pediatric ophthalmology to be subdivided into specialty categories. The field of oculoplastics was first identified in 1966. Oculoplastics encompasses the merging of plastic surgery and ophthalmology in an attempt to treat or repair the oculo-orbital region of the face. Surgeons may also focus their practice on corneal disorders, retinal disorders, or neuro-ophthalmology.

Eye Muscle Surgery for Strabismus

Any misalignment of the eyes is called strabismus. Strabismus is further subdivided into the categories listed in Box 26.5. Strabismus occurs as a result of poorly controlled neuromuscular eye movements. Any child can suffer from strabismus, but disorders that affect the brain (e.g., cerebral palsy, hydrocephalus, Down syndrome, brain tumors) are associated with an increased prevalence of the disorder. Additionally, strabismus may occur in conjunction with traumatic brain, nerve, or ocular injury.

The goal for treatment of strabismus is to straighten the eyes so that binocular vision functions appropriately. Nonsurgical treatments may include eyeglasses and eye exercises. Surgery may be recommended to change the alignment of the eyes relative to each other by strengthening, weakening, or repositioning the eye muscles. If a child presents with strabismus in addition to another eye disorder (e.g., amblyopia, cataract, ptosis), the other condition will be treated before corrective surgery.

Skin incisions are not necessary to repair strabismus. Instead the surgeon uses a lid speculum to retract the eyelid and incises the conjunctiva to expose the muscles (Fig. 26.52). Box 26.6 differentiates between the methods of muscle repair. The repaired muscles are sutured using a standard knot or adjustable suture. Adjustable sutures consist of temporary knots (bow or slip) placed in an accessible position so that eye alignment can be altered approximately 24 hours after surgery. The lateral rectus recession and lateral rectus resection procedures are described below.

BOX 26.5

Types of Strabismus

- *Esotropia:* inward turning of one or both eyes
- *Exotropia:* outward turning of one or both eyes
- *Hypertropia:* one eye higher than the other
- *Hypotropia:* one eye lower than the other

Modified from Lingua G et al: Techniques of strabismus. In Yanoff M et al, editors: *Ophthalmology*, ed 4, St Louis, 2014, Elsevier.

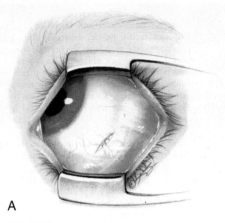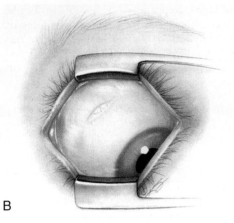

A   B

FIG. 26.52 Forniceal incisions for strabismus surgery. All six muscles can be isolated from these two incisions. (A) Inferotemporal incision: isolates the lateral rectus, inferior rectus, and inferior oblique muscles. (B) Superonasal incision: isolates the medial rectus, superior rectus, and superior oblique muscles.

BOX 26.6

Methods of Muscle Repair

Recession
- Is a weakening procedure.
- Alters the attachment site of the eye muscle on the eyeball.
- Muscle is cut from the surface of the eye and reattached at a point farther back from the front of the eye.

Resection
- Is a strengthening procedure.
- Extraocular muscle is reattached to the eyeball at its original site.
- A section of the muscle is removed and a stitch is placed in the muscle at the intended new attachment site.
- The segment of muscle between the stitch and the eyeball is removed.
- The shortened muscle is reattached to the eye.

Modified from Lingua G et al: Techniques of strabismus. In Yanoff M et al, editors: *Ophthalmology*, ed 4, St Louis, 2014, Elsevier.

Procedural Considerations

The patient receives a general anesthetic, and the full face above the nose is prepped with half-strength povidone-iodine. Both eyes are prepped so that the repair can be measured against the opposite eye for symmetry.

Operative Procedure: Lateral Rectus Recession

1. A lid speculum is placed in the affected eye and the unaffected eye is taped closed.
2. The surgeon grasps the infratemporal limbus using locking forceps, and then rotates the eye superonasally.
3. A conjunctival fornix incision is made posterior to the limbus in the infratemporal quadrant.
4. Tendons and episclera are dissected until bare sclera is reached, and the lateral rectus is isolated with a muscle hook.
5. The surgeon passes a suture through the original insertion of the lateral rectus muscle and locks it on superior and inferior aspects. The muscle is then cut from its insertion on the globe using scissors.

6. Calipers are used to mark a location posterior to the insertion point, and the surgeon passes a suture through the sclera using the "crossed swords" technique.
7. The muscle is pulled up firmly to the globe and tied into position. The location is measured again using calipers.
8. Conjunctiva is closed using plain gut suture.
9. The surface of the eye may be covered in neomycin/polymyxin/dexamethasone and tetracaine ophthalmic ointment.

Operative Procedure: Lateral Rectus Resection

1. Steps 1 through 4 of the lateral rectus recession procedure are performed.
2. A suture is passed through the original insertion of the lateral rectus muscle and locked on superior and inferior aspects. The central sutures are tied together, and a resection clamp is placed anteriorly.
3. The surgeon cuts the muscle anterior to the resection clamp, and then cuts the remaining muscle stump from its original insertion point.
4. The suture needles are passed through the original insertion in a perpendicular fashion and tied together.
5. The muscle is pulled up firmly to the globe and tied into position.
6. Conjunctiva is closed using plain gut suture.
7. The surface of the eye may be covered in neomycin/polymyxin/dexamethasone and tetracaine ophthalmic ointment.

Ptosis (Blepharoptosis) Surgery

Defined as a droopy eyelid, ptosis is either congenital or acquired (Fig. 26.53). Congenital ptosis is usually a result of a deficit in the levator palpebri muscle in the upper eyelid. Acquired ptosis occurs as a result of neurologic conditions that affect the nerves of the eye (e.g., myasthenia gravis, Horner syndrome, third nerve paralysis). It also can manifest in conjunction with movement disorders, resulting in double vision. Ptosis also may result from orbital tumors.

Ptosis is treated with corrective lenses if amblyopia with astigmatism is present. Surgery is indicated for cases in which the droopy eyelid is blocking normal vision or causes the child to position the head with the chin up in an attempt to compensate for the block in vision. The goal of surgery is to create as perfect an anatomic result as possible by elevating the position of the lid, creating

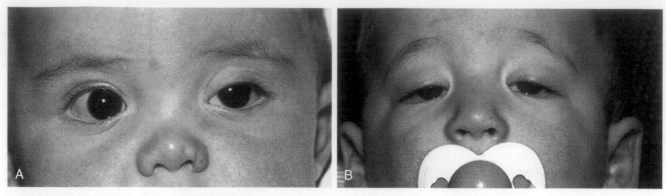

FIG. 26.53 Simple congenital ptosis. (A) Unilateral. (B) Bilateral.

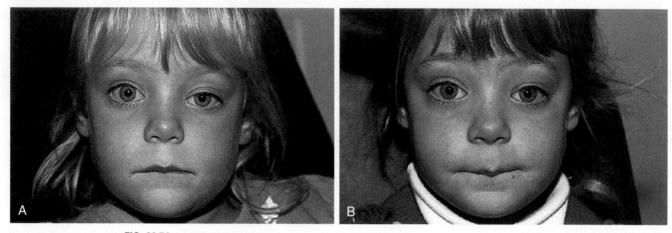

FIG. 26.54 Modified Fasanella–Servat procedure. (A) Preoperative. (B) Six months postoperative.

a lid fold, and preserving the contour and symmetry of both lids (Fig. 26.54).

Procedural Considerations

The patient is positioned supine with the head on a gel ring. The eyes are prepped with half-strength povidone-iodine. The patient is draped to expose both eyes for comparison during the procedure. Ophthalmic ointment is applied to the opposite eye, and the eye is taped shut for protective purposes during surgery.

Operative Procedure

1. The surgeon places a protective scleral shell into the affected eye to protect the globe.
2. The upper lid is everted and two curved hemostats are placed at the upper tarsal border.
3. Traction sutures are passed through the tissue at the nasal and temporal end below the clamps.
4. The tissue between the two clamps and traction sutures is excised.
5. A nylon suture is passed through the end of the lid crease out through the apex of the incision and run in a "serpentine" fashion. The suture reconnects the conjunctiva and Müller muscle to the cut edge of the tarsus
6. At the opposite end of the incision, the suture is passed through the apex of the incision and out through the crease and then buried beneath the conjunctival surface.
7. The surgeon removes the traction sutures and returns the lid to its normal position. A lid plate is used to smooth the incision line by pressing directly on the skin surface to flatten the tissues against the plate.
8. The nylon suture is tied snugly over the skin and remains in place approximately 1 week after surgery to allow for lid adjustment.
9. The surgeon removes the scleral shell and applies ophthalmic antibiotic to the eye and suture line. A dressing may be applied to the surgical site.

Cataract Surgery

Approximately 40% of acquired pediatric cataracts are secondary to trauma, and as many as approximately one-third of pediatric cataracts are inherited (Dahan, 2014) and are primarily classified as nuclear, posterior subcapsular, anterior polar, posterior polar, lamellar, or traumatic (Box 26.7). Unlike in adults, pediatric cataracts are soft and the lens can be easily aspirated through incisions that are 1 to 1.5 mm long at the limbus. Lensectomy, via the pars plana, may be another option. The limbal wound may need to be enlarged if the surgeon is planning to implant an intraocular lens (IOL). Wound dehiscence and iris incarceration are common complications after pediatric cataract surgery, so the surgeon must suture the wound securely to prevent these untoward events. Other options include wearing glasses or contact lenses to correct the deficit (Dahan, 2014).

Corneal Surgery

The cornea is only about 0.5 mm thick and consists of many layers. The stroma is the thickest part of the cornea. Diseases of the cornea

Types of Cataracts

- Nuclear: cloudiness in the center part of the lens
- Lamellar: cloudiness between the nuclear and cortical layers of the lens
- Traumatic: results from blunt or penetrating force that damages the lens
- Posterior subcapsular: affects the back surface of the lens cortex, inside the capsule
- Anterior polar: central opacity of the front part of the lens capsule; does not grow during childhood and does not require surgical management
- Posterior polar: central opacity of the back of the lens

Modified from Dahan E: Pediatric cataract surgery. In Yanoff et al, editors: *Ophthalmology*, ed 4, St Louis, 2014, Elsevier.

TABLE 26.4

Categories of Glaucoma

Category	Age at Presentation	Symptoms at Presentation
Congenital	Glaucoma present at birth	Excessive tearing Light sensitivity Large, cloudy cornea Dull-appearing iris
Infantile	Glaucoma presents between 1 and 24 months of age	Excessive tearing Light sensitivity Large, cloudy cornea Dull-appearing iris
Juvenile	Glaucoma presents after 36 months of age	No obvious symptoms; presents similar to adult-onset glaucoma

Modified from Brandt J: Congenital glaucoma. In Yanoff M et al, editors: *Ophthalmology*, ed 4, St Louis, 2014, Elsevier.

TABLE 26.5

Stages of Retinopathy of Prematurity (ROP)

Stages	Description	Intervention
Stage 1	Mildly abnormal growth of retinal vessels	Usually does not require treatment, no long-term affects
Stage 2	Moderately abnormal growth of retinal vessels	Usually does not require treatment, no long-term affects
Stage 3	Severely abnormal growth of retinal vessels	May require treatment Children with stage 3 ROP have a higher risk of long-term vision problems
Stage 4	Partial retinal detachment	Usually requires treatment May lead to long-term vision problems or blindness
Stage 5	Complete retinal detachment	Requires treatment May lead to long-term vision problems or blindness

Modified from Beard I: Neonatology. In Engorn B et al, editors: *The Harriet Lane handbook*, ed 20, Philadelphia, 2015, Saunders.

include, but are not limited to, allergies, conjunctivitis, corneal infections, dry eye, herpes zoster, ocular herpes, pterygium, and Stevens–Johnson syndrome. In some cases corneal surgery or a corneal transplant is necessary, particularly when high pressure from glaucoma allows fluid to accumulate in the stroma. When this occurs, it may lead to a cloudy cornea.

Trabeculotomy for Glaucoma

The pathophysiology of glaucoma is markedly different for infants and children than for adults, and its occurrence is rare. Pediatric glaucoma is categorized according to age of onset (Table 26.4). Cases of glaucoma are classified as primary (without specific identifiable cause) or secondary (occurring in conjunction with another disorder, medication use, or eye trauma). Children with glaucoma could have other eye abnormalities in addition to the glaucoma, including opacities of the cornea.

Pediatric glaucoma is treated by a combination of medical and surgical interventions because the goal of treatment is more than simply lowering intraocular pressure. Children diagnosed with congenital or infantile glaucoma often develop myopia and require glasses. There is also an increased occurrence of strabismus and amblyopia in children with glaucoma. Extreme cases may result in vision loss, supporting the need for early diagnosis and management of the disorder.

Pediatric glaucoma is commonly evaluated by examination under anesthesia (EUA). At this time the ophthalmologist measures intraocular pressure, corneal length, axial diameter, and refractive error and assesses corneal clarity and the optic nerve. If the intraocular pressure is elevated, it can be treated medically or surgically. The majority of primary pediatric glaucoma cases are treated surgically.

The most common surgical approach is trabeculotomy with goniometry, which opens the drainage canal and facilitates aqueous drainage. Other options, such as trabeculotomy with tube placement, create a bypass route to shunt aqueous drainage. Laser procedures are also effective in some cases of glaucoma. Successful management of the disease typically requires multiple examinations and procedures.

Retinal Disorders

Retinal diseases include retinopathy of prematurity (ROP). ROP is one of the most common causes of visual loss in childhood and can lead to lifelong vision impairment and blindness. It is classified according to stage (Table 26.5). The most effective proven treatments for ROP are laser therapy or cryotherapy. Both laser treatments and cryotherapy are performed only on infants with advanced ROP. Severe cases (stage 5) of this disorder are treated with scleral buckle and posterior vitrectomy (see Chapter 18).

Trauma

Principles governing surgical care of trauma patients are discussed in Chapter 28. However, when caring for the pediatric trauma patient in surgery, the perioperative nurse must possess additional knowledge to develop a detailed plan of action that effectively drives the delivery of safe patient care. During all episodes of patient care, it is necessary for the perioperative nurse to communicate with members of the surgical and interdisciplinary team in a fashion that best supports positive patient outcomes. The urgency of injury will dictate the timeliness of surgical intervention. In some instances, pediatric trauma patients may require transfer to a level I trauma center. The criteria for transfer are outlined in Box 26.8. The perioperative nurse should be prepared to administer care to any type of injury in a safe and effective manner that is appropriate across all age levels.

Unintentional and intentional injury and homicide cause more deaths in children and adolescents ages 1 to 18 years than all other causes combined. It is estimated that 1 in 4 children sustain an unintentional injury requiring medical care each year (AAP, 2016). Survivors of childhood trauma may suffer lifelong disability and require long-term skilled care. Several factors, such as age, gender, behavior, and environment, influence the risk of traumatic injury. For instance, infants and toddlers are more prone to falls resulting in severe injury, which may be related to the pliable nature of their skeletal system. If broken bones are present, a severe force of injury must be assumed. Older children and adolescents are at higher risk for sport-related, bicycle-related, and motor vehicle–related injuries. In this age group, blunt injuries resulting from motor vehicle accidents or direct blows (as with contact sports or child abuse) along with falls are the most common mechanisms of injury. It is not uncommon for pediatric traumatic injuries to occur in the home environment, stressing the importance of community awareness and education as it relates to trauma prevention. Some of the most significant prevention strategies focus on car seat safety as a means of preventing injury from motor vehicle accidents (Patient Safety).

Throughout the pediatric population neurologic injuries are the most common cause of traumatic death in children; the pediatric patient's head is proportionately larger in relation to his or her body mass and especially vulnerable to injury. Table 26.6 provides guidelines for using the Glasgow Coma Scale for infants and children. Because children have a much smaller reserve than adults, once a decline in vital functions is noted, demise is rapid. Information about commonly used medications in pediatric resuscitation is noted in the Surgical Pharmacology box.

IV access is often difficult in the pediatric patient, and an intraosseous line may be inserted by emergency rescue personnel before arrival at the hospital or in the emergency department (ED). These lines are inserted by use of an intraosseous needle or bone marrow aspiration needle and are placed slightly below the knee on the anterior aspect of the tibia at a 90-degree angle (Fig. 26.55). Stabilization of the line may be difficult, but the line can remain for up to 24 hours and provides rapid access when other routes are too time consuming or difficult to access. Fluid resuscitation levels for children experiencing hemorrhage, as well as types and dosages of medications, are based on body weight because weight provides a better mechanism of accuracy when calculating dosage.

Because of the nature of the trauma, it may be difficult for the healthcare team to obtain the patient's exact body weight. In these instances, body weight can be estimated using Broselow tapes or palmar methods. The body size of the patient determines the type

---

BOX 26.8

Trauma Transfer Criteria for Pediatric Patients Less Than or Equal to Age 14

A. Pediatric trauma patients, less than or equal to 14 years of age, who meet the following criteria should be transferred to a pediatric trauma center:

The decision to transfer should be consistent with the best practices of trauma care and under some circumstances may require immediate onsite neurosurgical treatment such as decompression of an expanding epidural hematoma or thoracic, abdominal, and pelvic or extremity procedures required to control hemorrhage, such as laparotomy for hemoperitoneum with hemodynamic instability.

1. Persistent physiologic derangements, shock, hemodynamically unstable, ongoing transfusion needs
2. Traumatic brain injury (significant structural abnormality on x-ray or CT, sustained GCS less than or equal to 13 for greater than 2 hours, or neurologic deterioration)
3. Intubation and mechanical ventilation not expected to be weaned and extubated within 24 hours
4. Children with special needs and those with other comorbid conditions such as congenital heart disease, chronic lung disease, or other disease processes that will benefit from the multidisciplinary care available at a pediatric trauma center

B. Pediatric trauma patients who meet the following criteria should be considered for transfer to a pediatric trauma center:

1. Nonoperative management of solid organ injuries
2. Any assessment of "negative points" on the Pediatric Trauma Score ("negative points are assigned for: less than 10 kg, airway unmaintainable, systolic blood pressure less than 50 mm Hg, coma, major open or penetrating wound, open or multiple fractures)
3. Injury Severity Score >9
4. Victim or nonaccidental injury that requires additional resources including a child protection team
5. When it is anticipated that the complexity of ongoing care will exceed the capabilities of the local resources at the adult trauma center

From Pennsylvania Trauma Systems Foundation: *Adult trauma center accreditation, Appendix C: transfer guidelines: adult trauma centers (level I, II, and III) to pediatric trauma centers,* Mechanicsburg, PA, 2016.

PATIENT SAFETY

Child Passenger Safety

Motor vehicle crashes are the number one killer of children older than the age of 4. Parents and caregivers should be encouraged to follow these best-practice recommendations to reduce the risk of injury or death for children who ride in motor vehicles:

1. All infants and toddlers should ride in a rear-facing CSS until they are 2 years of age *or* until they reach the highest weight or height allowed by the manufacturer of their CSS.
2. All children older than 2 years *or* children younger than 2 years who have outgrown the rear-facing weight or height limit for their CSS should ride in a forward-facing CSS with a harness for as long as possible, up to the highest weight or height allowed by the manufacturer of their CSS. The lowest maximum weight limit currently available in forward-facing CSSs is 40 pounds, but some seats can accommodate children up to 80 pounds.
3. All children whose height or weight is more than the forward-facing limit for their CSS should use a belt-positioning booster seat until the vehicle lap and shoulder seat belt fits properly (approximately 4 feet 9 inches in height and between 8 and 12 years of age).
4. Children who are old enough and large enough to use vehicle seat belts should use lap and shoulder seat belts for optimal protection.
5. All children younger than 13 years of age should be restrained in the rear seats of vehicles for optimal protection.

CSS, Car safety seat.

Modified from Centers for Disease Control and Prevention (CDC): *Child passenger safety* (website), 2016. www.cdc.gov/motorvehiclesafety/child_passenger_safety. (Accessed 18 February 2017).

TABLE 26.6
Pediatric Modification of Glasgow Coma Scale

Glasgow Coma Scale	Pediatric Modification	
Eye Opening		
Birth to 1 Year	**12 Months or Older**	
4 Spontaneous	4 Spontaneously	
3 To shout	3 To verbal command	
2 To pain	2 To pain	
1 No response	1 No response	
Best Motor Response		
Birth to 1 Year	**12 Months or Older**	
6 Purposeful movements	6 Obeys command	
5 Localizes pain	5 Localizes pain	
4 Flexion, withdrawal	4 Flexion, withdrawal	
3 Flexion, abnormal	3 Flexion, abnormal	
2 Extension, rigidity	2 Extension, rigidity	
1 No response	1 No response	
Best Verbal Response		
Birth to 1 Year	**1 to 5 Years**	**Older Than 5 Years**
5 Babbles, coos appropriately	5 Age-appropriate words, phrases	5 Oriented and converses
4 Cries, but consolable	4 Confusion, inappropriate words, phrases (for age)	4 Confused or disoriented conversation
3 Inconsolable crying	3 Cries, screams	3 Inappropriate words
2 Grunts	2 Grunts	2 Incomprehensible sounds
1 No response	1 No response	1 No response

Modified from Roskind et al: Acute care of the victim of multiple trauma. In Kleigman RM et al, editors: *Nelson textbook of pediatrics*, ed 20, St Louis, 2016, Elsevier; American Heart Association (AHA): *Pediatric advanced life support*, Dallas, 2016, AHA.

BOX 26.9
Estimating Blood Pressure (BP) for the Pediatric Patient

Systolic BP (mm Hg) = (2 × age in years) + 80

Diastolic BP (mm Hg) = ⅔ systolic BP

of instrumentation required. Pediatric trauma instrument sets, including vascular clamps and retractors, and suture supplies should be available and organized in a fashion that promotes easy and timely access when urgent situations arise. Creative problem-solving may be required of the perioperative nurse in adaptation of feeding tubes, drains, and other equipment.

Maintenance of body temperature is of utmost concern in the pediatric population, and undue skin exposure should be avoided. Fluids for irrigation and IV infusion should be warmed, and whenever possible, room temperature is elevated. Warming devices and head coverings and hats may be used to prevent heat loss; this is especially critical with children who have sustained burns.

Traumas are graded based on the severity of injury (Table 26.7). The perioperative nurse should attempt to obtain a trauma history from ED personnel or the family if the patient comes directly to the OR. Initial vital signs should be obtained and compared with those obtained during prehospital care or in the ED; Box 26.9 gives a formula for blood pressure estimation. When obtaining the initial

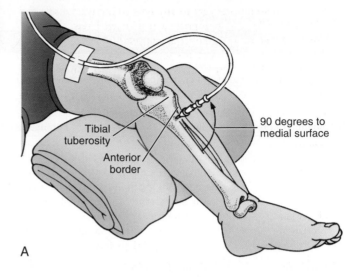

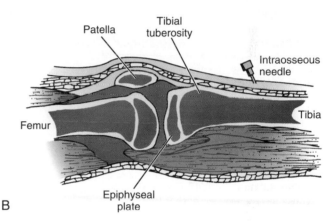

FIG. 26.55 (A) Intraosseous infusion technique. (B) Insertion.

assessment it is important to use a developmental approach to pediatric trauma patients, who respond differently from adults. During traumatic events it is also imperative to consider the well-being of patients, families, and caregivers. The perioperative nurse plays an integral role in preparing those associated with the child for outcomes associated with trauma surgery and may help facilitate consults from the departments of child life, social work, and clergy.

Airway and breathing are part of the primary survey for pediatric trauma victims. Anatomic variations of the upper airway related to age must be considered. Airway patency must be assessed and secured. Initial assessment for all pediatric trauma patients may best be obtained by application of the head tilt–chin lift or jaw-thrust method, depending on the age of the child and the nature of the injury. When the integrity of the spinal cord is questionable, in-line cervical traction should be applied. Collars and stabilizing devices must remain in place until cervical fracture has been ruled out and the spine declared free of injury by a radiologist. Airway equipment sizes may be selected based on age as well as whether the child is breathing spontaneously and whether the child is unconscious. An assessment of relevant systems will be performed on stabilization of the pediatric airway, and surgery will progress as planned.

Surgery for Congenital Heart Disease

Congenital heart disease (CHD) occurs in approximately 5 to 8 of every 1000 live births. Structural abnormalities of the heart and

Medications Used in Pediatric Resuscitation

Perioperative nurses must always be prepared in the event of a compromising cardiac or respiratory event in the pediatric patient. The information contained in this section provides several commonly used medications, their mode of action, and nursing implications for pediatric resuscitation.

Medication/Category	Dosage/Route for Infants and Children	Purpose/Action	Adverse Reactions	Nursing Implications
Adenosine Pharmacotherapeutic: Antiarrhythmic	IV: 0.1 mg/kg If not effective, give 0.2 mg/kg Do not exceed 6 mg in first dose and 12 mg in successive doses	Treatment of PSVT	• AV block, chest pain, facial flushing, hypotension • Dizziness, headache • GI discomfort, nausea • Dyspnea • Diaphoresis • Asystole, atrial fibrillation, bradycardia, bronchospasm (rare, but life-threatening)	Possible exacerbation of asthma in asthmatic patients Follow by rapid saline flush
Amiodarone Pharmacotherapeutic: Antiarrhythmic	IV bolus/IO: 5 mg/kg	Pulseless ventricular fibrillation or ventricular tachycardia	• AV block, bradycardia, cardiac arrhythmia, edema, hypotension • Dizziness, headache • Slate-blue skin discoloration • Abdominal pain, abnormal salivation • Coagulation abnormalities • Phlebitis with concentrations greater than 3 mg/mL • Acute intracranial hypertension, acute renal failure, acute respiratory distress syndrome (rare, but life-threatening)	Administer slowly in patients with diminished cardiac function
Atropine sulfate Pharmacotherapeutic: Antiasthmatic/ anticholinergic	IV/IT: 0.02 mg/kg, minimum dose 0.1 mg, maximum single dose 0.5 mg in children and 1 mg in adolescents May repeat in 5-min intervals to a maximum of 1 mg in children or 2 mg in adolescents	Treatment of sinus bradycardia	• Arrhythmia, hypotension, tachycardia • Ataxia, coma, disorientation • Urticaria • Delayed gastric emptying, nausea • Urinary retention • Weakness • Dyspnea, laryngospasm, pulmonary edema • Anaphylaxis	Monitor heart rate
Calcium gluconate Pharmacotherapeutic: Electrolyte supplement	IV: 30–100 mg/kg	Treatment of cardiac disturbances of hypocalcemia	• Arrhythmia, bradycardia, cardiac arrest, hypotension, syncope, vasodilation • Hypercalcemia • Tingling sensation	Contraindicated in ventricular fibrillation during cardiac resuscitation
Epinephrine Pharmacotherapeutic: Adrenergic agonist agent	IV/IO: 0.01 mg/kg of 1:10,000 solution, maximum single dose 1 mg ETT: 0.1 mg/kg of 1:1000 solution, maximum single dose of 2.5 mg Repeat every 3–5 min as needed to a maximum total dose of 10 mg	Treatment of bradycardia, asystole, or pulseless arrest	• Cardiac arrhythmia, chest pain, flushing, hypertension • Cerebral hemorrhage, restlessness • Nausea and vomiting • Dyspnea, pulmonary edema • Diaphoresis	Protect drug from light (do not use discolored or precipitated solutions); unstable in alkaline solution Most useful drug during cardiac arrest

SURGICAL PHARMACOLOGY

Medications Used in Pediatric Resuscitation—cont'd

Medication/Category	Dosage/Route for Infants and Children	Purpose/Action	Adverse Reactions	Nursing Implications
Lidocaine Pharmacotherapeutic: Antiarrhythmic agent	IV/IO/ETT: Loading dose 1 mg/kg May repeat in 10–15 min times two doses After loading dose, start IV continuous infusion 20–50 mcg/kg/min Use 20 mcg/kg in patients with shock, hepatic disease, cardiac arrest, or mild congestive heart failure	Treatment of ventricular arrhythmias from myocardial infarction or cardiac manipulation	• Bradycardia, hypotension, arrhythmias • Agitation, lethargy, seizures • Nausea and vomiting • Thrombophlebitis • Muscle twitching, paresthesias • Dyspnea, respiratory depression or arrest	For ETT administration, dilute with 1–2 mL normal saline before ETT administration
Sodium bicarbonate Pharmacotherapeutic: Alkalizing agent	IV push: 1 mEq/kg initially, may repeat with 0.5 mEq/kg in 10 min once as indicated by acid-base status Rate of administration should not exceed 10 mEq/min	Management of metabolic acidosis or life-threatening hyperkalemia	• Cerebral hemorrhage, edema • Tetany • Gastric distention • Hypernatremia, hypocalcemia, hypokalemia • Pulmonary edema	Patient should be adequately ventilated before administering sodium bicarbonate in cardiac arrest

AV, Atrioventricular; *ETT,* endotracheal tube; *GI,* gastrointestinal; *IO,* intraosseous; *IT,* intratracheal; *IV,* intravenous; *kg,* kilogram; *mEq,* milliequivalent; *PSVT,* paroxysmal supraventricular tachycardia.
Modified from the *Children's Hospital of Philadelphia emergency medication dosing book,* Philadelphia, 2016, Children's Hospital of Philadelphia.

TABLE 26.7
Trauma Grading

Level	Physiologic Considerations	Anatomic Considerations
Level I: Life-threatening injuries, unstable vital signs	Respiratory distress Artificial airway/unstable airway Cardiac arrest Hemodynamic instability Severe uncontrolled hemorrhage SBP less than 80 mm Hg that does not respond to fluid resuscitation GCS score <8 Lateralizing neurologic signs or worsening neurologic exam	Airway compromise Severe maxillofacial trauma Major vascular injury including significant crush or amputation above the elbow or knee with a high probability of operative intervention Significant penetrating injury to the head, neck, or torso Burns ≥25% total body surface area with or without inhalation injury Spinal cord injury with neurologic signs or symptoms Unstable vertebral fractures
Level II: Potentially life-threatening injuries, hemodynamically stable	GCS ≥9 and ≤13 Hypotension before transport, resolved during transport Transient neurologic changes	Blunt abdominal trauma with abnormal exam Blunt chest trauma with ≥2 rib fractures Significant penetrating trauma to upper extremities or distal to groin Significant crush or amputation distal to elbow or knee with high probability of operative intervention

GCS, Glasgow Coma Scale; *SBP,* systolic blood pressure.
Modified from Children's Hospital of Philadelphia: *2014–2015 Trauma program resident/fellow manual,* Philadelphia.

great vessels result in an embryologic failure in septation, malalignment, failure to develop, or failure to progress.

The etiology of CHD varies, although certain factors are associated with increased prevalence. For example, risk of CHD is increased secondary to environmental factors: rubella during the first 8 weeks of gestation may result in PDA and pulmonary artery stenosis. Other risk factors include maternal chronic illnesses such as diabetes or poorly controlled phenylketonuria (PKU), alcohol consumption, and exposure to environmental toxins. The incidence of CHD is also increased in certain chromosomal defects; for example, atrial septal defects (ASDs) are seen in children with trisomy 21 (Down syndrome). In addition, an increased prevalence is seen in small-for-gestational-age (SGA) babies and in children who have a positive family history of CHD.

Congenital cardiac abnormalities are classified as cyanotic or acyanotic as well as by their effect on pulmonary blood flow (Box 26.10). Of the acyanotic lesions, there are those that increase pulmonary blood flow, such as PDA, ASD, ventricular septal defect

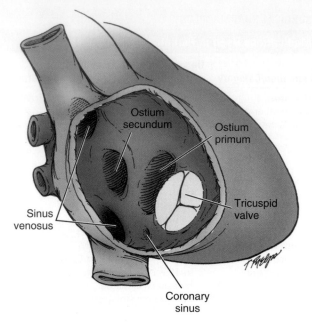

FIG. 26.56 Various types of atrial septal defects (ASDs) viewed through the right atrium (ostium secundum, ostium primum, sinus venosus). An unroofed coronary sinus may also act as an ASD.

(VSD), and atrioventricular canal (AVC) defects. With these abnormalities, blood flows from the high-pressure left side of the heart to the low-pressure right side of the heart because of an abnormal connection either between the septum or in the great arteries. The resultant increase in pulmonary blood flow causes the right side of the heart and lungs to become overloaded. HF may develop, pulmonary vascular resistance (PVR) may increase, and the pulmonary vessel walls may thicken; if left untreated, the condition may become irreversible.

Acyanotic obstructive lesions, such as AS, pulmonary stenosis, or coarctation of the aorta, increase the workload of the chamber that pumps against the obstruction (increases afterload). Cardiomegaly and ventricular hypertrophy may be seen in response to the increased workload, and if the obstruction is severe, HF may ensue.

The presence of cyanosis implies that one of the following conditions is present: right-sided heart obstruction with blood traveling right to left without passing through the lungs, mixing of venous and arterial blood within the heart or great vessels, or incorrect positioning of the great vessels. The degree of cyanosis depends on pulmonary blood flow and intracardiac mixing of blood through a shunt. This classification of lesions includes, but is not limited to, tetralogy of Fallot (TOF), pulmonary atresia with intact ventricular septum (PA/IVS), tricuspid atresia (TA), transposition of the great arteries (TGA), total anomalous pulmonary venous return (TAPVR), and HLHS. Treatment goals for these lesions include managing pulmonary blood flow or arterial oxygen saturation.

Repair of Atrial Septal Defect

ASDs are one of the most common forms of CHD. The classification within this group of defects is based on anatomic location and associated abnormalities (Fig. 26.56). The ostium secundum defect is located in the superior and central portions of the septum. The ostium primum defect is located in the lower portion of the atrial septum and is associated with other defects in the AVC, usually with a cleft of the mitral valve or occasionally of the tricuspid valve. An accompanying VSD may also be present. The sinus venosus defect is located at the right atrium–superior vena cava (SVC) junction and is associated with partial anomalous pulmonary venous return.

An ASD results in a left-to-right atrial shunt whose direction and magnitude are determined by the size of the defect and relative resistance to flow into the ventricles and great vessels (Fig. 26.57). ASDs are often tolerated well with no symptoms during childhood, especially if the defect is small. However, if the defect is large or of the ostium primum type, with a pronounced shunting of blood, the workload of the right side of the heart is increased. On assessment, there is a characteristic systolic pulmonary murmur at the second intercostal space at the left sternal border; a fixed splitting of the second heart sound also may be heard. The right side of the heart and the pulmonary artery and its branches become enlarged. The vascularity of the lung field is increased, with resulting pulmonary hypertension and subsequent failure of the right side of the heart. At this point the shunt may reverse. The initial symptoms may include fatigue, retardation of normal weight gain, and increased susceptibility to respiratory tract infections. Later signs and symptoms include those of failure of the right side of the heart and cyanosis with a reverse shunt. Asymptomatic children whose ASD is left unrepaired until adulthood may develop right atrial and right ventricular hypertrophy (RVH), atrial dysrhythmias, HF, embolic events, and pulmonary vascular disease. The defect is common in children with Down syndrome.

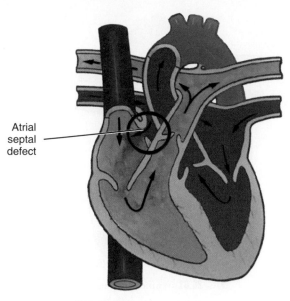

FIG. 26.57 Atrial septal defect.

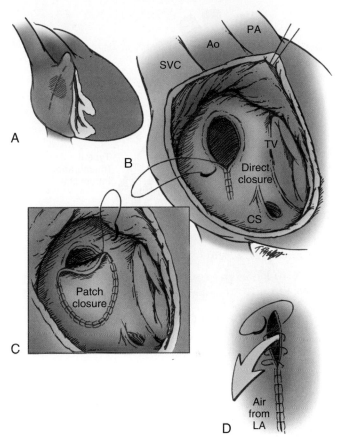

FIG. 26.58 Surgical procedure for atrial septal defect (ASD) closure. (A) Incision through right atriotomy. Direct suture closure (B) and patch closure (C) of secundum ASD. (D) De-airing of the left atrium. *Ao,* Aorta; *CS,* conduction system; *LA,* left atrium; *PA,* pulmonary artery; *SVC,* superior vena cava; *TV,* tricuspid valve.

Procedural Considerations

ASDs are closed, under direct vision, by a simple suture technique (primary closure) or by insertion of a synthetic prosthetic patch or pericardial patch.

The child is placed in the supine position for a median sternotomy or in a right anterior oblique position for an anterolateral thoracotomy. The instrument setup is the same as that described for basic open-heart surgery (see Chapter 25), with consideration given to the age and size of the child; intracardiac patch material, 2 × 2 inches or larger, also may be required.

Operative Procedure

1. The surgeon opens the chest with a median sternotomy incision and institutes cardiopulmonary bypass (CPB) (Fig. 26.58). (Infrequently, a right anterolateral incision is performed.) Many bypass strategies can be used. With bicaval cannulation, the child remains on bypass during the repair and blood is directed away from the right atrium through cannulae in the superior and inferior venae cavae. Occasionally with this method the cannulae may obstruct the view of the ASD. With single venous cannulation, a cannula is placed into the right atrium and the child remains on bypass during the repair. With this technique the venous line is clamped immediately before the right atrium is incised and pump suctions are placed into the inferior and superior venae cavae during ASD closure. Deep hypothermic circulatory arrest is sometimes used in more complicated repairs, such as ostium primum ASD or sinus venosus defects associated with anomalous pulmonary venous return.
2. The right atrium is incised, and the pathologic defect is determined.
3. The defect is closed with a continuous suture, or a patch of pericardium or prosthetic material may be used. By filling the atrium with blood before the atriotomy is completely closed, the surgeon can express air from the atrium. For the ostium primum defect with a cleft mitral valve, repair of the cleft is accomplished by approximation, with use of interrupted sutures.

Repair of Ventricular Septal Defect

One of the most common congenital cardiac anomalies, VSDs (Fig. 26.59) occur in approximately 2% to 7% of live births. Most VSDs are small with little physiologic importance. As with ASDs, the classification of VSDs depends on location and associated lesions (Fig. 26.60). Perimembranous VSDs (also called conoventricular, subaortic, infracristal, or membranous) are most commonly found. These defects occur directly adjacent to the membranous septum and the fibrous trigone of the heart, where the aortic, mitral, and tricuspid valves are in fibrous continuity. The tricuspid valve tissue sometimes forms an aneurysm of the membranous septum, which may be a mechanism of defect closure for this type of defect. Subpulmonary VSDs (also referred to as supracristal, infundibular, intracristal, outlet, conoseptal, or conal) are located above the crista supraventricularis within the outlet septum and border the semilunar valves. Muscular-type VSDs can be located anywhere in the muscular septum, including apical, anterior, or posterior, or in the midseptum inlet and outlet. Malalignment-type VSDs are created by a malalignment between the infundibular septum and the trabecular muscular septum. Canal-type or inlet defects are located posteriorly within the area confined by the tricuspid valve septal leaflet papillary muscles. The defect borders the tricuspid valve annulus.

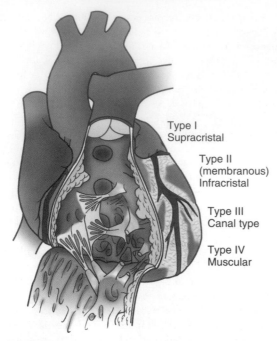

FIG. 26.59 Ventricular septal defects: anatomic classification.

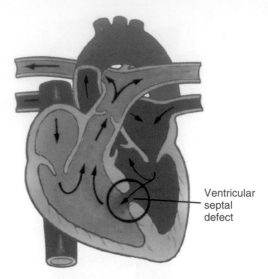

FIG. 26.61 Ventricular septal defect.

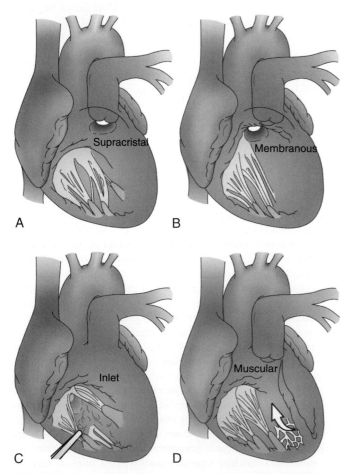

FIG. 26.60 Various types of ventricular septal defects viewed within the right ventricle. (A) Infundibular (supracristal). (B) Membranous. (C) Inlet (atrioventricular canal). (D) Muscular (trabecular).

The hemodynamics depend on the size and location of the defect as well as the PVR and systemic vascular resistance (SVR). Newborns are often asymptomatic until the PVR decreases and a left-to-right shunt occurs, and the corresponding murmur is auscultated. Small defects with moderate shunt and increased pulmonary blood flow but not increased pulmonary pressure may not produce any symptoms. A large VSD, however, may produce high pulmonary flow under high pressure and contribute to congestive heart failure (CHF). In this case the patient is at risk of developing pulmonary hypertension (Fig. 26.61). Surgical closure of the defect should be performed to prevent increased pulmonary hypertension. If PVR further increases and rises above SVR, shunt reversal (Eisenmenger syndrome, or shunting from right to left) and cyanosis may occur.

Operative Procedure

Under direct vision a congenital defect in the ventricular septum (Fig. 26.62) is closed by a simple suture technique or, in most instances, by insertion of a synthetic prosthetic or pericardial patch.
1. A median sternotomy is performed, and CPB is instituted.
2. The location of the defect determines the location of the incision. For membranous and canal defects, an incision is usually made in the right atrium, the atrium is retracted, and the VSD is identified by use of a pump suction through the tricuspid valve into the right ventricle. For supracristal VSDs, an incision is usually made in the pulmonary artery and may be extended into the right ventricle. A muscular VSD may require a ventriculotomy.
3. A patch (synthetic or pericardium) is most frequently used to close the defect. To place the patch, the surgeon uses a continuous 6-0 or 5-0 nonabsorbable suture on a small needle or an interrupted suture with or without pledgets. Rarely is the defect closed primarily.
4. CPB is discontinued, and the sternum is closed.

Correction of Tetralogy of Fallot

TOF, described initially in the early 19th century, includes the association of four anatomic findings: VSD, subpulmonic stenosis, aortic override of the ventricular septum, and RVH (Fig. 26.63). Occurring in approximately 10% of congenital heart defects, TOF is actually the result of a single anatomic abnormality: anterior malalignment of the infundibular septum with the muscular septum.

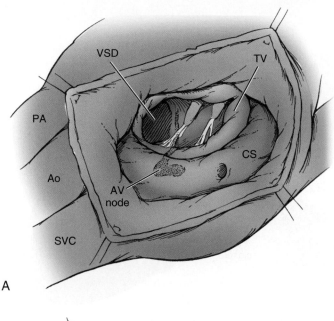

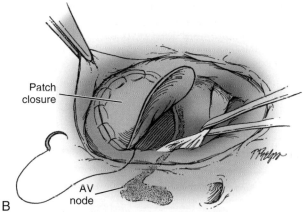

FIG. 26.62 Ventricular septal defect *(VSD)* closure through the tricuspid valve *(TV)*. (A) Open site. (B) Partial closure. *Ao*, Aorta; *AV*, atrioventricular; *CS*, conduction system; *PA*, pulmonary artery; *SVC*, superior vena cava.

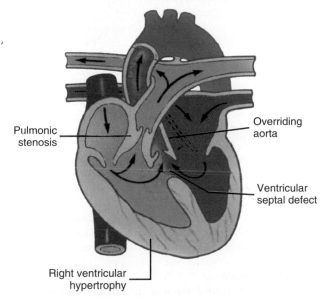

FIG. 26.63 Tetralogy of Fallot.

The preoperative hemodynamics or physiology depends mainly on the degree of pulmonary stenosis. In patients with minimal obstruction to pulmonary blood flow, the physiology is similar to that of a VSD with left-to-right shunting. These patients have pulmonary overcirculation and symptoms of HF. Occasionally labeled as "pink tetralogy" or "pink tets," these patients have little to no right-to-left shunting and do not exhibit cyanosis.

At the other end of the spectrum of this particular type of heart defect are children with severe pulmonary stenosis, who may have significant right-to-left shunting at the VSD level and exhibit hypoxemia with oxygen saturations in the 60% to 80% range. Cyanosis, as seen in the superficial vessels of the skin, is the result of shunting unoxygenated blood into the systemic circulation. Other clinical manifestations may include episodes of acute dyspnea with cyanosis, retarded growth, clubbing of extremities, reduced exercise tolerance, and increased prevalence of "tet," or hypercyanotic spells. A systolic murmur and secondary polycythemia are usually present in the cyanotic child. Echocardiography is performed to confirm the diagnosis of TOF; occasionally a cardiac catheterization and angiography may be necessary in delineating other anatomic abnormalities, such as with the coronary arteries, before surgical repair.

The selection of a palliative or corrective procedure is based on the age and general condition of the child and the severity of the pulmonary stenosis. The treatment of choice is primary repair; contraindications for primary repair include anomalous origin of the anterior descending coronary artery and presence of pulmonary atresia. Complete or primary repair consists of closure of the VSD and repair of the pulmonic stenosis under direct vision.

Procedural Considerations

The team positions the child on the OR bed in supine position. The setup is the same as that described for open-heart surgery, with consideration given to the child's age and size. Additional items to be added to the basic open-heart setup include the following: intracardiac patch, 2 × 2 inches; outflow cardiac patch, 2 × 2 inches; and a felt or polytetrafluoroethylene (PTFE) patch, 4 × 4 inches.

Operative Procedure

1. A median sternotomy is performed, and CPB with hypothermia is instituted.
2. A vertical ventriculotomy over the infundibular area may be performed (Fig. 26.64A).
3. The surgeon identifies the VSD. Closure requires an intracardiac patch in almost all instances. This can be of a synthetic material or a piece of pericardium.
4. Interrupted or continuous cardiovascular sutures are placed in the septum with caution because of the danger of suturing a branch of the neuroconductive system.
5. The surgeon excises the hypertrophied infundibular muscle as completely as possible, from the right ventricular outflow tract. If the pulmonic valve is stenosed, the fused commissures are incised.
6. An estimate is made about whether the right ventricle can be closed primarily or if a patch is necessary. If the pulmonic stenosis cannot be relieved adequately by valvulotomy and infundibulectomy, an outflow patch of synthetic material or pulmonary homograft tissue may be needed to enlarge the outflow tract (see Fig. 26.64B). If the pulmonary artery or valve annulus is small, it may be necessary to extend the patch across the valve ring to the proximal portion of the pulmonary artery (see Fig. 26.64C).
7. CPB is discontinued, and the sternum is closed.

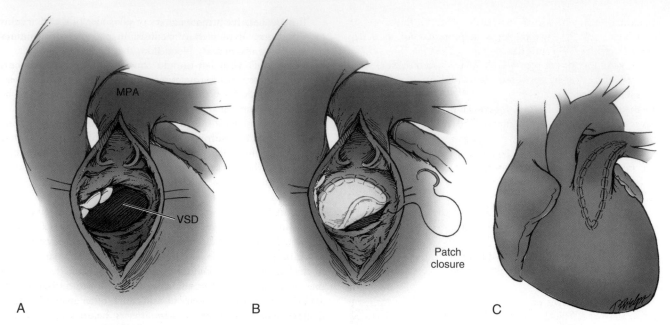

FIG. 26.64 (A) The most common ventricular incision used for repair of tetralogy of Fallot is vertical so that it can be extended as shown from the right ventricle across the pulmonary valve annulus and onto the main pulmonary artery *(MPA)*. It is possible to gain adequate exposure to the ventricular septal defect *(VSD)* by extending the incision a short distance beyond the infundibular septum. This "limited ventriculotomy" may help preserve late right ventricular function yet enable adequate enlargement of the hypoplastic area in the right ventricular outflow tract. (B) The VSD is closed with a prosthetic patch. Right ventricular outflow obstruction is relieved when the outflow tract is enlarged with a patch as shown. (C) In some cases it may be necessary to extend the incision onto the left pulmonary artery and to taper the patch at its most distal extent.

Closure of Patent Ductus Arteriosus

PDA occurs because of persistence of the fetal ductus arteriosus, which connects the pulmonary artery to the aorta. The condition is common in premature infants. In fetal life, blood bypasses the lungs, traveling directly to the systemic circulation through the PDA. This vessel normally closes shortly after birth as a result of the onset of respiration causing an increase in PaO_2 level and the release of circulating humoral substances. However, if this does not occur, the ductus arteriosus remains open (Fig. 26.65), creating a shunt from the aorta through the ductus into the pulmonary circulation. This increases the workload of the heart and causes subsequent enlargement and hypertrophy of the left atrium and ventricle. However, when persistent patency of the ductus is associated with other malformations such as TOF and extreme stenosis of the pulmonary orifice, it is a means of maintaining life. Surgery is not performed if the PDA is serving in a compensatory capacity.

Many children have few symptoms because of the small size of the shunt. A frequent clinical sign associated with this condition is a harsh, continuous murmur. Because the blood passing through the shunt is oxygenated, there is no cyanosis, clubbing, or reduction in peripheral arterial oxygen saturation. However, growth is retarded in children who have a large ductus. Other signs and symptoms may include dyspnea, frequent upper respiratory tract infections, palpitations, limited exercise tolerance, and cardiac failure.

Procedural Considerations

Closure of the PDA is achieved by suture ligation or by division of the ductus. For newborns, the surgeon and anesthesia provider may elect to perform this procedure in the intensive care nursery bed because the operation is short. However, after the newborn period,

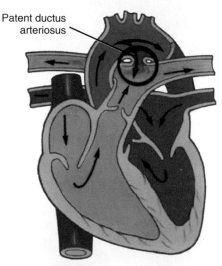

FIG. 26.65 Patent ductus arteriosus.

the surgery is done in the OR. The child is placed in a right lateral position. The setup is the same as that described for open-heart surgery, but with special patent ductus clamps and without items for CPB. Generally a left posterolateral approach is used; in some cases, however, a left anterolateral approach is used.

Operative Procedure

1. The incision is carried through the muscles over the fourth interspace. The chest wall is entered through the third or fourth

intercostal space, with use of items as described for thoracotomy (see Chapter 23). The wound edges are protected and retracted with a Finochietto rib spreader.

2. The surgeon incises the pleura with Metzenbaum scissors, and the left lung is protected and retracted with a moist pack and a malleable retractor.

3. The mediastinal pleura is opened between the phrenic and vagus nerves over the region of the ductus. The pleura is retracted by insertion of stay sutures. The recurrent laryngeal nerve is identified and protected. The aortic arch and pulmonary artery are dissected with fine scissors and dry dissectors. Fine arterial branches are divided and ligated with curved Crile or mosquito hemostats and nonabsorbable ligatures and cardiac suture ligatures.

4. The parietal pleura overlying the ductus is dissected with fine vascular forceps and scissors. Stay sutures may be inserted to facilitate retraction.

5. The surgeon dissects the adventitial layer of the ductus. A small portion of the obscure posterior ductus is carefully freed to admit a right-angle clamp.

6. The final step is performed in one of the following ways:
   a. For the suture-ligation method (Fig. 26.66A), two ligatures are placed around the ductus, one near the aorta and the other near the pulmonary artery side, both of which are tied in place. Between these two ligatures, two transfixion sutures may be inserted.
   b. For the division of the ductus method, the patent ductus clamps are applied as close to the aorta and pulmonary artery as possible. The ductus is divided halfway through and partially sutured with mattress cardiovascular sutures and continued back over the free edge with an over-and-over whip suture (see Fig. 26.66B). After both openings are sutured, a sponge is held on the area for compression while the patent ductus clamps are removed.

Repair of Hypoplastic Heart Syndromes

Hypoplastic heart syndromes can occur on both the left and right sides. Patients with hypoplastic right heart syndrome (HRHS) who fall on the milder end of the spectrum may respond. In premature infants only a hemoclip may be applied to the ductus because of the friable nature of the ductal tissue to biventricular repair, whereas those with more severe hypoplasia are managed with univentricular palliation or transplantation. Because HLHS (Fig. 26.67) is one of the most common forms of single ventricle malformation, it is described in further detail.

HLHS describes a range of congenital cardiac malformations that have in common underdevelopment of the left-sided heart structures, which include aortic valve atresia and stenosis with associated hypoplasia or absence of the left ventricle. The ascending aorta and arch are usually only a few millimeters in diameter and are functionally a branch of the ductus arteriosus–thoracic aorta continuum, with blood flowing retrograde through the aortic arch and into the small ascending aorta to the coronary arteries. Mitral valve atresia or stenosis also is present. Survival in the newborn period depends on a PDA to maintain systemic circulation; therefore these infants are maintained on an infusion of prostaglandin E_1 (PGE_1) to maintain ductal patency before surgical intervention.

Newborns with HLHS typically present with cyanosis, respiratory distress, and variable degrees of circulatory collapse during the first few days of life. If left untreated, a majority of these neonates will die within the first month of life; without surgical intervention, HLHS is fatal.

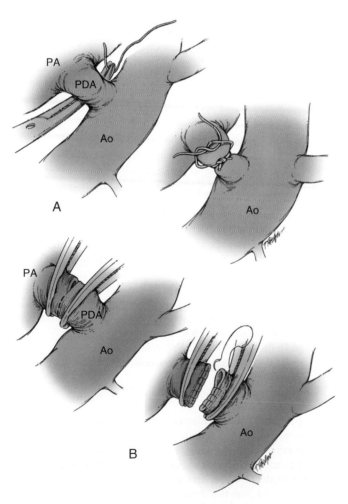

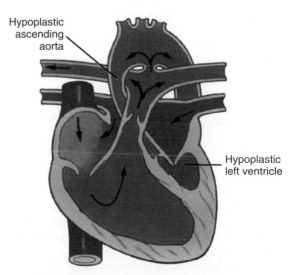

FIG. 26.66 Surgical correction of patent ductus arteriosus *(PDA)*. (A) Ligation of ductus arteriosus. (B) Division of ductus arteriosus. *Ao,* Aorta; *PA,* pulmonary artery.

FIG. 26.67 Hypoplastic left-sided heart syndrome.

It was not until the development of the Fontan procedure, a surgical correction for another form of single ventricle malformation (TA), that long-term survival in patients with HLHS was considered possible. However, because of the neonate's high PVR, the Fontan procedure is not a surgical option in the newborn period. A palliative repair (stage I) was developed in the late 1970s by Norwood to prepare the heart for the Fontan procedure.

Two surgical options for patients with HLHS exist: a series of reconstructive procedures or heart transplantation. The series of reconstructive procedures usually involves three stages. Stage I is performed during the newborn period. The goals of stage I are to (1) maintain systemic perfusion, (2) preserve the function of the only ventricle, and (3) allow normal maturation of the pulmonary ventricle. The first goal is met by creating unobstructed communication between the right ventricle and the systemic circulation. This is accomplished by transecting the main pulmonary artery and creating a neoaorta from the main pulmonary artery, native aorta, and pulmonary homograft tissue. The other two goals are met by creating a right modified Blalock-Taussig (BT) shunt and a nonrestrictive interatrial communication. These measures allow for adequate pulmonary blood flow and for the PVR to decrease as the child grows while the volume interposed on the single ventricle is limited.

The modified Fontan procedure was initially performed on a child at approximately 18 months of age. However, since 1989 a staged approach to the Fontan procedure has been undertaken to minimize the effect of rapid changes in ventricular configuration and diastolic function that can be associated with a primary Fontan procedure and its accompanying postoperative complications. In the stage II procedure (hemi-Fontan or the bidirectional Glenn shunt), SVC blood flow is directed to the lungs, and inferior vena cava (IVC) blood flow continues to flow to the right ventricle. The third and final stage, the modified Fontan procedure, separates the systemic and pulmonary circulations. These same procedures can be performed for patients with HRHS.

Procedural Considerations

Additional items for the open-heart setup include the following:
- Stage I: PTFE tube graft, 3.5 or 4 mm, and pulmonary homograft tissue
- Stage II: Oscillating saw and pulmonary homograft tissue
- Stage III: Oscillating saw and PTFE tube graft, 10 mm; a greater than usual supply of blood should be available

Operative Procedure

Stage I (Norwood Procedure)

1. The surgeon opens the chest with a median sternotomy incision (Fig. 26.68). The aortic cannula is placed into the main pulmonary artery rather than the diminutive aorta, and the venous cannula is placed into the right atrium. CPB is instituted, and the right and left pulmonary arteries are immediately occluded with tourniquets to force the blood through the ductus arteriosus to the systemic circulation.
2. When deep hypothermic circulatory arrest is about to be instituted, the innominate and left carotid arteries are occluded with tourniquets. The venous and aortic cannulae are removed.
3. The septum primum is excised through the venous cannulation site; occasionally a right atriotomy is necessary to facilitate the atrial septectomy.
4. The main pulmonary artery is transected immediately before the bifurcation of the right and left pulmonary arteries.

5. The surgeon closes the distal pulmonary artery with a small patch of homograft tissue.
6. The ductus arteriosus is then exposed and closed using a 2-0 nonabsorbable tie. The tie is left long to better expose the thoracic aorta. The ductus is transected.
7. At the point in which the ductus was attached to the aorta, the thoracic aorta is opened 1 to 2 cm, and the aortic arch and ascending aorta are opened to a point adjacent to the main pulmonary artery.
8. A gusset of homograft tissue is joined to the aorta starting at the thoracic end, and the pulmonary artery is incorporated at the proximal end of the ascending aorta. A continuous monofilament suture is used. Occasionally interrupted sutures are used to attach the main pulmonary artery to the aorta.
9. To perform a right BT shunt, the innominate artery is cross-clamped and incised and a 3.5-mm or 4-mm PTFE tube graft is interposed.
10. CPB is instituted, and the pulmonary end of the shunt is performed by incising the pulmonary artery and interposing the distal end of the tube graft.
11. Immediately after the shunt is completed, the surgeon occludes it with a bulldog clamp until termination of bypass.

Stage II (Hemi-Fontan Procedure)

1. The surgeon opens the previous chest incision using an oscillating saw to create the sternotomy (Fig. 26.69). An oscillating saw is used for safety because it allows the surgeon to gradually cut through the sternum and avoid any adhesions that may be present from the previous surgery.
2. The aorta, right atrium, and right BT shunt are exposed.
3. CPB is instituted, and the shunt is immediately occluded with a clip.
4. The surgeon exposes the branch pulmonary arteries.
5. Depending on the surgeon's preference, deep hypothermic circulatory arrest may be instituted.
6. The surgeon makes an incision in the confluence of the pulmonary arteries, extending to the pericardial reflections. A second incision is made in the dome of the right atrium, extending to the SVC.
7. The surgeon anastomoses the pulmonary artery to the SVC-right atrial junction.
8. The pulmonary arteries are augmented with a gusset of homograft tissue. In the hemi-Fontan procedure part of the homograft tissue is incorporated intra-atrially as a dam between the common atrium and the vena cava-pulmonary artery anastomosis. In the Glenn shunt, there is no intra-atrial incorporation.
9. CPB is reinstituted until the patient is normothermic. CPB is then discontinued, and chest closure is completed.

Stage III (Modified Fontan Procedure)

1. A median sternotomy is performed with an oscillating saw (Fig. 26.70).
2. The surgeon exposes the aorta and right atrium.
3. CPB is instituted.
4. Deep hypothermic circulatory arrest may be used.
5. A lateral incision is made in the right atrium.
6. A 10-mm PTFE tube graft is cut in half lengthwise and placed intra-atrially by suturing the inferior end of the graft around the orifice of the IVC and up the right lateral free wall of the right atrium to the superior dome of the right atrium. This creates a tunnel in which the inferior blood flow is directed to the pulmonary arteries. The SVC blood flow was directed to the pulmonary arteries during the stage II repair. (The surgeon may

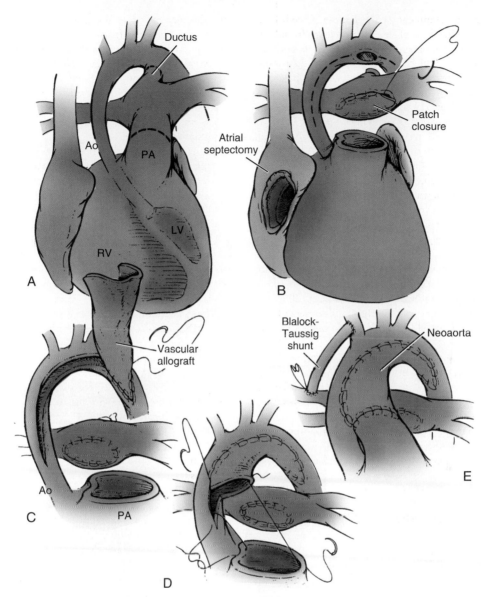

FIG. 26.68 Stage I Norwood procedure. (A) Transection points of the main pulmonary artery *(PA)* and ductus arteriosus. (B) Atrial septectomy to avoid pulmonary venous hypertension. Patch closure of the distal main PA. Division and ligation of the ductus arteriosus. (C and D) Construction of a "neoaorta" with use of the proximal main PA, diminutive ascending aorta, and vascular allograft. (E) Pulmonary blood flow supplied by a right modified Blalock-Taussig shunt connecting the right subclavian artery to the right PA. *Ao,* Aorta; *LV,* left ventricle; *RV,* right ventricle.

perform variations on this procedure, such as excluding a hepatic vein or performing a fenestrated Fontan by making a series of small openings in the PTFE tube graft or a single 4-mm opening with an aortic punch in the graft material.)

7. The atria are closed, and CPB is reinstituted until the patient is normothermic. CPB is then discontinued, and chest closure is completed.

Extracorporeal Membrane Oxygenation

ECMO is a therapy used on pediatric patients who have reversible pulmonary or cardiac disease. Many patients are neonates with respiratory disease syndrome (RDS), persistent pulmonary hyperten-

sion (PPH), meconium aspiration (MA), or CDH requiring adequate tissue oxygenation and waste removal from the body. In the cardiac patient it also may be used as a bridge to heart or lung transplantation until donor organs are available (Pellegrino, 2014). Adolescents and teenagers present with a larger variety of diagnoses necessitating ECMO treatment. These include respiratory causes such as pneumonia, status asthmaticus, acute respiratory distress syndrome (ARDS), near drowning, acute chest syndrome, and posttraumatic lung injury (Gehrmann et al., 2015). To perform ECMO, a facility must have an established ECMO service.

Most of the time patients are placed on ECMO in an ICU setting or in the ED during a resuscitative event. For venoarterial ECMO

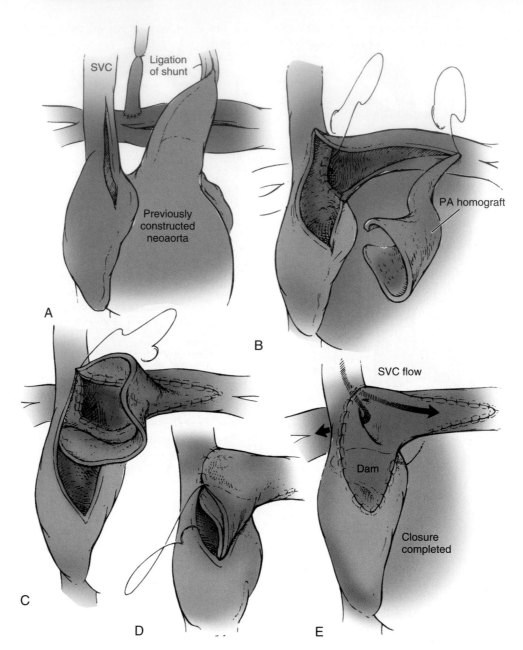

FIG. 26.69 Hemi-Fontan procedure in a patient with hypoplastic left-sided heart syndrome. (A and B) Ligation of the systemic-to-pulmonary artery shunt and side-to-side anastomosis of the superior vena cava *(SVC)* to the confluence of the pulmonary artery *(PA)* with allograft augmentation. (C–E) Placement of a dam to close the junction of the atrium with the SVC so that saturated pulmonary venous blood mixes in the common atrium with desaturated blood draining from the inferior vena cava. Pulmonary blood flow is supplied exclusively through the SVC.

the surgical approach is usually through the right carotid artery and internal jugular vein. This is the preferred treatment for conditions needing cardiac support. For the cardiac patient after surgical repair, cannulation of the carotid artery and jugular vein provides good venous drainage of the right atrium, and the incision site is remote from the sternotomy wound. However, the surgeon may choose to reopen the sternum on postoperative patients and cannulate the aorta and right atrium. Per Pellegrino (2014), veno-venous ECMO is the ECMO mode used for conditions that require respiratory support. Blood is removed from the great veins and returned to the right atrium, and the patient's native circulation is powered entirely by the heart. In the OR, for a patient who cannot be successfully weaned from bypass after surgery, the patient's bypass circuit may be switched to an ECMO circuit and the patient may be transferred on ECMO to the ICU.

Procedural Considerations

An area by the patient's bedside should be provided for the ECMO pump, surgical table and instrumentation, ESU, surgeon's headlight, and defibrillator with external and sterile internal paddles. A wall suction outlet should be available. Appropriate surgical attire must be provided for everyone involved with the procedure, and traffic should be limited.

Operative Procedure

For Neck Cannulation. A shoulder roll is placed under the patient, and the neck and chest to the nipple line are prepped and draped.

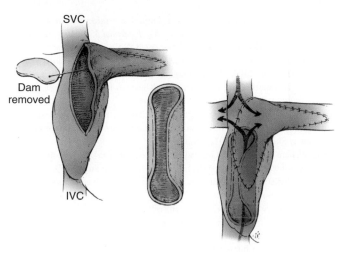

FIG. 26.70 Conversion of hemi-Fontan to completion of Fontan. Excision of the dam between the right atrium and the superior vena cava–pulmonary artery anastomosis. Inferior vena cava flow is directed to the inlet of the superior vena cava–pulmonary artery anastomosis by a baffle. *IVC,* Inferior vena cava; *SVC,* superior vena cava.

The ears should also be exposed and prepped for use as reference points.

1. An incision is made in the neck, and the right common carotid artery and right internal jugular vein are exposed for venoarterial ECMO. For veno-venous ECMO the jugular vein is used.
2. The surgeon may cannulate the vessels through a purse-string suture and then reconstruct these vessels at the time of decannulation.
3. After insertion of the arterial and venous cannulae, the clamped cannulae are connected to the ECMO circuit (Fig. 26.71). All the air is eliminated.
4. The cannulae are secured to the skin. The neck incision is closed and dressed. The surgical instruments are kept sterile until proper positioning of the venous and arterial cannulae is confirmed by x-ray examination.

For Median Sternotomy Cannulation. The patient is prepped from neck to umbilicus and draped.

1. The patient has usually had a prior sternotomy incision, so the sternum is opened with wire cutters.
2. A chest retractor is inserted, and purse-string sutures for cannulation are placed in the aorta and right atrium.
3. The surgeon inserts the aorta and venous cannulae and clamps them.
4. The clamped cannulae are connected to the ECMO circuit. All the air is eliminated.
5. The sternum is left open to prevent kinking of the cannulae and ECMO pump tubing. The wound is closed with a synthetic patch sutured to the skin. An antibiotic ointment may be applied and an "Open Chest" sign placed on top of the outer dressing to serve as a warning related to potential chest compressions.

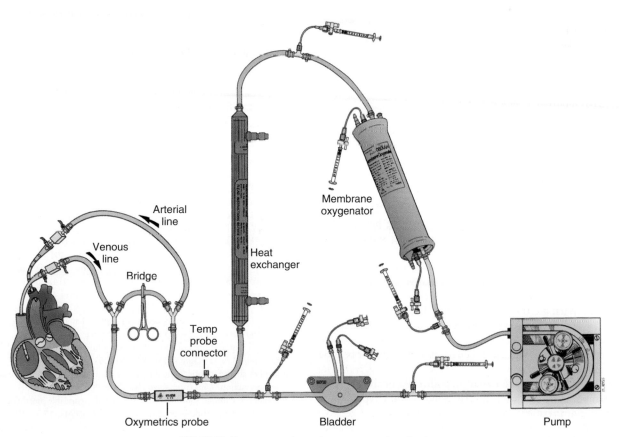

FIG. 26.71 Extracorporeal membrane oxygenation circuit.

Key Points

- Children require surgery for congenital malformations, an acquired disease, or trauma. The field of pediatric surgery is further subdivided into all the specialties.
- The difference between pediatric care and adult care is not just a size issue; from birth onward, the body and organs exist in a continual state of development, and multiple physiologic changes occur with age. Major areas of distinction are the airway and pulmonary status, cardiovascular status, temperature regulation, metabolism, fluid management, and psychologic development.
- Medical play items, audiovisual aids, puppets, and photographs are helpful in the perioperative education process. The nurse tailors interventions to suit the developmental level of the pediatric patient.
- Remaining with the child during induction, positioning, and prepping the surgical site; creating and maintaining a sterile field; collecting, documenting, and disposing specimens; and administering medications contribute to a safe environment for the pediatric surgical patient.
- Ensuring that the pediatric patient's family receives regular updates of the child's status will decrease their anxiety and help foster a sense of trust in the healthcare professionals caring for their child.
- For children younger than age 18, consent must be obtained from one of the following individuals: a legal parent (biologic parent whose parental rights have not been terminated) or an adoptive parent who has completed the adoptive process. Foster parents of children in the custody of a CYA are not permitted to give consent; rather, consent should be obtained from the CYA social worker. Legal guardians should be encouraged to bring any supporting documentation of legal guardianship or ability to consent for the child's medical care on the day of surgery.
- Every state has a child abuse law that dictates legal responsibility for reporting abuse and suspicion of abuse, and nurses are mandated reporters. Laws may differ from state to state.
- Pediatric instruments are usually shorter, have more delicate or less pronounced curves, and are smaller. A complete range of instrument sizes is necessary to make the appropriate size available for each child because pediatric patients can range in size from less than 1 kg to more than 100 kg.

Critical Thinking Questions

Several unique situations may arise when providing perioperative care to pediatric patients. Consider the following scenarios and determine the actions you would take:

1. Short-acting premedications are often administered to the pediatric patient before transfer from the preoperative area to the OR. What must the perioperative nurse consider when premedicating a patient? What are the safety considerations?
2. What are appropriate ways to facilitate parental presence in the OR for induction?
3. What considerations and safety behaviors are needed for bedside surgery?
4. What are some complications of hypothermia in the pediatric population? What are some interventions to avoid hypothermia of the pediatric patient?

ⅇvolve *The answers to the Critical Thinking Questions can be found at http://evolve.elsevier.com/Rothrock/Alexander.*

References

American Academy of Pediatrics (AAP): *Management of pediatric trauma, Management of pediatric trauma policy statement* (website), 2016. http://pediatrics.aappublications.org/content/early/2016/07/21/peds.2016-1569. (Accessed 18 February 2017).

Anderson D et al: Strategies to prevent surgical site infections in acute care hospitals: 2014 update, *Infect Control Hosp Epidemiol* 35(6):605–627, 2014.

Association of periOperative Registered Nurses (AORN): Guideline for prevention of unplanned patient hypothermia. In *Guidelines for perioperative practice*, ed 16, Denver, 2017, The Association.

Bales C et al: Intestinal atresia, stenosis. In Kliegman R, editor: *Nelson textbook of pediatrics*, ed 20, St Louis, 2016, Elsevier.

Campbell R: Vertical expandable prosthetic titanium rib (VEPTR) expansion thoracoplasty. In Kocher H, editor: *Operative techniques: pediatric orthopaedic surgery*, Philadelphia, 2011, Saunders.

Child Welfare Information Gateway: *Child abuse and neglect* (website), 2013. www.childwelfare.gov/topics/can/. (Accessed 18 February 2017).

Dahan E: Pediatric cataract surgery. In Yanoff M et al, editors: *Ophthalmology*, ed 4, St Louis, 2014, Elsevier.

Dominguez K et al: Necrotizing enterocolitis. In Holcomb G et al, editors: *Ashcraft's pediatric surgery*, ed 6, St Louis, 2014, Elsevier.

Ferrara C et al: Biomarkers of insulin for the diagnosis of hyperinsulinemic hypoglycemia in infants and children, *J Pediatr* 168:212–219, 2016.

Garg S et al: Variability of surgical site infection with VEPTR at eight centers: a retrospective cohort analysis, *Spine Deform* 4(1):59–64, 2016.

Gehrmann L et al: Pediatric extracorporeal membrane oxygenation: an introduction for emergency medicine physicians, *J Emerg Med* 49(4):552–560, 2015.

Jacob E: Pain assessment and management in children. In Hockenberry M, Wilson D, editors: *Wong's essentials of pediatric nursing*, ed 9, St Louis, 2013, Elsevier.

Jacob E et al: Adolescent pediatric pain tool for multidimensional measurement of pain in children and adolescents, *Pain Manag Nurs* 15(3):694–706, 2014.

Litman R: *Basics of pediatric anesthesia*, Philadelphia, 2016, Create Space.

Maki A et al: Intussusception. In Holcomb G et al, editors: *Ashcraft's pediatric surgery*, ed 6, St Louis, 2014, Elsevier.

Manga J et al: *Child abuse clinical presentation* (website), 2015. http://emedicine.medscape.com/article/800657-clinical. (Accessed 18 February 2017).

Mayer O et al: Thoracic insufficiency syndrome, *Curr Probl Pediatr Adolesc Health Care* 46(3):72–96, 2016.

McSweeney M et al: Advances in pediatric gastrostomy placement, *Gastrointest Endosc Clin North Am* 26(1):169–185, 2016.

Moldenhauer MS: Ex utero intrapartum therapy, *Semin Pediatr Surg* 22(1):44–49, 2013.

Murphy JP: Hypospadias. In Holcomb GW et al, editors: *Ashcraft's pediatric surgery*, ed 6, St Louis, 2014, Elsevier.

Panella J: Preoperative care of children: strategies from a child life perspective, *AORN J* 104(1):11–22, 2016.

Partridge EA, Flake AW: Maternal-fetal surgery for structural malformations, *Best Pract Res Clin Obstet Gynaecol* 26(5):669–682, 2012.

Pellegrino V: Extracorporeal membrane oxygenation (ECMO). In Bersten A, editor: *Oh's intensive care manual*, ed 7, St Louis, 2014, Elsevier.

Sala P et al: Fetal surgery: an overview, *Obstet Gynecol Surv* 69(4):218–228, 2014.

Schmitz M et al: Pediatric orthopaedics. In Miller M et al, editors: *Miller's review of orthopaedics*, ed 7, New York, 2016, Elsevier.

Segal I et al: Surgical site infections in infants admitted to the neonatal intensive care unit, *J Pediatr Surg* 49(3):381–384, 2014.

Tasain G et al: The robotic-assisted laparoscopic pyeloplasty: gateway to advanced reconstruction, *Urol Clin North Am* 42(1):89–97, 2015.

Waldhausen J: Complications in using the vertical expandable prosthetic titanium rib (VEPTR) in children, *J Pediatr Surg* 51(11):1747–1750, 2016.

CHAPTER 27
Geriatric Surgery

SHEILA L. ALLEN

The elderly contingent is growing in leaps and bounds in today's population, and, consequently, perioperative nurses must be proficient in meeting the needs of geriatric patients. As a geriatric patient, a different set of variables becomes important to maintain one's lifestyle. First and foremost, the older adult generation wants to live independently, care for themselves, and keep their quality of life intact.

Aging is a process that can be described in chronologic, physiologic, and functional terms. Human aging from a physiologic perspective has changed little in the past 300 years. Generally we age neither faster nor slower than we did in Colonial America. Chronologic age, the number of years a person has lived, is an easily identifiable measurement. Average or median life span, or life expectancy, is the age at which 50% of a given population survives. Maximum life span potential (MLSP) is the age of the longest-lived member or members of the population or species. Although the number of people living beyond their 90s has increased more recently, the MLSP, estimated at 125 years for women and somewhat less for men, has not changed significantly in recorded history. It is expected that by 2060 there will be 92 million people 65 or older, which is about 20% of the total population. Chronologic age or MLSP may not be the most meaningful measurement of age, however. Nevertheless, many people who have lived a long time remain physiologically and functionally young, whereas others are chronologically young but physiologically and functionally old (Williams, 2016).

Many aspects of our society will be affected by the growth of the population that is 65 years old or older. Policymakers, families, businesses, and healthcare providers will be challenged to meet the needs of this growing age group. With the aging of the baby boomers (born between 1946 and 1964), the gerontology boom will occur somewhere between 2010 and 2030, producing the most rapid increase in the older population. Every day, approximately 10 thousand baby boomers reach 65. Individuals older than 85 years now make up 4% of the entire US population and represent the fastest growing segment of the older population. Economics will play a factor because individuals born before 1937 will still qualify for full Social Security benefits at age 65 with incremental increases regarding benefit age for everyone born after that time. Those born in 1960 or after will have to wait until age 67 to qualify for full benefits, with reduced benefits calculated for individuals who apply for benefits after age 62 but before the specified retirement age (Williams, 2016). Nearly 40 million people 65 years and older lived in the United States in 2010, accounting for more than 13% of the total population, and they can be divided into subgroups (Box 27.1). The population considered oldest-old (age 85 years and older) increased from just more than 100,000 in 1900 to 4.2 million in 2000. In 2011 baby boomers started turning 65 years old; this segment of the population will increase at such a rate that the 2030 population is projected to be twice as large as it was in 2000. The 65-year and older population

will increase from 35 to 72 million, representing nearly 26% of the total US population. In 2014 there were 46 million people age 65 and older, accounting for 15% of the total population (FIFARS, 2016). The growth rate for this age group is expected to increase to 74 million, which is around 21% of the population after 2030, when the last of the boomers join the older population ranks. After 2030 the baby boomers will move into the oldest-old population (age 85 and older), which will grow accordingly (FIFARS, 2016; Fig. 27.1 provides population data). The US Census Bureau estimates that the population age 85 and older, in 2030, will be twice what it was in 2000 and grow from 6 million in 2014 to 20 million by 2060 (Williams, 2016; FIFARS, 2016). The proportion of the older population (65 and older) varies by state. This proportion is partly affected by the state fertility and mortality levels and partly by the number of older and younger people who migrate to and from the state. In 2014 Florida had the highest proportion of people ages 65 years and older at 19%. Maine, Pennsylvania, and West Virginia also had high proportions of more than 16%. The proportion of the population 65 years and older varies even more by county. In 2014, 53% of Sumter County, Florida, was 65 years and older, which is the highest proportion in the United States. In several Florida counties the proportion was more than 30%. At the other end of the spectrum was Chattahoochee County, Georgia, with only 4.1% of its population 65 years and older (FIFARS, 2016). As in most countries of the world, older women outnumber older men in the United States, and the proportion that is female increases with age. In 2014 women accounted for 56% of the older population and for 66% of the population 85 years and older. The United States is fairly young by comparison with other countries, with just more than 15% of its population age 65 years and older in 2015. Japan has 27% of its population 65 and older among countries of at least

BOX 27.1

Categorizing the Aging Population

- 65 to 74 years of age: The young-old
- 75 to 84 years of age: The middle-old
- 85 to 99 years of age: The old-old
- 100 years of age or more: The elite-old
  OR
- Older: 55 to 64
- Elderly: 65 to 74
- Aged: 75 to 84
- Extremely aged: 85 and older

Modified from Williams P: *Basic geriatric nursing*, ed 6, St Louis, 2016, Elsevier.

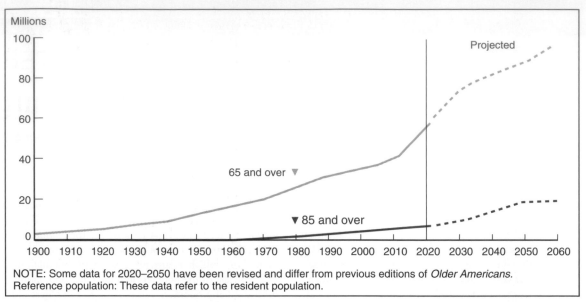

NOTE: Some data for 2020–2050 have been revised and differ from previous editions of *Older Americans*.
Reference population: These data refer to the resident population.

FIG. 27.1 Actual and projected population data for people age 65 years and older and 85 years and older. Selected years are 1900 to 2014; projected years are 2020 to 2060.

---

1 million. In most European countries the older population comprised more than 15% of the population, and it included nearly 20% of the population in both Germany and Italy in 2015 (FIFARS, 2016). Mirroring the total US population, the elder population is more racially diverse than ever (Box 27.2). By 2060 programs and services for older people will require greater flexibility to meet the needs of a more diverse population. In 2014 non-Hispanic whites accounted for 78% of the US older population; African Americans accounted for 9%; Asians 4%; and Hispanics (of any race), 8%. Projections are that by 2060 the composition of the older population will change to 55% non-Hispanic white, 22% Hispanic, 12% African American, and 9% Asian. The older Hispanic population is projected to grow the fastest, from just under 3.6 million in 2014 to 21.5 million in 2060, and to be larger than the older African American population. In 2014 over 2 million older Asians lived in the United States; by 2060 this population is projected to be 8.5 million (FIFARS, 2016).

Fig. 27.2 illustrates resident population by racial and ethnic composition.

Those older than 85 are the fastest growing age group in the US population. Improvements in medical care and healthier lifestyles have increased the ranks of US centenarians to 72,197 in 2014 from 50,281 in 2000, according to the Centers for Disease Control and Prevention report (Beasley, 2016). Those 85 and older could grow from 6 million in 2014 to 20 million in 2060 (FIFARS, 2016). Translating these demographics into healthcare trends produces even more startling implications for perioperative patient care. As a result of the "silver tsunami," healthcare will never be the same. A majority of older adults have at least one chronic condition, and many have multiple conditions that contribute to frailty and disability. Chronic diseases that are rarely cured, such as heart disease, stroke, cancer, and diabetes, are among the most common and costly health conditions. These long-term health conditions negatively affect quality of life, contributing to declines in functioning and the inability to remain in the community. Although chronic conditions can be prevented or modified with behavioral interventions, six of the seven leading causes of death among older Americans are chronic diseases (FIFARS, 2016). Fig. 27.3 lists the percentages of chronic diseases by gender. Between 1992 and 1999, the hospitalization rate in the older population increased from 306 hospital stays per 1000 Medicare enrollees to 365 stays per 1000. In 2013 the rate decreased to 276 stays per 1000 enrollees, and the average length of stay decreased from 8.4 days in 1992 to 5.3 days in 2013. The number of Medicare enrollees staying in skilled nursing facilities increased from 28 per 1000 in 1992 to 80 per 1000 in 2010 and 73 per 1000 beneficiaries in 2013. The utilization rates for many services change based on changes in medical technology and physician practice patterns (FIFARS, 2016). The dramatic growth in elderly surgical patients punctuates the necessity for perioperative nurses to recognize the special needs of these patients. Understanding how normal aging changes and chronic disease affect the successful outcome of any surgical procedure is critical; therefore it is the emphasis of this chapter.

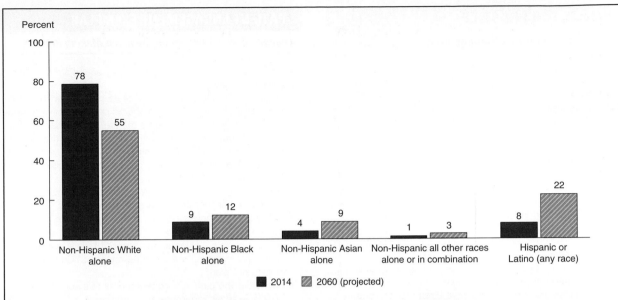

FIG. 27.2 Ethnic population data for people age 65 years and older for 2014 and projected for 2060.

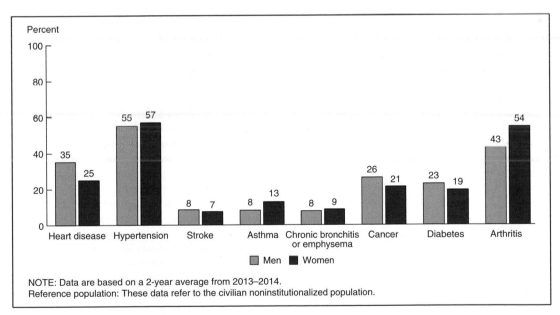

FIG. 27.3 Chronic disease by gender in people ages 65 years and older.

Perioperative Nursing Considerations

Preoperative Management

Before an elderly patient actually arrives in surgery, the healthcare team, patient, and his or her family or caregiver should ensure that the patient goals and treatment are understood before formulating a treatment plan. Usually this occurs in the physician's clinic in which fasting recommendations, prophylactic medications, and medication lists are included as the confirmation of the patient's preferences. Because checklists during surgery are important, the components of treatment must be ensured (Evidence for Practice). Although advances in monitoring techniques, technology, and anesthesia have made surgery safer for older adults, age remains a

EVIDENCE FOR PRACTICE

Checklist for Preoperative Management of Geriatric Surgery

The following checklist can be used when preparing the geriatric patient before surgery. In addition to a complete history and physical, this checklist can ensure that the treatment plan is comprehensive:

- Document and confirm patient goals and treatment preferences, including advance directives.
- Document and confirm patient's healthcare proxy or surrogate decision maker.
- Discuss new risks associated with the surgical procedure in patients with existing advance directives and an approach for potentially life-threatening problems consistent with the procedure.
- Consider shortened fluid fast (clear liquids up to 2 hours before anesthesia).
- Adhere to existing best practices regarding antibiotic and venous thromboembolism prophylaxis.
- Ensure nonessential medications have been stopped and essential medications have been taken.

From Mohanty S et al: *Optimal preoperative assessment of the geriatric patient: best practices guideline from the ACS NSQIP/American Geriatrics Society* (website). www.facs.org/~/media/files/quality%20programs/geriatric/acs%20nsqip%20geriatric%202016%20guidelines.ashx. (Accessed 25 August 2017).

PATIENT ENGAGEMENT EXEMPLAR

Engaging Older Adults in the Decision-Making Process

As noted throughout this chapter, older adults are a vulnerable population because of many factors.

The nurse's role as health advocate is the heart of patient-centered care, which fosters a shared decision-making model to involve the patient in all aspects of care. The presence of multiple morbidities in the elderly can hinder the provision of care. The AGS (2012) proposes the following list of concepts as a basis for involving the elderly patient in the decision-making process when multimorbidity is present:

- Inquire about the patient's primary concern (and that of the family and/or friends) and any other objectives.
- Conduct a complete review of the plan of care for older adults with multiple morbidities, or focus on a specific aspect of care, asking about current medical conditions and interventions. Is there adherence/comfort with the treatment plan?
- Consider the patient's preference. Is relevant evidence available regarding important outcomes?
- Consider the prognosis.
- Consider interactions within and among treatments and conditions.
- Weigh benefits and harms of components of the treatment plan.
- Communicate and decide for or against implementation or continuation of intervention/treatment.
- Reassess at selected intervals for benefit, feasibility, adherence, and alignment with the patient's preferences.

AGS, American Geriatrics Society.
Modified from American Geriatrics Society (AGS): *Patient-centered care for older adults with multiple chronic conditions: a stepwise approach from the American Geriatrics Society* (website), 2012. www.americangeriatrics.org/files/documents/MCC.stepwise.approach.pdf. (Accessed 28 November 2016).

---

significant risk factor. Nevertheless, adequate assessments of the functional age and the physiologic reserve of the elderly surgical patient are of significant importance.

According to the American Geriatrics Society (AGS), the occurrence of perioperative mortality in geriatric surgical patients is influenced by the following three factors:

1. *Emergency surgery.* Emergency surgery has an increased risk for all age groups. In a study of patients older than 90 years of age, in a 48-hour period, patients undergoing emergency procedures was 7.8% versus 0.6% in a similar group who had elective surgery.
2. *Site of surgery.* Major vascular, intrathoracic, and intra-abdominal procedures are reported to have a higher surgical risk than other surgical procedures in elders.
3. *Presence of coexisting disease as quantified by the American Society of Anesthesiologists (ASA) Physical Status Classification:* Patients with an ASA status of IV or V are consistently found to have greater mortality than those with a physical status of I or II. Current information supports the view that coexisting diseases outweigh age as a predictor of perioperative mortality (POGOE, 2014).

Surgical decision-making regarding elders can be challenging. As the baby boomers become seniors, they will be very different from healthcare consumers of the past because they will tolerate less and expect more. In clinical practice today, patients are increasingly involved in having a voice in their treatment plan. Emphasis on patient involvement in medical decision-making is a result of the growing amount of information available through the media, advertisements, the Internet, patient education materials, and access to public information. People are living longer, have better nutritional habits, and have healthier lifestyles. Older adult surgical patients have more allergies, slower metabolisms, higher risk of malnutrition, changes in physical and mental status, and decreased reserve capacity

of organs to respond to surgical stress (Penprase et al., 2014). What should be considered is the risk of not operating and the quality of life expected. There is no surgical specialty exempt from the challenge of decision-making for elderly, frail patients. The decision to proceed with an operative intervention may be irresistible in spite of the risk of postoperative complications. Important factors that need to be evaluated include the following:

- *Surgical risk versus medical management:* Deciding between the risks of medical or nonoperative management and surgical intervention can be difficult for elderly patients. Cultural and personal values of human life and the moral principles of abandonment shape influence decisions (Patient Engagement Exemplar). Surgical and anesthetic risks increase in proportion to the emergent nature of the patient's condition. When an acute emergency condition taxes an already overburdened physiologic state, survival is less likely. Patients may die even if the surgery was considered successful because of complications resulting from the complexity of the patient's comorbid conditions. Nonetheless healthcare providers need to be sensitive to this possibility when communicating with family members.
- *Disease course versus life expectancy:* Surgical intervention may not be appropriate if the prognosis of the disease is poor. However, if the patient has several years of life expectancy left and is likely to outlive the condition with minimal morbidity, surgical treatment may be the treatment of choice.

- *State of independence:* The patient's right to self-determination and making healthcare decisions should always be considered. The need for independence is of utmost importance to elderly adults, and most of them are far more interested in maintaining health and independence than longevity. Complications of surgery are not well tolerated by elders and can quickly develop into life-threatening situations. If surgical intervention will further incapacitate an already debilitated person, alternative treatment should be considered. However, if surgery will help alleviate debilitating conditions and improve or maintain independence, it should be considered an appropriate modality of care. The decision to proceed with surgery may be based on what the patient's life may be like postoperatively (Research Highlight).

RESEARCH HIGHLIGHT ‖

Investigation of Gene Expression and Serum Levels of PIN1 and eNOS With High Blood Pressure in Patients With Alzheimer Disease

An increased demand for surgical services can be anticipated with the aging of the population. As more elderly patients present for surgery, perioperative nurses may expect to see more patients with Alzheimer disease. Alzheimer disease is a serious neurodegenerative disease that reduces the cognitive capacity. Multiple studies have identified hypertension as a key factor in the development of Alzheimer disease. The object of the study examined the relationship between PIN1 and eNOS gene expression, as well as serum levels and hypertension in this patient population.

The PIN1 gene expression is reduced in patients with Alzheimer disease. eNOS is an isoform of nitric oxide, which influences vasodilator effects and cerebral vascularity. The enzyme has an important function in the control of blood pressure and protection from atherosclerosis. One of the most significant factors affecting the three-dimensional structure of eNOS is the enzyme PIN1, which is reduced in age-related neurodegenerative diseases such as Alzheimer disease.

Blood samples were gathered from subjects that were divided into four groups: the healthy group with only hypertension, the Alzheimer-sufferers group with hypertension, normotensive Alzheimer patients, and the control group. The inhibition of confounding factors was considered. PIN1 and eNOS genes expression with the serum levels were included in the study.

According to the results of the study, PIN1 and eNOS levels might contribute to blood pressure regulation. They may affect the risk of a person developing hypertension in addition to physiological vasodilatory and nitrite metabolism. Because there are statistical differences between the PIN1 and eNOS serum levels in the two groups of Alzheimer sufferers, the compounds can be measured to be used in early diagnostic biomarkers in early prognosis, prevention, and monitoring in Alzheimer disease. This would lead to a decrease in the mortality rate from cardiovascular disease in these patients. There is a recommendation that a study be conducted on a large scale to include patients with several stages of Alzheimer disease and patients with mild cognitive impairment.

eNOS, Endothelial nitric oxide.
Modified from Azimi M et al: Investigation of gene expression and serum levels of PIN1 and eNOS with high blood pressure in patients with Alzheimer disease, *J Clin Neurosci* 43:77–81, 2017.

- *Personal motivation:* Evaluation of the elderly patient's level of motivation must be considered when surgery is planned. Many elderly patients are reluctant to undergo surgery because of concerns that the surgery will not improve their quality of life or will make them more dependent or make them destined to life in a care facility. In addition, they do not want to withstand the pain, discomfort, and rigors of surgery and the recuperative period necessary to treat a condition that does not really bother them very much or that they have "learned to live with." This lack of motivation can have a negative influence on the results of the surgery. Conversely, some elders expect and in some cases demand the best of care. They believe that the money they spend on taxes and healthcare entitles them to the very best that healthcare has to offer, regardless of its practicality. Nonetheless, patients who show a strong sense of determination in doing all that is necessary to get well and stay well are better candidates for surgery than those who believe illness is a prelude to death. The outcome of surgery is enhanced if the patient is motivated to have a positive result.

The following questions should be considered when deciding to proceed with surgery in elders (Dunn, 2016):

- Is there a clear indication for surgery, considering the disease progression?
- What practical limitations will be imposed on the patient with the progression of the disease or the surgical intervention?
- How much improvement can be expected after the surgical procedure?
- What is the expectation for quality of life with or without surgery?
- How aware is the patient and the patient's family about the problem and proposed solutions?
- What risks are there for negative outcomes related to the procedure and the presence of comorbid conditions?
- Has an adequate preoperative assessment and preparation preceded an elective procedure?

There are many important considerations related to the extent of surgical treatment. Therefore the decision for surgery relies heavily on the patient's physical status at the time of surgery and on the extent of disease progression. When treating patients who are nearing the end of life, attention should shift from solely maximizing survival to maximizing the quality of life and dignity while minimizing suffering. Early identification of problems with aggressive, preventive surgical treatment is considered more appropriate than waiting for problems to develop. To prevent complications, the perioperative nurse must be the gatekeeper to help prevent complications through early identification of risk and appropriate interventions to address the risk to secure positive outcomes.

Assessment

In elderly people a preoperative medical assessment is conducted to determine present physiologic functioning. Consideration of the unique risks for older patient complications is important to include in a comprehensive assessment of that patient population. Key factors in the evaluation of the older surgical patient are assessing cognitive ability and capacity; existence of depression; risk for postoperative delirium; screen for alcohol and substance abuse; cardiac and pulmonary evaluations; documentation of functional status including falls, baseline frailty score, nutritional status, medication history, diagnostic tests, and understanding of treatment goals and expectations and their family/social support system (Oresanya et al., 2014). In 2015 the Association of periOperative Registered Nurse's position statement on care of the older adult asserts that cognitive decline can limit the understanding of informed consents and pain assessment and management, and identify the need for designated support. The risk factors for the postoperative concern of delirium and depression are increased age, coexisting medical comorbidities, underlying cognitive impairment, psychotropic medications, alcohol abuse, sensory loss, and poor mobility or functional impairment. The Mini-Cog test can be used as a tool for assessing cognitive impairment and indications for postoperative depression or delirium (Penprase et al., 2014). The assessment of cognition, function, nutrition, and frailty are outlined in Fig. 27.4. Depression and the lack of social support are also linked to adverse outcomes in older surgical patients. Several standardized tools exist for delirium screening. An evidence-based tool, the Confusion Assessment Method (CAM), is widely used because of its validity and reliability. The CAM short form takes 5 minutes to complete, whereas the 3D-CAM takes only 3 minutes (Bull, 2015).

In older patients, malnutrition is common and associated with poor surgical outcomes. Assessment of malnutrition can be determined by measuring body mass index, unintentional weight loss, a low preoperative serum albumin level, or a low Mini Nutritional Assessment score. The nurse's data collection includes the standard assessment information with considerations of coexisting conditions and a review of the patient's medication list including prescription, over the counter, herbal, diet, and recreational. Polypharmacy is an issue for many elderly patients and is a concern because of the physiologic changes associated with aging that lead to susceptibility to alterations in pharmacokinetics and vulnerability to adverse drug reactions.

Frailty. Chronic conditions may interfere with the elderly person's ability to distinguish between recent and long-standing ailments as the presence of multiple comorbidities will increase the risk of complications. Frailty has been used to predict how well a patient may recover from a surgical procedure. Five criteria are used to predict frailty: shrinking, weakness, poor endurance and energy, slowness, and low physical activity levels (Ogg, 2016). Although many centers may not make time for such assessments, researchers at Emory University have developed a 1-minute test. After testing the five-step method with their two-step version, they found that the patient's grip strength and weight loss were valid predictors of postoperative complications (McIsaac et al., 2016). Baylor College of Medicine in Houston, Texas, has developed a 20-second arm test that is easy to use and has proven validity. The upper extremity frailty (UEF) is performed by repetitive flexion and extension of the dominant elbow as quickly as possible in 20 seconds (Boggs, 2016).

Physiologic Changes. Aging is a biologic process characterized by the inevitable, progressive, predictable evolution and maturation until death. Aging is not the accumulation of disease, although the two are related in subtle, complex ways. A fundamental principle is that biologic age and chronologic age are not the same because different individuals age at different rates. Physical aging occurs in different organ systems at different rates, influenced by lifestyle choices and socioeconomic status. Generally the aging process imposes a decline in organ functions, atypical responses to pain and temperature, alterations in pharmacokinetics (Surgical Pharmacology), and atypical signs and symptoms of disease, all of which may vary from one elderly person to the next. Having a clear understanding of normal age changes helps establish appropriate nursing diagnoses and develop a plan of care (Box 27.3). The following review of systems focuses on age-specific changes of particular importance to the perioperative plan of care.

Integumentary System. The nails become thick and tough related to a decrease of circulation in the hands and feet. A nick or cut can lead to a serious infection. Color and texture of hair change, and the loss of pigmentation results in graying of hair. Decrease in oil content makes the hair dull and lifeless, and the amount of hair decreases. The skin loses elasticity and subcutaneous fat and becomes more prone to shear force and pressure injury. Because of the thinness of the skin and small-vessel fragility, bruising and hemorrhaging are common. Dry skin develops because of decreased oil and sweat production from sebaceous and sweat glands, respectively. As a result, skin breakdown and pressure ulcers, as well as wound infections, develop more easily. Therefore protection of bony prominences and appropriate positioning practices are important to reduce the chance of the development of pressure ulcers. The vascular system of the skin has nutritional and protective roles. It is necessary for body heat regulation, provides defenses against microbial and physical damage, provides nutrient supply to the avascular epidermis, and promotes wound healing. Having an intact vascular system to maintain these skin role characteristics is extremely important for a patient undergoing surgical intervention. However, papillary capillaries, responsible for epidermal nourishment and heat dissipation, degenerate with aging. What is left is only the horizontal arteriovenous plexus lying beneath the skin surface. This progressive impairment of vascular circulation and tissue nutrition and the loss of subcutaneous tissue predispose to a feeling of cold, especially in cool environments such as the operating room (OR). Therefore the ability to maintain thermoregulation is compromised in elders and must be controlled through external measures. The perioperative team can use the knowledge of these changes to prevent pressure ulcers, guard against inflammation and infection, and incorporate care to maintain an appropriate temperature for the elder patient in surgery.

Musculoskeletal System. Changes to the elderly person's skeleton, such as the loss of bone mass, contribute to skeletal instability and make fractures of the hip, rib, distal radius, and vertebrae common. Curvature of the spine and degenerative arthritis of the joints are also common. Pain as a fifth vital sign is routinely evaluated for all patients.

Osteoporosis is the most obvious skeletal change that occurs with advancing age. It leads to susceptibility to fracture, which doubles every 5 years after 50 years of age. An approximate loss of 25% to 40% of the mineral content of the bone must be present before detectable change is evident on x-ray films. To some degree, osteoporosis is related to a lessening of physical activity, but other risk factors are female gender, Northern European ancestry, multiparity, lean body build, and excessive alcohol intake (Ignatavicius, 2015). Osteoporosis is also related to decreased hormonal secretion; thus postmenopausal women are more prone to develop the condition and therefore more likely to sustain a hip fracture. Bone marrow density (BMD) is an assessment tool for osteoporosis. If medications are prescribed, testing of BMD may be done every 2 years to evaluate the patient's response to treatment (Williams, 2016).

In elders, long-standing conditions such as arthritis, neuralgia, and ischemic disorders produce chronic pain. Back pain is related to dehydration and decreased flexibility of the vertebral disks or may be the result of spondylosis (vertebral arthritis), stenosis, and mechanical or other causes (Jones et al., 2014). These changes result in a gradual loss of height, loss of strength, and decreased mobility. Poor posture tends to be proportional to the degree of back pain experienced and may greatly compromise internal organ function. Joint range of motion is impaired to varying degrees and may affect surgical positioning. The perioperative team should take extra care in

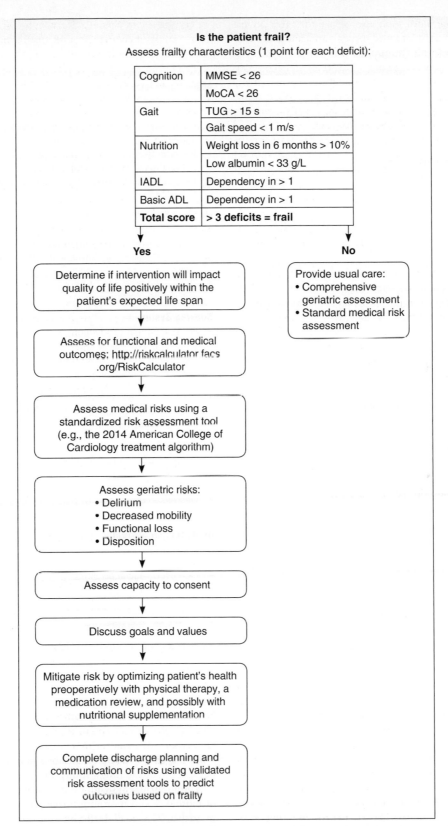

FIG. 27.4 Recommended model for preoperative assessment and decision making. *ADL,* Activities of daily living; *IADL,* instrumental activities of daily living; *MMSE,* Mini-Mental State Exam; *MOCA,* Montreal Cognitive Assessment; *TUG,* timed up and go test. (From Hill A, Alkeridy W: Preoperative assessment of the frail older adult, *BCMJ* 59(2):112–116, 2017.)

BOX 27.3

Age-Related Physiologic Changes

Integumentary System
- Decreased subcutaneous fat and thickness of epidermis
- Decreased vascularity of dermis and peripheral circulation
- Decreased sebaceous and sweat gland function
- Decrease in hair and nail growth

Hematopoietic and Lymphatic System
- Increased plasma viscosity and immature T cells
- Decreased red blood cell production

Respiratory System
- Decreased tissue elasticity, resulting in pooling of secretions in lower lung bases
- Increased calcification of cartilage, leading to increased rigidity of the rib cage, decreased lung capacity, and reduced cough efficiency
- Decreased ciliary activity by bronchial lining
- Reduction in number of capillaries, resulting in decreased gas exchange and drying of mucous membranes

Cardiovascular System
- Changes in cardiac muscle tone and blood vessel elasticity, leading to decreased tissue oxygenation and venous return
- Dysrhythmias; rapid or slow heartbeat
- High blood pressure related to atherosclerosis
- Chest pain or shortness of breath on exertion
- Decreased cardiac output, causing decreased circulation to extremities

Digestive System
- Dental issues (e.g., tooth loss, periodontal disease), leading to chewing issues
- Decreased saliva production
- Relaxation of esophageal muscle tone, increasing the prevalence of esophageal reflux
- Decreased gastric secretions
- Bowel dysfunction from decreased peristalsis

Urinary System
- Loss of nephron units
- Decline in renal tissue growth
- Reduced kidney size and bladder capacity
- Increased prostate size in men
- Weakened bladder muscles with consequent postvoid residual

Musculoskeletal System
- Progressive loss of muscle strength from decreased muscle mass
- Decreased fluid in intervertebral disks resulting in joint and back pain/stiffness
- Bone breakdown overcomes bone building, with resultant osteoporosis, and postural changes resulting in spine curvature
- Decreased tissue elasticity, resulting in decreased mobility and flexibility

Nervous System
- Loss of neurons, leading to decreased reflexes
- Slower reaction time from loss of nerve fibers
- Changes in sleep patterns; less rapid eye movement and deep sleep
- Decreased amounts of neuroreceptors, resulting in decreased perception of stimuli

Sensory System
- Decreased tear production
- Increased lens discoloration, which decreases color perception
- Decreased muscle tone in eye, leading to decreased pupil diameter, decreased night vision, increased refractive errors, increased sensitivity to glare
- Loss of hair cells in inner ear, leading to balance problems
- Decreased joint mobility in bones of inner ear
- Decreased number of papillae on tongue

Endocrine System
- Decreased pituitary secretions (growth hormone), leading to decreases in muscle mass
- Reduction in the production of thyroid-stimulating hormone
- Decreased production of parathyroid hormone
- Increased prevalence of diabetes mellitus

Reproductive System
Female
- Decreased estrogen levels and tissue elasticity
- Increased vaginal alkalinity

Male
- Decreased testosterone levels and circulatory changes
- Circulatory changes

Modified from Williams P: *Basic geriatric nursing*, ed 6, St Louis, 2016, Elsevier.

positioning elderly patients in the OR, ensuring appropriate padding and joint protection (Williams, 2016).

Respiratory System. As people age, lungs lose elasticity, which contributes to a decrease in functional residual capacity, residual volume, and dead space. Lungs increase in size and are lighter in weight with aging. A rigid chest wall is the result of calcification of costal cartilages, osteoporosis, and dorsal kyphosis. Muscles responsible for inhalation and exhalation may be weakened, resulting in a diminished ability to increase and decrease the size of the thoracic cavity. All these changes contribute to a minimal tidal exchange, which makes the elderly patient more susceptible to pulmonary complications, such as acute respiratory distress syndrome (ARDS), pneumonia, and aspiration. Lung changes are not usually obvious at rest. However, when the person becomes active, breathing may

be more difficult. As with other systems, in the elderly there is a reduced capacity to respond to sudden changes. If confronted with an increased demand for more oxygen or exposure to anesthetic or noxious agents, a respiratory insufficiency may occur and can quickly become life-threatening (Touhy and Jett, 2016).

Cardiovascular System. Cardiovascular disease is the leading cause of morbidity and mortality in the United States and accounts for more than 75% of all deaths in those over 65 years of age (Williams, 2016). Unlike other muscles, the heart does not atrophy with age; however, the mass of the heart and the thickening of the left ventricular wall may make the aging heart function less effectively. A decrease in coronary artery blood flow is more likely in older adults. Because of a shift in blood flow, there is a greater decrease in circulation to the kidneys and liver than to the brain and heart. Blood pressure

SURGICAL PHARMACOLOGY

Medication and the Elderly

Perioperative nurses caring for older adults must consider factors that affect the choice of medications and the effects of those medications on this population. Older adults may not tolerate the standard dosages used for younger adults and are at higher risk for side effects and toxicity. Dosages of drugs may initially be smaller than those used for the general adult population and then titrated based on the patient's response and therapeutic effect. Older adults have less reserve, and chronic disease may contribute to drug reactions. Physiologic changes may affect the absorption, distribution, metabolism, and excretion of medications. Older adults also have a higher prevalence of nonprescription drug use (e.g., analgesics, antacids, laxatives, supplements). A complete medication history should be obtained by the healthcare team to include prescription and over-the-counter medications such as vitamins and herbal products. The nurse should partner with the surgeon and anesthesia provider to ensure that drug therapy is individualized based on the patient's baseline condition, actual physiologic impairments, and severity of preexisting illness. Nonessential medications should be discontinued before surgery. Consider medications with withdrawal potential or those medically indicated throughout the perioperative time frame (i.e., cardiac medications, renal function medications). The nurse should monitor for polypharmacy and potential adverse interactions. The plan for continuation or discontinuation of the patient's medications should be in place before arrival into the preoperative holding area.

Common adverse drug reactions in older adults include the following:

- Edema
- Dizziness
- Nausea and vomiting
- Urinary retention
- Anorexia
- Diarrhea
- Dry mouth
- Constipation
- Fatigue
- Confusion
- Weakness

Expected age-related changes that may affect medication administration in the perioperative period are as follows:

- *Changes in Absorption*
  - Increased gastric pH
  - Decreased gastric blood flow
  - Decreased gastrointestinal motility
- *Changes in Drug Distribution*
  - Decreased amounts of total body water
  - Increased ratio of adipose tissue to lean body mass, causing storage of lipid-soluble drugs and decreased plasma drug levels
  - Decreased albumin levels
  - Decreased cardiac output
- *Changes in Metabolism and Excretion*
  - Decreased liver size
  - Decreased hepatic blood flow
  - Decreased liver enzyme activity
  - Decreased renal blood flow
  - Reduced glomerular filtration rate, leading to slower excretion times for medications and allowing serum drug levels to rise

For patients at increased risk for delirium:

- Avoid starting new prescriptions for benzodiazepines and reduce current prescriptions when possible.
- Avoid using meperidine (Demerol) for pain control. Make sure pain is well controlled to avoid postoperative delirium.
- Use caution when prescribing antihistamine H antagonists such as Benadryl and other medications with strong anticholinergic effects.

Modified from Hodgson BB, Kizior RJ: *Saunders nursing drug handbook 2015,* St Louis, 2015, Saunders; Ignatavicius DD: Common health problems of older adults. In Ignatavicius DD, Workman ML, editors: *Medical-surgical nursing: patient-centered collaborative care,* ed 8, St Louis, 2015, Saunders; Mohanty S et al: *Optimal preoperative assessment of the geriatric patient: best practices guideline from the ACS NSQIP/American Geriatrics Society* (website). www.facs.org/~/media/files/quality%20programs/geriatric/acs%20nsqip%20geriatric%20 2016%20guidelines.ashx. (Accessed 25 August 2017).

rises as a result of increased arterial resistance. When the elderly person is at rest, the heart rate remains approximately the same as that of a younger person. However, the older heart requires a longer recovery time after each beat, which means that it reacts poorly to stress and anxiety-produced tachycardia. Generally the capacity of the cardiovascular system to tolerate and buffer insults is limited. Activity, exercise, excitement, and illness increase the body's need for oxygen and nutrients. The older heart may be unable to meet these needs. Arteries lose their elasticity and become narrow, causing a weakened heart to work harder. As a result, less blood flows through the arteries, causing poor circulation in many parts of the body.

Elders have an increased risk for aortic arch disruption, myocardial contusion, ventricular hypertrophy, and aneurysm development. A complete, comprehensive cardiac workup (e.g., electrocardiogram [ECG], nuclear stress test, echocardiogram according to facility protocols within an appropriate time frame) should be performed before the elderly patient is scheduled for any surgical procedure (Workman, 2015).

Hematopoietic and Lymphatic Systems. The two major body fluids, blood and lymph, distribute nutrients, oxygen, essential protective factors, and electrolytes throughout the body in two parallel circulatory systems. Generally, the blood functions to transport nutrients, blood gases, waste products, and hormones. It also functions in the regulation of body temperature, acid-base balance, and fluid-electrolyte balance. The blood also serves as protection against pathogenic attack by the white blood cells and clotting mechanisms to guard against excessive bleeding. Lower serum albumin may cause edema, and decreased red and white blood cells can lead to anemia and less effective phagocytosis. The lymph system consists of the spleen, the thymus gland, fluid, nodes, nodules, and lymph vessels. The function of the system is to return fluids from the tissue to the circulation. Because of the changes related to aging, the changes in the immune response may alter the usual signs and symptoms of infection. Body temperature may not significantly change until infection is severe, and pain may not be present. For example, older adults with pneumonia may not have fever and chills or pain may be absent with appendicitis or peritonitis in spite of the patient being obviously ill. These factors may be important when assessing the patient's response to local anesthetics, antibiotics, and postoperative medications.

Gastrointestinal System. As a person ages digestive glands decrease the amount of secretions; mucus becomes thicker, causing dysphagia; and saliva becomes more alkaline. Loss of teeth or poorly fitted dentures make chewing difficult, resulting in digestion problems. Foods that are difficult to eat are avoided, and such avoidance can affect overall nutrition. Decrease in peristalsis and a reduction of gastric motility—the results of muscle tone loss—cause a delay in stomach emptying. Potential traumatic injuries to the bowel and mesenteric infarction are more likely to occur (Williams, 2016). The absorption of drugs is affected because of a reduction of blood flow to abdominal viscera, a reduction in the amount of hydrochloric acid secreted, and delayed gastric emptying. Decreases in the levels of total body water and plasma volume result in a smaller volume of distribution for water-soluble drugs. Because the percentage of body fat increases and the lean body mass decreases, the storage of lipophilic drugs, such as diazepam and lidocaine, is enhanced. These factors are of particular importance for assessing the patient's response to preoperative, anesthetic, and postoperative medications. Because of reduced peristalsis, fluid volume deficit, disease processes, and dietary changes, many older patients may have experienced problems with constipation. Patients who experience pain with defecation are more likely to delay or avoid the act. Chronic constipation increases the risk of a fecal impaction and is uncomfortable and traumatic to the rectal tissues. Examination of the patient's medications can assist in evaluating those that are constipation producing. Changes in diet, physical activity, positioning, and pharmacologic interventions may be required in addition to education of the patient, family, and caregiver for the patient's discharge.

Urinary System. The kidneys decrease in size by age 40 from 400 g to only 250 g by age 70. At 90 years of age, the glomerular filtration may be half of what it was at age 20. Nephrons decrease in function with age, so by 75 years of age a person has probably lost one-third to one-half of original nephron function. Elasticity and tone are lost in the ureters, bladder, and urethra, which lead to incomplete emptying of the bladder. Benign prostatic hyperplasia is the most common condition in men, with a significant increase in prevalence with age—from 20% in men ages 41 to 60 to 90% in men older than age 80 (Williams, 2016). Difficulty in voiding and retention of urine are common with this condition. Total bladder capacity also declines, so elderly persons experience a more frequent and urgent need to urinate. Because blood flow to the kidneys is decreased, patients are at greater risk for fluid overload, fluid and electrolyte imbalance, and alterations in the elimination of medications. During the perioperative phase of the patient's hospital stay, the greatest number and variety of drugs are given; the cumulative effect increases the chances for adverse and consequential results.

Nervous System. Although not functionally significant, a steady loss in the number of neurons begins at about 25 years of age. An inappropriate or slow response to stimuli is primarily a result of a decrease in some organ systems' ability to send reliable messages to the brain and spinal cord. Nerve cells are particularly sensitive to lack of oxygen. Brain tissue may decrease as much as 3% a decade from age 50 to 90. Motor responses take longer, reflexes become sluggish, and loss of coordination is common because older adults may have, in varying degrees, cerebral arteriosclerosis and atherosclerosis, and decreased blood flow and nervous system deficits, such as insomnia, irritability, visual motor deficits, and memory loss, may occur. These patients are more likely to experience subdural hematomas or closed head injuries because they are more prone to falls. Other neurologic changes significant to perioperative care include a loss of position sense in the toes, decreased tactile sense, and atypical response to pain. Neurologic changes that result in dementia, Parkinson disease, or Alzheimer disease can alter the way the perioperative nurse communicates with the patient. In addition, aging is associated with disruption of thermoregulation (Williams, 2016); inadvertent hypothermia (temperature less than 96.8°F [36°C]) is a common problem in elders (see Chapter 5 for a full discussion of preventing unplanned hypothermia in adult surgical patients). In the OR, maintaining a balance between heat gain (e.g., metabolic production, muscular contraction, hot ambient temperature) and heat loss (e.g., radiation, convection, evaporation, ventilation, cold fluid infusion, blood loss, antithermoregulatory drugs, impaired heat production) can be difficult in older surgical patients.

Endocrine System. The primary glands in the endocrine system are the thyroid, parathyroid, adrenal, pineal, pituitary, and thymus. The ovaries, testes, and pancreas are not glands; however, they contain endocrine tissue. In the elderly, signs and symptoms of a problem are often nonspecific and subtle. The decrease of the hormones of the pituitary, pancreas, thyroid, and parathyroid cause many of the comorbidities that can exacerbate previously existing conditions. Conditions of the endocrine system such as diabetes mellitus can cause changes in the function of other systems necessitating vascular surgical procedures to compensate for the changes in other organs. Reduced function of the thyroid can cause symptoms that may appear to be commonly observed in the aging such as constipation, dry skin, lack of energy, and depression when they may be hypothyroidism. Treatment with high thyroid hormone levels may reduce bone density in older women.

Sensory Changes. Changes in vision, hearing, taste, smell, and touch may influence the patient's response to care. Farsightedness, or presbyopia, in the aging person is a result of the lens becoming more rigid and less pliable. Consequently, visual acuity and accommodation are decreased. Color perception changes as a result of a yellowing of the lens, which makes distinguishing blue, green, and purple more difficult. By age 80, half of Americans have a cataract (Masterson, 2015). After the cataract is removed and a surgical lens implanted, the patient may still need contact lenses or glasses with appropriate correction (Williams, 2016). Of particular importance in the OR is an awareness of the older person's difficulty in adapting to changes in light. Moving patients from a dimly lit holding area to the bright lights of the OR can cause momentary "blindness."

Presbycusis, or loss of hearing sensitivity, is irreversible, bilateral, and primarily sensorineural, although metabolic and mechanical causes are also possible. It is the most frequent cause of hearing loss in the geriatric patient. Hearing loss, which appears to be greater in men than in women, is mostly within the higher frequencies (above 1000 Hz). In addition, cerumen thickens and the eardrum becomes less pliable, and such changes also contribute to diminished hearing. Often geriatric patients are labeled "confused" or "senile" because they respond inappropriately to questions they did not hear or they describe what they see inaccurately because of poor vision.

Changes in taste and smell begin to occur at approximately 60 years of age and become more pronounced with advanced age. Older adults have two to three times more difficulty in detecting flavors than do young adults. Oral hygiene, dental disease, and decreased salivary function may also alter tasting ability. There is a close association between the sense of smell and human behavior. Smell can affect emotions when a person recalls a particular odor. Other functions include protection of the individual by warning of danger in the air, such as smoke or gas fumes; assistance in digestion; and helping a person to remember or recollect. In elders, the sense of smell can be reduced, as well as the ability to identify odors (Williams, 2016).

Changes in sensitivity to touch often accompany the aging process, but the degree of change varies among individuals. In some cases, losses can be related to neuropathy caused by disease, injury, or circulatory problems. Decreased sense of touch can affect the elderly person's ability to localize stimuli and can reduce the speed of reaction to tactile stimulation. For example, an older person may have difficulty differentiating among coins, fastening buttons, or grasping small items. An important detail to remember in preparing the elderly patient for surgery is to remind the patient or family/caregiver to bring all aids for the patient (glasses, hearing aids, walkers, cane, or other devices needed for their care).

Psychologic Changes. Physiologic and psychologic stress may result in an acute state of confusion or delirium in the geriatric patient that is analogous to convulsions as a stress reaction in the pediatric patient. In elders, mental change can be a warning of some underlying problem. It is of pivotal importance to determine the patient's interpretation of pain in the assessment phase. Confusion or delirium should therefore not be dismissed as an expected behavior of the geriatric patient. Delirium occurs in more than 80% of intensive care patients and patients at the end of life and in as many as 50% of hospitalized elders. Recent evidence shows that it is an "independent predictor of 6 month mortality," specifically in hip fractures (Bellelli et al., 2014). It is associated with increased length of stay, increased morbidity, poorer functional outcomes, increased risk of nursing home placement, and increased patient care costs. Pain management is important to lessen the risk of delirium. The most important assessment factor is determining whether the confusion is chronic or acute. Chronic conditions, such as depression and Alzheimer disease, can make communication with the patient difficult. Depending on the stage of disease, patients may not be able to understand explanations. Family members are the best resource to determine the patient's ability to comprehend and respond to questions and instructions. Behavioral changes such as aggressiveness, agitation, and paranoia are not uncommon. Soft restraints may be necessary during local procedures in the OR to ensure patient safety. Taking the time to talk slowly, being deliberate in movements, getting to know the patient, and developing a trusting relationship before surgery can help to lessen the patient's anxiety and control the combative outbursts that occur in some Alzheimer patients (Box 27.4). The assessment of pain in the elderly can be difficult; therefore standardized, evidence-based tools and unbiased communication of the results can be the most effective in the cognitively intact and

the cognitively impaired. Tools such as the Numeric Rating Scale (NRS), the Verbal Descriptor Scale (VDS), and Faces Pain Scale-Revised (FPS-R) are generally used in the cognitively intact senior. Observational tools such as the Pain Assessment Checklist for Seniors with Limited Ability to Communicate (PACSLAC) and Pain Assessment in Advanced Dementia (PAINAD) can be valuable when assessing pain in the cognitively impaired senior (STTI, 2015). Because some elderly patients may fear becoming addicted to medications, sometimes comfort measures and nonpharmacologic measures may be effective to provide comfort (Box 27.5).

Acute confused states or delirium in elders can be precipitated by a number of conditions and may be the sole manifestation of a life-threatening complication. Delirium in elders may be evidenced by alteration in level of consciousness, inattention, disorganized thinking, or an acute onset of mental status change.

Some of the most common predisposing factors for confusion or delirium are noted in Box 27.6. Among the most predictive risk factors for delirium are immobility, functional deficits, use of restraints or catheters, medications, acute illness, infections, alcohol or drug abuse, sensory impairments, malnutrition, dehydration, respiratory insufficiency, surgery, and cognitive impairment. Even the disruption of relocation into the hospital, which brings the patient into an unfamiliar environment, can cause acute confusion, particularly during the postoperative period. Validation of the patient's previous mental state with a relative or significant other can help determine whether the onset occurred since hospitalization.

Routine Laboratory and Diagnostic Tests

The physiologic changes of aging do not significantly alter the diagnostic values of complete blood count (CBC), differential cell count, platelets, urinalysis, and blood chemistry results; therefore abnormalities should be evaluated. A slight increase may be noted in the levels of potassium, fasting blood glucose, postprandial blood glucose, oral glucose tolerance, total cholesterol, and thyroid-stimulating hormone. A decrease in the amounts of vitamin B_{12},

---

BOX 27.4

Strategies for Communicating With Impaired Elderly Adults

When communicating with elderly adults who have cognitive impairments, perioperative nurses and surgical technologists should consider the following strategies:

- Try not to startle the person when starting a communication.
- Approach from the front, knock, or announce your presence by addressing the person using their preferred name.
- Approach patients who have a left-sided hemiparesis from the right side and vice versa.
- Identify yourself.
- Eliminate or reduce noise and distractions.
- Make sure you have the person's attention before speaking.
- Try to use a variety of words or descriptions until meanings are clear.
- Ask clear, specific questions, one at a time.
- Pay attention to body language, yours and the patient's.
- Use pictures and gestures in addition to words if needed.
- Keep messages simple and repeat as needed.
- Be patient and do not interrupt. Slow down the pace of communication.

Modified from Williams P: *Basic geriatric nursing,* ed 5, St Louis, 2016, Elsevier.

BOX 27.5

Nonpharmacologic Measures for Pain Relief

- *Energy or touch therapies:* Touch therapy is a legacy of nursing. Contact therapy such as massage has long been recognized to provide comfort and relief. Noncontact therapies such as therapeutic touch and Reiki can also afford moderate pain relief. Because the acceptability of touch varies with individuals and cultures, the nurse should ask for permission to touch the patient.
- *Transcutaneous electrical nerve stimulation (TENS):* TENS units can be used for pain relief and now are available without prescriptions.
- *Acupuncture and acupressure:* Stimulate nerve clusters that block the pain from getting to the brain and prompt the release of endorphins. Can sometimes be performed by a trained anesthesia provider.
- *Relaxation, meditation, and guided imagery:* Reduce emotional stressors and lessens muscle tension and other physiologic indicators of pain.
- *Music:* With dementia and pain from osteoarthritis can serve as a distraction and provide some relief.
- *Cognitive behavioral therapy or biofeedback training:* Patient is taught to manage pain through concentration and defined process to mentally control pain.

Modified from Touhy TA, Jett K: *Ebersole and Hess' toward healthy aging: human needs and nursing response,* ed 9, St Louis, 2016, Elsevier.

BOX 27.6

Preoperative Risk Factors for Postoperative Delirium in Elders

Predisposing Factors
- Age 80 years or older and gender
- Malnutrition or dehydration
- Impairment of cognition or function
- Sensory impairment (hearing and vision)
- Comorbidities and health problems
- Drug interaction or more than three prescribed drugs

Precipitating Factors
- Depression
- Laboratory abnormalities such as anemia
- Hyponatremia or hypernatremia
- Drugs (opioids and anticholinergic)
- High risk: Emergent or urgent surgical procedures (hip fractures); vascular or thoracic procedures; longer procedures or excessive blood loss
- Moderate risk: Nonvalvular cardiac surgery, elective orthopedic surgery
- Uncontrolled pain

Modified from Nauert R: *Pre-op pain and depression put elders at risk for later delirium* (website). http://psychcentral.com/news/2014/11/04/pre-surgical-pain-and-depression-place-elders-at-risk-for-post-op-delirium/76959.html. (Accessed 4 November 2016); Suwanpasua S et al: Risk factors of delirium in elderly patients with hip fracture, *Asian Biomed* 8(2):157–165, 2014; Dasgupta M: *The operative setting: a unique opportunity for delirium prediction and prevention* (website). http://rgps.on.ca/files/The_Operative_Setting_a_unique_opportunity_for_delirium_prediction_and_prevention_Monidipa_Dasgupta.pdf. (Accessed 28 November 2016).

folic acid, magnesium, vitamin D, and albumin as well as decreased creatinine clearance also may be noted. A chest x-ray film may reveal increased anteroposterior diameter, osteopenia, and degenerative joint disease. The heart size should appear normal, even in elders. Cardiomegaly can contribute to postoperative complications and should be evaluated. The ECG may show P-wave notching, ST-segment depression or left ventricular hypertrophy, and T-wave flattening or inversion, which are associated with an increased risk of myocardial ischemia (Yeo et al., 2017). An increase in bundle branch block, hemiblock, and first-degree block also may be noted, largely as a result of degenerative disease of the conduction system. Opinion about the number of preoperative laboratory tests to be ordered varies. Use of a focused history and physical examination yields important information regarding which preoperative tests are indicated. The decision to perform preoperative testing should be based on the history and physical examination findings, perioperative risk assessment, and clinical judgment (Feely et al., 2013).

Medications

Because many elderly patients take several medications, assessing their drug history is important. A multidisciplinary approach, including surgeon, primary care provider, anesthesia, and cardiologist, will determine which medication should be withheld during the preoperative period and which should be administered with a sip of water the morning of surgery. Additional considerations for medications for the elderly surgical patient can be found in the Surgical Pharmacology box. Steroid therapy may have to be adjusted.

Control of diabetes is often difficult during the perioperative period. The general management principles to minimize the incidence of hypoglycemia and to limit the incidence of excessive hyperglycemia should guide surgical planning. For patients taking oral hypoglycemic agents, secretagogues (e.g., sulfonylureas, meglitinides) can cause hypoglycemia and may increase the risk of myocardial ischemia and infarction. Metformin is usually discontinued because of the risk of advancing to lactic acidosis. Depending on the type and duration of the surgery, short-acting insulin should be used for optimal glucose control (Loh-Trivedi, 2015). Diabetic patients treated with long-acting parenteral insulin typically reduce their bedtime dose of insulin the night before surgery, and regular insulin is given during the preoperative period. Diabetic patients who are fasting the morning of surgery should take their insulin as directed by the anesthesia provider and have an intravenous (IV) line inserted for infusion of 5% dextrose and water on admission to the OR.

Additional Assessment Data

Additional data regarding the patient can be gained from observing appearance, behavior, dress, and language. For instance, does the patient's apparent age (how old the patient looks) match the chronologic age? Facial expressions and contradictory behaviors can help the nurse assess the patient's mental status. Perioperative nurses in the preoperative area can gather additional data by noting the patient's clothing. For example, does the clothing size indicate signs of weight loss? Is clothing stained or burned? What is the condition of the patient's shoes? The patient's use of language and communication skills should also be assessed when formulating a teaching plan.

Another important but often overlooked area of assessment is dental and oral health evaluation. Disorders of the oral cavity can affect the patient's nutritional condition. Many elderly people simply do not attempt to eat because of ill-fitting dentures or poor oral health. In addition, the condition of the patient's temporomandibular joint and the presence of an oral disorder, including loose teeth and

---

BOX 27.7

Signs That May Indicate Elder Abuse

When abuse has occurred the older person may do the following:
- Demonstrate *excessive* agreement or compliance with the caregiver.
- Show signs of poor hygiene, such as body odor, uncleanliness, or soiled clothing or underpants.
- Have malnutrition or dehydration.
- Have burns or pressure sores.
- Have bruises in various stages of healing that may indicate repeated injury.
- Lack adequate clothing or footwear.
- Appear to have inadequate medical attention.
- Verbalize lack of food, medication, or care.
- Verbalize being left alone or isolated in some way.
- Verbalize fear of the caregiver.
- Verbalize his or her lack of control in personal activities or finances.

Modified from Williams P: *Basic geriatric nursing*, ed 6, St Louis, 2016, Mosby.

---

dentures, can make the difference between a smooth and safe anesthesia induction and a disastrous anesthesia experience.

The risk for impaired nutritional intake is exacerbated by other factors, such as reduced salivary gland activity, receding gums, and thinner tooth enamel, with concomitant brittleness in the teeth. Esophageal mobility is reduced, and a more relaxed cardiac sphincter slows emptying in the esophagus. Moreover, weakened intestinal musculature and slower peristalsis in the lower gastrointestinal (GI) tract may lead to constipation. The confluence of these factors often results in poor nutrition. For the elderly surgical patient this can have deleterious effects, especially for wound healing.

Life changes can also affect nutritional status. Of particular importance are the losses endured with aging, such as the loss of one's spouse, family, or friends through death or relocation; loss of a prior standard of living through retirement; and loss of physical or mental well-being. These changes can affect older people to the point that they either cannot afford to buy nutritious foods or lose the ability or interest to prepare food. The ultimate effect, among other things, is a nutritionally debilitated patient. Any nutritional deficits should be corrected before surgery because the success of the operative procedure, the rate of wound healing, and the length of hospital stay are directly related to the nutritional state.

Perioperative nurses have a unique opportunity to assess and screen for signs of emotional and physical abuse in elderly patients during their preoperative assessment and while assisting with surgical positioning. Box 27.7 lists signs that may indicate abuse. If such signs are present, the perioperative nurse should report the suspected abuse to the appropriate authority. Reporting laws and regulations vary by state and facility.

Determination of Operative Risk

After assessment of the patient is completed, conditions that can add to the patient's operative risk must be considered. Medical disorders (including cardiac, abdominal, and thoracic) as well as multiple operations performed on an emergency basis significantly increase operative risk. Whenever possible, medical conditions are treated before surgery. Sometimes correction is not possible, and the risk of forestalling surgery outweighs any other medical problem.

The determination of operative risk for the patient is generally based on the ASA Physical Status Classification. Although the anesthesia provider performs the actual classification of the patient, it is important for the perioperative nurse to understand the significance of the classifications. Refer to Chapter 5 for more information on ASA classifications. The American College of Surgeons and the National Surgical Quality Improvement Program (ACS NSQIP) team developed an operative risk calculator in 2013. In May 2016, the ACS NSQIP Risk Calculator underwent advances including improved analytics, additional postoperative outcomes, and a website redesign. Users can enter the Current Procedural Terminology (CPT) code for the planned procedure and 19 standard preoperative risk factors. The user views the risks for 15 postoperative outcomes based on the risk factors and the prediction equations imbedded in the calculator (i.e., complications, mortality, morbidity specific to the patient) (Carmichael et al., 2016).

The most common surgical diagnoses in the elderly population that pose a greater risk of death are as follows:
- Acute intestinal vascular insufficiency
- Fracture of neck or femur
- Malignant neoplasm of colon
- Perforated diverticulum of colon
- Peripheral arterial occlusive disease
- Ruptured abdominal aortic or thoracic aneurysm

The intraoperative management checklist and recommendations offered in the ACS NSQIP Best Practice Guideline for 2016 is as follows:
- Anesthetic approach with consideration of regional techniques to avoid postoperative complications and improve pain control
- Perioperative analgesic plan with components of directed pain history, multimodal or opioid-sparing techniques, and regional techniques
- Postoperative nausea risk stratification and prevention strategies
- Patient safety with strategies to prevent pressure ulcers and avoid nerve damage
- Prevention of postoperative pulmonary complications and hypothermia
- Fluid management and physiologic management with appropriate use of IV fluids and hemodynamic management and continuation of cardiac medications

Nursing Diagnosis

In evaluating, synthesizing, and prioritizing the data collected during the preoperative assessment, the perioperative nurse can formulate nursing diagnoses that will form the basis of the plan of care.

Nursing diagnoses related to the care of geriatric surgical patients might include the following:
- Risk for Deficient Fluid Volume
- Ineffective Thermoregulation
- Risk for Impaired Skin Integrity
- Risk for Perioperative Positioning Injury
- Risk for Injury related to medication safety
- Risk for Infection

Outcome Identification

Outcomes identified for the selected nursing diagnoses could be stated as follows:
- The patient will maintain adequate fluid volume levels intraoperatively and postoperatively.
- The patient will maintain normothermia ±1°F throughout the perioperative period.

- The patient's skin integrity will remain intact intraoperatively.
- The patient will be free from perioperative positioning injury.
- The patient receives appropriate medication or medications, safely administered during the perioperative period.
- The patient is free from signs and symptoms of infection.

Planning

As a result of anatomic and physiologic effects of aging, geriatric patients have, in varying degrees, a general decline in organ function and an altered ability to recover from stressful events. In addition to normal age changes, many older adults experience one or more chronic conditions that influence the risk of surgery. Successful surgical outcomes in the geriatric patient depend on elective versus emergency surgical procedures, optimum physical condition of the patient, thorough preoperative assessment, close intraoperative and postoperative monitoring, and preventive measures to decrease the likelihood of complications. Collaboration with the entire surgical team can create an environment that is safe, efficient, and caring and provides for a positive patient outcome.

A Sample Plan of Care for a geriatric surgical patient follows.

SAMPLE PLAN OF CARE

Nursing Diagnosis

Risk for Deficient Fluid Volume related to NPO status and intraoperative blood and body fluid losses secondary to age-associated decrease in total body water and plasma volume based on procedure, risk factors, and comorbidities.

Outcome

The patient will maintain fluid volume hemostasis intraoperatively and postoperatively.

Interventions

- Review medical history for presence and number of chronic diseases.
- Review, document, and communicate significant abnormal laboratory findings.
- Monitor and record intraoperative intake and output.
- Monitor and calculate estimated blood loss on sponges and in suction canisters.
- Distinguish between blood and irrigation fluid amounts in suction canister or canisters.
- Ensure visibility of the urine drainage bag.
- Ensure availability of blood and fluid replacement products as needed.
- Monitor and report intake and output to the anesthesia provider, surgeon, and PACU nurse.

Nursing Diagnosis

Ineffective Thermoregulation related to poikilothermy secondary to age-associated physiologic decompensation

Outcome

The patient will maintain normothermia (±1°F) throughout the perioperative period.

Interventions

- Identify risk factors for unplanned hypothermia.
- Use warm blankets during transport to the OR, and replenish as needed throughout the perioperative period (include the patient's feet within blanket covering).
- Adjust and maintain ambient room temperature at comfortable levels.
- Place a warmed sheet on the OR bed before patient transfer.
- Use active warming intraoperatively by applying a warming blanket.
- Monitor the patient's temperature.
- Provide additional head covering (cloth, plastic, or reflective) during surgical procedures.
- Minimize exposure of the patient.
- Use warmed irrigation and preparation solutions (as recommended by manufacturer).
- Administer warmed blood and blood products and intravenous fluids at room temperature.
- Remove wet linens before transport to the PACU.

Nursing Diagnosis

Risk for Impaired Skin Integrity related to preoperative and intraoperative procedures secondary to alterations in skin turgor, sensation, peripheral tissue perfusion, and skeletal prominence

Outcome

The patient's skin integrity will remain intact intraoperatively.

Interventions

- Review risk factors for intraoperative pressure ulcer development.
- Assess potential pressure areas before anesthesia induction and positioning, noting bruises, sores, skin tears, rashes, lesions, and pressure ulcers.
- Avoid friction and shearing forces by using a four-person lift, a lift sheet, or lifting device when transferring patient to or from the OR bed and turning the patient to the desired surgical position.
- Prevent wrinkling of linen under the patient or positioning devices.
- Place electrosurgical dispersive pad in the most appropriate area while avoiding bony prominences.
- Avoid pooling of solutions under the patient.
- Apply tape sparingly to prevent skin injury during removal. If tape must be used, consider paper tape or a nonadherent dressing on fragile skin. Gauze wrap, stockinette, or tape alternatives may also be considered.
- Position the patient.
- Evaluate for signs and symptoms of physical injury to skin and tissue.

Nursing Diagnosis

Risk for Perioperative Positioning Injury related to positioning procedures secondary to musculoskeletal changes and associated chronic pain

Outcome

The patient will be free from perioperative positioning injury.

Interventions

- Assess pain and skeletal/range-of-motion limitations before anesthesia induction and positioning.
- Assess potential pressure areas before anesthesia induction and positioning.
- Place safety strap above the knees; prevent undue pressure on the popliteal space and heels.
- Ensure that armboards are maintained at less than a 90-degree angle.
- Provide adequate padding to protect potential pressure areas including foam padding under bony prominences and possibly silicone foam sacral padding.
- Maintain body alignment within restrictions imposed by chronic pain and musculoskeletal age-related changes with pillow

SAMPLE PLAN OF CARE—cont'd

under knees if appropriate for supine positioning (to maintain knee flexion to reduce pressure on lumbar/sacral regions and protect popliteal nerves). For lateral position, consider an axillary roll to protect brachial plexus.
- Use gentleness during positioning and turning.
- Keep head and neck in a comfortable position that limits hyperextension.

Nursing Diagnosis
Risk for Injury related to medication safety

Outcome
The patient receives appropriate medications, safely administered during the perioperative period.

Interventions
- Administer prescribed antibiotic therapy and immunizing agents as ordered.
- Administer prescribed medications and solutions.
- Administer prescribed prophylactic treatments.
- Label all medications on the sterile field.

- Validate medication orders, allergies, and medication administration rights with perioperative team.

Nursing Diagnosis
Risk for Infection

Outcome
The patient is free from signs and symptoms of infection.

Interventions
- Implement aseptic technique and confirm with perioperative team prophylactic antibiotic, dose, time, and administration methodology.
- Assess for susceptibility of infection and monitor for signs and symptoms of infection.
- Initiate traffic control.
- Communicate with perioperative team the need for invasive catheters (i.e., vascular, urinary) and the possibility of discontinuing.
- Protect from cross-contamination.

NPO, Nothing by mouth; *PACU,* postanesthesia care unit.

Implementation

Perioperative geriatric patient care is very similar to the care provided to younger adults. However, modifications that involve consideration of age-specific differences between the two groups are made. The perioperative nurse who recognizes the special needs of the elderly patient during what may be the most critical period of hospitalization helps enhance the course of surgical intervention and postoperative recovery (Patient Safety). All members of the surgical team must work together in all phases of the perioperative continuum to provide an environment that focuses on the needs of the patient.

Preoperative Evaluation Guidelines

The American College of Surgeons and the AGS have issued best practice guidelines for preoperative evaluation of patients at least 65 years of age who are undergoing surgery. The major objective of these guidelines is to help surgeons and the entire perioperative care team improve the quality of surgical care for elderly patients. The evidence-based guidelines will enhance surgical practice by setting higher standards and performance measures for surgeons and the entire perioperative care team. Another impetus behind these recommendations is the number and severity of underlying medical conditions that often require multidisciplinary management. The guidelines highlight 13 important areas in geriatric patients: cognitive impairment and dementia, decision-making ability, postoperative delirium, alcohol and substance abuse, cardiac assessment, pulmonary assessment, functional status, mobility and fall risk, frailty and nutritional status, medication regimen, counseling, preoperative testing, and patient family and social support system. Caring for the elderly is a team approach. Everyone should be of same accord in providing good quality care.

The guidelines strongly recommend the following preoperative assessments for every geriatric patient:
- Performing complete history and physical examination
- Conducting cognitive assessment, including the patient's ability to understand the purpose and likely outcomes of the planned surgical procedure
- Screening for depression

- Determining risk factors for postoperative delirium
- Screening for substance abuse/dependence, including alcohol
- Performing cardiac evaluation following the American College of Cardiology/American Heart Association algorithm for patients undergoing noncardiac surgery
- Assessing risk factors for postoperative pulmonary complications and implementing suitable preventive strategies
- Documenting functional status and fall history
- Calculating frailty score at baseline
- Assessing nutritional status and considering implementation of preoperative interventions for high-risk patients
- Taking a complete medication history, making needed perioperative adjustments, and monitoring for polypharmacy
- Identifying the patient's treatment goals and expectations in light of anticipated and unexpected treatment outcomes
- Assessing the family and social support system
- Performing suitable diagnostic tests as needed for elderly patients (Yeo et al., 2017)

Preoperative Preparation

The preoperative period is an opportune time to evaluate the patient's psychosocial status and educational needs. As mentioned previously, the motivation of the patient can affect operative risk and successful surgical outcomes. Awareness of psychologic and emotional status is as important as awareness of physiologic status. Often the patient's concerns are focused on the spouse or other family members rather than on the impending surgery. An unexpected hospitalization can be very disruptive to an elderly patient who perhaps was the sole caretaker of an ill spouse, parent, or even a pet. In addition, the concern for quality of life and the fear of institutionalization after surgery can be extremely upsetting. This population has the highest morbidity and mortality in the adult population. Using the assistance of social services or a case manager to arrange for resources may help allay the patient's concerns and improve the odds of a successful discharge.

Sensory deficits, occurring either as a result of age-related changes or merely because eyeglasses and hearing aids are removed, can make

PATIENT SAFETY

Preventing Deep Vein Thrombosis in the Elderly

Providing safe care for older adults in the perioperative setting requires the nurse and scrub person to have a thorough knowledge of the changes associated with aging and the risk factors for surgical complications. One of the changes associated with aging is the increased risk for the development of DVT and VTE. The chances for developing DVT increase with age and double each decade of life over the age of 40 years. For example, a person who is 80 years old is twice as likely to develop DVT or VTE as someone who is 70 years old and 16 times more likely as someone who is 40 years old. The incidence of DVT is more than 150-fold higher among hospitalized patients than those in the community.

DVT is triggered by the Virchow triad: venostasis, hypercoagulability, and vessel wall injury/dysfunction, which leads to intravascular coagulation and the formation of a structureless mass of red blood cells, fibrin, and other cellular components. Several risk factors may increase the likelihood of DVT in an older person and include the following:

- Immobility; physical limitations that influence ambulation and movement
- Congestive heart failure
- Malignancy
- Hypertension
- Use of diuretics, which contribute to dehydration and hypercoagulability
- Obesity
- Smoking
- Varicose veins or history of VTE
- Atherosclerosis or coagulopathy

Prevention of DVT in the older person begins in the preoperative phase of care. Whenever possible, the nurse should contact the patient well in advance of the planned procedure to begin education on DVT precautions. Before surgery, patients should avoid long airline travel or immobility. Walking and increasing the activity level before surgery can improve the patient's venous return as well as overall health state. Unless contraindicated by the patient's condition or physician's order, the nurse should advise patients to drink adequate fluids up until the time of their NPO status to help maintain hydration. Whenever

possible, the patient should be instructed about leg exercises (e.g., ankle rolls, leg lifts) to be performed before and after the surgery.

When the patient arrives in the preoperative area, the nurse should consult with the surgeon to ensure that GCSs or IPCDs are ordered for the patient. GCS improve venous return by squeezing and closing venous valves, preventing pooling and stagnation of blood in the lower extremities. IPCD, which alternately inflate and deflate, serve to push the blood in the extremities back toward the heart.

Before anesthesia induction, the nurse ensures the patient's GCSs are placed correctly with no wrinkles or rolling that might impede venous return and verifies that the IPCD is functioning normally. Intraoperative measures for the perioperative nurse may include inspection and maintenance of applied mechanical prophylaxis and careful positioning and changing position during procedures of more than 4 hours' duration. Contraindications for use of these mechanical devices include dermatitis, cellulitis, infections, arteriosclerosis, massive edema, ischemic vascular disease; sensitivity to latex; thigh circumference that exceeds limits of instructions for use; and severe congestive heart failure.

The nurse encourages the patient to move his or her legs and perform the recommended exercises as soon as possible in the PACU. The PACU staff should reinforce preoperative teaching about DVT prevention and ensure that the patient's caregiver also understands the instructions.

Pharmaceutical prophylaxis for DVT and VTE may be considered in some patients and is ordered by the physician based on standardized protocols and an individual plan for the patient. The perioperative nurse's knowledge of complications and contraindications of this prophylaxis are important to patient safety.

The ANA Code of Ethics for nurses with perioperative explications provides the framework for the perioperative nurse's ethical obligation to participate in care to establish, maintain, and improve healthcare environments consistent with the values of the profession by collective and individual action. The perioperative nurse's knowledge and critical thinking skill facilitate the prevention of DVT.

ANA, American Nurses Association; *DVT*, deep vein thrombosis; *GCS*, graduated compression stockings; *ICPD*, intermittent pneumatic compression devices; *NPO*, nothing by mouth; *PACU*, postanesthesia care unit; *VTE*, venous thromboembolism.
Modified from McNamara SA: Prevention of venous thromboembolism, *AORN J* 99(5):642–647, 2014.

communication with geriatric patients more difficult. Unresponsive or uncooperative behavior may be inappropriately diagnosed as dementia, expected as part of aging, and ignored. As discussed earlier, acute confusion or delirium in elders is the most important indicator of possible underlying conditions that could seriously and adversely affect surgical intervention and outcomes. Knowing whether the patient's cognitive impairment is recent or chronic will provide direction for planning postoperative care.

The perioperative nurse should take advantage of the time spent in the preadmission interview, presurgical care unit, preoperative holding area, or the surgical corridor to introduce herself or himself and explain events to follow. Because a surgical mask is generally not required in these areas, this is the most opportune time for talking with the older adult. When the patient is taken into the OR, a reassuring touch and remaining close to the patient, particularly during anesthesia induction, can help decrease anxiety.

Anesthesia Induction

The perioperative nurse shares with the anesthesia provider any pertinent assessment data that may affect anesthesia. A medical history of asthma, previous patient or family anesthesia problems, abnormal laboratory data, and physical limitations affecting induction or airway management are important findings. The following anesthetic issues contribute to the morbidity and mortality of the older population:

- Active or unstable concurrent diseases
- Decreased mobility
- Intubation difficulties
- Gravity of the surgical procedure
- Myocardial depression from anesthetic agents
- Potentially altered respiratory and cardiac reserves

Elderly patients frequently have changes in airway anatomy that make appropriate ventilation difficult. Changes in facial contour from sunken cheeks or lack of dentition can result in an inadequately fitting anesthesia mask. Keeping dentures in place often offsets this problem; however, if intubation is planned, the anesthesia provider usually removes the dentures. The joints of the head and neck may exhibit limited range of motion, making intubation and airway management more difficult in elders. Identification of these potential problems before anesthetic administration facilitates a smooth induction period.

The choice of anesthesia in the elderly patient depends on physiologic status, length of the operative procedure, and preference of the anesthesia provider. IV sedation with local anesthesia may be selected for herniorrhaphy or other procedures that do not entail complicated manipulation of organs. Regional anesthesia (e.g., spinal, femoral, brachial, axillary, or peribulbar blocks) may be chosen over general anesthesia for specific surgical procedures (e.g., cataract extraction, transurethral resection of the prostate [TURP]) because blood loss, deep vein thrombosis, and pulmonary embolism are less likely to occur (Mohanty et al., 2016). The use of spinal anesthesia may be effective for orthopedic surgical procedures, such as hip fractures or knee replacements. Flexibility of the elderly patient or the presence of arthritic problems must be considered before attempting administration of a spinal anesthetic. In patients undergoing vascular or abdominal procedures, an epidural catheter may be considered for postoperative pain management.

Accurate predictions of how the elderly patient will respond to drugs or anesthetics are difficult to make because of a decrease in systems' function. Older patients have both an altered antiinflammatory (relationship between plasma concentration and drug effect) and an altered pharmacokinetic (distribution and elimination of drugs) response to drugs. These physiologic changes can affect medication administration because of a longer or shorter duration of action and less predictable effects. The increasing age of the patient decreases the dose requirement of anesthetic. This includes agents that induce anesthesia (e.g., thiopental sodium, etomidate, propofol) and narcotics. The induction dose of a barbiturate required for a 70-year-old patient will be less than that for patients 20 to 30 years old. Minimal blood levels of a drug may produce undesired side effects before therapeutic levels are reached. Likewise, reduced liver and kidney function, altered body composition, decreased albumin level, and decreased cardiac output all modify the aged person's ability to eliminate drugs from the body. Age-related changes in homeostatic mechanisms affect the older adult's ability to deal with physiologic stresses of surgery, such as fluid depletion, volume overload, or hypoxemia. Mild hypothermia of only 1°F to 3°F below normal can increase postoperative myocardial ischemia and ventricular tachycardia. The incidence of hypothermia is greatest with combined epidural-general anesthesia (Mohanty et al., 2016). The perioperative nurse should be prepared to respond quickly in assisting the anesthesia provider to stabilize the patient when adverse reactions occur.

Positioning

Protection of skin integrity is of utmost importance. Loss of subcutaneous fat, poor skin turgor, and tissue fragility can worsen a postoperative skin problem. Elderly patients should be lifted into position, rather than slid or dragged, to prevent shearing injuries. Aging changes in the musculoskeletal system accentuate bony prominences and decrease the range of motion. These skeletal changes coupled with limitations imposed by chronic pain make positioning one of the most important considerations of care. The provision of appropriate positioning devices is pivotal to the protection from injury for this population of surgical patients. The patient's arms are placed on padded armboards with the palms up and fingers extended. Armboards are maintained

at less than a 90-degree angle to prevent brachial plexus stretch. If there are surgical reasons to tuck the arms at the side, the elbows are padded with foam or gel padding to protect the ulnar nerve, the palms face inward toward the thighs, and the wrist is maintained in a neutral position (Hortman and Chung, 2015). A drape secures the arms. It should be tucked snugly under the patient, not under the mattress. This prevents the arm from shifting downward intraoperatively and resting against the OR bed rail.

Often, because of musculoskeletal deformity and chronic pain, elderly patients cannot fully extend the spine, neck, or upper and lower extremities. Using padding devices to compensate for these limitations not only makes the patient more comfortable during the procedure but also prevents residual pain or injury postoperatively. Depending on the situation, positioning the patient before anesthesia induction may be best so that the patient can direct positioning efforts in regard to comfort. Requirements for positioning should be tailored to the individual patient according to the risk factors for positioning-related injuries. Positioning devices should be used as the manufacturer defines. The perioperative nurse should continually assess the patient's respiratory, integumentary, circulatory, musculoskeletal, and neurologic structures (Oster and Oster, 2015).

Skin Preparation and Thermoregulation

Aging skin is more susceptible to rashes, infection, and inflammation. A common complaint of the elderly is dry skin that may be part of the natural aging process or can be related to diseases such as anemia, malignancy, kidney disease, or diabetes. Medications, such as corticosteroids, may cause skin to become more fragile. Changes in the dermal receptor cells can alter the ability of the elderly to perceive sensations of pressure and touch, as well as changes in temperature.

Decreased muscle tissue and activity, reduced subcutaneous fat, and diminished peripheral circulation are some of the changes in aging that can have a negative effect on thermoregulation (Williams, 2016). The perioperative environment can expose the elderly patient to cool temperatures and hazardous chemicals, requiring the perioperative registered nurse to assume extra caution in this environment.

Aseptic Techniques and Safety Measures

Age-related changes in functioning of the immune system and some age-associated diseases have a detrimental effect on the aging body's ability to appropriately respond to infection. One out of every 10 to 20 patients hospitalized in the United States develops a hospital-acquired infection. Central line–associated bloodstream infections, ventilator-associated pneumonia, catheter-associated urinary tract infections, and surgical site infections are targeted by hospitals' prevention efforts.

Immobility and drug therapy alter flora in the intestines. Infection and delayed wound healing are poorly tolerated and sometimes fatal in debilitated elderly patients. In addition to adherence to aseptic technique, there are other measures used in the OR to protect aging patients from the risk of infection. Because length of surgical procedure is related to incidence of infection, the nurse should ensure that needed supplies and equipment are readily available to avoid delays or prolonging the procedure. The scrub person, who may be a registered nurse or surgical technologist, should be familiar with the procedure being performed to maximize efficiency to prevent unnecessary delays, decrease exposure of the surgical site, and reduce the length of time the elderly patient is anesthetized.

Fluctuations in fluid volume are common in aging patients and can lead to impaired respiratory function, swelling of the extremities, and heart failure (Oster and Oster, 2015). Volume deficits occur as

TABLE 27.1

Important Clues in Initial Assessment of Dehydration in Older Adult Patients

Clinical Indicator	Water Deficiency	Water + Electrolyte Deficiency
Medical history	Recent >3% weight loss Impaired water intake Increased perspiration (fever, tachypnea, heat)	Recent >3% weight loss Vomiting, diarrhea, diuretic, drug use, diabetes, bleeding
Physical Examination		
Dry tongue; longitudinal tongue furrows; dry mucous membranes, mouth; upper body muscle weakness; confusion; speech difficulty; sunken eyes	Present	Present
Blood pressure	Unchanged or decreased	Highly decreased
Pulse rate	Unchanged or decreased	Highly decreased
Laboratory Tests		
Serum creatinine	Increased	Increased
Serum urea	Increased	Highly decreased
Tonicity	Highly decreased	Unchanged or decreased
Urinary output and urinary sodium concentration	Decreased	Decreased, unchanged, or highly decreased

Modified from Touhy TA, Jett K: *Ebersole and Hess' Toward healthy aging: human needs and nursing response*, ed 9, St Louis, 2016, Elsevier.

a natural course of aging, whereas volume excess can occur from intraoperative fluid replacement. The age-related failure of homeostasis to adjust for stressful disturbances has been demonstrated by changes in fluid balance. Large variability in the way different organs are affected by dehydration results in atypical symptoms in older adults. Table 27.1 provides important clues for assessing dehydration. Careful measurement of intake and output is essential. Communication among team members regarding blood loss during the procedure can prevent complications. The nurse and scrub person must collaborate to ensure accuracy in irrigation distributed to the sterile field and used during the procedure. The team closely monitors discarded sponges, suction canister contents, and urinary output as part of volume assessment. During the hand-off report, the nurse reports intraoperative IV fluid volumes, estimated blood loss, and other parameters to the postanesthesia care unit (PACU) staff for their continued assessment and evaluation.

Evaluation

Because of the relatively fine line between stability and development of postoperative complications, the elderly patient's response to surgery must be closely evaluated. Before transporting the patient to the PACU, the perioperative nurse should assess the care provided intraoperatively by evaluating expected versus actual outcomes. Specific outcome criteria established for each nursing diagnosis provide the basis for evaluation of care. Many of the nurse's actions at the end of the intraoperative phase provide data for evaluation of care.

The nurse collaborates with the anesthesia provider to complete and record the patient's intake and output measurements. Because of the consequences of postoperative dehydration or fluid volume overload in the elderly patient, fluids are increased or decreased accordingly. Blood loss is carefully evaluated, recorded, and reported.

The wound is closely observed for bleeding before dressing application and postoperatively because the elderly person's ability to recover from hemorrhage and shock is extremely poor. Anticipated frequency of dressing change, as in a draining wound, should govern the method used to secure the dressing. A minimal amount of tape should be used because its removal can cause additional skin trauma.

Depending on the wound site and character, rolled gauze, stockinette, or similar bandaging over the primary dressing may be the best choice so that tape is not applied directly to the skin. Another alternative is the use of Montgomery straps. For smaller wounds, the least possible amount of hypoallergenic tape should be used. Because infection is poorly tolerated, the choice of dressing should maximize wound protection while being minimally irritating to the skin.

The nurse examines the patient for signs of injury, particularly over bony prominences and under the electrosurgical dispersive pad. To prevent skin injury postoperatively the patient should be carefully lifted from the OR bed to the stretcher. Pain is assessed and compared with preoperative levels. Evaluation of musculoskeletal pain will determine intraoperative positioning effectiveness.

Evaluation of body temperature is particularly important in elders because postoperative hypothermia is quite common and can precipitate agitation and confusion or delirium. To prevent any adverse response, the nurse covers the patient with warmed blankets and uses a forced-air warming unit until the patient is transported to the PACU.

Depending on the patient's level of consciousness, the nurse should explain the impending transfer to the PACU as a form of reality orientation for the patient. As appropriate, the nurse should introduce the patient to the PACU nurse and explain what to expect in the unit. Explanations should always precede any procedure. Often the elderly person is reluctant to cooperate simply because no one has taken the time to explain what is going to happen.

Verbal communication between the perioperative and PACU nurses should include any pertinent preoperative and intraoperative information that could affect postoperative care outcomes. This information includes pain levels; physical and sensory limitations; intake and output measurements; allergies; type and location of catheters, drains, packing, and implantable devices; anesthetics and medications received; and any unusual occurrences that could affect the patient's recovery. Perioperative nurses should be aware of the risk for the phenomenon known as postoperative delirium, a condition that can occur in elderly patients. Box 27.6 (p. 1078) lists the most frequently identified preoperative risk factors for postoperative delirium.

Documentation of outcome evaluation can be phrased as follows:

- Fluid balance was maintained, urinary output was within normal limits, the patient's forehead skin was checked and had good turgor, and vital signs were stable.
- Temperature was ±1°F of normal range, skin was warm to touch, and the patient verbalized comfort.
- Skin integrity was maintained free from redness, bruises, and abrasions; patient reported no pain or impairment of the skin; and there were no apparent signs or symptoms of infection.
- The patient accurately perceived and interpreted environmental stimuli, expressed and demonstrated understanding of procedures, and responded appropriately to auditory and verbal stimuli.
- Perioperative positioning injury was effectively prevented and patient had no compromise in musculoskeletal ability or range of motion from preoperative levels. Patient had no complaints of increased pain.
- Medications used during the intraoperative procedure caused no apparent adverse reaction.
- Patient shows no signs or symptoms of infection.

The type and extent of surgery may affect postoperative pain. Elderly persons may not complain of pain, but this does not mean that pain does not exist. Those patients with cognitive impairment may experience pain but may be unable to verbalize it. Box 27.8 lists key elements of pain assessment and management in older adults.

Contemporary pain control delivery systems and techniques offer a variety of treatment routes and modalities. Various routes may be used to deliver medication for pain control: oral, intramuscular, IV, regional (i.e., spinal or epidural), or patient-controlled analgesia (PCA). Cognitive modalities that may be used are distraction, relaxation (i.e., biofeedback), or hypnosis. Physical modalities that may be used are cold, exercise, heat, immobilization/rest, massage, positioning, or transcutaneous electrical nerve stimulation (TENS).

Clinical management of pain should be multimodal and individualized for the patient, procedure, and circumstance. Evaluation of the balance between pain control and side effects should be documented, timely, routine, and specific.

Patient, Family, and Caregiver Education and Discharge Planning

Education should be conducted at a time when the patient is at rest rather than during preoperative or postoperative procedures. Too many stimuli from outside sources can interfere with the patient's ability to concentrate and motivation to learn. Education will be ineffective in the patient who is uncomfortable or in pain. Age-related changes can affect the elderly patient's ability to learn new material; therefore modification of traditional teaching approaches should be used to enhance effectiveness. Patient education should consider health literacy and be individualized based on how the patient will best understand the information.

Enhanced recovery pathways (ERPs) are multidisciplinary, standardized approaches with the collective goal of decreasing care

---

BOX 27.8

Pain and Older Adults

Prevalence of Pain
Recognize that older adults are at great risk for undertreated pain.

Beliefs About Pain
In addition to receiving less analgesia than younger adults, older adults tend to report pain less often. Many older people hold the following beliefs and concerns about pain:
- Pain is something that must be endured; it is part of life.
- Expressing pain is unacceptable or is a sign of weakness.
- Complaining of pain will result in being labeled as a "bad" patient.
- Nurses are too busy to listen to complaints of pain.
- Pain signifies a serious illness or impending death.
  Nurses should be aware of the beliefs of older patients regarding pain management. Nurses and other caregivers often undermedicate these patients and are sometimes reluctant to administer the prescribed analgesics.

Assessment
- Ask about present pain only.
- Use a standard scale, such as the numeric faces or Iowa thermometer rating scale.
- Explain the scale each time it is used.
- Use verbal descriptions other than pain, such as "ache," "sore," and "hurt."
- Use visual representations of pain measures rather than mental images of pain rating scales. Be sure that the patient is wearing glasses and hearing aids if needed and available.

- Alter a written pain scale to include large lettering, and so forth, for increased visualization.
- Provide adequate lighting and privacy to avoid distracting background noise.

Consideration for Cognitively Impaired Patients
- Assess for nonverbal indications of pain (facial expressions, grimacing, vocalizations, body movements, and behavioral changes).
- Remember to "assume pain is present" in cognitively impaired patients.
- Consider an analgesic trial.

Management of Pain
- Be aware of adverse effects of acetaminophen (hepatotoxicity and nephrotoxicity) and nonsteroidal antiinflammatory drugs (gastrointestinal bleeding and nephrotoxicity).
- Start low and go slow with opioid dosing.
- Avoid the use of meperidine and codeine.
- Use methadone and tramadol with caution.
- Older adults and those with renal disease should not take meperidine because of the prolonged half-life of its drug metabolite, normeperidine.
- Use nondrug pain-relief measures.

Modified from Pasero R, Ignatavicius DD: Pain: the fifth vital sign. In Ignatavicius DD, Workman ML, editors: *Medical-surgical nursing: patient-centered collaborative care*, ed 8, St Louis, 2015, Saunders.

costs without negatively impacting outcomes and decreasing the length of stay or increasing complications (Brady et al., 2015). Any comprehensive discharge plan should identify and address communication barriers, incorporate the patient's current mental and physical condition, address environmental issues that can be improved to support recovery, and diminish the social support challenges. Sensory changes in vision and hearing, cognitive impairment, and literacy level can be communication barriers that interfere with the patient's ability to understand and retain information. Giving the patient postoperative instructions in written form and modifications using large, easy-to-read typeface help with retention. It may be helpful to have a magnifying glass available and supplemental light on the object or surface involved in the teaching/learning activity. Family members or significant others who are present should be included in the educational session so that they can provide reinforcement at home.

The discharge plan should consider the patient's ability to perform activities of daily living (ADLs), ambulate, and manage his or her preexisting medical condition after surgery. The older person's basic medical condition does not change because of surgery. Content should focus only on relevant information about surgical procedures or postoperative recoveries; relating it to previous life experiences helps the patient grasp the concepts more readily. The nurse should provide the most important information first. If motor skills (i.e., crutch walking, dressing change) are involved, all steps should be taught one at a time, and mastery should be demonstrated before moving to the next step. Increased time is often necessary when teaching motor skills.

Discharge planning begins during the preoperative assessment. Sufficient time is needed to make appropriate decisions about postdischarge care to prevent complications, reduce the risk of rehospitalization, and minimize stress to the patient and the caregivers. The Re-Engineered Discharge (RED) project consists of 12 interrelated interventions performed during the patient's stay designed to ease the transition between healthcare settings (Mohanty et al., 2016). Consideration should be given to the environment to which the patient will be transferred after the surgery. The patient considers relocation as a disruption after discharge. Although the plan should consider that older adults prefer to keep their autonomy, the postoperative care may require special facilities, such as a rehabilitation center or long-term care facility, at least for a time.

Transitions between care settings are periods of vulnerability for the elderly. The reasons include the involvement of multiple caregivers and errors in communication and information transfer. Comprehensive communication and written information can ease the transfer and ensure the safety of the elder adult.

The type of surgery and expected postoperative recovery period determine the extent of resources and social systems needed, such as durable medical equipment, home health and homemaker services, extended care, social and community services, and physical rehabilitation. The success of postdischarge outcomes in elders is influenced by the patient's self-assessment of health as good or excellent, the complexity of the patient's medical condition, the patient's history of being able to maintain responsibility for his or her own health, and the patient's family or social networks. Many elders undergo procedures on an ambulatory basis (Ambulatory Surgery Considerations). Discharge needs of the patient should be evaluated as early as possible so that appropriate education, referrals, and home preparation can be completed before the patient leaves the hospital or ambulatory facility.

AMBULATORY SURGERY CONSIDERATIONS

Procedures of the Eye

Cataract surgery is among the most common ophthalmic surgical procedures performed in older adults. Some degree of cataract formation is expected in all people older than 70 years of age. The majority of these procedures are performed in an ambulatory setting, with patients returning home the day of surgery. Cataracts are associated with factors including trauma, inflammation, genetic predisposition, metabolic disease, and cigarette smoking, but aging is by far the most common factor. Most eye surgery patients make the decision to have the procedure done after months of deliberation and slow, progressive loss of vision. The overall risk of death is low and does not significantly change whether local or general anesthetic is used. Intraocular lenses can be safely implanted in the majority of patients. Microsurgical wound closure ensures a secure incision that allows immediate ambulation. The surgical stress is considered so low and visual rehabilitation so rapid that severe visual impairment is considered a reasonable indication to perform surgery even if the patient is debilitated (see Chapter 18 for an in-depth description of cataract surgery). Many older adults are healthy and an ASC is the appropriate setting for their procedure. These facilities have strict surgery scheduling criteria that can limit the types of procedures that can be performed in this setting.

ASC, Ambulatory surgery center.
Modified from Cunningham B: Ambulatory takeaways, *AORN J* 101(4):452–453, 2015.

Surgical Interventions

The elderly account for the majority of cancer patients. Cancer disproportionately affects those 65 years and older, and that number will increase substantially in the coming decades as a result of the increasing life expectancy, creating a challenge for cancer specialists. The optimum treatment must be determined while paying special attention to comorbidity, physical reserves, disabilities, and geriatric conditions. Colorectal cancer is one of the most common malignancies and the second cause of cancer death in the United States, with a great number of these patients being elderly (Yeo et al., 2017). Women 65 years and older have a rate of breast cancer of 404 per 100,000. Women 70 years and older comprise 30% to 40% of all breast cancer patients (Yeo et al., 2017).

Surgical procedures that are common among the geriatric population are governed more by pathologic condition than by anatomy and are directly related to the common diseases affecting older adults. Healing is an important consideration in the decision to perform surgery on this population. The level of tissue oxygen is the main factor in determining wound healing and is influenced by factors such as cardiovascular status, anemia, diabetes, hypothyroidism, malignancy, and renal failure. In the text that follows, some surgical procedures commonly seen in elderly patients are briefly discussed. Reference is made to other sections of the text for a more in-depth description of the technical aspects of the procedures. Surgical interventions take place in various types of venues. Operative and invasive procedures can be performed in the surgical department, cardiac catheterization laboratories, ambulatory surgical centers (ASCs), doctors' offices, and any other facility deemed appropriate for a surgical intervention.

Common Surgical Procedures in Geriatric Patients

It is becoming common for patients well past 85 years of age to have surgery with relatively good outcomes. Decisions are no longer based solely on surgical risk but rather on optimal disease management and the preservation of quality of life. This shift in thinking has taken us beyond just getting the patient through the surgery and has produced a genuine concern about what the surgery will do for patients in the remaining years of life.

The advent of advanced technology has led to a decreased length of time for surgical procedures for the elderly patient. Namely, an open abdominal aortic aneurysm (AAA) surgery has been replaced with an endoscopic AAA, an open coronary artery bypass graft (CABG) has been replaced with a minimally invasive CABG, and other procedures such as minimally invasive spine procedures and robotic-assisted laparoscopic cases are now frequently performed. These procedures also decrease infection rates and length of stay.

Thyroid Surgery

In the elderly population, thyroid gland dysfunction is common and associated with significant morbidity because the symptoms are often subtle, absent, or confused with coexisting diseases. Thyroid disorders are highly prevalent, with the highest incidence being in aging women (Yeo et al., 2017).

Typical symptoms of thyroid disorders may be absent or erroneously attributed to comorbid conditions or normal aging. The polypharmacy used in the treatment of elderly patients can interfere with normal thyroid function. Drugs such as lithium or amiodarone may cause primary hyperthyroidism. For example, an elderly man taking medication for hypertension, congestive heart failure, and atrial fibrillation with complaints of fatigue, weakness, constipation, and weight gain may be considered to have these symptoms because of medication or medical conditions, whereas the symptoms also could be caused by hypothyroidism.

A rare complication of hypothyroidism, myxedema coma, affects patients older than 75 years. Confusion, disorientation, lethargy, thinning eyebrows and hair, hoarse voice, bradycardia, cardiomegaly, pericardial effusion, hypothermia, hyponatremia, and pseudomyotonic reflexes characterize this condition.

Easily overlooked in the elderly population is hyperthyroidism and can easily be missed in patients older than 60 years. It can be severe and even life-threatening. Elderly patients may not have a goiter, exophthalmos, or other ophthalmopathy. Hyperthyroidism may also cause osteoporosis. Almost any condition that can make a person ill can cause euthyroid sick syndrome; thus elders are more susceptible because of their comorbid conditions. Medication to suppress hormone secretion by the gland, surgery to remove the hyperfunctioning tissue, and radioactive iodine (RAI) to destroy the gland are the three treatment options. Although surgery is a less attractive option, it must be used when RAI is ineffective in the presence of a single nodule or multinodular toxic goiter or when the patient has dysphagia, tracheal compression, or suspected malignancy (Yeo et al., 2017). The surgical team can consider the need for anesthesia assistive devices during intubation and extubation because of the proximity of pathology to the surgical site and the airway. After surgery, the perioperative nurse must be aware of the possibility of a hyperthyroid storm that can be precipitated by the stress of the procedure, systemic infections, and anesthesia induction (see Chapter 16 for an in-depth description of operations of the thyroid).

Abdominal Surgery

Accurate diagnosis of abdominal disease is important in elders to plan timely and appropriate surgical interventions. However, clinical signs of abdominal disease, such as tenderness, pain, muscle rigidity, and fever, are frequently less obvious in elderly patients. The common use of nonsteroidal antiinflammatory drugs (NSAIDs) may mask symptoms or even predispose elderly patients to acute abdominal disease.

The most common causes of acute abdominal complaints in older patients are biliary tract disease, peptic ulcers, intestinal obstruction, GI hemorrhage, inguinal and hiatal hernia, diverticulitis, and appendicitis. Common abdominal procedures in people older than 65 years include cholecystectomy, lysis of adhesions, appendectomy, and partial excision of the small bowel (Yeo et al., 2017).

Most often, surgery is performed for complications of calculus disease and less often for malignant obstruction of the bile ducts. The prevalence of gallstones increases with age. Because laparotomy is a stressor in older ill patients, laparoscopic cholecystectomy is considered the preferred surgical approach in elderly patients with both symptomatic and asymptomatic gallstone disease (see Chapter 12 for an in-depth description of operations of the biliary tract).

The age group older than 65 years has seen an increase of ulcer disease. Many believe that the higher incidence of *Helicobacter pylori* infection, prevalent use of NSAIDs, and prevalence of cigarette smoking in elders account for the age-related differences. Up to 80% of peptic ulcer–related deaths occur in patients older than 65 years (Yeo et al., 2017).

GI bleeding is a frequent indication for hospitalization affecting a substantial number of elderly people. A coordinated approach to diagnose and manage these patients can optimize favorable outcomes. Yeo and colleagues (2017) listed the following key points to remember:

- Immediate attention should be focused on hemodynamic stabilization followed by diagnostic assessment to identify the source of bleeding.
- Outcomes are influenced by the use of anticoagulant therapy, the presence of medical comorbidities, and the nature of the lesion.
- Peptic ulcer disease is usually the most frequent source of upper GI bleeding. Rebleeding and morbidity can be reduced with gastric acid suppression and endoscopic hemostatic therapy.
- Diverticular disease is the most frequent source of lower GI bleeding. Urgent colonoscopy to identify the bleeding site and perform hemostasis is indicated. Persistent, recurrent diverticular bleeding may necessitate emergency colectomy that is associated with higher morbidity and mortality.
- Tolerance of procedural sedation must be critically considered in providing safe, effective endoscopy for elderly patients.

In selecting the procedure to correct the source of GI bleeding, the surgeon considers the patient's overall condition, history of chronic versus acute symptoms, and bleeding location. Elderly patients tolerate a surgical procedure better than they tolerate prolonged or recurrent bleeding (see Chapter 11 for an in-depth description of ulcer surgery).

Hernia Surgery

The estimated incidence of abdominal wall hernia in persons older than 65 years is 13 per 1000, with a fourfold to eightfold increase in the incidence in men. Fifty percent of all hernias are indirect inguinal, 20% are direct inguinal, 10% are ventral, 6% are femoral,

3% are umbilical, and 1% are esophageal-hiatal (Yeo et al., 2017). The elective repair of inguinal and femoral hernias is strongly advised because of the risk of incarceration with subsequent emergency surgery. Many hernia repairs in elderly patients are emergency procedures because of incarcerations and small bowel obstruction. When elective, the operation may be performed as an ambulatory procedure; IV sedation and local anesthesia provide a very satisfactory alternative to general or spinal anesthesia.

Laparoscopic techniques for hernia repair have gained popularity because of associated shorter hospital stay, minimal pain postoperatively, and early recovery. However, the necessity for general anesthesia makes this approach one that may not be advisable in elders. Decisions for local versus spinal or general anesthesia are made based on the patient's overall physiologic status and surgical risk.

In elderly men the coexistence of inguinal hernia and prostatism is fairly common. Depending on the size of the prostate, the hernia repair should be postponed until after the prostate surgery.

Large, neglected scrotal hernias are not an unusual finding in elderly men. The repair of these hernias is not routine, in that the abdominal wall defect may be so large that primary repair cannot take place without tension. Synthetic abdominal wall replacements are helpful in the management of such large hernias. The repair of huge scrotal hernias can have a tremendous benefit on the personality of the geriatric patient, who is much relieved after removal of what can be considered an accessory appendage that is offensive, difficult to clean, and often an impedance to daily activities (see Chapter 13 for an in-depth description of herniorrhaphy).

Genitourinary Surgery

The predominant reason for urologic surgery in elderly men is benign prostatic hypertrophy (BPH). BPH may be silent or have minimal symptoms in the presence of severe bladder decompensation. As part of history taking, the nurse should determine whether symptoms such as dysuria, straining at micturition, and hematuria exist. Prostate surgery, especially TURP, is relatively safe and generally well tolerated. Other surgical procedures for prostate include high-intensity–focused ultrasound, prostatic stents, and transurethral electrovaporization. The majority of BPH operations are performed to relieve symptoms, such as nocturia, slow stream, intermittency, and double voiding. TURP is indicated if the surgeon believes that total resection can be accomplished in 1 hour and that no bladder disease or impairment to urethral access is present. Alternatives to TURP surgery are discussed in Chapter 15.

Genitourinary (GU) procedures may also be performed to correct incontinence. Incontinence in elderly men can result from nerve-damaging events such as radical prostatectomy and spinal cord injury. Surgical treatments can include artificial sphincter creation, formation of a bulbourethral sling, and a urinary diversion procedure (Touhy and Jett, 2016).

Older women experience urinary incontinence more frequently than younger women. Sneezing, coughing, and laughing may cause urine to leak from the bladder. The decision to have surgery should always be based on appropriate diagnosis, evaluation of all treatment modalities, and realistic expectations from surgical intervention. Surgical choices can include urethral sling, retropubic suspension, and tension-free vaginal tape surgery. Factors that can impair a positive outcome include, but may not be limited to, obesity, radiation therapy, aging, chronic cough, poor nutrition, low estrogen level, postmenopausal, and strenuous physical activity (Touhy and Jett, 2016) (see Chapter 15 for an in-depth description of GU procedures).

Ophthalmic Surgery

Because of elders' long life span, undergoing eye surgery (most commonly for cataracts) is more likely than other surgical procedures. Most ophthalmic procedures are minimally invasive and have a high success rate. Because elderly patients may have concurrent systemic disease, even a low-stress procedure should not be treated lightly. Age-related changes, such as hearing loss and musculoskeletal disease, may pose a challenge during ophthalmic surgery because the patient must lie still for long periods and be able to follow verbal instructions. Patients with chronic lung disease lying in the supine position may experience coughing, which can increase intraocular pressure and jeopardize the outcome of the surgery.

Orthopedic Surgery

Age-related changes in bone increase the prevalence of displaced femoral and intertrochanteric fractures of the upper femur. The prevalence of hip fracture increases with advancing age, is more common in women, and is higher in institutionalized patients (Research Highlight). Malnutrition (i.e., vitamin D, calcium) can contribute to osteoporosis because of the multitude of immunologic, endocrinologic, and hematologic pathologies (Stovall, 2013). Because the usual cause of death in patients with upper femur fracture is pulmonary embolus, surgery is designed to relieve the severe pain, allow movement in and out of bed, and return the patient to his or her former environment as quickly as possible with minimal debilitation. Only 50% to 60% of patients with hip fractures will recover their prefracture ambulation abilities in the first year postfracture. Older adults who fracture a hip have a five to eight times' increased risk of mortality during the first 3 months after the fracture (Touhy and Jett, 2016). A displaced femoral neck fracture must be surgically

---

RESEARCH HIGHLIGHT

New Guidelines Address Hip Fractures in Older Adults

Hip fractures are associated with high incidences of complications. Delirium is a common complication of a hip fracture, and it has been associated with a greater mortality and morbidity rate, longer hospital stay, and greater risk of institutionalization. The guideline developed by the Academy of Orthopaedic Surgeons Clinical Practice Guideline for treatment of hip fractures diagnosis and treatment in patients aged 65 or older is based on the research information evaluated. This guideline outlines the following recommendations:

- Preoperative regional analgesia to reduce pain in patients with hip fracture
- Hip fracture surgery within 48 hours of hospital admission
- Intensive physical therapy after hospital discharge to improve functional outcomes
- Osteoporosis workup after hip fracture, with vitamin D and calcium supplementation as needed
- Use of a cephalomedullary device for subtrochanteric or reverse obliquity fracture
- Blood transfusion threshold no higher than 8 g/dL in asymptomatic postoperative hip fracture patients
- Multimodal pain management after hip fracture surgery

Modified from Barclay L: *New guidelines address hip fractures in older adults* (website), 2014. www.medscape.com/viewarticle/831690. (Accessed 15 September 2014); American Academy of Orthopaedic Surgeons (AAOS): *Management of hip fractures in the elderly, summary* (website), 2014. www.aaos.org/cc_files/aaosorg/research/guidelines/hipfxsummaryofrecommendations.pdf. (Accessed 27 November 2016).

repaired (i.e., bipolar hemiarthroplasty) or healing will not occur. In patients 70 years and older, prosthetic replacement is usually done because it allows for early ambulation and will last throughout the remaining years of the patient's life. Intertrochanteric and subtrochanteric fractures are best treated with internal fixation (i.e., intermedullary nail). These methods also allow for early mobility.

Degenerative joint disease (osteoarthritis) and inflammatory polyarticular disease (rheumatoid arthritis) are the primary indications for total joint replacement in the hip and knee. In these patients, pain that disrupts normal daily activities and interrupts sleep is the major reason for surgery regardless of the patient's age. Octogenarians and nonagenarians achieve successful pain relief and report satisfaction after the procedure. Methyl methacrylate bone cement is often used in orthopedic procedures in spite of its cardiotoxic effect. Cardiac arrest from cement insertion is a possible risk for frail patients. Supplemental inspired oxygen at the time of insertion, irrigation of the bone to remove excessive marrow elements, and retrograde insertion of the cement are methods to prevent the risk of adverse effects (Yeo et al., 2017). Usually knee replacement procedures are elective, and patients have better functional status and a higher bone mass than those with hip fracture (see Chapter 20 for an in-depth description of hip and knee surgery).

Vascular and Cardiovascular Surgery

The most frequent vascular conditions treated surgically in the older population are AAAs, carotid artery disease, and peripheral vascular disease. In patients 65 and older, the mortality from elective aneurysm repair is less than 5% in spite of existing comorbidities. Emergency repair for ruptured aneurysm carries an operative mortality of more than 50% (Yeo et al., 2017). Peripheral vascular surgery for limb salvage can be safely performed in patients older than 80 years and may be indicated for ischemic rest pain and nonhealing ulcers.

Cardiovascular disease is a significant cause of death in older patients. More than 55% of CABG procedures are performed on patients older than 65 years. Several risk factors associated with increased mortality include emergency procedure, severe left ventricular dysfunction, mitral insufficiency requiring combined procedure, elevated preoperative creatinine level, chronic obstructive pulmonary disease (COPD), anemia, and prior vascular surgery. Factors associated with morbidity in the elderly population include obesity, diabetes mellitus, aortic stenosis, and cerebrovascular disease (Yeo et al., 2017) (see Chapters 24 and 25 for a more in-depth description of vascular and cardiac surgery, respectively).

Additional Considerations

Regardless of the age of the patient every surgical procedure possesses a certain amount of risk. With increasing life expectancy, the number of surgical procedures performed on older adults will increase. Nonetheless, just as comorbidity and emergent surgery increase surgical risk, so do the physiologic deficits of aging. Procedures that are performed in the thorax or the peritoneal cavity are considered high risk. Procedures of moderate risk include vascular and hip procedures, and lower risk procedures include prostatectomy and mastectomy. However, any procedure, even those considered low risk, can have poor outcomes, depending on the patient's overall condition. Caution is advised even with the ever-increasing numbers of minimally invasive surgeries (e.g., laparoscopy). It seems logical that elders would benefit from smaller incisions that produce less postoperative pain, atelectasis, and ileus. However, the extent of hemodynamic and pulmonary consequences of CO_2 pneumoperitoneum is still unclear. In patients with severe cardiac or pulmonary disease, recommendations include invasive monitoring to maintain adequate volume loading and use of alternate gas sources or gasless techniques.

An ethical consideration with elderly surgical patients centers on the dilemma of do not resuscitate (DNR) orders. The organization's policy must give the patient a voice in the intraoperative area. Even though the patient may have made end-of-life decisions, the fact that the patient has signed the surgical informed consent implies that he or she seeks to improve quality of life, which is incompatible with withholding cardiopulmonary resuscitation (CPR). The guiding principle in the decision to maintain or suspend DNR orders should be respect for the patient's autonomy. Elderly patients have the right to participate in the process for making end-of-life decisions.

The Physician Orders for Life-Sustaining Treatment (POLST) Paradigm is an approach to end-of-life planning that focuses on patients' wishes about the medical treatments that they are to receive. The patient, healthcare professional, and loved ones participate in informed shared decision-making so that the patient's treatment wishes are honored. Table 27.2 compares the POLST Paradigm and Advanced Directives.

As more procedures are performed, there are ways to assist perioperative nurses to prepare for the care of the elderly population:

- Educate staff members by reviewing the special needs of this age group.
- Develop a separate process for preoperative assessment, and use multiple screens for evaluation of older patients.
- Improve communication and collaboration among healthcare providers.

Understanding the age-specific needs of the older surgical patient is critical to successful outcomes for these patients. High rates of medical errors have become serious challenges in the healthcare industry. As a result of their role in providing the majority of direct patient care, a nurse's performance is closely tied to the quality of healthcare services. Fatigue has been associated with stress, safety, and the nurse's performance. Nurses who work more than 12.5 hours per day are three times more likely to commit an error (ANA, 2014). Challenges in the healthcare system such as nursing shortages, increased patient loads, and decreased resources place a high demand on nurses. Understanding the relationship between the work environment, fatigue, and the environment is essential.

An organizational culture of safety must include a blame-free response to medical mistakes. Potential for errors must be recognized as opportunities to review processes and policy to prevent future mistakes. Perioperative nurses have the responsibility to contribute to the creation of a culture of safety in the workplace and to improve safety in the workplace for patients and nurses.

To ensure that older Americans receive high-quality appropriate care, the Institute of Medicine recommends the following steps:

1. Enhance the competence of all healthcare personnel involved in the delivery of geriatric care instead of depending on specialists.
2. Provide stronger incentives to recruit and maintain geriatric practitioners.
3. Apply more flexible models of care to enable self-care for patients and informal caregivers (Supiano and Alessi, 2014).

Technical advances in surgery and anesthesia will continue to provide for beneficial surgery performed on older and older patients. The perioperative nurse who approaches the care of elders with this in mind will enhance the surgical outcome and significantly affect the patient's overall quality of life.

TABLE 27.2

Physician Orders for Life-Sustaining Treatment Versus Advanced Directives

	POLST Paradigm Form	Advanced Directive
Type of Document	**Medical Order**	**Legal Document**
Who completes	Healthcare professional (and patient or surrogate)	Individual
Who needs one	Seriously ill or frail (any age) for whom the healthcare professional has reasonable expectation will die within a year	All competent adults
Appoints a surrogate	No	Yes
What is communicated	*Specific* medical orders for treatment wishes	*General* wishes about treatment wishes
		May help guide treatment plan after a medical emergency
Can EMS use	Yes	No
Ease of locating	Very easy to find	Not as easy to find
	Patient has the original	Depends on where patient keeps it and if he or she has
	Copy is in medical record	told someone where it is, and/or has given a copy to
	Copy may be in a registry (if the patient's state has a registry)	surrogate or healthcare professional to put in their record

EMS, Emergency medical services; *POLST,* Physician Orders for Life-Sustaining Treatment.
Modified from the National POLST Paradigm. www.polst.org. (Accessed 2 November 2016).

Key Points

- Although the age of 65 is often used for reporting demographics of older patients, being 65 or older does not make a person necessarily "old."
- The majority of patients 65 or older have one or more chronic health conditions that may be a risk factor for perioperative mortality.
- Perioperative nursing assessment should take into consideration normal age-related changes.
- Age alone should not be a barrier to surgery in elders.
- Elderly persons with conditions treatable by surgery have as much right as younger patients to benefit from modern surgery, anesthesia, and medical and intensive care techniques.
- Medical and surgical techniques that can enhance the older person's life should be equally available to patients regardless of age.
- Elderly patients have special needs because of their atypical presentation of disease, multiple medical disorders or comorbidity, impaired homeostasis, and altered drug response.
- Most elderly patients are mentally competent and should therefore always be involved in making decisions about their plan of care.

Critical Thinking Question

When reviewing the surgery schedule, you note you are caring for a 91-year-old female who is scheduled for removal of a skin lesion with a possible local flap. When you interview her in the preoperative area, you discover she is alert, oriented, a good health historian, and generally experiencing only normal age-associated changes. What factors would you incorporate in your perioperative plan of care? Note the critical assessment factors you would include and perioperative nursing interventions to address them.

℮volve *The answer to the Critical Thinking Question can be found at http://evolve.elsevier.com/Rothrock/Alexander.*

References

American Geriatrics Society (AGS): *Patient-centered care for older adults with multiple chronic conditions: a stepwise approach from the American Geriatrics Society* (website), 2012. www.americangeriatrics.org/files/documents/MCC.stepwise.approach.pdf. (Accessed 27 November 2016).

American Nurses Association (ANA). *Addressing nurse fatigue to promote safety and health: joint responsibilities of registered nurses and employers to reduce risks* (website), 2014. http://nursingworld.org/MainMenuCategories/Policy-Advocacy/Positions-and-Resolutions/ANAPositionStatements/Position-Statements-Alphabetically/Addressing-Nurse-Fatigue-to-Promote-Safety-and-Health.html. (Accessed 30 October 2016).

Beasley D: *Ranks of U.S. centenarians growing rapidly: report* (website), 2016. www.reuters.com/article/us-usa-centenarians-idUSKCN0UZ2IR. (Accessed 24 January 2016).

Bellelli G et al: Duration of postoperative delirium is an independent predictor of 6-month mortality in older adults after hip fracture, *J Am Geriatr Soc* 62(7):1335–1340, 2014.

Boggs W: *Simple arm test identifies frailty in older trauma patients* (website), 2016. www.medscape.com/viewarticle/863129. (Accessed 13 May 2016).

Brady KM et al: Successful implementation of an enhanced recovery pathway: a nurse's role, *AORN J* 102(5):469–481, 2015.

Bull MJ: Managing delirium in hospitalized older adults, *American Nurse Today* 10(10):1–5, 2015.

Carmichael M et al: *JACS CME and the ACS NSQIP surgical risk calculator* (website), 2016. http://bulletin.facs.org/2016/06/jacs-cme-and-the-acs-nsqip-surgical-risk-calculator/. (Accessed 28 October 2016).

Dunn G: Shared decision-making for the elderly patient with a surgical condition, *Br J Surg* 103(2):19–20, 2016.

Federal Interagency Forum on Aging-Related Statistics (FIFARS): *Older Americans 2016: key indicators of well-being, Federal Interagency Forum on Aging-Related Statistics*, Washington DC, 2016, US Government Printing Office.

Feely MA et al: Perioperative testing before noncardiac surgery, guidelines and recommendations, *Am Fam Physician* 87(6):414–418, 2013.

Hortman C, Chung S: Positioning considerations in robotic surgery, *AORN J* 102(4):434–439, 2015.

Ignatavicius DD: Care of patients with musculoskeletal problems. In Ignatavicius DD, Workman ML, editors: *Medical-surgical nursing: patient-centered collaborative care,* ed 8, St Louis, 2015, Saunders.

Jones L et al: Back pain in the elderly. A review, *Maturitus* 78(4):258–262, 2014.

Loh-Trivedi M: *Perioperative management of the diabetic patient* (website), 2015. http://emedicine.medscape.com/article/284451. (Accessed 3 November 2016).

Masterson M: Cataracts, risks, prevention, treatment, *Kansas Nurse* 90(2): 16–17, 2015. http://c.ymcdn.com/sites/ksnurses.com/resource/resmgr/The _Kansas_Nurse/The_Kansas_Nurse_March-April.pdf. (Accessed 5 December 2016).

McIsaac DI et al: Association of frailty and one-year postoperative mortality following major elective noncardiac surgery a population based cohort, *JAMA Surg* 151(6):538–545, 2016.

Mohanty S et al: *Optimal perioperative assessment of the geriatric surgical patient: best practices guideline from the ACS NSQIP/American Geriatrics Society* (website), 2016. www.facs.org/~/media/files/quality%20programs/geriatric/ acs%20nsqip%20geriatric%202016%20guidelines.ashx. (Accessed 25 August 2017).

Ogg MJ: Using a frailty index to assess surgical patients, *AORN J* 104(2):169–170, 2016.

Oresanya LB et al: Preoperative assessment of the older patient, *JAMA* 311(20): 2110–2120, 2014.

Oster KA, Oster CA: Special needs population: care of the geriatric patient population in the perioperative setting, *AORN J* 101(4):444–459, 2015.

Penprase B et al: Optimizing the perioperative nursing role for the older adult surgical patient, *OR Nurse* July:26–33, 2014.

Portal of Geriatrics Online Education (POGOE): *Common surgical procedures in the elderly* (website), 2014. www.pogoe.org/sites/default/files/gsr/7_Common_Surgical _Procedures_in_the_Elderly.pdf. (Accessed 29 October 2016).

Sigma Theta Tau International (STTI): *Geriatric pain* (website), 2015. www .geriatricpain.org/Content/Assessment/Pages/default.aspx. (Accessed 28 November 2016).

Stovall DW: *Osteoporosis: diagnosis and management,* Chichester, West Sussex, 2013, Wiley-Blackwell.

Supiano M, Alessi C: Older adults and the health care workforce, *Health Aff (Millwood)* 33(5):907–908, 2014.

Touhy TA, Jett K: *Ebersole and Hess' Toward healthy aging: human needs and nursing response,* ed 9, St Louis, 2016, Elsevier.

Williams P: *Basic geriatric nursing,* ed 6, St Louis, 2016, Elsevier.

Workman ML: Assessment of the eye and vision. In Ignatavicius DD, Workman ML, editors: *Medical-surgical nursing: patient-centered collaborative care,* ed 8, St Louis, 2015, Saunders.

Yeo H et al: Surgery in the geriatric patient. In Townsend CM et al, editors: *Sabiston textbook of surgery,* ed 20, Philadelphia, 2017, Saunders.

CHAPTER 28
Trauma Surgery

DAVID P. GAWRONSKI

Trauma is the number one cause of death in the United States for age groups 1 to 46 years and is the third leading cause of death for all age groups (NTI, 2017). Whether the injury is a result of a motor vehicle collision (MVC), violence, crime, or is a work-related injury, trauma occurs unplanned and without warning. The unpredictable nature of trauma poses a major challenge to the perioperative nurse and the patient care team.

The potential for injury has existed since the beginning of humanity. Many of the major advances in care of critically injured patients have been accomplished through experience in the military. Clearly the shorter the response time, the greater is the survival rate for casualties. This was demonstrated by the success of the mobile army surgical hospital (MASH) units during the Korean conflict and again during the Vietnam conflict; MASH brought the necessary supplies, equipment, and personnel closer to the battlefields and consequently improved patient outcomes.

Eventually this concept was applied to the civilian population and is commonly referred to as the "golden hour" of trauma care. More specifically, the golden hour refers to the time immediately after the injury when rapid and definitive interventions can be most effective in the reduction of morbidity and mortality. The golden hour starts at the scene, where prehospital personnel determine the severity of injury, initiate medical treatment, and identify the most appropriate facility to which the patient should be transferred. Traumatic deaths may occur in three phases, or time frames. The first occurs immediately after the injury. In this phase, death is usually a result of lacerations to the heart or aorta or brainstem injury. These patients rarely survive transport to the hospital, and die at the scene. The second phase occurs within the first 1 to 2 hours after the injury. These patients have injuries to the spleen, liver, lung, or other organs that result in significant blood loss. This is the group in which definitive trauma care (i.e., appropriate and aggressive resuscitation with adequate volume replacement) may have the most significant effect (the golden hour). The third phase occurs days to weeks after the injury, often during the intensive care phase, and is usually caused by complications or a failure of multiple organ systems.

The wars in Iraq and Afghanistan have resulted in some changes in the way traumatic injuries are managed; the military has not set up convalescence centers as in Vietnam and Desert Storm. Rather, the doctrine of "essential care in theater" is followed. Physicians and nurses have been trained to provide immediate care, keeping in mind the treatment resources that will be available at the next level of care. Soldiers with upper body injuries are surviving because of body armor. However, there is no protection for upper extremities; therefore many amputations are performed, including above-elbow and shoulder disarticulations. The new philosophy is to stress continuity of care with the goal of returning the soldier to the highest possible level of function.

Time is of the essence in providing definitive care to the critically injured person. A significant number of patient deaths can be prevented if rapid transport is provided from the scene to a facility equipped to provide resuscitation and treatment in an efficient and timely manner. This concept is reflected in the national development of the emergency medical services (EMS) system. Facilities and resources are allocated and coordinated to provide specific interventions for a group of patients. For example, facilities that meet certain criteria to accommodate the specialized needs of the critically injured patient are designated as *trauma centers*. Communities establish transfer and triage protocols that allow for a trauma patient to reach the appropriate facility with the least out-of-hospital time possible. This may be accomplished by a helicopter with a specially trained flight crew or by the use of ground transport with an advanced life support (ALS) ambulance team (Fig. 28.1).

Trauma centers (TCs) are classified based on the scope of available services and resources. A level I TC is capable of providing total care for every type of injury. Accepting this designation commits the TC to providing qualified personnel and equipment necessary for rapid diagnosis and treatment on a 24-hour basis. A level II TC provides comprehensive care for all injuries but lacks some of the specialized clinicians and resources required for the level I designation. A level II facility may provide surgical intervention if the critical nature of the injury dictates immediate intervention before transfer to a level I facility. A level III facility provides prompt evaluation, resuscitation, emergency surgery, and stabilization, as needed, before transfer to a higher level facility. The American College of Surgeons (ACS) recommends that in level II and III centers, an operating room (OR) team be readily available at all times. Depending on the

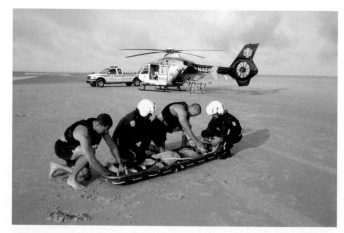

FIG. 28.1 New Hanover Health Network EMS Air Link rescue at the beach.

population served and the volume of urgent cases, this requirement may be met with on-call staff. A level IV TC has the ability to provide advanced trauma life support (ATLS) before patient transfer. These facilities may be located in rural areas with limited access and may be a clinic or a hospital.

Although the risk for death is 25% lower for a severe injury when treated in a level I TC (McCoy et al., 2013), not all patients require the services of a level I TC and thus may be transported to the closest emergency department (ED) for care. New guidelines and recommendations for triage, first developed as a position statement by the ACS in 1986, have been published (McCoy et al., 2013). Known as the Decision Scheme, this algorithm guides EMS personnel through the following four decision points: physiologic parameters, anatomic parameters, mechanism of injury (MOI), and other special considerations. Personnel review physiologic parameters. Patients with a Glasgow Coma Scale (see Table 21.2) score less than 14, systolic blood pressure less than 90 mm Hg, or respiratory rate less than 10 breaths/min or greater than 29 breaths/min should be transported to the highest level facility available. The anatomic parameters include specific types of injuries, such as penetrating injuries of the neck or torso, flail chest, or proximal long bone fracture; these patients are also transported to the highest level facility available. The MOI and other special considerations, such as age or prior medical history, are also reviewed to determine to what level facility the patient is transported.

Trauma patients require immediate access to the OR 24 hours per day, 365 days per year. A sudden influx of a large number of trauma patients to a TC may necessitate triage or classification of those less seriously injured as less urgent, allowing immediate access for the critically injured patients. The elective surgery schedule may need to be interrupted to expedite care for the trauma patient or patients. Scheduling policies and procedures are established collaboratively by the departments of surgery, trauma, anesthesia, and perioperative nursing services. Consequently the perioperative nurse and scrub person (who may be a registered nurse or surgical technologist) need to be familiar with supplies and equipment located in the OR designated for trauma or in the ORs that are used most frequently for these patients.

Perioperative Nursing Considerations

Preliminary Evaluation: Mechanism of Injury

Because of the unpredictable timing of trauma, it is often the on-call perioperative nursing team who cares for injured patients requiring surgical intervention. In contrast to an elective surgical procedure, little information may be known about trauma patients, and preparation time is often abbreviated. A working knowledge of the MOI is essential to assist the perioperative nurse in rapid patient assessment.

MOI, or kinematics, involves the action of forces on the human body and their effects. Knowing the forces applied provides valuable information in evaluation of the patient and injuries that may be present. The first EMS team to respond to the scene of an injury must carefully evaluate the patient in relation to the MOI. For example, the position of the victim in a car, whether the person was the driver or a passenger seated in the back seat or front seat, estimated velocity of the vehicle, location of impact, and use of a seat belt or airbag are all pieces of information used to determine the index of suspicion about the probable causes of injuries to the patient. After immediate threats to life are addressed, the MOI can provide valuable

clues as to probable cause of injuries. This systematic approach can reduce morbidity and mortality.

The MOI is a product of the type of injuring force and the resulting tissue response. The velocity of the collision, the shape of the object, and the tissue's flexibility influence the magnitude of the injury sustained. For example, long bone tissue has little or no flexibility. A strong collision involving a long bone most often results in a fracture of some type. In contrast, soft tissue injury from a colliding force may result in a contusion because this tissue has greater flexibility.

Blunt trauma is injury resulting from a combination of forces, such as acceleration, deceleration, shearing, and compression that do not result in a break of the skin. Morbidity and mortality may be greater than with penetrating trauma because identification of injuries is more difficult when injuries are less obvious. Causes of blunt trauma include MVCs, contact sports injuries, aggravated assault, and falls. Even low-energy trauma, such as that associated with low-level falls, can produce significant injuries.

Acceleration and deceleration injuries occur most frequently in blunt trauma. A ruptured thoracic aorta is an example of an injury that occurs as a result of these types of forces. In an MVC the large vessels are stopped or decelerated rapidly, resulting in vessel damage caused by stretching that exceeds the vessel's elastic ability. This affects the aorta at the ligamentum arteriosum, which is the anatomic point where it is affixed tightly to the chest wall, just below the origin of the subclavian artery. This shearing below the attachment site causes a rupture as the aorta continues to move in a forward motion after the chest wall motion has stopped.

MVCs account for a high degree of blunt trauma. During an MVC, actually three collisions occur (Fig. 28.2). The first collision

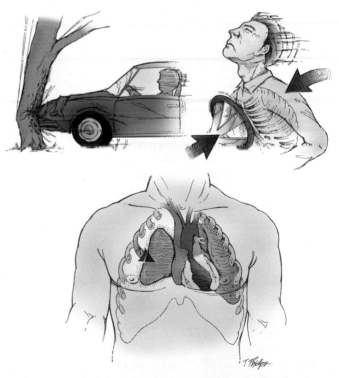

FIG. 28.2 Three collisions of a head-on motor vehicle crash: the car hits an object, the occupant's body impacts on some surface within the motor vehicle, and the result is a collision between internal tissues and the rigid body surface structures.

is that of a car into another object. The second collision is the impact of the occupant's body on the vehicle's interior. The third collision occurs when an internal body structure hits a rigid bony surface. A coup-contrecoup injury of the brain, for example, is the result of an acceleration force to one area of the brain and a deceleration force to an opposite area. Front and side airbag deployment along with the use of seat belts can decrease the severity of traumatic injury.

Falls also cause a significant number of traumatic deaths in the United States. Injuries are most commonly associated with children experiencing falls more than twice their height. In adults, falls more than 10 to 15 feet are usually accompanied by significant injury. Deceleration forces in falls produce forces of stretching, shearing, and compression. Consequently aortic injuries are also suspect in this group of patients. Skeletal injuries occur as well, because of the compressive forces present.

Penetrating trauma is a result of the passage of a foreign object through tissue. The degree or extent of tissue injury is a function of the energy that is dissipated to the tissue and the surrounding areas. The anatomic structures most often injured include the liver, intestines, and vascular system. The extent of the injury relates to the nature of the foreign object (e.g., bullet caliber, knife size), distance from the weapon, structures penetrated, and amount of energy dissipated to the structures.

The velocity of a bullet is responsible for the degree of injury or cavitation to the tissue. A low-velocity bullet is one that travels at a lower speed (1000 feet per second or less) and disrupts only the bullet tract and its immediate surrounding area. A high-velocity weapon, such as used by the military, fires a bullet traveling at a greater speed (3000 feet or more per second) and causes significantly more damage and tissue destruction because the bullet tract involves more extensive surrounding tissue (Fig. 28.3). The distance from

the weapon also influences the degree of injury because the velocity is greatest when the bullet leaves the weapon and decreases as it travels. In addition, the type of bullet (e.g., shotgun shells with multiple pellets and hollow-point bullets, which mushroom on impact) influences the degree of injury. Commonly the entrance wound is smaller than the exit wound because of the dissipation of energy, but an exit wound may not always be present. If the bullet completely fragments or is lodged in an internal structure, there will not be an exit wound. Depending on the position of the bullet and any injury that could be caused by attempting to remove it, bullets are not always removed.

Stab and impalement wounds are considered to be low-velocity wounds. The associated injuries usually correspond to the path of the penetrating object. Factors such as the object's width and length assist in identifying the possible occurrence of injuries. A single injury site may penetrate several different organs or cavities. Penetrating injuries located at or below the nipple line may cause both chest and abdominal injuries. This is attributable to the diaphragmatic excursion that occurs with inspiration and expiration. Impaled objects should not be removed at the scene or in the ED. The impaled object provides a tamponade effect to injured blood vessels and is removed only when the ability to control potential bleeding from those vessels is present. Wound debridement may also be necessary. Therefore these objects are removed in the OR, where the needed supplies and instrumentation are located.

Injuries that result from explosions are related to the effects of the blast. With the threat of terrorism, bombing, and mass murderers in our cities on the rise, the treatment of blast victims may become more frequent in trauma settings (Ambulatory Surgery Considerations). Blast injuries are capable of inflicting a variety of injuries. Primary blast injury is the result of a direct pressure wave on the body, most likely to affect the lungs, gastrointestinal (GI) tract, tympanic membrane, or blood vessels. Secondary blast injuries are often present as penetrating organ injuries and result from airborne shrapnel and debris. Tertiary injuries result from the blast wind moving bodies and debris, which may cause traumatic amputation of a limb (Beaven and Parker, 2015). The type of injury sustained and its intensity are directly related to factors such as the size of the blast and the proximity of the victim or victims. Patients from a blast explosion may present with penetrating injury, contusions, lacerations, amputations, abrasions, avulsions, evisceration, and various degrees of burns (Table 28.1).

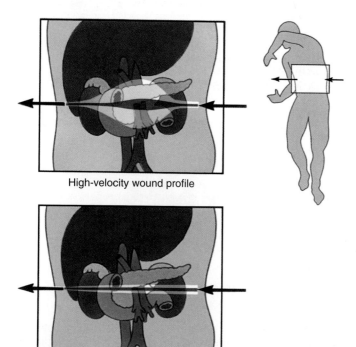

High-velocity wound profile

Low-velocity wound profile

FIG. 28.3 Potential injury path of high- and low-velocity bullets.

AMBULATORY SURGERY CONSIDERATIONS

Emergency Preparedness

The Centers for Medicare & Medicaid Services (CMS) is requiring surgery centers to be prepared in the event of natural and man-made disasters such as hurricanes, pandemics, and terrorist attacks. The four elements required for compliance are risk assessment and emergency planning, policies and procedures, communication plan, and training and testing. The CMS ruling ensures healthcare systems have a foundation of emergency preparedness and will be prepared to respond to disasters.

Modified from O'Connor D: *Is your facility disaster-ready?* (website), 2016. www.outpatient surgery.net/surgical-facility-administration/legal-and-regulatory/is-your-facility-disaster -ready--e-10-25-16. (Accessed 19 November 2016).

TABLE 28.1

Mechanisms of Blast Injuries

Category	Characteristics	Body Part Affected	Types of Injuries
Primary	Unique to HE results from the impact of the overpressurization wave with body surfaces	Gas-filled structures are most susceptible: lungs, GI tract, and middle ear	Blast lung (pulmonary barotrauma) TM rupture and middle ear damage Abdominal hemorrhage and perforation Globe (eye) rupture Concussion (TBI without physical signs of head injury)
Secondary	Results from flying debris and bomb fragments	Any body part may be affected	Penetrating ballistic (fragmentation) or blunt injuries Eye penetration (can be occult)
Tertiary	Results from individuals being thrown by the blast wind	Any body part may be affected	Fracture and traumatic amputation Closed and open brain injury
Quaternary	All explosion-related injuries, illnesses, or diseases not caused by primary, secondary, or tertiary mechanisms Includes exacerbation or complications of existing conditions	Any body part may be affected	Burns (flash, partial, and full thickness) Crush injuries Closed and open brain injury Asthma, COPD, or other breathing problems from dust, smoke, or toxic fumes Angina Hyperglycemia, hypertension

COPD, Chronic obstructive pulmonary disease; *GI*, gastrointestinal; *HE*, high-order explosives; *TBI*, traumatic brain injury, *TM*, tympanic membrane.
From Centers for Disease Control and Prevention (CDC): *Explosions and blast injuries: a primer for clinicians* (website). www.cdc.gov/masstrauma/preparedness/primer.pdf. (Accessed 24 July 2016).

TABLE 28.2

Decision Scheme Recommendations[a]

Steps	Transition	Recommendations
Step 1		Transport to TC for any of the following: GCS <14, systolic BP <90 mm Hg, respiratory rate <10 or >29 breaths/min, or need for ventilatory support
	1 to 2	These patients have potentially serious injuries and should be transported to highest level TC available
Step 2		Transport to TC for any of the following: penetrating injuries of head, neck, torso, and extremities proximal to elbow or knee; chest wall instability or deformity (e.g., flail chest); two or more proximal long bone fractures; crushed, degloved, mangled, or pulseless extremity; amputation proximal to wrist or ankle; pelvic fracture; open or depressed skull fracture; paralysis
	2 to 3	If yes to any criteria, transport to highest level TC available; if patient does not meet step 2 criteria, proceed to step 3
Step 3		Transport to TC for any of the following: falls >20 feet for adults, >10 feet or two to three times child's height; high-risk auto crash: intrusion, including roof, ejection, death in same compartment; auto versus pedestrian/bicyclist thrown; motorcycle crash at speeds >20 mph
	3 to 4	If yes to any criteria, transport to closest TC
Step 4		Consider transport to TC for the following: age >55, SBP <110, or <15, anticoagulation and bleeding disorders, burns, pregnancy, or provider judgment

[a]The Decision Scheme is an essential component of the trauma system, guiding EMS providers in transporting injured patients to the most appropriate facility, ensuring proper treatment, and thus reducing death and disability.
BP, Blood pressure; *GCS*, Glasgow Coma Scale; *SBP*, systolic blood pressure; *TC*, trauma center.
Modified from Centers for Disease Control and Prevention (CDC): *Guidelines for field triage of injured patients: recommendations of the National Expert Panel on Field Triage, 2011, MMWR 61(1):1–20, 2012* (website). www.cdc.gov/mmwr/preview/mmwrhtml/rr6101a1.htm. (Accessed 21 August 2016).

Thermal and electrical tissue damage and inhalation injuries may occur from an explosion or as a sole MOI. These patients are usually resuscitated and require operative intervention for debridement on a nonemergent basis, unless the injury is limb-threatening or life-threatening.

Injuries can be scored objectively according to their severity. This scoring system assists medical personnel in more effective triage and provides a universal method of communication among facilities, departments, and nursing personnel. The ACS guidelines, as published by the National Expert Panel on Field Triage, now recommend the use of the Decision Scheme (Table 28.2).

Assessment

The resuscitative process begins with arrival of emergency personnel on the scene and ends when the patient has been stabilized, received definitive care, and undergone a complete and thorough physical examination to determine all injuries sustained. When the patient arrives in the ED, the trauma team initiates a primary assessment and secondary assessment. This is a logical, orderly process of patient assessment for potential life threats. These assessment activities are based on established protocols for ATLS. The mnemonic used for the primary assessment is "ABCDE," representing assessment of the following:

- *A*irway (with cervical spine precautions)
- *B*reathing
- *C*irculation
- *D*isability (brief neurologic examination)
- *E*xposure (to reveal all life-threatening injuries) and *E*nvironmental control (thermoregulation)

Airway interventions may include manual maneuvers (chin lift, jaw thrust), insertion of oral or nasopharyngeal airways, or intubation. The trauma team may also perform emergent procedures, such as tracheotomy or needle cricothyrotomy, to secure the patient's airway. Pulse oximetry and capnography monitoring are used. If cervical spine precautions were not implemented before arrival at the hospital, the team initiates them before performing any other procedures on the patient. A trauma team member can stabilize the head and neck, if necessary, until a cervical collar is placed. Once placed, the team does not remove it until an examination and cervical radiograph confirms there is no neck injury.

During this time, the surgeon or ED physician and trauma team identify and correct life threats that are present before progressing to the next part of the examination. A patient requiring immediate surgery is transported to the OR, undergoes surgical intervention, and then is transferred to the postanesthesia care unit (PACU) or intensive care unit (ICU), depending on his or her condition. On the other hand, a patient may have a penetrating wound with evisceration of abdominal contents. However, correcting the obvious defect, which is currently not life-threatening, is postponed until the trauma team is assured that the patient has a patent airway and an effective breathing pattern and cervical spine precautions have been implemented. An evisceration needs to be corrected, but an inadequate airway is an immediate life threat and assumes priority.

Depending on the patient's injury, the surgeon may order an arterial blood gas (ABG) measurement. This test provides an accurate assessment of the ventilatory status of the patient and evaluates resuscitative airway and breathing interventions. Metabolic acidosis or a large base deficit (pH <7.35 or >7.45), with all other causes ruled out, may indicate internal bleeding. The surgeon may check for coagulopathy using thromboelastography (TEG). Rapid TEG testing has demonstrated a decrease in the morbidity and mortality of trauma patients because it provides valuable information about hemostatic function and clot formation and assists anesthetists in transfusion management (Collins et al., 2016).

After the trauma team completes the primary assessment and corrects any immediate life threats, they perform a secondary assessment. The purpose of the secondary assessment is to identify all injuries present. Sometimes the secondary assessment may be completed by the perioperative nurse, the PACU nurse, or the critical care nurse. The mnemonic used for the secondary assessment is "FGHI," representing assessment of the following:

- *F*ull set of vitals/focused adjuncts/facilitate family presence
- *G*ive comfort measures
- *H*istory/head-to-toe assessment
- *I*nspect posterior surfaces

This assessment begins with a full set of vital signs, including a rectal or tympanic temperature, unless contraindicated, and placement of noninvasive monitoring devices. Often during resuscitation the nurse will insert a Foley catheter to monitor urine output and fluid resuscitation efforts. The nurse should inspect the urinary meatus for the presence of blood before inserting the catheter. If blood is noted, the nurse notifies the surgeon and does not insert the catheter. The patient may have a ruptured bladder or a urethral injury, either of which is commonly associated with a fracture of the pelvis. The surgeon may wish to perform a retrograde urethrogram to examine the bladder and urethra for the presence of tears or disruption. After catheter insertion, urine is obtained for a urinalysis and urine drug screen. The identification of specific drugs in the urine may assist in further diagnosis and treatment. The urine will also be tested to determine the presence of red blood cells (RBCs). Depending on the amount of hematuria present, a renal contusion or other renal injury may be present. In addition, a nasogastric tube may be inserted at this time. The nurse prepares to provide comfort measures by assessing the patient's pain by using a pain scale (if indicated, orders for pain medication should be obtained).

The history and past medical history begin with information generated from the patient; if the patient is unable to provide the history, the team obtains the information from the family or significant others when possible (ENA, 2014). This history is referred to as the "SAMPLE" history and may be obtained even after the patient is transferred to the OR by the ED personnel. The history includes the following:

- *S*ymptoms
- *A*llergies
- *M*edications
- *P*ast medical history
- *L*ast oral intake
- *E*vents or *E*nvironment leading to the accident or injury

If the history is obtained after the initiation of surgery, it is important to communicate it to the surgeon and the anesthesia providers.

The head-to-toe evaluation of the patient (inspection, palpation, percussion, and auscultation) is used in the complete head-to-toe assessment to reveal any deformities, open injuries, tenderness, or swelling. The assessment begins at the head and face and then moves to the neck (including the spine), the chest, the abdomen, and the pelvis. The four extremities are next; distal pulses, motor function, and sensation are assessed. The final check is the back; the patient is carefully log-rolled to the side for a full visual and tactile assessment (Evidence for Practice).

Routine Laboratory Tests

Laboratory values aid the trauma team in evaluating the patient's status (see Appendix A). Appropriate laboratory tests include a minimum of a complete blood count (CBC), hemoglobin and hematocrit (H&H) value, blood alcohol level (BAL), and a blood type and screen; other tests may be requested during evaluation. The results of the laboratory studies should be reviewed and communicated as appropriate. An abnormal level of RBCs may signify dehydration, hypovolemia, or fluid overload (dilutional). An elevated white blood cell (WBC) count, indicating the presence of infection, may be related to inflammation, tissue necrosis, or that the patient is immunocompromised. H&H values also are important to note. Caution is recommended when evaluating an H&H drawn in the ED. The time delay between bleeding and a drop in the H&H value can be significant. It is only after hemodilution occurs (from shock compensation or crystalloid replacement) that the hematocrit level drops. Frequently, abnormal values in the patient with blunt trauma alert the team to the possibility of internal bleeding.

EVIDENCE FOR PRACTICE

Assessing Neurovascular Status in Patients With Musculoskeletal Trauma

Trauma patients frequently present to the OR with fractures or other musculoskeletal injuries. A thorough assessment of the patient's neurovascular status is imperative to establish a baseline for nursing and surgical interventions.

Assessment Technique	Normal Findings
Skin Color	
Inspect the skin distal to the injury	There is no change in pigmentation compared with other parts of the body
Skin Temperature	
Palpate the area distal to the injury (the dorsum of the hands is the most sensitive to temperature)	The skin is warm
Movement	
Ask the patient to move the affected area or the area distal to the injury (active motion)	The patient can move without discomfort
Move the area distal to the injury (passive motion)	There is no difference in comfort compared with active movement
Sensation	
Ask the patient if numbness or tingling is present (paresthesia)	There is no numbness or tingling
Palpate with a paper clip (especially in the web space between the first and second toes or the web space between the thumb and forefinger)	There is no difference in sensation between the affected and unaffected extremities (loss of sensation in these areas indicates perineal nerve or median nerve damage)
Pulses	
Palpate the pulses distal to the injury	Pulses are strong and easily palpated; there is no difference between the affected and unaffected extremities
Capillary Refill (Least Reliable)	
Press the nailbeds distal to the injury until blanching occurs (or the skin near the nail if nails are thick and brittle)	Blood return (to usual color) is within 3 s (5 s for older people)
Pain	
Ask the patient about the location, nature, and frequency of the pain	Pain is usually localized and is often described as stabbing or throbbing (pain out of proportion to the injury and unrelieved by analgesics may indicate compartment syndrome)

s, Seconds.
Modified from Ignatavicius DD: Care of patients with musculoskeletal trauma. In Ignatavicius DD, Workman ML, editors: *Medical-surgical nursing: patient-centered collaborative care,* ed 8, St Louis, 2016, Saunders.

BAL also assists the trauma team in their evaluation. If the patient's level is significantly high, the physical examination and response may be unreliable. In addition, the neurologic status of patients with high BALs is very difficult to assess. Abnormal clotting studies are of obvious significance in trauma patients. These results may be attributable to any anticoagulant medications the patient is taking or the effects of profound hypothermia. Clotting times may also be prolonged in the presence of excessive alcohol ingestion or the use of anabolic steroids. Clotting times may decrease with the use of antihistamines and diuretics.

A blood type and screen shortens the time needed by the blood bank to obtain a crossmatch, if needed later. Most TCs have several units of type O-negative blood (universal donor) available in the event that a blood transfusion is required before a type and crossmatch (T&C) can be performed. Because of regional shortages of O-negative blood, O-positive blood can be used in male patients and adult female patients of nonchildbearing age. Initially, trauma patients are fluid resuscitated with warmed crystalloid solutions, such as lactated Ringer's solution or normal saline solution. If the patient's blood pressure responds, the diagnostic examination continues. However, if the hypotension returns, blood transfusions may be initiated and the patient may be transported immediately to the OR for exploratory surgery.

Many TCs are implementing massive transfusion policies for the clinical management of patients experiencing massive hemorrhage and to coordinate interdisciplinary and interdepartmental resources. Massive transfusion is defined as the replacement of 10 units of red cells within a 24-hour period, or three units over 1 hour (Hess, 2016). Transfusion guidelines recommend a balanced administration of blood products. Replacing a patient's circulating volume with fresh frozen plasma, platelets, and RBC with ratios of 1:1:1 decreases mortality, improves oxygen-carrying capacity, and restores circulating volume and clotting factors (Stephens et al., 2016). This simple ratio not only is easy to use but also has the benefit of the administration of higher plasma and platelet volumes.

Diagnostic Procedures

Radiology. Depending on the TC protocol, a blunt trauma radiographic series may be ordered during the resuscitative phase. The series minimally includes a lateral view of the cervical spine and an anteroposterior (AP) view of the chest. In addition, the patient also undergoes lateral thoracic and lumbar spine films and an AP view of the pelvis. Any area with deformity, swelling, or pain may also be examined by x-ray. Trauma patients are always treated as if they have a cervical spine injury until proven otherwise. When reviewing the cervical spine films for cervical spine injury clearance, the clinician should consider any existing factors that place the patient at high risk for spine injury. These include age older than 65 years, a dangerous MOI, and paresthesias in the extremities. Patients with penetrating trauma injuries usually are transferred immediately to the OR for exploratory laparotomy.

If the resources are available, the TC protocol may also include a computed tomography (CT) scan as a diagnostic or screening tool. Depending on the MOI, such as a fall, CT scans of the head and abdomen may be performed. Because injuries in blunt trauma are very difficult to diagnose, the CT scan is frequently done before patient transfer to the OR. A high index of suspicion is maintained for other injuries until proven otherwise. Bowel injuries may be missed during initial scanning. A CT scan of the brain revealing an injury incompatible with life may alter the course of definitive treatment for a patient.

A CT-angiogram may be indicated in diagnosis of vascular injuries. If the patient is hemodynamically stable, this test is of great value in determining the extent of the injury. It is particularly beneficial in the diagnosis of a ruptured thoracic aorta, in which extravasation of the dye at the area of aortic fixation to the chest wall is noted. Other uses include evaluation of penetrating wounds, especially in the extremity. Vessel injury can be noted and the need for surgical intervention determined.

Other Diagnostic Tests. Cardiac monitoring is another component of the initial phase of trauma care and is particularly important in blunt trauma. Early detection of ventricular dysrhythmias may indicate a myocardial contusion, or bruising of the heart. An electrocardiogram (ECG) is obtained when indicated by the MOI or the patient's symptoms. Undiagnosed heart disease, as evidenced by an abnormal ECG, is noteworthy in a patient requiring operative intervention.

Focused assessment with sonography in trauma (FAST) may assist with diagnosis in difficult situations. FAST is a portable, noninvasive scan that can determine the presence of free fluid in the chest or abdomen. The typical FAST scan consists of chest, pelvic, and four abdominal scans. The chest scan examines right and left chest views and can determine the presence of pericardial fluid. The upper right abdominal scan evaluates the hepatorenal area, which is the first area that shows the presence of air. The left upper scan examines the splenorenal area. The left and right paracolic gutters are also scanned. The pelvic scan assesses for free fluid near the bladder. FAST is also used in pregnant patients; it is fast, reliable, and does not use iodinated contrast medium and ionizing radiation (Boutros et al., 2016).

Although FAST is useful in diagnosing free fluid, it cannot determine damage to solid organs; therefore it complements rather than replaces other imaging scans. Diagnostic peritoneal lavage (DPL) may be performed to determine the presence of abdominal injury. This tool is of particular benefit when evaluation of the abdomen is difficult, such as when the patient is intoxicated, unconscious, or hemodynamically unstable. DPL can be performed in the ED, OR, PACU, or ICU. Nonetheless, retroperitoneal blood may be missed with a DPL, whereas the FAST approach may be quicker and visualize more structures, even pericardium; it is also less expensive and noninvasive. Additionally, DPL detects bleeding without identifying

the injured organ (ENA, 2014). Thus FAST may be used with patients who are unstable and need a quick approach without the risk of a false-positive tap.

Internal compartment pressures may be measured with an injury to the extremity as well as to the abdomen. Swelling of the muscles below the fascia covering may compromise circulation and result in the eventual loss of the extremity because of tissue necrosis. This is known as *compartment syndrome*. There are multiple compartments in the lower extremity that may be affected (Fig. 28.4). Surgeons may measure compartment pressures with a manometer/stopcock/syringe or a commercial compartment pressure–measuring device. Normal compartmental pressures are less than 20 mm Hg. Pressures more than 30 mm Hg require a fasciotomy. Symptoms include severe pain, paresthesia, and a decrease in motor movement in the involved extremity, especially on passive movement (Table 28.3).

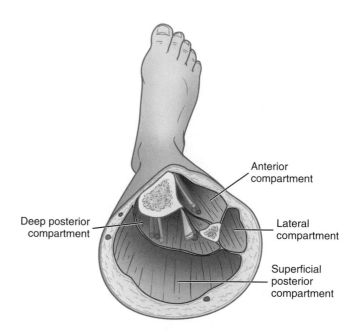

FIG. 28.4 Compartments of the lower leg.

TABLE 28.3

Signs and Symptoms Associated With Compartmental Syndromes

Compartment	Location of Sensory Changes	Movement Weakened	Painful Passive Movement	Location of Pain or Tenseness
Lower Leg				
Anterior	Deep perineal nerve	Toe extension Tibialis anterior	Toe flexion	Anterior aspect of the leg
Superficial posterior	None	Soleus and gastrocnemius	Foot dorsiflexion	Calf
Deep posterior	Posterior tibial nerve	Toe flexion Tibialis posterior	Toe extension	Distal medial part of the leg between the Achilles tendon and tibia
Forearm				
Volar	Ulnar, median nerves	Digital flexors	Digital extension	Volar forearm
Dorsal	None	Digital extensors	Digital flexion	Dorsal forearm
Hand				
Intraosseous	None	Interosseus	Abduction/adduction	Between metacarpals on dorsum of hand

Modified from Carter MA: Compartment syndrome evaluation. In Roberts JR et al, editors: *Roberts & Hedges' clinical procedures in emergency medicine*, ed 6, Philadelphia, 2014, Elsevier Saunders.

Massive intestinal edema may occur with trauma patients, causing compromise to internal organs and development of a different type of compartment syndrome. Abdominal compartment syndrome, also called abdominal hypertension, is characterized as an intra-abdominal pressure (IAP) greater than 20 mm Hg with a new organ dysfunction (Chopra et al., 2015). In healthy individuals a normal abdominal pressure is 0 to 5 mm Hg; an increase in IAP can have negative effects on the cardiovascular, respiratory, and neurologic systems, and the abdominal organs and structures (ENA, 2014). IAP is graded from I to IV based on a 12 to more than 25 mm Hg scale. Adverse effects on organ function may manifest as decreased cardiac output, oliguria, and hypoxia. Elevated intrathoracic pressure reduces left ventricular compliance, causing limitations in effective ventilation, often requiring ventilator support. Elevated IAP may cause an increase in intracranial pressure (ICP) related to obstruction of cerebral venous blood outflow and increased intrathoracic and central venous pressure. Delay in treatment of IAP may lead to brain deterioration and damage.

Management involves a decompressive laparotomy. After a decompression the greatest nursing priority is wound management. The swelling may render the abdomen difficult or impossible to close. If the abdomen is closed, IAP may rise to a level greater than 25 cm of H_2O, at which point it may lead to significant organ dysfunction (Kulaylat and Dayton, 2017). IAP monitoring is accomplished with the use of a nasogastric tube in the stomach or a Foley catheter in the bladder. Simple water-column manometry is done at 2- to 4-hour intervals, although it is possible to connect a pressure transducer to a Foley catheter by way of the sampling port (Fig. 28.5). By establishing a water column of urine in the Foley catheter with a clamp distal to the port, a pressure gradient is established. After zero-balancing the transducer, an 18-gauge needle is placed on the end of the pressure tubing and inserted into the sampling port. Using the pressure tubing and a 60-mL syringe, 50 to 60 mL of normal saline is then instilled into the Foley. On instillation of the saline, the waveform on the monitor is correlated to the existing bladder pressure. Normal IAP is zero, or subatmospheric. A pressure ≥20 mm Hg is considered diagnostic of abdominal compartment syndrome (Kulaylat and Dayton, 2017). Postoperatively these patients are susceptible to fluid and heat loss. Continuous

hemodynamic monitoring is essential in the critical care phase of treatment.

Admission Assessment

The perioperative nurse may not obtain information concerning the trauma patient until the patient arrives in the OR for surgical intervention. If the patient's condition permits, the perioperative nurse should obtain a brief, precise report from the ED nurse that contains the following information: MOI, a SAMPLE history (if available), condition on arrival (e.g., level of consciousness), availability of and prior administration of blood or blood products, spine clearance, injuries present, and any other pertinent information (e.g., family present, completion of secondary assessment). If the injury is life-threatening or limb-threatening, implied surgical consent is assumed (i.e., if the patient were able, consent would be given).

Additional data are collected as the perioperative nurse accompanies the patient to the OR. The status of the airway, as well as breathing patterns and circulatory condition, can be observed. The ED record also provides information concerning amount and type of intravenous (IV) fluid received, vital signs, core temperature, and laboratory and other diagnostic examinations performed. A quick visual and physical survey of the patient when the perioperative nurse is preparing the patient for the procedure enables identification of other sites of injury that might require attention.

The patient's psychologic status also can be assessed. If the patient is conscious, the perioperative nurse is challenged to allay fear and anxiety. The trauma patient has endured a very frightening experience and is in need of support. The perioperative nurse is often the best member of the surgical team to communicate with the patient and explain the interventions occurring before anesthesia induction. A touch or handhold is an important aspect of this communication process, demonstrating the nurse's caring behaviors and offering comfort.

Nursing Diagnosis

Nursing diagnoses related to the care of trauma patients undergoing operative intervention might include the following:
- Anxiety and Fear (patient, family, and caregiver) related to unpredictable nature of condition
- Deficient Fluid Volume related to hemorrhage, fluid shifts, alteration in capillary permeability, alteration in vascular tone, or myocardial compromise
- Hypothermia related to rapid infusion of IV fluids, decreased tissue perfusion, and exposure
- Acute Pain related to effects of trauma/injury agents, experience during invasive procedures or diagnostic tests
- Risk for Aspiration related to reduced level of consciousness secondary to injury or concomitant substance abuse; impaired cough and gag reflex; trauma to head, face, or neck; and secretions and debris in airway

Outcome Identification

Outcomes identified for the selected nursing diagnoses could be stated as follows:
- The patient, family, and caregiver will experience decreasing anxiety and fear, as evidenced by orientation to surroundings, ability to verbalize concerns and ask questions of the healthcare team, decreased fear-related behaviors (e.g., crying, agitation), and use of effective coping skills.
- The patient will have an effective circulating volume as evidenced by strong, palpable peripheral pulses; warm, dry skin of normal

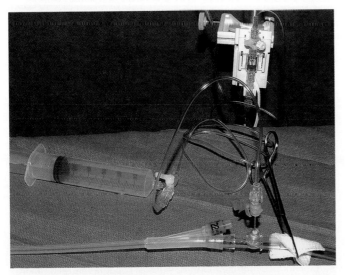

FIG. 28.5 Setup for measuring abdominal compartment syndrome using a two-way Foley catheter and a pressure monitoring system.

color; stable vital signs appropriate for age; maintenance of hematocrit level of 30 mL/dL or hemoglobin level of 12 to 14 g/dL or greater; and control of external hemorrhage.

- The patient will maintain a normal core body temperature, as evidenced by a core temperature measurement of 98°F to 99.5°F (36.6°C to 37.5°C) and warm, dry skin of normal color.
- The patient will experience relief of pain, as evidenced by diminishing or absent level of pain through his or her self-report, absence of physiologic indicators of pain (e.g., tachypnea, pallor, diaphoretic skin, increasing blood pressure), and ability to cooperate with care as appropriate.
- The patient will not experience aspiration, as evidenced by a patent airway; clear and equal bilateral breath sounds; regular rate, depth, and pattern of breathing; clear chest radiograph without evidence of infiltrates; and ability to handle secretions independently.

Planning

Because of the unexpected nature of trauma, planning perioperative care is of the utmost importance. Equipment, instruments, and supplies that have a high probability of use must be immediately available. Autologous blood salvage units should also be considered during patient care preparation, because blood salvage will be done if not contraindicated by the nature of the injury. (A Sample Plan of Care for a trauma patient follows.)

Implementation

Multiple Operative Procedures

Depending on the severity of the injuries, the multiple trauma patient may require many surgical interventions. Some of these procedures may be performed simultaneously. This is determined through a collaborative effort among the surgeons, anesthesia provider, and perioperative nurse. If a patient has sustained severe head and abdominal trauma, a surgeon will need to place an ICP monitoring device (Surgical Pharmacology). However, the abdominal exploration is also emergently indicated. Consequently the severe condition of the patient may require performance of both of these procedures at the same time.

Multiple procedures, either simultaneously or in succession, require a great deal of preparation by the perioperative nurse, scrub person, and the trauma team. The order of procedures is determined by the presence or absence of life threats. The usual order of priority is chest, abdomen, head, and extremities. However, this priority is determined for each patient's situation and adjusted accordingly.

SAMPLE PLAN OF CARE

Nursing Diagnosis
Anxiety and **Fear** (patient, family, and caregiver) related to unpredictable nature of condition

Outcome
The patient, family, and caregiver will experience decreasing anxiety and fear, as evidenced by orientation to surroundings; ability to verbalize concerns and ask questions to healthcare team; decreased fear-related behaviors (e.g., crying, agitation); and use of effective coping skills.

Interventions
- Monitor the patient's level of anxiety by assessing the state of alertness, ability to comprehend, and ability to comply with requests.
- Facilitate the family's presence.
- Assist the family in identifying coping mechanisms; facilitate and support their use.
- Reassure the patient, family, and caregiver during interactions by touch (when welcomed) and empathic verbal and nonverbal communication.
- Explain the perioperative environment to patient and what to expect to assist in reduction of anxiety.
- Discuss the patient's postoperative appearance (i.e., drains, tubes, equipment) with the patient, family, and caregiver.

Nursing Diagnosis
Deficient Fluid Volume related to hemorrhage, fluid shifts, alteration in capillary permeability, alteration in vascular tone, or myocardial compromise.

Outcome
The patient will have an effective circulating volume as evidenced by strong, palpable peripheral pulses; warm, dry skin of normal color; stable vital signs appropriate for age; maintenance of hematocrit level of 30 mL/dL or hemoglobin level of 12 to 14 g/dL or higher; and control of external hemorrhage.

Interventions
Manage any uncontrolled bleeding by doing the following:
- Applying direct pressure over bleeding site
- Elevating extremities
- Applying pressure over arterial pressure sites
- Ensuring that trauma profile laboratory work is complete
- Verifying that requested blood and blood replacement components are available in the OR
- Preparing laboratory request slips as required, and documenting time and type of analysis requested
- Collaborating with anesthesia provider in monitoring cardiovascular changes suggestive of hypovolemia
- Assisting in accurate monitoring of intake and output during the surgical procedure
- Administering blood and blood components as indicated

Nursing Diagnosis
Hypothermia related to rapid infusion of intravenous (IV) fluids, decreased tissue perfusion, exposure

Outcome
The patient will maintain a normal core body temperature, as evidenced by a core temperature measurement of 96.8°F to 99.5°F (36°C to 37.5°C) and warm, dry skin of normal color.

Interventions
- Warm IV solutions and blood products using approved warming devices.
- Minimize body exposure during all phases of perioperative care.
- Use forced-air warming units and warm blankets to facilitate normothermia.
- Ensure irrigant solutions are warm.
- Monitor body temperature for signs of hypothermia, and report to anesthesia provider.

SAMPLE PLAN OF CARE—cont'd

Nursing Diagnosis
Acute Pain related to effects of trauma/injury agents, experience during invasive procedures or diagnostic tests

Outcome
The patient will experience relief of pain, as evidenced by diminishing or absent level of pain through self-report, absence of physiologic indicators of pain (e.g., tachypnea, pallor, diaphoretic skin, increasing blood pressure), and ability to cooperate with care as appropriate.

Interventions
- Collaborate with anesthesia provider and surgeon regarding pain management therapy to increase the patient's level of comfort if condition permits.
- Assess nonverbal cues regarding level of pain and discomfort.
- Assume that pain is present or that procedures will cause pain if the patient is unable to provide verbal or nonverbal cues.
- Use a visual or numeric pain scale to assess pain levels and change in comfort if the patient is conscious and able to respond.

Nursing Diagnosis
Risk for Aspiration related to reduced level of consciousness secondary to injury or concomitant substance abuse; impaired cough and gag reflex; trauma to head, face, or neck; and secretions and debris in airway

Outcome
The patient will not experience aspiration, as evidenced by a patent airway; clear and equal bilateral breath sounds; regular rate, depth, and pattern of breathing; clear chest radiograph without evidence of infiltrates; and ability to handle secretions independently.

Interventions
- Ensure operation of suction apparatus preoperatively, and maintain one open suction line solely for use by the anesthesia provider.
- Provide assistance with cricoid pressure under the direction of the anesthesia provider.
- Assist with placement of nasogastric or orogastric tube to evacuate stomach contents.

SURGICAL PHARMACOLOGY

Commonly Used Medications by the Anesthesia Provider to Decrease Intracranial Pressure

Medication/Category	Dosage/Route	Purpose/Action	Adverse Reactions	Nursing Implications
Thiopental (Pentothal) *Pharmacotherapeutic:* Barbiturate	Adults: 1.5–3.5 mg/kg IV bolus	Reduce intraoperative elevations of ICP	Respiratory depression, hypotension, bronchospasm, and cardiac arrhythmias	Monitor for hypotension, ECG
Propofol (Diprivan) *Pharmacotherapeutic:* General anesthetics	Adults: Induction 1–2 mg/kg, administer 20 mg every 10 s until induction onset	For general anesthesia induction, reduce cerebral blood flow and the cerebral metabolic rate for oxygen	Respiratory depression, apnea, hypotension, and sinus bradycardia	Monitor respiratory rate, BP, heart rate, O_2 saturation, ABGs
Esmolol (Brevibloc) *Pharmacotherapeutic:* Beta blocker	Adults: Initially give a loading dose of 250–500 mcg/kg IV over 1 min, then begin a maintenance infusion of 50–100 mcg/kg/min IV for 4 min	Reduce systemic hypertension caused by laryngoscopy	Hypotension, bradycardia, dizziness, syncope, drowsiness, breathing difficulty, bluish fingernails or palms of hands, seizures	Monitor hypotension, ECG, heart rate; assess pulse for quality, irregular rate, bradycardia
Mannitol (Osmitrol) *Pharmacotherapeutic:* Osmotic diuretic	Adults: Initial dose 1–2 g/kg IV, followed by 0.25–1 g/kg IV q4h	Elevates osmotic pressure of glomerular filtrate, inhibiting tubular reabsorption of water and electrolytes, resulting in increased flow of water into interstitial fluid/plasma	Pulmonary edema, CHF, excessive diuresis may produce hypokalemia, hyponatremia	Monitor urinary output to determine therapeutic response Monitor serum electrolytes, BUN, renal/hepatic function tests, assess vital signs
Furosemide (Lasix) *Pharmacotherapeutic:* Diuretic	Adults: 0.5–1 mg/kg IV	Excretion of sodium, chloride, and potassium by direct action at ascending limb of loop of Henle; produces diuresis; lowers BP, ICP	Hypokalemia, hyponatremia, dehydration, sudden volume depletion may result in increased risk of thrombosis, circulatory collapse, sudden death	Check vital signs, BP, pulse; assess baseline serum electrolytes, especially for hypokalemia

ABGs, Arterial blood gases; *BP,* blood pressure; *BUN,* blood urea nitrogen; *CHF,* congestive heart failure; *ECG,* electrocardiogram; *ICP,* intracranial pressure; *IV,* intravenous; *s,* seconds.
Modified from ClinicalKey: *Esmolol* (website). www.clinicalkey.com/#!/content/drug_monograph/6-s2.0-228. (Accessed 11 November 2016); ClinicalKey: *Furosemide* (website). www.clinicalkey.com/#!/content/drug_monograph/6-s2.0-270. (Accessed 11 November 2016); ClinicalKey: *Mannitol* (website). www.clinicalkey.com/#!/content/drug_monograph/6-s2.0-363. (Accessed 11 November 2016); ClinicalKey: *Propofol* (website). www.clinicalkey.com/#!/content/drug_monograph/6-s2.0-519. (Accessed 11 November 2016); ClinicalKey: *Thiopental* (website). www.clinicalkey.com/#!/content/drug_monograph/6-s2.0-604. (Accessed 11 November 2016); Keech BM: Increased intracranial pressure and traumatic brain injury. In Duke JC, Keech BM, editors: *Anesthesia secrets,* ed 5, Denver, 2016, Elsevier Saunders.

Performance of simultaneous procedures is preferable when physically possible. Anesthesia time is decreased for the critically ill patient, and definitive surgical interventions are accomplished more rapidly.

Increased Risk for Infection

Many trauma patients have wounds that are contaminated with roadside debris, dirt, grass, or automobile parts. Others have a perforated full stomach, and food particles are released into the peritoneum, increasing the risk of peritonitis. Consequently many patients are at high risk for infection. Sterile technique may be compromised secondary only to immediate life threat. Pouring an antimicrobial solution across the surgical site may be the only surgical skin prep undertaken when an immediate life threat exists. The use of antimicrobial prophylaxis shortly before the skin incision has become the standard of care for surgical procedures. Perioperative nurses are in a position to ensure the timely administration of antibiotics.

Wounds may need to be grossly decontaminated before the surgical skin prep. Sterile scrub brushes or a mechanical irrigation-under-pressure device may be used preoperatively and intraoperatively. Care must be exercised to remove as much contamination as possible, without creating further damage to the wound or body part. Perioperative personnel must wear personal protective equipment (PPE) during irrigation under pressure to prevent splashes and contamination from the lavage system. Traffic in the OR should be limited to essential personnel. Increased traffic in the room increases the chances for contamination in an already compromised patient, as well as potentially interferes with the delivery of expedient care.

Procedure Preparation

Most level I TCs have a designated trauma OR that contains all equipment and supplies potentially needed for trauma patients. Many hospitals maintain an emergency abdominal procedure set, craniotomy procedure set, and chest procedure set either obtainable in the OR's sterile supply area or immediately available in the central supply department. This streamlines preparation for the surgical procedure and allows for rapid preparation in those instances in which the patient bypasses the ED on arrival and is transported directly to the OR.

After the perioperative nurse is notified of the surgical procedure, OR determination is made in consultation with the anesthesia provider and surgeon. Considerations include the following:

- Equipment required by the surgeon or surgeons to perform the surgical procedure
- Room availability
- Room size (to accommodate equipment, staff, and multiple procedures)
- Need for additional staff
- Capability for autologous blood salvage
- Availability of emergency procedure supplies (including power equipment)
- Selection of OR bed

Additional diagnostic procedures are often required during multiple trauma procedures. A fluoroscopic electric OR bed provides increased flexibility in patient management. The bed can be rotated on its base to facilitate two teams operating at once. The fluoroscopic capabilities allow for additional radiographs and arteriograms as needed. The bed should easily accommodate different positions, such as lithotomy or lateral rotation. If a fluoroscopic bed is not available, arrangements must be made in advance to perform diagnostic radiologic procedures intraoperatively.

Before transfer of the patient to the OR bed, the perioperative nurse must ascertain if the spinal column has been cleared by the surgeon or attending physician as free from injury. If the spine has not been cleared, the surgeon must be consulted before removal of the patient from the backboard. Safe transfer of the patient from the transport vehicle to the OR bed can be accomplished using the log-rolling technique.

Positioning the patient is based on the surgical approach. Ascertaining the type and location of the wound (anterior or posterior) and type of operative procedure dictates the patient's position. For example, an aortic injury may be approached through a thoracotomy or a median sternotomy incision. The thoracotomy requires lateral positioning devices, and the sternotomy necessitates a supine position.

If several procedures are being performed, positioning may change intraoperatively. Changing the anesthetized patient's position is accomplished under the supervision of the anesthesia provider, with particular attention to maintaining the airway. The patient is moved slowly, allowing for assessment of vital sign changes in response to the position change. All precautions regarding positioning are re-executed, with special attention given to the electrosurgical dispersive pad. This pad may loosen during patient repositioning and require replacement to ensure adequate pad contact.

When the trauma patient is transferred to the OR, the extent of injury is not always known. The perioperative nurse should prep the patient from the suprasternal notch to the midthigh. This allows for rapid access to the chest to clamp the aorta should massive hemorrhage control be indicated; it also allows for exposure of the femoral arteries for potential cannulation and access to the thigh for harvesting a saphenous vein.

Established policies for counting soft goods, instruments, and sharps should address surgical procedures of an emergent nature within the institution. Every attempt is made to verify appropriate numbers of counted items without compromising the timeliness of intervention in a life-threatening situation. If a preprocedural count is not performed, the perioperative nurse must document the occurrence and rationale used in accordance with established hospital policies and procedures. Some institutions require an x-ray examination postoperatively to examine the patient for the presence of a retained object. If counted soft goods are intentionally left in the patient (e.g., in a damage control procedure at a level II, III, or IV center before transfer to a level I facility), the number and type of soft goods left in the wound should be documented on the perioperative nursing record and communicated when there is a transfer in patient care (AORN, 2016). The operative dictation by the surgeon should also verify the presence of any retained soft goods, their type, and their number. This allows for accurate counts in subsequent procedures and prevents the potential for inadvertently retained soft goods.

In the presence of clotting difficulties or specific types of organ injuries with continuous oozing of blood, the surgeon may elect to pack the surgical site with soft goods and close the site as a temporary measure. After a period of 24 to 48 hours, the patient returns to the OR for removal of the soft goods and primary closure if possible. In such instances the perioperative nurse must document and record accurately the number of soft goods used for packing, as noted. When the soft goods are removed, the exact number is verified and they are isolated and contained in accordance with established hospital policy and procedure.

Autotransfusion

Considering the high blood loss associated with traumatic injuries, autotransfusion has become a vital asset in trauma care. Preoperative blood loss that is associated with an isolated hemothorax is collected in a designated chest-drainage device for reinfusion within 4 hours to avoid bacterial contamination. Intraoperative blood loss is collected, filtered, and reinfused to the patient. This provides immediate volume replacement, decreases the amount of bank blood used, and reduces the possibility of transfusion reactions or risk of transfusion with bloodborne pathogens.

The autologous blood salvage unit requires specialized training for operation. Institutional policies vary regarding appropriate personnel designated for operation of the equipment. Capabilities for autotransfusion should be considered during procedure preparation because additional qualified personnel may be required.

During autologous blood salvage the scrub person squeezes out additional blood and fluid from saturated soft goods before discarding them from the surgical field. The blood salvage suction is used whenever possible to maximize the amount of blood salvaged. However, care must be taken to ensure that the blood collected in the salvage unit is free from contamination. For instance, if the abdomen is contaminated with free food particles or colonic perforation is present, the blood cannot be used. Similarly, once antibiotic irrigation is initiated, the blood salvage unit is not used.

Evidence Preservation

If the injury to the patient is a result of a violent crime, the team must give special attention to preservation of evidence during the course of patient care. Physical evidence (e.g., bullets, bags of powder, weapons, pills, and other foreign objects), trace evidence (e.g., hair and fibers), biologic evidence (e.g., body fluids and blood), and clothing are types of evidence to be preserved. Specific procedures on handling of evidence may differ by institution and law enforcement agencies.

Clothing must be handled properly. When clothing is removed from the patient, the person removing it should cut along the seams or around the bullet or stab wound holes. The shape of the hole may help identify the weapon used. Clothing is placed in paper bags, labeled appropriately, and given to law enforcement personnel. Plastic bags trap moisture and may facilitate growth of mold, which could destroy evidence. The transport vehicle sheet should also be handled in a similar manner because evidence may be present. The nurse must ensure that descriptions of wound appearances, body markings consistent with gang or cult activity, and statements from the patient are accurately recorded.

The chain of custody for all evidence, including clothing, is followed. This process allows for identification of all people handling the evidence. Documentation must verify that the evidence has been in secure possession at all times. Records should be kept of all evidence discovered, including its site of origin and when and to whom the evidence was given. A system of documentation using receipts or a specific form should be established to ensure appropriate compliance.

Gunpowder residue, tissue, hair, or other valuable information may be present on the hands of a trauma patient. This evidence can be preserved by placing the patient's hands in a paper bag and securing it with tape. Washing the hands should be avoided until evidence is collected, or until directed to do so by the police.

Bullets and retained implements offer valuable evidence and may assist in identifying the assailant. The weapon firing the bullet and the bullet itself can be matched by the specific grooves and markings placed on the bullet when the gun was fired. Most bullets are composed of soft lead, and handling with metal instruments can interfere with the markings. Therefore the surgeon should avoid using metal instruments to handle bullets. Some of the newer exploding types of bullets can present a risk to perioperative team members during wound exploration. Care should be exercised to avoid sterile glove tears because these types of bullets are extremely sharp. Once a bullet is removed, the scrub person should place it in dry, clean gauze in a plastic specimen container and pass it off the sterile field to the perioperative nurse. Using the chain-of-custody procedures, the perioperative nurse should label the container appropriately and dispose of the bullet according to established institutional policies.

Deep Vein Thrombosis Prophylaxis

Because of the prolonged immobilization anticipated for the trauma patient, along with the frequency of orthopedic or lower extremity surgery, trauma patients are at high risk for developing venous thromboembolic events (VTE). Placement of an intermittent pneumatic compression device preoperatively is ideal. These pneumatic compression devices assist in decreasing the possibility of deep vein thrombosis (DVT), and their effect is optimized when applied before surgical intervention. Preoperative placement is subject to the physician's preference; clinical research regarding similar devices and demonstrated product effectiveness is ongoing. The incidence of DVT and pulmonary embolism (PE) in trauma patients varies widely. In the approximately 290,000 cases of traumatic brain injury (TBI) that occur every year, up to 54% who do not receive any intervention will develop VTE, DVT, or PE (Sadaka et al., 2013).

Currently, in patients with TBI, the only recommended prophylaxis is the use of an intermittent pneumatic compression device because of concerns with the use of heparin leading to bleeding complications. Subsequently, an inferior vena cava filter (VCF) may be inserted in high-risk patients to prevent pulmonary embolus. Risk factors for PE include prolonged immobility, multiple pelvic and lower extremity fractures, previous history of PE, severe head trauma, and incomplete spinal cord injury with paralysis. However, the placement of a VCF is associated with inferior vena cava obstruction and recurrent DVT. Contraindication to pharmacologic prophylaxis is generally limited to a short period after the initial trauma, and long-term vena cava filtration is rarely necessary.

Anesthesia Implications

Depending on institutional protocol, the anesthesia team may be directly involved in resuscitation of the trauma patient immediately after arrival at the ED. The anesthesia provider maintains the airway and intubates the patient if necessary. A critically injured patient may be transferred directly to the OR, whereas some interventions may be performed in the ED of a TC. These interventions vary from insertion of an ICP monitor to an emergent exploratory thoracotomy.

However, if diagnostic evaluation can be accomplished without intubation and sedation, the patient may be conscious on arrival in the OR. A trauma patient is assumed to have a full stomach; thus these patients are at high risk for aspiration and resultant pneumonia. Under the direction of the anesthesia provider, the perioperative nurse applies cricoid pressure (Sellick maneuver) (see Fig. 5.4). This pressure is maintained over the cricoid area until the cuff on the endotracheal tube (ETT) is inflated and tube placement verified by the anesthesia provider. This type of intubation is often referred to as a "crash induction."

In addition, the patient may require intubation for protection of the airway before radiologic examination of the cervical spine. If the cervical spine is not cleared or if the radiographic screening examination is not performed before intubation, ETT intubation is done while cervical spine precautions (i.e., in-line intubation) are maintained. The anesthesia provider may decide to use rapid-sequence intubation (RSI), which involves administering 100% oxygen, an analgesic, and a neuromuscular relaxant, and inserting a cuffed ETT tube. The perioperative nurse can facilitate RSI by ensuring availability of all intubation and resuscitation equipment, assisting with monitoring devices, and confirming correct ETT placement (Box 28.1).

In injuries of the face where midface fractures are present, nasal intubation and nasogastric tube placement are avoided. Tube placement in the brain through a fracture of the cribriform plate is a well-known complication. To avoid this, oral ETT intubation is the technique of choice. The anesthesia provider places an oral gastric tube to achieve stomach decompression. An oral intubation on a conscious patient is often necessary because anesthetics and muscle relaxants can result in the loss of any remaining airway in the presence of facial trauma.

Large-bore IV access used with rapid-infusion fluid warmers may be used in the ED. These fluid warmers can deliver high volumes of crystalloid solution at body temperature. Use of the fluid warmer may continue during the intraoperative phase to facilitate volume replacement and help maintain normothermia. A number of factors may influence a trauma patient's response to fluid loss. These factors include age, severity of injury, type and location of injury, time lapse from injury to treatment, prehospital fluid therapy, prehospital use of a pneumatic antishock garment (PASG), and medications taken for chronic conditions. Fluid resuscitation should be initiated when early signs of blood loss are suspected. A classification system can be useful in determining the needs of the patient (Table 28.4).

Pregnancy

Trauma in pregnancy is a leading cause of nonpregnancy-related maternal deaths and complicates 1 in 12 pregnancies (Murphy and Quinlan, 2014). Traumatic injuries include MVCs, falls, poisonings, burns, and assaults (Murphy and Quinlan, 2014). It is most important to remember that two patients are being treated.

The normal physiologic changes that occur during pregnancy increase the challenge of evaluation and treatment when these individuals are victims of trauma. The pelvis protects the uterus and fetus during the first trimester; during the second trimester, increases in amniotic fluid volume protect the fetus (Murphy and Quinlan, 2014). In the third semester the uterus is at an increased risk for injury from blunt and penetrating abdominal trauma (Murphy and Quinlan, 2014).

It is also important to note that the pregnant trauma patient has a much larger circulatory volume (Table 28.5). The cardiac output may be increased by as much as 40%. Oxygen requirements are increased. Heart rate increases over the prepregnant state. The usual clinical indicators of hypovolemic shock are unreliable in the pregnant trauma patient (Table 28.6). The team must assume that the pregnant trauma victim is in shock until proven otherwise. Early aggressive treatment is essential. The uterus is enlarged and no longer a pelvic organ, and it elevates the bladder out of the pelvis as well. Supine position for the pregnant patient can result in a decrease in cardiac output as a result of compression of the inferior vena cava. If the patient is close to term, cardiac output can be reduced by as much as 30% as a result of compression on the inferior vena cava.

BOX 28.1

Rapid-Sequence Intubation Steps

Preparation	Assist anesthesia care provider as needed; ensure all equipment is available
Preoxygenation	Provide high-flow oxygen at the highest concentration
Pretreatment	Assist anesthesia provider in medication administration, as indicated (lidocaine, opioids, atropine, and defasciculating dose of neuromuscular blocking agent)
Paralysis with induction	Stand by while anesthesia is induced (etomidate, ketamine, midazolam, propofol); provide support while patient loses consciousness and neuromuscular agent is administered (succinylcholine)
Protection and positioning	Protect the airway from aspiration and provide manual ventilation
Placement with proof	Inflate cuff; check placement with exhaled carbon dioxide detector, watch for symmetric rise and fall of the chest, and by listening to lungs with stethoscope
Postintubation management	Secure tube and monitor per routine

Data from Blair,[7] Kahn et al.,[18] Chan et al.,[22] Skidmore-Roth. *Mosby's 2012 nursing drug reference*, ed 25, St Louis, 2012, Elsevier. In Dixon MD, McAninch JW: *American Urological Association updates series, traumatic renal injuries, part 1: assessment and management*, Houston, 1991, The Association.

TABLE 28.4

Estimated Fluid and Blood Losses Based on Patient's Initial Presentation[a]

	Class I	Class II	Class III	Class IV
Blood loss (mL)	Up to 750	750–1500	1500–2000	>2000
Blood loss (% blood volume)	Up to 15%	15%–30%	30%–40%	>40%
Pulse rate (beats/min)	<100	>100	>120	>140
Systolic blood pressure	Normal	Normal	Decreased	Decreased
Pulse pressure	Normal or increased	Decreased	Decreased	Decreased
Respiratory rate (breaths/min)	14–20	20–30	30–40	>35
Urine output (mL/h)	>30	20–30	5–15	Negligible
Central nervous system/mental status	Slightly anxious	Mildly anxious	Anxious, confused	Confused, lethargic
Initial fluid replacement	Crystalloid	Crystalloid	Crystalloid and blood	Crystalloid and blood

[a]The guidelines are for a 70-kg man.
Modified from American College of Surgeons (ACS): *Advanced trauma life support student course manual*, ed 9, Chicago, 2012, ACS.

TABLE 28.5

Physiologic Changes of Pregnancy on Trauma Patients

Parameter	Adaptation	Impact
Plasma volume	50% increase	Relative resistance to limited blood loss
RBC mass	30% increase	Dilutional anemia (plasma volume increase >RBC mass increase)
Cardiac output	30%–50% increase	Relative resistance to limited blood loss
Heart rate	10–15 beat increase	May be interpreted as hypovolemia
Blood pressure	Fall in second trimester	May be interpreted as hypovolemia
Coagulation factors	Increased	Increased risk of DVT
Uteroplacental blood flow	20%–30% shunt	Uterine injury may predispose to increased blood loss
Uterine size	Dramatic increase	Compression of vena cava or aorta (supine hypotension); shifting of abdominal contents
Minute ventilation	25% increase	Decreased $PaCO_2$; decreased buffering capacity
Functional residual capacity	Decreased	Increased propensity for atelectasis and hypoxemia
Gastric emptying	Slowed	Increased risk of aspiration
Bladder	Displaced cephalad in second and third trimesters	Increased risk of bladder injury in abdominal trauma

DVT, Deep vein thrombosis; *$PaCO_2$*, partial pressure of carbon dioxide; *RBC*, red blood cell.
From Yadava SM: Trauma in pregnancy. In Mularz A et al, editors: *OB/GYN secrets*, ed 4, Philadelphia, 2017, Elsevier.

TABLE 28.6

Signs of Hypovolemic Shock in Pregnancy

	Circulating Blood Volume Deficit	
	Early (20%)	Late (25%)
Pulse rate	<100 beats/min	>100 beats/min
Respiratory rate	12–20 breaths/min	>20 breaths/min
Blood pressure	Normal	Hypotensive
Skin perfusion	Warm, dry skin	Cool, ashen skin
Capillary refill time	<2 s	>2 s
Level of consciousness	Alert	Agitated, lethargic
Urine output	>30–50 mL/h	<30–50 mL/h
Fetal heart rate (normally 120–160 beats/min)	High, low, late decelerations	High, low, absent, late decelerations

s, Seconds.

Consequently patients who are 20 weeks or more into their pregnancy should be placed in the left lateral decubitus position to avoid a hypotensive episode and maintain blood flow to the uterus and placenta. If this is not possible, manual displacement of the uterus by lateral abdominal pressure should be attempted. As a result of the physiologic changes just described, the pregnant patient is at risk for aspiration. Rapid-sequence induction, along with the Sellick maneuver, is the preferred method for intubation.

Ultrasound studies are conducted to determine viability of the fetus when possible. In the event of a ruptured uterus, a cesarean delivery and hysterectomy may be required if the fetus is viable. Neonatal resuscitation is of the utmost importance immediately on delivery of the fetus.

Pregnant patients requiring surgery also need fetal assessment performed intraoperatively. Any fetal movement should be noted. In addition, fetal monitoring is continuous. This includes fetal heart rate and uterine contractions. Fetal monitoring provides information on the condition of the fetus and the response to uterine contractions, if present. Fetal heart rate can usually be obtained after 10 weeks'

gestation. Abnormalities in fetal heart rate can be an early sign of maternal compromise because the pregnant uterus is viewed as a nonessential peripheral organ in states of hypovolemic shock. Personnel qualified in the interpretation of fetal heart rate patterns must be present. This expertise may be provided by the obstetric nursing staff.

Perimortem (postmortem) cesarean delivery may be performed in the event of the sudden death of the mother and the presence of a viable fetus.

Pediatric Trauma Patients

Special considerations related to the care of infants and children who have sustained a trauma are described in Chapter 26. Table 26.6 details a modified Glasgow Coma Scale for children.

Elderly Trauma Patients

As the number of adults older than 65 years continues to grow, so does the number of elderly patients requiring surgical intervention related to trauma. The physiologic effects of aging combined with the preinjury health status of many elderly patients significantly affect their ability to respond to initial treatment for traumatic injuries and subsequent surgical intervention. Consequently the mortality for elderly trauma patients is significantly higher than that in younger patients with the same level of injury because of preexisting medical conditions, medication use, and the physiologic effects of aging (Stevens, 2016). (See Chapter 27 for the physical and psychologic changes that occur in elderly patients.)

Bariatric Trauma Patients

There has been a notable increase in admissions of bariatric patients in all healthcare facilities. Bariatric medicine is defined as the care of the extremely obese patient, as measured by body mass index (BMI). The World Health Organization and the National Institute of Health define obese as a BMI equal to or greater than 30, and morbidly obese as a BMI of 40 or greater (Ditillo et al., 2015). Obesity is considered a risk factor for trauma patients because it is associated with other comorbid conditions, including cardiac disease, hypertension, respiratory disease, diabetes, and osteoarthritis (Research

Infection Risk for Obese Patients

Bell and colleagues (2016) conducted a retrospective analysis to examine the link between obese patients and infectious complications after trauma using 2012 data from the National Trauma Data Bank. They compared infectious complications between obese and nonobese patients; they found differences in rates of deep SSI, organ and/or space SSI, pneumonia, superficial SSI, UTI, severe sepsis, and infectious complication. The development of any hospital compilation was common in obese patients. Obesity increased the risk of developing an infectious complication by 60%. Additionally, obese patients are twice as likely to develop sepsis, UTI, or respiratory infections in the trauma or ICU setting.

The rate of obesity is rising in the United States, and TCs and ICUs will see an increase with this patient population. The authors suggest that protocols should be developed to reduce the infection risk in the obese population. Antibiotic guidelines need to be defined and adhered to along with the timing of administration for the obese patient with a traumatic injury. Blood glucose levels should be screened preoperatively with glucose control postoperatively. The patient may require additional staff to assist with mobilization, which is known to lower the risk of infection after surgery.

ICU, Intensive care unit: *SSI,* surgical site infection; *TCs,* trauma centers; *UTI,* urinary tract infection.
Modified from Bell TM et al: Infectious complications in obese patients after trauma, *J Surg Res* 204(2):393–397, 2016.

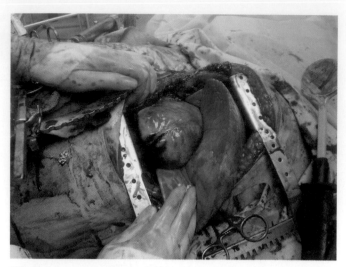

FIG. 28.6 Emergency clam shell thoracotomy performed in the emergency department.

Highlight: Infection Risk for Obese Patients) (Bell et al., 2016). After a trauma the patient may develop in-house complications including sepsis, pneumonia, urinary tract infections, DVT, disseminated intravascular coagulation (DIC), acute respiratory distress syndrome (ARDS), and decubitus ulcer (Ditillo et al., 2015). Additionally, obesity is a risk. Intraoperative injuries for the morbidly obese patients include pressure sores and nerve injuries; therefore care must be taken to safely position the patient (Fencl et al., 2015).

Invasive Emergency Department Interventions

If a patient has shown a very recent deterioration of vital signs, either en route to the hospital or on arrival at the ED, the surgeon may elect to perform an aortic occlusion with resuscitative endovascular balloon occlusion of the aorta (REBOA) (Research Highlight: Resuscitative Endovascular Balloon Occlusion of the Aorta) or an emergency thoracotomy in the ED. A left-sided thoracotomy approach is usually performed because this allows rapid access to the heart for external cardiac massage and exposure of the great vessels for clamping in the event of severe blood loss (Fig. 28.6). The incision can be extended to the right side by cutting across the sternum; this approach is commonly referred to as the clam shell thoracotomy. This procedure can be used to gain control of hemorrhage of the great vessels; to access the heart; or, in a grave situation, as a final effort to save a life. The procedure is used more often in penetrating injuries in which a laceration to a ventricle or other potentially treatable, life-threatening injury may be present.

Because of the perioperative nurse's knowledge of surgical instrumentation and procedures, his or her assistance in this procedure in the ED is often required. Rapid access to the heart and great vessels is the goal. The patient is then transported to the OR for additional interventions when hemorrhage is controlled.

In a similar fashion, an exploratory laparotomy can be initiated in the ED to control abdominal hemorrhage, especially when a splenic rupture is suspected and the patient is severely compromised.

If all other techniques of airway access are unsuccessful, the surgeon performs a cricothyrotomy. The surgeon makes a vertical incision through the skin, and incises the cricothyroid membrane. An ETT or tracheostomy tube can be inserted through the membrane to create an airway. In the event a tube is not immediately available, a large-bore needle can be inserted into the membrane and the catheter left in place. This provides a temporary airway access measure but is inadequate to effectively ventilate the patient without a jet oscillating ventilator.

Successive Surgical Interventions

Often the multiple trauma patient requires a multitude of surgical procedures, either specialty-related or as a stepwise progression in the primary treatment of the initial injury. Initially the trauma patient is critically ill and requires intensive care facilities. When surgery is scheduled, the perioperative nurse may need additional assistance in transporting the patient as transport monitoring of the ECG, arterial line, and blood pressure is performed. Oxygen administration and mechanical ventilation with an Ambu bag are necessary for the intubated patient. Acalculous cholecystitis is often a secondary complication of the trauma patient's postoperative course that requires cholecystectomy. Fixation of initially undiscovered fractures, debridements, secondary wound closures, flap constructions, and other reconstructive procedures make up the majority of follow-up procedures. Depending on the patient's condition, some procedures may be performed after discharge on an outpatient basis.

Evaluation

The evaluation of the patient should reflect the effectiveness of the interventions. Did the patient remain free from untoward complications? Was there progress toward the expected outcomes as described in the perioperative plan of care? The following are examples of evaluation statements in relation to the sample plan of care:

- The patient demonstrated a decreased level of anxiety; he or she verbalized less apprehension, maintained eye contact, and was able to comply with requests even though anxiety persisted.

RESEARCH HIGHLIGHT ▮▮

Resuscitative Endovascular Balloon Occlusion of the Aorta

Aortic occlusion can be used for resuscitation and hemorrhage control. REBOA is a minimally invasive endovascular approach that supports perfusion of vital organs until hemostasis can be achieved. The indications for REBOA in trauma have not been clearly defined, but patients who are not candidates for resuscitative thoracotomy should not be considered for REBOA. However, there is evidence supporting patients with abdominal or pelvic hemorrhage with a pulse and systolic blood pressure of 80 mm Hg or less should be considered for REBOA.

Three functional zones are used to facilitate balloon placement in the aorta. Zone I extends from the left subclavian artery to the celiac trunk; this zone controls inflow to the abdominal viscera to the pelvis and lower extremities. Zone II is between the celiac trunk and the lowest renal artery; this zone is considered a zone of no occlusion. Zone III consists of the infrarenal aorta; occlusion in this area controls pelvic and lower extremity inflow. Thoracic aortic occlusion (Zone I) should be considered in exsanguinating abdominal injury. Infrarenal aortic occlusion (Zone III) should be considered in hypotensive patients with severe pelvic fractures. In patients with torso trauma at risk for hemorrhagic shock, access for REBOA can be obtained in the ED or OR.

REBOA technique consists of five steps: arterial access and sheath placement, balloon catheter insertion, balloon inflation, deflation, and sheath removal. Arterial access to the common femoral artery can be achieved though one of three methods: percutaneous access with a needle and wire using a Seldinger technique, surgical cutdown, or a wire exchange through an existing arterial line. After a wire has been passed retrograde from the common femoral artery into the external iliac artery, a sheath will be passed over the wire. The sheath should be secured in place, the wire and introducer can be removed, and blood should be withdrawn from the sheath and flushed with 0.9% saline with heparin (10 units heparin/ mL saline). A long working wire with intermediate stiffness can be inserted through the sheath and advanced into the aorta under fluoroscopic guidance. The balloon catheter can then be advanced on the wire into position. Inflate the balloon using a 30-mL Luer lock syringe filled with a 50:50 mix of 0.9% saline and iodine-based contrast; this should be performed with fluoroscopy. The balloon should be inflated while using fluoroscopy.

According to Morrison and colleagues (2016), REBOA significantly reduced mortality; however, prolonged occlusion times are associated with increased mortality. Reported complications include arterial injury, thromboembolic complications resulting in limb ischemia, and end-organ failure. Further studies are needed to determine the ideal timing, duration of balloon inflation, and patient who may benefit from REBOA.

ED, Emergency department; *REBOA*, resuscitative endovascular balloon occlusion of the aorta.
Modified from Morrison J et al: *Endovascular methods for aortic control in trauma* (website). www.uptodate.com/contents/endovascular-methods-for-aortic-control-in-trauma?source=machineLearning&search=resuscitative%20endovascular%20balloon%20occlusion%20of%20the%20aorta&selectedTitle=1~4&sectionRank=1&anchor=H351707551#H351707551. (Accessed 16 October 2016.)

- The patient remained hemodynamically stable; fluid resuscitation was undertaken, blood pressure and pulse rate measurements were adequate considering the patient's status, and the H&H values were within acceptable ranges.
- The patient achieved and maintained normothermia in the OR.
- The patient reported reasonable relief from pain during preparatory maneuvers in the OR.
- The airway was maintained, and induction of anesthesia proceeded without complication.

On completion of the procedure or procedures, the perioperative nurse is afforded an opportunity to further assess the trauma patient as well as evaluate the plan of care implemented. If the patient sustained numerous injuries and remains critically injured, the PACU may be bypassed and the patient may be transferred directly to the ICU. The perioperative nurse should accompany the patient, along with the anesthesia provider, to the ICU. When the anesthesia report is given, the perioperative nurse can provide a wealth of information to the critical care nurse. At this point, family members may have been contacted or are present, allowing more specific medical history information to be obtained. However, the MOI and events surrounding the trauma are still significant. A high index of suspicion remains during postoperative care of the patient sustaining multiple injuries. Attention can be diverted from a less significant injury in the presence of a highly visible or obvious trauma. Once the obvious trauma undergoes intervention, pain or discomfort from other injuries becomes more apparent. In the care of a patient with neurologic deficit, physical assessment and continued evaluation are essential because patient self-report is nonexistent.

The nurse should also report the status of progress in the secondary assessment. Any additional laboratory work or interventions that have yet to be completed should be discussed. It is imperative in a thorough examination to view the back of the patient in an effort to locate all injuries.

Additional diagnostic procedures may be required after completion of the surgical procedure if the patient's condition is stable. The perioperative nurse may be requested to accompany the patient to the diagnostic department with the anesthesia provider. In addition, respiratory care personnel may assist in patient transport and maintenance of the airway.

Patient, Family, and Caregiver Education and Discharge Planning

Traumatic injury to a family member or significant other occurs without warning. Patients may be traveling or visiting out of town or state at the time of injury. Families or friends involved in an MVC may be triaged to several different facilities based on severity of injury or age. A family member or significant other may not be contacted until several hours or even days after the injury. Sometimes the patient's identity either is unknown or must be kept confidential to prevent further harm. Both the patient and the family member are truly victims of traumatic injury. Consequently patients and family members are in a time of crisis.

Some families may handle the crisis with ease, whereas others become dysfunctional. Coping strategies may be inappropriate at times as the patient, family, and caregiver attempt to reestablish patterns of function. A family system already taxed before the event may be overwhelmed with the additional stress of a sudden traumatic event. On the other hand, family members may wish to be present during resuscitation efforts. Family presence requires a facilitator to explain procedures and the accompanying sights, sounds, and smells that may occur. Nurses base their decisions on medical concerns, which may be very different from patient and/or family concerns. In trauma situations, nurses do not know their patient's preferences and may even be unaware that differences in opinion exist. The care team should identify a family member to be present, provide an explanation of the situation, answer any questions, and stay with the family (Strasen et al., 2016).

The perioperative nurse must be prepared for a variety of responses, both from the patient and from the family or significant others. Interaction with the patient before surgical intervention may be impossible because of the severity of the injury, prior intubation, or hemodynamic instability. The perioperative nurse will need to offer brief, simple instructions and explanations if the patient is conscious. These may include the following:

- Background noise as caregivers prepare for emergent intervention
- Perception of cold within the OR room
- Placement of safety and restraining straps, armboards, warming devices, and pneumatic compression stockings, for example
- Invasive interventions, such as additional IV access or arterial line monitoring

A reassuring touch or holding the patient's hand may be the only communication possible. Touch, placement of warm blankets, a gentle squeeze of the hand, and softly spoken words of reassurance are important comfort measures.

In accordance with hospital policies and procedures, the perioperative nurse may call the surgical waiting room with periodic updates on the patient's condition. The information shared is subject to the surgeon's discretion and is usually concise in nature, such as, "At this time the extent of injury is unknown; his or her condition is critical." When implemented, these contacts with family members are appreciated because frequently they were unable to see or speak with the patient before surgery.

All of the patient's injuries and possible subsequent complications may not be known at the time of operative intervention. The multiply injured patient frequently requires rehabilitation or an extended stay in a skilled nursing facility before discharge to home. In addition to coping with physical changes, some patients may experience posttraumatic stress disorder. Continued therapy, such as neuropsychology (for cognitive impairment) or occupational and physical therapy, may be provided on an outpatient basis. Consequently information regarding recovery and rehabilitation is limited on admission to the hospital. Many facilities have access to or provide support groups for patients and families related to the type of injury and its subsequent lifelong effects.

End-of-Life Care

Unfortunately some accidental injuries result in death. Many facilities have a chaplain or social worker available to assist family members during this time of crisis. These caregivers assist in the initial family contact and provide immediate support. Providing end-of-life care for patients and family is relevant, even in trauma situations. Trauma is different in that the patient, family, and caregiver do not have a prior relationship with the healthcare team. This makes it difficult for the team to know and/or understand the wishes and values of the patient, family, and caregiver. End-of-life care should be focused on communication with family regarding pain and symptom management; bereavement support; and assessment, planning, and implementation of palliative care (Cocanour, 2015).

Critical Incident–Stress Debriefing

When the end result of a traumatic injury is death, it can be particularly difficult for the perioperative team because most surgical interventions are of a curative or restorative nature. Many emergency medical systems have a critical incident–stress debriefing (CISD) team. The goal of the CISD team is to prevent or reduce the signs of traumatic stress, assist the team in recovering, and returning to normal function (Tuckey et al., 2014). The CISD team is composed of mental health professionals and specially trained volunteers who are also professionals and peers in the healthcare field. Police officers, firefighters, paramedics, ED nurses, and ICU nurses also may be on the team. In the event of a particularly tragic death of a patient, the team can be contacted, and a meeting with that patient's care providers is arranged. The benefit of this team is enhanced when intervention is timely for the care providers. Opportunity for them to discuss their feelings and emotions is provided and encouraged as each provider discusses feelings related to personal participation in the care of the patient. The CISD facilitator must adhere to the structured phases of this crisis intervention to ensure participants benefit from the group sessions (Pender et al., 2016).

Surgical Interventions

Damage Control Surgery

Damage control surgery is a well-recognized surgical strategy that sacrifices complete, immediate repair to adequately address the physiologic impact of trauma and surgery. Damage control surgery is a series of operations performed to accomplish definitive repair of abdominal injuries with consideration of the patient's physiologic tolerance. The focus is on control of hemorrhage and contamination to stop bleeding and control any intestinal, biliary, or urinary leak into the abdominal cavity. Indications for the potential need for damage control surgery include hemodynamic instability, hemorrhagic shock, coagulopathy, hypotension, tachycardia, tachypnea, inaccessible major anatomic injury, concomitant major injury, and altered mental status.

Abdominal packing is the foundation principle of damage control surgery, first reported in the early 20th century. Later reports detailed survival of patients with severe liver injuries that were packed. In 1971 a report described staged laparotomy procedures to repair vessels necessary for survival followed by packing the abdominal cavity (Roberts et al., 2017). The term *damage control* was first used in 1993 along with a detailed approach. The components are stop bleeding, close perforations; continue resuscitation, emphasizing correction of coagulopathy, acidosis, and hypothermia; and plan reoperation for definitive repair.

There are five decision-making stages for damage control.

- *Stage 1:* Patient selection and decision to perform damage control: The emphasis is on early recognition for potential damage control surgery, including rapid transport to the hospital and early decisions related to control of hemorrhage.
- *Stage 2:* Operation and intraoperative reassessment of laparotomy: This consists of control of hemorrhage and contamination with rapid packing and temporary abdominal closure.
- *Stage 3:* Physiologic restoration in the ICU: The focus here is on restoration of physiologic status, which may include rewarming and fluid replacement.
- *Stage 4:* Return to OR for definitive procedures: The focus is on removal of packing, repair of injuries, and closure. Indications

for emergency reoperation include massive ongoing bleeding, evidence of bowel leak or ischemic organ, and presence of abdominal compartment syndrome.

- *Stage 5:* Abdominal wall closure/reconstruction: It is not always possible to close the abdominal wall in stage 4, necessitating further repair.

Injuries of the Head and Spinal Column

Trauma to the head is responsible for half of all trauma deaths. Brain injury occurs either as a direct result of the trauma to the tissue or as a complication. Often forces of energy from the impact are tolerated by the rigid skull, but the soft tissue of the brain is traumatized, resulting in the formation of subdural (Fig. 28.7), epidural, or intracerebral hematomas. Blood clots are classified by their location in the brain and range from mild to life-threatening. A clot under the skull but on top of the dura is an epidural hematoma, which often results from a tear in an artery under the skull. A clot under the skull and dura but outside the brain is a subdural hematoma, often resulting from a tear in a vein or from a cut on the brain itself (Patient Engagement Exemplar). An injury to the brain itself, a contusion, is an intracerebral hematoma, which is a result of a skull fracture or other blood clot causing swelling inside the brain. In addition, cerebral swelling can result in herniation of the brain despite treatment (Fig. 28.8).

A baseline neurologic examination is extremely important. The pupils are examined, and the presence or absence of posturing is noted. The Glasgow Coma Scale (see Table 21.2) provides a universally accepted mechanism with which to assess the baseline data for the trauma team. However, in the presence of alcohol or drug intoxication or chemical paralysis, the scale cannot be used. For patients with a score of 8 or less, intubation with controlled ventilation is the immediate treatment of choice. In the highly combative patient,

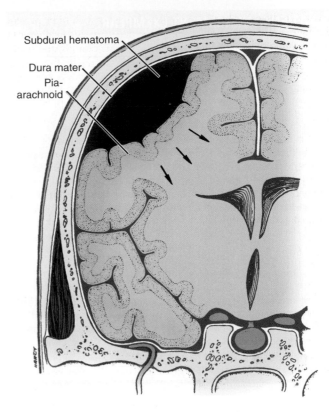

FIG. 28.7 Subdural hematoma causing increased intracranial pressure with shifting of tissue.

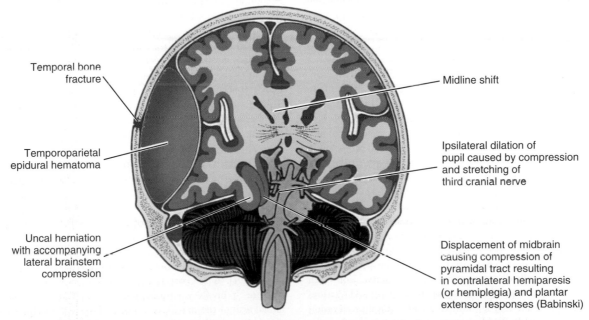

FIG. 28.8 Cross section showing herniation of lower portion of temporal lobe (uncus) through tentorium caused by temporoparietal epidural hematoma. Herniation may also occur in cerebellum. Note mass effect and midline shift.

intubation may also be performed to allow adequate assessment of the extent of injury.

Previously, hyperventilation was routinely used to decrease ICP in the initial management of patients with neurologic deterioration. No studies have shown improved outcomes for these patients, and other methods of assessment have shown that hyperventilation can cause significant constriction of cerebral vessels and may reduce cerebral blood flow to an ischemic level. Occasionally, hyperventilation may be necessary with persistently high ICP unresponsive to other treatment modalities.

An osmotic diuretic, such as mannitol, can be used to treat increased ICP. The diuretic effects take place in 15 to 30 minutes and inhibit water and electrolytes absorption (Kizior and Hodgson, 2017). Osmotic diuretics such as mannitol have proven benefits in lowering ICP without reducing cerebral blood flow. They are given by bolus administration to create an acute reduction phase in ICP. These agents are excreted in the urine and cause a rise in serum and urine osmolality (Surgical Pharmacology). Mannitol will not be given if a patient's serum osmolality is higher than 320 mOsm/kg, and hypertonic saline or high-dose barbiturate therapy may be advised (Ortega-Barnett et al., 2017). Hypovolemia should be avoided with the infusion of isotonic fluids as necessary. Because such agents act quickly, fluid intake and output and the potential for fluid and electrolyte imbalances mandate close hemodynamic monitoring. Elevating the head of the bed 30 degrees and keeping the patient's head midline (to promote venous drainage) also can be beneficial.

Skull fractures usually do not require operative intervention when there is no displacement and the fracture is linear. Depressed fractures or the presence of bone in the brain frequently requires elevation and debridement (Fig. 28.9). Hematoma evacuation is based on the location as well as the size and number of hematomas present. Before performing a craniotomy or drilling a burr hole, the CT scan, the

neurologic status of the patient, the morbidity or mortality associated with the procedure, and the presence of other injuries or underlying medical problems, if known, are evaluated. An ICP monitor may be placed in the patient who is at risk for increased ICP. (Chapter 21 discusses neurosurgical procedures.)

The patient with a cervical spine injury at or near C3 to C5 is at great risk for respiratory difficulties because this is the area of diaphragmatic innervation. There is also the possibility of swelling above the area of injury, and the perioperative nurse should be alert for the potential of respiratory distress even if it is not initially present. A 24- to 48-hour dose of methylprednisolone (Solu-Medrol), calculated by body weight, is considered to decrease initial cord swelling.

The standard indicators of possible cord injury are absence of rectal tone and bradycardia in the presence of hypotension. The body's normal response is to increase heart rate in the presence of decreased blood flow or hypotension. These responses are not present in injury of the spinal cord, and vagal control results in bradycardia.

Injuries involving the spinal cord can range from a contusion of the cord to complete transection, without hope of recovery. Fractures or dislocation of a vertebra can result in the protrusion of small pieces into the spinal canal. This is known as a *burst fracture.* Several vertebrae may be fractured or have fractured components. The decision to surgically treat vertebral fractures is based on many factors. In patients with minimal compression and no neurologic signs or symptoms, spinal bracing may be an option. Cerebral arteriography may be used to screen patients with cervical vertebral fractures for blunt vertebral artery injuries (BVIs). According to Payabvash and colleagues (2013), CT angiography will identify symptomatic BVIs. Patients are treated with anticoagulant therapy if not contraindicated because of severity of trauma injuries and bleeding potential (Payabvash et al., 2013).

Treating spinal column fractures can involve surgery (Patient Safety). Stabilizing the fracture may be necessary, depending on the severity of the injury. For cervical spine fractures, traction may be used initially to reduce the fracture, followed by surgical intervention as soon as the patient's condition permits. Internal fixation devices are discussed in Chapter 20.

Injuries of the Face

MVCs account for about 60% of maxillofacial injuries. Mandibular fractures alone are highly associated with assault as the MOI. In the patient who presents with facial injury, the airway must be secured. This requires ensuring patency and removing any items that pose the threat of aspiration. If a midface fracture is present, the anesthesia provider avoids nasogastric tube placement and nasotracheal intubation. A tracheostomy may need to be performed before initiation of the operative procedure. Control of scalp or facial hemorrhage can be achieved through a pressure dressing until surgical intervention is possible because exsanguinations can occur. Treatment of the fracture may be delayed until the immediate life threats have been successfully managed. Goals of operative intervention are to reduce and immobilize the fracture, prevent infection, and restore facial cosmesis and function.

Facial fractures can be categorized into Le Fort I, II, or III (see Fig. 22.24). A Le Fort I fracture is the most common maxillary fracture. It involves a horizontal interruption of the anterior and lateral wall of the maxillary sinus. Le Fort II is a pyramidal fracture along the maxilla and lacrimal bones and through the infraorbital rim. Le Fort III is otherwise known as *craniofacial disjunction.* The midface is completely disengaged from the cranial base, resulting

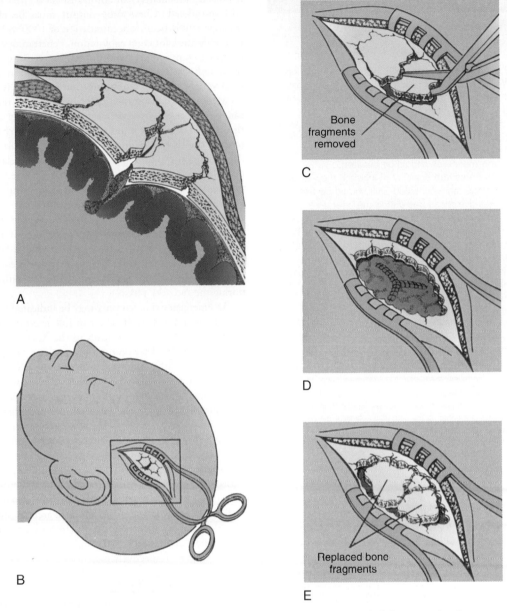

FIG. 28.9 Treatment of compound depressed fracture of skull. (A) Depressed skull fracture and scalp injury. (B) Incision to expose fracture and remove the portion of the scalp that is devitalized. (C) Removal of impacted bone by burr hole to locate and identify normal dura, followed by resection of bone fragments. (D) Watertight closure of dura after brain debridement. (E) Replacement and fixation of bone fragments.

from a fracture across the frontomaxillary sutures. (Specific information regarding these injuries is in Chapter 22.)

Injuries of the Eye

Eye injuries can result from blunt or penetrating types of trauma. Penetrating objects in the globe are stabilized and not removed until the patient is in the OR. These injuries threaten loss of vision because of the injury itself, inflammation, or infection. Blunt injury to the eye can result in hematomas and accompanying fractures. A blow-out fracture is the result of a blunt force to the eye that pushes soft tissue through the thin bony orbital floor. The eye recedes into the orbit and the patient loses the ability to gaze upward. Surgical repair is often indicated. (Chapter 18 discusses ophthalmic procedures.)

Injuries of the Neck

Injury to the neck and soft tissue structures is most commonly a result of penetrating trauma. The neck can be divided into three zones with respect to injury and consequence. Zone I is the base of the neck below the clavicles. Anatomic structures located in this region are the great vessels and aortic arch, innominate veins, trachea, esophagus, and lungs. Zone II is the area in the middle of the neck between the clavicles and the mandible. Structures located in this area include the carotid artery, internal jugular vein, trachea, and esophagus. Zone III is located between the angle of the mandible and the base of the skull. The primary target of evaluation in these injuries is vascular structures.

PATIENT SAFETY

Risk Factor: Development of Pressure Ulcers in Trauma Patients

Spinal cord injury patients are five times more likely to develop a pressure ulcer. Pressure ulcers are expensive to treat and may lead to increased pain, additional surgeries, increased length of hospital stay, and increased mortality and morbidity rates. Additionally, the development of a pressure ulcer is considered a never-event because it is considered a hospital-acquired condition. Therefore when a high-risk patient has been identified aggressive prevention measures should be initiated.

Trauma patients with severe spinal cord injuries, mechanical ventilation, increased age, and increased BMI should be treated with aggressive preventive measures during the operative procedure. Bedside skin care, skin protective pads, and frequent repositioning are routinely used to prevent pressure ulcers. The patient may be placed on a low-air-loss specialty mattress as soon as the spinal fracture has been stabilized.

AORN's position statement on perioperative pressure ulcer prevention recommends collaboration among the entire healthcare team to prevent pressure ulcer formation. The prevention should begin before the patient enters the OR. Every patient going to the OR should be assessed for risk factors, which should be communicated during patient handoffs. Education related to pressure ulcers should be performed annually.

AORN, Association of periOperative Registered Nurses; *BMI,* body mass index.
Modified from Association of periOperative Registered Nurses (AORN): Position statement on perioperative pressure ulcer prevention in the care of the surgical patient, *AORN J* 104(5):437–438, 2016; Raff LA et al: Identification of risk factors for the development of pressure ulcers despite standard screening methodology and prophylaxis in trauma patients, *Adv Skin Wound Care* 29(7):329–334, 2016.

Zone II injuries may necessitate an otorhinolaryngologist. Penetrating injuries to the larynx and trachea can be primarily repaired. Blunt force to the larynx can result in a fracture and impose immediate airway obstruction. These patients require immediate tracheotomy followed by repair of the fracture when it is unstable or displaced. Chapter 19 provides specific information concerning otorhinolaryngologic procedures.

Injuries of the Chest and Heart

Trauma to the chest area is the primary cause of death in approximately 20% to 25% of trauma victims (Roodenburg and Roodenburg, 2014). Blunt trauma is most often associated with high-speed MVCs. Penetrating traumas may be associated with violent crimes. Penetrating injuries at or immediately below the nipple line or level of the scapular tips are evaluated for both chest and abdominal involvement. Diaphragmatic injury is also a possibility.

Deceleration injury, such as that occurring from a fall or from striking the steering wheel in an MVC, may cause contusions of the chest wall, fractures of the ribs or sternum, contusions of the heart or lungs, or rupture of the aorta and other major vessels. Rib fractures are also associated with a hemothorax or pneumothorax. A flail-chest segment may result when two or more adjacent ribs are broken in two or more places. This results in paradoxical chest wall movement as a result of loss of bony support; that is, the affected segment of the chest wall moves in the opposite direction. If respiratory distress and diminished breath sounds are present, a chest tube is indicated immediately; an autotransfusion chest drainage device is also considered. Chest tube output must be closely monitored intraoperatively because accumulation of 1000 to 1500 mL of blood is an indication for chest exploration. Penetrating wounds, as a result of either gunshot or stab injuries, may cause hemothorax and pneumothorax as well. Lacerations or perforation of the lung, heart, great vessels, trachea, esophagus, and bronchus is possible.

Myocardial contusion usually involves the right ventricle and can be evidenced by dysrhythmias on patient arrival or shortly thereafter. The patient is monitored on a telemetry unit, and surgical intervention is not required. Rupture of a heart valve can occur, depending on the timing of the contusion in relation to the phase of the cardiac cycle. If valve rupture has occurred, surgical repair is necessary. Heart sounds should be evaluated during the secondary assessment to document the presence or absence of murmurs. Heart valve rupture can occur as a late complication of myocardial contusion. Pericardiocentesis is performed for signs and symptoms of pericardial tamponade (Fig. 28.10), which include jugular venous distention, muffled heart sounds, and a narrowing pulse pressure. Patients may present to the OR for a pericardial window either emergently or during the recovery phase.

An emergency thoracotomy may be indicated in the patient with penetrating trauma to the chest in full arrest or pulseless electrical activity on ECG. If a laceration to the heart is suspected and the patient is rapidly deteriorating, the surgeon may perform a thoracotomy in the ED. The laceration may be primarily repaired and the patient transferred to the OR for irrigation, wound debridement, and closure. Otherwise, surgical intervention is initiated in the OR. Wounds located across the mediastinum accompanied by hemodynamic instability; massive penetrating lung injuries; and disruption of the trachea, bronchus, or esophagus also require surgical intervention. Rupture of the thoracic aorta is another injury requiring surgical intervention and includes the use of extracorporeal bypass. This injury is an obvious life threat but may be difficult to diagnose. An arch aortogram is indicated in trauma patients who may have sustained such an injury. Rupture of the thoracic arch is associated with first rib or sternal fractures. (Chapters 23 and 25 provide additional information about associated surgical procedures in thoracic and cardiac surgery, respectively.)

Injuries of the Abdomen

The spleen is the most common organ injured in blunt trauma, and the liver, because of its large size, is the most common organ injured in penetrating trauma. Historically, initial efforts were aimed at performing splenectomy in response to splenic injury. However, because of the role of the spleen in the body's defense against infection, the surgeon makes every effort to control hemorrhage in the spleen and avoid its removal. Treatment is determined by the condition of the spleen and of the patient. Injury to the spleen occurs with deceleration injuries, resulting in fracture of the organ because of its multiple fixation points. Splenic injury may be associated with fractures of the left tenth through twelfth ribs. The patient may exhibit left shoulder pain (Kehr sign), upper left quadrant tenderness, abdominal wall muscle rigidity, spasm or involuntary guarding, or signs and symptoms of hemorrhage and hypovolemic shock. Splenic injuries (Table 28.7) range from laceration of the capsule to ruptured subcapsular hematomas or parenchymal laceration. The most serious injury is a severely fractured spleen or vascular tear, producing massive blood loss and splenic ischemia. Rupture of the spleen can be immediate or delayed. Splenic lacerations may be treated nonoperatively by close monitoring and bed rest or operatively for lacerations

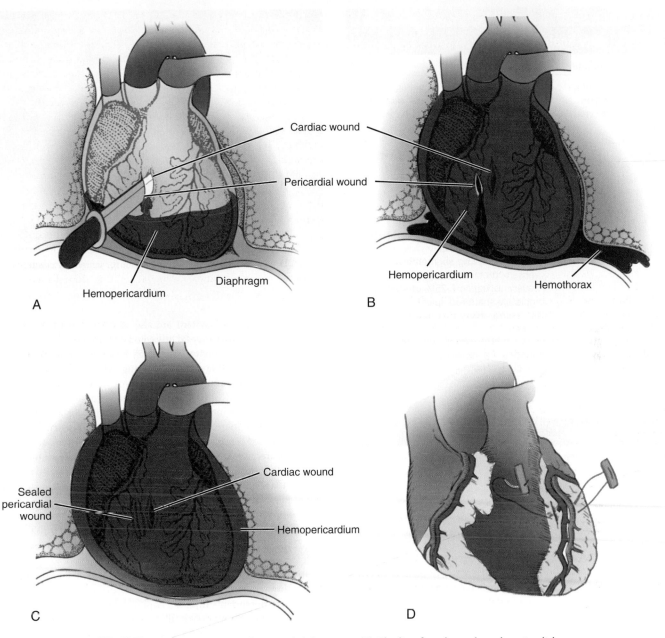

FIG. 28.10 (A) Cardiac injury with pericardial disruption. (B) Bleeding from heart through pericardial tear into pleural space. (C) Self-sealing of pericardial wound resulting in pericardial tamponade. (D) Sutured cardiac wound.

of a more severe nature. The surgeon creates a midline incision, which allows for exposure of all abdominal contents. Topical hemostatic agents are also used with success, as well as suturing and the use of the argon laser in some instances. In some cases, angiographic embolization may be attempted. A laceration involving the splenic hilum or complete shattering of the organ usually necessitates splenectomy.

The severity of hepatic injury ranges from controlled hematoma to severe vascular injury of the hepatic veins or hepatic avulsion (Table 28.8). Because liver tissue is so friable and has an extensive blood supply as well as blood storage capacity, hepatic injuries often result in profuse hemorrhage and require surgical control of bleeding. The patient usually exhibits upper quadrant pain, abdominal wall muscle rigidity, involuntary guarding, rebound tenderness, hypoactive

or absent bowel sounds, and signs of hemorrhage or hypovolemic shock. Nonoperative treatment is indicated in minor capsular and subcapsular injuries. This can be accomplished with bed rest and close monitoring. Topical hemostatic agents and suturing are used in management of minor injuries. Fibrin glue is also used in some institutions as a topical hemostatic agent. Some surgeons may request to use a kaolin-based gauze. This type of gauze speeds up the clotting cascade process and hemostasis is usually achieved within minutes (Z-Medica, 2014). More severe injuries with active expanding hematomas or lobe disruption require surgical exploration and may necessitate hepatic resection or ligation of associated vasculature. With massive hemorrhage, control of bleeding is the primary concern. Packing with soft goods may be indicated, along with manual compression of the organ if intraoperative hypotension becomes

TABLE 28.7

Splenic Injury Scale

Grade	Type of Injury	Description of Injury
I	Hematoma	Subcapsular: <10% of surface area
	Laceration	Capsular tear: <1 cm parenchymal depth
II	Hematoma	Subcapsular: 10%–50% of surface area; intraparenchymal: <5 cm in diameter
	Laceration	Capsular tear: 1–3 cm; parenchymal depth that does not involve a trabecular vessel
III	Hematoma	Subcapsular: >50% of surface area or expanding; ruptured subcapsular or parenchymal hematoma; intraparenchymal hematoma: >5 cm or expanding
	Laceration	>3 cm parenchymal depth or involving parenchymal vessels
IV	Laceration	Laceration involving segmental or hilar vessels, producing major devascularization (>25% of spleen)
V	Laceration	Completely shattered spleen
	Vascular	Hilar vascular injury that devascularizes spleen

From Martin RS, Meredith JW: Management of acute trauma. In Townsend CM et al, editors: *Sabiston textbook of surgery*, ed 20, Philadelphia, 2017, Saunders.

TABLE 28.8

Liver Injury Scale

Grade	Type of Injury	Description of Injury
I	Hematoma	Subcapsular: <10% of surface area
	Laceration	Capsular tear: <1 cm parenchymal depth
II	Hematoma	Subcapsular: 10%–50% of surface area; intraparenchymal: <10 cm in diameter
	Laceration	Capsular tear: 1–3 cm parenchymal depth; <10 cm in length
III	Hematoma	Subcapsular: >50% surface area of ruptured subcapsular or parenchymal hematoma; intraparenchymal hematoma: >10 cm or expanding
	Laceration	>3 cm parenchymal depth
IV	Laceration	Parenchymal disruption involving 25%–75% of hepatic lobe or 1–3 Couinaud segments
V	Laceration	Parenchymal disruption involving >75% of hepatic lobe or >3 Couinaud segments within a single lobe
	Vascular	Juxtahepatic venous injuries (i.e., retrohepatic vena cava/central major hepatic veins)
VI	Vascular	Hepatic avulsion

From Martin RS, Meredith JW: Management of acute trauma. In Townsend CM et al, editors: *Sabiston textbook of surgery*, ed 20, Philadelphia, 2017, Saunders.

severe. The surgeon may apply a pressure dressing and temporary wound closure until associated coagulopathies, hypothermia, and hemodynamic instability can be corrected. The patient usually returns to the OR within 24 to 72 hours postoperatively or when his or her condition permits further exploration and removal of the soft goods.

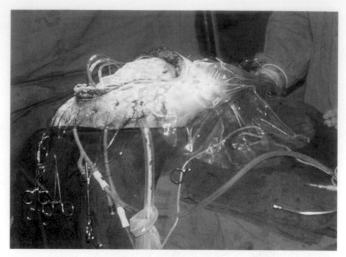

FIG. 28.11 Alternative technique using plastic for temporary closure of the abdomen.

Injuries to the GI system are also associated with abdominal trauma. Bowel injuries may be missed on abdominal CT scan during the initial diagnostic period. The small bowel is frequently injured because deceleration may lead to shearing, which causes avulsion or tearing. The most commonly affected areas of the small bowel are areas relatively fixed or looped. Associated with any perforation of the GI tract is a chance for peritonitis and sepsis or compartment syndrome from increased pressure. Crystalloid resuscitation and capillary leakage contribute to tissue swelling. The resulting abdominal edema creates a pressurized compartment that must be explored to render relief to the compromised organs.

If the abdomen is difficult to close, alternative wound closure techniques may be used to prevent the occurrence of abdominal compartment syndrome. One such method is to use a silo-bag closure, in which heavy plastic is trimmed to fit and sutured to skin edges (Fig. 28.11). A sterile absorbent drape may also be placed inside the abdomen to absorb fluid.

In the event of a penetrating injury, the trajectory of the missile or the implement is examined, and organs within the area are considered potentially injured. Exploration is indicated, and the surgeon thoroughly examines all components of the GI system for any perforations, contusion, hemorrhage, or compromise of vasculature, such as a mesenteric hematoma. When an injury is identified, suturing, stapling, or segmental excision may be indicated. (Chapter 11 discusses GI surgery, and Chapter 12 addresses surgery of the biliary tract, pancreas, liver, and spleen.)

Diagnostic laparoscopy is frequently used for direct visualization of abdominal organs to decrease the need for open abdominal exploration. This procedure allows the surgeon to effectively evaluate the presence of any injury and develop an appropriate plan of treatment in the stable patient. However, there is some concern that bowel injuries may not always be identified. Some therapeutic interventions may also be performed through the laparoscope so that the more invasive open approach is avoided. Increased IAP required in laparoscopic insufflation may create an adverse ventilatory effect. In the presence of abdominal vein injury with low pressures, CO_2 could leak into the vasculature and result in CO_2 emboli to the heart or lungs. Tension pneumothorax may be created in patients with a diaphragmatic injury. Consequently indications for these procedures in the trauma setting continue to be evaluated.

Injuries of the Genitourinary System

Laceration of the kidney is closely associated with fracture of the ribs and transverse vertebral processes (Table 28.9). Because the kidney is retroperitoneal, the presence of bleeding may not be observed on DPL. Renal contusions often produce hematuria. Gross clots may also be seen in more serious injury, but it should be noted that hematuria is not present in a complete avulsion injury. Management of renal contusions can be nonoperative with monitoring of hematuria. Lacerations involving the collecting system, severe crush injuries, or pedicle injuries necessitate surgical intervention (Fig. 28.12). Nephrectomy may be indicated with severe injury of the pedicle or massive hemorrhage.

Rupture of the bladder and urethral injury are most often associated with pelvic fractures. Both blunt trauma and penetrating trauma are causative factors. The type of bladder injury is a direct result of the amount of urine present in the bladder at the time of injury. Blunt forces applied to a full bladder result in an intraperitoneal rupture. This type of rupture is closely associated with alcohol consumption because of alcohol's diuretic effect. Pelvic fracture is associated with

an extraperitoneal bladder rupture. Most often these patients present with gross hematuria. A small extraperitoneal rupture may be managed by urinary catheter drainage. A large extraperitoneal rupture and intraperitoneal rupture require surgical intervention. The surgeon may place a suprapubic cystostomy tube, and repair the bladder. Pelvic fracture reduction and fixation are also performed.

Urethral injuries require exploration and primary repair. These types of injuries are more common in the male because the male urethra is longer and less protected than the female urethra (Fig. 28.13). A fall or straddle type of injury is usually responsible. This injury is detected by the presence of blood at the urinary meatus. In these instances an indwelling urethral catheter should not be inserted. Blood at the urinary meatus may indicate a tear in the anterior urethra. A retrograde urethrogram may be performed to evaluate for extravasation of urine and potential injury. Suspicion of a pelvic fracture raises the index of suspicion of a concomitant urethral injury. (Chapter 15 provides additional information on urologic procedures.)

Skeletal Injuries

Trauma to the skeletal system usually results in contusion or fracture. After stabilization of the patient, radiographs are taken of any body part that is distorted, edematous, painful, or highly suspicious for fracture or dislocation. Treatment of fractures is aimed at restoring function with a minimum of complications. Immobilization of fractures can be accomplished by casting, bracing, splinting, application of traction, or hardware fixation. Femur fractures in particular can be associated with a high risk of hemorrhage and require traction before surgical repair. Closed and open reductions, application of internal and external fixators, and some types of traction may be performed in the OR (Patient, Family, and Caregiver Education).

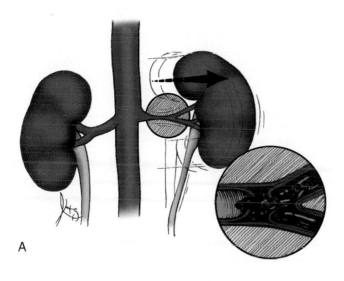

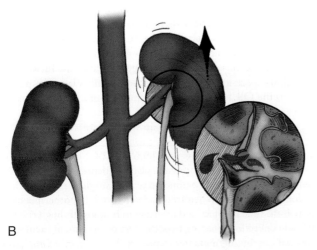

FIG. 28.12 Renal injuries. Acceleration-deceleration injury may produce disruption of the (A) renal artery and (B) the ureteropelvic junction.

TABLE 28.9

Renal Injury Scale

Grade*	Type of Injury	Description of Injury†
I.	Contusion:	Microscopic or gross hematuria; urologic studies normal
	Hematoma:	Subcapsular, nonexpanding without parenchymal laceration
II.	Hematoma:	Nonexpanding perirenal hematoma confined to renal retroperitoneum
	Laceration:	<1.0 cm parenchymal depth of renal cortex without urinary extravasation
III.	Laceration:	>1.0 parenchymal depth of renal cortex without collecting system rupture or urinary extravasation
IV.	Laceration:	Parenchymal laceration extending through the renal cortex, medulla, and collecting system
	Vascular:	Main renal artery or vein injury with contained hemorrhage
V.	Laceration:	Completely shattered kidney
	Vascular:	Avulsion of renal hilum, which devascularizes kidney

*Advance one grade for multiple injuries to the same organ.
†Based on the most accurate assessment at autopsy, laparotomy, or radiologic study.
From Moore E et al: Organ injury scaling: spleen, liver, and kidney, *J Trauma* 29(12):1664–1666, 1989.

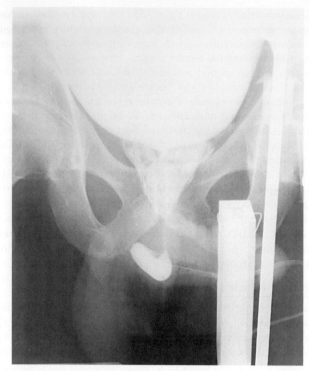

FIG. 28.13 Complete urethral injury as demonstrated on urethrogram.

The perioperative nurse involved in care of the trauma patient must have a working knowledge of orthopedics. Fractures must be repaired in a timely manner to avoid untoward complications; however, immediate life threats are corrected first. Open fractures are at an increased risk of infection. (Chapter 20 contains information on the surgical procedures used in fracture management.)

Pelvic fractures may pose an additional challenge to the perioperative team. Fractures within the pelvic ring are associated with significant internal blood loss and shock. Systemic peripheral vascular resistance is increased. A method to quickly minimize or tamponade blood loss in severe pelvic fractures is the application of a PASG or PASG trousers to provide stabilization of the fracture and reduce associated hemorrhage. The use of PASG trousers may be effective in patients who are 20 to 40 minutes away from the hospital and have pelvic fracture, hypotension, and decompensated shock (Adler et al., 2015). If a PASG is applied, the patient may be transported to the OR with the trousers still inflated. The perioperative nurse must be familiar with deflation procedures. The attending anesthesia provider directs deflation in collaboration with the surgeon. Blood pressure and other vital signs are closely monitored. The abdominal compartment is deflated first. Deflation continues slowly while IV fluids are infused to maintain blood pressure. A 5 mm Hg drop in the systolic blood pressure or an increase in heart rate of 10 beats/min or more requires fluid resuscitation before deflation of the next compartment. If the patient remains stable after 5 minutes of rest, each leg compartment is deflated slowly, assessing the systolic blood pressure and heart rate. The legs must be deflated one at a time, with a resting period of 5 minutes between deflations; if one leg is injured, the team begins deflating the uninjured leg first (Adler et al., 2015).

Some TCs apply external fixator devices in the ED during initial resuscitation. A pelvic C-clamp, sheet wrap, or a commercially available support binder may be used for initial stabilization of pelvic fractures. Severe hemorrhage associated with the fracture may be controlled by arterial embolization performed in the radiology department if surgical intervention for fracture fixation must be delayed.

Soft tissue injuries of an extremity are subject to compartment syndrome. This is a result of swelling of the soft tissues and muscles encased in the fascia. With a significant amount of swelling, pain is increased and the surrounding circulation may be compromised. The patient may experience a decrease in motor and sensory function. This injury must be treated surgically by a fasciotomy. Incising the fascia allows space for tissue swelling. Several days later the patient returns to the OR for closure, which may require skin grafting for complete coverage.

Hypothermia

A core body temperature less than 89.6°F (32°C) is associated with a 100% mortality rate. Hypothermia places patients at risk for massive bleeding and respiratory, pulmonary, and surgical site infections (Vardon et al., 2016). When trauma is involved, hypothermia often begins at the time of injury and is related to heat loss through conduction and convection. Starting hypothermia prevention at the trauma scene and continuing measures to prevent hypothermia throughout surgery and into the ICU continue to be the recommended best practices.

PATIENT, FAMILY, AND CAREGIVER EDUCATION

Home Care Instructions for External Fixation Devices

In many cases trauma patients may be discharged to home with external fixators in place. The nurse is responsible for providing education to the patient, family, and caregiver regarding the care of these devices. A best practice for patient teaching is to have the patient, family, and caregiver teach-back the information to the nurse so the nurse can gauge comprehension and learning.

External Fixator Home Care Instructions
- Examine the fixation device every day; check for loose pins and nuts. Pain at the site may indicate looseness. You may tighten loose nuts. Do not make any adjustments to the device.
- Clean the frame twice a week with a clean gauze sponge and rubbing alcohol mixed with water. After cleaning the frame, dry it with a clean towel. You may clean your frame in the shower after your physician tells you it is okay to shower.
- Clean your pin sites twice a day after you wash your hands thoroughly with antibacterial soap. Make a cleaning solution in a sterile container with equal parts hydrogen peroxide and saline solution. Use a sterile cotton swab dipped in the solution; around the base of your pin site, use a circular motion. Gently push down any skin that is moving up onto the pin and remove any crusts that may have formed. After the base of the pin is clean you may continue to clean the upper portion of the pin. Use a new sterile swab for each pin and dry each pin with a clean swab.
- Seek medical attention when
  - A pin moves or loosens
  - You experience pain at a pin site
  - The pin site is red or swollen
  - Fluid leaks around the pin site
  - You are experiencing pain where the bone was broken

Modified from ClinicalKey: *Patient education* (website). www.clinicalkey.com/#!/content/patient_handout/5-s2.0-pe_ExitCare_DI_External_Fixator_en. (Accessed 12 October 2016).

For purposes of definition, generalized hypothermia is considered to be present when the core temperature is below 96.8°F (36°C). (See Chapter 10 for a discussion of the prevention of inadvertent hypothermia in adult surgical patients.) Hypothermia can be classified into three types. *Mild hypothermia* is a core temperature between 89.6°F and 96.8°F (32°C and 36°C). These patients may appear gray and are cool to the touch. Some alterations in level of consciousness can be present. If the patient's clothing is wet, the nurse should remove it and cover the patient with warm blankets. Treatment is aimed at passive rewarming of the patient by means of warm ambient room temperature, warm fluids, and infrared radiant energy lights. *Moderate hypothermia* is characterized as core temperatures between 86°F and 89.6°F (30°C and 32°C). Warmed fluids are given by IV line and also by gastric or peritoneal lavage. In addition, a warming blanket, such as a forced-air warming device, may be used. Immersion in a Hubbard tank filled with warm water has also been successful. An irritable myocardium may cause dysrhythmias to be present. Shivering may or may not be present. If the patient is intubated, then warmed, humidified gases can be administered. *Severe hypothermia* is diagnosed in the patient with a temperature below 86°F (30°C). The heart rate and the respiratory rate are greatly decreased. This patient is comatose, often appears deceased, and requires active rewarming processes. It is advisable to warm the core first to avoid complications associated with rewarming. This can best be accomplished by using cardiopulmonary bypass (CPB), which directly warms internal vital organs, including the heart. The patient should be handled gently during transfers to avoid further tissue injury and stimulation of an irritable myocardium.

In the trauma patient, hypothermia may be potentiated by hypovolemia, hypotension, and shock. Cold hemoglobin cannot release oxygen to tissue as readily as normothermic hemoglobin, and decreased circulating volume related to hemorrhage reduces oxygen delivery to the tissues. The combination of hypothermia, acidosis, and coagulopathy is known as the "lethal triad" (Credland, 2016). The three parts of the triad have a complex relationship; each may be influenced by the other and often results in high mortality if not interrupted. In hypoperfusion, cells burn glucose for energy (lactic acidosis), which increases total blood acidity (metabolic acidosis). Hypoperfusion may also halt the coagulation cascade (coagulopathy), triggering the triad. Hypothermia also affects other body systems already compromised by the trauma. At a core temperature of less than 82.4°F (28°C) the risk for atrial fibrillation increases, which may convert to tachycardia or ventricular fibrillation (Vardon et al., 2016). Cerebral blood flow is highly sensitive to hypothermia, and the patient may appear to be dead. Resuscitation measures are ceased if the patient is rewarmed to at least 97°F (35°C) and cardiac functions remain nonexistent.

Thermal Injuries

Heat and cold exposure injuries require prompt initial management in the ED setting. Some institutions transfer pediatric burn patients and severely burned adult patients to a burn center for treatment once the patients' conditions are stabilized. In addition to treatment of the site of injury to decrease further tissue damage, fluid management is of the utmost importance in these patients. After hemodynamic stabilization of the patient, burn and frostbite wounds usually require a series of procedures. These patients may have multiple surgical debridement procedures before skin grafting and cosmetic interventions. Restoration of function is important. Circumferential burns may restrict the neurovascular structures during eschar formation. Chest burns with eschar may restrict movement of the chest wall and ventilatory function. An escharotomy (incision of the eschar) may be performed to alleviate the constriction. If necessary, this procedure may be performed at the bedside and the perioperative team may be asked to assist.

Organ and Tissue Procurement

As noted, trauma primarily affects young people. In the event that resuscitation efforts or surgical interventions are not successful, the patient may be declared dead. Depending on the cause of death and preexisting medical conditions, the patient may be an organ donor candidate. Both federal and state laws mandate that local organ procurement facilities are notified of potential donors and that families are informed that organ donation exists as an option. Organ donation agencies can be contacted early and will assist in assessing the potential donor, as well as provide a protocol for donor management once the patient is declared dead. The organ donation agency will also confirm the patient's enrollment in the organ donation registry. The organ donation agency will assist the family members in understanding the organ donation process and convey the patient's consent for organ donation if wishes were unknown to the family.

Brain death criteria for organ donation began around 1968, which are attributed to the Harvard Ad Hoc Committee on Brain Death. Most organ donations in this country are from patients who experience brain death. In 1980 the Uniform Declaration of Death Act offered an additional option: cardiopulmonary death, defined as irreversible cessation of circulatory and respiratory function. This may present an ethical dilemma to some perioperative nurses. With brain death, the physician declares the patient dead in the ICU and the family is offered an opportunity to say goodbye. The patient arrives in the OR on a ventilator, which is deactivated when the organs have been retrieved. Withdrawal of support can occur in the ICU or the OR depending on hospital policy. In cardiopulmonary death, organs may be procured after the ventilator is disconnected, the heart stops functioning, and the patient is declared dead (Shapiro et al., 2016). Definitions of brain and cardiopulmonary death are not uniform throughout the United States. The perioperative nurse should be familiar with the state's definitions of brain and cardiopulmonary death and the institution's criteria for the declaration.

After a patient is declared dead and becomes a potential organ donor, the patient's family does not incur any financial costs acquired from that point. The patient is not disfigured in any way that will interfere with bereavement rituals.

A transplantation coordinator assists in managing the organ donor patient in the ICU setting until the procurement teams arrive. The perioperative nurse must prepare for the organ procurement procedure. The procurement of organs and tissue may take several hours. Different organ procurement agencies will provide a surgical team, but additional scrub and circulating personnel are needed. The transplantation coordinators actively seek tissue and organ recipients during the procurement procedure. Most organ transplantation agencies contact the institution and provide follow-up information regarding the ultimate success of the transplantation procedures and information about the recipients.

The heart is removed first, followed by the lungs, pancreas, liver, and kidneys. Tissue dissection is performed in such a manner as to allow for optimal organ transplantation. Sterile technique remains important. In addition, traffic control is of concern during these procedures. Traffic should be limited to essential personnel. Bone, skin, and corneas can also be removed. Some procurement agencies remove bone and corneas in the morgue rather than in the OR.

Key Points

- Understanding the MOI will assist the perioperative nurse with patient assessment.
- A pregnant trauma patient who is 20 weeks or more into pregnancy should be placed in the left lateral decubitus position to avoid a hypotensive episode and maintain blood flow to the uterus and placenta. If this is not possible, manual displacement of the uterus by lateral abdominal pressure should be attempted.
- Osmotic diuretics such as mannitol have proven benefits in lowering ICP without reducing cerebral blood flow.
- The perioperative nurse must become familiar with the primary and secondary assessments performed with trauma patients. There may be times when the perioperative nurse has to complete the secondary assessment following the interventions to correct the immediate life threats.

Critical Thinking Questions

You are the on-call nurse working in the OR when the trauma surgeon calls over to tell you a patient is arriving for an exploratory laparotomy, now. The ED charge nurse calls to give a report and explains the patient was an unrestrained driver involved in a high-speed, frontal impact MVC. The vehicle's airbag did not deploy and the patient has bruises on the chest and abdomen. The OR was just opened, and you hear the trauma team entering the holding area. What information would you expect to be reported during the transfer of patient care? How would you assess this patient? Note the critical assessment factors you would include and perioperative nursing interventions to address them.

evolve *The answers to the Critical Thinking Questions can be found at http://evolve.elsevier.com/Rothrock/Alexander.*

References

Adler A et al: *Pneumatic anti-shock garment: deflating and removing* (website; CINAHL Nursing Guide), 2015. http://web.b.ebscohost.com/nup/detail/detail?vid=2&sid=a294ff08-b846-472a-9b1b-44bab3f0ee46%40sessionmgr104&hid=115&bdata=JnNpdGU9bnVwLWxpdmUmc2NvcGU9c2l0ZQ%3d%3d#db=nup&AN=T706101. (Accessed 24 July 2016).

Association of periOperative Registered Nurses (AORN): Guideline for prevention of retained surgical items. In *Guidelines for preoperative practice*, Denver, 2016, The Association.

Beaven A, Parker P: Treatment principles of blast injuries, *Surgery (Oxford)* 33(9):424–429, 2015.

Bell TM et al: Infectious complications in obese patients after trauma, *J Surg Res* 204(2):393–397, 2016.

Boutros SM et al: Blunt abdominal trauma: the role of focused abdominal sonography in assessment of organ injury and reducing the need for CT, *Alexandria Med J* 52(1):35–41, 2016.

Chopra S et al: Pressure measurement techniques for abdominal hypertension: conclusions from an experimental model, *Crit Care Res Pract* 2015:278139, 2015.

Cocanour CS: End-of-life care in trauma, *J Trauma Acute Care Surg* 79(6):891–896, 2015.

Collins S et al: Thromboelastography: clinical application, interpretation, and transfusion management, *AANA J* 84(2):129–134, 2016.

Credland N: Managing the trauma patient presenting with the lethal triad, *Int J Orthop Trauma Nurs* 20:45–53, 2016.

Ditillo M et al: Morbid obesity predisposes trauma patients to worse outcomes: a National Trauma Data Bank analysis, *J Trauma Acute Care Surg* 76(1):176–179, 2015.

Emergency Nurses Association (ENA): *Trauma nursing core course*, ed 7, Des Plaines, IL, 2014, The Association.

Fencl J et al: The bariatric patient: an overview of perioperative care, *AORN J* 102(42):116–131, 2015.

Hess JR: *Massive blood transfusion* (website), 2016. www.uptodate.com/contents/massive-blood-transfusion?source=machineLearning&search=massive+transfusion&selectedTitle=1%7E87&sectionRank=2&anchor=H15#H2. (Accessed 11 September 2016).

Kizior RJ, Hodgson BB: *Saunders nursing drug handbook*, St Louis, 2017, Saunders.

Kulaylat MN, Dayton MT: Surgical complications. In Townsend CM et al, editors: *Sabiston textbook of surgery*, ed 20, Philadelphia, 2017, Saunders.

McCoy CE et al: Guidelines for field triage of injured patients: in conjunction with the morbidity and mortality weekly report published by the Center for Disease Control and Prevention, *West J Emerg Med* 14(1):69–76, 2013.

Murphy NJ, Quinlan JD: Trauma in pregnancy: assessment, management, and prevention, *Am Fam Physician* 90(10):717–724, 2014.

National Trauma Institute (NTI): *Trauma statistics* (website), 2017. www.nattrauma.org/what-is-trauma/trauma-statistics-facts/. (Accessed 11 August 2017).

Ortega-Barnett J et al: Neurosurgery. In Townsend CM et al, editors: *Sabiston textbook of surgery*, ed 20, Philadelphia, 2017, Saunders.

Payabvash S et al: Screening and detection of blunt vertebral artery injury in patients with upper cervical fractures: the role of cervical CT and CT angiography, *Eur J Radiol* 83(3):571–577, 2013.

Pender DA et al: Exploring the process: a narrative analysis of group facilitators' reports on critical incident stress debriefing, *The Journal for Specialists in Group Work* 41(1):19–43, 2016.

Roberts DJ et al: History of the innovation of damage control for management of trauma patients: 1902–2016, *Ann Surg* 265(5):1034–1044, 2017.

Roodenburg B, Roodenburg O: Chest trauma, *Anaesth Intens Care* 15(9):411–414, 2014.

Sadaka F et al: Safety and efficacy of early pharmacologic thromboprophylaxis in traumatic brain injury, *J Neurol Res* 3(6):169–172, 2013.

Shapiro R et al: *Management of the potential deceased donor* (website), 2016. www.uptodate.com/contents/management-of-the-potential-deceased-donor?source=machineLearning&search=donation+after+cardiac+death&selectedTitle=1%7E14&sectionRank=1&anchor=H7#H6. (Accessed 5 September 2016).

Stephens CT et al: Trauma-associated bleeding: management of massive transfusion, *Curr Opin Anesthesiol* 29(2):250–255, 2016.

Stevens CL: Geriatric trauma: a clinical and ethical review, *J Trauma Nurs* 23(1):36–41, 2016.

Strasen JH et al: Family presence during resuscitation, *Crit Care Nurse* 11(4):42–46, 2016.

Tuckey MR et al: Group critical incident stress debriefing with emergency services personnel: a randomized controlled trial, *Anxiety Stress Coping* 27(1):38–54, 2014.

Vardon F et al: Accidental hypothermia in severe trauma, *Anaesth Crit Care Pain Med* 35(5):355–361, 2016.

Z-Medica: *What is QuikClot? Innovation in hemostasis* (website), 2014. www.quikclot.com/About-QuikClot. (Accessed 24 July 2016).

CHAPTER 29

Interventional and Image-Guided Procedures

BETH FITZGERALD

Interventional Radiology

Interventional radiology (IR) is a branch of radiology which involves minimally invasive procedures performed under image guidance. An interventional radiologist uses radiographs (x-rays), magnetic resonance imaging (MRI), ultrasound and computerized tomography (CT) to advance a catheter into the body, usually into an artery, to treat the source of the disease internally. Interventional radiologists are board-certified physicians with additional advanced training in minimally invasive, targeted treatments using imaging-guided technology with less risk, less pain, and less recovery time compared with open surgery (SIR, 2016).

The Society of Interventional Radiology (SIR) is a national organization of physicians, scientists, and allied health professionals dedicated to improving public health through disease management and minimally invasive, image-guided therapeutic interventions (SIR, 2016). Image-guided procedures use medical imaging to plan, perform, and evaluate surgical procedures and therapeutic interventions. Interventional techniques began in 1953 when Dr. Sven-Ivar Seldinger performed percutaneous vascular access using a hollow-core needle guidewire and catheter. This development led to the specialties of IR and interventional cardiology and was the catalyst for today's minimally invasive procedures. IR is the medical subspecialty of radiology using minimally invasive, image-guided procedures to diagnose and treat disease. IR procedures include vascular, neurologic, gynecologic, and treatment of cancer (Box 29.1).

Although this chapter focuses on IR, vascular procedures are not exclusive to IR and vice versa. Depending on the institution, interventional radiologists, vascular surgeons, and interventional cardiologists also perform peripheral vascular work, endovascular aortic stenting, filter placement, arteriovenous (AV) fistulas, and other similar procedures. Interventional radiologists have expertise in diagnostic imaging, radiation safety, radiation physics, the biologic effects of radiation and injury prevention, image-guided minimally invasive techniques, patient evaluation, and management associated with these procedures (SIR, 2016). SIR publishes guidelines for minimally invasive treatments including criteria for adequate training for specific interventional procedures, as well as positive outcomes. Interventional radiologists complete a residency in diagnostic radiology, then a fellowship in vascular and IR. Further specialization includes interventional neuroradiology and pediatrics. IR team members include registered nurses (RNs), nurse practitioners, physician assistants, radiology technologists (RTs), radiology assistants, cardiovascular technologists, and anesthesia providers. IR also includes nuclear medicine (NM), which is typically a distinct specialty and is not discussed in this chapter.

Interventional Radiology Nursing

The role of the imaging nurse in radiology varies according to the site, modality, and department organization as well as the level of expertise. Imaging nurses are involved in the assessment, care planning, and direct care of patients before, during, and after diagnostic and therapeutic imaging procedures. Imaging nurses use evidence-based practice to provide quality nursing care. The imaging nurse meets the physical, psychologic, cultural, and education needs of patients. IR staff members work as a team and are not interchangeable with nurses from other units in the hospital. Nursing staff must meet jurisdictional regulatory requirements, including those of moderate sedation and basic and advanced life support, in addition to compliance with The Joint Commission (TJC) standards (Baerlocher et al., 2016).

The Association of Radiologic and Imaging Nursing (ARIN) was founded in 1981 as the professional organization representing nurses who practice in diagnostic, interventional neuro/cardiovascular, ultrasonography, CT, NM, MRI, and radiation oncology. ARIN's mission is to provide radiology nurses with the knowledge and resources to deliver safe quality patient care in the imaging environment.

The functions of the imaging nurse include the following:

- Assess patient and plan care.
- Review laboratory, clinical, and critical test results.
- Administer, monitor, and evaluate therapeutic interventions.
- Ensure safety in medication management.
- Act as a patient advocate.
- Protect and monitor patient from excess radiation.
- Monitor the critically ill patient.
- Provide a safe, supportive, and therapeutic environment.
- Manage emergency situations.
- Teach the patient, caregiver, and family.
- Participate in quality assurance improvement activities.
- Participate in facility interdisciplinary activities including clinical, legal, and ethical issues (ARIN, 2014c).

There is no specific academic education preparation for radiology nursing. Typical qualifications are prior experience in perioperative nursing, critical care nursing, emergency nursing, moderate sedation, advanced cardiac life support (ACLS), and pediatric advanced life support (PALS). Nursing practice should be in accordance with the American Nurses Association (ANA) and ARIN standards, as well as other established nursing guidelines. The ANA recognizes ARIN as a specialty with its own certifying exam, using the credentials Certified Radiology Nurse (CRN). Nurses should receive specific training in the full spectrum of IR procedures offered by their respective institutional practice, including indications for procedures,

Interventional Radiology Procedures

Ablations
- Endovenous
- Sclerotherapy
- Radiofrequency
- Tumor (renal and hepatic)

Abdominal aortic aneurysm repair

Angiography, angioplasty (see stents)

Biopsies
- Abdominal
- Breast
- Chest, lung, and mediastinum
- Kidney
- Liver
- Musculoskeletal
- Thyroid

(Central) venous access procedures peripherally inserted central catheter

Coiling: aneurysms (cerebral)

Dialysis
- Grafts, studies, and repairs

Drainage
- Abscess
- Cysts
- Intrathoracic
- Lymphocele

Embolizations
- Chemoembolization
- Uterine fibroid
- Solid organ
- Radioembolozation
- Vessel (pulmonary, uterine, varicocele, portal vein)

Ischemic stroke: clot retrieval

Pain management

Percutaneous
- Biliary interventions
- Gastrostomy, jejunostomy, cecostomy
- Nephrostomy

Thrombectomy and thrombolysis
- Acute limb ischemia
- Dialysis grafts
- Deep vein thrombosis
- Shunts
- Transjugular intrahepatic portosystemic shunts

Stents (angioplasty)
- Hepatic
- Mesenteric
- Renal
- Pelvic
- Lower limb

Vena cava filter insertions

expected postprocedural signs and symptoms, and potential adverse advents (Baerlocher et al., 2016).

There is a clear delineation between the physician practice of diagnostic radiology and IR, but not necessarily for nursing. Depending on the institution, physician expertise, and case load, nurses may rotate or float from diagnostic radiology to IR. In other institutions, diagnostic and IR RNs are separate departments, with different

reporting structures, physician oversight, and dedicated staff. Nurses working within radiology may also work in the preprocedure unit. Because IR is procedure-based, it requires a higher standard of patient care than general radiology. The scope of IR nursing practice is diverse and includes patient education, preprocedure planning, circulating, scrubbing, administering moderate sedation, patient recovery, and postprocedure discharge planning. The procedures performed encompass many different organ systems, various pathologies, and disease processes and are performed in different environments using a variety of imaging technology. As with traditional surgery, patient safety, procedural setup, instrumentation, medications, moderate sedation monitoring, patient assessment, and complication management are IR nursing responsibilities. In IR, the concomitant use of various imaging modalities creates a different environment and new dimension of patient care (ARIN, 2014a).

Imaging Overview

The field of IR incorporates the same imaging technology (modalities) inherent to diagnostic radiology (e.g., radiography, CT, ultrasound, MRI, and fluoroscopy). IR is therapeutic and requires a higher standard of care than diagnostic radiology. In many instances the modality establishes nursing practice. Hence, a high-level understanding of each imaging technology, contrast agents, and radiation physics is important for the perioperative nurse.

Imaging and the Operating Room

The most common imaging in the operating room (OR) is ultrasound and portable C-arm fluoroscopy. The use of imaging during the procedure allows the provider to visualize the procedural area as they work. An ultrasound wand can be covered with a sterile drape to be used during the procedure to improve visualization of the site. The wand is favored for use in pelvic, prostatic, testicular, abdominal, obstetric, and pediatric studies. Other applications of ultrasound include transcranial Doppler, intravascular ultrasound (IVUS), and transesophageal echo (TEE). The traditional angiography system in the OR is a portable C-arm, used primarily as an adjunct to surgical procedures, producing limited imaging and quality views (Sloan et al., 2016). Relative to intraoperative CT and MRI, a few large academic centers have these in an OR. Potential applications are for trauma, neurosurgery, and stroke treatment, but the cost and facility constraints limit their overall adoption. The traditional care path for imaging and surgery is diagnostic imaging, surgery, repeat imaging with discharge, or additional surgery. Advances in imaging and percutaneous techniques have changed this sequenced care path to an integrated single episode, theoretically meaning a shorter length of stay, less-invasive procedures, customized care at the point of diagnosis, quicker recovery time, and a single anesthesia encounter. This integrated care requires effective collaboration of multiple staff members and physicians on all levels and interdisciplinary cooperation surrounding the new technology. As the adaption matures and becomes conventional in more specialties, some procedure overlap occurs.

Radiology Terminology

The specialty of radiology has its own vernacular, which is detailed here and in the text (Box 29.2). Terminology differences include the use of *physician* rather than surgeon or interventionalist because various specialists perform these procedures. IR uses the term *procedure* when referring to a case, rather than surgery. Many faculties use the term *special procedures* or *specials lab* versus IR. This terminology carries through in patient communication as well. Staff in the holding

---

BOX 29.2

Glossary of Terms

Absorbed dose: energy imparted per unit mass by ionizing radiation; unit is the gray (Gy).

CIN (contrast-induced nephropathy): most commonly defined as acute renal failure occurring within 48 hours of exposure to intravascular radiographic contrast material not attributable to other causes.

Contrast media: substances used to enhance the visibility of blood vessels, fluid, and other structures.

Control room: separate, nonsterile room for data processing.

CT (computed tomography): an imaging method that uses x-rays to create cross-sectional pictures of the body.

CTA (computed tomographic angiography): a test combining a CT scan with angiography to create detailed images of the blood vessels in the body.

CTDI and CTDIvol (CT dose index): metric to quantify the radiation output from a CT examination.

DAP (dose area product): a surrogate measure for the entire amount of energy delivered to the patient by the beam. The dose multiplied by the area of the tissue irradiated; expressed as $Gy \times cm^2$.

Deterministic effect: radiation effect characterized by a threshold dose; the effect is not observed unless the threshold dose is exceeded.

Dosimeter: small portable device recording the total accumulated dose of ionizing radiation received.

DSA (digital subtraction angiography): computer-assisted fluoroscopy technique that subtracts images of bone and soft tissue to view the vessels only.

Effective dose: sum of weighted equivalent doses, over specified tissues, of the products of the equivalent dose in a tissue and its tissue weighting factor; unit is the sievert (Sv).

Equivalent dose: measures the biologic damage to living tissue as a result of radiation exposure. Also known as the "biologic dose"; unit is the sievert (Sv).

Fluoroscopy: type of medical imaging showing a continuous x-ray image on a monitor, much like a movie.

Gauss: historic unit for magnetic field strength, the unit tesla (T) is used. (1 tesla = 10,000 gauss).

Gray (Gy): International System Unit (SI) of radiation dose, expressed as absorbed energy per unit mass of tissue. Gray describes any type of radiation (e.g., alpha, beta, neutron, gamma), but it does not describe the biologic effects of different radiations.

High-osmolarity contrast media (HOCM): media composed of salts dissociating into cations and anions.

Kerma: acronym for kinetic energy released in matter; the amount of energy transferred from the x-ray beam to charged particles per unit mass in the medium of interest (air, tissue, and bone); unit is the gray (Gy).

Low-osmolarity contrast media (LOCM): contrast media not composed of salts; does not dissociate.

MRA (magnetic resonance angiogram): type of magnetic resonance imaging (MRI) scan to image blood vessels.

MRI (magnetic resonance imaging): test using a magnetic field, pulses of radio wave energy, and a computer to image organs and structures inside the body.

PACS (picture archiving and communication systems): hardware and software to store, retrieve, manage, distribute, and view images; PACS replace film with digital images.

Peak skin dose: highest radiation dose at any portion of the patient's skin; includes scatter radiation.

Reference dose: approximation of the total radiation (gray) dose to the skin.

RIS (radiology information system): software for managing radiology, imaging, and scheduling.

Roadmapping: overlaying of a stored image superimposed on a current fluoroscopic image.

Rotational angiography: imaging technique in which a fixed C-arm rotates around the patient and acquires a series of x-ray images manipulated by software algorithms.

Scatter radiation: radiation occurring when the x-ray beam intercepts an object, causing the scatter of x-rays.

Sievert (Sv): measures the biologic effects of radiation (former term, "rem"); sievert is calculated as follows: gray multiplied by the radiation weighting factor (also known as the quality factor) associated with a specific type of radiation.

Stochastic effect: radiation effect in which probability of occurrence increases with increasing dose; severity of effect is independent of total delivered dose; example is radiogenic cancers.

Tesla: SI unit for magnetic field strength approximately 20,000 times as strong as the Earth's magnetic field (1 tesla = 10,000 gauss).

Threshold dose: minimum radiation dose at which a specific deterministic effect can occur.

Transient erythema: mild observable skin reaction to radiation resembling sunburn.

---

room area prepare and recover patients. *Modality* is a general term meaning imaging technology. Radiology does not use the term *table;* modalities have tables and table tops. The term *scanner* means either a CT scanner or an MRI scanner; likewise, *scanning* refers to the process of image acquisition for a CT or MRI. *Magnet* is another term for MRI scanner. Fluoroscopy is an imaging technique displaying continuous x-ray imaging of blood flow in vessels (angiography). A fluoroscope is the modality inherent to the IR suite or specials lab, as well as the cardiac catheterization lab, electrophysiology (EP) lab, neurointerventional labs, and hybrid ORs.

Radiography

Radiography is the most common study ordered in hospitals. The correct terminology for radiologic images is radiography or images, not x-ray. Historically, radiography studies required film. Today most

radiography systems are filmless, and are known as computed radiography (CR) or digital radiography (DR). Instead of film, a photosensitive layer on a flat detector absorbs the energy and converts it into photons captured for interpretation as a pixel. A computer converts the digital data into an image. Radiography is a proven and useful modality to evaluate human anatomy and pathology. The goal is to establish the presence or absence and nature of disease by demonstrating normal anatomy or the effects of the disease process on anatomic structures. The study should be performed with the minimal radiation dose necessary to achieve a diagnostic study (ACR-SIR, 2014).

Computed Tomography Scan

A CT scan enables the clinician to review anatomic cross-sections (slices) and three-dimensional images of the body using a combination of x-rays, x-ray detectors, and a computer. X-ray beams pass through sections of the patient as the patient traverses through the scanner. The detectors rotate, collecting a large amount of data reconstructed via computer to generate an image. CT studies are fast and rule out or determine the extent of any type of acute trauma, bleed, or injury as well as ongoing progression or resolution of a disease or condition. CT imaging assists with the planning and administering of radiation cancer treatments, surgical planning, guiding biopsies, and other minimally invasive procedures. CT contrast agents are either barium, for GI studies, or an iodine-based contrast injection given intravenously.

Fluoroscopy

Fluoroscopy is real-time continuous x-ray. Ionizing radiation passes through the patient and is collected by an intensifier or flat detector and digitally recorded and transmitted into moving images on a screen. Cardiac catheterization labs, EP labs, IR, and vascular and hybrid ORs use fluoroscopy for diagnostic and therapeutic procedures to determine catheter and device placement using iodine-based contrast agents.

Magnetic Resonance Imaging

MRI is a radiology technique using magnets, radio waves, and a computer to produce images of body structures. The MRI scanner is a tube surrounded by an oversized circular magnet with the patient placed on a movable table inserted into the magnet. The magnet creates a strong magnetic field aligning the protons of hydrogen atoms, which are then subject to radio waves. This spins the various protons of the specific body part being imaged producing a faint signal detected and amplified by coils. A computer receives and processes these signals generating an image. A magnetic resonance angiogram (MRA) is a type of MRI scan using a magnetic field and pulses of radio wave energy to image blood vessels. MRI scan times range anywhere from 30 minutes to several hours depending on the number of studies, requirement for contrast, and area of the body imaged. It is excellent for soft tissue anomalies and musculoskeletal studies as well as the abdomen, pelvis, brain, and spine and in other diagnostic applications. The generation of a magnetic field requires a closed space, resulting in noise. Claustrophobic patients may require sedation. Contraindications for MRI include patients with implanted metal devices (e.g., pacemakers, defibrillators, plates, screws, and aneurysm clips or any foreign body such as shrapnel). Although MRI does not use ionizing radiation, it is crucial for those working in the environment to adhere to the ferrous metal guidelines protecting the patient and staff from injury (Patient Safety).

Ultrasound

Ultrasound produces sectional images or slices in multiple planes much like CT and MRI. Ultrasound uses the interaction of high-frequency sound waves to form the image. As these sound waves strike different tissue densities, a transducer measures the sound waves and an image results by converting the echoes into electrical impulses. Ultrasound does not use ionizing radiation. Color flow Doppler uses ultrasound technology to quantify the direction and velocity of blood flow in vascular and cardiac diagnostic and surgical applications.

Radiation Physics

Ionizing Radiation

Radiation is present naturally in the environment and can be artificial. Radiation refers to kinetic energy (moving an object against resistance)

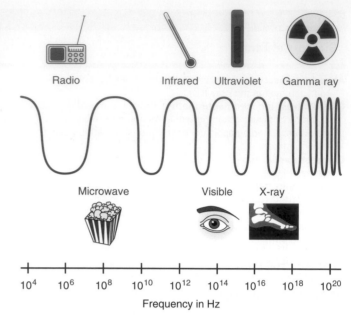

FIG. 29.1 Electromagnetic spectrum.

that passes from one location to another. During a radiographic examination (x-ray), high energy passes through the body to produce an image. The transfer of energy causes excitation (ionization) of atoms and molecules. Frequency and wavelengths of electromagnetic waves are known as the electromagnetic spectrum (Fig. 29.1).

Ionizing radiation damages living cells, which can repair themselves, die, or undergo a mutation. The effects of radiation on biologic tissue are generally classified as two types: deterministic effects and stochastic effects. Deterministic effects are dose dependent and result in cell death (Table 29.1). It is an acute event when a threshold level of radiation has been exceeded, and the higher the dose is, the greater the injury. The threshold is not absolute and can vary among individuals. Stochastic effects cause DNA damage to single cells, which results in mutation. The probability of occurrence increases as the cumulative radiation exposure increases. Stochastic effects refer to the probability of suffering a disease caused by the cumulative exposure of radiation over years, for example, radiation-induced cancers, such as leukemia (Cheng, 2014). Appropriate precautions must be taken to safeguard staff members and patients (Evidence for Practice).

Units of Measurement

It is important for the perioperative nurse to understand the basics of radiation physics and radiation dose metrics to effectively communicate with colleagues and patients, as well as for documentation, monitoring, and quality assurance. Different units of measure describe radiation dose. Dose refers to radiation to the tissues. The Health Physics Society (HPS) defines the use of the International System of Units (SI) for radiologic quantities, which are the gray (Gy), sievert (Sv), and millisievert (mSv). The gray is the unit of radiation dose expressed in terms of absorbed energy per unit mass of tissue, or the unit of absorbed dose. (Absorbed dose is the amount of energy deposited in any substance by ionizing radiation per unit mass of the substance.) The gray does not take into account the type of radiation or tissue damage. The sievert is a derived unit of ionizing radiation dose in the SI. It is a measure of the radiation dose and refers to the damage caused by the type of radiation on a specific

PATIENT SAFETY

Magnetic Resonance Imaging Safety

There is no ionizing radiation exposure with MRI; however, the MRI suite is potentially dangerous subsequent to the strong magnetic field. Ferromagnetic objects (mainly containing iron, nickel, or cobalt), when near to a magnet, experience a force of attraction toward the magnet bore (magnetic isocenter). Fatalities have resulted during the use of MRI. All patients, visitors, non-MR personnel, and pieces of equipment should be screened appropriately before entry into the controlled area. In practice, particular attention should be paid to oxygen cylinders, wheelchairs, stretchers, cardiac pacemakers, and intracranial aneurysm clips of ferromagnetic/unknown composition. There may be an occasion when the magnet needs to be shut down in an emergency (or *quenched*) if a person becomes trapped between the magnet and a ferromagnetic object. When the ERDU button is depressed, liquid helium will vaporize and there should be a pressure-release disk/pipe system to vent this gas to the outside. However, as a matter of caution, all personnel should exit the magnet room and the door should be kept closed. Magnetic field gradients can cause unpleasant peripheral nerve stimulation. This is an acute effect and not harmful. Modern system software should alert the operator when there is risk of attaining such levels. Protective ear plugs/headphones should be worn by patients and accompanying personnel.

The MR suite is conceptually divided into four zones. Zone I is the region including all areas that are freely accessible to the general public. This area is typically outside the MR environment itself and is the area through which patients, healthcare personnel, and other employees of the MR suite access the MR environment. Zone II is the area that interfaces between the publicly accessible, uncontrolled Zone I and the strictly controlled Zones III and IV. Typically, patients are greeted in Zone II, but are not free to move throughout Zone II at will. Preprocedure preparation occurs in this zone. Zone III is the area around the MR scanner room itself. Access to Zone III is to be strictly restricted. The Zone IV area contains the MR scanner magnet. Zone IV is located within Zone III. Zone IV should be demarcated and clearly marked as being potentially hazardous because of the presence of the very strong magnetic fields. As part of the Zone IV site restriction, the facility should provide for direct visual observation by personnel to access pathways into Zone IV. Zone IV should be clearly marked with a red light and lighted sign stating, "The Magnet Is On." Ideally, signage should inform the public that the magnetic field is active even when power to the facility is deactivated. In case of cardiac or respiratory arrest or other medical emergency within Zone IV, appropriately trained and certified MR personnel should immediately initiate basic life support or CPR as required by the situation while the patient is being emergently removed from Zone IV to a predetermined, magnetically safe location. All priorities should be focused on stabilizing and then evacuating the patient as rapidly and safely as possible from the magnetic environment. It is also important to ensure the patient's tissues do not form large conductive loops. Therefore care should be taken to ensure that the patient's arms or legs are not positioned in such a way as to form a large loop within the bore of the MR imager during the imaging process. For this reason, it is preferable that patients be instructed not to cross their arms or legs in the MR scanner. There have been reports of thermal injuries that seem to have been associated with skin-to-skin contact such as in the region of the inner thighs. Ensure skin-to-skin contact instances are minimized or eliminated in or near the regions undergoing radiofrequency energy irradiation.

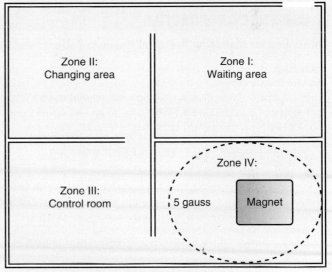

The four zones of a magnetic resonance imaging (MRI) suite. Zone I is the patient registration area, Zone II is the changing area, Zone III is the control room, Zone IV is in the MRI suite, and the 5 gauss line is around the magnet.

CPR, Cardiopulmonary resuscitation; *ERDU,* emergency run-down unit; *MRI,* magnetic resonance imaging.
Modified from Kanal E et al: ACR Guidance Document on MRI Safe Practices: 2013. Expert panel on MR Safety, *J Magn Reson Imaging* 37(3):501–530, 2013.

tissue. The millisievert is the international unit used to measure the amount of radiation (1 Gy = 1 Sv) (1 mSv = 0.001 Sv) (HPS, 2016).

Radiation dose varies by modality, with CT and fluoroscopy higher than radiography. For example, the adult effective dose from a CT examination of the head is equivalent to the adult effective dose from roughly 100 chest x-rays. The adult effective dose from a CT examination of the abdomen is roughly equivalent to the adult effective dose from roughly 400 chest x-rays (Table 29.2). The portion of the x-ray passed through the patient is the primary source. However, x-rays scatter on contact when interacting with various materials, producing scatter radiation, which is known as secondary radiation.

Fluoroscopic Dose Measurement. Fluoroscopy equipment should report three parameters: fluoroscopy time; radiation dose (air kerma, in Gy), a measure of deterministic injury potential; and the dose-area product (in cGy × cm²), which is a measure of stochastic injury potential (Haines et al., 2014).

Peak skin dose, measured in gray, is the highest radiation dose at any portion of the patient's skin during the procedure. This measurement includes radiation from the primary x-ray beam and scatter. The skin dose varies by procedure as well as other factors (Table 29.3). Reference dose measured in gray is the approximation of the total radiation dose to the skin and does not incorporate scatter. All fluoroscopes sold in the United States must display the

TABLE 29.1

Approximate Threshold Doses for Mild Deterministic Effects

Organ/Tissue	Effect	Approximate Threshold Dose (Single Exposure) Gy (Sv)	Latency Time
Eye lens	Detectable lens' changes (opacities)	0.2–0.5	Years
Skin	Transient erythema	2	2–24 hours
Reproductive system (male)	Transient oligozoospermia	0.1–0.2	2–3 months

Deterministic Effects at Various Acute Absorbed Doses

Skin erythema	2 Gy
Hair loss	3 Gy
Cataracts	5 Gy
Sterility	2–3 Gy
Lethality (whole-body radiation)	3–5 Gy

Modified from Geleijns J, Tack D: Medical physics: radiation risks. In Adam A et al, editors: *Grainger & Allison's diagnostic radiology*, ed 6, Philadelphia, 2015, Elsevier; Herring W: *Learning radiology: recognizing the basics*, ed 3, Philadelphia, 2016, Elsevier.

EVIDENCE FOR PRACTICE

Strategies for Managing Radiation Doses to Patients and Operators

Immediate

Optimize Dose to Patient
- Radiologists should ensure the proper dosing protocol is in place for the patient being treated.
- Keep extremities out of the beam.
- Maximize the distance between the x-ray tube and patient.
- Minimize the distance between the patient and image receptor.
  - Dose rates and scatter dose rates will be greater and dose will accumulate faster in larger patients.
- Minimize fluoroscopy time.
- Vary the beam angle to minimize exposure to any single skin area.
- Use last-image-hold and stored fluoroscopic image settings to review findings.
- Use collimation to the fullest extent possible.
- If the procedure is unexpectedly prolonged, consider options for positioning the patient or altering the x-ray field or other means to alter beam angulation so that the same area of skin is not continuously in the direct x-ray field.
- Consider the use of other diagnostic technologies such as MRI and ultrasound.

Minimize Dose to Operators and Staff
- Keep body parts out of the field of view at all times.
  - Position yourself in a low-scatter area whenever possible.
- Use movable shields; wear adequate protection, such as a lead apron, leaded eyeglasses, surgical radiation safety gloves, and thyroid shield.
- Strictly adhere to dosimetry and monitoring using a monitoring badge worn at the abdomen/waist under personal protective lead.
- Maximize the distance from the x-ray source; when possible use remote hand switch for acquisitions.

- Institute a process for annual education review and competency testing for physicians and technologists.
  - Use appropriate imaging equipment whose performance is controlled through a quality-assurance program.
  - Obtain appropriate training on radiation dose, ALARA techniques, and overall radiation safety practices.

Long Term
- Incorporate dose-reduction technologies and dose-measurement devices in equipment.
- Establish a facility quality improvement program that includes an appropriate x-ray equipment quality assurance program that is overseen by a medical physicist.
- Ensure that the recommended quality control testing (daily functional tests) and scheduled preventive maintenance is performed in accordance with the manufacturer's guidelines.
- Review dosing protocols annually or every 2 years.
- Establish appropriate dose ranges for high-volume and high-dose diagnostic imaging studies.

Documentation and Follow-Up
Measure and record patient radiation dose as part of the study summaries report findings:
- Inform patients who have received high doses to examine the x-ray beam entrance site for skin erythema.
- Develop methods to quantify late effects.
- Design medical records to clearly document the number and types of interventional procedures received by the patient.
- Maintain a database of all patients with procedure and dose information.
- Investigate patterns outside the range of appropriate doses.
- Participate in a national registry to track radiation doses as the start of a process to identify optimal and reference doses.

ALARA, As low as reasonably achievable; *MRI*, magnetic resonance imaging.
Modified from Dauer L et al: Occupational radiation protection of pregnant or potentially pregnant workers in IR: a joint guideline of the Society of Interventional Radiology and Cardiovascular and Interventional Radiological Society of Europe, *J Vasc Interv Radiol* 26(2):171–181, 2015; Association of periOperative Registered Nurses (AORN): Guideline for radiation safety. In: *Guidelines for perioperative practice*, Denver, 2016, The Association.

reference dose at the operator's working position. The dose area product (DAP) is a measure of the entire amount of x-ray energy delivered to the patient by the beam and is expressed as Gy × cm². The DAP uses a device in front of the x-ray tube to measure radiation entering the body (Fig. 29.2). Fluoroscopy time is a surrogate measure

for documenting approximate radiation dose. Fluoroscopy time measures the time the x-ray beam is on and does not incorporate information about dose rate or entrance ports.

Computed Tomography Dose Measurement. The radiation dose from CT is reported using different parameters. The CT dose index (CTDI) is the energy/dose absorbed from the acquisition slice. The absorbed dose of a patient depends on the longitudinal range of the scan. The CTDI is multiplied with the scan length to obtain the dose-length product (DLP). Because some tissues are more sensitive to radiation than others, the DLP can estimate the effective dose of the CT scan (Nieman et al., 2015). Current CT scan technology uses multiple slices and spiral rotations of the x-ray tube to acquire an image. The CTDI measures ionizing radiation exposure per slice of data acquisition. The CTDIvol represents the total absorbed dose in and outside the slices with a unit of milligray (mGy). The DLP factors in dose along the actual length of the body part being scanned (units are mGy × cm). As an example, the DLP for a CT

TABLE 29.2
Radiation Dose to Adults From Common Imaging Examinations

Procedure	Approximate Effective Radiation Dose (mSv)[a]	Comparable to Natural Background Radiation for
CT: abdomen and pelvis	10	3 years
Radiography (x-ray): spine	1.5	6 months
Radiography (x-ray): extremity	0.001	3 hours
CT: head	2	8 months
CT: chest	7	2 years
Radiography: chest	0.1	10 days
Intraoral x-ray	0.005	1 day
Coronary CTA	12	4 years
Bone densitometry (DEXA)	0.001	3 hours
Mammography	0.4	7 weeks

[a]The effective doses are typical values for an average-sized adult. The actual dose can vary, depending on a person's size as well as differences in imaging practices. Pediatric patient dose will vary significantly from those given to adults, since children vary in size.
CT, Computed tomography; CTA, computed tomographic angiography.
Modified from American College of Radiology (ACR): Radiation dose to adults from common imaging examinations (website). www.acr.org/~/media/ACR/Documents/PDF/QualitySafety/Radiation-Safety/Dose-Reference-Card.pdf?la=en. (Accessed 7 January 2017)

TABLE 29.3
Radiation Dose Comparisons

Diagnostic Procedure	Typical Effective Dose (mSv)
Chest x-ray (PA film)	0.02
Lumbar spine	1.5
CT: head	2
CT: chest	7
CT: abdomen	8
Coronary artery calcification CT	3
Coronary CT angiogram	16

CT, Computed tomography; PA, posteroanterior.
From McCollough CH et al: Average effective dose in millisieverts: answers to common questions about the use and safety of CT scans; Mayo Clin Proc 90(10):1300–1392, 2015.

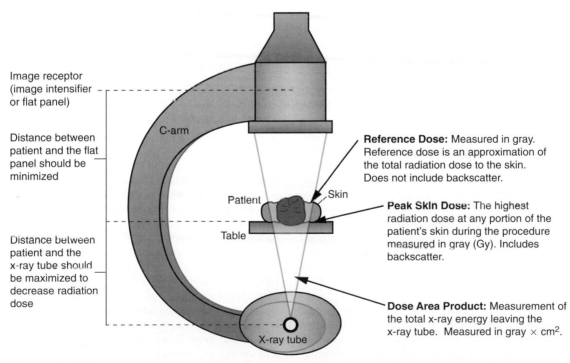

FIG. 29.2 Components of a C-arm fluoroscopy system and key terms relating to radiation dose and fluoroscopy.

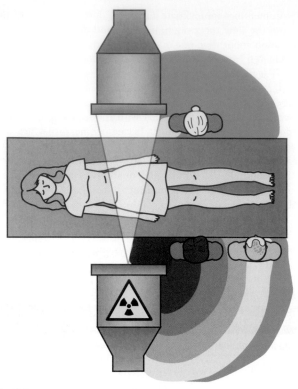

FIG. 29.3 Effect of scatter radiation on the operator and other personnel in the room.

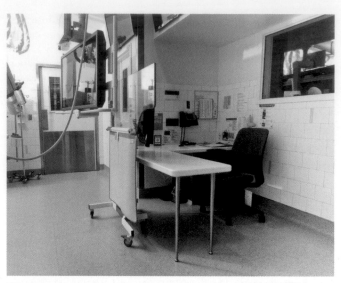

FIG. 29.4 Ceiling-mounted lead shield at the nurse's station in a hybrid operating room.

scan of the head will be smaller than the DLP for a CT scan of the chest and abdomen because the surface area is smaller (Nieman et al., 2015).

Radiation Dose Factors. Patient size is a key factor governing the dose of radiation. Obese patients, as well as those with larger chests, require higher radiation doses to adequately penetrate tissues to yield a quality image. Radiation exposure to staff occurs as a result of radiation scatter (Fig. 29.3). The amount of scatter radiation varies directly with patient size (i.e., the scatter produced from pediatric procedures is lower than adult procedures), duration of radiation exposure, the field of view, the intensity of the x-ray beam, and the angulation of the x-ray beam. The primary approaches used to reduce radiation exposure to the operator and team members are increasing distance from the source, scatter reduction, and dose limitation. Radiation dissipates in proportion to the square of the distance from the source. A modest effort to move away from the tube will significantly reduce exposure. Radiation scatter occurs as radiation from the generator tube enters the patient and is partially reflected, or by body tissues. Scatter from the patient is the main source of radiation exposure to the patient outside the imaging field and to the operator. The operator and laboratory personnel must be protected from exposure to the scatter radiation with shielding (Haines et al., 2014).

ALARA

As defined in Title 10, Section 20.1003, of the Code of Federal Regulations (10 CFR 20.1003), ALARA is an acronym for "as low as reasonably achievable," which means making every reasonable effort to maintain exposures to ionizing radiation as far below the dose limits as practical, consistent with the purpose for which the licensed activity is undertaken, taking into account the state of technology, the economics of improvement in relation to the state of technology, the economics of improvements in relation to benefits to the public health and safety, and other societal and socioeconomic considerations, and in relation to utilization of nuclear energy and licensed materials in the public interest (USNRC, 2014). Time, distance, and shielding measures minimize exposure to radiation in much the same way people protect themselves against overexposure to the sun.

The three major principles inherent to ALARA are the following:
1. *Time:* Minimizing the time of exposure directly reduces radiation dose. Minimizing the time of exposure (also known as "on beam" time) directly reduces radiation dose to the patient as well as the staff exposure to scatter radiation.
2. *Distance:* The intensity and dose of radiation decreases dramatically as the distance from the source increases.
3. *Shielding:* Barriers of lead, or absorber materials such as Plexiglas, concrete, or water, provide protection from penetrating radiation. Therefore inserting the proper shield between the person and a radiation source will greatly reduce or eliminate the dose of radiation. The procedure team ensures the patient is positioned as far from the x-ray tube and as close to the image intensifier as possible (USNRC, 2016).

These principles apply to ionizing radiation in general but are more relevant to fluoroscopy than CT. Regarding time and distance, CT scans take seconds, with the distance between the CT's x-ray source and the patient remaining relatively constant. The technologist is in a control room outside the CT scanner, shielded from radiation by lead-lined walls and doors. In contrast, exposure to fluoroscopy is longer (minutes) and varies by procedure. Prolonged procedures using fluoroscopy should change the beam's entry point to reduce repeated exposure to the same area. Staff members in the control room do not wear lead. Staff members in the procedure room during fluoroscopy wear lead in addition to radiation protection provided by table-side lead apron drapes, ceiling-suspended lead acrylic shields, and movable lead acrylic shields (Fig. 29.4). Wraparound lead aprons and thyroid shields with a minimum of 0.5 mm of lead must be worn by personnel in the room during fluoroscopy. Leaded eyeglasses provide protection against cataract development for the equipment operator and personnel adjacent to the operator (USNRC, 2016).

Protection and Regulation

Protective wraparound aprons with thyroid shields are the principal personal radiation protection tools. Properly fitted aprons are of particular importance for female staff members to provide adequate shielding of breast tissue. Consideration should be given to the overall weight of the lead apron because the weight can cause fatigue and strain and increase the potential for musculoskeletal and back issues. Personnel radiation monitoring is an important part of radiation safety. Personal radiation dosimeters are worn on the trunk (under the apron) and at the collar level (outside the apron) to measure exposure. The dosimeters should not be left on aprons because this would cause inaccurate readings when an apron is worn by another user. Team members need to know their occupational dose to ensure they are working safely and within regulatory limits. Dose data will not be accurate unless workers always wear their dosimeters, wear them correctly, and turn them in to be read at each monitoring frequency (typically monthly). All equipment should be properly maintained and periodically inspected for radiation safety. Radiation output should be monitored and radiation scatter surveys conducted by a qualified medical physicist/medical physics expert according to local regulations and hospital policy (Dauer et al., 2015). The US Nuclear Regulatory Commission (USNRC) states an annual limit of the total effective dose equivalent is equal to 5 rems (0.05 Sv), or the sum of the deep-dose equivalent and the committed dose equivalent to any individual organ or tissue other than the lens of the eye is equal to 50 rems (0.5 Sv) (USNRC, 2016).

Dosimeter frequency monitoring depends on the institution's policies and procedures and governing laws. Outside the hospital, regulatory and manufacturer initiatives exist to reduce radiation exposure. Real-time dosimetry is an emerging technology (Research Highlight). The US Food and Drug Administration (FDA) requires that fluoroscopy equipment produce an audible warning sound after 5 minutes of fluoroscopy. Other radiation reduction techniques and applications include beam collimation, pulsed versus continuous fluoroscopy, digital fluoroscopy imaging techniques, and specific dose-reduction protocols for CT and fluoroscopy (Dauer et al., 2015). Staff members who have declared their pregnancy should be monitored monthly and provided with their monthly dose record. A single personal dosimeter should be worn under the protective apron by the pregnant worker at waist level from the date the pregnancy is declared until delivery. An additional dosimeter can be placed on the pregnant woman's abdomen, under any radiation-protective clothing. If two dosimeter monitoring systems are used, staff members who may become pregnant should wear the "inside" dosimeter at waist level (Dauer et al., 2015). The preferred modality for the pregnant patient does not use ionizing radiation (e.g., ultrasound and MRI). All efforts should be made to minimize the exposure, with consideration of risk versus benefit for each clinical scenario. Each facility should have a written radiation safety policy or program for pregnant and potentially pregnant team members. There is potential for embryo or fetal radiation exposure during diagnostic or therapeutic procedures for pregnant women undergoing x-ray, fluoroscopy, or CT scans. Risk depends on the gestational age at the time of exposure and the absorbed radiation dose level (Dauer et al., 2015).

Hybrid Operating Room

A hybrid OR combines advanced imaging capabilities with a fully functioning sterile operating suite. The hybrid OR allows surgeons

RESEARCH HIGHLIGHT

Personnel Real-Time Dosimetry in Interventional Radiology

The number of IR procedures has increased steadily over the past decade. This increase has raised concerns about the absorbed ionizing radiation for patients and for healthcare personnel. Because personnel are not always wearing protective glasses or gloves, the radiation diffused by the patient's body may present a problem, especially to the staff's extremities and eye lenses. This study describes the calibration and validation of a wireless real-time prototype dosimeter.

The self-education of operators is the most efficient way to reduce the absorbed dose during a single operation by changing the procedures, if possible. Passive dosimetry integrates dose measurement over a period of 1 to 2 months, making it impossible to correlate peaks of radiation with specific activities. APDs have been developed to attain this goal, but present problems related to wearability and/or presence or cables.

This project studied the RAPID completely wireless real-time prototype dosimeter, worn by medical staff together with passive dosimeters in more than 40 procedures for comparison with a certified dose.

The validation campaign demonstrated the prototype capability of measuring dose rates with a frequency in the range of 5 Hz and an uncertainty of less than 10%, which are characteristics that are equal or better than other ADPs now available. Furthermore, the dose-rate signal trace during a procedure can be recorded and coupled with a video of the procedure. Synchronization of the data log of the machine, actions performed by the operators, and the dose received by the sensor allow an analysis of the process of each individual operator. This information can be used to assist in self-training, reducing unnecessary exposure while maintaining procedure quality. Given the type of sensor and the electronic components, miniaturization of the dosimeter to the size of a wristwatch is possible.

APD, Active personal dosimeter.
Modified from Servoi L et al: Personnel real time dosimetry in interventional radiology, *Phys Med* 32(12):1724–1730, 2016.

to use advanced diagnostic imaging during surgery to eliminate the transfer of high-risk patients from the OR to an imaging center, resulting in comprehensive patient care during minimally invasive surgeries, which typically leads to shorter lengths of hospital stay and faster recovery than open procedures (Schaadt and Landau, 2013).

The hybrid OR has a fixed angiography system (versus mobile C-arm) for performing open surgical and catheter-based interventions (Fig. 29.5). Multidisciplinary surgical procedures such as neurosurgery, orthopedics, and trauma, cardiac, and vascular surgery can be performed in the hybrid OR. Hybrid ORs vary in equipment configuration; however, the universal element inherent to a hybrid OR is its advanced imaging and reconstruction capabilities. These applications enable physicians to optimize their approach percutaneously, distinguish organ pathology, navigate instrument placement, ensure accurate device implantation and function, and convert to an open procedure if warranted. The image processing is done by a skilled RT or physician. Some of the advanced imaging techniques used in a hybrid OR include digital subtraction angiography (DSA), roadmapping, and rotational angiography. DSA is a computer-assisted fluoroscopy technique subtracting out the images of bone and soft tissue to view the vessels. DSA is useful in the diagnosis and treatment

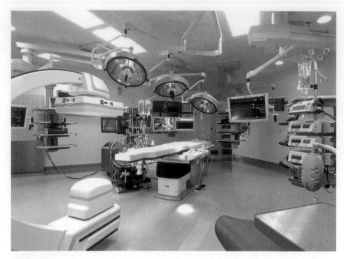

FIG. 29.5 Hybrid operating room containing a fixed angiography system.

of peripheral arterial and venous occlusions, carotid artery stenosis, pulmonary embolisms, acute limb ischemia, renal arterial stenosis, and cerebral aneurysms and arteriovenous malformations (AVMs). Roadmapping is the superimposition of a live fluoroscopic image on a previously stored digitally subtracted angiogram. Roadmapping facilitates catheter and wire placement in complex and small neuroendovascular procedures such as aneurysm coiling, advanced stroke interventions, AVMs, and carotid stenting. Rotational angiography uses the rotation of the C-arm around the patient to reconstruct three-dimensional, cross-sectional CT-like images from standard two-dimensional angiography. Uses for rotational angiography include visualization of endovascular stent placement, complex surgeries of the aortic arch, transcatheter aortic valve replacement (TAVR), atrial fibrillation ablations, embolization techniques for tumor treatment, punctures, and drainages. Additional procedures performed in a hybrid OR requiring basic fluoroscopy include arteriograms or venograms, angioplasty and stenting, thrombectomies, arrhythmia device implantation, high-risk percutaneous coronary intervention (PCI) for unprotected left main coronary artery disease, and other complex and high-risk morphology. Combination interventional and surgical procedures performed in a hybrid OR include hybrid revascularization cardiac bypass graft (CABG) and PCI in the same setting as well as congenital, structural, and heart valve interventions.

Location

The location of a hybrid OR depends on the facility design, physicians, and procedures. New construction tends to locate a hybrid OR near the cardiac catheterization lab, IR, OR, or vascular lab. Such adjacencies bring economies of scale because these services use the same support space, imaging equipment, anesthesia, recovery, and supplies, as well as shared expertise (Schaadt and Landau, 2013).

Personnel and Staffing Requirements for a Hybrid Operating Room

Hybrid ORs are complex work environments. There are no specific regulations or practices regarding skill sets and staffing patterns for a hybrid OR. Team members typically have a blended skill set of IR, surgery, and radiology. Although team members vary, an underlying key success factor is the interdisciplinary collaboration required to work in the room and optimize patient care. The personnel profile should include an open-minded attitude toward innovation, excellent

communication skills, and a willingness to change traditional processes. Process change is perhaps the biggest obstacle to overcome because the standard workflow and processes inherent to each specialty must merge. There may be significant changes regarding the procedure approach, equipment, and environment depending on the core skill sets of staff. Moreover, in some cases the procedures are evolving, and best practice or standard workflow has not yet been established. When the processes, roles, and responsibilities become defined and standardized the benefits of a hybrid OR can be realized.

Nursing Care of the Interventional Radiology Patient

Preliminary Evaluation

Depending on the institution, the perioperative nurse initiates patient contact to schedule the procedure and perform an assessment, either by telephone or at the hospital. The nurse provides clear verbal instructions regarding preprocedure laboratory work or special studies: the time, date, and place to arrive on the day of the procedure; advance directives; insurance information; and nothing by mouth (NPO) status. Most patients are NPO after midnight, although angiography patients receiving contrast may continue water as prophylaxis against the dehydrating effects of contrast. Patients undergoing MRI have additional metal screenings. Same-day procedure patients must adhere to the prerequisites for same-day discharge. The determination of special needs (e.g., interpreters, claustrophobia, transportation, etc.) and the corrective or preventive actions are also components of the preprocedure phone call or visit. Most institutions use a checklist for the initial screening.

Assessment

The assessment and preparation for IR patients includes a complete medical history and physical, nursing assessment with plan of care, informed consent, patient teaching, and the development of procedural sedation or analgesia planning. Because of the broad scope of IR, it is important to establish interdisciplinary patient preparation protocols. These include the requirement and completion of specific consultations (e.g., nephrology, oncology, anesthesia, orthopedics, gynecology, urology, etc.) as well as specific laboratory testing, urinalysis, and other required screenings and tests. Previous radiologic studies should be available for evaluating and planning procedure specifics. The physician performing the procedure determines protocol specifics including the access site, side and approach, imaging modality, contrast use, and device selection. Other considerations include specific medications, anesthesia plan, premedication for history of contrast reactions, antibiotic requirements, blood products, and use of closure devices.

Assessment includes obtaining the patient's height and weight, a brief history of the present illness, and past history, including renal dysfunction, coagulopathies, and allergies (including contrast medium allergy). The nurse verifies the patient's current weight for medication dose calculation and to ensure compliance with the manufacturer's modality table weight tolerance.

For bariatric patients, the ARIN position statement on bariatric patient safety states preadmission planning for the bariatric patient includes careful screening for comorbidities and determining special equipment needs and history of past procedure sedation. Preadmission information includes height, weight, and body mass index (BMI) calculation (ARIN, 2014b). Depending on the patient's body habitus, he or she may be within weight tolerance but the girth prohibits the scan. The average CT and MRI gantry size (bore opening) is 70 cm but does not factor in the table or instruments for a procedure.

The nurse or technologist can use an appropriate diameter hula hoop to determine whether a patient will fit in the scanner. The nurse performs and marks the initial distal pulse assessments' presence or absence and quality for patients undergoing angiography before and after the procedure. An 18- or 20-gauge intravenous (IV) catheter is standard for administrating medications, contrast, and hydration. IV placement is usually antecubital but varies depending on the procedure, patient positioning, and vascular access. For neuroangiography procedures, the nursing neurologic assessment should include notation of difficulty with speech, visual disturbances, facial weakness, and any motor or sensory loss in the extremities, before the procedure start. This assessment provides a comparison during the procedure and recovery. Timing and selection of preprocedure antibiotics should be in accordance with regulatory agencies and facility and professional association guidelines.

Labs

Please refer to Appendix A for standard labs. ARIN states that the nurse reviews serum laboratory results, including, but not limited to, coagulopathy studies for levels before invasive procedures. Serum creatinine and estimated glomerular filtration rate (eGFR) should be documented before iodinated contrast studies because this ensures that appropriate precontrast regimen is implemented in cooperation with the radiologist. If performed, the 12-lead electrocardiogram (ECG) and chest radiography reports should be reviewed. All abnormal or critical results must be communicated to the physician or designee.

The referring physician and interventionalist will collaborate to determine when and if to stop anticoagulants. Physician collaboration is essential regarding the use of aspirin-containing medication, nonsteroidal antiinflammatory drugs (NSAIDs), and antiplatelet medications. Some patients require bridging protocols (e.g., short-acting injected low-molecular-weight heparin) to wean oral anticoagulants while maintaining necessary anticoagulation until the procedure. The nurse provides clear instructions to the patients on continuing and discontinuing medications before the procedure. On admission the nurse reviews the appropriate coagulation profiles before the start of the procedure according to hospital policy.

Cardiopulmonary

All patients undergoing cardiac or pulmonary procedures and patients with a history of cardiopulmonary disease should have ECGs. The nurse gives specific dosing instruction to patients taking any hypertensive, antiarrhythmic, and cardiac medications before surgery. Patients with asthma should take their medications the day of the procedure and bring their inhalers. When appropriate, the anesthesia department should be consulted regarding airway management. The nurse should note any history or suspected problems with sleep apnea.

Patients using continuous positive airway pressure (CPAP) or bilevel positive airway pressure (BiPAP) at home should bring their own device because of the possibility of inducing sleep during sedation. Patients receiving sedation should undergo evaluation for obstructive sleep apnea (OSA) as per the American Society of Anesthesiologists (ASA) guidelines to identify adverse sedation reaction risk (Gross et al., 2014).

Diabetes

Diabetic patients who take oral hypoglycemic medications should take their routine dose on the morning of the procedure. The nurse obtains blood glucose on arrival to the procedure room via a fingerstick

---

BOX 29.3

Medications Containing Metformin

- Actoplus Met (metformin and pioglitazone)
- Avandamet (metformin and rosiglitazone)
- Glucovance (metformin and glyburide)
- Janumet (metformin and sitagliptin)
- Kombiglyze XR (metformin and saxagliptin)
- Metaglip (metformin and glipizide)
- PrandiMet (metformin and repaglinide)

Modified from Hodgson BB, Kizior RJ: *Saunders nursing drug handbook 2017*, St Louis, 2017, Saunders.

---

and consults the appropriate physician for insulin adjustment if the blood sugar is greater than 200 mg/dL. Additional screening of diabetic patients for metformin and medications containing metformin is critical (Box 29.3). These medications should be discontinued for 48 hours after the procedure in patients receiving contrast because of the risk of lactic acidosis. The ARIN clinical practice guideline for Metformin Therapy and Lactic Acidosis Risk (ARIN, 2014d) recommends evaluating renal function before resuming metformin or metformin-containing medications. It is not necessary to discontinue metformin or drugs containing metformin before gadolinium-enhanced MRI studies using normal dosage regimens (0.1–0.3 mmol/kg of body weight). The ARIN clinical practice guideline also recommends withholding metformin and drugs containing metformin with large doses of gadolinium because of potential nephrotoxicity (ARIN, 2014d).

Renal Disease

Preexisting renal disease and hydration status increase the risk of nephrotoxicity. The nurse reviews serum creatinine and eGFRs before contrast administration in patients with a history of kidney disease or surgery; family history of kidney failure, diabetes, paraproteinemia syndromes or diseases (e.g., multiple myeloma); collagen vascular disease (e.g., scleroderma, systemic lupus erythematosus); metformin-containing medications; chronic or high doses of NSAIDs; or regular use of nephrotoxic medications, such as aminoglycosides. Preprocedural considerations for renal disease patients include adequate hydration, coordination of contrast media volume, and preprocedure kidney function tests. If risk exceeds benefit, the physician may substitute another imaging modality (Reekers, 2015).

Contrast Allergies and Other Considerations

The nurse determines and documents any prior exposure to, or history of, contrast media allergic reactions. Predisposing allergic risk factors include asthma; renal insufficiency; significant cardiac disease; anxiety; and paraproteinemia, particularly multiple myeloma. Common pretreatment protocols for contrast allergies are 50 mg prednisone orally 13 hours, 7 hours, and 1 hour before procedure. Beta-blockers may increase the risk of reaction to contrast media or increase the severity of a reaction. Thyroid disease may increase the risk of delayed hyperthyroidism, and contrast media may be a contraindication in patients with thyroid cancer. The physiologic and emotional status of the patient contributes to the incidence and severity of adverse reactions. Often the procedure diagnosis is the source of anxiety more so than the procedure. Patients may experience claustrophobia when undergoing CT or MRI or any IR procedure in which sterile draping around the head, face, and neck occurs.

Reassurance that sedation and analgesia may be available may help to allay fears. Other alternatives include complementary or alternative therapies, such as verbal relaxation techniques, music distraction, and therapeutic presence.

Consent

Informed consent is required for invasive diagnostic and therapeutic procedures requiring moderate sedation. The physician or other qualified personnel assisting the physician should explain the procedure, intended benefits and alternatives, risks, answer all questions, and arrange for appropriate documentation of informed consent. In the consent discussion, the physician should explain the likelihood and characteristics of radiation injury, particularly for procedures associated with higher levels of radiation (e.g., transjugular intrahepatic portosystemic shunt [TIPS], embolization, stroke therapy, biliary draining, visceral angioplasty, stent placement, vertebroplasty, radiofrequency ablation [RFA]). Special consideration is required for the pregnant patient regarding fetal exposure, and should include a discussion of potential effects of radiation exposure to the fetus as part of the consent process (ACR-SIR, 2016).

TJC Universal Protocol is a requirement for correct patient, procedure, and site. The preprocedure verification process verifies the correct patient, correct procedure, and correct site. The time-out is performed immediately before the start of the procedure and involves the patient (whenever practical) and immediate members of the procedure team, including physicians, RTs, and nurses. The time-out should be initiated by a designated member of the team and is best standardized. During the time-out, the team members agree on correct patient identity, correct procedure, and correct site (Rafiei et al., 2016).

Nursing Diagnosis

Nursing diagnoses related to the care of patients undergoing IR procedures might include the following:

- Acute Pain
- Anxiety related to the procedure
- Deficient Knowledge related to the procedure and postprocedure period
- Ineffective Breathing Pattern related to pain or conscious sedation
- Risk for Ineffective Peripheral Tissue Perfusion related to sedation, procedural fluid imbalance, or postprocedure bleeding
- Risk for Injury related to radiation exposure

Outcome Identification

Outcomes for the selected nursing diagnoses could be stated as follows:

- The patient will verbalize relief of pain, and demonstrate less autonomic responses to pain.
- The patient will verbalize decreased anxiety.
- The patient will verbalize understanding of the procedure and postprocedure expectations.
- The patient's airway will be maintained and oxygen saturation will be within normal limits.
- The patient will maintain vital signs within acceptable limits, maintain peripheral pulses as expected, and demonstrate no evidence of excessive bleeding.
- The patient's skin will remain intact, not be reddened, and be free from blistering.

Planning

Planning for an interventional procedure consists of the standard elements of perioperative care as well as considerations relevant to

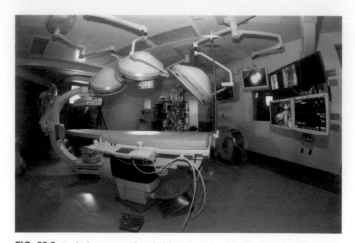

FIG. 29.6 Radiolucent nonbreakable imaging table fixed to the floor, with table controls mounted tableside.

the imaging modality. Some procedures, such as vascular access, drainage procedures, and biopsies, are done bedside with ultrasound. Sterile techniques for bedside procedures vary by facility. Because ultrasound incorporates the imaging unit and probes near or within the sterile field, additional sterile drapes are used when required as different configurations, probe sizes, and length and position of the probes may drape over the field. The nurse ensures the imaging screen is within the operator's line of sight. Procedures performed in the CT or MRI suites must consider the space required for the sterile field. Planning should include accommodation for appropriate clearance of needles and catheters during scanning and movement of the imaging table. When planning for interventional procedures the nurse must consider the table and the modality (CT, MRI, or fluoroscopy) as "integrated." The table is a specific component of the imaging system. Tables have a dedicated motor, are fixed to the floor, and are not interchangeable. Imaging tables are significantly longer and narrower than standard OR beds, with minimal or no padding (Fig. 29.6). CT and angiography tables are made of radiolucent carbon fiber containing no metal joints to reduce imaging artifacts. MRI tables contain no metal. In a standard IR suite that performs only interventions, the table is a nonissue. However, the table becomes an important planning consideration for hybrid ORs if the intent is to do interventional and open surgeries (Schaadt and Landau, 2013). Surgeries requiring elaborate patient positioning are not compatible with an imaging table. Alternatives include bringing in an articulated surgical bed while pivoting the radiolucent table out of the way, or purchasing a core table base with changeable table tops to accommodate various surgeries and interventions. As with traditional OR beds, imaging tables and table tops have weight tolerances. The mobility and range of movement of imaging tables for fluoroscopy is extensive, including vertical, float, stepping, tilt, and cradle rotation to accommodate visualization of the vasculature. Table controls are modular consisting of table side panels, touch screens, and joysticks to position the table, as well as the C-arm and detectors. Physicians may operate the table via table side controls, or the RT may use a remote trolley or foot-mounted controls (outside the sterile field). Because of the table's power and extensive range of motion, the nurse ensures nothing is underneath the fluoroscopy table that could cause significant damage to the table, carts, or supplies. For rotational angiography cases, the C-arm rotates around the patient for image acquisition. Before the rotation, all IV poles, tables, patient lines, monitoring equipment, and ventilator tubing must be out of the path of the C-arm. The scrub person should use a plastic sterile drape to cover the image intensifier or flat detector if it will be in the sterile field during the procedure. The nurse places imaging-acquisition foot pedals in waterproof plastic bags to prevent damage from inadvertent fluid leakage from the field. A best practice is to use a wireless foot switch to reduce tripping hazards and charge foot switches when not in use. ESU dispersive pads must be as close to the operative site as possible but not in the field of view because they impair image quality. Adequate planning for these issues at case setup is optimal because the physician may request to dim the lights during image acquisition. A Sample Plan of Care follows.

Implementation

The perioperative nurse verifies that all equipment, instrumentation, supplies, and radiation safety precautions are in place before the procedure.

SAMPLE PLAN OF CARE

Nursing Diagnosis
Acute Pain

Outcome
The patient will verbalize relief of pain, and demonstrate less autonomic responses to pain.

Interventions
- Assess characteristics of pain: location, severity on a scale of 1 to 10, type, frequency, precipitating factors, relief factors.
- Eliminate factors that precipitate pain.
- Offer analgesics per physician's orders.
- Teach the patient to request analgesics before pain becomes severe.
- Explore nonpharmacologic methods for reducing pain and promoting comfort.

Nursing Diagnosis
Anxiety related to the procedure

Outcome
The patient will verbalize decreased anxiety.

Interventions
- Monitor the patient's level of anxiety by assessing the state of alertness, ability to comprehend, and ability to comply with requests.
- Facilitate the family's presence.
- Assist the family in identifying coping mechanisms; facilitate and support their use.
- Reassure the patient, family, and caregiver during interactions by touch (when welcomed) and empathic verbal and nonverbal communication.
- Explain the IR environment to patient and what to expect to assist in reduction of anxiety.
- Discuss the patient's postoperative appearance (e.g., drains, tubes, equipment) with the patient, family, and caregiver.
- Have the interventional team, including the physicians and technologists, meet the patient, family, and caregiver before the procedure, and allow ample time for questions.

Nursing Diagnosis
Deficient Knowledge related to the procedure and postprocedure period

Outcome
The patient will verbalize understanding of the procedure and postprocedure expectations.

Interventions
- Assess the patient's desire to learn.
- Assess the preferred learning mode (e.g., auditory, visual) and literacy level.
- Provide orientation to the preprocedure unit, procedural area, and postprocedure unit.

- Provide health teaching and written or video/DVD instructions.
- Plan and share necessity of learning outcomes with the patient.

Nursing Diagnosis
Ineffective Breathing Pattern related to pain or conscious sedation

Outcome
The patient's airway will be maintained and oxygen saturation will be within normal limits.

Interventions
- Note risk factors for respiratory compromise.
- Assess for signs and symptoms of respiratory distress.
- Administer oxygen as ordered.
- Monitor respiratory rate, pulse oximetry, and capnography (when available) parameters.

Nursing Diagnosis
Risk for Ineffective Peripheral Tissue Perfusion related to sedation, procedural fluid imbalance, or postprocedure bleeding

Outcome
The patient will maintain vital signs within acceptable limits, maintain peripheral pulses as expected, and demonstrate no evidence of excessive bleeding.

Interventions
- Monitor the patient's vital signs and assess cardiac rhythm.
- Assess peripheral pulses and compare to preprocedure pulse assessment.
- Observe for signs of bleeding.
- Assess the patient for the underlying cause and contributing factors.
- Correct the underlying cause.
- Maintain patency of all IV and other invasive lines.
- Provide psychosocial support for the patient, family, and caregiver.

Nursing Diagnosis
Risk for Injury related to radiation exposure

Outcome
The patient's skin will remain intact, not be reddened, and be free from blistering.

Interventions
- Implement protective measures to prevent injury caused by radiation sources.
- Minimize the time of exposure to radiation.
- Maximize the distance from the radiation source if possible.
- Evaluate patient for signs and symptoms of radiation injury.

IR, Interventional radiology; *IV*, intravenous.

Positioning

Patient positioning for interventional and image procedures depends on the procedure and modality. Positioning is key because the quality of imaging depends on proper patient positioning and minimal patient movement. Complications from positioning include nerve injury, dyspnea, eye or ear injury, hemodynamic compromise, and soft tissue injury. Patients are positioned supine for abdominal, pelvic, chest, cervical and thoracic spine, skull, and peripheral procedures. The nurse pads all bony prominences and uses pillows to relieve pressure points and support the lower back. The arms are tucked at the sides in a neutral position to prevent brachial plexus stretch and ulnar nerve injuries. Patients are placed prone for nephrostomy tube placement or certain spinal procedures, either with the head turned to one side or facing down. When patients are prone, their arms should be placed in a neutral position at their side or next to their head, extended less than 90 degrees. The nurse pads and flexes the legs slightly at the knee and hips. Pressure points include the ear or eye on the dependent side of the head, or on the forehead or eyes if the patient is face down. This position may be difficult for elderly or acutely ill patients to tolerate and may cause hemodynamic changes in patients with pre-existing cardiac or pulmonary disease. The lateral recumbent position is used for procedures involving the skull, femoral head and neck, hips, shoulder, pelvis, and sacrum as well as biopsies and drainages (affected side up). The patient lies on his or her side balanced with anterior and posterior support with a pillow or padding to protect bony prominences (e.g., the knees and ankles). Additional pressure points include the shoulder, pelvis, and trochanter. When positioning patients the nurse checks to make sure no tension exists on drainage tubes, IV lines, or catheters to accommodate anticipated table movement. All sponges, wedge pillows, or other positioning or monitoring devices and ESU dispersive pads must be out of the field of view for imaging (AORN, 2016). Any equipment used during an MRI must be MRI compatible or be kept a certain distance from the magnet.

Prepping

For femoral access the nurse preps the skin with a solution of chlorhexidine gluconate 2% and isopropyl alcohol 70%. Manufacturers' drying time should be observed. The physician drapes the patient in the standard fashion using a disposable interventional drape. For nonvascular IR procedures (e.g., biopsies, ablations, embolizations) the patient is positioned, prepped, and draped per the specific site and procedure.

Equipment

Control Room. A separate lead-lined room for data processing of the images outside the scanner (CT or MRI) or fluoroscope (Fig. 29.7), the control room is a nonsterile area containing various computers accessing the picture archiving and communication system (PACS), radiology information systems (RISs), and imaging processing software. Control rooms are standard in CT, MRI, cardiac catheterization labs, and IR suites. Many institutions position two IR suites with a shared control room between them. Hybrid ORs or EP labs may or may not have a separate control room.

Angiography Equipment Configuration. In the angiography suite the C-arm(s) and the table move for image acquisition; however, the base of the system does not. The "system configuration" refers to the base location, either the floor or ceiling. Physician preference, procedure, facility structural limitations, and other regulations determine system configuration. Cardiac catheterization labs and IR typically use ceiling-mounted systems resulting in more floor space and easier foot traffic. For hybrid ORs, however, ceiling-mounted

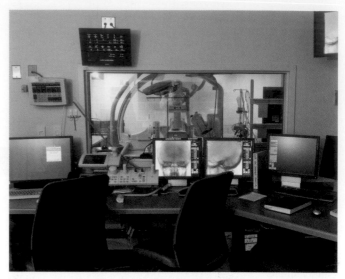

FIG. 29.7 Control room is a nonsterile room adjacent to the procedure area that is used for image processing and data archiving.

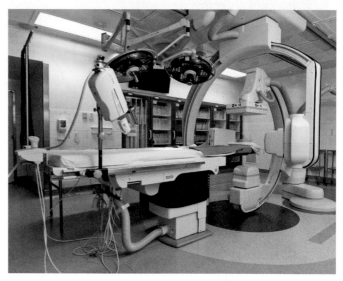

FIG. 29.8 Hybrid operating room containing a biplane (two C-arms) angiography system.

systems compete with "air space" subsequent to monitors, lights, and booms. Effects on positive air pressure and air exchange may also prohibit ceiling-mounted systems. Other concerns specific to a ceiling-mounted system in a hybrid OR are the location and cleaning of the support rails that extend over the open operative field. Floor-mounted systems eliminate ceiling congestion and potential airflow issues. Placement of floor-mounted systems is at the head of the bed, and generally offset at an angle to permit anesthesia workflow. A biplane configuration has two C-arms, one on the ceiling and one on the floor (Fig. 29.8). Biplane, as the name suggests, acquires images from two reference points at the same time. Clinical settings for biplane imaging include neuroangiography, congenital and/or structural cardiac abnormalities, and complex EP mapping procedures.

Contrast Injectors. Radiographic contrast is administered by a handheld syringe or a power injector. A power injector allows the operator to bolus contrast media at a rapid preset flow rate, triggered by a hand or foot switch. The physician selects the quantity, type of contrast media, dilution, and injection rate. Location of the power injectors is either free-standing or table-mounted.

Imaging Monitors. Image displays for CT and MR are on computers in the procedure and control room. In IR suites, typically two monitors provide live fluoroscopy and reference imaging. Another monitor displays C-arm positioning and angulation, or this information is integrated into an existing monitor. Monitor placement in IR and the catheterization lab is usually across from the operating physician. This is not necessarily the case with the hybrid OR. In the hybrid OR there are additional monitors displaying ultrasound, reconstructed images, vital signs, and hemodynamics in addition to the standard monitors. The number and arrangement of monitors varies by procedure, physician(s), and approach. Monitors must be easily movable, particularly in hybrid ORs. Staff members must be cognizant when working in the room to avoid collisions involving monitors, operating lights, booms, and other ceiling-mounted equipment.

Supply Space. IR suites and hybrid ORs need additional supply space for catheter-based interventions (Fig. 29.9). A reasonable number of various-sized sheaths, catheters, guidewires, and implants must be available in the room, control room, or in an adjacent clean core. In dedicated IR suites or newly constructed hybrid ORs, custom cabinetry accommodates a large variety of catheter, introducer, and sheath lengths. In smaller rooms or hybrid ORs, mobile carts transport interventional supplies into the room, reducing storage space requirements. Because some interventional suites and hybrid ORs are

the end destination for stroke patients, emergency supplies and medications are specifically set aside or available in the room for timely setup.

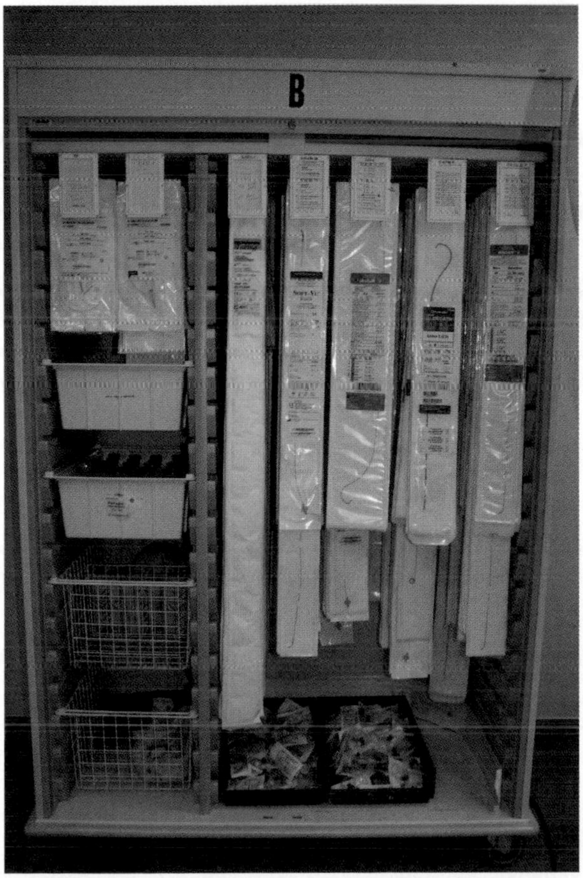

Supplies and Instrumentation. Needles, guidewires, sheaths, catheters, and vascular closure devices are inherent to most interventions. A Seldinger needle (18 gauge, $2\frac{3}{4}$ inches) is standard for groin access (Fig. 29.10). Smaller gauge needles or micropuncture sets are used for axillary or brachial artery punctures or pediatric cases. Guidewires range from 0.010 to 0.038 inches in diameter and 5 to 300 cm in length. Guidewire selection depends on its purpose and physician preference. Guidewires have tapered tips easing insertion. There are steerable and nonsteerable guidewires, as well as introducing and exchange guidewires. Coated guidewires decrease friction when wet, facilitating advancement. Flexible-tipped guidewires navigate past tortuous vessels. After each introduction into the body, the scrub person wipes the guidewire with saline solution–soaked gauze. The buildup of blood, clot, fibrin, or dried contrast impedes the guidewire's ability to advance or results in sticking inside the catheter and possible emboli. Because guidewires can dislodge during catheter exchanges, frequent fluoroscopy verifies proper guidewire position.

Placement of sheath and dilator assemblies at the arterial or venous puncture sites is over the guidewire as described in the Seldinger technique. Sheaths protect the puncture site and vessel from damage and increase patient comfort during multiple sheath and dilator exchanges. Sheaths have a valved end to prevent backflow of arterial blood and a side arm to infuse heparinized saline solution. Selection of dilators depends on the procedure, vessel, and anatomy. After the appropriate dilation and sheath insertion the physician removes the dilator and guidewire together while retaining the sheath hub in place. If a sheath is to be left in place for another procedure or thrombolysis, the physician sutures it to the skin and covers it with a sterile dressing.

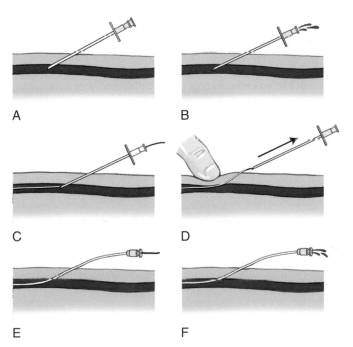

FIG. 29.9 Mobile cart for a hybrid operating room to store sheaths, catheters, and guidewires.

FIG. 29.10 Seldinger technique using a hollow needle and guidewire to obtain vessel access for percutaneous procedures. (A) Insertion of needle. (B) Placement of needle in lumen of vessel (inner cannula removed). (C) Insertion of guidewire. (D) Removal of needle (guidewire remains in place). (E) Threading of catheter over guidewire. (F) Removal of guidewire.

Catheters are made from a variety of materials in ranges of lengths and shapes sized by the French system. Generally the French size is the size in millimeters divided by 3. Flow rates vary according to catheter types, configuration, and lumen size. A pigtail catheter delivers a larger amount of contrast medium because of additional side holes, compared with a catheter with one end hole. Microcatheters (coaxial catheters) provide access to very small vessels. Balloon catheters have angioplasty balloons. Careful technique during the procedure prevents the introduction of inadvertent air or coagulation of blood in the catheter, resulting in thrombus. Thrombus formation depends on the size of the catheter's outer diameter, with respect to the vessel's inner diameter and indwelling time. The physician flushes the catheters frequently; usually after removing the wire and every few minutes while in the vessel and again on removal to reduce the incidence of thrombus. Interventional procedures require pressure bags with heparinized normal saline, high-pressure tubing, connectors, and three-way stopcocks and manifolds within the flush line for the drawing up and discarding of flush, contrast medium, or blood (Bakal and Flacke, 2014).

Medications and Contrast Agents

A variety of medications are used in IR (Surgical Pharmacology). In addition to becoming familiar with standardized medications, the perioperative nurse working in IR must also have a broad knowledge of contrast agents and their possible adverse effects.

Contrast. Various forms of contrast media are used to improve medical imaging. Like all other pharmaceuticals, these agents are not completely devoid of risk. Although adverse side effects are infrequent, side effects from the administration of contrast media vary from minor physiologic disturbances to rare severe life-threatening situations (ACR, 2017). Contrast visualizes blood flow and structures such as a blood vessel, part of the urinary tract, or body cavities. The healthcare professional (e.g., certified and/or licensed RT, nurse, physician assistant, physician, or other appropriate credentialed professional) under the supervision of the radiologist or physician designee may give contrast if the practice is in compliance with institution or state regulations (Box 29.4). State regulations, institutional policy, and licensure status govern who administers contrast. The total rate, volume, and type of contrast depend on the procedure, physician preference, and injection site. Contrast agent classification is, by effect, either positive or negative. A positive contrast agent has a higher density than the body tissue being investigated (e.g., iodine-based–contrast media, barium sulfate, and gadolinium). A negative contrast agent is a substance with a lower density than the body tissues being investigated (e.g., carbon dioxide, air).

Carbon Dioxide. Carbon dioxide (CO_2) is a contrast agent for arterial and venous studies and assists in a variety of endovascular interventions. CO_2 is considered an alternative contrast agent in patients with contraindication to iodine contrast medium (ICM) (de Almeida Mendes et al., 2017). CO_2 is used for procedures including central venography of the upper extremity, aorta, and wedged hepatic venography to visualize the portal venous system before TIPS (ACR-SIR, 2014). There are no nephrotoxic or allergic reactions with CO_2; after it is injected into the blood, CO_2 metabolizes into bicarbonate and bicarbonate reverts to CO_2, which the lung exhales. Contraindications include arterial studies above the diaphragm because of the risk of gas embolization of the spinal, coronary, and cerebral arteries. Likewise CO_2 may enter the arterial system in the presence of cardiac defects, resulting in embolism. CO_2 is used with caution in patients with pulmonary insufficiency or pulmonary hypertension because it may increase pulmonary artery pressure.

BOX 29.4
Administering Contrast Agents: Qualifications and Responsibilities

Personnel

The healthcare professional performing the contrast agent injection must be a certified and/or licensed radiologic technologist, magnetic resonance imaging technologist, registered radiologist assistant, nurse, physician assistant, physician, or other appropriately credentialed healthcare professional under the direct supervision of a radiologist or his or her physician designee. The injection technique must be in compliance with relevant institutional, state, and federal regulations. Training and proficiency in cardiopulmonary resuscitation are recommended for those who attend to patients undergoing contrast-enhanced examinations.

Physician

The physician should be a licensed physician with certification in radiology, diagnostic radiology, or radiation oncology to include imaging training on all body areas. The physician should be familiar with the various contrast media available and the indications and contraindications for each and risk factors that might increase the likelihood of adverse events. The physician is responsible for defining the examination protocol, including specifying the type, timing, dosage, rate of injection, and route of administration of contrast media.

Registered Radiologist Assistant

A registered radiologist assistant is an advanced-level radiographer who is certified and registered as a radiologist assistant by ARRT.

Registered Nurse

The certified and/or licensed nurse should be in compliance with the existing operating policies and procedures required by the imaging facility, and must be in compliance with state and federal regulations.

Technologist

Technologists performing injections of contrast media should be in compliance with existing operating policies and procedures required by the imaging facility. At a minimum, the technologist should understand the general benefits of contrast media administration, follow protocols that involve intravascular injection of contrast media, understand contraindications to intravascular injection of contrast media, and recognize adverse events after contrast media administration. Certification by ARRT, ARMRIT, or an unrestricted state license is required.

Pharmacist

In some settings, a pharmacist may review the contrast medium order for appropriateness and/or dispense the contrast media. The reviewing pharmacist should be familiar with the various contrast media available and the indications and contraindications for each.

ARMRIT, American Registry of Magnetic Resonance Imaging Technologists; *ARRT,* American Registry of Radiologic Technologists.
Modified from American College of Radiology (ACR): *ACR-SIR-SNIS-SPR practice parameter for interventional clinical practice and management, resolution 18* (website), 2014. www.acr.org/~/media/ACR/Documents/PGTS/guidelines/Interventional_Clinical_Practice.pdf. (Accessed 11 October 2017).

The nurse avoids excess sedation and monitors ECG, pulse oximetry, blood pressure, respiratory rate, and heart rate. End-tidal CO_2 ($ETCO_2$) is monitored in intubated patients.

Iodinated Contrast. Fluoroscopy and CT use iodine-based media. Iodine absorbs x-rays, resulting in a lighter appearance in areas containing contrast. Classification of iodine contrast is by

SURGICAL PHARMACOLOGY

Classification of Severity and Manifestations of Adverse Reactions to Contrast

The following describes a classification system for acute adverse reactions to iodinated and gadolinium–containing contrast media. Acute adverse reactions can be either allergic-like or physiologic. Sound clinical judgment should be used to determine when and how aggressively an acute reaction should be treated. However, many mild reactions resolve during a period of observation without treatment.

Mild

Signs and symptoms are self-limited without evidence of progression. Mild reactions include the following:
Allergic-like:

- Limited urticaria/pruritus
- Limited cutaneous edema
- Limited "itchy"/"scratchy" throat
- Nasal congestion
- Sneezing/conjunctivitis/rhinorrhea

Physiologic:

- Limited nausea/vomiting
- Transient flushing/warmth/chills
- Headache/dizziness/anxiety/altered taste
- Mild hypertension that resolves spontaneously

Treatment: Requires observation to confirm resolution or lack of progression but usually no treatment. Patient reassurance is usually helpful. The patient should be monitored for 20 to 30 minutes to ensure that the symptoms do not worsen.

Moderate

Signs and symptoms are more pronounced and commonly require medical management. Some of these reactions have the potential to become severe if not treated. Moderate reactions include the following:
Allergic-like:

- Diffuse urticaria/pruritus
- Diffuse erythema, stable vital signs
- Facial edema without dyspnea
- Throat tightness or hoarseness without dyspnea
- Wheezing/bronchospasm, mild or no hypoxia

Physiologic:

- Protracted nausea/vomiting
- Hypertensive urgency
- Isolated chest pain
- Vasovagal reaction that requires and is responsive to treatment

Treatment: Clinical findings in moderate reactions frequently require prompt treatment. These situations require close, careful observation for possible progression to a life-threatening event. Moderate reactions require close monitoring (frequent vital signs, pulse oximeter in place, and continuous observation by staff). Treatment may include diphenhydramine for symptomatic hives, leg elevation for hypotension, use of a beta-agonist inhaler for bronchospasm, or epinephrine for laryngeal edema.

Severe

Signs and symptoms are often life-threatening and can result in permanent morbidity or death if not managed appropriately. Pulmonary edema is a rare severe reaction that can occur in patients with tenuous cardiac reserve (cardiogenic pulmonary edema) or in patients with normal cardiac function (noncardiogenic pulmonary edema). Severe reactions include the following:
Allergic-like:

- Diffuse edema, or facial edema with dyspnea
- Diffuse erythema with hypotension
- Laryngeal edema with stridor and/or hypoxia
- Wheezing/bronchospasm, significant hypoxia
- Anaphylactic shock (hypotension + tachycardia)

Physiologic:

- Vasovagal reaction resistant to treatment
- Arrhythmia
- Convulsions, seizures
- Hypertensive emergency

Treatment: Requires *prompt* recognition and aggressive treatment and frequently requires hospitalization.

Modified from ACR Committee on Drugs and Contrast Media: *ACR manual on contrast media version 10.3* (website), 2017. www.acr.org/~/media/37D84428BF1D4E1B9A3A2918DA9E27A3. pdf. (Accessed 6 January 2017).

chemical structure, iodine content, osmolarity, and ionization in solution. Iodinated contrast agents are among the most widely used and safest of all medications (ACR, 2017). Types of iodinated contrast media are ionic high-osmolarity contrast media (HOCM) and both ionic and nonionic low-osmolarity contrast media (LOCM). HOCM dissociates in solution, yielding an anion and cation and producing undesirable side effects (e.g., vascular pain, nausea and vomiting, bradycardia, and disturbances in the blood-brain barrier). These adverse effects led to the development of LOCM. There are three types of LOCM: high osmolar (>1200 mOsm/kg H_2O); low osmolar (600–1000 mOsm/kg H_2O); and iso-osmolar (280 mOsm/kg H_2O), which is the approximate osmolarity of blood. Although LOCM reduces side effects, serious contrast reactions and complications still occur. Patients likely to benefit from LOCM are those with a previous adverse effect from contrast media; patients with asthma; patients with renal insufficiency, particularly those with diabetes; patients with known cardiac dysfunction; and severely debilitated patients as determined by a physician. Other circumstances warranting consideration for LOCM are patients with sickle cell disease, pheochromocytoma, or myasthenia gravis; patients very anxious about receiving contrast; and patients at risk for aspiration (ACR, 2017).

Gadolinium-Magnetic Resonance Imaging Contrast. Gadolinium is a magnetically active compound and is the contrast medium for MRI. Although the type of contrast agents used in CT, fluoroscopy, and MRI differ (x-ray absorbing versus magnetic), the outcome is similar. Gadolinium-based contrast agents (GBCA) increase the conspicuity of diseased tissues. GBCA agents can lead to nephrogenic systemic fibrosis (NSF) in some patients who have renal dysfunction. Gadolinium should be used in these patients only when no viable alternatives exist, and then should be used in as low a dose as possible. Patients should be evaluated for diagnostic efficacy, relaxivity, rate of adverse reactions, dosing/concentration, and propensity to deposit in more sensitive organs such as the brain (ACR, 2017).

Contrast Complications

Contrast-Induced Nephrotoxicity. Contrast-induced nephrotoxicity (CIN) results from administering iodine contrast agents. The exact mechanism is not well understood. Serious complications are rare but require rapid appropriate treatment. CIN is a risk in patients with diminished renal function, even when this is not reflected in serum creatinine levels. Hydration is important for all patients, particularly those with renal dysfunction. IV normal saline is superior to all other hydration.

If the patient cannot tolerate oral hydration it is appropriate to infuse 0.9% sodium chloride at 100 to 200 mL/h as early as 24 hours before contrast and continue the infusion 24 hours after administering contrast. The glomerular filtration rate (GFR) is the rate the glomeruli filter impurities in the blood per unit of time, and it estimates renal function. Creatinine levels remain normal until the GFR decreases. Direct GFR measurement is not possible. The GFR is estimated (eGFR) using the modification of diet in renal disease (MDRD) formula (Box 29.5). The severity of CIN depends on the baseline renal function, dehydration status, and other risks. Patients may develop permanent renal failure, particularly in the setting of multiple risk factors. The current approach to prevent CIN is to limit volume and pretreat with *N*-acetylcysteine, perhaps in combination with sodium bicarbonate, and to avoid iodinated contrast when possible (ACR, 2017).

Iodine-Based Contrast Reactions. Determining the incidence of adverse effects after the administration of iodine-based contrast

BOX 29.5

Reference for Population Mean Estimated Glomerular Filtration Rates

The MDRD study equations are serum creatinine–based equations used to estimate GFR. In adults, the recommended equation for the eGFR from serum creatinine is the MDRD study equation and is reported in mg/dL.

$$\text{GFR (mL/min/1.73 m}^2) = 175 \times (S_{cr})^{-1.154} \times (\text{Age})^{-0.203}$$
$$\times (0.742 \text{ if female}) \times (1.212 \text{ if African American})(\text{conventional units})$$

Population Mean eGFRs

Age (Years)	Mean eGFR (mL/min/1.73 m²)
20–29	116
30–39	107
40–49	99
50–59	93
60–69	85
70+	75

eGFR, Estimated glomerular filtration rate; *GFR*, glomerular filtration rate; *MDRD*, modification of diet in renal disease.
Modified from National Institute of Diabetes and Digestive and Kidney Diseases: *Glomerular filtration rate (GFR) calculators* (website), 2015. www.niddk.nih.gov/health-information/health-communication-programs/nkdep/lab-evaluation/gfr-calculators/Pages/gfr-calculators.aspx. (Accessed 4 January 2017).

media is difficult because signs and symptoms are synonymous with local anesthetic administration, needle, sheath and catheter insertions, and anxiety. There are three categories of contrast reactions: mild, moderate, and severe (see Surgical Pharmacology, page 1135). Fortunately serious contrast reactions are rare. Severe reactions are life-threatening if not recognized and treated promptly. Although most serious reactions occur in the immediate postinjection period, delayed reactions can occur. Thorough documentation of all contrast reactions, as well as notification of the patient's primary care provider and referring physicians, is advisable. The nurse informs the patient of the reaction and emphasizes the importance in communicating his or her history of reaction and verbalizing contrast when asked about allergies. Pretreatment with steroids and diphenhydramine (Benadryl) is recommended for patients with known or suspected past reactions to contrast media; however, premedication does not guarantee against a reaction. All patients are observed for the possibility of a contrast reaction after injection, and the nurse should maintain IV access until there is reasonable certainty that there is none. If the nurse suspects a reaction, the contrast injection should be stopped and no additional fluids or medications administered in tubing containing residual contrast media. All personnel in the area should be knowledgeable about, and know their role in, treating reactions (ACR, 2017).

Gadolinium-Based Contrast Reactions. Gadolinium-based contrast media (GBCM) reactions are extremely well tolerated by the vast majority of patients in whom the media are injected. Acute adverse reactions are encountered with a lower frequency than is observed after administration of iodinated contrast media (ACR, 2017). The majority of contrast reactions are mild and include coldness at the injection site, nausea with or without vomiting, headache, warmth or pain at the injection site, paresthesias, dizziness, and itching. Reactions of this type manifest as a rash or urticaria and very rarely bronchospasm. The adverse event rate for GBCM administered at clinical doses (0.1–0.2 mmol/kg for most GBCM) ranges from 0.07% to 2.4% (ACR, 2017). Allergic-like reactions are uncommon and vary in frequency from 0.004% to 0.7%. The manifestations of an allergic-like reaction to a GBCM are similar to those of an allergic-like reaction to an iodinated contrast medium. Severe life-threatening anaphylactic reactions occur but are exceedingly rare (0.001%–0.01%) (ACR, 2017). GBCM administered to patients with acute kidney injury or severe chronic kidney disease can result in a syndrome of NSF. Gadolinium is radio dense and can be used at much higher doses than that of iodinated contrast media in CT and angiography, but it should still be used with caution when extrapolating the lack of nephrotoxicity. Treatment of moderate to severe acute gadolinium reaction is similar to that for reactions with iodinated contrast. NSF is a fibrosing disease primarily of the skin and subcutaneous tissues but also involves the lung, esophagus, heart, and skeletal muscles. Initial symptoms develop rapidly and include skin thickening and/or pruritus. The relative risk of NSF development after the use of GBCM is unknown. The incidence of NSF occurs in patients receiving high contrast doses, as well as in patients receiving higher cumulative lifetime doses, and in patients with chronic kidney disease, severe renal failure, and transient acute renal failure. The highest risk patients are those between the ages of 30 and 70, with chronic kidney disease level IV or V, or recently on dialysis (ACR, 2017). Treatment of acute adverse reactions to GBCM is similar to that for acute reactions to iodinated contrast media. In a facility in which contrast media is injected, it is imperative that personnel trained in recognizing and handling reactions and the equipment and medications to do so be on site or immediately available. Some facilities take the position that patients requiring treatment should be taken out of the imaging room immediately and away from the magnet so that none of the resuscitative equipment becomes a magnetic hazard (ACR, 2017).

Contrast Media Extravasation of Iodinated Contrast. Extravasation is contrast medium injection into or leakage into soft tissue. Tissue damage is a result of the toxicity of the agent or through pressure (e.g., compartment syndrome). The use of power injectors increases the risk for extravasation as do certain medical conditions such as circulatory problems of an extremity, history of radiation, or surgery. Infiltration risk increases with IV lines in place longer than 24 hours. To prevent extravasation, the nurse establishes a reliable peripheral injection site and assesses the site before injection. Commercial extravasation detector devices are available but are not a substitute for patient site assessment, observation, and communication. The nurse should instruct the patient to report any burning, stinging, swelling, or tight feeling occurring with the injection of the contrast agent. The American College of Radiology (ACR, 2017) recommends close follow-up for any extravasation because the initial evaluation may not reveal the extent of the problem. Treatment includes limb elevation and warm or cold compresses as per the physician. It may take up to 2 weeks for tissue damage, discoloration, blistering, and sloughing to occur after extravasation. Compartment syndrome is often identifiable within 24 hours. Symptoms include coolness in the extremity and continuing swelling after the initial extravasation. Loss of pulse is a medical emergency, requiring a fasciotomy.

Contrast Media Extravasation of Gadolinium-Based Contrast. Extravasation events to GBCM are rare, with one series demonstrating a rate of 0.05% (28,000 doses). Laboratory studies in animals have demonstrated that gadolinium is less toxic to the skin and subcutaneous tissues than equal volumes of iodinated contrast media. The small volumes typically injected for MR studies limit the chances of developing compartment syndrome. For these reasons, the likelihood of a significant injury resulting from extravasated MR contrast media is extremely low (ACR, 2017). All extravasation events and treatment should be documented in the medical record, and the referring physician should be notified.

Moderate Sedation and Analgesia

The amount and type of analgesia and sedation depend on patient and procedure factors. Moderate sedation and analgesia (conscious sedation) facilitate imaging acquisition during the procedure by decreasing patient movement and preventing motion artifact, distorted images, and repeat scans. In many cases the level of sedation must be appropriate to enable the patient to comprehend and perform specific breathing instructions and repositioning or tolerate a painful maneuver (e.g., dilation or catheter advancement). ACR-SIR (2015) practice parameters as well as the ASA practice parameters for analgesia and sedation state that emergency and monitoring equipment must be available to accommodate all ages and sizes of patients. Additional equipment includes oxygen delivery equipment with a backup oxygen supply, airway maintenance, intubation, emergency medications, defibrillators, and physiologic monitoring. Selection of only MRI-compatible monitoring and emergency equipment is mandatory in the MRI environment (ASA, 2015).

Universal Protocol

TJC's Universal Protocol, which includes preprocedure verification, site marking, and time-out, is used in the IR setting. All procedures involving an incision, percutaneous puncture, or insertion of an instrument require site marking. The individual performing the site marking is the physician or other credentialed/privileged clinician or a physician in training who is part of the team performing the procedure. In the event of a life-threatening emergency, the site may not be marked before patient transport; however, the radiology team must affirm the site before beginning the procedure. All clinicians present and the patient (when appropriate) perform final verification immediately before the procedure, using active, verbal participation. The team verbally verifies patient identity, the procedure to be performed, and the site of the procedure (noting the current position of the patient). The team member responsible for documenting the final verification must verbally verify that all relevant information such as study reports, x-ray images, and any special equipment needed are present in the room before starting the procedure. Procedures involving laterality, multiple structures (fingers, toes, and lesions), or multiple levels (spine) should be identified by physicians' initials. In addition to preprocedure skin marking of the general spinal region, specific intraprocedural radiographic techniques are used for marking the exact vertebral level. Other procedures requiring site marking include biopsies (where there is more than one organ or laterality is involved), chest tube placement, thoracentesis, discogram, joint injection, vertebroplasty, extremity procedures specific to that extremity (angiogram, angioplasty, or thrombolysis), and percutaneous nephrostomy (PCN) tube placement. Exemptions to site marking may include cardiac catheterization and interventional cases for which the catheter insertion site is not predetermined (access site is determined using intraprocedural imaging to identify the lesion). For these procedures in which site marking is not required, the other requirements for preventing wrong-site, wrong-procedure, and wrong-person surgery still apply (ARIN, 2014a).

Documentation

The nurse documents patient identification, allergy assessment, surgical procedure verification, and any other intervention performed. A brief mental status and neurologic assessment is important for patients with neurologic conditions or those at high risk for stroke. Documentation should include the integrity of the patient's skin, presence or absence of peripheral pulses, positioning, use of positioning devices, fluid intake, output measurements, contrast usage, and the achievement of patient goals. If moderate sedation and analgesia is administered, then the nurse documents the patient's level of consciousness, anxiety and pain levels, and incremental doses of sedative medication. The nurse ensures all medications, medication containers, and other solutions on and off the sterile field in perioperative and other procedural settings are labeled (TJC, 2017). The labels should be verified by two qualified individuals if the person preparing the medication is not administering it. The nurse is responsible for documenting the type, size, serial number, and lot number of implantable devices according to institutional policy. The nursing report should include information about the procedure; all procedure-specific instructions; and information about possible equipment, device, and catheter care.

Radiation Dose Documentation. After each procedure, the measured or estimated radiation dose should be reviewed. Patient follow-up may be required if the patient received a radiation skin dose of 2 Gy or more. A postskin assessment at 30 days may be performed. If technically possible, all radiation dose data provided by the fluoroscopy unit or CT scanner should be transferred and archived with the images from the procedure. This is usually an automatic electric data transfer from the fluoroscopy unit or CT scanner to the PACS done by the technologist or physician on study completion. Archiving of radiation dose data is of particular importance if repeat procedures are probable or the patient received a clinically significant radiation dose. The use of PACS to record doses has several drawbacks. PACS are typically radiology department specific and do not interface with the facility's electronic medical record (EMR). In some institutions the cardiac catheterization lab, EP lab, hybrid OR, special procedures, and IR each have their own PACS, with no interdepartmental access. System configurations such as this do not offer insight into a patient's total exposure across hospital departments. Other forms of documentation include the radiology technician manually recording radiation doses into log books or the nurse documenting in the patient's medical record the dose information provided by the physician or RT. Exposure time, type of procedure area exposed, and safety precautions should also be recorded. Radiation dose monitoring, auditing, and reporting should be a component of the facility's quality assurance and quality improvement processes along with periodic reviews of protocols for radiation dose optimization. A process should also be in place to notify patients receiving significant radiation doses and a mechanism for patient follow-up of potential adverse effects (McEnery, 2015).

Evaluation

During the evaluation phase of care the nurse determines whether the outcomes established for the patient were met and revises outcomes and interventions accordingly. The evaluation period provides opportunities to improve nursing interventions through careful reflection and analysis of outcomes. The following are possible evaluation statements relating to the Sample Plan of Care (see page 1131):

- The patient verbalized an acceptable level of pain as defined with a 1 to 10 pain scale.
- The patient demonstrated a decreased level of anxiety, verbalized less apprehension, maintained eye contact, and was able to comply with requests even though anxiety persisted.

- The patient verbalized understanding of the procedure and described the actions to take after discharge.
- The patient's airway was maintained and oxygen saturation was within preprocedure baseline limits.
- The patient's vital signs were within acceptable limits, peripheral pulses returned to baseline, and there was no evidence of excessive bleeding.
- The patient's skin was intact with no reddened areas or lesions.

Postprocedural Care

Postprocedural nursing care involves ensuring hemostasis of the puncture site through patient discharge. After the procedure the nurse monitors vital signs and assesses the puncture site and distal pulses with the patient remaining flat as per institutional protocol. The catheter or sheath removal time, closure method, and catheter size are documented. Time to ambulation and elevation of the head of bed (HOB) depends on the procedure, whether it is diagnostic or interventional, if there is vascular access, if it is arterial or venous, and location of the puncture site. If the femoral artery was accessed, the nurse checks the groin site frequently for evidence of bleeding or hematoma. Hemostasis methods include manual pressure, compression devices, vascular suturing, or collagen plug devices according to procedure and physician preference. Compression should be firm but should not obliterate the distal pulses. The nurse monitors the appropriate distal pulse based on the access vessel (e.g., radial or femoral artery). If brachial access was used for the procedure, blood pressure measurement is not undertaken in the affected arm. The nurse observes the affected limb for changes in color, temperature, pain, and prepulse and postpulse quality to detect acute arterial occlusion. Pseudoaneurysm formation, nerve damage, and infection are complications from arterial punctures. The nurse monitors neurologic function in patients undergoing head and neck arteriography. Observation is increased to 6 hours in patients with hypertension, or those with a hematoma postprocedure. The nurse encourages patients receiving contrast to drink large amounts of clear liquids and/or increases the administration rate of IV fluids. Contrast agents act as an osmotic diuretic, thus, additional fluid counteracts dehydration as well as prevents contrast-induced nephropathy. Patients receiving contrast or experiencing contrast-related complications must receive appropriate discharge instructions and follow-up directions. Patient recovery and monitoring are in accordance with the amount of sedation and analgesia received, pain level, and vital signs. The type of interventional procedure performed determines additional monitoring criteria, including distal pulses for angiography; neurologic, motor, and sensory signs of the lower extremities after vertebroplasty; urine output after nephrostomy; and bleeding postbiopsy.

Patient, Family, and Caregiver Education and Discharge Planning

Patient, family, and caregiver education includes providing basic information about the procedure, table, room, and staff members and the identification and procedure verification process when appropriate. The nurse discusses the use of sedation (if planned for the procedure) and informs the patient of the need to remain still to avoid motion artifact resulting in the need to repeat the study. Included in the discussion is information about the procedure process and requirements for cooperation (e.g., breath holds, positioning, contrast administration, and staff activities). The nurse explains, during CT and MRI procedures, that staff members will exit the room during scanning, and voice communication with the patient

PATIENT, FAMILY, AND CAREGIVER EDUCATION

Discharge Instructions for Contrast Media Injection

Acute contrast media reactions remain rare, but can range in severity from mild discomfort to life-threatening anaphylaxis. The patient should call his or her physician if symptoms such as hives, rash, itching, or irritation in the region that was imaged occur. Medications may be provided such as diphenhydramine 25 to 50 mg PO (Benadryl). Diazepam 5 to 10 mg PO can be prescribed for anxiety, and anaphylaxis can be treated with epinephrine 0.01 mg/kg subcutaneous. Mild bronchospasm may require inhaled albuterol, or if severe, hydrocortisone 100 mg IV and epinephrine 0.05 to 0.1 mg subcutaneous may be administered. Severe reactions are life-threatening and include convulsions, unconsciousness, laryngeal edema, severe bronchospasm, pulmonary edema, severe cardiac arrhythmias, and cardiovascular collapse. Treatment of these life-threatening reactions is urgent. The airway must be secured, and oxygen, mechanical ventilation, external cardiac massage, and electrical cardiac defibrillation must be administered as required. Patients should inform their healthcare providers about allergies before any other procedures are performed, and obtain and wear a Medic Alert bracelet, in addition to carrying an identification card describing the allergy (Rathmell, 2014).

Before discharge:
- Provide the patient and the caregiver with verbal and written instructions.
- Discuss drain care instructions if applicable and remind the patient to schedule a follow-up appointment with the physician.
- Review medications and pain prevention.
- Provide the patient, family, and caregiver with the name and telephone number of the physician, nurse, or interventional radiology department to call if questions arise.
- Instruct the patient to notify the physician if any observable skin effects occur.
- Review the physician's explanation of postdischarge care and evaluate the patient's response to the instructions provided.

PO, By mouth.
From Rathmell J: Radiation safety and the use of radiographic contrast agents in pain medicine. In Benzon H, editor: *Practical management of pain*, ed 5, Philadelphia, 2014, Elsevier.

AMBULATORY SURGERY CONSIDERATIONS

Discharge Criteria

The following criteria should be met before patients are discharged after ambulatory surgery interventional radiologic procedures:
- Patient has stable vital signs (resembling baseline vital signs), including SpO_2 level.
- Patient shows no evidence of respiratory depression.
- Patient is oriented per baseline to person, place, and time.
- Patient can take fluids, if appropriate, without nausea.
- Patient can void, if a procedure-specific criterion.
- Patient can ambulate with or without assistance as appropriate and has no dizziness.
- Pain has been addressed and/or managed.
- Bleeding is not present; drainage is per procedure expectation.
- Written discharge instructions including medication reconciliation with phone number to call have been given to patient (patients are informed about how to obtain necessary supplies, if applicable).
- A responsible person is available to escort patient to home or stay with patient.

with the patient (or responsible caregiver) and provides supplies and written prescriptions if needed. The patient is provided with the physician's name and emergency contact numbers for problems or questions for 24 hours postprocedure.

Discharge instruction forms should be procedure specific and include activity restrictions, possible complications and when and whom to call for help, diet, medications, specific care related to the procedure, driving restrictions, signs of infection, and follow-up care plan and appointment. Patients with arterial punctures receive precise instructions in case of hemorrhage or other puncture site complication. Patient, family, and caregiver teaching with return demonstrations for procedures such as tube care, drainage bags, tube-catheter flushing, and sterile technique is essential.

The decision to admit a patient after an ambulatory surgery procedure is at the discretion of the physician. Indications include the following:
- Complication resulting from the procedure including any significant change in pulse in the affected extremity, neurologic changes, persistent bleeding, or persistent nausea and vomiting postprocedure.
- Significant findings on the diagnostic examination warranting further therapy requiring an inpatient admission.

Procedures

Interventional Access With the Seldinger Technique

The Seldinger technique changed IR because it provided a less invasive and safer means of access to vessels. Most IR procedures are initiated with the Seldinger technique (see Fig. 29.10). After sterile preparation and draping, the physician administers a local anesthetic over the intended entry site, usually the groin, for an angiogram that uses the retrograde femoral artery approach. A needle (Seldinger 18-gauge, 2¾ inch or other) with a stylet is used to gain vascular access, and then the stylet is removed. A pulsatile backflow of blood will be noted with arterial access. The physician passes a guidewire several

will be maintained via intercom. Additional information that is reviewed includes anticipated recovery time, discharge criteria, postprocedure care, and follow-up instructions (Patient, Family, and Caregiver Education).

Discharge assessments should be in accordance with facility policy. For inpatients, appropriate discharge criteria include stable cardiovascular and airway status; stable vital signs; and no evidence of bleeding, drainage, or hematoma at the puncture site. On stabilization, inpatients are transferred to the designated location per institutional policy. Neurointerventional procedure patients may go to intensive care. The IR nurse provides written documentation and verbal report to the receiving unit as well as notifies them of special patient needs, equipment, supplies, level of care, and expected time of transfer.

The nurse reviews postprocedure instructions with the patient, family, and caregiver if teaching is appropriate. A discharge criterion for ambulatory surgery patients is according to assessment criteria as per the facility's policy and procedure (Ambulatory Surgery Considerations). The physician or nurse reviews discharge instructions

centimeters into the needle, then removes the needle while compressing the puncture site and leaving the guidewire in place. A small incision is made, and the surgeon places an introducer with a dilator over the guidewire. The guidewire and dilator are removed and an introducer sheath is used to advance the catheter. Puncture location is crucial. High arterial punctures above the inguinal ligament may result in bleeding, whereas low arterial punctures may yield pseudoaneurysm. Fluoroscopy over the femoral head helps confirm access. Ultrasound facilitates vessel access in patients with altered anatomy, obesity, or scarring caused by previous vascular surgeries, multiple catheterizations, and previous insertion of intra-aortic balloon pumps. Femoral access alternatives include brachial or axillary artery punctures. Translumbar punctures are rare. The nurse documents the presence and quality of the distal extremity pulse before the procedure. Potential complications of arterial puncture and catheterization include hemorrhage, distal embolization, and pseudoaneurysm development. Complications of femoral venous puncture–catheterization include puncture-site infection, phlebitis, and hematoma.

Diagnostic Procedures

Angiography

Angiography uses fluoroscopy and contrast to image anatomic and pathologic changes in vascular anatomy. Angiography determines occlusive disease, aneurysms, AVM, and AV fistulae, as well as localizes small vascular tumors. Angiography may be performed as a single procedure or may precede an intervention. Classification of angiography is either coronary or noncoronary. Only interventional cardiologists perform PCI. Noncoronary angiography procedures include peripherally inserted central catheters (PICCs), vascular access procedures, organ-based therapies using fluoroscopic guidance for biopsies, tumor ablations, and various embolizations. Angiography and interventions on the cerebral vessels remain exclusive to the neurointerventionalist and usually use a biplane system.

Preoperative screening for angiography patients includes coagulation status, contrast allergies, metformin use, existing renal dysfunction or failure, anemia, and diabetes. Generally all patients are NPO except for extra fluids for hydration and renal dysfunction prevention subsequent to contrast. To avoid accidental contamination during the procedure, the nurse secures the patient's arms at the sides using wristbands or armboards. Good image quality requires a motionless field; thus a variety of soft restraints and bands ensure minimal patient movement. The nurse performs baseline assessment of the appropriate pulse site including axillary, brachial, radial, femoral, popliteal, and dorsalis pedis before needle entry. Arterial access sites include the femoral artery, as well as brachial, radial or axillary, translumbar, and subclavian. Venous access routes include brachial, femoral, internal jugular, and subclavian. Contrast injection occurs after the catheter is in the target vessel for catheter navigation. With an arterial puncture the injector system, tubings, and catheters must be free of air bubbles. Patients may feel a transient warmth or hot sensation in the injection area, or the sensation of incontinence with catheters positioned in vessels near or in the lower abdomen or pelvis.

Biopsy

Imaging used for biopsies include fluoroscopy, ultrasound, CT, and MRI. Modality selection is per the physician, site, and results of prior imaging studies. Specimens undergo preparation and handling according to established policy and procedures. After administering a local anesthetic the physician makes a small puncture with a scalpel to aid the passage of the needle followed by imaging to check for placement. Biopsy needle selection depends on the lesion location, size, and depth; the suspected diagnosis; the access route; and the amount of tissue required for study. Biopsies involving a specific area or small lesion are more labor intensive than random tissue sampling. Complications vary depending on the biopsy site.

Chest Biopsy

Thorax needle biopsies rule out suspicion of malignancy; evaluate nodules, lesions, and masses; obtain tissue staging samples; and determine localized infections. Patient positioning depends on the location of the lesion and the path the physician uses to reach it. Modality selection is CT, fluoroscopy, or ultrasound based on the biopsy site and lesion size. Access is via the Seldinger technique. Adequate anesthesia levels are essential to minimize discomfort and chest wall motion. Common complications include pneumothorax confirmed by CT or x-ray and minor bleeding resulting in hemoptysis. Patients must abstain from strenuous exercise for several days and go to the emergency department if dyspnea develops.

Liver Biopsy

Transcutaneous liver biopsies diagnose tumors and determine etiology. Some physicians perform liver biopsies at the bedside, but an increasing number use ultrasound or CT for image guidance. Indications for liver biopsy are patients with massive ascites and coagulopathies. Access is by the jugular vein using angiography. Bleeding is a common complication subsequent to the impaired clotting mechanisms in liver disease. Serious bleeding or bile leaks are complications causing acute abdomen, hypovolemia, and sepsis.

Kidney Biopsy

Kidney biopsies determine disease and rejection status in transplant patients as well as adrenal gland tumors. The physician isolates the tumor by CT scan or ultrasound guidance and obtains a sample for analysis. Caution is advised with adrenal biopsies because of the possibility of a pheochromocytoma. This tumor secretes adrenaline and other catecholamines resulting in paroxysms of hypertension, tachycardia, headache, nausea, and diaphoresis. Bleeding is the most common complication subsequent to the long sampling needles.

Therapeutic Interventions

Percutaneous Transluminal Angioplasty

Angioplasty is a nonsurgical means to open atherosclerotic vessels using fluoroscopy guidance to inflate a balloon-tipped catheter compressing atherosclerotic plaque. Peripheral angioplasty refers to vessels outside the coronary and cerebral vasculature, most notably the aortoiliac, infrapopliteal, superior femoral artery, and other lower extremity vessels. Indications for peripheral angioplasty include lifestyle-limiting claudication, chronic leg ischemia, restenosis of a previous graft anastomoses, treatment prebypass or postbypass surgery, tissue ulceration, and necrosis. Evolving technology for peripheral vascular procedures may also use endovascular robotic technology (Robotic-Assisted Surgery). After establishing vessel access, the patient receives heparin to achieve the desired anticoagulation status. The surgeon advances the appropriate guidewire across the stenosis or occlusion and positions the balloon catheter in the affected area using radiopaque markers and fluoroscopy. The balloon is inflated with a mixture of sterile saline and contrast medium to a specific atmosphere of pressure. Dilation may require several inflations. A postprocedure angiogram is performed to assess the technical success of the procedure and vessel patency. Complications are rare and include vessel trauma, hematoma, thrombosis, and vessel reocclusion.

ROBOTIC-ASSISTED SURGERY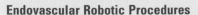

Endovascular Robotic Procedures

The remotely controlled robotic system used in ORs is comprised of a console and computer, which allows surgeons to control a bedside surgical cart consisting of robotic arms to perform a procedure remotely. Robotic surgery provides physicians with a remote system allowing increased control, precision, dexterity, and range of motion. Endovascular robotic procedures are in the early stages of development and will provide the physician with remote catheter control in EP procedures in the cardiovascular system. Robotically steerable catheter systems have been designed for use in peripheral blood vessels. The Magellan system is a CE-marked and FDA-approved robotically steerable endovascular catheter system for use in the peripheral vasculature. The concept of this robotic technology is built on the potential ability to drive a wire and catheter directly into the vessel, providing 360-degree control of the catheter tip. The physician is able to remotely control a catheter under live fluoroscopic imaging. The catheter and guidewire move immediately, but slowly, in response to the physician's commands. The catheters are designed to provide control at the catheter tip, in addition to the ability to deflect the tip in all configurations. A significant disadvantage of robotic endovascular procedures is the cost, in addition to the location of the remote physician's inability to monitor the patient. Therefore patients undergoing robotic-guided procedures may require increased monitoring by the nursing team members to assess vital signs and adequacy of sedation. The robotic system is also limited to selection of the target vessel. Delivery of medications/embolic materials, contrast injection, and insertion of therapeutic devices (e.g., balloons, stents, etc.) must be done manually. The advantages of robotic guided procedures provide the physician beneficial ergonomic positioning, without having to stand during a procedure while wearing a lead apron. The physician will also benefit from low radiation exposure because of the distance from the console to procedure bed. Endovascular robotic procedures with robotically steerable catheters continue to evolve to provide patients with safe and high-quality outcomes.

CE, Conformite Europeenc; *FDA,* US Food and Drug Administration.
Modified from Rao S: Endovascular robotic catheters: an emerging transformative technology in the interventional radiology suite, *J Radiol Nurs* 35(3):211–217, 2016.

Peripheral Vascular Stents

Stents are common adjuncts to angioplasty, acting as a mechanical scaffold to maintain vessel patency. Vascular stents come in various sizes, lengths, and materials and include a variety of coatings as well as drug-eluting capabilities. After angioplasty the physician directs the stent to the desired location using an introducer catheter with radiopaque markers under fluoroscopy and then deploys the stent. Contraindications include patients with bleeding disorders, patients not able to take anticoagulants, circumstances in which stent placement would exacerbate arterial leakage, and when stenoses prohibit the passage of the delivery catheter. Complications include hematoma formation, thrombosis, pseudoaneurysm formation, and stent migration.

Dialysis and Fistula Graft Repair

Long-term dialysis requires a surgical AV shunt, composed of native vessels or synthetic grafts or a combination of both, bridging an artery and vein. Problems inherent to maintaining vascular access include poor flow, increased resistance during dialysis, prolonged bleeding, arm swelling, and collateral vein development. Restoring patency by percutaneous transluminal angiography (PTA) is possible through the graft itself or via arm or femoral venous access. Strictures at venous anastomoses may be particularly severe, warranting prolonged inflation with high-pressure balloons and higher doses of IV analgesics and sedatives. Other options to restore patency include mechanical thrombectomy devices to aspirate blood clots, or injection of thrombolytic agents such as recombinant tissue plasminogen activator (rt-PA) to lyse, or dissolve, the clot. Complications include vein rupture, bleeding subsequent to thrombolysis, and pulmonary artery or arterial embolization.

Peripherally Inserted Central Catheters

A PICC is a long, thin venous access device inserted into the brachial or cephalic vein, terminating in the superior vena cava or right atrium. PICC lines provide long-term therapies such as antibiotic and narcotic administration and total parenteral nutrition (TPN). Physicians, physician assistants, radiology assistants, nurse practitioners, or specially trained RNs and RTs may insert PICC lines. PICC placement is a sterile procedure but can be done at the bedside. After placement, the position of the catheter tip is confirmed using fluoroscopy or chest x-ray. Patients receive instruction on how to care for the PICC line, including flushing the line, when to change the dressing, and when to shower. Patients must inspect the site daily for any irregularities such as swelling, redness, leakage, or pain and report them to a healthcare professional immediately.

Drainage Procedures

The development of cross-sectional imaging enables drainage of deep body cavities without open surgery. Image guidance for abdominal, pelvic, or other soft tissue fluid collections and abscesses use CT, ultrasound, or fluoroscopy. Indications include diagnostic fluid evaluation, treatment of abscess or sepsis, and palliation of symptoms for patients with tense ascites resulting in dyspnea, pain, or compromised renal function. Visceral collections include treatment for abscess and cysts of the liver, spleen, and pancreas. Depending on the drainage site, the approach can be subphrenic, transgluteal, transrectal, or transvaginal. A preliminary CT determines the optimal path for catheter placement. For therapeutic drainage two techniques are used, depending on the size of the collection, location, physician preference, and imaging modality. For large superficial drainage a trocar technique in conjunction with CT or ultrasound imaging is used. Small collections remotely situated or with limited access use the Seldinger technique. Catheter size and configuration selection depend on the site and fluid drained. Imaging is performed immediately before catheter removal to document emptying of the cavity, and then the catheter is withdrawn and the site covered with a dry, sterile dressing. Drainage catheters left in place must be safely secured and dressed by the nurse or IR technologist. Physician orders specify catheter care and measurement and emptying of the drainage chambers. Patients discharged with the catheter in place receive instructions on catheter care and an appointment for catheter removal.

Percutaneous Transhepatic Cholangiography

Percutaneous transhepatic cholangiography (PTC) visualizes drainage of the biliary system and accesses the biliary tree in cases in which endoscopic retrograde cholangiopancreatography (ERCP) is unsuccessful. PTC is characteristically palliative for patients with nonresectable malignant disease, although percutaneous treatment of biliary stone disease with or without choledochoscopy occurs in selected cases. Other applications include cholangioplasty for biliary strictures, biopsy of the biliary duct, and management of complications from laparoscopic cholecystectomy and liver transplantation. Contraindications include diffuse hepatic metastasis, liver failure, or a shortened life expectancy. After the initial workup, ultrasonography, MRI, or CT is done to determine the etiology of the obstruction. Patients receive prophylactic antibiotics 24 hours before a PTC. The patient is positioned supine, prepped, draped, and administered a local anesthetic. The physician selects the level to insert the needle between adjacent ribs, avoiding the lung. A 21-gauge or 22-gauge needle is guided along into the liver under fluoroscopy, with the exact position determined by contrast injection. PTC is more invasive and painful than ERCP, warranting additional doses of sedatives and opioids before the liver capsule is punctured. The physician exchanges various wires and introducers under fluoroscopy until the proper drainage catheter is in place. Bile may be sent to the laboratory for culture and sensitivity. Drainage may be external or internal. The bile drains into the duodenum and an external bag, or internally via stent placement in the small intestine. Initial drainage can be external until the bile is clear and debris free; it is then capped for internal drainage only. Catheters are changed every 4 to 6 weeks in an ambulatory setting, and oral antibiotics are given before catheter changes. Complications include sepsis, peritonitis, hemorrhage, and pneumothorax when using a right-sided approach.

Uterine Fibroid Embolization and Adenomyosis

Uterine fibroid embolization (UFE) treats uterine leiomyomata, adenomyosis, or fibroids by blocking perfusion to the benign tumors, resulting in degeneration, scar tissue formation, and fibroid shrinkage. This procedure appeals to many women because of its minimally invasive nature, ambulatory setting, and rapid recovery and return to work. A complete blood count, electrolytes, and pregnancy test are obtained before the procedure. Moderate sedation and local anesthesia or epidural anesthesia may be used. The radiologist performs arteriography of the pelvic vasculature under fluoroscopy to determine uterine artery blood flow and then embolizes the uterine arteries by injecting the agent through the catheter until proximal arterial flow or reflux of contrast material no longer occurs. Collateral circulation maintains the blood supply to the myometrium. Pain is moderate to severe depending on the degree of occlusion. Some institutions add pretreatment with steroids as well as the use of an epidural and intraoperative ketorolac or ketorolac tromethamine administration. Patient-controlled anesthesia with IV narcotics is standard in the immediate postoperative phase, transitioning to oral medications before discharge. Procedure success is according to patient symptomatology before and after the procedure, 6 weeks, and 6 months at gynecologic follow-up (Patient Engagement Exemplar). Fibroid embolization usually requires a hospital stay of one night. Analgesic medications and drugs that control swelling typically are prescribed after the procedure to treat cramping and pain. The most commonly reported complications of UFE are permanent amenorrhea and prolonged vaginal discharge. Less commonly reported complications include delayed expulsion of leiomyoma tissue, prolonged or poorly controlled pain, infection (pyomyoma, endometritis, or tuboovarian abscess), urinary tract infection or urinary retention, and vessel or nerve injury at the access site. Many women resume light activities in a few days, and the majority of women are able to return to normal activities within 7 to 10 days. In most instances, reduction in uterine and leiomyoma volumes becomes noticeable several weeks after embolization and continues for 3 to 12 months (Dariushnia et al., 2014).

PATIENT ENGAGEMENT EXEMPLAR

It's the Little Things

Mrs. G is a 38-year-old patient diagnosed with symptomatic uterine fibroids and is considering uterine fibroid embolization. She has the following questions:

- Am I a candidate for this treatment?
- Will it be successful?
- What are my options?
- What does this procedure entail?
- What will my recovery be like?
- What is the success rate for this procedure?
- What are the risks involved with this procedure?
- Can I get pregnant after this procedure?

Her physician does an excellent job answering her questions, and she understands her condition and has watched a video provided by her physician, which gave her extensive education about the procedure and decides to proceed. When Mrs. G is admitted to the Interventional Radiology suite she is greeted by her perioperative nurse, who asks her, "Can you tell me what problem you are being treated for with this procedure? Mrs. G states that she had fibroid tumors in her uterus that were causing her heavy bleeding and pain. Mrs. G clearly understands her procedure when she states that she knows that a catheter will be put in her groin and particles would be injected through it to block blood flow to the fibroid causing it to shrink. The perioperative nurse asks her, "What do you expect to happen after your procedure?" Mrs. G responds that she knows she may have some pain and there is a chance she would need to spend the night at the hospital. She goes on to say that she knows she will need to lie flat for 6 hours after the procedure to prevent bleeding from the puncture site. She states that she will be glad to see a resolution to her symptoms. The procedure is completed as planned without complications. A few weeks after her procedure the perioperative nurse receives the patient satisfaction survey form given to Mrs. G after surgery and was surprised to discover that, although Mrs. G thought she received great care during the procedure, she had been cold and no one offered her a warm blanket. Patient needs are of the utmost importance, and it is important to identify what is important to them. Patients can be extensively educated and know what to expect, but sometimes the only thing that is important to them is a warm blanket, and the only way to identify what is important to patients is to remember to ask.

Modified from Women's Health: *Uterine fibroids* (website), 2017. www.womenshealth.gov/a-z-topics/uterine-fibroids. (Accessed 7 January 2017).

Embolization for Obstetric Hemorrhage

Potential life-threatening hemorrhagic conditions amenable to embolization include abdominal and cervical pregnancy, placenta previa, and placenta accreta. Postpartum hemorrhage (PPH) remains a common health problem and is the main cause of pregnancy-related maternal death worldwide. Uterine embolization has a role in the treatment of PPH, and once a PPH diagnosis has been acknowledged, prompt management should be initiated. Uterine artery embolization (UAE) is an alternative treatment because the uterus and patient fertility can be preserved. The technique is similar to UFE: bilateral catheterization of the internal iliacs and uterine arteries is performed in a sequential manner. Multiple embolic materials can be used. Gelatin pledgets are the most commonly used agent because of their availability and distal embolization and temporary occlusion effect (Sentilhes et al., 2016).

Transjugular Intrahepatic Portosystemic Shunt

TIPS is a nonoperative therapeutic option for management of variceal bleeding from portal hypertension. Mostly commonly seen in patients with cirrhosis, these vessels enlarge, become tortuous, and bleed because of pressure buildup. A percutaneous stent is placed to dilate a tract between the hepatic and portal vein. The stent creates a shunt, lowering the portal vein pressure. All patients undergoing TIPS receive prophylactic broad-spectrum antibiotics. The physician confirms portal vein patency preoperatively by ultrasound and assesses coagulation profiles. Vascular access is through the internal jugular vein using ultrasound guidance. A guidewire is placed into the right atrium followed by a sheath for pressure recording. The physician then places a catheter into the hepatic vein under fluoroscopy. A balloon forming a shunt from the portal vein to the hepatic vein creates a dilated tract. Stent deployment occurs using angiographic verification to assess stent position. Repeated serial dilation of the stent occurs until pressures are satisfactory, followed by catheter removal. Major complications include hemorrhage and bile duct trauma. Other complications include hepatic encephalopathy, recurrent portal hypertension, and shunt thrombosis or stenosis.

Balloon-Occluded Retrograde Transvenous Obliteration

Gastric variceal (GV) bleeding is a major complication of portal hypertension and is associated with high morbidity and mortality. Balloon-occluded retrograde transvenous obliteration (BRTO) is a safe and effective interventional procedure for treating GV and reducing the risk of rebleeding by obliterating the gastric varix using direct sclerotherapy (Research Highlight). The clinical indications for BRTO are impending, prior, or active GV bleeding and GV with hepatic encephalopathy refractory to medical management. Although esophageal varices are more common, gastric varices are often more challenging to treat. It is imperative to conduct preprocedural CT imaging to document the presence of a portosystemic shunt and assess the patency of the portal vein. BRTO involves occlusion of the portosystemic outflow veins with a balloon catheter, followed by injection of a sclerosing agent into the varix. The venous access site is the common femoral vein or internal jugular vein. The occlusion balloon is kept in place for hours to ensure that there is sufficient dwelling of the sclerosing material within the varix and to minimize complications caused by reflux into systemic or portal vessels. The sclerosant results in thrombosis of the GV and draining portosystemic shunt, which marks the endpoint of the procedure.

Relative contraindications include severe coagulopathy (often associated with liver failure), splenic vein thrombosis, portal vein thrombosis, and uncontrolled esophageal varices. Technical failure may result if balloon rupture occurs early (before thrombosis and complete sclerosis is achieved); therefore a C-arm (cone-beam) CT is performed with the occlusion balloon inflated to outline the varices with trapped contrast confirming filling of the GV with the sclerosing agent. With the occlusion balloon left in place, the patient is transferred to the postprocedure unit and monitored during the sclerosant dwell time. Repeat fluoroscopy and C-arm CT is preformed 6 hours later. One of the greatest advantages of BRTO over TIPS is that it improves hepatic blood flow and liver function, improving hepatic encephalopathy. However, BRTO also increases the risk of new-onset or worsening esophageal variceal bleeding by closing the portal outflow shunt, altering local hemodynamics and collateral flow. Therefore patients should be closely monitored with upper endoscopy post-BRTO for detection and management of esophageal varices. Increased portal pressure may also increase the risk of ascites and pleural effusion in some cases. Complications

| RESEARCH HIGHLIGHT |

Prediction for Improvement of Liver Function After Balloon-Occluded Retrograde Transvenous Obliteration for Gastric Varices to Manage Portosystemic Shunt Syndrome

BRTO is an endovascular procedure developed for the treatment of GV. Recent reports have demonstrated improvement in liver function in some patients after BRTO for GV, but predictive factors for improved liver function were unknown. TE (with resulting liver stiffness measurement) is used worldwide in fibrosis testing and predicting the risk of death or hepatic complications in patients with chronic liver disease. This retrospective analysis investigated the predictive value of TE to identify patients who would experience improved liver function after BRTO.

PSS results in the gradual worsening of hepatic function, which may end in hepatic failure. To prevent progression, endovascular treatments such as BRTO may be considered to obliterate the portosystemic shunt. Because BRTO may potentially worsen portal hypertension, factors predictive of improved liver function after BRTO would be of value in the management of PSS.

Retrospective analysis was performed on 50 consecutive patients who had undergone TE before BRTO and who were followed for greater than 3 months after the procedure. Liver function studies were compared before and 3 months after BRTO. The correlation between change in liver function (total bilirubin, album, and prothrombin time) and baseline liver function values and LMS was evaluated. Liver stiffness was expressed in kilopascals (kPa), with LSM <6 kPa considered normal. Liver function was more improved in patients whose LSM was ≤22.9 kPa.

In conclusion, the study showed that LMS as obtained by TE, which is a rapid and noninvasive technique, was useful in predicting which patients would experience improved liver function after BRTO. The cutoff value for improvement was ≥22.9 kPa, with a sensitivity and specificity value of 78.4% and 69.2%, respectively.

BRTO, Balloon-occluded retrograde transvenous obliteration; *GV,* gastric varices; *LMS,* liver stiffness measurement; *PSS,* portosystemic shunt syndrome; *TE,* transient elastography. Modified from Yamamoto A et al: Prediction for improvement of liver function after balloon-occluded retrograde transvenous obliteration for gastric varices to manage portosystemic shunt syndrome, *J Vasc Interv Radiol* 27(8):1160–1167, 2016.

post-BRTO include fever; epigastric, chest, and/or back pain; transient systemic hypertension, pleural effusion, and hemoglobinuria (Basseri and Lightfoot, 2016).

Image-Guided Tumor Ablation

The term *tumor ablation* is defined as the direct application of chemical ablation (nonenergy ablation) or energy-based ablation (thermal and nonthermal ablation) therapies to eradicate or substantially destroy focal tumors. Most therapies can be performed using a host of imaging modalities such as ultrasonography, CT, MRI, positron emission tomography (PET), and fluoroscopy. However, virtually all available ablation techniques can be used with more than one image-guiding modality. Chemical ablation therapies are chemical agent(s) such as ethanol or acetic acid. Energy-based ablation includes modalities that destroy a tumor either through thermal (heat or cold) or nonthermal mechanisms. RFA ablation is a device using monopolar energy with a single "active" or "interstitial" electrode, with current dissipated at one or more return dispersive pads. High-intensity focused ultrasound allows more than one "focused" ultrasound beam to create an ablation. Laser ablation uses light energy; laser energy is applied with fibers directly inserted into the tissue. Cryoablation is used to destroy tissue by the application of freezing temperatures, or alternating freezing and thawing, or slight heating. Rapid tissue freezing and thawing produce the greatest cytotoxic effects by disrupting cellular membranes and inducing cell death. In the neck, chest, abdomen/pelvis, and extremities, cryoablation is generally performed using one or more closed cryoprobe(s) that are placed in close proximity to, or inside of, the target tumor. The most common clinically available cryoablation systems use the Joule–Thomson effect, which relies on the expansion of a cryogen (argon gas or liquid nitrogen) at the cryoprobe tip to cause internal temperature fluctuation. Cell death is the end result of the repeated application of short-duration high-voltage electrical pulses that create "irreversible" injuries to cellular membranes (Ahmed et al., 2014).

Intraoperative Magnetic Resonance Imaging

The advantages of an intraoperative MRI (iMRI) suite are especially evident for delicate intracranial neurosurgical procedures because the neurosurgeon receives timely feedback about progress or confirmation of completeness of tumor resections (Lebak et al., 2015). Using iMRI during neurosurgery gives neurosurgeons the most accurate information, which is important because it can be difficult to distinguish the edges of a brain tumor and separate normal tissue from abnormal tissue (Mayo Clinic, 2016). The iMRI configuration is a ceiling-mounted MRI scanner housed in a diagnostic room adjacent to a standard OR separated by a locked sliding door. In these procedures a standard craniotomy and tumor resection occurs in the OR. After the resection, preparation of the room and patient for the MRI scan begins. On completed preparation, the MRI technologist opens the door and the MRI scanner moves into the OR via ceiling rails. The MRI scan lasts about 30 minutes and is done with or without contrast. If the resection is complete, the MRI scanner returns to the diagnostic room, the door closes, and surgery proceeds. If additional pathology remains, subresections or partial resections may warrant further tissue removal and reimaging. The MRI and the OR remain separately functioning areas when not being used for iMRI. As with traditional MRI, safety considerations with iMRI require extensive training, preparation, and teamwork throughout all aspects of the case. All clinical staff must be current in iMRI safety training (indicated by stickered badges) to access this room. During case setup, the nurse ensures that all non–MRI-compatible equipment is tagged and placed underneath the scanning table with string for visibility and easy removal before bringing in the magnet and performs an additional instrument count before prepping and draping the patient for the scan. The anesthesia provider performs a separate instrument-needle count for all needles, angiocaths, syringes, stylets, blades, and other related equipment, and stores used needles and syringes in needle mats. All counts must be reconciled; scanning does not proceed if any counts are incorrect. The perioperative nurse and the MRI technologist position, pad, and prep the patient. ESU dispersive pads, hypothermia, and compression devices are removed. MRI coil cables must be off the floor and attached to bed rails. All IV lines, leads, Foley catheters, and wires must not be looped or in contact with the skin (Fig. 29.11). The nurse tapes the patient's earplugs into place. The urinary catheter system is positioned as far away from the magnet as possible and tucked under the mattress (many contain metal). With the patient

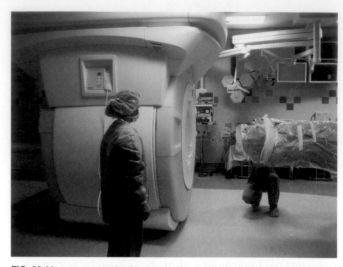

FIG. 29.11 Patient specifically prepped for intraoperative magnetic resonance imaging (iMRI) scan. MRI is mounted on ceiling rails and travels into the operating room after careful room and patient preparation.

prepped, the technologist and nurse check the diameter of the patient using a 70-cm hula hoop to confirm that the patient will fit into the 70-cm bore (opening) of the magnet before unlocking the doors. Before opening the door, the team moves all booms, lights, tables, microscopes, kick buckets, foot pedals, and other metal equipment that is not MRI safe behind the 5-gauss line. All anesthesia carts, supply carts, and IV infusion pumps are locked and secured. With additional staff, this preparation takes between 20 and 45 minutes to complete. The nurse documents and verbalizes the completion of all checklists and counts. The MRI travels into the OR on ceiling rails. All other doors providing OR access are locked during scanning. The anesthesia provider, an additional MRI tech, and the perioperative nurse remain in the room safe behind the 5-gauss line.

Percutaneous Nephrostomy

PCN is a procedure to drain the renal collecting system in cases of obstruction and is often performed in partnership between a urologist and IR physician. PCN refers to an external drainage catheter and collection system placed via a flank approach positioned in the renal pelvis. This procedure may also be performed before an intraoperative lithotripsy for kidney stones if the stones are unreachable by cystoscopy. Nephroureteral or nephroureterostomy catheters drain externally and internally via a catheter in the bladder. Ureteral stents are internal and extend from the renal pelvis to the bladder. Indications for PCN include obstructive uropathy (kidney and bladder stones, tumor obstructions) or tract creation for device insertion (e.g., antegrade ureteral stenting), extracorporeal shock wave lithotripsy, tumor biopsies, and stricture dilation. For concurrent procedures the interventionalist establishes drainage, and the urologist proceeds with stone removal via the PCN tract. Nephrostomies performed for future stone removal may plug the drainage until stone removal. Preprocedural imaging includes ultrasound of the kidney along with NM and CT scans. Local anesthesia with moderate sedation is typical; however, excessive dilation may warrant general anesthesia. Prophylactic antibiotic treatment varies with clinical practice and bacterial culture status. The nurse positions the patient prone with both arms above the head or one arm up and the other at the noninvolved side. Catheter insertion site is via the right, left, or bilateral flank;

pubis; or right or left lower quadrant of the abdomen of renal transplant patients. The site is prepped and draped and local anesthetic is infiltrated. The physician makes a small puncture, and then using ultrasound or fluoroscopic guidance directs the needle toward a lower calyx of the kidney. When the tip of the needle is in a dilated portion of the collecting system, urine flows back from the needle on stylet removal. If urine does not flow, the needle is retracted in small increments while aspirating with a 20-mL plastic syringe until urine emerges. The needle is exchanged over a guidewire, followed by upsizing of various dilator and introducer systems. The final trocar and catheter assembly, typically an 8F, terminates in the renal pelvis. The trocar and the guidewire are removed when the catheter is positioned correctly. Internal or external drainage determines catheter selection. Additional criteria, such as catheter material, configuration, coating, and locking mechanism, are per physician preference. If PCN was performed for obstruction, the nurse should be aware that a profuse diuresis may result, warranting IV volume replacement and monitoring of input and output. Antibiotic therapy is administered after the procedure to prevent infection. Hematuria may be present up to 48 hours postprocedure. Complications include hemorrhage, but the risk decreases with smaller needle sizes, as well as catheter dislodgement, blockage, or infection. Tube changes are scheduled for every 6 to 12 weeks. If the PCN is for decompression, the external drainage continues until achievement of the desired outcome occurs and urine flows naturally down the ureter.

Antegrade Ureteral Stent Placement

A ureteral stent functions both as a splint and a conduit for natural flow. In the urinary tract, it is an alternative to a nephrostomy. Although a stent is free of the complications of an external drain (external bag, leakage, skin irritation, accidental removal, and infection) and better for home care, it has disadvantages. The urinary tract does not tolerate artificial materials well. Stents can irritate the bladder or become infected. All stents, irrespective of their design or material of construction, will eventually become occluded, necessitating replacement. The common indications of antegrade ureteral stent placement are relief of ureteric obstruction or leakage, and splinting of the ureter after balloon dilatation of ureteric strictures or after ureteric surgery. Stenting before stone therapy is now a relative indication. Antegrade ureteric stenting may be performed either as a primary stenting procedure or as a second procedure after several days of external drainage. The technical success rate for the former is around 85% and near 100% for the latter. Primary stenting is contraindicated with infected obstructed systems (Patel et al., 2015). Preparation is similar to a PCN.

The physician obtains guidewire access and places a sheath through the skin into the renal pelvis to reduce friction when passing guidewires, dilators, and stents. A guidewire is placed distal to the obstruction and advanced into the bladder. This may require various guidewires because of the configuration of the ureter and obstruction type. The physician sizes the stent and positions it using contrast injection and fluoroscopy. Additional sedation may be required for supplemental dilations or balloon angioplasties if the stent cannot pass a stricture. When the stent is in the proper location, the physician deploys it, removes the sheath and guidewire, and replaces the nephrostomy tube. The draining nephrostomy catheter remains for 1 to 2 days after internal stent placement, allowing draining urine to flush normal operative debris from the stent. Postprocedure follow-up consists of an antegrade contrast injection through the nephrostomy tube to assess patency of the ureter and implanted stent. Contrast seen traversing the stent and collecting in the bladder justifies

nephrostomy tube removal. Complications include perforation of the renal collecting system or ureter. After the site heals, the urologist removes the stent in the cystoscopy room with urologic instruments. When the stent must remain in place, the urologist may be able to exchange it through a retrograde cystoscopy procedure.

Key Points

- Because of the broad scope of IR, it is important to establish interdisciplinary patient preparation protocols, according to procedure and modality selection. Imaging selection is according to physician; however, distinct nursing considerations exist for each modality.
- Radiography exposes the patient to ionizing radiation and is the most common imaging diagnostic modality.
- Fluoroscopy is a moving x-ray used to determine catheter placement in various procedures and clinical settings by different physician specialties. It requires iodinated contrast agents, which may result in an allergic reaction. The nurse needs to understand precipitating factors as well as management and prophylaxis regarding these reactions.
- CT scans also use ionizing radiation, and some scans require iodinated contrast agents. Diagnostic CT scans are very short in duration. Those using CT for procedures require preoperative planning to accommodate patient positioning and equipment positioning as well as potential contrast allergies.
- MRI scans are much longer in duration. This modality does not require ionizing radiation; however, MRI-guided procedures warrant meticulous monitoring because ferrous objects are attracted to the magnet and represent a safety issue. Some MRI studies and procedures use contrast. MRI contrast issues, however, are much less frequent than CT.
- Ultrasound is a portable technology and it uses sound waves. Ultrasound does not emit ionizing radiation. The use of ultrasound is common in urogynecologic and obstetric procedures. Considerations when using ultrasound are the use of probes and cables and their location to the sterile field.
- Depending on the procedure, the approach, and modality selection, patient positioning is highly variable. Because the quality of imaging is contingent on the patient being still, adequate procedure knowledge and preparation by the nurse to ensure patient comfort and positioning tolerance is important.
- Radiation safety is an important aspect in IR nursing. A basic understanding of the principles of radiation is needed to safely work in this environment as well as provide patient care.

Critical Thinking Question

When reviewing the special procedures schedule you learn you are scheduled to care for a 65-year-old female transferred to your institution to have an AV node ablation with pacemaker insertion. The electrophysiologist ordered an upper extremity venogram before the ablation procedure because the patient had an upper extremity thrombus approximately 6 months ago after a PICC placement. Her past medical history includes atrial fibrillation–flutter with uncontrolled ventricular response, moderate chronic obstructive pulmonary disease (COPD), insulin-dependent diabetes, and renal insufficiency. Her creatinine was 1.2 with a GFR of 45 mL/min/1.73 m² on her preadmission testing performed yesterday. Routine medications include aspirin, insulin, Coumadin, prednisone, metoprolol, and a metered-dose inhaler. She is allergic to sulfa and lorazepam. You need to set up her prescreening call. What factors would you incorporate in your perioperative plan of care?

ⓔvolve *The answer to the Critical Thinking Question can be found at http://evolve.elsevier.com/Rothrock/Alexander.*

References

Ahmed M et al: Clinical practice guideline Society of Interventional Radiology, Image-guided tumor ablation: Standardization of terminology and reporting criteria—a 10-year update, *J Vasc Interv Radiol* 25(6):1691–1705, 2014.

American College of Radiology (ACR): *ACR manual on contrast media: ACR committee on drugs and contrast media (version 10.3)* (website), 2017. https://www.acr.org/-/media/ACR/Documents/PDF/QualitySafety/Resources/Contrast-Manual/Contrast_Media.pdf?la=en. (Accessed 18 October 2017).

American College of Radiology (ACR) Society of Interventional Radiology (SIR) (ACR-SIR): *ACR–SIR–SPR practice parameter for the creation of a transjugular intrahepatic portosystemic shunt (TIPS)* (website), 2014. www.acr.org/-/media/ACR/Documents/PGTS/guidelines/TIPS.pdf?db=web. (Accessed 23 January 2017).

American College of Radiology (ACR) Society of Interventional Radiology (SIR), (ACR-SIR): *ACR–SIR practice parameter for sedation/analgesia* (website), 2015. www.acr.org/-/media/ACR/Documents/PGTS/guidelines/Adult_Sedation.pdf?db=web. (Accessed 23 January 2017).

American College of Radiology (ACR) Society of Interventional Radiology (SIR), (ACR-SIR): *ACR–SIR–SPR practice parameter on informed consent for image-guided procedure* (website), 2016. www.acr.org/-/media/1A03224CA4894854800C516012B6DB5A.pdf. (Accessed 23 January 2017).

American Society of Anesthesiologists (ASA): Practice advisory on anesthetic care for magnetic resonance imaging: an updated report by the task force on anesthetic care for magnetic resonance imaging, *Anesthesiology* 122(3):495–520, 2015.

Association of periOperative Registered Nurses (AORN): Guideline for positioning the patient. In *Guidelines for perioperative practice*, Denver, 2016, The Association.

Association for Radiologic & Imaging Nursing (ARIN): *ARIN clinical practice guideline: universal protocol for procedures in radiology* (website), 2014a. www.arinursing.org/practice-guidelines/ARINCPGUnversalProtocol.pdf. (Accessed 14 January 2017).

Association for Radiologic & Imaging Nursing (ARIN): *ARIN position statement: bariatric patient safety in the imaging environment* (website), 2014b. http://www.arinursing.org/practice-guidelines/arinpsbariatricsafety.pdf. (Accessed 18 October 2017).

Association for Radiologic & Imaging Nursing (ARIN): *ARIN position statements* (website), 2014c. www.arinursing.org/practice-guidelines. (Accessed 14 January 2017).

Association for Radiologic & Imaging Nursing (ARIN): *Clinical practice guideline: metformin therapy and lactic acidosis risk* (website), 2014d. www.arinursing.org/practice-guidelines/ARINCPGMetformin.pdf. (Accessed 14 January 2017).

Baerlocher M et al: Society of Interventional Radiology position statement: staffing guidelines for the interventional radiology suite, *J Vasc Interv Radiol* 27(5):618–622, 2016.

Bakal CW, Flacke S: Diagnostic catheters and guidewires. In Mauro M et al, editors: *Image-guided interventions*, ed 2, Philadelphia, 2014, Saunders.

Basseri S, Lightfoot CB: Balloon-occluded retrograde transvenous obliteration for treatment of bleeding gastric varices: case report and review of literature, *Radiol Case Rep* 11(4):365–369, 2016.

Cheng S: Radiation safety. In Cronenwett J, Johnston KW, editors: *Rutherford's vascular surgery*, ed 8, Philadelphia, 2014, Saunders.

Dariushnia SR et al: Quality improvement guidelines for uterine artery embolization for symptomatic leiomyomata, *J Vasc Interv Radiol* 25(11):1737–1747, 2014.

Dauer L et al: Occupational radiation protection of pregnant or potentially pregnant workers in IR: a joint guideline of the Society of Interventional Radiology and Cardiovascular and Interventional Radiological Society of Europe, *J Vasc Interv Radiol* 26(2):171–181, 2015.

de Almeida Mendes C et al: Carbon dioxide as contrast medium to guide endovascular aortic aneurysm repair, *Ann Vasc Surg* 39:67–73, 2017.

Gross JB et al: Practice guidelines for the perioperative management of patients with obstructive sleep apnea: an updated report by the American Society of Anesthesiologists task force on perioperative management of patients with obstructive sleep apnea, *Anesthesiology* 120(2):268–286, 2014.

Haines D et al: Heart rhythm society expert consensus statement on electrophysiology laboratory standards: process, protocols, equipment, personnel, and safety, *Heart Rhythm* 11(8):e9–e51, 2014.

Health Physics Society (HPS): *Radiation dose units* (website), 2016. hps.org/publicinformation/ate/faqs/radiationdoses.html. (Accessed 4 January 2017).

Lebak K, Lee J: Designing safety and engineering standards for the nonoperating room anesthesia procedure site. In Weiss M, editor: *Non-operating room anesthesia*, Philadelphia, 2015, Saunders.

Mayo Clinic: *Intraoperative magnetic resonance imaging (iMRI)* (website), 2016. www.mayoclinic.org/tests-procedures/intraoperative-magnetic-resonance-imaging/basics/definition/prc-20013344. (Accessed 5 January 2017).

McEnery KW: *Radiology information systems and electronic medical records* (website), 2015. www.acr.org/-/media/ACR/Documents/PDF/Advocacy/IT%20Reference%20Guide/IT%20Ref%20Guide%20RISEMR.pdf. (Accessed 5 January 2017).

Nieman K et al: Computed tomography. In Nieman K et al, editors: *Advanced cardiac imaging*, Philadelphia, 2015, Elsevier.

Patel U et al: Genitourinary tract intervention. In Adam A et al, editors: *Grainger & Allison's diagnostic radiology*, ed 6, Philadelphia, 2015, Elsevier.

Rafiei E et al: Society of Interventional Radiology IR pre-procedure patient safety checklist by the safety and health committee, *J Vasc Interv Radiol* 27(1):695–699, 2016.

Rathmell J: Radiation safety and the use of radiographic contrast agents in pain medicine. In Benzon H, editor: *Practical management of pain*, ed 5, Philadelphia, 2014, Elsevier.

Reekers J: Basic clinical requirements of interventional radiology, diagnostic radiology. In Adam A et al, editors: *Grainger & Allison's diagnostic radiology*, ed 6, Philadelphia, 2015, Elsevier.

Schaadt J, Landau B: Hybrid OR: a primer for the nurse, *AORN J* 97(1):81–100, 2013.

Sentilhes L et al: Postpartum hemorrhage: guidelines for clinical practice from the French College of Gynaecologists and Obstetricians (CNGOF), *Eur J Obstet Gynecol Reprod Biol* 198:12–21, 2016.

Sloan M et al: Closed cephalomedullary nailing with patient in lateral decubitus position for repair of peritrochanteric femoral fracture, *JBJS Essent Surg Tech* 6(1):e6, 2016.

Society of Interventional Radiology (SIR): *Diseases and conditions* (website), 2016. https://www.sirweb.org/patient-center/. (Accessed 6 January 2017).

The Joint Commission (TJC): *2017 national patient safety goals* (website), 2017. www.jointcommission.org/npsg_presentation/. (Accessed 5 January 2017).

US Nuclear Regulatory Commission (USNRC): *ALARA* (website), 2014. www.nrc.gov/reading-rm/basic-ref/glossary/alara.html. (Accessed 5 January 2017).

US Nuclear Regulatory Commission (USNRC): *Minimize your exposure* (website), 2016. www.nrc.gov/about-nrc/radiation/protects-you/protection-principles.html. (Accessed 14 January 2017).

CHAPTER 30

Integrative Health Practices: Complementary and Alternative Therapies

RACHAEL LARNER

Energy Therapies History and Background

An accurate presentation of the history of medicine in the United States needs to include influences from the botanic cultural traditions of Asia, India, Europe, and the First Nations. Our current medical system, referred to as *biomedicine,* began to dominate sometime in the mid-1800s with the discovery that microorganisms were responsible for disease and pathologic damage and that antitoxins and vaccines could improve the body's ability to oppose the effects of pathogens. Armed with this knowledge, scientists and clinicians were able to treat previously serious and fatal infections and refine surgical procedures.

As biomedicine dominated the healthcare system, it became the mainstream or "conventional" approach, establishing the standards for diagnosis and treatment of illness. By the 1990s, however, consumer faith and trust in this system began to falter, and many Americans sought complementary or alternative treatments for their healthcare. Complementary and alternative medicine (CAM), known currently as "integrative health practices," has grown to constitute a significant percentage of American healthcare dollars and visits. This growth is sustained by patients who desire to be more empowered healthcare consumers and the availability of media information about the many alternatives to mainstream, conventional Western biomedical approaches to healthcare. Because of this, there has been an increased use of CAM throughout hospitals and doctor offices within the United States since the mid-2000s.

Myths and misconceptions initially prevented investigation and development of promising therapies outside the biomedical regimen. In response to growing consumer pressure, anecdotal evidence, and a small body of published scientific results, the US Congress established the Office of Alternative Medicine (OAM) within the office of the director, National Institutes of Health (NIH), in 1992. This office was responsible for (1) facilitating fair, scientific evaluation of alternative therapies that showed promise in health promotion, and (2) reducing barriers to the acceptance and utilization of those alternative therapies that showed promise.

In 1998 the OAM became the National Center for Complementary and Alternative Medicine (NCCAM), which in turn is now recognized as the National Center for Complementary and Integrative Health (NCCIH) (NCCIH, 2016c). This expansion into a center allowed more substantial funding for and initiation of research projects, providing more sound information about integrative health practices. The annual budget for NCCIH has grown significantly, as has the sophistication of research designs of studies being funded by the center. The NCCIH adheres to guidelines set forth in public policy.

Many integrative health practices and therapies stem from a philosophy of wholeness, with the intent to treat the entire person (body-mind-spirit) (Evidence for Practice). This is in contrast to the current gold standard of randomized, controlled clinical trials, which may not be the best, or indeed appropriate, way to measure the effectiveness of many integrative health practices and therapies. Conventional scientists and physicians and the proponents of integrative health practices and CAM often debate the appropriate forms of research to determine efficacy and safety of alternative therapies. A reason for this disparity stems from divergent theoretic models. The *comprehensive approach* takes into account multidimensional factors that may not easily or appropriately be studied independently. The comprehensive approach is more congruent with the philosophic underpinnings of most integrative health practices and CAM. The *biomedical approach,* on the other hand, is concerned with a disease orientation, suggesting that a specific agent or variable is responsible for a specific disorder or illness.

There are five major domains used to categorize CAMs: alternative medical systems, mind-body medicine, biologically based therapies, manipulative and body-based methods, and energy therapies. Numerous treatments and systems are within each category. The remainder of this chapter discusses the major domains and provides examples of each.

Major Categories of Integrative Health Practices and Complementary and Alternative Medicine

Alternative Medical Systems

The National Health Interview Survey (NHIS), conducted most recently in 2012, by the National Center for Health Statistics (part of the Centers for Disease Control and Prevention) gathered information on roughly 90,000 American adults and 17,300 children. This survey found that about 33% of adults and 11% of children in the United States used some form of complementary health approach and spent roughly $30.2 billion out of pocket for these treatments. According to the NCCIH, most complementary health approaches fall into one of two subgroups, natural products or mind and body practices. Natural products consist of herbs, vitamins and minerals, and probiotics. Mind and body practices include a large and diverse group of procedures or techniques taught by a practitioner or teacher (NCCIH, 2016d). This survey, which included a comprehensive survey on the use of complementary health approaches by Americans, showed that natural products and deep breathing are the most popular complementary health approaches used today. Yoga, chiropractic and osteopathic manipulation, meditation, and massage therapy are among the most popular mind and body practices used by adults (Fig. 30.1).

EVIDENCE FOR PRACTICE

Evaluating Complementary and Alternative Medicine Therapies

According to the NCCIH, millions of Americans use some form of CAM. In discussing the use of CAM with perioperative patients, nurses have a unique opportunity to advise patients on best practices to adopt when considering using CAM therapies and should include the following advice:

- Take charge of your health by being an informed consumer. Investigate what studies or research has been done on the safety and effectiveness of any health approach that is recommended or interests you. Choose a complementary health practitioner as carefully as you would a conventional healthcare provider. The NCCIH's website has resources and tips to help choose a complementary health provider. Make sure to tell all your health providers about the health approaches you use, so that the safest complementary care can be given to you.
- Visit the FDA online (www.fda.gov) to see if any information is available on this alternative medicine or practice. You can also access any recalls or safety alerts on the FDA webpage at www.fda.gov/Safety/Recalls.
- Know the difference between "complementary," "alternative," and "integrative."
  - Complementary and integrative refer to the use of such nonmainstream approaches together with conventional medical approaches.
  - Alternative health approaches refer to the use of nonmainstream approaches in place of conventional medicine.
  - NCCIH advises against using any product or practice that has not been proven safe and effective.
- The Internet can be a good source to find information about CAM. In evaluating information on the Internet you should always ask the following questions:
  - Who runs the website? Is it a government, university, or reputable medical or health-related association? Is it

sponsored by a manufacturer of products, drugs, and so on? It should be easy to clearly identify the sponsor.
  - What is the purpose of the site? Is it to educate the public or sell a product? The purpose should be clearly stated.
  - What is the basis of the information? Is it based on scientific evidence with clear references?
  - Are any enforcement actions for deceptive advertising for this therapy called out by the FTC (www.ftc.gov)?
  - How current is the information? Is it reviewed and updated frequently?
- Visit the NCCIH website (https://nccih.nih.gov) for information on specific CAM therapies with links to other online services and information. You can also find information from NCCIH on Facebook, Twitter, YouTube, and Pinterest.
- If you do not have access to the Internet, contact the NCCIH clearinghouse at 1-888-644-6226 for assistance.
- Visit your local library or medical library to search for scientific information about CAM.
- Discuss CAM with your healthcare provider before making any decision about care. Ask questions about any possible interactions with medications you currently take or therapy you are undergoing. If your physician cannot answer your questions, he or she may be able to refer you to someone who can.
- Before taking herbal supplements:
  - Talk to your physician.
  - Talk to a licensed pharmacist if you have questions about the supplement, and discuss any potential reactions with any prescription or nonprescription medications (OTC medications) you currently take.
  - Buy only supplements that are approved by the American Botanical Council's Commission E. Read labels carefully.
  - Buy products from a reputable herbal company. Be cautious about products for sale through magazines, TV, radio, or the Internet.

CAM, Complementary and alternative medicine; *FDA,* US Food and Drug Administration; *FTC,* Federal Trade Commission; *NCCIH,* National Center for Complementary and Integrative Health; *OTC,* over the counter.
Modified from National Center for Complementary and Integrative Health (NCCIH): *Are you considering a complementary health approach?* (website), 2016. https://nccih.nih.gov/health/decisions/consideringcam.htm. (Accessed 1 August 2016).

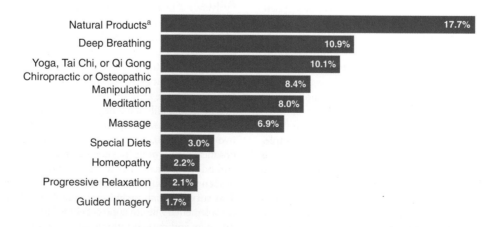

aDietary supplements other than vitamins and minerals.

FIG. 30.1 Ten most common complementary health approaches among adults according to the National Health Interview Survey, done most recently in 2012.

Cultural Characteristics Related to the Balance of "Hot" and "Cold"

A naturalistic or holistic approach often assumes that there are external factors (some good, some bad) that must be kept in balance if we are to remain well. The balance of "hot" and "cold" is a part of the belief system in many cultural groups, such as the Arab, Chinese, Filipino, and Hispanic cultures. To restore a disturbed balance (i.e., to treat) requires the use of opposites (e.g., a hot remedy for a cold problem). Different cultures may define hot and cold differently. It is not a matter of temperature, and the words used might vary; for example, the Chinese have named the forces yin (cold) and yang (hot). Western medicine cannot ignore the naturalistic view if many of its patients are to have appropriate treatment for illness as well as disease.

Hot Conditions and Their Corresponding Treatments

Hot Conditions	Cold Foods	Cold Medicines and Herbs
Fever	Fresh vegetables	Orange flower water
Infection	Tropical fruits	Linden
Diarrhea	Dairy products	Sage
Kidney problem	Meats such as goat,	Milk of magnesia
Rash	fish, chicken	Bicarbonate of soda
Skin ailment	Honey	—
Sore throat	Cod	—
Liver problem	Raisins	—
Ulcer	Bottle milk	—
Constipation	Barley water	—

Cold Conditions and Their Corresponding Treatments

Cold Conditions	Hot Foods	Hot Medicines and Herbs
Cancer	Chocolate	Penicillin
Pneumonia	Cheese	Tobacco
Malaria	Temperate-zone fruits	Ginger root
Joint pain	Eggs	Garlic
Menstrual period	Peas	Cinnamon
Teething	Onions	Anise
Earache	Aromatic beverages	Vitamins
Rheumatism	Hard liquor	Iron preparations
Tuberculosis	Oils	Cod liver oil
Cold	Meats such as beef,	Castor oil
Headache	waterfowl, mutton	Aspirin
Paralysis	Goat's milk	—
Stomach cramps	Cereal grains	—
	Chili peppers	—

Modified from Ball JW et al: *Seidel's guide to physical examination*, ed 8, St Louis, 2015, Mosby.

Many of these integrative health therapies are culturally, ethnically, spiritually, or religiously derived. Among the diverse values, beliefs, and practices found in the many cultural groups in the United States are those relating to health, illness, professional healthcare, and folk healthcare (Box 30.1). They include well-known and respected Asian systems of medicine. Many Asian medicine techniques or systems are widely known in the United States. The most well-known and popular of these include herbal medicines, massage, energy therapy, acupressure, acupuncture, qi gong, and cupping (Fig. 30.2). This integrative, alternative medicine system has a wide range of applications from health promotion to the treatment of illness. A significant

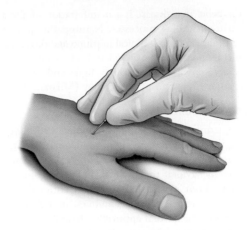

FIG. 30.2 Acupuncture is one tool a traditional Chinese medical doctor uses to shift a person's vital energy. It involves the insertion of thin, solid, stainless steel needles into specific points on the body. Acupuncture points can also be stimulated manually without the use of needles; this approach may be better suited for children or the elderly.

aspect of Asian medicine is an emphasis on diagnosing and treating disturbances of *qi* (pronounced "chee"), or vital energy, and restoring its proper balance (Micozzi, 2015).

Ayurveda is a traditional system from India that strives to restore the innate harmony of the individual while placing equal emphasis on body, mind, and spirit. Ayurvedic practitioners use many products and techniques to cleanse the body and restore balance. Key foundations are universal connectedness (e.g., that all living and nonliving things are joined together, health will be good if one's mind and body are in harmony, disease arises when a person is out of harmony with the universe), the body's constitution or *prakriti* (e.g., the person's unique physical and psychologic characteristics and how the person functions to maintain health), and life forces, or *doshas*. Each person has a combination of three doshas; each dosha has a particular relationship with a bodily function and can be upset for a variety of reasons. Treatment is tailored to each person's constitution and predominant dosha. Practitioners expect patients to be active participants because many Ayurvedic treatments require changes in diet, lifestyle, and habits.

Native American, Middle Eastern, Tibetan, Central and South American, and African cultures have developed other traditional medical systems (Micozzi, 2015). Additional examples of complete integrative health practice and alternative medicine systems are naturopathic and homeopathic medicine systems. Homeopathic medicine is based on the principle that "like cures like" (i.e., a substance that in large doses produces the symptoms of a disease will, in a very diluted dose, cure the patient). Small doses of plant extracts and minerals specially prepared are given to stimulate the body's defense mechanisms and encourage healing processes. Careful evaluation of symptoms enables the practitioner to determine a patient's specific sensitivity and to select the appropriate remedy.

Naturopathic medicine is one of the most recent alternative approaches to have developed as a health system across North America. In practice, modern naturopathic medicine is eclectic, drawing on different systems and models (e.g., Chinese medicine, homeopathy, and manual therapies) to fit the patient profile and clinical problem with the appropriate techniques (Micozzi, 2015). Naturopathic medicine emphasizes health restoration as well as disease treatment based on the belief that disease is a manifestation of alterations in the body's natural healing processes. Naturopathic physicians use multiple modalities, including clinical nutrition and diet; acupuncture; herbal medicine; homeopathy; spinal and soft tissue manipulation; physical therapies involving ultrasound, light, and electric currents; therapeutic counseling; and pharmacology (Micozzi, 2015).

Mind-Body Interventions

A growing scientific movement has explored the mind's ability to affect the body. The clinical application of this relationship is categorized as *mind-body medicine*. Some mind-body interventions (e.g., cognitive-behavioral therapy), formerly categorized as CAM therapies, have been assimilated into conventional mainstream medicine. Progressive relaxation techniques, biofeedback, meditation, and cognitive-behavioral approaches have a well-documented theoretic basis with supporting scientific evidence. Other mind-body interventions still considered "alternative" by some include hypnosis, music, dance, art therapy, prayer, and mental healing.

Yoga is one of the leading complementary health approaches used by adults in the United States. A mind-body practice with origins in ancient Indian philosophy, yoga consists of various styles (e.g., Bikram, Hatha) combining physical postures, breathing techniques, and meditation or relaxation. According to the most recent study done by the NCCIH in 2007, yoga is used by more than 13 million adults. The two main reasons yoga is used are to maintain health and well-being and to reduce back pain. Back pain was found as the number one reason that people use complementary health practices (NCCIH, 2016e).

Biologically Based Therapies

The integrative health practices category of biologically based therapies includes biologically based and natural-based practices, products, and interventions, some of which overlap with mainstream medicine's use of dietary supplements. Herbal, orthomolecular (i.e., a form of alternative medicine that aims to maintain human health through nutritional supplementation), individual biologic therapies, and special dietary treatments are encompassed in biologically based therapies.

Herbs are plants or parts of plants that contain and produce chemical substances that act on the body. Some diet therapies are believed to promote health and prevent illness. Proponents of diet therapies include religious factions such as Seventh-Day Adventist or Jewish Kosher. Veganism, vegetarianism, raw food diets, and diets promoted by Drs. Atkins, Pritikin, and Weil are other examples of therapeutic nutrition. Orthomolecular therapies use differing concentrations of chemicals or megadoses of vitamins aimed at treating disease. Many biologic therapies are available but not currently accepted by mainstream medicine, such as the use of cartilage products from cattle, sheep, or sharks for treatment of cancer and arthritis, or the use of bee pollen to treat autoimmune and inflammatory diseases.

Manipulative and Body-Based Methods

Methods that are based on the movement or manipulation of the body include chiropractic, osteopathy, and massage. Touch and manipulations with the hands have been used in healing and medical practice since the beginning of the history of medicine. At one time, the physician's hands were considered the most important diagnostic and therapeutic tool. This remains true today, despite sophisticated diagnostic equipment and modalities (Box 30.2). Manual healing methods are based on the principle that dysfunction of a part of

---

BOX 30.2

Use of Palpation in Physical Examination

Palpation involves the use of your hands and fingers to gather information through the sense of touch. Certain parts of your hands and fingers are better than others for specific types of palpation. The palmar surfaces of the fingers and finger pads are more sensitive than the fingertips and are used whenever discriminatory touch is needed for determining position, texture, size, consistency, masses, fluid, and crepitus. The ulnar surfaces of the hand and fingers are the most sensitive area for distinguishing vibration. The dorsal surface of the hands is best for estimating temperature; of course, this estimate provides only a crude measure and is best used to detect temperature differences in comparing parts of the body.

Touch is in many ways therapeutic, and palpation is the actuality of the "laying on of hands." It is the moment at which health practitioners begin their physical invasion of the patient's body. The oft-repeated advice that the approach to palpation be gentle and the practitioner's hands be warm is not only practical but also symbolic of respect for the patient and for the privilege the patient gives.

Modified from Ball JW et al: *Seidel's guide to physical examination*, ed 8, St Louis, 2015, Mosby.

---

the body often affects secondarily the function of other discrete, possibly indirectly connected body parts. Theories have developed for correction of these secondary dysfunctions by realigning body parts or manipulating soft tissues. Chiropractic science is concerned primarily with the relationship between structure (spine primarily) and function (nervous system primarily) of the human body to preserve and restore health. Osteopathic medicine incorporates an extensive body of work that supports the use of osteopathic techniques for both musculoskeletal and nonmusculoskeletal problems. Massage therapy is one of the oldest methods known in the practice of healthcare. Many different massage techniques are aimed at helping the body heal itself through the use of manipulation of the soft body tissues (Perlman, 2016).

Energy Therapies

Energy therapies have been categorized into two groups: biofield therapies (those that focus on fields believed to originate within the body) and electromagnetic fields (those that originate from other sources). The existence of energy fields that originate within and around the body has not yet been definitively proven. However, many studies have examined the experiences of the recipient or practitioner and the outcomes of this type of energy therapy. Examples of therapies with a biofield basis include acupuncture, Reiki, qi gong, therapeutic touch (TT), and healing touch. Therapies that involve electromagnetic fields use unconventional pulsed fields, magnetic fields, alternating current fields, or direct current fields.

Integrative Health Practices Use and Surgery

Energy Therapies

Patients have choices in how to manage their healthcare. However, surgery is the most invasive of all options. As healthcare consumers become more knowledgeable about their health they often seek complementary modalities to augment traditional Western medical therapies. Using the term *alternative* is actually misleading, which is why the field formerly known as CAM is more appropriately termed integrative health practices. Many progressive medical facilities embrace a holistic patient focus, exploring and integrating nontraditional healing modalities to support an individualized surgical experience. Biofield therapies represent a nonpharmacologic anxiolytic for surgical patients that may be integrated with an allopathic treatment plan.

Many ancient cultures refer to a human biofield or "life force." Sometimes referred to as "energy work," biofield therapeutics are a range of interventions sharing common beliefs. First is the existence of a "universal force" or "healing energy" arising from God (as the person understands this being), the cosmos, the Earth, or another supernatural source. Second, the human biofield, as part of the "universal field," is dynamic, open, complex, and pandimensional. Human biofields are constantly changing and interacting with each other, the environment, and the universal force field. Third, the ability to use one's biofield for healing is considered to be universal, although few people are aware of it without specific training. Last, practitioners intend to positively affect the patient's biofield, either by direct contact or by using the hands in proximity, similar to the ancient practice of laying on of hands (Dossey and Keegan, 2016) (Table 30.1).

Reiki is a complementary health approach in which the practitioner places his or her hands lightly on or just above the person, with the goal of facilitating the person's own healing response. Reiki is based on an Eastern belief in an energy that supports the body's innate or natural healing abilities. Reiki has been studied for a variety of conditions, including pain, anxiety, fatigue, and depression (NCCIH, 2016b). One pilot study showed that the use of Reiki postoperatively on total knee arthroscopy patients showed a decrease in pain and anxiety, thus resulting in a Reiki program at that specific hospital (Notte et al., 2016).

Therapeutic Touch

TT is the contemporary interpretation of several ancient healing modalities. Dolores Krieger and Dora Kunz developed TT in the early 1970s. The practice, like others that form part of the body of CAM, consists of learned skills for the conscious manipulation of human energies. In practice it is not necessary for the practitioner (healer) to actually touch the recipient (healee), because the energy field can be "felt" several inches away from the physical body. TT helps aid in relaxation, reduces pain, promotes deeper and easier breathing, improves circulation of blood and movement of lymph fluids, reduces blood pressure, and strengthens the immune system.

To work within biofields, the practitioner uses a model or map to focus the healing energy. Chakras, or energy centers, described by the Upanishads in the Vedas, the oldest literature of the East Indian people, are often used as a reference point. Although the most detailed descriptions are in the Upanishads' teachings, the attributes are found in the teachings of other cultures as widely geographic as the Sufis of the Middle East to the First Nations, particularly from the North American Southwest (Fig. 30.3).

TT practice lends itself well to the fast-paced surgical environment. The skills learned through study of TT provide a trained practitioner with the ability to center quickly and use intention to calm both himself or herself and others nearby in stressful situations. Research design, methods, techniques, and sample sizes are considerations for future studies into how biofield therapeutics may benefit surgical patients. Replicating past studies, as well as new research based on physiologic data and quantitative studies, is necessary (Research Highlight). It has become evident that the concepts involved in energy therapies need consistent definitions. If the concepts do not have preestablished definitions, they cannot be quantified or measured in meaningful ways. However, interest is high and research continues

TABLE 30.1

Comparisons of Selected Biofield Therapies

Therapy	Practice Initiated	Developers	Hand Placement	Theoretic Basis and Intent
Healing touch	1981	American Holistic Nurses Association	Both on and off the body	Uses elements of healing science and therapeutic touch in conjunction with crystal and dowsing to treat whole person and specific disorders
Qi gong	Traditional	Chinese	At meridian points or a short distance from the body	Qi follows meridians and body patterns to heal biologic disorder
Reflexology	Traditional	Ancient method of treatment for ailments dating back to Egyptians and earlier	Application of pressure to sites on feet, hands, ears, and so on that correspond with organs and nerves to cause a reflex arc of stimulation to area in need	Promotes balance and wellness through nerve stimulation
Reiki	Traditional 1800s 1936	Buddhist Japan: Hawayo Takata United States: Mikao Usui	A few standardized hand placements on the body	Spiritual energy from universe is channeled by "masters" to heal the spiritual body, which in turn heals the physical body
Therapeutic touch	1972	Dolores Krieger and Dora Kunz	Primarily off the body 2–4 inches	Aligning Kunz's Human Energy Field model with Martha Rogers's Science of Unitary Human Beings, the centered practitioner assesses, directs, and modulates biofield energy to achieve relaxation response for healing of whole person

Modified from Oschman JL: *Energy medicine the scientific basis*, ed 2, Philadelphia, 2016, Elsevier; National Center for Complementary and Integrative Health (NCCIH): *Health topics A-Z* (website). https://nccih.nih.gov/health/atoz.htm. (Accessed 8 August 2016).

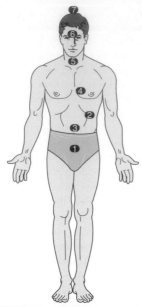

	English Name	Situation
1	Root or basic chakra	At the base of the spine
2	Spleen or splenic chakra	Over the spleen
3	Navel or umbilical chakra	At the navel, over the solar plexus
4	Heart or cardiac chakra	Over the heart
5	Throat or laryngeal chakra	At the front of the throat
6	Brow or frontal chakra	In the space between the eyebrows
7	Crown or coronal chakra	On the top of the head

FIG. 30.3 Chakras.

in an effort to better understand a phenomenon that seems to provide meaningful relief to the patient.

Perioperative Medical Hypnotherapy

Use of medical hypnotherapy in hospitals and clinics for perioperative care is not uncommon. Patients are seeking an active role in their treatment and are better informed regarding surgical options. Participating in perioperative medical hypnotherapy allows patients to take shared responsibility for their healing process, giving them a measure of control, because all hypnosis is self-hypnosis. Meaningful and active participation empowers a patient to enter into anesthesia and surgery with confidence.

Surgery is a life-changing event, and each perioperative medical hypnotherapy patient is unique. The initial assessment serves to determine goals and explore questions relative to emotional as well as physical concerns. The hypnotherapist, working within the patient's belief system, helps acknowledge areas of the patient's concern as a multidisciplinary partnership of healing is forged in a patient-centered manner.

As the hypnotherapist guides the patient into relaxation and induces hypnosis, both therapist and patient journey into the body, together addressing predetermined issues. One study found that by providing surgical patients with preparatory information regarding their procedure, postoperative discomforts and operative care, in combination with realistic, positive expectations of the surgical experience, they showed a decreased amount of postoperative anxiety, request for medication, and length of hospital stay (Kitaeff, 2013).

RESEARCH HIGHLIGHT

Effect of Structured Touch and Guided Imagery for Pain and Anxiety in Elective Joint Replacement Patients—A Randomized Controlled Trial: M-TIJRP

This study looked at the use of the "M" technique, which is a form of structured touch and massage, compared with guided imagery and usual care, for the reduction of pain and anxiety in patients undergoing elective total hip or knee replacement surgery. At a community hospital, over 2 years, 225 male and female patients, from ages 38 to 90 years, undergoing elective total hip or knee replacement surgery, were randomly assigned to one of three groups (75 patients in each group): M technique, guided imagery, or usual care. They were blinded to the assignment until the intervention.

The M technique is a registered method of structured touch created by Jane Buckle, PhD, who describes this as a series of gentle, slow, stroking movements done in a set sequence that causes the receiver a sense of relaxation. M technique was performed on the hands and feet for 18 to 20 minutes, with touch equally distributed among available extremities, paralleling the length of the guided imagery audio program and the mirroring the duration that other studies have shown for massage to be best effective at anxiety and pain reduction. This technique was done by licensed massage therapists who were trained in the use of M technique along with the use of guided imagery equipment.

This study evaluated the use of M technique, guided imagery, and usual care at four specific times during the hospital stay, using the NVAS for anxiety and PNRS for pain, administered before and after interventions. These were collected preoperative day 0, postoperative day 0, postoperative day 1, and postoperative day 2. A patient satisfaction questionnaire was completed at the time of discharge.

In conclusion, this study yielded positive results for the management of pain and anxiety in patients undergoing elective joint replacement using M technique and guided imagery compared with usual care. M technique showed the largest decreases in pain and anxiety between both groups. Patient satisfaction survey ratings were highest for M technique, followed by guided imagery.

NVAS, Numeric Visual Anxiety Scale; *PNRS*, Pain Numeric Rating Scale.
Modified from Forward JB et al: Effect of structured touch and guided imagery for pain and anxiety in elective joint replacement patients—a randomized controlled trial: M-TIJRP, *Perm J*, 19(4):18–28, 2015.

Hypnosis compassionately allows a patient to explore emotions without judgment or expectation of those feelings. The practice of emotional awareness, of being present with feelings, and of holding those feelings sacred can bring a sense of peace and healing insights during a time of profound stress, such as that experienced by many surgical patients. Predetermined suggestions or affirmations may increase confidence in the healthcare team, increase compliance with the treatment plan, decrease blood loss, maintain intraoperative homeostasis, reduce the need for sedation or pain medication, decrease postoperative nausea or vomiting, and increase patient satisfaction. It has been found that relaxation techniques used in the perioperative setting can greatly decrease anxiety of the patient (Chou et al., 2016).

Postoperative hypnotherapy sessions reinforce continued participation of patients in their healing process. This may take the form of establishing metabolic gauges in the "control room" or show a symbolic shield of protection, holding or sending color, light, or a certain feeling of safety to a specific part of the body. It may be expressing gratitude to and confidence in the medical and nursing community. Follow-up sessions allow both patient and hypnotherapist to evaluate attainment of preoperative goals, consider postoperative outcomes, and explore issues relevant to the ongoing healing process.

Guided Imagery

Another therapy closely related to hypnosis is guided imagery. Imagery, or thinking in pictures, is the natural language of the unconscious mind and is used by the autonomic nervous system as a primary mode of communication. The autonomic nervous system controls unconscious body functions such as heart rate, immune function, digestion, blood flow, smooth muscle tension, and pain perception (Fig. 30.4). Guided imagery for surgical patients may be in the form of prescripted tapes that lead the patient through relaxation exercises and provide healing suggestions. In other instances the perioperative nurse may assist the patient with guided imagery through the use of a calming, monotone voice; a smooth speaking delivery; and the use of relaxing images, such as a place in nature. The perioperative nurse coaches the patient to see, feel, smell, sense, and hear the imagined scene. Imagery may help patients build a "tool" to help in the postoperative period and lead to quicker recovery. According to Chou et al. (2016), benefits of guided imagery for surgery patients may include the following:

- Decreased anxiety
- Decreased pain scores
- Decreased or declined use of analgesics

Aromatherapy in Perioperative Services

Aromatherapy involves the therapeutic use of fragrance (e.g., aromatic plant extracts and essential oils) applied to the patient's body through inhalation or topical methods, or rarely ingestion. Clinical aromatherapy developed within the concept of Western medicine, before World War I in France (Lindquist et al., 2014). Today, clinical aromatherapy is gaining acceptance with the consent and participation of patients. It is practiced by certified clinical aromatherapy practitioners (CCAPs), knowledgeable about the specific properties of essential oils and how they interact with patients and the therapeutic environment. CCAPs use clinical-grade essential oils in a controlled way for specific, measurable outcomes. These may affect the patient on a psychologic, physiologic, or cellular level. The choice of essential oil is based on the chemistry of that essential oil and its proven effects (Table 30.2).

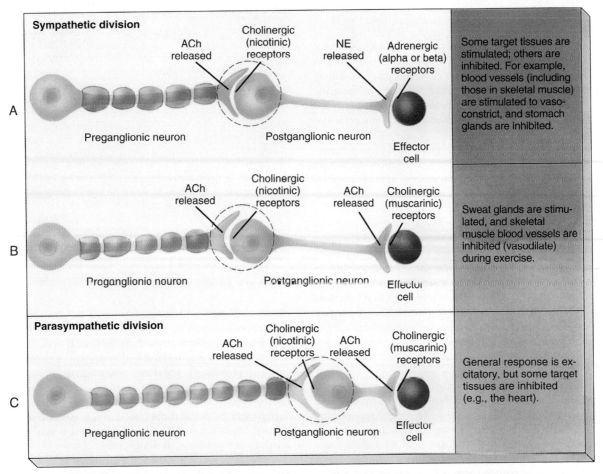

FIG. 30.4 Locations of neurotransmitters and receptors in the autonomic nervous system. In all pathways, preganglionic fibers are cholinergic, secreting acetylcholine *(Ach),* which stimulates nicotinic receptors in the postganglionic neuron. Most sympathetic fibers are adrenergic (A), secreting norepinephrine *(NE),* thus stimulating alpha- or beta-adrenergic receptors. A few sympathetic postganglionic fibers are cholinergic, stimulating muscarinic receptors in effector cells (B). All parasympathetic postganglionic fibers are cholinergic (C), stimulating muscarinic receptors in effector cells.

TABLE 30.2
Essential Oils and Their Properties

Essential Oils	Property
Chamomile, lavender, lemon, peppermint, ginger	Antiemetic
Bergamot, clove, eucalyptus, lavender, juniper, thyme, tea tree	Antiseptic
Benzoin, bergamot, chamomile, jasmine, lavender, neroli, rose, sandalwood, verbena, ylang-ylang	Anxiolytic
Lavender, West Indian lemongrass, peppermint, Turkish oregano, Brazilian mint	Analgesic
Bergamot, chamomile, jasmine, lavender, neroli, rose, ylang-ylang	Sedating
Basil, black pepper, eucalyptus, peppermint, rosemary	Stimulating
German chamomile, rosemary, black pepper, helichrysum	Antiinflammatory

Modified from Hass DJ: Complementary and alternative medicine. *Sleisenger and Fordtran's gastrointestinal and liver disease: pathophysiology, diagnosis, management*, ed 10, Philadelphia, 2016, Saunders; Medline Plus: *Drugs, herbs and supplements* (website). https://medlineplus.gov/druginformation.html. (Accessed 19 August 2016); National Center for Complementary and Integrative Health (NCCIH): *Herbs at a glance* (website). https://nccih.nih.gov/health/herbsataglance.htm. (Accessed 19 August 2016).

As pharmacology combines medications to potentiate effect, aromatherapy may act synergistically with traditional treatment, or it may be offered in concert with other complementary modalities to relieve discomfort, reducing dosages of analgesics or sedatives. One study found that the use of peppermint along with controlled breathing helped to decrease nausea and/or vomiting postoperatively (Sites et al., 2014).

The nursing process of aromatherapy begins with obtaining consent for use of aromatics and collecting pertinent information. Assessment of the patient, the physical environment, and the team of caregivers defines the healing environment (Patient Engagement Exemplar). Along with review of the medical and nursing histories, allergies, vital signs, and laboratory values, subjective data are relevant, such as how to offer treatment. The plan of therapy may include direct inhalation (on a cotton ball or through a diffuser), compresses, topical application, or massage. The main uses of aromatherapy in the clinical setting are to help address pain, anxiety, nausea, sleeplessness, or agitation. This can also be used to prevent or treat infections (Lindquist et al., 2014). As with all nursing interventions, postprocedure follow-up with the patient is imperative to assess efficacy of this intervention (Research Highlight).

Music and Surgery

The therapeutic and healing properties of music have been recognized throughout history. Music has been shown to reduce stress and can block out unwanted noises around the patient during all perioperative phases, which makes the environment more enjoyable for the patient. Music can be used to stimulate the left and right sides of the brain simultaneously, stimulating and organizing muscle response, which can be a large benefit to patients with neuromuscular disorders.

Music has been shown to increase metabolism; increase or decrease muscular energy, breathing rate, blood volume, pulse rate, and blood pressure; and lower sensory stimuli thresholds. Music can touch patients deeply and thus transform their anxiety and discomfort into relaxation and healing.

PATIENT ENGAGEMENT EXEMPLAR
Aromatherapy

Aromatherapy has become very popular among many people and its use in surgical patients has been proven to be effective for reducing anxiety, relieving pain, and controlling nausea and vomiting (Stea et al., 2014). Patients who are experiencing anxiety and fear before surgery can be offered lavender or orange essential oils to help them relax. These same oils have also been shown to be effective for decreasing postoperative pain. Ginger and peppermint oil have been successful at reducing postoperative nausea and vomiting (Stea et al., 2014). Some patients are open to receiving aromatherapy while others might not be. Before offering essential oils to patients, have a discussion about how aromatherapy works and what scents are available, respecting the patient's wishes and personal preference. Some patients may think aromatherapy is a great addition to their care while others may not like certain scents or see it as quackery. Consider this scenario:

Mr. Black is admitted to the preoperative holding area to be prepared for his left knee arthroscopy. His nurse, Jim, notes that he appears to be very anxious, constantly looking around, irritable, and short of breath. Jim gets Mr. Black changed into a gown and assists him onto the stretcher. Jim takes the time to sit down with Mr. Black and tell him exactly what is happening and what he can expect. Jim says, "Mr. Black, many patients feel anxious over having surgery, let's talk about what it is that you are worried about." After discussing Mr. Black's concerns and addressing each one, Jim explains to Mr. Black that the facility has an aromatherapy program that has been shown to reduce anxiety. Mr. Black seems very skeptical and says, "I have never heard of this before, but if you think it might help me relax then I am open to trying it." Jim offers Mr. Black lavender or orange essential oils, and Mr. Black asks to smell both before choosing the orange. Jim puts the orange essential oil on Mr. Black's pillow case and tells him to close his eyes and breathe in the scent. After about 15 minutes, Jim notices that Mr. Black is much more relaxed, his breathing has slowed, and he is able to close his eyes while he waits. Giving patients choices, even if they are small things such as this, helps them to feel like they have some control over what is happening to them, and the essential oils can help patients feel more relaxed and able to cope.

From Stea S et al: Essential oils for complementary treatment of surgical patients: state of the art, *Evid Based Complement Alternat Med* 2014:726341, 2014.

Anxiety and pain are common perioperative nursing diagnoses identified in the sample plans of care in Unit II in this book. Because anxiety and pain lead to increased stress and stress may cause detrimental physiologic reactions, many nursing interventions are undertaken to reduce patients' anxiety. According to the AORN (2016) Guideline for Complementary Care Interventions, music therapy can be implemented to decrease perioperative pain and anxiety. Music is a nursing intervention that is easy to administer, relatively inexpensive, and noninvasive.

Music is therapeutic if used in a manner that enables its elements and their influences to aid in integration of the body, mind, and spirit of the patient during the treatment of an illness or disability. When selecting music to invoke physiologic and psychologic changes, it is important to note the attributes of music. Factors that need to be considered are the various elements of music (e.g., tempo, mode, pitch, rhythm, harmony, melody); listener characteristics (e.g., age,

Lavender Fleur Oil and Unscented Oil Aromatherapy Reduce Preoperative Anxiety in Breast Surgery Patients: A Randomized Trial

This study was conducted on patients in the preoperative holding area who were to undergo breast surgery. This was a single-site, randomized study comparing the effect of LFO to UO. The objective was to determine whether LFO aromatherapy would reduce anxiety when administered to women before undergoing breast surgery.

Ninety-three women, all aged 18 years and older, participated in this study. Before the application of the essential oil, the women were given an STAI questionnaire to determine their level of preoperative anxiety. Vital signs were also obtained. The subjects were then given 2 drops of 2% LFO or UO placed inside of a nonrebreather oxygen mask, and then inhaled this scent for 10 minutes. During the aromatherapy, vital signs were checked at 5-minute increments, and after the aromatherapy subjects completed another STAI survey. STAI questions were divided into positive and negative emotions for analysis.

Subjects were randomized to either the LFO or the UO group on a 1:1 basis using a random number generator, in blocks of 20, ahead of time. Only the patients were blinded.

Before aromatherapy there was no significant difference between the two groups. The use of both LFO and UO increased the positive STAI scores, with the LFO group having a slightly, but statistically significant, greater increase. Both resulted in a decrease in negative score totals after treatment.

In conclusion, although there were no changes in vital signs with the LFO aromatherapy, both LFO and UO treatments were associated with an improved sense of well-being and a decrease in anxiety before the surgery. The authors state this could be due to the fact that the subjects were given more attention preoperatively, which in turn lowered anxiety.

LFO, Lavender fleur oil; *STAI*, Speilberger State Anxiety Inventory; *UO*, unscented oil. Modified from Franco L et al: Both lavender fleur oil and unscented oil aromatherapy reduce preoperative anxiety in breast surgery patients: a randomized trial, *J Clin Anesth*, 33:243–249, 2016.

as increased cardiac workload. High levels of preoperative anxiety may result in postoperative complications such as depression, fear, and anger, and the use of music during the preoperative phase can decrease anxiety and significantly lessen complications in the postoperative phase of recovery. Emotions are altered, apprehension and tension are reduced, and sympathetic stimulation and adrenocortical activation are more controlled. Therefore changes in vital signs, such as elevated blood pressure and increased heart rate, are minimal. In a recent study by Labrague and McEnroe-Petitte (2016) it was found that the use of music therapy helped to decrease preoperative anxiety in women undergoing gynecologic surgery.

Patients undergoing surgery in which local or regional anesthetics are administered have an acute awareness of the environment found within the OR. The OR may appear threatening, with unfamiliar machines, equipment, noises, and smells. Physical positioning and exposure of body parts intensify anxiety. Unfamiliar sounds, bright lights, and technical language add to the stressors of the surgical experience. During surgery, patient-selected music reduces anxiety by providing the patient some autonomy through self-selected musical choices, while distracting the patient from what is happening within the environment. The music not only blocks the various sounds in the room but also provides an escape through imaginative thought. Researchers support the idea that musical vibrations have an effect on the subconscious mind. Older patients have reported comfort and strength by listening to hymns and other music of spiritual or psychologic support. Daydreaming, imagery, escape, and fantasizing are common to listeners. This creates a release of tension and is a way of focusing attention away from threats. Intraoperative music may decrease the patient's anxiety and consequently minimize the need for patient-controlled conscious sedation and analgesia. Music can have a positive effect during general anesthesia when delivered through headphones or earpieces, as long as care is exerted to prevent pressure points and volume increases.

Pain is a common problem in the postanesthesia care unit (PACU). Pain results in negative respiratory, cardiovascular, gastrointestinal, renal, neuroendocrine, and autonomic nervous system consequences for patients. The traditional means to provide pain relief in the PACU has been through medication administration. Because the effects of medication differ from person to person, it is important to use both pharmacologic interventions along with nonpharmacologic ones.

Noise levels contribute to the patients' discomfort (Nightingale, 1859). The level of noise typically encountered during the surgical experience is potentially harmful to patients because of the undesirable effects of a release of stress hormones on the cardiovascular system, including increased vasoconstriction, heart rate, and blood pressure. Noise also increases psychologic stress and discomfort, and patients' ability to cope is reduced. Soothing music delivered through headphones or earpieces can block out external noises and can serve as a distraction from the noise of the PACU.

When using music as a nursing intervention to promote physiologic and psychologic well-being, the nurse prepares both the patient and the environment. The nurse should inform the patient of the purpose of the music experience and interview the patient about musical preferences, allowing the patient to listen to portions of selected music to ensure the music will afford the therapeutic purpose. The use of music therapy is documented in the medical record. A library of different types of music selections should be available. When compiling these collections, it is important that attention is given to the tempo, rhythm, melody, and harmony of the music (as noted earlier). In addition to implementing the music intervention,

language, culture, education, musical preferences); and the mode of delivery (e.g., headphones, speakers). Slow, quiet music without lyrics tends to lower the physiologic responses associated with stress and anxiety. Fast tempos tend to increase tension, and slow tempos can cause suspense. A tempo of 60 to 72 beats per minute appears to promote relaxation and decrease anxiety, as theorized by matching the normal heart rate of humans. Research also demonstrates the importance of patient-selected music that is familiar, desirable, and meaningful, which often leads to positive responses from patients. The use of headphones blocks unpleasant environmental sounds, which is a common occurrence in busy preoperative holding areas and operating room (OR) suites. CDs or streaming music from a phone provide consistent, uninterrupted music, which is critical to the success of the ongoing therapeutic reactions that music affords. Best of all, music therapy can be used preoperatively, intraoperatively, and postoperatively.

Anticipation of surgery commonly produces anxiety. The preoperative waiting period may be more stressful and anxiety-provoking for some patients than the anticipated surgical intervention. High levels of anxiety cause negative physiologic manifestations, such as elevated blood pressure, which can lead to postoperative complications, such

nurses monitor patients' responses to ensure that intended outcomes are achieved, making adjustments as necessary.

Psychoneuroimmunology

Psychoneuroimmunology studies the relationship between the brain and immune function. Thus perioperative nursing interventions that seek to reduce stress influences have the potential to improve immune system function, which helps the recovery process. This involves how perioperative nurses communicate with patients as well as their behaviors, the attitudes they convey, the language they use, and their being "present" and totally engaged with their patients. Good communication between the nurse and patient is essential for positive outcomes related to healing (Table 30.3).

Early animal conditioning studies showed links on a molecular level (immune regulators: neurotransmitters, and hormones) that act to stimulate nerves or trigger physiologic changes. Further, the perception of stress is known to lead to a reduced ability to fight infection. Because measurement of immune function is a complicated process, much remains to be learned about the precise mechanism of how psychosocial or emotional factors affect susceptibility to disease.

Consideration and awareness of the mind-body relationship is important to immediate and long-term surgical outcomes. According to Tagge et al. (2013), it is clear that emotions, thoughts, stress, and other psychosocial factors have an important role in the recovery process, making it important that all who care for perioperative patients become familiar with these factors.

Herbs and Surgery

The use of herbal and botanic products is common. An estimated four billion people throughout the world use over-the-counter herbal preparations to treat a range of illnesses and ailments, as well as maintain general health (Ujam et al., 2014). However, many patients do not communicate this information to their conventional medical physicians or nurse caregivers, because they are unsure of the reaction of conventional caregivers to their use of alternative substances. According the NCCIH (2016a), the most used supplement in the United States with adults is fish oil.

Botanicals are marketed as food supplements in the United States. Manufacturers are not allowed to make claims about health benefits for these products because they are not approved by the US Food and Drug Administration (FDA). Since 1994, when the Dietary Supplement Health and Education Act (DSHEA) was passed, the definition of dietary supplements has broadened. A product that contains a vitamin, mineral, herb, amino acid, or other botanic or dietary substance used to supplement the diet is considered a dietary supplement; this includes concentrates, metabolites, constituents, extracts, and combinations of listed ingredients. These supplements are no longer subject to premarket safety evaluations by the FDA. Once a supplement is marketed, under the DSHEA, the FDA can restrict its use only if it can be shown that the product is unsafe.

There are no regulations establishing criteria for purity, manufacturing procedures, or identification of ingredients for these supplements. Therefore the potential exists for high variability in the potency of different batches of the same botanic product. In addition, impurities and unknown substances may also be present in these products. Because herbal products are so readily available and have such widespread media attention, many people think that they can safely self-medicate (Patient, Family, and Caregiver Education). Another mistaken assumption is that dietary supplements are safer than prescribed or over-the-counter drugs.

Botanicals may initiate a pharmacologic response within the body and therefore should be considered as medications from a medical or nursing perspective. Many herbal products have effects that could be dangerous during surgery. Some herbal supplements may accentuate the toxicity of anesthetics or interfere with drug metabolism or clearance or even cause increased bleeding (Surgical Pharmacology). Herbal supplements may also have a role in the perioperative setting and are an important consideration for nurses.

Coagulation Interactions

Perioperative providers are concerned about the potential increased risk of instability intraoperatively resulting from inhibition of coagulation with the use of ginger, ginseng, ginkgo, and garlic (Wang et al., 2015). One difficulty with analyzing case reports is the lack of laboratory analysis of the purported botanicals. In some reported cases in which prolonged or excessive bleeding occurred, the patient had been taking multiple herb supplements and drugs. Many plants contain anticoagulant components, including ginger, ginseng, and others (Box 30.3); however, it is unknown if the danger posed is clinically significant.

TABLE 30.3

Languaging for Nurses: Enhancing Patient-Centered Communication

Positive, Therapeutic Language	Negative, Toxic Language
We're giving you the medication that will let you gently go to sleep.	We're going to put you to sleep now.
We are well trained in how to take care of you.	Don't be afraid.
I'll be with you the entire time to make sure you stay asleep and comfortable.	Don't worry; you won't wake up during surgery.
Focus your energy on healing.	Don't give up.
You might feel pressure; some people don't feel anything.	This isn't going to hurt. Just a little bee sting.

Data from Kourkouta L, Papathanasiou IV: Communication in nursing practice, *Mater Sociomed* 26(1):65–67, 2014.

BOX 30.3

Herbs That Affect Bleeding

Certain herbal preparations are known to affect bleeding. Careful preoperative screening for the following substances is essential:
- Dong quai
- Feverfew
- Garlic (high dose)
- Ginger
- *Ginkgo biloba*
- Ginseng
- Omega 3-fatty acid (high dose)
- Vitamin E (high dose)

Modified from University of Wisconsin Hospitals and Clinic Authority: *Medications, herbs and vitamins which affect bleeding* (website). www.uwhealth.org/healthfacts/cardiology/6404 .html. (Accessed 8 August 2016); Blumenthal RS et al: *Preventive cardiology: companion to Braunwald's heart disease*, Philadelphia, 2011, Elsevier; Miller R: *Miller's anesthesia*, ed 8, Philadelphia, 2015, Elsevier.

PATIENT, FAMILY, AND CAREGIVER EDUCATION

Advising Patients About Integrative Therapies

Nurses traditionally act as guides for patients as they navigate through the healthcare system, providing support, counseling, and advice. When providing education to patients about integrative therapies, the nurse should consider the overwhelming amount of information available via the Internet and popular media. The Internet is a popular source of information regarding the use of herbal and dietary supplements and other integrative therapies, but caution must be used in evaluating the validity of the information that is accessed. Nurses can use the following tips to educate their patients on accessing reliable information from the Internet. These tips are also useful for nurses to use when evaluating consumer information from the Internet.

Consider the Source: Use Recognized Authorities
- Know who is responsible for the content. Websites should have a way to contact the organization or webmaster. Use caution if you cannot find out who runs the website.
- Look for an "about us" page. Check to see who runs the site: Is it a branch of the federal government, a nonprofit institution, a professional organization, a health system, a commercial organization, or an individual?
- Scrutinize the source of the content. There is a big difference between a site that says, "I developed this site after my heart attack" and one that says, "This page on heart attack was developed by health professionals at the American Heart Association."

Focus on Quality: All Websites Are Not Created Equal
- Question whether the site has an editorial board. Is the information reviewed before it is posted? This information is often on the about us page, or it may be under the organization's mission statement or be part of the annual report.
- Determine whether the board members are experts in the subject of the site. For example, a site on osteoporosis whose medical advisory board is composed of attorneys and accountants is not medically authoritative.
- Look for a description of the process of selecting or approving information on the site. It is usually in the about us section and may be called "editorial policy," "selection policy," or "review policy." Sometimes the site will have information "about our writers" or "about our authors" instead of an editorial policy. Review this section to find out who has written the information.

Be a Cyberskeptic: Quackery Abounds on the Web
- Be skeptical if the site makes health claims that seem too good to be true. Does the information use deliberately obscure, "scientific"-sounding language? Does it promise quick, dramatic, miraculous results? Is this the only site making these claims?
- Beware of claims that one remedy will cure a variety of illnesses, that it is a "breakthrough," or that it relies on a "secret ingredient."

- Use caution if the site uses a sensational writing style (lots of exclamation points, for example). A health website for consumers should use simple language, not technical jargon.
- Get a second opinion! Check more than one site.

Look for the Evidence: Rely on Medical Research, Not Opinion
- Check to see if the site identifies the author for the content. Does it rely on testimonials?
- Look for the author of the information, either an individual or an organization. Good examples are "Written by Jane Smith, RN," or "Copyright 2017, American Cancer Society."
- Use caution when reading case histories or testimonials on the website. Look for contact information such as an email address or telephone number. If the testimonials are anonymous or hard to locate (e.g., "Jane from California"), be watchful.

Check for Currency: Look for the Latest Information
- Determine whether the information is current.
- Look for dates on documents. A document on coping with the loss of a loved one does not need to be current, but a document about the latest treatment of AIDS does.
- Click a few links on the site. If there are many broken links, the site may not be kept up to date.

Ask Who Pays for the Site, Beware of Bias: What Is the Purpose? Who Is Providing the Funding?
- Who pays for the site? Check to see if the site is supported by public funds, by donations, or by commercial advertising.
- Review any advertisements carefully. Advertisements should be labeled and should say "Advertisement" or "From Our Sponsor."
- Look at a page on the site, and see if it is clear when content is derived from a noncommercial source and when an advertiser provides it. For example, if a page about treatment of depression recommends one drug by name, see if you can tell if the company that manufactures the drug provides that information. If it does, you should consult other sources to see what they say about the same drug.

Protect Your Privacy: Health Information Should Be Confidential
- There should be a link saying "Privacy" or "Privacy Policy." Read the privacy policy to see if your privacy is really being protected. For example, if the site says "We share information with companies that can provide you with useful products," then your information is not private.
- If there is a registration form, check what questions you must answer before you can view the content. If you must provide personal information (such as address, date of birth, gender, mother's maiden name, credit card number) you should refer to the site's privacy policy to see what they can do with the information.

Modified from MedlinePlus: *MedlinePlus guide to healthy web surfing* (website). https://medlineplus.gov/healthywebsurfing.html. (Accessed 0 August 2016).

SURGICAL PHARMACOLOGY

Herbs: Effects and Precautions/Recommendations

The use of HDS has become increasingly popular as people become more educated consumers and take a more active interest in their health. Because herbal supplements and other nutraceuticals are available without prescription, patients may not reveal their use of these therapies unless specifically questioned. The perioperative nurse must always consider the possibility that the patient is taking supplements, and assess for their use. As with other medications the patient may be taking, the nurse is responsible to know the potential for interaction with medications used in the perioperative period. The information that follows offers a source for broadening the perioperative nurse's knowledge of commonly used herbal supplements.

Herb (Scientific Name) and Other Names	Dosage/ Route	Purpose/Action	Adverse Reactions	Nursing Implications
Black cohosh (*Cimicifuga racemosa*) Rattle root Squaw root	Oral	Antihypertensive; lowers cholesterol; reduces mucus production; induces labor to aid in childbirth; relieves menopausal symptoms (hot flashes)	May lead to premature labor if used in pregnancy	Avoid use in pregnancy
Cayenne (*Capsicum annuum*) Hot chili pepper Paprika	Topical or oral	External use: Muscle spasm or soreness Internal use: GI disorders	External: Skin irritation, especially if used longer than 2 days Internal: Lower GI discomfort; overdose may cause hypothermia	—
Dong quai (*Angelica polymorpha*)	Oral	Relieves menstrual disorders; increases effects of ovarian and testicular hormones	Dizziness, headache, nausea, miscarriage, dermatitis, GI upset, photosensitivity	Avoid use in pregnancy
Echinacea (*Echinacea purpurea, E. pallida, E. angustifolia*) Purple coneflower	Oral	Antiinfective; antiinflammatory; enhances immune function; may prevent or minimize symptoms and duration of common cold, URI; enhances wound-healing and burn-healing process	May activate T cells Cross allergic reaction Immune suppression if taken a long time	Discontinue as far in advance of surgery as possible Should not be used by patients with autoimmune diseases Should not be used by patients with allergy to sunflower Avoid use for transplant patients or those with liver dysfunction
Ephedra (*Ephedra sinica*) Ma Huang Mexican or Mormon tea Desert tea Natural ecstasy Natural fen-phen Ephedrine Chinese joint fir	Oral	Stimulant; bacteriostatic; antitussive; decongestant; bronchodilator; used for weight loss	HTN, tachycardia, dysrhythmias, cardiac arrest, myocardial infarction, nausea, vomiting, decreased GI motility, mydriasis, diuresis, anxiety, constipation, dizziness, headache, insomnia, psychosis, urine retention, seizure, stroke, uterine contractions	Do not use with cardiac glycosides, guanethidine, MAOI medications Do not use for patients with anxiety, HTN, glaucoma, enlarged prostate, or heart disease Discontinue use at least 24 h preoperatively Limit use to 7 days
Feverfew (*Tanacetum parthenium*) Featherfew Midsummer daisy	Oral	Antipyretic; relieves arthritis, fever, headache, and migraine pain; increases fluidity of respiratory mucus; promotes menses and uterine contractions	Oral lesions, GI tract irritation Rebound headache with sudden cessation Hypersensitive reaction in those allergic to ragweed, asters, chrysanthemums, or daisies May increase clotting time	Causes increased bleeding risk Avoid use preoperatively
Garlic (*Allium sativum*) Clove garlic Ajo Poor man's penicillin	Oral or topical	Antioxidant; antibiotic; lowers LDLs to prevent atherosclerosis; has antihypertensive, antiplatelet, and antithrombolytic properties	May prolong bleeding or clotting time, potentiate effects of antihypertensive or anticoagulant drugs	Large doses (>5 cloves) may cause GI upset, garlic breath/flatus Discontinue use at least 7 days preoperatively
Ginger (*Zingiber officinale*) African ginger Black ginger	Oral	Prevents nausea caused by motion sickness, pregnancy, chemotherapy, and anesthesia; antispasmodic	Heartburn Inhibition of platelet aggregation	Causes increased bleeding risk Avoid use preoperatively

SURGICAL PHARMACOLOGY

Herbs: Effects and Precautions/Recommendations—cont'd

Herb (Scientific Name) and Other Names	Dosage/ Route	Purpose/Action	Adverse Reactions	Nursing Implications
Ginkgo (*Ginkgo biloba*) Duck foot Kew tree Maidenhair tree Silver apricot Fossil tree	Oral	Antioxidant; anticlotting; enhances blood flow (especially to brain); reduces cellular lesions, retinal edema; treats symptoms of peripheral vascular disease and dementia; inhibits platelet-activating factors; used to enhance brain function and memory; treats headaches, depression, vertigo, and tinnitus	Headache, GI upset, palpitations, dizziness, or skin reactions	Causes increased bleeding risk Avoid use preoperatively Causes increased bleeding risk by inhibiting platelet activity, lowering fibrinogen levels, and decreasing plasma viscosity May potentiate anticoagulant therapy Discontinue use at least 36 h preoperatively
Ginseng American ginseng (*Panax quinquefolius*) Chinese ginseng or Korean ginseng (*Panax ginseng*) Siberian ginseng (*Eleutherococcus senticosus*)	Oral	Antioxidant; enhances memory and immune function; increases stamina; decreases fatigue; reduces stress response; lowers blood glucose level; inhibits clotting	Usually mild and dose-related: nervousness, dizziness, mastalgia "Ginseng abuse syndrome" (>15 g/d) = insomnia, hypotonia, and edema Siberian ginseng may falsely elevate digoxin levels; potentiate MAOIs	Contraindicated for patients with hypoglycemia, HTN, and cardiac disorders Avoid with other stimulants; may lead to tachycardia or HTN May decrease effectiveness of warfarin (decreased INR) May cause postmenopausal bleeding Discontinue use at least 7 days preoperatively
Goldenseal (*Hydrastis canadensis*) Orange or yellow root Ground raspberry Turmeric root Eye root	Oral	Antibacterial, antiinflammatory properties; diuretic (no sodium excreted); laxative; improves immune function; aids digestion; regulates menses	Hypotension, nausea, vomiting, abdominal cramping May exacerbate edema or hypertension May potentiate effects of insulin	May cause electrolyte imbalance, seizures, respiratory paralysis Avoid use preoperatively
Hawthorn (*Crataegus oxyacantha*) May bush May blossom Whitethorn	Oral	Antihypertensive; dilates coronary blood vessels; improves cardiovascular function (inotropic and beta-blocking effect); lowers cholesterol	Nausea, fatigue, sweating, headache, hypotension, mild CNS depression	Use caution with cardiac glycosides, CNS depressants, antihypertensives, and nitrates
Huang qi (*Astragalus membranaceus*)	Oral	Antibacterial; increases production of WBCs; immunostimulant; cardiotonic; energy tonic (strengthens wei qi); regulates water metabolism	Inhibits platelet aggregation and fibrinolysis	Causes increased bleeding risk
Kava kava (*Piper methysticum*) Awa, kawa Intoxicating pepper Tonga	Oral	Anxiolytic; mild sedative; muscle relaxant; sleep aid	Adverse effect on motor reflexes and judgment	Potentiates sedatives/ hypnotics Discontinue use at least 24 h preoperatively
Licorice (*Glycyrrhiza glabra*) Sweet root	Oral	Antipyretic; antiviral; demulcent; expectorant; beneficial for chronic fatigue, allergies, asthma, bronchitis, depression, emphysema, herpes, and hypoglycemia; treats gastritis and gastric and duodenal ulcers	May cause headache, muscle flaccidity, lethargy, edema, HTN, hypokalemia, or other electrolyte imbalance, and ECG changes (prolonged QT interval) Pseudoprimary aldosteronism a possible complication	Contraindicated for chronic liver conditions, renal insufficiency, hypertonia, or existing hypokalemia Avoid use for more than 7 consecutive days
Melatonin (Circadin, Melatol)	Oral	Sleep aid May be used in combination with cancer care	Drowsiness, headache, dizziness, or nausea	Can interact with various medications, including: blood-thinning medications, immunosuppressants, diabetes medications, birth control pills

Continued

SURGICAL PHARMACOLOGY

Herbs: Effects and Precautions/Recommendations—cont'd

Herb (Scientific Name) and Other Names	Dosage/Route	Purpose/Action	Adverse Reactions	Nursing Implications
Saw palmetto (*Serenoa repens*) Sabal cabbage palm	Oral	Relieves benign prostatic hypertrophy; has antiandrogenic and antiexudative properties	Headache, increased appetite	Causes additive effects with other hormone therapies
Senna (*Cassia senna*)	Oral	Stimulating laxative	Abdominal cramping; affects absorption in GI system	Causes potential electrolyte imbalance
St. John's wort (*Hypericum perforatum*) Amber touch-and-heal Goatweed Klamath weed	Oral and topical	Anxiolytic; antidepressant (mild to moderate symptoms), may take 4–6 wk for effect; relieves dyspepsia and insomnia; mechanism: inhibits uptake of neurotransmitters	Photosensitization, skin irritation, restlessness, fatigue May prolong effects of anesthesia and potentiate meperidine or other narcotics Possible peripheral neuropathy, serotonergic crisis	—
Valerian (*Valerian officinalis*) All heal Setwell Vandal root	Oral	Mild anxiolytic, muscle relaxant, hypnotic and sedative; may ease symptoms of benzodiazepine withdrawal	Headache, excitability, nausea, visual disturbance Potentiates sedative/hypnotics Long-term use may increase anesthesia tolerance Sudden cessation may cause withdrawal symptoms	Potentially prolongs anesthesia recovery time Treat withdrawal symptoms with benzodiazepines If possible, taper dose over 1–2 wk preoperatively; if not, continue use until surgery
Vitamin E (D-α-tocopherol)	Oral or topical	Oral: Antioxidant used for cardiovascular disease Topical: Reduce scars	Reduced platelet adhesion and aggregation	Causes increased bleeding risk
Yohimbe (*Pausinystalia yohimbe*)	Oral	Increases blood flow (particularly to genitalia) and libido	Anxiety, hallucinations, HTN, elevated heart rate, headache, dizziness, flushing	Avoid use by patients with psychologic or renal disorders

CNS, Central nervous system; *ECG*, electrocardiogram; *GI*, gastrointestinal; *HDS*, herbal and dietary supplements; *HTN*, hypertension; *INR*, international normalized ratio; *LDL*, low-density lipoprotein; *MAOI*, monoamine oxidase inhibitors; *URI*, urinary tract infection; *WBCs*, white blood cells.
Modified from Braun L, Cohen M: *Herbs and natural supplements, volume 2: an evidence-based guide*, ed 4, Sydney, Australia, 2015, Elsevier; Wang C et al: Commonly used dietary supplements on coagulation function during surgery, *Medicines (Basel)* 2(3):157–185, 2015; National Center for Complementary and Integrative Health (NCCIH): *Herbs at a glance* (website), 2016. https://nccih.nih.gov/health/herbsataglance.htm. (Accessed 25 August 2016).

Sedative Interactions

Some botanicals have significant sedative actions. Anesthesia providers are concerned about the potential for valerian and St. John's wort to prolong or potentiate the sedative effect of anesthetic agents. Valerian has been associated with central nervous system (CNS) depression and muscle relaxant effects in animals; large doses of valerian may contribute to delirium and high-output cardiac failure on emergence from general anesthesia. Although St. John's wort has been found to inhibit the binding of naloxone, no cases have been reported of excessive sedation when combined with narcotics. In addition, there is concern about the monoamine oxidase inhibitor (MAOI) activity of St. John's wort, although no cases of MAOI effects in humans have been reported (Wang et al., 2015).

Cardiovascular Interactions

Hypertension and cardiac dysrhythmias are potential adverse events that may result from the sympathetic stimulation that occurs during intubation and surgery. Ephedra has been associated with cardiovascular effects, including hypertension, palpitations, tachycardia, stroke, and seizures. Severe consequences of licorice use include hypertension and hypokalemia, which can case paralysis and torsades de pointes ventricular arrhythmia (White, 2014).

Because the use of botanic supplements may increase the risk of adverse herb–drug interactions, patients should be counseled to discontinue herbs preoperatively. Generally anesthesia providers recommend that patients stop taking any herbal supplement at least 2 weeks preoperatively (Wang et al., 2015). Most patients, however, do not see an anesthesia provider until the day of surgery or a few days before surgery, so the implementation of this recommendation is challenging. Clinical research is insufficient to quantify the actual dangers of these herbal supplements. Nonetheless, because individuals vary in their absorption, distribution, and clearance of the drugs administered during anesthesia, adding unknown chemicals into an already complex and fast-acting mix of drugs is likely an unnecessary risk.

Integrative Health Practices and Perioperative Patient Care

A variety of factors influence the perioperative patient's experience. Well-informed healthcare consumers increasingly choose a blend of traditional and nontraditional healing modalities with sensitivity to cultural, spiritual, and health education needs. Public involvement and legislative policy decisions are just beginning to equalize emphasis between the traditional biomedical model of care and a holistic comprehensive focus. Integrating health and wholeness incorporates

PATIENT SAFETY

Encouraging the Patient/Physician Relationship

Perioperative nurses can encourage safety in patients who use integrative health practices by promoting the National Center for Complementary and Integrative Health (NCCIH) Time to Talk education campaign. The goal of the campaign is to ensure safe and coordinated care for patients while helping minimize the risks of interaction with any conventional therapy in which the patient may be engaged. The campaign also seeks to inform and educate patients so they are empowered to make better healthcare decisions and more effectively manage their health. Videos are used online for patients to view as part of this campaign. Nurses can provide the following advice from NCCIH to patients as a starting point:

- Include all therapies and treatments you use when completing patient history forms. Make a list in advance. Also note all medical specialists or integrative practitioners you see. Take the list with you whenever you visit a healthcare provider.
- Tell your healthcare providers about all therapies or treatments, including over-the-counter and prescription medicines as well as herbal and dietary supplements.
- Take control. Do not wait for your providers to ask about your use of integrative therapies.
- Ask questions any time you are considering a new therapy; ask your healthcare providers about its safety, effectiveness, and possible interactions with medications (both prescription and over the counter).

Modified from National Center for Complementary and Integrative Health (NCCIH): *Time to talk campaign* (website). https://nccih.nih.gov/news/multimedia/gallery/asktell.htm. (Accessed 8 August 2016).

AMBULATORY SURGERY CONSIDERATIONS

Supporting Integrative Health Practices in the Ambulatory Surgical Setting

As advocates using the holistic approach, perioperative nurses play an important role in supporting patients who desire to use integrative health practices in ambulatory perioperative settings. It is important to balance the use of conventional and nonconventional interventions in respecting the patient's wishes and providing safe care. Many integrative interventions are well suited to the ambulatory setting, including music therapy, relaxation exercises, aromatherapy, and energy interventions. The perioperative nurse ensures that any healthcare personnel using integrative practices do so under the institution's policies and procedures. The nurse also documents use of these interventions in the perioperative nursing record along with the patient's response.

In the educator role, the nurse may be able to partner with patients to empower them to research the safety and efficacy of the techniques they are using. The preoperative assessment offers a prime opportunity for the nurse to identify possible safety risks for the perioperative patient. Whenever possible, the preoperative assessment should be conducted a few days before the planned surgical procedure to allow ample time to gather data and begin patient teaching in a controlled, unhurried setting versus the typical fast pace that occurs on the patient's day of admission to the ambulatory surgery setting. The nurse can use this time to educate patients about the effect of integrative health practices in the perioperative period and beyond. By obtaining information in advance about the patient's use of medications, herbs, vitamins, dietary supplements, and the like, the nurse can effect safe care by advising the patient to consult with the surgeon and modify the treatment regimen to avoid anesthetic complications.

Preoperative assessments also allow a forum to educate patients about the need to obtain reliable information about integrative health practices. The nurse reminds the patient that results should be supported by clinical trials and that information on the Internet may be commercial in nature rather than scientific (see Patient, Family, and Caregiver Education box on p. 1157). Patients who use integrative practices need to notify their physician if any side effects occur.

Modified from Association of periOperative Registered Nurses (AORN): Guideline for complementary care interventions. In Burlingame B et al, editors; *Guidelines for perioperative practice*, vol. 1, Denver, 2016, The Association; Dossey BM, Guzzetta CE: Holistic nursing practice. In Dossey BM et al, editors: *Holistic nursing, a handbook for practice*, ed 7, Burlington, MA, 2016, Jones & Bartlett.

elements of self-responsibility for wellness and self-awareness to inner changes on the part of the patient.

A collaborative partnership of professionals involved in an individual's care optimizes resources that promote comprehensive, effective, less-invasive, and nonpharmacologic adjuncts to allopathic medical treatment (Patient Safety). Perioperative nurses using available resources on interactions among prescriptions, dietary supplements, and herbals ensure preoperative medication safety. Seeking out and participating in appropriate research methodologies are essential for grounding the diverse components of our practice in evidence-based knowledge.

Documenting integrative health practices may involve noting herbals or the dietary supplement regimen the patient followed preoperatively. The nurse should also note whether these were discontinued and, if so, when. Nurse energy work practitioners who comply with a patient's request for energy treatment may refer to the North American Nursing Diagnosis Association (NANDA International) diagnosis Disturbed Energy Field when comfort measures such as TT, healing touch, or Reiki are provided by the perioperative nurse.

Integrative health practices and therapies have a place in each perioperative nurse's practice (Ambulatory Surgery Considerations). Nursing history demonstrates a philosophic attitude of altruism and compassion, founded in creating an environment of healing. Awareness of how vital self-care practices are to sustaining a caregiver role may ultimately benefit the practice. Self-care learning and meditative experiences may come full circle by enhancing the caregiver's therapeutic use of self through presence, compassion, and holistic assessment skills.

Key Points

- The *comprehensive approach* takes into account multidimensional factors that may not easily or appropriately be studied independently. The comprehensive approach is more congruent with the philosophic underpinnings of most integrative health practices.
- The *biomedical approach* is concerned with a disease orientation, suggesting that a specific agent or variable is responsible for a specific disorder or illness.

- The NCCIH generally uses the terms "complementary health approaches" when discussing practices and products of nonmainstream origin, and uses "integrative health" when talking about incorporating approaches into mainstream healthcare.

- Most complementary health approaches fall into one of two subgroups: natural products (herbs, vitamins, and minerals) or mind and body practices (yoga, chiropractic manipulation, meditation, massage therapy, acupuncture, Reiki, healing touch, guided imagery, and music therapy). Traditional healing practices such as Ayurvedic medicine, traditional Chinese medicine, homeopathy, and naturopathy may not neatly fit into these subgroups but are also other complementary health approaches.

- Naturopathic medicine emphasizes health restoration as well as disease treatment based on the belief that disease is a manifestation of alterations in the body's natural healing processes.

- Touch and manipulations with the hands have been used in healing and medical practice since the beginning of the history of medicine.

- To use the term *alternative* is actually misleading. Many progressive medical facilities embrace a holistic patient focus, exploring and integrating nontraditional healing modalities to support an individualized surgical experience.

- As pharmacology combines medications to potentiate effect, aromatherapy may act synergistically with traditional treatment; or it may be offered in concert with other complementary modalities to relieve discomfort, reducing dosages of analgesics or sedatives.

- Because the use of botanic supplements may increase the risk of adverse herb–drug interactions, patients should be counseled to discontinue herbs preoperatively. Generally anesthesia providers recommend that patients stop taking any herbal supplement at least 2 weeks preoperatively.

- Well-informed healthcare consumers increasingly choose a blend of traditional and nontraditional healing modalities with sensitivity to cultural, spiritual, and health education needs.

- Documenting integrated care may involve noting herbals or the dietary supplement regimen the patient followed preoperatively. The nurse should also note whether these were discontinued and, if so, when.

Critical Thinking Question

While assessing your preoperative patient undergoing a right total knee replacement, you notice he is visibly upset about the operation. He will not make eye contact, seems to have a slight tremor in his hand, and is sweating. Further discussion with the patient reveals that he is particularly upset about having nausea and vomiting in the PACU stating "after my gallbladder surgery I was sick to my stomach for hours." He is also worried about postoperative pain and the effects of pain medication. What type of holistic intervention can you offer this patient in the perioperative setting?

evolve *The answer to the Critical Thinking Question can be found at http://evolve.elsevier.com/Rothrock/Alexander.*

References

Association of periOperative Registered Nurses (AORN): Guideline for complementary care interventions. In Burlingame B et al, editors: *Guidelines for perioperative practice*, vol 1, Denver, 2016, The Association.

Chou R et al: Management of postoperative pain: a clinical practice guideline from the American Pain Society, the American Society of Regional Anesthesia and Pain Medicine, and the American Society of Anesthesiologists' Committee on Regional Anesthesia, Executive Committee, and Administrative Council, *J Pain* 17(2):131–157, 2016.

Dossey BM, Keegan L: *Holistic nursing: a handbook for practice*, ed 6, Burlington, MA, 2016, Jones & Bartlett Learning.

Kitaeff R: Nonpharmacologic control of pain. In Pizzorno JE, Murray MT, editors: *Textbook of natural medicine*, ed 4, St Louis, 2013, Churchill Livingstone.

Labrague LJ, McEnroe-Petitte DM: Preoperative anxiety and physiologic parameters in women undergoing gynecologic surgery, *Clin Nurs Res* 25(2):157–173, 2016.

Lindquist R et al: *Complementary and alternative therapies in nursing*, ed 7, New York, 2014, Springer.

Micozzi MS: Translation from conventional medicine. In Micozzi MS, editor: *Fundamentals of complementary and integrative medicine*, ed 5, St Louis, 2015, Saunders.

National Center for Complementary and Integrative Health (NCCIH): *Complementary, alternative, or integrative health: what's in a name?* (website), 2016a. https://nccih.nih.gov/health/integrative-health. (Accessed 6 October 2016).

National Center for Complementary and Integrative Health (NCCIH): *Reiki: In depth* (website), 2016b. https://nccih.nih.gov/health/reiki/introduction.htm. (Accessed 25 August 2016).

National Center for Complementary and Integrative Health (NCCIH): *The NIH almanac* (website), 2016c. www.nih.gov/about-nih/what-we-do/nih-almanac/national-center-complementary-integrative-health-nccih. (Accessed 1 August 2016).

National Center for Complementary and Integrative Health (NCCIH): *The use and cost of complementary health approaches in the United States* (website), 2016d. https://nccih.nih.gov/about/strategic-plans/2016/use-cost-complementary-health-approaches. (Accessed 2 August 2016).

National Center for Complementary and Integrative Health (NCCIH): *Yoga as a Complementary Health Approach* (website), 2016e. https://nccih.nih.gov/news/multimedia/infographics/yoga. (Accessed 3 August 2016).

Nightingale F: *Notes on nursing*, London, 1859, JB Lippincott.

Notte BB et al: Reiki's effect on patients with total knee arthroscopy: a pilot study, *Nursing* 46(2):17–23, 2016.

Perlman A: Complementary and alternative medicine. In Goldman L, Schafer AI, editors: *Goldman-Cecil medicine*, ed 25, Philadelphia, 2016, Elsevier.

Sites DS et al: Controlled breathing with or without peppermint aromatherapy for postoperative nausea and/or vomiting symptom relief: a randomized controlled trial, *J Perianesth Nurs* 29(1):12–19, 2014.

Stea S et al: Essential oils for complementary treatment of surgical patients: state of the art, *Evid Based Complement Alternat Med* 2014:726341, 2014.

Tagge EP et al: Psychoneuroimmunology and the pediatric surgeon, *Semin Pediatr Surg* 22(3):144–148, 2013.

Ujam A et al: Herbal preparations in head & neck surgery—friend or foe?, *Br J Oral Maxillofac Surg* 52(8):e61–e62, 2014.

Wang C et al: Commonly used dietary supplements on coagulation function during surgery, *Medicines* 2(3):157–185, 2015.

White JD: Complementary and alternative medicine. In *Abeloff's clinical oncology*, ed 4, Philadelphia, 2014, Elsevier.

Laboratory Values

Reference Intervals^a for Clinical Chemistry (Blood, Serum, and Plasma)

Analyte	Conventional Units	SI Units
Acetoacetate plus acetone		
Qualitative	Negative	Negative
Quantitative	0.3–2 mg/dL	30–200 µmol/L
Acid phosphatase, serum (thymolphthalein monophosphate substrate)	0.1–0.6 units/L	0.1–0.6 units/L
ACTH (see Corticotropin)		
Alanine aminotransferase (ALT), serum (SGPT)	1–45 units/L	1–45 units/L
Albumin, serum	33–52 g/L	33–52 g/L
Aldolase, serum	0–7 units/L	0–7 units/L
Aldosterone, plasma		
Standing	5–30 ng/dL	140–830 pmol/L
Recumbent	3–10 ng/dL	80–275 pmol/L
Alkaline phosphatase (ALP), serum		
Adult	35–150 units/L	35–150 units/L
Adolescent	100–500 units/L	100–500 units/L
Child	100–350 units/L	100–350 units/L
Ammonia nitrogen, plasma	10–50 µmol/L	10–50 µmol/L
Amylase, serum	25–125 units/L	25–125 units/l
Anion gap, serum calculated	8–16 mEq/L	8–16 mmol/L
Ascorbic acid, blood	0.4–1.5 mg/dL	23–85 µmol/L
Aspartate aminotransferase (AST), serum (SGOT)	1–36 units/L	1–36 units/L
Base excess, arterial blood, calculated	0 ± 2 mEq/L	0 ± 2 mmol/L
Bicarbonate		
Venous plasma	23–29 mEq/L	23–29 mmol/L
Arterial blood	21–27 mEq/L	21–27 mmol/L
Bile acids, serum	0.3–3 mg/dL	0.8–7.6 mmol/L
Bilirubin, serum		
Conjugated	0.1–0.4 mg/dL	1.7–6.8 µmol/L
Total	0.3–1.1 mg/dL	5.1–19 µmol/L
Calcium, serum	8.4–10.6 mg/dL	2.10–2.65 mmol/L
Calcium, ionized, serum	4.25–5.25 mg/dL	1.05–1.30 mmol/L
Carbon dioxide, total, serum or plasma	24–31 mEq/L	24–31 mmol/L
Carbon dioxide tension (Pco$_2$), blood	35–45 mm Hg	35–45 mm Hg
β-Carotene, serum	60–260 mcg/dL	1.1–8.6 µmol/L
Ceruloplasmin, serum	23–44 mg/dL	230–440 mg/L
Chloride	96–106 mEq/L	96–106 mmol/L
Cholesterol, serum or EDTA plasma		
Desirable range	<200 mg/dL	<5.20 mmol/L
Low-density lipoprotein (LDL) cholesterol	60–180 mg/dL	1.55–4.65 mmol/L
High-density lipoprotein (HDL) cholesterol	30–80 mg/dL	0.80–2.05 mmol/L
Copper	70–140 mcg/dL	11–22 µmol/L
Corticotropin (ACTH), plasma, 8 AM	10–80 pg/mL	2–18 pmol/L
Cortisol, plasma		
8:00 AM	6–23 mcg/dL	170–630 µmol/L
4:00 PM	3–15 mcg/dL	80–410 µmol/L
10:00 PM	<50% of 8:00 AM value	<50% of 8:00 AM value

Continued

Reference Intervals[a] for Clinical Chemistry (Blood, Serum, and Plasma)—cont'd

Analyte	Conventional Units	SI Units
Creatine, serum		
Males	0.2–0.5 mg/dL	15–40 µmol/L
Females	0.3–0.9 mg/dL	25–70 µmol/L
Creatine kinase (CK), serum		
Males	55–170 units/L	55–170 units/L
Females	30–135 units/L	30–135 units/L
Creatine kinase MB isoenzyme, serum	<5% of total CK activity	<5% of total CK activity
	<5 ng/mL by immunoassay	<5 ng/mL by immunoassay
Creatinine, serum	0.6–1.2 mg/dL	50–110 µmol/L
Erythrocytes	145–540 ng/mL	330–120 nmol/L
Estradiol-17 β, adult		
Males	10–65 pg/mL	35–240 pmol/L
Females		
Follicular	30–100 pg/mL	110–370 pmol/L
Ovulatory	200–400 pg/mL	730–1470 pmol/L
Luteal	50–140 pg/mL	180–510 pmol/L
Ferritin, serum	20–200 ng/mL	20–200 mcg/L
Fibrinogen, plasma	200–400 mg/dL	2–4 g/L
Folate, serum	3–18 ng/mL	6.8–41 nmol/L
Follicle-stimulating hormone (FSH), plasma		
Males	4–25 mU/mL	4–25 units/L
Females, premenopausal	4–30 mU/mL	4–30 units/L
Females, postmenopausal	40–250 mU/mL	40–250 units/L
Gastrin, fasting, serum	0–100 pg/mL	0–100 mg/L
Glucose, fasting, plasma or serum	70–115 mg/dL	3.9–6.4 nmol/L
γ-Glutamyltransferase (GGT), serum	5–40 units/L	5–40 units/L
Growth hormone (hGH), plasma, adult, fasting	0–6 ng/mL	0–6 mcg/L
Haptoglobin, serum	20–165 mg/dL	0.20–1.65 g/L
Immunoglobulins, serum (see table, Reference Intervals for Tests of Immunologic Function)		
Iron, serum	75–175 mcg/dL	13–31 µmol/L
Iron-binding capacity, serum		
Total	250–410 mcg/dL	45–73 µmol/L
Saturation	20%–55%	0.20–0.55
Lactate		
Venous whole blood	5–20 mg/dL	0.6–2.2 mmol/L
Arterial whole blood	5–15 mg/dL	0.6–1.7 mmol/L
Lactate dehydrogenase (LD), serum	110–220 units/L	110–220 units/L
Lipase, serum	10–140 units/L	10–140 units/L
Lutropin (LH), serum		
Males	1–9 units/L	1–9 units/L
Females		
Follicular phase	2–10 units/L	2–10 units/L
Midcycle peak	15–65 units/L	15–65 units/L
Luteal phase	1–12 units/L	1–12 units/L
Postmenopausal	12–65 units/L	12–65 units/L
Magnesium, serum	1.3–2.1 mg/dL	0.65–1.05 mmol/L
Osmolality	275–295 mOsm/kg water	275–295 mOsm/kg water
Oxygen, blood, arterial, room air		
Partial pressure (PaO$_2$)	80–100 mm Hg	80–100 mm Hg
Saturation (SaO$_2$)	95%–98%	95%–98%
pH, arterial blood	7.35–7.45	7.35–7.45
Phosphate, inorganic, serum		
Adult	3–4.5 mg/dL	1–1.5 mmol/L
Child	4–7 mg/dL	1.3–2.3 mmol/L
Potassium		
Serum	3.5–5 mEq/L	3.5–5 mmol/L
Plasma	3.5–4.5 mEq/L	3.5–4.5 mmol/L
Progesterone, serum, adult		
Males	0–0.4 ng/mL	0–1.3 mmol/L
Females		
Follicular phase	0.1–1.5 ng/mL	0.3–4.8 mmol/L
Luteal phase	2.5–28 ng/mL	8–89 mmol/L

Reference Intervals[a] for Clinical Chemistry (Blood, Serum, and Plasma)—cont'd

Analyte	Conventional Units	SI Units
Prolactin, serum		
Males	1–15 ng/mL	1–15 mcg/L
Females	1–20 ng/mL	1–20 mcg/L
Protein, serum, electrophoresis		
Total	6–8 g/dL	60–80 g/L
Albumin	3.5–5.5 g/dL	35–55 g/L
Globulins		
α_1	0.2–0.4 g/dL	2–4 g/L
α_2	0.5–0.9 g/dL	5–9 g/L
β	0.6–1.1 g/dL	6–11 g/L
γ	0.7–1.7 g/dL	7–17 g/L
Pyruvate, blood	0.3–0.9 mg/dL	0.03–0.10 mmol/L
Rheumatoid factor	0–30 IU/mL	0–30 kIU/L
Sodium, serum or plasma	135–145 mEq/L	135–145 mmol/L
Testosterone, plasma		
Men	300–1200 ng/dL	10.4–41.6 nmol/L
Women	20–75 ng/dL	0.7–2.6 nmol/L
Pregnant	40–200 ng/dL	1.4–6.9 nmol/L
Thyroglobulin	3–42 ng/mL	3–42 mcg/L
Thyrotropin (hTSH), serum	0.4–4.8 μIU/mL	0.4–4.8 mIU/L
Thyrotropin-releasing hormone (TRH)	5–60 pg/mL	5–60 ng/L
Thyroxine free (FT_4), serum	0.9–2.1 ng/dL	12–27 pmol/L
Thyroxine (T_4), serum	4.5–12 mg/dL	58–154 nmol/L
Thyroxine-binding globulin (TBG)	15–34 mcg/mL	15–34 mg/L
Transferrin	250–430 mg/dL	2.5–4.3 g/L
Triglycerides, serum, 12-h fast	40–150 mg/dL	0.4–1.5 g/L
Triiodothyronine (T_3), serum	70–190 ng/dL	1.1–2.9 nmol/L
Triiodothyronine uptake, resin (T_3RU)	25%–38%	0.25%–0.38%
Troponin I	0.05–0.50 ng/mL	0.05–0.50 ng/mL
Urate		
(FT_4) Males	2.5–8 mg/dL	150–480 μmol/L
(FT_4) Females	2.2–7 mg/dL	130–420 μmol/L
Urea, serum or plasma	24–49 mg/dL	4–8.2 nmol/L
Urea nitrogen, serum or plasma	11–23 mg/dL	8–16.4 nmol/L
Viscosity, serum	1.4–1.8 ∞ water	1.4–1.8 ∞ water
Vitamin A, serum	20–80 mcg/dL	0.70–2.80 μmol/L
Vitamin B_{12}, serum	180–900 pg/mL	133–664 pmol/L

EDTA, Ethylenediaminetetraacetic acid; *SI*, International System of Units.
[a]Reference values may vary depending on the method and sample source used.

Reference Intervals[a] for Clinical Chemistry (Urine)

Analyte	Conventional Units	SI Units
Acetone and acetoacetate, qualitative	Negative	Negative
Albumin		
Qualitative	Negative	Negative
Quantitative	10–100 mg/24 h	0.15–1.5 μmol/d
Aldosterone	3–20 mcg/24 h	8.3–55 nmol/d
δ-Aminolevulinic acid (δ-ALA)	1.3–7 mg/24 h	10–53 μmol/d
Amylase	<17 units/h	<17 units/h
Amylase-to-creatinine clearance ratio	0.01–0.04	0.01–0.04
Bilirubin, qualitative	Negative	Negative
Calcium (regular diet)	<250 mg/24 h	<6.3 nmol/d
Catecholamines		
Epinephrine	<10 mcg/24 h	<55 nmol/d
Norepinephrine	<100 mcg/24 h	<590 nmol/d
Total free catecholamines	4–126 mcg/24 h	24–745 nmol/d
Total metanephrines	0.1–1.6 mg/24 h	0.5–8.1 μmol/d
Chloride (varies with intake)	110–250 mEq/24 h	110–250 mmol/d

Continued

Reference Intervals[a] for Clinical Chemistry (Urine)—cont'd

Analyte	Conventional Units	SI Units
Copper	0–50 mcg/24 h	0–0.80 μmol/d
Cortisol, free	10–100 mcg/24 h	27.6–276 nmol/d
Creatine		
Males	0–40 mg/24 h	0–0.30 mmol/d
Females	0–80 mg/24 h	0–0.60 mmol/d
Creatinine	15–25 mg/kg/24 h	0.13–0.22 mmol/kg/d
Creatinine clearance (endogenous)		
Males	110–150 mL/min/1.73 m²	110–150 mL/min/1.73 m²
Females	105–132 mL/min/1.73 m²	105–132 mL/min/1.73 m²
Cystine or cysteine	Negative	Negative
Dehydroepiandrosterone		
Males	0.2–2 mg/24 h	0.7–6.9 μmol/d
Females	0.2–1.8 mg/24 h	0.7–6.2 μmol/d
Estrogens, total		
Males	4–25 mcg/24 h	14–90 nmol/d
Females	5–100 mcg/24 h	18–360 nmol/d
Glucose (as reducing substance)	<250 mg/24 h	<250 mg/d
Hemoglobin and myoglobin, qualitative	Negative	Negative
Homogentisic acid, qualitative	Negative	Negative
17-Hydroxycorticosteroids		
Males	3–9 mg/24 h	8.3–25 μmol/d
Females	2–8 mg/24 h	5.5–22 μmol/d
5-Hydroxyindoleacetic acid		
Qualitative	Negative	Negative
Quantitative	2–6 mg/24 h	10–31 μmol/d
17-Ketogenic steroids		
Males	5–23 mg/24 h	17–80 μmol/d
Females	3–15 mg/24 h	10–52 μmol/d
17-Ketosteroids		
Males	8–22 mg/24 h	28–76 μmol/d
Females	6–15 mg/24 h	21–52 μmol/d
Magnesium	6–10 mEq/24 h	3–5 mmol/d
Metanephrines	0.05–1.2 ng/mg creatinine	0.03–0.70 mmol/mmol creatinine
Osmolality	38–1400 mOsm/kg water	38–1400 mOsm/kg water
pH	4.6–8	4.6–8
Phenylpyruvic acid, qualitative	Negative	Negative
Phosphate	0.4–1.3 g/24 h	13–42 mmol/d
Porphobilinogen		
Qualitative	Negative	Negative
Quantitative	<2 mg/24 h	<9 μmol/d
Porphyrins		
Coproporphyrin	50–250 mcg/24 h	77–380 nmol/d
Uroporphyrin	10–30 mcg/24 h	12–36 nmol/d
Potassium	25–125 mEq/24 h	25–125 mmol/d
Pregnanediol		
Males	0–1.9 mg/24 h	0–6 μmol/d
Females		
Proliferative phase	0–2.6 mg/24 h	0–8 μmol/d
Luteal phase	2.6–10.6 mg/24 h	8–33 μmol/d
Postmenopausal	0.2–1 mg/24 h	0.6–3.1 μmol/d
Pregnanetriol	0–2.5 mg/24 h	0–7.4 μmol/d
Protein, total		
Qualitative	Negative	Negative
Quantitative	10–150 mg/24 h	10–150 mg/d
Protein-to-creatinine ratio	<0.2	<0.2
Sodium (regular diet)	60–260 mEq/24 h	60–260 mmol/d
Specific gravity		
Random specimen	1.003–1.030	1.003–1.030
24-h collection	1.015–1.025	1.015–1.025
Urate (regular diet)	250–750 mg/24 h	1.5–4.4 mmol/d
Urobilinogen	0.5–4 mg/24 h	0.6–6.8 μmol/d
Vanillylmandelic acid (VMA)	1–8 mg/24 h	5–40 μmol/d

d, Day; *h,* hour; *SI,* International System of Units.

[a]Values can vary depending on the method used.

Reference Intervals for Tests Performed on Cerebrospinal Fluid (CSF)

Test	Conventional Units	SI Units
Cells	<5/mm^3; all mononuclear	<5 × 10^6/L; all mononuclear
Glucose	50–75 mg/dL	2.8–4.2 mmol/L
	(20 mg/dL less than in serum)	(1.1 mmol less than in serum)
IgG		
Children less than 14 yr	<8% of total protein	<0.08 of total protein
Adults	<14% of total protein	<0.14 of total protein
IgG index	0.3–0.6	0.3–0.6
Oligoclonal banding on electrophoresis	Absent	Absent
Protein electrophoresis	Albumin predominant	Albumin predominant
Pressure, opening	70–180 mm H$_2$O	70–180 mm H$_2$O
Protein, total	15–45 mg/dL	150–450 mg/L

IgG, Immunoglobulin G; *SI,* International System of Units.

From *Mosby's dictionary of medicine, nursing, and health professions,* ed 10, St Louis, 2017, Elsevier.

Illustration Credits

Chapter 1

1.1, Courtesy University of Pennsylvania School of Medicine, Philadelphia; **1.3,** From Christiana Care Health System, Newark, DE; **1.4,** From Titler MG et al: The Iowa model of evidence-based practice to promote quality care, *Crit Care Nurs Clin North Am* 13(4):497–509, 2001.

Chapter 2

2.1, From Robinson NL: Promoting patient safety with perioperative handoff communication, *J Perianesth Nurs* 31(3):245–253, 2016; **2.2,** From Seifert PC, Peterson E, Graham K: Crisis management of fire in the OR, *AORN J* 101(2):250–263, 2015.

Chapter 3

3.1, From Waters T et al: AORN ergonomic tool 1: lateral transfer of a patient from a stretcher to an OR bed, *AORN J* 93(3):334–339, 2011; **3.2,** From Nancy Hughes, 2009, American Nurses Association.

Chapter 4

4.1, Courtesy Charleston Area Medical Center, Charleston, WV; **4.3,** From Fuller JR: *Surgical technology,* ed 6, St Louis, 2013, Saunders; **4.4,** From Fuller JR: *Surgical technology,* ed 4, St Louis, 2005, Saunders; **4.5, 4.7, 4.9C,** Courtesy STERIS Corp., Mentor, OH; **4.9A and B,** Reprinted with permission from Advanced Sterilization Products. STERRAD is a registered trademark of Advanced Sterilization Products, Division of Ethicon, Inc.

Chapter 5

5.4, Redrawn from Whitten C: *Anyone can intubate,* ed 4, San Diego, 1997, K-W Publications.

Chapter 6

6.1, From Loeper JM et al: *Therapeutic positioning and skin care,* Minneapolis, 1986, Sister Kenny Institute; **6.2, 6.3, 6.4,** Courtesy Molnlycke Health Care US, LLC; **6.5, 6.6, 6.12, 6.13,** Courtesy Kendall-LTP; **6.9, 6.16, 6.27, 6.32, 6.38,** From Miller RD et al: *Miller's anesthesia,* ed 7, Philadelphia, 2009, Churchill Livingstone; **6.10,** Modified from Martin JT: *Positioning in anesthesia and surgery,* ed 2, Philadelphia, 1987, Saunders; **6.17,** From Munro D: The perioperative nurse's role in table-enhanced anterior total hip arthroplasty, *AORN J* 90(1):57, 2009; **6.18,** Courtesy Mizuho OSI, Unionville, CA; **6.21,** Courtesy HoverTech International, Fountain Hill, PA; **6.23,** From Chitlik A: Safe positioning for robotic-assisted laparoscopic prostatectomy, *AORN J* 94(1):39, 2011; **6.24,** From Shveiky D et al: Brachial plexus injury after laparoscopic and robotic surgery, *J Minim Invasive Gynecol* 17(4):419, 2010; **6.29,** From Bennicoff G: Perioperative care of the morbidly obese patient in the lithotomy position, *AORN J* 92(3):297–312, 2010; **6.30,** Courtesy Allen Medical Systems,

Acton, MA; **6.31, 6.35, 6.36,** From St-Arnaud D: Safe positioning for neurosurgical patients, *AORN J* 87(6):1167, 2008; **6.37,** Courtesy SchureMed, Abington, MA.

Chapter 7

7.2, From Mitchell R et al: Clinical applications of barbed suture in aesthetic breast surgery, *Clin Plast Surg* 42(4):595–604, 2015; **7.3,** From Robinson JK, Hanke CW, Siegel DM: *Surgery of the skin,* ed 3, Philadelphia, 2015, Elsevier; **7.4, 7.8,** From Pfenninger JL, Fowler GC: *Pfenninger and Fowler's procedures for primary care,* ed 3, Philadelphia, 2011, Elsevier. **7.5, 7.6, 7.10,** From Davis and Geck: *Surgical atlas and suture guide,* ed 2, Wayne, NJ, 1992, American Cyanamid Co.; **7.7,** From Phillips N: *Berry & Kohn's operating room technique,* ed 12, St Louis, 2013, Mosby; **7.9,** From Meehan JJ, Sawin R: Robotic lateral pancreaticojejunostomy (Puestow), *J Pediatr Surg* 46(6):e5–e8, 2011; **7.11,** Courtesy 3M, St Paul, MN; **7.12,** From Toriumi DM, Chung VK, Cappelle QM: Surgical adhesives in facial plastic surgery, *Otolaryngol Clin North Am* 49(3):585–599, 2016; **7.13, 7.14, 7.15, 7.16, 7.17, 7.18, 7.19,** From Baggish MS, Karram MM: *Atlas of pelvic anatomy and gynecologic surgery,* ed 4, St Louis, 2016, Elsevier; **7.20,** From Falcone T, Goldberg JM: *Basic, advanced, and robotic laparoscopic surgery,* Philadelphia, 2010, Elsevier; **7.21,** From Nogueira JF, Stamm A, Vellutini E et al: Evolution of endoscopic skull base surgery, current concepts, and future perspectives, *Otolaryngol Clin North Am* 43(3):639–652, 2010; **7.24,** From Roberts JR: *Roberts and Hedges' clinical procedures in emergency medicine,* ed 6, Philadelphia, 2014, Elsevier.

Chapter 8

8.2, 8.5, 8.8, 8.9, 8.11, 8.14, 8.15, 8.17, 8.57, 8.59, 8.65, From Ball KA: *Endoscopic surgery,* St Louis, 1997, Mosby; **8.3, 8.32, 8.39,** Courtesy Gyrus-ACMI, Southborough, MA; **8.4,** Courtesy HGM Medical Laser Systems, Santa Clara, CA; **8.6, 8.26, 8.27, 8.30,** Courtesy Olympus Surgical America, Orangeburg, NY; **8.7,** Courtesy Endoscopy Support Services, Inc., Brewster, NY; **8.10,** From Tighe SM: *Instrumentation for the operating room,* ed 8, St Louis, 2012, Mosby; **8.12, 8.16, 8.18, 8.21, 8.24,** Copyright © 2010 Covidien. All rights reserved. Used with the permission of Covidien; **8.13,** From Applied Medical Inc., Rancho Santa Margarita, CA; **8.19, 8.20, 8.47, 8.64,** Courtesy Ethicon Endo-Surgery, Cincinnati; **8.25,** Courtesy Medivators, a Minntech Corporation Business Group, Minneapolis, www.medivators.com; **8.31,** From New Wave Surgical Corp., Coral Springs, FL; **8.33, 8.34, 8.35, 8.36, 8.37,** From Intuitive Surgical, Inc., Sunnyvale, CA; **8.40, 8.41, 8.43,** Courtesy Valleylab, Inc., Boulder, CO; **8.42,** From Spruce L, Braswell ML: Implementing AORN recommended practices for electrosurgery, *AORN J* 95(3):373–384, 2012; **8.44,** From Megadyne Medical Products Inc., Draper, UT; **8.45, 8.46,** Courtesy Megadyne Medical Products Inc.,

Draper, UT; **8.49, 8.50,** Courtesy Encision, Boulder, CO; **8.60,** Courtesy I.C. Medical Inc., Phoenix, AZ; **8.61,** From ConMed Electrosurgery, Centennial, CO.

Chapter 9

9.1, From Herlihy B: *The human body in health and illness*, ed 5, St Louis, 2014, Saunders; **9.2,** From Ignatavicius DD, Workman ML: *Medical-surgical nursing: patient-centered collaborative care*, ed 8, St Louis, 2016, Elsevier; **9.3,** From Townsend CM, et al: *Sabiston textbook of surgery*, ed 20, Philadelphia, 2017, Elsevier; **9.4,** From Harkreader H et al: *Fundamentals of nursing: caring and clinical judgment*, ed 3, St Louis, 2007, Saunders; **9.5,** Courtesy KCI, San Antonio, TX; **9.6,** From Ignatavicius DD, Workman ML: *Medical-surgical nursing: patient-centered collaborative care*, ed 7, St Louis, 2013, Saunders; **9.7C and D,** Courtesy CR Bard, Inc., Murray Hill, NJ.

Chapter 10

10.1, 10.2, From Litwack K: *Post anesthesia care nursing*, ed 2, St Louis, 1995, Mosby; **10.3, 10.4,** From Monahan FD et al: *Phipps' medical-surgical nursing: health and illness perspectives*, ed 8, St Louis, 2007, Mosby; **10.5,** Reproduced with permission. Copyright © 2017 3M. All rights reserved; **10.6,** From Nagelhout JJ, Elisha S: *Nurse anesthesia*, ed 6, St Louis, 2018, Saunders; **10.7,** From Gan T, Meyer T, Apfel C et al: Consensus guidelines for the management of postoperative nausea and vomiting, *Anesthes Analg* 118(1):85–113, 2014; **10.8,** From Apfel CC: Postoperative nausea and vomiting. In Miller RD et al: *Miller's anesthesia*, ed 8, Philadelphia, 2015, Saunders; **10.9,** From Acute Pain Management Guideline Panel: *Acute pain management in adults: operative procedures: quick reference guide for clinicians*, AHCPR Pub No. 92-0019, Rockville, MD, 1992, Agency for Health Care Policy and Research; **10.10A–C,** From Acute Pain Management Guideline Panel: *Acute pain management in adults: operative procedures: quick reference guide for clinicians*, AHCPR Pub No. 92-0019, Rockville, MD, 1992, Agency for Health Care Policy and Research; **10.10D,** From Hockenberry MJ, Wilson D, Rodgers CC: *Wong's essentials of pediatric nursing*, ed 10, St Louis, 2017, Elsevier. Used with permission. Copyright Mosby; **10.11,** From Prospect Working Group: PROSPECT: Procedure Specific Postoperative Pain Management at www.postoppain.org; **10.12,** From Long BC et al: *Medical-surgical nursing: a nursing process approach*, ed 3, St Louis, 1993, Mosby.

Chapter 11

11.3, 11.4, 11.14, 11.17, 11.18, From Thompson JC: *Atlas of surgery of the stomach, duodenum, and small bowel*, St Louis, 1992, Elsevier; **11.6, 11.10, 11.25, 11.26, 11.27, 11.28, 11.29, 11.30, 11.31, 11.32,** From Bauer JJ: *Colorectal surgery illustrated*, St Louis, 1993, Mosby; **11.8,** Modified from Thibodeau GA, Patton KT: *Anthony's textbook of anatomy and physiology*, ed 20, St Louis, 2013, Mosby; **11.19,** Courtesy Inamed Health, Inc., Santa Barbara, CA. In Townsend CM et al: *Sabiston textbook of surgery: the biological basis of modern surgical practice*, ed 17, Philadelphia, 2004, Saunders; **11.20, 11.21, 11.22,** From Townsend CM et al: *Sabiston textbook of surgery: the biological basis of modern surgical practice*, ed 18, Philadelphia, 2007, Saunders; **11.23, 11.24,** From Marceau P et al: Malabsorptive obesity surgery, *Surg Clin North Am* 81(5):1113–1127, 2001. In Townsend CM et al: *Sabiston textbook of surgery: the biological basis of modern surgical practice*, ed 17, Philadelphia, 2004, Saunders.

Chapter 12

12.6, From Townsend CM et al: *Sabiston textbook of surgery*, ed 16, Philadelphia, 2001, Saunders; **12.7,** From Daly JM, Cady B: *Atlas of surgical oncology*, St Louis, 1993, Mosby; **12.13,** From Zuidema G, editor: *Shackelford's surgery of the alimentary tract*, ed 3, Philadelphia, 1996, Saunders; **12.17,** Modified from Moody FG, editor: *Surgical treatment of digestive disease*, ed 2, St Louis, 1990, Mosby; **12.18,** Modified from Larson-Wadd K, Belani KG: Pancreas and islet cell transplantation, *Anesthesiol Clin North Am* 22(4):663, 2004; **12.19, 12.20, 12.21,** Copyright © 1990 Lahey Clinic, Burlington, MA; **12.22,** From Simmons RL et al, editors: *Manual of vascular access, organ donation, and transplantation*, New York, 1984, Springer-Verlag.

Chapter 13

13.1, From Sahani DV, Samir AE: *Abdominal imaging*, ed 2, Philadelphia, 2017, Elsevier; **13.2, 13.6,** From Paulsen F, Waschke J: *Sobotta atlas of human anatomy*, vol 1, ed 15, Philadelphia, 2013, Urban & Fischer; **13.3,** From Ball JW, Dains JE, Flynn JA et al: *Seidel's guide to physical examination*, ed 8, St Louis, 2015, Elsevier; **13.4,** From Netter FH: *Atlas of human anatomy*, ed 6, Philadelphia, 2014, Elsevier; **13.5, 13.12,** From Garden OJ, Parks RW: *Principles and practice of surgery*, ed 7, Philadelphia, 2018, Churchill Livingstone; **13.7,** From Baggish MS, Karram MM: *Atlas of pelvic anatomy and gynecologic surgery*, ed 4, Philadelphia, 2016, Elsevier; **13.8,** From Rosen MJ: *Atlas of abdominal wall reconstruction*, ed 2, Philadelphia, 2017, Elsevier; **13.9,** From Wein AJ, Kavoussi LR, Partin AW et al: *Campbell-Walsh urology*, ed 11, Philadelphia, 2016, Elsevier; **13.10,** From Yeo CJ, Matthews JB, McFadden DW et al: *Shackelford's surgery of the alimentary tract*, ed 7, Philadelphia, 2013, Elsevier; **13.14,** From Kulacoglu H: Mini-mesh repair for femoral hernia, *Int J Surg Case Rep* 5(9):574–576, 2014; **3.17,** Illustration by Steven P. Goldberg. In DiCocco JM, Magnotti LJ, Emmett KP et al: Long-term follow-up of abdominal wall reconstruction after planned ventral hernia: a 15-year experience, *J Am Coll Surg* 210(5):686–695, 2010.

Chapter 14

14.1, From Ball JW, Dains JE, Flynn JA et al: *Seidel's guide to physical examination*, ed 8, St Louis, 2015, Elsevier; **14.2, 14.8,** From Lowdermilk DL, Perry SE, Cashion K: *Maternity and women's health care*, ed 11, St Louis, 2016, Elsevier; **14.4,** From Dalrymple NC et al: *Problem solving in abdominal and pelvic imaging*, Philadelphia, 2009, Mosby; **14.5,** From Standring S: *Gray's anatomy*, ed 40, London, 2008, Churchill Livingstone; **14.6,** From Gabbe SG, Niebyl JR, Simpson JL et al: *Obstetrics: normal and problem pregnancies e-book*, ed 7, Philadelphia, 2017, Elsevier; **14.7,** From DiSaia PJ, Creasman WT, Mannell RS et al: *Clinical gynecologic oncology*, ed 9, Philadelphia, 2018, Elsevier; **14.9,** From Bristow R, Armstrong DMD: *Early diagnosis and treatment of cancer series: ovarian cancer*, Philadelphia, 2010, Saunders; **14.10, 14.30, 14.41,** From Bieber EJ et al: *Clinical gynecology*, Philadelphia, 2006, Churchill Livingstone; **14.11,** From Townsend CM et al: *Sabiston textbook of surgery: the biological basis of modern surgical practice*, ed 18, Philadelphia, 2008, Saunders; **14.12,** From Ignatavicius DD, Workman ML: *Medical-surgical nursing: patient-centered collaborative care*, ed 6, St Louis, 2010, Saunders; **14.13B, 14.14B,** Lemmi FO, Lemmi CAE: *Physical assessment findings CD-ROM*, Philadelphia, 2000, Saunders; **14.15,** Redrawn from Symmonds RE: Relaxation of pelvic supports. In Katz VL et al: *Comprehensive gynecology*, ed 5, Philadelphia, 2007, Mosby; **14.16, 14.17,** From Lobo RA, Gershenson D, Lentz GM et al: *Comprehensive gynecology*, ed 7, St Louis, 2017, Elsevier; **14.23, 14.27, 14.35, 14.43,** From Ball TL: *Gynecologic surgery and urology*, ed 2, St Louis, 1963, Mosby. Daisy Stillwell, medical illustrator; **14.24,** From Nucci MR, Oliva E: *Gynecologic pathology*, London, 2009, Churchill Livingstone; **14.26,** Courtesy Dr. Henry J. Norris, Orlando, FL. From Robboy SJ et al: *Robboy's pathology of the female reproductive tract*, ed 2, London, 2009, Churchill Livingstone; **14.28,** From Emond RT: *Colour atlas of infectious diseases*, ed 4, St Louis, 2003, Mosby; **14.31,** From Hacker NF et al: *Essentials of obstetrics and gynecology*, ed 4, Philadelphia, 2004, Saunders; **14.32, 14.33, 14.34,** From Edwards SK et al: Surgery in the pregnant patient, *Curr Prob Surg* 38(4):213–292, 2001; **14.36,** From Ignatavicius DD, Workman ML: *Medical-surgical nursing: patient-centered collaborative care*, ed 8, St Louis, 2016, Elsevier; **14.37, 14.44, 14.45,** From Nichols DH: *Gynecologic and obstetric surgery*, St Louis, 1993, Mosby; **14.39,** From Hacker NF, Gambone JC, Hobel CJ: *Hacker & Moore's essentials of obstetrics and gynecology*, ed 6, Philadelphia, 2016, Elsevier; **14.42,** From Voet RL: *Color atlas of obstetric and gynecologic pathology*, St Louis, 1997, Mosby; **14.48, 14.49,** Courtesy Marjorie Pyle, RNC, Lifecircle, Costa Mesa, CA. In Lowdermilk DL, Perry SE, Cashion K: *Maternity and women's health care*, ed 11, St Louis, 2016, Elsevier.

Chapter 15

15.1, 15.6, 15.7, Modified from Ball JW, Dains JE, Flynn JA et al: *Seidel's guide to physical examination*, ed 8, St Louis, 2015, Elsevier; **15.3, 15.10, 15.18, 15.22, 15.28, 15.33, 15.34, 15.44, 15.56,** From Nagle GM: *Genitourinary surgery*, St Louis, 1997, Mosby; **15.8,** Courtesy Bard Urological, Covington, GA; **15.11, 15.41,** Courtesy Gyrus-ACMI, Southborough, MA; **15.12,** Courtesy Circon Corp., Santa Barbara, CA. In Nagle GM: *Genitourinary surgery*, St Louis, 1997, Mosby; **15.14B,** From Tighe SM: *Instrumentation for the operating room*, ed 4, St Louis, 1994, Mosby; **15.17, 15.19, 15.20, 15.50A,** Courtesy American Medical Systems, Minnetonka, MN; **15.23,** From Williamson MR, Smith AY: *Fundamentals of uroradiology*, Philadelphia, 2000, Saunders; **15.26,** Courtesy Ethicon, Inc., Somerville, NJ; **15.29,** Courtesy Omni-Tract Surgical, St Paul, MN; **15.30, 15.31, 15.35, 15.36, 15.48, 15.49, 15.50B, 15.55, 15.57,** From Droller MJ: *Surgical management of urologic disease*, St Louis, 1992, Mosby; **15.39,** Courtesy Circon Corp., Santa Barbara, CA; **15.42, 15.43,** From Raz S: *Atlas of transvaginal surgery*, ed 2, Philadelphia, 2002, Saunders; **15.51, 15.52,** From Gillenwater JY et al: *Adult and pediatric urology*, ed 3, St Louis, 1996, Mosby; **15.53,** From Gray M: *Genitourinary disorders*, St Louis, 1992, Mosby; **15.54,** Copyright © Karl Storz Endoscopy America, Inc.

Chapter 16

16.2, From Drake RL, Vogl AW, Mitchell AWM: *Gray's anatomy for students*, ed 3, Philadelphia, 2015, Churchill Livingstone; **16.3,** From Wein RO, Weber RS: Parathyroid surgery: what the radiologists need to know, *Neuroimaging Clin North Am* 18(3): 554–555, 2008; **16.4,** From Netter Anatomy Illustration Collection, © Elsevier, Inc. All rights reserved, www.netterimages.com; **16.5,** From Goldman L, Schafer AI: *Goldman's Cecil medicine*, ed 24, Philadelphia, 2012, Saunders; **16.6,** From Fakhran S et al: Parathyroid imaging, *Neuroimaging Clin North Am* 18(3):538, 2008; **16.7,** From Kukora JS et al: Thyroid nodule. In Cameron

JL, editor: *Current surgical therapy*, ed 7, St Louis, 2001, Mosby; **16.8, 16.9, 16.10, 16.11,** From Dhingra JK, Raval T: Minimally invasive surgery of the thyroid, eMedicine.com, June 13, 2008, WebMD; **16.12,** From Healy J, Hodge J: *Surgical anatomy*, ed 2, Philadelphia, 1990, BC Decker.

Chapter 17

17.1, 17.11, 17.13, From Townsend CM et al: *Sabiston textbook of surgery*, ed 19, Philadelphia, 2012, Saunders; **17.2, 17.3,** From Isaacs JH: *Textbook of breast disease*, St Louis, 1992, Mosby; **17.4,** From Standring S et al, editors: *Gray's anatomy*, ed 41, London, 2016, Elsevier; **17.5,** From Townsend CM: *Sabiston textbook of surgery*, ed 16, Philadelphia, 2001, Saunders; **17.6,** Courtesy Wende W. Logan, MD, Rochester, NY, and the Breast Clinic of Rochester; **17.7A,** From Don Bliss, artist, National Cancer Institute (NCI), www.cancer.gov; **17.7B,** From Ignatavicius DD, Workman ML: *Medical-surgical nursing: critical thinking for collaborative care*, ed 5, St Louis, 2006, Saunders; **17.8,** From Townsend CM et al: *Sabiston textbook of surgery: the biological basis of modern surgical practice*, ed 18, Philadelphia, 2008, Saunders; **17.9,** From Hueske RD: *Mosby's PDQ for surgical technology*, St Louis, 2008, Mosby; **17.10,** From Focal Therapeutics, Aliso Viejo, CA; **17.12,** From Ignatavicius DD, Workman ML: *Medical-surgical nursing: patient-centered collaborative care*, ed 7, St Louis, 2013, Saunders; **17.14,** Redrawn from Zollinger RM: *Atlas of surgical operations*, ed 6, NY, 1988, MacMillan.

Chapter 18

18.1, 18.2, 18.4, Courtesy Eyemaginations, Towson, MD; **18.5,** From Thompson JM et al: *Mosby's clinical nursing*, ed 4, St Louis, 1997, Mosby; **18.6,** From Thompson JM et al: *Mosby's clinical nursing*, ed 5, St Louis, 2002, Mosby; **18.7A and B, 18.8, 18.11, 18.12, 18.15,** Courtesy Todd Bauders; **18.7C, 18.13, 18.14, 18.18, 18.24,** Courtesy National Eye Institute, National Institutes of Health; **18.16,** Courtesy Alcon Laboratories, Inc., Fort Worth, TX; **18.17, 18.25, 18.26,** From Lindquist TD, Lindstrom RL: *Ophthalmic surgery: looseleaf and update service*, St Louis, 1990, Mosby; **18.19, 18.21,** From Federman JL et al: *Retina and vitreous*, London, 1994, Mosby; **18.22,** From Ryan SJ et al: *Retina*, ed 4, St Louis, 2006, Mosby; **18.30,** From Swartz MH: *Textbook of physical diagnosis*, ed 7, Philadelphia, 2014, Elsevier; **18.33, 18.34, 18.36, 18.37,** From Tenzel RR: *Textbook of ophthalmology*, vol 4, *Orbit and oculoplastics*, London, 1993, Gower; **18.35,** From Massry GG: Ptosis repair for the cosmetic surgeon, *Facial Plast Surg Clin North Am* 13(4):533–539, 2005; **18.38,** Courtesy June Nichols, Board Certified Ocularist, Diplomate, American Society of Ocularists.

Chapter 19

19.1, 19.2, From Ignatavicius DD, Workman ML: *Medical-surgical nursing: patient-centered collaborative care*, ed 8, St Louis, 2016, Elsevier; **19.3,** From DeWeese DD et al: *Otolaryngology: head and neck surgery*, ed 7, St Louis, 1988, Mosby; **19.5, 19.17A and C,** From Saunders WH et al: *Nursing care in eye, ear, nose, and throat disorders*, ed 4, St Louis, 1979, Mosby; **19.7,** From Seidel HM et al: *Mosby's guide to physical examination*, ed 8, St Louis, 2015, Mosby; **19.8,** Redrawn from Thompson JM et al: *Mosby's clinical nursing*, ed 5, St Louis, 2002, Mosby; **19.9,** From Marino LB: *Cancer nursing*, St Louis, 1981, Mosby; **19.10, 19.16, 19.17B,** From Myers EN: *Operative otolaryngology: head and neck surgery*, ed 2, St Louis, 2008, Saunders; **19.11, 19.22, 19.31, 19.32,**

19.33, 19.43, From Cummings CW et al: *Otolaryngology: head and neck surgery,* ed 3, St Louis, 1993, Mosby; **19.13,** Courtesy Medtronic Xomed; **19.19,** Courtesy Cochlear, Ltd.; **19.21, 19.27,** From DeWeese DD, Saunders WH: *Textbook of otolaryngology,* ed 6, St Louis, 1982, Mosby; **19.24,** From Schuller DE, Schleuning AJ: *Otolaryngology: head and neck surgery,* ed 8, St Louis, 1994, Mosby; **19.25, 19.26,** Courtesy Entellus Medical, Plymouth, MN; **19.35,** Modified from LaFleur Brooks M, LaFleur Brooks D: *Exploring medical language: a student-directed approach,* ed 10, St Louis, 2018, Elsevier; **19.36,** From Luckmann J: *Medical-surgical nursing,* ed 3, Philadelphia, 1987, Saunders; **19.38, 19.39,** From Ignatavicius DD, Workman ML: *Medical-surgical nursing: critical thinking for collaborative care,* ed 5, St Louis, 2006, Saunders.

Chapter 20

20.1, 20.4A and B, 20.8, From Patton KT, Thibodeau GA: *Anatomy and physiology,* ed 9, St Louis, 2016, Elsevier; **20.2,** From Patton KT, Thibodeau GA: *Anatomy and physiology,* ed 7, St Louis, 2010, Mosby; **20.3,** Redrawn from Lewis RC: *Primary care orthopedics,* New York, 1988, Churchill Livingstone; **20.4C, 20.5, 20.6, 20.9,** Courtesy Vidic B, Suarez FR: *Photographic atlas of the human body,* St Louis, 1984, Mosby; **20.7A, 20.12, 20.13, 20.83,** From Thibodeau GA, Patton KT: *Anatomy and physiology,* ed 3, St Louis, 1996, Mosby; **20.11, 20.37, 20.64, 20.67,** Courtesy Zimmer, Inc., Warsaw, IN; **20.14,** Courtesy Tenet Medical, Dallas, TX; **20.15,** Courtesy Innomed, Savannah, GA; **20.16, 20.57,** Courtesy Acufex Microsurgical, Inc., Mansfield, MA; **20.17,** Courtesy OSI, Union City, CA; **20.18, 20.25, 20.34, 20.35, 20.44, 20.55, 20.69, 20.71,** From Gregory B: *Orthopaedic surgery,* St Louis, 1994, Mosby; **20.19, 20.48,** Courtesy Zimmer Traction Handbook, 1989, Zimmer, Inc., Warsaw, IN; **20.21,** From Mourad LA: *Orthopedic disorders,* St Louis, 1991, Mosby; **20.23,** From Monahan FD et al: *Phipps' medical-surgical nursing,* ed 8, St Louis, 2007, Mosby; **20.24,** Courtesy EBI, Parsippany, NJ; **20.26,** Courtesy Synthes USA, Paoli, PA; **20.27,** Courtesy Prototech AS, Bergen, Norway; **20.28, 20.46, 20.47,** From Gustilo RB et al: *Fractures and dislocations,* vol 2, St Louis, 1993, Mosby; **20.29,** Courtesy LTI Medica and the Upjohn Co. Illustration by Beverly Kessler, 1982, Learning Technology, Inc.; **20.30, 20.39, 20.50,** From Canale ST, Beaty JH: *Campbell's operative orthopaedics,* ed 11, St Louis, 2008, Mosby; **20.31,** Courtesy Biomet, Inc., Warsaw, IN; **20.33,** Redrawn from Rockwood CA et al: *Fractures in adults,* ed 2, Philadelphia, 1984, Lippincott; **20.36,** Redrawn from Neerii CS: Displaced proximal humeral fractures: part I: classification and evaluation, *J Bone Joint Surg Am* 52(6):1077–1089, 1970; **20.40, 20.42,** From Crenshaw AH: *Campbell's operative orthopaedics,* ed 8, St Louis, 1992, Mosby; **20.41,** From Knight RA: The management of fractures about the elbow in adults, *Instr Course Lect* 14:123, 1957; **20.43, 20.59,** From Muller ME et al: *Manual of internal fixation: techniques recommended by AO-ASIF group,* ed 3, Berlin, 1990, Springer-Verlag; **20.45,** Redrawn from Sprague HH, Howard FM: Herbert screw for treatment of scaphoid fractures, *Contemp Orthop* 16:19–25, 1988; **20.49,** Courtesy OsteoMed, Addison, TX; **20.51,** Courtesy Exactech, Inc., Gainesville, FL; **20.52,** From Gustilo RB: *The fracture classification manual,* St Louis, 1991, Mosby; **20.53,** Redrawn from Muller ME et al: *The comprehensive classification of fractures of long bones,* Berlin, 1990, Springer-Verlag; **20.54,** Redrawn from Schatzker J et al: The tibial plateau fracture. The Toronto experience 1968-1975, *Clin Orthop Relat Res* 138:94–104, 1979; **20.56,** From DePuy ACE Medical Co., El Segundo, CA; **20.58,** From Canale ST: *Campbell's operative orthopaedics,* ed 9, St Louis, 1998, Mosby; **20.60,** From Richards V: *Surgery for general practice,* St Louis, 1956, Mosby; **20.62, 20.68,** Courtesy Howmedica, Inc., Rutherford, NJ; **20.65,** Courtesy Stryker, Kalamazoo, MI; **20.66,** Redrawn from Gristina AG, Webb LX: *Proximal humeral and monospherical glenoid replacement: surgical technique,* Rutherford, NJ, 1983, Howmedica, Inc.; **20.70,** Courtesy College of Southern Idaho, Twin Falls; **20.72, 20.73, 20.74,** Courtesy ConMed Linvatec, Utica, NY; **20.75,** From Canale ST, Beaty JH: *Campbell's operative orthopaedics,* ed 12, Philadelphia, 2013, Mosby; **20.76,** Courtesy Johnson & Johnson; **20.80,** Courtesy Smith & Nephew Dyonics, Andover, MA; **20.81,** From Kim DH et al: *Surgical anatomy and techniques to the spine,* St Louis, 2006, Saunders; **20.82,** Courtesy NuVasive, Inc., San Diego, CA; **20.84,** Courtesy Medtronic Sofamor Danek, Memphis, TN; **20.85, 20.86,** Reprinted with permission from Synthes Spine LP.

Chapter 21

21.1, 21.24, From Thibodeau GA, Patton KT: *Structure and function of the body,* ed 13, St Louis, 2008, Mosby; **21.2, 21.3, 21.4, 21.6,** From Thibodeau GA, Patton KT: *Anatomy and physiology,* ed 3, St Louis, 1996, Mosby; **21.5,** Photograph by Sarah-Jane Smith. Artwork modified from Lumley JSP: *Surface anatomy,* ed 3, Edinburgh, 2002, Churchill Livingstone; **21.7, 21.9, 21.10, 21.12, 21.26,** From Conway-Rutkowski BL: *Carini and Owens' neurological and neurosurgical nursing,* ed 8, St Louis, 1982, Mosby; **21.8, 21.19,** From Anthony CP, Thibodeau GA: *Textbook of anatomy and physiology,* ed 11, St Louis, 1983, Mosby; **21.11,** Photograph by Kevin Fitzpatrick on behalf of GKT School of Medicine, London. In Standring S: *Gray's anatomy,* ed 41, Edinburgh, 2016, Churchill Livingstone; **21.13,** Modified from Thibodeau GA, Patton KT: *Anatomy and physiology,* ed 5, St Louis, 2003, Mosby; **21.14, 21.28, 21.29, 21.31, 21.43, 21.44, 21.45, 21.50,** From Rengachary SS, Ellenbogen RG: *Principles of neurosurgery,* ed 2, Edinburgh, 2005, Mosby Ltd.; **21.15, 21.16, 21.17,** From Rengachary SS, Wilkins RH: *Principles of neurosurgery,* London, 1994, Wolfe/Mosby Europe Ltd.; **21.18,** From Patton KT, Thibodeau GA: *The human body in health and disease,* ed 7, St Louis, 2018, Elsevier; **21.20,** From Standring S: *Gray's anatomy,* ed 40, Edinburgh, 2008, Churchill Livingstone; **21.21, 21.22,** From Mettler FA: *Neuroanatomy,* ed 2, St Louis, 1948, Mosby; **21.30,** Provided by Shaun Gallagher, GKT School of Medicine, London; photograph by Sarah-Jane Smith. In Standring S: *Gray's anatomy,* ed 40, Edinburgh, 2008, Churchill Livingstone; **21.32,** Courtesy Dr. Justin Lee, Chelsea and Westminster Hospital, London. In Standring S: *Gray's anatomy,* ed 40, Edinburgh, 2008, Churchill Livingstone; **21.33,** Courtesy Integra LifeSciences Corp., Plainsboro, NJ; **21.35,** From Barker E: *Neuroscience nursing,* St Louis, 1994, Mosby; **21.40, 21.41, 21.42,** Courtesy Codman, a Johnson & Johnson Co., Raynham, MA; **21.46, 21.47, 21.48,** From Ellenbogen RG, Abdulrauf SI, Sekhar LN et al: *Principles of neurological surgery,* ed 3, Philadelphia, 2012, Elsevier; **21.49,** From Sachs E: *Diagnosis and treatment of brain tumors and the care of the neurosurgical patient,* ed 2, St Louis, 1949, Mosby; **21.51,** From Carini E, Owens G: *Neurological and neurosurgical nursing,* ed 6, St Louis, 1974, Mosby.

Chapter 22

22.1, From Townsend CM et al, editors: *Sabiston textbook of surgery,* ed 18, Philadelphia, 2008, Saunders; **22.2, 22.3, 22.10, 22.19,**

22.20, 22.26, 22.30, 22.34, From Fortunato N, McCullough SM: *Plastic and reconstructive surgery*, St Louis, 1998, Mosby; **22.4,** Courtesy Carl Zeiss, Oberkochen, Germany; **22.5,** © 2017 Allergan. Used with permission; **22.6, 22.16, 22.17, 22.21,** Courtesy Ramasamy Kalimuthu MD, FACS, Oak Lawn, IL; **22.7,** From Thibodeau GA, Patton KT: *The human body in health and disease*, ed 5, St Louis, 2010, Mosby; **22.8, 22.12,** From Ignatavicius DD, Workman ML: *Medical-surgical nursing: patient-centered collaborative care*, ed 8, St Louis, 2016, Elsevier; **22.9,** From Patton KT, Thibodeau GA: *The human body in health and disease*, ed 7, St Louis, 2018, Elsevier; **22.15,** Courtesy Inamed Aesthetics, Santa Barbara, CA; **22.18, 22.39, 22.40,** Courtesy Marc A. Drimmer, MD; **22.22,** From Weinzweig N, Weinzweig J: *The mutilated hand*, St Louis, 2005, Mosby; **22.24,** From Flint PW, Haughey BH, Lund VJ, et al: *Cummings otolaryngology head and neck surgery*, ed 6, Philadelphia, 2015, Elsevier; **22.25,** From Fonseca RJ et al: *Oral and maxillofacial trauma*, ed 3, Philadelphia, 2005, Saunders; **22.27, 22.33,** From Kaminer MS et al: *Atlas of cosmetic surgery*, ed 2, St Louis, 2009, Saunders; **22.35,** From Capella JF: Body lift, *Clin Plast Surg* 35(1):28, 2008; **22.36,** From Aly A et al: Brachioplasty in the massive weight loss patient, *Clin Plast Surg* 35(1):146, 2008; **22.37,** From Cram A, Aly A: Thigh reduction in the massive weight loss patient, *Clin Plast Surg* 35(1):170, 2008; **22.41,** From Wilkinson TS: *Atlas of liposuction*, Philadelphia, 2005, Saunders.

Chapter 23

23.4, From Schottelius BA, Schottelius DD: *Textbook of physiology*, ed 18, St Louis, 1978, Mosby; **23.5,** From Townsend CM et al: *Sabiston textbook of surgery*, ed 16, Philadelphia, 2001, Saunders; **23.7,** From Johnson J, Kirby CK: *Surgery of the chest*, ed 4, Chicago, 1970, Year Book; **23.8,** Courtesy Teleflex Medical, Research Triangle Park, NC; **23.9,** From Baumgartner FJ: Surgical approaches and techniques in the management of severe hyperhidrosis, *Thorac Surg Clin* 18(2):167–181, 2009; **23.10,** From Damjanov I, Linder J, editors: *Anderson's pathology*, ed 10, St Louis, 1996, Mosby; **23.11,** From McCance KL, Huether SE: *Pathophysiology—the biologic basis for disease in adults and children*, ed 7, St Louis, 2014, Elsevier; **23.17,** In McCance KL, Huether SE: *Pathophysiology—the biologic basis for disease in adults and children*, ed 7, St Louis, 2014, Elsevier. Modified from Des Jardins T, Burton GG: *Clinical manifestations and assessment of respiratory disease*, ed 3, St Louis, 1995, Mosby. **23.20,** From Sellke F et al: *Sabiston & Spencer's surgery of the chest*, ed 8, Philadelphia, 2010, Saunders.

Chapter 24

24.1, From Patton KT, Thibodeau GA: *The human body in health and disease*, ed 7, St Louis, 2018, Elsevier; **24.2,** From Thibodeau GA, Patton KT: *Anatomy and physiology*, ed 5, St Louis, 2003, Mosby; **24.3,** From Kumar V, Abbas AK, Aster J: *Robbins and Cotran pathologic basis of disease*, ed 9, Philadelphia, 2015, Elsevier; **24.4,** From Patton KT, Thibodeau GA: *Anatomy and physiology*, ed 9, St Louis, 2016, Elsevier; **24.5,** From Dettenmeier PA: *Radiographic assessment for nurses*, St Louis, 1995, Mosby; **24.10,** From Townsend CM et al: *Sabiston textbook of surgery*, ed 17, Philadelphia, 2004, Saunders; **24.11,** From Haimovici H: *Vascular surgery: principles and technique*, ed 4, Oxford, 1995, Blackwell Science; **24.13, 24.16,** From Hershey FB, Calman CH: *Atlas of vascular surgery*, ed 3, St Louis, 1973, Mosby; **24.14, 24.15,** From MacVittie BA: *Vascular surgery*, St Louis, 1998, Mosby;

24.20, 24.22, 24.23, From Wilson SE: *Vascular access: principles and practice*, ed 3, St Louis, 1996, Mosby; **24.21,** From Calne R, Pollard SG: *Operative surgery*, London, 1992, Gower; **24.24,** From Ballinger PW: *Merrill's atlas of radiographic positions and radiologic procedures*, ed 8, vol 2, St Louis, 1995, Mosby; **24.25, 24.26,** From Townsend CM et al: *Sabiston textbook of surgery*, ed 20, Philadelphia, 2017, Elsevier.

Chapter 25

25.1A, 25.6A, From Thibodeau GA, Patton KT: *Anatomy and physiology*, ed 5, St Louis, 2003, Mosby; **25.2, 25.6B and C,** From Seifert PC: *Cardiac surgery*, St Louis, 1994, Mosby. Drawings by Peter Stone; **25.4,** From Pappano AJ, Wier GW: *Cardiovascular physiology*, ed 10, St Louis, 2013, Mosby; **25.5,** From Thompson JM et al: *Mosby's clinical nursing*, ed 5, St Louis, 2002, Mosby; **25.8, 25.11,** From Canobbio M: *Cardiovascular disorders*, St Louis, 1990, Mosby; **25.9A,** From Braunwald E et al, editors: *Heart disease*, ed 6, Philadelphia, 2001, Saunders; **25.9B, 25.32B and C, 25.43A,** From Seifert PC: *Cardiac surgery*, St Louis, 1994, Mosby; **25.10,** Courtesy Edward A Lefrak, MD, Annandale, VA; **25.12,** From Kinney M, Packa D: *Andreoli's comprehensive cardiac care*, ed 7, St Louis, 1995, Mosby; **25.13,** Courtesy Lakeland Regional Health and Creative Contractors, Lakeland, FL; **25.14,** Courtesy Scanlan International, St Paul, MN; **25.15,** Courtesy Rultract, Inc., Cleveland; **25.16,** Courtesy Pilling Co., Fort Washington, PA; **25.17,** Courtesy Hewlett-Packard Co., Medical Products Group, Andover, MA; **25.18, 25.40, 25.44, 25.47, 25.53, 25.61, 25.62, 25.64, 25.65, 25.69, 25.73, 25.75, 25.76,** From Waldhausen JA et al: *Surgery of the chest*, ed 6, St Louis, 1996, Mosby; **25.19, 25.20,** Courtesy Meadox Medicals, a division of Boston Scientific Co., Natick, MA; **25.21,** Courtesy WL Gore & Associates, Inc., Flagstaff, AZ; **25.22,** Courtesy St. Jude Medical, Inc., St Paul, MN; **25.23,** Courtesy Sulzer Carbomedics, Inc., Austin, TX; **25.24, 25.25, 25.31,** Copyright Medtronic, Inc., Minneapolis; **25.26, 25.32A,** Courtesy Baxter Healthcare Corp., Edwards CVS division, Santa Ana, CA; **25.27, 25.77,** Courtesy ATS Medical, Minneapolis, MN; **25.28, 25.66,** From Medtronic Cardiovascular, Mounds View, MN; **25.29, 25.30,** Courtesy CryoLife, Inc., Marietta, GA; **25.33, 25.34, 25.36, 25.37, 25.38, 25.39, 25.45, 25.56, 25.57, 25.59, 25.70, 25.71, 25.72, 25.74,** From Doty JR, Doty DB: *Cardiac surgery: operative technique*, ed 2, Philadelphia, 2012, Elsevier; **25.35, 25.42,** Courtesy Terumo Cardiovascular Systems Corp. All rights reserved; **25.41, 25.46, 25.49, 25.55, 25.58,** From Townsend CM et al: *Sabiston textbook of surgery*, ed 20, Philadelphia, 2017, Elsevier; **25.48,** Courtesy Heartport, Inc., Redwood City, CA; **25.50,** From Doty DB: *Cardiac surgery: operative technique*, St Louis, 1997, Mosby; **25.51,** From Lytle BW et al: Coronary artery bypass grafting with the right gastroepiploic artery, *J Thorac Cardiovasc Surg* 976:826, 1989; **25.52, 25.68,** From Zipes DP et al: *Braunwald's heart disease: a textbook of cardiovascular medicine*, ed 7, Philadelphia, 2005, Saunders; **25.60,** From David TE et al: Long-term results of mitral valve repair, *J Thorac Cardiovasc Surg* 115(6):1279–1286, 1998; **25.67,** From Cleveland Clinic Center for Medical Art & Photography © 2006-2013. Reprinted with permission. All rights reserved; **25.78,** From Seifert PC et al: Surgery for atrial fibrillation, *AORN J* 86(1):23–40, 2007.

Chapter 26

26.3, 26.4, 26.5, 26.8, 26.9, 26.10, From Children's Hospital of Philadelphia; **26.6,** From Schalamon J et al: Minimally invasive correction of pectus excavatum in adult patients, *J Thorac Cardiovasc Surg* 132(3):524–529, 2006; **26.7,** From Tasian GE, Casale P: The robotic-assisted laparoscopic pyeloplasty: gateway to advanced reconstruction, *Urol Clin North Am* 42(1):89–97, 2015; **26.11, 26.12, 26.13, 26.22,** From Coran AG et al: *Surgery of the neonate*, Boston, 1978, Little, Brown; **26.14, 26.15A and B, 26.17, 26.18, 26.27, 26.29, 26.32, 26.34, 26.35, 26.36, 26.71,** From Holcomb III GW, Murphy JP, Ostlie DJ: *Ashcraft's pediatric surgery*, ed 6, Philadelphia, 2014, Elsevier; **26.16, 26.24, 26.25, 26.28, 26.38,** From Spitz L et al: *A colour atlas of paediatric surgical diagnosis*, London, 1990, Mosby Ltd.; **26.19,** In Kliegman RM, Stanton BF, St. Geme III JW et al: *Nelson textbook of pediatrics*, ed 20, Philadelphia, 2016, Elsevier. From Welch KJ, Randolph JG, Ravitch MM, eds: *Pediatric surgery*, ed 4, Chicago, 1986, Year Book Medical Publishers; **26.20,** Modified from Boley SJ: An endorectal pull-through operation with primary anastomosis for Hirschsprung's disease, *Surg Gynecol Obstet* 127(2):253, 1986; **26.21,** From Chessell G et al: *Diagnostic picture tests in clinical medicine*, vol 2, St Louis, 1984, Mosby; **26.23,** From DeVries PA: Posterior sagittal anorectoplasty. In Holmann von Kap S, editor: *Anorektale fehlbildungen*, Stuttgart, 1984, Gustav Fischer-Verlag; **26.26,** Courtesy Dr. David Clark, NeoPIX, Albany, NY; **26.30,** From Davenport KP et al: Pediatric malignancies: neuroblastoma, Wilms tumor, hepatoblastoma, rhabdomyosarcoma and sacrococcygeal teratoma, *Surg Clin* 92(3):745–767, 2012; **26.31,** From Townsend CM et al: *Sabiston textbook of surgery*, ed 18, Philadelphia, 2008, Saunders; **26.33,** Courtesy H. Gil Rushton, MD, Children's National Medical Center, Washington, DC. In Hockenberry MJ, Wilson D: *Wong's nursing care of infants and children*, ed 10, St Louis, 2015, Elsevier; **26.37,** Copyright Andrew F. Inglis, Jr. In Fuhrman BP, Zimmerman J: *Pediatric critical care*, ed 5, Philadelphia, 2017, Elsevier; **26.39,** Courtesy Albert Biglan, MD, Children's Hospital of Pittsburgh. In Zitelli BJ, McIntire S, Nowalk AJ: *Zitelli and Davis' atlas of pediatric physical diagnosis*, ed 7, Philadelphia, 2018, Elsevier; **26.40,** From Neurosurgery wound closure, Ethicon, Inc.; **26.41,** From Shnorhavorian M, Song K, Zamilpa I et al: Spica casting compared to Bryant's traction after complete primary repair of exstrophy: safe and effective in a longitudinal cohort study, *J Urol* 184(2):669–674, 2010; **26.42,** From Miller MD, Thompson SR: *Miller's review of orthopaedics*, ed 7, Philadelphia, 2016, Elsevier; **26.43, 26.44,** From Kocher M, Millis MB: *Operative techniques: pediatric orthopaedic surgery*, Philadelphia, 2011, Elsevier; **26.48,** Courtesy Joseph Imbriglia, MD, Allegheny General Hospital, Pittsburgh, PA. In Zitelli BJ, McIntire S, Nowalk AJ: *Zitelli and Davis' atlas of pediatric physical diagnosis*, ed 7, Philadelphia, 2018, Elsevier; **26.49,** From Zitelli BJ, McIntire S, Nowalk AJ: *Zitelli and Davis' atlas of pediatric physical diagnosis*, ed 7, Philadelphia, 2018, Elsevier; **26.50,** Courtesy Wolfgang Loskin, MD, University of North Carolina, Chapel Hill, NC. In Zitelli BJ, McIntire S, Nowalk AJ: *Zitelli and Davis' atlas of pediatric physical diagnosis*, ed 7, Philadelphia, 2018, Elsevier; **26.51,** Courtesy Emory University School of Medicine, Atlanta, GA; **26.52, 26.53, 26.54,** From Katowitz JA, editor: *Pediatric oculoplastic surgery*, Philadelphia, 2002, Springer; **26.55A,** Redrawn from Chameides L: *Pediatric advanced life support*, Dallas, 1988, American Heart Association; **26.55B,** From Barkin RM, Rosen P: *Emergency pediatrics: a guide to ambulatory care*, ed 3, St Louis, 1990, Mosby; **26.56, 26.58, 26.60, 26.62, 26.66,** From Nichols DG, Cameron DE: *Critical heart disease in infants and children*, ed 2, St Louis, 2006, Mosby; **26.57, 26.61, 26.63, 26.65, 26.67,** From Hockenberry MJ, Wilson D: *Wong's nursing care of infants and children*, ed 10, St Louis, 2015, Mosby; **26.59,** From Cooley DA, Norman JC: *Techniques in cardiac surgery*, Houston, 1975, Texas Medical Press; **26.64, 26.68, 26.69, 26.70,** From Nichols DG et al: *Critical heart disease in infants and children*, St Louis, 1994, Mosby.

Chapter 27

27.1, 27.2, 27.3, From Federal Interagency Forum on Aging-Related Statistics, *Older Americans 2016: key indicators of well-being*, Federal Interagency Forum on Aging-Related Statistics, Washington, DC: U.S. Government Printing Office, August 2016, available at https://agingstats.gov/docs/LatestReport/Older-Americans-2016-Key-Indicators-of-WellBeing.pdf.

Chapter 28

28.1, Courtesy New Hanover Health Network EMS Air Link, EMS, Emergency Medical Services, Wilmington, NC; **28.2, 28.12,** From McQuillan KA et al: *Trauma nursing*, ed 4, St Louis, 2009, Saunders; **28.3, 28.10,** From Neff JA, Kidd PS: *Trauma nursing: the art and science*, St Louis, 1993, Mosby; **28.6,** From Cothren CC, Moore EE: Emergency department thoracotomy for the critically injured patient: objectives, indications, and outcomes, *World J Emerg Surg* 1(4):1–13, 2006; **28.7,** From Cosgriff II, Jr, Anderson DL: *The practice of emergency care*, ed 2, Philadelphia, 1984, Lippincott; **28.8,** Redrawn from Kintzel KC: *Advanced concepts in clinical nursing*, ed 2, Philadelphia, 1997, Lippincott; **28.9,** Redrawn from Becker DP et al: Diagnosis and treatment of head injury. In Youman JR, editor: *Neurological surgery*, ed 3, Philadelphia, 1990, Saunders; **28.11,** Courtesy Haim Paran, MD; **28.13,** From Townsend CM et al: *Sabiston textbook of surgery*, ed 18, Philadelphia, 2008, Saunders.

Chapter 29

29.5, 29.6, 29.9, From St. Peter's Hospital, Albany, NY; **29.4, 29.7, 29.8,** From Massachusetts General Hospital, Boston, MA; **29.10,** From Lampignano JP, Kendrick LE: *Bontrager's textbook of radiographic positioning and related anatomy*, ed 9, St Louis, 2018, Elsevier; **29.11,** From University of Utah Medical Center, Salt Lake City, UT.

Chapter 30

30.1, From Clarke TC, Black LI, Stussman BJ et al: Trends in the use of complementary health approaches among adults: United States, 2002–2012, *Natl Health Stat Report* 79:1–16, 2015, https://nccih.nih.gov/health/integrative-health; **30.3,** From Jonas WB: *Mosby's dictionary of complementary and alternative medicine*, St Louis, 2005, Mosby; **30.4,** Modified from Patton KT, Thibodeau GA: *Anatomy and physiology*, ed 9, St Louis, 2016, Elsevier.

Index

A

AA. *see* Anesthesiologist's assistant

Abbreviations, "do not use," 29

ABC assessment, in postanesthesia care unit, 261

ABCDE assessment, in traumatic injury, 1095–1096

ABCDE characteristic, of melanoma, 820*b*–821*b*

Abdomen, traumatic injury of, 1112–1114, 1114*f*, 1114*t*

Abdominal adhesions, 306*b*

Abdominal aortic aneurysms (AAAs), 883–884, 885*b*, 885*f*
  repair of
    endovascular, 899–901, 901*f*
    patient and family education in, 897*b*–898*b*
    resection of, 898–899, 900*f*
    surgical skin prep for, 892, 892*f*

Abdominal compartment syndrome, 1099*f*

Abdominal hysterectomy, total, 436–437, 437*b*, 438*f*

Abdominal incisions
  for abdominal aortic aneurysm resection, 899, 900*f*
  complications in, 304
  oblique, 302–303
  open, 299–301, 300*f*
  transverse, 303–304, 304*f*
  vertical, 301–302, 302*f*

Abdominal packing in damage control surgery, 1108

Abdominal surgery
  abdominoplasty, 844–845
  in geriatric patients, 1087
  pediatric, 1026–1030

Abdominal wall
  horizontal section of, 300*f*
  muscles of, 301*f*

Abdominoperineal resection (APR), 333–335, 334*f*

Abdominoplasty, 844–845

Abducens nerve, 768, 769*f*, 770*t*

Abduction, patient positioning for orthopedic surgery and, 676

Abduction pillow, 682

Ablation
  for conduction disturbances, 993
  endometrial, 413*b*–414*b*, 430
  image-guided, 1143–1144
  microwave, 241
  radiofrequency, for Barrett esophagus, 311

Abortion, 424*b*

Above-knee popliteal artery, exploration of, 902

Abscess
  Bartholin duct, 427–428, 427*f*
  breast, 563–564
  liver, 366–367
  spinal epidural, 774–775

Absorbable collagen, 350*t*

Absorbable gelatin, 350*t*

Absorbable gelatin sponge, 789, 790*t*

Absorbable sutures, 177–178, 178*t*
  synthetic, 177–178

Absorbed dose, 1121*b*, 1122–1123

Absorption, in laser-tissue interaction, 229*f*, 230

Abuse
  child, 1003–1004, 1004*b*
  elderly, 1079*b*

AC. *see* Alternating current

Accelerated partial breast irradiation (APBI), 552–553

Acceleration injury, 1093

Accessories, for patient positioning, 160–163, 162*f*–163*f*, 164*t*

Accessory instruments, 190–192, 192*f*
  endoscopic, 210

Accessory nerve, 769*f*

Accessory reproductive glands, 459

ACDF. *see* Anterior cervical decompression and fusion

Acellular extracellular matrix scaffolds, 255–256, 255*t*–256*t*

Acetabulum, 669–670
  cups of, total hip arthroplasty and, 722
  fractures of, 702–704, 704*f*

Acetaminophen, 272, 276*t*

Acetazolamide sodium, 580*t*–584*t*

Acetylcholine (ACh), 123–124

Acetylcholine chloride, 580*t*–584*t*

Achalasia, esophageal, 314

ACL. *see* Anterior cruciate ligament (ACL) repair

Acoustic nerve, 769, 770*t*

Acoustic neuroma, 644

Acromioclavicular (AC) joints, 668
  separation of, correction of, 691–692, 693*f*

Acromion process, 668

Action Plan tool, 17*b*

Active electrode monitoring (AEM), 227, 227*f*

Active shooter, 52

Active transport, 137

Acucise endopyelotomy, 518–519

Acupuncture, 1149*f*

Acute arterial insufficiency, 885

Acute graft rejection, of liver transplantation, 370*t*

Acute otitis media (AOM), 638, 639*f*

Acute renal failure, after liver transplantation, 370*t*

Acute venous insufficiency, 886

Adam's apple, 621

Adapters (couplers) in video technology, 215–216, 215*f*–216*f*

Adduction, patient positioning for orthopedic surgery and, 676

Adenoidectomy, 657

Adenoids, 619

Adenomas
  pituitary, 763
  thyroid, 530, 531*f*

Adenomyosis, 1142

Adenosine triphosphate (ATP), 136

Adherents, 580*t*–584*t*

Adhesions, 250*b*
  abdominal, prevention of, 306*b*

Adhesives
  in cardiac surgery, 941*t*–942*t*
  surgical, 185–186, 186*b*

Adjustable gastric band, 323, 323*f*, 325*t*

Adjustable pressure-limiting (APL) valve, 107*b*

Admission
  assessment of trauma patient upon, 1099
  to operating room, 939
  to postanesthesia care unit, 261
  to surgical unit, 280

Page numbers followed by *f* indicate figure; *t*, tables; *b*, boxes.

Special Features

Continued